Seminars in General Adult Psychiatry

College Seminars Series

For details of available and forthcoming books in the College Seminars Series please visit:
www.cambridge.org/series/college-seminars-series/

Seminars in General Adult Psychiatry

Third Edition

Edited by

David Kingdon
University of Southampton

Paul Rowlands
Derbyshire Healthcare NHS Foundation Trust

George Stein
Emeritus Consultant Psychiatrist, Oxleas NHS Foundation Trust

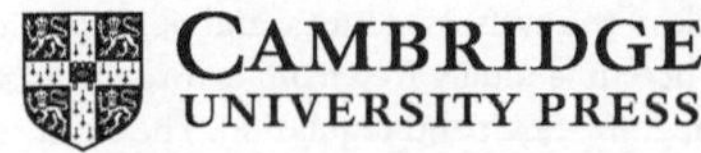
CAMBRIDGE
UNIVERSITY PRESS

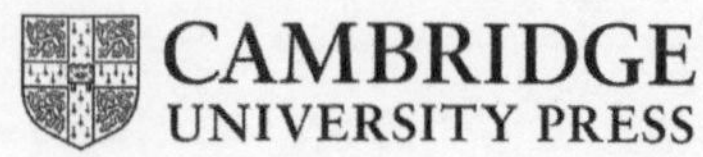

Shaftesbury Road, Cambridge CB2 8EA, United Kingdom

One Liberty Plaza, 20th Floor, New York, NY 10006, USA

477 Williamstown Road, Port Melbourne, VIC 3207, Australia

314–321, 3rd Floor, Plot 3, Splendor Forum, Jasola District Centre, New Delhi – 110025, India

103 Penang Road, #05-06/07, Visioncrest Commercial, Singapore 238467

Cambridge University Press is part of Cambridge University Press & Assessment, a department of the University of Cambridge.

We share the University's mission to contribute to society through the pursuit of education, learning and research at the highest international levels of excellence.

www.cambridge.org
Information on this title: www.cambridge.org/9781911623854

DOI: 10.1017/9781911623861

First published 1998

Second edition 2007

Third edition 2024

Printed in the United Kingdom by CPI Group Ltd, Croydon CR0 4YY

A catalogue record for this publication is available from the British Library

Library of Congress Cataloging-in-Publication Data
Names: Kingdon, David G., editor. | Rowlands, Paul (Psychiatrist), editor. | Stein, George, editor.
Title: Seminars in general adult psychiatry / edited by David Kingdon, Paul Rowlands, George Stein.
Other titles: College seminars series.
Description: Third edition. | Cambridge, United Kingdom ; New York, NY : Cambridge University Press, 2023. | Series: CGSS college seminars series | Includes bibliographical references and index.
Identifiers: LCCN 2023033727 (print) | LCCN 2023033728 (ebook) | ISBN 9781911623854 (paperback) | ISBN 9781911623861 (epub)
Subjects: MESH: Mental Disorders | Psychiatry–methods
Classification: LCC RC454 (print) | LCC RC454 (ebook) | NLM WM 140 | DDC 616.89–dc23/eng/20231026
LC record available at https://lccn.loc.gov/2023033727
LC ebook record available at https://lccn.loc.gov/2023033728

ISBN 978-1-911-62385-4 Paperback

'A genuinely comprehensive textbook of general psychiatry with contributions from psychiatrists with a wide range of academic and clinical backgrounds, offering experience from both specialist and generalist practice. The historical perspective given to many of the controversies in modern psychiatry is highly valuable, but the text also remains bang up to date in referencing the Community Mental Health Framework and recent treatment guidelines, and is aligned to the latest UK psychiatry curriculum. This is the perfect companion to training for UK psychiatric trainees and a helpful reference guide for practising clinicians.'

Dr Lenny Cornwall, MD FRCPsych, Consultant Psychiatrist, Tees, Esk and Wear Valleys NHS Foundation Trust, UK

'This 3rd edition of seminars in general adult psychiatry is a must-read for all those new to and currently working in adult mental health services. This book covers all the core mental health illnesses seen by general adult psychiatrists, but crucially now includes neurodevelopmental disorders such as ADHD and autism. In addition, the authors critically cover the significant changes in how general adult mental health services are now delivered in modern healthcare via specialised and functional teams, with the impact on continuity of care for patients, carers and clinical professionals. Finally, psychiatrists play a critical role within their clinical teams and local populations, and so I was delighted to see quality improvement and outcomes, public mental health, data and digital literacy also being discussed within this seminal text.'

Dr Asif Bachlani, Consultant Psychiatrist, Priory Group and Associate Non-executive Director, Kent and Medway NHS and Social Care Partnership Trust, UK

'This is a comprehensive and scholarly textbook; the first in the post-DSM-5 and post-ICD-11 era to be mapped to the new RCPsych curriculum and syllabus, making it an ideal text for trainees in psychiatry. The person-centred focus of this new edition blends academic evidence with the practical and lived experience of both clinicians and patients/carers to provide a handy guide to the specialist practice of general adult psychiatry.'

Professor Subodh Dave, Dean, Royal College of Psychiatrists, Consultant Psychiatrist and Deputy Director of Undergraduate Medical Education, Derbyshire Healthcare Foundation Trust and Professor of Psychiatry, University of Bolton, UK

Contents

List of Contributors ix

Introduction 1
David Kingdon, Paul Rowlands and George Stein
Appendix I.1 3
Veryan Richards and Paul Rowlands

1 **Clinical Epidemiology** 6
James B. Kirkbride and Annie Jeffery

2 **Assessment, Formulation and Diagnosis** 30
David Kingdon, George Stein and Paul Rowlands

3.1 **Clinical Features of Depressive Disorders** 64
Ian M. Anderson and Kate Williams-Markey

3.2 **Causes of Depression** 89
Glyn Lewis, Gemma Lewis and Ramya Srinivasan

3.3 **Drug and Physical Treatments of Depression** 108
Ryan Williams and Anthony Cleare

3.4 **Psychological and Social Treatment of Depression** 147
Stirling Moorey

4.1 **Bipolar Disorder: Diagnosis, Clinical Features, Outcome and Treatment** 162
Jennifer Burgess, Alan Currie, Stuart Watson, Aditya Sharma, David Cousins, John Cookson and R. Hamish McAllister-Williams

4.2 **Bipolar Disorder: Treatment, Psychological, Social and Physical Health Approaches** 183
Richard Morriss

5.1 **Schizophrenia and Other Primary Psychoses: Clinical Features** 198
Peter F. Liddle

5.2 **Causes and Outcome of Psychosis** 224
Cecilia Casetta, Adrianna P. Kępińska, Simona A. Stilo and Robin M. Murray

5.3 **Drug Treatment of the Psychoses** 241
Jonathan Rogers, Edward Chesney, Paul Morrison and Fiona Gaughran

5.4 **Psychosocial Management of Psychosis** 282
David Kingdon

6.1 **Anxiety Disorders** 293
David S. Baldwin, Bethan Impey and Vasilios Masdrakis

6.2 **Post-traumatic Stress Disorder** 314
Jonathan I. Bisson

6.3 **Specific Phobias** 324
Julius Burkauskas, Naomi A. Fineberg, Arun Enara, Giovanna Cirnigliaro and Lynne M. Drummond

6.4 **Obsessive-Compulsive and Related Disorders** 334
Lynne M. Drummond, Arun Enara, Giovanna Cirnigliaro, Julius Burkauskas and Naomi A. Fineberg

6.5 **Functional Neurological Disorder** 366
Matt Butler and Timothy R. Nicholson

6.6 **Bodily Distress Disorder, Chronic Pain and Factitious Disorders** 387
David Kingdon

7.1 **Clinical Features and Implications of New Classification of Personality Disorders** 404
Peter Tyrer

7.2 **Clinical Approaches to Personality Disorder (AKA Complex Emotional Needs)** 414
Oliver Dale and Andrew Howe

7.3 **Antisocial and Other Personality Disorders, Impulse Control Disorders, and Non-substance Addictive Disorders** 444
George Stein

8 **Neuropsychiatric Disorders** 460
Andrea E. Cavanna and Alan Carson

9 **Autism** 527
Ian A. Davidson, Mary Doherty and Clair Haydon

10 **Attention-Deficit/Hyperactivity Disorder** 539
Marios Adamou

11 **Sleep Disorders and Psychiatry** 546
Hugh Selsick

12 **Eating Disorders** 565
Agnes Ayton

13 **Perinatal Psychiatry** 598
Joanna Cranshaw, Gertrude Seneviratne and George Stein

14 **Substance Use Disorders** 636
Ed Day and Zainab Bashir

15 **Suicide and Self Harm** 654
George Stein

16 **Physical Health Care** 688
Paul Rowlands and John Wass
Appendix 16.1 697

17 **Culture, Mental Health and Mental Illnesses** 699
Dinesh Bhugra, Max Pemberton, Sam Gnanapragasam and Daniel Poulter

18 **Psychiatry in Primary Care** 726
Linda Gask and Safi Afghan

19 **Psychiatry in the General Hospital** 739
Parashar Ramanuj and Alice Ashby

20 **Adult Mental Health Services** 767
David Kingdon and Paul Rowlands

Index 805

Contributors

Marios Adamou
School of Human and Health Sciences, University of Huddersfield, West Yorkshire, England and South West Yorkshire Partnership NHS Foundation Trust, Wakefield, England

Safi Afghan
Black Country Healthcare NHS Foundation Trust, Dudley, UK and University of Wolverhampton, Wolverhampton, England

Ian M. Anderson
Faculty of Biology, Medicine and Health, The University of Manchester, Manchester, UK

Alice Ashby
West London NHS Trust, Southall, England

Agnes Ayton
Faculty of Eating Disorders, RCPsych, HOPE PC, University of Oxford, Oxford, UK

David S. Baldwin
Faculty of Medicine, University of Southampton, Southampton, UK and Department of Psychiatry and Mental Health, University of Cape Town, Cape Town, South Africa and Mood and Anxiety Disorders Service, Southern Health NHS Foundation Trust, Southampton, UK

Zainab Bashir
Department of Psychiatry, Birmingham and Solihull Mental Health Foundation Trust, Birmingham, UK

Dinesh Bhugra
Institute of Psychiatry, Psychology and Neuroscience, King's College London, London, UK

Jonathan I. Bisson
Division of Psychological Medicine and Clinical Neurosciences, Cardiff University School of Medicine, Cardiff, UK

Jennifer Burgess
Northern Centre for Mood Disorders, Translational and Clinical Research Institute, Newcastle University, Newcastle upon Tyne, UK and Regional Affective Disorders Service, Cumbria, Northumberland Tyne and Wear NHS Foundation Trust, Newcastle upon Tyne, UK

Julius Burkauskas
Laboratory of Behavioral Medicine, Neuroscience Institute, Lithuanian University of Health Sciences, Palanga, Lithuania

Matt Butler
Institute of Psychiatry, Psychology and Neuroscience, King's College London, London, UK

Alan Carson
Centre for Clinical Brain Sciences, University of Edinburgh, Edinburgh, Scotland

Cecilia Casetta
Department of Psychiatry, South London and Maudsley NHS Foundation Trust, London, UK

Andrea E. Cavanna
Department of Neuropsychiatry, Birmingham and Solihull Mental Health Foundation Trust and University of Birmingham, Birmingham, UK and School of Life and Health Sciences, Aston University, Birmingham, UK and Institute of Neurology, University College London, London, UK

Edward Chesney
Institute of Psychiatry, Psychology and Neuroscience, King's College London, London, UK

Giovanna Cirnigliaro
Hertfordshire Partnership University NHS Foundation Trust, Hertfordshire, UK and Department of Biomedical and Clinical Science Luigi Sacco, University of Milan, Italy

Anthony Cleare
Institute of Psychiatry, Psychology and Neuroscience, King's College London, London, UK

John Cookson
Royal London Hospital and East London NHS Foundation Trust, London, UK

David Cousins
Northern Centre for Mood Disorders, Translational and Clinical Research Institute, Newcastle University, Newcastle upon Tyne, UK and Regional Affective Disorders Service, Cumbria, Northumberland Tyne and Wear NHS Foundation Trust, Newcastle upon Tyne, UK

Joanna Cranshaw
South London and Maudsley NHS Foundation Trust, London, UK

Alan Currie
Regional Affective Disorders Service, Cumbria, Northumberland Tyne and Wear NHS Foundation Trust, Newcastle upon Tyne, UK

Oliver Dale
H&F Community and Recovery Mental Health Services and South H&F Mental Health Integrated Network Team (MINT)

Ian A. Davidson
Cheshire and Wirral Partnership NHS Foundation Trust and Crisis/Acute Mental Health GIRFT (Getting It Right First Time England)

Ed Day
School of Psychology, University of Birmingham

Mary Doherty
University College Dublin School of Medicine

Lynne M. Drummond
University of Hertfordshire and South West London and St George's NHS Trust

Arun Enara
Hertfordshire Partnership University NHS Foundation Trust, Hertfordshire, UK

Naomi A. Fineberg
University of Hertfordshire and Hertfordshire Partnership University NHS Foundation Trust, Hertfordshire, UK and School of Clinical Medicine, University of Cambridge, Cambridge, UK

Linda Gask
Centre for Primary Care, The University of Manchester, Manchester, UK

Fiona Gaughran
Professor of Physical Health and Clinical Therapeutics in Psychiatry, King's College London, Lead Consultant Psychiatrist, National Psychosis Service and Director of Research and Development, South London and Maudsley NHS Foundation Trust, London, UK

Sam Gnanapragasam
South London and Maudsley Foundation NHS Trust, London, UK

Clair Haydon
Adult Autism Team, Cheshire and Wirral Partnership NHS Foundation Trust and Mental Health Complex Care, NW Region England

Andrew Howe
Department of Psychiatry, South London and Maudsley NHS Foundation Trust, London, UK

Bethan Impey
University Department of Psychiatry, University of Southampton, Academic Centre, College Keep, Southampton, UK

Annie Jeffery
Division of Psychiatry, University College London, London, UK

Adrianna P. Kępińska
Institute of Psychiatry, Psychology and Neuroscience, King's College London, London, UK

David Kingdon
Emeritus Professor of Mental Health Care Delivery, University of Southampton, Southampton, UK

James B. Kirkbride
Division of Psychiatry, University College London, London,UK

Gemma Lewis
Division of Psychiatry, University College London, London, UK

Glyn Lewis
Division of Psychiatry, University College London, London, UK

Peter F. Liddle
Division of Psychiatry and Applied Psychology, Institute of Mental Health, University of Nottingham Innovation Park, Nottingham, UK

Vasilios Masdrakis
First Department of Psychiatry, School of Medicine, Eginition Hospital, National and Kapodistrian University of Athens, Athens, Greece

R. Hamish McAllister-Williams
Northern Centre for Mood Disorders, Translational and Clinical Research Institute, Newcastle University, Newcastle upon Tyne, UK and Regional Affective Disorders Service, Cumbria, Northumberland Tyne and Wear NHS Foundation Trust, Newcastle upon Tyne, UK

Stirling Moorey
South London and Maudsley NHS Foundation Trust, London, UK

Paul Morrison
Institute of Psychiatry, Psychology and Neuroscience, King's College London, London, UK

Richard Morriss
Department of Psychiatry, University of Nottingham, Nottingham, UK

Robin M. Murray
Institute of Psychiatry, Psychology and Neuroscience, King's College London, London, UK and Psychosis Unit, South London and Maudsley NHS Foundation Trust, London, UK

Timothy R. Nicholson
Institute of Psychiatry, Psychology and Neuroscience, King's College London, London, UK

Max Pemberton
Camden and Islington NHS Foundation Trust, London, UK

Daniel Poulter
All-Party Parliamentary Group on Global Health, Houses of Parliament, London, UK and South London and Maudsley NHS Foundation Trust, London, UK

Parashar Ramanuj
Royal National Orthopaedic Hospital NNS Trust, London, UKAQ

Veryan Richards
Associate Lay Consultant
veryanrichards@aol.com

Jonathan Rogers
Division of Psychiatry, University College London, London, UK

Paul Rowlands
Consultant General Adult Psychiatrist, Derbyshire Healthcare NHS FT, Derbyshire, England

Hugh Selsick
University College London Hospitals NHS Foundation Trust, London, UK and Insomnia Clinic, Royal London Hospital for Integrated Medicine, London, UK

Gertrude Seneviratne
South London and Maudsley NHS Foundation Trust, London, UK

Aditya Sharma
Northern Centre for Mood Disorders, Translational and Clinical Research Institute, Newcastle University, Newcastle upon Tyne, UK and Regional Affective Disorders Service, Cumbria, Northumberland Tyne and Wear NHS Foundation Trust, Newcastle upon Tyne, UK

Ramya Srinivasan
Division of Psychiatry, University College London, London, UK

George Stein
Emeritus Consultant Psychiatrist, Oxleas NHS Foundation Trust, London, UK

Simona A. Stilo
Institute of Psychiatry, Psychology and Neuroscience, King's College London, London, UK

Peter Tyrer
Lincolnshire Partnership NHS Foundation Trust, Lincolnshire, England

John Wass
Oxford University Hospitals NHS Foundation Trust, Oxford, UK

Stuart Watson
Northern Centre for Mood Disorders, Translational and Clinical Research Institute, Newcastle University, Newcastle upon Tyne, UK

Kate Williams-Markey
Secondary Care Psychological Therapies Service, Ashton-under-Lyne, Manchester. OL6 6QQ

Ryan Williams
Division of Psychiatry, Imperial College London, London, UK

Introduction

David Kingdon, Paul Rowlands and George Stein

Psychiatry, according to Johann Christian Reil (1759–1813), the German anatomist who first coined the term, consists of the meeting of two minds, the mind of the patient with the mind of the doctor. As the patient's story unfolds, the doctor's task is to recognise the pattern and to do so with compassion. Pattern recognition lies at the heart of the diagnostic process throughout medicine and none more so than in psychiatry, which lacks almost all the special investigations that help clarify diagnosis in other medical specialities. Thus, detailed knowledge of the key features of all the psychiatric disorders, both common and rare, is the core body of information that the psychiatrist will need to acquire during their training years. Because of this, we have provided detailed descriptions of each and every disorder as well as their diagnostic criteria according to DSM-5 and ICD-11.

Diagnostic acumen separated from therapeutic skill is of little use to patients or their families. When Reil first introduced the term 'psychiatry', he used the term in the therapeutic sense so that the mind of the doctor would act as a healing agent on the mind of the patient. Whilst the initial consultation serves to reach a diagnostic formulation and to establish a therapeutic alliance, all the later meetings between doctor and patient involve 'treatment' in the broadest sense: the development of a collaborative management plan. At one time, particularly in the first half of the twentieth century, the skills of psychotherapy were shrouded in the mystery of psychoanalysis and were very difficult to acquire without years of training, but today a large array of therapies for almost every condition exist, the necessary skills are far easier to learn, and their descriptions are distributed throughout this book. Drug therapy, which is also an essential component of good psychiatric practice in many cases, is well covered in Chapter 3.3 for depression and Chapter 5.3 for schizophrenia. An understanding of social, cultural, historical and economic factors influencing mental health is also essential, and in all chapters, we would emphasise that the disorders described are seen in this context. All planning of 'treatment' is founded on an ongoing effort to establish a collaborative therapeutic alliance with a unique individual person using this broad holistic framework.

The 2nd edition of this textbook was published more than 15 years ago in 2008. Since then, much has changed but also much has remained the same. What has barely changed are the core descriptions of all the psychiatric disorders. This body of knowledge is unlikely to change much in the coming period and, as this is the crucial body of knowledge needed for making psychiatric diagnoses, trainees will find acquiring this body of information will serve them well throughout all their years in practice. Minor changes in diagnostic criteria, nomenclature and classification are to be expected in both the DSM and ICD systems as more knowledge is acquired.

Psychiatric research, once the concern of a few elite institutions in Europe and the USA, has expanded rapidly, and today, numerous universities the world over have large and productive academic departments of psychiatry. Thus, for the first and second editions of this book, many scientific articles on most topics were available. However, in the last few years, there has been an explosion in both the quantity and quality of scientific psychiatry (see Chapter 1). There are now systematic reviews and meta-analyses on almost every specific intervention in psychiatry. These have been included in this book, making the factual basis for psychiatry widely available and far more solid than for our previous editions.

At the same time, specific psychiatric interventions can only take place in the context of a therapeutic relationship and a service delivering psychiatric interventions. Psychiatric services, by their very nature, involve numerous skilled professionals and others, and for most of their existence, there has been a struggle to secure adequate funding. There was an expansion of services in the early part of the millennium, but since that time, austerity has restricted the implementation of new developments. The closures of psychiatric beds released some, but insufficient, funding for community developments in the 1960s, 1970s and 1980s, and a similar process in recent decades has also occurred. This has placed pressure on a shrinking stock of inpatient beds leading to increased use of the private sector and numerous out-of-area placements. At times, a sense of crisis has enveloped the whole system, and this suggests this process of bed closure has perhaps gone too far (Chapter 20). Despite this, mental health now has a higher profile, and parity with physical health care is accepted. Though this has yet to be achieved, a spirit of seeing opportunities for improvement and working towards these opportunities is required. Doctors have had an important role in leading these changes over many decades. Supporting their patients and services through challenging times is a crucial role and is based on this combination of practical clinical experience, detailed theoretical knowledge and an ability to work alongside others.

There have also been substantial changes in the classification of disorders, with DSM-5 released in 2013 and even more radical changes in ICD-11 in 2019. In particular, changes in approaches to personality disorder have considered alternative terminology as well as a move to a dimensional rather than a categorical approach (Chapter 7.1).

Assessment, formulation and diagnosis are discussed as the basis for clinical skills (Chapter 2), and this is essential reading for those at the start of their careers. Then, each of the major disorders are explored in relation to clinical features, causation and treatment (Chapters 3–7). Some new categories have emerged with ICD-11, such as functional neurological disorder (previously, conversion disorder) and bodily distress disorder (previously, somatisation disorder; Chapters 6.5 and 6.6). Catatonia is now classified under its own heading in ICD-11, and its presentation is discussed in various chapters, including those on affective disorders, schizophrenia and neuropsychiatric conditions. Two new chapters have been added on neurodevelopmental problems, including autism and ADHD. The growing realisation (or rediscovery) that serious psychiatric disorder is associated with a high all-cause mortality and a shorter lifespan has led us to include a separate chapter on the physical health of psychiatric patients. The subspecialities of neuropsychiatry (Chapter 8), sleep disorders (Chapter 11), eating disorders (Chapter 12) and perinatal psychiatry (Chapter 13) are then covered. The book ends with a group of topics that are common to all disorders: suicide (Chapter 15), cultural and international psychiatry (Chapter 17), psychiatry in general practice (Chapter 18), psychiatry in the general hospital (Chapter 19) and finally mental health services (Chapter 20).

This is a substantial book, and reading it cover to cover would appear to be a daunting prospect for any trainee starting out in psychiatry. However, there is no need to digest its contents in the first month of the first placement, and it is intended that the greater bulk of it can be read well into the second year of the three-year core training programme and beyond. We hope it can also be used by anyone else interested in the subject. We would recommend that those new to psychiatry and mental health services focus first on understanding the organising principles of assessment (Chapter 2) and the core common conditions of depression (Chapter 3.1), bipolar disorder (Chapter 4.1), schizophrenia and its clinical features (Chapter 5.1) and their respective drug treatments (Chapters 3.3 and 5.3). The development of a therapeutic alliance is at the core of psychiatric practice, and the complexities sometimes encountered are discussed in chapters on personality disorder, body distress disorder and neuropsychiatric disorders. Other chapters deal with commonly encountered conditions as well as those less-often seen. Learning in psychiatry, as in medicine more widely, is based on the blend of clinical experience and the acquisition of theoretical knowledge, supervised by experienced clinicians. A consistent and reliable assessment technique can only be acquired by practice. Learning from the individual patient by reading the theoretical background to their problems brings an increase in understanding and meaning to the individual case. It enriches the knowledge base with which the clinician then approaches each new clinical encounter. We learn psychiatry from our individual patients and not from a book – but a book can provide a framework to organise this learning. As such, we hope that reading the whole book, sometime in the 2nd or 3rd year of a three-year training programme, will provide a feel for the breadth and depth of psychiatry as well as provide a summary of the current known facts of our discipline.

Psychiatry is however far more than a body of facts to be memorised. It is a skill, a mode of healing and an empathic profession that include a variety of differing capabilities. Defining these more diffuse qualities needed to practise successfully has proved a challenge, but the Royal College of Psychiatrists in the United Kingdom has drawn up a syllabus to form the basis of the necessary values and skills required to practise. The new curriculum has guided the selection of content included in this book, and further details are given in Appendix I.1.

We are extremely grateful to the authors who have either fully updated or provided completely new chapters for this edition. These chapters are erudite, concise and readable. Each contain a wealth of information drawn from the considerable expertise of these leaders in their field, providing evidence and practical guidance which, we're sure, will be of great value to readers in their clinical practice – and for their exams.

Appendix I.1: Broad Themes for Psychiatry within the Revised Curricula

Veryan Richards and Paul Rowlands

The Purpose of a Curriculum in Psychiatry

'The purpose of the core and higher psychiatry curricula is to train medical doctors to specialise in the assessment, diagnosis, treatment, management of patients with mental disorders in a wide range of clinical settings in collaboration with the patient, other health professionals and relevant others including families and carers of all ages.'[1]

One of the great strengths that psychiatry brings to the diagnosis, care and treatment of patients is the fact that psychiatrists come from an extended, holistic training background that takes into account the psychological, biological, social, cultural, spiritual and gender context in which all these issues are embedded. 'This holistic person-centred care approach underpins the speciality of psychiatry and the key role of psychiatrists in multi-disciplinary teams.'[1] Psychiatrists also work with capacity and risk issues and address prevention, advocacy and the reduction of stigma.

A person-centred and recovery-oriented approach to clinical practice is now an explicit part of health service policy in the UK: 'Person-centred care focuses on the patient as a person, with 'personhood' being its superordinate principle'.[2] This forms the key message of *Person-Centred Care: Implications for Training in Psychiatry* (CR215) and reminds us that the language we use in clinical practice is of crucial importance.[2,3] Person-centred care is now a central feature of the revised curricula, comprising a number of different but related components.

Generic Professional Capabilities and Specific Speciality Curricula

Good Medical Practice[4] and *Core Values for Psychiatrists* (CR204)[5] are the foundation documents for the revised curricula. There is a new curricula structure that aligns to the General Medical Council (GMC) frameworks *Excellence by Design*[6] and *Generic Professional Capabilities*[7] and in line with the principles of the *Shape of Training Review* [8] with implementation in autumn 2022.

There are nine **Generic Professional Capability** domains:

1. Professional values and behaviours
2. Professional skills
3. Professional knowledge
4. Health promotion and illness prevention
5. Leadership and team-working
6. Patient safety and quality improvement (QI)
7. Safeguarding vulnerable groups
8. Education and training
9. Research and scholarship

Each domain is shaped by a 'why, what, how' model – higher learning outcomes (HLO) provide the 'why', key capabilities (KC) provide the 'what', and illustrations provide the 'how'. The domains are supported by a separate updated illustrations document. The new curriculum framework aims to provide a flexible and adaptable approach to training, and the broad capabilities will ensure that trainees draw on a breadth of experience to achieve them. The curricula continue to be outcome based and capability focused.

Implementation of the Curricula in Psychiatry

Training in psychiatry, as in all areas of medicine, is explicitly experiential, learning through doing. Supervised 'workplace based' learning is the keystone to developing safe practice, and this is blended with the expectation that psychiatrists develop a wide and deep theoretical knowledge base from a range of perspectives. Doctors progressing through psychiatric training progress through a blend of completing work in real workplace settings, undertaking workplace-based assessments with experienced supervisors, developing a portfolio demonstrating their working practice – including feedback from others – and testing their theoretical knowledge via examinations.

Since the second edition of *Seminars in General Adult Psychiatry,* the health, wellbeing and service delivery landscapes in the UK have evolved significantly. This is reflected in the revised curricula by some existing themes becoming more prominent and the introduction of some new themes into the training and assessment programmes for core and higher trainees. Going forward, the following themes are fundamental to the practice of modern psychiatry; they will enhance the delivery of person-centred care and treatment for patients of all ages:

- A values-based and evidence-based clinical approach
- Multi-disciplinary model of person-centred care
- Shared responsibility and shared decision-making
- Integration of social psychology developments and interventions, with biological advances and interventions, particularly in neuroscience
- Integrating approaches to addressing the physical and mental health needs of patients
- Ensuring safe, effective prescribing of medicines and other interventions
- Developing sustainable approaches to health and health care
- Developing a sophisticated understanding of their duties as a doctor and a psychiatrist and the rights and duties of the people with whom they work
- Developing a sophisticated understanding of how medicine and psychiatry impact on and interact with society and how systems impact on individuals, including psychiatrists
- The need to develop psychiatrists and others, including people who use services, to adapt and shape developments in the service and future legal landscapes

Two themes in particular merit highlighting as they have significant implications for future training and will impact positively on the delivery of person-centred care in clinical practice.

The core values and principles that are outlined in *Core Values for Psychiatrists* (CR204)[5] underpin the therapeutic relationship between the patient and the doctor, which in turn influences the quality of recovery. This key thread is embedded into the revised curricula and training, ensuring the balance of a values-based and evidence-based approach to clinical practice. Domain 1 (HLO 1)[1]: 'Demonstrate the professional values and behaviours required of a medical doctor in Psychiatry, with reference to *Good Medical Practice*[4] and *Core Values for Psychiatrist* (CR204)'.[5]

Shared decision-making is a model of consent mandated by the *Montgomery* ruling[8] and is clarified in the updated GMC guidance *Decision Making and Consent*[9]. Shared decision-making and consent is a collaborative process, based on the evidence and values through which a doctor supports a person to reach a decision about their treatment. In person-centred care, alongside the relevant evidence, this process requires advanced communication skills to support a dialogue with the patient and to identify and manage any values conflicts that may arise. The dialogue should include explaining the outcome of the assessment and discussing the patient's ideas, values, concerns and expectations as well as informing the patient of the material risks and benefits of available treatment options. Domain 2 (HLO 1)[1]: 'Consistently use active listening skills and empathic language which respects the individual, removes barriers and inequalities, ensures partnership and shared decision-making and is clear, concise, non-discriminatory and non-judgemental'.

How Does This New Edition of *Seminars* Fit with the Continued Development of Training in Psychiatry?

This edition of *Seminars in General Adult Psychiatry* aims to describe some of the practical aspects of general adult psychiatry blended with the theoretical background for the main conditions found in its practice, particularly within a UK context. In the spirit of quality improvement, it is intended as a 'work in progress'. It seeks to synthesise the knowledge of experienced academics with the practical experience of people with the lived experience of the conditions described and people with experience in delivering and developing services. As such, we hope it will provide a readable and helpful manual to aid the present and coming cohorts on their journey.

Person-centred care is the principle at the heart of good medicine and psychiatry; this is demonstrated through the professional values and behaviours shown by practitioners. Like all crafts, experience and skill are gained over time. The blend of supervised broad practical experience, theoretical knowledge across the domains and personal reflection enables psychiatrists to acquire the necessary values, behaviours, knowledge and skills through their training. The process of learning, however, never reaches an end point as psychiatrists are dealing with complexity and uncertainty. They are always in a state of 'incomplete knowledge', and good psychiatry requires the humility to recognise this. With the right support and training, psychiatry provides an unequalled opportunity for a career in which the holistic person-centred approach to the care of people with mental illness can bring the greatest of rewards.

References

1. Royal College of Psychiatrists. *2022 Curricula Implementation Hub.* www.rcpsych.ac.uk/training/curricula-and-guidance/curricula-implementation (accessed 23 March 2023).
2. Royal College of Psychiatrists. *College Report 215. Person-Centred Care: Implications for Training in Psychiatry.* www.rcpsych.ac.uk/docs/default-source/improving-care/better-mh-policy/college-reports/college-report-cr215.pdf (accessed 23 March 2023).

3. Richards V. The power of language: The importance of shaping language as a constructive tool in health care. *Journal of Evaluation in Clinical Practice* 2019;25(6):1055–56.
4. General Medical Council. *Good Medical Practice: Protecting Patients, Guiding Doctors.* www.gmc-uk.org/ethical-guidance/ethical-guidance-for-doctors/good-medical-practice (accessed 23 March 2023).
5. Royal College of Psychiatrists. *College Report CR204: Core Values for Psychiatrists.* www.rcpsych.ac.uk/improving-care/campaigning-for-better-mental-health-policy/college-reports/2017-college-reports/core-values-for-psychiatrists-cr204-sep-2017 (accessed 23 March 2023).
6. General Medical Council. *Excellence by Design.* www.gmc-uk.org/education/standards-guidance-and-curricula/standards-and-outcomes/excellence-by-design (accessed 23 March 2023).
7. General Medical Council. *Generic Professional Capabilities Framework.* www.gmc-uk.org/education/standards-guidance-and-curricula/standards-and-outcomes/generic-professional-capabilities-framework (accessed 23 March 2023).
8. Adshead G, Crepaz-Keay D, Deshpande M, et al. Montgomery and shared decision-making: implications for good psychiatric practice. *British Journal of Psychiatry* 2018;213(5):630–32.
9. General Medical Council. *Decision Making and Consent.* www.gmc-uk.org/ethical-guidance/ethical-guidance-for-doctors/decision-making-and-consent (accessed 23 March 2023).

Chapter

1 Clinical Epidemiology*

James B. Kirkbride and Annie Jeffery

Introduction

Epidemiology is typically defined as the study of the *frequency*, *distribution* and *determinants* (causes) of health-related states and events in a defined population. These may include disease, disorder, symptoms, wellbeing, causes of death, behaviours and the provision and utilisation of health services.[1] Unlike most other branches of medical science, it is chiefly concerned with understanding and improving the health and disease status of populations rather than individuals, though public health interventions to prevent disease or promote wellbeing may be targeted at a variety of levels, including the individual (e.g. smoking cessation programmes, early detection services for people at risk of psychosis), familial (e.g. parenting interventions for mental, emotional and behavioural problems in children and young people) or societal levels (fluoridation of water supplies to reduce dental caries, folic acid fortification in non-wholemeal wheat flour to reduce birth defects in children).

The concept of *epidemics* – from the Greek *epi*', meaning 'upon'; *demos*, meaning 'people' and *ic*, meaning 'pertaining to' (literally 'pertaining to what is upon the people') – dates back at least to Hippocrates's writings in 400 BCE,[2] who described the relation of the seasons to various diseases occurring in the population at the time. However, the study or discourse – *logos*, in Greek – of epidemics – that is, epidemi*ology* – first arose in the nineteenth century following the identification of bacteria and subsequent observations that epidemics were strongly associated with infectious diseases. Indeed, the study widely credited to be the first epidemiological inquiry of its kind – *On the Mode of Communication of Cholera* – famously saw Dr John Snow remove the pump handle from the Broad Street pump in Soho, London, on 8 September 1854, following a groundbreaking investigation that helped prove cholera was transmitted via contaminated water and not through the air – the prevailing theory at the time.[3]

It soon became clear that many of the methods used for tracking infectious diseases, such as accurate case identification and determining precisely when and where cases had occurred, as well as their frequency in different settings, had a far wider application across population health, extending to our understanding of non-communicable diseases including mental health problems.

Cooper and Morgan[4] provide a brief overview of the history of psychiatric epidemiology, and they credit Émile Durkheim, the French sociologist, as among the first to apply epidemiological methods in psychiatry, in his studies of suicide. Durkheim examined successive five-year average suicide rates in different European countries and showed these were remarkably constant within each country but differed widely between countries, with the Protestant North European countries having rates that were three to four times higher than the Mediterranean and presumably Catholic countries such as Italy. To test his hypothesis further, Durkheim investigated how suicide rates varied within just one country, Germany, where some provinces were strongly Catholic while others were predominantly Protestant. He showed that the Protestant provinces (less than 50% Catholic) had a relatively high mean suicide rate, of 192 per 100,000 population, while the rate for provinces with 90% or more Catholics had rates less than half this, at 75 per 100,000. Those provinces that were 50–90% Catholic fell between these values, with 135 suicide deaths per 100,000 population. Durkheim conducted similar analyses comparing suicides rates between married and divorced people or between those who were fertile against those who were childless and, even without the help of modern statistical tests, found large differences between these different social groups. This led him to conclude that suicide, as a phenomenon, was a collective act, in that it was related to societal forces, and that the Catholic religion in some way appeared to offer a degree of protection.

Although the epidemiology of suicidality is complex and multifaceted,[5] (for a comprehensive introduction), recent evidence confirms that suicide rates are influenced by societal and cultural factors. For example, in Sweden, Hollander et al.[6] have observed that rates of suicides amongst first-generation migrants were over 60% lower than in the Swedish-born comparison population, after taking into account differences in age, natal sex and family income. This suggests that migrants import a range of protective factors that lower their risk of death by suicide, including sociocultural and religious beliefs, behaviours and customs and attitudes to suicide. Most strikingly, however, in this study, rates of suicide in migrants were dependent on the length of time lived in Sweden; no deaths by suicide were reported in migrants living in Sweden

* We are grateful to Matthew Hotopf for allowing us to revise a previous edition of this chapter.

for less than five years, while rates then began to increase in a dose-response manner, with no differences in suicide rates observed for those who had lived in Sweden for over 21 years. These findings lend further evidence to suggest that societal forces to which people are exposed can influence risk of suicide (and potentially other adverse health outcomes[7]), as Durkheim first suspected in the nineteenth century.

In the early twentieth century, in the southern United States, there was an alarming rise in the prevalence of pellagra, a debilitating neuropsychiatric disease presenting with neurasthenic symptoms, occasionally psychoses and dementia, as well as skin rashes. It was thought the cause was a specific communicable disease, possibly because of its known association with unsanitary conditions. In 1914, the US public health authority appointed Joseph Goldberger to investigate the cause of pellagra. Goldberger first observed that, in institutions where pellagra was rife, all the cases seemed to occur only among the inmates, and none of the staff were affected. He wrote that 'this pattern seemed to be no more comprehensible on the basis of an infection than is the absolute immunity of the asylum employees'.[8] Furthermore, new cases seemed to occur among inmates who had been there for a long time and who had little contact with the outside world rather than amongst new arrivals who had recent contact with the outside world. In a more detailed survey of an orphanage in Jackson, Mississippi, Goldberger found that the pellagra cases seemed to be confined to those aged 6–12 years. He noted that the younger children (below 6 years old) received a daily ration of fresh milk, while most of those aged 12 years or over were sent out to work on the farms, where they received supplementary food. Meanwhile, those aged 6–12 years subsisted only on the orphanage diet. To confirm his hypothesis that a dietary deficiency was responsible, Goldberger then conducted a dietary survey of households in seven villages in South Carolina, where the prevalence of pellagra was known to be very high. There were no cases of pellagra in households consuming more than 19 quarts of fresh milk per fortnight, but there was a 22.5% rate among households consuming less than one quart per fortnight. A similar pattern was found for the consumption of fresh meat.

This simple but well-designed survey, based only on good case identification and the ascertainment of the age and occupational distribution of cases and non-cases followed by a basic dietary survey, led to the identification of the probable cause of pellagra as a specific dietary deficiency. The disease was then easily prevented by ensuring an adequate supply of fresh milk and meat protein, and all this was clarified long before laboratory scientists had isolated vitamin B6 and identified its deficiency as the definitive biochemical cause of pellagra.

There are two main branches of epidemiology. The first branch provides a framework to *describe* diseases (or, more correctly for psychiatry, disorders, syndromes or dimensions) as they arise in the population. This branch encompasses studies that characterise the *frequency* and *distribution* of disorders such as psychotic disorders, anorexia or depression, or suicide rates as in Durkheim's studies. It is important to know whether disorders are on the increase or in decline and whether they vary dramatically between countries or regions. Having this knowledge allows services to be planned but also helps develop hypotheses about possible causes. Further, it is especially important for patients and their families that their clinical team is able to describe the prognosis of disorders. How many people with first-episode psychosis make a full recovery and never require psychiatric treatment again? How many will develop severe symptoms and require psychiatric care for the rest of their lives?

The second main branch of epidemiology deals with identifying and establishing the *determinants* of a disorder, using *analytic* study methods. It is centrally concerned with establishing whether a putative risk (or protective) factor is causally related to changes in the risk of experiencing a disorder or disease characteristic under study at the population level. Does removal or prevention of exposure to a given risk factor, such as high-potency cannabis, reduce the risk of a disorder, such as psychosis? The studies by Goldberger on pellagra described earlier are one early example of analytic studies in epidemiology. Such analytic studies test hypotheses that exposures (or risk factors) cause disorders or, once the disorder is established, examine whether the exposure (such as different forms of health care or treatment interventions) causes better or worse outcomes. As such, randomised controlled trials, which primarily assess whether an intervention (typically a therapeutic intervention but sometimes extending to social interventions) improve health outcomes, are a special type of analytic study design used in epidemiology. These *experimental* study designs (see 'Randomised Controlled Trials (RCTs)' later in the chapter) are differentiated from *observational* studies in epidemiology based on how the exposure is assigned to the population under study. In experimental designs, the investigator assigns the exposure (often randomly); in all other observational designs, the exposure is not assigned by the investigator, who instead observes what has occurred (or will occur) in the population under study. Inferring causal effects from observational studies requires great care, because of hidden differences that are often present between those who are, and are not exposed to a given risk factor under study. We will explore this critical issue in greater detail throughout this chapter.

As common to many scientific disciplines, analytic epidemiology is centrally concerned with establishing whether an association between two measured variables (typically referred to as exposures and outcomes) is causal. As in all quantitative disciplines, such associations are estimated statistically, but as the old adage goes, correlation does not imply causation, and special *causal inference* techniques are required to evaluate the likelihood that any given relationship is causal. While a vital issue for all analytic studies, causal inference is a particular challenge in observational epidemiology due to the inherent limitations of different study designs along with the (often hidden) roles played by various *biases*, which can nullify or even reverse apparently causal relationships between a risk factor and disorder. Later in this chapter, we provide an overview of both *traditional* and *contemporary* causal inference methods in epidemiology that can be used to investigate causality. The last two decades have seen an explosion in the development and application of contemporary causal inference methods (for an excellent primer, see for example, Hernan & Robins[9]), which – under certain (strong) assumptions – can be applied to observational data to strengthen the plausibility that a given association between an exposure and outcome is causal (see 'Causation', later in this chapter).

Exposures and Outcomes

In most studies, investigators measure three main things:

- Exposures
- Outcomes
- Potential confounders, which are other factors that may influence both the exposure and the outcome

The term 'exposure' encompasses a wide range of different factors that might be important in the aetiology of a disorder. These can include simple demographic variables such as age and gender; biological entities such as genotype, intra-uterine infection and brain abnormalities; psychological variables such as experiences of parenting; or social factors such as life events, deprivation and income inequality. Clearly, these exposures may be measured in many different ways, but the methodological principles behind linking exposure to outcome are essentially similar.

The term 'outcome' is also used broadly – to psychiatrists, the most obvious outcomes are diagnostic categories such as schizophrenia, depression or anorexia nervosa. While some researchers may choose to 'split' psychiatric categories into diagnostic groups as defined in ICD-11[10] or DSM-V, others may 'lump' together broad categories (e.g. 'psychotic disorders', 'common mental disorders' or 'eating disorders'). Increasingly, it is common in both clinical practice and in research to investigate the *dimensions* underlying different presentations, recognising that there are continua of experiences in the population (from no mental health symptoms to mild, moderate or severe symptoms) and that there is often phenomenological overlap in symptom dimensions across traditional categorical diagnostic boundaries. Further, in some countries, clinical practice increasingly seeks to avoid formal diagnoses in the early stages of mental illness to avoid stigma (particularly as most psychiatric conditions begin in adolescence) and allow a clear clinical presentation to unfold. The latest iteration of the *Diagnostic and Statistical Manual*, DSM-V[11], explicitly recognises dimensional approaches to mental illness. Thus, depending on the research question, investigators may choose to study clinical disorders, sets of psychiatric conditions or dimensions of psychopathology.

Potential *confounders* are described in more depth later but are essentially any variable that may present alternative explanations for the observed relationship between exposure and outcome; in causal language, they are referred to as common causes of the exposure and outcome.

Development of Measures: Reliability and Validity

All quantitative research involves the measurement of variables, which may be outcomes or exposures. In physical science, there are often objective criteria on which to base measurement (weight, length, electrical resistance, etc). In psychiatry (and much of medicine besides), such objective, external measures are lacking, and our measurement is therefore particularly prone to error. In developing questionnaires, rating scales or diagnostic interviews, it is necessary to assess their reliability and validity.

Reliability

There are two main types of reliability: inter-rater reliability and test–retest reliability. The term is also used, though, to describe the 'internal' integrity of an instrument – that is, inter-item reliability.

Inter-rater Reliability

Inter-rater reliability indicates whether two or more researchers using the same measure on the same subject will gain similar answers. The measurement of inter-rater reliability depends on the type of variable generated by the questionnaire. If it generates a binary outcome, such as the presence or absence of a specific diagnosis, reliability could be described as the *percentage agreement* between the two researchers. However, this would not take into account agreements that happened just by chance. Instead, *Cohen's kappa* takes into account that some of the observed agreements would be expected by chance. Kappa can vary anywhere between −1 and +1, where positive values indicate above-chance agreement (1 indicates perfect agreement) and negative values indicate below-chance agreement.

If the measure generates an ordered categorical outcome – for example, levels of certainty about the presence of a diagnosis (definite, probable, possible, absent) – a *weighted kappa* can be used. This gives more emphasis to serious levels of disagreement between raters than to trivial ones.

If the measure is a continuous variable, such as a symptom score, the *intraclass correlation coefficient* may be used, which will take a value between 0 and 1, with 1 again indicating perfect agreement.

Test–Retest Reliability

Test–retest reliability involves the same rater using the same measure to assess the same subject twice over an interval of time. The same parameters can be used as for inter-rater reliability. Test–retest reliability is important for measures that assess stable psychological traits, such as personality or intelligence, but is less useful for gauging the reliability of psychological symptoms, as these fluctuate over time.

Inter-item Reliability

Split-half reliability describes the integrity or coherence of a questionnaire and assesses whether the questions assess the same underlying construct. It can be measured by calculating a correlation between the scores of the first and second half of the questionnaire or between odd-numbered versus even-numbered questions. Alternatively, Cronbach's α can be used, which provides the average correlation between all possible ways of splitting the items.

Validity

Validity refers to the extent to which an instrument (which in this context usually means a questionnaire or interview) *actually* measures what it sets out to measure. There are three main types of validity:

- *Content validity* (which includes 'face validity') refers to the degree to which the measure covers what it is meant to cover – for example, one would expect a measure of depression to include items on low mood, anhedonia and fatigue.
- *Construct validity* is a more abstract term meaning the degree to which results from a measure fit with underlying theoretical constructs pertaining to that measure. For example, if the phenomenon under study changes with age, one would expect the results of the test to reflect this.
- *Criterion-related validity* (*concurrent* or *predictive*) is the degree to which the measure compares with an alternative criterion. In concurrent validity, the measure is compared with a 'gold standard', and the results are summarised as the sensitivity and specificity of the measure (these are discussed further in the chapter). Predictive validity is assessed by how well the measure is able to *predict* a subsequent outcome that fits into the construct being examined – for example, an IQ test used in children should go some way to predict future academic performance, or a measure of suicidal ideas should be able to predict future suicide attempts to some extent.

Concurrent Validity: Sensitivity and Specificity

Table 1.1 gives the overall framework for calculating a range of common parameters for assessing the concurrent validity of an instrument against a gold standard, including *sensitivity* and *specificity*.

Table 1.1 Definitions of sensitivity and specificity

		Gold standard		
		Positive	**Negative**	**Total**
Our instrument	**Positive**	a	b	a + b
	Negative	c	d	c + d
	Total	a + c	b + d	a + b + c + d

The formula for these measures are given below:

$$Sensitivity = \frac{a}{a+c}$$

$$Specificity = \frac{d}{b+d}$$

$$Positive\ predictive\ value = \frac{a}{a+b}$$

$$Negative\ predictive\ vale = \frac{d}{c+d}$$

$$Likelihood\ ratio\ (LR)\ of\ positive\ result = \frac{sensitivity}{(1-specificity)}$$

$$Pretest\ odds\ of\ disorder = \frac{a+c}{b+d}$$

$$Post\ test\ odds\ of\ disorder = \frac{a+c}{b+d} \cdot LR$$

$$Post\ test\ probability\ of\ disorder = \frac{Post\ test\ odds}{(1+post\ test\ odds)}$$

It will be easiest to define and discuss sensitivity and specificity in relation to an example and some actual numbers. Say a general practitioner (GP) decided to screen all attenders with the 12-item General Health Questionnaire (GHQ-12) to improve their detection of common mental disorders. It would be important to know the concurrent validity of the questionnaire – in other words, how it performs against a 'gold standard' psychiatric interview. The GP might therefore compare the results of the GHQ-12 with those on the 'gold standard' Revised Clinical Interview Schedule (CIS-R), which is a structured diagnostic interview. It is then possible to give the sensitivity and specificity of the GHQ-12 (in relation to the CIS-R). Say the doctor uses both measures on 49 patients, and the results are as shown in Table 1.2.

Note, first, that the frequency of psychiatric disorders rated on the CIS-R is high (nearly half the patients score positive). Note also that the frequency of patients who are positive on the GHQ-12 is higher still – this is usually the case when a questionnaire is being used to detect possible cases and indicates that at least some of the 'positives' on the questionnaire are false positives. *Sensitivity* is a measure of the ability of an instrument to pick up genuine cases – in this instance, the sensitivity is close to one (0.96, see below), indicating that the GHQ-12 identifies nearly all those who are true cases.

Table 1.2 Example calculations of sensitivity and specificity for a sample of 49 patients

		CIS-R (Gold standard)		
		Positive	**Negative**	**Total**
GHQ-12	**Positive**	23	9	32
	Negative	1	16	17
	Total	24	25	49

Specificity is a measure of the ability of an instrument to identify correctly those who are free from the disorder. Here the specificity is much lower (0.64), indicating that the GHQ-12 was performing less well. There is a play-off between sensitivity and specificity: the more sensitive a measure is, the more likely it is to also pick up false positives, and *vice versa*. The positive predictive value (0.72) describes the chances that an individual scoring positive on the test will actually have the disorder when the gold standard is applied. Similarly, the negative predictive value (0.94) is the chance that an individual who tests negative will be free from the disorder. Note that the positive and negative predictive values are sensitive to the frequency of the disorder under study. If the disorder is very rare, it is likely that a higher proportion of those who test positive will not have the disorder compared with when it is very common.

$$Sensitivity = \frac{23}{24} = 0.96$$

$$Specificity = \frac{16}{25} = 0.64$$

$$Positive\ predictive\ value = \frac{23}{32} = 0.72$$

$$Negative\ predictivevale = \frac{16}{17} = 0.94$$

The Odds, the Likelihood Ratio and Proportion

The GP knows from past experience that a high proportion (in fact, 49 per cent) of his patients have a psychiatric disorder. How much of a difference does the test make? The likelihood ratio of a positive value gives us an idea of the 'added value' that the test makes, but to use it, we also have to calculate the *odds* of a patient having a disorder. As per the formulae above, this leads to the following values:

$$Likelihood\ ratio\ (LR)\ of\ positive\ result = \frac{0.96}{0.36} = 2.67$$

$$Pretest\ odds\ of\ disorder = \frac{24}{25} = 0.96$$

$$Post\ test\ odds\ of\ disorder = 0.96 \cdot 2.67 = 2.56$$

Note that the odds are different from the probability, and the odds are calculated as the proportion with the disorder divided by the proportion without a disorder (here, 24/25=0.96). The *likelihood ratio* of a positive test is defined as the amount by which a positive test result increases the odds of a patient having the disorder – in this case, 2.67. If a patient scores positive on the GHQ-12, the odds that they have a disorder now increases by 2.67-fold to 2.56. What does this mean in terms of proportions? As above, we now use the formula for the post-test probability of disorder, given as:

$$Post\ test\ probability\ of\ disorder = \frac{2.56}{3.56} = 0.72$$

Hence, the positive test result on the GHQ-12 has changed the probability that the patient has a disorder from 49% to 72%.

Measures of Disorder Frequency: Prevalence and Incidence

One of the basic functions of epidemiology is to describe the frequency of disorders in the population. Knowledge about the burden of disorders in a given population should be the founding principle on which clinical and public health resources are based. There are two main measures of frequency: *prevalence* and *incidence*.

Prevalence

Prevalence is the total number of individuals with the disorder divided by the population from which they are drawn:

$$Prevalence = \frac{Total\ cases}{Total\ population}$$

Prevalence estimates will include some patients who have had the disorder for many years and others who have only just developed it. Prevalence is therefore a function of the number of new cases developing the disorder over a given time period (i.e. the incidence rate) and the average chronicity of the disorder (i.e. its average duration). It is worth noting, therefore, that the prevalence of the disorder will be affected by both recovery and death rates as a result of the disorder – two pertinent and pernicious issues in psychiatry; a higher recovery rate (fewer cases) would reduce prevalence as, paradoxically, would a higher death rate as a result of the disorder (fewer cases).

Two subtypes of prevalence exist: *point prevalence*, which is the proportion of the population who have the disease at the point in time when it is measured, and *period prevalence*, which is the proportion of the population who have experienced the disorder over a defined interval. In psychiatry, there are advantages to using period prevalence as many disorders relapse and remit, and a point prevalence may not reflect the true proportion of the population who have been affected by the condition under study. The two most common timescales for estimating period prevalence in psychiatric epidemiology are annual and lifetime prevalence.

Lifetime prevalence is the proportion of people in the total population who have ever experienced a disorder in their lifetime. There has been considerable controversy over the accuracy of lifetime prevalence estimates when obtained from psychiatric interviews. The problem with such estimates is that they depend on the recall of clusters of symptoms (e.g. for depression: low mood, anhedonia, sleep disturbance) many years before. Recall of such complex information is likely to be very inaccurate. Alternative sources – such as prospectively recorded cases in case registers – may be free from issues of recall bias (see 'Bias') but may still lead to underestimates of lifetime prevalence if case identification is based purely on clinical contact and diagnosis.

Lifetime prevalence is frequently confused with morbid risk of a disorder. Lifetime prevalence is an estimate of the total proportion of people alive at a given point in time (or at a given age) who have ever experienced the disorder of interest (that is, it is dependent on survivorship to that point in time or age). Morbid risk, by contrast, is an estimate of the proportion of disease-free people at a given point in time or age who will go on to experience the disorder of interest over a certain time period or by a certain age.

Finally, a common error in reporting prevalence estimates in the literature is to describe them as prevalence rates; any estimate of prevalence is a proportion in a fixed population (denominator), such as the percentage of people surveyed today who have ever experienced depression.

Incidence, Incidence Rates and Cumulative Incidence

In epidemiology, the term '*incidence*' strictly describes the *number* of individuals in an initially disease-free population who develop the disorder of interest for the first time within a specific time period. For example, there were 80 new cases of schizophrenia in the at-risk population of 400,000 people in 2022. Colloquially, however, *incidence* is used synonymously with the term *incidence rate*, which estimates the rate at which new cases occur within a population:

$$\textit{Incidence rate} = \frac{\textit{Number of new cases}}{\textit{Population at risk} * \textit{time at risk}}$$

For example, in the aforementioned population, the incidence rate was 20 new cases of schizophrenia per 100,000 people at risk in 2022. Note here the important concept of the 'population at risk', which includes only individuals who have never had the disorder. It excludes people who have previously had the disorder or those who would not be at risk of developing the disorder. The latter issue may seem trivial, but if someone with an organic brain disorder were to develop psychosis symptoms in the earlier example, there may be a high probability that those symptoms were caused by the organic disorder. Since that person would not meet diagnostic criteria for non-organic psychotic disorders, they could never have been 'at risk', and they should not be included in the estimation of either the numerator (new cases) or denominator (population at risk) when estimating incidence rates.

Cumulative incidence, sometimes referred to as incidence risk, estimates the proportion of new cases in an initially disease-free population at risk over a given length of time. Unlike an incidence rate, the denominator for cumulative incidence is the initial disease-free population at risk, ignoring the time at risk:

$$\textit{Cumulative incidence} = \frac{\textit{Number of new cases}}{\textit{Initial population at risk}}$$

Conceptually, cumulative incidence is similar to morbid risk. To illustrate the difference between these measures, we use a simplistic example of 10 individuals in a population, as depicted in Figure 1.1. These individuals are followed for one year to determine who develops a disorder. Three possible outcomes are possible for each individual: remain well, develop the condition under study, or be censored – in other words, stop contributing to the study because of death, emigration or other loss to follow-up. When calculating cumulative incidence, the problem of censoring is ignored. The numerator is all new cases of the disorder, and the denominator is the population at risk. In the study illustrated in Figure 1.1, we would state that two cases (4 and 7) developed the disorder, so the risk is 2/10 or 0.2.

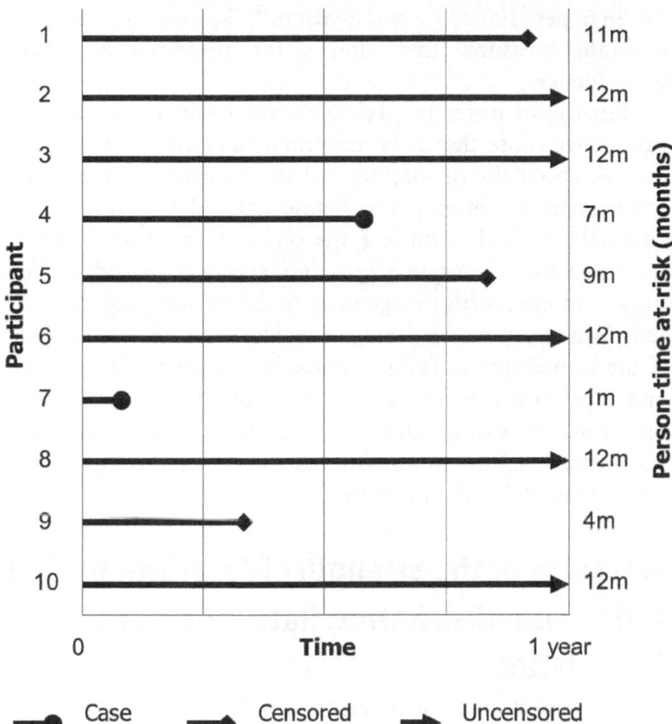

Figure 1.1 Calculation of incidence measures (see text for explanation).

When calculating the rate, a more precise estimate is made to take into account the differing amounts of time each individual spends 'at risk' of the outcome. Individuals who become ill can no longer contribute to 'time at risk', nor can individuals who die or who are otherwise censored. The denominator for the rate is the total 'person-time' at risk in the study. From Figure 1.1, only five individuals (2, 3, 6, 8 and 10) contribute an entire year of time at risk. Case 7 hardly contributes any time, becoming ill after 1 month. Case 4 becomes ill at 7 months, and cases 1, 5 and 9 are all censored, at 11, 9 and 4 months, respectively. The total person-time at risk here is 7.7 years, and the rate is 2 per 7.7 person-years at risk. Typically, we then re-express rates on a common person-years scale, such as per 100 person-years, per 1,000 person-years or even per 100,000 person-years to make it easier to compare between studies or groups. The scale is arbitrary and a function of the frequency of the disorder in the population. Here, we could express 2.0 per 7.7 person-years as 26.0 per 100 person-years, but for rarer disorders, such as psychotic disorders, we typically express incidence rates on a larger scale (i.e. a recent meta-analysis of the incidence of psychotic disorders placed this to be 26.6 per 100,000 person-years).[12] Because it is a more accurate measure, this rate is the preferred expression of incidence.

Finally, in order to precisely estimate incidence rates or prevalence, note that it is important to have accurate information about the denominator. Denominator error occurs if the investigator attempts to define a population using some routinely available data (e.g. the census or electoral register), but these are inaccurate because not everyone provided information in the census or signed up to the electoral register. This may lead to an over-estimate of incidence or prevalence, even if the numerator is being accurately recorded. The strength and effect of this *bias* (see further in this chapter) will depend on the accuracy of the denominator source, whether such bias was differential or non-differential across subgroups and the absolute rarity of the disorder.

Measures of the Strength of Associations: Risk Difference, Risk Ratios, Rate Ratios and Odds Ratios

In analytical studies, an attempt is usually made to describe the *strength* of an association between an *exposure* (or risk factor) and an *outcome* (or disorder). These are referred to as *measures of effect* or *measures of association*. In cohort studies, the incidence of a disorder is compared in two groups - one exposed to a risk factor, the other not exposed. The study estimates incidence risks or rates for each group. The risk or rate difference (sometimes *excess risk* or *rate*) is the difference in risks (or rates) between the exposed and unexposed group, expressed as:

$$Risk\ difference = Risk_{Exposed} - Risk_{unexposed}$$

and

$$Rate\ difference = Rate_{Exposed} - Rate_{unexposed}$$

Risk (rate) ratios are ratios of the risk (rate) in the exposed population divided by the risk (rate) in the unexposed population, as follows:

$$Risk\ ratio = \frac{Risk_{Exposed}}{Risk_{unexposed}}$$

and

$$Rate\ ratio = \frac{Rate_{Exposed}}{Rate_{unexposed}}$$

A risk ratio of 3, for example, indicates that individuals with the exposure are three times more likely to have the outcome as those unexposed.

Use of ratio measures is more common in clinical epidemiology than difference measures, although the choice will depend on the intended goal of the researcher when setting the research question and designing the study. Risk (or rate) differences can be useful in quantifying the absolute excess incidence or risk of disorder in one group compared with another, providing valuable clinical or public health information. Difference measures are particularly useful when reporting the results from RCTs, since they provide valuable information about the absolute magnitude of benefit or harm of the treatment in those who received the intervention. These should be reported alongside ratio-based measures of effect.[13]

Another widely used measure of impact is the odds ratio, which is used especially in case-control studies. The relationship between the odds ratio and risk or rate ratios is described in detail elsewhere,[14] but it can be illustrated in the following example.

Imagine that we are interested in determining the effect of unemployment on suicide rates in men of working age. We might identify a population of 1 million men for whom we know their employment status. Assume that 5 per cent of the population are unemployed and we follow the population for one year assessing suicide rates to obtain the figures shown in Table 1.3.

From these figures, it is possible to calculate the rate ratio:

$$Rate\ ratio = \frac{36\ per\ 100{,}000}{12\ per\ 100{,}000}$$

$$Rate\ ratio = 3$$

Now let us assume that it was impossible to identify the employment status of the entire population at the start of the study, and instead a case-control design was used. In the case-control study, the exposure status for cases (i.e. people who die by suicide) and controls (i.e. people who do not die by suicide) are compared. Assuming that it was possible to identify all 132 suicides in the population and compare them with a randomly selected sample of individuals who did not commit suicide, and assuming that the rate of unemployment in this randomly selected group of controls was similar to that of the general population, we could compare the odds of exposure in the cases with that in the controls. This might generate a table like Table 1.4.

Table 1.3 Illustration of rate of suicide by employment status

	Employed	Unemployed
Number of suicides	114	18
Denominator	950,000	50,000
Suicide rate	12 per 100,000 per year	36 per 100,000 per year

Table 1.4 Illustration of rate of unemployment by suicide status in a case-control study

	Cases of suicide	Controls	Total
Total	132	264	396
Employed	114	251	365
Unemployed	18	13	31
Odds of exposure	0.158	0.052	-

From this, it is possible to calculate the odds ratio, where the odds ratio is defined by the odds of exposure in cases divided by the odds of exposure in controls:

$$Odds\ ratio = \frac{Odds_{Cases}}{Odds_{Controls}}$$

$$Odds\ ratio = \frac{0.158}{0.052}$$

$$Odds\ ratio = 3.05$$

In the above example, we calculated the 'exposure' odds ratio, that is, the increased relative odds of exposure (being unemployed) in cases relative to controls. In a case-control study, we could have equally calculated the 'disease' odds ratio, that is, the increased relative odds of suicide in those who were unemployed (the exposed) relative to those who were employed. This yields the same odds ratio ([18/13]/[114/251] = 3.05).

The odds ratio in this example is a close approximation to the rate ratio estimated in Table 1.3; however, the two are not identical. The odds ratio approximates to the rate or risk ratios where the outcome under study is rare, as is often the case for many psychiatric disorders. When it is not rare, the odds ratio is higher than the risk ratio. See Box 1.1 for a technical note as to why we should not estimate risk (or rate) ratios in case-control studies. An exception to this rule exists for nested case-control studies in which controls are sampled by a method called incidence density sampling; here, provided conditional logistic regression is used, the odds ratios will be equivalent to incidence rate ratios (for further introduction to this advanced issue, see Lubin and Gail).[15]

Box 1.1 Use of odds ratios and not risk ratios in case-control studies

In the example in Table 1.4, we saw how the exposure odds ratio and disease odds ratio yielded the same effect size of 3.05.

The same property does not hold if one were to estimate the 'disease' risk ratio and 'exposure' risk ratio using case-control data. For example, in Table 1.4, the risk of suicide in the unemployed group is 18 of 31 (risk = 0.581) while the risk of suicide in the employed group is 114 of 365 (risk = 0.312), leading to a 'disease' risk ratio of 0.581/0.312=1.86. However, the 'exposure' risk ratio would be estimated as (18/132)/(13/264) = 2.77.

This situation arises in case-control studies because the researcher artificially constrains the number of controls in the study by design (for example, often one control per case). Because of this, risk of disease in both the unexposed and exposed group will change as a function of the proportion of controls to cases.

Suppose now we decide to sample 10 times as many controls for our study, which, under consistent sampling to the data generated in Table 1.4, would yield 130 unemployed and 2,510 employed controls. Now, the risk of suicide in the unemployed group would be 18/148 = 0.122, and the risk of suicide in the employed group would be 114/2624 = 0.043, yielding a 'disease' risk ratio of 2.80, compared with 1.86 previously. Thus, calculation of the risk ratio is a function of the number of controls, which is decided in advance by the researcher in case-control studies, while calculation of the odds ratio remains unchanged ([18/130]/[114/2510] = 3.05).

Assuming that the proportion of exposed to unexposed controls remains consistent as the number of controls increases, the odds of exposure in controls will be unaffected by the total sample size (which is constrained by design), leading to a valid measure of effect in case-control studies.

Measures of Impact

A key question for preventive medicine is determining how much impact a risk factor has on the overall rate of a disorder. Thus, *measures of impact* provide a useful way of understanding how much disease, disorder or burden could – theoretically – be prevented in the population, if a given risk factor or exposure could be removed (e.g. if we could stop everybody from being exposed to bullying in childhood, what proportion of psychiatric disorders in the population would we prevent?). Note, that *measures of impact* are predicated on several assumptions, including that there is a *causal* association between the exposure and outcome, the exposure can be prevented and that removal of the exposure would lead to removal of the outcome in a given population. The extent to which these assumptions are valid is of considerable debate, particularly given the multi-factorial causal structure of most psychiatric conditions, where any single risk factor may be neither sufficient nor necessary to cause morbidity. We return to issues of *causation* later in this chapter.

Returning to the unemployment and suicide example in Table 1.3, we might want to know how much unemployment contributes to the total suicide rate and whether removing the exposure (i.e. providing conditions of full employment) would have a sizeable impact on suicide rates. The population attributable risk (PAR) gives an estimate of this:

$$PAR\% = \left[\frac{P_e(I_e - I_u)}{P_t I_t}\right] \cdot 100$$

where:

P_e = Number of persons exposed = 50,000

P_t = Total population = 1,000,000

I_e = Incidence in the exposed = 36 per 100,000 per year

I_u = Incidence in the unexposed = 12 per 100,000 per year

I_t = Incidence in the total population = 13.2 per 100,000 per year

Leading to a PAR estimate of:

$$PAR\% = \left[\frac{50{,}000 \cdot (36 - 12)}{(1{,}000{,}000 \cdot 13.2)}\right] \cdot 100$$

$$PAR\% = \left[\frac{1{,}200{,}000}{13{,}200{,}000}\right] \cdot 100$$

$$PAR\% = 9.1\%$$

In other words, this shows us that, of the 132 suicides that occurred in the year, 9.1% were attributable to unemployment. This implies that if unemployment was removed as a risk factor, the suicide rate would fall by this amount. Thus, the population attributable risk can be defined as the proportion of a population's experience of a disorder that can be explained by the presence of a risk factor. As noted earlier, PAR has major practical limitations. In this example, it may not be feasible to remove unemployment entirely from the population, or the risk factor itself may not be a cause of suicide. For example, people may be unemployed because of other underlying health conditions, including mental health issues such as depression, and these issues may remain even if someone returned to work.

For a more comprehensive overview of the strengths and limitations of such measures of impact and to learn more about various methods for estimating the PAR (and other measures of impact) that exist, we refer the reader elsewhere.[14]

Study Designs

Ecological Studies

The ecological study design looks for population-level associations between the rates of a disease or disease outcome and the rates of a given exposure. This type of study design can be used to compare associations between different geographical locations, across time or between different groups such as migrant groups or social class. This approach requires routinely available estimates of prevalence or incidence as well as data on exposure. The problem in psychiatry, and the reason that ecological studies are not a common design, is that there are relatively few reliable estimates of prevalence or incidence that apply between many populations. Two key exceptions are suicide rates and hospital admissions. An example of an ecological study assessing suicide is that by Helbich et al.,[16] who assessed the relationship between suicide rates and the proportion of green space across different municipalities in the Netherlands. The authors found that municipalities with more green space had lower rates of suicide compared to municipalities with less green space. Another example of an ecological study assessing time trends in involuntary psychiatric hospital admissions is that by Keown et al.[17] The authors assessed the relationship between annual changes in the state provision of mental illness beds in the United Kingdom and involuntary admission rates. They found that reductions in mental illness beds were associated with increases in involuntary psychiatric admissions.

Ecological studies can be useful to generate hypotheses on the aetiology of a disorder at a relatively low cost. However, because they do not measure the exposure or the outcome at the level of the individual, it is not possible to use them to link exposures and outcome at the level of the individual. Therefore, they only provide weak evidence of causal relationships. This is referred to as the *ecological fallacy*. Another problem with ecological studies is *ecological bias*. There are two ways in which ecological bias may occur. Firstly, ecological bias may occur when associations described in ecological studies can be explained by factors that might link the exposure and outcome (confounding). For example, if it was found that suicide rates were highest in areas with the most developed mental health services, a naive interpretation would be that mental health services are bad for mental health and have caused this excess. An alternative explanation is that there are unmeasured confounders, such as social deprivation or urban environments, which are associated with both suicide and the extent of local mental health services.

The second way in which ecological bias may occur is when the effect of the exposure is modified by another factor that varies between populations (effect modification). For example, if a study found that suicide rates were lowest in areas with more green space, this could be modified by the level of perceived safety – areas with high perceived safety may benefit from more green space, whereas this may not be the case in areas with low perceived safety where green space is not utilised.

Despite these concerns, ecological studies can reveal important trends in psychiatric outcomes at a population or group level and across time. This information can be valuable for the planning of health services and public health initiatives, as well as hypothesis generation.

Cross-sectional Studies

Cross-sectional studies examine health outcomes within a defined population at a particular point in time. They are usually survey-based and are conducted on individuals, rather than at the group level like ecological studies. They can be used to assess the frequency of disease occurrence (prevalence) and the distribution of disease occurrence (e.g. by sex, age, ethnicity or social class). There are several important examples of large cross-sectional studies in psychiatry, such as the UK Adults Psychiatric Morbidity Survey[18] and the WHO World Mental Health Survey.[19]

The first step in the design of a cross-sectional study is the identification of a population. For the purposes of most studies, population means individuals living within a defined geographical area. However, it can be any group of individuals of interest to the researchers, as long as that group can be defined in a reproducible way. Thus, cross-sectional studies may be carried out within specific settings, such as primary care or general hospital outpatient departments, and specific populations in these settings, such as among employees of a firm or pupils within a school. In some circumstances, the researcher may be interested in defining a population of individuals with a disorder – such as patients with schizophrenia – and measuring the prevalence of another disorder – such as tardive dyskinesia – within this group.

As it is not always possible to survey an entire population, cross-sectional surveys are typically conducted using samples from an accessible subset. The key to making valid inferences using a study sample is to ensure that it is representative of the *target population*. Thus, if a cross-sectional study of school refusal was carried out, it would clearly be important not to limit the interviews to those children attending school as the group of most interest are those least likely to be there! Another example might be a cross-sectional study that interviewed individuals within their own home. If the survey was performed during working hours, it is likely that the healthiest members of the community would be at work, and the survey would exaggerate rates of illness as a consequence. Relevant groups (e.g. children who do not attend school or household members in full-time employment) should be identified in advance so that efforts can be made to ensure their inclusion. Random sampling is then preferable to maximise the representativeness of the sample.

Although cross-sectional studies can be used to measure associations between risk factors and disease outcomes, because both exposure and outcomes are measured at the same time point, the direction of causation may not be clear. However, there are a number of important examples where cross-sectional studies have been repeated with the same participants over time (e.g. the UK Household Longitudinal Study ('Understanding Society'), the English Longitudinal Study of Ageing). These are termed *panel studies* and are in essence, a hybrid form of cross-sectional and cohort study.

Cohort Studies

Cohort studies examine the relationship between exposures and subsequent health outcomes. In a cohort study, the sample is defined according to its *exposure status* and followed up over time to determine who develops the disorder(s) of interest. The key strength of the cohort study is its longitudinal design, which means that participants are assessed for the exposure before the onset of the disorder. Thus, cohort studies can usually give an insight into the direction of causation (see later) and are not susceptible to recall bias. Cohort studies allow rare exposures to be studied and can assess the effect of such exposures on multiple outcomes. In psychiatric epidemiology, cohort studies identify groups of people exposed to risk factors (such as childhood maltreatment, substance abuse, workplace stress or a history of depression) and compare the incidence of mental health outcomes with that among a non-exposed group. The analysis of a cohort study then involves the calculation of a risk ratio or rate ratio (see previous discussion).

The cohort study is best suited to situations where the outcome is common. For rarer outcomes (such as suicide and schizophrenia), cohort studies, unless very large, may have more limited utility. To illustrate this, suppose that a research team designs a cohort study to determine the effect of birth asphyxia on schizophrenia. They may identify babies with birth asphyxia (the 'exposed' group) and babies without such a history (the 'unexposed' group). They then have to follow the babies until adulthood in order to see whether any of them have developed schizophrenia. Assuming that by 25 years of age, the risk of schizophrenia is 0.5 per cent in those without birth asphyxia, the team would have had to follow (on average) 200 babies for each individual with schizophrenia in the unexposed cohort. In order to have a reasonable chance of detecting a twofold increase in the risk of schizophrenia over the course of the study, they would have had to follow over 10,000 individuals for 25 years. This example illustrates that cohort studies can be very expensive and time-consuming, especially if the outcome is rare. Cohort studies need to follow-up as many of the original sample as possible. *Non-response bias* (see 'Non-response Bias' in this chapter) is therefore a major concern in psychiatric cohort studies, as the individuals who cannot be traced may be the ones of most interest. For example, individuals with schizophrenia frequently become homeless or may not be cooperative with requests to participate in research. In the reporting of these studies, the investigators should describe the characteristics of those who could not be traced and how they differ from those who were traced.

Two approaches can be used to overcome some of these difficulties. The first is the use of large population-based cohort studies. In the UK, there are several large birth cohort studies that follow individuals born in a certain year over the course of their lives.[20–22] There is also, for example, the English Longitudinal Study of Ageing, which identified a sample of 11,391 people over the age of 50 in the year 2002 and continues to follow-up these individuals every two years. These cohort studies have looked at many different aspects of health, and because of their size and inclusion of relevant exposures, they have provided important data for psychiatric epidemiologists.[23,24] The second common approach is the retrospective cohort study. To return to the example of birth asphyxia and schizophrenia, instead of following babies born now, the investigators could examine the hospital records of babies born 25 years ago, and – provided sufficient information on asphyxia was available – could then trace the babies to identify individuals who had developed schizophrenia. This is a cheaper approach because the long follow-up time is not required. Population registers, such as those in the Nordic countries,[25] contain health information for all citizens stored under a unique personal identity number – these registers enable easier tracing of whole populations over long periods of time and are ideal data sources from which to conduct retrospective cohort studies. For more detail about the design, strengths and limitations of cohort studies, see Chapter 3.2 on the 'Causes of Depression' by Lewis, Lewis and Srinivasan.

Prognostic Studies

Studies on prognosis essentially use a cohort design in which the participants are patients with a disorder who are followed over time. There is usually no comparison group, as such studies are essentially descriptive – giving insights into the natural history of the disorder rather than its cause. The main methodological consideration is ensuring that an *inception cohort* is defined, meaning that to be included, patients must be as close as possible to the start of their first episode of illness. Most psychiatric disorders have a fluctuating course, with relapses and remissions. If a study assessing the prognosis of psychotic illness gathered a sample of individuals at different stages of their illness, it would tend to give an overly pessimistic view of prognosis because it would preferentially include individuals whose illness had an established chronic course. Determining that the cohort of individuals are all in their first episode ensures that those who get better quickly and never suffer further symptoms are included.

Another consideration with such studies is that the sample should be truly representative of the general population. If patients are recruited from specialist centres, there may be important *referral biases*, where more unusual cases are included, perhaps with a poorer outcome. For example, many of the earlier prognostic studies in the UK, for example of depression, were conducted from the Maudsley Hospital, which is not only a tertiary referral centre but also has an inner-city catchment area, both factors that may skew the outcome in a negative direction.

Case-Control Studies

Like cohort studies, case-control studies examine the relationship between exposures and health outcomes. Unlike the cohort study, where the sample is defined according to its exposure status, in a case-control study, the sample is defined according to its *outcome status*.

Cases with a disorder or outcome of interest are compared with individuals who are free from the disorder or outcome. An example of a case-control study in psychiatric epidemiology is that of Jongsma et al.,[26] where the authors recruited 1,130 cases with schizophrenia and 1,497 controls without schizophrenia, then compared a range of exposures between these groups, including ethnicity and social disadvantage. Unlike cohort studies, case-control studies are useful for rare disorders, and it is possible to determine the relationship between many different exposures and the disorder under study. Case-control studies are usually quicker and cheaper to perform than cohort studies because the disorder has already occurred, and it is not necessary to follow individuals over many years. Unless very large, case-control studies are not useful for rare exposures because insufficient cases and controls will have experienced them to make useful comparisons. The analysis of the case-control study involves a comparison of the odds of exposure in the cases compared with the controls – and is expressed as the odds ratio (see previous discussion).

The most important issue in case-control studies is the selection of both cases and controls. The key problem is *selection bias*, which occurs when the risk factor under study has an effect on the likelihood that the individual will be recruited to the study. This can work for both cases and controls. For example, some neuroimaging studies in psychiatry involve selecting patients with severe chronic psychotic illness from 'centres of excellence' and comparing them with controls who may be PhD students from the same centres. For both cases and controls, equal and opposite selection factors may generate misleading results. Cases may be unlikely to give a true representation of psychotic illness because those most readily available tend to be those with chronic symptoms (an instance of *prevalence bias*, discussed later). The controls are unlikely to represent the typical 'normal' brain because they have been drawn from a highly educated sample. For this reason, much emphasis is placed on attempting to select as representative a sample of cases as possible. The key to the selection of controls is that they should be drawn from a similar population and be similar to the cases in all respects apart from the disorder under study.

Depending on how and when the exposure is assessed, case-control studies may be unable to determine the direction of causality and may be susceptible to recall bias. However, this may not be the case when there is a clear temporal sequence (e.g. exposure to childhood maltreatment and the outcome of substance abuse in adolescence or the exposure to domestic violence and the outcome of suicide). Recall bias may also be overcome if exposures are identified through, for example, medical records.

Randomised Controlled Trials

In the randomised controlled trial (RCT), interventions to treat (or sometimes prevent) a disorder are compared to a placebo or to one or more other active treatments. RCTs can be used to evaluate intervention efficacy, acceptability and adverse effects. RCTs randomly assign participants to an intervention as part of the trial. To perform an RCT, the investigator should demonstrate that there is no evidence to suggest that a treatment is better than placebo or another active intervention. If one treatment was already known to be far superior to another, it would not be ethical to randomise. Unlike studies of risk factors, where it would be unethical for the investigator to assign individuals to receive a potentially harmful exposure, RCTs are ethical because the intervention is expected to do good.

Appropriately designed RCTs are the most robust research method for determining causal relationships between an intervention and outcome (for a more detailed discussion of this, see the 'Causation' section later in this chapter). The key methodological feature of the RCT is randomisation with concealed allocation. The rationale behind randomisation is that each participant has an identical chance of receiving each treatment. Then, if the trial is sufficiently large, potential confounders will be evenly distributed between the groups; this process should theoretically remove *confounding* by both observed and unobserved variables, as well as avoid *selection bias*.

In *simple randomisation*, the participants are assigned to groups in sequence according to a randomly generated number. The problem with this method is that the random

Simple randomisation of 48 subjects

abbaaaababbaaabbaaaaaabbabaabaabbabbbabbaaaabaab

Allocated to a = 28

Allocated to b = 20

Balanced randomisation: block size 8

abbaaabb

Figure 1.2 Distinction between simple randomisation and balanced randomisation. In the simple randomisation, the total in each group is unlikely to be balanced. In balanced randomisation, the investigator has decided to randomise within blocks of eight. In each block of eight, there must be four participants on each treatment.

groups may not be balanced: it is possible that, simply by chance, the two groups are of different size, and this is statistically inefficient. *Balanced randomisation* overcomes this by allocating participants in blocks. A typical block size would be eight, and the investigator would arrange that within this block, four participants would receive the intervention and four would be the control condition (see Figure 1.2).

Randomisation usually ensures an even distribution of important confounders between groups. However, in smaller trials, this cannot be guaranteed – by chance, there may be big differences in the distribution of confounders. To get around this, the investigator can perform a *stratified randomisation*, where the sample is divided according to the presence of the variable. For instance, in a trial of sertraline to treat depression, the baseline severity of depression was considered to be a key variable, and so, the investigators stratified the randomisation on this.[27] In *minimisation*, this process is taken a step further, and a wide range of key variables are identified; participants are then effectively matched on each of these variable to ensure that they are as similar as possible.

Concealment of allocation refers to the degree to which it is predictable to the researcher which treatment the patient will receive. If the investigator had considerable faith in a new treatment, they might consciously or unconsciously manipulate the randomisation process in order to ensure that patients with a good prognosis were assigned to the experimental treatment. Thus, the trial would be more likely to report 'positive' results. The best method is to have randomisation performed by an independent third party who is not aware of the study questions.

RCTs usually have a list of inclusion and exclusion criteria to ensure that patients entered are similar. The rationale for exclusion criteria may be to prevent the following groups from participating:

- People with contraindications for the treatments
- Clinical subtypes with particular profiles that might confuse the results (e.g. having psychiatric comorbidities with similar symptoms)
- Certain groups who are considered 'high risk' (e.g. patients with suicidal ideation – this may prevent embarrassment of the investigators and sponsors, but it is not useful to clinicians, who see such patients all the time)
- Those who might be considered to have difficulties consenting or following trial protocol (e.g. individuals with learning disabilities or cognitive impairment)

It is good practice for trials to report the number of individuals approached, the number who refused to participate or were excluded, and the number randomised. The CONSORT statement provides a widely endorsed checklist of standard reporting items for RCTs.[25]

As with cohort studies, dropouts from RCTs are a major problem. The investigators should attempt to follow everyone up, including patients who drop out of treatment. Many trials simply compare those in the two groups who have completed the trial according to protocol. This may mean that a sizeable proportion of those randomised (one-third in average antidepressant trials) are left out. This is misleading and can be a source of potential bias. A better approach is to use *intention to treat* analysis, where all randomised participants, no matter how long they were on treatment, are included in the analysis.

The analysis of RCTs depends on the nature of the outcome. Many RCTs describe results in terms of change of scores on symptom-rating scales. In these cases, it is preferable to present results as differences in the changed scores from the baseline. For categorical outcomes (e.g. recovery or admission to hospital), the approach will be similar to cohort studies, and a relative risk or rate ratio may be calculated. The number needed to treat, which expresses the number of individuals whose recovery can be attributed to the intervention, can also be calculated. This is a clinically useful measure that describes the number of individuals who would have to be placed on a treatment in order to produce one good outcome. For example, in a meta-analysis (see Box 1.2) of the antidepressant fluoxetine versus a placebo to treat depression, 45.8% of those treated with fluoxetine were considered to be in remission after six weeks, compared with 30.2% of those treated with the placebo.[25] The number needed to treat is then the inverse of the risk difference (see Box 1.2). In other words, a doctor would have to prescribe antidepressants to more than six patients (at least seven, in fact) in order for one to meet criteria for remission.

Systematic Reviews and Meta-analysis

Reviews aim to synthesise evidence on a topic of interest and are an important source of information for policy makers,

Box 1.2 Example calculation of number needed to treat

Risk of recovery on antidepressant	45.8/100
Risk of recovery on placebo	30.2/100
Risk difference	15.6/100
Number needed to treat (NNT)	6.41

clinicians and researchers. While narrative reviews are sometimes used to summarise a body of knowledge, this approach has been criticised because the methods are not reproducible: important articles may be missed, and the reviewer may overemphasise results that confirm his or her point of view. *Systematic reviews*, on the other hand, involve a systematic effort to identify all relevant literature; inclusion and exclusion criteria are then applied to that literature, and results are extracted in a systematic way.

Just as with primary research, systematic reviews should aim to answer a specific question and state their aims and objectives explicitly. Systematic reviews also include a 'methods' section that describes the search strategy. The reviewer performs a literature search, which will usually involve a combination of searching databases of published research (e.g. MEDLINE), tracing other articles in the reference lists of identified studies, searching clinical trial databases for unpublished trial results and so on. The results section should include information on the number of studies identified from the literature search, the numbers excluded and included, and the characteristics of the studies included. Several reporting guidelines now exist for systematic reviewing and meta-analyses, including the Preferred Reporting Items for Systematic Reviews and Meta-Analyses (PRISMA; www.prisma-statement.org) and the Meta-Analyses of Observation Studies in Epidemiology (MOOSE) reporting guidelines (https://jamanetwork.com/journals/jama/fullarticle/192614). Like other forms of research, prospectively registering systematic reviews, on databases such as PROSPERO (https://www.crd.york.ac.uk/PROSPERO/), is also encouraged.

Meta-analysis is a statistical synthesis of the main results from the studies identified by a systematic review. Because randomised trials in psychiatry are often too small to give reliable information, pooling the results of many similar studies will improve the precision of the effect size. When the effect size varies between studies, meta-analysis can also be used to identify the reason for the variation. For example, different trials of the same intervention may take place in different settings (outpatient, inpatient, primary care), with disorders of differing severity or chronicity. For pharmacological treatments, the drug prescribed in different trials may have been identical, but the dosage may have been different. For non-pharmacological treatments, such as psychotherapy or trials of the way in which community care is delivered, the treatment may differ radically between trials. It is possible to use a statistical test of heterogeneity to assess whether all the trials included in a meta-analysis are 'pulling the same way'. If this test indicates that significant heterogeneity between trials exists, the researchers should investigate why this might be.

Publication Bias

An important problem with meta-analysis is *publication bias*. It is a fact of life that researchers and journal editors like to have 'positive' results. There is considerable evidence that papers that show that one treatment has a clear advantage over another are more likely to be published than those that do not. Substantial publication bias could radically alter the conclusions of a meta-analysis. Publication bias is best avoided by a comprehensive search strategy – unpublished results may be publicly available in clinical trial databases or databases of 'grey literature' (e.g. OpenGrey).

The role of publication bias can then be assessed using a funnel plot.[28] If researchers complete a large RCT, they are likely to want to see it published even if the result is negative because of the effort involved. If publication bias does exist, it is most likely to be due to small negative trials not being published. The funnel plot is a graphical representation of the size of trials plotted against the effect size they report. As the size of trials increases, they are likely to converge around the true, underlying effect size. For the large trials, one would expect to see an even scattering of trials on either side of this true, underlying effect. When publication bias occurs, one expects an *asymmetry* in the scatter of small studies, with more studies showing a positive result than those showing a negative result.

Choosing a Study Design

The choice of a study design depends on the type of question being asked, the nature of the disorder/outcome and the exposure, and the time and resources available. The first question a researcher should ask is whether the question has been answered already, and the step before any serious research project should be to identify systematic reviews on the topic or to perform one. For some types of questions, the study design may be obvious. Studies on treatment efficacy are usually best answered by an RCT or a systematic review and meta-analysis of RCTs. When the researcher wants to describe the prevalence of a disorder, cross-sectional studies provide the obvious solution. However, it is more difficult to settle a question about the aetiology of a disorder, or the potential harmful effect of an exposure (including exposure to different treatments), and the study design will often be a trade-off between methodological considerations and resources.

The question next to ask is whether there are existing sources of data. Previous research studies may have collected the data necessary to answer the question. Kandola et al.[29] were able to use data from the Avon Longitudinal Study of Parents and Children to determine whether sedentary behaviour between the ages of 12 to 16 was associated with depressive symptoms at age 18, which the study showed to be the case. This was an extremely economical way of answering a well-focused question, which would otherwise have required major resources. Sometimes routinely collected data exist that are not part of a research study but which still allow the question to be answered. For rare side effects of drugs, large databases such as the UK Clinical Practice Research Datalink are an ideal resource.

If existing data do not exist, the choice of whether to use a case-control, cohort or cross-sectional study will depend on the relative frequency of the outcome and exposure and how easy they are to measure. Case-control studies manipulate the frequency of the outcome (by sampling according to participants' disorder status), and cohort studies manipulate the frequency of the exposure (by sampling according to the participants' exposure status). Thus, case-control studies are best for rare disorders and cohort studies for rare exposures.

Causation

The observational (e.g. cohort, case-control) and experimental (e.g. trial) study designs in epidemiology described earlier share the common goal of identifying whether an association between two variables is causal. This fundamental tenet of epidemiology then forms and informs the basis of effective clinical and public health intervention and policy. In observational studies, the researcher attempts to understand whether an association between exposure (a risk or protective factor) and disorder is causal; in experimental studies, the researcher attempts to understand whether an association between an intervention or treatment (a protective factor) and effect is causal. In this section, we provide a theoretical overview to help the reader understand important conceptual issues around causation and how they apply particularly to studies in psychiatric epidemiology and psychiatry more generally. In other chapters of this book, for example, Chapter 3.2 on the "Causes of Depression" by Lewis, Lewis and Srinivasan, more direct application of causal theory to specific issues is given.

As would be expected of this cornerstone issue, causal inference in epidemiology has received substantive theoretical and empirical attention, particularly given the controversies and harms that potentially arise from incorrect inferences; one of the most infamous (and since debunked[30] and retracted[31]) recent examples in psychiatric epidemiology was the erroneous conclusion – based on a very weak study design and (as it later turned out) falsified data and unethical procedures – that a combined measles, mumps and rubella (MMR) vaccine caused an increased risk of autism in children. Subsequent research has demonstrated the profound impact on public health this had, increasing both measles susceptibility in young children[32] in the years after publication until the partial retraction (1998–2004) and in increases in vaccine hesitancy in the population.[33]

Causal inference has been central to the development and evolution of epidemiology as a discipline. In his seminal President's Address to the Royal Society of Medicine in 1965, Sir Austin Bradford Hill outlined nine criteria (Box 1.3) of any exposure-outcome association that we should 'especially consider before deciding that the most likely interpretation of it is causation'.[34] These *traditional causal inference* criteria remain useful today, while recognising that establishing causation requires careful triangulation of a range of evidence across a variety of settings, study designs and methodological disciplines. For example, recent randomised trial evidence that the drug lecanemab can delay cognitive impairment and lead to reductions in amyloid burden in those with early Alzheimer's disease over an 18-month period[35] builds on decades of biomedical, neuroscientific and other observational and experimental research that has identified the agglomeration of amyloid beta (Aβ) in plaques as one of the core features of the pathology of Alzheimer's disease. Indeed, several influential epidemiologists have proposed modern *triangulation* criteria to strengthen *causal inference* in aetiological epidemiology,[36,37] which seek to incorporate and assess evidence generated by different methodological approaches that – although not free from bias – will likely contain different sources of biases that may (or may not) counteract each other to strengthen (or weaken) the plausibility of a causal association.

Box 1.3 Bradford Hill criteria for causation

1. *Strength* – Stronger associations are more likely to be causal
2. *Consistency* – The finding replicates across different studies in different samples by different researchers
3. *Specificity* – Evidence that a single risk factor has a specific effect on one disorder but not others may increase the likelihood of causality (though Hill also recognised that most disorders would have multiple causes, or the so-called *multifactorial aetiology*)
4. *Temporality* – The exposure should precede the outcome
5. *Dose-response* – The greater the level of exposure, the greater the risk of disorder
6. *Plausibility* – The finding agrees with accepted biological understanding
7. *Coherence* – Triangulation of findings across different designs and disciplines. Here, epidemiological evidence would cohere evidence from other disciplines such as neurobiology, psychology and animal evidence
8. *Experimental evidence* – Observational findings are supported by RCT evidence and natural experiments
9. *Analogy* – Analogous exposures and outcomes show similar effects. For example, if low socioeconomic status (SES) was a determinant of schizophrenia, we would expect to see this association across validated measures of education, income, occupation and social class

Complementing these approaches, a set of more statistically based *contemporary causal inference* methods in epidemiology have also been developed over the past two decades to strengthen the plausibility that associations between exposure and outcome from observational epidemiology are causal. A causal effect would be established if we could prove that an individual exposed to a risk factor for disease developed the disease following their exposure (i.e. the *factual* scenario) but would not have developed the disease had they not been exposed (i.e. the *counterfactual* scenario). In other words, if we could observe the outcome status that a single individual would experience if they were both exposed or unexposed to a given risk factor or treatment, we could estimate the individual causal effect of the exposure on the outcome. This is an example of counterfactual reasoning, where any individual has two potential outcomes: the outcome they would have received if exposed versus the outcome they would have received if they had remained unexposed. The difficulty here, however, is that we can never simultaneously observe the factual and counterfactual outcomes for a single individual, meaning that individual causal effects are not identifiable. As discussed previously, the great advantage of experimental epidemiology study designs, such as randomised controlled trials, is that provided certain assumptions are satisfied, the process of randomisation ensures that both measured and unmeasured confounders are similarly distributed in both the intervention and control arms of the trial. Given this, the two groups become exchangeable such that the average outcome experienced in the intervention arm (i.e. the factual scenario) would be the same as the average outcome experienced in the control arm, had the control arm been the intervention arm (i.e. the counterfactual scenario), and vice versa. Thus, at the population or group level, it is possible to estimate the average causal effect in an RCT design under certain assumptions; for example, provided that the trial achieves a sufficient sample size, has true randomisation and is free from attrition bias, the effect size (i.e. the odds ratio) becomes equivalent to the causal odds ratio.

Unfortunately, establishing counterfactual effects under a potential outcomes framework from observational study designs is much more difficult. This is particularly problematic for applied research in mental health (as most disciplines), where randomised controlled trials are often infeasible or unethical for testing exposure to putatively harmful effects. *Contemporary causal inference* methods, including genetically informed studies (e.g. twin and sibling designs, Mendelian randomisation (MR)), the broader class of instrumental variable approaches of which MR is a special case, inverse probability weighting and propensity scoring have been developed as statistical techniques to mimic the fundamental concept of exchangeability that is achieved in an RCT through randomisation. Thus, these methods – under certain strong assumptions – recover the *average causal effect* between exposure and outcome in an observational study design. It is beyond the scope of this chapter or book to provide a detailed introduction to this class of causal inference methods in epidemiology, but for excellent introductions on theory and critique of causal inference, see Rothman and Greenland;[38] causal inference methods, see Hernan and Robins;[9] and on contemporary approaches to triangulation, see Lawlor et al.[36] and Munafò et al.[37] In this book, Lewis, Lewis and Srinivasan also provide more details about Mendelian randomisation, its advantages and limitations, and how it has been used in depression research in Chapter 3.2 on the 'Causes of Depression'.

In addition to these approaches, the use of causal diagrams provide a further *contemporary causal inference* technique to aid transparent identification of causal effects from observational data. Causal diagrams, such as Directed Acyclic Graphs (DAGs), have been developed in parallel to more statistically based approaches to estimating causal effects under a potential outcomes framework using observational (or experimental) data in epidemiology. DAGs provide a useful and transparent tool to declare the theoretical model and assumptions underlying any causal effect of interest to be estimated.[39] Since correct causal inference requires the identification and removal of all potential *threats to validity*, including the

Box 1.4 Directed Acyclic Graphs (DAGs)

DAGs are causal diagrams that can help researchers identify and declare the hypothesised causal data structure underpinning the association between an exposure and outcome. These graphical tools can help researchers identify a minimal set of confounders that would need to be controlled for in the design or analysis of a study to estimate the causal effect of exposure on outcome, as well as to help identify any potential biases that may be introduced in the design or analysis of the study. In this way, DAGs provide a useful conceptual tool to design, conduct and report transparent and reproducible research. All potential variables relevant to the causal model should be included, regardless of whether they can be (or have been) collected.

A DAG includes *nodes* (variables) and *edges* (arrows). They are *directed* because they must indicate the assumed causal direction from one variable to another, and they are *acyclic* because a variable cannot cause itself; no node should have a path via edges that points back to itself.

In a DAG, we are usually interested in estimating the *direct causal effect* of the exposure, A, on the outcome, Y. Many other *paths* between A and Y may exist, via other nodes, including a set of confounders, L. These are so-called *biasing paths* because they are alternate, non-causal paths through which the association between A and Y exists. Failure to account for these biasing paths will result in biased estimation of the direct effect of A on Y. Biasing paths are said to be *open* when a confounder is not controlled for, as depicted in Figure 1.3, and *closed* or *blocked* when a confounder is controlled for – or *conditioned on* – in some way. Note that a potential biasing path is any path between A and Y, regardless of the directionality of the arrows (e.g. A←L→Y is a biasing path between

Box 1.4 (cont.)

A→Y in Figure 1.3). Conditioning on L, as shown in Figure 1.4, blocks the biasing path of this confounder.

Some variables in the assumed causal model may not be confounders but so-called colliders, C – that is, variables that are common effects (or common descendants) of two other variables, as depicted in Figure 1.7. Here, unlike with confounders, conditioning on a collider will *open* a biasing path, while leaving a collider as unconditioned will block that path.

The open access software 'DAGitty' (www.dagitty.net) provides a helpful tool for researchers to build their hypothesised causal model and understand the potential biasing paths that need to be blocked in the design and analysis of their study.

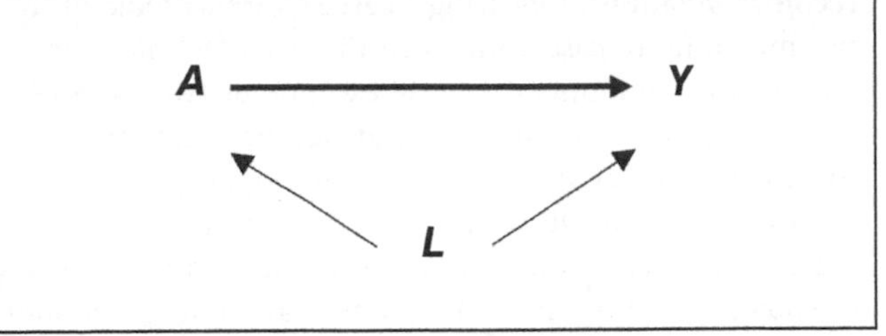

Figure 1.3 Basic confounding structure, represented in a causal diagram. The potentially causal association between the putative exposure, *A*, and the outcome, *Y*, may not be causal in the presence of a confounder, *L*, which is not taken into account during the design or analysis phase of a study.

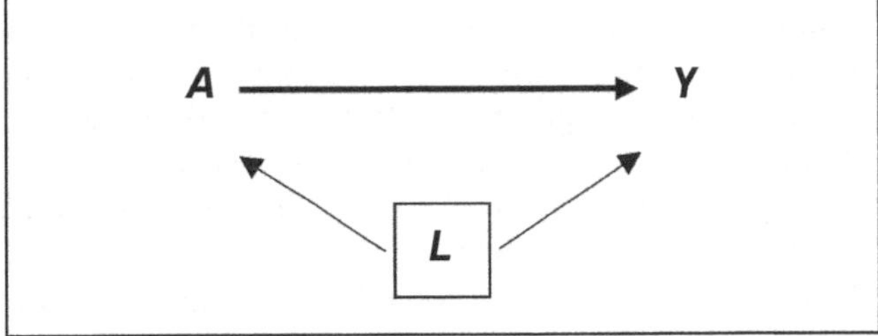

Figure 1.4 Controlling for a confounder, *L*, blocks the potential alternate causal path between *A* and *Y* that travels from *A*←*L*→*Y*, allowing the direct causal effect of *A*→*Y* to be estimated.

critical issues of *confounding, bias* and *chance* (discussed in detail later), we use simplified DAGs (see Box 1.4 for an elementary introduction) in the remainder of this section to highlight how these issues can affect our ability to infer causation from estimated associations of measures of effect (e.g. odds ratios, rate ratios) in observational epidemiology. For a comprehensive introduction to causal diagrams, see both Hernan and Robins[9] and Tennant et al.[39]

Confounding

Confounders are variables that are common causes of both the exposure and the outcome and can lead to a spurious association or eliminate a real one (Figure 1.3). Importantly, this implies that a confounder must temporarily precede the occurrence of both the exposure and the outcome. For example, we might be interested in understanding whether cannabis use (*A*, in the causal diagram in Figure 1.3) was causally associated with the risk of developing psychosis (*Y*, in Figure 1.3). A common cause of both cannabis use and psychosis (i.e. a potential confounder) may be (lower) socioeconomic status (SES) (*L*, in Figure 1.3). Since cannabis use may, theoretically, also change your subsequent SES, any study investigating the potentially causal association between cannabis use and psychosis would need to include methods to control for SES that was measured *prior* to the measurement of cannabis use; this may mean taking measurements of SES in childhood or at birth, for example, parental SES. Note that confounding is a reflection of the relationship between variables in real life – unlike bias (see later in this chapter), confounding is not a result of error in the design or analysis of studies.

When planning a study, we must identify, measure and decide on methods to deal with (control for) all potential confounders that may stop us from concluding that there is a direct causal effect of *A*→*Y*. In causal diagrams, we represent a confounder that has been controlled for (or in statistical terms 'conditioned on') by placing a box around the confounder (Figure 1.4). This indicates that the potential alternate causal pathway from *A* to *Y* that travels between *A*←[*L*]→*Y* has been blocked. Subject to assumptions (including the perfect measurement of the confounder, no other confounding, and correct specification of the causal model), this would allow estimation of the direct causal effect, *A*→*Y*.

There are five main methods of dealing with confounding:

1. *Restriction* is a method by which individuals with the confounding variable are removed from the study altogether. In the previous example, one could restrict the study to those from the lowest SES group (or highest) and determine whether psychosis is still more common amongst those who smoke more cannabis.
2. *Matching* involves artificially making the two groups similar in terms of the confounding variable. The investigator might ensure that, in a case-control study, each case with psychosis of a given SES was matched with a control of the same SES. Matching in case-control studies is intuitively easy to understand but has some disadvantages in terms of greater sample size requirements as well as difficulty in finding suitable matched participants when matching on several variables. Furthermore, recent epidemiological theory demonstrates that matching alone does not control for the matched factors included in the design and that these still need controlling for via other methods (see the later discussion) at the analysis stage.[40] Older textbooks also suggest that a matched design requires specific statistical methods to take into account the matching, though this is no longer considered necessary and indeed can introduce bias to the results. Our

recommendations, following Pearce,[40] are to judiciously use matching in case-control studies as a technique to control for confounders, limited to one or two variables (e.g. age, gender); ensure the matched variables are included in the analysis stage; and use appropriate ('unmatched') analytical methods during the analysis. Matching is also sometimes used in cohort studies, where the object goal is to make the exposed and unexposed more similar to each other on certain confounders. Advanced methods such as *propensity scoring techniques* attempt to match participants on their propensity to be exposed (often, their propensity to receive treatment) in an attempt to improve the conditions under which the assumption of *exchangeability* is satisfied.

3. *Stratification* is a method used at the analysis stage, where instead of lumping all subjects together, the sample is split according to the presence of the confounder – thus those from different SES groups would be analysed separately. It is possible using stratification to calculate a combined estimate of the size of the effect (e.g. the odds ratio) using specific statistical techniques.
4. *Regression adjustment* is a general term for multivariable modelling techniques used at the analysis stage, where the confounders of interest are included as covariates in the regression model to control for their effects on the statistical association between exposure and outcome. Like with stratification, all confounder variables must be identified from theory and empirical evidence before the start of the study and measured appropriately using reliable and valid instruments. Under any of the earlier methods (1–4), failure to perfectly measure a confounder may result in only partial control for the variable, thus only partially blocking the alternate causal path in Figure 1.3; this could lead to *residual confounding* biasing inferences about the direct causal effect of $A \rightarrow Y$.
5. The final approach to confounding is *randomisation*, which is dealt with in the section on RCTs. Under randomisation, all participants in a trial are randomly assigned to receive the intervention or control, meaning that the distribution of the confounding factors, L – whether measured or unmeasured – will be the same in each arm and thus cannot be common causes of the treatment, A, or the outcome, Y, as assumed in Figure 1.5. In practice, one would wish to check whether randomisation achieved balance (or *exchangeability*) of confounders between the two arms of the trial and take additional steps to control for variables in the presence of imbalance. However, randomisation is considered as the strongest method to demonstrate causal effects between exposure and outcome because it will theoretically deal with unknown or unmeasured confounders, which cannot be taken into account by any of the other methods. Nonetheless, because it is not ethical to assign participants in studies on risk factors to receive a potentially hazardous exposure, randomisation is limited to treatment or preventive studies. This means that studies investigating risk factors are generally limited to observational epidemiology, and special causal inference methods have been developed that attempt to strengthen the *counterfactual* strengths that are implicit to unbiased RCTs.

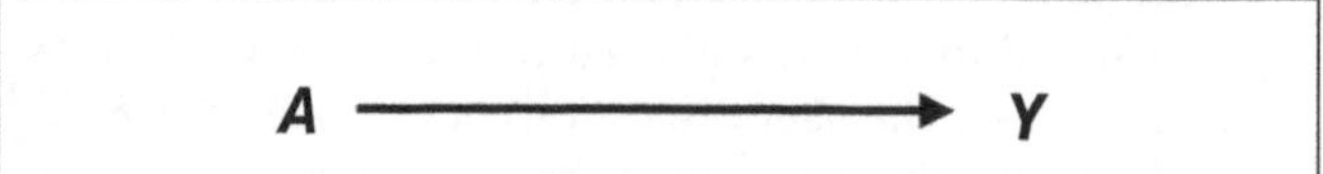

Figure 1.5 Causal diagram of the association between an exposure, *A*, and outcome, *Y*, under the assumption of no confounding, as may arise following randomisation in a randomised controlled trial.

As mentioned earlier, as common causes of exposure and outcome, confounders must temporarily precede the exposure (and outcome). Variables that proceed the exposure but precede the outcome are on the *causal pathway* (Figure 1.6); that is, they are not common causes of the exposure and outcome (i.e. confounders) but potential *mediators* of the relationship. From our example earlier, measuring someone's SES after their cannabis use but before the outcome, psychosis, would make SES a mediator, not a confounder. Inadvertent control for a variable on the causal pathway may induce bias (Figure 1.6) into the results since you are no longer estimating the total *causal effect* of $A \rightarrow Y$.

Typically, more complex confounding structures frequently exist in the causal relationship between an exposure and outcome, including *confounding-by-indication*. For example, in investigating the possible causal role of antidepressants on dementia risk, confounding-by-indication would arise if depression status was an indicator for an antidepressant prescription and if depression was a cause of dementia. For more complex examples of confounding structures in observational data, see Hernan and Robins.[9]

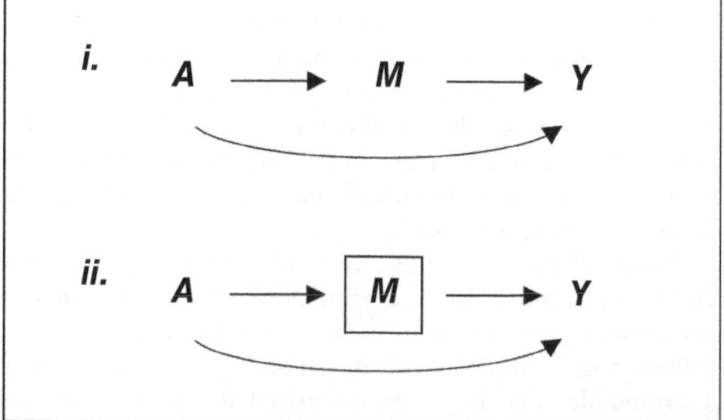

Figure 1.6 ***i.*** When a variable, *M*, lies on the causal pathway, it is not a common cause of the exposure, *A*, and outcome, *Y*. ***ii.*** Inadvertent control for the mediator, *M*, would induce bias in estimation of the total causal effect of $A \rightarrow Y$ by blocking the part of the causal effect that travels via $A \rightarrow M \rightarrow Y$.

Bias

Bias refers to systematic errors in the design of a study that may generate misleading results. Unlike confounding, bias comes about as a result of the study design or execution. Bias is classified into selection bias and information bias.

Selection Bias

Selection bias refers to the way in which participants in a study are selected and the impact this may have on the study's results. It occurs when there are systematic differences between those who take part in a study and those who do not. It is a particular problem in case-control studies but is not exclusive to them. An example was given under the 'Case-Control Studies' section. Selection bias tends to be a particular problem when studies identify cases from clinical populations, especially in specialist settings, since these cases may differ in important ways to cases that do not present to services. For example, a case-control study of the relationship between bullying and disordered eating restricted to clinically diagnosed cases may bias the results because those who have presented to services may differ systematically to those cases who do not present to services (but still have an undiagnosed eating disorder) in terms of their exposure or confounding factors.

From a causal inference perspective, *restriction* to clinical cases in this example is a form of conditioning on that variable (clinical presentation) as discussed in the previous section on *confounding*. Conditioning on a common effect of both the exposure, the bullying, as well as the outcome, eating disorders, may induce a spurious – biased – association between the exposure and outcome via a phenomenon called *collider bias* (Figure 1.7).

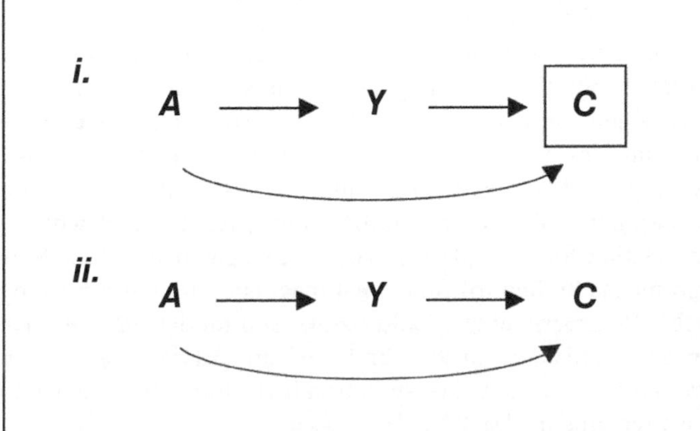

Figure 1.7 ***i.*** Selection bias occurs when those who took part are systematically different to those who did not: the exposure, *A*, and outcome, *Y*, such that selection into the study, *C*, is a common effect of *A* and *Y*. Restriction to those who took part conditions on *C*, inducing a biasing path between $A \rightarrow \boxed{C} \leftarrow Y$, an example of *collider bias*. ***ii.*** If participation is unrelated to exposure or outcome status, there is no conditioning on the common effect, *C*, and the non-causal path $A \rightarrow C \leftarrow Y$ is blocked, allowing correct estimation of the causal effect, $A \rightarrow Y$.

In this example, collider bias occurs because, via restriction, we have conditioned on the common effect (the *collider*) of clinical presentation; in causal inference theory, conditioning on a collider opens an alternate non-causal path between the exposure and outcome via the common effect, *C*, of the form $A \rightarrow \boxed{C} \leftarrow Y$, biasing the true *causal effect* of $A \rightarrow Y$. To estimate the true causal effect of bullying on eating disorders, one would need to obtain a representative sample of cases from the target population, such that there was no conditioning on the collider of clinical presentation. In causal inference theory, the non-causal path between $A \rightarrow C \leftarrow Y$ is blocked when unconditioned, allowing estimation of the causal effect, $A \rightarrow Y$. Various types of *selection bias* exist, including two important ones discussed next.

Non-response Bias

Non-response bias is a form of selection bias of particular importance in cohort studies (but relevant to all study designs), where the individuals of greatest interest may be those who are least likely to participate. This can cause misleading results if the exposure (or outcome) under study also influences participation. In cohort studies, non-response over time is known as loss to follow-up, attrition or censoring.

As a motivating example, consider the long-standing observation that many migrant groups are at increased risk of psychosis.[41] Cohort studies of this association may be affected by differential non-response bias, as depicted in Figure 1.8. In such studies, genetic liability for psychosis is unmeasured (or at best, imperfectly measured), as represented by *U*, but is known to increase both later risk for psychosis[42], *Y*, and drop-out or censoring[43], *C*, in cohort studies. Reasons for this differential loss to follow-up may include greater cognitive impairment or paranoia, *M*, as shown via the mediating path $U \rightarrow M \rightarrow C$. At the same time, migrants, *A*, may also be more likely to be lost to follow-up,

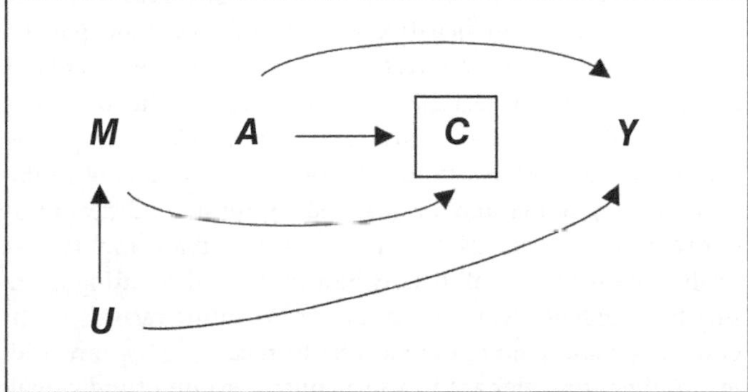

Figure 1.8 Differential non-response bias is induced when censoring (loss to follow-up). C is a common effect of both the exposure, A, and other unmeasured factors, U, which are also related to risk of the outcome, Y. Analyses restricted to those with complete data, indicated by conditioning on censorship, C, would induce a non-causal open path between $A \rightarrow \boxed{C} \leftarrow M \leftarrow U \rightarrow Y$, biasing the estimated association between $A \rightarrow Y$. M represents a set of mediating variables that may be caused by unmeasured factors, U, and may influence non-response, C, such as cognitive impairment, paranoia or other symptoms of disorder.Adapted from Hernan and Robins.[9]

C, for a variety of reasons including returning to their home country. If we let drop-out from the study be denoted by C=1, and we restrict the analysis to those who do not drop out from the study (i.e. C=0), then we have conditioned the analysis on the descendant of a common effect, C, which, as in Figure 1.8, induces a non-causal path between $A \rightarrow \boxed{C} \leftarrow M \leftarrow U \rightarrow Y$ resulting in biased estimation of the causal effect of migrant status on psychosis risk, $A \rightarrow Y$.

Various other patterns of selection bias may exist (see Hernan and Robins).[9] Careful consideration of design features of the study should be made before the start of a new study, while methods that attempt to mitigate selection bias at the analysis stage, including inverse probability weighting and multiple imputation, exist though require strong assumptions and theoretical considerations and may not overcome all issues arising from selection bias.

Prevalence Bias

Prevalence bias is a subtype of selection bias that is a problem in case-control and cross-sectional studies where investigators identify prevalent cases, some of whom may have had the disorder for many years. With disorders such as depression, where relapse and remission are the rule, prevalent samples will be biased because they will over-represent those with chronic depression. It is then difficult to determine whether exposures act to cause or maintain the disorder.

Information Bias

Information bias refers to errors made in the gathering of information from participants. There are two main types of information bias – recall bias and observer bias.

Recall Bias

Recall bias particularly occurs when a disorder has an impact on the participant's recall. For example, patients with depression, when asked about recent life events, may be more inclined to dwell on negative events and over-look positive ones, as this is a feature of depressive thinking. In schizophrenia research, it is notoriously difficult to gain reliable information on early experiences via retrospective recall, such as obstetric complications, and mothers of people with schizophrenia may be inclined to put a good deal more effort into remembering remote events than mothers of healthy controls. Recall bias is best prevented by using documentary evidence (e.g. clinical or other routine records) or by choosing a study design less prone to recall (e.g. cohort studies). Other strategies are to use a control group of individuals with another disorder not thought to be associated with the risk factor under study, where similar recall effects would be expected, serving as a *negative control outcome*.

Observer Bias

In its most general sense, observer bias arises whenever the way in which something in a study (exposure, outcome, confounder) is measured leads to a systematic departure from the true value of that variable. As such, observer bias comes in many guises.

It can relate to the way in which researchers ask questions of participants in studies. If the researcher is aware of the hypothesis under study and also knows which group the participant is from, they may ask questions in subtly different ways. For example, if the study was assessing the efficacy of cognitive therapy versus standard care for depression, the researcher may probe depressive symptoms in a less persistent way to the group who have had cognitive therapy. 'Blinding' is an important approach to prevent this type of observer bias, but it is not always possible to blind the researcher – in case-control studies it may be very obvious which participants have a psychiatric disorder and which do not. This type of observer bias may be overcome by using highly structured interviews or self-completed questionnaires so that every participant is asked the same question in the same way.

Observer bias may also relate to some other systematic error in data collection that we have already come across; for example, many epidemiological studies that rely on diagnoses made as part of someone's routine care will implicitly include (or ignore) between-clinician variance – or *inter-rater reliability* – as a result of the way that different clinicians formulate and apply the same diagnostic criteria to patients. Without consideration, this could introduce bias into the results. For example, in the Social Epidemiology of Psychoses in East Anglia (SEPEA) study of the epidemiology of first-episode psychosis in a rural part of the east of England,[44] the authors used clinical diagnoses made in routine Early Intervention in Psychosis (EIP) care to identify potential cases before asking a panel of clinicians – all trained in the same way with good inter-rater reliability – to make diagnoses using a standardised research instrument; this ensured both reliable and valid diagnoses were used to define the epidemiology of psychotic disorders in this study as well as minimise possible observer bias.

In other situations, systematic errors in observation may arise during the analysis phase of the study if the measures, techniques or observers introduce incorrect data, have faulty readings or fail to correctly interpret information. Classic examples of this exist, including the so-called dead salmon experiment in which the authors demonstrated that without correction for multiple comparisons, results from (though by no means limited to) functional magnetic resonance imaging (fMRI) experiments would show substantial *post-mortem* neural activation in the brain of an Atlantic salmon in response to socially stressful stimuli (to humans, whether to fish remains unclear).[45]

Ascertainment bias is another form of observer bias, whereby the methods used to detect cases may systematically fail to identify and include relevant cases in the target population from different groups equally. For example, studies in which hospitalised cases of depression were over-represented compared with community cases (who may be harder to find) would underestimate the true incidence or prevalence of depression in a population; moreover, if hospitalised cases differed from those in the community in terms of the frequency of the exposure of interest, this would introduce differential bias, leading to inaccurate estimation of the true effect size (i.e. the odds ratio) between exposure and outcome. For example, if hospitalised cases were more likely to have a family history of depression than community cases, this would lead to an overestimation of the true effect of family history of depression on the depression risk in this example.

Reverse Causation

In reverse causation, the association between the risk factor and the disorder is a valid one, but the interpretation is turned around. For example, a study might find that there is a strong association between job loss and depression, and this might be interpreted as indicating that those who lose their jobs are at greater risk of becoming depressed. However, an alternative hypothesis is that depression is an important cause of job loss – individuals who become depressed perform less well at work and are therefore more at risk of losing their jobs.

From a causal inference perspective,[9] *reverse causation* is effectively a special form of confounding, when an unmeasured factor – say the prodromal symptoms of psychotic disorder – is a common cause of both a decline in SES (because people in the prodromal phases of psychotic disorder can no longer hold down a job due to their symptoms) and a clinical diagnosis of psychotic disorder (Figure 1.9).

In psychosis research, reverse causation is a long-standing problem[46] in understanding whether the higher rates of schizophrenia and other non-affective psychotic disorders seen in city dwellers is due to features of urban life ('social causation'), or whether those suffering from non-affective psychotic disorders are more likely to migrate to the cities ('social drift'). These issues can be partially addressed using longitudinal study designs, such as cohort studies, where the risk factor is measured many years *before* the onset of the disorder to decrease the likelihood that prodromal symptoms could be related to exposure (i.e. effectively removing the arrow between *U* and *A* in Figure 1.9). There is now strong evidence from such studies that an association persists between urbanicity at birth[47] or during upbringing[48] and later schizophrenia risk. Nonetheless, more complex – intergenerational – social drift patterns may still explain such an association if parental genetic liability for schizophrenia (now *U* in Figure 1.9) was a common cause of both child genetic liability for schizophrenia (now *L* in Figure 1.9) and urbanicity at child birth (now *A* in Figure 1.9). Evidence to support this possibility is currently equivocal (see Colodro-Conde et al., Solmi et al. and Paksarian et al.[49–51] for further reading on this issue).

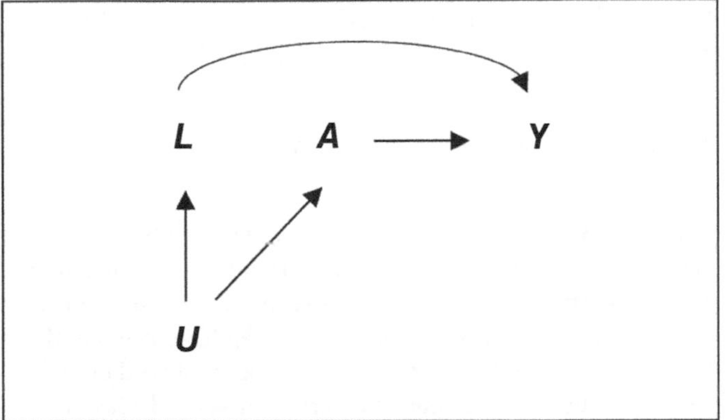

Figure 1.9 *Reverse causation* is effectively a form of confounding, where the putative relationship between an exposure, *A* (for example, SES), and outcome, *Y* (for example, psychotic disorder), is actually due to the prodromal symptoms of psychosis which are unmeasured, *U*, and which may be a common cause of SES (for example, loss of a job due to the prodromal symptoms of psychosis) and which increase the risk of psychotic disorder, *Y*, via some unobserved pathway, *L*, for example, cognitive impairment. Since *U* and *L* are unobserved, reverse causation may provide an alternate non-causal path between *A*→*Y*.

Chance

Type 1 and Type 2 Error

Most studies aim to describe reality by taking a *sample* of the total population. However, the sample will not exactly describe the true underlying population distribution: there is always a degree of *sampling error*. Tossing a coin 10 times will yield different combinations of heads and tails. Statistically the *most likely* result would be five heads and five tails, but any combination of heads and tails is possible. More extreme results (e.g. all tails or all heads) become less probable with increasing numbers of tosses of the coin. In other words, increasing the number of tosses increases the *precision* with which the underlying 'true' situation can be estimated.

In any analytic study, we hope that the results of our study reflect reality. Nevertheless, if 10 identical studies were performed, they would all come up with slightly different results. The size of the difference would depend on the size of the sample in each study. Studies that report an association between two variables may either be describing the true underlying situation or, by chance, have committed a *type 1 error* (see Table 1.5). A type 1 error occurs where a spurious association is detected by chance (a 'false positive'), and the probability that this has occurred is assessed by statistical testing. By convention, the type 1 error rate is often set at the arbitrary level of $P < 0.05$.

Studies that report a 'negative finding' (i.e. do not show an association between two variables) may either be describing the

Table 1.5 The relationship between the results of a study and 'true life'

	'True life'	
Study	**Association exists**	**No association exists**
Association demonstrated	*	Type 1 error ('false positive')
No association demonstrated	Type 2 error ('false negative')	*

* Indicates where the study results represents 'true life'

true underlying situation or may, by chance, have committed a type 2 error. A type 2 error occurs when a genuine association is missed by chance (a 'false negative'). In designing a study, the power calculation takes into account an acceptable type 2 error rate, usually set at 10–20%, meaning that most studies accept that there is a 10–20% chance that they will fail to detect a true effect. Statistical power is the converse of the type 2 error rate (and is therefore usually set at 80–90%). While the type 1 error rate can be set as an arbitrary threshold beyond which statistical significance is inferred, the type 2 error rate is determined by the power the study has to detect an effect size of a pre-specified magnitude in a sample of a given size. This means that power and sample size calculations are required before starting a study to understand how big a study needs to be to detect an effect should one of (at least) that size exist in reality. More powerful studies require bigger sample sizes.

Hypothesis Testing, Statistical Significance and Uncertainty

Most epidemiological studies seek to test whether there is an association or effect between a hypothesised exposure and outcome. Implicitly, this is a hypothesis test that the association differs from what would be expected under the null condition – that is, there being no association between the two variables. Conventionally, a test of the 'statistical significance' of this association is made, with the test being appropriate to the type of data and model used. If the estimated P-value is smaller than an arbitrary threshold (often, $P < 0.05$, though smaller in genetic studies due to multiple comparisons), conclusions are drawn that the observed effect differs from the null and is 'unlikely to be due to chance' (type 1 error).

The received wisdom presented in the previous paragraph is, however, a bastardisation of the use of statistics in medical research. There is no P-value that can 'prove' an association is true. The misuse and misinterpretation of statistical testing, P-values and related measures such as confidence intervals are one of the most endemic and enduring issues in medical statistics, and we encourage readers of this chapter to develop a deeper understanding of the correct use and interpretation of statistics in epidemiology and other fields of medicine (see Greenland et al.[52] for an excellent primer on this topic).

Briefly, though, any statistical model we construct defines a set of assumptions we, as researchers, make about the relationship between exposures, confounders and outcomes. We collect data from a (hopefully unbiased and representative) sample of our target population, and we test the extent to which that model provides an accurate representation of the data collected. Effect sizes between the outcome and other variables in our model – including any exposure(s) of interest – are estimated alongside the level of uncertainty around them. This statistical uncertainty codifies the probability or likelihood of the observed data, given the effect size(s) estimated, and is often represented as confidence intervals around the estimated effect size. Models produced from smaller datasets will estimate effect sizes with greater statistical uncertainty (and wider confidence intervals). P-values and confidence intervals are intimately linked in statistics (a type 1 error alpha level of 0.05 corresponds to a 95% confidence interval, or 1 – 0.05), and P-values should more correctly be thought of 'as a statistical summary of the compatibility between the observed data and what we would . . . expect to see if we knew the entire statistical model . . . were correct' (Lewis, Lewis and Srinivasan, p.339).[48]

Table 1.6 Parameters and their null values

Parameter	Null value
Differences in means, risk difference	0
Odds ratio, rate ratio, risk ratio, hazard ratio	1
Number needed to treat	∞

Confidence intervals provide us with a more intuitive measure of the likelihood or probability that the estimated interval from our study sample contains the true effect size in our target population, or the precision of our effect. If one were to repeat our study 100 times in another valid (i.e. comparable) population, on 95 of those 100 occasions we would expect the confidence interval around our effect size to contain the true effect size. Confidence intervals may be calculated for most parameters we estimate. For example, it is possible to calculate a confidence interval around purely descriptive statistics like a mean or a proportion. It is also possible to show a confidence interval around a comparative parameter such as a difference between two means, a relative risk or a number needed to treat. When the 95% confidence interval crosses the null value of a parameter, this indicates that there is no difference at the P=0.05 level between the groups compared. It is important here to know the null value (see Table 1.6).

We recommend de-emphasising the reliance on P-values, arbitrary thresholds of 'significance testing' or the reporting of 'statistically significant' results (or worse, 'significant' results) in favour of interpretation of effect sizes alongside 95% confidence intervals, which tells us about the level of uncertainty in our observed data given the model.

Points to Consider If a Study Reports One or More Positive Associations

Uncertainty around any estimate and the possibility of a type 1 error mean that no single study will provide sufficient evidence to demonstrate a causal effect between an exposure and outcome. This is why researchers seek to replicate one another's results and triangulate evidence from a body of studies around causation. Positive findings may arise for several reasons.

First, it may be that the study is very big, and even differences that are in clinical terms trivial appear 'statistically significant'. Here, it is important to consider the effect size (i.e. how big the odds ratio is) and its potential clinical relevance instead of reliance on the P-value.

Second, the more statistical comparisons made, the greater the likelihood that a 'statistically significant' association will be found by chance. If researchers collected data on 40 possible risk factors for schizophrenia, they could expect two to be associated at $P < 0.05$ *just by chance*.

There is a balance to be reached between wasting data and 'data trawling'. The best way to overcome this dilemma is to set out with one or two main hypotheses that form the centre of the research protocol and on which the power calculation is based. All additional findings can be labelled 'secondary analyses' and be seen as a useful by-product of the main research, potentially for follow-up in other future studies. Further, in keeping with contemporary causal inference methods, defining one or two main hypotheses *a priori* and specifying the theoretical model you assume to be relevant (for example, via construction of a DAG, see previous discussion) also reduces the reliance on data trawling and multiple testing; instead, one constructs a theoretical model for the hypothesised relationship, designs the study, collects the data and tests that model.

An alternative approach to multiple statistical testing is to use a *Bonferroni correction*. This works on the principle that the level of statistical significance set should be adjusted to take account of the number of tests performed. Thus, if we set $P < 0.05$ for a single significance test, this should be reduced to $P < 0.005$ if we perform 10 comparisons. This approach is generally considered too conservative and may lead one to miss significant positive findings. A better approach is to express results in terms of their *precision* (see the previous section on confidence intervals).

Another way of getting spurious P-values is by using subgroup analyses. Here, the researcher breaks down the statistical analysis according to certain characteristics of the participants. For example, a researcher may have performed a randomised trial comparing a new atypical antipsychotic with haloperidol in patients with treatment-resistant psychosis. The main results show no overall difference, but the researcher may investigate whether there are any particular subgroups of patients in whom there was a difference. For example, the researcher might hypothesise that patients with pronounced positive symptoms will respond better to the atypical antipsychotic. Such analyses are often reported as showing positive evidence for the new intervention but are best avoided as it is notoriously easy to generate a type 1 error in this way.

Points to Consider If the Study Reports a Negative Finding

The key question to consider when a negative finding is presented is whether the sample size was sufficient to detect a true difference if it really existed – that is, are the results due to a type 2 error? For example, in evaluations of new antidepressants, the new treatment is often pitted against a reference compound. Studies often report no difference in treatment effect between the two drugs, suggesting perhaps that the new treatment is as good as the old one. However, comparisons between two active treatments require large samples. If one assumes that two-thirds of patients treated with imipramine respond within 6 weeks, Table 1.7 indicates the sample size required to detect differing levels of recovery rates for a new treatment at 95% confidence and 80% power. It indicates that a sample size of 82 would be able to detect only a very big difference between the treatments and that to detect a difference of 10 percentage points in recovery rates (which would be a clinically meaningful difference) would require over 650 participants. Thus, an underpowered study that demonstrates no difference between two treatments *does not* indicate that the treatments have similar efficacy!

Table 1.7 Power calculations for different effect sizes: sample size required to detect differing levels of recovery rates for a new treatment at 95% confidence and 80% power

Recovery rate on new antidepressant (compared with 66% improvement on imipramine)	Number required to be randomised
33%	82
40%	128
50%	320
55%	654
60%	2096

Internal versus External Validity

Most of the previous discussion has concentrated on threats to the *internal validity* of research studies. However, a common complaint about research is that participants may be so dissimilar from patients seen in normal clinical practice that it is impossible to generalise from the research findings. This complaint particularly applies to RCTs, which are indeed performed in different settings and with different patient groups to those seen in standard practice. In general, complaints about lack of generalisability of RCTs have been misplaced. There are very few examples of treatments working on one group of patients with a disorder but not on others. In some circumstances, the practicalities of recruiting patients make it difficult to ensure that those entered into the study are similar to those seen in clinical practice; this particularly applies to patients with psychotic or manic illness, where the most severely affected are least likely to give their consent to participate. In other circumstances, RCTs impose unnecessarily long lists of exclusion criteria. It is now more common in psychiatric epidemiology to see pragmatic RCTs, which apply standard trial methodology on representative samples of patients to reduce potential issues affecting external validity.[53,54]

Critical Appraisal

This chapter has discussed a number of aspects of clinical epidemiology, with particular emphasis on developing understanding of the principal study designs and their associated flaws. Critical appraisal is the approach of putting this knowledge into practice when assessing research findings. While some knowledge of study designs and common flaws helps, critical appraisal is a skill that requires practice. This is best gained by:

- Reading new research with a sceptical frame of mind, including assessment of the major 'threats to validity' of the reported findings (chance, bias, confounding)
- Following correspondence about published studies
- Discussing studies with colleagues
- Presenting and attending journal clubs
- Being prepared to ask 'what's your evidence?' when given a 'fact' (even in this book!)

References

1. Last JM. *A Dictionary of Epidemiology*, 4th ed. Oxford: Oxford University Press; 2001.
2. Hippocrates. *Hippocrates, Volume I: Ancient Medicine*, Loeb Classical Library. Cambridge, MA: Harvard University Press; 2022.
3. Snow J. *On the Mode of the Communication of Cholera*, 2nd ed. London: John Churchill, New Burlington Street; 1855 (reprinted New York; 1936).
4. Cooper B, Morgan HG. *Epidemiological Psychiatry.* Springfield, IL: Charles C Thomas Pub Ltd; 1973.
5. Wasserman D (ed.). *Oxford Textbook of Suicidology and Suicide Prevention*, 2nd ed. Oxford: Oxford University Press; 2021.
6. Hollander A-C, Pitman A, Sjöqvist H, et al. Suicide risk among refugees compared with non-refugee migrants and the Swedish-born majority population. *The British Journal of Psychiatry* 2020;217(6):686–92. doi.org/10.1192/bjp.2019.220.
7. Harris S, Dykxhoorn J, Hollander A-C, et al. Substance use disorders in refugee and migrant groups in Sweden: a nationwide cohort study of 1.2 million people. *PLoS Medicine* 2019;16(11): e1002944. doi.org/10.1371/journal.pmed.1002944.
8. Goldberger J, The cause and prevention of Pellagra on JSTOR. *Public Health Report* 1914;29(37):2354.
9. Hernan M, Robins J. *Causal Inference: What If.* Boca Raton: Chapman & Hall/CRC; 2020.
10. World Health Organization. *International Statistical Classification of Diseases and Related Health Problems* (11th ed.). https://icd.who.int/ Geneva: World Health Organization; 2019.
11. American Psychiatric Association. *Diagnostic and Statistical Manual of Mental Disorders (DSM-V)*, 5th ed. Washington DC: American Psychiatric Association; 2013.
12. Jongsma HE, Turner C, Kirkbride JB, et al. International incidence of psychotic disorders, 2002–17: a systematic review and meta-analysis. *The Lancet Public Health* 2019;4(5): e229–e244. doi.org/10.1016/S2468-2667(19)30056-8.
13. Moher D, Hopewell S, Schulz KF, et al. CONSORT 2010 explanation and elaboration: updated guidelines for reporting parallel group randomised trials. *BMJ* 2010;340:869. doi.org/10.1136/BMJ.C869.
14. Lash TL, VanderWeele TJ, Haneuse S, et al. *Modern Epidemiology*, 4th ed. Philadelphia: Lippincott Williams & Wilkins; 2021.
15. Lubin JK, Gail MH. Biased selection of controls for case-control analyses of cohort studies. *Biometrics* 1984;40(1):63. doi.org/10.2307/2530744.
16. Helbich M, de Beurs D, Kwan MP, et al. Natural environments and suicide mortality in the Netherlands: a cross-sectional, ecological study. *The Lancet Planetary Health* 2018;2(3):e134–e139. doi.org/10.1016/S2542-5196(18)30033-0.
17. Keown P, Weich S, Bhui KS, et al. Association between provision of mental illness beds and rate of involuntary admissions in the NHS in England 1988–2008: ecological study. *BMJ* 2011;343:d3736. doi.org/10.1136/BMJ.D3736.
18. McManus S, Bebbington PE, Jenkins R, et al. Data resource profile: adult psychiatric morbidity survey (APMS). *International Journal of Epidemiology* 2020;49(2):361–62e. doi.org/10.1093/IJE/DYZ224.
19. Scott KM, de Jonge P, Stein DJ, et al. (eds.). *Mental Disorders around the World: Facts and Figures from the WHO World Mental Health Surveys.* Cambridge: Cambridge University Press; 2018.
20. Wadsworth M, Kuh D, Richards M, et al. Cohort profile: the 1946 national birth cohort (MRC National Survey of Health and Development). *International Journal of Epidemiology* 2006;35(1):49–54. doi.org/10.1093/IJE/DYI201.
21. Elliott J, Shepherd P. Cohort profile: 1970 British Birth Cohort (BCS70). *International Journal of Epidemiology* 2006;35(4):836–43. doi.org/10.1093/IJE/DYL174.
22. Boyd A, Golding J, Macleod J, et al. Cohort profile: the 'children of the 90s'—the index offspring of the Avon Longitudinal Study of Parents and Children. *International Journal of Epidemiology* 2013;42(1):111. doi.org/10.1093/IJE/DYS064.
23. Solmi F, Lewis G, Zammit S, et al. Neighborhood characteristics at birth and positive and negative psychotic symptoms in adolescence: findings from the ALSPAC birth cohort. *Schizophrenia Bulletin* 2020;46(3):581–91. doi.org/10.1093/SCHBUL/SBZ049.
24. Geoffroy MC, Arseneault L, Girard A, et al. Association of childhood bullying victimisation with suicide deaths: findings from a 50-year nationwide cohort study. *Psychological Medicine* 2022. doi.org/10.1017/S0033291722000836.
25. Laugesen K, Ludvigsson KF, Schmidt M, et al. Nordic health registry-based research: a review of health care systems and key registries. *Clinical Epidemiology* 2021;13:533–4. doi.org/10.2147/CLEP.S314959.
26. Jongsma HE, Gayer-Anderson C, Tarricone I, et al. Social disadvantage, linguistic distance, ethnic minority status and first-episode psychosis: results from the EU-GEI case-control study. *Psychological Medicine* 2021;51(9):1536–48. doi.org/10.1017/S003329172000029X.
27. Lewis G, Duffy L, Ades A, et al. The clinical effectiveness of sertraline in primary care and the role of depression severity and duration (PANDA): a pragmatic, double-blind, placebo-controlled randomised trial. *The Lancet Psychiatry* 2019;6(11):903–14. doi.org/10.1016/S2215-0366(19)30366-9.
28. Egger M, Smith GD, Schneider M, et al. Bias in meta-analysis detected by a simple, graphical test. *BMJ* 1997;315:629–34. doi.org/10.1136/BMJ.315.7109.629.

29. Kandola A, Lewis G, Osborn DPJ, et al. Depressive symptoms and objectively measured physical activity and sedentary behaviour throughout adolescence: a prospective cohort study. *The Lancet Psychiatry* 2020;7 (3):262–71. doi.org/10.1016/S2215-0366 (20)30034-1.
30. Godlee F, Smith J, Marcovitch H. Wakefield's article linking MMR vaccine and autism was fraudulent. *BMJ* 2011;342:64–6. doi.org/10.1136/BMJ .C7452.
31. Wakefield AJ, Murch SH, Anthony A, et al. Retracted: Ileal-lymphoid-nodular hyperplasia, non-specific colitis, and pervasive developmental disorder in children. *Lancet* 1998;351 (9103):637–41. doi.org/10.1016/S0140-6736(97)11096-0.
32. Napier G, Lee D, Robertson C, et al. A model to estimate the impact of changes in MMR vaccine uptake on inequalities in measles susceptibility in Scotland. *Statistical Methods in Medical Research* 2016;25 (4):1185–200. doi.org/10.1177/ 0962280216660420.
33. Motta M, Stecula D. Quantifying the effect of Wakefield et al. (1998) on skepticism about MMR vaccine safety in the U.S. *PLoS ONE* 2021;16(8): e0256395. doi.org/10.1371/JOURNAL .PONE.0256395.
34. Hill AB. The Environment and Disease: Association or Causation? *Proceedings of the Royal Society of Medicine* 1965;58 (5):295–300.
35. van Dyck CH, Swanson CJ, Aisen P, et al. Lecanemab in early Alzheimer's disease. *The New England Journal of Medicine* 2023;388(1):9–21. doi.org/10 .1056/nejmoa2212948.
36. Lawlor DA, Tilling K, Smith GD. Triangulation in aetiological epidemiology. *International Journal of Epidemiology* 2016;45(6):1866–86. doi .org/10.1093/IJE/DYW314.
37. Munafò MR, Higgins JPT, Smith GD. Triangulating evidence through the inclusion of genetically informed designs. *Cold Spring Harbor Perspectives in Medicine* 2020;1:11. doi.org/10.1101/ CSHPERSPECT.A040659.
38. Rothman KJ, Greenland S. Causation and causal inference in epidemiology. *American Journal of Public Health* 2005;95:S144–S150. doi.org/10.2105/ AJPH.2004.059204.
39. Tennant PWG, Murray EJ, Arnold KF, et al. Use of directed acyclic graphs (DAGs) to identify confounders in applied health research: review and recommendations. *International Journal of Epidemiology* 2021;50 (2):620–32. doi.org/10.1093/IJE/ DYAA213.
40. Pearce N. Analysis of matched case-control studies. *BMJ* 2016;352:i969. doi .org/10.1136/bmj.i969.
41. Henssler J, Brandt L, Müller M, et al. Migration and schizophrenia: meta-analysis and explanatory framework. *European Archives of Psychiatry and Clinical Neuroscience* 2020;270:325–35. doi.org/10.1007/ S00406-019-01028-7.
42. Pardiñas AF, Holmans P, Pocklington AJ, et al. Common schizophrenia alleles are enriched in mutation-intolerant genes and in regions under strong background selection. *Nature Genetics* 2018;50:381–9. doi.org/10.1038/s41588-018-0059-2.
43. Martin J, Tilling K, Hubbard L, et al. Association of genetic risk for schizophrenia with nonparticipation over time in a population-based cohort study. *American Journal of Epidemiology* 2016;183(12):1149–58. doi.org/10.1093/aje/kww009.
44. Kirkbride JB, Hameed Y, Ankireddypalli G, et al. The epidemiology of first-episode psychosis in early intervention in psychosis services: findings from the social epidemiology of psychoses in East Anglia [SEPEA] study. *American Journal of Psychiatry* 2017;174 (2):143–53. doi.org/10.1176/appi.ajp .2016.16010103.
45. Bennett C, Miller M, Wolford G. Neural correlates of interspecies perspective taking in the post-mortem Atlantic Salmon: an argument for multiple comparisons correction. *NeuroImage* 2009;47:S125. doi.org/10.1016/S1053-8119(09)71202-9.
46. Faris R, Dunham H. *Mental Disorders in Urban Areas: An Ecological Study of Schizophrenia and Other Psychoses.* Chicago/London: The University of Chicago Press; 1939.
47. Lewis G, Dykxhoorn J, Karlsson H, et al. Assessment of the role of IQ in associations between population density and deprivation and nonaffective psychosis. *JAMA Psychiatry* 2020;77 (7):729–36. doi.org/10.1001/ jamapsychiatry.2020.0103.
48. Lewis G, David A, Andreasson S, et al. Schizophrenia and city life. *Lancet* 1992;340(8812):137–40. doi.org/10 .1016/0140-6736(92)93213-7.
49. Colodro-Conde L, Couvy-Duchesne B, Whitfield JB, et al. Association between population density and genetic risk for schizophrenia. *JAMA Psychiatry* 2018;75(9):901–10. doi.org/10.1001/ jamapsychiatry.2018.1581.
50. Solmi F, Lewis G, Zammit S, et al. Neighborhood characteristics at birth and positive and negative psychotic symptoms in adolescence: findings from the ALSPAC birth cohort. *Schizophrenia Bulletin* 2020;46 (3):581–91. doi.org/10.1093/SCHBUL/ SBZ049.
51. Paksarian D, Trabjerg BB, Merikangas KR, et al. The role of genetic liability in the association of urbanicity at birth and during upbringing with schizophrenia in Denmark. *Psychological Medicine* 2018;48 (2):305–14. doi.org/10.1017/ S0033291717001696.
52. Greenland S, Senn SJ, Rothman KJ, et al. Statistical tests, P values, confidence intervals, and power: a guide to misinterpretations. *European Journal of Epidemiology* 2016;31:337–50. doi.org/10.1007/ S10654-016-0149-3.
53. Ford I, Norrie J. Pragmatic trials. *New England Journal of Medicine* 2016;375:454–63. www.nejm.org/doi/10 .1056/NEJMra1510059.
54. Hotopf M, Churchill R, Lewis G. Pragmatic randomised controlled trials in psychiatry. *The British Journal of Psychiatry* 1999;175(3):217–23. doi.org/ 10.1192/BJP.175.3.217.

Chapter 2

Assessment, Formulation and Diagnosis

David Kingdon, George Stein and Paul Rowlands

Canst thou not minister to a mind diseased,
Pluck from the memory a rooted sorrow,
Raze out the written troubles of the brain
And with some sweet oblivious antidote
Cleanse the stuff'd bosom of that perilous stuff
Which weighs upon the heart?
—Macbeth *Act V Scene 3*

The psychiatrist as a practitioner deals with individuals, with the human being as a whole.
***—Karl Jaspers,* General Psychopathology**

The wit of man has rarely been more exercised then in the attempt to classify the morbid phenomena covered by the term insanity - and the result has been disappointing.
—Daniel Hack Tuke (1892)

Daniel Hack Tuke (1827–1895) was a descendent of William Tuke, a Quaker and a progressive asylum physician of the nineteenth century and, for 18 years, the editor of the *British Journal of Mental Science*, the predecessor of the *British Journal of Psychiatry*. The difficulties and debates over classification in the diagnosis of mental disorders in the late nineteenth century are described in detail in J C Bucknill and Daniel Tuke's classic textbook *A Manual of Psychological Medicine.*[1] Despite vast amounts of work refining this over the years since, the topic of psychiatric diagnosis remains subject to heated debate to this day.

Yet, diagnosis and classification are fundamental to the way we organise our approaches to medicine and psychiatry. As human beings, we organise our understanding of the world by grouping and naming phenomena, experiences and objects. At a fundamental cognitive level, we apply 'categories' to the world. The philosopher Immanuel Kant described this in terms of our minds processing and holding together the incoming chaos of perceptual information through applying organising concepts and categories to it, the most basic being Space and Time. A human mind develops a myriad of other organising principles for the world. At a prosaic level, classifications of 'things in the world' have been developed for flowers, animals, furniture and music (classical, rock, folk, etc.). Humans have also developed language-based classifications of both physical and mental diseases and illnesses. Acceptance is needed of the limitations of such processes as well as the benefits. The advantages are that such processes ease communication and define groups that can be investigated, creating a common language. This, in turn, allows research into groups to be conducted, treatments to be developed and prescribed, and outcomes to be evaluated. Patients themselves can find out more about specific described diagnoses, for example, about treatment of depression or an eating disorder. However, all such classifications, it could be argued, merely represent products of the human mind organising the chaos of phenomena and may not represent either an underlying reality or distinct natural forms: there may also be no clear distinctions between described 'diagnoses'.

Nonetheless, the doctor's human task is not primarily philosophy: it is to assess, diagnose and treat their patients. For the physically ill, the suffering is frequently obvious; there are often characteristic symptoms and objective physical signs, and the diagnosis can usually be confirmed by blood tests, X-rays or other investigations. An appropriate physical treatment, if available, will commonly follow. The general physician may therefore be less likely to be troubled by semantic issues such as the nature of disease and its definition, the boundary between normality and pathology or even the overall value of diagnosis. However, causes of many physical illnesses remain elusive. Diagnoses may therefore also be descriptive (e.g. chronic headache, fatigue, back pain or dementia) and dimensional (e.g. hypertension), and treatments may be palliative rather than curative.

For the psychiatrist, however, the issue of diagnosis is usually more complex – for most patients, assessment is more time-consuming and the formulation more multidimensional. Comorbidities are common, and diagnoses therefore involve consideration of a broad range of factors. Sometimes there is no overt suffering on the part of the patient, who may not regard themselves as 'ill' or in need of attention for their health. There may be disagreement amongst professionals and wider society as to whether the person's condition should be regarded as a 'health' problem worthy of attention from health services, as more of a moral or social problem or as a legitimate personal lifestyle choice. Whilst similar issues regarding the boundaries and definitions of health and disease are present across the landscape of medical practice, it is within psychiatry that these issues are most acutely expressed. There are rarely unequivocal physical signs – though the observation of verbal and non-verbal expressions gives valuable information on the emotional state. There are few, if any, objective biological tests for most of the conditions encountered. Psychiatric diagnosis is therefore not easy. In this chapter, we explore how psychiatric diagnoses are made today, how they evolved to reach their current format, what they consist of and their usefulness. We describe as well the development of the two main classificatory schemes in use today – the International Classification of Diseases (ICD-11) and the American scheme, *The Diagnostic and Statistical Manual of Mental Disorders*, 5th edition (DSM-5) – and the criticisms of the very process of diagnosis. We then outline an approach to assessment and the communication of the outcome of this assessment within present-day services.

Human beings have an intrinsic need to make sense of the information that confronts them. Different diagnostic approaches have evolved for medicine and specifically psychiatry: phenomenological psychopathology described, defined and classified mental phenomena as independent entities[2] seeking an approach that would enable the development of scientific approaches to subjective mental phenomena, describing without assuming aetiology. Other systems were more theoretically driven, either by biological theory (e.g. somato-aetiological theories of brain disorder) or by psychological theory and experimental psychopathology (e.g. psychodynamic theories of the mind).

All approaches should be undertaken with humility and a recognition that, in psychiatry, this is a complicated construct. Diagnosis should be viewed as a process rather than an isolated act[3]: a patient's symptoms and signs are assessed and investigated with a view to the categorisation of his or her experience with others of a similar sort that have been studied in the past. The patient can then benefit from a collaborative application of established knowledge to the problem[4] to plot a way forward.

History of Classifications

Aristotle (384–322 BCE) set out a scheme of taxonomy of living things with a binomial scheme that was influential for two thousand years until the Swedish botanist and physician Carl Linnaeus (1707–1778) developed the modern scientific approach. His major work, *System Naturae* (1735),[5] classified all the known flora and fauna according to their shared physical characteristics, and he developed the modern binomial scheme of nomenclature whereby every plant or animal is assigned a name according to its genera and then its species. By the time his book reached its 10th edition in 1858, it contained 4,400 species of animals and 7,700 species of plants with each given a brief description, often an illustration and, most importantly, a two-word Latin name. Linnaeus was also a physician and published *Genera morborum*,[6] a catalogue of diseases. François Bossier de Lacroix (1706–1777) of Montpellier in France, better known as Sauvages, was the first to attempt to classify diseases systematically. His classificatory system was mainly symptom based. It was published in his book *Nosologica methodica* (1763)[7] and included over 2,400 separate species of disease, although many of these conditions were just single symptoms. This system is highly detailed and highlights the dilemma of modern nosology – whether to have a vast number of individual categories, or whether to opt for fewer but larger categories within which there are numerous subtypes, genera and species as in the Linnaean system.

One of the greatest medical textbooks to emerge in the late eighteenth century, which also included chapters on neurological and mental disorders, was William Cullen's *Synopsis Nosologica Methodica*,[8] published in Latin in 1769. Cullen adapted Linnaeus's botanical approach and used classes, genera, species and subspecies in his work, which included a neurological chapter. Thus, within his class of neurosis were the *comate* (coma, apoplexy and paralysis), the *adynamia* (syncope, dyspepsia and hypochondriasis), the *spasmii* (tetanus, chorea, epilepsy and diabetes) and the *vesanii*, which included all the insanities.

From the nineteenth century until the middle of the twentieth, psychiatrists from different countries in Europe developed their own nosologies of mental disorders. Shorter[9] summarises how this evolved to the modern day. In the nineteenth century, the spread of ideas was through textbooks rather than journals, and through proceedings of learned societies rather than social media. Within Europe, there was a Balkanisation of psychiatric nosology governed more by the authority of a particular professor in each region and his self-authored textbook than by any peer-reviewed process. Kendler[10] asserted that such nosologies were predominantly determined by the 'famous professor principle', and as the profession grew in numbers in the twentieth century, this could be said to have been replaced by the 'committee of famous professors' principle, for example, in the development of the ICD and DSM. Stengel, quoting Zilboorg, observed that to produce a well-ordered classification seemed to have become the unspoken ambition of almost every psychiatrist of industry and promise of the nineteenth century. Stengel's 1959 paper[11] for the World Health Organization (WHO) describes over 20 different nosologies.

In France, the 'famous professors' who shaped ideas about psychopathology from the late eighteenth century into the nineteenth century included Philippe Pinel, Jean-Étienne Dominique Esquirol, Jean-Pierre Falret, Valentin Magnan, Bénédict Morel and Jean-Martin Charcot. Morel was a French psychiatrist who, in his book *Traitsé des Maladies Mentales,*[12] saw 'mental deficiency' as the end point of an inherited degenerating process that included passing through a phase of mental illness. He was the first to apply the term *Dementia Precoce* to this degenerating process. In England, Bucknill and Tuke wrote an influential text[13] that went into several editions and classified disorders following the International Congress of Alienists meeting in Paris in 1867, which met to agree on a classificatory framework. Bucknill and Tuke refined this classification within the third edition of their textbook into the following:

- Undeveloped intellectual power
- Dementia
- Delusional insanity
- Mania
- Emotional insanity

with each potentially comorbid with epilepsy or general paralysis. Bucknill and Tuke were mainly describing asylum populations, and within this context, it is clear that their classification is not wholly removed from the most recent iterations of ICD and DSM.

Symptom-Based Classification versus Aetiologically Based Classification

By the latter part of the nineteenth century, Germany became dominant in psychiatric nosology, following alongside the dramatic advances in understanding of neuropathology and brain function. Wilhelm Griesinger, based in Berlin, published in 1845 the first edition of an influential textbook, *Pathology and Treatment of Mental Diseases*.[14] He argued that 'all mental illness is disease of the brain'. He also put forward the principle of the *Einheit psychosen*, or unitary psychosis, which proposed that all the different psychoses were simply different manifestations of one and the same condition. Recent genomic studies have shown that this idea may not be so far from the truth as the major functional psychoses seem to share many genetic variants in common, though most mental disorders do not have clear and obvious pathophysiological abnormalities.

There had emerged two broad ways of classifying mental disorders: the symptom based or 'symptomatological', based on a description of the symptoms the patient reports and the signs the doctor observes, and the causation based or 'somatoetiological', in which the classification is based around physiological and pathological underlying mechanisms. The latter, of course, is preferable, as nosology in the rest of medicine is usually based on causation. Causation-based nosologies had to be discarded because aetiology was unknown in most cases, although a large minority of patients clearly did have identifiable coarse pathophysiological abnormalities. Even in those without observable pathology, eminent neurologists such as Carl Wernicke proposed elaborate biological theories such as 'transcortical aphasia', in which fibre tracts were theorised to be disrupted to explain all the observed phenomena of a serious mental illness. If an aetiology was uncovered, such as the various avitaminoses and general paresis, some diseases became regarded more as a part of general medicine, though the patient might remain within the asylum. Nineteenth-century textbooks, such as that of Bucknill and Tuke,[13] contain detailed historical review and discussion of the different schemes that had been suggested over the years.

The Case History Approach

By the late nineteenth century, the scheme and case history approach developed in Heidelberg, Germany, and, promulgated by Emil Kraepelin, held sway throughout much of Europe. This approach was 'symptomological' but also longitudinal, based on a combination of symptoms and course over time, gathering together different syndromes of non-affective psychosis (hebephrenia, catatonia and dementia paranoids) and periodic-affective psychoses (manic-depressive insanity). Based on meticulous descriptions and longer-term follow-up of hundreds of individual cases, Kraepelin's scheme became the dominant influence on psychiatric nosology moving into the twentieth century and beyond. Karl Jaspers, a young psychiatrist working in Heidelberg under the professorial supervision of Franz Nissl, Kraepelin's successor, was given the task of producing a textbook summarising the state of psychiatric knowledge in the first decade of the twentieth century. Jaspers, going far beyond Nissl's expectations, produced a work that sought a way of approaching mental disorders that incorporated the idea of meaningful understanding of the patient's perspective with objective description of the symptoms they reported. The systematic 'phenomenological' approach to descriptive psychopathology, summarised by Jaspers in his *General Psychopathology* (1913),[15] emphasised the approach of examining the subjective, objective and somatic features of a case in an attempt to understand the meaning of objective phenomena and the individual's personal world ('Weltanschauung'). Influenced by philosophers interested in the subjective world of the individual person, such as Wilhelm Dilthey and Max Weber, Jaspers was critical of the dogmatic approaches then competing for dominance in psychiatry. He described psychiatrists with biological psychiatric approaches, such as Wernicke, as promoting 'brain mythologies', on the one hand, and Freud and the growing group of psychoanalysts of mistaking

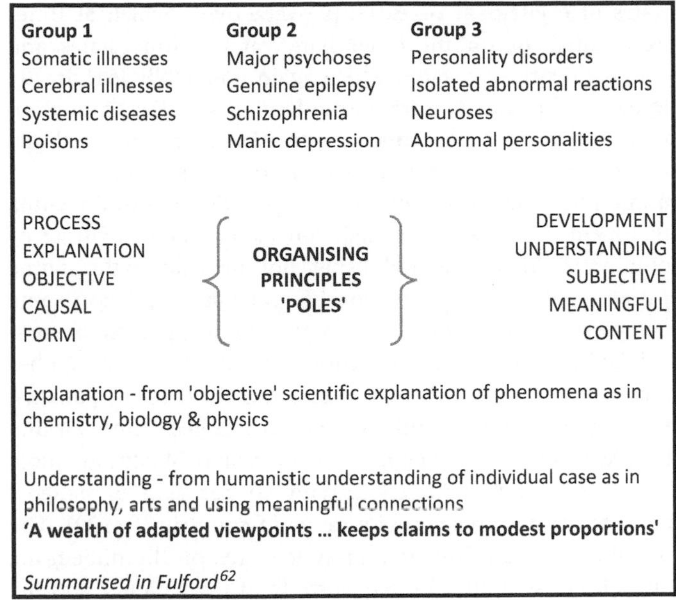

Figure 2.1 Classification of psychiatric disorders(Jaspers[2]).

'meaningful connections for causal connections', on the other, promoting in their own way an account of the individual every bit as deterministic as that of the 'biological' psychiatrists with their 'brain mythologies'.

Jaspers was concerned with the 'ill person as a whole': 'the chaos of phenomena should not be blotted out with some diagnostic label ... Psychiatric diagnosis is too often a sterile running round in circles'. Whilst Jaspers stated that 'conversation with the patient' is the most important method, he emphasised gathering information from many sources, including written personal accounts from patients and collateral histories, to arrive at a 'full biographical account'. Within this empathic approach, the psychiatrist is tasked to describe particular aspects of subjective experience, phenomenology, that inform an understanding of the mental life of the patient. He suggested 'introducing fairly the different viewpoints' rather than offering 'a list of symptoms for parrot-like repetition' – advice that probably remains sound. In his nosology, developing the Kraepelinian approach, he separated conditions into three broad groups: Groups I, II and III (see Figure 2.1). He emphasised the need for approaching psychiatric diagnosis by not only recognising its limitations but also seeing its usefulness and, at the same time, the importance of seeking an understanding from the ill person's perspective of 'walking in their shoes'.

Kraepelin's Contribution to Classification

A series of editions of Kraepelin's textbooks,[16] which started to attract world attention with the fourth edition in 1893 and concluded with the renowned eighth edition – published in its five volumes between 1909 and 1915 – grew to be anticipated similarly to new editions of the DSM are today. Translations and synopses of editions of his *Lehrbuch der Psychiatrie* became important teaching volumes in the United States at the turn of the century, establishing his approach that included a 'definite routine method of examination', including 'anamnesis [the patient's personal account] of the family ... personal history previous to the disease ... anamnesis of the disease ... and status praesens'. Karl Jaspers[15] summarised this nosology in the first edition of *General Psychopathology* describing how 'the greatest influence [on psychiatry] came from Kraepelin ... Kraepelin's impact has extended from year to year ... his textbook is the most read of all psychiatric textbooks' (p. 332).

Following on from Karl Ludwig Kahlbaum, the genius of Kraepelin's classification was not that it was somato-aetiological or cross-sectionally syndromic, but clinical, looking longitudinally as well as cross-sectionally. The groupings of 'major psychoses' without definite organic pathology in the Kraepelinian system – manic-depressive insanity and dementia praecox (later 'schizophrenia') – were not included for biological, or pseudo-biological, reasons. Rather, it was because Kraepelin had studied the patients in detail and followed them up over long time periods. He believed that he had discerned two starkly different courses and outcomes. Manic-depressive insanity was a fluctuating illness that did not necessarily deteriorate into 'dementia'. Patients were admitted, commonly recovered to the point of being discharged, but might then later relapse. Dementia praecox, by contrast, commonly had its onset in adolescence or early adulthood and, within a short period of time, progressed to appear to simulate 'dementia' and institutionalisation:

> As the patients neither quickly die off like the paralytics, nor become in considerable number again fit for discharge like the manic-depressive cases, they accumulate more and more in the institutions and thus impress on the institution its peculiar stamp.[17]

Even though the two great diseases might share some symptoms, it was based on this course that he believed them to differ. He was not however dogmatic – he accepted that whether it represented '*one uniform disease* cannot be decided at present with certainty'.

His approach to classification has had, and continues to have, considerable influence on classifications of mental disorders into the twentieth and twenty-first centuries. He observed not only the pattern of his patients' symptoms but also their longitudinal course, in order to try and discover common features that would help to distinguish between patient groups. His three groups are shown below, with Jaspers' summary added, which uses the same groupings and incidentally remain the same broad groupings used in the National Health Service (NHS):

Group I organic psychosis: 'Known Somatic Illnesses with psychic disturbances'

Group II endogenous psychosis: 'the three major psychoses: Genuine Epilepsy, Schizophrenia, Manic-depressive illnesses'. Epilepsy was included here as it often has no obvious associated organic lesion, and Kraepelin and Jaspers were writing before the advent of EEGs.

Group III deviations of personality and reactive states: 'Isolated abnormal reactions, Neuroses . . . Abnormal personalities . . .' Jaspers emphasised here the interaction of the individual predisposition, however constituted, and events in the person's life.

These three main groups of disorders remain relevant today. The definition of 'organic psychosis' can be applied to the dementias, general paresis of the insane (GPI) and confusional states and other conditions with clear 'organic' contributions. The definition of 'endogenous psychosis' includes present-day schizophrenia and psychotic affective disorders, while that of 'reactive states' could apply to nonpsychotic unipolar depression, anxiety and personality disorders.[18] The phrase 'dementia praecox' was gradually dropped in favour of the newer term 'schizophrenia', largely as a result of Eugene Bleuler's influential work, originally published in 1911, entitled *Dementia Praecox or the Group of Schizophrenias*.[19] Bleuler's concept of 'the group of schizophrenias' was a much broader concept than the narrower concept of Kraepelin's and had far-reaching consequences, particularly influencing different rates of diagnosis between the United States and Europe.

Advances in Diagnosis in the Mid-Twentieth Century

The use of sedatives and stimulants dates back millennia in human societies. In the eighteenth and nineteenth centuries, trade in opium became an issue associated with colonialism and war. Laudanum, a tincture containing 10 per cent opium, was widely available 'over the counter' as an aid to sleep and a pain killer. Cocaine was a constituent of many medicinal preparations and even soft drinks. Huge advances in the understanding of organic chemistry during the nineteenth century, particularly in Germany, led to the isolation of compounds such as morphine and the synthesis of others such as di-acetyl morphine (heroin), oxycodone and methamphetamine.[20] All became easily available and widely used. In the 1950s, further major pharmacological discoveries and 'repurposing' of existing compounds revolutionised treatment of serious mental illness.[21] Anti-psychotics, derived from methylene blue which had been used to treat malaria earlier in the century, were introduced for schizophrenia, and anti-depressants were introduced for the treatment of severe depression. Iproniazid, a monoamine oxidase inhibitor, had originally been developed as a treatment for tuberculosis (TB), chlorpromazine as a pre-anaesthetic agent for the management of trauma and associated surgical shock and lithium as a treatment for gout. Prior to the introduction of effective pharmacological treatments, treatments for acute serious mental illness often had a vivid and sometimes brutal physicality. These treatments might be targeted, on the one hand, at states of excitement or extreme overactivity, which at times were lethal, or on the other hand, at catatonic states and extreme depressive states, which again potentially led directly to death. Treatments were, to modern sensibilities without an understanding of this context, sometimes extreme: malarial treatment for neurosyphilis; Cardiazol shock treatment and unmodified electroconvulsive therapy (ECT); insulin coma treatment and leucotomy; sedation using chloral hydrate or opium; or 'hydrotherapy' using hot or cold baths. Some patients got better spontaneously, and others did not; some got worse or died; sometimes, the treatment appeared to work. Whilst 'incurable' patients accumulated and the total number increased over time, there was in fact a turnover of patients, with many people admitted and discharged after varying lengths of stay. Bucknill and Tuke, in their 1874 edition, quote recovery rates of between 25 and 50 per cent of patients admitted to asylums across a range of countries (p.129). The initial emphasis in the asylum system was on the milieu, the attitudes of staff and the safe custody of the patients, and the 'doctor–patient' relationship. Apart from the physical treatments, specific interventions of the doctor for the most severe conditions appeared to have little effect though a range of treatments were tried. Despite the fact that around half of admissions might improve and be discharged, the numbers in asylums rose dramatically. Overwhelmed by the increase in numbers, the initial ideals of 'traitement moral' – a 'talking treatment' in a humane setting – receded. Now, with the new drugs, diagnosis began to matter more: the diagnosis might determine the drug treatment, and the ease, tolerability and effectiveness of drug treatment for severe cases pushed and extended the boundaries of what would be regarded as a case requiring treatment and the acceptability of that treatment, building on the trends in this direction apparent before the Second World War.

Throughout the asylum era, there had been a parallel system – largely accessed by the more wealthy – involving treatment for less-severe conditions, where the predominant features did not involve gross disturbance of behaviour, mood and thought. These symptoms might include non-specific fatigue, anxiety, low mood, listlessness and other features. New York neurologist George Beard popularised the term 'Neurasthenia' to describe this syndrome, which has been described using different terms across cultures for millenia. Although the term has now slipped out of modern classifications, along with words such as 'neurosis', it was applied to a large group of patients who sought treatment for their mental and physical ailments through sources other than the asylum system, for example through general physicians, psychoanalysts, the use of patent medicines as well as active pharmacological compounds such as opiates, and the use of health spas and cures. Diagnosis in these patient groups was not precisely defined. Jaspers, describing these conditions as Group III, emphasised the developmental, subjective and situational ways in which these conditions needed to be understood.

Operational Criteria

Within the seriously ill population, it was noted that in the early 1950s, schizophrenia was much more commonly diagnosed in the USA than in Europe.[22] Was there truly an increased rate of schizophrenia in the USA, or was this due to some artefact? 'The US-UK study'[23] explored this question using a new psychiatric interview known as the Present State Examination (PSE).[24] Diagnoses were generated by a computer programme known as CATEGO, which had an algorithm that yielded diagnoses of schizophrenia or manic depression according to the ICD-8 criteria. The research psychiatrists played no part in making the diagnosis after gathering the data. Their role was confined to asking symptom-based questions, and if a symptom was present, then this was entered into the computer.

The results showed that the computer-based diagnoses did not differ between the two countries, but the diagnoses made by the admitting psychiatrists (i.e. not the research doctors), in contrast, confirmed that American psychiatrists diagnosed schizophrenia twice as often as their British counterparts. This meant that, while there was no real difference between rates in the USA and the UK using defined symptom-based approaches, the differences lay in the way the condition was diagnosed in each country. That is, the application of the diagnostic criteria used in the two nations was different. The teams went on to verify these findings in a much larger study (n=1,000) in the International Pilot Study of Schizophrenia,[25] which examined diagnostic practices in nine different cities around the world. This showed that in two locations (Washington, DC, and Moscow), schizophrenia was diagnosed more frequently than in the other seven locations. Generally, UK and European psychiatry was working towards a diagnostic approach that reflected the diagnostic approach of Kraepelin, Jaspers and Kurt Schneider, with a narrow construct, and which had influenced the development of the PSE, whereas the US psychiatrists were more heavily influenced by Bleuler and psychobiological/psychoanalytic approaches with a much wider and looser definition. USSR psychiatrists were influenced by the context in which they practised and had been trained.

The US–UK studies had shown that reliable diagnoses could be made by a computer algorithm. However, in the 1960s and subsequently, such availability and use of computers was not practical for everyday clinical work. Instead, a series of rules or 'operational criteria' were devised for the definition of disorder to form the basis for more reliable diagnoses within and between countries. The operational approach to scientific definitions was originally proposed by Percy Williams Bridgman (1927),[26] a physicist:

> An operational definition of a scientific term (S) is a stipulation to the effect that S is to apply to all and only those cases for which the specific test (T) yields a specific outcome (O).

The advantage of such an operational definition is that, provided the specific test (T) is sufficiently clearly defined, any person can apply it one or more times to confirm or refute the reliability of the definition of the scientific term (S). This is the basis of modern inter-rater reliability tests commonly used to check for the reliability of diagnostic criteria and rating scales used in both psychology and psychiatry.

The application of operational definitions to mental disorder was actively discussed by many prominent psychiatrists in the 1950s, most notably Erwin Stengel and Aubrey Lewis. The logical positivist philosopher Carl G. Hempel (1961) also argued for its application to psychiatry.[27] Thus, instead of saying 'The typical features of a disorder are A, B, C and D', each of these features must be clearly and *quantitatively* defined. Thus, for the A in depression, a low mood on its own would be much too vague to serve as a diagnostic criterion, but something like 'low mood every day consecutively for two weeks' is quantifiably defined and is sufficiently clear to become one of the criteria for the new operational definition of major depression. Similarly, an important criterion for hypochondriasis is that 'it fails to respond to reassurance to alleviate the condition'. This gives the clinician a test to conduct – namely, to try and reassure the patient – and if reassurance does not alleviate the patient's distress, then one of the main criteria for hypochondriasis is satisfied. A great deal of work over many decades has gone into attempting to delineate diagnostic criteria for each category of disorder, and these are constantly revised as new knowledge appears. Note that his approach does not make any assumptions about the underlying reality or otherwise of the diagnostic construct 'S': 'S' is defined as those cases where outcome 'O' meets the defined criteria when test 'T' is applied.

> The first set of operational criteria used in psychiatry were the St. Louis Criteria (also known as the Feighner Criteria) published in 1972 by John P. Feighner,[28] at the time a trainee at Washington University in St. Louis, Missouri. There were 15 categories and, by using these operational criteria, his team could reliably classify 75 per cent of patients admitted to the hospital.

A few years later, Robert Spitzer published a more sophisticated set of criteria known as the Research Diagnostic Criteria,[29] and this was soon to herald the arrival of the DSM-III in 1980, in which Spitzer played a leading role.

Diseases and Disorders, Medicine and Psychiatry

Advances in general medicine have often led to changes in thinking in psychiatry. Thus, towards the end of the nineteenth century, the discovery of bacteria and the application of microscopy led to much greater understanding of the aetiology of many physical diseases. Rudolf Virchow, a German pathologist, considered the presence of a lesion an essential prerequisite for a condition to qualify as a disease entity. He wrote:

> In my view, the disease entity is an altered part of the body, in principle an altered cell or organ . . . that disease is a

> living entity which has a parasitic relationship with the otherwise healthy body to which it belongs, and at the expense of which it lives.[30]

Apart from the clearly organic conditions, such as the dementias and conditions such as neurosyphilis/GPI and other neuropsychiatric conditions, no 'lesions' have been found in any of the common mental illnesses. This fact, that the term 'disease' in Virchow's sense – a 'somato-aetiological' approach – could not be applied to mental illnesses, has been used to minimise at times the obvious fact that mental illness can wreak huge devastation on people's lives. We would argue that 'mental illness' is rightly worthy of attention from doctors and health services and that it cannot be seen as purely a social construct. Rather, it is a complex phenomenon arising from interaction across a range of different levels in the vastly complex biological, psychological and social domains making up an individual person and their sense of self.[31] At its apex, mental illnesses affect an individual person and those around them, sometimes devastatingly so, and looking to ameliorate this suffering is rightly seen as firmly within the remit of medicine and health services across the world. Nowadays, both the major glossaries therefore apply the term *disorder* to the syndromes they describe and broadly take a symptomological approach.

Dimensions and Disease Definition

Another advance in how to approach psychiatric nosology came from the field of chest medicine and was made by a London chest physician, John Scadding.[3] The problem for diagnosis in chest medicine is that it has many rather vague non-specific symptoms such as cough, sputum and shortness of breath, which are also quite common in the general population. None of these are pathognomonic for any particular condition, and this makes it difficult to delineate morbid conditions from what is 'normal'. Psychiatry has a similar problem; symptoms such as low mood, anxiety, irritability, tension and so forth are all common and distributed as a continuum in the general population, and as in chest medicine, there is no clear demarcation between what is 'normal' and what is pathological. Scadding offered some guidance as to what exactly should go into the definition of a disease. He made no attempt to define disease in general, which he believed to be impossible, but arrived at a definition of what the contents of a specific disease definition might be, and this could apply to all the fields of medicine, as well as to animal and plant diseases.

> A disease is the sum of all abnormal phenomena displayed by a group of living organisms in association with specified common characteristics by which they differ from the norm of their species in such a way as to place them at a biological disadvantage.

Essentially, this definition implies a specific syndrome resulting in some sort of harm. However, what did the term 'abnormal phenomena' mean? Firstly, it signified something that does not occur in 'normal healthy people', such as a shadow on the lung in chest medicine or persistent auditory hallucinations in psychiatry. Secondly, it refers to statistical abnormality with regard to the general population. Thus, most people can experience a depressed mood for a couple of hours, but a depressed mood every day for two weeks continuously is statistically abnormal and hence became one of the agreed criteria of a 'major depressive episode' in the DSM scheme.

Scadding's definition also included the term 'biological disadvantage'. In chest medicine, this might be obvious, but in psychiatry, perhaps less so. Kendell[32] proposed that 'biological disadvantage' meant increased mortality and lowered fertility. Frederick Kräupl Taylor,[33] a psychiatrist who specialised in treating people with severe personality disorder, a group regarded as difficult to diagnose and treat, accepted Scadding's concept of statistical abnormality as a key component of disease definition but could not envisage how the notion of biological disadvantage could be applied to his population group of people with severe personality disorder. Instead, he opted for the concept of 'therapeutic concern', and his definition was the first to include any subjective criteria into disorder definition:

> The attributes of disease must be abnormal by the standards of the population or the norms of the individual and must be associated with at least three criteria:
> (a) Therapeutic concern for the patient himself and experienced by the person
> (b) Concern for the person experienced by the social environment
> (c) Medical concern for the person

Kräupl Taylor's definition thus retained the presence of statistical abnormality but discarded the notion of biological disadvantage. This definition was immediately criticised by Kendell of being nothing short of a tautology: 'Doctors treat diseases, therefore diseases are what doctors treat'.

Despite Kendell's criticism, the subjective element has been retained in almost all later definitions of psychiatric disorder in both the ICD and DSM systems, and the theme of therapeutic concern remains central to the concept of a mental disorder today. All the more recent definitions place a much greater emphasis on *subjective* personal suffering and pain occurring as a result of the condition in contrast to the rather soulless earlier formulation of 'biological disadvantage'. In recent years, however, evidence has accumulated documenting the shortened life expectancy of people with serious mental illness, which perhaps suggests at some level this biological disadvantage construct has some validity.

Why Diagnose?

Despite the challenges, it is widely acknowledged that there is a need for a universal language that can help professionals to communicate with each other and with their patients. Cawley (1992)[4] wrote about a psychiatric world completely lacking in any psychiatric diagnoses.

> Without categories or dimensions and some system of classification all psychiatric knowledge would be reduced to the memorisation of multiple single case histories and we would be doomed to slosh around in some impressionistic garbage.

Apart from the impossibility of doing clinical work without some sort of diagnostic system, implicit or explicit, diagnosis and classification are fundamental to the way we organise our worlds. We bring our prior knowledge, assumptions and cognitive structures to the things we experience and then process this combination into a judgement upon which we may then act to make sense of the world. Any approach to diagnosis without explicit categorisation will have an implicit judgement system even though an individual professing that they do not 'categorise' may not be aware of this. This process enables us as individuals to interpret a world that would otherwise seem chaotic, every new experience requiring a completely new response.

Taxonomy and Nosology in Psychiatry

In the scientific approach, taxonomy is the science of naming, describing and classifying objects and concepts. Taxonomy when applied to medicine and diseases is known as nosology. A good nosological system should ease communication and define groups and patterns that can be investigated and managed using a common language. It should enable research into groups with characteristics in common to be conducted, knowledge to be shared and treatments to be developed and prescribed. It should facilitate education and understanding.

Psychiatric diagnoses are not based on blood tests or brain scanning or other objective tests (excluding the neuropsychiatric conditions in Group I previously) but on clinical observation and the patient's expressed experience of reality. Including an individual's subjective experience of the world in the diagnostic process is no less valid, *per se*, although inevitably it does involve an indirect judgement and is not accessible to direct empirical measurement. Psychiatric diagnosis allows knowledge gained from an individual case, unique though that person is, to be generalised across a group with similar characteristics so that the management of each individual can be informed by this wider grouping of knowledge. This in turn can be used to inform understanding of the longitudinal outcomes of patients sharing these clinical forms. At a service level, it can be used to plan services and measure outcomes, always bearing in mind that the focus of an intervention must always be around the individual patient. It can also inform discussions on prognosis. Diagnostic groupings are not, however, 'persons'. A diagnostic category or label should never be used to describe a person (e.g. 'a schizophrenic') as opposed to the problems that they are encountering. Language is important – 'a person with schizophrenia' emphasises personhood first. It is essential that we recognise first and foremost a 'person', and 'person-centred care' should be the fundamental bedrock of all medicine including psychiatry.[34] Outdated words and phrases such as 'a schizophrenic', 'just EUPD', 'PD' and others are demeaning and stigmatising, not only to the person being so described but arguably also to the professional using such terms. Jaspers,[15] drawing from a Kantian perspective, describes this as: 'the idea of the disease-entity never reaches realisation in the individual case' (p.569). It indicates 'the path for fruitful research and supplies a *valid* point of orientation for particular empirical investigations' but 'a personal history . . . in its entirety provides the setting for every individual life' (p.46).

Diagnosis is therefore, generally, a prerequisite for research, although symptom-based phenomenological research – for example, on 'auditory hallucinations', or the subjective experience of 'hearing voices' – is sometimes undertaken. Understanding epidemiology, interventions and planning and costing services requires some diagnostic framework. In recent decades, mental health services have been commissioned through block contracts in the UK; this has disadvantaged funding as better data on diagnostic groupings and outcomes would better address and identify need and service planning and subsequently support more equitable resource allocation (see Chapter 20 on funding).

Criticisms and Disadvantages of Diagnosis

There are a multitude of potential criticisms of diagnosis:

Diagnosis Is Too Reductionist

The first and foremost criticism of a simple ICD-11 or DSM-5 diagnosis based solely on the current clinical picture, course, symptoms and phenomenology is that such a diagnosis is far too reductionist or simplistic. It fails to provide a holistic view of the individual, potentially reducing the person to a mere 'label'. The use of a single label to describe the individual's problems will inevitably omit a vast amount of biographical information that the assessment interview will have revealed, and more often than not, this will conceal the complexity of the person's situation. Jaspers recognised the danger of this – 'The chaos of phenomena should not be blotted out with some diagnostic label'; he cautioned against seeing mental disorders as consisting of 'mosaic like' fragments that simply needed piecing together mechanistically to produce a diagnosis: ' a list of symptoms for parrot-like repetition'. At the same time, some diagnostic framework is necessary – a fact also recognised by Jaspers. The task of the clinician is to ensure wise and compassionate use of whichever framework they are using, setting it within the context of the person's life.

Diagnosis Lacks Validity

'Validity' may also be a problem (see Chapter 1). The 'reliability' of a diagnosis must be distinguished from its 'validity'. Validity, as part of the theory of knowledge or epistemology, can be considered very simply as 'content related' (face validity and construct validity) and 'criterion related' (predictive validity and concurrent validity).

A further 'validity', that of 'epistemic' validity, might also be considered.

Thus, both the main schemes could be accused of creating an illusion of discrete 'valid' entities or categories ('lacking construct validity'), whereas many mental disorders exist on a spectrum and are variants, often at the extreme, of individual lifestyles, beliefs and behaviours existing within a social and interpersonal context. Although these constructs may have 'concurrent validity' – the 'test' measures well against another 'test' of the same construct – the construct itself may be invalid, not describing anything meaningful in terms of something 'real' in the world ('lacking face validity') or even something 'real' of the service user experience ('lacking epistemic validity'). It may thus capture nothing of the individual's needs and may not indicate anything helpful about the interventions needed to assist that individual or the likely course of the illness ('lacking predictive validity'). Underpinning this are deep philosophical questions relating to how human beings may come to know the world.

Thus, diagnosis, it could be argued, may be positively harmful, creating a sense of 'something' being present when in fact there may be 'nothing' beyond that the condition 'exists' because it is defined in the classification. Thus, echoing Kendell, a tautologous loop is established in which the construct is established by virtue of being in the classification and this is then used to reinforce its 'criterion validity'. The criterion validity is then used to establish the supposed validity of the original construct. Sixteenth-century witch finders would no doubt have had a good degree of inter-rater reliability for their construct of 'witch' along with a range of diagnostic tests – the vivid metaphor employed by Thomas Szasz[35] to challenge the whole premise of psychiatric diagnosis as a valid construct.

Diagnosis Lacks Reliability

Reliability refers to how consistently a method measures something (see Chapter 1). It can be considered in various ways: inter-rater reliability considers the extent that different observers agree, test-retest reliability considers the consistency of the same test over time, and intra-rater reliability considers the extent to which there is agreement from the same rater completing the test at different time points. Application of diagnostic criteria may therefore not be reliable within the same rater and between raters. This is termed 'unreliability'. The consequences may be serious: they may yield different diagnoses between different assessors and between the same observer at different times in the person's episode of illness. The use of modern diagnostic criteria – particularly the operational criteria in the DSM system – has to some extent reduced this problem of reliability for some conditions, and operational definitions used for phenomena such as delusions, obsessions, hallucinations and passivity experiences have a high inter-rater reliability amongst trained clinicians, comparable to the reliability found in general medicine for many clinical signs. It leaves open the question of validity and the question of what should be regarded as a 'mental disorder'. ICD-11 acknowledges these boundary issues though, considering 'boundary with normality' and 'boundary with other conditions' in its condition descriptors.

Depersonalisation/dehumanisation

Diagnosis has certainly been misused to categorise and depersonalise individuals with a dismissal of their complex unique individual histories. Diagnosis has been used in repressive political regimes such as the former Soviet Union, where terms such as 'sluggish schizophrenia' or 'reformist delusions' were used to incarcerate and invalidate dissidents.[36] This also makes an independent contribution to stigma. Such problems discredit diagnosis in the eyes of some professionals and some service users: for example, in the Soviet Union, such constructs may have had 'reliability' in that state psychiatrists agreed on the presence of 'reformist delusions' but did not have 'validity' as constructs suitable for health services to use for the good of individual patients.

The Views of the Anti-psychiatrists That Mental Illness Itself Was a Myth

The anti-psychiatrist movement, developing amidst the post-modernist counter-cultural wave of the 1960s, objected to the whole concept of 'mental' illness. This movement included a wide range of perspectives, from Michel Foucault – a figure whose critique has profoundly affected the post-modern world – to, in the USA, Thomas Szasz (1920–2012), a Professor of Psychiatry in Syracuse University in New York. Szasz was a prominent anti-psychiatrist. A psychoanalyst, a libertarian, a believer in free will and a prolific and opinionated author, he was particularly opposed to all forms of coercive treatment. In his books, including *The Myth of Mental Illness*[35] and *The Manufacture of Madness*,[37] he criticised the whole notion of mental illness, diagnosis and labelling:

> Labelling individuals displaying or disabled by problems in living as being mentally ill has only impeded the understanding of the moral and political nature of the phenomena to which psychiatrists address themselves.
>
> Mental illness is a myth ... Psychiatrists are not concerned with mental illnesses but in actual practice deal with personal, social and ethical problems of daily living ... Individuals who want to reject the reality of free will and responsibility can medicalise their life and thereby entrust its management to the health professionals.

He was amongst the first US psychiatrists to criticise the notion of homosexuality as a 'disease', then the dominant view amongst the psychoanalytically oriented North American psychiatrists of that time. During the 1950s and 1960s, Szasz linked this to a wider thesis encompassing the mentally ill and other groups as subject to processes akin to the hunting of witches in an earlier era. The French philosopher Michel

Foucault (1926–1984), still the world's most cited academic in the social sciences and humanities, constructed a sweeping narrative of the 'Great Incarceration' in which he saw the development of the psychiatric systems from the seventeenth century onwards as part of a wider system of power, knowledge and social oppression linked to the rise of Capitalism.[38] Foucault, in particular, writing with vivid metaphor and imagery, has had a profound impact on the study of the humanities and social sciences and beyond. However, the application of the anti-psychiatry approach to the individual care of patients potentially results in therapeutic nihilism and in approaches that neglect the most vulnerable in our societies.

Szasz was however early in identifying the tendency towards medicalising problems of daily living, and this remains an important issue today – where are the boundaries? An early striking example of this is related to the benzodiazepine addiction epidemic that developed from the 1950s with the introduction of meprobamate (Miltown) in 1955. Within a year of its introduction, 5 per cent of Americans had used it (pp.35–39).[39] Patients sought counsel from their GPs for a wide range of social and personal problems that had made them anxious. Recommendations at the time included the prescription of small doses of benzodiazepines such as diazepam or related drugs such as meprobamate, diazepam and related drugs grouped as 'minor tranquillisers' in the advertising to help treat this anxiety. Pharmaceutical advertisements from that era describe benzodiazepines as 'versatile . . . dependable . . . easy to use', and their use became ubiquitous. By the 1970s, around 15 per cent of American women were reporting use of these drugs in the past year, and benzodiazepines were amongst the most prescribed drugs. Most prescribing was done in primary care and for a broad range of indications. The addictive potential for these drugs for certain individuals was not fully appreciated, but it resulted in large numbers of people who initially presented with relatively minor ailments taking their benzodiazepines for years or even decades after their original problem had been resolved.

More recently, the potential over-prescribing of antidepressants and potential withdrawal effects have been raised as significant issues with clear parallels. The marketing strategy for selective serotonin re-uptake inhibitors (SSRIs) and other drugs in the 1990s sought to increase the numbers of people diagnosed with conditions such as 'depression', succeeding to the point that Public Health England estimated that in 2017 to 2018, 17 per cent of the adult population were prescribed antidepressants, and around a quarter of the population were prescribed one or more of antidepressants, gabapentinoids, benzodiazepines or opioid analgesics.[40] These rates of prescribing indicate that, to some degree, this 'medicalisation' of distress, and maybe even personal problems, has, rightly or wrongly, become part of our culture, though as noted earlier, the nineteenth century had its own issues with opiates. The potential risks of prescribing, as well as the benefits, are perhaps now better understood, and there has been a huge expansion in the availability and accessibility of brief psychological therapies through the 'Increasing Access to Psychological Therapies' (Talking Treatment) programme, increasing the range of options available for people presenting with common mental health problems or social difficulties. Nonetheless, over-prescribing remains an often heated and polarised area of public debate.[41]

RD Laing and David Cooper in the UK in the 1960s were associated with anti-psychiatry but rejected the label. Their approach to psychosis in particular challenged prevalent, generally biological, thinking in many ways, and their clinical descriptions[42] and theoretical contributions influenced many psychiatrists in examining interpersonal and other social influences more closely. From a different but similarly challenging perspective, Anthony Clare's *Psychiatry in Dissent*[43] also sought to stimulate less reductionist thinking.

Culture and Classification

The role of culture in diagnosis and classification systems has been acknowledged, and an outline for cultural formulation was first introduced in DSM-IV based on the recommendations of an independent National Institute of Mental Health (NIMH) workgroup on culture.[44] However, there was no method for collecting the required information. Subsequently, guidelines and practical approaches to develop a cultural formulation were proposed.[45] DSM-5 describes five aspects of culture that need to be taken into account in the formulation of any case: cultural identity of the individual, cultural conceptualisation of illness, psychosocial factors and cultural stressors, cultural features of relationship between the individual and the physician and overall cultural assessment.

'*Culture*' and its impact on mental health is a complex subject. There are stark differences between ethnic groups in relation to diagnosis and management – for example, detention under the Mental Health Act. The impact of a culture and diversity is discussed in detail in Chapter 17.

Mental Health, Disorder and Illness

Having discussed theoretical considerations around diagnosis, the next stage is to discuss the terms used, starting with mental health, illness and mental disorder – the broad descriptions. The World Health Organization defines health in its constitution:

> Health is a state of complete physical, mental and social well-being and not merely the absence of disease or infirmity.

According to the WHO concept of mental health, it should include subjective well-being, perceived self-efficacy, autonomy, competence, intergenerational dependence and recognition of the ability to realise one's intellectual and emotional potential. It has also been defined as

> a state of well-being in which every individual realizes his or her own potential, can cope with the normal stresses of life, can work productively and fruitfully, and is able to make a contribution to her or his community.[46]

Mental health is about enhancing the competencies of individuals and communities and enabling them to achieve their self-determined goals.[47]

The converse of a state of mental health is however not a state of mental illness because there also exists a large population of people who fall far short of this state of bliss but who do not have a diagnosable psychiatric disorder. These are people who are struggling at work in a job they hate, students who dislike school, people unhappy in their personal life, and those who have clinically sub-threshold mental disorder. Mental disorder is therefore a state where mental health is impaired to the point of causing distress or disability. People can often maintain good functioning and may not even be distressed by what to others may seem to be a mental disorder. For example, some people hear voices and value the experience. 'Normal' stresses – for example, bereavements – can cause distress, but this can be accepted as an inevitable response to the development of close relationships. There have been persisting arguments about whether these should be defined as disorders: bereavement can be distressing but not abnormal, or it can trigger other issues related to previous experiences, persistent low mood, dependency or anger, and so be 'disordered'. One route to differentiate has been to exclude anything that has an understandable cause, but this has meant that many people with distress and disability from the consequences of life experiences do not receive the help they could benefit from. The degree and impact of distress rather than the understandability becomes more important in determining 'disorder' or at least whether treatment and support is appropriate.

Mental ill health describes where health is affected by a mental disorder (however caused), and a response by society is appropriate. A core problem is the confusion about how mental disorder relates to mental illness. The *Diagnostic and Statistical Manual* (DSM-5)[48] particularly has struggled with this in its apparent attempts to define illness rather than disorder. Defining who is ill is really a societal function, based on but not the same as a classification of disorders. The concept of illness is used to describe situations where support to individuals is appropriate. This is where their human experiences have caused, and may continue to cause, distress to them or otherwise interfere with their lives. They are consequently excused from some or all of their responsibilities – for example, to go to work or attend to their usual duties – whilst they receive help to cure or cope with their problems – their illness. It can therefore relate to physical but also mental functioning. Society, in a range of ways often involving health professionals, determines receipt of the 'sick role'. Mental health professionals may guide but do not determine this. On that basis, it would be reasonable, as earlier, to say that bereavement may cause distress (mental disorder) but may not be an illness as most people accept and work through it. In some circumstances, the reaction to bereavement is so distressing and disabling that support is given – time off work and maybe psychological help until recovery occurs.

Stigma

There are disadvantages of a diagnosis specific to mental health that do not seem to apply to diagnoses in physical health. The stigma of mental illness continues to be a problem in society today, especially for patients/people who use services (see Chapter 20). To a limited degree, this is linked to misunderstandings surrounding diagnoses and labelling, which is an integral part of making a diagnosis. However, as an unwanted byproduct of the diagnostic process, it has become a major contributor to the problem of stigma.

The stigmatising effect of a label is best shown in how almost all the labels for people with intellectual disabilities have changed many times over the last 200 years. Once a new name entered into common usage, it soon also became a term of abuse. These changes in terminology can most clearly be seen in the wording in legislation for intellectual disabilities over the last 200 years. Thus, the 1886 *Idiots* Act made a very clear distinction between the definition of a *lunatic* on one hand and *idiots* and *imbeciles* on the other. Into the twentieth century, the 'care' of such individuals was investigated by the Royal Commission on the Care and Control of *the Feeble Minded* (1908). In the *Mental Deficiency* Act (1913), these clients were still being classified as *imbecile, idiot* or *feeble-minded. Moral imbeciles* were described as having both 'mental defect' as well as 'vicious or criminal propensities'. In 1946, the National Association of Parents of *Backwards Children* (now known as Mencap) was founded to support these *'uneducable' children.* It would be unthinkable nowadays to apply any of these terms to this group of people – these terms have all acquired pejorative connotations, and this social process continues. DSM-5 uses the term 'Intellectual Disability' (Intellectual Developmental Disorder), and the relevant college faculty is now the Faculty for People with Intellectual Disabilities, a move rightly emphasising personhood first.

Most psychiatric labels start off as purely medical terms with little or no apparent stigmatising intention or effect. However, once the term enters into common usage, it may become a term of abuse and become stigmatising on its own. An example from general psychiatry is the word 'psychopath', originally applied broadly to describe people with abnormal personalities, but which came to be used more narrowly. It became a term of abuse with unpleasant connotations long before World War II. To compensate for this, in 1930, the term *sociopath* was proposed by George Partridge, an American psychologist, with little difference in clinical meaning. Accompanying this desire to rename is sometimes the wish that by so doing, the underlying condition or at least its impact may somehow soften. In practice, if the new term enters common usage and it becomes apparent that nothing has really changed in its presentation or management, the new name itself becomes a term of abuse, well illustrated by the example of 'sociopath'. On the other hand, the replacement of manic depression with bipolar disorder seems to have been well received such that, anecdotally, patients (including celebrities) frequently ask for a review of diagnoses which they find less acceptable, including personality disorder, addictions and schizophrenia.

So there remain concerns about the terminology that is used, and 'schizophrenia'[49] and 'personality disorder'[50] have been particularly criticised in this context as stigmatising or even, for the latter, a term of abuse. Alternatives that seem more acceptable to some include 'psychosis' and 'emotional dysregulation/difficulties' or trauma-related terms. The manner of use is clearly important with this. A 'person with schizophrenia' emphasises first the 'personhood' of the individual. Any diagnostic formulation should not define the person.

Diagnostic Systems

Diagnosis and classificatory systems for mental disorders have raised controversy over many hundreds of years with debate from often entrenched positions accompanying the discussion. However, organising the world of phenomena is an inevitable part of engaging in seeking to understand the world. Categories rarely have 'pure' or 'ideal' forms but rather tend to have 'fuzzy' boundaries. Thus a 'good-enough' classification will accept this limitation and always be a 'work in progress', attempting to further understanding of the world but rarely reaching a point of complete understanding – in Wittgenstein's phrase, 'tracing around the frame'. The psychiatrist embarks with humility and trepidation on the task of diagnostic formulation, holding in mind Jaspers' advice that the psychiatrist should adopt a position bearing in mind the 'problems, questions and methods' and attempting to take an overview, watching for dogmatic expressions of 'personal opinion, school or fad' and all the time seeking understanding of the individual case.

A further issue is whether mental disorders are appropriately classified, and the controversy over DSM suggests that there remain doubts about this. Despite this, practitioners, psychiatrists and therapists have grouped individuals together for the purpose of research and teaching, and broad categories such as those used in treatment guidelines, for example, from the UK National Institute of Clinical Excellence (NICE) and US PORT have been widely accepted.

Jablensky and Kendell[51] defined the criteria for assessing a classification system in psychiatry as:

1. **Reliability**: Reliability shows how far errors of measurement have been excluded from assessment (see Chapter 1). Diagnostic reliability can be improved by operational diagnostic criteria and by using structured interview schedules. Reliability establishes a ceiling for validity. Lower reliability means lower validity, but the converse does not hold true.
2. **Validity**: Validity establishes how far a test actually measures what it is supposed to measure, meaning 'the nature of reality', the 'thing in itself'.
3. **Utility**: Utility is a graded concept and is partially context dependent. The clinical utility of a classificatory system can be assessed empirically by taking into account its impact on three domains: its use in practice, its use in the decision-making process and its relationship to clinical outcome.
4. **Ease of use**: A classification system will only be used if it is convenient and relevant to clinical staff.
5. **Applicability across settings and cultures**: As we have mentioned, psychopathology and diagnosis can be influenced by culture, and generalisability is important.
6. **Ability to meet needs of various users**: If a classification system is a language for communication, it should meet the needs of clinicians, researchers and users of mental health services.

Formulation and Diagnosis

Once DSM-III and ICD-10 came into common usage – and making the diagnosis in the context of either of these two schemes became the focus of the assessment interview – then rigorous and comprehensive formulation, arguably, was neglected, especially in communication with patients and carers. Description of the patients as if they 'were' their diagnosis – schizophrenic, depressive, etc. – occurred too frequently and has rightly been criticised by team colleagues and, most importantly, patients themselves. Increased recognition of the need for holistic assessment and collaborative person-centred management planning in all cases is occurring. A case has recently been made by some that 'diagnosis' should be replaced by 'formulation', which is individualised and addresses the range of biological, psychological and social issues.[52] This is in fact a re-emphasising of the approach described by Jaspers, Kraepelin and others. It is however a reminder for psychiatrists and others to not lose sight of the rich work of our predecessors and to avoid 'parrot-like' approaches to diagnosis.

Kleist accused Jaspers of 'diagnostic nihilism' and said that under this approach 'psychiatry will degenerate into a psychiatry of individual cases'. At its most extreme, each case would need to be considered as entirely novel, with no prior experience brought to bear on what is to be considered as part of the management plan. However, combined with diagnosis, the formulation approach has much in common with that of the Heidelberg School as summarised by Karl Jaspers in *General Psychopathology* and later articulated by William Mayer-Gross and others, which has had a profound impact on the development of psychiatry across many decades, particularly in the UK. The importance of the individual perspective applies in all medicine, in that ultimately we are dealing with an individual in a particular life situation and particular circumstances.

Formulation, by definition, applies to an individual, and as in Kleist's criticism, it does not provide a simple descriptor to guide treatment. For example, an individual formulation cannot have its own treatment guidelines or the body of research and language to communicate with others. This is why diagnosis is also required, and the two can complement each other if used sensibly. Patients frequently speak of the power of diagnosis in enabling them to seek information to help themselves, such as through books and websites, to communicate with others and explain their situation to employers, friends and family, and to access the correct help and support. Essentially diagnosis and formulation serve complementary functions and are both essential, and a phrase such as 'diagnostic formulation' probably best captures this, within the modern reworking of the holistic, phenomenological or biopsychosocial approach, as described by Bolton.[53]

Weaving the information gathered during the assessment interview into a statement of no more than a few paragraphs has become known as a 'formulation'. Thus, candidates for public examinations such as the MRCPsych were expected to produce a formulation for their 'long case'. Whilst 'long cases' no longer form part of the examination schedule – instead replaced by 'Objective Structured Clinical Examinations' (OSCE) – fragments of the full assessment, Work Place Based Assessments (WPBAs) such as observed clinical encounters, and case-based discussions may at some level be the modern equivalent of the 'long case', and seeking holistic understanding remains the bedrock of good psychiatric approaches.

A good formulation would focus, non-dogmatically, on any aetiological factors contributing to the present situation, namely the predisposing factors, the current diagnosis in phenomenological terms and its precipitants, the current social situation and potential maintaining or protective factors. Formulation of an assessment in such a way using the '5Ps' – presenting complaint and predisposing, precipitating, perpetuating and protective factors – provides a basis for synthesising assessment information and commencing management. A management plan might follow on.

Categories, Dimensions, Hierarchies and Comorbidity

A categorical approach assumes that all members of a class are relatively homogeneous in some chosen respect and that different categories are mutually exclusive. A nosological system should therefore have sufficient categories to cover all possible disorders. Both ICD-11 and DSM-5 systems can be defined as 'categorical classifications', though both now also incorporate some level of dimensional approach. In the dimensional approach, it is assumed (and probably correctly) that clinical phenomena are distributed on a continuum, whereas in a true categorical system, the assumption is that these phenomena are distributed in a binary, all-or-none fashion.

In nature, it is more likely that most mental phenomena are distributed as a continuum. Dimensions have the theoretical advantage that there is no loss of information and so maximum flexibility is preserved. There are no typical or atypical forms: most cases will fall near the centre position, and only a few 'outliers' will occupy positions at the extremes of the axis. Attributes such as intelligence, memory and personality traits are distributed on a continuum. A more dimensional approach for personality disorder that allows clinicians to rate along a continuum of severity has been adopted for ICD-11. Dimensional approaches are more likely to reduce the need for the 'not otherwise specified (NOS)' conditions, now termed 'not elsewhere defined (NED)' conditions, which in practice had become very commonly used categories. A dimensional diagnostic system also better correlates with treatment planning.

It is still possible at some level to create a binary system with a dimensional approach. Thus, most symptoms can be quantified; indeed, symptoms like low mood or anxiety can be readily conceptualised as continuous dimensions, running from mild and within the normal range through to severe and pathological. Kraepelin, often seen wrongly as very categorical in his approach, described how in his view 'the slighter and slightest forms of manic-depressive insanity pass over quite imperceptibly into the forms of morbid predisposition'. Within this range, it is possible, though, to impose a cut-off or threshold to the important question of 'how much' or 'how severe' it is. A severity-criterion or a duration-criterion or both can be applied to form the threshold between health and disorder for most mental symptoms.

All of us have had some experience of mental symptoms such as feeling anxious or depressed. In clinical interviews for depression, some psychiatrists might ask, 'On a scale of 0-10, with 0 being no depression and 10 being very severe depression, where would you place yourself today?' Even symptoms that appear to be clear dichotomies (present or absent), such as delusional beliefs, can usually also be quantified (e.g. how much of the time they dominate thought or behaviour).

Despite the obvious theoretical advantages of a dimensional approach, most clinicians use a blending of dimensional and categorical approaches. For any patient assigned a categorical diagnosis as part of their diagnostic formulation, the clinician will also have a sense of the dimension of just how 'unwell' this particular individual is compared to all patients, as well as compared to other patients with this particular condition. Some clinical work at times will involve making binary decisions – for example, whether to admit to hospital or not, to prescribe a drug or not, or to support a medicolegal or insurance claim or not. The wording in the Mental Health Act, 'Mental Disorder ... of a nature or a degree ...', combines both a dimensional and a categorical understanding of mental disorder. Thus, 'Mental disorder' is a category and 'of a degree' is a dimension, and both are seen in the context of the individual circumstances of the case as well as the wider construct of 'Mental disorder' itself.

Comorbidity

Patients may often have two or more psychiatric diagnoses. A patient with dementia may become depressed; a person with schizophrenia may use recreational drugs. Are these two conditions independent, or has one led to the other? Jaspers[15] (see Figure 2.1) was the first to describe an explicit diagnostic hierarchy with his division into 'disease groups', and in his scheme, the more severe and pervasive disorder was regarded as primary and causal, and the less-severe disorder as secondary. Organic disorder took precedence over all other disorders, followed by schizophrenia; manic depression was at the third level, and at the fourth and lowest level were the neuroses and personality disorders. Both ICD-11 and DSM-5 systems promote a hierarchy in selecting diagnoses with certain categories tending to be more dominant. For example, if someone meets criteria for an organic disorder and psychosis or a common mental disorder, the diagnosis of the organic disorder is made, which is assumed to be the primary condition. Similarly, psychosis takes precedence over depression and over a personality disorder. This hierarchy generally makes sense in that, for example, in a case of delirium or dementia, anxiety or depressive symptoms are common but making the delirium the primary diagnosis enables treatment to focus on the organic disorder first. However, as this example illustrates, this hierarchy is limited and has meant that 'secondary' diagnoses – for example, depression – are sometimes ignored when frequently the secondary diagnosis will require treatment in its own right.

This problem with hierarchies is that, in the real clinical world, it may not be possible to determine which is the primary disorder and which is the secondary. Thus, in the above example of an association between drug taking and schizophrenia, we know that taking amphetamines can trigger psychotic episodes in some people, suggesting the drug abuse 'caused' the psychosis. However, in the real world, the situation is more complex than a direct line of 'causation'. It is possible that people with schizophrenia may be more sensitive to the effects of drugs such as amphetamine or may be more likely to become impoverished and mix in circles where they might be offered illicit drugs. Here, it is the schizophrenia that has led to the substance misuse problems, or the drugs have compounded the effects of an underlying diathesis towards mental illness. Thus, the assumption that one condition has always caused the other may sometimes be mistaken. Far simpler and more likely to reflect the true situation is just stating that both conditions have occurred together, or are *comorbid*, without invoking the notion of diagnostic hierarchies to explain this or assuming that one has caused the other. This notion has proved useful and, in psychiatry, dates at least back to the nineteenth century (see Bucknill and Tuke's[1] qualifier of 'with or without epilepsy or general paralysis'). This approach is now extensively applied throughout other branches of medicine. Thus, for example in the recent Covid pandemic, mortality was found to be higher among subjects who were also comorbid for diabetes and obesity – a statement that can be readily understood by all. Similarly, those who have schizophrenia comorbid with (or 'associated with') substance misuse are, *as a group*, less likely to engage in treatment and have worse outcomes than those without substance misuse. Again, the non-dogmatic stance of Jaspers can help – think less in terms of simple causation and recognise the complexity: a cause, not **the** cause.

Models of Mental Illness

Treatments are determined by what elements the psychiatrist believes have caused the patient's condition. From the nineteenth century, a divergence between 'biological' and 'psychological' paradigms developed: Freudian psychoanalysis, rooted in a theory of unconscious drives and conflicts, pitted itself against 'brain' pathology. Both approaches had their adherents, and there were often heated debates and rivalries, although severe mental illness remained predominantly within the remit of the asylum doctors rather than the analysts. Private neurology services, often focused around spas and 'rest cures', emerged to treat wealthier patients with non-psychotic conditions such as 'neurasthenia' and 'hysteria'. For the severely mentally ill, in contrast, the asylum or the home remained the location of their management, and the analysts showed little if any interest in actually managing them. For those with serious mental illness (SMI), the Heidelberg School approach – blending biographical and phenomenological description and description of longitudinal course – critiqued the scientific pretensions of the psychoanalytic approach whilst moving away from biological reductionism.

Jaspers, amongst his 'organising principles', emphasised two important concepts fundamental to practising person-centred psychiatry: 'Erklaren', 'Explanation', in the sense of a natural sciences 'causal' explanation and 'Verstehen', 'Understanding', in the sense of understanding the individual subjective psychological development of a particular psychopathological state. Within this approach, the 'meaningful connections' of the individual's life are seen as of central importance. In the United States and later in the UK and Australia, the development of this narrative approach was extended by Swiss emigre Adolph Meyer, who became a dominant figure in US psychiatry before World War II. His typewritten 'Clinical Guides' were summarised by George Kirby[54] in *Guides for History Taking and Clinical Examination of Psychiatric Cases* in 1921 and adopted in many hospitals. A line can be traced from this approach to the modern biopsychosocial approach articulated by George Engel and others and the modern curriculum in which this is described as the holistic person-centred approach.

The middle of the twentieth century brought the psychopharmacological revolution and from this a renewed confidence in biological approaches: Erklaren rather than Verstehen perhaps came to dominate for a time, whether from a biological or a psychoanalytic perspective. Some psychiatrists reverted to a wholly biological approach and worked on the simple hypothesis that patients had a medical 'brain' disorder and appropriate drug treatment was the answer. This became known sometimes pejoratively as the 'medical model'. Clare[43] identified the particular characteristics of the medical model as 'specific aetiology, predictable course, manifestations including predictable symptoms and a predictable outcome and prognosis as well as known responses to a designated treatment', an approach originally described by Emminghaus (1878) and later critiqued by Jaspers.

Psychiatrists with a more psychotherapeutic orientation from Jaspers onwards were reluctant to subscribe to such a mechanistic view of the world and often preferred to work within more psychological models, particularly with non-organic and non-psychotic conditions. Psychodynamic models, following from Freud and others, became the dominant psychotherapeutic approach, particularly for people with non-psychotic conditions. The psychodynamic models often postulated that aetiology was largely rooted in early childhood. Emotional deprivation or distorted relationships in childhood, perhaps as a result of abuse or other trauma, superimposed on some biological vulnerability would result in developmental fixations. Conflicts in later life might arise in the patient's subconscious between the internal representations of the parents and the instinctual forces, their ego or the reality of the outside world. Such conflicts might result in symptoms or breakdowns. Therapy consisted of exploring the meanings of events, emotions, impulses and current behaviours in the light of past or forgotten events especially through the mechanism of the transference. The psychodynamic world developed a multitude of different schools and so there are several different versions of the psychodynamic formulation. With its elaborate theoretical framework, psychoanalysis is itself a form of 'Erklaren', at times every bit as reductionist and deterministic as any purely 'biological' approach.

From the early part of the twentieth century arose another strand of psychological understanding that would in its turn become a strong presence, namely Cognitive Behavioural Therapy. The application of the animal models of behaviour from Pavlov, Skinner and Watson to human conditions led to the rise of behavioural therapy and associated theory, formulations and treatments. The development of psychological approaches examining the accessible thought processes and beliefs of patients, whilst having deep philosophical roots in the work of Stoic philosophers and other religious and spiritual traditions, led to the modern approaches described by Albert Ellis, Aaron Beck and others in the form of 'Cognitive Behavioural Therapy' and 'Rational Emotive Therapy'.

From a sociological perspective, it has been established for many years now that many common mental disorders in the community are associated with adverse life events. Adverse Childhood Events (ACEs) are associated with an increased risk of developing later adult mental disorders, and throughout the adult period, new life events are associated with development of many mental disorders. Events associated with the onset of depressive disorders are typically loss events, such as deaths, separations, unemployment (see Chapter 3.2), whilst improvements or resolutions for some of these episodes of depression may be related to new positive life events such as finding a new partner or obtaining a new job. The effect of adverse life events appears to be greater in the presence of specific vulnerabilities that might relate to earlier experiences, including trauma and disrupted attachments, and social vulnerabilities, such as poverty or the absence of a close confiding relationship. The social model holds that people fall ill because bad things happen to them in the form of adverse life events, especially if they are in a socially vulnerable position, such as poverty. The role of intangible biological predispositions or unconscious intrapsychic conflicts plays no part in the pure social model though modern approaches to the biopsychosocial model are able to integrate understanding of the impact of adverse life events at multiple different levels, including the biological.

Case Example

How then do these models interact in practice? The fictitious example below illustrates how multiple perspectives can be combined:

> John is a 40-year-old mechanic who has recently lost his job because the Covid-19 pandemic has led to a loss of trade at his garage. He has just been admitted to hospital in a state of agitation, believing that he is in touch with Bill Gates and says he has developed a vaccine that will cure billions of people. He has not slept for a week and is constantly running around the ward, at times stripping off his clothes, alternately agitated and laughing, talking in a disjointed way about his discoveries and insisting on an audience with the Prime Minister. Detailed history taking reveals he stopped taking lithium two weeks previously.

Bio-medical Approach

The simple bio-medical model describes him as a having an illness with a characteristic form and course, caused by physical brain dysfunction – 'chemical imbalances' perhaps – and suggests that this is specifically treated by lithium. The cause of his relapse is the cessation of his medication, and treatment requires no more than restoration of his daily lithium intake. No more attention or understanding ('Verstehen') to his particular circumstances is required than determining how to administer his daily lithium effectively as his diagnosis – 'Mania' – is sufficient explanation ('Erklaren').

Psychodynamic Model

However, the assessment interview and review of his records reveals that he had a poor relationship with his father, who used to verbally and physically abuse and humiliate him, and since his teenage years, he has often displayed anti-authority behaviour. At one level, is it a rebellion against authority that has contributed to his non-adherence? Is his mania a defence against the experience of humiliation rooted in his childhood? Does the process of engaging with John in exploring this help John and our understanding ('Verstehen')? The psychodynamic model goes beyond the 'understanding' to postulate an 'explanation' ('Erklaren') rooted in the unconscious drives and conflicts from his earliest childhood. Difficulties in compliance are explained by his early childhood experiences, his ongoing unresolved conflicts and his anti-authority sentiments. Therapy directed at the early father-son relationship will hopefully remove such tendencies – though in the short term, it might be a challenge to attempt such therapy even if this were thought the best option.

Social/Interpersonal Model

During further discussions, John confides to one of the nurses on the ward that his wife became upset at the lack of money coming into the household and had left to commence a relationship with one of John's friends. Dwelling on this had made him miserable. The social model postulates that it is the loss of his employment, his wife's affair and the misery associated with this that has tipped John over into a state of distress and non-adherence, and this resulted in his admission in what the doctors label a state of 'mania'. His powerlessness is indicative of the power imbalance for him within the wider society, and the 'mania' is a legitimate statement of his rage. Should the 'mania' in this situation be viewed as 'illness'? Or is it simply a reasonable statement of his dissatisfaction with his own situation and the wider society in which he lives? Is 'society to blame' and the cure a complete reworking of the power relationships within the society? Is John's detention and treatment in hospital the response of an authoritarian state to this overt challenge to its hegemony with the doctors and other professionals involved acting as the coercive arm of the state?

The Non-dogmatic Holistic Approach

Whilst the earlier descriptions caricature the respective positions, it is intended to illustrate the incompleteness of any one approach and to show how all three models, and others, may be relevant. All may express some truth (or none), but none of them offer the whole truth. Dogmatic approaches favouring one 'explanation' at the expense of all others are at best potentially unhelpful. Better understanding ('Verstehen') may be achieved by combining elements of all the above models and trying to seek an empathic understanding from the individual perspective. Today, the 'holistic' model – formerly termed the *biopsychosocial model* – is the favoured explanatory framework. Although the term 'biopsychosocial' has now been replaced by the word 'holistic' within the college curriculum (see Appendix I.1), it encourages the assessor to look at diverse explanations for the patient's condition with none excluded on dogmatic or *a priori* theoretical grounds. A model is necessary because only with a model can a treatment plan be formulated.

The Main Classification Systems: ICD-11 and DSM-5

There are currently two widely established classification systems for mental disorders—the International Classification of Diseases (ICD-11)[55] by the World Health Organization (WHO) and the *Diagnostic and Statistical Manual of Mental Disorders* (DSM-5)[48] by the American Psychiatric Association (APA). There are other national classification systems such as the Chinese (Chinese Classification of Mental Disorders, CCMD) and French systems. In both countries, there is a convergence towards the main international classifications, with some important differences.

The ICD Scheme

The ICD- 11 was ratified in 2019 and involved the efforts of hundreds of psychiatrists from over 50 countries, and its history is outlined in its introduction. It had its origins in Britain, France and Switzerland. Thus, at its inception in 1837, the 'General Register Office of England and Wales for the registrations of Births Deaths and Marriages' employed William Farr (1807–1883) as its first medical statistician. Farr attempted to apply Cullen's classification to all the deaths in England.[56] He found this to be an almost impossible task because, at the time, a single disease might have had three or four different names, disease descriptions were vague and varied in different accounts, and sometimes the same medical term was applied to several different diseases.

Farr attended the International Statistical Congress in Brussels in 1853, and the Congress directed Farr to team up with Marc D'Espine,[57] a Swiss physician from Geneva who was the only other doctor with an interest in tabulating the causes of death. D'Espine and Farr failed to agree on a common nomenclature and continued a creative rivalry for many years. Farr's classification of diseases was arranged under five groups:

> Epidemic diseases, constitutional diseases, local diseases, developmental disease and diseases that were the direct result of violence.

D'Espine classified diseases according to their nature:

I Still births
II Indeterminate deaths
III Violent deaths
IV Deaths by morbid accidents
V Deaths from acute diseases
VI Deaths from chronic diseases
VII Congenital malformations
VIII Old age.

The 1855 Congress in the end adopted a compromise list of 139 rubrics. In 1893, the topic of an international classification of the causes of death was again raised by the French father and son L. A. and J. Bertillon. They extended its scope to cover not just deaths but diseases and injuries as well. In the Vienna meeting of 1891, its Chairmanship was taken over by Jacques Bertillon (1851–1922), the chief of the statistical service to the city of Paris, and this list came under the auspices of the French government and became known as 'The Bertillon Classification of the Causes of Death', which was widely adopted internationally.[58] Decennial meetings organised by the French government continued until 1928 when the task was given over to the health division of the League of Nations, whose commission drafted the proposals for the 4th revision (1929) and the 5th revision (1938).

After World War II, the League of Nations was replaced by the United Nations, which had its own health division, the World Health Organization (WHO), which took over this task and published the 6th revision, by then known as the *Manual of the International Statistical Classification of Diseases, Injuries and Causes of Death (WHO, ICD-6, 1948)*. The scope expanded from only recording causes of death to making it suitable for recording morbidity as well. This, for the first time, also incorporated a section on mental health conditions (Chapter 5 of ICD-6).

It was soon found that ICD-6 and the first edition of the American *Diagnostical and Statistical Manual* (DSM-I) were little-used in routine psychiatric practice. The WHO commissioned Erwin Stengel, Professor of Psychiatry at Sheffield University, to investigate approaches to classification. Stengel[11] concluded the main problem was the inclusion of aetiological factors mainly of a psychodynamic nature in the definitions of disorders and suggested that these were impossible to ascertain reliably in routine clinical assessments. He made two recommendations for the next revision: firstly, there should be no aetiology in any of the clinical descriptions, and secondly, all the definitions should be operationally defined. Neither of his recommendations were followed in the ICD-8 (1968) and, apart from removing the term 'reaction', there was little improvement. However, there was some change in ICD-9 (1979), where aetiology was removed, and again in ICD-10, where disorder definitions were sharpened, and a separate volume was published that incorporated operational criteria, the DCR-10.

The ICD-11, which appeared in 2018, is published in an online version (ICD-11 for Mortality and Morbidity Statistics (version: 02/2022), 2022). This format was selected because it is more readily amenable to continuous revision as new knowledge becomes available, instead of having to wait for the decennial revisions. The ICD-11 site allows access and download of pdfs if required. Sleep disorders, which were included in Chapter 5 in ICD-10 and were officially a part of psychiatry, are no longer included in this chapter but are allocated a separate chapter on their own in the ICD-11 system.

Although many doctors prefer to have a reference work as a book on their shelves to be ready at hand, most are able to appreciate the benefits of an online reference in the form of the ICD-11 browser. Chapter 6 of the ICD-11 (in previous versions of the ICD, this was Chapter 5) is entitled 'Mental, Behavioural or Neurodevelopmental Disorders' (see Box 2.1), and this is the relevant section for psychiatry, consisting of 203 pages and therefore much shorter than DSM-5, which has 946 pages. It contains 20 chapters, starting with neurodevelopmental disorders, proceeding to schizophrenia, then down through further diagnostic groupings. Catatonia is separated out from schizophrenia, breaking a confusion in classification going back to Kraepelin's time.

Box 2.1 **ICD-11: 06 Mental, behavioural or neurodevelopmental disorders (6A00–6E8Z)**

1. Neurodevelopmental disorders
2. Schizophrenia or other primary psychotic disorders
3. Catatonia
4. Mood disorders
5. Anxiety or fear-related disorders
6. Obsessive-compulsive or related disorders
7. Disorders specifically associated with stress
8. Dissociative disorders
9. Feeding or eating disorders
10. Elimination disorders
11. Disorders of bodily distress or bodily experience
12. Disorders due to substance use or addictive behaviours
13. Impulse control disorders
14. Disruptive behaviour or dissocial disorders
15. Personality disorders and related traits
16. Paraphilic disorders
17. Factitious disorders
18. Neurocognitive disorders
19. Mental or behavioural disorders associated with pregnancy, childbirth or the puerperium
20. Psychological or behavioural factors affecting disorders or diseases classified elsewhere

The definitions in the ICD system are all written in precisely worded paragraphs. These are easy to read, it is easy to grasp the sense of the meaning, and such descriptions are similar to descriptions found in textbooks. They are termed prototypal and can be readily matched with the patient currently under review. They are not operational definitions in the same sense as the DSM-5: the ICD-11 criteria do not have a list of criteria that must be fulfilled in a checklist fashion. The ICD-11 allows clinical judgement to inform on the diagnoses and includes discussion of the boundaries with normality and other diagnostic constructs.

The American Diagnostic and Statistical Manual (DSM-5)

The history of the DSM has been summarised in a number of clear accounts from different perspectives, including Shorter[9] and Horwitz[39] and the introduction to DSM-IV itself. The origins of the DSM date back to 1840 when the US government began to collect data on mental illness for its census. This included only one category for mental conditions, namely idiocy/insanity. By the time of the 1880 census, seven separate categories of mental illness were distinguished: mania, melancholia, monomania, paresis, dementia, dipsomania and epilepsy. In 1917, the Committee on Statistics of the American Medico-Psychological Association, soon to become the American Psychiatric Association (the APA), formulated a list of diagnoses for use in mental hospitals.

The immediate origins of the modern DSM lay not in the statistical classification for the mental hospitals, but in a nosology directed by psychoanalyst William Menninger, who, during World War II, was a brigadier-general and the head of psychiatry in the Office of the Surgeon General.[9] The military nosology appeared in October 1945 as the *War Department Technical Bulletin Medical*[59] of the United States Army, and it was thereafter referred to as *Medical 203*. The bulletin breathed the spirit of psychoanalysis, describing 'psychoneurotic disorders' as 'resulting from the exclusion from the consciousness (i.e. repression) of powerful emotional charges, usually attached to certain infantile and childhood developmental experiences'. Drawing on Johns Hopkins psychiatrist Adolf Meyer, as well as on Freud, the disorders were referred to as 'reactions'. Of 'dissociative reaction' it was said, 'in acute cases, the personality (ego) disorganization appears to permit the anxiety to overwhelm, and momentarily govern the total individual. The repressed impulse, giving rise to the anxiety, may be either discharged or deflected into various symptomatic expressions such as fugue, amnesia, etc'.[9] This document became the basis of psychiatric classification in post-war America.

In 1952, the APA published the *Diagnostic and Statistical Manual for Mental Disorders*, which subsequently became known as the DSM-I. It was very much based around *Medical 203*. The wording of the sections on 'anxiety reaction' and 'depressive reaction' (in DSM-I, the latter became termed 'neurotic depressive reaction') was virtually identical. In any event, such was the prestige of psychoanalysis at this point that there was an extensive section on psychoneurosis.

DSM-I included ten categories for psychoses, nine for psychoneuroses and seven categories for disorders of character, behaviour and intelligence. It also contained a glossary of the descriptions of mental disorders and was the first official manual of mental disorders to focus on its clinical utility. Many conditions were called 'reactions', reflecting Adolph Meyer's psychobiological views that mental disorders represented reactions of the personality to psychological, biological and social stressors. The concept of 'reactions' was dropped in its first revision to the DSM-II (1968), but otherwise there were no major changes.

The change from DSM-II to DSM-III was however far bigger in scope and more fundamental in its philosophy and had major implications for both the practice of clinical psychiatry and research. Thus, both DSM-I and DSM-II had been heavily influenced by psychoanalytic and Meyerian 'psychobiology' thinking that was dominant in the USA in the middle decades of the twentieth century. In DSM-II, conditions were described in paragraphs as was the case in all versions of the ICD system. These conditions were loosely defined so they were unsuitable for research, lacking reliability. The APA specified to the task force, headed by Robert Spitzer, that the new DSM-III should be atheoretical (not include any items appertaining to aetiology) in its definitions, and all the conditions should be defined by operational criteria, similar but not identical to those developed by Feighner and as earlier advocated in Europe by Stengel. This had the advantage of reliability, but validity was compromised as the experiences that are described as mental illnesses or disorders often lie on a continuum or spectrum with 'normality' without precise cut-off points dictated by using fixed criteria.

Nevertheless, with DSM-III in 1980, psychiatry in the USA marked the switch from approaches dominated by psychoanalytic constructs and a disdain for symptomatic diagnosis to the operational, largely symptom-based definitions of DSM-III with an emphasis on reliability. The authors believed that with improved reliability, validity and underlying brain-based mechanisms for disorders would emerge. This perhaps did not turn out as might have been wished: it could be argued that the creation of operationally defined 'categories' has not really led to increased deep understanding of the construct of 'mental disorder', though reliability in diagnosis has improved. Rather than further incremental refinement, the development of DSM-V was riven by infighting and conflict, with the primary drivers of DSM-III and DSM-IV, Robert Spitzer and Allen Frances, excluded from the development of DSM-5 (see Box 2.2).[39]

Some of the conditions included in the DSM-II scheme were rejected for inclusion in DSM-III. One such disorder – emblematic in many ways of the clash between paradigms – was homosexuality, and this provoked a passionate debate within the APA. Attitudes to homosexuality have changed dramatically over the last 150 years. Prior to the Sexual Offences Act (1967), homosexuality was a crime as well as being a mental disorder. Although homosexuality lost its criminal associations, it

Box 2.2 DSM-5 – Diagnostic categories

1. Neurodevelopmental disorders
2. Schizophrenia spectrum and other psychotic disorders
3. Bipolar and related disorders
4. Depressive disorders
5. Anxiety disorders
6. Obsessive-compulsive and related disorders
7. Trauma and stressor related disorders
8. Dissociative disorders
9. Somatic symptoms and related disorders
10. Feeding and eating disorders
11. Sleep-wake disorders
12. Sexual dysfunction
13. Gender dysphoria
14. Disruptive, impulse control and conduct disorders
15. Substance related and addictive disorders
16. Neurocognitive disorders
17. Paraphilic disorders
18. Personality disorders

Note: Sleep disorders are included amongst the psychiatric disorders in DSM-5 but not in ICD-11, where they are classed separately.

remained a psychiatric disorder despite widespread changes in society that by this time had become far more tolerant and had come to view it as a normal variant of sexuality. Spitzer, who was tasked with revising the DSM-II, took an interest in its medical status and interviewed a number of homosexuals and found that almost none of them expressed any distress about their homosexuality. It was on this basis he argued it could not be considered a 'psychiatric disorder' since the presence of 'distress' was a key element to qualify as a disorder. There were furious debates within the APA with strong opposition to dropping homosexuality from the new manual coming mainly from senior psychotherapists, and the matter came to a vote in the APA in 1973, which Spitzer won. Thus, homosexuality was dropped from the new manual. The new DSM-III was published in 1980, and although there have been many changes between DSM-III and later versions, these have been of a lesser magnitude and are generally of a more technical nature. The expansion in size and number of categories in DSM-IV led Chodoff, a president of the American Psycho-analytical Association reflecting on his 60-year career, to say:[60]

> As new diagnoses proliferate in each successive DSM . . . I feel concern about a burgeoning *furor diagnosticus* – offering a name and number for every untoward feeling or behaviour in a way that trivialises the human condition by denying its inescapable, somber, and even tragic elements.

Diagnostic categories that require further research and more time for clinicians to become acquainted with before being formally recognised as diagnosable psychiatric disorders are described in Section 3 of DSM-5. These include eight possible disorders illustrating the mutability of the diagnostic constructs and their boundaries:

Attenuated Psychotic Syndrome: where there are only mild or transient psychotic symptoms with the preservation of insight

Depressive Episodes with Short Duration Hypomania: these are people with major depression followed by a brief episode of hypomania, but which fails to meet the four day criteria for hypomania

Persistent Complex Bereavement Disorder: this can only be diagnosed in a bereaved person after at least 12 months following on after the death that caused the bereavement, the 12 month clause being inserted to exclude normal bereavement and refers to continued distress, psychiatric symptoms and impaired function over a prolonged period. Previously, this was referred to as morbid grief reaction

Caffeine Use Disorder: although 'Caffeine Intoxication' and 'Caffeine Withdrawal' are included in the main body of the text of the DSM-5, this is a chronic disorder of addiction amongst people who are getting adverse symptoms from their caffeine addiction but who have difficulty in stopping it

Internet Gaming Disorder. Persistent and recurrent use of the internet to play games with others associated with some distress and difficulties in stopping (see Chapter 7.3)

Neurobehavioural Disorder Associated with Prenatal Alcohol Exposure: this is effectively Foetal Alcohol syndrome 'grown up'. There is usually a history of maternal alcohol consumption, learning difficulties and foetal alcohol syndrome in childhood

Suicidal Behaviour Disorder: at least one Suicide attempt in the last 24 months

Non-suicidal Self Injury: at least five or more days engaged in self-inflicted damage to the surface of the body

Diagnostic criteria are set out for all of the above, and field trials will determine whether any of these criteria yield a coherent disorder with reliable diagnostic criteria for inclusion in the next DSM revision. Thus, in the previous generation, the DSM-IV (1994) included a condition 'Pre-menstrual Dysphoric Disorder' amongst one of its 'conditions for further study', and this seems to have succeeded in the field trials as it now appears in the main body of the text in the depression chapter under the same name and is assigned a code 625.4.

The final section of the DSM manual consists of several Appendices, these being:

(i) The changes from DSM-IV to DSM-5, and these are given in the individual chapters of this book
(ii) A glossary of technical terms. This is a very useful explanation of the majority of psychiatric symptoms and other technical terms
(iii) A glossary of cultural concepts of disease. This covers a number of well-known syndromes in cross-cultural psychiatry, and they are covered in Chapter 17 in this book
(iv) An alphabetical listing of all DSM-5 conditions together with their numerical codes according to the ICD-9-CM and ICD-10-CM codes as well as the corresponding ICD-10 'F' number codes.

The Development of Schemes for Clinical Assessment

Psychiatrists are likely to spend the bulk of their working week assessing, diagnosing and managing patients referred to them and working with teams charged with delivering person-centred holistic care to these patient groups. The vast majority of psychiatrists the world over follow a similar assessment scheme and spend the greater part of their professional time conducting their initial interviews applying this same scheme, which has been called the 'case history' approach.

So where did this scheme come from? It probably originated in Europe, notably Great Britain, France and Germany in the nineteenth century but was not formalised in English-speaking countries until the early twentieth century in America. Many nineteenth-century alienists made meticulous clinical descriptions of their patients and the course of their illnesses. For example, Bucknill and Tuke[13] (p.782) describe their case histories using a standard scheme of 'History of onset' and background 'Mental state', 'Bodily condition' and 'Treatment', often including vivid personal details:

They describe Case J.N.G. No 555: 'Acute mania subsiding into quiet melancholia; recovery'. He is described as 'an engineer; a clever, industrious man of steady habits ... [who] experienced a great disappointment, in not getting an order for a certain steam engine ... he became excited and irritable ... neglected his work ... acute mania gradually came on'. They describe 'Mental state': 'Extreme excitement; believes that he going to be shot ... shouting all night long ... wets and dirties his bed ... miscalls persons, fancying he has seen every one before ...' and go on to describe 'Bodily condition': 'Expression pale, wild, haggard ... clammy ... cold extremities ... pulse small and quick'. They move on to describe 'Treatment': tincture of opium, Aether sulphuricus, and purgatives, under which treatment he 'improved greatly' but remained 'occasionally violent ... muttering to himself, and swearing ...' After five months, he is described as 'improved considerably' and is 'employed in the engine house but requires careful watching ...', under this 'agreeable occupation' he improves further such that he is 'discharged recovered, seven months from the time of his admission'.

Clinical description and the course over time was brought to a fine art by Kraepelin who undertook detailed evaluations of the patients presenting through his central clinic in Heidelberg, 'walking on the sure foundation of direct experience'. He ascertained detailed medical and biographical details for each patient before the patients were dispersed to local asylums. Taking an approach rooted in natural sciences, he would subsequently follow them up using a card system to establish their longitudinal course. Karl Jaspers, also a product of the Heidelberg system, described the approach as one in which the practitioner learns to 'observe, ask questions, analyse, and think in psychopathological terms'. Writing an initially small volume published in its first edition in 1913, this grew into the highly influential, deeply nuanced textbook *General Psychopathology*,[2] described by the late Andrew Sims as the 'bedrock of much of our practice'. The 1959 seventh edition of *General Psychopathology* was translated and published in English in 1963 by Hoenig and Hamilton, working in Manchester, but its influence had spread before then through others including psychiatrist refugees from Nazi Germany and Central Europe such as Wilhelm Mayer-Gross and Martin Roth, as well as other prominent British psychiatrists including Aubrey Lewis. Jaspers' summary of this approach can be best understood as a way of ordering our thinking about the clinical situations we encounter. It includes phenomenological approaches to understanding subjective experiences including the approach now termed 'descriptive psychopathology', with important contributions to this from Hans Gruhle and Kurt Schneider ('First Rank symptoms of schizophrenia'), with whom Jaspers had a 50-year correspondence, and others. Subjective experiences are defined, and the 'form' of the experiences is delineated alongside 'content' to try to reach an empathic understanding of the person's experience. His work, however, encompasses far more than descriptive psychopathology alone, and Jaspers[15] makes clear that all 'acts of understanding' are embedded within a broader 'comprehensive understanding' including cultural, existential and metaphysical understanding:

> Understanding is constantly in touch with *something more comprehensive in which all acts of understanding lie embedded.* (p.307)

He emphasised the importance of 'conversation' with the patient and obtaining information from multiple sources to inform a biographical account of the patient's life in a case history. Jaspers' organising principles are a powerful tool[62] for approaching the task of diagnostic formulation (see Figure 2.1), and 'phenomenology' is rooted in seeking an understanding of an individual's unique experience and perspective on the world. His initially modest aim of a short summary textbook introduced a revolutionary way of thinking about mental illness, mental disorders, the processes of psychiatry and human experience itself, borrowing from a philosophical tradition including amongst others Kant, Hegel, Schopenhauer, Nietzsche, Dilthey, Husserl and Weber.

Adolf Meyer in the United States, originally a Swiss pathologist who later became a psychoanalyst and a psychiatrist, had worked in Heidelberg with Kraepelin. He also emphasised the importance of biographical details for his own 'case history' approach, urging his staff to compile detailed biographical histories as part of an ongoing, documented, longitudinal review. There was no formal publication of his scheme until George Kirby, a student of Meyer's, published *Guide for History Taking and Clinical Examination of Psychiatric Cases* through the New York State Hospital Commission in 1921.[54] The manual went into seven editions and is recognisably the basic scheme for psychiatric history taking the world over today. He was greatly influenced by Meyer's psychobiological approach,[62] which influenced the development and practice of psychiatry in the UK and was referenced in major textbooks.

The textbooks written by Frank Fish, first Professor of Psychiatry at Liverpool until his untimely death in 1968, also gave clear descriptions of 'Method in Psychiatric Case-taking' based around this approach, which he described as 'Neo-Meyerian', with an emphasis on descriptive psychopathology and consideration of all factors that may be relevant, an approach which is directly drawn from Jaspers.[63]

A Scheme for Psychiatric Assessment

'Every good case-history grows into a biography'
Karl Jaspers

The Structure and Process of a Psychiatric Assessment

Psychiatrists develop a 'standard approach' to how they conduct therapeutic assessments based on repeated practice combined with a theoretical template. This account gives a brief description of how this operates in practice and a scheme of broad headings. Jaspers describes this approach in a beautifully written piece published as the Appendix to *General Psychopathology*[15]

> One must devote oneself to the individuality of the patient ... but also conduct this with 'guiding goals'.

The variation of the approach is 'a matter of art' and the process is not simply the 'running through of a questionnaire'.[64]

Introduction to the Assessment and Presenting Issues

The assessment should begin with a polite, respectful introduction and clarification of the reasons for the meeting (see further discussion in Chapter 16). The time-frame available for the assessment and the main issues from the patient's perspective should be clarified. The setting for the interview needs to be considered – for example, office, home, community, ward or at bedside – to balance practical convenience and efficiency with making the patient feel safe and relaxed – or simply agreeable to be interviewed. Safety considerations also need to be taken into account.

History

History of the Present Complaint

The opening questions aim to explore the 'complaint' – the reason for the person coming to the attention of the mental health service. The history of the presenting complaint needs to be explored in as much detail as necessary in the allotted time permitting. If possible, the assessor should adopt a conversational style and refrain from interrupting the flow of the patient during this opening phase of the interview, enabling the patient to tell their story freely: 'Let the patient speak and say as little as possible'. Within the patient's account of their distress, many mental symptoms of diagnostic importance such as depressed mood, episodes of anxiety or panic and so forth may be declared and should be noted. The doctor should be alert to any distress and seek to demonstrate accurate empathy to the patient's distress. Done authentically, this will help facilitate rapport, opening the doors for a later therapeutic relationship.

Sometimes a story of a series of events and characters cascades out of the patient, in which case simply recording this story will help in understanding the patient's predicament. In other instances, only a series of symptoms are declared, and their onset, severity and the degree of distress they cause needs to be recorded. As each symptom is mentioned, the interviewer should use the patient's own words to explore the symptoms in more detail – for example, 'You mentioned you felt panicky. Can you tell me a little more about that?', 'Can you give me an example of when this happened?'. Reflecting back and using open questions will usually achieve a better understanding than the use of closed questions. However, after identifying the initial problem and how long it has been present, it can often be helpful to work through the personal history as this often clarifies and organises the history of the presenting problem.

However, where obtaining a neat history with the usual headings is impossible because the patient is in a distressed, disorganised or psychotic state, it may be best to abandon systematic questioning but just record verbatim the patient's speech and ensure there is a thorough documentation of the mental state at presentation. The history of the events leading up to the consultation/admission may be obtained from an informant – if possible, a close relative and other records and sources – and then confirmed with the patient. In other patients, even if acutely unwell, it is still possible for the experienced interviewer to obtain the details that will inform a good holistic assessment – and this in itself can be therapeutic and reduce distress. A degree of flexibility needs to be maintained because it is simply not possible to document the myriad of different ways in which patients' unique stories unfold. The interview is conducted, nonetheless, holding in mind a mental template of the required domains to be covered whilst imposing as little as possible on the patient's subjective description. The following describes the main domains, but experienced interviewers will be flexible in how they order this in the interview. Most will then summarise in a written form following a standard approach.

Personal History

Once the initial free-flowing phase is over, the interviewer may thank the patient for sharing details of their problem with frankness and then add something along the lines of 'Now if it's ok, can I ask a little about your background . . .? But if there's anything you'd prefer not to talk about that's fine . . .' and then proceed to explore the items in the personal history listed in Box 2.3. To cover all the areas listed with all patients in detail would be a fruitless task, and accumulation of too much irrelevant information can impede the overall assessment, leading to a 'chaos of detail'. Thus, there may be little point in eliciting details of the developmental milestones in an elderly patient with depression or a detailed relationship chronology in a person with dementia, though even in such cases, the biographical information will always inform the holistic assessment. With time and experience, each psychiatrist will build up their own knowledge base on each broad category of disorder and learn which fields of enquiry will assist in the assessment process and the development of therapeutic alliance as well as those domains that fail to add anything relevant. The refining of history taking by making it more focused is a skill that cannot be taught but can only be acquired by seeing a large number of patients over several years. The ultimate aim is to develop a fluency in assessment that gathers necessary information whilst simultaneously developing a therapeutic alliance from which an initial diagnostic formulation and collaborative plan can be developed. This must be accomplished in a finite time without exhausting either the doctor or the patient. The experienced practitioner develops a systematic mental template ensuring that all relevant domains are explored but is able to do this in a relaxed, empathic, non-judgemental, conversational manner that facilitates the development of a shared understanding of the problems and the therapeutic alliance. The patient should feel heard, and the psychiatrist should listen. It is most definitely not a checklist; however, the following domains are important and an 'aide memoire' can be helpful especially early in one's career:

Prenatal development and birth include details of the patient's antenatal environment, such as maternal alcohol and substance misuse, birth and early infancy. Prematurity or perinatal hypoxia might suggest possible minor brain damage affecting later development. The early years and milestones may shed light of the possibility of neuro-developmental disorders such as autistic spectrum disorder and ADHD. Informant histories, for example from a parent, are important here.

Family history provides information about key individuals in the family, the nature of early relationships and whether there was also a history of parental mental health problems or other illnesses. Sometimes there are relationship difficulties in childhood; a history of bullying; emotional, physical or sexual abuse; or otherwise disrupted parenting. Family warmth or closeness and parental marital disharmony or divorce may be disclosed early on. This may open the door to the exploration of attachment issues, wider trauma and later problems in relationships in adult life. In other instances, the family history data reveals a family history for one or more other family members having a similar or related condition to the patient, indicating there is a familial or hereditary diathesis. This commonly applies to affective disorders and major psychoses but is seen in many other problems as well. An attempt should be made to work out how many other relatives demonstrate such similar or related conditions and how closely related they are to the individual being assessed.

Educational history will highlight if there are literacy difficulties whilst the patient's academic achievements in terms of public examinations may indicate specific or general difficulties or issues with their social engagement or home life impacting on their schooling. There is nothing diagnostic in this, but it builds understanding of the individual's life story and their experience. A history of having identified Special Educational Needs or Disabilities may point to developmental or intellectual disabilities. The astute clinician may explore from this knowledge further to obtain old reports including formal psychological and other assessments that are likely to have been conducted in such cases, all of which might further inform the ongoing assessment process. Socialisation in school as indicated by having friends might indicate important aspects of their premorbid personality, whereas behavioural difficulties such as fights, being disciplined, suspended or excluded point to an early onset of possible conduct disorder and antisocial behaviours, which may be associated with disruptions or trauma in the home background and conditions such as ADHD. They may also correlate with later development of adult antisocial personality traits.

Occupational history gives pointers to the patient's social class as well as to their degree of wealth or their levels of poverty and disengagement from the wider social milieu. The work record may reveal long continuous periods of work providing some indication of aspects of their health and adaptation to the world whereas prolonged gaps may indicate periods of previous illness or other aspects of their being in the world.

The relationship and psychosexual history offer clues as to the patient's capacity to form and sustain relationships or otherwise. Because a great deal of non-psychotic mental disorder may revolve around the nature and quality of interpersonal relationships – whether these are supportive or abusive, or rapidly changing or sustained – this can provide important information. If difficulties are present, these can then become the focus of a later more detailed exploration. Issues around sexual development and gender identity are considered as are issues around menstruation and menopause.

Premorbid Personality

This provides a picture of interaction style and interests occurring prior to the 'complaint' emerging, and this can be very important in understanding how problems have developed – for example, isolation and introversion – which also reduces supports available for recovery. Unless a personality disorder is suspected, this section need not be overlong. Where personality disorder is suspected, further clues and history should be sought from an informant if available. Comorbid Personality disorder makes treatment more difficult for many conditions; hence, it is important to consider its presence or otherwise. It is important to understand also that cross-sectional judgements of personality are notoriously difficult to make, and caution should be exercised in reaching such diagnostic conclusions. It is important to consider the individual's strengths and how they regard other people's views of them. The ICD-11 approach of grading personality in a more dimensional way and shifting away from identifying particular subtypes except in a broad way is likely to be helpful to clinicians moving forward (see Chapter 7.1).

The Previous Medical and Psychiatric History

A brief history of any medical conditions is important and may be extensive, especially with increasing age. The decision to conduct a physical examination may be dependent on this history. For the majority of younger patients seen in outpatient clinics, a history of a serious medical conditions requiring immediate examination is uncommon, and so it is unusual to conduct a full physical examination in routine outpatient practice. It is simple and acceptable to weigh almost all patients and ask for or check height. This should be standard practice leading to calculating the body mass index (BMI). Targeted examination – for example of blood pressure, pulse – may be required and is appropriate for some patients. A full physical examination is mandatory for hospitalised patients on admission and should form part of the standard processes of inpatient admission. Collaboration with primary care over physical health issues is essential, ensuring that necessary examinations, investigations and management occur.

Current medication and any allergies must be recorded at the initial meeting and updated in all patients.

The past psychiatric history should briefly outline the chronological course that the individual's mental health problems have followed, including brief details of admissions, detentions under the Mental Health Act and any significant events, such as incidents of self harm or other potential serious incidents, that have occurred. Understanding is needed of what has worked in the past to aid recovery and how the patient and their family view this. Sometimes the patient can recall which approaches and particular medications were helpful as well as which medications gave severe or unpleasant adverse effects, and this should be recorded. Entitlement to Section 117 aftercare might be noted along with the patient's involvement with this process.

Alcohol and Drug History

Both alcohol and drug misuse are associated with mental disorder; if either is present, then aim to quantify and describe the pattern. How much is drunk in a week, quantifying using units of alcohol? What is the preferred drink, and what is the pattern of drinking? The pattern over the past month is a useful way of further exploring, moving on to explore the pattern over time from when alcohol was first consumed (see also Chapter 14). With drugs, other areas need exploring including the range of drugs used, the method (oral, inhaled, IV) and other associated problems. Discussions around alcohol and drug use can sometimes be difficult. A patient may be reticent or ashamed to disclose the pattern, and sophisticated interviewing may be required to obtain an accurate account. The CAGE questionnaire[65] provides an acronym to recall a series of open questions that can enable the conversation to proceed in a balanced and helpful way. A series of open questions provide a stem into exploring the alcohol history and creating a dialogue:

1. Have you thought of **cutting** down? (C)
2. Do you ever become **angry** if others criticise your drinking? (A)
3. Do you ever feel **guilty** after you have been drinking? (G)
4. Do you ever need to have a drink first thing in the day to settle things down? (E, '**Eye-opener**')

Whilst the yes/no answers to this could be scored, it is far more helpful to use them as openers leading on to further exploration. They can be helpful in gauging whether the individual recognises a problem in themselves and can provide a route allowing a person to open up more fully about a problem that they may feel initially they cannot share.

A part of this assessment would explore whether there are any medical or psychiatric complications of the drinking (see also Chapter 14). With regards to drugs of abuse, it is important to list which drugs have been used, what effect they had on the subject; the extent and duration of the usage and whether true dependency has occurred. Sometimes drugs and alcohol are being used in an attempt to alleviate low mood or anxiety whilst cannabis is sometimes used as a hypnotic or for pain relief. Sometimes, their usage is purely recreational.

Forensic History and History of Violence

An initial inquiry as to whether there has been any substantive contact with the criminal justice system will often be appropriate – for example, 'Have you had any significant contact with the police?'. If so, this needs to be explored in as much detail as necessary.

Current Social Situation

This describes briefly where the person is living, their housing situation, with whom they are living, who the children in the house are if any (names, dates of birth, parentage, schools), what the individual does with their time, what their financial situation is and what support networks are available. What are the things they usually enjoy? How would they like things to be different? Cultural background and experiences, any intergenerational conflicts and other related issues also need to be noted. Further aspects of cultural diagnosis and formulation are considered in Chapter 17.

Mental State Examination

This includes both an attempt to describe the subjective conscious experience of the patient and objective expressions of this.

The mental state examination is a description and categorisation in a structured way of how the individual appeared, behaved and talked during the interview and whether there were any particular phenomenological (subjective psychic) features or behaviours. Conventionally, it is broken down into a number of separate headings, but in writing letters, these headings are often omitted by experienced clinicians, and the same information is incorporated into a series of descriptive sentences with the headings implied rather than explicit. This is easier to read and usually conveys the information more clearly, but both approaches are acceptable. When commencing training, keeping the headings may be useful in embedding the approach. The areas that are covered include:

Appearance and behaviour: As far as possible, this should be a neutral description and, for the majority of outpatients, appearance and behaviour is generally unremarkable, but care and sensitivity must still be exercised in describing this. Disparity between what the patient expresses and how they appear and behave can give valuable clues to underlying issues and mood (e.g. 'smiling depression' or restlessness when discussing specific events or relationships). However, it is important not to read too much into non-verbal communication – for example, a statement of suicidal feelings can be conveyed without much emotion but still be an indication of intent.

Amongst inpatients, abnormalities are more common especially during the initial assessment. The patient may appear neglected, dirty or dishevelled, which may be associated with a range of conditions with no great diagnostic specificity, though indicating important information about how the individual is caring for themselves. Alcohol or drug problems, persistent psychosis, or organic mental states such as a dementia may be associated with extreme levels of self-neglect, sometimes with apparent lack of awareness on the part of the patient. In depression, there may be classical depressive facies with the outer corners of the lips turned downwards combined with a furrowed brow. The anxious individual may have a tremor or be obviously sweating as well as looking worried. A fixed stare may suggest Parkinsonism, possibly drug induced, whilst an absence or delay of any speech may suggest the psychomotor retardation of severe depression or the mutism of catatonia and other conditions. Constant movement or agitation may suggest mania or an elated state, or it may suggest the agitated states sometimes seen with severe mixed affective disorders and akathisia, an adverse effect secondary to antipsychotic medication. Twitches or bizarre movements such as tics, choreiform movements, grimacing and dystonias may be features of many conditions and were described in schizophrenia/dementia praecox by Kraepelin and others before the advent of antipsychotic medication associated with tardive dyskinesia.

Mood: Objective indicators of a depressed mood include the depressed facies or weeping during the interview, and subjective indicators are the patient's account of their depressive symptoms, including low mood itself. If a suggestion of depression is present, then the examiner should explore the other key symptoms of major depression: anhedonia, appetite and weight changes, insomnia, agitation, low energy, poor concentration and decision-making, guilt or other depressive thoughts. Any suicidal thoughts or plans should be noted and if present will need to be explored in more detail (see Chapter 15).

An elated mood as a result of mania or psychosis may be associated with distractibility, irritability and other features of mania. Moods can also be rapidly changing ('labile'), and overactivity or agitation may be accompanied by dysphoria, as in 'mixed affective disorder'. When the predominant affect is anxiety, then symptoms and signs such as sweatiness or tremor may be observed. The mood may sometimes be bizarrely out of tune with the circumstances and, if so, is said to be incongruous – for example, giggly at some sad occasion. Incongruous laughter and giggling can occur in schizophrenia, and other conditions – including cerebrovascular disease – can be associated with marked lability, the patient switching between tears and a normal countenance with little provocation. In psychotic depression, the delusions may be termed 'mood congruent' if their content is also depressive (e.g. 'I am the most wicked person who has ever lived, and I am going to be taken to prison because of my crimes') but 'mood incongruent' when their content has a very different, more neutral or bizarre theme.

Speech: Quiet, delayed or slowed speech is found in depression and with negative symptoms of psychosis, particularly in the presence of psychomotor retardation, whereas rapid loud speech may indicate mania or hypomania or other psychoses. The complete absence of speech is termed mutism, and examination of the mute patient is described in Chapter 8.

Loudness of speech can indicate mania or anger, and this may presage an outburst of violence. Experienced clinicians develop an almost intuitive sense of when the clinical interaction is escalating in this way and will pre-emptively seek to de-escalate such situations if possible. Nonetheless, it is important to avoid developing an over-confidence around this and continue to cultivate safe approaches to conducting all clinical interviews – for example, by ensuring that one can leave the room easily.

Thoughts: Abnormalities of thought lie at the heart of making the diagnosis of psychotic conditions, especially schizophrenia. By convention, abnormalities are described in terms of (i) the form of the thought and (ii) the content of the disordered thoughts. The main syntactic abnormalities of the form of thought include the way sequential thoughts are connected – for example, jumping from one idea to another rapidly with some connection between the thoughts is known as 'flight of ideas', as in mania. If there is no apparent connection, with syntactic breakdown of the thought process, the phrase 'formal thought disorder' is used. There may be a 'knights move' thought disorder, so called because of the way the knight chess piece moves off at a diagonal. However, when sequences seem to be completely random, it may be described as a 'word salad' or verbigeration, whereby there is a complete syntactic breakdown of the structure of the expressed thoughts. Both these latter types of thought disorder occur in schizophrenia. When there is little or no output at all, the term 'poverty of thought' is used, although this may indicate a lack of desire to communicate thoughts.

Particular variants of experience can occur in schizophrenia and in some other conditions whereby the individual experiences a breakdown of the normal sense of a mind-body or self enclosed within a subjective space. The term 'ego-boundary disturbance' can be used to group these experiences, and in the absence of intoxication with drugs or 'coarse brain disease', Kurt Schneider described them as symptoms of the 'first rank' in diagnosing schizophrenia. These symptoms still have a prominence within the two main classification systems though their lack of diagnostic specificity means that, within ICD -11, their emphasis has been removed from the schizophrenia definitions. These experiences include thought withdrawal, thought insertion, thought broadcast, thought echo ('Gedankenlaudwerden' or 'Echo de la pensee'), passivity experiences (experiences of external influence on the body) and 'delusional perception' – a description of the process of formation of a 'primary delusion'. Because these experiences are in many ways bizarre and hard to make sense of, they are often associated with the development of explanatory delusional beliefs. However, there are also analogies with telepathy and thought control that can be used to understand the experiences. Delusions that 'explain' a prior abnormal mental experience – for example, an explanation of symptoms of anxiety such as paraesthesia as electric shocks or gastric discomfort as poisoning – are termed 'secondary' delusions. The term 'thought block' refers to a sensation of a completely empty mind such as occurs with anxiety or public speaking. However, when the patient believes his thoughts have been taken away or stolen from him, it may constitute a symptom of psychosis/schizophrenia. The first rank symptoms are described in detail in Chapter 5.1.

Exploration of thought content around suicidal or violent thoughts is required, again in as much detail as necessary.

Delusions: Long considered one of the characteristic defining feature of major mental illness, delusions present issues with definition that raise profound philosophical questions that are explored in eloquent detail by Jaspers in his *General Psychopathology*. The process and preceding state in which an individual arrives at a belief is important as well as the certainty with which the belief is held. In schizophrenia and related psychotic conditions, there is often a heightened sense of meaning or 'salience' to ordinary events – a 'delusional atmosphere' – for the individual, and this can lead to 'false relations between events' forming into fixed beliefs, sometimes via an epiphanous experience, a delusional perception, whereby everything 'falls into place'. Delusions often have idiosyncratic, bizarre colourings that cannot be counter-argued (although may be possible to discuss) and which are out of keeping with the person's sub-cultural background. Delusions and other symptoms seen in schizophrenia are described in more detail in Chapter 5.1 and for depression in Chapter 3.1. The assessor will need to clarify whether any seemingly bizarre beliefs might even be true, how strongly they are held, whether they might be culturally appropriate, and if not bizarre, whether or not they are overvalued ideas and whether they have led on to any actions.

Abnormal perceptions (e.g. hallucinations or passivity phenomena): Hallucinations can occur in any modality. In schizophrenia, auditory hallucinations are most common, but they can occur in other psychiatric – and non-psychiatric – conditions also.

Auditory hallucinations, if present, should be described as far as possible. Record the description given by the patient: What do they say? Do they make sense to the patient? Is it one voice or many? Do the voices talk to each other? Do they recognise the voices? Do they comment on or discuss the patient? Are they loud or screaming? Do they wake the patient out of their sleep? Where is their origin or location in space? Are they distressing or confusing? If so, how much? What is their explanation for them? A good mental state examination will gather this information through open questioning and through recording the patient's own description of their experience with as little prompting as is required: 'Do you hear voices?' is a loaded, leading question, whereas 'Can you tell me what you have been experiencing?' is less so; 'Have you been experiencing things you find hard to explain?' is a little more leading but not too bad; 'Can you give me an example?' is very open. An empathic interview style conducted with patience can elicit a lot of relevant information with very little talking on the part of the interviewer and is at the heart of the phenomenological approach.

Visual hallucinations again should be described as clearly as possible. They are common in psychosis but also may be associated with organic neuropsychiatric conditions, including drug intoxication and particularly alcohol withdrawal or alcohol hallucinosis.

Olfactory hallucinations can occur. The subject reports that he or she is experiencing unpleasant smells and may describe secondary delusions associated with the smells such as beliefs that he or she is being poisoned or tortured (usually associated with schizophrenia). In other cases, the person reports that he himself smells or is giving off an unpleasant odour (usually associated with psychotic depression).

In gustatory hallucinations, the subject reports the food he eats tastes unpleasant or has a strange or metallic taste. There may be delusional explanations of these hallucinations – the patient believes that somebody who passed him in the street put some poison in his mouth or his food has been contaminated by his neighbour who is determined to kill him. In tactile hallucinations (also called haptic), there are strange and unpleasant sensations in their skin. Delusional elaboration may also be present, and dermatologists are familiar with the syndrome of delusional parasitosis, 'formication', in which the patient is convinced that small creatures are crawling over the skin, sometimes even producing 'evidence' of the little creatures for the doctor. Such presentations may also be seen as part of drug-associated states, classically in the chronic use of cocaine.

The examiner should attempt to also clarify when the abnormal phenomena are occurring in relation to sleep. If they occur on waking (hypnopompic) or if in the transitional state on falling asleep (hypnogogic), they may be a normal phenomena. They can also be interpreted as part of spiritual or traumatic experiences.

Cognitive function: In most working-age outpatients, this is usually essentially normal, but with certain conditions seen in general adult psychiatry such as comorbid alcohol misuse or cardiovascular disease, there may be abnormalities. Some cognitive decline is common in people with longer-term serious mental illness as in the general population but occurring typically at an earlier age. In persistent schizophrenia, cognitive impairment may form a core part of the syndrome. Amongst the elderly and those admitted to hospital especially for confusional states due to any cause, cognitive impairment is frequent, and with increasing age, there is increased likelihood of a progressive dementia being present. Assessing cognitive function covers orientation in space, time, and person; concentration; and memory, both recent and remote. How to do this assessment is described in Chapter 8. All psychiatrists – indeed, all doctors – should understand an approach to assessing this quickly and appropriately.

Insight: This is a traditional part of the mental state examination and can be caricatured as to whether the patient agrees with the psychiatrist or not. It is more nuanced than this but is best described in terms of the patient's views on the issues: Do they agree that they have an illness or that their troublesome experiences – for example, voices or delusions – are originating from themselves? How do they view it all? Regardless of any points of disagreement, of possibly the most importance is whether they will accept support or treatment?[67] They may not agree with any of the clinician's views but may still accept that things are not right and be prepared to engage. What is their general willingness to collaborate on developing an approach to management? Stating this in neutral, descriptive terms is a better approach than attempting to quantify it in some way or asserting simply that the patient 'lacks insight'. Having said this, a lack of a shared, common understanding of their problems is a characteristic of some people with severe mental disorders, including both psychotic conditions and disturbances of personality and behaviour. Amongst those with severe personality disorders, there may sometimes be little awareness or sense of remorse for the impact their behaviour may have had on others, but such individuals retain a sense of the world that does not have the same delusional quality seen in acute and sometimes chronic psychosis.

Physical Assessment and Investigations

As judged appropriate, physical assessment and investigations will inform the assessment in collaboration with primary care. An understanding of the person's physical health is an essential component of the holistic assessment. All inpatients should have a full physical and neurological examination, and most will require a standard set of blood investigations. In outpatient settings, accessing blood tests already taken or ordering new ones required should be done. Avoiding duplication is of course sensible, but assuming 'someone else' is doing what is required is not an acceptable way of approaching this issue. Modern electronic patient records should enable clinicians to have a clear view of what has and has not been done.

Diagnostic Formulation and Summary

At some point, the gathering of data must pause, and the clinician must synthesise the data into an informative summary. From this, important judgements may be needed, such as the assessment of risk and what should be done next. Whether shared directly with the patient (e.g. in a letter summarising the contact) or with a letter to the GP, the transparency of modern health care records systems means that all clinicians should work from the assumption that what they write will be shared with the patient.

Risk Issues

Although a separate form may need to be completed depending on local policies, risk assessment is complex in nature and difficult in practice. There is a lack of evidence that risk assessment tools, as such, are helpful, and current guidance is that a full holistic psychiatric assessment is made taking into account known risk factors with consequent management following logically from this[67] (see further discussion of the assessment of suicidal risk in Chapter 15). The clinician must ask themselves three fundamental questions when facing the challenge of assessing and managing risk in this individual: What can I know? What should I do? What may I hope for?

Some judgement of immediate risks must be made alongside the documentation of historic or 'static' risks. On the basis that knowledge of the past can inform our understanding of the present and the future, details of past episodes of dangerous, violent, or suicidal behaviours should be sought out as they will inform the assessment of potential 'worst case' scenarios. Some hospitals require trainees to record risks in a tabular format covering specific categories of risk. These include risk to themselves, to others, of suicide, of self harm, risks of neglect, risk to children, exploitation, absconding or other vulnerabilities.

Understanding the 'historical risk' runs alongside understanding the current 'dynamic risk': 'What has happened in the past?' and 'What is happening now?'. This can be combined, and applying this blended information will help shape the clinical judgement that lies at the heart of good clinical risk assessment: 'what should be done now?' Although the past cannot be changed, it can guide what may happen in the future and aid understanding of what is happening now. This can assist determining what elements of the risk profile can be subject to change or treatment as well as those elements that are unlikely to be amenable to change.

Risk assessment needs to be embedded within the wider assessment and should be linked to the actions following on in the management plan. For the majority of outpatients, risks are usually low, and it is an error to imagine that the risks can be quantified with any degree of exactness in an individual patient. The focus should be on developing a standard approach to assessment that includes collaborative person-centred approaches to the resulting management plan and a discussion and plan around any potential safety issues. Clinicians must be conscious that they are always in a state of incomplete knowledge that will remain incomplete regardless of how much data is gathered. In the same way that a weather forecast even a few days in advance is almost always expressed in percentage terms ('10 per cent chance of rain'), so it is with most judgements of risk in psychiatry and indeed in life. On rare occasions would any degree of certainty approaching 100 per cent be possible. In general, assigning a numerical value to a particular risk should be avoided as it gives a false reassurance that an assessor can actually predict events in individual patients. To use an example given by Jaspers, I might know the percentage mortality for a particular operation, but this does not tell me whether I as an individual will survive the operation. It may be better to use adjectives such as 'high', 'medium' or 'low' to any particular risk,[68] but this needs to be within a comprehensive assessment – see the discussion in the report from Healthcare Safety Investigation Branch.[67] Comparison of the current risk estimate can be made using the concept of a putative 'baseline' risk for that individual patient, based around their history and demographics. An assessor is then assigning a vaguer probabilistic judgement that will then potentially shape their proposed management plan. The nature of the statistics of rare events, though, is that identifying a small 'high-risk' subset may lead to missing the majority of actual cases occurring in those not identified as 'high-risk'.[68,69] Thus the judgement one is making refers to whether the risk for this individual is raised from the baseline that would be expected for the group of patients sharing the same characteristics and if so whether this should alter the proposed management.

By the fact that inpatient beds have fallen greatly over many decades, inpatient admission is now reserved predominantly for those judged to be presenting a significant risk to themselves or others – in many services now, the majority are detained under the Mental Health Act. Despite the inexact nature of the art of risk assessment, ongoing assessment of this risk judgement is central to decision-making around step-down of care to less-dependent settings as much as it is to the decisions around who should be subjected to compulsory treatment in the first place.

The lot of psychiatrists and other mental health staff is that they are obliged to make these judgements in real situations involving the lives of real people and the lives of the families and communities within which everyone lives. Even if the risk assessment is imperfect on admission, it is nevertheless vital to record something about risk at this stage and then to refine this judgement as new information comes to light and to attempt to work with the patient and others to mitigate any potential risks that may be identified, bearing in mind that the benefit of hindsight is something that emerges after events have occurred.

Box 2.3 Summary of assessment structure

History Items

- Presenting issues (presenting complaint)
- History of presenting complaint
- Past psychiatric history
- Past medical history
- Alcohol and substance use history
- Family history
- Personal history (background history)
- Forensic history
- Premorbid personality
- Current social situation

Mental State Examination (MSE) Items

- Appearance
- Behaviour
- Mood
- Speech
- Thoughts, including particular forms such as obsessions and compulsions, delusions, misinterpretations, phobias; and suicidal or violent thoughts.
- Abnormal perceptions, including illusions, hallucinations, 'ego-boundary disturbances' such as passivity experiences and the Schneiderian First Rank symptoms, depersonalisation/derealisation
- Cognitive function, including orientation, concentration, memory etc.
- Insight/patient's perspective

Physical Evaluation

A physical evaluation is part of a full psychiatric evaluation.

Any immediate issues arising from the history must be addressed.

In inpatient settings, a full standard physical examination forms a standard part of the initial evaluation.

In clinic-based settings, targeted examination may be required and a review of physical health, usually through primary care, should form part of the management plan. Basic parameters such as BMI should be calculated.

Review of any blood tests or recent investigations should be completed. In modern settings, checking the online results systems should be straightforward.

Diagnostic Evaluation and Formulation

A diagnostic formulation in the context of the individual narrative/biographical history should be developed. A diagnosis on its own is insufficient – a good formulation should personalise and contextualise any diagnostic hypothesis that is suggested.

The diagnostic formulation lays the basis for the development of the individual plan of management and for judgements about likely course and the appropriate setting for management.

May use approaches such as '5Ps'

May include rating scales, outcome measures

Management Plan

This should be simple, clear and as broad as required.

It should be collaborative and 'co-produced'.

Box 2.3 (*cont.*)

It should be possible to print it out as a clear document.
It should be regarded as a 'work in progress', subject to review and revision

See possible domains to consider and the process of delivery further in the chapter (also see Figure 2.2).

Risk Assessment/Safety Assessment

Making judgements about 'risk' is inevitably a core expectation on psychiatrists. It should be conducted with sufficient humility to accept that all such judgements are potentially flawed. At best, they are a probabilistic statement with a judgement about a threshold that might indicate a certain course of action as opposed to another. They should be part of the broad holistic assessment of the person, their relationships and their environment; 'collaborative'; and understanding of the demographics of risks and relative risks with particular patient groups. An assessor must have a clear knowledge of the demographics of risk and the course of the conditions seen in psychiatric practice and act accordingly.

Group-based Risks

Demographics
Particular conditions

Individual Factors

Historical
Current dynamic factors
Future planning/risk management

Risk judgements are made forward in time, always in a state of 'incomplete knowledge'. Psychiatrists should resist the temptation of behaving like a 'Monday morning quarter back' after the event but should be willing to engage collaboratively with the process of mitigating any potential probabilistic risks identified during an evaluation.

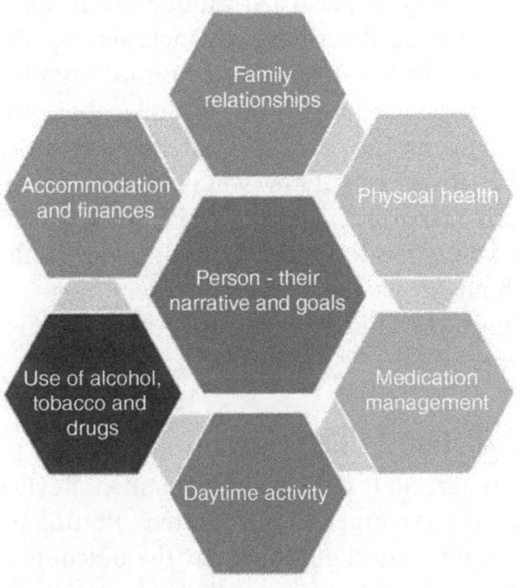

Figure 2.2 Management plan.

Interviewing Style

The style of gathering the information will often initially be free-flowing to develop trust and fluency, and then focused on gathering data likely to contribute to reaching the main diagnosis and formulation. This can be further supplemented by appropriate assessment questionnaires and outcome measures. The aim is to retain an open mind whilst using guided questioning and a systematic approach. This may be supplemented by further examination – for example, neurological examinations (see Chapter 8), physical investigations, psychological testing and further exploration of social aspects. The pattern emerging is compared to diagnostic criteria, and those most closely matching provide a differential diagnosis or set of comorbidities.

It is important to gather this information as systematically as possible for all patients, especially for a first assessment. For follow-up, it is not necessary to repeat the same assessment but important to ensure that previous records are effectively examined and all relevant information is available. For many, it should then be possible to focus on recent events and situations, a review of the collaborative plan, including medication and physical health and the present mental state. Patients find it frustrating having to repeat their story endlessly to different people but may want to confirm – or otherwise – important information in records.

For this reason, whilst the full summary does not need to be repeated each time, the clinician should be aware of the full history and know where to locate it in the clinical record. Modern electronic patient records (EPRs) should make this much more straightforward than written, often illegible records, but they can may make it worse where information is not entered appropriately or swamped by material irrelevant to the assessment. Whilst old 'paper' notes were far from perfect, it was usually straightforward to locate a reasonable typed letter summarising a full background assessment. Sometimes, modern EPRs have been implemented without any transfer of such old important information or the user is unaware of where information is stored in EPRs or does not have previous written records available – or the time to search them. A task of the initial assessment is therefore identifying where the best past summaries are located – or recreating a summary of it, if necessary. It's often quicker, but important information can be missed.

Communicating Assessments in Psychiatry

Good communication is crucial to ensure that the raw material ('data') of the assessment described earlier is synthesised into a meaningful summary that can convey 'useful information'. The collection of raw data on its own does not of itself enable information to be conveyed, nor does the completion of a tick box form that might waste much time in its completion. The sequence of tasks required before a meaningful assessment is completed is given in Figure 2.3.

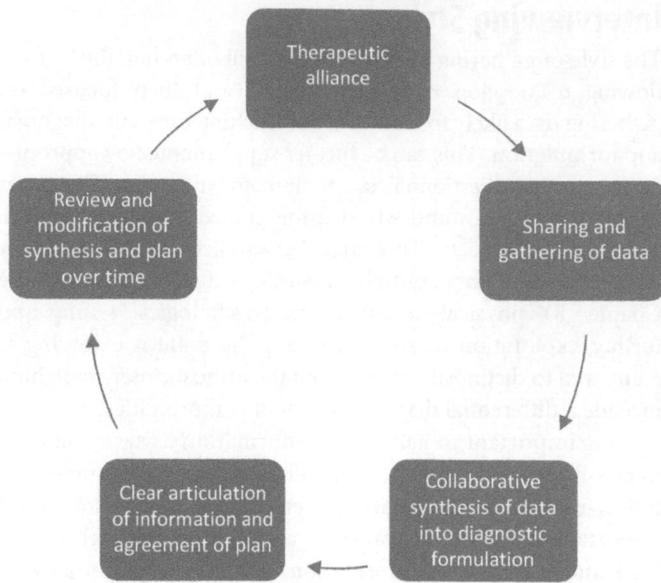

Figure 2.3 Assessment: tasks and their order.

The 'plan' resulting from the synthesis is adjusted but always remains 'a work in progress'.

Summarising Assessments in Letter Form to Patients, Primary Care and Others

Up until a few years ago, the psychiatric synthesis was sent in a letter to the GP who might or might not choose to read it, and a copy was retained in the notes and EPR. Some psychiatrists developed an approach of also sending the GP letter to the patient with or without a covering letter. Even if the psychiatrist was not in the habit of doing this, the patient could still request a copy but could become embroiled in a bureaucratic process to obtain the release of this information, which was still at the discretion of the consultant to release. Access for patients to their own medical records has shifted hugely over recent years in line with wider societal moves encapsulated in the Freedom of Information Act (2005) regarding the entitlement of people to see what data is held about them by all organisations. Health care is not exempt. The Academy of Royal Colleges (2018) suggested that doctors in outpatient settings should write directly to patients,[70] and this now appears to be preferred by both patients and their GPs. This recommendation was supported by the Paterson Inquiry.[71] Paterson was a breast surgeon who was convicted of assaulting hundreds of his patients. One of the issues that emerged in the inquiry was how he conveyed different information to patients compared to their GPs. Some of this difference would have been readily apparent if the patients had received the same letters as their GPs.

The Paterson Inquiry therefore recommended:

> We recommend that it should be standard practice that consultants in both the NHS and the independent sector should write to patients, outlining their condition and treatment, in simple language, and copy this letter to the patient's GP, rather than writing to the GP and sending a copy to the patient.

It would be fair to say that, at the time of writing, this practice is not widely embedded within psychiatric practice in the UK, although the Royal College of Psychiatrists has recently endorsed this approach.[72] One of the authors (Paul Rowlands) is a general psychiatrist in a Community Mental Health Team (CMHT) with a typical caseload who has followed the practice of writing directly to all patients in all situations since 2018, having previously sent copies of the GP letter to patients. This forces the issue of attempting to clarify thought into understandable language and, perhaps most importantly, seeks immediate clarification from the patient of any factual inaccuracies or points of disagreement. Psychotic symptoms can be described non-judgementally and the psychiatric interpretation explained:

> *You described to me hearing your neighbours discussing how they would mutilate you during the night. I do understand how distressing this was to you and how you cannot see any other explanation for this other than that your neighbours wish to kill you and are discussing how to do this. As a psychiatrist, however, I have met other people with similar experiences and I believe that such experiences, utterly real as they seem, can arise in certain conditions which can be helped greatly by support and treatment from my service. We do not need to agree on the details of this and I hope that we can continue to discuss approaches to the immense distress which we both agree you are experiencing at the moment.*

Patient feedback is almost always supportive of the approach, and it helps to develop a sense of managing a collaborative venture in both psychiatrist and patient. The vast majority of patients support this approach, but adaptations may be needed for some patient groups such as those with dementia, those with literacy problems, those with intellectual disabilities or those who do not want this approach. Here, involving carers and advocates may be helpful, and respecting patient choice is important. The use of some words may require particular caution or qualification. An example would be describing a conclusion by the psychiatrist that somebody has 'paranoid delusions': quoting verbatim the words the patient used – for example, about the conspiracy against them or the certainty that they are being poisoned – can lead to an account of how you reach any conclusions that differ from them, an explanation of any diagnostic terms you use and a willingness to continue working respectfully with the person without necessarily agreeing on everything.

This is an area of practice that will inevitably evolve further over the coming years.

Reviewing the Agreed Plan

Once a plan has been agreed, it must be implemented. Review of this implementation is sometimes forgotten. Putting in place a plan is one thing – checking to review the outcome is another. It is easy to assess and recommend, harder to implement and review.

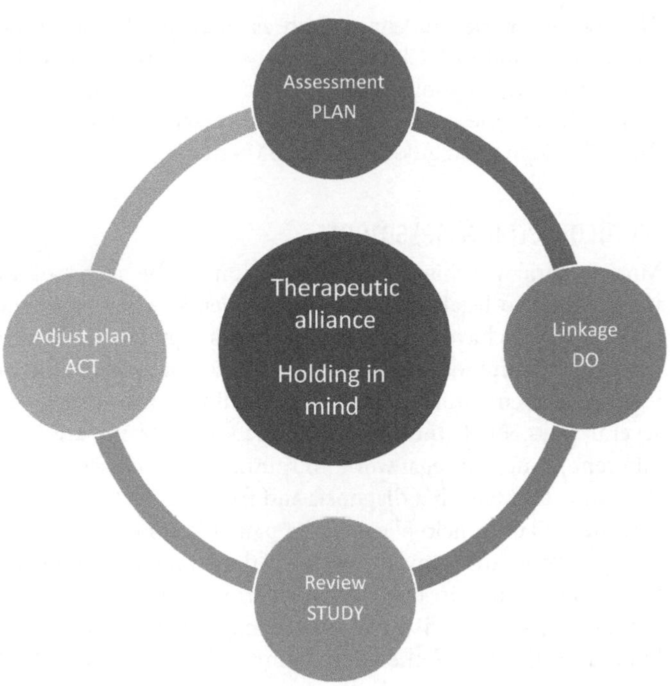

Figure 2.4 Plan-do-study-act (PDSA) cycle.

Therefore, clarity around who will review the plan with the patient is needed from the outset. The timescale needs to be specified and contingency plans agreed in case of any need to bring forward the review. These issues should be explicitly spelled out and likely timeframes agreed. Consistency is a key goal, and it should not be assumed that others will do what has not been agreed with them (e.g. 'GP to review in 2 weeks'; 'CMHT to offer psychodynamic psychotherapy').

Viewing this as a plan-do-study-act (PDSA) cycle is helpful (see Figure 2.4).

Other Types of Psychiatric Assessments: Non-medical Diagnosis and Legal Reports

In the later sections, we consider two further types of assessments: first, assessments carried out by non-medical personnel such as nurses, occupational therapists and social workers, and second, medico-legal assessments for the court.

Advanced (Clinical) Practice Involving Professions Other Than Doctors

Demand for health care across the world is high and rising in all countries. This is the case in the UK, and even prior to the Covid-19 pandemic, health services faced challenges with recruitment, retention of staff and management of workload demands. Shortages of general psychiatrists are not new. The NHS Plan sets out a strategy to improve recruitment and retention alongside approaches intended to empower people and their communities to meet these challenges. The workforce strategies include ambitious plans to extend the clinical roles of existing non-medical clinical staff and to establish new roles and career pathways. For clinical-facing roles, there have been a plethora of different terms describing these, but Advanced (Clinical) Practitioner has become a preferred term to describe people from non-medical backgrounds (for example, nurses, occupational therapists, physiotherapists) working at this level, alongside the psychiatrists, psychologists, psychotherapists and some social workers who might regard themselves as already at an 'advanced' level of clinical practice. All are graduate professions with their own approaches to assessment that have evolved over many years. Health Education England, in partnership with NHS Improvement and NHS England, has developed a multi-professional framework for Advanced Practice in England,[73] which includes a national definition and standards to underpin the multi-professional advanced level of practice. It is intended that these will become a common framework across all disciplines in health care, with specific curriculum and competence frameworks for the various specialities.

> A national definition and framework of what advanced clinical practice is and what the requirements for entry are . . . will ensure that there is national consistency across the role and . . . ensure that advanced clinical practitioners, colleagues, employers and patients clearly understand the role.[73]

Multi-disciplinary Working

Paul Rowlands, who is the psychiatrist for a typical neighbourhood catchment area CMHT of 100,000 population, shares the area with one other consultant. This team over many years has received around 80–100 new referrals a month, the majority from primary care but some as internal referrals or transfers. A small 'Single Point of Access' team looks at each referral every day and is empowered to make judgements about the appropriate pathway and to offer assessment slots with nurses, available without any waiting list. Some cases are straightforward to allocate, and the pathway is obvious, but sometimes cases need further discussion, which usually occurs at a short weekly team referral meeting. During the day, discussion with a consultant is occasionally needed. Some cases are allocated directly to other professions within the CMHT, others to a range of group-based approaches, others to further ongoing assessment or care co-ordination or to social care-based interventions. Some are directed elsewhere – for example, to other teams such as the local Increasing Access to Psychological Therapy services (now Talking Therapies), third sector organisations or 'specialist' teams such as the Eating Disorders team, Perinatal team, the Early Intervention in Psychosis team or, very occasionally, to the Forensic team. A few are referred back, after discussion with the referrer, as not being appropriate for the CMHT. Using this approach, the two consultant psychiatrists, the speciality doctor and their junior staff might see between them 20–30 new cases per month as well as providing follow-up care and treatment to a (changing) caseload of around a thousand patients alongside their other team colleagues.

In a previous generation, all referrals had to come via the GP and were made to the consultant who would then share the load with the junior doctors and perhaps a speciality doctor and the wider team. However, by the early millennium, a workload of 100 new cases a month became intolerable and contributed to exhaustion, early burnout and poor recruitment. In response, in the early 2000s, the UK guidance on *New Ways of Working for Psychiatrists*[74] was developed as a previous generation's response to recruitment and retention issues in psychiatry, and this has evolved in various ways to the current situation. Whatever the drawbacks of the present system may be, no one wishes to revert back to the previous system. Issues of consultant burnout and poor recruitment remain, however, as challenges for existing and coming generations of psychiatrists. It is not simply about workload but must also address the demands inherent in a role where at times much uncertainty and risk are present.

In the past, diagnosis had always been considered a medical responsibility, but service development and increased demand has meant that increasingly non-medically trained people have made diagnostic judgements. Today, the reality is that the vast majority of initial assessments for NHS psychiatric services are made by non-medical personnel, predominantly nurses but also social workers, occupational therapists and others. Anyone doing such assessments should have been trained to an appropriate level and work within the local governance systems of their employer and their own professional guidelines. Whether or not they regard themselves as making 'diagnoses', they should be aware that they cannot escape the fact that the management plans they make are based on a 'diagnostic' judgement.

Local training in the mental health assessment is now provided in many Trusts for their registered mental health staff. The agreed curriculum framework for Advanced Practice requires such individuals to have an understanding of diagnostic frameworks. However, the diagnostic detail given in the ICD-11 and DSM-5 is at a level not required for most routine psychiatric practice, and generally broad diagnostic groupings have been used instead.

The guideline groupings are relatively self-evident and map to the broad headings of ICD-11 and DSM-5. Major groupings that any training should cover would include:

- Psychosis and schizophrenia
- Psychosis with substance misuse
- Common mental disorders (with specific guidelines for anxiety, depression, OCD and PTSD)
- Personality disorders (including 'borderline', complex PTSD and trauma)
- Bipolar disorder
- Eating disorders
- Substance misuse
- Developmental disorders
- Intellectual disability

The use of clinical guidelines, such as those produced by the National Institute of Clinical Excellence, is now required by monitoring organisations such as the Care Quality Commission in the UK, and these are all diagnostically based – some, such as the NICE depression guideline, on DSM criteria.

Medico-Legal Assessments

Most general psychiatrists will occasionally be required to write a medico-legal report on their patients. A few, particularly those who have retired or are in private practice, will also write reports on those who are not their own patients. Medico-legal assessments differ from ordinary clinical assessments in several ways. First, the aim and direction of travel are very different in medico-legal work. In routine clinical assessments, the aim is to establish a diagnosis and from this to formulate a treatment plan to help alleviate the patient's condition.

By contrast, the primary purpose of the psychiatrist reporting to the court is to assist the court in securing justice. This may be for the patient, but in the case of crime, this may be for the injured parties or for the wider community. Second, medical reports are commissioned by the court or by solicitors acting for the patient or other parties, such as a local authority. Irrespective of who has requested the report, the duty of the psychiatrist is to the court, which is the representative of justice and the rule of law. This raises issues of confidentiality as court documents are usually shared between the parties, that is between prosecution and defence or plaintiff and defendant. Even though court documents retain overall confidentiality, this is not sacrosanct in the same way as the patient's medical meetings with their doctors are. Patients must therefore be forewarned that whatever they tell the assessor, it may be made public to the court and so to others associated with the case. Thus, if they wish to keep an item confidential, they should decline to discuss it and indicate this to the examiner. Third, terminology in the legal world is also different; thus, there are no service users although the word patient is still sometimes retained.

A further cautionary note is given in the DSM-5 in that the medical criteria for a disorder may not be the same as the legal criteria for that particular problem. Legal categories will vary between different jurisdictions whereas medical criteria as in ICD-11 and DSM-5 are the same everywhere. Also, although making a diagnosis in the NHS today is frequently made by non-medical personnel, the DSM-5 cautions against this practice in legal settings. In the UK, in court liaison schemes, the person writing the report is often a psychiatric nurse or social worker.

Certain issues are common to all medico-legal assessments. Questions of 'competence' and of 'fitness to plead' come up at potentially several points of an individual's journey through the criminal justice system. Thus, at the point of potential arrest, a police officer might make their own judgement that an individual should be diverted to a mental health setting rather than be arrested for any alleged offence, using Section 136 powers – the origins of which go back several centuries. If arrested, police procedures are laid down in legislation, and codes and questions may be raised regarding the 'fitness to be detained' of the detainee and their 'fitness to be interviewed'. Necessary safeguards that might be required such as the presence of an 'appropriate adult' must be considered by the custody staff and medical assessors such as the forensic medical examiner. Any deviation from the proper processes can lead to evidence being challenged or disregarded in court proceedings. Different criteria may be needed at each step and not all relate to mental health issues. A person in severe pain from an injury, for example, or an intoxicated person would not be 'fit for interview' at that point. A person with a psychotic mental illness would not necessarily be unfit for detention or for interview simply by virtue of this fact, an issue that sometimes causes confusion in the acute setting of a custody suite. Any decision to divert a person alleged to have committed a serious criminal offence to the mental health system – for example, by using civil sections such as Section 2 or Section 3 – and discontinuing the criminal investigation is a very serious matter. It is often better in these circumstances to ensure that the criminal process continues in parallel.

Later, in the course of the journey through the justice system, questions around fitness to plead may be raised. The Criminal Procedure (Insanity and Unfitness to Plead) Act 1991 codified aspects of the existing Common Law and other statutes which dated from the nineteenth century and the Pritchard case. Thus, in England and Wales, the legal test of fitness to plead is based on the ruling of Alderson B. in the case of *R v Pritchard* (1836). In this case, Pritchard was a deaf-mute man charged with a capital felony. The judge asked the jury to consider whether he was 'Mute of malfeasance, or mute by visitation of an Act of God', and the jury assented to the latter. The judge then asked whether in the light of Pritchard's poor intellect he was fit to plead, and the judge gave the following criteria on which to test this matter as shown in Box 2.4.

The level of proof must be on the balance of probabilities. The answer to the question is determined by a jury. In Scotland, the requirement is only that the person can follow proceedings and can instruct their representatives.

These straightforward and readily understandable criteria can be applied to many cases including, for example, people with conditions likely to be permanent, such as severe dementia or severe intellectual disability, as well as those with conditions that may be temporary, such as acute psychosis.

Box 2.4 Fitness to plead, according to the Pritchard criteria

The defendant must have the capacity to:

(i) Understand the charges
(ii) Follow the course of the proceedings in the trial so as to make a proper defence
(iii) Challenge any juror to whom they might object
(iv) Comprehend any evidence
(v) Give proper instructions to their representatives

The court usually delegates the issue of whether there is a lack of legal capacity to the psychiatrist. Common law holds that every person is responsible for their actions, and a defence of 'lack of capacity' should only be used sparingly. Thus, in cases of serious crime where this is used in the defence, the prosecution may hire their own psychiatrist to test the issue. If the two psychiatrists disagree, the judge will direct them to come to a common opinion although eventually the issue may be decided by the jury. A lack of capacity can be present one day and then change the next according to the patient's mental state. A person may have legal capacity yet still be unable to go to court as in cases of overwhelming anxiety, and the two will need to be distinguished. Capacity in other legal settings usually only refers to capacity in the specific area of interest of the court – for example, a person may be quite capable of managing their day-to-day responsibilities but fail to comprehend the legal issues involved in a complicated hire purchase agreement on which he or she has now defaulted.

In criminal cases, once a decision around fitness to plead has been reached by the court, psychiatric evidence may later be sought on other matters – including in homicide cases, around the issue of 'diminished responsibility' – prior to conviction. In some cases, the court will make a finding of fact without the individual pleading to the indictment, seeking reports to aid its deliberations, such as it might under provisions in Part III of the Mental Health Act such as Section 35.

With the exception of homicide cases, where the psychiatric evidence may have a bearing on the ultimate verdict, psychiatric evidence is generally not provided in the course of the trial but mostly provided post-conviction. Reports might be requested to help determine the ultimate disposal of a case. This is not simply a question of 'hospital or prison' but might nowadays include consideration of whether or not a community-based (Probation) Order should include a Mental Health Treatment Requirement (MHTR).

In each instance, psychiatrists requested to provide reports must bear in mind their overarching duty to the court and justice and put aside any individual duty they might feel to their patient or the person commissioning the report.

Conclusions

Good assessment, formulation and diagnosis lies at the heart of psychiatric practice, and every case represents a new challenge to the psychiatrist. Each case is a unique individual in their own right. Diagnostic criteria and disorder definition have undergone a lengthy journey over the last 200 years starting with brief lists of terminology, some of which have now passed into oblivion. These early lists have been transformed and matured into the sophisticated glossaries we have today in the ICD-11 and DSM-5, but they remain works in progress. Diagnosis and classification of mental disorders has inevitably created confusion and controversy, and some of the terminology used is unnecessarily stigmatising. When official coding is needed, the DSM-5 is used in America, and the ICD-11 is used in the UK and the rest of the world. However, being able to apply this knowledge depends on the ability to perform high-quality assessments, a skill that is usually acquired through years of experience. While scientific endeavour has had a major and beneficial impact on diagnostic practices, our ability to get the best outcome for an individual patient depends on getting as full an understanding of the person as possible and developing a shared diagnostic formulation within the setting of a therapeutic alliance. This is not so much a science as an art: the art of psychiatry.

References

1. Tuke DH. *A Dictionary of Psychological Medicine: Giving the Definition, Etymology and Synonyms of the Terms Used in Medical Psychology with the Symptoms, Treatment, and Pathology of Insanity and the Law of Lunacy in Great Britain and Ireland*. Philadelphia: Blakiston; 1892.
2. Jaspers K. *General Psychopathology* (trans. J Hoenig and MW Hamilton 1963). Manchester: Manchester University Press; 1959:826.
3. Scadding JG. Diagnosis: the clinician and the computer. *Lancet* 1967;2 (7521):877–82.
4. Mindham RH, Scadding JG, Cawley RH. Diagnoses are not diseases. *British Journal of Psychiatry* 1992;161:686–91.
5. Linnaeus C. *Systema naturae*. Leiden; 1735.
6. Linnaeus C. *Genera morborum*. Upsaliae: CE Steiner; 1763.
7. de Sauvages FB. *Nosologie metodique, dans la quelle les maladies sont rangées par classes, suivant le systême de Sydenham & l'ordre des botanistes*. Tome second. chez Hérissant, le Fils; 1771.
8. Cullen W. *Synopsis nosologiae methodicae, exhibens clariss. virorum Sauvagesii, Linnaei, Vogelii, Sagari, et Macbridii systemata nosologica*. Sumptibus Joannis Antonii Pezzana; 1787.
9. Shorter E. The history of nosology and the rise of the *Diagnostic and Statistical Manual of Mental Disorders. Dialogues in Clinical Neuroscience* 2015;17 (1):59–67.
10. Kendler KS. Toward a scientific psychiatric nosology: strengths and limitations. *Archives of General Psychiatry* 1990;47(10):969–73.
11. Stengel E. Classification of mental disorders. *Bulletin of the World Health Organization* 1959;21(4–5):601.
12. Morel B. Traitsé des Maladies Mentales. *American Journal of Psychiatry* 1860;17 (2):199–211.
13. Bucknill JC, Tuke DH. *A Manual of Psychological Medicine, Containing the Lunacy Laws: the Nosology, Aetiology, Statistics, Description, Diagnosis, Pathology, and Treatment of Insanity, with an Appendix of Cases*. Philadelphia: Lindsay and Blakiston; 1879.
14. Griesinger W. *Mental Pathology and Therapeutics*. London: New Sydenham Society; 1845.
15. Jaspers K. *General Psychopathology* (trans. J Hoenig and MW Hamilton 1963). Manchester: Manchester University Press; 1959.
16. Kraepelin E. *Psychiatrie: Рипол Классик*. Leipzig: Verlag Von Johan Ambrosius Barth; 1927.
17. Kraepelin E. *Dementia Praecox and Paraphrenia* (trans. RM Barclay and GM Robertson). Edinburgh: Livingstone; 1919.
18. Jablensky A. The 100-year epidemiology of schizophrenia. *Schizophrenia Research* 1997;28(2–3):111–25.
19. Bleuler E. *Textbook of Psychiatry* (trans. AA Brill). New York: Macmillan; 1951.
20. Ohler N. *Blitzed: Drugs in Nazi Germany*. London: Penguin; 2016.
21. Healy D. *The Creation of Psychopharmacology*. Harvard: Harvard University Press; 2002.
22. Kramer M. Some problems for international research suggested by observations as differences in first admission rates to mental hospitals of England & Wales, and of the United States. *Proceedings of the Third World Congress of Psychiatry* 1961;3:153–60.
23. Kendell RE, Cooper JE, Gourlay AJ, et al. Diagnostic criteria of American and British psychiatrists. *Archives of General Psychiatry* 1971;25(2):123–30.
24. Wing JK. The use of the Present State Examination in general population surveys. *Acta Psychiatrica Scandinavica* 1980;62:230–40.
25. World Health Organization. *Report of the International Pilot Study of Schizophrenia*: Geneva: World Health Organization; 1973.
26. Bridgman PW. *The Logic of Modern Physics*. New York: Macmillan; 1927.
27. Hempel CG. *Paper delivered by Carl G. Hempel. Morning Session: Introduction to Problems of Taxonomy. Field Studies in the Mental Disorders: Proceedings of the Work Conference on Problems in Field Studies in the Mental Disorders, February 15–19, 1959, under the Auspices of the American Psychopathological Association*. Grune & Stratton; 1961.
28. Feighner JP, Robins E, Guze SB, et al. Diagnostic criteria for use in psychiatric research. *Archives of General Psychiatry* 1972;26(1):57–63.
29. Spitzer RL, Endicott J, Robins E. Research diagnostic criteria: Rationale and reliability. *Archives of General Psychiatry* 1978;35(6):773–82.
30. Virchow R. *Über die culturgeschichtliche Stellung des Kaukasus: unter besonderer Berücksichtigung der ornamentirten Bronzegürtel aus transkaukasischen Gräbern*. Königl: Academie der Wissenschaften; 1895.
31. Bolton D, Gillet G. *The Biopsychosocial Model of Health and Disease*. London: Palgrave Macmillan; 2019.
32. Kendell RE. *The Role of Diagnosis in Psychiatry*. Oxford: Blackwell Scientific; 1975.
33. Kräupl Taylor F. *The Concepts of Disease, Illness and Morbus*. Cambridge: Cambridge University Press; 1979.
34. Royal College of Psychiatrists. *Core Values for Psychiatrists CR204*. London: Royal College of Psychiatrists; 2017.
35. Szasz TS. *The Myth of Mental Illness*. New York: Harper & Row; 1961.
36. Bloch S. Delusions of reformism – Dissent or madness? *World Medical Journal* 1979;26(3):36–8.
37. Szasz T. *The Manufacture of Madness: A Comparative Study of the Inquisition and the Mental Health Movement*. Syracuse: Syracuse University Press; 1997.
38. Foucault M. *Madness and Civilization: A History of Insanity in the Age of*

Reason (trans. R Howard). New York: Vintage; 1965.

39. Horwitz A. *DSM: A History of Psychiatry's Bible.* Baltimore: Johns Hopkins University Press; 2021.
40. Shorter E. *The Rise and Fall of the Age of Psychopharmacology.* New York: Oxford University Press; 2021.
41. Moncrieff J, Cooper RE, Stockmann T, et al. The serotonin theory of depression: a systematic umbrella review of the evidence. *Molecular Psychiatry* 2022;20. doi.org/10.1038/s41380-022-01661-0.
42. Laing RD, Esterson A. *Sanity, Madness and the Family. Vol. 1, Families of Schizophrenics.* London: Tavistock; 1964.
43. Clare A. *Psychiatry in Dissent: Controversial Issues in Thought and Practice*, 2nd ed. London: Routledge; 2012.
44. Mezzich JE, Kirmayer LJ, Kleinman A, et al. The place of culture in DSM-IV. *Journal of Nervous and Mental Disease* 1999;187(8):457–64.
45. Mezzich JE, Caracci G, Fabrega H, et al. Cultural formulation guidelines. *Transcultural Psychiatry* 2009;46 (3):383–405.
46. World Health Organisation. *Fact Files.* www.who.int/news-room/facts-in-pictures/detail/mental-health (accessed May 2014).
47. World Health Organisation. *Investing in Mental Health.* Geneva: WHO; 2013.
48. American Psychiatric Association. *Diagnostic and Statistical Manual of Mental Disorders: DSM-5.* American Psychiatric Association; 2013.
49. Kingdon D, Taylor L, Ma K, et al. Changing name: changing prospects for psychosis. *Epidemiology and Psychiatric Sciences* 2013;22(4):297–301.
50. Kingdon D. DSPD or 'don't stigmatise people in distress'. *Advances in Psychiatric Treatment* 2007;13(5):333–5.
51. Jablensky A, Kendell R. Criteria for assessing a classification in psychiatry. In: Maj M, Gaebel W, López-Ibor J, et al. (eds.) *Psychiatric diagnosis and classification.* West Sussex: John Wiley and Sons Ltd.; 2002: 1–24.
52. Johnstone L. Psychological formulation as an alternative to psychiatric diagnosis. *Journal of Humanistic Psychology* 2018;58(1):30–46.
53. Bolton D, Gillet G. *The Biopsychosocial Model of Health and Disease.* Switzerland: Palgrave Macmillan; 2019.
54. Kirby G. *Guide for History Taking and Clinical Examination of Psychiatric Cases.* Albany: New York State Hospital Commission; 1921.
55. World Health Organization. *ICD-11: International classification of diseases (11th revision).* Geneva: World Health Organization, 2019.
56. Farr W. Letter to the registrar general. *First Annual Report of the Registrar General*; 1839.
57. d'Espine M. *Essai analytique et critique de statistique mortuaire compare.* Geneva: Cherbuliez & Leidecker; 1858.
58. American Public Health Association. *The Bertillon Classification of Causes of Death.* Lansing: R. Smith Print Company; 1890.
59. War Department. Nomenclature of psychiatric disorders and reactions: War Department Technical Bulletin, Medical 203. *Journal of Clinical Psychology* 1946;2:289–96.
60. Chodoff P. *Psychiatric Diagnosis: A 60-Year Perspective.* psychnews.psychiatryonline.org/doi/full/10.1176/pn.40.11.00400017a (accessed 20 March 2023).
61. Fulford B. Karl Jaspers and General Psychopathology. In: Fulford B, Thornton T, Graham G (eds.) *Oxford Textbook of Philosophy and Psychiatry. Oxford*: Oxford University Press; 2006: 160–79.
62. Meyer A. *Psychobiology; a Science of Man.* Oxford, England: Charles C Thomas; 1957.
63. Fish FJ. *Fish's Clinical Psychopathology: Signs and Symptoms in Psychiatry.* Bristol: John Wright; 1985.
64. Mayer-Gross W, Slater E, Roth M (eds.). *Clinical Psychiatry*, 3rd ed. London: Williams and Wilkins; 1969.
65. Ewing JA. Detecting alcoholism: the CAGE questionnaire. *Jama* 1984;252 (14):1905–07.
66. David A, Buchanan A, Reed A, et al. The assessment of insight in psychosis. *British Journal of Psychiatry* 1992;161 (5):599–602.
67. Healthcare Safety Investigation Branch (HSIB). *Care Delivery within Community Mental Health Teams.* www.hsib.org.uk/investigations-and-reports/care-delivery-within-community-mental-health-teams/care-delivery-within-community-mental-health-teams/ (accessed 25 March 2023).
68. Sanati A. Matthew Large. *BJPsych Bulletin* 2021;45(3):190–2.
69. McHugh CM, Corderoy A, Ryan CJ, et al. Association between suicidal ideation and suicide: meta-analyses of odds ratios, sensitivity, specificity and positive predictive value. *BJPsych Open* 2019;5(2):e18.
70. Academy of Medical Royal Colleges. *Please, Write to Me: Writing Outpatient Clinic Letters to Patients.* London: Academy of Medical Royal Colleges; 2018.
71. James G. Report of the Independent Inquiry into the Issues Raised by Paterson. London: Government of the United Kingdom; 2020.
72. Royal College of Psychiatrists. *Writing Clinic letters: College Guidance on Improving Engagement with Patients.* London: Royal College of Psychiatrists; 2021.
73. Health Education England. *Multi-professional Framework for Advanced Clinical Practice in England.* www.hee.nhs.uk/sites/default/files/documents/multi-professionalframework foradvancedclinicalpracticeinengland.pdf (accessed 5 March 2023).
74. Department of Health. *New Ways of Working for Psychiatrists: Enhancing Effective, Person-Centred Services through New Ways of Working in Multidisciplinary and Multiagency Contexts.* London: Department of Health; 2005.

Chapter

3.1 Clinical Features of Depressive Disorders

Ian M. Anderson and Kate Williams-Markey

Introduction

Depressive disorders have been recognised since antiquity, although how they have been described and understood has changed considerably over time. In this chapter, we outline key aspects of the history of depression and some of the limitations in its current classification in ICD-11 and DSM-5-TR. We describe the range of symptoms experienced in depressive disorders, together with the recognised variations in clinical presentation and how these are conceptualised and classified. The relationship between depression and related disorders – including anxiety disorders, premenstrual dysphoric disorder and grief – is discussed, as well as boundary issues with bipolar disorder and primary psychotic disorders. We review current knowledge about depression's considerable psychiatric and medical comorbidity as well as its epidemiology, natural history and health burden. A brief practical guide to assessing depressive disorders is given, together with rating scales that are useful for clinical assessment and monitoring.

History of Depression

Antiquity to the Renaissance

The Greek physician Hippocrates wrote in the fifth century BCE that 'fears and despondencies, if they last a long time' were symptomatic of melancholia. However, melancholy also included what are now considered non-affective psychoses, obsessive-compulsive disorders and anxiety disorders, with states of grandiosity, increased energy and exaltation not recognised as a separate condition. Melancholy was also associated with intellectual ability or even genius, rather as bipolar disorder has been linked with creativity today. Historical melancholy is therefore best seen as a broad, inconsistently applied term that could include much of today's mental illness.

The humoural theory of illness, based on four humours (blood, yellow bile, black bile and phlegm), was systematised in Ancient Greece around the fifth century BCE and influenced medicine for the next 2,000 years. Deficiencies or excesses of humour could cause disease, with melancholia as the state associated with an excess of black bile. Galen, in the second century, proposed that moderate imbalances in humours (dyscrasias) produced different temperaments, meaning both psychological dispositions (sanguine, melancholic, etc.) and susceptibility to bodily illness. His writings influenced the Islamic world and were rediscovered in Europe in the second millennium. In contrast, supernatural causes of illness were invoked in many ancient civilisations and by Christianity in the Middle Ages. Psychological explanations were also entertained in antiquity; the Roman orator and statesman Cicero, in the first century, suggested that melancholy could be caused by excessive anger, fear or pain.

One of the most famous works on melancholy, *The Anatomy of Melancholy* by Robert Burton (1577–1640), is a culmination of the classical view written towards the end of the Renaissance. It is a vast wide-ranging book, extensively revised between 1621 and 1638, written to avoid and treat Burton's own melancholy. It is full of quotations from classical to contemporary times, comprising a haphazard literary and medical encyclopaedia of types of melancholy and their symptoms, causes and treatments, drawing on the range of sciences of the day including theology and astrology. He distinguished dispositional or transitory melancholy – reactive to 'occasions' and from which 'no living man is free' – from melancholy as a habit, a serious ailment 'not errant, but fixed', a distinction still relevant today.

Seventeenth to Nineteenth Centuries

As observational and empirical methods of understanding nature gained ground in the Western world, the humoural system gave way to theories of disturbances of the brain and nervous system. A phase of viewing melancholy as a disorder of the intellect or judgement (i.e. characterised by delusions) independent of mood changes, exemplified by William Cullen (1710–1790) and Phillipe Pinel (1745–1826), was challenged in the nineteenth century when the core of affective symptoms was reasserted, and non-delusional melancholy closer to our current idea of depression was described by Joseph Guislain (1789–1860) and Daniel Tuke (1827–1895).[1] By the end of the nineteenth century, melancholy was accepted as primarily a mood disorder, in which delusions arose from the mood change, as described by Richard von Krafft-Ebing (1840–1902) and Emil Kraepelin (1856–1926) among others, laying the foundation for our modern concept of mood-congruent psychosis.[1] Melancholic and non-melancholic forms of mood disorder (such as neurasthenia) were recognised by the end of the nineteenth century, with Carl Lange (1834–1900) among the earliest to use the term 'depression' to describe a condition of low mood, enervation, difficulty making decisions, loss of joy in life and often anxiety, which he contrasted with melancholy.[2] In parallel, psychodynamic theories were developing, beginning with Sigmund Freud (1856–1939), who proposed that conflict within the unconscious results in emotional difficulties in adulthood. Freud theorised that melancholy is a pathological reaction to loss in which internally directed anger leads to guilt and self-loathing.

Twentieth Century to Today

Around the start of the twentieth century, Kraepelin famously distinguished dementia praecox (schizophrenia) from manic depressive illness (psychotic and non-psychotic depression, along with mania), although he also recognised a psychogenic form of depression reactive to social circumstances. By the second half of the twentieth century, there were a plethora of different terms applied to depression including endogenous, vital, involutional, neurotic, reactive and depressive personality, with attempts to identify differential clinical and biological determinants and treatment response. The World Health Organization, in the ninth revision of the International Classification of Diseases (ICD-9, 1970s to 1990s), followed Kraepelin in distinguishing 'manic depressive psychosis, depressed type' from neurotic depression and other neurotic disorders such as anxiety states and neurasthenia. In response to the psychoanalytic dominance in American psychiatry and a general lack of reliability in psychiatric diagnoses, operationalised diagnostic criteria were developed in the 1970s. The resulting Feighner criteria, based on observations in psychiatric populations, informed the Research Diagnostic Criteria (RDC) that were subsequently adopted by the American Psychiatric Association in the third edition of the *Diagnostic and Statistical Manual of Mental Disorders* (DSM-III) in 1980. DSM-III also distinguished between depression and bipolar disorder, originating from Karl Leonhard's (1904–1988) re-evaluation in the 1950s of manic depressive illness according to polarity based on distinct family genetics. This distinction, together with the failure to be able to reliably identify depressive subtypes based on aetiology, or treatment response, led to the diagnosis we recognise today: eliminating the distinction between psychotic and neurotic disorders, putting depressive disorders together in a single group of mood disorders based on a limited number of features, and separating 'unipolar' from 'bipolar' depression. This change, continuing through subsequent editions of the DSM, was largely adopted by ICD-10 in 1992 and is now fully implemented in ICD-11 (2022). Criteria that were developed from a relatively small group of severely ill hospitalised patients have become applied to community settings, increasing the recognition of depression, which is now the most common mental health diagnosis. Different presentations of depression are identified by symptom profiles. The vertical hierarchical structure deals with horizontal symptom overlap by allowing comorbidity, so that a person can have more than one disorder at the same time (e.g. both a depressive and an anxiety disorder), or by using specific exclusions (e.g. a history of mania places a depressive episode under bipolar disorders).

Current Controversies and Implications

Whether depression is better viewed descriptively/phenomenologically or understood in terms of aetiology/causation is a dilemma still present today. Although the definition of depression is now relatively stable, the distinction between normal and pathological sadness and between different types of depression has become less clear. There remain tensions between depression as a dimension and as a category, uncertainty about how it relates to other disorders – especially anxiety disorders and bipolar disorder – little progress in identifying underlying pathology, no diagnostic clinical test or truly specific treatment, and no coherent conceptualisation of its likely multifactorial aetiologies.

Kendler[3] argues that the current criteria for depression are useful as a rapid and reliably applicable index for a condition that has been recognised throughout history but that it is a category mistake to equate the limited criteria with the underlying condition, and the criteria do not capture the broader symptomatology present nor lived experience. In the continuing search for subtypes that might allow the identification of specific pathology and guide treatment, a meta-review identified five broad approaches based on symptom profile, aetiology, time of onset, gender and treatment resistance, but the meta-review argues that these approaches need to be integrated to enable the progress that has so far been elusive.[4] Population surveys show an exponential distribution of depressive symptoms, with no evidence of bimodality or any 'point of rarity' that would suggest a pathological category of depression. However Parker[5] argues that melancholia is a distinct categorical depressive disorder if defined by key psychomotor features and that there is suggestive evidence for bimodality using this restricted symptom set.

These uncertainties have contributed to a wider questioning of the value of diagnosis in psychiatry. The aim of the Research Domain Criteria, developed by the US National Institute of Mental Health, is to characterise mental disorders trans-diagnostically according to patterns of variation in six higher-level neurobehavioural domains (positive and negative valence, cognition, social processing, arousal/regulatory, and sensorimotor systems) in order to investigate their multilevel biological and psychological underpinnings. It has been criticised for being a top-down approach with no account taken of natural history,[6] and the integration of biological and psychological constructs remains a challenge. Another approach, which overtly rejects diagnoses and causal biological pathology, is the Power Threat Meaning Framework.[7] This proposes that social factors and trauma (Power, Threat) lead to emotional distress and behaviour (Threat Responses) that can be addressed by enabling someone to make sense of their experiences through the creation of more helpful narratives (Meaning), instead of seeing themselves as blameworthy, weak, deficient or mentally ill. It is suggested that, for some people, depression and anxiety are better seen as synonyms for a 'general pattern' of expressing distress, provisionally identified as 'surviving defeat, entrapment, disconnection and loss'. Whatever the value of this approach for individuals, it is debatable whether what the authors describe as "broad [...] patterns that synthesise the influences of Power, Threat, Meaning and associated Threat Responses" can replace diagnoses at a public health level.

What can we learn from this? First, a diagnosis of depression is primarily a cross-sectional description of a limited range of symptoms, providing an index of mood disturbance rather than representing the disorder itself, and therefore only a starting point. Second, the diagnosis doesn't explain the mood symptoms or the person's lived experience, with no distinction between responses to life difficulties and specific underlying pathology (the popular 'scientific' explanation of a chemical imbalance in the brain is essentially the humoural imbalance theory of old). Third, a diagnosis of depression does not by itself imply a particular, or even any, treatment, and management needs to be based on a broader clinical assessment and approached pragmatically and collaboratively. Finally, given that depression and its symptom profiles do not describe homogeneous populations, taking these as categories is likely to be unfruitful for research.

Symptoms and Signs

Depressive disorders include a range of possible symptoms and signs that are inter-related, interact with each other, and can change over time, with each person having an individual experience and pattern. Table 3.1.1 shows the frequency of a range of symptoms found in individuals seeking help for depression in studies in two settings[8,9]; they show a similar prevalence pattern of common symptoms in spite of the difference in the severity of depression. Notable is the high prevalence of fatigue/lack of energy and anxiety as well as low mood. A recent systematic review investigating possible gender differences found that depressed women are more likely than depressed men to report standard symptoms used for diagnosis, but the difference was small and the pattern broadly similar. Men did however show more risk taking, impulsive behaviour and alcohol and drug use, which may reflect a fundamental difference in presentation (so-called male depressive syndrome) or different self-medicating and coping behaviours.[10]

Affective Symptoms

Depressed Mood

Lowered mood is unsurprisingly a central feature of depressive disorders and the most commonly reported symptom (Table 3.1.1), although it doesn't have to be present for the diagnosis to be made. For many, their depressed mood is qualitatively different to feelings of unhappiness or sadness

Table 3.1.1 Frequency of different symptoms in individuals seeking help for depression in community and psychiatric settings

	Community sample (N = 1,884)[a]	Depressed psychiatric outpatients (N = 196)[b]
Diagnosis (DSM-IV criteria)		
Major depressive episode	57%	84%
(Melancholic depression)	(-)	(59%)
Other depressive disorders	10%	16%
≥2 Depressive symptoms with minimal impairment	33%	-
Symptoms/behaviours when depressed		
Depressed mood	76%	94%
Emotional/cry a lot/want to cry	59%	-
Fatigue/tired/listless/no energy	73%	74%
Anhedonia/reduced interest	37%	76%
Impaired sexual desire	‡	49%
Apathy/lack of motivation	39%	-
Decreased activity/productivity	-	82%
Social withdrawal	-	77%
'Psychic' anxiety - tension/worry/fear	-	93%
Anxious/nervous/fearful	57%	-
Constant worry	38%	-
'Somatic' anxiety - autonomic/respiratory	34%	62%
Panic	18%	18%
Agoraphobia	‡	16%
Subjective irritability	50%	-
Concentration/memory difficulties	51%	-
impaired concentration	-	82%
impaired memory	-	30%
Inappropriate guilt/loss of self-esteem	29%	52%
Feeling worthless/inadequate	40%	-
Hopelessness	-	55%
Feeling life not worth living	34%	-
Suicidal thoughts	‡	29%
Broken sleep/sleep less than normal	63%	-
Early insomnia/hypersomnia	-	31%
Early morning waking	-	47%
Change in appetite	40%	-
Weight loss	-	33%
Weight gain/bulimia	-	6%
Agitation	-	59%
Subjective slowing	-	30%
Motor retardation	-	29%
Intrusive thoughts	37%	-
Obsessive thoughts	-	28%
Compulsions	‡	10%
Hypochondriacal preoccupations	-	40%
Dramatic attention-seeking behaviour	-	8%
Delusions	-	8%
Hallucinations	-	3%
Suspiciousness	-	4%
Feeling worse in the morning	-	49%

Table 3.1.1 *(cont.)*

	Community sample (N = 1,884)[a]	Depressed psychiatric outpatients (N = 196)[b]
Somatic complaints	-	57%
Concomitant medical condition	65%	-

- Not specifically assessed/reported; ‡ occurred in <30% but figure not given.

[a] Community participants (70% female) who had sought professional help for depression in the last six months. Some assessed symptoms are not reported if <30% (adapted with permission from Tylee et al. *International Clinical Psychopharmacology* 1999;**14**: 139–51).

[b] Sequential psychiatric outpatient referrals (69% female) with a depression diagnosis (11% bipolar depression) (adapted with permission from Faravelli et al. *Comprehensive Psychiatry* 1996;**37**: 307–15).

(e.g. after experiencing a loss) although the experience is individual; one person might describe a general, persistent, oppressive feeling of misery and despair, whilst another might describe a highly unpleasant dark emptiness or hopeless numbness, and others as a 'black dog', 'black days' or a 'dark cloud'. Some people will be tearful or easily moved to tears, whereas others may be unable to cry and feel that their ability to do so is blocked. Depressed mood may lead to a feeling of being disconnected from emotions and from others (see 'Depersonalisation/Derealisation'). Typically, the depressed mood is unremitting and unreactive (or changing only minimally) in response to usually pleasurable events. Diurnal variation, in which mood and other symptoms are worse in the morning and lift somewhat as the day goes on, is not uncommon, but this may be lost in the most severe depression. In contrast, some individuals experience 'atypical' low mood similar to unhappiness or sadness, which is temporarily reactive to circumstances, and can improve in response to something positive, such as meeting a friend. This picture may also be accompanied by a worsening of mood as the day progresses and can be associated with sleeping more, increased appetite and anxiety (see section on 'Atypical Depression'). In some, the predominant presentation may be anxiety, agitation or health preoccupations, and the depressed mood may be 'masked' by these features.

Anhedonia

Anhedonia is viewed as a core symptom of depression alongside low mood, although for a substantial minority, the intensity is below the symptom threshold (Table 3.1.1). Anhedonia is loss of interest in, and an inability to derive pleasure from, daily activities such as spending time with loved ones or enjoying activities they would typically enjoy (e.g. exercise, reading) and not caring about tasks, activities or others as much as they may have done previously. It may also be experienced as an inability to feel an improvement in mood despite positive things happening around them. Others may notice that the person is less engaged or interested in conversations and social activities. Anhedonia can also be closely linked to thoughts of worthlessness, diminished drive and energy, loss of libido, reduced engagement in activities, apathy and social withdrawal. It can also overlap, or be conflated with, depersonalisation/derealisation in which detachment from emotions is experienced (see later in the chapter).

Hopelessness

Hopelessness may be expressed as the future appearing dark, uncertain and unpleasant, with little or no hope that the situation can improve and the feeling of powerlessness to change things. It appears as an inability to think of positive future events rather than anticipating negative events, and it is often accompanied by feelings of worthlessness or inadequacy, with a sense of feeling trapped or defeated, and suicide may be seen as the only way out. Hopelessness is one of the strongest predictors of suicidal thoughts but with weaker effects on suicide attempts and death from suicide, so that the absolute effect is small and of limited use on its own to predict suicide risk.[11]

Worthlessness, Shame and Guilt

Worthlessness can involve feeling useless, inadequate or unlovable, as well as thinking they have no worth as a human being or that they have failed in life. This often involves unfavourable comparison with others, believing that they are inferior – or worth less – than others around them. Low self-esteem and lack of self-worth may be pre-existing traits with childhood origins that become more intense and pervasive when depressed. This can lead to internalising feelings of self-blame, being defective and unlovable, being responsible for one's own suffering and failure, and being a burden to others. Closely related is shame (not emphasised in the diagnosis of depression), which together with guilt, can arise in response to an experience of failure or wrongdoing. Shame typically involves attributing this failure or wrongdoing to the whole self, rather than a particular action, with a focus on being flawed as a person, whereas guilt tends to be directed towards the impact on others, attributing failure or harm to others to one's intentions and actions. Guilt in normal circumstances is often adaptive and leads to a motivation to change behaviour or make amends. In depression, these emotions can be unwarranted and excessive and become generalised beyond specific events; shame leads to feelings of worthlessness, inadequacy and humiliation, and the guilt often magnifies perceived wrongdoings or past events, which may progress to the feeling that others know what they have done and are blaming or accusing them (ideas of reference). In severe depression, feelings of guilt may become delusional – for example, feeling responsible for disasters or evil events or of having committed a crime and needing to be punished for it. Worthlessness can also become delusional – for example, holding delusions of poverty or being bankrupt. In assessing whether guilt is excessive for someone, it is important to determine whether it is disproportionate given their situation and background; feeling guilty about letting other people down or causing financial difficulties may not be inappropriate. Shame, guilt and their interaction may lead to someone being fearful of rejection or judgement, as well as being reluctant to seek help, talk about their feelings or reveal their difficulty in coping. They can also manifest in statements that are self-critical and self-judgemental, in anger, and in suicidal thoughts and behaviour.

Anxiety

Anxiety is very common (Table 3.1.1) and an important aspect of depressive disorders (see section on 'Anxious Depression'). The symptoms are often divided into psychic (or psychological) and somatic (or physical). Psychological symptoms include the feeling of tension, the inability to relax, being 'on edge', irritability, apprehension about the future, worry or churning thoughts that won't stop regarding things that might happen or that seem minor to others. Sometimes, there can be catastrophic thoughts leading to panic attacks. Physical symptoms are largely related to autonomic system activation and muscle tension, including headaches, dry mouth, tingling, tremulousness, palpitations, chest pain, sweating, dizziness, shortness of breath, nausea, abdominal pain, cramps, a feeling of 'butterflies' in the stomach, heavy limbs, diarrhoea and urinary urges and frequency. Anxiety may be evident from worried or fearful facial expressions and motor overactivity (see 'Agitation'). For some, the physical symptoms might lead to a preoccupation with physical health (see 'Hypochondriasis') and even obscure the depressive symptoms.

Irritability and Anger

Those who are depressed commonly describe a low threshold for annoyance or anger in the face of frustration, both in relation to their own perceived failings or the actions of others. This may be purely subjective or expressed by being 'short' or argumentative with others, in outbursts of temper or even physical violence to things or other people. Anger has long been believed to be integral to the experience of depression and, psychoanalytically, depression has been interpreted as anger turned inwards onto the self. In depressed people who deny anger, irritable feelings may present as self-criticism and self-blame, whereas those who admit irritability may feel guilt about the way they 'take it out' on their partner or family. In adults, irritability and anger are no longer emphasised in the diagnosis of depression, but they are recognised as important in the presentation of children and adolescents.

Cognitive Symptoms

Thought content in depression is usually congruent with, and integral to, the affective symptoms described earlier. Aaron Beck described a 'cognitive triad' of negative thoughts – occurring automatically – about self, the world and the future, which forms a central focus of cognitive therapy. Typically, these thoughts reflect self-criticism, self-blame, self-disgust and self-hatred, extending to automatic negative beliefs and assumptions about the motives and actions of others, obstacles being too difficult or demanding, and the future being without hope. As well as these 'affective cognitions' there is also impairment in attention, concentration and cognitive function more broadly.

Thoughts of Death and Suicide

Thoughts that life seems pointless and not worth living are common and may not involve any active wish to end life, although fleeting suicidal ideas can occur even when acting on them is not contemplated. Some may even find comfort in thinking of suicide as an option. Sometimes, rather than suicidal thoughts, mental images of one's own death, or that of others, are experienced in an intrusive and distressing way. Underlying suicidal thoughts may be a desire to escape intolerable feelings, pain or situations; a method of punishing others; a belief that others would be better off without them; an atonement for perceived sins or wrongdoing; an apparently logical solution to a life that has nothing left in it worth living for; or the desire to join loved ones who have died. Depression is one of the most common associations with completed suicide, and the more persistent and planned the suicidal intent, the higher the risk; these include 'final acts' such as putting affairs in order, writing a suicide note and taking precautions against being found. However, suicidal impulses often occur unpredictably and can appear to be without warning. Evidence of risk to others needs to be taken seriously, although murder in the context of suicide – such as infanticide by a mother who then kills herself – is rare. There is no evidence that asking about suicidal ideation increases the risk of suicide; on the contrary, being given the opportunity to talk about it may bring relief, particularly if they have not felt able to discuss it with others. However, suicidal intent may be concealed, and a final decision to act on plans may be accompanied by apparent calm or an improvement in mood.

Self harm with suicidal intent needs to be distinguished from non-suicidal self injury (NSSI, sometimes called deliberate self harm), defined as 'self-directed, deliberate destruction or alteration of bodily tissue in the absence of suicidal intent', commonly manifest through cutting, head banging, scratching, picking at wounds or burning. It is not uncommon for both to co-exist in an individual – predisposing factors have been found to be similar for both – and the distinction can sometimes be unclear. NSSI is typically more common in those who are younger and female and, as well as occurring in mood disorders, is particularly associated with a diagnosis of borderline personality disorder. The motives for NSSI include self-punishment, release of psychic tension, distraction from emotional turmoil and the communication of internal distress to others. Self harm with suicidal intent frequently follows NSSI, with its risk being greater the higher the frequency and severity of NSSI.[12]

Repetitive, Intrusive and Distressing Thoughts

Worry and Rumination

Worry and rumination appear to share similar psychological processes and often occur together, differing in time orientation and some aspects of content. Worry is perseveration on future experiences and associated with apprehension about future consequences, whereas rumination is typically more related to brooding on past experiences and the meaning and causes of negative emotions and thoughts, often involving self-criticism, self-blame and thoughts of worthlessness. Both can be attempts to problem solve, cope or understand the situation but instead they reinforce repetitive thought patterns that further entrench negative thoughts, feelings and behaviours.

Hypochondriasis (Illness Anxiety)

Hypochondriasis refers to a persistent, distressing and disproportionate preoccupation, or fear about the possibility, that one has a serious illness. This may relate to excessive focus on physical symptoms or involve checking for signs of illness, often accompanied by a lack of awareness or insight that the concerns are unreasonable. Hypochondriasis is now seen as a derogatory term, and many prefer health, or illness, anxiety. People with depression experience multiple physical symptoms (see 'Anxiety' earlier and 'Somatic Symptoms' later), and awareness of these may become heightened and preoccupying in the context of low, anxious and pessimistic mood. In severe depression, this can become a conviction of having a fatal disease or lead to beliefs of delusional intensity that the body is unhealthy or rotting, sometimes with a fantastic or nihilistic quality such as having no bowels that or other body parts are rotting, absent or don't exist (i.e. Cotard delusion/syndrome, named after the neurologist who described it).

Obsessive-Compulsive Phenomena

Obsessions are thoughts, images or urges that are recognised as one's own but are intrusive or unwanted, cause distress and anxiety, and lead to attempts to ignore, resist or neutralise them. They are often, but not always, experienced as being without foundation. They may be part of a pre-existing obsessive-compulsive disorder but can arise as part of a depressive episode, in which depression-related content pervades with themes of contamination, harm to self or others, aggression or obscenity. Compulsions are repetitive and time consuming behaviours that may arise as a means of coping with, or neutralising, obsessions – for example, repeated checking, handwashing or cleaning, hiding dangerous implements, or avoiding places that could trigger these obsessions. They may also be a ritualistic way of warding off anxiety or something bad happening even if the activity is perceived as pointless. Usually, the obsessional nature of the thoughts or urges protects against acting on them (e.g. violently harming someone), but change to a more delusional quality can increase the risk.

Impaired Cognitive Function

An inability to concentrate and stay focused on tasks (e.g. reading, watching television, talking with others) is common and may be described as a 'fog' or 'cloud', impairing the capacity to process and retain information. This affects daily tasks, work requirements and engaging in interpersonal relationships, with impairment ranging from maintaining performance with effort through to failing to be able to carry out even simple tasks. Objective testing confirms impairments not only of attention and concentration but also memory, planning, problem solving and cognitive flexibility. There are also more subtle effects, such as tending to preferentially remember more negatively biased memories or having difficulty in recalling the specific details of memories (overgeneral memory). Memory and cognitive difficulties can be a focus of concern and even raise the question of dementia. Apparent dementia that resolves with improvement in depression has been called pseudodementia, a term now out of favour given the complex relationship between depression (particularly of late onset) and dementia, as well as the recognition that some aspects of cognitive impairment can persist even after depression has remitted.

Impaired cognitive function may lead to difficulty weighing up alternatives and making choices and may present as indecision. However, indecision is also strongly influenced by emotional factors such as low self-esteem, lack of self-belief, obsessional thinking and fear of making the wrong decision.

Delusions

Delusions, false beliefs not amenable to change on the basis of evidence and not culturally explicable, often relate to emotional and cognitive content (mood congruency), with some examples given earlier. In practice, the boundaries between intrusive themes, overvalued ideas (where there may be some doubt entertained) and delusions can be difficult to draw; in addition, the content may not be admitted due to embarrassment, suspiciousness or persecutory beliefs. Mood congruence is also not always clear (e.g. in some delusions of persecution) and may only apply to a proportion of the psychotic phenomena. Non-mood-congruent or bizarre delusions can raise the possibility of bipolar or schizoaffective disorder (see section on 'Boundary Disorders'). Delusions have been viewed as a feature indicating severe depression but recently this has been questioned, and psychotic phenomena may be an independent aspect (see section on 'Psychotic Depression'). Sometimes, there is a 'delusional mood' in which an unshakeable belief that something terrible, but not identified, is occurring and from which specific delusions may develop. The following broad types of mood-congruent delusions have been described:

- Delusions of guilt
- Delusions of poverty
- Hypochondriacal delusions
- Delusions of catastrophe
- Nihilistic (Cotard) delusions

Persecutory delusions (e.g. being under surveillance or poisoned) and delusions of reference (e.g. believing they are being referred to by newsreaders on the media) may relate to feelings of guilt and worthlessness, but they sometimes can be seen as unjust or unwarranted.

Physical Symptoms

Reductions in sleep and appetite/weight in depression are sometimes called 'neurovegetative symptoms'. However, caution is needed as, in some circumstances, the term is used more broadly to include anhedonia, loss of libido, diurnal variation, motor retardation and even fatigue. Hypersomnia and increased appetite are on occasion referred to as 'reversed neurovegetative symptoms'.

Fatigue and Lack of Energy

Fatigue, encompassing tiredness and lack of energy, is one of the most common symptoms in depression (Table 3.1.1) and was included in ICD-10 as one of the three most typical features. It has a considerable impact on daily functioning, appears to improve more slowly than affective symptoms, and is a common residual symptom. Descriptions include feeling drained, physically weak, sluggish, lethargic and 'heavy'. Activities that seemed small or easily managed previously may now feel like huge undertakings and necessitate great effort (e.g. taking a shower, getting dressed, cooking, walking or talking with others). 'Leaden paralysis' describes a physical feeling of heavy limbs that can only be moved with great effort (see section on 'Atypical Depression'). Care may be needed to distinguish fatigue from overlapping symptoms such as anhedonia, difficulty with concentration and mental effort, and motivational deficits. Fatigue is a common feature of other medical and psychiatric disorders – and associated with some medications – so differential diagnoses need to be carefully considered, especially when fatigue is predominant, and care needs to be taken when ascribing causality.

Appetite and Weight

Changes in appetite, and consequently in weight, are not uncommon. Some may describe having no interest in food and feeling unable to derive any pleasure or taste from it; others may find they have so little energy or motivation that eating is no longer a priority. In more severe cases, there may be no desire for food at all, and people may miss meals or need to force themselves to eat, with failure to eat (and drink) an indication for urgent intervention. In contrast, some people find they turn increasingly to food as a way to bring relief or pleasure, with food offering some temporary form of contentment or self-soothing or a means of distraction/disconnection from difficult emotions or thoughts; in this situation, weight gain may occur. A change of at least 5 per cent in body weight in a month is often taken as an indication of significant weight change.

Sleep

Sleep disturbance is common and traditionally divided into initial insomnia (difficulty getting to sleep), middle insomnia (waking in the night and finding it difficult to get back to sleep) and late insomnia (early morning awakening and not getting back to sleep again). Anxiety, racing thoughts and not being able to 'switch off' are common in initial insomnia, whereas early morning awakening is viewed as a feature of typical depression, associated with diurnal mood variation and other melancholic features (see section on 'Melancholic Depression'). Nightmares are particularly common in those with terminal insomnia and in those with melancholia.[13] Insomnia occurs in spite of feelings of exhaustion, and at night, increased rumination and feelings of isolation and aloneness are often prominent. In contrast, others – most commonly, younger adults – may report increased sleep, sleepiness, naps during the day and difficulty waking up. Sleep may be seen as a way of finding respite or escape from low mood or negative thoughts. A change in time asleep of at least two hours is often taken as an indication of a significant change, although for some people the experience is of sleep being of poor quality, broken or unrefreshing, rather than a change in duration. There are objective abnormalities in sleep electroencephalographic measures associated with insomnia in depression. As well as the expected changes in sleep amount and continuity, sleep structure is altered with decreased rapid eye movement (REM) latency, increased REM sleep and REM density, and decreased slow-wave sleep. In contrast, those with hypersomnia have been found to have a normal sleep structure.[14] Sleep difficulties impact cognition and daily functioning, impair the ability to regulate emotions and are associated with an increased risk of suicidal behaviour.

Somatic Symptoms

Pain, such as headaches, muscular, joint, stomach and back pain, is a common feature of depression, is more likely with greater depression severity, and may be the reason for seeking help or become a focus for illness anxiety. Also common are gastrointestinal symptoms such heartburn, diarrhoea and constipation and physical symptoms related to anxiety (discussed earlier). Given that depression is also associated with medical illness (see section on 'Medical Comorbidity') and medication can cause physical adverse effects, the direction of causation for somatic symptoms may be difficult to determine or be bidirectional.

Loss of Libido

Sexual function is affected by many aspects of depression, with loss of interest in sex often related to a general loss of motivation and interest in things, as well as changes in intimate relationships. There may also be an inability to become physical sexually aroused, including difficulties reaching orgasm or erectile dysfunction. Loss of libido has been seen as a loss of a basic drive, akin to loss of appetite, and sometimes included under neurovegetative symptoms. It was listed as one of the somatic (melancholic) symptoms in ICD-10 but no longer features in ICD-11 or DSM-5. Sexual dysfunction can also be a direct consequence of some antidepressant drugs, especially selective serotonin re-uptake inhibitors, which can complicate assessment.

Perceptual Symptoms

Hallucinations

Hallucinations (perceptions that appear real in the absence of a stimulus) are less common than delusions. When they occur, they are usually auditory and in the second person, consistent with depressive themes such as worthlessness, guilt, punishment or death. They can be indistinct or often simple phrases such as 'you deserve to die' and may be attributed to God or the Devil. It can be unclear whether or not they come from external space, and they may be experienced inside the head. Simple auditory hallucinations (noises) or those in other modalities, such as olfactory hallucinations of putrefaction, are relatively rare. It may be difficult to distinguish visual hallucinations from illusions, such as distortion of faces or visions of death. Command hallucinations can occur, including telling the person to kill themselves, and if the person feels compelled to act on them as though controlled by an external power (passivity phenomenon), the situation is extremely dangerous.

Non-mood-congruent hallucinations, including third person, running commentary, bizarre hallucinations or experiences such as thought insertion, may occur but, as with non-mood-congruent delusions, raise the possibility of schizoaffective disorder or schizophrenia, particularly if they are prominent.

Depersonalisation/Derealisation

Depersonalisation/derealisation (DPDR) describes an altered experience of oneself (depersonalisation) or of the external world (derealisation) in a way that is unpleasant and anxiety provoking. DPDR occurs on a continuum, from transient occurrences in healthy individuals to being a debilitating independent disorder highly comorbid with neurological and psychiatric conditions, including mood and anxiety disorders.[15] Information on DPDR in depressive disorders is limited, and it may be under-recognised, especially in those severely ill. The description of being cut off from feelings overlaps with the black numbness of severe depressed mood. It can appear similar to anhedonia but, rather than a loss of interest or pleasure, the experience is of being detached, feeling 'cut off' or 'like a robot', lacking emotions, not feeling affection for loved ones, or everything seeming unreal, distant, flat, lifeless, colourless or confusing. It may also need to be distinguished from nihilistic delusions, in which there is a fixed belief rather than an experience. DPDR has been proposed as a shutdown response to emotional overload.

Behavioural Features

Appearance

Appearances can be deceptive in a consultation, especially in less severe depression when a good 'social front' can be put on. There can be an apparent mismatch between expressed and observed mood. Some patients can present with 'smiling' depression, and it is only when they are caught off guard or don't know that they are being observed that lowered mood is apparent.

Depressed affect can be observed in facial expression with a lack of expression or a miserable appearance and downturned mouth and furrowed brow (depressive facies). Sometimes, worry or fear may be apparent. Eye contact may be poor with a downward gaze, and there may be hopeless gestures such as sitting with head in hands and slumped shoulders. There may be tearfulness or crying, and often an empathic response is elicited in others of the despair and hopelessness that is being experienced. At other times, there may be hostility or reluctance. Talk may be soft, slow and sparse, with alteration in motor movements (see later). In severe depression there can be grey, dry or waxy look to the skin, perhaps contributed to by self-neglect and poor nutrition/hygiene.

Lack of Motivation and Apathy

Lack of motivation overlaps with fatigue, lack of energy and anhedonia, but it refers to a lack of will, volition or initiative to engage in tasks, rather than the physical effort involved or lack of enjoyment. It is included here because of its behavioural consequence of impairment in goal-directed behaviour with, at the extreme, apathy and failing to carry out basic daily activities such as a self care. This may be linked with feelings of hopelessness, pessimism and self-criticism over failure to find the will to do things that should be done. It has long been believed clinically that the risk of suicide may be elevated in the early stages of recovering from depression, due to an early increase in motivation and energy that allow suicidal impulses to be acted upon; however, empirical evidence tends not to support this period being associated with more risk than at other times. This does not detract from the need to be vigilant for suicidal risk, which can occur throughout the course of a depressive episode.

Altered Psychomotor Function

Retardation

Feeling slowed up (and also that time is moving slowly) is not uncommon in depression, but psychomotor retardation requires the slowing to be observable by others in speech, facial expression, movements and posture. Speech may be slow, quiet, low in pitch, hesitant, with pauses, delay before answering questions, and monosyllabic or impoverished content. There may be a lack of facial expression, fixed gaze and poor eye contact with slumped posture and little spontaneous movement, although increased self-touching of the face may occur. Psychomotor retardation is associated with both greater depression severity and, by definition, with melancholic depression, but the nature of the relationship remains unclear; as mentioned earlier, Parker[5] has argued for this feature being the defining characteristic of melancholia rather than just one symptom of it.

Agitation

Agitation is increased motor activity including pacing, handwringing, inability to sit still, fidgeting with objects or picking or pulling at hair, skin or clothing, which may be accompanied by verbal outbursts, irritability or inability to stop talking while not able to focus on any specific topic. In contrast to the situation in mania, these are an expression of intolerable inner tension, anxiety and worry in which the person doesn't know what to do to relieve their distress, rather than being goal directed or due to elation or excess energy. The distinction between agitation in unipolar depression and mixed states as a presentation of bipolar disorder may be difficult (see also sections on 'Agitated Depression' and 'Bipolar Disorders'). Apparently, paradoxically, psychomotor retardation and agitation are not mutually exclusive, and intense inner tension can be experienced by someone barely moving whereas someone who cannot sit still may only move slowly; depressive episodes with both psychomotor agitation and retardation may be more likely in bipolar disorder.[16]

Agitation also needs to be distinguished from akathisia as an extrapyramidal adverse effect of medication, in which motor restlessness in the absence of severe anxiety is usual, and from catatonic excitement or stereotopies (see next section).

Catatonic Features

Catatonia refers to a cluster of abnormal motor features including an absence of response, negativity, overactivity and unusual muscle tone and behaviours. How these are conceptualised in the context of depression is discussed in the section 'Psychotic Depression and Catatonia'. Periods of inactivity may be interspersed with excitement, and it is difficult to access thought content. The boundary between severe psychomotor retardation and catatonic stupor can be unclear, the latter consisting of immobility while apparently awake and conscious as well as lack of response to even painful stimuli. Abnormal muscle tone and control can be evident with catalepsy (rigidity with limbs remaining where moved to), waxy flexibility (slight but even resistance to movement) and posturing (adoption of unnatural positions). There may be mannerisms (caricatured goal-directed movements), stereotopies (repetitive movements that are not goal directed), echopraxia (mirroring another's movements), grimacing or excitement/agitation without obvious cause. Negativism may range from non-response to requests or physical guidance or to opposition or resistance. Speech abnormalities include mutism, echolalia (repeating another's speech), perseveration or verbigeration (repetition of random words or phrases without a prompt). A case series found that immobility and mutism were the most common features, closely followed by staring, withdrawal and refusal to eat, with echolalia/echopraxia and verbigeration least common.[17]

Dissociative and Histrionic Behaviour

Descriptions of melancholia and severe depressive states from the early twentieth century included dramatically altered behaviour including 'hysterical' convulsions, fainting fits, attention seeking, extreme dependency, melodramatic or exaggerated complaints, inappropriate intimacy or provocative acts. Today, these features are little mentioned in the context of depressive disorders, with possible explanations including decreased frequency due to a move from institutional inpatient care, societal changes in the expression and understanding of distress, less recognition or re-conceptualisation as part of comorbid personality disorders. Depression can exaggerate pre-existing personality traits and trigger uncharacteristic behaviour that disappears on recovery, so it is important not to assume that disturbances in behaviour are due to pre-existing personality or behavioural disorders rather than the depressive disorder. This is particularly the case when depression fails to improve or is persistent.

General Functioning

An impact on function and behaviour is an intrinsic feature of depression although, at milder severity, this may be hidden from, or not obvious to, others. Withdrawal from social life, impaired efficiency at work, and struggles with maintaining care for self and others, a daily routine and financial commitments may all become apparent and cause conflict. Irritability and emotional distance may cause strain and discord in close relationships, with at times cause and effect difficult to disentangle in the relationship problems. As described in the previous section, there can be changed behaviour, which can include shoplifting, taking sexual risks and causing violence, which may be combined with alcohol and drug misuse.

Types of Depressive Disorders and Their Classification

The classification of depressive disorders in the two major systems, ICD-11 (with implementation from 2022)[18] and DSM-5 (implemented in 2013, with text revision [DSM-5-TR] in 2022),[19] are very similar. The previous classification, ICD-10,[20] will continue to be used in a transitional period varying by country. We focus on ICD-11 (at the time of writing, the detailed clinical descriptions and diagnostic guidelines had not been published) and describe differences from ICD-10. For simplicity DSM-5 is used in the text where DSM-5 and DSM-5-TR are identical.

Depressive disorders are defined in relation to a core depressive syndrome, called a major depressive episode in DSM-5. We will use the term (major) depressive episode when not specifying the classification system. 'Clinical depression' is a term best avoided, as it can be taken to imply that milder degrees of depression are not important and suggests a particular threshold for professional treatment. Depressive disorders are predominantly distinguished by duration, severity and longitudinal course (Tables 3.1.2 and 3.1.3); whether or not different symptom profiles denote discrete subtypes of depression is contentious, and they are identified by the use of added descriptions, specifiers or qualifiers (Table 3.1.4).

The symptoms in depressive disorders should not be better accounted for by another psychiatric diagnosis such as bipolar disorder or schizophrenia. When a depressive syndrome is present but accounted for by the physiological effects of a physical illness or drugs, it is not identified as a primary depressive disorder but considered secondary or induced (Table 3.1.2). However, in the context of physical illness or substance use, careful clinical assessment and judgement are

Table 3.1.2 An outline of the classification of depressive disorders in ICD-10/11 and DSM-5-TR

ICD-10	ICD-11	DSM-5-TR
F32 Depressive episode	6A70 Single episode depressive disorder	F32 Major depressive disorder single episode
F33 Recurrent depressive disorder	6A71 Recurrent depressive disorder	F33 Major depressive disorder recurrent episode
F34.1 Persistent mood [affective] disorders: dysthymia	6A72 Dysthymic disorder	F34.1 Persistent depressive disorder (dysthymia)
F41.2 Mixed anxiety and depressive disorder	6A73 Mixed depressive and anxiety disorder	-
F38 Other mood [affective] disorders	6A7Y Other specified depressive disorders	F32.89 Other specified depressive disorder
F39 Unspecified mood [affective] disorder	6AYZ Depressive disorders, unspecified	F32.A Unspecified depressive disorder F39 Unspecified mood disorder
-	-	*F.34.81 Disruptive mood dysregulation disorder (note: under age 18 years)*
-	*GA34.41 Premenstrual dysphoric disorder*	*F32.81 Premenstrual dysphoric disorder*
‡	*6C4x Substance-induced mood disorders*	*_._ Substance/medication-induced depressive disorder*
F06.32 Organic depressive disorder	*6E62.0 Secondary mood syndrome, with depressive symptoms*	*_._ Depressive disorder due to another medical condition*

- not included; ‡ not specifically identified, coded under substance involved or as organic mental disorder depending on picture; x number used to identify substance; _._ coding based on substance/condition
Disorders in *italics* have primary classification elsewhere or are not consistently agreed primary (adult) depressive disorders.

Table 3.1.3 Summary of requirements for a (major) depressive episode

ICD-11 Depressive 'Episode'[a]	DSM-5-TR Major Depressive Episode (A-C required)
At least five of the following, almost daily for at least 2 weeks: 1. Depressed mood* 2. Diminished interest in activities* 3. Difficulty concentrating 4. Feelings of worthlessness or excessive or inappropriate guilt 5. Hopelessness 6. Recurrent thoughts of death or suicide 7. Changes in appetite 8. Changes in sleep 9. Psychomotor agitation or retardation 10. Reduced energy or fatigue * At least one should be present	**A** Five or more of the following during the same 2-week period, most of the day, nearly every day, representing a change from normal: 1 Depressed mood (subjective or observed)* 2 Markedly diminished interest or pleasure (subjective or observed)* 3 Significant decreased or increased weight (e.g. ≥5% in a month) or appetite 4 Insomnia or hypersomnia 5 Psychomotor agitation or retardation (observed only) 6 Fatigue or loss of energy 7 Feelings of worthlessness or inappropriate guilt 8 Diminished ability to think or concentrate, or indecisiveness 9 Recurrent thoughts of death, suicidal ideation or suicide attempt * At least one must be present
The symptoms significantly affect an individual's ability to function	**B** The symptoms cause clinically significant distress or impaired functioning
	C Not attributable to physiological effects of a drug or a medical condition

[a] Not independently defined and only included in description of individual disorders

often required to decide the best way to account for the clinical picture (see section on 'Comorbid Disorders').

ICD-10 and ICD-11 use 'diagnostic guidelines' to retain the flexibility to apply clinical judgement whereas DSM-5 applies stricter diagnostic criteria and more exclusions in an attempt to maximise reliability.

Definition of a (Major) Depressive Episode

ICD-11 describes depressive episodes as part of individual disorders, whereas ICD-10 defined a depressive episode separately; we retain this in Table 3.1.3 for clarity. The term 'major' depressive episode in DSM was used to distinguish it from a 'minor' depressive episode, now called a depressive episode with insufficient symptoms in DSM-5 (see 'Other Specified Depressive Disorders').

A (major) depressive episode is polythetic with no single symptom needed for the diagnosis, although low mood or diminished interest in activities must be present – sometimes called 'core symptoms'. Table 3.1.1 shows that low mood is not always present, the recognition of which led to anhedonia being incorporated into DSM-III and subsequently into ICD-10. The diagnostic definitions/criteria are aimed at discriminating depressive from other disorders and therefore only partially capture the clinical picture,[3] with non-criteria symptoms such as anxiety and somatic complaints equally prominent. Both systems emphasise the need for the depressive symptoms to be present for the majority of the time, but ICD-10 was more specific in stating that the lowered mood varies little from day to day, is often unresponsive to circumstances, and may show diurnal variation.

Table 3.1.4 The principal severity and course descriptors for (major) depressive disorders in ICD-11 and DSM-5-TR

ICD-11		DSM-5-TR	
Single episode depressive disorder	**Recurrent depressive disorder** (at least two episodes separated by several months without significant mood disturbance)	**Major depressive disorder single episode**	**Major depressive disorder recurrent episode** (at least two months between separate episodes when major depressive episode criteria not met)
Meets definition of a depressive episode. Bipolar disorder diagnosed if previous history of a manic, mixed or hypomanic episode.		Meets criteria A–C of depressive episode. D: Not better explained by schizophrenia, schizoaffective or other psychotic disorder. E: There has never been a hypomanic or manic episode (does not apply if attributable to a substance or medical condition).	
6A70.0 Mild	**6A71.0 Current episode mild**	**F32.0 Mild**	**F33.0 Mild**
None of the symptoms are present to an intense degree. Some, but not considerable, difficulty with ordinary activities. No delusions or hallucinations.		Few, if any, symptoms in excess of the minimum, which cause distress of manageable intensity and minor impairment of functioning.	
Moderate: **6A70.1 without psychotic symptoms** **6A70.2 with psychotic symptoms**	**Current episode moderate:** **6A71.1 without psychotic symptoms** **6A71.2 with psychotic symptoms**	**F32.1 Moderate**	**F33.1 Moderate**
Several symptoms to a marked degree, or a large number of lesser severity, are present. Considerable difficulty in continuing with usual activities but still able to function in some areas. With or without delusions or hallucinations.		The number and intensity of symptoms, and functional impairment are between mild and severe.	
Severe: **6A70.3 without psychotic symptoms** **6A70.4 with psychotic symptoms**	**Current episode severe:** **6A71.3 without psychotic symptoms** **6A71.4 with psychotic symptoms**	**F32.2 Severe**	**F33.2 Severe**
Many or most symptoms are present to a marked degree, or a smaller number of symptoms to an intense degree. Inability to function except to a very limited degree. With or without delusions or hallucinations.		Substantially more symptoms than the minimum, which cause severe and unmanageable distress and markedly interfere with functioning.	
60A70.5 Unspecified severity	**60A71.5 Current episode unspecified severity**	**F32.34 With psychotic features**	**F33.34 With psychotic features**
Insufficient information to determine severity. At least some difficulty with ordinary activities.		Delusions and/or hallucinations present irrespective of severity. Specify if mood congruent or incongruent.	
6A70.6 Currently in partial remission	**6A71.6 Currently in partial remission**	**F32.4 In partial remission**	**F33.4 In partial remission**
Definitional requirements for depressive episode not now met but some significant mood symptoms remain.		Symptoms of preceding major depressive episode present but below threshold, or less than two months without significant depressive symptoms following the episode.	
6A70.6 Currently in full remission	**6A71.6 Currently in full remission**	**F32.5 In full remission**	**F33.5 In full remission**
Definitional requirements for depressive episode met in the past but no longer any significant mood symptoms.		A previous major depressive episode but no significant depressive symptoms in the past 2 months.	
6A70.Y Other specified	**6A71.Y Other specified**		
6A70.Z Unspecified	**6A71.Z Unspecified**	**F32.9 Unspecified**	**F33.9 Unspecified**

The symptom lists in ICD-11 and DSM-5 are almost identical, apart from the former retaining hopelessness about the future (present in ICD-10) as it performs well in differentiating depressive from non-depressed individuals.[21] ICD-10 required two symptoms from low mood, anhedonia or fatigue to be present with a threshold of four symptoms for mild depression, although inter-rater reliability is low at this severity.[20] Other changes from ICD-10 are the inclusion in ICD-11 of psychomotor symptoms and the recognition of increased – as well as decreased – appetite or weight as well as the omission of reduced self-esteem and self-confidence.

In distinguishing between a depressive episode and an understandable or appropriate reaction to significant loss or life event, DSM-5 requires judgement based on the individual's history and cultural norms in expressing distress to loss. ICD-11 differentiates depressive disorders from normal reactions to adverse life events by the severity, range and duration of symptoms.

(Major) Depressive Disorders

ICD-11 and DSM-5 both identify three levels of severity for the current depressive episode, further classified by the absence or presence of psychotic symptoms (Table 3.1.4). The severity categories in both classifications have little empirical basis, and their relationship to rating scales scores, which are often used as a proxy, is imprecise and variable. Both ICD-11 and DSM-5 use symptom number and severity together with functional impairment to determine severity, although with slightly different emphases. ICD-10 had similar functional impairment requirements but was more prescriptive with regard to symptom numbers (at least 4 in mild, 6–7 in moderate, at least 7 in severe), and psychotic symptoms were only linked with severe depression. ICD-11 allows psychotic symptoms to also occur in moderate depression, whereas DSM-5 dissociates them from severity entirely. The UK NICE clinical guidelines on depression[22] divides depression into less severe (subthreshold and mild) and more severe (moderate and severe) in order to guide treatment.

ICD-11 now follows DSM-5 in recognising partial and full remission (defined in Table 3.1.4) in contrast to ICD-10, where only the latter was described. The diagnosis of recurrent (major) depressive disorder is less strict in DSM-5 than in ICD-11 in requiring only two months of partial remission between episodes rather than several months without significant mood symptoms. It should be noted that even a single episode of depression now becomes a lifetime diagnosis in both systems.

Table 3.1.5 Mood episode qualifiers and specifiers in ICD-11 and DSM-5-TR

ICD-11	DSM-5-TR
Episode qualifiers/second condition (coded in addition to main code: e.g. 6A7x.x/6A8x.x)	Episode specifiers
6A80.0 Prominent anxiety symptoms in mood episodes 6A80.1 Panic attacks in mood episodes	With anxious distress
6A80.2 Current depressive episode persistent	Persistent episodes classified under Persistent depressive disorder
6A80.3 Current depressive episode with melancholia	With melancholic features
-	With atypical features
-[a]	With mixed features
-	With mood congruent psychotic features or With mood-incongruent psychotic features
6A40 Catatonia associated with another mental disorder	With catatonia
6E20/6E21 Mental or behavioural disorders associated with pregnancy, childbirth or the puerperium	With peripartum onset
6A80.4 Seasonal pattern of mood episode onset	With seasonal pattern

- no qualifier in ICD-11

[a]The term mixed is reserved for the co-existence of prominent manic and depressive symptoms during bipolar type I disorder (6A60)

Symptom Profiles in the Clinical Presentation of (Major) Depression

DSM-5 uses specifiers to describe different symptom profiles, and ICD-11 introduces qualifiers for the first time (Table 3.1.5), with both also applicable to other depressive disorders and to bipolar and related disorders. The presence of subsyndromal hypomanic symptoms (e.g. increased energy or elevated mood) in individuals with (major) depressive disorder raises a debate about the boundary between depression and bipolar II disorder, and DSM-5 has introduced a mixed features specifier (discussed in the section 'Bipolar Disorders').

Psychotic Depression and Catatonia

Historically, psychotic depression has been viewed as being at the highest end of a continuum of severity of (major) depression and associated with melancholia and severe impairment (as exemplified in ICD-10). However, psychotic and non-psychotic depression can be equally severe, and – in an individual presenting with psychotic depression – psychosis and severity often behave independently over subsequent episodes.[23] Therefore, the view that psychosis is an independent trait has gained ground.

Catatonia, since its early description in the nineteenth century, has been linked primarily with psychosis – in particular, schizophrenia. Recently, however, it has become apparent that it is more commonly associated with affective disorders, as well as being a feature of organic disorders, substance misuse and autism. Stupor was included under psychotic symptoms in ICD-10 but not in ICD-11 and DSM-5, which describe catatonia separately (see Table 3.1.5). Different presentations of catatonia have been described, including a more common retarded type (including immobility and stupor) and excited type (with severe psychomotor overactivity – see also the section on 'Agitated Depression'). It can be differentiated from psychosis in its response to benzodiazepines but not to antipsychotics. There remains uncertainty about the nosological status of catatonia as it is only seen in association with other conditions;[5] in ICD-11, it is a separate diagnostic category; ICD-10 diagnosed it under schizophrenia, whereas in DSM-5, it is a specifier. Catatonia is associated with severe mood episodes and psychosis, although delusions and hallucinations can be difficult to assess. ICD-11 requires the simultaneous occurrence of several symptoms such as stupor, catalepsy, waxy flexibility, mutism, negativism, posturing, mannerisms, stereotypies, psychomotor agitation, grimacing, echolalia and echopraxia. In DSM-5, at least three of these 12 symptoms are required.

The prevalence of psychotic symptoms has been estimated to occur in 10–19% of adults with (major) depression, rising to 25–45% of those hospitalised. Compared with non-psychotic depression, it is associated with an earlier age of onset, greater severity and chronicity, more and longer hospital admissions, greater psychiatric comorbidity and a poorer prognosis. It is also more likely to have a bipolar outcome than non-psychotic depression (especially in early onset illness), a risk that appears greater if the psychosis is mood incongruent.[23] Knowledge about the prevalence of catatonia in depression is hampered by varying definitions, study settings and diagnoses; a recent meta-analysis reported a prevalence of about 8% in psychiatric inpatients and 3% in outpatients, less common in unipolar depressive disorder than bipolar disorder.[24]

Anxious Depression, Mixed Depressive and Anxiety Disorder

Separating anxiety and depression has been compared to trying to disentangle wind and rain in stormy weather,[25] and their high rate of co-occurrence is a problem in their classification as separate disorders, with a mixture of anxiety and depression by far the most common presentation in primary care.[25] It was only in DSM-III and ICD-10 that they were completely separated; since then, it has become increasingly recognised that higher levels of anxiety in (major) depressive episodes are associated with poorer functioning and quality of life, higher suicide risk, more depressive episodes, a worse longitudinal course and poorer treatment response. This has led to DSM-5 and ICD-11 adding anxiety as a specifier/qualifier, but as this is the most common presentation of depression (and anxiety disorders do not have a depression specifier), the conceptual problem of their relationship is not resolved.[25]

The ICD-11 anxiety qualifier for depressive disorders requires prominent and clinically significant anxiety symptoms (e.g. feeling nervous, anxious or on edge; not being able to control worrying thoughts; fearing that something awful will happen; having trouble relaxing; having motor tension; having autonomic symptoms) to be present for most of the time during the episode and, for separate diagnoses, if diagnostic requirements are also met for an anxiety or fear-related disorder. ICD-11 also has a separate panic attack qualifier (at least two panic attacks in the last month related to anxiety-provoking depressive cognitions). The future primary care version of ICD-11 (ICD-11 PHC) may include a new category of anxious depression in which case-level requirements (i.e. scoring above a threshold on rating scales) are met for a depressive and an anxiety disorder but using the same two-week duration requirement for both.

The DSM-5 anxious distress specifier requires the presence, during the majority of days in an episode, of a least two of: (1) feeling keyed up or tense, (2) feeling unusually restless, (3) difficulty concentrating because of worry, (4) fear that something awful might happen or (5) feeling that the individual might lose control of themself. In addition, severity is specified by the number of symptoms present: mild (2 symptoms), moderate (3 symptoms), moderate-severe (4–5 symptoms) or severe (5 symptoms with motor agitation). If anxiety symptoms meet the criteria for a specific anxiety disorder, then that is given as a comorbid diagnosis. DSM-5 appears at first sight to differ from ICD-11 in not having a panic attack specifier, for depressive disorders, but in fact it is described in the section on anxiety disorders.

A separate mixed depressive and anxiety disorder is recognised in ICD-11, when the two occur together but requirements for neither a full anxiety nor a depressive disorder diagnosis are met (it was called mixed anxiety and depressive disorder in ICD-10, classified with anxiety disorders). DSM-5 found the diagnosis insufficiently reliable to include.

Psychological distress not meeting specific criteria for an anxiety or depression diagnosis accounted for nearly half of the psychological problems found in England in 2014, over twice that of depression,[26] but the prevalence of mixed anxiety and depressive disorder is highly variable in epidemiological studies, ranging from less than 1% to 10%,[27] presumably related to poor reliability. About three quarters of patients with DSM-5 major depressive disorder in both psychiatric and community samples also have anxious distress,[28] consistent with the symptom profile in Table 3.1.1.

Melancholic Depression

There is agreement that there are depressed patients with a cluster of symptoms now designated melancholic, but evidence that this reflects a distinct subgroup remains elusive, and it has only a modest tendency to repeat across different episodes; an alternative view has been that it is a manifestation of more severe illness and older age. There is large overlap between melancholic and depression historically described as 'endogenous/endomorphogenic', 'biological', 'vital' or 'neurovegetative'. Endogenous/endomorphogenic (originating from within) and biological refer to presumed aetiology whereas the concept of vital depression, arising in Continental Europe, stems from a theoretical contrast between vital (somatic) and sensuous (stimulus-related) feelings and, like neurovegetative, focuses on early morning waking, loss of appetite and weight, physical fatigue and diurnal variation.

The ICD-11 melancholic qualifier requires several of the following symptoms during the worst period of the current episode: pervasive anhedonia, lack of emotional reactivity to normally pleasurable stimuli, waking at least two hours before the usual time, depressive symptoms worse in the morning, marked psychomotor retardation or agitation, or marked loss of appetite or loss of weight. In ICD-10, the somatic syndrome was the equivalent of melancholia and required 'usually' at least symptoms (from the above list plus marked loss of libido).

DSM-5 criteria are broadly similar, requiring a minimum of four of eight features occurring together at the most severe stage of the episode:

A. At least one from (1) near complete loss of pleasure in (almost) all activities or (2) lack of reactivity to usually pleasurable stimuli
B. At least three from (1) distinct quality of depressed mood (qualitatively different to sadness, 'emptiness', profound despair), (2) depression worse in the morning, (3) early

morning awakening (at least 2 hours earlier than usual), (4) marked psychomotor agitation or retardation observable by others (noted as almost always present), (5) significant anorexia or weight loss or (6) excessive or inappropriate guilt.

In two large naturalistic studies including primary care and psychiatric outpatients with major depressive disorder, 16–24% were reported to have melancholic features according to DSM criteria. Compared with non-melancholic patients, those with melancholia had more severe depression and poorer response to antidepressant treatment.[29,30]

Atypical Depression

The term atypical depression was first used in the middle of the last century based on a distinction from typical (i.e. endogenous or melancholic) depression, but confusingly it has had at least eight different definitions,[31] many with overlapping features including anxiety, reversed neurovegetative features, mood reactivity to circumstances and prominent fatigue; some early definitions also emphasised preferential response to monoamine oxidase inhibitors over tricyclic antidepressants. There remains uncertainty about its value and definition as discrete presentation within the non-melancholic group, particularly with regard to the roles of mood reactivity and anxiety.

ICD-11 does not have an atypical features qualifier while the use of atypical in ICD-10 referred to presentations that do not fit the usual description, noted to be particularly common in adolescence. The atypical features specifier in DSM-5 first appeared in DSM-IV and has not been changed in spite of uncertainty about the usefulness of the mood reactivity criterion, and it does not include anxiety symptoms. The criteria are that for the majority of the days of the episode:

A. There is mood reactivity (mood brightening in response to actual or potential positive events, even including euthymia for extended periods of time in favourable circumstances)
B. There are at least two of (1) significant weight gain or increase in appetite, (2) hypersomnia (at least 10 hours/2 hours more than usual a day which may include daytime naps), (3) leaden paralysis (heavy lead-like feeling in arms or legs) or (4) a long-standing pattern of interpersonal rejection sensitivity not limited to mood disorders causing functional impairment
C. Criteria for melancholic features or catatonia are not met in the same episode

The atypical specifier uniquely includes a criterion related to personality – that of long-standing interpersonal rejection sensitivity – and is clearly demarcated as a non-melancholic presentation of depression. However, it also illustrates considerable overlap with personality disorders (e.g. avoidant personality disorder) and has a high comorbidity with anxiety disorders, binge eating disorders and bulimia nervosa, ICD-10 neurasthenia (fatigue and weakness, muscular aches and pains, autonomic and depressive symptoms) and seasonal affective disorder (see later), and is commonly found in bipolar disorder.[31]

Major depressive disorder with atypical features has been found to be only modestly stable over time, and patients can fluctuate between melancholic and atypical episodes more frequently than reliably repeating either type. Nevertheless, atypical features are consistently associated with younger age of onset and a greater female preponderance that non-atypical depression; anxiety is common and a family history of depression more frequent. Atypical features are found in 15–29% of depressed patients[31] and, in a naturalistic study, were associated with milder severity, fewer depressive episodes and higher rates of remission than melancholic patients.[30] However, other studies have reported that depression with atypical features is associated with a more chronic course than melancholic depression.

Agitated Depression

Agitated depression is not a recognised diagnosis but is a term commonly used clinically, and it has been associated with more severe illness, poorer prognosis and suicide risk.[32] Before the delineation of bipolar and unipolar disorders, it was recognised that presentations featuring both excitement and inhibition ('excited depression') could occur, as described by Kraepelin and others in the nineteenth century, derived from the concept of melancholia agitata. Agitated depression was included in RDC criteria and in DSM-III, but it disappeared in subsequent versions of the DSM. In ICD-10, it was included in severe depressive episodes, but it does not appear in ICD-11. DSM-5-TR gives acute agitation as an example of the reintroduced diagnosis of 'Unspecified mood disorder' in which a mood disorder is suspected but criteria for a specific bipolar or depressive disorder are not met.

One of the problems is that agitated depression is not clearly defined. At the core are physical restlessness and psychic tension; however, it can include emotional lability, talkativeness and crowded or racing thoughts, rumination, impulsive behaviour, suicide attempts and verbal outbursts. There has been debate about the degree to which agitated (or activated) depression is a mixed state on the bipolar disorder spectrum (see also the section on 'Bipolar Disorders') as opposed to a potentially distinct manifestation of unipolar depression. In practice, it is likely that agitation can be a feature of a number of overlapping presentations ranging through psychosis, catatonia, melancholia and severe anxiety to mixed features or mixed states. One potentially useful distinction is whether the agitation is a reflection of inner tension with anxious overactive thoughts and behaviours that are weakly goal directed (e.g. hand wringing, pacing, ruminations) or a reflection of disinhibited, disorganised, goal-oriented behaviour together with racing thoughts or flight of ideas; the former is more suggestive of unipolar (major) depression and the latter of a bipolar disorder. In assessing agitation, it is therefore important to examine its nature and the range of accompanying symptoms to guide diagnosis and treatment options.

(Major) Depressive Episodes Defined by Timing of Onset

Seasonal Affective Disorder

Seasonal affective disorder (SAD) (predominantly onset in autumn/winter and recovery in spring/summer, less commonly associated with the summer period) was first described in the 1980s and characterised by low mood associated with hypersomnia, increased appetite and overeating (with carbohydrate craving) and extreme loss of energy. SAD of the winter type, which has a strong female preponderance and higher prevalence in younger people,[33] has become widely accepted, with an apparently plausible link to chronobiology and congruent with beliefs about 'winter blues', hibernation, and the mood-elevating effects of sunlight (and bright light therapy). It has however been difficult to identify a clear aetiology, and epidemiological studies do not substantiate a general effect of season or latitude on the overall prevalence of depression. SAD has symptomatic overlap with atypical features, but a seasonal pattern has been found in only about 10 per cent of the latter,[31] consistent with the finding that major depression with seasonal pattern has a low prevalence.[33,34] The apparent specificity of bright light treatment for SAD has been challenged by evidence of its efficacy in non-seasonal depression, with the evidential quality poor for both. Beliefs about seasonal depression appear influenced by cultural perceptions and self-selection, and instruments assessing seasonality of depression have methodological problems.[34] There is therefore considerable uncertainty about the status of the seasonal pattern specifier/qualifier for depressive disorders, and some evidence that feeling worse in winter may apply generally across mental disorders, and indeed to non-clinical mood states.

ICD-11 requires a regular seasonal pattern of onset and remission of depressive episodes with a substantial majority corresponding to the seasonal pattern. They should not be related to a psychological stressor (e.g. seasonal unemployment) that regularly occurs at that time of the year. ICD-10 only included SAD as a diagnosis of uncertain status in its research version.

The DSM-5 seasonal pattern specifier requires:

A. A regular temporal relationship between the onset of a major depressive episode and particular time of year (e.g. winter)
B. Full remission occurring also at a characteristic time of year (e.g. spring)
C. Two major depressive episodes with this pattern having occurred in the last two years with no non-seasonal pattern episodes in the same period
D. A lifetime seasonal pattern of major depressive episodes substantially outnumbering non-seasonal pattern episodes

In addition, the seasonal pattern should not be better explained by seasonal stresses. Specific symptoms are not required, but it is noted that they are often those of SAD as described at the start of this section.

Peripartum Depression

Peripartum onset of a (major) depressive episode refers to onset in pregnancy or in a defined period after delivery (puerperium), which is four weeks in DSM-5 and about six weeks in ICD-11 (and ICD-10). Its importance is related to its consequences for maternal and infant health and the safety of treatment options, which likely explains why the commonly used term of postpartum (or postnatal) depression (PPD) for non-psychotic (major) depression occurring after childbirth covers the subsequent period of six months or even a year. However, PPD is not a diagnostic category in either classification system and is often used more broadly to cover the whole range and severity of mood changes that can occur after childbirth.[35]

Although there is some debate, (major) depression after childbirth has not been clearly established as a separate type of depression given that the weight of evidence does not find a distinct symptomatic profile, its risk is strongly increased if there is a history of depression, and in about 50 per cent of cases, the episode starts during pregnancy.[35] In spite of the profound hormonal and bodily changes during pregnancy and after childbirth, their contribution to the risk of depression appears less than that of psychosocial factors (both general and related to transition to parenthood). The prevalence of depression in the postpartum period may be elevated, especially in the first few months, but the evidence for this is weak, and assessment is complicated by variation in the assessment tools used, and the overlap of some depressive symptoms with those related to pregnancy and the postpartum period (including loss of energy, disturbed sleep and appetite and weight changes).[36] A recent meta-analysis found the pooled prevalence of perinatal depression to be 11.9% but considerably lower if diagnostic instruments – rather than symptoms scales – had been used and also lower in high- versus low- and middle-income countries.[37]

(Major) depression with peripartum onset is distinct from postpartum (puerperal) psychotic episodes, which typically occur in the first two postpartum weeks. These have clearer evidence for a specific relationship to childbirth (prevalence about 1–2 per 1,000 births) and are usually a presentation of bipolar disorder characterised by fluctuating and mixed-mood symptoms.[35]

Depression with Onset in Later Life

Kraepelin originally distinguished between involutional melancholia and manic depressive illness but abandoned this distinction in later editions of his textbook. The term 'involutional melancholia' nevertheless persisted in psychiatry, describing a depression of gradual onset occurring during the involutional years (around the menopause in women and a decade later in men) characterised by agitation, somatic concerns and hypochondriasis, often with a prolonged course and poor prognosis. The term fell out of use in the second half of the twentieth century due to lack of evidence for a specific type of depression associated with the menopause. However, the question has remained as to whether depression with onset later in life differs from earlier onset disorder given the effects of ageing on the brain, greater medical comorbidity and the possibility of organic brain disease. A systematic review of studies comparing early- and late-onset depression (age 60 years as the typical cut-off) reported that some inpatient cohorts reported a more severe presentation, hypochondriasis, somatic delusions and gastrointestinal symptoms in those with late onset. However, this was not consistently replicated nor found in community samples, suggesting possible selection bias, and overall phenomenological differences were not supported, apart from some evidence of more pessimistic/suicidal thinking in early onset depression.[38] The same review also found little evidence for differences in response to antidepressants, risk factors or aetiology (apart from a reduced family history of depression in those with late-onset depression). The current evidence is that potential neurobiological/aetiological differences between early- and late-onset depression do not translate into consistent differences in clinical presentation or management.

Persistent Depressive Disorders

Traditionally, mood disorders have been viewed as episodic, remitting disorders, but it was recognised in the 1970s that many patients with depression had a chronic course. This has proved difficult to satisfactorily describe and is reflected in differences between the ICD and DSM classifications. The term 'dysthymia' was introduced in DSM-III (and subsequently in ICD-10), bringing together older, overlapping concepts of depressive neurosis and depressive personality, with continuing debate about the degree to which low-grade persistent symptoms dating back to childhood or adolescence reflect a personality disorder or style rather than a mood disorder. This has contributed to dysthymia having relatively little clinical recognition or adoption. Dysthymia is associated with higher rates of personality disorders and neuroticism than non-chronic (major) depressive disorder but also has strong similarities with the latter in terms of a positive family history of depression, the development of (major) depressive episodes and response to antidepressants. To add to the confusion, a number of different clinical pictures are seen in the longitudinal course in individuals with chronic/persistent depressive symptoms related to the presence or absence, pattern, timing and degree of recovery of (major) depressive episodes, influenced by age of onset. It is estimated that 20–30% of depressive disorders have a chronic course, rising to 33–50% in clinical settings.[39]

ICD-11 includes a current depressive episode persistent qualifier for episodes that have lasted at least two years. These are distinguished from dysthymic disorder, which is characterised as persistent (i.e. lasting two years or more) depressive mood for most of the day, for more days than not, accompanied by additional symptoms from the list for a depressive episode (except ideas of self harm or suicide) but not sufficient to meet the diagnosis of a depressive episode. Dysthymic disorder is excluded if there has been a depressive episode during the first two years of the depressed mood. In children and adolescents, depressed mood can manifest as pervasive irritability. The ICD-10 diagnosis of dysthymia was broadly similar, although it allowed a mild depressive episode to have occurred at the start. It noted that onset was typically early (late teenage/early 20s) and lasts for several years, sometimes indefinitely, but that late onset can occur, often in the aftermath of a depressive episode and associated with bereavement or other stress. Full depressive episodes can also be superimposed during the course of dysthymic disorder/dysthymia (sometimes called double depression).

DSM-5 takes a more radical approach and consolidates all chronic depression into a broad category of persistent depressive disorder. The rationale is that the different presentations have more in common than they differ in terms of comorbidity, personality, impairment, personal and family history and treatment response and that, in naturalistic follow-up, there is shifting between different forms over the course of the illness. In addition, there are differences between chronic and non-chronic major depression, including greater childhood adversity, earlier onset, higher rates of depression in relatives, greater functional impairment and a higher suicide rate in the former, with the distinction between the two remaining stable over time.[39] In spite of this apparent simplification, a complex array of types/specifiers are applied to chart the clinical presentation. The criteria for persistent depressive disorder are:

A. Depressed mood most of the day, for more days than not, for at least two years
B. At least two of (1) poor appetite or overeating, (2) insomnia or hypersomnia, (3) low energy or fatigue, (4) low self-esteem, (5) poor concentration or difficulty making decisions or (6) hopelessness
C. During the two years, the individual has never been without these symptoms for more than two months at a time. In children and adolescents the required duration is reduced to 1 year.

In addition, the symptoms cause clinically significant distress or impaired functioning, and it is possible to meet criteria for a major depressive episode throughout the two years. As for all depressive disorders, a lack of history of mania or hypomania is required, and the symptoms are not better explained by another psychiatric or medical disorder or effects of a substance.

There are four types specified based on the symptom profile of the pattern of major depression in the last two years: (1) pure dysthymic disorder (full criteria for a major depressive episode have not been met), (2) persistent major depressive episode (full criteria met throughout), (3) with intermittent major depressive episodes, with current episode (periods of at least 8 weeks not meeting threshold criteria, but currently meets criteria) and (4) with intermittent major depressive episodes, without current episode (not currently meeting threshold criteria but met in the last two years).

Onset is specified as early (before 21 years) and late (21 years or older), and current severity and atypical and anxious distress episode specifiers can be applied (Tables 3.1.3 and 3.1.4), as discussed in the last section. It is worth noting that the severity requirements for persistent depressive disorder are therefore lower (between three and seven symptoms) than for major depressive disorder (five to nine).

Other Specified Depressive Disorders

The category is primarily concerned with other presentations that fail to meet the duration or severity criteria for (major) depression but cause significant distress or impairment. At the time of writing, ICD-11 had not published the details of disorders included here.

Recurrent Brief Depression

Recurrent brief depression remains somewhat of an enigma and has made little impact on clinical practice, possibly because it is poorly represented in clinical samples and due to uncertainty or pessimism about its effective treatment. Descriptions of short but severe episodes of mood disorder date back to the middle of the nineteenth century, but the current concept of recurrent brief depression – in which full syndromal (major) depressive episodes last less than eight days – was first published in the 1980s by Jules Angst based on a longitudinal epidemiological cohort.[40] Some studies have reported this picture in conjunction with borderline personality disorder, but this comorbidity is reportedly rare in epidemiological studies, which generally report an annual prevalence between 5–8%, an overlap with (major) depressive disorder and an increased risk of suicide.[40]

ICD-10 included recurrent brief depressive disorder in which sometimes intense depressive episodes last less than two weeks (typically 2–3 days) about once a month over the period of a year with full recovery in between, unrelated to the menstrual cycle (although those linked to the menstrual cycle can be specified). DSM-5 retains the name of recurrent brief depression and specifies depressed mood and at least four other depressive symptoms lasting 2–13 days at least once a month for at least 12 consecutive months, unrelated to the menstrual cycle. The criteria for another mood disorder must never have been met nor those for an active or residual psychotic disorder met currently.

Other Specified Disorders

DSM-5 also includes 'short-duration depressive episodes', lasting 4–13 days that have similar requirements to recurrent brief depression apart from the frequency and recurrence criteria, as well as 'depressive episodes with insufficient symptoms' equivalent to minor depression (mentioned earlier), which requires depressed mood and at least one other symptom and lasting at least two weeks but not meeting criteria for any other mood, psychotic or mixed anxiety and depressive disorder. DSM-5-TR now includes major depressive episodes superimposed on primary psychotic disorders (see section below) under this category, apart from for schizoaffective disorder where an additional depressive disorder diagnosis is not warranted.

Related and Boundary Disorders

Related disorders (premenstrual dysphoric disorder and complicated grief) have similarities to depressive disorders with some debate as to whether to include them in the group, whereas boundary disorders have manifestations in which the syndromal criteria for a depressive episode are met, but the diagnoses are mutually exclusive. We briefly consider key aspects here and how they are dealt with in the two classification systems.

Premenstrual Dysphoric Disorder

Reports of a link between the menstrual cycle and disturbance in mood have a long history, but it was only in 1931 that Frank described premenstrual tension, subsequently renamed as premenstrual syndrome in 1953 by Greene and Dalton.[41] Premenstrual syndrome consists of at least one affective symptom (mood changes, anger, confusion, social withdrawal) or somatic symptom (swelling/bloating of abdomen, breast or extremities; breast tenderness; weight gain; headache; joint or muscle pain) in the second half of the menstrual cycle and relieved after menses, with the syndrome associated with identifiable dysfunction. Premenstrual dysphoric disorder (PMDD) overlaps with it but emphasises psychiatric symptoms and has more stringent criteria (see later). The debate about whether PMDD is a distinct disorder or a depressive disorder has been both cultural (including gender political aspects) and scientific.[41] Support for it being a distinct diagnosis include its menstrual-cycle pattern – which is stable over time – cessation at the menopause, cross-cultural occurrence, reasonably high heritability (which is distinct from major depression) and rapid response to serotonin reuptake inhibitors (SSRIs) and hormonal treatments (see below). The evidence for it being a type of depression is based on mood disturbance being a key feature, with major depression the most frequently reported previous disorder. However, the pathophysiology remains obscure, it is not simply related to peripheral hormonal levels and, at least in some studies, depressed mood and anhedonia are less common than mood lability, irritability, anxiety and lethargy. In addition, physical symptoms such as bloating and breast tenderness are among the most common symptoms.[42]

Unlike ICD-10, ICD-11 now includes premenstrual dysphoric disorder (distinct from premenstrual tension syndrome), classified as a genitourinary system disease, although cross-referenced with depressive disorders. It requires, in the majority of menstrual cycles within the past year, a pattern of mood symptoms (depressed mood, irritability), somatic symptoms (lethargy, joint pain, overeating) or cognitive symptoms (concentration difficulties, forgetfulness) that begin several days before the onset of menses, start to improve within a few days after the onset of menses, and then become minimal or absent within approximately one week following the onset of menses. The symptoms should cause significant distress or functional impairment and not represent the exacerbation of a mental disorder. The pattern should ideally be confirmed by a prospective symptom diary over at least two symptomatic menstrual cycles.

PMDD was identified as a proposed disorder needing further research in both DSM-III-R in 1987 (called late luteal phase disorder) and DSM-IV, finally moving into the main text as a depressive disorder in DSM-5.[41] The DSM-5 diagnostic criteria for PMDD are that, for the last year:

A. At least five symptoms occur in the majority of menstrual cycles, are present in the final week before menses, start to improve within a few days after menses and are minimal or absent in the week after menses
B. At least one symptom of (1) marked affective lability (mood swings or sensitivity to rejection), (2) marked irritability or anger or increased interpersonal conflict, (3) marked depressed mood, hopelessness or self-deprecation or (4) marked anxiety, tension or feeling keyed up or on edge
C. At least one symptom, to make at least five combined with those from (B) of (1) decreased interest in usual activities, (2) subjective difficulty in concentration, (3) lethargy, easy fatigability or marked lack of energy, (4) marked change in appetite, overeating or specific food cravings, (5) hypersomnia or insomnia, (6) a sense of being overwhelmed or out of control or (7) physical symptoms such as breast tenderness or swelling, joint or muscle pain, bloating or weight gain.

D-E. The symptoms are associated with significant distress or interference with usual activities or relationships and are not merely an exacerbation of symptoms of another disorder such as a depressive, anxiety or personality disorder (but may co-exist with them). The symptoms should be confirmed by prospective ratings in at least two symptomatic cycles and not be attributable to the physiological effects of a substance or medical disorder.

Whereas about 80 per cent of premenopausal women report at least one physical or psychiatric symptom in the luteal phase, most do not report significant impairment in their daily life. PMDD (by self-report ratings only) has an annual prevalence of about 5 per cent and is most highly comorbid with anxiety disorders but also with depressive and somatoform (somatic symptom) disorders.[42,43]

Randomised, controlled, trials (RCTs) have shown that SSRIs administered continuously, and intermittently in the 14 days before menses, are effective in the treatment of PMDD, with the latter not associated with significant antidepressant withdrawal symptoms. Intermittent SSRIs started at symptom onset appears less consistently beneficial. Hormonal treatments are viewed as second line in view of more limited evidence. The oral contraceptive pill in standard dosing (21 days active, 7 placebo) has not been shown to be beneficial, but continuous treatment, or reducing the placebo to 4 days in the cycle, has some RCT support for efficacy. Ovarian suppression using the gonadotrophin releasing hormone agonist, leuprolide, has also been shown to be effective given as a monthly depot but has a significant side-effect burden. There is current interest in drugs targeting progesterone and allopregnanolone, with preliminary evidence for efficacy.[44] Cognitive behavioural therapy has its proponents but robust evidence is lacking for significant benefit.

Grief and Bereavement-Related Depression

Grief is a universal emotional and cognitive reaction to bereavement, with mourning (bereavement-related behaviour and customs) strongly culturally influenced. It is a normal experience that will affect nearly everyone, with most people coming to terms with their loss without the need for professional intervention. The symptomatology of grief has many similarities to that of depression; bereavement was given as a cause of melancholy by Burton in his *Anatomy of Melancholy*, with descriptions of overwhelming despair experienced after the death of a loved one going back to antiquity, and Freud in *Mourning and Melancholy* proposed that the former is a healthy, and the latter a pathological, response to loss. The relationship between grief, complex grief and bereavement-related depression is however not straightforward and illustrates the difficulty in determining the threshold between normal and pathological experience, and this is reflected in different emphases in the classification systems.

'Normal' Grief

Following bereavement, many people experience a period of intense suffering in which there is an increased risk of mental and physical health problems, with adjustment highly variable between individuals and cultures and not simply dictated by a specific time period. Recovery for many is not 'getting over it' but rather learning to live with it over time. The experience of grief can include the range and severity of affective, cognitive, somatic and behavioural features seen in depressive disorders, but the difference is the focus on the deceased with yearning and the preoccupying thoughts and rumination about the person who has died. These can be associated with guilt and self-blame related to the person who has died, a sense of their presence, even briefly seeing or hearing the deceased as well as feelings of unreality, hopelessness or emptiness about the future without them. Grief often comes in waves triggered by thoughts or reminders of the person and can be interspersed with positive emotions or memories. Bowlby's theory of attachment has influenced much of the current thinking about the process of grief, stating that once an attachment has been formed, as between a child and parent, a response is unavoidable if the bond breaks – commonly with fear, anger, frustration or grief. A number of models of grief have been described, including those of Parkes and Bowlby (four phases of initial shock and numbness, yearning and searching, disorganisation and despair, and reorganisation and recovery), Kübler-Ross (five phases of denial, anger, bargaining, depression and acceptance), with others such as Worden emphasising tasks of grieving rather than phases (acceptance of loss, processing the pain, adjusting to a world without the deceased, and retaining a connection with them while embarking on a new life). However, grieving doesn't follow a prescribed or predictable route, and although these descriptions can be useful, there has been a move away from understanding grief as a sequential process – or a set of stages or tasks – and individuals experience qualitatively different paths through grief. In addition, grief is not just about pain but also about happy memories and positive feelings as well as finding meaning in the life of the deceased and in their legacy.[45]

Bereavement is associated with an increased risk of mortality – highest in the first year – from suicide, accidents, alcohol-related causes and physical illness, in particular cardiovascular disease. The last is sometimes called 'broken heart' syndrome (also applied to acute stress-related cardiomyopathy) due to psychological distress and loneliness, as well as the secondary consequences of this such as changes in social ties, living arrangements, eating habits and economic support.[46] Morbidity due to physical health problems is increased, and there are elevated rates of psychiatric disorders, especially depressive, anxiety and post-traumatic stress disorders, especially if the loss of life has been great or the death traumatic or horrific.[46,47]

In spite of the associated morbidity professional intervention is generally neither justified nor effective for uncomplicated forms of grief, with the necessary support received from family, friends and community groups. Societal resources (such as CRUSE bereavement support) are available to provide information, counselling and practical advice for those seeking further help.

Complicated Grief

Complicated grief refers to a deviation from what is considered the 'normal' experience of grief in a particular individual's cultural and social context, either in time course, intensity or both. Many different terms have been used including abnormal grief, inhibited or delayed grief, prolonged or chronic grief, pathological grief, traumatic grief and persistent complex bereavement disorder. Chronic/prolonged grief is the most common type of complicated grief, typically defined as intense symptoms persisting beyond six months, with an overall prevalence of about 10 per cent after bereavement,[48] although much higher prevalence in parents after the traumatic death of a child. However, these figures are dependent on the definition of what is normal, and individuals vary in their experience of grief. Risk and resilience factors related to developing complicated grief can be grouped into events related to the death (e.g. cause, circumstances, type and quality of relationship, pre-existing strains, subsequent conflict and hardship), intrapersonal factors and coping style (e.g. personality, attachment style, belief system, emotion regulation, grief work) and interpersonal or external (e.g. social and economic support).[46]

Complicated grief is not categorised as a depressive disorder but clearly has overlap with bereavement-associated depression, and the distinction is made on the nature of the symptoms and their severity. Under 'Disorders specifically associated with stress' ICD-11 has a diagnosis of prolonged grief disorder based on core symptoms of longing or persistent preoccupation with the deceased, as well as at least one additional symptom of intense emotional pain or another grief-related symptom, associated with significant psychosocial impairment and lasting at least six months. In ICD-10, grief reactions judged to be abnormal in form, content or duration are classified as adjustment disorders. DSM-5-TR also includes prolonged grief disorder as a 'Trauma- and stressor-related disorder' involving intense yearning/longing and/or preoccupation with thoughts or memories of the deceased together with at least 3 of 8 further symptoms (including clinically significant emotional distress, numbness, identity disruption, social integration difficulties) in response to the death, associated with clinically significant distress or functional impairment outside sociocultural norms, and a duration of at least 12 months.

Evidence is lacking that preventive interventions are beneficial but targeted psychotherapy for complicated grief once it occurs has RCT evidence for efficacy.[45] This is aimed at helping to find ways to think about the loss without experiencing intense distress, together with encouraging restoration of function and enthusiasm/planning for the future. Other psychotherapies that incorporate adaptation to grief, together with strategies to reduce avoidance of reminders of loss and behavioural activation, may also be helpful. While non-randomised trial evidence has suggested a benefit from antidepressants, an RCT found that citalopram was not significantly better than placebo in reducing symptoms of chronic grief, and did not enhance targeted psychotherapy, although in the latter case it did show a small significant additional benefit in improving depressive symptoms.[49]

Bereavement-Related (Major) Depression

In the immediate period following a bereavement, changes in mood that have the symptomatic features and course characteristic of 'normal' grief (as described earlier) have traditionally not been diagnosed as a psychiatric disorder, even though it not uncommon to have sufficient symptoms for a (major) depressive episode. Bereavement nonetheless can result in depression similar to other stressors, but given the overlap in symptoms, there is often difficulty in distinguishing between the two, especially in the early months after bereavement. This may be important in offering the appropriate support or treatment and in avoiding pathologising a normal human process. Those arguing against excluding depression in the early stages after a death (i.e. arguing against a 'bereavement exclusion') point to the similarities between bereavement-related depression and depression after other stresses in terms of clinical features, number of previous depressive episodes and comorbidities, and response to treatment. In contrast, those supporting the bereavement exclusion point out that, after bereavement, there is less treatment seeking and impairment, lower levels of guilt and neuroticism, and a lower risk of subsequent depressive episodes, which is similar to those without a history of depression.[50,51]

While ICD-10 did not directly address the issue, ICD-11 identifies a depressive episode during a period of bereavement by persistence of constant depressive symptoms a month or more following the loss and severe depressive symptoms such as extreme beliefs of low self-worth and guilt not related to the loss of the loved one, presence of psychotic symptoms, suicidal ideation or psychomotor retardation.[51]

DSM-IV had a bereavement exclusion and diagnosed major depression based on symptom duration (>2 months) or nature (similar to those in ICD-11). DSM-5, controversially, has removed this, noting that for all types of stressor, the decision about whether symptoms are an understandable or appropriate reaction to stress or are due to a major depressive episode requires clinical judgement based on the individual's pattern of symptoms and history, and cultural norms in the expression of distress after loss.

The occurrence of a major depressive episode in the year following bereavement due to loss of a partner has been found to be about 20 per cent (by DSM-IV criteria) with a relative risk of 4–6 compared to a non-bereaved comparison group.[47]

Bipolar Disorders

Bipolar disorders form an important boundary with depressive disorders as the presence of manic symptoms excludes the latter, making them exclusive diagnoses. Although, as we have seen, historically this distinction was not made, it has yet to have a firm aetiological basis, and causes classificatory challenges at the boundary. Cyclothymia (instability of mood with numerous periods of sub-threshold mild depression and elation) was classified with dysthymia as a persistent mood disorder in ICD-10 but is included under bipolar disorders in both ICD-11 and DSM-5. Mood presentations meeting criteria for neither a bipolar nor depressive disorder are classified as 'Unspecified mood disorder' in DSM-5-TR.

Depression in Bipolar Disorder

Unrecognised, or yet to occur, episodes of hypomania or mania not infrequently lead to the initial 'misdiagnosis' of bipolar disorder as unipolar depression (see section on the 'Natural History of Depressive Disorders'). Although differences have been proposed between depression occurring in the two disorders, these are not sufficiently established or distinctive to allow confident diagnosis at the level of the individual. Some features may raise the level of suspicion of bipolarity such as a family history of bipolar disorder, early onset, psychotic symptoms, frequent episodes and mixed features or mood states.[52] It has also been suggested that bipolar depression should be considered in non-responders to antidepressant treatment, given the lack of evidence for antidepressant efficacy in bipolar disorder and the availability of alternative treatment options (see Chapter 4.1).

Mixed Features

It is now recognised that manic symptoms exist on a continuum with no natural cut-off between depressive disorders and bipolar spectrum/bipolar II disorder. One long-term follow-up study of patients presenting with a depressive episode found that 22% had at least one sub-threshold manic symptom at baseline, and each additional symptom increased the risk of subsequent hypomania or mania by 29% over a median 20 years follow-up.[52] However, the optimal cut-off of ≥3 manic symptoms only had a positive predictive value of 42%, with 17% of those without any manic symptoms at initial presentation subsequently progressing to bipolar disorder.

ICD-10 and ICD-11 do not directly address this issue, and the presence of significant mixed-mood symptoms generally leads to classification with the bipolar disorders. DSM-5 has taken a different approach and, given the evidence that sub-threshold manic symptoms only weakly predict bipolar disorder, has added a mixed features specifier to major depressive disorder, consisting of at least three of (1) elevated expansive mood, (2) inflated self-esteem or grandiosity, (3) more talkative than usual or pressure of speech, (4) flight of ideas or subjective racing thoughts, (5) increase in goal-directed activity (social, work or sexual), (6) increased or excessive involvement in activities with a high potential for painful consequences or (7) decreased need for sleep (sleeping less but feeling rested). These symptoms need to be a change in usual behaviour observable by others, not meet criteria for mania or hypomania, nor be attributable to the physiological effects of a substance. A US national survey found that 15.5% of individuals with major depressive disorder met criteria for the mixed features specifier.[28]

Primary Psychotic Disorders

Schizophrenia, and related disorders including schizoaffective disorder (called here primary psychotic disorders), are the other main boundary group in which prominent non-affective psychotic features during an acute episode of illness excludes a depressive disorder. However, the high prevalence of depression at all stages of primary psychotic disorders causes conceptual, aetiological and classificatory challenges. Mood disturbance during an acute psychotic illness is usually seen as an intrinsic dimension of psychosis. At other times, depression could also potentially reflect common aetiological factors or a psychological reaction to the psychosis, better viewed as a comorbid disorder (although assessment is complicated by the overlap with negative symptoms); a recent systematic review reported the prevalence of major depression to be 33% in patients with stabilised schizophrenia.[53]

Apart from schizoaffective disorder where depressive episodes are included in the diagnosis, ICD-10, 1CD-11 and DSM-5 retain a hierarchical structure when there are active or residual symptoms from a primary psychotic disorder and do not diagnose comorbid depression in this situation. ICD-11 has a depressive mood symptoms qualifier for primary psychotic disorders, including when they are in remission, whereas ICD-10 allowed an additional depressive disorder diagnosis if the psychotic disorder had fully resolved. DSM-5-TR has introduced a comorbid diagnosis of major depressive episode, superimposed (classified under `Other specified depressive disorder) in this situation.

Comorbidity in Depressive Disorders

Comorbidity refers to the co-occurrence of different disorders in an individual, but this apparently simple term hides the potential complexity of their relationship in terms of chronology (e.g. which occurred first, occurring at the same time or at different times), aetiology/risk factors (e.g. chance/independent risk factors, common risk factors, one disorder directly causing the other, interaction between common risk factors) and even whether the apparently different disorders are facets of the same underlying condition (e.g. depressive and anxiety disorders, as discussed earlier). The use of the term 'secondary' for depression occurring in the course of another disorder, or physical illness, has now largely fallen out of use in favour of an agnostic stance on causation. However, the concept of direct causation is retained for depressive disorders that are better explained as direct manifestations of the physiological effects of physical illness or substances, and ICD-11 retains the term secondary mood syndrome for the former. In general, the greater the number of comorbidities, the poorer is the clinical outcome.

Psychiatric Comorbidity

A comprehensive worldwide study shows the pervasive nature of comorbidity within mental disorders, highest in those disorders more closely related and when starting before the age of 20 years with the greatest risk of developing a second disorder in the first two years after onset and slowly decreasing over time or plateauing after about 10 years. Although the first onset of a depressive disorder can precede the onset of other disorders, the risk is much higher for it to follow them; for example, bulimia nervosa is hardly ever first diagnosed after a first episode of depression whereas about 60% of those with bulimia nervosa will have a subsequent major depressive episode, and for panic disorder, the figures are 7% versus 50% respectively.[54]

Surveys and claims data find that 60–67% of people with depression also meet criteria for another mental disorder – most of these anxiety disorders – with the risk increasing with depression severity.[55] One important aspect is that even when the depressive disorder has resolved, anxiety symptoms/disorder may persist. Substance use disorders are the second most common comorbidity, with a systematic review finding a prevalence of 25%, with similar rates in major depression and dysthymia and nearly twice as high in men (36%) as women (19%). It is most commonly comorbid with alcohol misuse disorder (21%) with illicit drug use disorder occurring in 12% of cases.[56]

The prevalence of comorbid personality disorder has been reported to be 45% in major depression and 60% in dysthymia in a systemic review of studies using predominantly DSM criteria.[57] The greatest comorbidity was with cluster C disorders (most commonly avoidant) followed by cluster B disorders (mostly borderline); in contrast, a study using German national health insurance claims data and ICD-10 criteria reported the prevalence of comorbid personality disorders to be much lower at 10%,[55] which is likely to reflect both methodological and classification differences.

Medical Comorbidity

A wide range of diseases have been shown to have an elevated prevalence of depressive disorders, often varying according to the activity of the disease, with the prevalence of major depression usually greater than 10% and not infrequently above 20%.[58] The mechanisms of the association are usually obscure and, in practice, likely to be multifactorial, combining physiological and psychosocial factors, with direction of effect often going both ways (note this is also true for comorbid substance use disorders in the previous section). This can make a clear distinction between primary and secondary depressive disorders difficult, if not impossible. The emphasis is usually on comorbid depressive disorders in established physical conditions, but a recent large population-based national cohort examined the risk of subsequent medical conditions following the diagnosis of mental disorders. It found that for all mental disorders, including mood disorders, there was an increased risk of developing medical illnesses, highest early on and persisting beyond 15 years of follow-up, with only the cumulative incidence of cancers not increased.[59] One of the highest was the cumulative incidence of a circulatory condition after the diagnosis of a mood disorder, which reached 41% after 15 years compared to 33% in a reference group without a mood disorder. These data do not prove causation but highlight the complexity that lies behind comorbidity.

Epidemiology

The reported prevalence of depressive disorders is influenced by the classification, instruments and methodology used, as well as variation in geography, cultural and social factors, so great caution is needed in interpreting different studies. A survey of European studies carried out at the end of the last century found a median annual prevalence for (major) depression of 6.9% (range 3.1–10.1%)[60] while a systematic review reported a global point prevalence of 4.4% in 2010, varying between 2.5% in East Asia and 7.4% in North Africa/Middle East and about 5% in Western Europe.[61] Lifetime prevalence of depression found in surveys is about twice that of the annual prevalence (i.e. 10–20%). Whether or not the overall prevalence of (major) depression has been increasing in recent decades is debated. In England, an increase in the point prevalence of (major) depression from 2.2% in 1993 to 3.8% in 2014 has been reported for 18–64 year olds,[26] whereas no change in age-adjusted estimates was found between 1990 and 2010, either globally or regionally, in the systematic review previously cited.[61] An increase in psychological distress measured by symptom checklists had increased however, possibly due to greater public awareness and a wider use of terms such as depression to describe distress.[61]

About one-and-a-half to two times as many women compared with men experience (major) depressive episodes, with the peak age of onset between adolescence and 29 years and the highest prevalence between ages 18–64 years. In women, the perimenopausal period is associated with around twice the risk of depression compared to the pre-menopause but only in those with a previous history of depression.[62] It is sometimes claimed that depression is more common in the elderly, but national surveys show a lower prevalence above 65 years compared to earlier ages,[26,28] although it may rise again after the age of 75 years.

Less is known about persistent depressive disorders, but the lifetime prevalence of dysthymia has been estimated as 1–6% and that of DSM-5 persistent depressive disorder (i.e. dysthymia together with persistent major depression) as 4–6%.[39]

Natural History of Depressive Disorders

Long-term outcomes of depressive disorders vary between studies and settings; a systematic review of prospective cohorts who were followed over the course of 3 and 49 years in community and primary care settings found that 35–60% of participants had a single episode with stable recovery, and 10–17% had a chronic course. Recurrence rates were 35–65% in studies with follow-up over 20 years.[63] The median duration of depressive episodes was between 12 and 24 weeks in one extended follow-up study (those with higher rates of recurrence at the shorter end of the range), and another study estimated that over the course of 23 years of follow-up – for a patient who has received a diagnosis of depression – 15% of the time on average was spent in a major depressive episode. Given that up to half of patients with bipolar disorder present initially with depression, a proportion of those with an apparent (unipolar) depressive disorder will 'convert' to bipolar disorder, with the rate estimated to be about 1% a year in the early years after diagnosis[64]; one study of psychiatric patients presenting with a major depressive episode and followed for a median length of 20 years found that about 20% were re-diagnosed as having bipolar disorder (about twice as many with bipolar II compared with bipolar I disorder).[52] However, a lower figure of 10–15% had received a bipolar diagnosis up to 40 years after the onset of a depressive disorder in a comprehensive analysis of nationally representative epidemiological studies.[54]

Depression is associated with considerable morbidity, and in 2019, the WHO reported that depressive disorders ranked highest of all psychiatric disorders in its global disease burden measured by disability-adjusted life years (DALYs, the number of years lost due to ill-health, disability or early death). It ranked seventh in non-communicable diseases in all age groups combined but between second and fourth in age groups under 50 years. Its burden has remained essentially unchanged between 1990 and 2019 as measured by the age-standardised DALY rate, although the percentage of global DALYs that are attributable to depression increased from 1.1% to 1.8% over this period.[63] It has been suggested that impairment due to depression is usefully conceptualised along two orthogonal axes of severity and chronicity – the latter historically over-looked, meaning that the distress and impairment associated with dysthymia tends to be relatively unrecognised. The highest impairment and suffering are found with the combination of high severity and high chronicity.[39]

Systematic reviews have found that depressive disorders are associated with twelve-fold increase in the risk of suicide compared with the general population,[66] with a 2.2% lifetime prevalence of suicide in mixed inpatient/outpatient depressed patients (compared with less than 0.5% in the non-affectively ill population) rising to 4% in those hospitalised and 8.6% if hospitalised for suicidality.[67] Depression is also associated with an increased risk of dying from natural causes (typically 1.5–2 times), although a causal link has been questioned. A recent large population-based cohort study found that the mortality rate ratio was raised for all mental disorders; for mood disorders (unipolar and bipolar disorder combined), it was 1.9 (increased for all types of illness apart from cancer), translating into about seven life years lost. Also highlighted was the high mortality rate ratio in mood disorders for deaths from external causes, especially due to accidents.[68]

Assessment

The general approach to the psychiatric clinical interview is covered elsewhere (see Chapter 2). It is important to try and understand the person as well as the features of the disorder. Finding out the wider picture involving developmental, personal and past history, strengths and vulnerabilities, social support, and their beliefs and expectations about their condition and treatment can help put the flesh on the skeletal diagnostic structure and give context and meaning to what is being experienced. Table 3.1.6 outlines relevant features to assess to determine the type of depressive disorder, which in its turn may give some general guidance about prognosis and treatment.

Rating Scales

Rating scales allow a quantitative assessment of symptoms. Some self-report scales are used for screening and for epidemiological studies, but it is important to realise that these do not accurately reflect clinical assessment and so should not be viewed as

Table 3.1.6 A brief guide to assessing some relevant features of someone presenting with mood symptoms

• Establish presence of persistently lowered mood and/or anhedonia, and impact on function
• Assess for other symptoms – depressive and non-depressive (especially anxiety)
• Are these better explained by another disorder, caused directly by physical illness or substance, or appropriate to the context (e.g. bereavement, stressful event)?
• Could the picture be part of bipolar disorder (presence or history of hypomanic/manic/mixed symptoms)?
• How severe are the symptoms (subsyndromal, mild, moderate, severe)?
• What is/was the duration (very recent onset/established/chronic) and evolution (worsening/improving/partially remitted) of symptoms during this episode?
• Are there psychotic symptoms in current episode?
• Main symptom profile in current episode (anxious/melancholic). May also be useful to note atypical or mixed features
• Other prominent features in current episode (e.g. agitation/ depersonalisation/catatonia)
• Have there been previous episodes? Note age of first episode/how many/severity/usual duration/response to treatments/degree of inter-episode recovery
• Is there a particular temporal pattern (perinatal/seasonal/recurrent brief episodes)?
• Assess risks (suicide/neglect/violence/acting on psychotic symptoms) and mitigating factors

Table 3.1.7 Some rating scales useful for the assessment of depression

Scale	Description	Comment
Observer-rated		
Hamilton Depression Rating Scale (HRSD or HAM-D)[69]	Core scale has 17 items (+ sexual function, hypochondriasis, diurnal variation and depersonalisation in 21-item version). Symptom severity rated (9 items on a 5-point, 8 items on a 3-point scale) over last 1–2 weeks. Weighted towards somatic features and only scores reduced sleep and appetite/weight.	Developed to quantify severity in diagnosed depressed patients. Remains a primary outcome measure in antidepressant treatment trials. Other versions of the scale are available that also rate increased sleep and appetite.
Montgomery Åsberg Depression Rating Scale (MADRS)[69]	10 items rating depression symptom severity on a 7-point scale. Time interval can be specified. Only scores reduced sleep and appetite/weight.	Items selected to be sensitive to change with treatment. There is a 9-item self-rated version (MADRS-S) omitting observed mood item and rated over the last 3 days.
Quick Inventory of Depressive Symptomatology Clinician-Rated (QIDS-C)[69]	16 items rating severity of DSM-IV/5 depression criteria on a 4-point scale over the last 7 days. Only the highest score taken from 4 items on sleep and 4 on appetite/weight to score each criterion once (i.e. 9 items contribute to score).	Developed to provide a clinically useful scale reflecting DSM-IV criteria with matched clinician and patient ratings.
Self-Report		
Beck Depression Inventory (BDI-II)[69]	21 items rating severity of DSM-IV/5 depression criteria plus additional items on a 4-point scale, over the last 2 weeks. Weighted towards cognitive features.	Revised from original BDI to make consistent with DSM-IV. Often the primary outcome measure in psychological treatment trials. Copyrighted, fee for use.
Hospital Anxiety and Depression Scale (HADS)[70]	14 items (7 depression, 7 anxiety) rating severity on a 4-point scale over last 7 days. Emphasises affective, and avoids somatic, features.	Designed to be used with medically ill outpatient populations. Copyrighted, fee for use.
Quick Inventory of Depressive Symptomatology Self-Report (QIDS-SR)[69]	As QIDS-C.	Most commonly used version.
Patient Health Questionnaire (PHQ-9)[69]	9 items rating 'how often bothered' by DSM-IV/5 depression criteria on a 4-point scale over the last 2 weeks.	The first 2 items (depressed mood, little interest, PHQ-2) can be used for screening. Epidemiological studies often omit 'thoughts of being better off dead/hurting yourself' item (PHQ-8).
Generalised Anxiety Disorder Assessment (GAD-7)[71]	7 items rating 'how often bothered' by generalised anxiety symptoms on a 4-point scale over the last 2 weeks.	Complements, and correlates highly with, the PHQ-9 but provides a separate anxiety dimension.
Hypomania Check-List (HCL-16)[72]	16 items rated yes/no occurring during a period of being in a 'high' state. Score of $\geq$8 gave best balance of specificity (71%) and sensitivity (83%) for bipolar disorder.	Developed to screen for hypomania to help distinguish between unipolar depression and bipolar disorder.

diagnostic instruments. Although sensitivity and specificity are important features of rating scales used for screening or as a proxy for diagnosis, ease of use, reliability and face validity are much more important when used to monitor symptoms in clinical care. Table 3.1.7 describes some of the more common and useful rating scales for use with depressive disorders.

Given differences in choice and wording of scale items, and sometimes weighting of different symptoms, the constructs measured by each rating scale vary, and correlation between scales may only be moderate. As rating scales cannot cover the whole range of an individual patient's symptoms and concerns, they do not replace clinical assessment. Self-rating scales are increasingly favoured as providing the patient's own perspective, and they offer clear advantages in terms of feasibility and time in clinical practice as they can be completed before a consultation; they do however need to be interpreted in light of the whole clinical picture, as responses may be influenced by illness factors, personality and circumstances. Rating scales are of great value in recording the overall severity of depression, anxiety and individual symptoms over time, assessing response to treatment, helping communication between professionals and between professionals and patients, and self-monitoring. However, they are woefully underused in clinical practice, even though recommended by NICE guidance.[21]

References

1. Kendler KS. The origin of our modern concept of depression – the history of melancholia from 1780–1880: a review. *JAMA Psychiatry* 2020;77 (8):863–8.
2. Shorter E. The doctrine of the two depressions in historical perspective. *Acta Psychiatrica Scandinavica Supplementum* 2007;433:5–13.
3. Kendler KS. The phenomenology of major depression and the representativeness and nature of DSM criteria. *American Journal of Psychiatry* 2016;173(8):771–80.
4. Baumeister H, Parker G. Meta-review of depressive subtyping models. *Journal of Affective Disorders* 2012;139(2):126–40.
5. Parker G, McClure G, Paterson A. Melancholia and catatonia: disorders or

specifiers? *Current Psychiatry Reports* 2015;17(1):536.

6. Ross CA, Margolis RL. Research Domain Criteria: strengths, weaknesses, and potential alternatives for future psychiatric research. *Molecular Neuropsychiatry* 2019;5(4): 218–36.
7. Johnstone, L, Boyle, M, Cromby, J, et al. *The Power Threat Meaning Framework: Overview*. Leicester: British Psychological Society; 2018.
8. Tylee A, Gastpar M, Lépine JP, et al. DEPRES II (Depression Research in European Society II): a patient survey of the symptoms, disability and current management of depression in the community. DEPRES Steering Committee. *International Clinical Psychopharmacology* 1999;14(3):139–51.
9. Faravelli C, Servi P, Arends JA, et al. Number of symptoms, quantification, and qualification of depression. *Comprehensive Psychiatry* 1996;37(5): 307–15.
10. Cavanagh A, Wilson CJ, Kavanagh DJ, et al. Differences in the expression of symptoms in men versus women with depression: a systematic review and meta-analysis. *Harvard Review of Psychiatry* 2017;25(1):29–38.
11. Ribeiro JD, Huang X, Fox KR, et al. Depression and hopelessness as risk factors for suicide ideation, attempts and death: meta-analysis of longitudinal studies. *British Journal of Psychiatry* 2018;212(5):279–86.
12. Griep SK, Mackinnon DF. Does nonsuicidal self-injury predict later suicidal attempts? A review of studies. *Archives of Suicide Research* 2020;26 (2):428–46. DOI: 10.1080/13811118.2020.1822244.
13. Akkaoui MA, Lejoyeux M, d'Ortho MP, et al. Nightmares in patients with major depressive disorder, bipolar disorder, and psychotic disorders: a systematic review. *Journal of Clinical Medicine* 2020;9(12):3990.
14. Plante DT, Cook JD, Barbosa LS, et al. Establishing the objective sleep phenotype in hypersomnolence disorder with and without comorbid major depression. *Sleep* 2019;42(6): zsz060.
15. Mula M, Pini S, Cassano GB. The neurobiology and clinical significance of depersonalization in mood and anxiety disorders: a critical reappraisal. *Journal of Affective Disorders* 2007;99 (1–3):91–9.
16. Swann AC. Activated depression: mixed bipolar disorder or agitated unipolar depression? *Current Psychiatry Reports* 2013;15(8):376.
17. Rasmussen SA, Mazurek MF, Rosebush PI. Catatonia: our current understanding of its diagnosis, treatment and pathophysiology. *World Journal of Psychiatry* 2016;6(4):391–8.
18. World Health Organization. *ICD-11 for Mortality and Morbidity Statistics (Version : 05/2021)*. 2021. icd.who.int/browse11/l-m/en. (Accessed 26 May 2021).
19. American Psychiatric Association. *Diagnostic and Statistical Manual of Mental Disorders, Fifth Edition, Text Revision (DSM-5-TR)*. Washington DC: American Psychiatric Association; 2022.
20. World Health Organization. *The ICD-10 Classification of Mental and Behavioural Disorders. Clinical descriptions and Diagnostic Guidelines*. Geneva: World Health Organization; 1992.
21. Stein DJ, Szatmari P, Gaebel W, et al. Mental, behavioral and neurodevelopmental disorders in the ICD-11: an international perspective on key changes and controversies. *BMC Medicine* 2020;18(1):21.
22. National Institute for Health and Care Excellence. *Depression in adults: treatment and management*. www.nice.org.uk/guidance/ng222. (Accessed 20 November 23).
23. Dubovsky SL, Ghosh BM, Serotte JC, et al. Psychotic depression: diagnosis, differential diagnosis, and treatment. *Psychotherapy and Psychosomatics* 2021;90(3):160–77. DOI: 10.1159/000511348.
24. Solmi M, Pigato GG, Roiter B, et al. Prevalence of catatonia and its moderators in clinical samples: results from a meta-analysis and meta-regression analysis. *Schizophrenia Bulletin* 2018;44(5):1133–50.
25. Demyttenaere K, Heirman E. The blurred line between anxiety and depression: hesitations on comorbidity, thresholds and hierarchy. *International Review of Psychiatry* 2020;32(5–6): 455–65.
26. McManus, S, Bebbington, P, Jenkins, R, et al. *Mental Health and Wellbeing in England: Adult Psychiatric Morbidity Survey*. Leeds: NHS Digital; 2016.
27. Möller H-J, Bandelow B, Volz HP, et al. The relevance of 'mixed anxiety and depression' as a diagnostic category in clinical practice. *European Archives of Psychiatry and Clinical Neuroscience* 2016;266(8):725–36.
28. Hasin DS, Sarvet AL, Meyers JL, et al. Epidemiology of adult DSM-5 major depressive disorder and its specifiers in the United States. *JAMA Psychiatry* 2018;75(4):336–46.
29. McGrath PJ, Khan AY, Trivedi MH, et al. Response to a selective serotonin reuptake inhibitor (citalopram) in major depressive disorder with melancholic features: a STAR*D report. *Journal of Clinical Psychiatry* 2008;69 (12):1847–55.
30. Gili M, Roca M, Armengol S, et al. Clinical patterns and treatment outcome in patients with melancholic, atypical and non-melancholic depressions. *PLoS ONE* 2012;7(10):e48200.
31. Łojko D, Rybakowski JK. Atypical depression: current perspectives. *Neuropsychiatric Disease and Treatment* 2017;13:2447–56.
32. Sampogna G, Del Vecchio V, Giallonardo V, et al. Diagnosis, clinical features, and therapeutic implications of agitated depression. *Psychiatric Clinics of North America* 2020;43(1):47–57.
33. Meesters Y, Gordijn MC. Seasonal affective disorder, winter type: current insights and treatment options. *Psychology Research and Behavior Management* 2016;9:317–27.
34. Traffanstedt MK, Mehta S, LoBello SG. Major depression with seasonal variation: is it a valid construct? *Clinical Psychological Science* 2016;4(5): 825–34.
35. Jones I, Cantwell R. The classification of perinatal mood disorders – suggestions for DSMV and ICD11. *Archives of Women's Mental Health* 2010;13(1):33–6.
36. O'Hara MW, McCabe JE. Postpartum depression: current status and future directions. *Annual Review of Clinical Psychology* 2013;9:379–407.
37. Woody CA, Ferrari AJ, Siskind DJ, et al. A systematic review and meta-regression of the prevalence and incidence of perinatal depression. *Journal of Affective Disorders* 2017;219:86–92.
38. Grayson L, Thomas A. A systematic review comparing clinical features in early age at onset and late age at onset late-life depression. *Journal of Affective Disorders* 2013;150(2):161–70.
39. Schramm E, Klein DN, Elsaesser M, et al. Review of dysthymia and persistent depressive disorder: history,

correlates, and clinical implications. *Lancet Psychiatry* 2020;7(9):801–12.

40. Pezawas L, Angst J, Kasper S. Recurrent brief depression revisited. *International Review of Psychiatry* 2005;17(1):63–70.
41. Zachar P, Kendler KS. A diagnostic and statistical manual of mental disorders history of premenstrual dysphoric disorder. *Journal of Nervous and Mental Disease* 2014;202(4):346–52.
42. Epperson CN, Steiner M, Hartlage SA, et al. Premenstrual dysphoric disorder: evidence for a new category for DSM-5. *American Journal of Psychiatry* 2012;169(5):465–75.
43. Wittchen H-U, Becker E, Lieb R, et al. Prevalence, incidence and stability of premenstrual dysphoric disorder in the community. *Psychological Medicine* 2002;32(1):119–32.
44. Carlini SV, Deligiannidis KM. Evidence-Based Treatment of Premenstrual Dysphoric Disorder: A Concise Review. *J Clin Psychiatry* 2020;81(2):19ac13071.
45. Stroebe, M, Schut, H, Boerner, K Bereavement. In: Wright J (ed.) *International Encyclopedia of the Social & Behavioral Sciences,* 2nd ed., Vol. 2. Amsterdam: Elsevier Ltd; 2015: 531–6.
46. Stroebe M, Schut H, Stroebe W. Health outcomes of bereavement. *Lancet* 2007;370(9603):1960–73.
47. Onrust SA, Cuijpers P. Mood and anxiety disorders in widowhood: a systematic review. *Aging & Mental Health* 2006;10(4):327–34.
48. Lundorff M, Holmgren H, Zachariae R, et al. Prevalence of prolonged grief disorder in adult bereavement: a systematic review and meta-analysis. *Journal of Affective Disorders* 2017;212:138–49.
49. Shear MK, Reynolds CF, III, Simon NM, et al. Optimizing treatment of complicated grief: A randomized clinical trial. *JAMA Psychiatry* 2016;73:685–94.
50. Wakefield JC, First MB. Validity of the bereavement exclusion to major depression: does the empirical evidence support the proposal to eliminate the exclusion in DSM-5? *World Psychiatry* 2012;11(1):3–10.
51. Zachar P, First MB, Kendler KS. The bereavement exclusion debate in the DSM-5: a history. *Clinical Psychological Science* 2017;5(5):890–906.
52. Fiedorowicz JG, Endicott J, Leon AC, et al. Subthreshold hypomanic symptoms in progression from unipolar major depression to bipolar disorder. *American Journal of Psychiatry* 2011;168(1):40–8.
53. Etchecopar-Etchart D, Korchia T, Loundou A, et al. Comorbid major depressive disorder in schizophrenia: a systematic review and meta-analysis. *Schizophrenia Bulletin* 2021;47 (2):298–308.
54. McGrath JJ, Lim CCW, Plana-Ripoll O, et al. Comorbidity within mental disorders: a comprehensive analysis based on 145 990 survey respondents from 27 countries. *Epidemiology and Psychiatric Sciences* 2020;29:e153.
55. Steffen A, Nübel J, Jacobi F, et al. Mental and somatic comorbidity of depression: a comprehensive cross-sectional analysis of 202 diagnosis groups using German nationwide ambulatory claims data. *BMC Psychiatry* 2020;20 (1):142.
56. Hunt GE, Malhi GS, Lai HMX, et al. Prevalence of comorbid substance use in major depressive disorder in community and clinical settings, 1990–2019: systematic review and meta-analysis. *Journal of Affective Disorders* 2020;266:288–304.
57. Friborg O, Martinsen EW, Martinussen M, et al. Comorbidity of personality disorders in mood disorders: a meta-analytic review of 122 studies from 1988 to 2010. *Journal of Affective Disorders* 2014;152–154:1–11.
58. Gold SM, Köhler-Forsberg O, Moss-Morris R, et al. Comorbid depression in medical diseases. *National Review. Disease Primers* 2020;6(1):69.
59. Momen NC, Plana-Ripoll O, Agerbo E, et al. Association between mental disorders and subsequent medical conditions. *New England Journal of Medicine* 2020;382(18):1721–31.
60. Wittchen HU, Jacobi F. Size and burden of mental disorders in Europe – a critical review and appraisal of 27 studies. *European Neuropsychopharmacology* 2005;15(4):357–76.
61. Baxter AJ, Scott KM, Ferrari AJ, et al. Challenging the myth of an "epidemic" of common mental disorders: trends in the global prevalence of anxiety and depression between 1990 and 2010. *Depression and Anxiety* 2014;31 (6):506–16.
62. Maki PM, Kornstein SG, Joffe H, et al. Guidelines for the evaluation and treatment of perimenopausal depression: summary and recommendations. *Menopause* 2018;25 (10):1069–85.
63. Steinert C, Hofmann M, Kruse J, et al. The prospective long-term course of adult depression in general practice and the community. A systematic literature review. *Journal of Affective Disorders* 2014;152–154:65–75.
64. Baldessarini RJ, Faedda GL, Offidani E, et al. Antidepressant-associated mood-switching and transition from unipolar major depression to bipolar disorder: a review. *Journal of Affective Disorders* 2013;148(1): 129–35.
65. GBD 2019 Diseases and Injuries Collaborators. Global burden of 369 diseases and injuries in 204 countries and territories, 1990-2019: a systematic analysis for the Global Burden of Disease Study 2019. *Lancet* 2020;396(10258):1204–22.
66. Too LS, Spittal MJ, Bugeja L, et al. The association between mental disorders and suicide: a systematic review and meta-analysis of record linkage studies. *Journal of Affective Disorders* 2019;259:302–13.
67. Bostwick JM, Pankratz VS. Affective disorders and suicide risk: a reexamination. *American Journal of Psychiatry* 2000;157(12):1925–32.
68. Plana-Ripoll O, Pedersen CB, Agerbo E, et al. A comprehensive analysis of mortality-related health metrics associated with mental disorders: a nationwide, register-based cohort study. *Lancet* 2019;394(10211):1827–35.
69. Furukawa TA. Assessment of mood: guides for clinicians. *Journal of Psychosomatic Research* 2010;68 (6):581–9.
70. Zigmond AS, Snaith RP. The hospital anxiety and depression scale. *Acta Psychiatrica Scandinavica* 1983;67 (6):361–70.
71. Spitzer RL, Kroenke K, Williams JB, et al. A brief measure for assessing generalized anxiety disorder: the GAD-7. *Archives of Internal Medicine* 2006;166(10):1092–7.
72. Forty L, Kelly M, Jones L, et al. Reducing the Hypomania Checklist (HCL-32) to a 16-item version. *Journal of Affective Disorders* 2010;124 (3):351–6.

Causes of Depression

Glyn Lewis, Gemma Lewis and Ramya Srinivasan

Depression is a leading cause of disability in high- and middle-income countries and is of increasing relative burden in low-income countries. The Global Burden of Disease study illustrates how depression is increasing as a proportion of all the disability resulting from illness.[1] This is because we know how to prevent other major causes of disability such as cardiovascular disease and infection so their incidence is on the decline. Meanwhile, there is evidence that rates of depression are rising slightly. In order to have an impact on this major public health burden, we will need to devise preventive strategies to reduce the incidence. As depression is a continuum, much of the disability is experienced by larger numbers of those with mild and moderate levels of depression who might not seek treatment for themselves. Therefore, effective preventive strategies applied to the whole population will have more widespread benefits than interventions simply targeted to those at high risk.[2] In order to develop preventive interventions, we need to know what causes depression.

Causation and What It Means

Before we can answer the question 'What causes depression?', we need to define 'cause'. This is not quite as straightforward as it might seem, and we have to distinguish the use of 'cause' in everyday language and its use when applied to disease and illness. Epidemiology is particularly concerned with causes, and so we will explain the concept of causation from that perspective.

The term 'risk factor' is often used in relation to causes. Risk factor sounds a bit ambiguous, and that is no doubt intentional, given the difficulty of establishing causation. However, in this chapter, we will use 'risk factor' synonymously with a cause or hypothesised cause of illness.

Knowing the causes of illness are important for several reasons. Most important is that once we have identified a risk factor or cause, then we can often devise and evaluate interventions to reduce the frequency of risk factors in the population, and that should then reduce the incidence of illness. Our patients often ask us what has caused their own illness, a question that is usually difficult to answer. Medicine is a highly pragmatic discipline, but we should not underestimate the importance of understanding illness and providing explanations to patients even if there is little we can do to affect the outcome. Knowing about causes can also sometimes tell us about mechanisms of illness that in turn might suggest treatments or interventions.

Causes and Mechanisms

Epidemiology tends to be primarily concerned with causes outside the individual or with genetic causes (see Chapter 1). This is in contrast to the mechanisms of disease within an individual. For example, early stressors (a likely risk factor for depression) might lead to changes in reward pathways in the brain. There is still a likely chain of 'causal events' within the brain, and these then lead to the symptoms of depression such as anhedonia or lack of motivation. In a similar way, there are genes that increase the risk of depression. Those genes will code for proteins that will in turn influence molecular mechanisms and so ultimately, through a chain of mechanisms, affect the risk of depression. In both these examples, we think it is helpful to distinguish between the cause that resides in the environment or in our genes and the mechanisms or neurobiology of illness that then explain, within the individual, how those causes lead to illness. It can sometimes be more difficult to disentangle causal relationships in the realm of neurobiology. In this chapter, we will primarily be concerned with causes outside the individual, though we will also discuss possible mechanisms.

'Neither Necessary nor Sufficient'

The dominant model of cause in medicine and psychiatry is often referred to with the phrase 'multifactorial aetiology'. Perhaps single-gene disorders can have a single cause, but this is uncommon. Most illnesses have a wide range of causes. One definition of a cause is 'something that increases the incidence of illness', though something that reduces the incidence also has a causal relationship. If a cause is 'sufficient', it means that illness is inevitable. A 'necessary' cause means that the illness cannot occur unless the cause is present (but the illness might not be inevitable). The measles infection is a good example of a necessary cause as the measles illness has to require the measles virus, but the virus alone is not a sufficient cause. Many people are exposed to the virus without developing the illness. It is difficult to give examples of sufficient single causes except for single-gene disorders.

If we take the example of heart disease, there is good evidence that most causes are neither necessary nor sufficient.

Someone can smoke cigarettes all their life without developing heart disease while people who do not smoke can develop heart disease. If we stop people smoking, their risk (or probability) of developing heart disease will be reduced. This pattern of causes that are neither necessary nor sufficient is the norm when causation is understood within medicine.

It seems very likely that depression will also have a multifactorial aetiology in which causes are neither necessary nor sufficient. The potential risk factors include, for example, such things as genes, early adversity and unemployment, and all the evidence suggests these fit the usual multifactorial model. The evidence also suggests that such risk factors combine so that someone who has all three is much more likely to develop illness than someone with just a single risk factor.

Patients often ask us about the causes of their own illness and might have their own thoughts of past events that might be important. Explaining that causes are multifactorial could be helpful in putting less emphasis on particular events and identifying other current problems that could be addressed. Patients want to understand why they have become ill, and of course, we have few answers at present. Nevertheless, we think explaining the overall model of many causes – none of which are overwhelmingly important – is helpful as a way of framing their illness.

How Do We Identify Causes?

Epidemiology is concerned with identifying causes or risk factors. This is almost always done using observational studies, a term used to contrast with randomised controlled trials. In other words, we study the association between potential risk factors and the later incidence of depression in a group of people. We cannot intervene or carry out a randomised trial, for example, by increasing level of stress or making people unemployed. So, we have to rely upon observing what happens to those who have experienced stress or become unemployed and investigating whether they have a higher rate of depression.

The use of observational data leads to an important and universal problem when interpreting results of such studies. Without randomisation, the possibility of confounding is always present. So, people who experience stress or become unemployed will be different from people without those experiences in many different ways. Those other differences could confound the relationship between unemployment and depression and lead to a spurious association (or sometimes hide an association that is really there). Epidemiologists go to great lengths to adjust for confounders, but there is always a residual doubt about being certain that a risk factor does cause an illness. In general, we can probably never be certain that something does cause illness because we can never be certain that we have adequately adjusted for all confounders (not to mention other methodological problems such as bias and the role of chance).

Depression is common, and there have been many cross-sectional surveys of the general population that have studied associations between the prevalence of depression and a range of potential risk factors. However, cohort or longitudinal data will be much more persuasive in trying to infer causation.

Why Do We Need Longitudinal Studies to Investigate the Determinants of Illness?

The answer to this question relates to the complex issue of disentangling cause and effect. Why can't we take people who currently have depression and ask them about their history of exposure to potential causal risk factors? Case-control and cross-sectional studies do exactly this. Case-control studies recruit a group of people with a certain illness (cases) and a group of people without this illness (controls). These people are asked about their previous exposure to potential determinants. Case-control studies have many advantages. As people with the outcome are purposely selected, case-control studies are often used for rare illnesses (like schizophrenia). Cross-sectional surveys identify a population of people – for example, all adults living in private households in an area – and then assess depression and possible risk factors in those individuals.

The main limitation of this approach is that once a person has an illness, it can affect their recollection of the events that preceded it, called recall bias. Any effect of the illness on recall would occur in those with the illness but not in those without. This recall bias can distort and invalidate the results of a study. In a cohort study or longitudinal study, participants are recruited ideally before they develop illness so recall bias does not affect cohort studies as the potential risk factor can be assessed before the illness has developed. Birth cohorts in which participants are recruited shortly after (or before) birth are particularly valuable in this respect because we can start collecting data on potential risk factors at the beginning of life.

Another potential source of bias in case-control studies occurs because of how the controls may have been selected. Controls should be representative of the population that the cases were selected from (i.e. the population at-risk of becoming cases). If they are not, selection bias can occur. For example, there is evidence that obstetric complications increase the risk of schizophrenia in case-control studies but not in cohort studies, probably due to selection biases that case-control studies are prone to.[3] Though, when case-control studies can be designed to minimise selection bias, they can provide more accurate answers.[4]

Only a small proportion of those with depression are identified or receive treatment in the health service so this makes case-control studies for depression very difficult, if not impossible, to carry out without the risk of introducing selection bias. Cross-sectional designs, which are less susceptible to selection bias, are a better design when investigating depression. Cross-sectional studies recruit a cross-section of the population, and an investigation is conducted at a single point in time. These studies are useful for assessing how many people have an illness at a certain point in time (prevalence). The Adult Psychiatric Morbidity Survey (APMS) is a large-scale national survey of private households conducted every seven years in Britain. The aim is to monitor the prevalence of mental health problems in order to inform the development of health policy and service provision. Four APMS surveys have been conducted (in 1993 and 2000, of the British population, and in 2007 and 2014, in England only). These repeated cross-sectional surveys use nationally representative samples and similar measures. They can therefore monitor changes in the prevalence and distribution (e.g. by gender, ethnicity or socio-economic status) of mental health problems over time. The APMS has shown that, since 1993, the prevalence of depression has increased. This increase has been larger and more consistent in women than men and particularly among young women (16–24 years of age).

Despite their value for monitoring prevalence and distribution, it is impossible for cross-sectional studies to provide valid estimates of cause and effect. Although cross-sectional studies often collect data on potential determinants, it is usually impossible to know whether the determinant preceded the outcome. For example, a researcher may want to investigate whether physical activity reduces the risk of depression. However, people with depression are likely to be less physically active than people without depression. If we measure physical activity and depression at the same time, we cannot exclude the possibility that the depression caused the levels of physical activity, instead of vice versa.

What Are Longitudinal Studies?

Longitudinal (or cohort) studies are large, time consuming and expensive. They often take many years to deliver answers to pressing research questions. Yet, they are often regarded as the bedrock of research on aetiology because they are the best method of identifying potential causes of illness. So, what are longitudinal studies, and why are they so valuable? The answer to this question relates to the complex task of disentangling cause from effect.

Longitudinal studies that investigate causes of illness start with a cohort of people without the illness and follow them over time to identify who develops illness. When the study begins, data on the potential risk factors (often called exposures in epidemiology) are collected. Participants are classified as exposed or unexposed for a potential risk factor and then followed as they age. As the study progresses, data is subsequently collected on outcomes (i.e. the illness under investigation, such as depression). The occurrence of the outcome is then compared among participants who were exposed to the determinant and those who were not. The hypothesis is usually that the participants exposed to the risk factor will experience higher rates of the outcome. For example, if unemployed people are more likely to develop depression, then that supports the hypothesis that unemployment has a causal relationship with depression.

The term 'cohort' was originally used to describe a standard military unit of Roman soldiers (the equivalent of a modern military battalion). In epidemiology, it refers to a group of people with a characteristic in common – for example, period of birth. Britain is renowned for its national birth cohort studies. The first was the 1946 National Birth Cohort study, later known as the National Survey of Health and Development (NSHD). NSHD began a few months after the Second World War and set out to answer questions about health and social policy before the National Health Service (NHS) was established in 1948. The study aimed to recruit all women who had given birth in England, Scotland and Wales during one week in March 1946. It successfully recruited 13,687 women (91 per cent of births that week). The study was originally intended as a one-off project to answer certain questions: Why had the national fertility rate in Britain been dropping? Were the costs of giving birth a deterrent to having children? How well were midwifery and obstetric services working? Despite these initial interests, NSHD continued to track participants as they aged and is now the longest continually running birth cohort in the world. It has been used for several studies identifying possible risk factors for depression. One study found that childhood deprivation, childhood stressors (e.g. parental separation) and low birth weight increased the risk of depression by age 54. Another study demonstrated an increased risk of premature mortality by age 68 among people with adolescent onset symptoms of depression.

Other British birth cohort studies include the 1958 National Child Development Study (NCDS), the 1970 British Birth Cohort study (BCS70), the Millennium Cohort Study (MCS) and the Avon Longitudinal Study of Parents and Children (ALSPAC). ALSPAC differed in recruiting pregnant women in the area around Bristol in the west of the United Kingdom. In 2017, researchers used the MCS to investigate whether depressive symptoms in fathers increased the risk of depression in their teenage children. The link between depression in mothers and depression in children was already well known. The researchers measured symptoms of depression among fathers when their children were nine years of age. Symptoms of depression in the children were measured at 13 years of age. The results showed an association between depressive symptoms in fathers and depressive symptoms in their children that was similar in magnitude to the effect of a mother's depression. These findings suggested that fathers should be included in family-based interventions to prevent or reduce adolescent depression.

The Limitations of Cohort Studies

Of all the observational study designs (e.g. cohort, case-control, cross-sectional), cohort studies provide the strongest evidence of cause and effect. However, they are not without limitations.

One limitation is that cohort studies often need to be large as the statistical power will depend upon the number of people who develop the illness during the follow-up period. Even in large cohorts, rare outcomes would only affect a small number of people, and this would limit the statistical power of the study. For example, there were only 30 people with schizophrenia in the 1946 Birth Cohort. Depression is of course much commoner than schizophrenia, and so this is less of a problem when studying depression as an outcome.

There are three main threats to the validity of any observational study including cohorts: chance, bias and confounding. The possibility that a finding is due to chance can be assessed through hypothesis testing (P-values) and should be reduced in large samples, but we still need to be cautious especially if results have not been repeated. The most common and potentially influential source of bias in cohort studies occurs because some people drop out over time (attrition), introducing missing data. As cohorts are often followed for decades, participants often drop out and are consistently different from those who remain. For example, people from poorer backgrounds are less likely to be followed up. These differences can distort the estimate of cause and effect. However, there are now advanced statistical methods to replace missing data, which should reduce the potential consequences of attrition bias.

The most concerning threat to the validity of cohort studies is likely to be confounding. A confounding variable can lead to a spurious association between exposure and outcome or reduce the size of the association. To be considered as a potential confounder, a variable must be associated with both the exposure and outcome but not be on the causal pathway between them. For example, researchers may observe that an unhealthy diet during childhood is associated with an increased risk of mental health problems, indicating a potential role for diet in the aetiology of depression.[5] However, after statistical adjustment for socioeconomic status, the association between unhealthy dietary patterns and symptoms of depression disappears.[5] This is because lower socioeconomic status is a cause of both unhealthy dietary patterns and depression. Statistical adjustments can be made for all potential confounders that the researcher knows about and has measured in their data set. However, statistical adjustment for confounders will usually be incomplete. Confounders may not have been measured in the data set, and those that were are likely to have been measured imperfectly. Confounding is eliminated in randomised controlled trials (RCTs), which are the best design for inferring causality in medicine and public health.

How Can We Strengthen Estimates of Cause and Effect in Observational Cohort Studies?

On rare occasions, natural experiments arise, and exposure to potential risk factors is almost randomly distributed (analogous to how the treatment is assigned in an RCT). This enables researchers to provide evidence of causal effects more convincingly. A well-known example occurred when British gas companies started decreasing the carbon monoxide content of gas in 1963. During the 1950s, carbon monoxide poisoning from coal gas used for cooking and heating was the most common form of suicide in the United Kingdom. After the gas companies started switching to natural gas without carbon monoxide, there was a sharp decline in suicide rates. Importantly, this decline only occurred in suicides due to carbon monoxide poisoning. Another example is the introduction of a casino in a community of Native Americans in North Carolina who were already part of the Great Smoky Mountains longitudinal study.[6] The Native American population received an annual income supplement from the casino during the study, and there was a reduction in the prevalence of psychiatric disorders in the young people after this point, though there was no apparent association in adults. This is good evidence to support a causal relationship between improved income and better mental health.

Modern epidemiology is continually improving the methods by which the causes of human illness can be inferred. This is important because, if an association is spurious or biased, any prevention effort that it informs is likely to be ineffective. Most methods of advanced causal inference aim to reduce the possibility of confounding. One example of these methods is instrumental variable analysis, which originates from economics. Instrumental variable analyses use a proxy for the exposure (i.e. an instrument) that, in principle, should provide an unconfounded estimate of the causal effect. For example, month of birth has been used as an instrumental variable for educational attainment at age 16 (exposure) to examine the association with drug abuse in adulthood. Month of birth is randomly distributed with respect to the outcome and all potential confounders. It is associated with the exposure because children born later in the school year tend to have lower attainment levels than those born earlier. Month of birth should therefore only show an association with drug abuse if this association operates through educational attainment. In this study, there was strong evidence that month of birth increased the risk of drug abuse, supporting a causal role for low educational attainment in the causal pathway to drug abuse.

In research on depression, most examples of instrumental variable analysis use genetic variants as instruments, a method known as Mendelian randomisation.[7] According to Mendel's laws, genetic variants should be randomly distributed in the process of producing the gametes that create the embryo. So, if a gene that causes, for example, a change in age of menarche is also associated with depression, that association cannot be a result of confounding. In effect, the gene variants are being randomly allocated at birth. One study used Mendelian randomisation to test the hypothesis that an earlier onset of puberty in girls caused an increase in the risk of later depression. The instrument was a genetic risk score for age at menarche.[8] This study found strong evidence that early menarche was associated with higher levels of depressive symptoms at 14 years of age and supported the association seen in observational studies. There is also evidence from

Mendelian randomisation studies that higher body mass index and obesity increases the risk of depression.[9] Sleep disturbances such as insomnia have also been found to increase the risk of depression in Mendelian randomisation studies.[10]

Mendelian randomisation is a potentially powerful approach towards studying causality. However, it does have limitations. It relies upon the assumption that the genetic markers can only be associated with depression via the intermediate variable. This can work well when the biological system is well understood and a single gene alters a potential risk factor. For example, there are genes that affect the cytokine IL-6, and Mendelian randomisation analyses support that these genes might cause depression, supporting some observational associations.[11] However, there are also many studies that generate polygenic risk scores involving tens or hundreds of genetic markers that might be associated with fairly complex potential risk factors. For example, polygenic risk scores have been generated for educational achievement. One large study found that a polygenic risk score for educational achievement was associated with a reduced risk of depression, indicating a potentially causal role for low educational achievement in the aetiology of depression.[12] In those circumstances, there is a real possibility that some of the genetic markers included in the educational achievement genetic score might themselves be directly associated with depression and not via educational achievement. However, there are now methods that aim to overcome this problem of pleiotropy, such as those used in the study by Yuan, Xiong, Michaëlsson, et al.[12] Mendelian randomisation studies also need very large samples to provide accurate estimates of association.

Differences by Gender and Age

Understanding differences in how depression is distributed within the population can inform hypotheses about causal risk factors. Depression is very common in the population overall, in women and men. However, one of the most consistent and robust findings in psychiatric epidemiology is that women are twice as likely to experience depression as men. This gender disparity in rates of depression first emerges at around 12–13 years of age. Before the age of 12 or 13, there is little evidence of a difference in depression between boys and girls. A few studies have even found that, during childhood, boys are more likely to develop depression than girls, though depression is fairly uncommon at that age. However, around the age of 12–13, the rate of first-onset depression increases sharply in girls but not boys. Later in adolescence, around the age of 16, there is a sharp increase in the rate of first-onset depression among boys. However, incidence rates remain higher in girls throughout adolescence and early adulthood. Around the age of 55, the prevalence of depression decreases in women and men, and though the gender disparity remains, it narrows slightly. However, even among older adults, women still have a higher prevalence of depression than men.

There are few studies that compare gender differences in depression across cultures and countries. In lower-income countries, studies of the epidemiology of mental health problems in general are sparse. However, the general pattern is that – in low-, middle- and high-income countries – women are more likely to experience depression than men. There is some evidence that, although women are consistently more likely to experience depression than men, the size of this gender difference varies across countries. This could be due to differences in the samples and methods used across studies. However, the possibility that the gender difference in depression truly varies in magnitude across countries (and is not due to a methodological artefact) cannot be ruled out. Poverty, unemployment and exposure to discrimination, violence and crime are more common in women than men, and these risk factors increase the risk of depression. These factors vary within and between countries. Geographical variation in the size of the gender difference in depression therefore seems plausible, though there is little evidence for this at present.

One study pooled data from representative studies of almost two million people in over 90 countries.[13] Women were twice as likely to experience depression as men. However, perhaps unexpectedly, there was some indication that this gender difference was slightly larger in countries that were wealthier. The researchers examined three indicators of gender equality (the percentage of women who use contraception, the percentage of women in executive positions and the ratio of women to adult men who are literate). For all three indicators, greater gender equality was associated with a larger gender difference in depression. The reasons for this finding were unclear, and methodological explanations cannot be ruled out. For example, gender equality indicators were only available for a subset of nations, and depression is likely to be interpreted and measured differently across countries. All studies in this analysis used measures of depression that were created in Western countries, with limited cross-cultural adaptations. Another study pooled estimates from European studies and produced a different finding. Across Europe, higher national gender equality is related to a lower prevalence of depression and a smaller gender difference in depression for some groups.

The reasons underlying the gender difference in depression are poorly understood. There are many theories, although the mechanisms are difficult to study empirically. It has been suggested that women are more likely to disclose symptoms of depression than men and that the gender difference is artefactual. Women are more likely to seek treatment for depression than men, but this is the case for most health problems. The gender difference in depression is present in general population (non-clinical) samples when people complete confidential self-report questionnaires. Observer bias (e.g. men not wanting to report emotional symptoms that are culturally stereotyped as female) is less likely to operate with self-report measures. It is worth mentioning that even though depression is commoner in women than men, suicide, substance abuse and schizophrenia are more common in men than women.

Potential explanations for the gender difference in depression can be divided into two broad categories, internal and external.[14] Internal factors refer to biological or psychological characteristics such as sex hormones or differences in cognitive vulnerability. External factors are environmental or societal such as poverty, bullying, violence, harassment, abuse or discrimination. Several risk factors for depression are more commonly experienced by girls and women, compared with boys and men, including physical and emotional abuse. However, the distinction between internal and external factors is an artificial one. The external environment in which people develop could also influence their own vulnerability to future stressors.

Difference by Socioeconomic Background

In high-income countries, unemployment, neighbourhood deprivation, and lower levels of income, education and social class have been consistently associated with depression. High levels of income inequality are also associated with mental health problems.

Theories to explain the relationship between the various indicators of socioeconomic status and mental health can be divided into social causation and social drift hypotheses. Social causation hypotheses state that exposure to lower socioeconomic status causes the onset of subsequent mental health problems. For example, poverty can lead to stress, adverse life events, physical health problems, social exclusion, stigma, discrimination, and reduced access to health, educational, economic and social resources. These risk factors can then increase the risk of mental health problems. The theory of social comparison has been used to explain associations between income inequality and depression. People may experience shame, helplessness and hopelessness, which leads to negative self-concepts. There is also the potential for social exclusion and segregation after exposure to income inequality. People may experience stigma, discrimination and mistrust in their community or social groups. This might reduce social cohesion within a community. The social drift hypothesis has generally been considered more relevant to schizophrenia and other forms of psychosis (often referred to as severe mental illness, SMI) compared with depression and anxiety (often referred to as common mental disorders, CMD). The social drift hypothesis states that a range of negative consequences result from the mental health problem, which leads to downward social mobility or stagnation. People with mental health problems might therefore drift into or remain in positions of lower socioeconomic status.

The social causation hypothesis is particularly relevant to understanding the determinants of depression. Cohort studies are needed to adequately test this hypothesis. Cohort studies have examined socioeconomic status at birth or during childhood and risk of depression during adolescence and young adulthood. One study of the ALSPAC cohort in the South-West of England measured socioeconomic status using four indicators: parental occupational social class, parental education, standard of living (material hardship, home ownership, car access) and financial problems in the family. Early exposure to low socioeconomic status (considered cumulatively across all indicators) was associated with an increased risk of first-onset depression between 10 and 20 years of age. When considered individually, each indicator of socioeconomic status was itself associated with an increased risk of subsequent depression. These results cannot be explained by social drift (or reverse causation) because the socioeconomic markers were all recorded at the birth of the child and so could not be influenced by the young person's mental health.

Poverty

Family poverty has been associated with a variety of physical and mental health outcomes, including depression. One birth cohort study in Australia investigated the association between exposure to family poverty and subsequent depression and anxiety. Poverty was measured according to total annual household income during the mother's pregnancy and when the child was 6 months, 5 years and 14 years old. The lowest income group was selected to represent families at or below the poverty level. Family poverty was associated with an increased risk of adolescents developing depression and anxiety at 14 and 21 years of age. The longitudinal relationship between exposure to family poverty during childhood or adolescence and an increased risk of subsequent depression has been reported in other cohort studies. In one randomised controlled trial, boys who were aged 8–13 years moved from public housing in high-poverty neighbourhoods to private housing in low-poverty neighbourhoods. Those who moved from high-poverty areas to wealthier areas experienced a reduction in depressive and anxiety symptoms compared to boys who did not move.

Poverty can be thought of as multidimensional (e.g. income, expenditure, assets, education, employment, food security, access to health resources, inequality). Absolute poverty uses a fixed level of income, and people at or below that level are classed as living in poverty. Relative poverty refers to a person's income in relation to the average income of the population in which they live. The effects of absolute and relative poverty on mental and physical health generally seem undisputable. However, understanding which components of poverty are the most important contributors to mental health inequalities could help refine public health strategies. There is also a lack of research in low- and middle-income countries compared with high-income countries. In one review of studies from low- and middle-income countries, a variety of dimensions of poverty were found to be associated with depressive and anxiety disorders. Factors such as education, food insecurity, housing, social class, socioeconomic status and financial stress were consistently associated with depression and anxiety. However, results were more inconsistent for other dimensions such as income, employment and household per capita expenditure. It is also likely that these factors operate in combination as part of a complex causal pathway.

Deprivation and Neighbourhood Environments

Studies have shown that high levels of deprivation in the area where people live can increase the risk of mental health problems. This effect of area deprivation has been observed irrespective of individual factors such as education and social class. For example, even if people have relatively high levels of education or income, area-level deprivation can still increase their risk of developing a mental health problem. Deprivation has been distinguished from poverty, though there is a strong overlap between the two. Deprivation has been defined as a person's unmet needs whereas poverty refers to a lack of resources to meet those needs. For example, a person who is financially wealthy could live in an area characterised by high levels of deprivation (e.g. poor local access to services, high rates of crime and unemployment) and vice versa. The Townsend index is a widely used measure of material deprivation within a population. It was first described by sociologist Peter Townsend in 1988.

The original Townsend index incorporated four variables:

- Unemployment (as a percentage of those aged 16 and over who are economically active)
- Non-car ownership (as a percentage of all households)
- Non-home ownership (as a percentage of all households)
- Household overcrowding

The Index of Multiple Deprivation (IMD) is now used in the UK as the government measure of deprivation. Seven domains of deprivation are considered and weighted as follows:

- Income (22.5%)
- Employment (22.5%)
- Education (13.5%)
- Health (13.5%)
- Crime (9.3%)
- Barriers to housing and services (9.3%)
- Living environment (9.3%)

Each domain has multiple components. For example, the 'barriers to housing and services' domain consists of levels of household overcrowding, homelessness, housing affordability and the distance to key amenities.

One longitudinal study of 30,445 people aged 40 years and older and living in England found that higher levels of area-level deprivation, assessed with the Townsend index, increased the risk of depression. This effect was observed independent of individual characteristics such as education and income and was stronger in men than women. There is some mixed evidence across studies, and this might depend upon the length of follow-up time in longitudinal studies (studies with longer follow-up periods tended to find less evidence of an association). However, based on longitudinal evidence, the effect of area-level deprivation on the risk of depression generally seems consistent and plausible. Another area-level factor that seems to contribute to the risk of depression is social cohesion. Social cohesion refers to neighbours knowing, helping and trusting each other. Lower levels of social cohesion in an area have been associated with an increased risk of depression. It is also possible that lower levels of social cohesion result from higher levels of deprivation, forming a causal pathway to depression.

Differences by Ethnicity

Evidence on whether the prevalence of depression differs according to ethnicity is largely inconsistent, particularly in the UK. A recent study found that, at age 14 or 15, ethnic minority children in the UK and Australia had lower levels of depressive symptoms than their white majority peers. A similar pattern was found in the Children and Young People's Mental Health Surveys in England. However, these studies combined all minority ethnic groups into one category, due to small numbers in some groups. When examined in five categories, rates of probable mental disorder were higher among 6- to 23-year-olds in the White British (18.9%) and the mixed or other (22.5%) groups than in the Asian/Asian British (8.4%) and Black/Black British (8.3%) groups. In the most recent APMS, the prevalence of depression was lower in men who reported their ethnicity as white other (1.7%) and black (1.85%) compared with other groups (Asian, 3.3%; mixed/multiple/other, 3.1%; White British, 3.0%). In women, the prevalence of depression was higher in black women (7%) than in other groups (Asian, 2.6%; mixed/multiple/other, 1.9%; White British, 3.9%).

In the USA, the distribution of depression according to ethnicity shows a more consistent pattern, though there are still some mixed findings. Non-Hispanic black and Hispanic people have been found to have a higher prevalence of depression than non-Hispanic white people. One study examined the intersection between ethnicity and socioeconomic characteristics (income, home ownership, marital status and education). Non-Hispanic black and Hispanic people had lower income and education levels and were less likely to be married or own their own home. Before accounting for these socioeconomic differences in the statistical models, non-Hispanic black and Hispanic people had 1.3 greater odds of depression than non-Hispanic white people. However, this association reduced in size and the direction reversed after accounting for socioeconomic differences between the ethnic groups. In these adjusted models, non-Hispanic black and Hispanic people had 0.8 times lower odds of depression than non-Hispanic white persons. This suggests that, in the USA, the higher prevalence of depression in certain minority ethnic groups could be partially due to socioeconomic inequalities.

Exposure to racism is a plausible risk factor for the development of depression since it can result in psychological, emotional and physical harm; trauma; marginalisation; discrimination; and a range of adverse social, educational and economic consequences. One review found that, among Black American adults, self-reported exposure to racism was associated with higher levels of depression and anxiety. Another review included data from all over the world on multiple ethnic groups (although over 80 per cent of studies were done in the USA). Exposure to racism increased the risk of depression and other mental health problems in cross-sectional and longitudinal studies. In the UK, one study used the UK Household Longitudinal Survey. Minority ethnic participants were classified as: Indian, Pakistani, Bangladeshi, Black African, Black Caribbean or non-white from other minority backgrounds including Chinese, Arab and mixed ethnic backgrounds. These participants were classified as having experienced or not experienced racial discrimination in the past 12 months. Cross-sectionally, participants who reported racial discrimination had higher levels of depressive symptoms than those who did not report racial discrimination. In longitudinal analyses, those who reported racial discrimination had higher levels of depressive symptoms two years later than those who did not report racial discrimination. It was unclear from this study whether effects differed according to ethnicity, and few studies have had large-enough samples to investigate this robustly.

One review applied a life-course lens to examine evidence for a longitudinal association between racial discrimination during childhood and adolescence and later mental and physical health outcomes. There was evidence that exposure to racial discrimination during childhood and adolescence increased the risk of subsequent depression.

Differences by Sexual Orientation and Gender Identity

Sexual minorities (e.g. people who are lesbian, gay, bisexual, queer or attracted to the same gender) are approximately twice as likely to experience depression, compared with heterosexuals.[15] Compared with heterosexuals, sexual minorities are also more likely to experience other mental health problems including anxiety, self harm, psychosis and suicidality. This mental health disparity between sexual minorities and heterosexuals has been observed across the life course and across countries though there is a lack of research from low- and middle-income countries.

The mental health disparity between sexual minorities and heterosexuals has been found to emerge early in adolescence. One birth cohort study in England measured sexual orientation at age 16 and examined the natural history of depressive symptoms in sexual minorities compared with heterosexuals.[16] The mental health disparity between sexual minorities and heterosexuals was found to emerge at around 11–12 years of age. A similar finding was observed in a Dutch cohort. It could be that, during early adolescence, young people who will later identify as sexual minority are perceived as different, or feel different, to their peers, even if the reasons for this are unclear. In the same birth cohort, gender nonconformity (rated by parents during early childhood) was associated with later sexual-minority orientation and mental health. An analysis of successive waves of the APMS showed that the mental health disparity between sexual minorities and heterosexuals has not reduced in magnitude over recent years.[17]

Most studies combine all sexual minorities into one group because there are often relatively small numbers within individual groups. The added rationale, from a clinical and public mental health perspective, is evidence that all sexual-minority groups are at increased risk of mental health problems compared with heterosexuals. The limitation of this approach is that sexual-minority groups have been found to have different mental health outcomes. Bisexuals, and bisexual women in particular, are consistently found to have worse mental health outcomes than lesbians and gays. One potential explanation for this is exposure to what has been described as double discrimination; in qualitative studies, bisexual people report experiencing discrimination from within the LGBTQ+ community as well as from heterosexual populations and wider society.

In contrast to the amount of research on the mental health of sexual minorities, there have been few high-quality population-based studies of mental health in trans people (transgender, non-binary, gender diverse) compared with cisgender people.[18] However, there is evidence that, compared with cisgender people, trans people are at increased risk of depression along with anxiety, self harm and suicidality.

Minority stress theory hypothesises that the primary cause of mental health problems among sexual-minority and trans people is exposure to stigma, prejudice and discrimination, in a society that promotes being heterosexual and cisgender as normal. There is evidence that, in schools, sexual-minority and trans young people experience higher levels of bullying, discrimination, exclusion and marginalisation than their heterosexual and cisgender peers. As adults, sexual-minority and trans people are more likely to experience many risk factors that are associated with depression. These include discrimination; loneliness; physical, sexual and emotional abuse; and barriers to accessing sexuality or gender-affirming health care.

Risk Factors

Origins in Early Life

It is often challenging to establish the impact of any single risk factor because risk factors are often linked to each other as well as with future adverse experiences. However, there is good evidence that certain risk factors for depression can be identified early in life; these include family history of depression, childhood adverse experiences and stressful life events.

Family History of Depression: Perinatal Risk Factors and Parental Depression

There is evidence that antenatal (i.e. before birth), perinatal (around the time of birth, before or after) and postnatal (after birth, usually within the first year of life) factors can influence the risk of future depression.

In-utero or perinatal factors such as low weight, premature birth, having younger (<20 years) or older (>35 years) parents and parental smoking have all been associated with an increased risk of subsequent depression in the offspring. Associations between these early risk factors and depression have been observed when the offspring are children, adolescents and adults.

Perinatal maternal stress and anxiety have also been associated with increased risk of offspring depression. There is also strong evidence that perinatal and postnatal depression in mothers as well as postnatal depression in fathers increases the risk of depression in their offspring. There has been less research on the effect of paternal depression and later offspring depression, but this association appears to be as important as maternal depression. The association between parental depression during the perinatal period and offspring depression is likely to be due to the influence of early-life environmental factors including parenting, underlying genetic susceptibilities towards low mood and – in the case of maternal antenatal depression – possible in-utero effects that increase the risk of future low mood.

There is also evidence that parental depression during childhood can influence childhood development and the future risk of depression. Some studies find that up to 50 per cent of children whose parents have depression will go on to develop depression, with the risk of depression highest in those with both a parent and grandparent with depression. A family history of depression has also been associated with an earlier onset of depression and, therefore, a worse prognosis.[19]

Whilst genetic factors are likely to contribute to the increased risk of depression associated with family history, there is evidence that environmental and psychosocial factors play an important role. Such factors include parental mood, inconsistent parenting and development of a negative attributional style (see later). Parental depression could also lead to unemployment, poverty or parental conflict. Parental depression is more likely to be associated with offspring depression when these other psychosocial factors are present, as well as when parental depression is of greater severity or duration. Also, factors associated with depression such as temperament, emotional regulation and reward responsiveness have been associated with parental psychopathology and parenting. Maternal interactions with children have also been linked to neural activity during reward-related cognitive tasks, and different areas of neural activity have been linked to low parental warmth. There is less research on fathers in this area, but the effects of paternal depression on parenting interactions are likely to be as important.

Adverse Childhood Experiences

Adverse childhood experiences (ACEs) are associated with an increased risk of future depression. ACEs tend to refer to traumatic or frequent events, including child abuse (physical abuse, emotional abuse, sexual abuse and both emotional or physical neglect) as well as parental conflict or separation, domestic violence, family substance use or mental health difficulties, familial criminality or incarceration, and loss of a parent. ACEs are common, with approximately half of UK adults reporting having experienced at least one ACE. Abuse and neglect may be experienced at home, school or as part of wider society. ACEs are strongly associated with future risk of mental illness, including depression. Some studies suggest that ACEs may account for approximately half of adult cases of depression. ACEs may play a role in the intergenerational transmission of depression risk with research suggesting that parental experience of ACEs is associated with child depressive difficulties. Research also suggests that parental depression may be a mechanism in this causal pathway; ACEs could increase the risk of parental depression which, in turn, increases the risk of depression in the offspring.

Stressful Life Events

Stressful life events during adolescence are also associated with depression risk and may play a role in precipitating depressive episodes. For example, one study found that half of depression onset in a cohort of adolescents was preceded by a stressful life event during the past 12 months. In another study, stressful life events included serious illness or accidents, peer victimisation, moving school or home, changes to the family environment, relationship or friendship breakdowns or loss of a significant other. These stressful life events, experienced at or before 14 years of age, were associated with depression at age 17 in girls but not in boys. It is possible that these life events impact girls more strongly than boys, although this difference might also be due to methodological issues. It is also important to consider that anything that might be considered stressful (e.g. deployment to war, environmental events such as earthquakes) appears to be associated with depression and that these events can include those that are positive but involve significant upheaval.

ACEs and stressful life events might increase the risk of subsequent life events such as bullying, which is strongly associated with depression. Bullying is associated with family risk factors such as socioeconomic disadvantage, childhood maltreatment, more negative parenting practices as well as maternal depression during early childhood.

The Role of the Stress Response and Inflammation

The Stress Response

Many of the neuromodulators involved in the stress response affect brain function, and differences in the hormonal systems involved in the stress response have been associated with depression. Corticotrophin releasing hormone (CRH) is released in response to stress and activates the hypothalamic-pituitary-adrenal (HPA) axis, resulting in release of adrenocorticotrophic hormone (ACTH), which is neuroactive and stimulates the productions of glucocorticoids, such as cortisol from the adrenal glands. Glucocorticoid receptors are widely located in multiple tissues as well as within the HPA axis itself as part of the inhibitory feedback loops involved in homeostatic regulation of the system. In addition to metabolic effects and immune actions, the HPA system has effects on brain function. Glucocorticoids are involved in neuronal processes including neurogenesis, neuronal survival and the sizes of neuroanatomical structures such as the hippocampus. There is also evidence that glucocorticoids are involved in cognitive functions such as memory formation, emotional appraisal and reward processing. Depression has been linked with increased HPA-axis activity; for example, it has been associated with elevated cortisol levels and altered cortisol reactivity, as well as increased activity of the adrenal and pituitary glands. This is thought to be partly related to reduced inhibition of the HPA system. The theory of allostatic load proposes that exposure to chronic stress, such as childhood adversity, leads to the overload of the homeostatic mechanisms that regulate the HPA axis. In addition to HPA-axis dysregulation in those with depression, there is evidence that early stress can alter the function of the HPA axis, and that alterations in HPA-axis function may be associated with an increased risk of developing depression. This may explain why stress experienced much earlier in life may result in an increased risk of experiencing depression much later. Cortisol levels have been proposed as a potential biomarker for depression, though the evidence for this is inconsistent. The potential role of cortisol is also complicated by the interaction between glucocorticoids and sex steroids, which undergo significant changes during adolescence – a time when depression increases substantially. Early-life stress and the HPA axis can affect the function of the monoamines associated with mood and affect (i.e. noradrenaline, NA, dopamine, DA and 5HT) via proposed epigenetic changes to transporters, receptors and those of associated neuromodulators. Much of the evidence for a relationship between the HPA axis and depression has relied upon cross-sectional and case-control studies, and there is little support for the hypothesis that abnormal function of the HPA axis is associated with depression in longitudinal data.

Inflammation

The immune/inflammatory response is another area that has been linked to environmental stress and depression in both adults and adolescents.[20] Higher levels of inflammatory markers have been reported in people with depression. Risk factors for depression such as ACEs are also associated with increased levels of inflammatory markers such as Interleukin 6 (IL-6) and c-reactive protein (CRP). This suggests a potential causal role for inflammation and the immune system in depression. There is also some evidence suggesting that inflammation may be associated with altered brain development or function and depression onset in adolescence; environmental risk factors, immune changes and altered brain development leading to vulnerability to depression may therefore be connected. This interaction between environmental stress and alterations in biological pathways may help us understand how prior experiences of early stressors can lead to vulnerability to depression. There is now evidence that earlier raised inflammatory markers are longitudinally associated with later depression, and as mentioned, Mendelian randomisation studies also support the hypothesis that this is a causal relationship.

Bullying

There is strong evidence that bullying is a causal risk factor for physical and mental health problems, which can also affect longer-term psychosocial and socioeconomic functioning.[21] Bullying is defined as a systematic abuse of power and intentional harm-doing or aggressive behaviour. Bullying can be direct (e.g. physical or verbal aggression) or indirect (e.g. social exclusion or spreading of rumours) and can be conducted in person or online (cyberbullying). Bullying is the most common form of abuse that children experience, with up to a third having experienced some form of bullying at some points in their lives. Young people who experience bullying are at increased risk of a range of adverse physical and mental health outcomes, and the effects can last into adulthood. Mental health problems associated with bullying include anxiety, depression, psychosis, self harm and suicidal ideation. Those who experienced chronic bullying or multiple forms of bullying are at the highest risk of depression, suggesting a dose-response relationship. Bullying may result in an increased risk of depression via a number of potential pathways. Bullying is a stressful experience and may therefore affect the stress response and may also result in an altered inflammatory response. Being bullied may also affect cognitive processing, such as the response to threat and social cognition, which may affect social relationships. Bullying is also likely to affect self-esteem and self-efficacy; bullying is also linked to poor school attendance, which may affect educational attainment and longer-term socioeconomic functioning.

Physical Activity and Sedentary Behaviour

There is good evidence that physical activity can prevent depression.[22] 'Physical activity' can be defined as any bodily movement that requires energy expenditure whereas the term 'exercise' tends to refer to more structured or planned activities where the goal is to improve physical fitness, such as running or weight training. There is evidence that even small amounts of physical activity (e.g. walking less than 150 minutes per week) can reduce the risk of future depression in people of all ages and genders. Structured physical activity or exercise has been found to reduce depressive symptoms in those with depression with moderate effect sizes. Related to physical activity, there is strong evidence that increased sedentary behaviour is associated with an increased risk of future depression. This is important to consider because, whilst physical activity and sedentary behaviour are related and might be considered extremes of a spectrum, it is important to understand and quantify the relationship between these behaviours. For example, it is possible to engage in high-intensity physical activity whilst also spending the majority of time engaged in sedentary behaviour. There is some evidence in other disorders, such as cardiovascular disorders, that these two types of behaviour have independent effects. In addition, it is important to understand whether there are differences in the types of sedentary behaviour given how common sedentary behaviours are. Sedentary behaviours are sometimes divided into mentally passive and mentally active. Mentally passive sedentary behaviours might include activities such as watching TV, listening to the radio or scrolling through social media, whereas mentally active sedentary behaviours would include activities such as using a computer for work purposes, reading books, attending a meeting or engaging in arts and crafts. This is a potentially important distinction, which requires further exploration. There is some evidence that mentally passive sedentary behaviours may be more likely to increase the risk of depression, whilst mentally active sedentary behaviours do not.

Physical activity may reduce depressive symptomatology and prevent depression via several complementary mechanisms. Physical activity not only initiates multiple biological changes within the body but also in the brain, and these changes are likely to act via multiple pathways that are relevant to depression as well as other disorders. There is evidence that physical activity can induce neuroplasticity and that disruptions in this process are related to depression. Physical activity is also involved in the regulation of the stress response and HPA axis, which, as previously mentioned, is dysregulated in depression. There is also evidence linking exercise to a reduction in inflammation levels, which have been associated with depression; in addition, low levels of physical activity have been associated with higher levels of inflammation. Further work is required to understand how exercise may be involved in the relationship between depression and inflammation. Physical activity also provides psychological benefits that are likely to be beneficial in relation to depression. For example, physical activity may improve low self-esteem, self-efficacy, negative self-perception, goal setting, sense of purpose, reward and poor body image, all of which have been associated with depressive symptoms. As well as these, engaging in regular, structured physical activity may help to improve social support, the lack of which has been linked to an increased risk of depression.

It is important to note that even though it is helpful to advise patients on taking regular physical activity, just giving advice is unlikely to have a positive impact on their mental health. The successful trials have always provided a good deal of supervised physical activity – for example, attending a gym class three times a week. Unfortunately, it seems people often stop the physical activity when the supervision is withdrawn. Nevertheless, some people can maintain regular physical activity, and this could have longer-term benefit.

Obesity

Obesity is associated with an increased risk of subsequent depression. This association is bidirectional in that depression is also associated with the development of obesity. Obesity has been found to be associated with inflammation, physical health problems and HPA-axis dysregulation that are also associated with depression. In addition, there is considerable evidence that obesity is associated with stigma, and this may cause psychological distress both via direct experiences of discrimination and the internalisation of weight stigma resulting in low self-esteem and body dissatisfaction. Obesity is also a known risk factor for eating disorders such as anorexia nervosa and bulimia nervosa, which are associated with depression. The relationship between obesity and depression has also been studied using Mendelian randomisation methods. These studies have generally supported the hypothesis that obesity plays a causal role in the development of depression.

Physical Health Problems

Depression is associated with a broad range of physical health problems, with an estimated 20 per cent of those with a chronic physical health problem experiencing symptoms of depression. Depression is also associated with poorer outcomes in those with physical health difficulties. Higher rates of depression are found in those with diabetes and metabolic syndrome, cardiovascular disease, autoimmune conditions, asthma, stroke, cancer, chronic pain syndromes and multiple sclerosis. There are bidirectional relationships between physical health problems and depression, with depression increasing the risk of physical health problems as well as physical health problems increasing the risk of future depression. It is also important to note that low mood can be a side effect of some medical interventions (e.g. steroids, hormonal treatments). In addition to the hardship associated with experiencing a physical health problem, experiencing physical health difficulties may affect motivation, self-esteem and the ability to engage with activities that reduce the risk of depression – for example, by limiting social relationships and physical activity. Physical health problems are also a source of potential stress and may affect the ability to work and socioeconomic status. There is also the possibility that some physical health problems and depression have overlapping causes – for example, that inflammatory mechanisms might cause both, resulting in their association.

Sleep Problems

Sleep problems such as insomnia, difficulties falling and staying asleep, night waking, and excessively short or long sleep durations are common and are associated with depression. Sleep difficulties are a common symptom of depressive episodes, a possible prodromal symptom of depression and an independent risk factor for future depression. Depressed people with sleep difficulties often experience more severe depression and can be harder to treat with poor sleep being a risk factor for relapse. There is evidence that patients with depression experience changes across all phases of sleep, with changes in REM sleep being the most obvious characteristic.

Sleep problems are more common in women than in men, and it is well established that depression is more common in women than men. The differences in sleep problems between women and men first become apparent from puberty onwards, at a similar stage to the differences in depression. It has been proposed that female sex hormones (such as oestrogen and progesterone) may be involved. The potential involvement of female sex hormones is supported by evidence that changes in sleep are associated with changes in the hormones associated with premenstrual syndromes (PMS) and menopause. Low testosterone levels may also be associated with poor sleep and depression.

There is evidence that non-pharmacological sleep interventions are effective at reducing depression severity and that sleep interventions may reduce the risk of depression. However, there seems to be a reciprocal relationship between sleep and depression in longitudinal data. People with sleep problems and without depression are more likely to develop later depression while people with depression and without sleep problems are more likely to develop sleep problems later.

Potential mechanisms that have been considered in relation to sleep difficulties and depression include inflammation and the HPA axis. Poor sleep has been associated with increased levels of inflammatory markers, and elevated inflammatory markers are also associated with poor sleep. Poor sleep may result in a chronic stress response and might also lead to heightened sensitivity to stressful life events. The circadian rhythm, a 24-hour biological rhythm of animal physiology and behaviour, plays an important role in the regulation of the sleep/wake cycle. Disruptions in the circadian rhythm and its regulatory systems have been found to exist in depression although the exact mechanisms underlying these relationships are not clear. Poor sleep can affect eating behaviour and is associated with weight gain and obesity; however, there is little research examining the causal associations in this area. There is also potential overlap in the genetic factors underlying both depression and sleep that require further investigation. It is also possible that existing studies have not adequately controlled for the fact that stressful life events might confound associations between sleep and depression.

Social Relationships and Loneliness

There is good evidence that social relationships have an impact on physical and mental health, with good social relationships being related to better overall health and reduced mortality. There is strong evidence that poor social relationships are a risk factor for depression. The components of social relationships that have been found to be associated with depression include social support, social networks, social connectedness and loneliness. Loneliness is experienced as a painful emotional state and can be defined as a discrepancy between an individual's desired social relationships and those they have. Loneliness is distinct from other aspects of social relationships and can be experienced even in the context of objectively good social support, contact and networks.

High perceived social support is associated with a lower risk of depression, whilst low levels of perceived social support are associated with higher levels of depression and poorer outcomes, with evidence for causal associations. Most of the evidence for social support relates to perceived emotional support, whilst evidence for instrumental support, work-related social support and objectively measured received social support (in contrast to perceived social support) is more contradictory. Similarly, a larger social network has been found to be a protective factor for depression with a more diverse social network (i.e. comprising family relationships as well as different peer networks relating to different contexts) being more beneficial. Evidence for social connectedness is overall more limited but does appear to be linked to a lower risk of depression, particularly in older adults. Related to this, social isolation is associated with future depression and loneliness and seems to be particularly common in older adults. However, there is also evidence that social isolation is associated with depression in young adults.

A number of factors may explain associations between depression and social relationships. Positive social experiences are rewarding and help people cope with stress, perhaps by increasing social support and reducing time for rumination. Poorer social relationships, including isolation and loneliness, might lead to reduced self-esteem and negative cognitions about the self, world and future. There are also potential biological consequences of positive social relationships, including on the HPA axis. More research on how perceptions of social relationships and loneliness as well as the interplay between such characteristics and social relationships is required; more focus on younger age groups is also required. Given the potential importance of social relationships in preventing depression and other health problems, there has been growing interest in social interventions and so-called social prescribing. There is some evidence to suggest that social interventions can reduce depression in adults. However, there is limited evidence thus far for social prescribing, and further research in this area is required.

Alcohol and Cannabis Use

Alcohol use increases during adolescence and young adulthood, and alcohol abuse and dependence have been associated with a range of adverse outcomes including premature death, accidental injuries, sexual assault, cognitive and memory impairments, and physical health complications. Alcohol abuse and dependence are prospectively associated with future depression. There is evidence that high levels of alcohol consumption (i.e. frequency and quantity of use) do not increase the risk of depression, unless there are features of abuse and dependence involved. There have been some findings suggesting that there may be gender differences in the relationship between alcohol use and depression, with stronger associations between alcohol use and depression in females than males; however, these findings are inconsistent. There is, as yet, limited research on the mechanisms underlying this association. However, potential mechanisms include disruptions in reward processing, along with potentially widespread biological, psychological and social consequences of alcohol abuse and dependence. Cannabis is another commonly used substance and is frequently used by adolescents and adults; in the UK, 4% of 14- to 19-year-olds report having used cannabis in the past month, and 26% of all 15- to 64-year-olds in the EU had tried cannabis during their lifetimes. Related to this, there is evidence that cannabis use – in particular, heavy use – is prospectively associated with depression. With regard to the use of other substances, whilst their use is highly likely to be linked to depression, the evidence base is less robust; this is likely due to lack of research in this area and the difficulty of carrying out any population-based studies because most other forms of substance use are less common.

Theories of Vulnerability

Psychological

Many environmental factors are associated with the onset of depression. For example, recent life events, intimate partner violence, bullying, low socioeconomic status, unemployment and deployment to war are all associated with depression. What is striking is that there is considerable variation in how individuals respond to these environments. It is impossible to eliminate all stressors in the environment, and even when reduction is possible, it often relies upon political and social change that is itself difficult to influence. Understanding more about how individuals might respond to stressors may be a fruitful way of informing potential preventive strategies.

Aaron T. Beck, the inventor of cognitive behavioural therapy (CBT), formulated a theory of depression that was published in 1967 alongside his therapeutic innovations.[23] His theory proposes that early experiences lead to the development of schema, rules or dysfunctional assumptions – these are all the same thing, but the nomenclature varies. These dysfunctional assumptions can be very idiosyncratic but often have a perfectionistic theme – for example, 'if I don't get top grades in my exam, then I am a failure, and other people will look down on me'. Cognitive behaviour therapists will often spend time eliciting and describing these dysfunctional assumptions, and patients will often have an account of early experiences that led to such beliefs. For example, the dysfunctional assumption mentioned earlier could arise if someone grew up in a family that emphasised success and achievement in exams or was in a school that created a great deal of academic pressure.

Beck's theory suggests that the dysfunctional assumptions are present irrespective of whether someone is ill or well. They only become important if an event arises that conflicts with the rule. In the earlier example, if someone carries on getting top grades, then they will be fine. The problems only arise if they were to get poor marks or, sometimes, when people leave school and university and find the environment at work is much less clearcut about what is or is not a success.

Another influential theory of depression arises from the concept of learned helplessness. Learned helplessness was a term that originally described a situation where experimental animals were given a series of uncontrollable electric shocks. The animal will then find it more difficult to learn a future contingency that allows them to escape those shocks. It seems that the animal has learned that nothing they do will allow them to escape the shock. Martin Seligman, the experimental psychologist who coined this term, argued for a parallel between this observation and depression in humans.

Some years later, in collaboration with two clinical psychologists, Abramson and Teasdale, a revised theory based loosely on learned helplessness was proposed. They suggested that the underlying vulnerability to depression resulted from an attributional style that attributed adverse life events to global, internal and stable causes. For example, if someone failed an exam, they would be more likely to develop depression if they thought this meant they would never succeed in anything (global), that it was due to a lack of drive or intelligence (internal) and that these characteristics would be unchangeable going forward (stable). This theory concerning attributional style now looks quite dated, and there is also a marked overlap with Beck's cognitive theory. For example, under Beck's theory, someone with a rule based on the importance of achievement would respond to a poor exam mark by explaining it as due to a personal failure. In effect, they will be attributing the cause of the poor exam mark to an internal cause, possibly with both global and stable characteristics. It seems likely that both theories are describing a similar kind of vulnerability to future depression. The learned helplessness theory though is less specific about how these attributional styles might have arisen in contrast to Beck's developmental emphasis.

There is now empirical research that supports both these theories. As explained, longitudinal evidence is very important here if we are to build evidence for a causal relationship. One problem experimentally has been how to measure these dysfunctional assumptions in research studies. One method is to ask people to endorse statements such as "My life is wasted unless I am a success" as used in the Dysfunctional Attitudes Scale and based upon Beck's theory. In contrast, the Cognitive Styles Questionnaire arises from the learned helplessness theory and asks people to imagine certain life events have happened (e.g. failing an exam) and then rate the cause of that according to the dimensions described earlier (global, internal, stable). Both these kinds of measure are associated longitudinally with later depressive symptoms, and most importantly, this association is independent of any pre-existing depressive symptoms. At present though, there is much less empirical evidence to support the idea that depressive symptoms arise as a result of early experience though there is evidence that there is a genetic influence on dysfunctional assumption measures from twin studies.

Genetics of Depression

There is now very good evidence for a genetic influence on depression incidence. Studies have indicated that depression is more common in the offspring of people who are depressed, but this could be due to shared environments rather than genes. The most convincing evidence comes from two sources: twin studies and genome-wide association studies.[19]

Twin studies compare monozygotic twins that have identical DNA and dizygotic twins that only share 50% of their DNA. Dizygotic twins have the same genetic relationship as ordinary siblings. Quantitative genetic modelling can compare the association between depression in the monozygotic and dizygotic twins and estimate what proportion of the variation can be attributed to genes. This results in an estimate of genetic heritability, and for depression, it seems the heritability is about 30–40%. This is much lower than for schizophrenia and bipolar disorder, where heritabilities of over 60% have been reported. So, in this sense, depression is less genetic than schizophrenia, though genes are still an influence.

Heritability is a difficult statistic to interpret and is also dependent upon the influence of the environment. If the environments were completely identical for twins, then the overall heritability would rise. These analyses also usually find that shared familial environment has a small influence on rates of depression. This also seems unlikely from a clinical perspective and might be because families tend to treat children differently. Nevertheless, the twin studies have found moderate genetic influences as described earlier.

Since the revolution in molecular genetics, scientists have tried to identify so-called candidate genes – such as those associated with the serotonin system – and see if these are associated with illness in case-control studies comparing those with depression and those without. Unfortunately, candidate gene studies have been very unreliable in their findings and so have been superseded by genome-wide association studies (GWAS). There is also now evidence that the serotonin system is unlikely to be a causal factor in the development of depression.

GWAS involve identifying genetic markers called single nucleotide polymorphisms (SNP) over the whole genome. This might involve several hundred or even thousands of markers over the 23 pairs of chromosomes. The distribution of markers can be compared between people with depression and those without. The method relies upon linkage disequilibrium. If the SNP is near a gene that is causal for depression, then you would expect a higher proportion of the people with depression to have that SNP. The results are then provided as a 'Manhattan' plot, where the statistical significance for the association with each SNP is on the y-axis and all the hundreds of SNPs are ordered according to their position on the genome on the x-axis (see Figure 3.2.1).[24,25]

GWAS is a highly robust approach towards identifying genetic markers. It is a hypothesis-free approach, and the main problem is that the large number of SNPs means many statistical tests are performed. This leads to a very high type-1 error rate. We usually have a level of $p=0.05$ for 'statistical significance'. When we have many thousands of tests, as we do in GWAS, the level of statistical significance has to be made much more rigorous and is usually set at $p=10^{-8}$. This reduces the power of the study, and so, very large sample sizes are required in order to detect real associations. A GWAS study for depression published in 2018 included 135,458 cases and 344,901 controls and identified 44 genetic markers.[24] These studies are only possible through a worldwide collaboration, with over 180 scientists contributing towards this major effort. The latest analyses now include 340,591 cases and 1,154,267 controls and have identified over 200 markers associated with depression.[25] This increase in identified markers with increased sample size is to be expected.

One of the limitations of the method is that we are not studying genes, meaning that we rely upon markers that may be near genes. However, the markers can then be used to identify likely genes nearby. What is also clear is that many hundreds of genes are likely to be involved in conferring the genetic risk of depression. The association between a single marker and the illness is very small. Each one of the markers confers a very small increase of risk. The odds ratios for individual variants are under 1.05; in other words, someone with the variant has an increased risk of depression of less than 5 per cent. So, it is only when all the markers are taken together that the increased risk of depression becomes important. Nevertheless, these methods are beginning to identify particular molecular pathways as playing a role in depression aetiology. The results so far indicate that pathways to do with immunity and inflammation could be important in addition to genes that affect synaptic function. Further work on identifying the pathways related to these genes could aid our understanding of depression and potentially lead to new interventions, but this is likely to take many years, perhaps decades, before these new interventions bear fruit. GWAS studies can also be used to generate 'polygenic risk scores' though, at present, these only account for a small proportion of the total genetic heritability of depression. Polygenic risk scores use markers across the whole genome to provide a measure of the overall genetic risk for depression. In aggregate, the genetic markers are much more predictive, though we are still far away from any clinical use.

One major concern of the current genetic studies is that they are almost exclusively studying people of European heritage.[26] There is now increasing evidence that the genetic markers associated with depression differ in other populations.

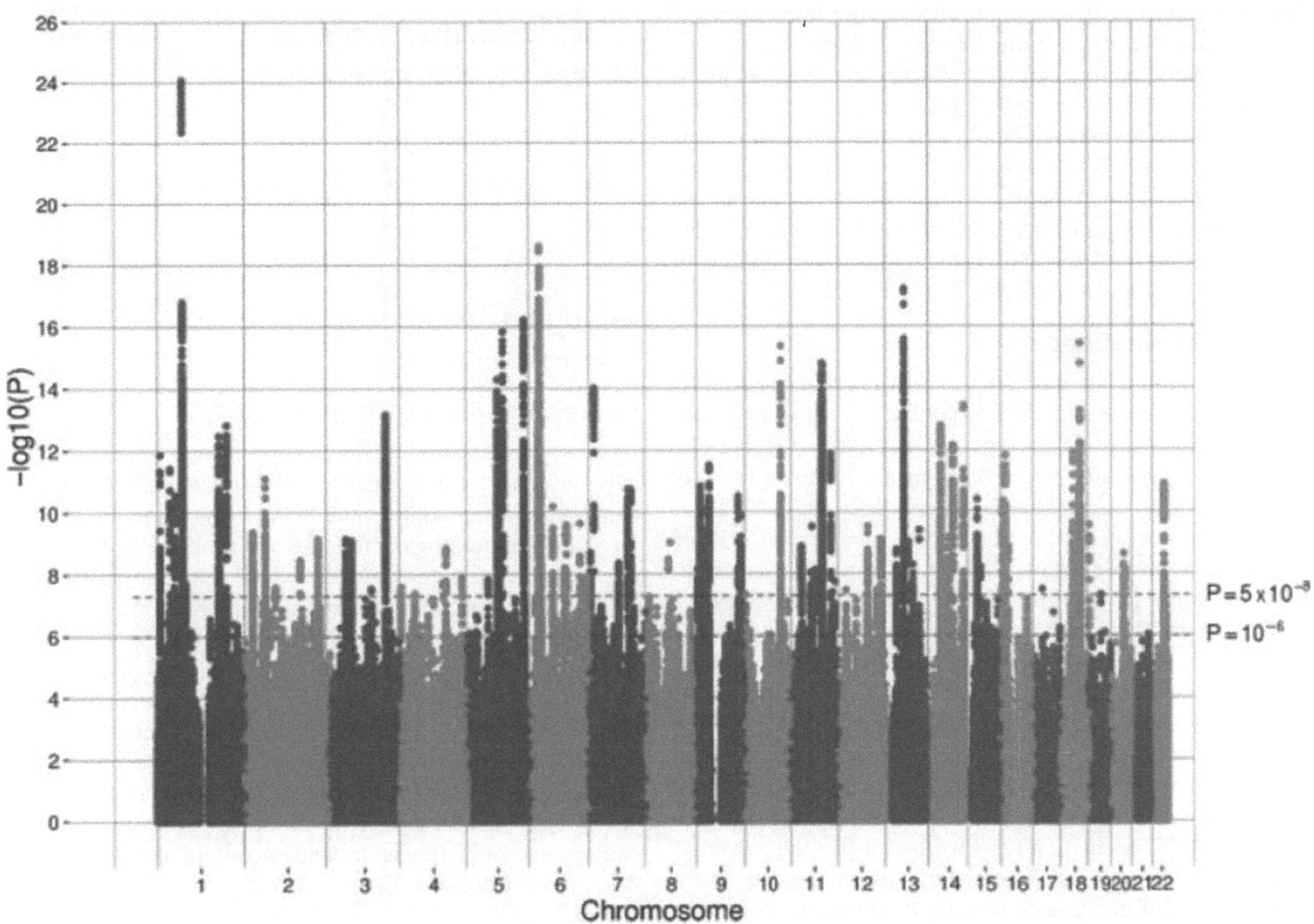

Figure 3.2.1 Manhattan plot of the observed -log$_{10}$ P-values of each variant for an association with depression in the meta-analysis (n=807,553; 246,363 cases and 561,190 controls).From: www.ncbi.nlm.nih.gov/pmc/articles/PMC6522363/pdf/emss-80873.pdf.

An important part of future genetic research will be to study how the association between genetic markers differs amongst people from backgrounds outside Europe. This will help us understand more about the genetic architecture of depression.

In other psychiatric disorders such as schizophrenia and autism, rare copy number variants, deletions and duplications of the genome have proved to be important. At present, these seem to be less important in depression, but further research is needed. Likewise, there is no convincing evidence at present that any single genes confer an important risk. These might be present but are likely to be exceptionally rare if they do exist.

Genes and Environments

Genes and environments are often contrasted as complementary causes of illness, but the relationship between the two can be more complex. There are two concepts that have acquired some importance in depression research: gene-environment correlation and gene-environment interaction.

Gene-environment correlation describes the phenomenon whereby measures that seem – superficially, at least – to be of the environment are also substantially affected by our genetic make-up. Twin studies have established a genetic influence on the reporting of adverse life events, parenting styles, social support and marital quality. This might arise for a number of highly plausible reasons. Firstly, an individual's genes and subsequent behaviour might elicit environmental responses from parents and others in the environment. For example, someone with a tendency for rebelliousness might affect the behaviour of parents and others towards them. A second possibility is that individuals might choose different environments as a result of their genetic make-up. If someone was more risk taking, they might select more risky environments. Finally, genetic influences could also lead to rating your environment as worse, even if the reality was less adverse.

The existence of gene-environment correlation has implications when we are looking for causes of illness. When we observe associations between supposed environmental measures and depression, we have to consider the possible role of genetic factors. Genes could confound that relationship – in other words, causing both the disease and environment. Genes could also lead to behaviours that influence environments that themselves increase the risk of illness.

That distinction is clearly important for the implications of research and how to intervene to prevent depression. A good example might be that bullying in adolescence has a strong longitudinal association with depression. There are anti-bullying interventions for schools, and in principle, this might be a good target for prevention. However, some recent research has suggested that there might be genetic factors that increase the risk of bullying; so, if there is a causal association between the experience of bullying and depression, it might be less strong than it at first seems.

Gene-Environment Interaction

Gene-environment interaction has also been investigated in relation to depression. In 2003, Caspi and colleagues published a widely cited paper that reported an interaction between adverse life events and a genetic polymorphism in the promoter region of the serotonin transporter gene (SLC6A4).[27] In this context, an interaction means that the association between adverse life events and depression is larger in the presence of the polymorphism than when the polymorphism is not present. This area has proved very controversial, and there is still an absence of consensus about whether the life event and serotonin transporter interaction is supported by empirical studies and also whether gene-environment interactions are potentially useful in understanding causation.[28]

There have been a number of attempts to replicate this finding, and overall, the empirical data does not support the existence of the interaction reported by Caspi. One possibility is that this finding of an interaction varies according to the precise way that depression and environments are measured. However, there is no evidence that the serotonin transporter polymorphism is associated with depression from GWAS studies, yet this would be expected given the pattern of the interaction observed.

A more fundamental criticism of this area concerns the proposition that all human disease relies upon an 'interaction' between the environment and our genetic make-up. The use of interaction here is to indicate that disease occurs because particular environments do not suit our specific genetic make-up – that our genes are not adapted to all environments, and when they are poorly adapted, an illness might result. This proposition must be true. This observation is using interaction in its everyday use. In contrast, empirical studies are using interaction in a very specific statistical way that is dependent upon the precise assumptions of the regression model used in the research. As a result, it seems unlikely that the study of statistical interaction between genes and environment will advance the field.

Biopsychosocial Causation: Integrating Stressors and Vulnerability

One way of formulating the relationship between stressors and vulnerability is to consider stressors, interpretation of stressors and the physical response to stressors as three separate levels (see Figure 3.2.2). There is good evidence to support the

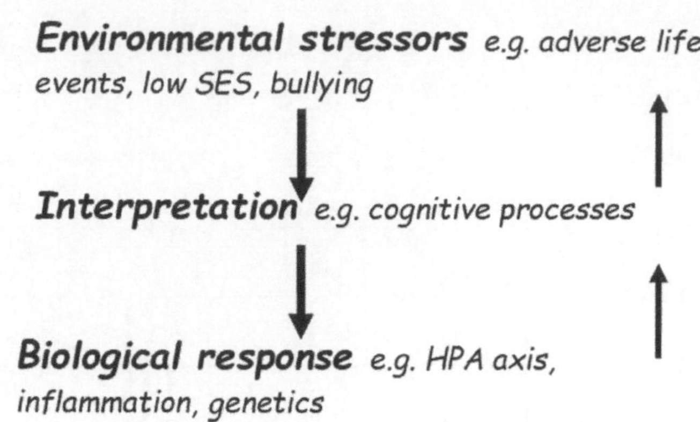

Figure 3.2.2 Environmental stressors and response.

hypothesis that environmental stressors increase the risk of depression. Beck argues that there is variation in how we interpret the meaning of stressors, and that variation will alter our emotional response. Finally, even if someone has the same stressor and same interpretation, then there is likely to be variation in our response. Of course, if we are the sort of person who has a large psychological or biological response to stressors, that will also influence our interpretation of stressors and could change our behaviour and change the stressors we are exposed to. This approach is one way of integrating the biological, psychological and social factors that are thought to cause depression and puts environmental stressors as a central theme in understanding the aetiology of depression (Figure 3.2.2).

Preventing Depression

The prevention of depression is an important public health priority, but at present, preventive strategies have not been widely adopted. This is due to various complexities. The risk factors for depression are complex, involving the interplay of biological, psychological and social factors. Also, some actions require changes in policy, long-term commitment and funding across a broad range of sectors including health, education and social care. There is also still some uncertainty about evidence for causation and the best kind of intervention that could reduce those causes.

There have been RCTs that have contributed to meta-analyses of interventions that aim to prevent, rather than treat, depression. These studies consistently report small effect sizes however; the numbers needed to treat (NNT) are sometimes comparable to those for medications used to prevent cardiovascular disease, such as statins. A problem with this evidence is, however, that most trials tend to involve psychological interventions delivered to those deemed high risk or with mild/sub-threshold symptoms. This kind of strategy is often called a 'high risk' approach towards prevention and is relevant to the prevention paradox, first described in 1981 by the epidemiologist Geoffrey Rose.[2] According to the prevention paradox, most cases of an illness will arise from the populations who are at relatively low risk of that illness. Only a minority of cases will arise from the populations at high risk of the illness because high-risk populations are usually much smaller than low-risk ones. As such, offering preventive psychological interventions for those at higher risk or with milder symptoms may not be the most effective large-scale preventive strategy and will be unable to prevent most cases of depression as they will likely occur in the 'low risk' part of the population.

For physical health problems such as heart disease and certain cancers, universal interventions aimed at the entire population have succeeded at prevention. These large-scale interventions aim to reduce exposure to common, modifiable causal risk factors. Universal interventions for mental health problems could transform prevention, but their development continues to lag behind those for physical health. The UK government has aimed to 'close the prevention gap' between mental and physical illness, stating that high-quality research on modifiable causal risk factors is essential to achieving this. The most effective universal preventive strategies are likely to be those that are embedded within existing health, education and social care structures.

Adolescence is a critical window for preventing mental health problems. Half of all mental health problems begin by age 14 and three-quarters by age 24. Most adolescents attend school, and schools are therefore one potential setting for universal interventions to prevent mental-health problems. A number of universal approaches have been investigated, but they target students as individuals (e.g. psychoeducation) and have failed to reduce symptoms of depression. For example, one trial investigated the effectiveness of classroom-based CBT for 12- to 16-year-olds attending secondary schools in England.[29] The intervention was the resourceful adolescent programme: a universal depression-prevention programme, which was delivered during personal, social and health education lessons. The intervention focused on emotion-regulation capacities, coping mechanisms and thinking styles, which are reported to protect against the development of depression. The programme consisted of nine modules and two booster sessions, each lasting about 50–60 minutes. Two trained facilitators led each session, working alongside the class teacher. However, there was no evidence that this intervention had reduced depressive symptoms 12 months later. Mindfulness interventions in schools have also been found to be ineffective. The recent MYRIAD trial was a very large effort to reduce emotional symptoms in secondary school children on the grounds that intervention at that age would help to reduce mental health problems in adulthood. The researchers compared a school-based group mindfulness intervention with the usual educational provision on mental health. They did not find their intervention had any influence on symptoms, and there was very low engagement of students with the mindfulness approach.[30]

It could be that 'whole-school' interventions, increasingly advocated by the UK Department for Education, would provide a better approach to preventing health problems. Whole-school interventions aim to change the school climate, culture and values by involving staff, students, families and communities rather than just concentrating on teaching coping mechanisms to individuals. By focusing on the wider system rather than the individual, whole-school interventions could be more effective. There are some evidence that whole-school interventions improve mental health, but many interventions are unsuccessful, and we need a better understanding of which risk factors to target. Aspects of the school environment that could be important to target to prevent depression include academic pressures, bullying, discrimination, social connectedness and inclusion. Other modifiable risk factors associated with future depression risk that may potentially be open to modification in large-scale universal prevention strategies include physical activity, physical health problems, body image, obesity, sleep problems, social isolation or loneliness, and alcohol or substance use.

Early recognition and intervention are often defined as secondary prevention. Sub-threshold or mild depression may be amenable to treatment with interventions that are generally considered preventive. A trial of a health-visitor-based intervention found that the risk of developing depression postnatally was reduced in women with sub-threshold symptoms who were not depressed.[31] Similarly, there could be scope to prevent intergenerational depression by identifying parental depression early on and treating it effectively. In addition, all parents could be offered high-quality early-years parenting advice, including on how to develop their child's emotional regulation, self-regulation, problem-solving and prosocial skills; such early-years interventions have strong long-term evidence for reducing the risk of depression alon with a broad range of other adult health and economic outcomes. For example, there is evidence that the Sure Start early-years intervention in England reduced hospitalisations among primary school children in disadvantaged areas. Related to this, children with neurodevelopmental differences and early-onset emotional or conduct disorders would be identified early and their families offered appropriately tailored intervention and holistic support as part of intervention and prevention of future mental health difficulties.

References

1. Walker ER, McGee RE, Druss BG. Mortality in mental disorders and global disease burden implications: a systematic review and meta-analysis. *JAMA Psychiatry* 2015;72(4):334–41. www.ncbi.nlm.nih.gov/pubmed/25671328 (accessed 17 June 2019).
2. Rose G. Sick individuals and sick populations. *International Journal of Epidemiology* 1985;14(1):32–8. academic.oup.com/ije/article-abstract/14/1/32/694724 (accessed 14 June 2020).
3. Geddes JR, Lawrie SM. Obstetric complications and schizophrenia: a meta-analysis. *British Journal of Psychiatry* 1995;167(6):786–93. pubmed.ncbi.nlm.nih.gov/8829748 (accessed 18 August 2022).
4. Lewis G, Pelosi AJ. The case-control study in psychiatry. *British Journal of Psychiatry* 1990;157(2):197–207. www.cambridge.org/core/journals/the-british-journal-of-psychiatry/article/

abs/casecontrol-study-in-psychiatry/D1AE628DFCF1A8F4F026FE30E72E350D (accessed 17 February 2022).

5. Peacock PJ, Lewis G, Northstone K, Wiles NJ. Childhood diet and behavioural problems: results from the ALSPAC cohort. *European Journal of Clinical Nutrition* 2011;65(6):720–6. pubmed.ncbi.nlm.nih.gov/21427741 (accessed 18 August 2022).

6. Costello EJ, Erkanli A, Copeland W, et al. Association of family income supplements in adolescence with development of psychiatric and substance use disorders in adulthood among an American Indian population. *JAMA* 2010;303(19):1954–60. pubmed.ncbi.nlm.nih.gov/20483972 (accessed 18 August 2022).

7. Wootton RE, Jones HJ, Sallis HM. Mendelian randomisation for psychiatry: how does it work, and what can it tell us? *Molecular Psychiatry* 2022;27(1):53–7. pubmed.ncbi.nlm.nih.gov/34088980 (accessed 19 August 2022).

8. Sequeira M-E, Lewis SJ, Bonilla C, et al. Association of timing of menarche with depressive symptoms and depression in adolescence: Mendelian randomisation study. *British Journal of Psychiatry* 2016;2010(1):39–46.

9. Tyrrell J, Mulugeta A, Wood AR, et al. Using genetics to understand the causal influence of higher BMI on depression. *International Journal of Epidemiology* 2019;48(3):834–48. academic.oup.com/ije/article/48/3/834/5155677 (accessed 19 August 2022).

10. Sun X, Liu B, Liu S, et al. Sleep disturbance and psychiatric disorders: a bidirectional Mendelian randomisation study. *Epidemiology and Psychiatric Sciences* 2022;31:e26. www.cambridge.org/core/journals/epidemiology-and-psychiatric-sciences/article/sleep-disturbance-and-psychiatric-disorders-a-bidirectional-mendelian-randomisation-study/91F50 052232BF115FED4DC4E1CD97D1B (accessed 19 August 2022).

11. Khandaker GM, Zuber V, Rees JMB, et al. Shared mechanisms between coronary heart disease and depression: findings from a large UK general population-based cohort. *Molecular Psychiatry* 2020;25(7):1477–86. pubmed.ncbi.nlm.nih.gov/30886334 (accessed 18 August 2022).

12. Yuan S, Xiong Y, Michaëlsson M, et al. Genetically predicted education attainment in relation to somatic and mental health. *Scientific Reports 2021* [Internet]. 2021;11(1):1–11. www.nature.com/articles/s41598-021-83801-0 (accessed 19 August 2022).

13. Salk RH, Hyde JS, Abramson LY. Gender differences in depression in representative national samples: Meta-analyses of diagnoses and symptoms. *Psychological Bulletin* 2017;143(8):783–822. www.ncbi.nlm.nih.gov/pubmed/28447828 (accessed 23 March 2020).

14. Bone JK, Lewis G, Lewis G. The role of gender inequalities in adolescent depression. *The Lancet Psychiatry* 2020;7(6):471–2. www.thelancet.com/article/S221503662030081X/fulltext (accessed 3 August 2021).

15. Plöderl M, Tremblay P. Mental health of sexual minorities. A systematic review. *International Review of Psychiatry* 2015;27(5):367–85. www.tandfonline.com/doi/full/10.3109/09540261.2015.1083949 (accessed 23 March 2018).

16. Irish M, Solmi F, Mars B, et al. Depression and self-harm from adolescence to young adulthood in sexual minorities compared with heterosexuals in the UK: a population-based cohort study. *Lancet. Child & Adolescent Health* 2018;3(2):91–8.

17. Pitman A, Marston L, Lewis G, et al. The mental health of lesbian, gay, and bisexual adults compared with heterosexual adults: results of two nationally representative English household probability samples. *Psychological Medicine* 2021;February 17:1–10. pubmed.ncbi.nlm.nih.gov/33592165 (accessed 13 April 2021).

18. Reisner SL, Poteat T, Keatley JA, et al. Global health burden and needs of transgender populations: a review. *Lancet* 2016;388(10042):412–36. pubmed.ncbi.nlm.nih.gov/27323919 (accessed 7 December 2021).

19. Thapar A, Eyre O, Patel V, et al. Depression in young people. *Lancet* 2022;400(10352):617–31. pubmed.ncbi.nlm.nih.gov/35940184 (accessed 18 August 2022).

20. Khandaker GM, Dalman C, Kappelmann N, et al. Association of childhood infection with IQ and adult nonaffective psychosis in Swedish men. *JAMA Psychiatry* 2018;75(4):356–62. archpsyc.jamanetwork.com/article.aspx?doi=10.1001/jamapsychiatry.2017.4491 (accessed 31 October 2018).

21. Bowes L, Joinson C, Wolke D, et al. Peer victimisation during adolescence and its impact on depression in early adulthood: prospective cohort study in the United Kingdom. *BMJ* 2015;350(June 2):h2469–h2469. www.ncbi.nlm.nih.gov/pubmed/26037951 (accessed 23 April 2019).

22. Kandola A, Lewis G, Osborn DPJ, et al. Depressive symptoms and objectively measured physical activity and sedentary behaviour throughout adolescence: a prospective cohort study. *The Lancet Psychiatry* 2020;7(3):262–71. www.thelancet.com/article/S2215036620300341/fulltext (accessed 27 June 2020).

23. Beck AT. The evolution of the cognitive model of depression and its neurobiological correlates. *American Journal of Psychiatry* 2008;165(8):969–77. ajp.psychiatryonline.org/doi/10.1176/appi.ajp.2008.08050721 (accessed 19 August 2022).

24. Wray NR, Ripke S, Mattheisen M, et al. Genome-wide association analyses identify 44 risk variants and refine the genetic architecture of major depression. *Nature Genetics* 2018;50(5):668–81.

25. Howard DM, Adams MJ, Clarke TK, et al. Genome-wide meta-analysis of depression identifies 102 independent variants and highlights the importance of the prefrontal brain regions. *Nature Neuroscience* 2019;22(3):343–52. www.nature.com/articles/s41593-018-0326-7 (accessed 22 August 2022).

26. Fatumo S, Chikowore T, Choudhury A, et al. A roadmap to increase diversity in genomic studies. *Nature Medicine* 2022;28(2):243–50. www.nature.com/articles/s41591-021-01672-4 (accessed 23 August 2022).

27. Caspi A, Sugden K, Moffitt TE, et al. Influence of life stress on depression: moderation by a polymorphism in the 5-HTT gene. *Science* 2003;301(5631):386–9. pubmed.ncbi.nlm.nih.gov/12869766 (accessed 19 August 2022).

28. Zammit S, Owen MJ, Lewis G. Misconceptions about gene-environment interactions in psychiatry.

Evidence-Based Mental Health 2011;13 (3):65–8. ebmh.bmj.com/cgi/doi/10.1136/ebmh1056 (accessed 21 January 2018).

29. Stallard P, Sayal K, Phillips R, et al. Classroom based cognitive behavioural therapy in reducing symptoms of depression in high risk adolescents: pragmatic cluster randomised controlled trial. *BMJ* 2012;345(7878): e6058. www.bmj.com/content/345/bmj.e6058 (accessed 2 March 2022).
30. Kuyken W, Ball S, Crane C, et al. Effectiveness and cost-effectiveness of universal school-based mindfulness training compared with normal school provision in reducing risk of mental health problems and promoting well-being in adolescence: the MYRIAD cluster randomised controlled trial. *BMJ Mental Health.* 2022;25(3):99–109. ebmh.bmj.com/content/25/3/99 (accessed 19 August 2022).
31. Brugha TS, Morrell CJ, Slade P, et al. Universal prevention of depression in women postnatally: cluster randomized trial evidence in primary care. *Psychological Medicine* 2011;41 (4):739–48. pubmed.ncbi.nlm.nih.gov/20716383/ (accessed 19 August 2022).

Chapter 3.3

Drug and Physical Treatments of Depression

Ryan Williams and Anthony Cleare

Classification of Drug Treatments for Depression

Antidepressants

A Word on Terminology

Current nomenclature for psychotropic medications is confusing, inconsistent and likely outdated!

Some examples:

- As 'SSRI' refers to a 'selective serotonin re-uptake inhibitor', 'SNRI' might reasonably be expected to refer to a 'selective noradrenaline re-uptake inhibitor' – NOT the case (SNRI = 'serotonin + noradrenaline re-uptake inhibitor').
- A number of antidepressants are 'tricyclic' (containing three connected rings of atoms in their chemical structure). However, so are a number of antipsychotics (chlorpromazine, clozapine), antiepileptics (carbamazepine), antihistamines (promethazine, loratadine) and beta blockers (carvedilol).
- What makes an antipsychotic 'typical' as opposed to 'atypical'?

In addition, drug classes are generally named according to descriptors based on indication (e.g. antidepressants, antipsychotics, mood stabiliser). However, during the course of this book, it will be apparent that these indications are fluid – 'antidepressants' are used to treat anxiety, 'antipsychotics' are used to treat depression and so on.

In recognition of the potential for confusion, efforts are underway to standardise the nomenclature based specifically on a drug's pharmacology and its mode of action. The traditional groupings have been used in this chapter as they will be familiar to prescribing clinicians. However, the inconsistencies in using this approach should be acknowledged. The moves towards a standardised nomenclature based on pharmacology and mode of action, such as that proposed by the Neuroscience-based Nomenclature group, should be welcomed. We would also caution at the outset that the exact mechanisms by which all pharmacological agents exert antidepressant effects remain uncertain. However, the mechanisms presented here represent the best understanding based on current available evidence.

SSRI (Selective Serotonin Re-uptake Inhibitor)

Examples

Citalopram, escitalopram, fluoxetine, fluvoxamine, paroxetine, sertraline

Background

First licensed as a treatment for depression in 1982 (zimeldine), SSRIs were felt to represent a major advance from previous available treatments due to their 'selective' method of action – resulting in fewer side effects and reduced toxicity in overdose. By 1993, fluoxetine was one of the most widely used medications in the world, prescribed to some 10 million people. Their popularity has persisted, and they remain so prevalent that metabolites are detectable in trace amounts in public water supplies.[1]

Mechanism of Action

All SSRIs act as selective inhibitors of serotonin (5-HT) re-uptake at the synaptic cleft. In broad terms, this results in an increase in synaptic serotonin and potentiation of post-synaptic 5-HT effects. The actual pharmacokinetics are somewhat more complex than this – initially, the increased synaptic 5-HT actually triggers inhibitory auto-receptors, resulting in the <u>reduced</u> release of 5-HT by pre-synaptic cells. However, repeated administration of SSRIs results in downregulation of these inhibitory auto-receptors over time, restoring 5-HT release and resulting in an overall increase (after around two weeks of regular dosing). As a group, SSRIs are all structurally quite similar, and most SSRIs have some minor degree of action on other neurotransmitter systems in addition to 5-HT.

Pharmacokinetics

All SSRIs are hepatically metabolised. They have relatively long elimination half-lives (see Table 3.3.1).

Low concentrations of SSRIs are found in breast milk (highest with fluoxetine and citalopram, lowest with sertraline and paroxetine).

Side Effects

Frequent side effects are headache and gastrointestinal disturbance – nausea, vomiting and diarrhoea have been reported in up to 20 per cent of clinical trials. Sleep disruption and insomnia are possible and may be clinically relevant, complicating symptoms

Table 3.3.1 SSRI elimination half-lives and cytochrome P450 inhibition

Agent	Elimination half-life	Cytochrome P450* inhibition
Fluvoxamine	15 hours	1A2, 2C19
Paroxetine	20 hours	2D6
Sertraline	26 hours	Minimal
Escitalopram	27–33 hours	2C19, 2D6, 3A4
Citalopram	36 hours	Minimal
Fluoxetine	146 hours**	2D6, 3A4

* 'Cytochrome P450' refers to a family of enzymes united by a common mechanism of action. Found primarily in the liver in humans, they are of singular importance in the metabolism and clearance of exogenous compounds (as well as playing a role in hormone production). Around 70–80% of all drugs in clinical use are metabolised by CP450 enzymes![2] Agents that act as 'inhibitors' or 'inducers' of these pathways can therefore result in significant changes (increase or decrease respectively) in the circulating levels of other drugs. An exhaustive list of substrates, inducers and inhibitors is beyond the scope of this chapter, but where these medications are introduced for patients already taking other medication, use of an interaction checker is recommended (there are many available online).

** N.B. While the half-life of fluoxetine itself is only 72 hours, it has a pharmacologically active metabolite (norfluoxetine) with a long half-life of 146 hours – necessitating a five-week wash-out period before the effects of the medication fully dissipate. This can complicate medication switches involving other agents that affect the 5-HT system.

resulting from underlying depressive illness – the effect can be mitigated by taking medication earlier in the day. Sexual side effects are common, may also be clinically relevant and are probably under-reported – anorgasmia is common in both sexes, delayed ejaculation is seen in men, and reduced sexual desire and satisfaction have also been described.

'Discontinuation' symptoms are possible – particularly with shorter half-life drugs (paroxetine and fluvoxamine) – and can be quite unpleasant (flu-like symptoms, insomnia, agitation, nausea, 'electric-shock'-like sensory disturbances), necessitating gradual down-titration when treatment is stopped. These are generally considered distinct from 'withdrawal' symptoms (seen with many classes of medication with addictive potential). Antidepressant use does not lead to dependence in the clinical sense, as key features such as craving/compulsion, tolerance and dose escalation are absent.[3] Usually discontinuation symptoms are short-lived (5–8 days) and self-limiting, as well as associated with higher doses and longer duration of use. However, a minority of patients may experience severe or prolonged symptoms and require extremely gradual reductions with small-dose decrements (see 'when and how to stop effective treatment').

There has been much debate regarding the physiological basis of so-called SSRI activation syndrome – a state of agitation, anxiety and emotional lability experienced by some within the first couple of weeks of commencing treatment with an SSRI. Current hypotheses have suggested a causative mechanism in the initial decrease in synaptic 5-HT resulting from auto-inhibition of pre-synaptic cells following SSRI initiation. Whatever the cause, an initial deterioration in mental state (followed by later improvement) is a recognised phenomenon that has been linked to increased suicidality, particularly in young people.

For the elderly, or those with physical comorbidities or polypharmacy, there are several other risks that must be addressed. SSRIs have been associated with 'syndrome of inappropriate anti-diuretic hormone' (SIADH) – resulting in hyponatraemia – and citalopram and, to a lesser extent, escitalopram are associated with a dose-dependent QTc increase. There is an increased risk of bleeding due to disruption of 5-HT dependent mechanisms in clotting pathways; gastroprotective agents are therefore recommended in those considered at high risk (see 'managing side effects' later).

Interactions

Over-stimulation of serotonergic pathways can result in serotonin toxicity – so-called serotonin syndrome – a medical emergency, classically described as a clinical triad of locomotor, autonomic and cognitive abnormalities. In practice, presentation can be diverse – with clinical features including restlessness (45%), confusion (42%), myoclonus (34%), hyper-reflexia (29%), diaphoresis (26%), shivering (26%), tremor (26%), hypomania (21%), diarrhoea (16%) and incoordination (13%).[4] In addition, delineation of the syndrome can be unclear because of both variation in the severity and overlap with another 'psychotropic toxicity' syndrome – 'neuroleptic malignant syndrome' (NMS), which classically occurs in association with antidopaminergic agents (e.g. antipsychotics). Where agents of both classes have been used, it may be possible to differentiate NMS by its slower onset (24–72 hours versus serotonin syndrome, which makes its appearance over a few hours) and specific neurological signs (Parkinsonian motor features, such as akathisia, bradykinesis, leaden rigidity and occasionally stupor).

Technically, serotonin syndrome is possible with any serotonergic agent (including most antidepressants as well as some antiepileptics, analgesics, anti-emetic agents, anti-migraine medications, St John's Wort and recreational drugs such as ecstasy and LSD). However, the risk is increased if multiple drugs are co-prescribed – and particularly high for specific combinations (e.g. SSRI plus MAOI). Lithium may also enhance the serotonergic effects of SSRIs through unknown mechanisms, thereby also increasing this risk. If such co-prescriptions are unavoidable, clinicians and patients should be vigilant for the signs of serotonin syndrome, particularly after dose increases, and seek medical attention urgently, if required.

SSRIs can inhibit cytochrome enzymes (see Table 3.3.1), resulting in increased levels of many other drugs that are metabolised via these pathways (including some antipsychotics, tricyclic antidepressants and opiates).

Contraindications

An absolute contraindication exists with co-prescription of MAOIs and serotonergic agents (SSRIs, SNRIs) due to the particularly high risk of serotonin syndrome. At least one week is required between discontinuation of an SSRI and the initiation of a MAOI (five weeks for fluoxetine, given the long half-life described earlier) – see 'switching treatment'.

SSRIs are contraindicated in patients experiencing mania as they tend to exacerbate manic symptoms. Indeed, they should be used only with caution for patients with bipolar affective disorder even during depressive episodes, due to their tendency to induce 'switches' to manic states and the association with mixed states, rapid cycling and cycle acceleration. Cautious use with adequate anti-manic cover is possible, although there is a relative lack of evidence demonstrating their efficacy specifically for bipolar depression. SSRIs may induce manic episodes even in those not otherwise predisposed to affective symptoms (so-called type 3 bipolar affective disorder).

Citalopram specifically is contraindicated in patients with pre-existing QT-interval prolongation.

Toxicity in Overdose

SSRIs have a low toxicity when taken in overdose. The greatest risks are of serotonin syndrome or QTc interval prolongation with associated cardiotoxicity. This risk may be more pronounced for citalopram compared to other SSRIs and relevant for those with cardiac comorbidities. However, in the majority of cases, toxicity is considered to be so modest as to be clinically insignificant.

Overdose is usually treated conservatively – except in the case of serotonin syndrome, which may require treatment with cyproheptadine (a powerful antihistamine that also has anti-serotonergic properties) and other interventions to prevent deadly hyperthermia.

SNRI (Serotonin and Noradrenaline Re-uptake Inhibitor)

Examples

Desvenlafaxine, duloxetine, venlafaxine

Background

Following their discovery in the 1980s, the huge popularity of SSRIs amongst prescribers led to concerted efforts to develop new antidepressant drugs. A 'middle ground' was sought between SSRIs (where the single method of action caused issues for those who could not tolerate serotonergic side effects) and older antidepressants (which were viewed as non-specific and caused a spectrum of adverse effects due to their broad mechanisms of action). In 1993, venlafaxine was introduced with the suggestion that selectively inhibiting both noradrenaline and serotonin re-uptake without significant other pharmacological actions may enhance efficacy but with fewer adverse effects than older drugs.

Interestingly, some SNRIs have proven to have rather diverse effects besides their psychotropic properties. Duloxetine has been associated with (admittedly modest) benefits in neuropathic pain and fibromyalgia[5] – it carries a specific licence for these indications and is often prescribed even in the absence of depression. Venlafaxine has been shown to be effective at treating vasomotor symptoms (hot flushes, night sweats) resulting from menopause. A further SNRI, 'sibutramine', was approved as an appetite suppressant for the treatment of obesity in the USA, before being withdrawn after it was associated with an increased risk of cardiovascular events.

Mechanism of Action

SNRIs (also known as 'dual action' uptake inhibitors) combine the 5-HT re-uptake inhibition of SSRIs with various degrees of inhibition of noradrenaline (NA) re-uptake. Whether this broader mechanism of action actually confers an additional benefit over SSRIs in terms of antidepressant efficacy has not been conclusively established, despite much research and debate, although meta-analyses do suggest a small benefit in efficacy.[6] It is possible that different 'clusters' of symptoms involved in depressive illness respond differentially to treatments targeting specific monoamine pathways (with noradrenaline specifically implicated in fatigue, apathy and anhedonia).[7]

Pharmacokinetics

Venlafaxine and desvenlafaxine show preferential 5-HT action at lower doses – their additional effect of NA re-uptake inhibition is dose-dependent. At lower doses, these drugs essentially function entirely as SSRIs, with NA re-uptake inhibition occurring only at higher doses (equivalent to >150 mg venlafaxine daily).

Duloxetine's relative affinity for 5-HT and NA re-uptake inhibitor is similar throughout its dose range.

All SNRIs may also result in increased dopamine (DA) neuro-transmission in specific brain areas (e.g. frontal cortex) due to reciprocal pathways involving the inactivation of DA by NA re-uptake (inhibited by SNRIs). The clinical relevance of these effects remains unclear.

Compared to SSRIs, the SNRIs have relatively short half-lives (see Table 3.3.2) and fewer active metabolites, necessitating the use of multiple daily dosing or extended-release formulations. The shorter half-life of venlafaxine is probably related to the somewhat higher incidence of discontinuation symptoms.

Side Effects

In line with their mechanism of action, SNRIs can cause many of the same serotonergic side effects as SSRIs, including headache, GI upset, sleep disturbance, discontinuation symptoms

Table 3.3.2 SNRI elimination half-lives and cytochrome P450 inhibition

Agent	Elimination half-life*	Cytochrome P450 inhibition
Venlafaxine	6 hours	2D6 (less than SSRIs)
Desvenlafaxine	10 hours	2D6 (less than SSRIs)
Venlafaxine (extended-release)	12 hours	2D6 (less than SSRIs)
Duloxetine	12 hours	2D6

* Varies between individuals

and issues with sexual function. In addition, elevation in noradrenaline from SNRI use can result in (usually mild) tachycardia, increased sweating and changes in blood pressure.

For venlafaxine, increases in blood pressure are dose-dependent, and regular blood pressure monitoring is recommended, particularly following dose increases or at high doses (>300 mg/daily). Duloxetine is less likely to cause such dose-related increases.

Interactions

See SSRIs – note that SNRIs on the whole are less potent inhibitors of the cytochrome P450 system.

Contraindications

See SSRIs – SNRIs are similarly contraindicated in patients taking MAOIs or experiencing manic symptoms.

In addition, pre-existing hypertension should be controlled before treatment with SNRIs and blood pressure monitored after initiation and dose changes. Other agents may be preferable for patients with a history of cardiovascular disease.

Duloxetine specifically should not be prescribed to patients with chronic liver disease due to an association with liver failure in this group (it may cause deranged liver function tests even in patients without pre-existing disease)[8] nor to patients with uncontrolled narrow-angle glaucoma, as it has been shown to increase the incidence of mydriasis.

Toxicity in Overdose

See SSRIs – venlafaxine may be more toxic in overdose compared with other SNRIs or SSRIs (fatal toxicity index of 12.7 deaths per million prescriptions compared with ~2 deaths for most primarily serotonergic antidepressants).[9,10]

Tricyclics

Examples

Amitriptyline, amoxapine, clomipramine, desipramine, dosulepin, doxepin, imipramine, lofepramine, protriptyline, nortriptyline, trimipramine

Background

Tricyclic antidepressants (TCAs) were one of the great innovations of psychopharmacology in the early 1950s. Derived from the revolutionary first-generation antipsychotics or so-called major tranquilisers (the first TCA, imipramine, was an analogue of the antipsychotic chlorpromazine), they were intended as sedatives but were repurposed as antidepressants after clinicians noticed an increase in mania amongst the patients they were trying to sedate! TCAs were widely used for decades before being supplanted by newer antidepressants with more favourable side-effect profiles. Their use in routine clinical practice is now largely restricted to patients with resistant symptoms that have not responded to other options, although they remain in wide usage for other indications such as pain management.

Mechanism of Action

TCAs are united by their similar (three-ringed) atomic structure rather than their mechanism of action per se. Pharmacologically, they are a rather diverse group with varying degrees of NA and 5-HT re-uptake inhibition. At one end of the spectrum, clomipramine has mostly serotonergic effects and behaves similarly to an SSRI; at the other end, lofepramine is almost entirely noradrenergic, via its active metabolite desipramine. The rest fall somewhere in between and may be considered similar to SNRIs.

However, TCAs are renowned for their lack of specificity in targeting other receptor systems – they have varying but typically high affinity for histamine receptors, muscarinic acetylcholine receptors and NMDA receptors (where they act as antagonists), opioid receptors (agonists) and sodium/calcium channels (blockers). The significance of this diversity is unclear – while it has been suggested that some or all of these effects may be instrumental in TCA's antidepressant efficacy, they also result in a range of side effects (including toxicity in overdose) that limit their usefulness.

Pharmacokinetics

Similar to their pharmacological profiles, the half-lives of TCAs vary widely (see Table 3.3.3). They are extensively hepatically metabolised, with tertiary amines (like imipramine) being metabolised to secondary amines (like desmethylimipramine or desipramine) via the removal of a methyl group. Many of the commercially available TCAs are metabolites of each other – amitriptyline is metabolised to nortriptyline, and both lofepramine and imipramine are metabolised to desipramine (this is important to bear in mind when considering half-lives and potential for accumulation).

The rate of metabolism is reduced in the elderly, leading to higher plasma levels and increased risk of toxicity.

Side Effects

TCAs have a broad and deterring range of side effects resulting from their action on multiple receptor systems.

As well as exerting serotonergic and noradrenergic effects (see SSRIs and SNRIs respectively), TCAs are potent antihistamines (resulting in sedation and increased appetite)

Table 3.3.3 TCA elimination half-lives and cytochrome P450 inhibition

Agent	Elimination half-life	Cytochrome P450 inhibition
Lofepramine	5 hours	Minimal
Imipramine	17 hours	Minimal
Desipramine	20 hours	Minimal
Amitriptyline	25 hours	Minimal
Lofepramine	36 hours	Minimal
Clomipramine	37 hours	2D6
Nortriptyline	38 hours	Minimal

and anticholinergics (blurred vision, dry mouth, hot flushes, constipation and urinary retention). Tolerance to these adverse effects may develop if treatment is continued, and side effects may also be less troublesome if treatment is initiated with low doses and then gradually increased. Postural hypotension can also be troublesome, particularly in the elderly. Tertiary amines tend to be more sedative than the secondary amines, which can be alerting in some patients. A comprehensive summary of the differing side-effect profiles of specific tricyclics has been published elsewhere.[11]

However, their blockade of sodium and calcium channels is particularly troublesome as it results in the potential for serious side effects at higher doses (or in overdose), including arrhythmias, rhabdomyolysis and metabolic acidosis. Although felt to be safe with long-term use, some recent research has suggested preliminary evidence of a link between long-term use of anticholinergic medication (including TCAs) and dementia.[12]

Interactions

TCAs are prone to interactions with a number of other medications due to their diverse mechanism of action, and we recommend using a dedicated 'interaction checker' such as that provided by the British National Formulary.[13]

As well as their potential for interaction with other serotonergic drugs (see SSRIs – particularly relevant for clomipramine as the most serotonergic TCA), the TCAs are highly metabolised by cytochrome P450 enzymes. Drugs that inhibit cytochrome P450 may therefore lead to increases in TCA blood concentrations and accompanying toxicity (particularly potent examples are cimetidine, paroxetine, fluoxetine, some antipsychotics and calcium-channel blockers).

Drugs that prolong the QT interval may increase the risk of cardiac arrythmias. Anticholinergic side effects may also be compounded by other drugs that have antimuscarinic properties. TCAs may enhance the sedative effects of alcohol, benzodiazepines and other CNS depressants.

Contraindications

See SSRIs – TCAs are similarly contraindicated in patients taking MAOIs or experiencing manic symptoms. Their risk of precipitating mania in vulnerable patients appears even higher than with SSRIs.[14]

In addition, TCAs are contraindicated for those with a history of myocardial infarction, arrhythmia, bundle branch block or QT prolongation, and they should be used only with extreme caution for patients with any pre-existing cardiovascular disease. Cautious use is advised for patients with epilepsy due to TCA's ability to lower seizure thresholds.

Toxicity in Overdose

TCAs are extremely dangerous in overdose, with well-documented cardiovascular and neurological toxicity (lofepramine is a possible exemption to this rule – it seems less toxic than other TCAs[15]). They are rapidly absorbed and result in arrythmias, seizures, metabolic acidosis, delirium, coma and death (usually due to ventricular fibrillation). The anticholinergic side effects of TCAs may provide early signs of a serious overdose (dry mouth, blurred vision, dizziness and vomiting). Emergency medical attention should be sought immediately if overdose is suspected. No antidote is available, but management of complications (correction of acidosis with hypertonic sodium bicarbonate, correction of hypoxia and electrolyte imbalance, benzodiazepines for seizures) may improve outcomes.

NaSSA (Noradrenergic and Specific Serotoninergic Antidepressant)

Examples

Mianserin, mirtazapine

Background

Mirtazapine was another product of the pharmacological developments that followed the discovery of SSRIs. The confusingly named NaSSAs have complex and still poorly understood pharmacodynamics, but they have become popular for their ability to be safely combined with SSRIs and SNRIs as well as for their complementary side-effect profile (useful for patients with insomnia and reduced appetite). They are widely used as an augmentory agent to treat patients whose symptoms have not responded to trials of monotherapy with other antidepressants – indeed, a recent meta-analysis suggests that the use of drugs antagonising the pre-synaptic α2 autoreceptor (largely mirtazapine, but also mianserin and trazodone) was the most effective combination strategy,[16] although it is worth noting that the efficacy of mirtazapine in this regard was not supported by a large recent RCT in UK primary care.[17]

Interestingly, NaSSAs have also found another niche as an appetite stimulant in veterinary medicine!

Mechanism of Action

NaSSAs selectively antagonise specific NA and 5-HT receptors (α2-adrenergic receptor, 5-HT2A, 5-HT2C, 5-HT3, 5-HT6, 5-HT7). The clinical significance of this selectivity is unclear. However, the net effect seems to be to enhance adrenergic and serotonergic activity in some brain areas (e.g. by blocking auto-inhibitory receptors) while avoiding the generalised increases responsible for serotonergic side effects. They also exert potent antihistamine effects.

Pharmacokinetics

Mirtazapine has an elimination half-life of 20–40 hours dependent on individual variation. It is hepatically metabolised by CYP2D6 and CYP3A4 cytochromes. Mirtazapine itself exerts minimal inhibitory effects on CYP isoenzymes.

Side Effects

NaSSA's favourable side-effect profiles are probably their greatest strength – their most common side effects result from their antihistaminergic properties, which cause sedation and increased appetite (with associated weight gain). However, these can often be turned to their advantage as many patients with depressive symptoms struggle with insomnia and reduced appetite (issues that can be compounded by the serotonergic side effects of other antidepressants). On the other hand, patients who are overweight or struggle with hypersomnia may be less well suited to these drugs.

Despite targeting 5-HT and NA systems, mirtazapine particularly is less likely than other antidepressants to cause common serotonergic and noradrenergic side effects (such as nausea, sexual dysfunction, sweating and blood pressure changes), probably due to its selective action on specific receptors.

Interactions

Compared to other antidepressant combinations, NaSSA + SSRI/ SNRI/ TCA are considered to be relatively safe augmentation strategies[18] and are widely used – the specific combination of venlafaxine + mirtazapine is so popular that it earned its own nickname among prescribers – 'California rocket fuel'.[19]

This is not to say that serotonin toxicity is not possible – there are (admittedly rare) case reports of serotonin syndrome resulting from many of these combinations (including venlafaxine-mirtazapine),[20] so clinicians should remain vigilant to this possibility – and combination with MAOIs is still contraindicated.

Concurrent use with cytochrome inhibitors or inducers can result in significant changes of up to 60 per cent in circulating levels of mirtazapine. A specific interaction exists between mirtazapine and clonidine that can result in hypertensive crisis – mirtazapine blocks clonidine's antihypertensive effects at $\alpha 2$ NA receptors.

Contraindications

Similarly to other antidepressants, NaSSAs are contraindicated in patients taking MAOIs or experiencing manic symptoms. NaSSAs are considered to be relatively safe in the event of an overdose – probably more toxic than most of the SSRIs (except citalopram), but less than TCAs or MAOIs.[21]

MAOI (Monoamine Oxidase Inhibitor)

Examples

Isocarboxazid, moclobemide, phenelzine, selegiline, tranylcypromine

Background

The first antidepressant, iproniazid, was discovered in 1952, during trials of potential treatments for tuberculosis. Proposed as an anti-mycobacterial agent (it is closely related in structure to isoniazid, which inhibits bacterial cell wall production), researchers noted that some patients treated with iproniazid became 'inappropriately cheerful' and more physically active.[22] On further exploration, it was shown to prevent the breakdown of 5-HT, DA and NA via inhibition of the enzyme monoamine oxidase (MAO) – this was suggested as a causative mechanism, and the 'monoamine hypothesis' of depression was born!

MAOIs are complex to use – iproniazid itself was withdrawn from markets due to its hepatotoxicity, and all MAOIs share the ability to trigger catastrophic 'hypertensive crises' when combined with specific foodstuffs and other medications, requiring regimented dietary control. As such, they are not widely used, although experience suggests that some patients respond to MAOIs when other antidepressants have proved ineffective.

Mechanism of Action

Monoamine oxidase (MAO) exists in two forms, MAO-A (which metabolises NA/5-HT/DA/tyramine) and MAO-B (DA/tyramine/phenylethylamine).

The traditional MAOIs (isocarboxazid, phenelzine, selegiline and tranylcypromine) irreversibly inhibit both MAOI-A and MAOI-B. This results in a potent and lasting increase in concentrations of NA, DA and 5-HT within synapses, as new enzymes have to be synthesised in order to relieve the blockade. This mechanism is responsible for the risk of dangerous interactions with other agents that affect the levels of these neurotransmitters.

Tranylcypromine has additional effects in that it acts as a NA re-uptake inhibitor and also stimulates DA release at higher doses, an amphetamine-like effect.

The newer MAOI moclobemide functions as a selective and reversible inhibitor of MAO-A only, and therefore has reduced propensity for interactions (although they are still possible).

Pharmacokinetics

MAOIs are extensively hepatically metabolised. They have short elimination half-lives (e.g. 1.5–4 hours for all agents). However, after irreversible blockade (i.e. use of any MAOI other than moclobemide), it takes around two weeks to re-synthesise MAO and restore normal enzyme function and catecholamine clearance. About half of the white population are 'fast acetylators', clearing these drugs and restoring normal MAO levels relatively quickly. A higher proportion of the population who have originated from East Asia are 'slow acetylators', which can be associated with higher plasma levels and a greater potential for side effects.

In practice, this means that a two-week 'wash-out' period should be implemented for all patients before the use of any other agents with a potential interaction (see 'Interactions'). This is not applicable for moclobemide.

In addition, they may exert some minimal (probably clinically insignificant) inhibitory effects on cytochrome p450 enzymes.

Side Effects

Side effects are fairly common, particularly with the older irreversible MAOIs, resulting from serotonergic (headache, nausea, insomnia, sexual dysfunction), noradrenergic (sweating, postural hypotension) and dopaminergic (tremor, agitation) effects. Peripheral oedema is also possible, especially with phenelzine.

However, the most dangerous side effect of MAOIs is the drastic increase in blood pressure ('hypertensive crisis'), which results from widespread vasoconstriction when they are combined either with other NA-increasing medication or sources of tyramine (which triggers NA release). This risk is greatly reduced with reversible MAOIs (moclobemide) or certain formulations of older MAOIs (e.g. selegiline slow-release transdermal patch), but it is not eliminated entirely.

People taking MAOIs generally need to change their diets to limit or avoid foods and beverages containing tyramine – see 'Interactions'.

Interactions

The MAOIs are infamous for interactions – not only with other medications but also food and other products that either:

1. are metabolised by MAO, as these can be boosted by several-fold.
2. impact the catecholamine systems to increase 5-HT, NA or DA activity – over-stimulation of these pathways can result in severe acute consequences (serotonin syndrome, hypertensive crisis and psychosis, respectively).

Between them, these categories encompass all other antidepressant medications, many commonly used recreational psychoactive drugs (including cocaine, opioids, amphetamine, mescaline, MDMA, PCP, DMT and ketamine) and many other medications, including local anaesthetic products (which commonly contain NA).

Tyramine-containing foods that should be avoided include strong or aged cheeses (aged cheddar, Swiss, parmesan, stilton, gorgonzola, camembert); cured, aged or smoked meats (dried sausages, hot dogs, bacon, corned beef, game); pickled foods (sauerkraut, kimchi, caviar, pickles); sauces (soy, fish, miso, teriyaki); dried or overripe fruits (raisins, prunes, overripe bananas or avocados, soybeans and fava beans); yeast-extract products (marmite, sourdough); and alcoholic beverages (beer, red wine, sherry, liqueurs).

We recommend using a dedicated 'interaction checker' such as that provided by the British National Formulary.[13]

Contraindications

Similarly to other antidepressants, MAOIs are contraindicated in mania. They should not be prescribed in combination with other antidepressants. The risk of hypertensive crisis prohibits their use for those with a history of cardiovascular or cerebrovascular disease. A rare contraindication also exists in phaechromocytoma (a catecholamine-secreting tumour), for obvious reasons.

Toxicity in Overdose

MAOIs are extremely dangerous in overdose, with a high propensity to cause serotonin syndrome or hypertensive crisis (this risk may be reduced for moclobemide specifically). Emergency medical attention should be sought immediately if overdose is suspected. No antidote is available, and management is largely supportive, but specific treatments for serotonin syndrome may be required (e.g. cooling for hyperthermia, cyproheptadine).

Other Antidepressants

Bupropion

Background -- Bupropion is a drug with a somewhat chequered past – shortly after its initial approval, it was withdrawn due to widespread incidence of seizures amongst those taking the drug at its (then) recommended dosage (600 mg/day). Subsequently, this side effect was found to be highly dose-dependent, and bupropion was re-introduced to markets with a lower maximum recommended daily dose of 450 mg/day. However, licensing agencies were rather cautious to re-welcome it, and it still does not hold a license as an antidepressant in many countries including the UK.

After further investigation showed that bupropion had additional beneficial effects as a smoking cessation aid (comparable in efficacy to nicotine replacement therapy),[23] it did gain a licence for this indication, making it available for off-label use as an antidepressant. This has been popularly adopted, and in many countries, bupropion now rivals SSRIs as a first-line treatment for depression.[24]

Unfortunately, it has not avoided further controversy completely – in 2012, manufacturers conceded a $3 billion fine for illegally promoting the unapproved use of bupropion for weight loss.

Mechanism of Action -- Bupropion acts as a NA and DA uptake inhibitor (unique amongst antidepressants) and an antagonist of nicotinic acetylcholine receptors.

Pharmacokinetics -- Bupropion has an elimination half-life of 15–25 hours (highly variable between individuals). It is hepatically metabolised by CYP2B6 cytochromes. Bupropion itself is a significant inhibitor of CYP2D6.

Side Effects -- One of the advantages of bupropion compared to other antidepressants pertains to its lack of involvement with serotonergic pathways, thereby avoiding sexual side effects.

Bupropion's most common troublesome side effects are headache, nausea and excessive sweating. Similar to SNRIs, it may result in (usually mild) changes in heart rate and blood pressure. It is alerting, which may result in sleep disruption and insomnia (but may also be useful for hypersomnolent patients or those who are oversedated by other medications).

However, it has several rare but serious side effects which must be taken into account. It lowers seizure thresholds and even causes seizures through unknown mechanisms – this is highly dose-dependent and very unlikely at currently recommended doses.[25] It is teratogenic – bupropion use by mothers in the first trimester of pregnancy is associated with increased risk of congenital heart defects. It has also been (rarely) associated with instances of hepatotoxicity and Stevens-Johnson syndrome.

Interactions -- Compared to other antidepressant combinations, bupropion is considered to be relatively safe when used alongside other medication targeting serotonergic pathways (e.g. SSRIs) due to its distinct method of action.

Combination with MAOIs is still contraindicated due to the potential for hypertensive crisis.

Concurrent use with cytochrome inhibitors or inducers can result in significant changes of up to 90 per cent in circulating levels of bupropion. As a significant inhibitor of CYP2D6, bupropion can result in an increased concentration of other drugs metabolised by this pathway.

Bupropion can potentially interact with other medications that affect seizure thresholds, including most antipsychotics.

Contraindications -- Similarly to other antidepressants, bupropion is contraindicated in patients taking MAOIs or experiencing manic symptoms. In addition, it is contraindicated in those with increased risks of seizures (epilepsy, increased intracranial pressure, acute alcohol or benzodiazepine withdrawal) or those with liver disease.

Toxicity in Overdose -- Bupropion is considered moderately dangerous in overdose, with potential for cardiotoxic effects as well as seizures. Large-scale investigations have found that bupropion is among those antidepressant agents with the highest potential for mortality in overdose (excluding TCAs and MAOIs).[26]

Agomelatine

Agomelatine is a novel antidepressant with an evidence base still very much under development. Preliminary studies did not produce convincing enough results to gain a license in the USA, where it is still not available, but it is used (albeit not commonly) in many other countries, and a recent meta-analysis indicated noteworthy effects.[27]

It acts on melatonin (a hormone that regulates the circadian rhythms involved in sleep-wake timing), and its intriguing pharmacodynamics have garnered interest regarding potential applications for patients with sleep-cycle disturbances. Agomelatine is an agonist at melatonin MT1 and MT2 receptors and a 5-HT antagonist specifically at 5-HT2C and 5-HT2B receptors. 5-HT2C is known to inhibit DA/NA release in the frontal cortex, so it is possible that agomelatine increases DA/NA transmission in a site-specific manner through a process of 'disinhibition' (blocking an inhibitory receptor), although the clinical significance is unclear.

Pharmacokinetics -- Agomelatine has a very short elimination half-life of 1–2 hours. It is hepatically metabolised by CYP1A2 cytochromes. Agomelatine itself exerts minimal effects on CYP isoenzymes.

Side Effects -- Similar to NaSSAs, agomelatine has a favourable profile in that it is sedating while avoiding the bulk of unfavourable side effects that come with non-selective stimulation of catecholamine pathways, and it is therefore potentially useful for patients with clinically significant insomnia.

Agomelatine's most common troublesome side effects are headache and nausea. It can also cause hepatotoxicity and elevation in liver function tests, necessitating monitoring at regular intervals (three weeks, six weeks, three months and six months after starting treatment). Limited evidence is available regarding the use of agomelatine in combination with other antidepressants – however, its distinct mechanism and lack of serotonergic activity means that troublesome interactions are unlikely. Combination with MAOIs is still contraindicated due to the potential for hypertensive crisis.

Concurrent use with cytochrome inhibitors or inducers can result in significant changes in circulating levels of agomelatine. Agomelatine can potentially interact with other agents that cause hepatotoxicity. Similarly to other antidepressants, agomelatine is contraindicated in patients taking MAOIs or experiencing manic symptoms. In addition, it should be avoided in those with histories of liver disease or ongoing alcohol abuse. Limited data are available on toxicity in overdose – however, based on its mechanism of action and short elimination half-life, agomelatine is expected to be relatively safe in overdose.

Reboxetine

Reboxetine is another novel agent that is not widely used, due primarily to a rather controversial evidence base. Independent meta-analysis of clinical trials revealed that some data had been omitted from early publications; analysis of complete datasets concluded that reboxetine was no more effective than placebo, with a significant side-effect burden.[28]

These results raised questions about reboxetine's efficacy that have still not been conclusively resolved. This, along with its relatively poor tolerability, has restricted its use – it is not licensed in the USA, and routine use elsewhere is not recommended. It may, however, be considered in patients where other strategies (particularly involving primarily serotonergic antidepressants) have failed.

Reboxetine functions primarily as a NA re-uptake inhibitor, although it may also slightly inhibit the re-uptake of serotonin at therapeutic doses.

Pharmacokinetics -- Reboxetine has an elimination half-life of 13 hours. It is hepatically metabolised by CYP3A4 cytochromes. Reboxetine itself is a moderate inhibitor of CYP2D6 and CYP3A4.

Side Effects -- Reboxetine unsurprisingly results in primarily noradrenergic side effects (see SNRIs), including increased sweating, tachycardia, dizziness and changes in blood pressure.

A 2009 meta-analysis found that reboxetine was the least tolerable of 11 antidepressants examined (not including TCAs and MAOIs).[28] Its distinct mechanism and lack of serotonergic activity means that troublesome interactions are unlikely. Combination with MAOIs is contraindicated due to the potential for hypertensive crisis. Concurrent use with cytochrome inhibitors or inducers can result in significant changes in circulating levels of reboxetine. As a moderate inhibitor of CYP2D6 and CYP3A4, reboxetine can result in an increased concentration of other drugs metabolised by this pathway. It has contraindications relevant to its noradrenergic method of action (see SNRIs) – cardiovascular disease, narrow-angle glaucoma and prostatic hypertrophy. However, similar to SNRIs, reboxetine is expected to be relatively safe in overdose.

Trazodone

Trazodone is an interesting case. Actually one of the earliest developed antidepressants (it was the first non-TCA or MAOI to be licensed), at the time it represented a significant advancement in specificity. Probably, it would be more widely used if not for the discovery of the SSRIs (and successors), which took this principle of specificity even further and largely supplanted trazodone in routine clinical practice. It lies somewhere between SSRIs and NaSSAs in its pharmacodynamic profile, with properties of both – and may be underused relative to these newer alternatives, despite evidence of comparable efficacy.[29]

Mechanism of Action -- Trazodone is sometimes referred to as a 'serotonin antagonist and re-uptake inhibitor' (SARI).

Similar to NaSSAs, trazodone is a selective antagonist at specific NA and 5-HT receptors (in its case, α1- and α2-adrenergic, 5-HT2A and 5-HT2B). However, unlike the NaSSAs, it is also a partial agonist at the 5-HT1A receptor and a weak 5-HT re-uptake inhibitor. It also exerts weak antihistaminergic effects.

Pharmacokinetics -- Trazodone has an elimination half-life of 10–12 hours. The metabolic pathways involved in its metabolism are not well characterised, although it is known to be hepatically metabolised, and CYP3A4, CYP2D6 and CYP1A2 are all likely to be involved. Trazodone itself is not known to exert inhibitory or inducing effects on CYP isoenzymes.

Interestingly, one of the metabolites of trazodone, meta-chlorophenylpiperazine (mCPP), is itself a serotonin-releasing agent with structural similarity to the recreational psychedelic MDMA ('ecstasy'). It is not known whether this is relevant to trazodone's clinical effects, but clinicians should be aware that patients administered trazodone may test positive for MDMA on urinary drug screens.

Side Effects -- See SSRIs – while trazodone is not an SSRI, it does share many side effects resulting from serotonergic activity (unlike NaSSAs), including nausea, headache, the potential for 'activation'/'discontinuation' symptoms and serotonin syndrome.

There are some notable differences – trazodone is sedating (due to its antihistamine effects), which may be beneficial for some cases and a reasonable indication to select trazodone over alternatives (e.g. SSRIs). It has a reduced propensity for sexual side effects. In fact, there is some evidence that it may be beneficial as a remedy for sexual side effects induced by other serotonergic medication,[30] and it has been associated (rarely) with incidences of 'overarousal', including priapism and spontaneous orgasm.[31,32] Postural hypotension can be problematic.

Interactions -- See SSRIs – note that trazodone is not known to inhibit or induce cytochrome P450 enzymes, but as a substrate, concurrent use with cytochrome inhibitors or inducers could result in significant changes in circulating levels of trazodone. Trazodone is similarly contraindicated in patients taking MAOIs or experiencing manic symptoms. It is also contraindicated during the acute recovery phase following myocardial infarction.

Toxicity in Overdose -- See SSRIs – trazodone is generally considered to be somewhat more toxic in overdose than most SSRIs (other than citalopram) but safer than TCAs and MAOIs. Similar to SSRIs, the greatest risks are of serotonin syndrome and cardiotoxicity, but uneventful recoveries have been reported after ingestion of doses some 20 times higher than the recommended daily dose, and most reported fatalities also involved other central nervous system depressants.[33]

Vortioxetine

Licensed in 2013, vortioxetine is the latest product of continued efforts to characterise the role of specific 5-HT receptors in depressive symptomatology. Vortioxetine benefits from advances in the understanding of serotonergic effects and exerts complex multimodal effects on 5-HT pathways. However, it is worth stating that the actual contribution of vortioxetine's various receptor interactions to its antidepressant effects remains to be established. Some uncertainty remains about whether it is indeed a clinically multimodal antidepressant – or rather, functionally equivalent to an SSRI – and to what degree it offers improvements on older, less-selective alternatives. There is some limited evidence that vortioxetine may have more beneficial effects than other antidepressants on the impaired cognition many patients with depression experience.

Mechanism of Action -- Vortioxetine exerts differential actions at a number of 5-HT receptors – acting as an antagonist (5-HT3, 5-HT1D and 5-HT7), a partial agonist (5-HT1B) and a full agonist (5-HT1A) simultaneously. It is also a 5-HT re-uptake inhibitor and has some as-yet poorly characterised affinity with β1-adrenergic NA receptors.

The clinical relevance of this pharmacodynamic complexity has not been established. To further complicate the picture, it has been suggested that vortioxetine indirectly modulates DA, NA, acetylcholine, GABAergic and glutamatergic systems.[34] Some early promising evidence of benefits for cognitive symptoms in depression has been proposed to be linked with specific activity at the 5-HT3 receptor.[35]

Pharmacokinetics -- Vortioxetine has an elimination half-life of 57–66 hours. It is extensively hepatically metabolised by cytochrome P450 enzymes – primarily CYP2D6. Vortioxetine itself is not known to exert inhibitory or inducing effects on CYP isoenzymes.

Side Effects -- See SSRIs – although with vortioxetine's specific interactions with 5-HT pathways, it was hoped that common troublesome side effects would be avoided (e.g. reducing nausea by employing 5-HT3 antagonism, a mechanism shared by some anti-emetic agents such as ondansetron); in practice, this did not turn out to be the case. Vortioxetine shares a very similar side-effect profile with SSRIs, including nausea, headache, sexual side effects, potential for 'activation'/ 'discontinuation' symptoms and serotonin syndrome – although side effects may be less common overall.

Interactions -- See SSRIs – note that vortioxetine is not known to inhibit or induce cytochrome P450 enzymes, but as a substrate, concurrent use with cytochrome inhibitors or inducers could result in significant changes in circulating levels of vortioxetine. Vortioxetine is similarly contraindicated in patients taking MAOIs or experiencing manic symptoms. There is only limited data available regarding the toxicity of vortioxetine in overdose. However, it is expected to be relatively safe and similar to SSRIs in terms of potential complications (serotonin syndrome, cardiotoxicity) and mortality.

Augmentory Medications

Antipsychotics (Dopamine Antagonists)

Examples

Aripiprazole, asenapine, brexpiprazole, cariprazine, lurasidone, olanzapine, quetiapine, risperidone, ziprasidone

Background

Antipsychotic medications have had a well-established role in the treatment of depression ever since it was first realised that mood was amenable to pharmacological interventions. In the early days of psychopharmacology, the first 'typical' (or 'first-generation') antipsychotics were found to be comparable to TCAs in terms of antidepressant efficacy,[36] but their risk of disabling, irreversible and dangerous side effects (extrapyramidal side effects, tardive dyskinesia and neuroleptic malignant syndrome) limited their use. However, they were always considered as an option (either as monotherapy or combined with TCAs) for those whose depressive symptoms were particularly severe, treatment-resistant or comorbid with psychosis.

Over time, older 'typical' antipsychotics were replaced by newer 'atypical' agents with lower rates of extrapyramidal effects, which only served to increase their popularity. The efficacy of many of these drugs as augmenting agents to antidepressants has been strongly supported by the developing evidence base. Along with other augmentation strategies, they are usually considered when depressive symptoms have failed to respond adequately to two or more adequate trials of antidepressant monotherapy (see 'treatment algorithms' in this chapter).

Studies have found little evidence for differential effects between different antipsychotics – one meta-analysis suggested there may be higher remission rates for quetiapine, risperidone and aripiprazole.[37,38] Another combination, olanzapine + fluoxetine, may be particularly effective for severe depressive episodes with psychotic symptoms.[39] Unfortunately, direct comparisons between specific atypical antipsychotics (or indeed, most augmenting agents) are lacking, and the choice between them is probably best made based on their side-effect profiles, which vary widely. Even with the atypical antipsychotics, side effects are a major consideration – studies have shown that discontinuation rates are four times higher in patients who are treated with antipsychotic augmentation alongside their antidepressant, despite the benefit for depressive symptoms.[40]

Note that depressive symptoms may respond to augmentation with atypical antipsychotics at lower doses than those typically used to treat primary psychotic disorders. For example, quetiapine was shown to be equally effective at 150 mg/day compared to 300 mg/day.[41] Recommended dose ranges for aripiprazole are 2.5–10 mg, for olanzapine 2.5–10 mg and for risperidone 0.5–2 mg/day.[42] Note that of these, only quetiapine actually holds a specific product licence for unipolar depression in the UK.

Also, note that clozapine – an atypical antipsychotic that is pharmacologically distinct from many others in this category and used specifically for treatment-resistant psychosis – does not currently have a role in the management of non-psychotic unipolar depression.

Mechanism of Action

All antipsychotics currently in use are united by their antagonism of DA D2 receptors (except for aripiprazole, which is a partial agonist but thought to exert antagonistic effects in situ). Different agents vary widely in their relative affinity for the D2 receptor and for various other receptors, both in DA systems and numerous others (NA, 5-HT, histamine, acetylcholine) – exact characterisation is beyond the scope of this chapter.

Clinical experience and the diverse pharmacodynamics of the atypical antipsychotics suggest that one agent may prove effective where another has failed; it is unclear the degree to which modes of antidepressant action are shared or differ between the individual drugs. Pharmacokinetics differ widely between specific antipsychotics. Differences in side effects may be the most important consideration when choosing between atypical antipsychotics as potential augmenting agents for an individual patient.

Most atypical antipsychotics are associated with some degree of sedation, increased appetite (with resultant weight gain and metabolic abnormalities) and sexual side effects. Notable exceptions are aripiprazole (which is generally considered to have the most favourable profile – it is activating rather than sedating, appetite-neutral and does not usually cause sexual side effects) and lurasidone (fewer sexual side effects and a more benign metabolic profile).

Most atypical antipsychotics also have the potential to cause lowered seizure thresholds and QTc prolongation to varying degrees, and so caution should be exercised when prescribing to patients with a history of cardiovascular disease or epilepsy. Regular monitoring of cardiovascular and metabolic parameters, as well as screening blood tests (full blood count, renal profile, liver function tests, prolactin), are recommended for all patients prescribed antipsychotic medication. Toxicity in overdose differs between specific antipsychotics. That being said, despite a range of potentially serious complications (including cardiotoxicity, seizures and neuroleptic malignant syndrome), most are considered fairly safe in overdose. Complications (other than sedation) are rare, and most do well with supportive management.

Lithium Salts (Lithium Carbonate, Lithium Citrate)

Lithium is the oldest psychotropic agent still in clinical use, although its mechanism of action remains as elusive today as in the 1800s! It has a rich history. Initially, it was applied therapeutically for its ability to dissolve uric acid crystals – hypotheses at the time linked these to a range of ailments from gout (correctly) to mania (probably wishful thinking). In the early twentieth century, it enjoyed a renaissance as a food additive (due to growing concerns about the adverse metabolic effect of sodium-based salts), replacing table salt and forming the main ingredient of a popular refreshment beverage (7-Up). Finally, in 1949, it was 'rediscovered' as an effective psychiatric treatment for mania after the incidental finding that it caused tranquility in lab animals.[43]

While its use as a mood-stabilising agent for disorders with a fluctuating affective component (e.g. bipolar disorder, schizoaffective disorder) is well established, its role in the treatment of unipolar depression is somewhat less certain. However, most available evidence indicates modest but significant efficacy as an augmenting agent alongside antidepressant therapy in treatment-resistant depression – in meta-analyses, 41% response rate with lithium vs 14% without[44,45] as well as a 59% response rate with lithium augmentation following failure of a trial of antidepressant monotherapy.[46]

Lithium did not perform particularly well in 'STAR*D' – 'Sequenced Treatment Alternatives to Relieve Depression', a massive trial sponsored by the US government (N=4,041) – which assessed different sequences of antidepressant augmentation, still considered one of the landmark studies in psychiatry – with only 16% remitting and a 23% rate of discontinuation due to side effects,[47] but this may have been confounded by patient characteristics or possibly inadequate dosing. While effective dose ranges and duration of treatment are not as well established for unipolar depression as for bipolar (where clear thresholds for manic and prophylactic phases exist), a growing body of evidence points towards greatest efficacy with plasma levels between 0.6–1.0 mmol/l[48] and a need to continue lithium for at least one year following remission to prevent early recurrence of symptoms.[49] Lithium may be particularly useful in relapse prevention. In a cohort of 120,000 patients admitted to hospital with depression in Finland, lithium use was associated with the lowest risk of readmission during long-term follow-up.[50] Lithium is also associated with lower suicide rates in both bipolar and unipolar patients.[49]

Mechanism of Action

Despite much investigation, the exact pharmacodynamics of lithium salts (to say nothing of the mechanisms by which they exert antidepressant effects) remain unknown. No lithium-specific receptors have been identified.

Lithium has been hypothesised to increase 5-HT synthesis and inhibit NA release via intracellular 'second messenger' systems, possibly resulting in modification of gene expression[51,52] or interaction with enzymes which are downstream intracellular targets of monoamine neurotransmitter pathways.[53,54] It may also potentiate antagonistic effects at NMDA receptors.[55]

Lithium is known to possess neuroprotective properties, inhibiting cell death and increasing cell longevity,[56] but the relevance of this is unknown.

Pharmacokinetics

Lithium carbonate has an elimination half-life of 18–27 hours (varies with age and renal function, can be significantly increased in renal impairment). It is almost entirely renally excreted (freely filtered in glomerulus, not protein-bound). It does not exert any effects on CYP isoenzymes.

Note that the two available formulations – lithium carbonate and lithium citrate (used where liquid preparation is required) – are NOT dose-equivalent (204 mg lithium carbonate is equivalent to 520 mg Priadel lithium citrate). In addition, specific preparations from different manufacturers vary widely in bioavailability – retitration (with suitable monitoring) is recommended after any change in preparation.

Side Effects

Lithium has an extremely broad potential for side effects. Commonly troublesome occurrences are tremor, dry mouth and increased thirst, ankle oedema, altered taste, increased appetite (with resultant weight gain), GI upset, hair loss, polyuria and skin reactions (acne and psoriasis).

Other more serious side effects may occur with prolonged use (renal impairment, hypothyroidism, hyperparathyroidism). The exact magnitude of these risks in real-world application is not clear, with some studies finding conflicting results[57] – a detailed review of lithium toxicity has been published elsewhere.[58] However, lithium-induced renal impairment in particular does seem to be a dose-dependent phenomenon, and the risk may be much reduced by maintaining plasma levels at the lower end of the therapeutic range. Routine monitoring of renal and thyroid function is recommended.

Additional adverse effects are associated with levels above the therapeutic window (see 'toxicity in overdose').

Lithium is a known teratogen, but it is effective in perinatal depression, both as a therapeutic and prophylactic agent (see Chapter 13).

Monitoring

Lithium salts require close monitoring due to their narrow therapeutic/toxic window and potential for serious and irreversible side effects.

Routine plasma level monitoring should be performed weekly after initiation and dose changes until concentrations are stable for two consecutive tests at the same dose, then every three months for the first year of treatment, then every six months thereafter. Renal and thyroid function should be checked before initiation and every six months during treatment.

Interactions

Lithium plasma concentrations can be increased with concurrent use of loop/thiazide diuretics, non-steroidal anti-inflammatory drugs, ACE inhibitors, theophylline, caffeine and acetazolamide. Conversely, increasing dietary sodium or water intake may reduce lithium levels by prompting the kidneys to excrete more lithium.

Lithium may potentiate the effects of serotonergic medications through unknown mechanisms, resulting in increased risks of serotonin syndrome. It has a similar potentiating effect with antipsychotic medication, and lithium co-treatment is a risk factor for neuroleptic malignant syndrome in people receiving high doses of (particularly typical) antipsychotics.

Contraindications

Lithium salts are contraindicated in patients with cardiovascular disease associated with arrythmia, untreated hypothyroidism and Addison's disease. They should be used with extreme caution only (and doses adjusted) for patients with renal impairment.

Toxicity in Overdose

Lithium has a narrow therapeutic/toxic window and is extremely toxic in overdose. Plasma levels >1.2 mmol/l can result in gastrointestinal disturbance and neurotoxicity (nystagmus, tremor, hyperreflexia, ataxia, delirium, seizures) with subsequent cardiovascular collapse. Emergency medical treatment should be sought if overdose is suspected.

Antiepileptics/Mood Stabilisers

Examples

Carbamazepine, lamotrigine, sodium valproate/valproic acid

Amongst the non-lithium antiepileptic/mood-stabilising agents, only lamotrigine is currently thought to have a significant role in the treatment of unipolar depression. Its use in this role stemmed from the finding that it is more effective at preventing depressive (rather than manic) relapses of bipolar affective disorder.

High-quality evidence is sparse, but some studies have indicated significant benefits for depressive symptoms when lamotrigine is added as an augmenting agent to SSRIs,[59] even outperforming lithium in one study (53% vs 41%, NNT 9).[60] As yet, however, these findings have not been consistently reproduced.

Mechanism of Action

Similar to other drugs in this category, lamotrigine is a voltage-gated sodium channel blocker. It also acts as a weak antagonist at the 5-HT3 receptor. It has minimal downstream effects on other monoamine neurotransmitter systems but is thought to suppress the release of glutamate and aspartate (the dominant excitatory neurotransmitters in the CNS). Lamotrigine has an elimination half-life of 29 hours. It is hepatically metabolised by glucuronyl transferase. Lamotrigine itself is not known to exert inhibitory or inducing effects on CYP isoenzymes. Lamotrigine is generally well tolerated, although possible side effects include sedation, headache, nausea and dizziness. Its main concerning adverse effect is the potential for serious and life-threatening skin reactions ('Stevens-Johnson syndrome'), which necessitate gradual initial titration with vigilant monitoring for any new rash.

Lamotrigine is not known to interact significantly with cytochrome P450 enzymes, but manufacturers advise that some decrease in circulating levels of lamotrigine can occur with co-prescription of P450 inducers (e.g. carbamazepine, phenytoin). Valproate significantly increases the level of lamotrigine and necessitates much lower dosing, titration and maximum dose. Lamotrigine has no absolute contraindications. However, it is not advised in pregnancy due to potential for teratogenic effects. In overdose, case reports indicate that most incidents result in mild or no toxicity, with potential for neurotoxic and cardiotoxic effects only at very high doses.[61]

Monitoring

Monitoring of lamotrigine levels is not routinely required. However, there is some evidence that a minimum therapeutic serum level exists at >6 mg/l, and if in doubt, then checking would be sensible. Note that there is no well-established safe upper level for serum lamotrigine – however, current research suggests toxicity may be more likely at levels exceeding 15 mg/l.

Thyroid Hormone – Levothyroxine Sodium, Liothyronine Sodium

The relationship between thyroid function and mood disorders was first described over 200 years ago.[62] Disturbances in emotion and cognition are well documented in thyroid disease, and subclinical abnormalities in thyroid hormones have been identified in sizeable proportions of patients with depressive symptoms.[63,64] However, the link is still poorly understood, and it has been hypothesised that there may be clinical benefits to adding supplementary thyroid hormone, even for patients without these demonstrable abnormalities.

There is some modest evidence to support this practice – STAR*D found comparable remission rates (and fewer discontinuations due to side effects) with augmentory thyroid hormone compared to lithium,[47] while a meta-analysis found significant improvements in objective measures of depressive symptoms (although no difference in overall remission rates).[65] In two network meta-analysis of all augmentation agents, thyroid hormones had the highest response, remission and tolerability rates.[66,67] Despite this, they remain relatively underused compared to other augmentation strategies.

Mechanism of Action

Thyroxine (T4) analogues are converted to the metabolically active triiodothyronine (T3). T3 exerts well-characterised effects on various organ systems via nuclear thyroid hormone receptors. How these effects relate to depressive psychopathology is not known. Liothyronine (the more commonly used preparation for depression) has an elimination half-life of 22 hours, although its effects are rather longer lasting than this would imply, due to downstream effects on gene expression and protein synthesis. It is hepatically metabolised by a process of deiodination. Nevertheless, the much shorter half-life of T3 compared to T4 allows for easier dose titration and more rapid alleviation of any adverse events. Thyroid hormones are generally well tolerated, but they have a side-effect profile that mirrors the consequences of hyperthyroidism – hot flushes, sweating, tremor, reduced appetite, menstrual irregularities and tachycardia. More serious side effects (arrhythmias, angina pectoris) are possible in those with pre-existing cardiovascular risk factors.

Liothyronine is not known to interact significantly with cytochrome P450 enzymes, but manufacturers advise that some decrease in circulating levels of liothyronine can occur with co-prescription of P450 inducers (e.g. carbamazepine, phenytoin). Further interactions are possible with some antiarrhythmic agents (digoxin, amiodarone). Thyroid hormones are obviously contraindicated in hyperthyroidism. For overdoses only, limited data are available, and most overdoses are thought to be fairly benign. However, a massive overdose of thyroid hormones can result in acute thyrotoxic crisis or 'thyroid storm' with associated fever, tachycardia, severe hypertension (leading to heart failure) and neurological abnormalities, so urgent medical attention is warranted. Unlike primary thyrotoxicosis, symptoms resulting from administration of exogenous T3 are not amenable to anti-thyroid drugs (which block the synthesis, release and activation of thyroid hormone) and must be managed supportively.

Because measurements of thyroid hormone levels are routine in the diagnosis of thyroid disease, monitoring of thyroid function tests is recommended when using liothyronine to augment antidepressant therapy. Although there is no well-defined therapeutic range, anecdotal evidence suggests that treatment should be titrated aiming for a free T3 at the upper end of the normal range and low normal or suppressed TSH (0.4 mU/L or lower). With longer-term use, monitoring for bone density may be appropriate.[68]

Buspirone

Buspirone is primarily used to treat anxiety disorders, and the degree to which it exerts antidepressant effects (either alone or as an augmenting agent) is questionable. It did not perform well (for either efficacy or tolerability) in STAR*D[69] or in dedicated RCTs,[70,71] although secondary analyses of data indicated that it may have been associated with improvements in a subset of patients with more severe depressive symptoms.[70] Based on its more convincing efficacy in treating anxiety disorders, it may have a role where prominent comorbid anxiety symptoms are present.

Mechanism of Action

Buspirone is primarily a 5-HT agonist with highest affinity for the 5-HT1A receptor and some lesser activity at 5-HT2A, 5-HT2B, 5-HT2C, 5-HT6 and 5-HT7 receptors.

It is also a weak antagonist of DA D2 receptors and has been investigated for possible antipsychotic properties (none have been identified).

A major metabolite of buspirone, 1-(2-pyrimidinyl)piperazine (1-PP), occurs at higher circulating levels than buspirone itself and acts as a potent α2-adrenergic receptor antagonist. Buspirone has an elimination half-life of 2–11 hours. It is hepatically metabolised by cytochrome P450 enzymes – primarily CYP3A4. Buspirone itself is not known to exert inhibitory or inducing effects on CYP isoenzymes. Side effects are similar to SSRIs, along with some distinct adverse effects including dizziness and tinnitus. Rarely, movement disorders have been reported, including dystonia, Parkinsonism, akathisia and myoclonus – possibly related to dopaminergic effects. Buspirone is not known to inhibit or induce cytochrome P450 enzymes, but as a substrate, concurrent use with cytochrome inhibitors or inducers could result in significant changes in circulating levels of buspirone. Buspirone is contraindicated in patients taking MAOIs and those with epilepsy. In overdose, it is expected to be relatively safe and similar to SSRIs in terms of potential complications (serotonin syndrome, cardiotoxicity) and mortality. In some early exploratory trials, subjects who received doses many times higher than those currently in clinical use experienced an increased risk of movement disorders but no serious cardiotoxicity or neurotoxicity, and all documented fatalities also involved numerous other CNS depressants.[72]

Pindolol

Pindolol was first investigated in the 1990s as a potential adjunct for SSRI treatment. During the early stages of treatment with SSRIs, the increase in 5-HT was known to result in auto-inhibitory effects, which had been linked to troublesome 'activation' symptoms. Proponents suggested that pindolol's specific 5-HT antagonism may be capable of preventing this, leading to greater therapeutic effect. Early results were encouraging,[73] including with rapidity of onset, but these were not validated by subsequent meta-analysis.[74] Critics have pointed to considerable variations in the methodology of studies included in this meta-analysis, and they have suggested that individual differences (such as in metabolism) may also be significant.[75] No definitive conclusion regarding efficacy has been reached, and use as an add-on to other serotonergic medication may be considered where other strategies have failed.

Side effects include bradycardia, dizziness, bronchospasm, fatigue, headache and cold peripheries. Pindolol can potentiate the effects of other antihypertensive/antiarrhythmic medications, resulting in bradycardia and hypotension. It is contraindicated in cases of clinically significant bradycardia or hypotension, arrythmias (e.g. AV block) and asthma (or other history of bronchospasm or obstructive airway disease).

Mechanism of Action

Pindolol is a non-selective 'beta blocker' (i.e. β-adrenergic receptor antagonist) that also acts as an antagonist at the 5-HT1A receptor. It appears to have some specificity for blocking inhibitory pre-synaptic 5-HT1A receptors, thereby increasing serotonin release through 'disinhibition'.[76]

Pindolol has an elimination half-life of 3–4 hours. Pindolol is around two-thirds hepatically metabolised by gluconuridation and one-thirds renally excreted. Pindolol itself is not known to exert inhibitory or inducing effects on CYP isoenzymes.

Toxicity in Overdose

Beta blockers are seriously toxic in overdose, resulting in severe bradycardia and associated circulatory collapse. Heart failure may be precipitated or exacerbated. Effects may be countered with the administration of anticholinergic medication (atropine), and urgent medical attention should be sought.

Ketamine

Ketamine is a recent, and somewhat controversial, addition to the arsenal of antidepressant treatments. Developed as an anaesthetic agent, tested on human prisoners[77] and first employed clinically during the Vietnam War,[78] ketamine later found widespread use as a safe option in settings where access to modern anaesthetic equipment and expertise were limited (including veterinary medicine). Popular for its broad therapeutic window, ketamine is able to induce a state of 'surgical anaesthesia' (sedation, catalepsy, somatic analgesia and bronchodilation) without suppressing respiratory drive or blood pressure, even at high doses.

Over time, it gained increased popularity as a recreational drug due to its additional ability to induce dissociative 'dream-like' states at sub-anaesthetic doses – concerns about unregulated use eventually resulting in its prohibition in many countries including the UK (where it is classified as 'class B' under the Misuse of Drugs Act).

However, in recent years, research has pointed towards a range of unrealised clinical applications, including anti-inflammatory and neuroprotective properties alongside antidepressant effects. It has demonstrated considerable efficacy in producing rapid (albeit often short-lived) improvements in both unipolar and bipolar depressive symptoms,[79,80] and efforts are underway to establish effective methods of maintaining these improvements.[81] Nevertheless, the rapid onset of antidepressant action and novel mechanism of action raise intriguing possibilities for future new developments in the field.

Mechanism of Action

Ketamine is a glutamate NMDA receptor antagonist. Its analgesic effects result from interference in pain-signalling pathways in the spinal cord dorsal horn, which rely on these receptors. It also has some agonistic effect at opioid receptors within the central nervous system as well as some as-yet poorly characterised interactions with nicotinic and muscarinic cholinergic receptors. The mechanism of antidepressant action of ketamine is not known, and it has been found to affect a variety of downstream-signalling pathways influencing neuro-transmission (e.g. upregulation of brain-derived neurotrophic factor). It is worth mentioning that multiple other NMDA receptor antagonists (e.g. memantine, lanicemine) have not demonstrated any efficacy in treating depression, suggesting that this may not be the primary mechanism by which ketamine exerts its antidepressant effects. Interestingly, co-administration with opioid receptor antagonists also attenuates its antidepressant effects, suggesting that its opioid receptor agonism is at least partly responsible for its clinical effects.[82]

Ketamine is a racemic compound; the S enantiomer (esketamine) now has a product licence in many countries for intranasal administration in combination with oral antidepressants, but the R enantiomer is likely to contribute to the efficacy of the racemic mixture and is also being investigated for stand-alone use.

Pharmacokinetics

Ketamine has an elimination half-life of 2–3 hours. It is hepatically metabolised by CYP3A4 and CYP2B6 isoenzymes. Ketamine itself is not known to exert inhibitory or inducing effects on CYP isoenzymes.

Side Effects

At doses usually used for treating depression (substantially lower than anaesthetic doses and also usually lower than those commonly used recreationally), ketamine's most common side effect is that sought by recreational users – an altered mental status frequently described as 'spacey' or 'floating', with associated dissociative symptoms, drowsiness, euphoria and sometimes confusion (an experience colloquially labelled a 'k-hole' with the more extreme symptoms associated with higher recreational doses).

Dizziness, blurred vision and nausea are also possible, although usually transient. Blood pressure needs to be monitored during clinical use.

Serious adverse effects are possible – urinary toxicity with associated ulcerative cystitis is known to occur, usually following repeated high-dose recreational use but also possible with treatment doses.[83]

Regular ketamine users may be at risk of developing dependence with physical tolerance and withdrawal symptoms (including tremors, sweating and palpitations), although this is thought to be unlikely with treatment doses.[84]

Interactions

Clinical observations suggest that benzodiazepines may diminish the antidepressant effects of ketamine through unknown mechanisms.[85]

Ketamine is known to potentiate the effects of other sedative medication, including anaesthetic agents such as propofol and midazolam.

Ketamine is not known to inhibit or induce cytochrome P450 enzymes, but as a substrate, concurrent use with cytochrome inhibitors or inducers could result in significant changes in circulating levels.

Contraindications

Ketamine (at doses used in treatment of depression) is contraindicated for those with a history of aneurysmal vascular disease, cardiovascular events or stroke.

Toxicity in Overdose

Ketamine is used as an anaesthetic agent in doses many times higher than those indicated for depression. At these levels, it will result in an anaesthetised state with complete sedation, catalepsy and somatic analgesia. Hypertonia and tonic-clonic movements are sometimes observed. Clearly, this can be extremely dangerous in specific circumstances, and deaths have occurred (e.g. from vomit aspiration). However, it has minimal direct cardiotoxic or neurotoxic effects and does not suppress respiration, even at extremely high doses, so outcomes are good with supportive management.

Other/Experimental Medications

Hypericum Perforatum (St John's Wort)

For some time, St John's Wort has occupied an uneasy niche at the interface of modern medicine and herbalism; it has a long and storied history as a mental health remedy (dating back to Ancient Greece). Among clinicians, reluctance to recommend its use probably stems from its classification as a 'dietary supplement' rather than a medicinal product, resulting in less-strict regulation and wide variation between manufacturers and even between batches of the same product – both in potency and in potential for interactions for other medications (which can be extreme). Some countries have more standardised products, and it is more widely prescribed.[86]

Results from studies (including a Cochrane review and recent meta-analysis), however, have been generally positive, with comparable efficacy to SSRIs and possibly fewer side effects.[87–89] The studies do vary in methodological quality, and few are long term. Reservations still exist regarding substantial variations in findings between countries where it is more or less widely used – these will need to be overcome if it is to find common use in mainstream practice, but it may be worth considering for patients opposed to more conventional medications.

The specific component(s) of St John's Wort relevant to its antidepressant effects have not been identified. Extracts can contain a number of bioactive compounds including flavonol derivatives, biflavones, proanthocyanidines, xanthones, phloroglucinols and naphthodianthrones. Combinations of these can variably induce re-uptake inhibition of 5-HT, NA and DA, as well as weak MAO inhibition. In addition, in vitro binding assays carried out using St John's Wort extract have demonstrated significant affinity for adenosine, GABA(A), GABA(B) and glutamate receptors.

Exact pharmacokinetic characterisation is not possible due to the multiple compounds involved, but elimination half-life is thought to be around 20 hours. Many components of St John's Wort are hepatically metabolised by cytochrome isoenzymes, and it is a potent inducer of CYP2C9 and CYP3A4. St John's Wort has been likened specifically to fluoxetine in its side-effect profile.[90] In addition, St John's Wort may cause photosensitivity. Discontinuation symptoms have been reported, but rates are unclear. St John's Wort shares the potential for serotonergic toxicity common to many antidepressants. Neurotoxicity has been reported in overdose.[91]Combination with MAOIs carries a potential for hypertensive crisis. It should not be used by those experiencing manic symptoms.

St John's Wort and its component compounds have complex interactions with cytochrome enzymes, and concurrent use with cytochrome inhibitors or inducers is probably best avoided. St John's Wort itself is a potent inducer of CYP2C9 and CYP3A4, with the potential to drastically reduce the concentration of other drugs metabolised by this pathway (e.g. anticoagulants, antiarrhythmics, immunosuppressants, antiretrovirals, birth control medications). This can have catastrophic results. Before prescribing an antidepressant, it is a sensible precaution to always add in a question as to whether the person is taking any other substances, such as St. John's Wort, to minimise the risks of harmful and unpredictable interactions.

Tryptophan (L-Tryptophan)

Tryptophan is the biochemical precursor of several endogenous neuroactive compounds including 5-HT and melatonin. It is an essential amino acid (must be obtained from diet). Theories involving tryptophan deficiency in the pathogenesis of depression became popular after deliberate 'tryptophan depletion' was shown to induce depressive symptoms in laboratory settings.[92] Unfortunately, this intriguing finding has not yet resulted in clinical advancement. Despite an appealing sense of logical validity, tryptophan supplementation has not been associated with convincing benefit in depression.[93,94] However, risks involved in taking tryptophan medicinally are low, and it may be considered when other options have been exhausted. Tryptophan exerts no direct effects. It is an amino acid involved in protein synthesis (of serotonin, as well as numerous other compounds). Tryptophan is unlikely to result in clinically significant side effects, but headache, nausea, dizziness and drowsiness have been reported. It has been rarely associated with eosinophilic myalgia syndrome, although this appears most likely to have been limited to certain contaminated batches. L-tryptophan may potentiate serotonergic effects resulting from other medications. Tryptophan is contraindicated for those with a history of eosinophilic myalgia.

Anti-inflammatories

Recent years have seen some diversification in biological models of mental illness, with researchers looking outside traditional monoamine neurotransmitter pathways and considering alternative mechanisms such as the HPA axis and neuroinflammatory processes.

These are still poorly understood but have some face validity in that they suggest a mechanism by which psychosocial stress may be translated into organic pathology. Additionally, inflammatory markers have been found to be reliably elevated in a range of mental disorders and may predict treatment resistance.[95] Investigations have yielded some intriguing research findings – for example, improved response and remission rates in depressed patients treated with anti-inflammatory medications such as celecoxib (an NSAID),[96] infliximab (a monoclonal antibody)[97] and minocycline (an antibiotic with anti-inflammatory properties)[98,99] alongside antidepressant therapy. Particular groups (for example, those with elevated inflammatory markers, a history of childhood trauma or treatment resistance) may be more likely to benefit.[97,98] These findings have yet to be translated into routine clinical practice.

Different anti-inflammatory medications that have been studied in an antidepressant context exert their actions through highly heterogenous pathways. The relation of these mechanisms to their possible antidepressant effects is not known.

Potential side effects vary considerably between specific anti-inflammatory agents (e.g. celecoxib, one of the more widely-studied, is an NSAID) – long-term use (for conditions other than depression) is associated with risks of gastric irritation, bleeding, renal impairment and cardiovascular events.

Nimodipine

So-called vascular depression is a recognised phenomenon, characterised by a distinct clinical presentation and an association with (sometimes subtle) cerebrovascular abnormalities.[100] Although there is little strong evidence for a vascular aetiology in the majority of depressive illness, the high incidence of depressive symptoms resulting from cerebrovascular pathology has resulted in investigation of vasodilating agents that increase cerebral perfusion. The calcium-channel blocker nimodipine (usually used to prevent neurological ischaemia in subarachnoid haemorrhage) is the best studied of these.

Nimodipine is a calcium-channel blocker. It appears to have some specificity for cerebral vasculature (as compared to widely used antihypertensive agents diltiazem and verapamil) – the reason for this is not clear. It induces vasodilation and improves cerebral perfusion.

Interestingly, calcium-channel blocking drugs had already received some psychiatric attention as potential mood-stabilising agents, due to similarities with effective antiepileptic mood stabilisers (e.g. sodium valproate). Although some evidence of benefits was found for patients with rapid-cycling bipolar illness, ultimately this was not convincing enough to result in widespread use or inclusion in clinical guidelines.[101] Side effects include flushing, dizziness, headache and peripheral oedema. Nimodipine can potentiate the effects of other antihypertensive medications, resulting in hypotension. Nimodipine is contraindicated in those with ischaemic heart disease. However, clinical interest has been renewed, with trials of nimodipine augmentation (e.g. of SSRIs) producing encouraging results.[102,103] Whether these benefits are restricted to those with identifiable vascular pathology remains to be seen.

Nutrients

N-acetyl cysteine, L-methyl-folate, curcumin, saffron, omega-3 fatty acids, S-adenosyl-O-methionine

The beneficial effects of micronutrient supplementation in those who have not been shown to have a specific deficiency is a controversial area, particularly as the sales and promotion of certain products involve large sums of money. In general, claims from the (thriving) 'wellness industry' regarding the mental benefits of various supplements should probably be viewed with suspicion, as many are unfounded, and few have any rigorous RCT backing. Their mechanism of action is uncertain because the pharmacodynamic profiles of various micronutrients are diverse and not well characterised. Various mechanisms with similarities to the profiles of more established antidepressants have been suggested (e.g. interactions with monoamine and glutamate neurotransmitter pathways).

However, tentative evidence exists for antidepressant effects resulting from all the agents listed here. Many of the studies involved are unreplicated and relatively low-quality. However, specific examples (particularly n-acetyl cysteine,[104] omega-3 fatty acids[105] and s-adenosylmethionine[106]) have garnered enough support to warrant their inclusion in guidelines with sections on alternative treatments.[107] They may be considered for patients opposed to more conventional medications.

Psychedelics

3,4-Methylenedioxymethamphetamine (MDMA), lysergic acid diethylamide (LSD), N,N-Dimethyltryptamine (DMT), psilocybin

The past decade has seen an explosive increase in research into the antidepressant effects of psychedelic agents. In some ways, the most surprising thing about this development is its recency, although in fact in the UK, research was thriving prior to the 1971 Misuse of Drugs Act, which proscribed any medicinal use for any of the psychedelic drugs. All of these agents have been revered amongst counterculture groups (and increasingly in the mainstream) for many years for their ability to induce revelatory changes in mental state and perspective amongst those experiencing emotional distress. The use of naturally occurring psychedelics in this manner may date back millennia![108]

Most of the trials so far have focused on the use of psychedelics in psychotherapeutic contexts – 'psychedelic-assisted psychotherapy', usually involving several sessions before and after the psychedelic experience, where they are thought to facilitate processes of insight, awareness and reflectiveness. Early results indicate significant improvements in anxiety and depressive symptoms, at least in the short to medium term.[109] Longer-term benefits have not yet been demonstrated, and it is unclear if repeated treatments might be necessary. Whether these results are reproducible across wider samples of patients and whether psychedelics also exert beneficial effects outside of these highly specialised settings remains to be established. The use of these interventions in other settings like 'retreats' is not recommended.[110]

Mechanism of Action

They differ between specific agents. However, all have been shown to exert varying degrees of agonistic activity at a number of different 5-HT receptors. 5-HT2A agonism is thought to be particularly significant for the psychedelics' mind-altering effects,[111] as their psychotomimetic (psychosis-mimicking) intoxication of psilocybin can be prevented by co-administration of 5-HT2A antagonists such as ketanserin and risperidone but were enhanced by the dopamine agonist Haloperidol.[112] However, they are pharmacologically diverse, also interacting to greater or lesser degrees with other neurotransmitter pathways (e.g. DA, glutamate), and the relevance to their antidepressant efficacy is unknown. Most have half-lives of a few hours and are initially broken down by MAO before being extensively hepatically metabolised. Side effects differ between agents. All psychedelic agents produce profound alterations in mental state, which underpin their mechanism of therapeutic action but can also be distressing and result in paranoia, confusion, increased anxiety, dissociative symptoms and even psychosis. Such side effects are managed with psychotherapeutic support and, if necessary, benzodiazepines until the effects wear off. At currently studied doses, other physical side effects seem to be rare but can include nausea, tachycardia, hot flushes and altered sensation. Most psychedelics are initially metabolised by MAO, with resulting drastic increases in potency and duration of effects if they are taken in conjunction with a MAOI. This is actually the intended effect with the compound 'ayahuasca' (a brew used ritualistically by various native Amazonian tribes), where DMT is mixed with 'harmala alkaloids', which contain naturally occurring MAOIs.

Deaths have been reported with illicit MDMA (ecstasy) use. Neurotoxicity to the serotonergic system in the brain has been reported with a possible link to later psychiatric problems. A 2010 literature review revealed over 87 'ecstasy'-related fatalities, caused by hyperpyrexia, rhabdomyolysis, intravascular coagulopathy, hepatic necrosis, cardiac arrhythmias, cerebrovascular accidents and drug-related accidents or suicide. The toxic or even fatal dose range appears to overlap with the range of recreational dosage,[113] although interestingly, such problems have not been encountered in research settings. Psilocybin appears to be less toxic – in one study of 33 cases admitted to hospital following ingestion, vomiting was the main presenting symptom, only two cases had to be ventilated and there were no deaths.

Classification of Physical Treatments for Depression

Neuromodulatory

Electroconvulsive Therapy

Background

The history of ECT is worthy of a book in its own right. Ever since they were first discovered in the 1700s, methods of inducing seizures have been used to varying degrees to treat a range of psychiatric and neurological complaints. Initially based on (misguided) theories about antagonistic relationships between mental disorders and epilepsy, ECT actually represented a significant advancement in safety over previous pharmacological agents (camphor and metrazol) used to induce seizures.

Camphor was first used by Ladislav Meduna in 1934 to induce fits – in his series of patients with schizophrenia, 10 recovered, 3 improved and 13 showed no change. This caused some excitement at the time, and Ugo Cerletti (professor of psychiatry in Rome) sent one of his associates to visit Meduna. Noting the unpleasant side effects of hallucinations caused by metrazol, he decided to try and induce the fits using electricity. Lucio Bini (a trainee psychiatrist with Cerletti at the time) worked out that a bi-temporal electrode placement would be safest, as only minimal current would go through the heart. Their first patient was a 39-year-old mute man who was found wandering around a Rome railway station. On 14 April 1938, he was given his first shock, which gave him a myoclonic reaction, and he began to sing loudly; after a total of 11 sessions of ECT, he was cured. The publication of this case in their famous paper 'Un nuevo metodo di shockterapie: "L'elettroshock"'[114] marked a major turning point in the history of psychiatry and was to usher in the modern era of effective physical treatments.[114]

Over the decades, the mechanisms underlying the efficacy of ECT (and other subsequently derived physical treatments) – or even the changes they induce in the brain – have yet to be satisfactorily described. Popularity has waxed and waned, although ECT has unfortunately never quite managed to shed its historical controversial image.

For depression, ECT has a well-established role in the management of severe, life-threatening or treatment-resistant symptoms, with significant superiority over placebo and all classes of pharmacological antidepressants (including TCAs and MAOIs).[115,116] Resistant postpartum psychoses may respond well, alongside a small number with recurrent depressive disorder who do not respond to any drug therapies. In cases of severe psychotic depression, some patients (particularly the elderly) stop eating and drinking and present with a medical emergency, which can be speedily reversed with ECT. Given its substantial evidence base, it is probably underused in this regard relative to other treatments.[117] Relapse rates following ECT may be high, and it is probably best used in combination with pharmacological options for this reason.[118] For most patients who successfully complete a course of ECT, provided they are sent home with a prophylactic antidepressant, relapse in the near term is unusual. However, there are a small number of individuals who have responded well to ECT who begin to relapse soon after their course is complete. For these individuals, continuing ECT as maintenance is sometimes helpful. A recent trial applying Spanish national ECT guidelines (weekly ECT for four weeks, every two weeks for two months, and then monthly for six months up to a total of 14 sessions in nine months) found that, after a successful course, those in the 'drugs + maintenance ECT' group had a significantly lower relapse rate (35%) compared to those in the 'drugs only' group (61%).[119] Numbers were small, mainly because such cases are unusual, but replication of these findings is clearly indicated.[117]

Practical considerations for treatment include the dose and duration of electrical stimulation, as well as the use of unilateral vs bilateral electrode placement. Unilateral is thought to cause fewer cognitive side effects but is also less effective unless administered at higher doses – generally, it is used when speed and completeness of response are less of a priority or when minimising cognitive symptoms is particularly crucial. These should all be determined on a per-patient basis.

In general, ECT-naïve patients have a seizure threshold between 50–100 mC (highly variable dependent on age, gender and psychotropic medications). Various methods exist to guide the process of establishing seizure threshold for a specific patient.[120] Once this has been established, the dose is titrated based on physiological parameters, with a seizure of >15 seconds duration considered optimal to achieve therapeutic effects while minimising risks (generally achieved at 50% above the seizure threshold dose for bilateral ECT, or 200% above for unilateral).

Modern ECT machines administer newer types of electrical pulse delivery designed to minimise side effects and allow EEG monitoring of seizures. Further details are given in the *Handbook on ECT* published by the UK Royal College of Psychiatrists.[121]

Mechanism of Action

Despite decades of research, the mechanism(s) of action of ECT are not known. Numerous theories have been proposed involving the release of neurotransmitters, neurotrophic factors and hormones – with resultant changes in blood flow, metabolism and even brain architecture[122] (these latter changes are unlikely to explain its relatively rapid, sometimes instantaneous, antidepressant effects). Beneficial effects do seem to be related to some degree to the occurrence of seizure activity,[123] rather than just the administration of electric current.

Side Effects

ECT's main troublesome side effect is memory loss – it is associated with variable degrees of retrograde and anterograde amnesia, usually limited to events occurring within weeks of treatment but sometimes more far-reaching.[124] A thorough systematic review of objective cognitive testing found significant reductions in cognitive performance zero to three days after ECT, but a recovery to pre-treatment levels thereafter; by day 15 after ECT, many areas of cognitive function were improved over baseline.[125] Thus, although most do recover lost memories over time, this does not appear to always be the case, and some patients report persistent autobiographical memory loss.[126]

These effects have led critics to postulate about lasting effects of ECT on brain tissue (making unfavourable comparisons with traumatic brain injury). However, to date, the evidence does not support these comparisons.[127] Cognitive impairments in those treated with ECT may be complicated by similar symptoms resulting from depressive illness, or other psychiatric pathology; effective treatment of depression can result in large benefits to cognition.[128]

ECT can (extremely rarely) cause cardiac arrythmia but probably only in those with underlying cardiac pathology.[129] Mortality is vanishingly rare, comparable to other minor procedures involving general anaesthesia – around 6 in every 100,000 treatments.

Other side effects of the procedure may result from ECT or the use of general anaesthetic itself – headache, myalgia and nausea.

Contraindications

There are no absolute contraindications for ECT. The main factors limiting its use pertain to the need for general anaesthesia (which may be associated with unacceptable risks, such as for those with severe pulmonary or cardiovascular disease).

There may be increased risks of adverse events from ECT itself for patients with cardiovascular disease, recent CVA/clinically significant head trauma or raised intracranial pressure, and it should be used only with caution (and probably as a last resort) for these groups.

Doses may need to be adjusted for patients who are prescribed medications that affect seizure threshold (e.g. antipsychotics, benzodiazepines), and it may be preferable to omit these medications on the day of treatment, if clinically appropriate.

Transcranial Magnetic Stimulation

Background

The early success of electroconvulsive therapy, coupled with uncertainty about underlying mechanisms, naturally led to attempts to reproduce the beneficial effects with less invasive alternatives. Initially, these involved administering lower electrical currents intended to manipulate specific brain areas without inducing seizure activity (and thereby avoiding the requirement for general anaesthesia). However, this proved intolerably painful at all but very low doses (which had no clear therapeutic effect), and so-called transcranial electrical stimulation is not currently used clinically – although it has continued to attract research interest.[130]

In the 1980s, attention turned to magnetic fields as a method of altering electrical signalling within the brain; it was some time, however, before any evidence of therapeutic potential was demonstrated,[131] and the use of 'transcranial magnetic stimulation' in clinical contexts is a recent development.

Trials to date have shown promise for treatment-resistant depressive disorders (as well as a host of other conditions including anxiety disorders, epilepsy, tinnitus and traumatic brain injury).[132] One meta-analysis found a convincing effect with an odds ratio of 4.76 for remission of depressive symptoms (compared to 'sham' TMS) and a NNT of 5, which compares favourably to results from pharmacological treatment.[133]

Many of these studies have suffered from limitations including short follow-up duration, questionable blinding/control procedures and uncertainty regarding the specificity with which specific brain areas are 'targeted'. In addition, questions about optimal dosing and durations of treatment have not been conclusively answered. These, along with issues of accessibility – patients need to attend daily for up to six weeks – and availability, have limited the adoption of TMS amongst most practitioners, but popularity looks set to increase as long as ongoing research continues to produce favourable results.[134] Improvements such as the use of an MRI to localise treatment and 'theta burst' protocols are being trialled.

Mechanism of Action

Similar to ECT, the effects of electrophysiological manipulation (whether achieved with magnetic fields or direct electrical current) within the brain are not known. In contrast to ECT, the occurrence of seizure activity is not involved. Various theories exist regarding the ability of TMS to induce differential brain activity (e.g. inhibiting vs stimulating cortical activation) by altering parameters such as the intensity of stimulation, magnetic coil orientation and frequency.[135]

Side Effects

Side effects with TMS are rare. Possible effects include vasovagal syncope, headache, transient changes in hearing or memory impairment. Serious adverse events have been reported including seizures and malfunction in implanted devices such as cardiac pacemakers.[136]

Contraindications

TMS is contraindicated for patients with implanted metal devices (pacemaker, spinal/bladder stimulators, foreign bodies). It should be used with caution in patients with epilepsy or histories of clinically significant head trauma.

Deep Brain Stimulation

Direct electrical stimulation of specific brain areas via implanted electrodes has been shown to be an effective treatment for some neurological disorders. The application of these techniques for depressive illness remains experimental, as an optimal neuroanatomical target has not been identified.[137] A wide range of potential areas have been investigated in the few trials conducted to date, and results have been variable even between studies where the same area was stimulated.[138,139] The most promising effect was obtained in a study targeting the superolateral branch of the medial forebrain bundle.[140] However, it remains unclear what the optimal stimulation parameters are and whether serial adjustments can be linked to enhancing clinical benefit over time. Needless to say, further reproduction and verification are required before any clinical application can be realised.

Mechanism of Action

See TMS. The mechanism of action of DBS is not known (even for those conditions where it has established efficacy, such as Parkinson's disease). A variety of hypotheses exist, involving both excitatory and inhibitory effects on neuronal outputs at or near the electrode site.

Side Effects

Implantation of electrodes for DNS involves major neurosurgery, with all the inherent associated potential for complications including infection and haemorrhage. Additional side effects are poorly characterised and include a wide range of neurological and psychiatric effects (e.g. cognitive dysfunction, personality changes, sensory changes, changes in ability to perform complex motor tasks such as swimming) – these are probably relative to electrode placement. In comparison to ablative surgical interventions, DBS has the advantage that the induced 'lesions' are mostly reversible.

DBS may be further complicated over time by device malfunction, breakage or disconnection. DBS is obviously contraindicated in those who are not able to undergo major neurosurgery for whatever reason (due to medical comorbidities) and those with structural brain abnormalities.

Vagal Nerve Stimulation

Background

Despite clear parallels with DBS, vagal nerve stimulation actually developed from independent lines of scientific enquiry. Initially, electroencephalogram changes were seen to result from stimulation of the vagus nerve during animal studies. This led to the development of implantable devices for use in treatment-refractory epilepsy and, subsequently, the observation of mood improvements (independent of seizure control) amongst those who used them.[141]

Since the early 2000s, VNS has developed a reasonable evidence base as an adjunctive therapy for treatment-resistant depression.[142,143] Although there is unfortunately a lack of good RCTs, recent follow-up of patients involved in early trials indicated substantial effect sizes and sustained benefits (with a remission rate of 43.3% for those treated with VNS vs 25.7% without).[144] Interestingly, there is some evidence that benefits accrue over time for up to 12 months, in contrast to pharmacological treatment. As with other novel neuromodulatory treatments, further randomised controlled trials (with close attention to methods of blinding and control interventions) are needed before definitive conclusions can be made about efficacy, and use is currently limited to tertiary specialist centres.

Mechanism of Action

See TMS. The mechanism of action of VNS is not known. The vagus nerve includes afferent fibres carrying sensory information, which eventually project to a wide array of different brain areas, including those historically implicated in depressive illness (e.g. dorsal raphe nucleus, hypothalamus, amygdala, limbic forebrain areas). Stimulation may result in localised changes in neurotransmitter pathways or possibly exert anti-inflammatory effects.[145]

Side Effects

Implantation of the stimulation device for VNS is possible as an outpatient procedure under local anaesthetic (although general anaesthetic is sometimes used). Surgical complications are possible (bleeding, infection, local pressure effects from implanted device). The stimulation process itself has been associated with headache, nausea, sensory changes and bradycardia (the vagus nerve supplies the parasympathetic innervation to the heart – this effect is minimised by targeting the left vagus rather than the right, which specifically innervates the sinoatrial node). Most notably, the patients may notice a change in tone or hoarseness of voice whilst the stimulator is active (e.g. for 30 seconds every 5 minutes).

Rare incidents of cardiac arrhythmias have been reported – pre-existing cardiovascular disease is suspected to have been implicated. VNS is contraindicated in patients who have undergone cervical vagotomy. It should be avoided in patients with a history of (particularly bradycardic) cardiac arrythmias.

Light Therapy (Phototherapy)

Background

The existence of a relationship between mood and circadian rhythm is fairly well established and directly observable in the case of seasonal affective disorder. Whether this relationship is relevant to other forms of depressive illness and, if so, the degree to which the underlying mechanism can be harnessed through the administration of artificial light is less certain.

Despite a previous favourable Cochrane review indicating some benefit for 'non-seasonal' depression,[146] two recent meta-analyses drew quite different conclusions from the available data. Their main point of agreement was that most studies to date have significant methodological flaws (including a lack of suitable control interventions).[147,148]

However, phototherapy benefits from widespread accessibility of necessary equipment, ease of use and relative lack of adverse effects, and it should be given due consideration as a fairly low-risk adjunct strategy, particularly for treatment-resistant patients.

Effective doses are not well defined, but typical recommendations involve a 10,000 lux light source used daily at a consistent time (usually the morning) for 20–30 minutes. The mechanism of action of phototherapy is not known. Current theories implicate various autonomic and hormonal pathways that display circadian patterns, suggesting that dysregulated rhythms may be corrected by CNS impulses elicited by bright light.[149] Side effects with phototherapy are rare. Prolonged exposures to sources of UV light are not recommended, but most commercially available phototherapy lamps either filter out or do not emit ultraviolet light. Skin reactions are still possible, but mainly with rare pre-existing conditions (lupus, porphyria) or concomitant use of photosensitising agents (e.g. retinols, St John's Wort). Other side effects include headache and eyestrain.

Rarely, phototherapy has been associated with manic 'switches' in bipolar affective disorder. There are no absolute contraindications to phototherapy. It should be used with caution for patients with a history of photosensitivity reactions or predisposing conditions (e.g. lupus, porphyria) and for patients with bipolar affective disorder.

Neuroablative

Stereotactic Psychosurgery

Examples

Anterior cingulotomy, subcaudate tractotomy, limbic leucotomy, anterior capsulotomy

Background

Neuroablative surgery has an undeniably troubled past in the treatment of psychiatric disorders. The widespread historical practice of leucotomy is (deservedly) remembered as a disastrous lapse in regulatory oversight and basic ethical principles. However, neurosurgery and psychiatry are irrevocably bound – some of the first indications for neurosurgical intervention involved treatment-refractory mental illness, and the need to develop safer and more effective psychiatric treatments directly led to surgical innovations such as gamma-knife radiosurgery.[150]

In recent years, there has been some renewed interest in this field, and the growing evidence base does suggest that a very select group of patients with highly treatment-resistant symptoms may benefit from the procedures listed here (cingulotomy is the best studied of these).[151] Theoretically, ablative techniques may offer advantages over modulatory alternatives by removing the risk of attenuating effects over time.

However, available studies are still limited by small sample sizes, inconsistent methods of determining optimal targets pre-operatively/confirming lesion placement postoperatively, and inconsistent recording of adverse events. Currently, neurosurgical treatment for mental illness remains rare, and a great deal more research is needed to establish whether these techniques will have a role in the future management of depressive disorders. Within the UK, strict procedures under the Mental Health Act need to be followed for any patient wishing to consider neurosurgery for a psychiatric indication.

Mechanism of Action

The mechanism of action of neuroablative procedures in depression is not known. Various neuroanatomical structures have been implicated in signalling pathways thought to be relevant to the pathogenesis of depressive symptoms. However, the exact effects of disrupting these structures (in terms of changes in cell signalling or overall brain architecture) are unclear. Various side effects have been described including personality changes, seizures, neuromotor abnormalities and cognitive impairment. Psychosurgery is obviously contraindicated in those who are not able to undergo major neurosurgery for whatever reason (due to medical comorbidities) and those with structural brain abnormalities.

Systematic Approach to Treatment/ Treatment Algorithms

General Principles

Making the Diagnosis

Accurate classification of depressive symptoms based on a holistic assessment is essential to guide effective management, inform escalation strategies and establish realistic expectations about treatment response. Note that many current guidelines emphasise the importance of a dimension of assessment relating specifically to functional impairment. There are many causes of low mood that do not equate to a depressive episode!

Most symptoms of depression exist on a continuum with everyday experience (which also encompasses pathological stress reactions and 'adjustment disorder'), and clinicians should endeavour not to overly medicalise grief and distress resulting from crises, losses and hardships. Although patients may be keen to trial pharmacological treatments – and in cases of diagnostic uncertainty, we would suggest these should not be withheld (to do so would be likely to damage therapeutic alliance) – supportive psychosocial interventions should also be sought and may ultimately be more important.

Note that even where a depressive episode is confidently established, NICE guidelines do not recommend the routine use of pharmacological interventions except for 'severe' symptoms[152] (a threshold which, admittedly, is inconsistently defined and applied elsewhere). In contrast, the BAP suggests that antidepressants are beneficial for moderate to severe episodes, for mild episodes that are chronic, or for mild episodes in the context of an established recurrent depressive disorder (i.e. not waiting for episodes to become more severe before starting treatment).[153]

Low mood may also occur as part of a spectrum of persistent 'emotional dysregulation' in personality disorder, often superimposed onto a 'dysthymic' baseline state (commonly described as feeling 'empty' or 'numb'). Personality disorder is widely prevalent, underdiagnosed and has implications for treatment selection. It should be suspected where symptoms are persistent and long-standing, dating back to adolescence or childhood. Histories of early complex trauma and relationship difficulties are frequently present. While it does not preclude comorbid depressive episodes (indeed, these are common), treatment approaches for depression are generally ineffective for the persistent or rapidly fluctuating affective symptoms that characterise personality disorder.

Primary 'dysthymia' – where (typically low-grade) depressive symptoms are chronic rather than delineated into episodes and periods of remission – has strong associations with personality disorder,[154] but it can also occur independently (recognised as 'persistent depressive disorder' in DSM-5). Contrary to historical opinion, research increasingly indicates that treatment approaches used for depressive episodes are effective for dysthymia[155] – although where symptoms are very long-standing, benefits may be modest, and aiming for a reduction in symptoms to tolerable levels (rather than complete remission) may be more realistic.

Finally, any presentation consistent with a clear-cut severe depressive episode must be further explored in order to exclude (where possible) the presence of underlying bipolar affective disorder as well as to identify the presence or absence of psychotic symptoms – due to different treatment approaches in these cases. Previous studies have indicated that amongst those presenting with a depressive episode, 16 per cent meet formal DSM-IV criteria for bipolar disorder and many more may have subsyndromal features.[156]

A more detailed discussion of the concept of a bipolar spectrum of affective disorders is out of the scope of this chapter (see Chapter 4.2). Nevertheless, the frequent presence of subsynromal hypomanic or mixed affective features has led to the addition of a 'mixed features' specifier in DSM-5. For such patients, the addition of mood stabilisers to an antidepressant may be of benefit, with clinical trials specifically supporting the efficacy of lurasidone and ziprasidone.[157]

As always, a crucial aspect of the diagnostic assessment is to establish risk. This encompasses not just risk of suicide, which may determine whether and how more toxic drugs can be used, but also many other aspects, including the risk of exacerbating comorbid medical conditions such as hypertension, cardiac disease, diabetes and epilepsy, to name but a few of the more commonly seen.

Dose Adjustment – Onset of Action, the 'Adequate Trial' and Level Monitoring

In our experience, many patients linger on low doses of ineffective treatments for extended periods (sometimes years) before alternative approaches are tried.[158] This is clearly not optimal – pharmacological treatment should be regularly reviewed (except where long-term maintenance use with an effective treatment has been agreed – see 'when to stop' and 'relapse prevention').

The existence of a delay in the onset of antidepressant action has become a widely-held belief, even among clinicians. This is not actually supported by research, which indicates significant antidepressant-placebo differences even in the first seven days,[159] and that up to 35 per cent of the eventual improvement can be expected during this period.[160] Possibly such beliefs stem from the existence of 'activation' symptoms with SSRI treatment (which prompt many clinicians to sensibly warn patients that they may feel worse before they feel better) or reflect the fact that it does take time to notice appreciable, clinically significant improvement.

A good response to treatment in the first two weeks strongly predicts final outcome. If there are no or minimal improvements at that point, a satisfactory therapeutic response with an extended trial of the same treatment is probably unlikely (although possible).[161,162]

As a result, current guidelines for treatment of depression stress the importance of an 'adequate trial' of antidepressant treatment before judgements are made about efficacy. Exact definitions differ: most refer to the minimum effective dose maintained for a period of four to six weeks with good adherence, although some specify the maximum tolerated dose of an antidepressant drug (within regulatory limits).[163]

The issue of dose increases remains controversial, at least in part due to the lack of good RCTs that increasing the dose above the starting dose is an effective strategy for many commonly used treatments – and for some evidence that it is ineffective.[153] For many drugs, however – escitalopram, venlafaxine, vortioxetine and TCAs, for example – there is evidence for a dose-response relationship within the therapeutic range. Metabolic status is also an issue; some patients are fast or slow metabolisers for certain treatments, which may in turn affect propensity to side effects and response rates and has led to the emergence of pharmacogenetic testing to help better target treatments.[164]

In practice, therefore, completing an 'adequate trial' involves initiating a standard dose, reviewing early, and – in non-responsive patients – considering titration to the maximum tolerated dose, which is maintained for several more weeks. Patients should be encouraged not to abandon treatment until this process is completed. Please note, the same concept of an 'adequate trial' does not apply to most augmentory treatments, where higher doses do not equate straightforwardly to better response.

Therapeutic drug monitoring is an established necessity for some augmentory agents (e.g. lithium, thyroid hormone), but while possible, it is not commonly used for antidepressants. Optimal plasma levels and therapeutic windows are not well established for many drugs. Individual variations in plasma levels at the same dose are also high, although efforts have been made to characterise this.[165] However, monitoring may be helpful in some cases, particularly where very high doses above regulatory limits are being considered (there is some evidence to support this practice for TCAs, although it is mainly employed at specialist centres).

Monitoring Treatment Response

Establishing treatment efficacy is not always a straightforward process, particularly where patients have comorbid issues that may complicate the assessment of their 'baseline' affective state (such as personality disorder). Formal quantification of symptoms may help identify changes in symptoms over time or partial responses, allowing incremental therapy benefits to be consolidated and built upon, as well as enabling a proactive approach to discontinuing and switching ineffective treatments. Standardised measurement-based assessments using validated rating scales – for example, the Montgomery-Asberg Depression Rating Scale (MADRS), Hamilton Depression Rating Scale (HAM-D), Quick Inventory of Depression Symptomatology Clinician Rating (QIDS-C) and Patient Health Questionnaire 9 (PHQ-9) – are recommended. There is some evidence that adopting such approaches (rather than relying on a general 'clinical impression') may result in improved quality of care and patient outcomes, even for experienced clinicians.[166]

Optimum frequencies of follow-up for patients with depression are not well established, but in general, increased contact seems to be associated with better outcomes.[167] This may be particularly important during the first few weeks of treatment, where side effects are likely to be most pronounced and risk of discontinuing treatment probably highest as a result. 'Crisis' presentations including suicide attempts are also commonest during this period – contingency plans and routes of accessing emergency support should be clearly established.[168]

The need to maintain good adherence should be an ever-present theme in antidepressant treatment, and both the Royal College of Psychiatrists and the NHS website provide reliable patient information to supplement the initial explanation provided by the clinician. This is known to be a significant issue – it is likely that a third of people will discontinue treatment after a month, often without consulting with their treating physician,[169] and only a minority of people will continue to take their recommended medication after six months.[170] Contrary to popular belief, this risk may be reduced in the elderly (although factors such as cognitive impairment and lack of appropriate care/supervision must be considered).[171] 'Adherence counselling' involving special educational sessions does improve adherence to antidepressants, but it is not standard in most services – clinicians should endeavour to incorporate these principles into their routine practice by addressing the following factors:[172]

Illness factors that contribute to non-compliance with antidepressants include lack of motivation, feelings of hopelessness or a mild degree of cognitive impairment leading to forgetfulness.

Drug factors include side effects. There is considerable variation between the tolerability of drugs, and certain side effects – notably sexual side effects – may not be reported yet result in drug discontinuation or delay in response, which needs to be explained to the patient.

Patient factors include a distaste for taking any medication or misinformation – for example, the belief that antidepressants are addictive or that taking a drug may lead to a change of personality. Life events may also contribute. Depressive episodes, whether or not precipitated by recent life events, respond equally well to antidepressants, but patients who have experienced a recent life event may find this difficult to understand. They may question how a tablet can help in a social crisis and be sceptical of the role of medication.

Managing Side Effects

Management of specific side effects for every available agent is beyond the scope of this chapter. However, there are some common issues that clinicians will encounter in their practice and general principles that might be applied to address these issues.

Firstly, care should be taken to differentiate medication side effects from symptoms related to underlying depressive pathology (particularly poor sleep, appetite and libido). This is not always possible, and of course, both may be contributing. Careful longitudinal histories are required to establish the onset, progression and dose-dependence of significant difficulties – where possible, choose agents with side effects that counteract presenting biological symptoms (e.g. SSRI/bupropion for hypersomnolence/hyperphagia; mirtazapine/trazodone for insomnia/poor appetite; mirtazapine/bupropion/agomelatine for low sex drive).

Once side effects are established, there is little good evidence for effective strategies to dispel them. Common approaches include altering timing of administration (e.g. in the case of insomnia or sedation), dose reduction, slower titration, a switch to a drug with less tendency to cause the same side effect, or symptomatic treatment with another drug.

Many common serotonergic side effects are self-limiting and attenuate over time (e.g. headache, nausea).[173,174] Unfortunately, this is not true of the sexual side effects that plague most serotonergic medication and may significantly impact adherence, particularly in younger people. This should be specifically asked about and addressed in cases of unexpectedly poor treatment response. Co-prescription of sildenafil may improve sexual functioning in men (and possibly women) with antidepressant-induced sexual dysfunction.[175,176]

Many antidepressants disrupt sleep patterns and cause insomnia; great caution should be taken in counteracting these effects with adjunctive hypnotic medication (particularly benzodiazepines and other Z-drugs). Clinicians should be mindful of risks of tolerance and 'rebound' phenomena resulting in dependence following regular use. Where possible, insomnia should be managed by adjusting dose timing, optimising conservative sleep hygiene measures and switching to alternative sedating antidepressants, if necessary.

'Activation syndrome' mentioned earlier in this chapter (see SSRIs) remains a controversial concept, but clinicians must be mindful of the possibility of increased suicidality following antidepressant initiation. One study found that 'suicidal adverse drug reactions' were associated with restlessness, ego dystonic thoughts of suicide and impulsiveness. Most cases (71%) occurred within the first 7 days of starting the antidepressant, 22% between days 7 and 14 and 7% thereafter – indicating that increased vigilance in at least the first two weeks after prescribing is sensible. These effects were found for all antidepressant groups but most frequently for SSRIs (although these were also the most frequently prescribed antidepressant group). Management varied from stopping the antidepressant, switching to another or adding in a benzodiazepine.[177]

The suggestion that antidepressants actually increase the risk of completed suicide has proven concerningly difficult to refute and remains unresolved. Clearly, antidepressant trial populations already have an increased rate of suicidality. Previous meta-analyses of antidepressant trials have actually showed little difference between placebo and active drug suicide rates. A more recent analysis of 12 placebo-controlled studies showed a 2.77-fold raised rate for the active drug for all suicide events over placebo. Understandably, this finding was controversial and was criticised for important limitations (not all the placebo-controlled trials had adequate follow-up periods or routinely collected comprehensive data on suicide attempts).[178] More recent data suggests that the rates of suicidal behaviour are highest in the 30 days before SSRI prescription and reduced thereafter,[244] and overall rates of suicide have reduced not increased despite vastly increased use of SSRI medication (see Cleare et al.[153] for review).

Probably less common still and possibly related to the 'activation syndrome' are episodes of severe unprovoked violence that are out of character for the individual concerned and can result in criminal justice involvement. One study obtained details of violent episodes reported to the FDA adverse events database for a five-year period and, for each drug, established a statistic 'proportional reporting ratio' indicating the association of each drug with violent episodes.[179] By this measure, the 'most dangerous' drug was varenicline (a smoking cessation aid), which had an 18-fold increased risk! Fluoxetine and paroxetine had a 10-fold increased risk, and many other psychotropic medications also demonstrated significant associations. Where such violent behaviour results in criminal charges, psychiatrists may be called upon to provide a court report to explain this side effect to the court and so effect a discharge. Notwithstanding this, the available evidence is of association rather than causation, and reverse causation (altered behaviour leading to medication use) or confounding (for example, psychiatric disorder leading to both medication use and altered behaviours) are just as plausible of an explanation for the observed associations, if not more so.

SSRIs are known to decrease platelet aggregability and activity and prolong bleeding time. The risk appears lower with other non-SSRI antidepressants, and the mechanism is almost certainly serotonin-dependent. Co-prescription of gastroprotective agents is not currently recommended routinely, but NICE recommends this should be considered if SSRIs are prescribed to those taking NSAIDs or anticoagulant medication, or are at high risk of GI bleeding.[153]

Switching Treatment

Switching treatment is not straightforward and, to avoid a withdrawal depression or hazardous interactions, is usually a two-stage process, starting with a wash-out of the initial antidepressant followed by the gradual introduction of the second antidepressant. A guide to switching regimes taken from *The Maudsley Prescribing Guidelines in Psychiatry, 14th Edition*,[11] is given below reproduced with permission (see Tables 3.3.4 and 3.3.5).

Advice given in these tables is partly derived from manufacturers' information and available published data and partly theoretical. There are several factors that affect individual drug handling, and caution is required in every instance. Cross taper cautiously – usually over 2–4 weeks as per example.

When and How to Stop Effective Treatment

Once satisfactory improvement in symptoms has been achieved, antidepressant treatment need not, and probably should not, continue long term for the majority of patients. This principle is variably applied in clinical practice – many patients do not think to ask their prescribers about stopping antidepressants and may assume they are intended to continue indefinitely.[180] Others may stop prematurely as soon as they feel better.

Cessation of treatment is clearly associated with a risk of relapse. Consistently, studies have found that continuing an effective treatment regimen for at least six months after remission (or satisfactory improvement) reduces this risk.[181] This 'six-month rule' is not set in stone, and it may be sensible to delay the decision to stop treatment if the six-month mark coincides with a period of increased psychosocial stress – for example, work deadlines or exams – as such stressors have been associated with risk of relapse.[182–184] The popular practice of avoiding stopping antidepressants in winter in favour of delaying until the summer is not particularly grounded in evidence (except in seasonal affective disorder).

Many antidepressants are associated with withdrawal symptoms on cessation – conventionally referred to as 'discontinuation syndrome' in order to distinguish them from 'addictive' drugs (antidepressants lack many of the other features of this category such as a 'high', cravings, or tolerance).[3] These can be unpleasant (flu-like symptoms, insomnia, agitation, nausea, 'electric-shock'-like sensory disturbances), and gradual down-titration over a period of several weeks (dependent on initial dose) is advised to minimise them. Whilst usually mild, these symptoms can be severe. Some patients do experience marked difficulty when stopping treatment and may need very gradual dose reductions with small increments (liquid formulations, where available, may assist with this).

The risk of discontinuation symptoms is greater with higher doses, with longer durations of treatment and with shorter half-life preparations (like venlafaxine and paroxetine), so that switching to longer half-life drugs may be beneficial. It is good practice to discuss the possibility of discontinuation symptoms prior to starting antidepressant treatment. The optimum rate for tapering is unknown, and opinions vary widely from weeks to months[185] – clinicians should be flexible in their approach.

When antidepressants are eventually stopped, the greatest risk of relapse falls in the following six months.[186] If relapse does occur, treatment should be reinstated and titrated back to previously effective doses as quickly as possible. Cessation can then be attempted again after a further 6–12 months.

Of course, even after a single episode, patients may prefer to continue treatment for longer than six months – even indefinitely – rather than risk relapse. This may be sensible for some – a number of factors have been shown to be associated with increased risk of relapse, including number of previous episodes,[187,188] length/severity/treatment resistance of episode,[189–191] presence of psychotic symptoms[192,193] or residual depressive symptoms.[183,194,195] Female patients[189,196,197] or those with comorbid medical illness[198,199] may also be particularly susceptible to relapse after a successful course of treatment. Frank discussion of risks and benefits is advised. Where

Table 3.3.4 Cross-tapering of antidepressants (1)

From \ To	Agomelatine	Bupropion	Clomipramine	Fluoxetine	Fluvoxamine	MAOIs Phenelzine Tranylcypromine Selegiline	Moclobemide	Mirtazapine	Reboxetine	Trazodone	Other SSRIs[f] Vortioxetine	SNRIs Duloxetine Venlafaxine Desvenlafaxine	TCAs (except clomipramine)
Agomelatine[a]		Stop agomelatine, then start bupropion	Stop agomelatine, then start clomipramine	Stop agomelatine, then start fluoxetine	Stop agomelatine, then start fluvoxamine	Stop agomelatine, then start MAOIs	Stop agomelatine, then start moclobemide	Stop agomelatine, then start mirtazapine	Stop agomelatine, then start reboxetine	Stop agomelatine, then start trazodone	Stop agomelatine, then start SSRI	Stop agomelatine, then start SNRI	Stop agomelatine, then start TCA
Bupropion[b]	Cross-taper cautiously		Cross-taper cautiously with low dose clomipramine	Cross-taper cautiously	Cross-taper cautiously	Taper and stop, wait 2 weeks, then start MAOIs	Taper and stop, then start moclobemide	Cross-taper cautiously	Cross-taper cautiously	Cross-taper cautiously	Cross-taper cautiously	Cross-taper cautiously	Cross-taper cautiously with low-dose TCA
Clomipramine	Cross-taper cautiously	Cross-taper cautiously		Taper and stop, then start fluoxetine at 10 mg/day	Taper and stop, then start low dose fluoxetine	Taper and stop, wait 3 weeks, then start MAOIs	Taper and stop, wait 1 week, then start moclobemide	Cross-taper cautiously	Cross-taper cautiously	Cross-taper cautiously	Taper and stop, then start low-dose SSRI	Taper and stop, then start low-dose SNRI	Cross-taper cautiously
Fluoxetine[c]	Cross-taper cautiously	Stop fluoxetine, wait 4–7 days, then start bupropion	Stop fluoxetine, wait 2 weeks, then start low-dose clomipramine		Stop fluoxetine, wait 4–7 days, then start fluvoxamine	Stop fluoxetine, wait 5–6 weeks, then start MAOIs	Stop fluoxetine, wait 5–6 weeks, then start moclobemide	Cross-taper cautiously	Cross-taper cautiously	Cross-taper cautiously	Stop fluoxetine, wait 4–7 days, then start low-dose SSRI	Stop fluoxetine, wait 4–7 days, then start SNRI	Stop fluoxetine, wait 4–7 days, then start low-dose TCA
Fluvoxamine[d]	Taper and stop, wait for 4 days, then start agomelatine	Cross-taper cautiously	Taper and stop, then start low-dose clomipramine	Direct switch possible		Taper and stop, wait 1 week, then start MAOIs	Taper and stop, wait 1 week, then start moclobemide	Cross-taper cautiously. Start mirtazapine at 15 mg/day	Cross-taper cautiously	Cross-taper cautiously	Direct switch possible	Direct switch possible	Cross-taper cautiously with low-dose TCA
MAOIs **Phenelzine** **Tranylcypromine** **Selegiline**	Cross-taper cautiously	Taper and stop, wait for 2 weeks, then start bupropion	Taper and stop, wait for 3 weeks, then start clomipramine	Taper and stop, wait for 2 weeks, then start fluoxetine	Taper and stop, wait for 2 weeks, then start fluvoxamine	Taper and stop, wait 2 weeks, then start MAOIs	Taper and stop, wait 2 weeks, then start moclobemide	Taper and stop, wait 2 weeks, then start mirtazapine	Taper and stop, wait 2 weeks, then start reboxetine	Taper and stop, wait 2 weeks, then start trazodone	Taper and stop, wait 2 weeks, then start SSRI	Taper and stop, wait 2 weeks, then start SNRI	Taper and stop, wait 2 weeks, then start TCA
Moclobemide	Taper and stop, wait 24 hours, then start agomelatine	Taper and stop, wait 24 hours, then start bupropion	Taper and stop, wait 24 hours, then start clomipramine	Taper and stop, wait 24 hours, then start fluoxetine	Taper and stop, wait 24 hours, then start fluvoxamine	Taper and stop, wait 24 hours, then start MAOIs		Taper and stop, wait 24 hours, then start mirtazapine	Taper and stop, wait 24 hours, then start reboxetine	Taper and stop, wait 24 hours, then start trazodone	Taper and stop, wait 24 hours, then start SSRI	Taper and stop, wait 24 hours, then start SNRI	Taper and stop, wait 24 hours, then start TCA
Mirtazapine	Cross-taper cautiously	Cross-taper cautiously	Cross-taper cautiously	Cross-taper cautiously	Cross-taper cautiously	Taper and stop, wait for 2 weeks, then start MAOIs	Taper and stop, wait 1 week, then start moclobemide		Cross-taper cautiously	Cross-taper cautiously	Cross-taper cautiously	Cross-taper cautiously	Cross-taper cautiously
Reboxetine[e]	Cross-taper cautiously	Cross-taper cautiously	Cross-taper cautiously	Cross-taper cautiously	Cross-taper cautiously	Taper and stop, wait 1 week, then start MAOIs	Taper and stop, wait 1 week, then start moclobemide	Cross-taper cautiously		Cross-taper cautiously	Cross-taper cautiously	Cross-taper cautiously	Cross-taper cautiously

Table 3.3.5 Cross-tapering of antidepressants (2)

	Agomelatine	Bupropion	Clomipramine	Fluoxetine	Fluvoxamine	MAOIs Phenelzine Tranylcypromine Selegiline	Moclobemide	Mirtazapine	Reboxetine	Trazodone	Other SSRIs Vortioxetine	SNRIs Duloxetine Venlafaxine Desvenlafaxine	TCAs (except clomipramine)
Trazodone	Cross-taper cautiously	Cross-taper cautiously	Cross-taper cautiously with low-dose clomipramine	Cross-taper cautiously	Cross-taper cautiously	Taper and stop, wait for 1 week, then start MAOIs	Taper and stop, wait for 1 week, then start moclobemide	Cross-taper cautiously	Cross-taper cautiously		Cross-taper cautiously	Cross-taper cautiously	Cross-taper cautiously with low-dose TCA
Other SSRIs[f] **Vortioxetine**[g]	Cross-taper cautiously	Cross-taper cautiously	Taper and stop, then start low-dose clomipramine	Direct switch possible	Direct switch possible	Taper and stop, wait for 1 week[h], then start MAOIs	Taper and stop, wait for 1 week, then start moclobemide	Cross-taper cautiously	Cross-taper cautiously	Cross-taper cautiously	Direct switch possible	Direct switch possible	Cross-taper cautiously with low-dose TCA
SNRIs[h] **Duloxetine**[i] **Venlafaxine** **–** **Desvenlafaxine**	Cross-taper cautiously	Cross-taper cautiously	Taper and stop, then start low-dose clomipramine	Direct switch possible	Direct switch possible	Taper and stop, wait for 1 week, then start MAOIs	Taper and stop, wait for 1 week, then start moclobemide	Cross-taper cautiously	Cross-taper cautiously	Cross-taper cautiously	Direct switch possible	Direct switch possible	Cross-taper cautiously with low-dose TCA
Tricyclics[j]	Cross-taper cautiously	Halve dose, add bupropion and then slow withdrawal	Direct switch possible	Halve dose, add fluoxetine and then slow withdrawal	Cross-taper cautiously	Taper and stop, wait for 2 weeks[j], then starts MAOIs	Taper and stop, wait for 1 week, then start moclobemide	Cross-taper cautiously	Cross-taper cautiously	Halve dose, add trazodone then slow withdrawal	Halve dose, add SSRI then slow withdrawal	Cross-taper cautiously starting with low-dose SNRI	Direct switch possible

[a] Agomelatine has no effect on monoamine uptake and no affinity for α, β adrenergic, histaminergic, cholinergic, dopaminergic and benzodiazepine receptors. The potential for interactions between agomelatine and other antidepressants is low, and it is not expected to mitigate discontinuation reactions of other antidepressants. Some crossover with other antidepressants might be cautiously attempted when switching from agomelatine.

[b] Bupropion is licensed for smoking cessation but unlicensed for the treatment of depression in the UK. It is a CYP2D6 inhibitor, and particular caution is required when cross-tapering with drugs metabolised by this enzyme.

[c] Beware: interactions with fluoxetine may still occur for five weeks after stopping fluoxetine because of its metabolite's long half-life.

[d] Fluvoxamine is a potent inhibitor of CYF1A2, and to a lesser extent of CYP2C and CYP3A4, and has a high potential for interactions; hence, extra precaution is required.

[e] Switching to reboxetine as antidepressant monotherapy is no longer recommended.

[f] Citalopram, escitalopram, paroxetine and sertraline.

[g] Limited experience with vortioxetine and extra precaution required. Particular care when switching to or from bupropion and other CYP2D6 inhibitors such as fluoxetine and paroxetine.

[h] Wait three weeks in the case of vortioxetine.

[i] Abrupt switch from SSRIs and venlafaxine to duloxetine is possible starting at 60 mg/day.

[j] Wait three weeks in the case of imipramine.

patients conclude that they would rather continue treatment long-term, this should not usually be opposed.

However, in most current guidelines, long-term treatment is only formally recommend for those with a diagnosis of recurrent depressive disorder (>2 depressive episodes) – see next section.

Relapse Prevention

For patients with recurrent depressive disorder, especially after three or more recurrences, long-term treatment is recommended. Some patients who do not fall in this category may also opt to continue with long-term treatment after a discussion of risks and benefits (see previous section). 'Maintenance treatment' has shown consistent efficacy over placebo in reducing relapse rates, with reductions in the order of two- to three-fold for as long as treatment is maintained, although few studies have been undertaken beyond five years.[200–202] The longer remission is maintained, the lower the subsequent risk of further relapse.[188,203]

Exactly what form this maintenance treatment should take is somewhat less clear – the most commonly used practice involves continuing with whatever regimen (and doses) successfully induced remission. This is supported by a number of studies indicating a reduction in relapses with continuation of the 'effective treatment' dose as compared to lower doses.[201,204–206] No individual antidepressants have been shown to be more effective than others at preventing relapse.[203,207–209]

However, this may not be ideal where adjunctive agents have been used. Drugs such as atypical antipsychotics are associated with significant side-effect burdens and monitoring requirements, and evidence for long-term benefits in unipolar depression is inconclusive.[210] In practice, treatment may involve a trial-and-error approach similar to that used in bipolar affective disorder, where adjunctive medications are cautiously reduced with the eventual aim of maintaining patients on the minimum possible doses necessary to prevent relapse.

It is an unfortunate fact that some patients will eventually experience relapse despite being maintained on the same medication regimen that achieved successful resolution of a previous episode. The causes for this are not understood and reflect our incomplete understanding of the mechanisms involved – attenuation of medication effects and altered pathogenesis of symptoms are both possible, although adherence should also be carefully checked.[186] Treatment escalation should resume as for any non-responsive episode.

Unipolar Depression (Without Psychotic Symptoms)

First-Line

- Any SSRI except citalopram. Preference may be given to sertraline (if gradual titration preferred) or escitalopram (if rapid titration preferred).

Rationale

SSRIs are generally considered a sensible first-choice treatment for depressive illness. Of these, sertraline and escitalopram may have a slight advantage, as established by extensive meta-research examining comparative efficacy, tolerability and safety.[29,211–213]

Sertraline's availability in smaller dose increments (25 mg increments with a max dose of 200 mg, compared to 5 mg increments with a max dose of 20 mg for escitalopram) theoretically allows for more gradual titration and greater fine-tuning in case of side effects (without splitting tablets). However, in practice, the difference is probably clinically insignificant.

If for some reason sertraline or escitalopram are not felt to be suitable, any SSRI other than citalopram could be substituted. Citalopram is not recommended first-line due to its slightly greater propensity for cardiac side effects.[214] If fluoxetine is selected, clinicians should be aware of its comparatively long half-life, which can complicate treatment switches if these are required at a later date. If paroxetine or fluvoxamine are selected, clinicians should be aware of their relatively short half-lives, which can lead to unpleasant discontinuation symptoms if doses are missed.

If SSRIs are not felt to be appropriate (e.g. due to side effects), see the second-line options below.

A possible future alternative to SSRI's first-line may be buproprion; although not currently licensed for depression in the UK, it compares favourably to SSRIs as a first-line option[24,215] and is widely used as such in much of the world – especially for patients who do not want to risk encountering the sexual side effects of SSRIs.

Second-Line

- SWITCH to a second SSRI

OR

- SWITCH to a non-SSRI antidepressant (not MAOI or tricyclic)

Rationale

There is no evidence-based, clear, single option to recommend after one failed adequate trial of an antidepressant. While many options have been demonstrated to be superior to placebo, there is very little data available from head-to-head trials of different alternatives.

A second trial of antidepressant monotherapy is suggested by NICE,[152] and in practice, most clinicians offer at least two trials of monotherapy before proceeding to the other options later, including antidepressant combinations or augmentation. However, it is worth re-stating that studies of switching to another single agent after a failed trial of antidepressant monotherapy have produced mixed results.

We would recommend involving the patient in the decision about which option to try after a failed trial of first-line treatment. Meta-analyses have demonstrated that switching to a second antidepressant of a different class (rather than a second SSRI) seems to result in a faster/greater reduction in depressive symptoms, at the cost of a greater side-effect burden and reduced tolerability.[216,217]

Sensible options for a non-SSRI antidepressant include a NaSSA (e.g. mirtazapine or mianserin), which may be preferred if appetite and sleep are poor, or an SNRI (e.g. venlafaxine or duloxetine), which may be preferred if appetite and sleep are preserved and the patient would prefer to avoid potential sedation or weight gain.

MAOI and tricyclic antidepressants are not recommended at this stage due to their relatively higher propensity for side effects.

Third-Line (Treatment-Resistant)

- AUGMENTATION treatment with an antidepressant and a non-antidepressant medication

OR

- COMBINATION treatment with two antidepressants from different classes

OR

- SWITCH to third antidepressant from a class not yet tried

Rationale

At this point, the patient should have completed two adequate trials of treatment. If the response in symptoms remains inadequate, this is a 'treatment-resistant' depressive episode by definition.

If they have not completed two adequate trials – or if they have but express a preference to not combine medications – a further trial of antidepressant monotherapy (from a class not yet tried) could be considered. However, the evidence to support the use of repeated trials of antidepressant monotherapy for treatment-resistant depression is relatively weak, and this is not our recommended approach.

Instead, we recommend adding a second drug to the current antidepressant, referred to as 'augmentation' when the second agent is not primarily an antidepressant and 'combination' when two antidepressants are used. Again, there is relatively little high-quality evidence from head-to-head studies to guide the choice between different augmentation and combination strategies. One such study (VAST-D) found that augmentation with aripiprazole was modestly more effective than either the addition of or the switch to bupropion in treatment-resistant patients.[218]

In practice, a pragmatic guide often used is that where there has been some response to the current antidepressant and it is well tolerated, augmentation is preferred, whilst if there has been no response or the current antidepressant is poorly tolerated, an antidepressant switch is preferred in the first instance. We would suggest involving the patient in making this decision via discussion of the options available and their relative side-effect profiles. Of note, the efficacy of augmenting antidepressants with a non-antidepressant agent is probably overall better established than combination treatment with two antidepressants. However, adverse effects also appear to be greater with augmentation rather than combination treatment, particularly if antipsychotics or lithium are used as the augmenting agents.

Reviewing available evidence, the BAP guidelines concluded that the best evidence of efficacy in augmentation of antidepressants is for quetiapine, aripiprazole and lithium, with less robust evidence for risperidone, olanzapine, thyroid hormone, buspirone or lamotrigine, or a combination treatment with supplementary bupropion or mirtazapine.[153] However, this may result from some options being more extensively researched than others. Even for the most popular options, NNT is modest, and side-effect burdens are relatively high.[219] The place of ketamine/esketamine is not yet clear and is only available in certain treatment settings in the UK, but it is another augmentation option that can be considered.

Additional Options

At this point, the patient's symptoms have failed to respond to at least two adequate trials of antidepressant monotherapy plus a trial of combination or augmentation treatment with two agents.

There are a wide range of options for further escalation but little evidence to suggest which is most likely to succeed. Even STAR*D offers little in the way of certainty, as it stops after four treatment trials.[218,220]

Before committing to a particular approach, consider the following questions – is the diagnosis certain? Have organic conditions that may present with depressive symptoms been excluded? Are you attempting to treat the core symptoms of personality disorder with antidepressants (this is unlikely to succeed)? Are there psychotic symptoms or features of bipolarity present, which may benefit from antipsychotics/mood stabilisers respectively? Is the patient compliant with treatment (if not, why not – are there side effects which can be addressed)? Are there psychosocial stressors present that may be amenable to non-pharmacological interventions? Is there comorbid substance use or medical problems that may be complicating the presentation?

Having considered these, possible options include:

- Further antidepressants from classes not yet tried. Less commonly used options – such as high-dose TCAs (with monitoring of plasma levels) or an MAOI – may be more efficacious for treatment-resistant patients than repeated trials of newer, more selective agents, at the cost of increased side effects.[221] However, endless trials of monotherapy (particularly of multiple agents from the same class) should be avoided.
- Additional augmentations/combinations. Newer antipsychotics with more favourable side-effect profiles,

such as lurasidone and cariprazine, may be worth trying where more conventional options (quetiapine, risperidone) have failed. The specific combination of venlafaxine + mirtazapine, if not yet tried, has a reasonable evidence base.[19] However, there is a risk of becoming mired in repeated switches, seeking an elusive cocktail that may not exist. Try to be pragmatic: change one agent at a time, complete adequate trials and quantify responses with validated outcome measures.

- Consider interventions with less supportive evidence but with a low risk of adverse effects. These include nutrients (check interactions carefully, avoid St John's Wort in combination with antidepressants), tryptophan (caution patients regarding potential serotonergic interactions) and phototherapy.
- Consider ECT – always an option, particularly if symptoms deteriorate to the point where severe suicidality or malnutrition/dehydration (due to self-neglect) emerge.
- Consider novel treatments such as ketamine augmentation, TMS or VNS. These may only be accessible through specialist tertiary centres, so establish contact/referral pathways early. More experimental treatments such as psychedelics or stereotactic psychosurgery may also be available as part of ongoing research protocols.
- Whilst it is beyond the scope of this chapter (see Chapter 3.4), we always recommend considering psychological interventions alongside pharmacological therapies in treatment-resistant patients, as well as patient with severe, chronic or recurrent depression. As discussed in the BAP guidelines, the strongest evidence is for cognitive, behavioural and interpersonal therapies. However, other therapeutic approaches such as couple therapy or family therapy do have a place in selected cases.

Unipolar Depression (With Psychotic Symptoms)

First-Line

Is the patient severely ill (e.g. with severe suicidality, or malnutrition/dehydration resulting from self-neglect)? Are they likely to be non-compliant with pharmacological treatment?

If YES:

- Consider ECT as a first-line treatment.

If NO:

- SSRI + AUGMENTATION with an atypical antipsychotic (preferred)

OR

- Tricyclic antidepressant (ideally with an antipsychotic but may be effective without)

Rationale

Depression with psychotic symptoms may necessitate very urgent improvement – risks of adverse outcomes, including completed suicide, are high.[222] ECT will often be seen as a controversial opening strategy, and in practice, organisational considerations will probably result in other treatments being initiated first. However, it has unparalleled efficacy, with remission rates as high as 95 per cent reported for psychotic depression (note that many studies were not controlled).[223] Think of ECT early – it is an option at any other stage in this algorithm if symptoms are deteriorating.

If the presentation is not associated with urgent risks, or ECT is not possible for some reason (there are relatively few), then pharmacotherapy alone can be tried first. A strong evidence base supports the use of an antidepressant (SSRIs are a good starting-point) and an antipsychotic (choose based on side-effect profile, avoid clozapine) started simultaneously and titrated to effective doses as rapidly as is practically possible.[224] Fluoxetine + olanzapine is a popular combination (to the degree that a single combined formulation is available in some areas) with a supportive evidence base,[225] although its actual superiority to other combinations is uncertain.

If the use of antipsychotics or combination treatment is not possible (patient reluctance is probably the most likely reason), there is some evidence to indicate that TCAs may be more effective than other forms of monotherapy.[226,227] However, they are almost certainly inferior to antipsychotic-augmented treatment, with some studies suggesting they can actually temporarily worsen psychosis[228] – patients should be made aware that this approach is not preferable.

Second-Line

- Antidepressant + AUGMENTATION with an atypical antipsychotic – switch antidepressant

OR

- Antidepressant + AUGMENTATION with an atypical antipsychotic – switch antipsychotic

Rationale

If antidepressant monotherapy (e.g. with a TCA) was chosen initially and was ineffective, an atypical antipsychotic should be added.

If the first trial was of SSRI + atypical antipsychotic, there is some evidence that switching the SSRI to an SNRI[229] or TCA may still be effective, although data from good quality head-to-head trials is lacking.

The other option is to switch the atypical antipsychotic to another agent from this class. The efficacy of this approach is unproven. The strongest evidence base is for olanzapine and quetiapine, although this probably just reflects the fact that they are better-studied for affective symptoms overall (both are commonly used in bipolar depression). If one of these was chosen as part of the first trial, switching to another agent is unlikely to confer much additional efficacy (although newer agents such as aripiprazole/lurasidone/cariprazine may have advantages in terms of side-effect profile and improved tolerability). If the first-line choice was aripirazole/lurasidone/cariprazine, though, a switch to quetiapine or olanzapine is worth attempting.

Third-Line

- Antidepressant + atypical antipsychotic + lithium

OR

- Antidepressant + clozapine

AND

- Reconsider ECT

Rationale

If a patient has failed to respond to a couple of antidepressant + antipsychotic combinations (ideally, including a TCA at some stage and either quetiapine/ olanzapine), then further switching between antidepressant and antipsychotic agents is not recommended. Time is likely to be of the essence.

Lithium has performed well as an additional augmenting agent in this situation (e.g. response rates of 40–60%, albeit based on sparse data).[230,231]

If lithium is contraindicated, another option is the pharmacologically unique atypical antipsychotic clozapine (most commonly used for treatment-resistant schizophrenia). High side-effect burden (including risk of serious, life-threatening adverse events) has limited its inclusion in the literature on affective disorders, but it does have some supportive evidence from case series and case reports.[232]

Typical antipsychotics may also still have a place, supported by older RCTS, but they obviously carry the additional risks of using these agents.

Regardless of the choice of pharmacotherapy, ECT should be revisited as an option. Despite negative connotations (stigma), it has clear advantages – both in terms of proven efficacy and side effects – over the other choices presented at this stage.

Additional Options

If all of the options presented above (including ECT) have proven ineffective, the choice of further options is beyond any available robust evidence base. Clinicians would be wise to seek advice from a tertiary-level specialist centre with experience in the management of treatment-resistant symptoms, if available. Potential options are rather experimental and may include augmentation with ketamine or stimulants[233] (possibly in combination with ECT).

Special Cases

Atypical Depression

- Explore carefully for comorbidities (personality disorder, anxiety disorders) and exclude bipolar affective disorder
- Consider bupropion early in treatment
- Consider MAOI

'Atypical' depression refers to a recognised subtype of depressive episode, where mood reactivity is preserved and 'vegetative symptoms' are prominent – hypersomnia, hyperphagia (classically with cravings for carbohydrate-rich foods) and specific psychomotor abnormalities (feelings of heaviness in the limbs, commonly referred to as 'leaden paralysis'). This contrasts with symptoms such as insomnia and poor appetite, which are more commonly seen in typical or 'melancholic' depressive illness.

Atypical depression is (unlike the name suggests) common; atypical presentations may account for up to 40 per cent of cases of depression.[234] It may be more likely to be comorbid with personality disorder and anxiety disorders. Patients with atypical depression are also more likely to have a history of childhood trauma, metabolic abnormalities, raised inflammatory markers and medical comorbidity, all of which have impact on treatment choices. Clinicians should also examine the history carefully for features of bipolarity, as 'atypical' presentations are common in fluctuating affective disorders such as bipolar affective disorder, cyclothymia and seasonal affective disorder.[235]

Regarding the need for treatment modifications, early perspectives favoured the use of MAOIs over TCAs (when these were the only two classes of antidepressant medication available). In more recent studies, including newer agents, the competitive advantage of MAOIs has not been reproduced – for example, one meta-analysis found negligible differences between SSRIs and MAOIs.[236] However, they may be more beneficial for atypical depression than other third-line options (e.g. TCAs) and should be considered where initial conventional strategies have failed.

Studies have also found selective advantages for some specific treatments, including bupropion[237] and, in one study, ECT,[238] although conventionally ECT is thought to be more effective in patients with the melancholic subtype of depression. Pragmatically, the use of augmentation drugs that are activating (like aripiprazole) would be preferred over those that are sedating (like quetiapine).

Renal Impairment

- SSRIs preferable to other classes – sertraline best – dose adjustments may be needed
- Avoid SNRIs/TCAs/MAOIs if possible
- Avoid lithium

Patients with moderate to advanced renal disease are often excluded from trials related to treatment of depression, and as a result, few studies exist to guide pharmacological management in this group.

The majority of antidepressant medications are highly protein-bound and hepatically metabolised, but many have active metabolites that are renally excreted and not removed by dialysis. This leads to the potential for accumulation and eventual toxicity. Dose adjustments are recommended by manufacturers for many antidepressants – a comprehensive summary of these has been published elsewhere.[239]

Sertraline is a good first-line choice as a relatively rare agent where a dose adjustment is not recommended (although it is worth noting that even sertraline has a renally-excreted active metabolite).

Agents that interfere with blood pressure control (SNRIs) and have high risks of medication interactions (TCAs/MAOIs) should generally be avoided. Lithium should obviously be avoided: it is renally excreted so it quickly accumulates if clearance is impaired, extremely toxic at high plasma levels and can adversely affect renal function.

Hepatic Impairment

- Almost all psychotropic medications are affected to some degree
- Use lower doses, monitor closely for side effects/interactions
- Avoid sedative agents

Hepatic enzymes are involved in the metabolism of essentially all antidepressant and augmentory medication. Adjustments are recommended both in initial doses and titration. A comprehensive summary has been published elsewhere,[240] but as a general rule, doses should be 50 per cent of that used for the healthy population.

Sedative agents (mirtazapine, trazodone, antipsychotics) should be avoided where possible due to the risk of complicating the assessment of emerging hepatic encephalopathy.

Strongly serotonergic agents (particularly SSRIs) should be prescribed only with gastroprotective cover, and co-prescription with NSAIDs and anti-platelet agents should be avoided due to bleeding risk.

Comorbid Chronic Pain

- Consider duloxetine early in treatment
- Consider tricyclics early in treatment

Chronic pain is associated with poor treatment outcomes for depressive illness and is a risk factor for suicide.[241]

Several antidepressants – most commonly SNRIs and tricyclics – are commonly used as adjunctive treatments for chronic pain syndromes. However, evidence for beneficial effects are modest at best,[5] even for duloxetine, which is specifically licensed for pain syndromes including diabetic neuropathy.[242] However, some studies found clomipramine in low doses to be helpful, particularly for co-existing anxiety symptoms,[243] although amitriptyline and nortriptyline are more widely used in chronic pain.

References

1. Brausch J, Connors K, Brooks B, et al. Human pharmaceuticals in the aquatic environment: a review of recent toxicological studies and considerations for toxicity testing. *Reviews of Environmental Contamination and Toxicology* 2012;218:1–99.
2. Zanger UM, Schwab M. Cytochrome P450 enzymes in drug metabolism: regulation of gene expression, enzyme activities, and impact of genetic variation. *Pharmacology & Therapeutics* 2013;138(1):103–41.
3. Haddad PM. Do antidepressants cause dependence? *Epidemiologia e Psichiatria Sociale* 2005;14(2):58–62.
4. Sternbach H. The serotonin syndrome. *American Journal of Psychiatry* 1991;148(6):705–13.
5. Gebhardt S, Heinzel-Gutenbrunner M, König U. Pain relief in depressive disorders: a meta-analysis of the effects of antidepressants. *Journal of Clinical Psychopharmacology* 2016;36(6):658–68.
6. MacHado M, Einarson TR. Comparison of SSRIs and SNRIs in major depressive disorder: a meta-analysis of head-to-head randomized clinical trials. *Journal of Clinical Pharmacy and Therapeutics* 2010;35(2):177–88.
7. Blier P, Briley M. The noradrenergic symptom cluster: clinical expression and neuropharmacology. *Neuropsychiatric Disease and Treatment* 2011;7(Suppl 1):15–20.
8. McIntyre RS, Panjwani ZD, Nguyen HT, et al. The hepatic safety profile of duloxetine: a review. *Expert Opinion on Drug Metabolism & Toxicology* 2008;4 (3):281–5.
9. Taylor D, Lenox-Smith A, Bradley A. A review of the suitability of duloxetine and venlafaxine for use in patients with depression in primary care with a focus on cardiovascular safety, suicide and mortality due to antidepressant overdose. *Therapeutic Advances in Psychopharmacology* 2013;3(3):151–61.
10. Fischer M, Unterecker S, Pfuhlmann B. Overdose of venlafaxine with mild outcome. *Neuroscience and Medicine* 2012;2012:327–9.
11. Taylor D, Barnes TRE, Young AH, et al. *The Maudsley Prescribing Guidelines in Psychiatry*, 14th ed. Hoboken, NJ: Wiley-Blackwell;2021.
12. Gray SL, Anderson ML, Dublin S, et al. Cumulative use of strong anticholinergics and incident dementia. *JAMA Internal Medicine* 2015;175 (3):401–7.
13. National Institute for Health and Care Excellence. *Interactions | BNF content published by NICE.* bnf.nice.org.uk/interaction/.
14. Gijsman H, Geddes J, Rendell J, et al. Antidepressants for bipolar depression: a systematic review of randomized, controlled trials. *American Journal of Psychiatry* 2004;161(9):1537–47.
15. Hawton K, Bergen H, Simkin S, et al. Toxicity of antidepressants: rates of suicide relative to prescribing and non-fatal overdose. *British Journal of Psychiatry* 2010;196(5):354–8.
16. Henssler J, Alexander D, Schwarzer G, et al. Combining antidepressants vs antidepressant monotherapy for treatment of patients with acute depression: a systematic review and meta-analysis. *JAMA Psychiatry* 2022;79 (4):300–12.
17. Kessler D, MacNeill S, Tallon D, et al. Mirtazapine added to SSRIs or SNRIs for treatment resistant depression in primary care: phase III randomised placebo controlled trial (MIR). *BMJ* 2018;363. DOI:10.1136/BMJ.K4218.
18. Fawcett J, Barkin RL. Review of the results from clinical studies on the efficacy, safety and tolerability of mirtazapine for the treatment of patients with major depression. *Journal*

of Affective Disorders 1998;51 (3):267–85.

19. Silva J, Mota J, Azevedo P. California rocket fuel: and what about being a first line treatment? *European Psychiatry* 2016;33(Supplement):S551.
20. Houlihan DJ. Serotonin syndrome resulting from coadministration of tramadol, venlafaxine, and mirtazapine. *Annals of Pharmacotherapy* 2004;38 (3):411–3.
21. White N, Litovitz T, Clancy C. Suicidal antidepressant overdoses: a comparative analysis by antidepressant type. *Journal of Medical Toxicology* 2008;4(4):238–50.
22. Maxwell RA, Eckhardt SB. *Drug Discovery: A Casebook and Analysis.* London: Springer Science & Business Media;1990.
23. Patnode CD, Henderson JT, Coppola EL, et al. Interventions for tobacco cessation in adults, including pregnant persons: updated evidence report and systematic review for the US Preventive Services Task Force. *JAMA* 2021;325 (3):280–98.
24. Zimmerman M, Posternak M, Attiullah N, et al. Why isn't bupropion the most frequently prescribed antidepressant? *Journal of Clinical Psychiatry* 2005;66 (5):603–10.
25. Pisani F, Oteri G, Costa C, et al. Effects of psychotropic drugs on seizure threshold. *Drug Safety* 2002;25 (2):91–110.
26. Nelson JC, Spyker DA. Morbidity and mortality associated with medications used in the treatment of depression: an analysis of cases reported to U.S. poison control centers, 2000–2014. *American Journal of Psychiatry* 2017;174 (5):438–50.
27. Taylor D, Sparshatt A, Varma S, et al. Antidepressant efficacy of agomelatine: meta-analysis of published and unpublished studies. *BMJ* 2014;348: g1888. DOI:10.1136/BMJ.G1888.
28. Eyding D, Lelgemann M, Grouven U, et al. Reboxetine for acute treatment of major depression: systematic review and meta-analysis of published and unpublished placebo and selective serotonin reuptake inhibitor controlled trials. *BMJ* 2010;341:c4737.
29. Cipriani A, Furukawa TA, Salanti G, et al. Comparative efficacy and acceptability of 21 antidepressant drugs for the acute treatment of adults with major depressive disorder: a systematic review and network meta-analysis. *Lancet* 2018;391(10128):1357–66.
30. Stryjer R, Spivak B, Strous RD, et al. Trazodone for the treatment of sexual dysfunction induced by serotonin reuptake inhibitors: a preliminary open-label study. *Clinical Neuropharmacology* 2009;32(2):82–4.
31. Abber JC, Lue TF, Luo JA, et al. Priapism induced by chlorpromazine and trazodone: mechanism of action. *Journal of Urology* 1987;137(5):1039–42.
32. Battaglia C, Venturoli S. Persistent genital arousal disorder and trazodone. Morphometric and vascular modifications of the clitoris. A case report. *Journal of Sexual Medicine* 2009;6(10):2896–900.
33. Martínez MA, Ballesteros S, Sánchez De La Torre C, et al. Investigation of a fatality due to trazodone poisoning: case report and literature review. *Journal of Analytical Toxicology* 2005;29(4):262–8.
34. Sanchez C, Asin KE, Artigas F. Vortioxetine, a novel antidepressant with multimodal activity: review of preclinical and clinical data. *Pharmacology & Therapeutics* 2015;145:43–57.
35. Bishop MM, Fixen DR, Linnebur SA, et al. Cognitive effects of vortioxetine in older adults: a systematic review. *Therapeutic Advance in Psychopharmacology* 2021;11:1–10. DOI: 10.1177/20451253211026796.
36. Robertson MM, Trimble MR. Major tranquillisers used as antidepressants. A review. *Journal of Affective Disorders* 1982;4(3):173–93.
37. Spielmans G, Berman M, Linardatos E, et al. Adjunctive atypical antipsychotic treatment for major depressive disorder: a meta-analysis of depression, quality of life, and safety outcomes. *PLoS Med* 2013;10(3):e1001403. DOI: 10.1371/JOURNAL.PMED.1001403.
38. Berman R, Marcus R, Swanink R, et al. The efficacy and safety of aripiprazole as adjunctive therapy in major depressive disorder: a multicenter, randomized, double-blind, placebo-controlled study. *Journal of Clinical Psychiatry* 2007;68 (6):843–53.
39. Brunner E, Tohen M, Osuntokun O, Landry J, Thase ME. Efficacy and safety of olanzapine/fluoxetine combination vs fluoxetine monotherapy following successful combination therapy of treatment-resistant major depressive disorder. *Neuropsychopharmacology* 2014;39(11):2549–59.
40. Nelson J, Papakostas G. Atypical antipsychotic augmentation in major depressive disorder: a meta-analysis of placebo-controlled randomized trials. *American Journal of Psychiatry* 2009;166(9):980–91.
41. Vieta E, Bauer M, Montgomery S, et al. Pooled analysis of sustained response rates for extended release quetiapine fumarate as monotherapy or adjunct to antidepressant therapy in patients with major depressive disorder. *Journal of Affective Disorders* 2013;150(2):639–43.
42. Taylor D, Cornelius V, Smith L, et al. Comparative efficacy and acceptability of drug treatments for bipolar depression: a multiple-treatments meta-analysis. *Acta Psychiatrica Scandandinavica* 2014;130(6):452–69.
43. Cade JFJ. Lithium salts in the treatment of psychotic excitement. *Medical Journal of Australia* 1949;2(1):349–52.
44. Crossley N, Bauer M. Acceleration and augmentation of antidepressants with lithium for depressive disorders: two meta-analyses of randomized, placebo-controlled trials. *Journal of Clinical Psychiatry* 2007;68(6):935–40.
45. Bauer M, Adli M, Ricken R, et al. Role of lithium augmentation in the management of major depressive disorder. *CNS Drugs* 2014;28(4): 331–42.
46. Birkenhäger T, van den Broek W, Moleman P, et al. Outcome of a 4-step treatment algorithm for depressed inpatients. *Journal of Clinical Psychiatry* 2006;67(8):1266–71.
47. Nierenberg AA, Fava M, Trivedi M, et al. A comparison of lithium and T(3) augmentation following two failed medication treatments for depression: a STAR*D report. *American Journal of Psychiatry* 2006;163(9):1519–30.
48. Bauer M, Dell'osso L, Kasper S, et al. Extended-release quetiapine fumarate (quetiapine XR) monotherapy and quetiapine XR or lithium as add-on to antidepressants in patients with treatment-resistant major depressive disorder. *Journal of Affective Disorders* 2013;151(1):209–19.
49. Cipriani A, Hawton K, Stockton S, et al. Lithium in the prevention of suicide in

mood disorders: updated systematic review and meta-analysis. *BMJ* 2013;346:f3646. DOI: 10.1136/BMJ.F3646.

50. Tiihonen J, Tanskanen A, Hoti F, et al. Pharmacological treatments and risk of readmission to hospital for unipolar depression in Finland: a nationwide cohort study. *Lancet Psychiatry* 2017;4(7):547–53.
51. Böer U, Cierny I, Krause D, et al. Chronic lithium salt treatment reduces CRE/CREB-directed gene transcription and reverses its upregulation by chronic psychosocial stress in transgenic reporter gene mice. *Neuropsychopharmacology* 2007;33(10):2407–15.
52. Scheuch K, Höltje M, Budde H, et al. Lithium modulates tryptophan hydroxylase 2 gene expression and serotonin release in primary cultures of serotonergic raphe neurons. *Brain Research* 2010;1307:14–21.
53. Einat H, Manji HK. Cellular plasticity cascades: genes-to-behavior pathways in animal models of bipolar disorder. *Biological Psychiatry* 2006;59(12):1160–71.
54. Gould T, Picchini A, Einat H, et al. Targeting glycogen synthase kinase-3 in the CNS: implications for the development of new treatments for mood disorders. *Current Drug Targets* 2006;7(11):1399–409.
55. Ghasemi M, Raza M, Dehpour AR. NMDA receptor antagonists augment antidepressant-like effects of lithium in the mouse forced swimming test. *Journal of Psychopharmacology (Oxford)* 2010;24(4):585–94.
56. Malhi GS, Tanious M, Das P, et al. Potential mechanisms of action of lithium in bipolar disorder. *CNS Drugs* 2013;27(2):135–53.
57. Gong R, Wang P, Dworkin L. What we need to know about the effect of lithium on the kidney. *American Journal of Physiology. Renal Physiology* 2016;311(6):F1168–71.
58. McKnight RF, Adida M, Budge K, et al. Lithium toxicity profile: a systematic review and meta-analysis. *Lancet* 2012;379(9817):721–8.
59. Barbosa L, Berk M, Vorster M. A double-blind, randomized, placebo-controlled trial of augmentation with lamotrigine or placebo in patients concomitantly treated with fluoxetine for resistant major depressive episodes. *Journal of Clinical Psychiatry* 2003;64:403–7.
60. Schindler F, Anghelescu I. Lithium versus lamotrigine augmentation in treatment resistant unipolar depression: a randomized, open-label study. *International Clinical Psychopharmacology* 2007;22(3):179–82.
61. Alyahya B, Friesen M, Nauche B, et al. Acute lamotrigine overdose: a systematic review of published adult and pediatric cases. *Clinical Toxicology (Philadelphia)* 2018;56(2):81–9.
62. D'haenen H, Boer J den, Willner P. *Biological Psychiatry*. Chichester: John Wiley & Sons Ltd; 2002. ndl.ethernet.edu.et/bitstream/123456789/12897/1/Hugo%20D%E2%80%99haenen.pdf.
63. Hage MP, Azar ST. The link between thyroid function and depression. *Journal of Thyroid Research* 2012;2012:590648. DOI: 10.1155/2012/590648.
64. Kirkegaard C, Faber J. Altered serum levels of thyroxine, triiodothyronines and diiodothyronines in endogenous depression. *Acta Endocrinologica* 1981;96(2):199–207.
65. Aronson R, Offman H, Joffe R, Naylor C. Triiodothyronine augmentation in the treatment of refractory depression. A meta-analysis. *Archives of General Psychiatry* 1996;53(9):842–8.
66. Nuñez NA, Joseph B, Pahwa M, et al. Augmentation strategies for treatment resistant major depression: a systematic review and network meta-analysis. *Journal of Affective Disorders* 2022;302:385–400.
67. Zhou X, Ravindran A v, Qin B, et al. Comparative efficacy, acceptability, and tolerability of augmentation agents in treatment-resistant depression: systematic review and network meta-analysis. *Journal of Clinical Psychiatry* 2015;76(4):487–98.
68. Rosenthal LJ, Goldner WS, O'Reardon JP. T3 augmentation in major depressive disorder: Safety considerations. *American Journal of Psychiatry* 2011;168(10):1035–40.
69. Trivedi MH, Fava M, Wisniewski SR, et al. Medication augmentation after the failure of SSRIs for depression. *New England Journal of Medicine* 2009;354(12):1243–52. dx.doi.org/10.1056/NEJMoa052964.
70. Appelberg BG, Syvalahti EK, Koskinen TE, et al. Patients with severe depression may benefit from buspirone augmentation of selective serotonin reuptake inhibitors: results from a placebo-controlled, randomized, double-blind, placebo wash-in study. *Journal of Clinical Psychiatry* 2001;62(6):448–52.
71. Landén M, Björling G, Fahlén T. A randomized, double-blind, placebo-controlled trial of buspirone in combination with an SSRI in patients with treatment-refractory depression. *Journal of Clinical Psychiatry* 1998;59(12):664–8.
72. Burkhart KK. *Medical Toxicology*. Philadelphia: Lippincott Williams & Wilkins; 2004.
73. Blier P, Bergeron R. The use of pindolol to potentiate antidepressant medication. *Journal of Clinical Psychiatry* 1998;59(Suppl 5):16–23, discussion 24–5.
74. Liu Y, Zhou X, Zhu D, et al. Is pindolol augmentation effective in depressed patients resistant to selective serotonin reuptake inhibitors? A systematic review and meta-analysis. *Human Psychopharmacology* 2015;30(3):132–42.
75. Segrave R, Nathan PJ. Pindolol augmentation of selective serotonin reuptake inhibitors: accounting for the variability of results of placebo-controlled double-blind studies in patients with major depression. *Human Psychopharmacology: Clinical and Experimental* 2005;20(3):163–74.
76. Celada P, Bortolozzi A, Artigas F. Serotonin 5-HT1A receptors as targets for agents to treat psychiatric disorders: rationale and current status of research. *CNS Drugs* 2013;27(9):703–16.
77. Domino EF. Taming the ketamine tiger. 1965. *Anesthesiology* 2010;113(3):678–84.
78. Mion G. History of anaesthesia: the ketamine story – past, present and future. *European Journal of Anaesthesiology* 2017;34(9):571–5.
79. Murrough JW, Iosifescu D v., Chang LC, et al. Antidepressant efficacy of ketamine in treatment-resistant major depression: a two-site randomized controlled trial. *American Journal of Psychiatry* 2013;170(10):1134.
80. Rot MA het, Zarate CA, Charney DS, et al. Ketamine for depression: where do we go from here? *Biological Psychiatry* 2012;72(7):537–47.

81. Canuso CM, Singh JB, Fedgchin M, et al. Efficacy and safety of intranasal esketamine for the rapid reduction of symptoms of depression and suicidality in patients at imminent risk for suicide: results of a double-blind, randomized, placebo-controlled study. *American Journal of Psychiatry* 2019;17(7):55–65. doi.org/10.1176/appi.ajp.2018.17060720.

82. Williams NR, Heifets BD, Blasey C, et al. Opioid receptor antagonism attenuates antidepressant effects of ketamine. *American Journal of Psychiatry* 2018;175(12):1205.

83. Smith HS. Ketamine-induced urologic insult (KIUI). *Pain Physician* 2010;13(6):E343–6.

84. Morgan CJA, Curran HV. Ketamine use: a review. *Addiction* 2012;107(1):27–38.

85. Andrade C. Ketamine for depression, 5: potential pharmacokinetic and pharmacodynamic drug interactions. *Journal of Clinical Psychiatry* 2017;78(7):e858–61.

86. Dörks M, Langner I, Dittmann U, et al. Antidepressant drug use and off-label prescribing in children and adolescents in Germany: results from a large population-based cohort study. *European Child & Adolescent Psychiatry* 2013;22(80):511–8.

87. Linde K, Berner MM, Kriston L. St John's Wort for major depression. *Cochrane Database of Systematic Reviews* 2008;2008(4):CD000448.

88. Apaydin EA, Maher AR, Shanman R, et al. A systematic review of St. John's wort for major depressive disorder. *Systematic Reviews* 2016;5(1):148.

89. Ng QX, Venkatanarayanan N, Ho CYX. Clinical use of Hypericum perforatum (St John's wort) in depression: a meta-analysis. *Journal of Affective Disorders* 2017;210:211–21.

90. Hoban CL, Byard RW, Musgrave IF. A comparison of patterns of spontaneous adverse drug reaction reporting with St. John's Wort and fluoxetine during the period 2000–2013. *Clinical and Experimental Pharmacology and Physiology* 2015;42(7):747–51.

91. Karalapillai DC, Bellomo R. Convulsions associated with an overdose of St John's wort. *Medical Journal of Australia* 2007;186(4):213–4.

92. Young SN. The effect of raising and lowering tryptophan levels on human mood and social behaviour. *Philosophical Transactions of the Royal Society B: Biological Sciences* 2013;368(1615):20110375. DOI:10.1098/RSTB.2011.0375.

93. Ravindran A v., da Silva TL. Complementary and alternative therapies as add-on to pharmacotherapy for mood and anxiety disorders: a systematic review. *Journal of Affective Disorders* 2013;150(3):707–19.

94. Shaw KA, Turner J, del Mar C. Tryptophan and 5-Hydroxytryptophan for depression. *Cochrane Database of Systematic Reviews* 2002;1:CD003198. DOI:10.1002/14651858.cd003198.

95. Miller AH, Maletic V, Raison CL. Inflammation and its discontents: the role of cytokines in the pathophysiology of major depression. *Biological Psychiatry* 2009;65(9):732–41.

96. Na KS, Lee KJ, Lee JS, et al. Efficacy of adjunctive celecoxib treatment for patients with major depressive disorder: a meta-analysis. *Progress in Neuro-psychopharmacology & Biological Psychiatry* 2014;48:79–85.

97. Raison CL, Rutherford RE, Woolwine BJ, et al. A randomized controlled trial of the tumor necrosis factor antagonist infliximab for treatment-resistant depression: the role of baseline inflammatory biomarkers. *JAMA Psychiatry* 2013;70(1):31–41.

98. Husain MI, Strawbridge R, Stokes PRA, et al. Anti-inflammatory treatments for mood disorders: systematic review and meta-analysis. *Journal of Psychopharmacology* 2017;31(9):1137–48.

99. Nettis MA, Lombardo G, Hastings C, et al. Augmentation therapy with minocycline in treatment-resistant depression patients with low-grade peripheral inflammation: results from a double-blind randomised clinical trial. *Neuropsychopharmacology* 2021;46(5):939–48.

100. Aizenstein HJ, Baskys A, Boldrini M, et al. Vascular depression consensus report – a critical update. *BMC Med* 2016;14:1–16.

101. Cipriani A, Saunders K, Attenburrow MJ, et al. A systematic review of calcium channel antagonists in bipolar disorder and some considerations for their future development. *Molecular Psychiatry* 2016;21(10):1324–32.

102. Taragano FE, Bagnatti P, Allegri RF. A double-blind, randomized clinical trial to assess the augmentation with nimodipine of antidepressant therapy in the treatment of 'vascular depression'. *International Psychogeriatrics* 2005;17(3):487–98.

103. Goodnick PJ. The use of nimodipine in the treatment of mood disorders. *Bipolar Disorders* 2000;2(3 Pt 1):165–73.

104. Dean O, Giorlando F, Berk M. N-acetylcysteine in psychiatry: current therapeutic evidence and potential mechanisms of action. *Journal of Psychiatry & Neuroscience* 2011;36(2):78–86.

105. Bozzatello P, Brignolo E, de Grandi E, et al. Supplementation with omega-3 fatty acids in psychiatric disorders: a review of literature data. *Journal of Clinical Medicine* 2016;5(8):67. DOI:10.3390/JCM5080067.

106. Cuomo A, Beccarini Crescenzi B, Bolognesi S, et al. S-Adenosylmethionine (SAMe) in major depressive disorder (MDD): a clinician-oriented systematic review. *Annals of Genera; Psychiatry* 2020;19:50. DOI:10.1186/S12991-020-00298-Z.

107. Ravindran A v., Balneaves LG, Faulkner G, et al. Canadian Network for Mood and Anxiety Treatments (CANMAT) 2016 clinical guidelines for the management of adults with major depressive disorder: Section 5. Complementary and alternative medicine treatments. *Canadian Journal of Psychiatry* 2016;61(9):576–87.

108. Akers BP, Ruiz JF, Piper A, et al. A prehistoric mural in Spain depicting neurotropic Psilocybe mushrooms? *Economic Botany* 2011;65(2):121–8.

109. Goldberg SB, Pace BT, Nicholas CR, et al. The experimental effects of psilocybin on symptoms of anxiety and depression: a meta-analysis. *Psychiatry Research* 2020;284:112749.

110. Rucker JJ, Young AH. Psilocybin: from serendipity to credibility? *Frontiers in Psychiatry* 2021;12:445.

111. Fantegrossi WE, Murnane KS, Reissig CJ. The behavioral pharmacology of hallucinogens. *Biochemical Pharmacology* 2008;75(1):17–33.

112. Vollenweider FX, Vollenweider-Scherpenhuyzen MFI, Bäbler A, et al. Psilocybin induces schizophrenia-like psychosis in humans via a serotonin-2 agonist action. *Neuroreport* 1998;9 (17):3897–902.

113. Kalant H. The pharmacology and toxicology of "ecstasy" (MDMA) and related drugs. *CMAJ: Canadian Medical Association Journal* 2001;165(7):917–28.

114. Cerletti U, Bini L. L'Elettroshock. *Archivio Generale di Neurologia, Psichiatria e Psicoanalisi* 1938;19:266–8.

115. Pagnin D, de Queiroz V, Pini S, et al. Efficacy of ECT in depression: a meta-analytic review. *Journal of ECT* 2004;20 (1):13–20.

116. Geddes J, Carney S, Cowen P, et al. Efficacy and safety of electroconvulsive therapy in depressive disorders: a systematic review and meta-analysis. *Lancet* 2003;361(9360):799–808.

117. Sackeim HA. Modern electroconvulsive therapy: vastly improved yet greatly underused. *JAMA Psychiatry* 2017;74 (8):779–80.

118. Sackeim HA, Haskett RF, Mulsant BH, et al. Continuation pharmacotherapy in the prevention of relapse following electroconvulsive therapy: a randomized controlled trial. *JAMA* 2001;285(10):1299–307.

119. Martínez-Amorós E, Cardoner N, Gálvez V, et al. Can the addition of maintenance electroconvulsive therapy to pharmacotherapy improve relapse prevention in severe major depressive disorder? A randomized controlled trial. *Brain Science* 2021;11(10):1340. DOI:10.3390/BRAINSCI11101340.

120. Kellner CH, Jørgensen MB. Dosing methods in electroconvulsive therapy (ECT): towards the modal ECT technique. *Nordic Journal of Psychiatry* 2021;76(3):159–61.

121. Ferrie IN, Waite J. *ECT Handbook*, 4th ed. Cambridge: Cambridge University Press; 2019.

122. Tsoukalas I. How does ECT work? A new explanatory model and suggestions for non-convulsive applications. *Medical Hypotheses* 2020;145:110337.

123. Jan Shah A, Wadoo O, Latoo J. Electroconvulsive Therapy (ECT): important parameters which influence its effectiveness. *British Journal of Medical Practitioners* 2013;6:634.

124. Lisanby SH, Maddox JH, Prudic J, et al. The effects of electroconvulsive therapy on memory of autobiographical and public events. *Archives of General Psychiatry* 2000;57(6):581–90.

125. Semkovska M, McLoughlin DM. Objective cognitive performance associated with electroconvulsive therapy for depression: a systematic review and meta-analysis. *Biological Psychiatry* 2010;68(6): 568–77.

126. Squire LR, Slater PC. Electroconvulsive therapy and complaints of memory dysfunction: a prospective three-year follow-up study. *British Journal of Psychiatry* 1983;142:1–8.

127. Jolly A, Singh S. Does electroconvulsive therapy cause brain damage: An update. *Indian J Psychiatry* 2020;62(4):339.

128. Semkovska M, McLoughlin DM. Measuring retrograde autobiographical amnesia following electroconvulsive therapy: historical perspective and current issues. *Journal of ECT* 2013;29 (2):127–33.

129. Duma A, Maleczek M, Panjikaran B, et al. Major adverse cardiac events and mortality associated with electroconvulsive therapy: a systematic review and meta-analysis. *Anesthesiology* 2019;130(1):83–91.

130. Reed T, Cohen KR. Transcranial electrical stimulation (tES) mechanisms and its effects on cortical excitability and connectivity. *Journal of Inherited Metabolic Disease* 2018;41(6):1123.

131. Horvath JC, Perez JM, Forrow L, et al. Transcranial magnetic stimulation: a historical evaluation and future prognosis of therapeutically relevant ethical concerns. *Journal of Medical Ethics* 2011;37(3):137–43.

132. Perera T, George M, Grammer G, et al. *TMS Therapy for Major Depressive Disorder: Evidence Review and Treatment Recommendations for Clinical Practice.* 2015. tmscenterofcolorado.com/wp-content/uploads/2015/09/Clinical-TMS-Society-WhitePaper_2015.pdf.

133. Berlim MT, van den Eynde F, Jeff Daskalakis Z. Clinically meaningful efficacy and acceptability of low-frequency repetitive transcranial magnetic stimulation (rTMS) for treating primary major depression: a meta-analysis of randomized, double-blind and sham-controlled trials. *Neuropsychopharmacology* 2012;38 (4):543–51.

134. Carpenter LL, Philip NS. The future is now? Rapid advances by brain stimulation innovation. *American Journal of Psychiatry* 2020;177(8):654–6. doi.org/10.1176/appi.ajp.2020 .20060844.

135. Cusin C, Dougherty DD. Somatic therapies for treatment-resistant depression: ECT, TMS, VNS, DBS. *Biology of Mood & Anxiety Disorders* 2012;2:14.

136. Fitzgerald PB, Daskalakis ZJ. *Repetitive Transcranial Magnetic Stimulation Treatment for Depressive Disorders: A Practical Guide.* London: Springer Science & Business Media; 2013.

137. Anderson RJ, Frye MA, Abulseoud OA, et al. Deep brain stimulation for treatment-resistant depression: efficacy, safety and mechanisms of action. *Neuroscience and Biobehavioral Reviews* 2012;36(8):1920–33.

138. Dougherty DD, Rezai AR, Carpenter LL, et al. A randomized sham-controlled trial of deep brain stimulation of the ventral capsule/ventral striatum for chronic treatment-resistant depression. *Biological Psychiatry* 2015;78(4):240–8.

139. Bergfeld IO, Mantione M, Hoogendoorn MLC, et al. Deep brain stimulation of the ventral anterior limb of the internal capsule for treatment-resistant depression: a randomized clinical trial. *JAMA Psychiatry* 2016;73 (5):456–64.

140. Schlaepfer TE, Bewernick BH, Kayser S, et al. Rapid effects of deep brain stimulation for treatment-resistant major depression. *Biological Psychiatry* 2013;73(12):1204–12.

141. Elger G, Hoppe C, Falkai P, et al. Vagus nerve stimulation is associated with mood improvements in epilepsy patients. *Epilepsy Research* 2000;42(2–3):203–10.

142. Cimpianu CL, Strube W, Falkai P, et al. Vagus nerve stimulation in psychiatry: a systematic review of the available evidence. *Journal of Neural Transmission (Vienna)* 2017;124 (1):145–58.

143. Carreno FR, Frazer A. Vagal nerve stimulation for treatment-resistant depression. *Neurotherapeutics* 2017;14 (3):716.

144. Aaronson ST, Sears P, Ruvuna F, et al. A 5-year observational study of patients with treatment-resistant depression treated with vagus nerve stimulation or treatment as usual: comparison of response, remission, and suicidality. *American Journal of Psychiatry* 2017;174(7):640–8.

145. Groves DA, Brown VJ. Vagal nerve stimulation: a review of its applications and potential mechanisms that mediate its clinical effects. *Neuroscience and Biobehavioral Reviews* 2005;29 (3):493–500.

146. Tuunainen A, Kripke DF, Endo T. Light therapy for non-seasonal depression. *Cochrane Database of Systematic Reviews* 2004;2004: CD004050.

147. Al-Karawi D, Jubair L. Bright light therapy for nonseasonal depression: Meta-analysis of clinical trials. *Journal of Affective Disorders* 2016;198: 64–71.

148. Mårtensson B, Pettersson A, Berglund L, et al. Bright white light therapy in depression: a critical review of the evidence. *Journal of Affective Disorders* 2015;182:1–7.

149. Oldham MA, Ciraulo DA. Bright light therapy for depression: a review of its effects on chronobiology and the autonomic nervous system. *Chronobiology International* 2014;31 (3):305–19.

150. Volpini M, Giacobbe P, Cosgrove GR, et al. The history and future of ablative neurosurgery for major depressive disorder. *Stereotactic and Functional Neurosurgery* 2017;95(4):216–28.

151. Shields DC, Asaad W, Eskandar EN, et al. Prospective assessment of stereotactic ablative surgery for intractable major depression. *Biological Psychiatry* 2008;64(6):449–54.

152. National Institute for Health and Care Excellence (NICE). *Depression in Adults: Recognition and Management (CG90).* 2009.

153. Cleare A, Pariante CM, Young AH, et al. Evidence-based guidelines for treating depressive disorders with antidepressants: a revision of the 2008 British Association for Psychopharmacology guidelines. *Journal of Psychopharmacology* 2015;29 (5):459–525.

154. Garyfallos G, Adamopoulou A, Karastergiou A, et al. Personality disorders in dysthymia and major depression. *Acta Psychiatrica Scandinavica* 1999;99(5):332–40.

155. Levkovitz Y, Tedeschini E, Papakostas GI. Efficacy of antidepressants for dysthymia: a meta-analysis of placebo-controlled randomized trials. *Journal of Clinical Psychiatry* 2011;72(4):509–14.

156. Angst J, Gamma A, Bowden C, et al. Diagnostic criteria for bipolarity based on an international sample of 5,635 patients with DSM-IV major depressive episodes. *European Archives of Psychiatry and Clinical Neuroscience* 2012;262(1):3–11.

157. Verdolini N, Hidalgo-Mazzei D, Murru A, et al. Mixed states in bipolar and major depressive disorders: systematic review and quality appraisal of guidelines. *Acta Psychiatrica Scandinavica* 2018;138(3):196–222.

158. Day E, Shah R, Taylor RW, et al. A retrospective examination of care pathways in individuals with treatment-resistant depression. *BJPsych Open* 2021;7(3):e101. DOI: 10.1192/BJO.2021.59.

159. Stassen HH, Angst J, Delini-Stula A. Delayed onset of action of antidepressant drugs? Survey of recent results. *European Psychiatry* 1997;12 (4):166–76.

160. Posternak MA, Zimmerman M. Is there a delay in the antidepressant effect? A meta-analysis. *Journal of Clinical Psychiatry* 2005;66(2):148–58.

161. Szegedi A, Müller MJ, Anghelescu I, et al. Early improvement under mirtazapine and paroxetine predicts later stable response and remission with high sensitivity in patients with major depression. *Journal of Clinical Psychiatry* 2003;64(4):413–20.

162. Farabaugh AH, Alpert J. Timing of onset of antidepressant response with fluoxetine treatment. *American Journal of Psychiatry* 2000;157(9):1423–8. DOI: 10.1176/appi.ajp.157.9.1423.

163. Sforzini L, Worrell C, Kose M, et al. A Delphi-method-based consensus guideline for definition of treatment-resistant depression for clinical trials. *Molecular Psychiatry* 2022;27 (3):1286–99. DOI: 10.1038/S41380-021-01381-X.

164. Bousman CA, Arandjelovic K, Mancuso SG, et al. Pharmacogenetic tests and depressive symptom remission: a meta-analysis of randomized controlled trials. *Pharmacogenomics* 2019;20(1):37–47.

165. Reis M, Aamo T, Spigset O, et al. Serum concentrations of antidepressant drugs in a naturalistic setting: compilation based on a large therapeutic drug monitoring database. *Therapeutic Drug Monitoring* 2009;31(1):42–56.

166. Xiang Y-T, Xiao L, Ungvari G. Measurement-based care versus standard care for major depression: a randomized controlled trial with blind raters. *American Journal of Psychiatry* 2015;172(10):1004–13. DOI: 10.1176/appi.ajp.2015.14050652.

167. Posternak MA, Zimmerman M. Therapeutic effect of follow-up assessments on antidepressant and placebo response rates in antidepressant efficacy trials: Meta-analysis. *The British Journal of Psychiatry* 2007;190:287–92.

168. Simon GE, Savarino J. Suicide attempts among patients starting depression treatment with medications or psychotherapy. *American Journal of Psychiatry* 2007;164(7):1029–34.

169. Hotopf M, Hardy R, Lewis G. Discontinuation rates of SSRIs and tricyclic antidepressants: a meta-analysis and investigation of heterogeneity. *British Journal of Psychiatry* 1997;170:120–7.

170. Sawada N, Uchida H, Suzuki T, et al. Persistence and compliance to antidepressant treatment in patients with depression: a chart review. *BMC Psychiatry* 2009;9:1–10.

171. Maidment R, Livingston G, Katona C. 'Just keep taking the tablets': adherence to antidepressant treatment in older people in primary care. *International Journal of Geriatric Psychiatry* 2002;17 (8):752–7.

172. Vergouwen ACM, Bakker A, Katon WJ, et al. Improving adherence to antidepressants: a systematic review of interventions. *Journal of Clinical Psychiatry* 2003;64(12):8795.

173. Greist J, McNamara RK, Mallinckrodt CH, et al. Incidence and duration of antidepressant-induced nausea: duloxetine compared with paroxetine and fluoxetine. *Clinical Therapeutics* 2004;26(9):1446–55.

174. Demyttenaere K, Albert A, Mesters P, et al. What happens with adverse events

during 6 months of treatment with selective serotonin reuptake inhibitors? *Journal of Clinical Psychiatry* 2005;(7):859–63.

175. Taylor MJ, Rudkin L, Bullemor-Day P, et al. Strategies for managing sexual dysfunction induced by antidepressant medication. *Cochrane Database of Systematic Reviews* 2013;2013(5): CD0033. DOI:10.1002/14651858.CD003382.PUB3.

176. Nurnberg HG, Hensley PL, Heiman JR, et al. Sildenafil treatment of women with antidepressant-associated sexual dysfunction: a randomized controlled trial. *JAMA* 2008;300(4):395–404.

177. Stübner S, Grohmann R, Greil W, et al. Suicidal ideation and suicidal behavior as rare adverse events of antidepressant medication: current report from the AMSP Multicenter Drug Safety Surveillance Project. *International Journal of Neuropsychopharmacology* 2018;21(9):814–21.

178. Baldessarini RJ, Lau WK, Sim J, et al. Suicidal risks in reports of long-term treatment trials for major depressive disorder. *International Journal of Neuropsychopharmacology* 2015;19(3):1–2.

179. Moore TJ, Glenmullen J, Furberg CD. Prescription drugs associated with reports of violence towards others. *PLoS ONE* 2010;5(12):e15337. DOI: 10.1371/JOURNAL.PONE.0015337.

180. Read J, Gee A, Diggle J, Butler H. Staying on, and coming off, antidepressants: the experiences of 752 UK adults. *Addictive Behaviors* 2019;88:82–5.

181. Kato M, Hori H, Inoue T, et al. Discontinuation of antidepressants after remission with antidepressant medication in major depressive disorder: a systematic review and meta-analysis. *Molecular Psychiatry* 2020;26(1):118–33.

182. Reimherr FW, Strong RE, Marchant BK, et al. Factors affecting return of symptoms 1 year after treatment in a 62-week controlled study of fluoxetine in major depression. *Journal of Clinical Psychiatry* 2001;62(Suppl 2):16–23.

183. Kanai T, Takeuchi H, Furukawa TA, et al. Time to recurrence after recovery from major depressive episodes and its predictors. *Psychological Medicine* 2003;33(5):839–45.

184. Ghaziuddin M, Ghaziuddin N, Stein GS. Life events and the recurrence of depression. *Canadian Journal of Psychiatry* 1990;35(3):239–42.

185. Greden J. Antidepressant maintenance medications: when to discontinue and how to stop. *Journal of Clinical Psychiatry* 1993;54(Suppl):46–7.

186. Thase ME. Preventing relapse and recurrence of depression: a brief review of therapeutic options. *CNS Spectrums* 2006;11:12–21.

187. Kessing L, Andersen P. Predictive effects of previous episodes on the risk of recurrence in depressive and bipolar disorders. *Current Psychiatry Reports* 2005;7(6):413–20.

188. Solomon DA, Keller MB, Leon AC, et al. Multiple recurrences of major depressive disorder. *American Journal of Psychiatry* 2000;157(2):229–33.

189. McGrath PJ, Stewart JW, Quitkin FM, et al. Predictors of relapse in a prospective study of fluoxetine treatment of major depression. *American Journal of Psychiatry* 2006;163(9):1542–8.

190. Dotoli D, Spagnolo C, Bongiorno F, et al. Relapse during a 6-month continuation treatment with fluvoxamine in an Italian population: the role of clinical, psychosocial and genetic variables. *Progress in Neuro-psychopharmacol & Biological Psychiatry* 2006;30(3):442–8.

191. Ramana R, Paykel ES, Cooper Z, et al. Remission and relapse in major depression: a two-year prospective follow-up study. *Psychological Medicine* 1995;25(6):1161–70.

192. Kessing LV. Subtypes of depressive episodes according to ICD-10: prediction of risk of relapse and suicide. *Psychopathology* 2003;36(6):285–91.

193. Flint AJ, Rifat SL. Two-year outcome of psychotic depression in late life. *American Journal of Psychiatry* 1998;155(2):178–83.

194. Dombrovski AY, Mulsant BH, Houck PR, et al. Residual symptoms and recurrence during maintenance treatment of late-life depression. *Journal of Affective Disorders* 2007;103(1–3):77–82.

195. Paykel ES, Ramana R, Cooper Z, et al. Residual symptoms after partial remission: an important outcome in depression. *Psychological Medicine* 1995;25(6):1171–80.

196. Mueller TI, Leon AC, Keller MB, et al. Recurrence after recovery from major depressive disorder during 15 years of observational follow-up. *American Journal of Psychiatry* 1999;156(7):1000–6.

197. Kessing LV. Recurrence in affective disorder: II. Effect of age and gender. *British Journal of Psychiatry* 1998;172:29–34.

198. Reynolds CFI, Dew MA, Pollock BG, et al. Maintenance treatment of major depression in old age. *New England Journal of Medicine* 2006;354:1130–8. dx.doi.org/10.1056/NEJMoa052619.

199. Iosifescu D v., Nierenberg AA, Alpert JE, et al. Comorbid medical illness and relapse of major depressive disorder in the continuation phase of treatment. *Psychosomatics* 2004;45(5):419–25.

200. Åkerblad AC, Bengtsson F, von Knorring L, et al. Response, remission and relapse in relation to adherence in primary care treatment of depression: a 2-year outcome study. *International Clinical Psychopharmacology* 2006;21(2):117–24.

201. Dawson R, Lavori PW, Coryell WH, et al. Maintenance strategies for unipolar depression: an observational study of levels of treatment and recurrence. *Journal of Affective Disorders* 1998;49(1):31–44.

202. Loonen AJM, Peer PGM, Zwanikken GJ. Continuation and maintenance therapy with antidepressive agents. Meta-analysis of research. *Pharmaceutisch Weekblad. Scientific Edition* 1991;13(4):167–75.

203. Franchini L, Gasperini M, Zanardi R, et al. Four-year follow-up study of sertraline and fluvoxamine in long-term treatment of unipolar subjects with high recurrence rate. *Journal of Affective Disorders* 2000;58(3):233–6.

204. Reynolds CF, Perel JM, Frank E, et al. Three-year outcomes of maintenance nortriptyline treatment in late-life depression: a study of two fixed plasma levels. *American Journal of Psychiatry* 1999;156(8):1177–81.

205. Frank E, Kupfer DJ, Perel JM, et al. Comparison of full-dose versus half-dose pharmacotherapy in the maintenance treatment of recurrent depression. *Journal of Affective Disorders* 1993;27(3):139–45.

206. Franchini L, Rossini D, Bongiorno F, et al. Will a second prophylactic treatment with a higher dosage of the

same antidepressant either prevent or delay new depressive episodes? *Psychiatry Research* 2000;96:81–5.

207. Pollock B. Paroxetine versus nortriptyline in the continuation and maintenance treatment of depression in the elderly. *Depression and Anxiety* 2001;13(1):38–44.

208. Walters G, Reynolds CF, Mulsant BH, et al. Continuation and maintenance pharmacotherapy in geriatric depression: an open-trial comparison of paroxetine and nortriptyline in patients older than 70 years. *Journal of Clinical Psychiatry* 1999;60(Suppl 20):21–5.

209. Montgomery SA, Reimitz PE, Zivkov M. Mirtazapine versus amitriptyline in the long-term treatment of depression: a double-blind placebo-controlled study. *International Clinical Psychopharmacology* 1998;13(2):63–73.

210. Mulder R, Hamilton A, Irwin L, et al. Treating depression with adjunctive antipsychotics. *Bipolar Disorders* 2018;20(Suppl 2):17–24.

211. Giakoumatos CI, Osser D. The Psychopharmacology Algorithm Project at the Harvard South Shore Program: an update on unipolar nonpsychotic depression. *Harvard Review of Psychiatry* 2019;27(1):33–52.

212. Cipriani A, Furukawa TA, Salanti G, et al. Comparative efficacy and acceptability of 12 new-generation antidepressants: a multiple-treatments meta-analysis. *Lancet* 2009;373 (9665):746–58.

213. Sung SC, Haley CL, Wisniewski SR, et al. The impact of chronic depression on acute and long-term outcomes in a randomized trial comparing selective serotonin reuptake inhibitor monotherapy versus each of 2 different antidepressant medication combinations. *Journal of Clinical Psychiatry* 2012;73(7):967–76.

214. Cooke MJ, Waring WS. Citalopram and cardiac toxicity. *European Journal of Clinical Pharmacology* 2012;69 (4):755–60.

215. Fava M, Rush AJ, Alpert JE, et al. Difference in treatment outcome in outpatients with anxious versus nonanxious depression: a STAR*D report. *American Journal of Psychiatry* 2008;165(3):342–51.

216. Thase M, Shelton R, Khan A. Treatment with venlafaxine extended release after SSRI nonresponse or intolerance: a randomized comparison of standard- and higher-dosing strategies. *Journal of Clinical Psychopharmacology* 2006;26 (3):250–8.

217. Papakostas G, Fava M, Thase M. Treatment of SSRI-resistant depression: a meta-analysis comparing within- versus across-class switches. *Biological Psychiatry* 2008;63(7):699–704.

218. Mohamed S, Johnson GR, Chen P, et al. Effect of antidepressant switching vs augmentation on remission among patients with major depressive disorder unresponsive to antidepressant treatment: the VAST-D randomized clinical trial. *JAMA* 2017;318(2): 132–45.

219. Pringsheim T, Gardner D, Patten SB. Adjunctive treatment with quetiapine for major depressive disorder: are the benefits of treatment worth the risks? *BMJ* 2015;350:h569. DOI:10.1136/ BMJ.H569.

220. Warden D, Rush AJ, Trivedi MH, et al. The STAR*D Project results: a comprehensive review of findings. *Current Psychiatry Reports* 2007;9 (6):449–59.

221. Amsterdam JD, Shults J. MAOI efficacy and safety in advanced stage treatment-resistant depression – a retrospective study. *Journal of Affective Disorders* 2005;89(1–3):183–8.

222. Gournellis R, Tournikioti K, Touloumi G, et al. Psychotic (delusional) depression and completed suicide: a systematic review and meta-analysis. *Annals of General Psychiatry* 2018;17:39. DOI:10.1186/S12991-018-0207-1.

223. Petrides G, Fink M, Husain MM, et al. ECT remission rates in psychotic versus nonpsychotic depressed patients: a report from CORE. *Journal of ECT* 2001;17(4):244–53.

224. Farahani A, Correll CU. Are antipsychotics or antidepressants needed for psychotic depression? A systematic review and meta-analysis of trials comparing antidepressant or antipsychotic monotherapy with combination treatment. *Journal of Clinical Psychiatry* 2012;73(4):486–96.

225. Meyers BS, Flint AJ, Rothschild AJ, et al. A double-blind randomized controlled trial of olanzapine plus sertraline vs olanzapine plus placebo for psychotic depression: the study of pharmacotherapy of psychotic depression (STOP-PD). *Archives of General Psychiatry* 2009;66(8):838–47.

226. Bruijn JA, Moleman P, Mulder PGH, et al. A double blind, fixed blood-level study comparing mirtazapine with imipramine in depressed in-patients. *Psychopharmacolog* 1996;127(3):231–7.

227. van den Broek WW, Birkenhäger TK, Mulder PGH, et al. A double-blind randomized study comparing imipramine with fluvoxamine in depressed inpatients. *Psychopharmacology* 2004;175:481–6.

228. Kantrowitz JT, Tampi RR. Risk of psychosis exacerbation by tricyclic antidepressants in unipolar major depressive disorder with psychotic features. *Journal of Affective Disorders* 2008;106(3):279–84.

229. Wijkstra J, Burger H, van den Broek WW, et al. Treatment of unipolar psychotic depression: a randomized, double-blind study comparing imipramine, venlafaxine, and venlafaxine plus quetiapine. *Acta Psychiatrica Scandinavica* 2010;121(3):190–200.

230. Price LH, Charney DS, Heninger GR. Variability of response to lithium augmentation in refractory depression. *American Journal of Psychiatry* 1986;143(11):1387–92.

231. Birkenhäger TK, van den Broek WW, Wijkstra J, et al. Treatment of unipolar psychotic depression: an open study of lithium addition in refractory psychotic depression. *Journal of Clinical Psychopharmacology* 2009;29(5):513–5.

232. Ranjan R, Meltzer HY. Acute and long-term effectiveness of clozapine in treatment-resistant psychotic depression. *Biological Psychiatry* 1996;40(4):253–8.

233. Huang CC, Shiah IS, Chen HK, et al. Adjunctive use of methylphenidate in the treatment of psychotic unipolar depression. *Clinical Neuropharmacology* 2008;31(4):245–7.

234. Łojko D, Rybakowski JK. Atypical depression: current perspectives. *Neuropsychiatric Disease and Treatment* 2017;13:2447–56.

235. Singh T, Williams K. Atypical depression. *Psychiatry* 2006;3(4):33–9.

236. Henkel V, Mergl R, Allgaier AK, et al. Treatment of depression with atypical features: a meta-analytic approach. *Psychiatry Research* 2006;141 (1):89–101.

237. Papakostas GI, Nutt DJ, Hallett LA, et al. Resolution of sleepiness and fatigue in major depressive disorder: a comparison of bupropion and the selective serotonin reuptake inhibitors. *Biological Psychiatry* 2006;60 (12):1350–5.

238. Husain MM, McClintock SM, Rush AJ, et al. The efficacy of acute electroconvulsive therapy in atypical depression. *Journal of Clinical Psychiatry* 2008;69(3):406–11.

239. Hedayati SS, Yalamanchili V, Finkelstein FO. A practical approach to the treatment of depression in patients with chronic kidney disease and end-stage renal disease. *Kidney International* 2012;81(3):247–55.

240. Mullish BH, Kabir MS, Thursz MR, et al. Review article: depression and the use of antidepressants in patients with chronic liver disease or liver transplantation. *Aliment Pharmacology & Therapeutics* 2014;40 (8):880–92.

241. Briley M, Moret C. Treatment of comorbid pain with serotonin norepinephrine reuptake inhibitors. *CNS Spectrums* 2008;13(7 Suppl 11):22–6.

242. Spielmans GI. Duloxetine does not relieve painful physical symptoms in depression: a meta-analysis. *Psychotherapy and Psychosomatics* 2008;77(1):12–6.

243. Bech P, Gormsen L, Loldrup D, et al. The clinical effect of clomipramine in chronic idiopathic pain disorder revisited using the Spielberger State Anxiety Symptom Scale (SSASS) as outcome scale. *Journal of Affective Disorders* 2009;119(1–3):43–51.

244. Lagerberg T, Fazel S, Sjölander A, et al. Selective serotonin reuptake inhibitors and suicidal behaviour: a population-based cohort study. *Neuropsychopharmacology* 2022;47:817–23.

Chapter 3.4

Psychological and Social Treatment of Depression

Stirling Moorey

Psychosocial intervention, in its broadest sense, is a vital component in the management of all types of depression, from mild depressive reactions to psychotic episodes. Even if pharmacological therapy or electroconvulsive therapy (ECT) is the main treatment, the way in which the clinician assesses and engages the patient, gives information about the illness and its treatment, and provides support contributes significantly to a successful outcome. In addition to this basic level of supportive work, many patients will benefit from more structured forms of psychotherapy. This chapter will consider the psychological and social therapies available for depression and the evidence for their effectiveness. Some general principles of psychological management for the depressed patient will be described.

Introduction

The last 40 years have seen significant changes in our view of depression and its treatment. Major depressive disorder is now recognised to be a chronic, recurring condition in many people:[1] once someone has had two depressive episodes, there is an 80 per cent chance they will have further episodes.[2] So, this puts the onus on any treatment to demonstrate that it has a long-term as well as short-term effect on depression. Prior to the randomised controlled trial (RCT) conducted by Rush et al in 1977, antidepressant medication and ECT appeared to be the only treatments that worked.[3] Cognitive therapy, the type of psychotherapy employed in that trial, holds its own as a treatment that is the equal of medication. Since then, other psychological therapies for depression have also emerged. In order to prove their cost effectiveness and to allow the RCTs to compare them with antidepressants, these therapies have tended to be brief (12–20 sessions) compared to more traditional long-term therapy. They seem to be as effective as medication in treating acute depression in an outpatient or community setting. Most exciting is the finding that all these treatments not only work in the short term but offer some degree of protection against relapse. The chapter will begin with a review of the brief psychological therapies: cognitive behaviour therapy (CBT), behavioural activation, third-wave CBT, interpersonal therapy and brief psychodynamic psychotherapy. The clinical practice of these therapies will be described, and the research evidence supporting them wil be reviewed. The application of psychological therapies for depression in groups and family systems will then be considered as well as the important, though often over-looked, role that social interventions can play in combatting depression. How the psychiatrist assesses, engages, informs and supports the patient contributes significantly to a successful outcome. Some of the principles from cognitive behavioural and interpersonal/psychodynamic therapies will be used to describe a framework for the psychological management of the depressed patient.

Evidence-Based Brief Psychological Therapies for Depression

A number of brief psychological therapies have proven efficacy for people with major depressive disorder. Most published research focuses on cognitive, behavioural and interpersonal therapy, but more recently, brief psychodynamic psychotherapy for depression has offered some promising results.

Cognitive Behaviour Therapy

Cognitive behaviour therapy is the term for a broad range of psychological interventions ranging from those that are learning theory based to those that give primacy to thoughts and beliefs. There are several types of empirically validated CBT for depression, including problem-solving therapy and behavioural activation (BA), but the most well known is Beck's cognitive therapy (CT). This therapy is based on Beck's cognitive model of depression.[4] Beck's theory is a tripartite one: consisting of cognitive structures (assumptions), which when activated, bias cognitive processing (cognitive distortions) and produce depressive cognitions (automatic thoughts). In depression, there is a depressive cognitive triad: a negative view of the self, the world and the future; depressed patients believe themselves to be inadequate and worthless (self), that their surroundings seem bleak and uninteresting (world), and that the future seems hopeless (future). Interpretations of current events and predictions about future events are distorted. Beck identifies particular biases in information processing, called cognitive distortions or thinking errors (See Box 3.4.1). These often take the form of faulty inferences. One of the most common thinking error is 'overgeneralisation', where a single negative event is seen as the beginning of a neverending pattern of defeats. For example, a depressed

Box 3.4.1 Thinking errors

All or Nothing Thinking
You see things in black and white, missing all the shades of grey in between. If you are depressed, you may think, 'If I can't do everything I used to do, then there's no point in doing anything.' If you do less well than usual, you may think, 'If I don't succeed, I must be a total failure.'

Overgeneralisation
From a single event, you predict a neverending pattern of loss or defeat that may be exaggerated and not based on fact.

Magnification and Selective Attention
You focus on the negative aspects of the problem and selectively attend to them. You tend to filter out or disqualify more positive information. For example, if you face an operation, you may remember all the possible side effects but fail to hear that they are extremely rare.

Arbitrary Inference
Instead of looking at the evidence available, you jump to conclusions. For instance, if a loved one is late coming home, you might conclude, 'He's had an accident!'

Labelling
Here, the distortion leads to a global, overgeneralised negative view of yourself. You label yourself as hopeless, incompetent and invalid or a victim.

person may forget to buy some items at the supermarket, concludes from this that his memory is beginning to fail, and becomes convinced that he is facing an inexorable decline into senility.

The depressed person's distorted view of the world manifests itself as frequent negative automatic thoughts. These are spontaneous, plausible thoughts and images that enter the mind unbidden and are associated with unpleasant emotions. When viewed logically, they appear to be exaggerated and unrealistic. For instance, if criticised for a small mistake at work, a depressed patient might have the following negative automatic thoughts:

- Negative view of self – 'I'm stupid; this job's beyond me. I never get anything right.'
- Negative view of world – 'Nobody likes me here; I just don't fit in.'
- Negative view of future – 'What's the point? It's useless even trying. They'll give me the sack soon.'

Other symptoms of depression are derived from this cognitive bias: behavioural symptoms such as social withdrawal and low activity levels, a loss of motivation and interest, or cognitive deficits such as poor concentration. Cognitive factors are not the cause of depression but mediate between various factors such as biological and environmental stressors and depressive symptoms. There are two vicious circles that maintain depression. Firstly, depressed mood is associated with more depressive thinking, which distorts reality, selectively attending to negative aspects of the environment and ignoring or disqualifying positive information. This causes further depression, and the mood spirals downwards. Secondly, depressive thinking influences behaviour. The future looks hopeless, and depressed people believe they are helpless and inadequate, so they give up trying to solve their problems and disengage from rewarding activities. This behavioural deactivation further depresses their mood and confirms their negative beliefs about themselves. Indeed, the interpersonal consequences of their depressive behaviour (friends being unsure of how to deal with them or partners becoming exasperated and critical) may confirm their negative self-image. Cognitive therapy is aimed at breaking into these vicious circles of negative thinking, depressed mood and maladaptive behaviour.

Vulnerability to depression is explained by the presence of depressogenic schemas. These are collections of idiosyncratic beliefs or rules derived from experiences in childhood and later life. At their root are unconditional core beliefs around the themes of helplessness and unlovability (e.g. I am inadequate; I am unloveable). More intermediate beliefs take the form of imperatives such as 'I must always be nice to people' or conditional statements such as 'I can only be happy if I'm a success at everything I do'.

> A woman presenting with depression had experienced the divorce of her parents at the age of six. She believed she was responsible for the break-up of the marriage and developed the assumption that she had to make the perfect marriage to make up for it. Whenever she got into a relationship, this assumption was activated, and she put so much effort into the affair that her partner backed off. She ended up rejected and depressed, feeling that her negative beliefs about herself were correct.

Like many assumptions, this one remained latent until activated by a critical event (the relationship) when its true maladaptive nature became apparent. It also illustrates the rigid, global and idiosyncratic characteristics of these silent rules. Often the conditional beliefs may protect the person from depression until a major life event occurs. A policewoman had a set of beliefs that if she did everything within the rules, she would never be criticised and her secret fear that she was inadequate would not be confirmed. When she was accused of wrongful arrest and her seniors did not support her, she became bewildered and deeply depressed because her rule system did not work.

Characteristics of Cognitive Therapy

Cognitive therapy aims to make the patient his own therapist. The emphasis is on teaching the patient to identify problems and learn strategies for coping with and resolving them.

The therapist is therefore more active and directive than in traditional psychotherapy, and the relationship is a collaborative partnership in problem solving. The focus is on how maladaptive thinking is maintaining current problems rather than on the origins of these problems. From the first session, patients are told that the therapy is time-limited and that it will involve learning and practising self-help skills that the patient will be able to continue to use after therapy ends. In addressing the problems, patients are encouraged to distance themselves from their thoughts and beliefs and to see them as hypotheses that can be examined and tested, rather than facts set in stone. In challenging these maladaptive beliefs, the therapist uses questioning and guided discovery rather than confrontation. Box 3.4.2 summarises some of the techniques used in cognitive therapy, which are described in more detail later.

Box 3.4.2 Cognitive therapy techniques

Behavioural Techniques

Activity scheduling – patients structure time to distract themselves from negative thoughts and to encourage pleasurable and rewarding activities.

Graded-task assignment – large or complex tasks are divided into smaller achievable ones to give graded success experiences.

Mastery and pleasure ratings – patients rate activities for mastery and pleasure on a 10-point scale. Tasks scoring high are scheduled more frequently over the coming weeks.

Behavioural experiments – homework tasks are assigned to test negative beliefs.

Cognitive Techniques

Identifying negative automatic thoughts – patients learn to monitor negative thoughts associated with the exacerbation of depressed mood as well as to link external events, thought and affect.

Challenging negative automatic thoughts – patients keep a mood diary and replace negative thoughts with more realistic alternatives. There are various methods for challenging thoughts:

- Labelling distortions
- Reality testing
- Searching for alternatives
- Decatastrophising

Preventative Strategies

Challenging assumptions – underlying assumptions and core beliefs are challenged using a cost-benefit analysis followed by cognitive challenging and experimental behaviour change.

Relapse prevention – risk factors for future relapses are identified, and strategies for coping are reviewed before the end of therapy.

Behavioural Techniques in Cognitive Therapy

In the treatment of depression, behavioural assignments are important in the early stages since they often lead to a rapid improvement in mood. The tasks are set up as experiments for testing negative beliefs and predictions. For instance, a depressed patient believed his family would be better off without him because he was useless and a burden to them. The therapist was aware that his relatives were very supportive, so he encouraged the patient to test the belief by asking them if they did indeed feel they would be better off if he were dead. The response was a very moving, open display of affection from his grown-up children, which they had not been able to show before. This convinced him that he was valued and needed and led to a marked improvement in his mood.

Activities that give a sense of pleasure or achievement are particularly useful in raising the depressed person's mood. The therapist establishes what activities the patient used to find rewarding and then helps him or her to plan these on a daily basis. A weekly activity schedule (Table 3.4.1) is used to log what is actually done and the degree of pleasure or achievement recorded. Sometimes, tasks need to be broken down into small manageable steps so that they are achievable – many depressed people have very high expectations of themselves even when they are ill, and they set themselves up for failure. For instance, if a patient has a problem with concentration, a graded-task programme would involve reading for increasing time spans, reading materials of increasing complexity and gradually increasing the amount of time spent on work-related activities. Success at a homework task helps to build self-esteem.

In grading tasks, care must be given to ensuring the task is not too difficult for the depressed patient. However, even if the patient is unable to carry out the assignment, it is not considered a failure but instead gives valuable information about the patient's negative thoughts.

A woman who had some difficulty deciding which problems she wanted to tackle in therapy was asked to write down three problems as homework and to fill out the assessment questionnaires. She came back despairing that the therapy could not help her because she had such difficulty in doing the homework. This gave information about the degree of her problems with concentration and decision-making; the therapist used her catastrophic reaction (based on the thought, 'If I can't do this homework, it means the therapy can't help me') to show her how she was overgeneralising from the failure on one task to conclude that she would never get anything out of cognitive therapy.

Strategies for Changing Cognition

Cognitive interventions are aimed at helping patients to identify and change the cognitive processes that are at the centre of their depression. This can be seen as a three-step process:

Step 1. Teaching the model. In the early stages of therapy, the patient is introduced to the cognitive model of

Table 3.4.1 Weekly activity schedule

Rate activites (0–10) for mastery and pleasure.							
Time	**Monday**	**Tuesday**	**Wednesday**	**Thursday**	**Friday**	**Saturday**	**Sunday**
9–10							
10–11							
11–12							
12–1							
1–2							
2–3							
3–4							
4–5							
5–6							
6–7							
7–8							
8–12							

emotion and the problems conceptualised using this framework. The patient is shown how his or her problems are part of the depressive syndrome, and the central role of negative thinking in depression is illustrated. The link between events, cognitions and emotion is described, and the patient is encouraged to look at how this fits in with their own experiences. For instance, the patient may be asked to recall a day during the week when the depression was more severe, then they are asked what events might have triggered this exacerbation. The negative interpretation made of the situation will then demonstrate how negative thinking increases depressed mood. If the patient became more depressed after a friend did not return a phone call, a link might be found between this trigger and negative thoughts such as 'She's not interested in me; if I was worth anything, people would want to be with me; I must be boring'. The material from behavioural assignments is often used to illustrate the model – for example, when thinking about a task, the patient may say, 'I won't be able to do it' or 'There's no point in trying'. The link between these negative thoughts and depressed mood and lack of motivation can then be demonstrated. Explanatory material is often given at the beginning of each session to explain the model.

Step 2. Identifying negative automatic thoughts. Once the patient understands the basic concepts involved, the next step is to identify their repetitive automatic thoughts. Initially, the therapist elicits negative automatic thoughts in the session, and then the patient records instances of these as homework. A daily form monitoring upsetting events, associated emotions and intervening thoughts can be used to structure this exercise. No matter how pervasive the mood disorder, there is usually a fluctuation with everyday events, and noticing this change is a step towards gaining control over the mood. Labelling the type of distortions in thinking can be helpful at this stage (Box 3.4.1), and this can be given as a handout to the patient. Most patients, if they are given clear instructions about how to monitor thoughts with examples, can catch their thoughts with a little practice. If they have difficulty, their thoughts about the monitoring itself can be examined. This may reveal negative thoughts about the therapist despising them if they reveal themselves, the fear of exposing themselves to the painful cognitions, or hopeless thoughts about the whole exercise being pointless. Once these cognitions are identified, they can be challenged with the usual cognitive techniques.

Step 3. Challenging negative automatic thoughts. As the behavioural work helps to lift the patient's mood and he or she becomes familiar with automatic thoughts, the therapy moves into a more cognitive mode. From session one, the therapist has used cognitive techniques to question the reality of the patient's negative thinking. Now the patient learns to do this for himself, recording the automatic thoughts as they occur and challenging them with rational responses (Table 3.4.2). The aim is not to think positively but to subject thoughts and beliefs to reality testing and thus overcome the depressive bias. This is known as cognitive restructuring. Several techniques are commonly used to challenge automatic thoughts. Patients can be taught to ask these as questions:

i. What's the evidence? This is one of the core cognitive techniques. It could be argued that the whole of cognitive therapy boils down to helping the patient to stop accepting thoughts at face value and instead to always ask the question, 'What's my

Table 3.4.2 Dysfunctional thought record

Situation	Emotions (Rate from 0 to 100)	Automatic Thoughts	Alternative Response	Action Plan
Contemplating writing a court report.	Anxious 50% Depressed 50%	I won't be able to concentrate. It will take hours, and I'm sure to make mistakes. I'm incompetent. I can't do my job properly. Belief 70% -> 30%	I'm depressed at the moment, and my concentration and energy levels are low. It will take time to get back to my old levels of functioning. If I avoid this, I'll only feel worse. I've written many reports before. If I take it steadily, I can do this. Belief 75% No one has ever criticised my work or complained about my efficiency.	Break the report into sections. Work on a section for 20 minutes so I don't lose concentration.

evidence?' A simple way of doing this is to draw a line down the centre of a piece of paper and list on one side the evidence for and on the other side the evidence against a particular belief. If you were a depressed psychiatrist, you might have the following automatic thought when you were faced with writing a court report: 'I'm incompetent; I can't do my job properly.'

Negative automatic thought: 'I'm incompetent; I can't do my job properly.'

Evidence for the thought:	Evidence against the thought:
– I keep putting off writing that court report. – I can't concentrate when talking to my patients. – My colleagues seem to look down on me. – I've taken weeks off work lately, and I'm letting people down.	– I know I'm depressed at the moment, and my concentration and motivation are badly affected by that. – Until six months ago, I never had any problems with my work. – I know I'm not the only person to procrastinate. – I've no evidence that my colleagues really look down on me; I'm just making assumptions. In fact, I know they value me for my contributions because they have told me so in the past. – Taking time off work is not a sign of incompetence. – No one has ever criticised my work or complained about my efficiency.

With practice, this questioning of evidence becomes automatic and gradually challenges the ingrained negative bias in the patient's thinking. Table 3.4.2 demonstrates how the depressed psychiatrist might use a thought record to identify the situation (writing the report), negative thoughts (I can't do this; I'm incompetent) and emotional reaction (anxious and depressed). They can then evaluate these negative thoughts and generate an alternative, more adaptive set of thoughts. In the final column, an action plan can be developed. In this case, breaking the task down into 20-minute segments might allow the psychiatrist to concentrate without getting too fatigued. Looking for evidence for the thoughts is the core cognitive technique. As well as learning this skill of 'reality testing' the situation, the patient can also learn some other questions that can help create a different perspective.

ii. What alternative views are there? Alternative interpretations of an event are considered. The depressed person usually chooses the most negative interpretation of an event and automatically assumes this is correct. The therapist teaches the patient to generate alternatives. At first, these are also quite negative, but as more and more alternatives are asked for by the therapist, the patient is forced to think of more positive ones. This starts to break up the depressive bias in interpretations. After practising in the session, the patient is able to question their immediate response to situations in the outside world. For instance, if a friend passes the patient in the street, rather than automatically thinking, 'He's deliberately ignoring me', the patient starts to consider other explanations such as 'He's busy, and he probably didn't notice me'. The likelihood of these various explanations being correct can then be assessed, and a less-biased judgement can be made about the situation.

iii. What are the advantages and disadvantages of this way of thinking? Even if a negative thought is accurate, it is not necessarily helpful. Looking at the usefulness of a belief or thought can help to change it. In this exercise, the patient can list the advantages and disadvantages of the negative belief or thought.

Ruminations about real-life problems such as unemployment, loss or even impending death may be accurate reflections of reality, but in depression, they rarely lead to effective problem solving or working through emotions. In fact, they have the disadvantage of making the person feel worse, preventing them from engaging in life and even alienating them from loved ones. Once patients see these disadvantages, they are often able to reduce the frequency of these thoughts themselves or to use distraction techniques.

iv. If my interpretation is correct, are things as catastrophic as they seem? Patients who are anxious and depressed often catastrophise, but they rarely think beyond the catastrophe. Facing up to the worst fear often reveals that it is not as terrible as it seems or that the person has the resources to cope with it. For example, a depressed student convinced he will fail his exam can explore what would be so terrible if he did. He may never have even thought about the fact that he would be able to retake it again without any bad effect on his career.

Preventative Strategies

These are aimed at changing the underlying assumptions about the world that make people vulnerable to psychological problems. The same cognitive change techniques that were applied to thoughts can be used with assumptions. Evidence for and against the reasonableness of these assumptions is sought, the advantages and disadvantages of the assumption explored, and its origins plotted. Finally, a more-flexible, less-punitive rule is developed, and behavioural assignments are set so the patient can experiment with acting differently. The final sessions of therapy usually involve some preparation for the future with the discussion of relapse prevention strategies.

Case Illustration

A patient had a very negative relationship with her mother, who had been critical and rejecting throughout her childhood. A typical painful memory was of her mother refusing to give her a goodnight kiss. The one way the patient did get acceptance was through achievement, and the patient developed the rule that she must do things perfectly or she would be rejected. A specific example of this rule applied in her relationship with her partner: she believed completely that if she was not a perfect partner, giving no cause for criticism, her lover would eventually leave her. The reality and usefulness of this assumption was challenged in the session. Then, the patient showed her partner the beliefs she had written down. She was astonished to find that her partner did not agree with her at all, and in fact, had a more-flexible rule that no one was perfect, and it was healthy to have the occasional row about the irritating things the other person did. As a result, her belief in her original rule diminished greatly, and with help from the therapist, she began to gradually give up her perfectionistic view of relationships.

Efficacy of CBT

Beck's cognitive therapy has been compared with antidepressants (originally tricyclics and now specific serotonin re-uptake inhibitors). The two treatments are equally effective (see reviews by Butler et al and Cuijpers et al.).[5–7] Combining CBT and medication adds to the effects of both.[8,9] CBT is more effective than waiting-list controls, treatment as usual, or placebo (effect size 0.71).[6] Direct comparisons with other evidence-based therapies, such as interpersonal therapy, have found both therapies to be equally effective.[10] If CBT is delivered by well-trained therapists, it can be effective with patients with more severe levels of depression.[11]

CBT for patients with bipolar disorder is more challenging than with unipolar depression. There are overall mild to moderate effects, with improvement in depressive symptoms and relapse rates and some suggestions that there is an effect on mania.[12,13]

Face-to-face sessions are costly and time consuming, and researchers have explored the potential of other methods of delivery such as computerised CBT (cCBT), internet-based CBT and telephone therapy. A review of cCBT found large within-group effect sizes averaging 1.23.[14] Rather than simply presenting the patient with a computer programme, cCBT works best when a clinician explains the procedure, monitors progress and is available to troubleshoot problems.[15] There is also research evidence for internet and telephone CBT for depression.[16–18] Meta-analysis suggests that these new formats are as effective as individual and group CBT.[19]

Relapse Prevention

If psychological therapy is no more effective than antidepressants, is it not more cost-effective to stick with the latter? The potential benefit of CBT and some other psychotherapies is their impact on relapse. Early RCTs, where antidepressant medication was withdrawn at the end of the trial, found relapse rates of 15–28% for CBT compared to 50–60% with a tricyclic.[20,21] If the medication is continued for a longer period, receiving continuation medication is equivalent (30%) to patients receiving a short course of CBT.[22] To further investigate this, patients who have recovered with CBT or medication were randomised to either receive maintenance medication or no medication for a year. When continuation medication was withdrawn, the relapse rates increased again to 60% whereas they remained at 30% for those who had initially received CBT.[23,24] In partially recovered depressed outpatients, adding cognitive therapy to maintenance medication reduces relapse rates more than maintenance medication alone, with effects of CBT persisting for more than three years.[25,26] There is strong support in these studies for an enduring relapse prevention effect from CBT.[27] However, Andrews has argued that rather than CBT preventing relapse, discontinuation of medication promotes it.[28] When SSRIs block serotonin re-uptake, the system responds by reducing serotonin synthesis in the pre-synaptic neurone and reducing post-synaptic receptor sensitivity. Stopping the SSRI would then in effect reduce the availability of serotonin in the synapse and would explain why it is often difficult to withdraw medication without triggering a relapse.[29] The current status of CBT and antidepressants is summarised in Box 3.4.3.

Box 3.4.3 CBT and antidepressant medication

CBT is as effective as antidepressant medication in outpatient depression, but in both treatments, 40% of patients remain depressed.

The combination of CBT and antidepressants is more effective than either alone in severe depression.

When both treatments are withdrawn, relapse rates are lower with CBT than antidepressants.

After a single course of CBT, only 30% of patients relapse – the same as if they received maintenance antidepressants.

Behavioural Activation

In 1996, Neil Jacobson and colleagues reported the results of a three-way dismantling study that compared the behavioural activation component of Beck's cognitive therapy for depression with behavioural activation plus thought challenging and also with the full cognitive therapy package. Each proved equally effective, and the results held up at follow-up.[30] This led to the development of a new therapy: behavioural activation. In this approach, thoughts are not central to depression. Instead, depression is said to result from reduced positive reinforcement, which leads to a reduction in behaviour and further low mood. An important component of this model is the negative reinforcement that is experienced through various types of avoidance. Avoiding responsibilities, withdrawing from social activities and ruminating bring temporary relief from painful emotions but result in more passivity and inactivity. Like Beck's cognitive therapy, BA uses activity monitoring and scheduling to encourage healthy behaviours. It also teaches the depressed person to identify triggers for avoidance (using the mnemonic TRAPs: trigger, reaction and avoidance pattern) and then replace them with more adaptive responses (TRACs: trigger, response alternative coping). Other techniques such as completing graded-task assignments (as in CBT), learning problem solving, rehearsing actions in imagination, and working on skills training are also used.[31] Although there are not as many trials of BA as Beck's CT, the results are promising. Behavioural activation is superior to controls (standardised mean difference (SMD) of -0.74) and may be superior to medication (SMD of -0.42).[32] BA is also simpler and easier to teach than cognitive therapy.[33]

Third-Wave CBT

One of the most influential developments in CBT in recent years has been mindfulness-based cognitive therapy (MBCT) for relapse prevention. Rather than working with the content of thoughts, MBCT helps people develop a 'meta-awareness' of their experiences so they identify with these experiences less. MBCT is delivered in groups of 8–15 people and uses a combination of regular formal and informal meditation practices and insights from CBT. For patients with three or more depressive episodes, MBCT reduces the relative risk of relapse by 43 per cent.[34] MBCT and other 'third wave' therapies focus more on cognitive processes rather than content. Well's meta-cognitive therapy[35,36] and Watkins's rumination-focused CBT[37,38] are examples of third-wave therapies.

Interpersonal Therapy

Interpersonal therapy (IPT) is a treatment that was developed by Weissman and Klerman in the New Haven-Boston Collaborative Depression Project. It is a brief (12–16 weeks) weekly treatment originally devised for outpatient, non-psychotic, unipolar depressives, which focuses on improving the patient's interpersonal functioning.

Theoretical Framework

IPT is based on the assumption that psychosocial and interpersonal factors are of major significance in the development and maintenance of depression, and they possibly contribute to vulnerability to further episodes. Two main areas of empirical evidence support the contention that problems with social roles are important in depression. Firstly, there is strong evidence that interpersonal relations are impaired in depression, and research shows that depressives behave in a way that elicits negative responses from others. Although these findings may be a result rather than a cause of the depression, their role in maintenance and relapse may still be significant. The second source of empirical support for the interpersonal theory is research on social stresses and social support. A close confiding relationship with a spouse is a buffer against depression (see also the earlier discussion on the vulnerability to depression).[39]

Role impairments in depression: IPT sees all roles – in the nuclear and extended family, work, friendship and community – as having a potential buffering effect. Any disruption of these roles may lead to depression. This psychosocial contribution will interact with the effects of biological factors to produce the final common pathway to depression. Four main problem areas are defined and become the focus of treatment: grief, interpersonal disputes, role transitions and interpersonal deficits.

Clinical Application of Interpersonal Therapy

This section will give a brief description of the techniques used in IPT. A manual describing the therapy in detail is available.[40] Like cognitive therapy, IPT is a here-and-now therapy. Current relationships, rather than childhood experiences, are the focus of attention. The therapeutic techniques are eclectic, incorporating reassurance, clarification of emotional states, improvement of communication, and reality testing of perceptions and performance. These methods are used to achieve two main goals: the alleviation of depressive symptoms and the development of strategies for dealing with the interpersonal problems associated with the depressive episode.

Managing the Depressive State

This phase is supportive and educational. Patients are educated about the nature of depression. The therapist reviews all the patient's symptoms and describes how they are all part of a syndrome of depression, which is a well-recognised and treatable condition. Information is then given about the prevalence of the condition. Hopelessness may be directly addressed by informing the patient that their belief that they will never recover is part of the depressive syndrome, just like symptoms of weight loss or sleep disturbance. Symptom management is another component of this phase and is similar in many ways to the behavioural techniques used in cognitive therapy. Situations that exacerbate the depression are identified, and strategies are devised to avoid these situations or reduce their impact. For instance, if the patient feels worse when alone, measures for increasing social contact can be explored, or if the patient is overwhelmed at work, they may be helped to reduce their expectations and plan essential tasks. Antidepressant medication may be considered in this symptom-reduction phase.

Targeting Interpersonal Problem Areas

Once there has been some reduction in depressive symptoms, the therapist adopts a more interpersonal focus. The initial assessment will show which of the four interpersonal problem areas are affected, and one or two of these will be dealt with in therapy. If an unresolved grief reaction is part of the problem, the therapist will help the patient to mourn by expressing feelings about the lost person – particularly suppressed anger – reconstruct the relationship more realistically and finally go on to re-establish interests and new relationships. This latter stage may involve the prescription of quite specific tasks such as joining social organisations. Dealing with role transitions involves a similar approach to handling the loss, plus developing a more positive attitude to the new role. Interpersonal role disputes most frequently occur with the spouse. During treatment, the patient is helped to identify the dispute, to make choices about a plan of action and then encouraged to modify maladaptive patterns of communication. IPT works individually with the patient to either change the patient's or spouse's behaviour or to change the patient's attitude to the problem. Finally, interpersonal deficits may contribute to depression. Social isolation, lack of social skills or low self-esteem may all be present. IPT reviews past relationship problems and adopts problem solving and role play to develop social skills. The therapeutic relationship is also used as a vehicle for demonstrating and working with the interpersonal problems in the session.

Efficacy of Interpersonal Therapy

Like CBT, IPT for acute depression has moderate-to-large effect sizes compared with control groups ($g = 0.60$; 95% CI = 0.45–0.75) and is as effective as other therapies ($g = 0.06$) and pharmacotherapy ($g = -0.13$). Combined IPT and medication treatment is more effective than IPT alone ($g = 0.24$). IPT in sub-threshold depression can prevent the onset of major depression, and maintenance IPT significantly reduces relapse.[7] Interpersonal therapy for bipolar disorder is combined with social rhythm therapy to help patients regulate their daily routines and comply with medication regimes.[41] This approach has been shown to stabilise depressive symptoms in bipolar patients.[13]

Psychodynamic Therapy

There is no single psychodynamic model of depression but rather a body of theoretical writings that build on each other to develop and expand various themes. Freud was the first to point out the similarities of depressive reactions to grief reactions.[42] He suggested that the depressed patient has high dependency needs for a parental figure, with consequent ambivalent feelings (love mixed with anger and frustration because of the dependency). In depression, the loss of a real or imagined object results in an introjection of the lost object (i.e. an internal unconscious representation of the lost person as an attempt to avoid the real loss). The anger towards this object then becomes unleashed on the ego itself, resulting in depression. Freud believed the depressive's self-reproaches were not really anger at the self but an indirect attack on the lost loved object. Similar themes can be found in subsequent psychoanalytic theories: loss, internal objects, dependence and ambivalence, and anger directed at the self (see later). Present day theories, influenced by the work of Klein, Bowlby and Winnicott, see depression as primarily an interpersonal problem, resulting from conflict, confusion or a deficit in the person's internal representations of significant others (object relations theory). Although different metaphors may be used, they share the idea that, as children, we build up working models of ourselves and other people derived from repeated interactions with caregivers. If there is an absence of loving, consistent parenting through loss, abandonment or lack of affective response, the child will not develop a sufficiently caring and soothing set of internal representations to call upon in times of crisis. Parental figures may be represented in the internal world as harshly critical, absent or unpredictable, and the child's rage against them may be disavowed because of guilt or fear of the consequences of rejection. Adult experiences of loss or failure may re-evoke these unresolved developmental representations, and the conflict can lead to anger being directed at the self, explaining the self-criticism and self-hatred seen in many depressive states.

A distinction should be made between psychoanalysis (a highly specialised form of psychotherapy carried out three to five times weekly for years) and psychoanalytically oriented therapies (lasting 3–12 months, with once-weekly sessions and a more active therapeutic stance). There are now a number of brief psychoanalytically oriented therapies for depression. One of the most promising is dynamic interpersonal therapy (DIT). This is a 16-session treatment developed by Peter Fonagy and colleagues.[43] It builds on the work of Luborsky and Kernberg and is heavily influenced by attachment and mentalisation theories.[44–46] As described earlier, we all have internal, non-conscious models of attachment figures from our past that guide our behaviour. Childhood experiences may make us vulnerable to loss, separation or rejection. DIT helps patients understand how their reactions to current interpersonal challenges are responses to unconscious threats to attachment. They learn to identify repetitive patterns of relating based on these attachments and to reflect on their own and others' thoughts and feelings (the process of mentalisation). The most important pattern becomes the 'interpersonal affective focus' of therapy. By becoming consciously aware of this pattern, the depressed person sees how it plays out in their life and is responsible for their depressive symptoms. They recognise its interpersonal costs and can begin to make changes. The therapist helps the patient see how this process takes place both in the therapeutic relationship and in relationships outside the therapy session. Meta-analyses generally show brief psychodynamic therapies to be as effective as other treatments.[9] A recent naturalistic pilot study of DIT has supported its potential as a treatment in the Improving Access to Psychological Therapies services (see later).[47]

Conclusions

It is encouraging that such a range of brief therapies is available to the clinician. Although CBT is the most researched approach, head-to-head trials do not show any one therapy to be superior to the others. In Cuijpers network meta-analysis, there was also no significant difference between any psychological therapy and pharmacotherapy (RR = 0.99; 95% CI: 0.92–1.08). Combined treatment was more effective than psychological therapy alone (RR = 1.27; 95% CI: 1.14–1.39) and pharmacotherapy alone (RR = 1.25; 95% CI: 1.14–1.37).[9] While psychological treatment may be less cost-effective in the short term than medication, it may have the advantage of reducing relapse rates with a single course of therapy. In comparison, medication would have to be continued to keep patients well. So, when psychological therapy is available – especially if the patient has recurrent depression – it should be considered as a treatment option. Despite the undoubted benefits of various treatment options, remission is achieved in only 60 per cent of patients, even in the best trials. When publication bias and use of waiting-list controls are accounted for, the effect size of randomised controlled trials of psychotherapy and antidepressants reduces considerably.[48–50] More research is needed to find treatment methods for the 40 per cent of patients who remain depressed after receiving psychotherapy or antidepressant medication.

Group and Systemic Therapies

One of the themes running through much depression research is the relevance of interpersonal factors to the vulnerability and maintenance of depression. The therapies described so far can all be applied in groups, which have the advantage that more patients can be treated in the same time as one patient can with individual therapy. Cognitive behavioural groups tend to be structured and educational in nature.[51] A meta-analysis found that individual CBT was slightly superior to group CBT post-treatment, but there was no difference at three months follow-up.[52] Skills-based groups (e.g. social skills and assertiveness training) can be used as an adjunct to other treatments. The indication for these treatments will depend upon the problems identified at assessment. Many depressed people have long-standing difficulties with assertiveness and may tend to suppress their own wishes and try excessively to accommodate and please others. This may predispose them to depression, and assertiveness training can help to make them less vulnerable to depression in the future.

Yalom was one of the pioneers of group therapy (Yalom and Leszcz, 2020).[53] His approach emphasises 'here and now' experiences: in a group, the patient's relationship with the therapist and other group members offers an opportunity for valuable interpersonal learning. The therapist's realistic, supportive and tolerant attitude replaces the patient's harsh self-criticism and allows the members of the group to gradually treat themselves in a more accepting way (in analytic terms, the members internalise the therapist's more tolerant superego, which replaces the depressive's punitive superego). The group also allows patients to express guilt and hostile feelings in a supportive atmosphere. The effectiveness of this type of group work in actively depressed patients has not been evaluated. An eclectic, interpersonal form of group therapy is often used with hospital inpatients. Ward groups are frequently led by inexperienced therapists, with little supervision. Group psychotherapy with inpatients demands quite specialised skills and modifications of techniques used with outpatients. Because the depressed inpatient may show psychomotor retardation, their capacity to engage in group work is limited. Inpatient groups need to be less challenging, less demanding and more focused than outpatient groups. Group therapy has more to offer after the resolution of the acute depressive phase. Recovered depressives can explore and change interpersonal patterns that predispose them to depression. Groups can also function as vehicles for support in chronic cases.

Like group therapy, couples therapy and family therapy are modes of delivery rather than specific models of therapy. Cognitive, behavioural and psychodynamic forms of therapy all exist, but they have as their focus the naturally occurring systems within which the depression develops. They all have in common the assumption that the interactional patterns in the family contribute to depression and can be used as a vehicle for change. Interactional patterns may include complementary role fits between a dependent depressive partner and a controlling caring partner or problems in distance regulation in the family. A range of couple-based interventions for depression have been reported.[54] Behavioural couple therapy (BCT), for instance, is a brief (12–20 sessions) intervention that can be applied when there is relationship distress and at least one partner is depressed. BCT seeks to improve the relationship through using communication training, fostering positive exchanges between partners and teaching joint problem-solving skills. BCT improves both depression and the quality of the relationship[55] and is recommended in a number of guidelines, such as the NICE guidelines for depression.

Social Interventions

Social factors have long been known to both predispose and protect people from depression. A systematic review found that perceived emotional support, perceived instrumental support, and large diverse social networks all buffered against depression.[56] In the United Kingdom, social interventions have traditionally been accessed via primary care referrals to a link worker or navigator who helps people find local sources of support, though mental health services are now increasingly using this model (see Chapter 20). This approach, known as social prescribing, is not directly aimed at relieving depression but has been shown to have a positive effect on mental health. Patients are more likely to take part in these programmes if they believe the social prescription will be of benefit, the referral is presented in an acceptable way that matches their needs and expectations, and if their concerns are addressed by the referrer. Referrals should not be perfunctory. Patients are more likely to engage if the activity is accessible and if attendance at the first session is supported, while the activity leader needs to be skilled and knowledgeable. There is a hope that social prescribing in mental health may prove more cost-effective than psychotherapy or medication. Nagy and Moore were able to identify seven types of social interventions for depression described in the literature: peer support (e.g. sharing and empathising with others), skill building (e.g. coping skills, action planning skills), group-based activities (e.g. team-building activities, community clubs, outings within the community), psycho-education (e.g. group-based education on contributors to stress, depressive symptoms and mental wellbeing), psychotherapy (e.g. cognitive behavioural therapy and interpersonal therapy), exercise (e.g. walking groups, football teams, yoga) and links to community resources (e.g. linking participants with various supports and resources in the community).[56] Most of the studies used a variety of these approaches in various settings such as community organisations, workplaces, outdoor green spaces, people's homes, health or mental health centres, online, by telephone and even in an out-of-town retreat. Seventeen out of 24 interventions showed significant reductions in depressive symptoms. Social interventions should therefore be considered in the treatment of anyone with depression.

The UK Improving Access to Psychological Therapies Initiative

The UK Improving Access to Psychological Therapies programme (IAPT) delivers local psychological therapy services for anxiety and depression.[57] The IAPT programme implements psychological treatments that have been shown to be effective and monitors their impact. CBT, IPT, DIT, BCT and MBCT are all available in IAPT. Patients with less-severe problems are initially treated with low intensity (LI) interventions, such as computerised CBT, and stepped up to high intensity (HI, i.e. formal therapy), if necessary. For those who receive these services, 36% of people receive only LI, 28% receive HI and 34% receive both.[57] IAPT services now treat nearly a million patients a year, achieving recovery in 50% of cases and reliable improvement in 66%.[57]

Principles of Psychological Management

Two major themes run through the psychological literature on depression and its treatment. One is the cognitive-behavioural axis, with substantial evidence that depressed patients show behavioural deficits and cognitive abnormalities. The second is the interpersonal axis. Critical losses of important relationships or current relationship difficulties are closely related to depression. These two lines of research and the treatment associated with them should inform the psychiatrist's clinical management of the depressed patient. No research has yet been done on the application of these techniques in a traditional outpatient psychiatric consultation. Antidepressant medication is likely to be the main treatment modality used by the psychiatrist. However, even in a series of 15-to-30-minute consultations at monthly intervals, it is possible to apply psychological understandings and interventions.

Psychological Aspects of the Assessment Process

The process of taking a history and assessing mental state can be therapeutic in its own right if it is done in a sensitive and respectful manner. To be able to tell your story and to have someone empathically listen is helpful. This can challenge beliefs such as 'I'm the only person like this' and 'no one can understand me'. A problem-oriented assessment can be more beneficial than one that simply focuses on symptoms. Defining problems and drawing up problem lists helps to diminish the idea that depression is overwhelming and starts to engender hope. Problems that the patient considers important can then become the focus of therapeutic work. For instance, if insomnia is particularly worrying for the patient, identifying this as a problem could lead to the selection of an appropriate antidepressant or giving direct information and advice about sleep hygiene. Risk assessment is obviously a primary concern at this stage. If a suicide risk is identified, then this should be the primary focus for any psychological work to be done in the first consultations. At the end of the assessment, a diagnostic formulation that both names the disorder as depression and provides some understanding of how biological and psychosocial factors interact to make the person depressed right now can help to give meaning to the depressed person's experience and encourage trust.

Engaging the Patient and Maintaining the Therapeutic Relationship

Challenging Hopelessness

Trust and hope are the most important concerns in establishing a helping relationship with a depressed patient. Hopelessness has been shown to correlate more strongly with suicide risk than severity of depression, so interventions that engender hope are of particular importance in the early stages of consultation with the depressed patient. Traditionally, the psychiatrist has used his status as a knowledgeable professional to give reassurance and information in order to instil hope in the depressed patient. In addition to this, there are some cognitive techniques which may be of help in this setting:

Cost-Benefit Analysis of Suicide

In actively suicidal patients, considering reasons for dying and reasons for living both gives information about the risk of self harm and can engender hope (see further in Chapter 15). The process involves first asking the patient for all the reasons that life is not worth living. It is important to do this before looking at the reasons for living because otherwise the psychiatrist will be seen as yet another person trying to convince the patient to think positively about a hopeless situation. Asking for more reasons for suicide will eventually take the person to the point where they run out of advantages; this realisation that there is a finite limit to the reasons for suicide can be therapeutic. Then, a list of reasons for living can be placed alongside the reasons for dying. By focusing on the benefits of living and establishing whether there are alternative ways out of the apparently hopeless situation, the clinician can often help the patient to feel more hopeful that it is worth holding on.

Reasons for dying	Reasons for living
This feeling will never go.	My mother would be devastated if I killed myself.
No one cares if I live or die.	I've been told I'll feel better.
I'll never pay off my debts.	Once I kill myself, it's final.
I'm useless, and I might as well admit it.	I'm trying a new medication; it might work.
It will be a way out of the pain.	I haven't always felt that I'm useless; perhaps this will pass.
	I might be able to get help with my debts.

Review of Past Depressive Episodes and Periods of Euthymia

In people who are depressed and also in people who self harm, there are deficits in problem-solving ability and distortions in autobiographical memory. It is difficult for these patients to gain access to specific positive memories to dispel their pessimistic view of the future. The psychiatrist can help by asking focused questions about the past:

Have you always felt this way, or were there times when you were not depressed?

How long did your last depression last?

Did you feel as hopeless then as you do now?

What did you do to recover?

Could the same things work again?

What would you have said to me about your life last year before you became depressed?

What are the strengths you have when well?

How could we help you find them again?

Time Projection

Negative thoughts about the future prevent the depressed patient from thinking beyond the present. Asking what life might be like when they recover from depression gives the message that there is a future and gets the patient thinking about it as a definite possibility. A time-projection exercise can help patients elaborate on what life might be like in a year's time or two years' time when their depression has remitted. Identifying possible goals for the future and looking at ways to achieve those goals can also engender hope.

The Therapeutic Relationship

The doctor–patient relationship is important in the management of all psychiatric disorders. In depression, the doctor needs to achieve a balance between under- and over-involvement with the patient. Too distant a stance will fail to engage the patient and confirm the depressed person's view that she is isolated and not understood. Over-involvement can lead the psychiatrist to 'buy into' the depressive person's negative world view and see the situation as hopeless and overwhelming. A warm, friendly, supportive and empathic manner is necessary, but this needs to be balanced with objectivity and professionalism. The patient's negative bias may influence the therapeutic relationship. He or she may think, 'He's not interested in me; I'm boring.' These automatic thoughts about the therapist can be checked out periodically and corrected with appropriate information.

Psychodynamic theory can inform the clinician of transference phenomena that may interfere with the supportive relationship. The depressed person's ambivalence towards important relationships means that the psychiatrist is likely to be perceived as both hostile and punishing as well as being nurturing at various times in the relationship. The negative thoughts described earlier illustrate a transference in which the therapist is seen as critical. When a good rapport exists, the therapist may be idealised, and a dependent transference may develop. This, and the depressed patient's sensitivity to loss, means that cancellations of appointments, holidays and other interruptions may be particularly difficult. The psychiatrist should also be aware of how his or her own feelings to the patient may be a sign of 'countertransference' that may be elicited when the therapist is drawn into a reciprocal role, unconsciously playing a real or fantasised relationship from the patient's childhood (e.g. the role of a critical parent). Strong feelings of anger or wanting to punish or get rid of the patient as well as positive urges to look after or rescue the patient are indications of possible countertransference reactions. If these occur, the clinician should discuss the patient with a colleague or obtain supervision.

Education about Depression and Medication

Education can be invaluable in giving the patient a sense of hope and trust in the clinician. The negative cognitive bias in depression can lead to the misinterpretation of symptoms – lack of motivation and loss of energy are seen as signs of weakness, failure or laziness – and so create a syndrome of 'depression about depression'. Giving the person information about depression can dispel these self-criticisms:

1. Depression is a syndrome with characteristic symptoms.
2. Depression is associated with negative views of the self, experience and the future.
3. Depression is treatable.

Similarly, education about the side effects of medication prevents misattribution of symptoms and improves compliance (see Chapter 3.3). Many patients expect antidepressants to work immediately and, if they are not told otherwise, become disillusioned and may give up taking the drugs before they can take effect. The treatment plan should be explained to the patient and the rationale for any intervention given.

Fatigue, poor concentration and a negative bias may all contribute to difficulties in decision-making and impairment of work performance. It is therefore wise to advise patients not to make any major life decisions and to delay large, difficult tasks until the depression has lifted.

It is vital to check the patient's understanding of information given. In severe depression, impairment of concentration may reduce the amount that is taken in. Even in less-severe cases, misunderstandings can occur. Information leaflets, books and websites can all reinforce the message that depression is a common, treatable disorder that need not carry a stigma. Boxes 3.4.4 and 3.4.5 give details of some self-help materials for patients.

Box 3.4.4 Self-help books

Cognitive Behaviour Therapy		
Mind Over Mood: Changing the Way You Feel by Changing the Way You Think	Dennis Greenberger and Christine Padesky	Guilford Press 2015
Cognitive Behavioural Therapy (CBT): Your Toolkit to Modify Mood, Overcome Obstructions and Improve Your Life	Elaine Foreman and Clair Pollard	Icon Books 2016
Behavioural Activation		
Overcoming Depression One Step at a Time	Michael Addis	New Harbinger 2004
Mindfulness-Based Cognitive Therapy		
The Mindful Way Through Depression: Freeing Yourself from Chronic Unhappiness	Mark Williams, John Teasdale, Zindel Segal and John Kabat-Zinn	Guilford Press 2007
Interpersonal Therapy		
Mastering Depression through Interpersonal Psychotherapy: Patient Workbook	Myrna Weissman	Oxford University Press 2005

Box 3.4.5 Websites and apps

Overcoming Apps: overcoming.co.uk/709/Overcoming-Apps

Overcoming Depression and Overcoming Low Self-Esteem apps are available free on iTunes and Google Play. They allow patients to track their moods and behaviour, set goals and monitor progress, and design behavioural experiments to test their beliefs.

Moodkit: apps.apple.com/ca/app/moodkit-mood-improvement-tools/id427064987

Moodkit is an app available for the iPhone that helps patients to track their mood, identify and change negative thoughts, and use activities to manage mood.

Headspace: www.headspace.com/

This is a popular meditation app for managing stress.

Interviewing Family Members

Partners, friends and relatives can not only give information about the patient and his or her relationships, but they can also be directly involved in treatment. Education about the nature of depression can be helpful for them too. If the relationship is good, the partner can be used as a co-therapist. If the relationship is poor, some simple work on communication combined with education about the nature of depression may be helpful. In assessing relationship problems, think of the IPT problem areas:

1. Grief
2. Role disputes
3. Role transitions
4. Interpersonal deficits

Utilising Specific Change Techniques

Cognitive Behavioural Techniques

It is obviously not possible to carry out a full course of CBT in a busy outpatient setting where time is limited, but some simple techniques can be used. These are best instituted in conjunction with a self-help programme. There is growing evidence for the effectiveness of CBT delivered through books and computer self-help programmes (see earlier). Psychiatrists should have a supply of these materials for use in outpatients. Some of these books are workbooks, which give exercises for patients to follow (e.g. Overcoming Depression by Paul Gilbert, 2009). The psychiatrist can select chapters from these books for patients to work on between appointments. Behavioural techniques may be easier for psychiatrists with no formal training in CBT to use in brief outpatient sessions. The self-monitoring, activity scheduling and graded-task assignment described earlier can easily be incorporated into the psychiatric interview, particularly when integrated with a self-help book. Patients can also be taught simple problem-solving skills.

Guidance and Advice

Advice on lifestyle changes such as attention to sleep hygiene, alcohol use and exercise can be helpful. A good assessment may indicate activities that can be discouraged (e.g. a depressed patient visiting a friend who overloads her with her own problems) or those that can be encouraged. If a support worker or 'navigator' is available, then they may be able to point the patient in the direction of local self-help groups, befriending schemes or other community activities that increase engagement and social networking.

In the long run, larger environmental changes may be indicated such as moving houses, changing jobs, divorce or medical retirement. Sometimes, it may be clear that environmental stresses are maintaining the depression, and the psychiatrist can contribute by helping to remove them.

A patient presented one month after a cot death with severe depression and suicidal thoughts. She reported that she was unable to go into the room where the baby had died. Despite classical biological features of depression, she refused antidepressant medication and confided little in her community psychiatric nurse. She insisted that the only thing that would help her would be for the council to arrange a move to another flat. The psychiatrist wrote a letter strongly supporting such a move, and once the patient had moved, she felt considerably improved.

The following case of a depressed police officer in a stressful job demonstrates the therapeutic role of medical retirement.

A 47-year-old Flying Squad officer worked in a very stressful job that involved waiting in banks that were thought to be the target of robberies. His teenage daughter had become delinquent because he was away for considerable periods of time, quite unpredictably, as part of his job. He presented with a classical depressive syndrome, but once he had been off sick for a month, he felt quite unable to return to his previous work. The psychiatrist offered to support retirement on medical grounds, and once this had been arranged, his depression cleared completely, indicating that the underlying cause had been great fear associated with his stressful job and the destructive effect it had on his family's life.

The psychiatrist can and should intervene on the patient's behalf whenever this is appropriate in order to diminish the external stresses on the patient.

Monitoring Change and Considering Referral for Specialist Psychological Therapy

In the UK, most psychological therapy for anxiety and depression now takes place within IAPT services. Psychiatrists in primary care will have access to these services, but they are often not open to patients attending community mental health teams (CMHTs). CMHTs will usually have their own psychologist or psychological therapist and possibly access to more centralised psychology/psychotherapy services, but these resources are sometimes limited. If the depressed patient has not responded to medication, a referral for conjoint CBT should be considered. Current problems within the family are indications for marital or family therapy. Wider-ranging relationship difficulties, particularly if associated with a disturbed early life (e.g. parental loss or family disruption in childhood), would make one consider a more interpersonally oriented therapy like IPT or individual or group psychodynamic therapy. We do not yet have empirical support for which therapy works for whom, but Table 3.4.3 summarises some of the clinical features that might guide your decision to refer to a specific treatment. CBT, BA, IPT and DIT are all effective treatments, but unfortunately, the limiting factor is often the availability of psychological treatment. The skills within the CMHT should not be underestimated. Often, basic behavioural activation by a keyworker can have a significant effect.

Table 3.4.3 Indications for therapies

PROBLEM	THERAPY
• Recurrent depression • Depression not responsive to adequate trials of antidepressants • Residual depression after severe depressive illness	COGNITIVE BEHAVIOUR THERAPY
• Current problems in marital relationship	COUPLES THERAPY
• Unresolved grief • Maladaptive relationship patterns: role conflicts or role transitions	INTERPERSONAL THERAPY
• Recurrent problems with relationships • Unresolved childhood trauma, conflict or deprivation • Patient wants exploratory/insight-focused therapy, rather than a symptom-focused approach	PSYCHODYNAMIC PSYCHOTHERAPY
• Chronic depressive illness	SUPPORTIVE PSYCHOTHERAPY

Conclusions

A variety of psychological therapies for depression are now available, and there is a growing research literature to support their efficacy. Cognitive and behavioural treatments are the most extensively researched, but there is also evidence for the effectiveness of interpersonal psychotherapy and brief, focal psychodynamic psychotherapy. There is growing evidence that these therapies have long-term effects on vulnerability to depression. A single course of CBT reduces relapse to the same degree as keeping someone on maintenance antidepressants. Some of the clinical insights from therapies demonstrated to be effective in depression can be used in the psychological management of depression even if formal psychotherapy is not being undertaken.

References

1. Burcusa SL, Iacono WG. Risk for recurrence in depression. *Clinical Psychological Review* 2007;27(8):959–85. www.sciencedirect.com/science/article/abs/pii/S027273580700058X (accessed 13 Feb 2021).
2. Kupfer DJ, Frank E, Wamhoff J, et al. Mood disorders: update on prevention of recurrence. In: Mundt C, Goldstein MJ, Hahlweg K, et al. (eds.) *Interpersonal Factors in the Origin and Course of Affective Disorders*. London: Gaskell; 1996: 289–302.
3. Rush AJ, Beck AT, Kovacs M, et al. Comparative efficacy of cognitive therapy and pharmacotherapy in the treatment of depressed outpatients. *Cognitive Therapy and Research* 1977;1(1):17–37.
4. Beck AT, Rush AJ, Shaw B, et al. *Cognitive Therapy of Depression*. New York: Guilford Press; 1979.
5. Butler AC, Chapman JE, Forman EM, et al. The empirical status of cognitive-behavioral therapy: a review of meta-analyses. *Clinical Psychology Review*. 2006;26(1):17–31.
6. Cuijpers P, Berking M, Andersson G, et al. A meta-analysis of cognitive-behavioural therapy for adult depression, alone and in comparison with other treatments. *Canadian Journal of Psychiatry* 2013;58(7):376–85. search.proquest.com/docview/1426313762?accountid=136549.
7. Cuijpers P, Donker T, Weissman MM, et al. Interpersonal psychotherapy for mental health problems: a comprehensive meta-analysis. *American Journal of Psychiatry* 2016;173(7):680–7. ajp.psychiatryonline.org/doi/abs/10.1176/appi.ajp.2015.15091141 (accessed 6 January 2021).
8. Cuijpers P, Sijbrandij M, Koole SL, et al. Adding psychotherapy to antidepressant medication in depression and anxiety disorders: a meta-analysis. *World Psychiatry* 2014;13(1):56–67.
9. Cuijpers P, Noma H, Karyotaki E, et al. A network meta-analysis of the effects of psychotherapies, pharmacotherapies and their combination in the treatment of adult depression. *World Psychiatry* 2020;19(1):92–107.
10. Luty SE, Carter JD, McKenzie JM, et al. Randomised controlled trial of interpersonal psychotherapy and cognitive-behavioural therapy for depression. *British Journal of Psychiatry* 2007;190(June):496–502.
11. DeRubeis RJ, Hollon SD, Amsterdam JD, et al. Cognitive therapy vs medications in the treatment of moderate to severe depression. *Archives of General Psychiatry* 2005;62(4):409–16.
12. Chiang KJ, Tsai JC, Liu D, et al. Efficacy of cognitive-behavioral therapy in patients with bipolar disorder: a metaanalysis of randomized controlled trials. *PLoS ONE* 2017;12(5): e0176849.
13. Miklowitz DJ, Efthimiou O, Furukawa TA, et al. Adjunctive psychotherapy for bipolar disorder: a systematic review and component network meta-analysis. *JAMA Psychiatry* 2020;78(2):141–50.
14. Hofman J, Pollitt A, Broeks M, et al. Review of computerised cognitive behavioural therapies: products and outcomes for people with mental health needs. *Rand Health Quarterly* 2017;6(4):12.
15. Andersson G, Cuijpers P. Internet-based and other computerized psychological treatments for adult depression: a meta-analysis. *Cognitive Behaviour Therapy* 2009;38(4):196–205. www.tandfonline.com/doi/abs/10.1080/16506070903318960 (accessed 1 December 2020).
16. Farrer L, Christensen H, Griffiths KM, et al. Internet-based CBT for depression with and without telephone tracking in a national helpline: randomised controlled trial. *PLoS ONE* 2011;6(11): e28099. dx.plos.org/10.1371/journal.pone.0028099 (accessed 10 February 2021).
17. Castro A, García-Palacios A, García-Campayo J, et al. Efficacy of low-intensity psychological intervention applied by ICTs for the treatment of depression in primary care: a controlled trial. *BMC Psychiatry* 2015;15(1):106. bmcpsychiatry.biomedcentral.com/articles/10.1186/s12888-015-0475-0 (accessed 10 February 2021).
18. Gili M, Castro A, García-Palacios A, et al. Efficacy of three low-intensity, internet-based psychological interventions for the treatment of depression in primary care: randomized controlled trial. *Journal of Medical Internet Research* 2020;22(6):e15845. www.jmir.org/2020/6/e15845 (accessed 10 February 2021).
19. Cuijpers P, Noma H, Karyotaki E, et al. Effectiveness and acceptability of cognitive behavior therapy delivery formats in adults with depression: a network meta-analysis. *JAMA Psychiatry* 2019;76(7):700–7. jamanetwork.com/journals/jamapsychiatry/fullarticle/2730724 (accessed 10 February 2021).
20. Simons AD, Murphy GE, Levine JL, et al. Cognitive therapy and pharmacotherapy for depression: sustained improvement over one year. *Archives of General Psychiatry* 1986;43(1):43–8.
21. Evans MD, Hollon SD, DeRubeis RJ, et al. Differential relapse following cognitive therapy and pharmacotherapy for depression. *Archives of General Psychiatry* 1992;49(10):802–8.
22. Cuijpers P, Hollon SD, van Straten A, et al. Does cognitive behaviour therapy have an enduring effect that is superior to keeping patients on continuation pharmacotherapy? A meta-analysis. *BMJ Open* 2013;3(4):e002542.
23. Hollon SD, DeRubeis RJ, Shelton RC, et al. Prevention of relapse following cognitive therapy vs medications in moderate to severe depression. *Archives of General Psychiatry* 2005;62(4):417–22.
24. Dobson KS, Hollon SD, Dimidjian S, et al. Randomized trial of behavioral activation, cognitive therapy, and antidepressant medication in the prevention of relapse and recurrence in major depression. *Journal of Consulting and Clinical Psychology* 2008;76(3):468–77.
25. Paykel ES, Scott J, Teasdale JD, et al. Prevention of relapse in residual depression by cognitive therapy. *Archives of General Psychiatry* 1999;56(9):829–35.
26. Paykel ES, Scott J, Cornwall PL, et al. Duration of relapse prevention after cognitive therapy in residual depression: follow-up of controlled trial. *Psychological Medicine* 2005;35(1):59–68. www.proquest.com/docview/57124896.
27. Clarke K, Mayo-Wilson E, Kenny J, et al. Can non-pharmacological interventions prevent relapse in adults who have recovered from depression? A systematic review and meta-analysis

of randomised controlled trials. *Clinical Psychology Review* 2015;39:58–70. pubmed.ncbi.nlm.nih.gov/25939032 (accessed 10 February 2021).

28. Andrews PW, Kornstein SG, Halberstadt LJ, et al. Blue again: perturbational effects of antidepressants suggest monoaminergic homeostasis in major depression. *Frontiers in Psychology* 2011;2(July):159.
29. Hollon SD, Cohen ZD, Singla DR, et al. Recent developments in the treatment of depression. *Behavior Therapy* 2019;50(2):257–69.
30. Jacobson NS, Dobson KS, Truax PA, et al. A component analysis of cognitive-behavioral treatment for depression. *Journal of Consulting and Clinical Psychology* 1996;64(2):295–304.
31. Martell CR, Dimidjian S, Herman-Dunn R. *Behavioral Activation for Depression: A Clinician's Guide*. New York: Guilford Press; 2013.
32. Ekers D, Webster L, van Straten A, et al. Behavioural activation for depression; an update of meta-analysis of effectiveness and sub group analysis. *PLoS ONE* 2014;9(6):e100100.
33. Ekers DM, Dawson MS, Bailey E. Dissemination of behavioural activation for depression to mental health nurses: training evaluation and benchmarked clinical outcomes. *Journal of Psychiatric and Mental Health Nursing* 2013;20 (2):186–92.
34. Piet J, Hougaard E. The effect of mindfulness-based cognitive therapy for prevention of relapse in recurrent major depressive disorder: a systematic review and meta-analysis. *Clinical Psychology Review* 2011;31(6):1032–40.
35. Wells A. *Metacognitive Therapy for Anxiety and Depression*. New York: Guilford Press; 2011.
36. Normann N, van Emmerik AAP, Morina N. The efficacy of metacognitive therapy for anxiety and depression: a meta-analytic review. *Depression and Anxiety* 2014;31(5):402–11.
37. Watkins ER. *Rumination-Focused Cognitive-Behavioral Therapy for Depression*. New York: Guilford Publications; 2018.
38. Watkins ER, Mullan E, Wingrove J, et al. Rumination-focused cognitive-behavioural therapy for residual depression: phase II randomised controlled trial. *British Journal of Psychiatry* 2011;199(4):317–22. www.cambridge.org/core/services/aop-cambridge-core/content/view/8A7837A95E24712C034EB101FD53F41A/S0007125000258352a.pdf/div-class-title-rumination-focused-cognitive-behavioural-therapy-for-residual-depression-phase-ii-randomised-controlled-trial-div.pdf (accessed 1 December 2020).
39. Brown GW, Harris T. *Social Origins of Depression: A Study of Psychiatric Disorder in Women*. New York: Free Press; 1978.
40. Weissman MM, Markowitz JC, Klerman GL. *The Guide to Interpersonal Psychotherapy: Updated and Expanded Edition*. Oxford: Oxford University Press; 2017.
41. Frank E, Swartz HA, Kupfer DJ. Interpersonal and social rhythm therapy: managing the chaos of bipolar disorder. *Biological Psychiatry* 2000;48 (6):593–604.
42. Freud S. *Mourning and Melancholia*. Collected Papers, Vol. 4. London: The Hogarth Press; 1925.
43. Lemma A, Target M, Fonagy P. *Brief Dynamic Interpersonal Therapy: A Clinician's Guide*. Oxford: Oxford University Press; 2011.
44. Luborsky L, Crits-Christoph P. *Understanding Transference: The Core Conflictual Relationship Theme Method*. Washington, DC: American Psychological Association; 1998.
45. Kernberg OF. Object relations theory in clinical practice. *The Psychoanalytic Quarterly* 1988;57(4):481–504.
46. Luyten P, Blatt SJ. Psychodynamic treatment of depression. *Psychiatric Clinics* 2012;35(1):111–29.
47. Fonagy P, Lemma A, Target M, et al. Dynamic interpersonal therapy for moderate to severe depression: a pilot randomized controlled and feasibility trial. *Psychological Medicine* 2020;50 (6):1010–9. doi.org/10.1017/S0033291719000928 (accessed 8 February 2021).
48. Turner EH, Matthews AM, Linardatos E, et al. Selective publication of antidepressant trials and its influence on apparent efficacy. *New England Journal of Medicine* 2008;358(3):252–60.
49. Driessen E, Hollon SD, Bockting CLH, et al. Does publication bias inflate the apparent efficacy of psychological treatment for major depressive disorder? A systematic review and meta-analysis of US National Institutes of health-funded trials. *PLoS ONE.* 2015;10(9):e0137864, journals.plos.org/plosone/article?id=10.1371/journal.pone.0137864.
50. Cuijpers P, Cristea IA, Karyotaki E, et al. How effective are cognitive behavior therapies for major depression and anxiety disorders? A meta-analytic update of the evidence. *World Psychiatry* 2016;15(3):245–58.
51. Whitfield G. Group cognitive-behavioural therapy for anxiety and depression. *Advances in Psychiatric Treatment* 2010;16(3):219–27. www.cambridge.org/core/journals/advances-in-psychiatric-treatment/article/group-cognitivebehavioural-therapy-for-anxiety-and-depression/458CD3360742FE9E90AEB107493E2F0C (accessed 10 February 2021).
52. Huntley AL, Araya R, Salisbury C. Group psychological therapies for depression in the community: systematic review and meta-analysis. *British Journal of Psychiatry.* 2012;200 (3):184–90.
53. Yalom ID, Leszcz M. *The Theory and Practice of Group Psychotherapy*. London: Hachette UK; 2020.
54. Whisman MA, Johnson DP, Be D, et al. Couple-based interventions for depression. *Couple and Family Psychology: Research and Practice* 2012;1(3):185–98.
55. Christensen A, Atkins DC, Yi J, et al. Couple and individual adjustment for 2 years following a randomized clinical trial comparing traditional versus integrative behavioral couple therapy. *Journal of Consulting and Clinical Psychology* 2006;74(6): 1180–91.
56. Nagy E, Moore S. Social interventions: An effective approach to reduce adult depression? *Journal of Affective Disorders* 2017;218:131–52.
57. Clark DM. Realizing the mass public benefit of evidence-based psychological therapies: the IAPT program. *Annual Review of Clinical Psychology* 2018;14:159–83.

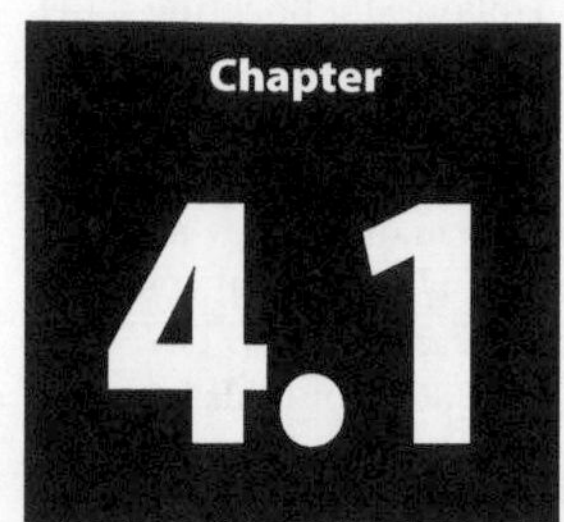

Bipolar Disorder

Diagnosis, Clinical Features, Outcome and Treatment

Jennifer Burgess, Alan Currie, Stuart Watson, Aditya Sharma, David Cousins, John Cookson and R. Hamish McAllister-Williams

- Bipolar disorder is an affective disorder defined on the basis of the presence of periods of elevated mood.
- Patients often present with depression, and previous episodes of elevated mood may be missed if not specifically explored during assessment.
- Bipolar disorder may be difficult to differentiate from other conditions which cause mood instability and impulsivity.
- It is important to identify comorbidities such as substance use, neurodiversity and physical illnesses.
- The first-line treatment for mania is antipsychotic medication. First-line pharmacological treatments for bipolar depression include quetiapine, lurasidone, olanzapine (with or without fluoxetine) and lamotrigine.
- Antidepressants are reported to have little to no efficacy in treating bipolar depression on average.
- Lithium is not the only long-term prophylactic agent, but it remains the gold standard with good evidence that it reduces mood episodes and adverse outcomes. Monitoring is required to ensure lithium level is optimised and potential side effects minimised.

History

The writers of ancient Greece used the terms 'mania' and 'melancholia'. For accounts of the origin of the words 'mania' and 'melancholia' and quotations of the original Greek descriptions, the best source is Angst and Marneros.[1] Hippocrates (fifth to fourth century BCE) argued that such disorders were due to physical (humoral) imbalance and not to supernatural forces. Aretaeus of Cappadocia (second century CE) was probably the first to see mania and depression as manifestations of the same disorder. Jean-Pierre Falret, who described folie circulaire, and Jules Baillarger, who described folie à double forme in 1854, recognised that mania and depression could occur in the same episode of illness – the modern concept of a 'cycle'. Karl Ludwig Kahlbaum described cyclothymia in 1874, as well as the association between states of excitement, some resembling mania and catatonia. Starting in 1893, Emil Kraepelin – basing his views upon both the pattern of symptoms and the longitudinal course – developed the concept of 'manisch–depressives Irresein' (manic-depressive insanity) in successive editions of his textbook. He unified various forms of depression and mania under this name in 1899 and later distinguished these from dementia praecox. Eugen Bleuler in 1920 used the term 'affective illness' to describe the condition. Kraepelin's concept of manic-depressive illness was too broad and, in 1957, Karl Leonhard proposed the distinction between bipolar depressed patients (those with a history of mania or hypomania) and unipolar depressed patients. Later, those patients with recurrent depression who have hypomanic episodes (not requiring hospitalisation) – especially on recovery from depression – were described as bipolar-II (bipolar), and those with a history of mania were described as bipolar-I.[2]

A landmark in the bipolar literature was the publication of a comprehensive monograph textbook *Manic Depressive Illness*.[3] Goodwin and Jamison emphasised the importance of cyclicity in recognising affective disorders. Jamison described the link between bipolar disorder and creativity in writers and other successful individuals in research articles and autobiographical accounts, which have helped to reduce the stigma of the condition.[4] The first parallel-group placebo-controlled randomised trial in mania with lithium and valproate was conducted by Bowden and colleagues,[5] paving the way for others to design informative studies of new antipsychotics and anticonvulsants in bipolar disorder. The revised APA guidelines of 2002 and 2005 confirmed the change in official advice to recommend antipsychotics as a first-line treatment for mania, rather than the earlier North American view that their use should be confined to managing severe agitation or psychotic symptoms while lithium and valproate were termed 'mood stabilisers' and recommended as first-line treatments.[6] Bipolar disorder has attracted the interest of numerous gifted clinicians, and their views are more easily found as chapters in textbooks.[7-9] The contributions by Hagop Akiskal (temperaments and the bipolar spectrum) and Athanasios Kukopoulos (the primacy of mania) are of particular note.

Diagnosis

'Bipolar disorder' encompasses a range of presentations and diagnoses. The 5th edition of the *Diagnostic and Statistical Manual* (DSM-5)[10] describes the bipolar and related disorders as bipolar I disorder, bipolar II disorder, cyclothymic disorder, substance/medication-induced bipolar and related disorders, bipolar and related disorders due to another medical condition, other specified bipolar and related disorders, and unspecified bipolar and related disorders. The key distinctions between each are summarised in Table 4.1.1.

Table 4.1.1 Types of bipolar spectrum disorder

Disorder	Distinguishing characteristics
Bipolar I disorder	At least one manic episode (full syndrome) Likely also to have had a depressive episode (full syndrome) Need not have experienced psychotic symptoms
Bipolar II disorder	At least one depressive episode (full syndrome) At least one hypomanic episode
Cyclothymic disorder	At least two years of hypomanic and depressive episodes Episodes do not meet criteria for mania, hypomania or depression
Substance/medication-induced bipolar and related disorder	History, examination or laboratory findings indicate symptoms related to exposure to, intoxication by or withdrawal from a substance or medication capable of producing mood disturbance Mood disturbance is not better explained by another bipolar or related disorder or delirium
Bipolar and related disorder due to another medical condition	History, examination or laboratory findings indicate that mood disturbance is a direct physiological consequence of another medical condition Mood disturbance is not better explained by another bipolar or related disorder or delirium
Other specified bipolar and related disorder	Symptoms do not meet full criteria for another bipolar or related disorder. Specific reasons include: - short duration hypomania - hypomania with subsynromal depressive episodes - hypomania without depressive episodes - short duration cyclothymia
Unspecified bipolar and related disorder	Symptoms do not meet full criteria for another bipolar or related disorder and the reason is not specified or cannot be specified

Bipolar I Disorder

In this disorder, in DSM-5, a manic episode must have been present. Hypomanic episodes may also be seen. Major depressive episodes are likely but not essential for the diagnosis. Neither is it necessary to have experienced psychotic symptoms to attract a diagnosis of bipolar I disorder. The disorder is sub-classified in three principal ways.

1. Whether the most recent episode was of mania, hypomania or major depression or mixed
2. By severity and whether the most recent episode was mild, moderate or severe. The presence or absence of psychotic symptoms is also specified. When present, psychotic symptoms are usually a reflection of severity and seldom if ever seen in mild or moderate episodes
3. Whether the patient is in full remission, partial remission or not in remission

Manic Episode

In DSM-5, the four principal features of a manic episode are:

1. Elevated mood with increased activity or energy
2. Associated symptoms such as grandiosity, reduced sleep, distractibility and over-talkativeness
3. Impaired functioning
4. The episode is not a consequence of substance abuse, medication or another medical condition

These features need to be present most of the time on most days for at least one week to constitute a manic episode.

Criterion 1. Elevated Mood with Increased Activity or Energy

The changes in mood might be towards elevated or irritable mood. The abnormality of mood is quite distinct from that usually experienced by the patient and is persistent. To meet this criterion, there should also be a persistent increase in activity or energy.

Criterion 2. Associated Symptoms

At least three of the associated symptoms need to be present to fulfil the second criterion. If the abnormality of mood is only one of irritability, then four or more associated symptoms need to be present. Seven symptoms are described:

- Grandiosity and increased self-esteem
- Diminished need for sleep. The emphasis here is on the reduced need. The individual may not experience tiredness and wake refreshed and energetic after only a few hours of sleep
- More talkative with pressure to keep talking
- The subjective experience of racing thoughts, which may be evident to others as flight of ideas
- Easily distracted by unimportant or irrelevant external stimuli
- Increased activity, which may be goal directed towards usual activities or purposeless as in psychomotor agitation
- Involvement in activities that may have harmful consequences, such as spending sprees or sexual indiscretions

Criterion 3. Impairment of Functioning

The severity of mood disturbance and associated symptoms lead to marked impairment in social or occupational functioning. This criterion is also met if hospitalisation is necessary to prevent harm or if psychotic symptoms are present.

Criterion 4. Not a Consequence of Substance Abuse, Medication or Another Medical Condition

If the episode is attributable to the physiological effects of a substance or is the consequences of another medical condition, then the episode should be classified separately as 'substance/medication induced' or 'due to another medical condition'.

Hypomanic Episode

The features of a hypomanic episode are very similar to a manic episode except that the episode is not severe enough to cause marked impairment in functioning, psychotic features are absent, and symptoms need to only be present for four days.

Criterion 1. Elevated Mood with Increased Activity or Energy

The changes in mood might be towards an elevated or irritable mood and are as described for a manic episode.

Criterion 2. Associated Symptoms

At least three need to be present (or four, if the abnormality of mood is only one of irritability). The seven symptoms or features are as described for a manic episode.

Criterion 3. Change in Functioning

There is an unequivocal change in the usual and characteristic functioning.

Criterion 4. Observable to Others

Changes in mood and functioning are observable to others.

Criterion 5. Impairment of Functioning

The impairment in social or occupational functioning is unequivocal and observable but not sufficient to cause marked impairment in functioning or necessitate hospitalisation. In addition, psychotic features are absent.

Criterion 6. Not a Consequence of Substance Abuse, Medication or Another Medical Condition

As with a manic episode, if the changes are attributable to the physiological effects of a substance or the consequences of another medical condition, then the episode should be classified separately as 'substance/medication-induced' or 'due to another medical condition'.

Antidepressant Drug Treatment and Manic/Hypomanic Episodes

If an episode emerges during antidepressant treatment with either medication or electroconvulsive therapy (ECT), then an episode is only diagnosed if symptoms persist beyond the expected physiological effect of that treatment. If only one or two symptoms are present (for example, agitation or irritability), this does not necessarily indicate a bipolar diagnosis. If hypomanic symptoms are only ever seen as a consequence of antidepressant prescription, then some classify this as bipolar III disorder.[11]

Major Depressive Episode

DSM-5 describes nine symptoms or groups of symptoms that constitute a major depressive episode. These are listed below. Note that in addition to these symptoms:

- Symptoms should be present for at least two weeks
- At least one of the first two symptoms of depressed mood or loss of interest or pleasure must be present
- At least five of the nine symptoms must be present
- The symptoms should not be attributable to another medical condition
- There is clinically significant distress or impairment in functioning (social occupational or any other important area)
- The episode is not attributable to another medical condition or to the physiological effects of a substance

The nine symptoms described are

1. Depressed mood, which is either subjective or observed by others. This could include describing sadness, emptiness or hopelessness or appearing tearful. The change in mood should be present most of the day and nearly every day.
2. A marked reduction in interest or pleasure from almost all activities. This change is noticeable most of the day and nearly every day.
3. Weight change of 5 per cent or more of body weight or a change in appetite. This might be weight loss (when not dieting) or weight gain or a sustained increase or decrease in appetite.
4. Reduced or increased sleep with insomnia or hypersomnia present nearly every day.
5. Psychomotor changes. This might be subjective or observed by others. The changes might include retardation and the feeling of being slowed down or, alternatively, agitation.
6. Loss of energy or feelings of fatigue on nearly every day.
7. Feeling worthless or with thoughts of excessive or inappropriate guilt. This does not include mere self-reproach about being sick. Thoughts might reach delusional intensity.
8. Reduced concentration, indecision and a diminished ability to think clearly. This can be subjectively reported or observed by others.
9. Recurrent thoughts of death or suicidal ideation or a suicide attempt or a specific plan for suicide.

Mixed States

Mixed states may occur when features of mania/hypomania and depression are seen during the same episode. This can occur with depressive symptoms seen during a predominantly manic/hypomanic episode and conversely with manic/hypomanic features during a predominantly depressive episode.

A manic or hypomanic episode with mixed features is characterised by a full manic or hypomanic syndrome and at least three depressive features present on most days during the episode. The depressive features can include:

- Prominent depressed mood or dysphoria
- Anhedonia

- Psychomotor retardation
- Anergia/fatigue
- Thoughts of worthlessness or feelings of excessive guilt
- Recurrent thoughts of death or suicide

A depressive episode with mixed features is characterised by a full depressive syndrome and at least three manic or hypomanic features present on most days during the episode. These features can include:

- Elevated mood
- Grandiosity or heightened self-esteem
- Over-talkativeness or with pressured speech
- Flight of ideas or racing thoughts
- Increased energy and activity
- Excess activities that may be harmful, such as spending large amounts of money or sexual disinhibition
- Reduced need for sleep

Rapid Cycling

Patients may also cycle rapidly from episode to episode. Rapid cycling is defined as four episodes of either mania or hypomania or depression within 12 months. There should be at least partial remission for a minimum of two months between episodes of the same polarity although episodes can occur in any order or combination. Rapid cycling is primarily an index of poor prognosis and does not appear to represent a distinct sub-population of patients with bipolar disorder. Patient's presentation can move into, and out of, the definition of rapid cycling over time.

Bipolar II Disorder

This is defined by the presence of at least one episode of hypomania but an absence of any history of manic episodes. Depressive episodes tend to predominate, but mixed episodes are also common. There is relatively little transition to bipolar I disorder over time, and there is some evidence of differences in genetics between bipolar I and II.[12]

Diagnostic Issues: DSM versus ICD

ICD-11 is almost identical to DSM-5 in its description of the mood episodes characteristic of bipolar I and II.[13] There are some minor differences. ICD-11 does not require a greater number of associated symptoms if only an irritable (rather than an elevated and irritable) mood state is present. The number of consecutive days of symptoms to diagnose a hypomanic episode is not specified and simply stated as 'several' as compared with the four-day minimum specified in DSM-5. There is also less emphasis on functional impairment, which in ICD-11 requires only that a change in mood is observable to those who know the patient well rather than unequivocal impairment of functioning.

Neither ICD-11 nor DSM-5 has unipolar mania as a distinct disorder. Unipolar mania has been proposed to differ from bipolar mania in several respects.[14,15] There is a weaker family history of depression and earlier onset of illness. There are fewer comorbidities with anxiety disorders, substance use disorders and bulimia/binge-eating disorder. Finally, the illness course has better remissions and fewer recurrencies but more psychotic symptoms.

Clinical Features

History

Assessment in bipolar disorder requires not just a careful evaluation of the current mental state but a detailed history of the course of the illness. A corroborative history from a close friend or family member can be invaluable in clarifying the illness course and the nature and frequency of episodes.

Mental State Examination in Bipolar Depression

The abnormalities in the mental state of a patient with bipolar depression are very similar to those seen in unipolar depression, though subtle differences may exist. However, bipolar depression is associated with a family history of bipolar disorder, an earlier age at onset and a greater previous number of depressive episodes.

Mental State Examination in Mania and Hypomania

The mental state examination is a structured tool in psychiatric practice. However, a major difficulty in the examination of a patient who may be in a hypomanic or manic state is that the features are unlikely to present in an orderly manner. Nonetheless, a systematic process is necessary, and the interviewer must keep their eyes and ears open to ensure that all the features are noted. There may need to be much organising and re-organising of information when the examination is complete to ensure that these features are presented in a structured and coherent manner.

As with any other disorder, a detailed account of the mental state is required. A diagnosis is not made on one feature alone, no matter how garishly dressed, garrulous or overfamiliar is the subject.

Appearance

This might be relatively unremarkable, which of course does not exclude the diagnosis. The patient's choice of clothing may vary with mood state, or they may be inattentive to aspects of personal hygiene. In severe cases, there may be physical health concerns, and the subject might look exhausted (whilst denying this) or have physical signs such as peripheral oedema. Be alert also for factors that may complicate the presentation such as alcohol or stimulants. Signs of stimulant use include increased arousal, dilated pupils and possibly tics.

Behaviour

Avoid stigmatising language such as 'attention seeking'. Be specific, and if the patient is, for example, overfamiliar or hostile, then say so and try to give examples. Aim to describe what can be seen in a manner that would allow a non-observer to easily conjure an image of the patient. The patient's level of arousal may be increased, and they may be unusually vigilant or distractible. Motor activity may be increased, with restlessness clearly evident. Eye contact may reflect distractibility and may not be sustained in the usual manner. Facial expressions may reflect the underlying mood state with excessive smiling, laughing or giggling. The patient may be disinhibited in social interactions with a degree of disregard for the usual conventions. Using the interviewers first name is not necessarily unusual but can be a little unconventional. Note that the interviewer is trying to build an overall picture, and one specific detail is insufficient to make a diagnosis. The patient may experience an increased sex drive or find that they are engaging in more sexual activity than is usual for them.

Mood

Mood should be rated both subjectively and objectively. Subjective ratings of mood may report feelings such as being full of energy and excitement or 'on top of the world'. This is usually described as a welcome and pleasant experience, but some patients report it as unpleasant or even dysphoric. An objective assessment of mood is largely based on appearance, behaviour and, to a lesser extent, other aspects of the mental state. The patient may appear elated or irritable. Lability may be evident with fleeting mood swings towards low mood or even tearfulness. Irritability can emerge as a feature of frustration when others do not share the patient's ideas and plans.

Speech

The rate of speech production is typically increased. There may be pressure of speech, and the patient may be hard to interrupt or seeking out others to listen to their ideas. Greater degrees of pressured speech merge into flight of ideas. When this is present, there are still connections between each element of the conversation, but they can be hard to follow, and the connections may be weak (e.g. rhymes or puns) or even lost in the rapidity of speech. This is to be distinguished from the thought-disordered speech of schizophrenia where there are no connections and conversation jumps from one topic to another unconnected topic (e.g. knight's move thinking). Recording verbatim examples of speech to illustrate these features is difficult but invaluable.

Thinking

Abnormalities of thinking can be present in both form and content. The rate or flow (form) of thoughts is often increased, and for some, this can be unpleasant. The content of the patient's thoughts will likely reflect their elevated mood state (mood congruence). They may report ambitious plans or schemes, and self-esteem can be elevated with an exaggerated estimation of abilities and status. Ideas may reach the intensity of delusions, but mood congruence is usually still evident. A patient may become convinced that they have been chosen for a special mission, have special powers or abilities, or a special relationship with those in high positions. It can sometimes be hard to establish mood congruence. If delusions are clearly incongruent and especially if psychotic symptoms were present before mood elevation or are protracted, then a diagnosis of schizoaffective disorder should be considered.

Perceptions

When psychotic symptoms such as hallucinations are present, they are usually a marker of illness severity. They are a feature of more severe manic states and are not seen in hypomanic states. Mood congruence is the norm as with other psychotic symptoms such as delusions. The patient may describe hearing a voice telling them that they have special powers or that they have been chosen for a special mission. This could be perceived as the voice of God or a person of high status.

Cognitive Abilities

If cognitive abilities are disturbed during a manic or hypomanic episode, this is most usually seen as deficits in sustaining attention. The patient may be easily distracted by external noise or other minor intrusions. This can extend to increased vigilance and even suspiciousness. The patient usually retains full orientation to time, place and person.

Around 40 per cent of people with bipolar disorder have some associated cognitive impairment,[16] and there may be problems with executive function and memory even when mood symptoms are relatively absent.[17] Deficits are more pronounced in bipolar I disorder and in those with psychotic symptoms[18] but are generally not as problematic as in schizophrenia.[19]

Insight

Insight is usually significantly impaired in manic states. It is common for patients not to recognise that they are ill or that their behaviour is unusual. However, they may recognise it as a change from their previous functioning – acknowledging their increased energy, reduced need for sleep and the novelty of their plans. Regaining insight during recovery can be a source of significant embarrassment for patients.

Self-Reports

The subject of the experience of mania is often difficult to express. Several public figures have been open about their diagnosis and experience of bipolar disorder, and their descriptions can be illuminating. Musician and singer Adam Ant (Stuart Goddard) describes some of the features of a manic episode:[20]

> The night after that, though, I stayed up all night working. I had more ideas for songs or scripts that night than I had had in six months. I started making lists of notes at half past midnight, and the ideas wouldn't leave me alone, so I went to the study in our house and jotted them down. It was like being hit by lightning with ideas racing across the page as

> if from nowhere. I created visuals for the album cover, wrote four letters, two of them for Heather. I telephoned Marco, Boz and EMI and then the sun came up and I was still rolling along.

Athlete Suzy Favor Hamilton has also written and published her experiences of bipolar disorder.[21] She has described the history of bipolar disorder in her family, the stigma attached to this and her own experiences of depression. She gives a graphic account of a manic episode in association with being prescribed antidepressant medication, which includes her report of uncharacteristic sexual behaviour.

> My doctor put me on another antidepressant. The effects were immediate. I felt great. I felt beyond great. I felt alive. I wanted to live. Time for my fantasies to now become a reality. Our 20th wedding anniversary was coming up. A nice dinner date out on the town with flowers perhaps? Not for me. I wanted to go to Vegas, jump out of a plane, hire an escort, have a threesome. Bucket list stuff I never thought I would actually do. Never. I wanted it now.

Differential Diagnosis

Other Medical Conditions and Medication-Induced Bipolar Disorder

These conditions are usually more of a consideration in older populations where the medical conditions associated with mood disturbance are more common. Examples of these conditions include thyroid disease, multiple sclerosis and cortical or subcortical brain lesions. A careful history and examination are essential, and further investigations including scanning studies may be required. Be especially wary of a late presentation of hypomania or mania whilst noting that a careful history (with corroboration) may occasionally identify earlier and subclinical episodes. A full medication history is also essential, with an awareness of which medications are especially associated with mood changes (e.g. corticosteroids and thyroid replacement therapy).

Substance Use Disorders

The use of substances may be acknowledged during a sensitive inquiry, and corroborative reports from family and friends may be helpful. Substance use disorders may be associated with relatively short-lived episodes of mood disturbance, which are often subsyndromal for either depression or hypomania. Episodes may self limit within a few days, and there is frequently a close temporal relationship between substance use and mood disturbance. The physical examination may also be revealing – for example, of the increased arousal, dilated pupils and motor tics that can be seen with stimulant use. The use of anabolic androgenic steroid (AAS) drugs by bodybuilders and athletes is an interesting example of how substance use can mimic the episodic mood disturbance of bipolar disorder. Hypomanic symptoms can emerge with AAS use and especially with high doses or multiple drugs. Depressive symptoms are associated with more chronic use and during withdrawal. Thus both 'poles' may be seen. Substance use disorders are also found comorbid with bipolar disorder, and a positive drug screen or history of use does not exclude a diagnosis of bipolar disorder.

Personality Disorder

Differentiating bipolar disorder, primarily bipolar II, from borderline personality disorder can be challenging. Impulsive acts without full consideration of the possible consequences can be a feature of borderline personality disorder, and marked changes in mood are also a feature of this condition. The mood changes of borderline personality disorder can be towards anger or irritability and are usually triggered very abruptly by an interpersonal cue. These changes tend to be less sustained than in bipolar disorder and can disappear just as quickly as they emerge. DSM-5 specifies that the intense emotions of borderline and other personality disorders should typically last only a few hours at most. Other features of the condition will also be apparent such as efforts to avoid real or imagined abandonment, an unstable self-image and chronic feelings of emptiness.

Other distinctions have been suggested.[22] Although there is an age co-incidence in presentation, borderline personality disorder evolves over time with some emotional dysregulation present in childhood and adolescence whilst bipolar II has an onset episode and discontinuity in presentation, from absence of symptoms to their clear presence. The nature of mood episodes may also be different. In borderline personality disorder, the dysregulated mood typically has salient anger and irritability, and the mood state is unpleasant, even painful. In contrast, whilst anger and irritability can be prominent in the elevated mood state of bipolar II disorder, the shift is usually to a more care-free state where anxiety and worry disappear and where euphoria, grandiosity and creativity are accompanied by feelings of invincibility.

It is important to note that the diagnoses of bipolar disorder and borderline personality disorder are not mutually exclusive.

Attention-Deficit/Hyperactivity Disorder (ADHD)

In ADHD, there may be features similar to mania or hypomania such as increased energy, distractibility and over-talkativeness with a tendency to interrupt others. However, the primary disturbances are in behaviour and attention. In bipolar disorder, the primary disturbances are in mood, and the other features of the disorder are congruent with this mood disturbance. In ADHD, there are persistent symptoms, which are evident from childhood, whilst in bipolar disorder, the illness usually runs an episodic course with an onset in early adulthood.

Unipolar Depression

The hallmark distinction between unipolar and bipolar depression is the course of the illness and the presence of at least one hypomanic or manic episode in the latter. The onset of illness is typically earlier in bipolar disorder and with more rapid recurrence of episodes. During a depressive episode, the symptoms and presentation show a great deal of overlap, although anxiety and agitation may be more common in episodes of unipolar depression.[23]

Bipolar Disorder in Young People and Neurodiverse Populations

The diagnostic criteria for bipolar disorder in young people are the same as that for adults.[10] There is an established consensus that when considering a diagnosis of (hypo)mania, caution must be exercised when using irritability on its own, especially in prepubertal children.[24] Assessing for discrete episodes (meeting the duration criteria) as outlined in diagnostic criteria over a prospective longitudinal period helps clinch the diagnosis. The course of bipolar disorder is frequently characterised by onset of short-lived but frequent depressive episodes before the onset of the first (hypo)manic episode. These depressive episodes continue to be the most frequent form of relapse but get longer in duration if not treated. Risk of suicide is particularly high in young people.

Neurodiversity

Bipolar disorder in a neurodiverse population, such as those with autism spectrum disorder, has only recently started to receive the focus it deserves. Most screening tools, psychiatric interviews and rating scales for bipolar disorder are not validated for use in a neurodiverse population. Biological features such as sleep, appetite, self care and activity may offer more utility in making a diagnosis than self-reported affect. Furthermore, neurodiverse populations are also more prone to side effects of medication. Any psychological interventions may also require adaptations to make them developmentally appropriate to the neurodiverse individual.

Measurement of Mania

The most commonly used observer rating scale for mania is the Young Mania Rating Scale.[25] This has 11 items, each with five-point sub-scales and defined anchor points. Completion of the scale requires a 15-to-30-minute interview. This instrument is convenient for following the progress of mania in an individual patient during treatment. The Altman Self-Rating Mania Scale[26] is a commonly used questionnaire that asks patients to rate how frequently they are experiencing five symptoms of hypomania or mania. This self-rated scale correlates well with observer rating scales, even in patients with psychosis or impaired insight. The measurement of depression is discussed elsewhere; its use in patients with bipolar depression extrapolated from unipolar depression.

Natural History

It is important to note that the natural history of bipolar disorder is extremely variable between patients. If a patient's presentation is very different from the mean or median, this is not a good indicator that the diagnosis may be in error.

Prevalence

The prevalence of bipolar disorder depends on its definition and what screening tools are used. Worldwide estimates range from 1–5%, and the Adult Psychiatric Morbidity Survey found that 2% of the English adult general population surveyed screened positive for a lifetime bipolar spectrum disorder.[27]

Age of Onset

The peak age of first hospitalisation for mania is in the late teens, the median in the mid-20s and the mean age of first hospitalisation about 26. There have often been earlier affective episodes sufficient to cause some impairment or for the patient to receive treatment outside hospital. There is a greater prevalence of affective illness among the first-degree relatives of those whose first episode of mania occurs by the age of 20 than among the relatives of patients whose mania begins later. There is a slight secondary peak of onset in women aged 45–50 years, and first episodes of mania continue to be seen in late life. An onset over the age of 60 is more likely to be associated with organic brain disease.

Number of Episodes

The great majority of patients have more than one episode of mania, confirming the view that bipolar disorder is a recurrent illness. The disorder follows a relapsing, often-chronic course, with, in some studies, an average of approximately eight episodes over the 10 years following diagnosis.

Duration of Episodes

The duration of manic episodes in the pre-treatment era was usually 3–12 months, with a mean of 6 months. Treatment shortens this duration. Remission from mania occurred in 50% of manic episodes by 12 weeks in one series.[28] After the first episode of mania, 93% had recovered within two years in terms of the syndrome of mania, but only 35% had recovered in terms of personal and occupational functioning.[29]

Frequency of Episodes

The interval from one episode to the next tends to decrease during the first five episodes.[30] For instance, in Kraepelin's series, the average time between the first and second episode was five years, but this had fallen to two years between the fifth and sixth episode. A series of patients with first-episode mania with two-year follow-up found that major depression had occurred previously in 24%, and further depression followed immediately after mania ('post-manic depression') in 16%.

There was a recurrence of mania or depression within 2 years in 36%, but 40% had no recurrence within five years.[31]

In an individual, there is great variability in the length between episodes and a tendency for episodes to be clustered at particular times in the patient's life – for instance, when he or she has difficulties coping with children or when relationships are ending. Antidepressant treatments may increase the tendency to switch from depression to mania and may have altered the natural course of the illness towards more frequent episodes.

Outcome

Mortality rates are significantly higher in patients with bipolar disorder, with relative risks of around 2.5 compared to the general population, a figure similar to that seen for schizophrenia.[32] Patients with bipolar disorder are at particular risk of death by suicide (3–6%), and up to half of the patients in secondary care will attempt suicide or self harm.[33] However, this is not the main driver for the overall increased mortality seen, which is due to an increase across all causes of death. The reasons for the increased physical health mortality are likely to be multifactorial.

Some patients become socially and economically disadvantaged, but a systematic review of studies found that 40–60% of patients with bipolar disorder are in employment.[34] Many patients do not have significant problems functioning at work; however, some studies found that approximately 50% of patients reduce their hours or change job role. Symptoms of depression and irritability are associated with poorer quality of life and functioning (as reported by patients), as were being female and having comorbid psychiatric diagnoses (except substance misuse). Manic symptoms were not associated with quality of life or functioning.[35]

Patients and their spouses report that bipolar disorder significantly affects their relationship and family, and there is a higher divorce rate than the general population. Both partners feel the emotional impact of the symptoms – especially their unpredictable nature – and worry about relapses, hospitalisation and compliance with treatment. Couples also report wanting to have more children but not doing so because of bipolar disorder.[36]

There is a commonly held view that bipolar disorder and artistic genius are related. Much of this discussion has centred on the lives and possible symptoms of eminent individuals, but there have also been attempts to study this empirically. A systematic review and meta-analysis found an association between patients with bipolar disorder and the patient's self-report of creative accomplishments and behaviour (but not creative cognition, self-concept or production). However, it should be noted that publication bias may affect these results.[37] Possible explanations for this link are that both creative individuals and people with bipolar disorder score more highly on the personality trait 'openness to experience' and sensitivity of the behavioural activation system. This association with creativity has been found in patients who are euthymic and in those who are taking medication.[38]

Aetiology

The prevalence of bipolar disorder does not appear to notably differ across gender and ethnicity.[39] High socioeconomic status has been associated with a higher risk of bipolar disorder,[40] but this is most likely accounted for by diagnostic bias. However, socioeconomic disadvantage – as demonstrated by low income, unemployment and being unmarried – particularly for bipolar disorder with psychosis, as well as living in an urban environment is associated with an increased risk of bipolar disorder.[41]

Family History and Genetics

Bipolar disorder runs in families, with a 5–10% risk of bipolar disorder among first-degree relatives, which is around sevenfold higher than in the general population.[42] Some clinical features also demonstrate familiarity, including age[43] and polarity[44] at onset, presence of psychosis,[45] cycle rate,[46] attempted suicide[47] and lithium responsivity.[48] Twin and adoption studies show that much of the shared familial risk can be explained by shared genes; heritability has been estimated to be between 70 and 90%. Multifactorial inheritance, heterogenous phenotype, absence of biological diagnostic markers and the presence of assortative mating hinders genetic elucidation. This complexity impairs the ability of genetic-linkage analysis to identify risk loci, and the lack of understanding of the pathophysiology of bipolar disorder has limited the value of candidate-gene approaches, with the best signals for the serotonin transporter, SLC6A4, d-amino acid oxidase and brain-derived neurotrophic factor.[49] Copy number variants (the duplication of DNA on a chromosome) is associated with neurodevelopmental disorder and schizophrenia but not so convincingly with bipolar disorder.[50] Genome-wide association studies hold more promise. Large samples comparing the rates of genetic variants in those with a clinical diagnosis of bipolar disorder have revealed susceptible loci, which can suggest potential biological mechanisms for bipolar disorder. However, the challenge remains to use pathway analysis and transcriptome imputation to move from the identification of loci to the elucidation of individual risk genes and pathways.[51] Together, the genetic data suggest that genetic risk factors – most likely multiple single nucleotide polymorphisms that are common in the general population – transcend diagnostic categories, and each exert a small increased risk of developing bipolar, schizophrenia, major depressive disorder and autism, and interaction with environmental risk factors may be relevant.

Neurodevelopmental and Psychosocial Factors

Cross-sectional studies support a link with previous – including prenatal – infection by Toxoplasma gondii,[52] with a pro-dopaminergic mechanism having been suggested. A role for other pre- or perinatal factors has been examined; first-trimester exposure to influenza has inconsistently been shown to be a vulnerability factor, and there is some evidence for extreme prematurity and large head size,[53] but the impact of obstetric complications is not as well supported as for schizophrenia. Childhood adversity, particularly emotional neglect,[54] is found at increased rates in people with bipolar disorder and appears to confer a worse prognosis.[55] Putative biological mechanisms are being examined, and it seems relevant that many of the biological abnormalities noted in bipolar patients are associated also with childhood trauma, such as dysregulation of the hypothalamic-pituitary-adrenal (HPA) axis,[56] increased levels of inflammatory cytokines[57] and reduced prefrontal-paralimbic system grey matter volume.[58] More recent stressful life events can also precipitate first and subsequent[41] episodes of bipolar disorder.

Comorbidity

Comorbid disordered substance use is relatively common in bipolar disorder,[59] but it can be difficult at a population and individual level to disentangle the extent to which this is cause, consequence, co-incidence, epiphenomenon or misdiagnosis. However, the evidence that cannabis use increases the risk of first, and subsequent, manic episode is robust.[60] Opiates, alcohol and stimulants such as cocaine are also implicated but less well studied.

Over a third of people with bipolar disorder, even when not in a fully syndromal bipolar episode, have a comorbid anxiety disorder.[61] Anxiety symptoms and anxiety disorders are associated with a higher likelihood of rapid switching, of suicidal behaviour, shorter periods of recovery, worse treatment response and a greater long-term depressive morbidity.[62] There is preliminary evidence for beneficial effects of targeting anxiety symptoms in bipolar patients who are not in an episode using modified CBT and pharmacotherapy.[63] Also, the awareness that anxiety symptoms precede and co-exist with bipolar disorder suggests the value of asking about manic symptoms in people with anxiety disorders.

Physical Illnesses

Increased rates of physical illness have been found in patients with bipolar disorder, including asthma, type 2 diabetes mellitus, hypercholesterolaemia, epilepsy, hypertension and renal and thyroid disease.[64] This did not appear to differ between people with bipolar I or II, but other features that increased the risk of medical illness were rapid-cycling pattern, acute onset of mood episodes, a history of anxiety disorder or suicide attempts. Sleep disorders – including insomnia, sleep apnoea and circadian rhythm disturbance – are seen at increased rates in people with bipolar disorder.[65] A recent study suggested that the cognitive impairment that is a feature of bipolar disorder may be confined to those with disturbed sleep.[66] Targeting insomnia using modified cognitive behaviour therapy improves sleep and reduces risk of relapse into an episode,[67] though it is not known it this improves cognition.

Drug Treatment

Treatment Guidelines

Numerous guidelines exist for the management of bipolar disorder (NICE,[68] BAP,[33] APA[69, 70] and SOBP[71]), perhaps reflecting the uncertainty that has prevailed about the efficacy and side effects of treatments.

A physical examination and blood and urine tests should, whenever possible, precede drug treatment in order to elucidate any intercurrent physical illness, especially to determine baseline renal, hepatic and thyroid function. An electrocardiogram (ECG) should be done if instructed by the drug's summary of product characteristics, the patient has cardiovascular risk factors, there is a family history of cardiovascular risk factors (including sudden collapse) or disease, or the person is an inpatient.[68]

Treatment of Manic Episodes

Guidelines generally recommend that severe mania is treated with an antipsychotic, with or without lithium or valproate. Some guidelines include starting with high doses of valproate alone. Less severe mania should usually be treated initially with monotherapy, with either an antipsychotic – preferably a second-generation drug – or valproate or lithium; carbamazepine is an alternative.[33,68]

The original investigations conducted by John Cade in Australia into the use of lithium were for acute mania,[72] with this efficacy confirmed in later placebo-controlled trials.[5] It is often argued that for lithium to be effective acutely, plasma levels of 0.8–1.0 mmol/l should be used. However, given that levels above 1.0 mmol/l are associated with an increased risk of renal damage[73] – which old data suggested for more activated and agitated patients – chlorpromazine is superior to lithium.[74] Generally, antipsychotics are preferred as first-line treatments of mania. Lithium tends to require two weeks or more to approach a full effect. Used alone, it is more useful in mild than in severe cases. Patients who respond tend to have classical mania rather than mixed episodes (including dysphoric mania), as well as non-rapid-cycling disorder. There is no data to confirm whether a family history of bipolar disorder predicts an anti-manic response as it does for prophylaxis. Patients who have benefited previously from lithium are more likely to do so again. If the patient has an episode whilst already taking lithium, treatment should be optimised, and an increase to achieve levels of 0.8–1 mmol/L can be considered as a short-term solution.

Similarly, there is data supporting the use of valproate for acute mania,[5] where it is used at high doses (20–30 mg/kg). However, given that valproate should be avoided in women (and potentially men) of childbearing potential, antipsychotics again tend to be preferred. Note that there is either a lack of data, or even negative data, for the use of other anticonvulsants (e.g. gabapentin, lamotrigine and topiramate) for the treatment of acute mania, with the exception of some lower-quality data for carbamazepine and oxcarbazepine. The former tends to not be recommended due to the dose needed to be anti-manic – potentially causing neurotoxicity – and because of problematic drug-drug interactions. However, oxcarbazepine does have placebo-controlled trial data supporting its use,[75] and it is less prone to interacting with other medications.

Mania is usually most rapidly controlled by antipsychotic drugs.[76, 77] Phenothiazines (e.g. chlorpromazine) and thioxanthines (e.g. zuclopenthixol) are effective but have generally in practice been replaced by newer second-generation antipsychotics. Those with proven efficacy in mania include olanzapine (15–20 mg/day), risperidone (up to 6 mg/day), quetiapine (at least 600 mg/day), aripiprazole (10–30 mg) and ziprasidone. Rapid improvement in mania usually starts occurring one to three days after antipsychotic medication is begun and then more gradually over the next two weeks or so. If a patient has a manic episode whilst already taking an antipsychotic, raising the dose may be sufficient. If they are already taking an optimised mood stabiliser, then adding an antipsychotic should be considered.

A proportion of patients with mania show only partial improvement or initial improvement followed by partial relapse with antipsychotic drugs. There is little evidence that increasing the dose will produce further improvement. Clozapine may exert effects through an action on a different subtype of DA receptors, and this drug may prove to be useful in resistant mania as in resistant schizophrenia.[78] While a systematic review of five randomised controlled trials of clozapine verses first- or second-generation antipsychotics in non-treatment-resistant mania found no difference,[79] a two-year Danish registry study found that patients with bipolar disorder who used clozapine experienced fewer admissions, bed-days and number of co-medications.[80] However, at present, the main alternatives or adjuncts to the antipsychotic drugs are lithium and the anticonvulsants valproate and carbamazepine.

Lithium and antipsychotics are often safely used together in combination, with the best data being for the combination of lithium together with risperidone, olanzapine, quetiapine and aripiprazole. However, combinations of high levels of lithium with high doses of antipsychotics, particularly conventional first-generation drugs including haloperidol, have been associated with severe neurological symptoms, hyperthermia, impaired consciousness and irreversible brain damage.[81,82] The conditions reported resemble both lithium toxicity and neuroleptic malignant syndrome.

For patients with mania who are not adequately calmed by antipsychotic drugs – or to avoid prescribing such drugs – diazepam (10–20 mg intravenously or 30 mg orally total daily doses) may be used. For intramuscular (IM) use, lorazepam (1–2mg orally or IM) is absorbed faster, causes less local pain and is the first-line treatment in the rapid tranquillisation of acutely disturbed patients. The patient must be monitored post-administration for respiratory depression, which can be reversed using the benzodiazepine antagonist flumazenil.

Patients may also have episodes of acute disturbance, where they are more emotionally distressed or agitated, perhaps aggressive or violent. There is little evidence for the efficacy of oral antipsychotics in this situation, and benzodiazepines are preferred.[83] If a patient declines oral medication, 'rapid tranquillisation' with an intramuscular medication may be required. If IM benzodiazepines are not effective, IM aripiprazole or olanzapine can be used (although olanzapine must be used at least one hour after benzodiazepines due to the risk of hypotension when combined). IM haloperidol is no longer given as monotherapy due to the risk of acute dystonia, which can be reduced in combination with promethazine.[83] It also prolongs the QTc interval and so should be avoided if a recent ECG is not available.

Treatment of Bipolar Depression

Naturalistic data demonstrates that time to response following treatment initiation is much slower for bipolar depression compared with mania.[28] Twenty per cent of patients presenting with bipolar depression do not achieve remission within 12 months.[28] Antidepressants, while commonly used in bipolar depression, have little or no evidence of efficacy.[84–86] There is limited evidence for the effect of lithium on depressive episodes in the context of bipolar disorder, but lithium may be useful if symptoms are less severe and long-term prophylaxis is also the intention. Current UK guidelines provide limited recommendations of evidence-based medication that include just quetiapine, olanzapine (with or without fluoxetine), lurasidone and lamotrigine (NICE and BAP). Recent data also suggests evidence for cariprazine.[87] Note that, in general, it appears that the dose of antipsychotic needed to treat bipolar depression is significantly lower than that needed to treat bipolar mania, with target doses being in the order of 300 mg of quetiapine, 10–15 mg olanzapine and 55.5 mg of lurasidone. Lamotrigine is a challenging drug to use for the acute treatment of bipolar depression. It requires slow dose up titration to reduce risks of serious adverse dermatological complications (e.g. Stevens-Johnson syndrome), and positive effects on mood are slow to occur and often not of great magnitude. However, it can be combined with either lithium[88] or quetiapine[89] with potential benefits. Aside from this, as also seen in unipolar disorder, there is some evidence for intravenous ketamine,[90] and studies with pramipexole are ongoing.[91]

Treatment of Mixed Episodes

In general, there is little in the way of recommendations for the management of mixed episodes in current guidelines.[33,68] This is in part due to a paucity of data. What data there is tends to be from post-hoc analysis of patients with significant depressive symptoms who had been recruited into studies of acute mania. This supports a perspective of treating such mixed episodes as per mania. DSM-5 criteria allow for both manic episodes with mixed features and depressive episodes with mixed features. The latter have rarely been studied. There is data from a randomised placebo-controlled trial showing efficacy of lurasidone in patients with unipolar depression and mixed features.[92] This supports the pragmatic notion of treating depression with mixed features with medication known to be efficacious for bipolar depression that also have known (quetiapine or olanzapine) or theoretical (lurasidone) anti-manic effects.

Prophylaxis of Mood Episodes

In terms of long-term prophylaxis, to date only five drugs have been shown to be effective in monotherapy in placebo-controlled trials lasting for one year or more: lithium, quetiapine, olanzapine, aripiprazole and lamotrigine. Valproate in monotherapy is only supported by equivalence to olanzapine in one study[93] but also showing inferiority to lithium in another.[94]

Lithium remains the gold standard long-term prophylaxis agent, with randomised data supported by a large naturalistic data set showing lower admission rates,[95] efficacy against both mania and depression[96] and reduction in the risk of suicide by 60 per cent versus placebo.[97] A key consideration when using lithium is the risk of rapid recurrence of mania upon sudden discontinuation.[98] Quetiapine also demonstrates efficacy against both depressive and manic relapse,[99] while olanzapine[100] and aripiprazole[101] appear to protect predominantly against manic relapse while lamotrigine appears to protect against depression.[102] In this regard, it appears that there is a close correlation between efficacy against acute episodes and prophylaxis.[103] Note that there is no randomised controlled trial data for carbamazepine as a prophylaxis in bipolar disorder, though naturalistic data suggest it may help prevent manic relapses.[95] Similarly, there is little or no data to support the use of antidepressants long term, and indeed an increase in manic switches is seen if they are used in the absence of a prophylactic agent efficacious against mania.[104]

For patients whose bipolar disorder relapses on monotherapy, there is some data demonstrating efficacy of the combination of olanzapine,[105] aripiprazole[106] and quetiapine[107] in combination with lithium or valproate being more effective than lithium or valproate alone, and more limited data shows a similar effect for lurasidone.[108]

For patients who decline treatment, or have difficulty regularly taking oral medication, long-acting injections (LAI) can be used. Both risperidone[109] and aripiprazole[110] LAI, added into ongoing treatment as usual, have been shown to reduce time to relapse and relapse rates in randomised controlled trials versus treatment as usual.

Prophylaxis in patients with rapid-cycling bipolar disorder is a particular challenge. There are limited studies in such patients, and naturalistic data demonstrates worse outcomes.[28] There is some suggestion that while outcome data with all treatments may be worse than in non-rapid-cycling patients, lithium might be particularly prone to being less effective.[111] As a general rule, antidepressants should be withdrawn, and often combinations of an antipsychotic plus lithium, valproate or lamotrigine are used.[33] Of interest, a small double-blind placebo-controlled trial has shown that levothyroxine (L-T4) decreased duration of ill health in patients with treatment-resistant rapid-cycling bipolar disorder when used as an adjunct to lithium.[112] Triiodothyronine (T3) had an effect in the same direction but did not reach significance versus the placebo. Both drugs were dosed to fully suppress thyroid stimulating hormone (TSH).

Drug Treatment of Bipolar Disorder in Children and Adolescents

Atypical antipsychotics, lithium and valproate (males only) are usually first-line treatment options. Young people are more prone to side effects, including but not limited to extrapyramidal metabolic syndrome as well as cardiac and endocrine side effects, and therefore require careful monitoring. There are very few RCTs studying the efficacy of agents to treat bipolar depression. The use of antidepressants poses considerable risks, including increasing the risk of suicidal ideation or switch. Once euthymic, management should focus on continuing mood stability and could employ the use of manualised family-based psychological interventions.

Using Medication for Bipolar Disorder

Lithium

Lithium is a monovalent cation with a long history of use in psychiatry. There are two salts that are not interchangeable: lithium carbonate and lithium citrate.

Dosage

The dose of lithium is determined by the desired concentration as measured by plasma levels. For most indications, aim for 0.4–1.0 mmol/litre, and there is a narrow therapeutic window. Take the level at 12 hours post-dose to avoid the absorption redistribution sampling. Lithium is usually started at a low dose and titrated to the correct level, but loading doses can be used in mania.

Contraindications

Lithium should not be prescribed to people who have cardiac disease that is associated with pathological rhythms, Brugada syndrome or a family history of Brugada syndrome, cardiac insufficiency, clinically significant renal impairment, uncontrolled hypothyroidism, Addison's disease, dehydration, hyponatraemia or a low-sodium diet.

Some clinicians withhold lithium for 48 hours prior to ECT to reduce the risk of delirium, although recent research found that delirium was less common in patients receiving ECT for bipolar disorder (0–3.4%) than for depression (7.8%).[113] However, they are often used concurrently with a low stimulus as lithium may lower the seizure threshold.

Side Effects

At therapeutic doses, lithium has actions on many bodily systems. These are important, as some require intervention, and they contribute to patients not taking medication as prescribed. The majority of patients on lithium will experience at least one side effect. All should be informed about side effects, signs of toxicity and the risks of abrupt discontinuation.

Gastrointestinal -- Mild gastrointestinal side effects such as nausea or abdominal discomfort are common but often settle after a few weeks of treatment. It is important to note that diarrhoea is a symptom and a risk factor for toxicity.

Kidney -- Lithium can affect the ability of the kidney to concentrate and filter urine.[114] Common side effects are polyuria (excessive urination) and polydipsia (excessive drinking), but it is difficult to estimate how many patients will develop this as the rates reported in the literature range from 20 to 90 per cent. Many patients will notice these effects in the first few months after commencing lithium. However, the risk increases with long-term treatment. It may become irreversible; however, it is less likely to contribute to discontinuation than other side effects. Polyuria is thought to be due to lithium's effect on the tubules, causing a nephrogenic diabetes insipidus that results in polydipsia. Higher serum levels and toxicity have been associated, and once-daily dosing can reduce the risk. If it becomes particularly problematic, specialist advice can be sought regarding the use of amiloride, with particular attention paid to monitoring serum lithium and potassium levels.

Lithium is also associated with renal impairment in approximately one-quarter of patients who take lithium long term.[115,116] However, this is not necessarily clinically significant or progressive. Risk factors for renal impairment are age, duration of treatment and periods of toxicity. The median time to development of Stage 3 chronic kidney disease (CKD) was over 20 years after the patient first took lithium, and only 0.3% of patients develop end-stage renal failure.[117] Decisions about whether to discontinue lithium should be made carefully, often in consultation with a renal physician, on the balance of risks and benefits for the individual patient. Research is ongoing. However, recent observational studies found no difference in the progression of CKD between patients who continued and discontinued lithium.[115]

The mechanism of renal impairment is debated. However, glomerular filtration is affected, and interstitial nephritis with fibrosis and focal nephron atrophy have been reported. There is a growing consensus that with modern standards of monitoring, such as regular blood tests, avoidance of toxicity and high levels, and avoidance of polypharmacy with other nephrotoxic drugs, development of end-stage renal failure can be avoided.

Thyroid -- Lithium tends to reduce thyroid function. The most sensitive laboratory index, increased TSH, occurs in up to 23% of patients. Thyroid enlargement (goitre) develops in about 5%, and clinical hypothyroidism develops in 8–19% of patients. Risk factors are the presence of anti-thyroid antibodies (risk increased eight-fold), female sex, older age and family history of hypothyroidism. Thyroid function (TSH and possibly T3/T4/anti-thyroid antibodies) should be checked prior to commencing lithium, at 3–6 months, and thereafter every 6–12 months or if features of hypothyroidism develop, depending upon the dose and duration of treatment. Patients with pre-existing thyroid antibodies or a family history of thyroid disease are at greater risk of developing hypothyroidism, and lithium treatment can increase antibody levels.

The development of hypothyroidism is often signalled by weight gain and lethargy and should be distinguished from depression. Treatment with L-thyroxine is usually straightforward. Thyrotoxicosis during lithium treatment has also been described, and there may be a rebound exacerbation when lithium is discontinued.

Central Nervous System -- A fine tremor of the hands occurs in about 25 per cent of patients and is similar to that in anxiety. Tricyclic antidepressants, selective serotonin reuptake inhibitors (SSRIs) and caffeine can worsen the tremor. Betablockers such as propranolol (starting at 10 mg twice daily) reduce this and are probably best taken intermittently.

Lithium can increase extrapyramidal (Parkinsonian) side effects in patients on antipsychotic drugs[118] and can itself produce cogwheel rigidity in a small minority of patients.[119] In contrast to antipsychotic-induced Parkinsonism, this does not improve with anticholinergic drugs. Cerebellar tremor and incoordination are signs of toxicity, as are more severe forms of fine tremor and Parkinsonism.

Mental and Cognitive Effects -- There have been reports of memory problems secondary to lithium. However, research suggests that performance on neurocognitive tests are not impaired by lithium,[120] and several observational studies have found a lower risk of dementia in patients with bipolar disorder who take lithium.

The possible effect of lithium upon creativity was explored by Schou (1979),[121] who interviewed 24 successful artists and professionals taking lithium. Some did not want to continue lithium because of this effect, but the majority – although missing some hypomanic swings – considered that their long-term productivity and creativity were higher under lithium treatment. Only six thought they were diminished.

In therapeutic doses, lithium does not impair psychomotor coordination and is not a bar to driving private motor vehicles, although patients must stop driving and notify the UK Driver and Vehicle Licensing Agency if they are diagnosed with bipolar disorder. Licensing will be considered after a period of mood stability, adherence to a treatment plan, no medication side effects that would impair ability to drive, and a favourable report from a suitable specialist.

Skin -- Lithium can produce or exacerbate acne and psoriasis. Tetracyclines should be used with caution because of their interaction with lithium, and retinoids can be used but also with caution due to the risk of exacerbating neuropsychiatric symptoms. Hair loss and altered hair texture may also occur in about 6 per cent of patients. Hair loss is sometimes associated with thyroid impairment but can occur in the presence of normal thyroid function. There may also be a golden discolouration of the distal nail plates or interruption of nail growth.

Metabolic Effects and Weight Gain -- About 25 per cent of patients gain more than 4.5 kg in weight. The mechanism is unknown and likely involves complex interactions with multiple genetic, environmental and pharmacological factors. However, weight gain has been found to be less common with lithium than other medications used in bipolar disorder, such as quetiapine.[122] Although increased consumption of sweet drinks is cited, an increase in food intake and altered metabolism are also possible. Lithium produces subtle alterations in glucose and insulin metabolism. It may occasionally worsen control of diabetes. Fluid retention and oedema may occur, especially with higher doses. Lithium may antagonise aldosterone and increase angiotensin levels.

Cardiovascular Effects -- Lithium can often produce benign reversible T-wave flattening or inversion and sinus bradycardia. However, these signs can also indicate cardiac ischaemia.[123] Cardiac dysrhythmias are rare at therapeutic doses, especially in younger patients, but sinus node arrhythmias have been described (sick sinus syndrome).[124] Long-term treatment has been associated with the development of sinoatrial and bundle branch blocks of varying severity. QTc prolongation has not been associated with lithium use within the therapeutic range, but it can be caused by lithium toxicity and increases the risk of torsades de pointe and sudden cardiac death. In rare cases, lithium unmasks Brugada syndrome through its action as a sodium channel blocker. If so, lithium should be discontinued, and the patient should be referred to cardiology. Caution should be exercised in using lithium in patients with cardiac failure and the elderly. Higher rates of arrhythmia should be expected when lithium is used in combination with carbamazepine than with either drug alone. Lithium treatment ameliorates the excessive cardiovascular mortality found in untreated patients with bipolar disorder.

Blood and Bone Marrow -- Lithium produces a benign reversible leucocytosis, probably by an effect on marrow growth factors. This effect can be useful in some patients on clozapine who have a benign lowering of the white cell count. A very small number of cases of acute lymphocytic and acute myeloid leukemias were published in the 1980s, but no subsequent significant concerns have been raised.

Parathyroid, Bones and Teeth -- Lithium produces mild increases in parathyroid hormone level, and the prevalence of hypercalcaemia is approximately one-quarter.[125] Clinical hyperparathyroidism in patients on lithium has been reported, and NICE recommends that serum calcium is measured at least every year and every 6 months if raised calcium is found.

No long-term effects on bone have been found in animals or humans, and lithium improved bone regeneration in rats.[126] It is unknown whether this applies to the growing bones of children. Severe dental decay has been reported in patients taking lithium, which may be related to a loss of dentin mineral.[127] Stomatitis, a metallic taste, and both hypersalivation and hyposalivation have been reported. Hyposalivation increases the risk of gum disease and dental caries.

Sexual Function -- Impairment of sexual drive, arousal, orgasm and ejaculation have been attributed to lithium but are thought to be rare. The LH response to luteinising hormone releasing hormone (LHRH) is potentiated by lithium treatment, as is the potentiation of the TSH response to TRH.

Neuromuscular Junction -- Lithium reduces acetylcholine release and impairs neuromuscular transmission. Some patients may experience muscle weakness early in therapy. Normally, the safety factor in neuromuscular transmission is sufficient to overcome these effects, and the weakness resolves. Lithium potentiates neuromuscular blocking agents, including succinyl choline, and in very rare cases, may cause, unmask or exacerbate myasthenia gravis.[128]

Respiratory Effects -- Lithium can produce hypercapnia and exacerbations of chronic obstructive pulmonary disease, especially at toxic blood levels. Lower therapeutic levels reduce the reactivity of bronchial smooth muscle and may benefit some patients with asthma.

Pregnancy

Lithium does not affect the ability to become pregnant, and it is unknown whether lithium increases the risk of miscarriage. Initial concern about the risk of teratogenicity was based largely on the frequency of abnormalities reported to the Lithium Information Center in Wisconsin. These voluntary reports included particularly high rates of Ebstein's cardiac anomaly and suggested that foetal exposure to lithium, especially in the first trimester, carried substantially greater risk of other malformations as well. However, in more recent studies, findings have been mixed, with some finding no increased risk and only a very small increase in others. Preconception counselling is advised.[129] No extra ultrasound scans are needed, but the midwifery or medical teams should be informed that the patient is taking lithium so the foetus can be screened for heart defects.

We do not know if lithium is associated with premature birth or low or high birth weight. Lithium levels should be measured more often than usual during pregnancy, as physiological changes can alter lithium levels. Perinatal toxicity has been reported, characterised by hypotonicity and cyanosis (sometimes termed 'floppy baby syndrome'). A naturalistic study, however, found no evidence of neonatal toxicity in the newborns exposed to lithium at the time of labour and delivery.[130] Before delivery, lithium should be restarted to reduce the risk of puerperal psychosis. A five-year follow-up of children with second and third trimester exposure to lithium born without congenital malformations found no significant physical or developmental problems.

Lithium is secreted in breast milk, and serum lithium levels in nursing infants are reported to be 10–50% of the mother's serum level. It remains unclear what effect this low lithium intake might have on well-hydrated, breast feeding infants. However, breastfeeding whilst taking lithium is not recommended. Women accepting this risk and wishing to breastfeed should be counselled to provide supplemental fluids and discontinue breast feeding under circumstances of increased fluid loss or decreased intake.

A switch from lithium to an anticonvulsant medication for prophylaxis during pregnancy is not recommended. The risks of teratogenicity associated with valproate and carbamazepine are higher than with lithium, and a lithium-responsive patient may not be protected by these anticonvulsants.

Even the remote possibility of teratogenicity or developmental effects upon the child causes understandable concern among those planning to conceive. Pregnancy in a patient with bipolar disorder may be managed acceptably without psychotropic drugs. However, the risk of lithium discontinuation mania applies even during pregnancy.[131] This risk is likely to be lowest in people with only one previous episode.[132] Patients choosing to discontinue lithium should be encouraged to taper medication gradually (over several weeks or months) and only after a euthymic period of one year or more. If alternative medication is needed when pregnancy is planned, antipsychotics or antidepressants are probably the safest. There is a risk of transient extrapyramidal side effects in the neonate if antipsychotics are continued up to delivery.

Lithium Toxicity

Clinical Features -- Lithium toxicity is indicated by the development of three groups of symptoms: gastrointestinal, motor (especially cerebellar) and mental (Table 4.1.2). Nausea and diarrhoea progress to vomiting and incontinence. Marked fine tremor progresses to a coarse (cerebellar or Parkinsonian) tremor, giddiness, cerebellar ataxia and slurred speech, and then to gross incoordination with choreiform movements and muscular twitching (myoclonus), upper motor neuron signs (spasticity and extensor plantar reflexes), abnormalities on electroencephalography (EEG) and seizures. In mild toxicity, there is impairment of concentration, but this deteriorates into drowsiness and disorientation. In more severe toxicity, there is marked apathy and impaired consciousness leading to coma. A Creutzfeldt- Jakob-like syndrome with characteristic EEG changes, myoclonus and cognitive deterioration has been described but was reversible in these cases.[133]

Diagnosis of Toxicity -- Lithium toxicity should be assumed in patients on lithium with vomiting or severe nausea, cerebellar signs or disorientation. Lithium treatment should be stopped immediately, and serum lithium, urea and electrolyte levels should be measured. However, the severity of toxicity bears little relationship to serum lithium levels,[134] and neurotoxicity can occur with serum levels in the usual therapeutic range.[135] Diagnosis should be based upon clinical judgement and not upon the blood level. Lithium should be restarted (at an adjusted dose) only after the patient's condition has improved or an alternative cause of the symptoms has been found.

Table 4.1.2 Symptoms of lithium toxicity

Severity	Gastrointestinal	Motor/cerebellar	Mental
Mild	Nausea Diarrhoea	Severe fine tremor	Poor concentration
Moderate	Vomiting	Coarse tremor Cerebellar ataxia Slurred speech	Drowsiness Disorientation
Severe	Vomiting Incontinence	Choreiform/Parkinsonian movement General muscle twitching (Myoclonus) spasticity and cerebellar dysfunction EEG abnormalities and seizures	Apathy Coma

Treatment of Lithium Toxicity -- Often, cessation of lithium and provision of adequate salt and fluids, including saline infusions, will suffice. In patients with high serum levels (greater than 3 mmol/l) or coma, haemodialysis can speed the removal of lithium and reduce the risk of permanent neurological damage.

Outcome -- Patients who survive episodes of lithium toxicity will often make a full recovery. However, some will have persistent renal or neurological damage with cerebellar symptoms, spasticity and cognitive impairment. This outcome is more likely if patients are continued on lithium while showing signs of toxicity or during intercurrent physical illnesses.[136] Those patients who develop persistent neurological damage have more severe signs of toxicity in their episode of toxicity.[134] Signs of toxicity develop gradually, over several days, during continued lithium treatment and, in some cases, continue to develop for days after treatment is stopped. Serum lithium levels may also continue to rise after treatment is stopped, probably because of the release of lithium from intracellular stores.[137]

Factors Predisposing to Lithium Toxicity -- Conditions of salt depletion (diarrhoea, vomiting and excessive sweating during fever or in hot weather) can lead to lithium retention. Drugs that reduce the renal excretion of lithium include thiazide diuretics (but not frusemide or amiloride), certain nonsteroidal anti-inflammatory drugs (ibuprofen, indomethacin, piroxicam, naproxen and phenylbutazone, but not aspirin, paracetamol or sulindac) and some antibiotics (erythromycin, metronidazole and probably tetracyclines) and calcium antagonists. These drugs should be avoided, if possible; if they are used, the dose of lithium should be reduced, and the blood levels should be monitored. In patients with serious intercurrent illnesses, especially infections, lithium should be stopped or reduced in dose and carefully monitored until the patient's condition is stable. Gastroenteritis is particularly liable to lead to toxicity. In the elderly, renal function is decreased, lower doses of lithium are required and toxicity can develop more readily.

Valproate

Valproate is a branched chain fatty acid. It is also available as a noncovalent dimer (two identical molecules held together by hydrogen bonding) called divalproex in the USA (Depakote©, known in the UK as semisodium valproate). This formulation was used in several clinical trials after the company was granted a patent separate from that for valproate.

Dosage

The starting dose is 750 mg in 2–3 divided doses, rising by 200 mg at 3-day intervals towards 2000 mg daily according to clinical response. For more rapid control, a starting dose of 20 mg/kg is used. The modified-release form is started at 500 mg daily and increased.

Side Effects

Valproate is generally well tolerated, but side effects include vomiting, tremor, ataxia, weight gain, rash, hair loss – usually transient – and, potentially, acute liver damage in children. A confusional state with asterixis (flapping tremor) occurs rarely, and high blood ammonia levels confirm the cause; liver damage is not involved. Pancreatitis has occasionally been reported, as has spontaneous bruising or bleeding. Valproate is associated with the development of polycystic ovarian syndrome. Generally, the modified-release form is associated with fewer side effects.

A foetal valproate syndrome has been identified with cardiac and other congenital abnormalities and with jitteriness and seizures in the neonate. There is also a significantly increased incidence of developmental delay and global reduction in IQ.

Pharmacokinetics

Valproate is metabolised in the liver and has a plasma half-life of 8–20 hours, which may be prolonged by cimetidine.

It inhibits cytochrome enzymes and thereby tends to raise the blood levels of lamotrigine.

Selection of Patients for Valproate and Combinations

Patients with mania who do not respond to antipsychotics alone can be tried on a combination with valproate or lithium. Those with mixed affective disorders may be given valproate in preference to lithium. Although side effects – including weight gain, tremor and drowsiness – may be greater, the combination is generally safe.

Because of the teratogenic and reduced IQ risks associated with in-utero exposure, the UK Medicines and Healthcare products Regulatory Agency has essentially banned the use of valproate for bipolar disorder during pregnancy. It must not be prescribed to girls, women or people of childbearing potential unless there is a pregnancy prevention programme (PPP) in place and a risk acknowledgement form signed by the patient at least annually.

Monitoring and Testing

The recommended plasma concentration is in the range 50–150 mg/l. In children and patients with a history of liver disease, metabolic or degenerative disorders, or organic brain pathology, liver function tests should be done before treatment and occasionally during the first six months.

Carbamazepine

Dosage

The dose of carbamazepine for prophylaxis in bipolar disorder is usually to start at 100 mg twice daily, increasing by 200 mg every two or three days, up to a daily dose of 400–600 mg. Gradual introduction reduces the incidence of side effects, discussed later. Unless immediate discontinuation is medically required, carbamazepine should be tapered over at least four weeks.

No clear relationship has been found between blood level and response. As a result, the dose should be determined mainly by clinical response and tolerance of side effects.

In patients of Han Chinese or Thai origin, prescreen for the HLA-B*1502 allele as this is associated with an increased risk of Stevens-Johnson syndrome. If present, carbamazepine should be avoided.

Side Effects

The most common side effects are nausea, dizziness, ataxia and double vision. Others include headache, drowsiness and nystagmus. At higher doses, confusion may occur.

Carbamazepine is associated with antiepileptic hypersensitivity syndrome, which usually occurs in the first two months of starting the drug. Symptoms include fever, rash, lymphadenopathy and multiorgan abnormalities. It can be fatal, and the drug must be immediately discontinued and should never be re-prescribed for that patient.

A generalised erythematous rash develops within two weeks in about 3% of patients and requires great caution and usually cessation of the drug, and a full blood count should be performed. Carbamazepine must be discontinued if the rash worsens, the blood count is abnormal or other symptoms develop. Serious toxic side effects are agranulocytosis, aplastic anaemia, Stevens-Johnson syndrome and water intoxication. A moderate leucopenia occurs in 1–2% of patients, often transiently at the start of treatment. Agranulocytosis and aplastic anaemia can develop suddenly and occur in about eight patients per million treated.

Carbamazepine regularly lowers the white cell count via a pharmacological effect on the marrow. Hyponatraemia and water intoxication may occur – due to potentiation of ADH – and may lead to malaise, confusion and fits. Fluid retention may occur.

Patients should be warned of side effects and advised particularly to report any rashes, fevers or severe sore throats, which may herald agranulocytosis and require immediate discontinuation of the drug.

Because of the possibility of foetal neural tube defects, carbamazepine should be avoided in pregnancy.[129]

Pharmacokinetics and Drug Interactions

Carbamazepine induces liver enzymes. This results in the lowering not only of its own blood levels after three weeks of treatment, but in also increasing the metabolism of other drugs such as haloperidol, risperidone, valproate, lamotrigine, oral contraceptives, clonazepam and tricyclic antidepressants. Its own plasma half-life may shorten from 48 hours to 7 hours during long-term treatment. The dose of oral contraceptives needs to be raised, or an alternative method of birth control should be used. The dose of warfarin may also need increasing. Thyroid hormone metabolism is increased, and blood levels are lowered; carbamazepine may precipitate hypothyroidism, particularly in combination with lithium.

Carbamazepine is itself metabolised by CYP IIIA4. A metabolite (carbamazepine 10,11 epoxide) has similar pharmacological activity. Barbiturates and phenytoin induce enzymes and lower plasma levels of carbamazepine. On the other hand, the blood level of carbamazepine is increased by some drugs, including erythromycin, verapamil, dextropropoxyphene (in co-proxamol), cimetidine, valproate and some SSRIs (e.g. fluoxetine).

Being of tricyclic structure, carbamazepine should not be given in combination with a monoamine oxidase inhibitor, as serotonin syndrome is a risk.

Oxcarbazepine

A related drug, oxcarbazepine, carries a lower risk of bone marrow toxicity. Its efficacy in bipolar disorder is poorly defined. However, it has an advantage over carbamazepine due to a lower propensity for pharmacokinetic drug interactions.

Other Physical Treatments

Electroconvulsive Therapy (ECT)

Early reports of the use of ECT in mania showed that about two-thirds of patients responded. In a retrospective study, 78% of patients treated with ECT showed marked improvement, compared with 62% on lithium.[138] There is only one randomised controlled trial in patients having a manic episode (concomitantly treated with chlorpromazine), which compared bilateral ECT with sham ECT.[139] Twelve out of 15 patients receiving bilateral ECT – and one out of 15 patients receiving sham ECT – were recovered after eight sessions.

A randomised controlled trial of unilateral ECT compared with pharmacological treatment in 73 patients with treatment-resistant depression in bipolar disorder found a significantly greater response rate in the ECT group. However, the remission rates did not differ.[140] A systematic review and meta-analysis of non-randomised trials came to a similar conclusion.[141]

The use of lithium during ECT is discussed earlier (under contraindications to lithium); neurotoxic complications have been reported.

In some countries, clinicians reserve ECT for patients with the most severe and drug-resistant mania, whereas elsewhere, it is regarded as generally helpful in mania and used often. ECT is not mentioned at all in current UK NICE guidelines[68] but is included as an option for difficult-to-treat bipolar mania and depression in the British Association for Psychopharmacology (BAP) guidelines.[33]

Transcranial Magnetic Stimulation

While there is a large evidence base supporting the use of transcranial magnetic stimulation (TMS) in unipolar depression, there is much less data in bipolar disorder. Very few studies have examined the effect of TMS in treating mania, and the results don't tend to show a clinically meaningful effect. There are more studies that have examined TMS for bipolar depression. Overall, these suggest TMS is well tolerated, but efficacy is unclear.[142] This suggests that it may not be as effective as it appears to be in unipolar depression.

Vagus Nerve Stimulation

Implanted vagus nerve stimulation (VNS) involves the surgical implantation of a pacemaker-like device in the left side of the chest wall, with a wire passing to the vagus nerve in the neck. The treatment was first introduced for treatment-resistant epilepsy. However, there is increasing data suggesting efficacy in difficult-to-treat depression. The largest data set comes from a non-randomised registry study comparing around 500 patients who received VNS combined with treatment as usual (TAU) versus around 300 who just received TAU.[143] This study included patients with both unipolar and bipolar depression. Although numbers of the latter were small, VNS seemed to be beneficial for both groups of patients. Further case series have shown benefits of VNS in patients with rapid-cycling bipolar disorder[144] and in patients with bipolar depression receiving maintenance ECT, where the need for ongoing ECT was significantly reduced.[145] A large randomised controlled trial of VNS for bipolar depression is currently underway in the USA.

Neurosurgery

Very few patients undergo ablative neurosurgery (anterior cingulotomy or anterior capsulotomy), and evidence for its use in patients with bipolar disorder comes from two small case series only. Deep brain stimulation may improve depression in patients with bipolar disorder; it can cause transient hypomania, which can be managed by adjusting the stimulation and the patient's medication.[146]

References

1. Angst J, Marneros A. Bipolarity from ancient to modern times: conception, birth and rebirth. *Journal of Affective Disorders* 2001;67(1–3):3–19.
2. Dunner D, Gershon ES, Goodwin FK. Heritable factors in the severity of affective illness. *Biological Psychiatry* 1976;11(1):31–42.
3. Goodwin FK, Jamison KR. *Manic-Depressive Illness: Bipolar Disorders and Recurrent Depression*. Oxford: Oxford University Press; 2007.
4. Cookson J. Bipolarity, creativity, stigma and authenticity in the work of Kay Redfield Jamison – reflection. *The British Journal of Psychiatry* 2018;212 (2):87.
5. Bowden CL, Brugger AM, Swann AC, et al. Efficacy of divalproex vs lithium and placebo in the treatment of mania. *JAMA* 1994;271(12):918–24.
6. Cookson J. Use of antipsychotic drugs and lithium in mania. *The British Journal of Psychiatry* 2001;178(S41): s148–s56.
7. Maj M, Akiskal HS, López-Ibor Jr JJ, et al. *Bipolar Disorder*. Chichester: Wiley; 2002.
8. Marneros A, Angst J. *Bipolar Disorders: 100 Years After Manic-Depressive Insanity*. Dordrecht, the Netherlands: Springer Science & Business Media; 2007.
9. Marneros A, Goodwin F. *Bipolar Disorders: Mixed States, Rapid Cycling and Atypical Forms*. Cambridge: Cambridge University Press; 2005.
10. American Psychiatric Association. *Diagnostic and Statistical Manual of Mental Disorders: DSM-5*. Washington, DC: American Psychiatric Association; 2013.
11. Akiskal HS, Hantouche E-G, Allilaire J-F, et al. Validating antidepressant-associated hypomania (bipolar III): a systematic comparison with spontaneous hypomania (bipolar II). *Journal of Affective Disorders* 2003;73 (1–2):65–74.
12. McIntyre RS, Berk M, Brietzke E, et al. Bipolar disorders. *Lancet* 2020;396 (10265):1841–56.
13. World Health Organization. *ICD-11 for Mortality and Morbidity Statistics*. Geneva: World Health Organization; 2018.
14. Angst J, Grobler C. Unipolar mania: a necessary diagnostic concept. *European Archives of Psychiatry and Clinical Neuroscience* 2015;265(4):273–80.
15. Angst J, Rössler W, Ajdacic-Gross V, et al. Differences between unipolar mania and bipolar-I disorder: evidence from nine epidemiological studies. *Bipolar Disorders* 2019;21(5):437–48.
16. Iverson GL, Brooks BL, Langenecker SA, et al. Identifying a cognitive impairment subgroup in adults with mood disorders. *Journal of Affective Disorders* 2011;132(3):360–7.
17. Robinson LJ, Thompson JM, Gallagher P, et al. A meta-analysis of cognitive deficits in euthymic patients with bipolar disorder. *Journal of Affective Disorders* 2006;93(1–3):105–15.
18. Bora E. Neurocognitive features in clinical subgroups of bipolar disorder: a meta-analysis. *Journal of Affective Disorders* 2018;229:125–34.
19. Bortolato B, Miskowiak KW, Köhler CA, et al. Cognitive dysfunction in bipolar disorder and schizophrenia: a systematic review of meta-analyses. *Neuropsychiatric Disease and Treatment* 2015;11:3111.
20. Ant A. *Stand and Deliver: The Autobiography*. London: Pan Macmillan; 2007.
21. Hamilton SF. *Fast Girl: A Life Spent Running from Madness*. New York: HarperCollins; 2015.
22. Parker G. Is borderline personality disorder a mood disorder? *The British Journal of Psychiatry* 2014;204(4):252–3.
23. Cuellar AK, Johnson SL, Winters R. Distinctions between bipolar and unipolar depression. *Clinical Psychology Review* 2005;25(3):307–39.
24. Morriss R, Kendall T, Braidwood R, et al. *The Assessment and Management of Bipolar Disorder in Adults, Children and Young People in Primary and Secondary Care*. London: NICE; 2014.
25. Young RC, Biggs JT, Ziegler VE, et al. A rating scale for mania: reliability, validity and sensitivity. *The British Journal of Psychiatry* 1978;133 (5):429–35.
26. Altman EG, Hedeker D, Peterson JL, et al. The Altman self-rating mania scale. *Biological Psychiatry* 1997;42 (10):948–55.
27. McManus S, Bebbington PE, Jenkins R, et al. *Mental Health and Wellbeing in England: The Adult Psychiatric Morbidity Survey 2014*. London: NHS Digital; 2016.
28. Kupfer D, Frank E, Grochocinski V, et al. Stabilization in the treatment of mania, depression and mixed states. *Acta Neuropsychiatrica* 2000;12 (3):110–4.
29. Tohen M, Hennen J, Zarate Jr CM, et al. Two-year syndromal and functional recovery in 219 cases of first-episode major affective disorder with psychotic features. *American Journal of Psychiatry* 2000;157(2):220–8.
30. Kessing LV, Bolwig TG, Andersen PK, et al. Recurrence in affective disorder: I. Case register study. *The British Journal of Psychiatry* 1998;172(1):23–8.
31. Tohen M, Zarate Jr CA, Hennen J, et al. The McLean-Harvard first-episode mania study: prediction of recovery and first recurrence. *American Journal of Psychiatry* 2003;160(12):2099–107.
32. Ali S, Santomauro D, Ferrari AJ, et al. Excess mortality in severe mental disorders: a systematic review and meta-regression. *Journal of Psychiatric Research* 2022;149:97–105.
33. Goodwin G, Haddad P, Ferrier I, et al. Evidence-based guidelines for treating bipolar disorder: revised third edition recommendations from the British Association for Psychopharmacology. *Journal of Psychopharmacology* 2016;30 (6):495–553.
34. Marwaha S, Durrani A, Singh S. Employment outcomes in people with bipolar disorder: a systematic review.

Acta Psychiatrica Scandinavica 2013;128 (3):179–93.

35. Sylvia LG, Montana RE, Deckersbach T, et al. Poor quality of life and functioning in bipolar disorder. *International Journal of Bipolar Disorders* 2017;5(1):1–8.
36. Granek L, Danan D, Bersudsky Y, et al. Living with bipolar disorder: the impact on patients, spouses, and their marital relationship. *Bipolar Disorders* 2016;18 (2):192–9.
37. Taylor CL. Creativity and mood disorder: a systematic review and meta-analysis. *Perspectives on Psychological Science.* 2017;12(6):1040–76.
38. Santosa CM, Strong CM, Nowakowska C, et al. Enhanced creativity in bipolar disorder patients: A controlled study. *Journal of Affective Disorders* 2007;100 (1):31–9.
39. Rowland TA, Marwaha S. Epidemiology and risk factors for bipolar disorder. *Therapeutic Advances in Psychopharmacology* 2018;8(9): 251–69.
40. Weissman MM, Myers JK. Affective disorders in a US urban community: the use of research diagnostic criteria in an epidemiological survey. *Archives of General Psychiatry* 1978;35 (11):1304–11.
41. Tsuchiya KJ, Byrne M, Mortensen PB. Risk factors in relation to an emergence of bipolar disorder: a systematic review. *Bipolar Disorders* 2003;5(4):231–42.
42. Craddock N, Sklar P. Genetics of bipolar disorder: successful start to a long journey. *Trends in Genetics.* 2009;25(2):99–105.
43. Strober M. Relevance of early age-of-onset in genetic studies of bipolar affective disorder. *Journal of the American Academy of Child & Adolescent Psychiatry* 1992;31 (4):606–10.
44. Kassem L, Lopez V, Hedeker D, et al. Familiality of polarity at illness onset in bipolar affective disorder. *American Journal of Psychiatry* 2006;163 (10):1754–9.
45. Potash JB, Chiu YF, MacKinnon DF, et al. Familial aggregation of psychotic symptoms in a replication set of 69 bipolar disorder pedigrees. *American Journal of Medical Genetics Part B: Neuropsychiatric Genetics* 2003;116 (1):90–7.
46. Fisfalen ME, Schulze TG, DePaulo Jr JR, et al. Familial variation in episode frequency in bipolar affective disorder. *American Journal of Psychiatry* 2005;162(7):1266–72.
47. Sokolowski M, Wasserman D. Genetic origins of suicidality? A synopsis of genes in suicidal behaviours, with regard to evidence diversity, disorder specificity and neurodevelopmental brain transcriptomics. *European Neuropsychopharmacology* 2020;37:1–11.
48. Senner F, Kohshour MO, Abdalla S, et al. The genetics of response to and side effects of lithium treatment in bipolar disorder: future research perspectives. *Frontiers in Pharmacology* 2021;12.
49. Gordovez FJA, McMahon FJ. The genetics of bipolar disorder. *Molecular Psychiatry* 2020;25(3):544–59.
50. Rees E, Kirov G. Copy number variation and neuropsychiatric illness. *Current Opinion in Genetics & Development* 2021;68:57–63.
51. Huckins L, Dobbyn A, Ruderfer D, et al. Novel bipolar and schizophrenia risk genes identified through genic associations in Transcriptome imputation. *European Neuropsychopharmacology* 2017;27: S487.
52. de Barros JLVM, Barbosa IG, Salem H, et al. Is there any association between Toxoplasma gondii infection and bipolar disorder? A systematic review and meta-analysis. *Journal of Affective Disorders* 2017;209:59–65.
53. Pugliese V, Bruni A, Carbone EA, et al. Maternal stress, prenatal medical illnesses and obstetric complications: risk factors for schizophrenia spectrum disorder, bipolar disorder and major depressive disorder. *Psychiatry Research* 2019;271:23–30.
54. Palmier-Claus J, Berry K, Bucci S, et al. Relationship between childhood adversity and bipolar affective disorder: systematic review and meta-analysis. *The British Journal of Psychiatry* 2016;209(6):454–9.
55. Agnew-Blais J, Danese A. Childhood maltreatment and unfavourable clinical outcomes in bipolar disorder: a systematic review and meta-analysis. *The Lancet Psychiatry* 2016;3(4):342–9.
56. Smart C, Strathdee G, Watson S, et al. Early life trauma, depression and the glucocorticoid receptor gene–an epigenetic perspective. *Psychological Medicine* 2015;45(16):3393–410.
57. Baumeister D, Akhtar R, Ciufolini S, et al. Childhood trauma and adulthood inflammation: a meta-analysis of peripheral C-reactive protein, interleukin-6 and tumour necrosis factor-α. *Molecular Psychiatry* 2016;21 (5):642–9.
58. Kirsch DE, Tretyak V, Radpour S, et al. Childhood maltreatment, prefrontal-paralimbic gray matter volume, and substance use in young adults and interactions with risk for bipolar disorder. *Scientific Reports* 2021;11 (1):1–12.
59. Cassidy F, Ahearn EP, Carroll BJ. Substance abuse in bipolar disorder. *Bipolar Disorders* 2001;3(4):181–8.
60. Marwaha S, Winsper C, Bebbington P, Smith D. Cannabis use and hypomania in young people: a prospective analysis. *Schizophrenia Bulletin* 2018;44 (6):1267–74.
61. Pavlova B, Perlis R, Mantere O, et al. Prevalence of current anxiety disorders in people with bipolar disorder during euthymia: a meta-analysis. *Psychological Medicine* 2017;47(6):1107–15.
62. Coryell W, Solomon DA, Fiedorowicz JG, et al. Anxiety and outcome in bipolar disorder. *American Journal of Psychiatry* 2009;166(11):1238–43.
63. Seeberg I, Nielsen IB, Jørgensen C, et al. Effects of psychological and pharmacological interventions on anxiety symptoms in patients with bipolar disorder in full or partial remission: a systematic review. *Journal of Affective Disorders* 2021;279:31–45.
64. Forty L, Ulanova A, Jones L, et al. Comorbid medical illness in bipolar disorder. *The British Journal of Psychiatry* 2014;205(6):465–72.
65. Bradley A, Webb-Mitchell R, Hazu A, et al. Sleep and circadian rhythm disturbance in bipolar disorder. *Psychological Medicine* 2017;47 (9):1678–89.
66. Bradley AJ, Anderson KN, Gallagher P, et al. The association between sleep and cognitive abnormalities in bipolar disorder. *Psychological Medicine* 2020;50(1):125–32.
67. Harvey AG, Soehner AM, Kaplan KA, et al. Treating insomnia improves mood state, sleep, and functioning in bipolar

disorder: a pilot randomized controlled trial. *Journal of Consulting and Clinical Psychology* 2015;83(3):564.

68. National Collaborating Centre for Mental Health. *Bipolar Disorder: the NICE Guideline on the Assessment and Management of Bipolar Disorder in Adults, Children and Young People in Primary and Secondary Care.* London: The British Psychological Society and the Royal College of Psychiatrists; 2014.
69. American Psychiatric Association. *Practice Guideline for the Treatment of Patients with Bipolar Disorder (Revision).* Washington, DC: American Psychiatric Pub; 2002.
70. Hirschfeld RM. *Guideline Watch: Practice Guideline for the Treatment of Patients with Bipolar Disorder.* Arlington, VA: American Psychiatric Association. 2005.
71. Grunze H, Vieta E, Goodwin GM, et al. The World Federation of Societies of Biological Psychiatry (WFSBP) guidelines for the biological treatment of bipolar disorders: update 2012 on the long-term treatment of bipolar disorder. *The World Journal of Biological Psychiatry* 2013;14 (3):154–219.
72. Cade JF. Lithium salts in the treatment of psychotic excitement. *Medical Journal of Australia* 1949;2(10): 349–52.
73. Kirkham E, Skinner J, Anderson T, et al. One lithium level> 1.0 mmol/L causes an acute decline in eGFR: findings from a retrospective analysis of a monitoring database. *BMJ Open* 2014;4(11): e006020.
74. Prien RF, Caffey EM, Klett CJ. Comparison of lithium carbonate and chlorpromazine in the treatment of mania: report of the Veterans Administration and National Institute of Mental Health Collaborative Study Group. *Archives of General Psychiatry* 1972;26(2):146–53.
75. Talaei A, Dastgheib MS, Soltanifar A, et al. Oxcarbazepine versus sodium valproate in treatment of acute mania: a double-blind randomized clinical trial. *International Clinical Psychopharmacology* 2022;37(3):116–21.
76. Cookson J. Haloperidol and risperidone in mania. In: Akiskal HS, Tohen M (eds.) *Bipolar Psychopharmacology: Caring for the Patient.* Chichester: Wiley; 2006: 105–25.
77. Cookson J. Treatment of mania. In: Hirschfeld R, Kasper S (eds.) *Handbook of Bipolar Disorder: Diagnosis and Therapeutic Approaches.* Boca Raton, Florida: Taylor & Francis, CRC Press; 2005: 157–79.
78. Suppes T, Webb A, Paul B, et al. Clinical outcome in a randomized 1-year trial of clozapine versus treatment as usual for patients with treatment-resistant illness and a history of mania. *American Journal of Psychiatry* 1999;156(8):1164–9.
79. Delgado A, Velosa J, Zhang J, et al. Clozapine in bipolar disorder: a systematic review and meta-analysis. *Journal of Psychiatric Research* 2020;125:21–7.
80. Nielsen J, Kane JM, Correll CU. Real-world effectiveness of clozapine in patients with bipolar disorder: results from a 2-year mirror-image study. *Bipolar Disorders.* 2012;14(8):863–9.
81. Cohen WJ, Cohen NH. Lithium carbonate, haloperidol, and irreversible brain damage. *JAMA* 1974;230 (9):1283–7.
82. Loudon JB, Waring H. Toxic reactions to lithium and haloperidol. *Lancet* 1976;2(7994):1088.
83. Patel MX, Sethi FN, Barnes TR, et al. Joint BAP NAPICU evidence-based consensus guidelines for the clinical management of acute disturbance: de-escalation and rapid tranquillisation. *Journal of Psychiatric Intensive Care* 2018;14(2):89–132.
84. Sachs GS, Nierenberg AA, Calabrese JR, et al. Effectiveness of adjunctive antidepressant treatment for bipolar depression. *New England Journal of Medicine* 2007;356(17):1711–22.
85. McElroy SL, Weisler RH, Chang W, et al. A double-blind, placebo-controlled study of quetiapine and paroxetine as monotherapy in adults with bipolar depression (EMBOLDEN II). *Journal of Clinical Psychiatry* 2010;71(2):163–74.
86. Sidor MM, MacQueen GM. Antidepressants for the acute treatment of bipolar depression: a systematic review and meta-analysis. *The Journal of Clinical Psychiatry* 2010;71(2):953.
87. Earley WR, Burgess MV, Khan B, et al. Efficacy and safety of cariprazine in bipolar I depression: a double-blind, placebo-controlled phase 3 study. *Bipolar Disorders* 2020;22(4):372–84.
88. van der Loos ML, Mulder PG, Erwin GTM, et al. Efficacy and safety of lamotrigine as add-on treatment to lithium in bipolar depression: a multicenter, double-blind, placebo-controlled trial. *The Journal of Clinical Psychiatry* 2009;70(2):6169.
89. Geddes JR, Gardiner A, Rendell J, et al. Comparative evaluation of quetiapine plus lamotrigine combination versus quetiapine monotherapy (and folic acid versus placebo) in bipolar depression (CEQUEL): a 2× 2 factorial randomised trial. *The Lancet Psychiatry* 2016;3 (1):31–9.
90. Zarate Jr CA, Brutsche NE, Ibrahim L, et al. Replication of ketamine's antidepressant efficacy in bipolar depression: a randomized controlled add-on trial. *Biological Psychiatry* 2012;71(11):939–46.
91. Azim L, Hindmarch P, Browne G, et al. Study protocol for a randomised placebo-controlled trial of pramipexole in addition to mood stabilisers for patients with treatment resistant bipolar depression (the PAX-BD study). *BMC Psychiatry* 2021;21(1):1–14.
92. Suppes T, Silva R, Cucchiaro J, et al. Lurasidone for the treatment of major depressive disorder with mixed features: a randomized, double-blind, placebo-controlled study. *American Journal of Psychiatry* 2016;173(4):400–7.
93. Tohen M, Ketter TA, Zarate CA, et al. Olanzapine versus divalproex sodium for the treatment of acute mania and maintenance of remission: a 47-week study. *American Journal of Psychiatry* 2003;160(7):1263–71.
94. Geddes JR, Goodwin GM, Rendell J, et al. Lithium plus valproate combination therapy versus monotherapy for relapse prevention in bipolar I disorder (BALANCE): a randomised open-label trial. *Lancet* 2009;375(9712):385–95.
95. Joas E, Karanti A, Song J, et al. Pharmacological treatment and risk of psychiatric hospital admission in bipolar disorder. *The British Journal of Psychiatry* 2017;210(3):197–202.
96. Nolen WA, Weisler RH. The association of the effect of lithium in the maintenance treatment of bipolar disorder with lithium plasma levels: a post hoc analysis of a double-blind study comparing switching to lithium or placebo in patients who responded to

quetiapine (Trial 144). *Bipolar Disorders* 2013;15(1):100–9.

97. Cipriani A, Hawton K, Stockton S, et al. Lithium in the prevention of suicide in mood disorders: updated systematic review and meta-analysis. *BMJ* 2013;346.

98. Suppes T, Baldessarini RJ, Faedda GL, et al. Risk of recurrence following discontinuation of lithium treatment in bipolar disorder. *Archives of General Psychiatry* 1991;48(12):1082–8.

99. Weisler RH, Nolen WA, Neijber A, et al. Continuation of quetiapine versus switching to placebo or lithium for maintenance treatment of bipolar I disorder (Trial 144: a randomized controlled study). *The Journal of Clinical Psychiatry* 2011;72(11):3707.

100. Tohen M, Calabrese JR, Sachs GS, et al. Randomized, placebo-controlled trial of olanzapine as maintenance therapy in patients with bipolar I disorder responding to acute treatment with olanzapine. *American Journal of Psychiatry* 2006;163(2):247–56.

101. Keck PE, Calabrese JR, McQuade RD, et al. A randomized, double-blind, placebo-controlled 26-week trial of aripiprazole in recently manic patients with bipolar I disorder. *The Journal of Clinical Psychiatry* 2006;67(4):626–37.

102. Goodwin GM, Bowden CL, Calabrese JR, et al. A pooled analysis of 2 placebo-controlled 18-month trials of lamotrigine and lithium maintenance in bipolar I disorder. *The Journal of Clinical Psychiatry* 2004;65(3):432–41.

103. Taylor MJ. Bipolar treatment efficacy. *The Lancet Psychiatry* 2014;1(6):418.

104. Ghaemi S, Wingo A, Filkowski M, et al. Long-term antidepressant treatment in bipolar disorder: meta-analyses of benefits and risks. *Acta Psychiatrica Scandinavica* 2008;118(5):347–56.

105. Tohen M, Chengappa KR, Suppes T, et al. Relapse prevention in bipolar I disorder: 18-month comparison of olanzapine plus mood stabiliser v. mood stabiliser alone. *The British Journal of Psychiatry* 2004;184(4):337–45.

106. Marcus R, Khan A, Rollin L, et al. Efficacy of aripiprazole adjunctive to lithium or valproate in the long-term treatment of patients with bipolar I disorder with an inadequate response to lithium or valproate monotherapy: a multicenter, double-blind, randomized study. *Bipolar Disorders* 2011;13 (2):133–44.

107. Suppes T, Vieta E, Liu S, et al. Maintenance treatment for patients with bipolar I disorder: results from a North American study of quetiapine in combination with lithium or divalproex (trial 127). *American Journal of Psychiatry* 2009;166(4):476–88.

108. Calabrese JR, Pikalov A, Streicher C, et al. Lurasidone in combination with lithium or valproate for the maintenance treatment of bipolar I disorder. *European Neuropsychopharmacology* 2017;27 (9):865–76.

109. Vieta E, Montgomery S, Sulaiman AH, et al. A randomized, double-blind, placebo-controlled trial to assess prevention of mood episodes with risperidone long-acting injectable in patients with bipolar I disorder. *European Neuropsychopharmacology* 2012;22(11):825–35.

110. Calabrese JR, Sanchez R, Jin N, et al. Efficacy and safety of aripiprazole once-monthly in the maintenance treatment of bipolar I disorder: a double-blind, placebo-controlled, 52-week randomized withdrawal study. *The Journal of Clinical Psychiatry* 2017;78 (3):324–31.

111. Swann AC, Bowden CL, Calabrese JR, et al. Mania: differential effects of previous depressive and manic episodes onresponse to treatment. *Acta Psychiatrica Scandinavica.* 2000;101 (6):444–51.

112. Walshaw PD, Gyulai L, Bauer M, et al. Adjunctive thyroid hormone treatment in rapid cycling bipolar disorder: a double-blind placebo-controlled trial of levothyroxine (L-T(4)) and triiodothyronine (T(3)). *Bipolar Disorders* 2018;20(7):594–603.

113. Patel RS, Bachu A, Youssef NA. Combination of lithium and electroconvulsive therapy (ECT) is associated with higher odds of delirium and cognitive problems in a large national sample across the United States. *Brain Stimulation* 2020;13 (1):15–9.

114. McKnight RF, Adida M, Budge K, et al. Lithium toxicity profile: a systematic review and meta-analysis. *The Lancet* 2012;379(9817):721–8.

115. Pahwa M, Joseph B, Nunez NA, et al. Long-term lithium therapy and risk of chronic kidney disease in bipolar disorder: a historical cohort study. *Bipolar Disorders.* 2021;23(7):715–23.

116. Schoretsanitis G, de Filippis R, Brady BM, et al. Prevalence of impaired kidney function in patients with long-term lithium treatment: a systematic review and meta-analysis. *Bipolar Disorder* 2021;24(3):264–74.

117. Aiff H, Attman P-O, Aurell M, et al. Effects of 10 to 30 years of lithium treatment on kidney function. *Journal of Psychopharmacology* 2015;29 (5):608–14.

118. Tyrer P, Alexander M, Regan A, et al. An extrapyramidal syndrome after lithium therapy. *The British Journal of Psychiatry* 1980;136(2):191–4.

119. Asnis G, Asnis D, Dunner D, et al. Cogwheel rigidity during chronic lithium therapy. *The American Journal of Psychiatry* 1979;136(9):1225–6.

120. Burdick KE, Millett CE, Russo M, et al. The association between lithium use and neurocognitive performance in patients with bipolar disorder. *Neuropsychopharmacology* 2020;45 (10):1743–9.

121. Schou M. Artistic productivity and lithium prophylaxis in manic-depressive illness. *The British Journal of Psychiatry* 1979;135(2):97–103.

122. Yaramala SR, McElroy SL, Geske J, et al. The impact of binge eating behavior on lithium-and quetiapine-associated changes in body weight, body mass index, and waist circumference during 6 months of treatment: findings from the bipolar CHOICE study. *Journal of Affective Disorders* 2020;266:772–81.

123. Mehta N, Vannozzi R. Lithium-induced electrocardiographic changes: a complete review. *Clinical Cardiology* 2017;40(12):1363–7.

124. Mitchell JE, Mackenzie TB. Cardiac effects of lithium therapy in man: a review. *The Journal of Clinical Psychiatry* 1982;43(2):47–51.

125. Meehan AD, Udumyan R, Kardell M, et al. Lithium-associated hypercalcemia: pathophysiology, prevalence, management. *World Journal of Surgery.* 2018;42(2):415–24.

126. Wang X, Zhu S, Jiang X, et al. Systemic administration of lithium improves distracted bone regeneration in rats. *Calcified Tissue International* 2015;96 (6):534–40.

127. Eduardo CdP, Simões A, de Freitas PM, et al. Dentin decalcification during lithium treatment: case report. *Special Care in Dentistry.* 2013;33(2):91–5.

128. Alevizos B, Gatzonis S, Anagnostara C. Myasthenia gravis disclosed by lithium carbonate. *The Journal of Neuropsychiatry and Clinical Neurosciences* 2006;18(3):427–9.

129. McAllister-Williams RH, Baldwin DS, Cantwell R, et al. British Association for Psychopharmacology consensus guidance on the use of psychotropic medication preconception, in pregnancy and postpartum 2017. *Journal of Psychopharmacology* 2017;31 (5):519–52.

130. Cohen LS, Sichel DA, Robertson LM, et al. Postpartum prophylaxis for women with bipolar disorder. *American Journal of Psychiatry* 1995;152 (11):1641–5.

131. Viguera AC, Nonacs R, Cohen LS, et al. Risk of recurrence of bipolar disorder in pregnant and nonpregnant women after discontinuing lithium maintenance. *American Journal of Psychiatry* 2000;157(2):179–84.

132. Cohen LS, Rosenbaum JF. Psychotropic drug use during pregnancy: weighing the risks. *Journal of Clinical Psychiatry* 1998;59(2):18–28.

133. Smith S, Kocen R. A Creutzfeldt-Jakob like syndrome due to lithium toxicity. *Journal of Neurology, Neurosurgery & Psychiatry* 1988;51(1):120–3.

134. Hansen HE, Amdisen A. Lithium intoxication: report of 23 cases and review of 100 cases from the literature. *QJM: An International Journal of Medicine* 1978;47(2):123–44.

135. West AP, Meltzer HY. Paradoxical lithium neurotoxicity: a report of five cases and a hypothesis about risk for neurotoxicity. *The American Journal of Psychiatry* 1979;136(7):936–6.

136. Schou M. Long-lasting neurological sequelae after lithium intoxication. *Acta Psychiatrica Scandinavica* 1984;70 (6):594–602.

137. Sellers J, Tyrer P, Whiteley A, et al. Neurotoxic effects of lithium with delayed rise in serum lithium levels. *The British Journal of Psychiatry* 1982;140 (6):623–5.

138. Black DW, Winokur G, Nasrallah A. Treatment of mania: a naturalistic study of electroconvulsive therapy versus lithium in 438 patients. *The Journal of Clinical Psychiatry* 1987;48(4): 132–9.

139. Sikdar S, Kulhara P, Avasthi A, et al. Combined chlorpromazine and electroconvulsive therapy in mania. *The British Journal of Psychiatry* 1994; 164(6):806–10.

140. Schoeyen HK, Kessler U, Andreassen OA, et al. Treatment-resistant bipolar depression: a randomized controlled trial of electroconvulsive therapy versus algorithm-based pharmacological treatment. *American Journal of Psychiatry* 2015;172(1):41–51.

141. Bahji A, Hawken ER, Sepehry AA, et al. ECT beyond unipolar major depression: systematic review and meta-analysis of electroconvulsive therapy in bipolar depression. *Acta Psychiatrica Scandinavica* 2019;139(3):214–26.

142. Konstantinou G, Hui J, Ortiz A, et al. Repetitive transcranial magnetic stimulation (rTMS) in bipolar disorder: a systematic review. *Bipolar Disorders* 2022;24(1):10–26.

143. Aaronson ST, Sears P, Ruvuna F, et al. A 5-year observational study of patients with treatment-resistant depression treated with vagus nerve stimulation or treatment as usual: comparison of response, remission, and suicidality. *American Journal of Psychiatry* 2017;174(7):640–8.

144. McAllister-Williams RH, Sousa S, Kumar A, et al. The effects of vagus nerve stimulation on the course and outcomes of patients with bipolar disorder in a treatment-resistant depressive episode: a 5-year prospective registry. *International Journal of Bipolar Disorders* 2020;8 (1):13.

145. Aaronson ST, Goldwaser EL, Kutzer DJ, et al. Vagus nerve stimulation in patients receiving maintenance therapy with electroconvulsive therapy: a series of 10 cases. *Journal of ECT* 2021;37 (2):84–7.

146. Graat I, van Rooijen G, Mocking R, et al. Is deep brain stimulation effective and safe for patients with obsessive compulsive disorder and comorbid bipolar disorder? *Journal of Affective Disorders.* 2020;264:69–75.

Bipolar Disorder

Treatment, Psychological, Social and Physical Health Approaches

Richard Morriss

Summary

This chapter will cover psychosocial and physical health approaches to the management of bipolar disorder. These include psychosocial and physical health approaches to the condition that should be offered by every psychiatrist, as well as specialist psychological treatments delivered by psychological therapists. The approach outlined here is supported by the National Institute for Care Excellence (NICE) in its 2014 clinical guideline for bipolar disorder[1] and other clinical guidelines for bipolar disorder more recently published from Canada, Australia and New Zealand. Overall, the current best standard of practice for bipolar disorder is to adopt a collaborative proactive holistic approach, attending to both mental health and physical health stability without the use of unnecessarily high doses of medication, particularly when they may impact on physical health. It should be consistent with the life goals and wishes of the person with bipolar disorder, convey a message of hope, and consider lifestyle and cognitive factors alongside symptoms and function. Bipolar disorder is a long-term condition where there is a potential for a normal function and a high quality of life for many. A psychologically informed approach to management enables people with bipolar disorder to be proactive in their care, practice self-management and do their best across all outcomes. Lifestyle factors such as keeping regular routines, healthy sleep, exercise, substance use and diet may play a big role in the stability of bipolar disorder and overall health. There are now a number of specific psychological therapies that may contribute to stability in bipolar disorder and a proactive, self-management approach to treatment. It is likely that digital monitoring and treatment delivery will enhance such care. Since the vast majority of people with bipolar disorder also have other forms of mental health, neurodevelopmental and physical comorbidity, then the management of each of these is just as important as the bipolar disorder itself.

Historical Development of Psychosocial Approaches to Bipolar Disorder

Before the 1980s, the mainstream view of psychiatrists was that bipolar disorder was primarily a genetic condition that would only respond to medication such as lithium, antidepressants and antipsychotic drugs, or physical treatments such as electroconvulsive therapy.

However, in the 1980s, people with bipolar disorder organised themselves into third-sector organisations providing psychological and pragmatic support as well as promoting holistic care and often also psychosocial interventions (e.g. Bipolar UK, which has branches in nearly every town or city in the United Kingdom plus a substantial online presence).

At the same time, there was a growing literature from psychology and sociology suggesting that psychosocial factors such as life events (both negative and positive goal attainment) might be associated with the onset of bipolar disorder and its course.

In the 1980s, psychological treatments focused on promoting concordance with medication, particularly lithium.

Starting with Perry et al. (1999),[2] many randomised controlled trials (RCTs) have shown the benefits of psychological treatment beyond concordance with medication, further cementing the importance of psychosocial factors in determining prognosis and outcome.

A Collaborative Recovery Focused Approach

Bipolar disorder has an onset usually in adolescence or early adulthood and tends to last for most of the rest of a person's adult life.

For most people, it is a relapsing-remitting condition, with periods of being quite well with the ability to function fully or near fully in almost aspects of their life punctuated with regular disruptive and sometimes life-threatening episodes of illness, either mania or depression.

Therefore, a person with bipolar disorder should be encouraged to live positively with this disability, making their own life choices with an understanding of how to do this in a way that does not lead to worsening their mental or physical health.

In order to do so, people with bipolar disorder usually benefit from gaining an understanding of bipolar disorder and how it affects them in their life context. In the United Kingdom – and now under similar legislation in most other legal jurisdictions – the Mental Capacity Act[3] allows people with bipolar disorder to make advance decisions about their welfare, treatment and those who are told about their illness or can act on behalf of them if they lose their mental capacity to make such decisions (e.g. in severe mania and depression).

However, under this legislation, people also have the right to make unwise decisions or not to take a responsible approach as long as that does not have a severe impact on other people. Interpretation of the latter can be challenging at times in clinical situations.

For these reasons, a positive proactive collaborative approach to care by the psychiatrist and the mental health team working with people with bipolar disorder is recommended.[1] Such an approach encourages hope, and a willingness to understand all psychosocial and biological factors are important not only to control symptoms but to improve social and occupational functioning as well as quality of life.

When asked, people with bipolar disorder point out that they have to live with the symptoms on most or many days so, for them, their ability to function well and their overall quality of life are a more important goal than being symptom or relapse free.

Determinants of social function and quality of life are not just symptoms and medication (benefits and side effects); a range of other psychosocial factors and physical health factors are important as well.

Sometimes, important therapeutic aims might include a reconsideration of life aims and goals to accommodate the underlying condition (e.g. negotiation with employers to avoid or manage shift work). Where possible, these might be seen as temporary and kept under review. In the past, psychiatrists have rightly been criticised for taking a very negative prognostic view such as suggesting that people give up their life goals and occupations completely.

People with bipolar disorder may progressively improve or decline in function. However, it is very difficult to predict with any certainty in any given individual what the prognosis might be beyond the short to medium term.

Given a proactive approach to care, many people with bipolar disorder achieve fulfilling lives, including almost complete recovery punctuated by brief periods of being unwell for a few days or weeks. However, such a prognosis is often hard-won through determination and persistence, by making incremental progress over time through learning by trial and error rather than achieved through a 'magic bullet' from treatment.[4]

A Holistic Approach

Even though the availability of psychological treatment for bipolar disorder in the United Kingdom and most countries remains patchy in implementation, modern approaches to the routine management of bipolar disorder need to be informed from a psychosocial perspective.[1]

A holistic approach does not ignore biological factors or drug approaches to treatment. However, a number of psychosocial factors have also been identified that may be relevant to understanding the development and progression of bipolar disorder or a particular individual's presentation.

Antecedent factors, such as childhood maltreatment,[5] may act as predisposing factors for developing the disorder.

Concurrent factors, such as social class, social support and self-esteem or variation in self-esteem, may act as course modifiers or as precipitants or relieving factors for episodes in established mood disorders.[6]

In the past, not only have the psychosocial needs of people with bipolar disorder been neglected, but there has also been little consideration of good physical health and lifestyle factors, which is also an essential feature of good holistic care.

There is excess and premature physical health mortality in bipolar disorder, particularly from cardiovascular and some respiratory causes.[7] Although much of the focus of such mortality has been related to medication such as antipsychotic drugs and lithium, the paradox is that the highest cardiovascular and overall mortality rates are among people who are not treated or have poor adherence to drug treatment.

A growing realisation is that bipolar disorder is rarely the sole clinical condition. Over 75 per cent of people with bipolar disorder have at least one other mental health condition.[8] However, many will have a physical comorbidity as well, with an increased prevalence of all physical health conditions except possibly cancer.[9]

People with bipolar disorder may have cognitive impairment – particularly in executive function – and there is an increased incidence of dementia in later life.[9]

Therefore, good holistic care of bipolar disorder – including care that promotes good psychosocial function, good physical health and personalised life goals – needs to consider all of the person's mental and physical health comorbidity in the context of what might be achievable and what the person's wishes may be.

Developmental and Life Course Perspectives

The approach must also take a neurodevelopmental and ageing perspective.

The incidence of bipolar disorder increases from puberty to young adulthood. Onset at an earlier age is associated with a poor outcome, especially if there is also a history of childhood maltreatment.[5]

Presentations are often atypical with mixed affective and rapid cycling presentations, often with irritability as a presenting feature. Bipolar disorder also usually evolves from mild fluctuating mood episodes to more severe and frequent episodes.[10]

Impulse control and other neurodevelopmental disorders, such as ADHD[8] and autistic spectrum disorders, are common in children and young people, but these may persist into adulthood as well. Often, children and young person's services recognise comorbidities of bipolar disorder rather than the bipolar disorder itself.

Insecure adult attachment[11] or the experience of childhood and early adult trauma are found in the majority of people with bipolar disorder attending mental health services. It is not helpful nor accurate to portray all of these patients as having an emotionally unstable personality disorder, a term that should be confined to those patients who persistently have most or all of these features between bipolar episodes.

Such neurodevelopmental experience may profoundly affect trust, behaviour and communication needs, and until recently, these needs have not been adequately addressed. If these needs are not recognised, there may be lasting consequences for interpersonal, educational and occupational attainment.

With older age, there is a greater possibility of poor physical health, cognitive decline and social isolation, complicating management. However, many people with bipolar disorder learn to live with their condition effectively through life experience and support. As a result, bipolar disorder can present challenges for management but are not over-represented in older people.

Cultural and Family Approaches

A psychosocial approach must consider cultural issues such as stigma against mental health, which may be particularly high in South Asian or other non-white cultures.[12] A family-centred approach rather than a focus exclusively on the individual with bipolar disorder may help.

There may be particular problems with late presentation and misdiagnosis of bipolar disorder in black African or Caribbean ancestry cultures due to a variety of possible factors including but not confined to racial bias and stereotyping.[13]

In bipolar disorder, there may be multigenerational affected individuals. The relationship to other family members and the nature of their family experience of bipolar disorder may either delay or facilitate the presentation to mental health services and the diagnosis of bipolar disorder.

For some people with bipolar disorder, there may be a need to accommodate and work positively with spiritual, religious or existential considerations.

Psychosocial Stressors

Psychosocial stressors may play an important role in the aetiology, clinical presentation and exacerbation of acute episodes in bipolar disorder.

Prolonged psychosocial stressors during childhood – such as physical or emotional neglect or physical, emotional or sexual abuse – are associated with hypothalamic-pituitary-adrenal (HPA) axis dysfunction in later life, which may result in hypersensitivity to stress.

In future years, such dysregulation may predispose an individual to affective disturbance, which may be coupled with a genetic propensity to develop a more progressive increase in severity and sometimes more intense fluctuation in positive or negative affect than other people.

The term 'positive affect' is used rather than positive emotion, which has a broader definition – it includes joy and love that are not necessarily associated with mood states or mood disorders. Positive affect consists of not just euphoria and elation, but also increased drive and energy and an increase in the propensity to take risks with little incentive.

Negative affect does not just include depressed mood but all types of negative emotion such as anxiety, irritability, emotional aspects of fatigue and pain.

The build-up of positive and negative affect to the development of mania and depression episodes is shown schematically in Figure 4.2.1.[14] Associated with changes in affect are mood-related changes in cognition (appraisals of self, the outside world and the future), perception (e.g. of sound, colour, behaviour) and physiology (e.g. need for sleep), all of which have the potential to either increase or decrease levels of affect until these reach a threshold when an episode starts. The speed of this build-up is sometimes fast (over a few days) or can be much slower (building up over weeks and months).

Psychological approaches such as cognitive behaviour therapy or even the coping strategies promoted in psychoeducation or more behaviourally focused family interventions would typically involve trying to identify early signs of this build-up of positive or negative affect.

With the build-up of affect, coping strategies are employed. These might involve modifications in appraisals (e.g. recognition that extreme beliefs are a feature of the disorder and can be challenged), behavioural responses (e.g. to stay at home in the face of the urge to socialise more as positive affect increases), social context (e.g. spending less time with people being critical) or approaches that might modify physiology (e.g. medication that might induce sleep or reduce drive in the face of the build-up of positive affect).

As well as intervention studies that are reviewed later, there is evidence that persistent cognitive responses to appraisals are associated with either increased or decreased frequency of mood episodes in bipolar disorder – rumination about the build-up of positive affect distinguishes people with bipolar disorder from those with unipolar major depression, who tend to dampen such thoughts when they occur.

There are long-established theories such as kindling or behavioural sensitisation[15] suggesting that, over time, some people with bipolar disorder develop more frequent relapses into depression and mania, and these relapses are less and less precipitated by psychosocial stress. The tendency to relapse becomes autonomous.

However, critics have pointed out that a course of increasing relapses precipitated by less and less stress over time is not universal and that such observations may not apply in a large proportion of people with bipolar disorder.

On a practical basis, there is a need to establish patterns of relapse in relation to stressors from each person's life history rather than make assumptions about the underlying course of the condition.

In some people with established bipolar disorder, acutely stressful life situations or hostility or criticism in a family may trigger episodes. The degree of negative emotionality expressed by close family members (termed 'expressed

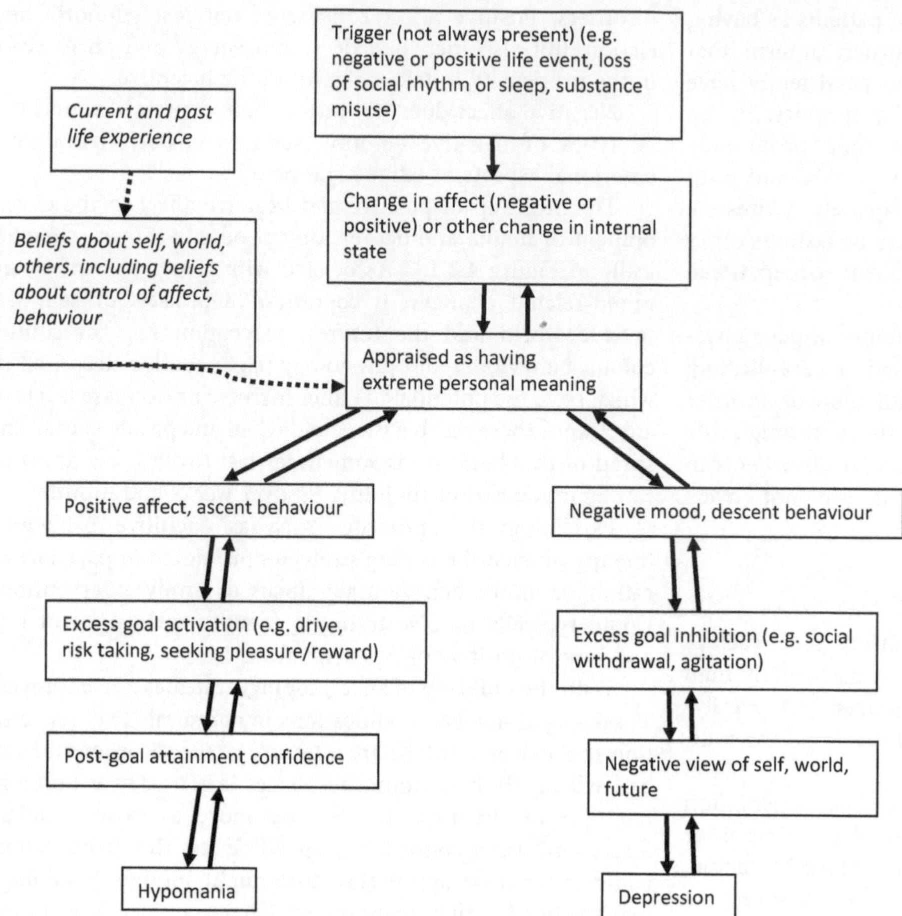

Figure 4.2.1 Cognitive behavioural model of factors leading to hypomania and depression relapse in bipolar disorder.

emotion') has been shown to predict future depressive episodes in patients with bipolar disorder[16] and levels of depressive and manic symptoms.[17]

Moreover, even if stressful life events play no direct role in the onset of mania or depression, they may have indirect effects such as disrupting sleep patterns or triggering a change in substance use, which in turn might lead to a mania or depression relapse.

In turn, the illness in itself is stressful and may contribute to negative life events (e.g. breakdown in relationships, loss of job), which may lead to further destabilisation, creating the possibility of a self-perpetuating cycle.

Traumatic experiences in childhood have been associated with an adverse course of bipolar disorder and the development of comorbid post-traumatic stress disorder (PTSD), borderline or emotionally unstable personality disorder, alcohol use disorders, anxiety or eating disorders in adult life.[5] All of these conditions have a higher prevalence with bipolar disorder than in the general population.

Compared to people with bipolar disorder without a history of traumatic events in childhood, people with bipolar disorder with a history of childhood trauma also have greater severity and frequency of mania and depression episodes, and they are more likely to have psychosis, rapid cycling and suicide attempts.[5] In bipolar disorder, psychotic symptoms following childhood trauma are often true mood congruent and mood incongruent psychotic features,[18] although there may also be dissociative experiences.

An uncomfortable truth is that rough or degrading treatment by mental health services can be seen as trauma capable of having similar effects on people with bipolar disorder as other trauma, as well as creating long-lasting mistrust of mental health services.

The diagnosis of bipolar disorder with all its implications can be a significant source of life stress for some people who have just received the diagnosis. They may need time and support to adjust to this news before they may be ready to embark on courses of management of the condition.

Other Types of Stressors

In addition to stressful and negative life events, other types of social stressors are related to the onset of mania-type episodes.

People with bipolar disorder often score high on sociotropy, a strong need for social acceptance and approval, compared to other patient groups.[19]

Positive life events related to goal attainment and especially the praise and social approval of that attainment is associated with the onset of episodes of mania-type episodes or mania symptoms, including drive and anger with increases in the behavioural activation system in subsequent days and weeks.[20,21] For instance, a person might become ill each time they receive a positive appraisal of their performance at work, so how this information is conveyed might have an important bearing on that employee's health.

As with all psychosocial factors, there is considerable heterogeneity between individuals so many people with bipolar disorder do not have sociotropy or a relationship between goal attainment and mania-type episodes. For some, goal attainment and other positive life events may help to relieve depression or give a short-term boost to self-esteem and confidence.

There is also a specific relationship between life stressors that may disrupt the early-morning routine of people with bipolar disorder and the onset of mania-type episodes. These may interplay with the behavioural activation system leading to increased drive.[22]

Approximately four hours before waking, the hypothalamus starts to prepare the body and mind for the day. There is a large release of stress hormones (e.g. around two-thirds of total daily cortisol, a peak of growth hormone release) from this time to up to four hours after waking time. These set the major circadian rhythms of the day, such as periods of alertness, hunger, energy and drive as well as even the ability to cope with unexpected injury, infection or stress. The hypothalamus computes the likely need for the day on the previous pattern of need in the previous four to seven days by monitoring a number of parameters, including the behaviour of the person in the last four to seven days. The hypothalamus monitors the time of waking and the routines followed, such as early-morning exercise and food intake, but does not monitor social factors, such as where the person is or who they are with.

Around two-thirds of people with bipolar disorder are sensitive to disruptions to daily early-morning routines from around four hours before waking to four hours after waking. Stressors in relation to early-morning routines such as shift working, travel across time zones or even early-morning travel – for work or to the hospital for an early appointment – or disruption in the home in the early hours might trigger mania-type episodes or periods of mood cycling within the subsequent eight weeks.

If such events are necessary, then some consideration might need to be given to travel plans (e.g. travel to a destination and stay overnight rather than travel in the early morning).

As in depression, there are seasonal effects on the onset of depression in the autumn and in the spring, but there is a relationship between the peak of summer and mania-type episodes in countries that are at some distance north or south of the equator.

The autumn peak in depression and the summer peak in mania are thought to be related to hours and intensity of light as well as possibly related factors such as ions, rather than heat. The reason for the spring peak in depression is less clear. Suicide attempts in bipolar disorder may also be related to the hours and intensity of light, although many interpersonal and other factors are also involved.

The only clinical approach that can be taken to determine if either positive life events, life events disrupting early-morning rhythms, or seasonal effects are relevant to an individual is through careful history taking in relation to such events and the onset of mania, depression or instability of mood.

Problem-solving approaches to addressing these issues can be helpful alongside other established management approaches for bipolar disorder.

Self-Esteem and Explanatory Style

Theories of the psychology of bipolar disorder have identified factors such as self-esteem and explanatory style that may contribute to mood symptoms.

The manic defence hypothesis explains the appearance of symptoms of mania as an attempt to avoid the negative and ego-destroying thought patterns associated with depression and anxiety. The ascent into feelings of omnipotence and triumph are thought to overcompensate for feelings of worthlessness and the underlying depression that are seen as the backdrop to the manic syndrome. This formulation suggests there is a degree of fragility to the manic state, and evidence of negative self-concept or thinking styles should be evident in both patients with mania and remitted patients. There is evidence that patients with bipolar disorder have a negative self-concept, highly variable self-esteem and increased drive, even during the remitted state with an absence of depressive symptoms.[19,23]

Moreover, self-esteem is a predictor of time to depressive or mania relapse even when treatment, sociodemographic, comorbidity and illness course are taken into account.[6]

One important difference between bipolar disorder and borderline personality disorder is that, in bipolar disorder, variability in self-esteem is not reflected in a lack of a sense of self identity as tends to occur in borderline personality disorder. People with bipolar disorder have a better developed sense of who they are and what they would like to strive for but may vary considerably in their sense of whether they can achieve what they wish and how it may turn out.

Overly optimistic or pessimistic beliefs about the consequences and controllability of the extremes of mood (depression and mania) may be associated with switching from depression to hypomania or the severity of depressive symptoms.[24]

Psychological theories of bipolar disorder may help observers understand some of the ideas and beliefs held by those suffering from mania and depression in everyday practice, as well as inform psychological treatments for bipolar disorder.

Early Warning Signs

Early detection of a mania-type (mania, hypomania, mixed affective episode) or depression episode in bipolar disorder is widely used by people as a self-management tool to remain

Table 4.2.1 Early warning signs (EWS) of relapse into mania and depression episodes in bipolar disorder

Feature	Mania	Depression
Content of EWS for each episode	Same	Same
Length of EWS	2–4 weeks before relapse	Variable before relapse
Difference of EWS from other inter-episode symptoms	Usually qualitatively different	Often an increase in severity, frequency and duration of existing inter-episode symptoms
Examples	Bright colours, decreased need for sleep, increased confidence, increased energy, great ideas that do not seem great 24 hours later	Dull colours and sounds, increased tiredness, lower confidence, increased rumination, intense anxiety, slow thinking, less interest in meeting people or usual hobbies

well. It is a strategy that has an empirical evidence base[2,25] and is promoted by third-sector organisations such as Bipolar UK.

Many people with bipolar disorder are fearful of relapses or at least recognise the need for proactive action. They may utilise a number of different methods to recognise early signs of relapse such as their use of their phone, sleep patterns, activity patterns and the use friends and family to judge when a relapse may be starting. There are also increasingly a range of digital tools such as apps or websites to enable the recognition of early warning signs, as well as face-to-face psychoeducation programmes in some NHS trusts and through the third sector such as Bipolar UK or privately.

Typically, if early warning symptoms of mania-type relapse or depression are detected, people with bipolar disorder will put in contingencies to either reduce the risk of escalation of symptoms to a full relapse or to mitigate any risk from their behaviour such as overspending, neglect of dependents, poor decision-making or suicide.

People with bipolar disorder may not tell their clinicians about such self-management approaches unless clinicians ask directly about them. Clinicians can play a role in improving the detection of early warning signs or improve the effectiveness of such strategies. Primary care clinicians are also keen to know about early warning signs and their management, and there is a NICE recommendation that such information is put into crisis plans and discharge letters to GPs.[1]

Often, mental health services and clinicians refer to early warning signs of relapse in care plans, but sometimes they are, in fact, describing signs of a severe established relapse – such as hallucinations – at which point it is too late to prevent a full episode. In this chapter, the term 'early warning signs' of bipolar disorder refers to changes in mood, thinking, perception or behaviour that indicate the early stages of an episode (Table 4.2.1).

Early warning signs typically occur within two to four weeks before a full mania-type episode or a few weeks to a few months before a depression episode. Early warning signs of mania-type episodes differ from those of early warning signs of depression in each individual. However, within each individual, they are consistent from mania episode to mania episode over a period of 10 years or more, however severe each episode is. They are also similar preceding each episode of depression within the same individual. However, they vary considerably between individuals with bipolar disorder.

Hence, each bipolar episode starts with a similar pattern of symptoms that is idiosyncratic and typical for that pole (mania type or depression) in each individual. Since there may be a variety of explanations or causes for any single early warning sign of mania or depression, a pattern of three or more early warning signs appearing together or close together in time is utilised.

Hence, a collection of such early warning signs of relapse into mania or depression is sometimes called 'relapse signatures'.

The term 'prodrome' is avoided since it is often used in relation to the build-up of symptoms and signs before the onset of a first episode of a mental health disorder.

Early warning signs can only be reliably identified through history taking among individuals who have had more than one episode of mania and more than one episode of depression.

Checklists of common early warning symptoms greatly improve the recognition of these early warning signs.[26]

Care has to be taken to distinguish early warning signs of mania-type episodes or depression from many other causes of inter-episode symptoms that may be present and have many other causes (e.g. partial remission from the last bipolar episode, comorbidity with another mental or physical disorder, side effects of medication, stress).

Relapse signatures can be helpful indicators to individuals themselves, family members, close friends or clinicians. They may be liberating to individuals and their families who may otherwise fear any change in mood, thinking or behaviour as an indicator of a forthcoming episode when most such changes have much more everyday causes.

Those people with bipolar disorder who are adept at recognising early warning symptoms and have contingencies in place are usually able to improve their function as well as taking on more risks with their life such as being prepared to take on a new job, role or go on holiday because they have a clear relapse plan that they can enact.

Many people with bipolar disorder place great store on identifying triggering life stressors or circadian or seasonal stressors that are associated with relapse. However, research tends to show that not all episodes of mania or depression are tiggered by such stressors, so recognition of early warning signs of mania-type episodes and depression are recommended alongside such stressors.

Positive Psychology, Resilience, Capability and Recovery

As well as an understanding of stressors to avoid or manage that may have a negative effect on mental health and early warning signs of relapse, there is a body of research indicating positive steps that people may take to improve their wellbeing and function.

It is important to recognise that mental wellbeing and function is more than the absence of symptoms and relapses and that to achieve personal recovery and wellbeing requires more than taking medication as a management plan.

Various studies have identified important characteristics of recovery including the maintenance of hope that there will be improvement, a sense of identity as a person separate from the conditions that the person suffers from, empowerment and the setting of personal goals.[27]

People who have achieved such recovery usually describe the process has a hard-won journey typically involving three or four approaches that they rely on and regularly utilise.[4]

Sometimes, patients who are challenging in the sense that they wish to take their own path rather than necessarily the one the clinician advises can make the most progress in the end if their empowerment can be channelled into taking the rights steps towards recovery.

Since bipolar disorder usually develops during adolescence or young adulthood, there are dangers that a person's identity and ability to set goals may be compromised, but it is also a basis for hope since people will change over time.

Recovery is also often a series of small incremental improvements in the personal understanding of their condition, in their confidence and in their function that sets up the possibility of further improvement.

Setbacks such as a further episode do not necessarily need to completely undo such progress, particularly if they are used as a basis for further understanding of their condition.

Therefore, it is more helpful to think of capability without a fixed ceiling or floor to personal recovery but as a set of realistic steps to a more complete personal recovery and fulfilment of life goals in the present and the future.

Another helpful concept is resilience – a sense of confidence based on experience of previous success of being able to find a way through setbacks and relapses. Resilience is obtained when a person is willing to take risk in their life to achieve life goals with contingencies to manage setbacks that are envisaged but also with the confidence that they will navigate their way through a relapse or a setback. It is not necessary to have a contingency for every possible setback. Thus, a relapse plan needs to be 'good enough' rather than perfect.

A key ingredient to interventions – such as psychoeducation – involving experts by experience or peer support schemes can be the instilment of hope into those with a more recent diagnosis by seeing examples of people with bipolar disorder living fulfilled lives.[28]

A further enabler for people with bipolar disorder to express their wishes is to use the Mental Capacity Act 2005[3] in England and Wales to establish advance directives in relation to not accepting some specific treatments that are binding on mental health services. Recently, in England and Wales, advance directives refusing treatment have become binding even when they are involuntarily detained. Other countries are increasingly likely to have similar legislation, although it is not universal and there may be important differences in what is permitted across different countries.

In England and Wales, people with bipolar disorder can also set up advance statements about their choices of which treatment to receive as well as who is to be informed about their welfare and can make decisions on their behalf if they are too unwell to make them, including welfare decisions about dependents (other than children, who are covered under separate legislation) and pets.

Since most people with bipolar disorder will wish to regain autonomy for their affairs as they recover from a bipolar episode, lasting or enduring power of attorney to enable another person to make choices on their behalf is rarely sought.

Neuropsychological Function

Research suggests that around a third of people diagnosed with bipolar disorder exhibit deficits in neuropsychological function independent of depression or mania symptoms, most often in executive function such as problems with attention, planning or working memory but also sometimes also in declarative memory.[29]

Such impairments in neuropsychological function may appear quite early in the course of bipolar disorder in some people, but in others, they develop later in the course of their illness, possibly as a result of multiple episodes of mania. There is some controversy whether neuropsychological deficits are present before the onset or diagnosis of bipolar disorder and to what extent they are progressive.[30]

The most common reason for deficits in neuropsychological function are the presence of persisting depression symptoms or episodes, unsuspected ADHD or autistic spectrum disorder, substance misuse, other mental comorbidity and the cognitive side effects of some medication used to treat bipolar disorder. Neuropsychological function can take up to one year to recover from a severe depression episode.

At present, we have no drug interventions that improve neuropsychological function, but there is some preliminary evidence that psychological interventions – such as cognitive or functional remediation – may improve some aspects of executive function with impacts on day-to-day life function.[31]

Advice on how to manage neuropsychological deficits so that they have less effect on function, such as concentrating for shorter periods with breaks in between, may also be important.

Mood Monitoring

Mood monitoring can be important, especially in younger people or those with atypical or complex presentations, to establish a diagnosis of bipolar disorder.

It can also help people with bipolar disorder to understand whether or not they have mania-type episodes so that they recognise the onset of these episodes.

Mood monitoring are especially useful in really complex mood cycling (e.g. cycling through the day, in relation to the menstrual cycle), for frequent relapses, to establish a relationship to substance use, in situations with high expressed emotion and criticisms, or to establish seasonal patterns.

Digital methods have enabled mood monitoring to become relatively easy to carry out. There are many apps available with a variety of digital completion tools such as validated rating scales or simple visual analogue rating on a weekly, daily or more frequent basis with summaries of mood ratings over time such as graphs, numerical presentations, colours charts or emojis to suit personal preference.

In some people, mood monitoring of depression symptoms might lead to negative rumination that in turn leads to a worsening of depression. In such people, mood monitoring is not recommended unless they are taught methods of challenging negative automatic thoughts that emerge during mood monitoring. Mood monitoring alone has been shown sometimes to reduce mania symptoms and improve function, with reflection on the mood monitoring.[32] It can also be used to reduced unnecessary routine outpatient visits and to target clinical contacts that occur when clinical decision-making is required.

Psychological Interventions for Bipolar Disorder

While there are still some authors who dispute the effectiveness of psychological treatments for bipolar disorder on the basis of methodological weaknesses in randomised controlled trials examining their effectiveness,[33] treatment guidelines around the world – including NICE[1] – accept that many types of psychological intervention now have an evidence basis demonstrating their effectiveness in bipolar disorder.

Moreover, there are now RCTs from every continent in the world demonstrating the effectiveness of psychological treatments – sometimes also backed by evidence from real-world observational studies.

Effective psychological interventions for bipolar disorder differ in their underlying theoretical basis (e.g. cognitive behaviour therapy, interpersonal therapy, psychoeducation), method of delivery (e.g. individual, group, family, digital), complexity requiring little training (e.g. psychoeducation) or a considerable amount of supervised training (e.g. cognitive behaviour therapy) and also the phase of the condition in which they should be used (e.g. depression or remission).[1]

There are no effective psychological treatments for people who have mania, although psychosocial interventions such as moving patients from a busy, noisy inpatient ward to one that is calmer may improve the severity of mania.[1]

Generally, randomised controlled trials comparing different modes of therapy for bipolar depression have shown no differences in outcome, and that they are all more effective than usual care.

There is a recognition that effective psychological treatments for bipolar depression or for secondary prevention of further relapse tend to have a number of techniques in common:[1]

- Education about bipolar disorder
- Mood charting by patient
- Problem solving to promote coping
- Regularity in sleep/wake cycle and morning routine
- Medication adherence
- Stress reduction (e.g. in the family)
- Early warning signs of relapse

Factors that determine the quality of psychological treatments in bipolar disorder are similar to those for other mental disorders, namely that the therapist is adequately trained, supervised and experienced in the therapy; that they keep to an established manualised form of therapy rather than practice an eclectic mixture of different approaches within the same therapy; and that there is a good trusting therapeutic alliance or relationship between patient and therapist.

Problems with the quality of the evidence from randomised controlled trials of psychological treatments for bipolar disorder are similar to those in other mental disorders as well such as the nature of the control group – inflated effect sizes with waiting list controls, poor standard of usual care when usual care is the control, blinding, quality of the therapy and its consistency from therapist to therapist. Also, many RCTs are small and may select participants who are mildly ill.

Most psychological interventions are studied in addition to usual care, but sometimes, usual pharmacological care might be suboptimal.

Psychological interventions tend to be more effective earlier in the illness course and in less complex cases without personality disorder or other comorbidity. Although, there are also examples of trials showing effectiveness in specific comorbidities with bipolar disorder such as people with bipolar disorder and harmful alcohol use or bipolar disorder and cardiovascular disease comorbidity or risk factors.

There is also more evidence of their benefit in bipolar I disorder (at least one episode of mania) with fewer participants in trials with bipolar II disorders (at least one hypomania and one depressive episode) and few trials limited to those with bipolar II disorder.

Whether a RCT demonstrates that a psychological treatment is effective may therefore be due to the case mix of participants, with a greater likelihood of showing the effectiveness of psychological treatments if there is a greater proportion earlier in the course of their illness and with less comorbidity with personality disorder.

However, there is also evidence of a similar effect with pharmacological and service delivery interventions as well, so these may be markers of overall treatment resistance rather than a specific reduced effectiveness of psychological interventions.

Psychoeducation

The simplest psychological interventions for bipolar disorder are individual, group and family psychoeducation. These can be delivered to people with bipolar disorder by staff after a relatively brief training, but nevertheless, there are still important competencies that the therapist should achieve.

The evidence demonstrating the effectiveness of group and family psychoeducation is more robust than for individual psychoeducation.[34,35] This does not necessarily mean that group or family psychoeducation are superior in effectiveness to individual psychoeducation.

The most thoroughly investigated intervention is the Barcelona group psychoeducation programme (Table 4.2.2), which delivered over 21 sessions added to usual care, where there is evidence of effectiveness in comparison with attention-delivered controls also meeting in groups added to usual care for two to five years.[28,36]

Table 4.2.2 Weekly topics of 21-week group psychoeducation course in modified Barcelona protocol

Session no.	Topic
1	Introduction to the group and defining bipolar disorder
2	What causes and triggers bipolar disorder
3	Symptoms 1: mania and hypomania
4	Symptoms 2: depression and mixed episodes
5	Evolution of bipolar disorder and the future
6	Treatment 1: mood stabilisers
7	Treatment 2: anti-manic drugs
8	Treatment 3: antidepressants
9	Pregnancy, genetic counselling and effects on families
10	Prescribed drugs and alternative therapies
11	Risks associated with treatment withdrawal
12	Alcohol, smoking, diet and street drugs
13	Early detection of mania and hypomania 1
14	Early detection of mania and hypomania 2
15	Early detection of depression and mixed episodes 1
16	Early detection of depression and mixed episodes 2
17	What to do when a new phase is detected
18	Regularity of habits
19	Stress-control techniques
20	Problem-solving strategies
21	Finalisation of stay well plan and closure

It is important to recognise that although the intervention is taught as a group, each person develops their own individual relapse prevention programme, and this entails reviewing their own history of relapses and factors (e.g. medication, psychosocial stress, substance use, sleep, disruption of routines and social rhythms) that might have contributed to them. There is a consideration of protective factors, life goals and early warning signs of relapse into mania and depression.

If expert patients are used as therapists, their role is often to share their own life chart and show how their own personal experience relates to the development of a relapse prevention plan. The involvement of health professionals as therapists encourages people with bipolar disorder to develop the confidence to discuss relapse prevention strategies and life goals rather than just accounts of symptoms and medication.[28]

The overall meta-analysis of RCTs show benefits of group psychoeducation on all types of bipolar episodes – including improved function, improved hope and proactive approaches to managing their illness – and the intervention is both cost-effective and cost-saving.[1]

The cost of the intervention is recouped if one in 15 participants spends less than seven days in the next two years as an inpatient or in one of the intensive community alternatives to admission.

RCTs tend to show benefits are greater in people who are earlier in the course of their illness (i.e. fewer than seven previous bipolar episodes or three previous admissions), particularly in terms of improvements in depression in one large UK trial.[28]

There is inconsistent evidence on the benefits of psychoeducation on symptoms and the adherence to medication.

Group processes may be important, not just in terms of efficiency but also in terms of the participants being able to relate to other people in the same position rather than feeling isolated, as well as spending time with positive role models of people living successfully with their condition.

Importantly, these benefits are confirmed by service evaluation studies in routine practice carried out in the UK and a number of other countries, especially across Europe. A national study from Sweden showed substantial improvements in terms of admissions to hospital, compulsory admission and mania and depression episodes but not in terms of self harm and suicidality.[37]

There are now a number of follow-up studies of four years or more showing that the benefits of psychoeducation are maintained without any evidence of any diminution of effect. If so, then the cost savings from such an approach may be vastly underestimated.

One RCT from Denmark of a service pathway that included a brief intervention for people admitted to an inpatient unit with bipolar disorder delivering clinical guideline medication and physical care and group psychoeducation cost two-thirds of what a community mental health team offering standard mental health care to a locality would typically cost in the UK NHS over six years.[38]

There is also robust evidence of the effectiveness of family psychoeducation, although most of these studies have been conducted in the United States.[34,35]

The content of such programmes is similar to other psychoeducation, but there is also attention paid to family communication and attitudes. These can be important since many people come from families with multiple affected individuals.

Individual psychoeducation has tended to involve shorter courses of psychoeducation focusing on particularly understanding the condition, promoting agency and hope, recognising early warning signs, and creating a relapse prevention plan with coping and risk reduction strategies tailored to each individual.[2] Shorter courses of individual or group psychoeducation retain participants in the psychological treatment better but may be less effective overall.[35]

There are fewer RCTs examining the effectiveness of individual psychoeducation. It is unclear whether individual psychoeducation is less effective per se; there is evidence that short courses of psychoeducation are ineffective, possibly because they do not give enough time for participants to emotionally and cognitive process the important change in approach to their illness from a reactive, clinician-driven approach to a proactive, self-management one, as well as understanding the various techniques and how they might be integrated in their overall life goals.

There is also some evidence for the effectiveness of psychoeducation for primary carers of people with bipolar disorder without the person with bipolar disorder being present or receiving psychoeducation directly.

There are also a number of digitally delivered psychoeducation programmes for bipolar disorder involving apps. On the whole, these have not shown greater benefit as compared to face-to-face programmes on relapses, although improvements are demonstrated in function and quality of life.[32] They may play an important role in maintaining well-being among patients who no longer access or infrequently access mental health services.

There are also culturally adapted approaches to psychoeducation for bipolar disorder designed for communities (e.g. South Asian) where mental health is more stigmatised and where consideration of the family may have greater priority on the needs of any given individual.[12]

Cognitive Behaviour Therapy

There are now a number of specific cognitive behaviour therapy (CBT) models of bipolar disorder that show important differences from CBT for unipolar depression. They address the role of positive affect, cognitions and behaviour (Figure 4.2.1).

Early studies of cognitive behaviour therapy for bipolar disorder tended to slightly modify the established Beckian approaches to CBT for depression. On the whole, these were not successful, especially with more severe and more complex disorders, where they seemed ineffective compared to usual care.

More recent CBT for bipolar disorder, whether for depression or to prevent relapse, that consider more specific models of positive affect, cognition and behaviour have been associated with more convincing evidence of clinically important effectiveness.[35] Like other psychological treatments, they are more effective earlier in the course of a bipolar illness.

Later trials have accommodated general developments in CBT such as mindfulness and compassion-based approaches. There is preliminary evidence that mindfulness CBT adapted for bipolar disorder may be effective, especially for bipolar depression.[39]

There are other interesting developments such as recovery-based CBT focusing on the recovery process as the primary focus of treatment and only incorporating approaches to manage symptoms of depression and mania if these block progress to recovery.[27] Such approaches merit further research.

Cognitive or Functional Remediation

Cognitive remediation or functional remediation has been developed with some success for people with non-affective psychosis.

There is a growing realisation that there are important impairments in function in people with bipolar disorder that are underpinned by deficits in neuropsychological impairment independent of mood or medication.

Cognitive remediation or functional remediation interventions have now been trialled in bipolar disorder versus usual care or group psychoeducation. It has been delivered in individual, group and digital formats with some benefits on function, quality of life and neuropsychological symptoms but with more limited effects on mood symptoms or mood episodes. Since these benefits are not robust and sometimes do not last,[31] they are currently subject to further research and evaluation.

Interpersonal and Social Rhythm Therapy (ISRT)

A psychological therapy that has been specifically developed for bipolar disorder is interpersonal and social rhythm therapy.

It is a hybrid approach taking evidence on social rhythms on mood symptoms and relapse in bipolar disorder and fusing it with the management of interpersonal problems found in unipolar depression that are effectively treated with interpersonal therapy. Interpersonal therapy for bipolar disorder has been adapted to address interpersonal issues that are common in bipolar disorder, particularly within relationships and in relation to communication.

There is some empirical evidence to support its effectiveness in reducing bipolar depression symptoms,[35] but it is a treatment that is not widely available outside some centres in North America.

Family Therapy and Prevention Programmes

As well as family psychoeducation, there are RCTs demonstrating the effectiveness of family-based therapies addressing stigma, expressed emotion and communication within families rather than having a focus on the bipolar disorder symptoms. These tend to show improvements in family communication and reductions in depression symptoms.[35]

There is also some preliminary evidence for digital or face-to-face interventions targeted at parents with bipolar disorder to improve the adjustment, behaviour and functioning of school-age children.[40] There is evidence that the children of parents with bipolar disorder may develop more childhood mental disorders and function less well than children with parents who do not have mental health problems. Such strategies may be important in preventing mental ill-health and promoting mental wellbeing in adults who had parents with bipolar disorder.

Some studies have focused on identifying which children at higher genetic risk of developing bipolar disorder or depression might show early signs of bipolar or unipolar relapse with a view to delaying or even preventing the onset of bipolar disorder or depression. While there are some promising early results from longitudinal observational studies, there is no robust evidence from intervention studies that the onset of bipolar disorder can be delayed or prevented.

Psychodynamic and Other Psychological Treatment Approaches

Despite the long-standing concept of the manic defence, which has some empirical evidence to support it in experimental psychology studies, there is no RCT evidence to support the use of psychodynamic therapy, cognitive analytic therapy or any similar therapy.

There is also no RCT evidence to support the effectiveness of counselling or supportive therapy, although in clinical practice, patients sometimes find such approaches helpful in terms of personally adjusting to the diagnosis of bipolar disorder. Sometimes this diagnosis is devastating to a young person, especially one from a background where mental ill-health is stigmatised or unrecognised or where there is family experience of the devastating consequences that bipolar disorder may have for some individuals and their family as a whole.

For these people, they need support to work through this adverse life event in a similar manner to the needs of people who receive other devastating news about their health and wellbeing.

It may be appropriate for the clinician to hold off medication or more active psychological treatment until the person recently diagnosed with bipolar disorder has received such help. They are likely to adhere badly to such medication, and some medications such as lithium and other mood stabilisers may be associated with more relapses in people who adhere intermittently to medication than they would have had without any medication.

Another common group of patients are people who require psychological treatments for comorbid mental disorders. Mental and physical comorbidity may be present in over 75 per cent of people with bipolar disorder.[8]

However, most practitioners of psychological treatment have had little clinical experience with bipolar disorder. Frequently, people with bipolar disorder who require psychological treatment for comorbid conditions such as PTSD, anxiety disorders, substance use disorders, eating disorders or obsessive-compulsive disorders are denied them because of the complexity of their mental disorder and perceptions of instability and increased risk.

Unfortunately, this comorbidity often generates high levels of negative affect and destabilises the bipolar disorder as well. The job of the clinician managing bipolar disorder is to prepare the person with bipolar disorder as best they can by trying to stabilise the bipolar disorder as much as possible, maybe treating the comorbidity with medication and non-psychological approaches as an interim measure and matching as best they can the needs of the patient to the psychological treatment resources that are available.

There is some evidence that adaptations of usual psychological approaches for trauma-induced psychopathology and substance use in people with bipolar disorder are effective in terms of reducing the adverse effects of trauma or substance misuse. There is little evidence that such approaches improve specific bipolar outcomes, but they may improve overall function and quality of life.

Physical Health Care

Bipolar disorder has been estimated to reduce healthy life by 12 years and total length of life by nine years. It is associated with a standardised mortality ratio of two for cardiovascular disease compared to age and gender matched controls, even when all risk factors for cardiovascular disease such as smoking, exercise, diet and alcohol are controlled for.[7]

Although people with bipolar disorder may have a standardised mortality ratio from suicide of 10–20, around half of the people with bipolar disorder will die from cardiovascular disease compared to around one-third of the general population. There is also an excess of early mortality from respiratory disease – particularly pulmonary embolus – renal disease and accidents. There may be a small excess of cancer deaths, but this association is disputed.

All physical illness, except possibly cancer, shows an increased prevalence in bipolar disorder.[9] Research shows that more minor physical illness that is unlikely to lead to death is also more common almost across the board in bipolar disorder compared to the general population.

Of particular note is that there is a four- or five-fold increase in migraines compared to the general population, and the prevalence of conditions such as irritable bowel syndrome and fibromyalgia is also inflated.

Endocrine disorders, particularly thyroid disease or even subclinical hypothyroidism (raised thyroid-stimulating hormone (TSH) but normal free T4 and free T3), can be associated with increased frequency of relapse and are an important cause of rapid cycling bipolar disorder.

An intriguing possibility is that some systemic inflammation from a physical health cause might precipitate or improve bipolar episodes but, at present, we have only a rudimentary understanding of such possibilities.

There are also complex relationships between bipolar disorder and common neurological disorders such as epilepsy and Parkinson's disease. These conditions or their underlying treatment may increase, decrease, modify or have no direct effect on the course of bipolar disorder, the effect varying from person to person. They require an individualised management plan given this complex prognosis.

Some treatments for physical disorders, particularly parenteral or oral corticosteroids, may precipitate bipolar disorder for the first time and precipitate bipolar episodes in established bipolar disorder. Alternatives to systemic corticosteroids (e.g. their topical use or steroid-sparing treatments) might play a role, especially if distress and poor function from bipolar disorder is more important than the underlying physical disorder.

It is important to review whether drug treatments for physical disorders might have precipitated or exacerbated the bipolar disorder. For instance, some antibiotics such as erythromycin may be associated with mania.

In some women, the initiation or sudden withdrawal of high doses of oestrogens or progesterone might precipitate bipolar episodes.

A similar issue can occur with the initiation or sudden withdrawal of prescribed or illicit opioid drugs in any person with bipolar disorder. These medications can have powerful direct or indirect effects on brain dopamine with possible implications for the onset of mania-type symptoms or mood cycling.

The reasons for the poor prognosis of bipolar disorder in terms of cardiovascular and other health conditions are complex.

Although many of the drugs used to manage bipolar disorder might lead to weight gain and poorer glycaemic control (e.g. antipsychotic drugs such as quetiapine and olanzapine) or the potential for decline in renal function (e.g. lithium), the risk of greater morbidity and mortality from poorer cardiovascular health is associated with poor concordance with medical and other therapies.

Since the association is not unique to bipolar disorder but is also seen in unipolar depression and non-affective psychosis, then it is possible that chaotic and unhealthy lifestyles contribute. It is thought that lifestyle factors contribute greatly to the onset of diabetes mellitus and overall poor cardiovascular health.

People with bipolar disorder have higher rates of smoking, alcohol (binge and non-binge) use disorders and other substance use disorders. Substance use may increase during mania with increased socialisation and risk taking and increase during depression episodes as a form of avoidance of negative affect and thinking.

Especially during depression episodes or persistent depression symptoms, which are three times as common as mania-type episodes and symptoms in bipolar disorder, resting metabolic rate and the energy expended in activity are reduced.

During depression, there is less motivation to cook healthy food so convenience food with high calorie and sugar content may be consumed. Even if the appetite is reduced, calorie and sugar content may be increased at a time of low energy expenditure, in which case weight gain is likely to occur.

Some people during depression episodes overeat or binge eat to relieve distress or sometimes as an act of self harm. Ensuing guilt and poor body image can further exacerbate depression symptoms.

There is evidence that people with mental health problems are less likely to receive timely health care or certain types of intervention for cardiovascular health or other physical health problems.

There may also be a range of underlying biological processes that contribute to the poor cardiovascular process. Although some are supported with evidence, the mechanisms are not fully understood or robustly tested.

The association of bipolar disorder and indeed other serious mental illness with increased mortality from cardiovascular disease means that all NHS organisations in England have to report the proportion of such patients who are receiving adequate monitoring of their cardiovascular health.[1]

The NICE Guideline for Bipolar Disorder[1] has made the following key recommendation for practice – mandatory in England – for people with bipolar disorder aged over 40 years whether or not they are taking medication:

- Monitor the physical health of people with bipolar disorder when monitoring is transferred from secondary care, and then at least annually
- The health check should be comprehensive and focus on cardiovascular disease, diabetes, obesity and respiratory disease
- A copy of the results should be sent to the care coordinator and GP and put in the secondary care records. The psychiatrist should check if GP has done this, and if not, the psychiatrist does this.

In England and Wales, primary care practitioners are incentivised to keep practice lists of people with serious mental illness (non-affective psychosis and bipolar disorder) and to perform an annual review. Recent audits have suggested around 85 per cent of people with bipolar disorder over the age of 40 years are offered such checks.

Table 4.2.3 National Institute for Care Excellence recommendations for physical health monitoring for people with bipolar disorder

• Weight or BMI, diet, nutritional status and level of physical activity
• Cardiovascular status, including pulse and blood pressure
• Metabolic status, including fasting blood glucose or glycosylated haemoglobin (HbA1c) and blood lipid profile
• Liver function
• Renal and thyroid function, and calcium levels, for people taking long-term lithium
• Primary care should keep a practice register or people with serious mental illness (including bipolar disorder)
• Secondary care should ensure adequate primary care monitoring and perform it if primary care has not completed physical health monitoring
• Healthy eating and physical activity programme provided by mental health care provider
• Treatment available for any physical health problem that is detected
• Annual audit and report on physical health monitoring and management to the board of any mental health provider

Many NHS mental health organisations have employed nurses to ensure that their mandatory obligation is fulfilled in people with bipolar disorder and often with all patients in continuing care of mental health services.

Recommendations for monitoring in the annual health checks for bipolar disorder are shown in Table 4.2.3.[1]

Key Learning Points

A collaborative, proactive and holistic approach to care with patients with bipolar disorder seems to promote effective self-management and overall optimal outcomes.

Management of lifestyle and overall physical health is required to address historical gaps in life expectancy due to twice the standardised mortality ratio from cardiovascular disease and elevated risk of all physical disease except possibly cancer.

People with bipolar disorder should receive an annual physical review of cardiovascular and other physical health factors, especially if they are over the age of 40 years, whether or not they are taking psychotropic medication (which may require additional monitoring).

In England and Wales, there are mandatory checks on mental health organisations to ensure that annual health checks are made in people with serious mental illness, including bipolar disorder.

Negative life events and high expressed emotion are associated with more frequent depression, especially early in the course of bipolar disorder.

Positive life events associated with goal attainment, high sociotropy and drive from activation of the behavioural activation system may lead to mania episodes and symptoms.

Low or variable self-esteem as well as life events leading to the disruption of the usual daily social rhythm may lead to mania or depression episodes.

Early warning symptoms of relapse into mania and depression are idiosyncratic to the individual and pole of illness; early recognition of these provide the opportunity for the person with bipolar disorder to intervene to prevent or lessen the severity and consequences of bipolar episodes.

Psychoeducation is effective, especially longer courses. The evidence base of effectiveness is more robust for group or family psychoeducation than individual or digital psychoeducation.

Specific cognitive behaviour therapy models of bipolar disorder are developed. Although there is evidence for the effectiveness of cognitive behaviour therapy to reduce depressive symptoms and prevent relapse, some still dispute that evidence.

People with bipolar disorder may show problems with executive function and declarative memory affecting daily function. Optimising treatment for depression and medication as well as cognitive or functional remediation therapy may help.

References

1. National Collaborating Centre for Mental Health. *Bipolar disorder: The NICE Guideline on the Assessment and Management of Bipolar Disorder in Adults, Children and Young People in Primary and Secondary Care. Updated Edition. CG185.* London: British Psychological Society and Gaskell; 2014.
2. Perry A, Tarrier N, Morriss R, et al. Randomised controlled trial of teaching bipolar disorder patients to identify early symptoms of relapse and obtain early treatment. *BMJ* 1999;318 (7177):149–53.
3. Ministry of Justice. *Mental Capacity Act.* London: Ministry of Justice; 2005.
4. Russell SJ, Browne JL. Staying well with bipolar disorder. *Australia and New Zealand Journal of Psychiatry* 2005;39 (3):187–93.
5. Agnew-Blais J, Danese A. Childhood maltreatment and unfavourable clinical outcomes in bipolar disorder: a systematic review and meta-analysis. *Lancet Psychiatry* 2016;3 (4):342–9.
6. Pavlickova H, Varese F, Turnbull O, et al. Symptom-specific self-referential cognitive processes in bipolar disorder: a longitudinal analysis. *Psychological Medicine* 2012;30:1–13.
7. Osby U, Brandt L, Correia N, et al. Excess mortality in bipolar and unipolar disorder in Sweden. *Archives of General Psychiatry* 2001;58(9):844–50.
8. Merikangas KR, Jin R, He J-P, et al. Prevalence and correlates of bipolar spectrum disorder in the World Mental Health Survey Initiative. *Archives of General Psychiatry* 2011;68 (3):241–51.
9. Kessing LV, Ziersen SC, Andersen PK, et al. A nation-wide population-based longitudinal study mapping physical diseases in patients with bipolar disorder and their siblings. *Journal of Affective Disorders* 2021;282:18–25.
10. Howes OD, Lim S, Theologos G, et al. A comprehensive review and model of putative prodromal features of bipolar

affective disorder. *Psychological Medicine* 2011;41(8): 1567–77.

11. Morriss RK, van der Gucht E, Lancaster G, et al. Adult attachment in bipolar 1 disorder. *Psychology and Psychotherapy* 2009;82(Pt 3):267–77.
12. Husain MI, Chaudhry IB, Rahman RR, et al. Pilot study of a culturally adapted psychoeducation (CaPE) intervention for bipolar disorder in Pakistan. *International Journal of Bipolar Disorders* 2017;5(1):3.
13. Akinhanmi MO, Biernacka JM, Strakowski SM, et al. Racial disparities in bipolar disorder treatment and research: a call to action. *Bipolar Disorders* 2018;20(6):506–14.
14. Mansell W, Morrison AP, Reid G, et al. The interpretation of, and responses to, changes in internal states: an integrative cognitive model of mood swings and bipolar disorders. *Behavioural and Cognitive Psychotherapy* 2007;35(5): 515–39.
15. Post RM. The kindling/sensitization model and early life stress. *Current Topics in Behavioral Neuroscience* 2021;48:255–75.
16. Yan LJ, Hammen C, Cohen AN, et al. Expressed emotion versus relationship quality variables in the prediction of recurrence in bipolar patients. *Journal of Affective Disorders.* 2004;83(2–3):199–206.
17. Miklowitz DJ, Wisniewski SR, Miyahara S, et al. Perceived criticism from family members as a predictor of the one-year course of bipolar disorder. *Psychiatry Research* 2005;136(2–3):101–11.
18. Hammersley P, Dias A, Todd G, et al. Childhood trauma and hallucinations in bipolar disorder: a preliminary investigation. *British Journal of Psychiatry* 2003;182:543–47.
19. Van der Gucht E, Morriss R, Lancaster G, et al. Psychological processes in bipolar affective disorder: negative cognitive style and reward processing. *British Journal of Psychiatry* 2009;194 (2):146–51.
20. Johnson SL, Cueller AK, Ruggero C, et al. Life events as predictors of mania and depression in bipolar I disorder. *Journal of Abnormal Psychology* 2008;117(2):268–77.
21. Johnson SL, Edge MD, Holmes MK, et al. The behavioral activation system and mania. *Annual Review of Clinical Psychology* 2012;8:243–67.
22. Boland EM, Stange JP, Labelle DR, et al. Affective disruption from social rhythm and behavioral approach system (BAS) sensitivities: a test of the integration of the social zeitgeber and BAS theories of bipolar disorder. *Clinical Psychological Science* 2016;4(3):418–32.
23. Lyon HM, Startup M, Bentall RP. Social cognition and the manic defense: attributions, selective attention, and self-schema in bipolar affective disorder. *Journal of Abnormal Psychology* 1999;108(2):273–82.
24. Banks FD, Lobban F, Fanshawe TR, et al. Associations between circadian rhythm instability, appraisal style and mood in bipolar disorder. *Journal of Affective Disorders* 2016;203:166–175.
25. Jackson A, Cavanagh J, Scott J. A systematic review of manic and depressive prodromes. *Journal of Affective Disorder.* 2003;74(3):209–17.
26. Lobban F, Solis-Trapala I, Symes W, et al. Early warning signs checklists for relapse in bipolar depression and mania: utility, reliability and validity. *Journal of Affective Disorders* 2011;133 (3):413–22
27. Jones SH, Smith G, Mulligan LD, et al. Recovery-focused cognitive-behavioural therapy for recent-onset bipolar disorder: randomised controlled pilot trial. *British Journal of Psychiatry* 2015;206(1):58–66.
28. Morriss R, Lobban F, Riste L, et al. Clinical effectiveness and acceptability of structured group psychoeducation versus optimised unstructured peer support for patients with remitted bipolar disorder (PARADES): a pragmatic, multicentre, observer-blind, randomised controlled superiority trial. *Lancet Psychiatry.* 2016;3(11):1029–38.
29. Cotrena C, Damiani Branco L, Ponsoni A, et al. Executive functions and memory in bipolar disorders I and II: new insights from meta-analytic results. *Acta Psychiatrica Scandinavica* 2020;141:110–130.
30. Szmulewicz A, Valerio MP, Martino DJ. Longitudinal analysis of cognitive performances in recent-onset and late-life bipolar disorder: a systematic review and meta-analysis. *Bipolar Disorders* 2020;22(1):28–37.
31. Tamura JK, Carvalho IP, Leanna LMW, et al. Management of cognitive impairment in bipolar disorder: a systematic review of randomized controlled trials. *CNS Spectrums* 2021:1–22. DOI: 10.1017/S1092852921000092
32. Liu JY, Xu KK, Zhu GL, et al. Effects of smartphone-based interventions and monitoring on bipolar disorder: a systematic review and meta-analysis. *World Journal of Psychiatry* 2020;10 (11):272–85.
33. Jauhar S, McKenna PJ, Laws KR. NICE guidance on psychological treatments for bipolar disorder: searching for the evidence. *Lancet Psychiatry* 2016;3 (4):386–8.
34. Oud M, Mayo-Wilson E, Braidwood R, et al. Psychological interventions for adults with bipolar disorder: systematic review and meta-analysis. *British Journal of Psychiatry* 2016;208 (3):213–22.
35. Miklowitz DJ, Efthimiou O, Furukawa TA, et al. Adjunctive psychotherapy for bipolar disorder: a systematic review and component network meta-analysis. *JAMA Psychiatry* 2021;78(2):141–50.
36. Colom F, Vieta E, Sanchez-Moreno J, et al. Group psychoeducation for stabilised bipolar disorders: 5-year outcome of a randomised clinical trial. [Erratum appears in *British Journal of Psychiatry* 2009;194(6):571]. *British Journal of Psychiatry* 2009;194(3):260–5.
37. Joas E, Bäckman K, Karanti A, et al. Psychoeducation for bipolar disorder and risk of recurrence and hospitalization – a within-individual analysis using registry data. *Psychological Medicine* 2020;50:1043–49.
38. Kessing LV, Hansen HV, Hvenegaard A, et al. Treatment in a specialised out-patient mood disorder clinic v. standard out-patient treatment in the early course of bipolar disorder: randomised clinical trial. *British Journal of Psychiatry* 2013;202(3):212–9.
39. Xuan R, Li X, Qiao Y, et al. Mindfulness-based cognitive therapy for bipolar disorder: a systematic review and meta-analysis. *Psychiatry Research* 2020;290(5):113116.
40. Jones SH, Jovanoska J, Calam R, et al. Web-based integrated bipolar parenting intervention for parents with bipolar disorder: a randomised controlled pilot trial. *Journal of Child Psychology and Psychiatry* 2017;58(9):1033–41.

Further Reading

Alloy LB, Ng TH, Titone MK, et al. Circadian rhythm dysregulation in bipolar spectrum disorders. *Current Psychiatry Reports* 2017;19(4):21.

Gallagher P. Neuropsychology of Bipolar Disorder. *Current Topics in Behavioral Neuroscience* 2021;48:239–253.

Jones SH, Lobban F, Cooke, A. *Understanding Bipolar Disorder – Update.* Leicester: British Psychological Society; 2020.

Saraf G, Moazen-Zadeh E, Pinto JV, et al. Early intervention for people at high risk of developing bipolar disorder: a systematic review of clinical trials. *Lancet Psychiatry.* 2021;8:64–75.

Tremain H, Fletcher K, Scott J, et al. The influence of stage of illness on functional outcomes after psychological treatment in bipolar disorder: a systematic review. *Bipolar Disorder* 2020;22(7):666–92.

Chapter 5.1

Schizophrenia and Other Primary Psychoses

Clinical Features

Peter F. Liddle

Schizophrenia is a psychotic illness that erodes the ability to initiate and organise self-directed mental activity and to recognise oneself as the source of such activity. It can produce a diverse array of disturbances within the domains of thought, perception, affect and volition. Typically, the illness follows a course in which acute episodes of hallucinations, delusions and florid disorganisation of thought are superimposed upon more persistent and subtle disorders of the initiation and organisation of thought and behaviour. These persistent disorders can profoundly disrupt occupational activities and social relationships. However, the severity of persisting disorder varies greatly between cases.

The disorder we think of as schizophrenia is the archetypal exemplar of a spectrum of disorders that extends to schizoaffective disorder, delusional disorder and schizotypal disorder. While there have not been major changes in the specific diagnostic criteria for any of these specific disorders in the 11th edition of International Classification of Diseases, ICD-11,[1] nor the fifth edition of the *Diagnostic and Statistical Manual* of the American Psychiatric Association, DSM-5,[2] compared with the immediately preceding editions, a shift towards emphasis on regarding schizophrenia as one pole of a spectrum of psychotic disorders reflects an ongoing debate about the utility and validity of the concept of schizophrenia itself. Some authorities argue that it is time to abandon the concept of schizophrenia as the paradigm exemplar of psychotic illness.[3] We will therefore start with a brief discussion of the shift towards describing schizophrenia as part of a spectrum.

The Spectrum of Psychotic Disorders

Despite the enduring influence of Emil Kraepelin's subdivision of psychotic disorders into dementia praecox and manic-depressive insanity over a century ago,[4] a satisfactory framework for the classification of psychotic illnesses has remained elusive. The first challenge was the implication of progressive decline implied by the term 'dementia praecox'. This was partially addressed by Eugen Bleuler's recognition that progressive decline was not inevitable.[5] Bleuler renamed the illness 'schizophrenia', a name denoting the fragmentation of the mind. While Bleuler's concept of fundamental symptoms still implied a degree of persistence, he recognised variability in outcome. The second challenge was the difficulty of delineating a distinct boundary between schizophrenia and bipolar mood disorder. This overlap led Jacob Kasanin to introduce the concept of schizoaffective disorder.[6] In recent diagnostic manuals (e.g. ICD-11 and DSM-5), the Kraepelinian distinction between affective and non-affective psychosis has been maintained and the overlap dealt with by specifying operational criteria for the diagnosis of schizoaffective disorder.

In recent decades, evidence from several sources has provided a powerful impetus to place even greater emphasis on the concept of a spectrum of psychotic disorders, at least within the domain of the non-affective disorders. This evidence has arisen from epidemiological and clinical observations on the one hand and from molecular genetics and neuroscientific evidence on the other. One relevant epidemiological observation is that psychotic phenomena, including apparently genuine hallucinations, occur commonly in non-clinical samples of individuals who neither seek nor require mental health services.[7] Perhaps of even greater clinical importance is the observation that a noteworthy number of young people who seek support from mental health services exhibit attenuated psychotic symptoms. An appreciable proportion of these cases, typically 20 per cent, develop an overt psychotic illness within the following year. This has led to the establishment of early intervention services that provide clinical care for these 'at risk' individuals or for individuals in the very early stages of overt illness. Many clinicians argue that due to uncertainty in outcome at this early phase, it is difficult and probably not helpful to make a formal diagnosis of a specific psychosis according to conventional DSM or ICD criteria.[8]

Molecular genetics also supports the concept of a psychotic spectrum. More than 100 different genetic variations contribute to the risk of psychotic illness: some are specific for schizophrenia, others for bipolar mood disorder and yet others for both disorders.[9] This diversity of predisposing genetic risk factors, together with a multiplicity of social and environmental risk factors, implies that every individual with a psychotic disorder is unique. While assigning diagnostic labels based on clusters of clinical features that tend to occur together may have value in facilitating management decisions, the diversity of causal factors suggests that the underlying boundaries between diagnostic categories are likely to be indistinct.

Furthermore, evidence from neuroscience reveals that many of the neuronal abnormalities that are observed in mental disorders are not unique to a specific diagnosis. Increased pre-synaptic levels of dopamine are observed in both schizophrenia and psychotic bipolar disorder.[10] Structural brain abnormalities transcend diagnostic boundaries to an even greater extent. There is compelling evidence that a transdiagnostic psychopathological factor known as the p factor is associated with a diverse range of mental disorders.[11] The severity of the p factor is correlated with decreased thickness of the cerebral cortex, especially those regions of cortex engaged in higher mental functions.[12]

The evidence discussed in this section might be grounds for identifying a psychotic continuum that embraces schizophrenia, other non-affective psychoses and affective psychoses. Antipsychotics are at least partially effective in the treatment of an acute psychotic episode irrespective of whether it is in the setting of an affective or non-affective psychotic illness. However, from the point of view of both patients and professionals, in many cases of psychotic mood disorder, much of the therapeutic focus is on the management of mood symptoms. Hence, in both ICD-11 and DSM-5, affective psychotic disorders in which the abnormalities of mood predominate are classified as mood disorders. Nonetheless, in regard to non-affective psychotic illnesses, both diagnostic manuals recognise that schizophrenia is part of a spectrum. In both manuals, the schizophrenia spectrum extends to schizotypal disorder, characterised by schizophrenia-like symptoms that do not reach full psychotic intensity. In many instances, these attenuated psychotic symptoms might be described as prominent manifestation of features discernible in the general population.

The hallmark of the disorders in the schizophrenia spectrum is distortion of reality. This is manifest as delusions or hallucinations. The observation that the disorders embraced by this spectrum vary widely in their outcome might help reduce unhelpful therapeutic pessimism and stigma attached to psychotic illnesses. However, there is risk in focusing unduly on reality distortion as the hallmark of the psychotic spectrum. Many patients with psychotic illness continue to suffer substantial persisting disability despite effective treatment of their delusions and hallucinations. If we are to minimise the risk of persisting disability, we need to understand the processes that lead to persisting disability. We should not let undue focus on reality distortion distract attention from the core features of the classical concept of schizophrenia as it was described by Kraepelin and Bleuler.[13]

In this chapter, we will review key features in the historical origins of the concept of schizophrenia and also the criteria of diagnosis presented in ICD-11 and DSM-5. We will then present a comprehensive description of the clinical features of schizophrenia and provide a brief account of other disorders in the schizophrenia spectrum with a focus of what they contribute to the concept of the spectrum.

The Origins of the Concept

The concept of schizophrenia emerged in a complex manner from nineteenth-century attempts to describe the psychotic illnesses of young and middle adult life. Berrios and colleagues have provided a comprehensive account of the patchwork of concepts regarding psychotic illnesses that preceded Kraepelin's concept of dementia praecox.[14,15] In 1860, the French psychiatrist Bénédict Morel described a condition that he referred to as *demence precoce,* which had its onset in late adolescence with odd behaviour and self-neglect and a subsequent deterioration in mental function. However, the major developments that led to the concept of schizophrenia occurred in Germany – in the three decades that extended from Wilhelm Griesinger's formulation of the concept of a unitary psychosis in 1867 to Kraepelin's conclusion in 1896 that the two major types of psychotic disorder should be separated on the grounds of their tendency to differ in course.

A major figure of these three decades was Karl Kahlbaum. He described two chronic psychotic conditions: catatonia and hebephrenia. He is best known for his description of catatonia, a condition dominated by disturbances of voluntary motor activity. Kahlbaum emphasised the importance of evaluating not only the current symptoms but also the course of an illness. Catatonia runs a course that includes atonic or stuporous periods of underactivity and periods of excitement and overactivity. In some instances, it progresses to a demented state. Kahlbaum also emphasised the association between affective symptoms and catatonic motor symptoms, thus foreshadowing the notion that there are pathophysiological processes common to affective and non-affective psychoses. Kahlbaum's colleague Ewald Hecker provided the classic description of hebephrenia, a condition beginning in young adult life with 'silly' behaviour, inappropriate affect, disordered form of thought and fragmentary delusions.

Kahlbaum's ideas provided threads that Kraepelin drew together when he separated manic-depressive psychosis – which tends to be episodic, with the restoration of virtually normal mental function between episodes – from the chronic psychoses – hebephrenia and catatonia. He added a third chronic psychosis: dementia paranoides, characterised by delusions in a setting of deteriorating personality. He amalgamated these three chronic psychoses to form a single illness, which he named dementia praecox, in recognition of its tendency to begin in early adult life and its propensity to lead to a state of mental enfeeblement. In a later essay, he described the essential feature of this illness as[16]

> that destruction of conscious volition . . . which is manifest as loss of energy and drive, in disjointed volitional behaviour. This rudderless state leads to impulsive instinctual activity: there is no planned reflection which suppresses impulses as they arise or directs them into proper channels.

Although Kraepelin regarded impaired volition and loss of unity of mental processes as cardinal features of the illness, he also emphasised the prevalence of auditory hallucinations – especially in the acute phase.

The illness was renamed schizophrenia by Eugen Bleuler in 1911.[5] He wished to discard the name 'dementia praecox' because he recognised that many cases did not show progressive deterioration. He regarded fragmentation of mental functions as the hallmark of the illness and chose the name 'schizophrenia' to denote this fragmentation of mental activity. He specified a number of fundamental symptoms that he considered to be present in every case, including affective flattening, looseness of associations, ambivalence and autism. He assigned a special prominence to looseness of associations:

> Of the thousands of associative threads which guide our thinking, this disease seems to interrupt, quite haphazardly, sometimes such single threads, sometimes a whole group, and sometimes even large segments of them. In this way thinking becomes illogical and often bizarre. (Bleuler,[5] p.14)

He considered than many of the other symptoms arose from looseness of associations. Bleuler regarded hallucinations and delusions as accessory symptoms:

> Besides these specific permanent or fundamental symptoms we can find a host of other more accessory manifestations such as delusions, hallucinations or catatonic symptoms. The fundamental symptoms are characteristic of schizophrenia, while the accessory symptoms may also appear in other types of illness. (Bleuler,[5] p.13.)

To summarise: in the evolution of the concept of schizophrenia, the emphasis was initially on the fragmentation of mental functions and relatively enduring deficits. Delusions and hallucinations were recognised as concomitant of the disorder but were considered to be a transient, though potentially recurring, feature. However, as attempts were made to improve the reliability of diagnosis, delusions and hallucinations – especially those identified as 'first- rank symptoms' by Kurt Schneider[17] – assumed greater importance, and the emphasis shifted from the enduring deficits to the acute phases of the illness, during which delusions and hallucinations are usually prominent. This shift in emphasis was reinforced in the second half of the twentieth century by the development of pharmacological treatments that were relatively successful in alleviating the symptoms of the acute phase. However, these treatments do not cure the illness: the chronic deficits present a persisting challenge.

Current Diagnostic Criteria

The fifth edition of the Diagnostic and Statistical Manual (DSM) of the American Psychiatric Association, DSM-5, was published in May 2013.[2] As in preceding editions of the DSM since the third edition published in 1980, diagnosis in the fifth edition is based on operational criteria: sets of explicit criteria that should be satisfied to justify the diagnosis. Operational criteria facilitate agreement between clinicians regarding diagnosis. However, the distinctions between different conditions do not necessarily identify naturally occurring boundaries between discrete diseases. The evidence regarding the diverse genetic and environmental factors that contribute to the cause of the major mental disorders, with some of these causal factors contributing to several disorders, indicates that a degree of overlap in the underlying pathological mechanisms is an intrinsic feature of these disorders. The goal of employing operational criteria is to facilitate reliable classification of individuals into groups in a manner that is clinically useful.

The chapter of DSM-5 describing psychotic disorders is entitled 'The Schizophrenia Spectrum and Other Psychotic Disorders'. This chapter places schizophrenia within a spectrum of disorders that extends from schizophrenia to schizoaffective disorder, delusional disorder and schizotypal disorder. The spectrum also embraces brief psychotic disorder and schizophreniform disorder, as well as psychosis associated with substance use or medical conditions. The criteria for the disorders were proposed by the Psychosis Work Group, who analysed data from relevant field trials testing the proposed criteria over a period of several years preceding 2012.

The 11th edition of the World Health Organization (WHO) International Classification of Disease (ICD-11)[1] was approved by the World Health Assembly in May 2019. The transition from ICD-10 to ICD-11 for reporting health statistics began on January 1, 2022. Like DSM-5, ICD-11 specifies operational criteria for the diagnosis of mental disorders. The revision of the ICD was a broad international, multilingual, multi-disciplinary and participative process over a period of a decade, with the goal of providing clinically useful descriptions and diagnostic guidelines with global applicability. This goal included harmonisation with the DSM-5 as far as was feasible. The aim was to minimise arbitrary differences between ICD-11 and DSM-5, although justified conceptual differences were permitted. Some of the members of the DSM-5 Psychosis Work Group also served on the WHO Psychotic Disorders Working Group.

In ICD-11, the non-affective psychotic disorders are in a block entitled 'Schizophrenia and Other Primary Psychotic Disorders'. The term 'primary' implies that the psychotic disorder is not attributable to another identifiable cause such as a primary mood disorder, drug toxicity or a general medical condition. Mental disorders due to substance abuse or medical conditions are described elsewhere in ICD-11. However, the cross-linked framework for recording diagnosis does allow psychosis due to substance abuse or a general medical condition to also be recorded in the section on schizophrenia and other primary psychotic disorders. The other primary psychotic disorders include acute and transient psychotic disorder (ATPD), schizoaffective disorder, delusional disorder and schizotypal disorder.

Both ICD-11 and DSM-5 place schizophrenia within a spectrum of disorders that extends from schizophrenia to schizotypal disorder. Thus, both manuals reflect a hybrid description of the status of schizophrenia as a disease. On the one hand, the specific operational criteria describe schizophrenia as a distinct medical condition. On the other hand, the concept of the schizophrenia spectrum treats schizophrenia as one pole of a continuum that extend beyond psychotic disorders to non-psychotic schizotypal disorder, which itself is characterised by prominent expression of features that can be discerned in the non-clinical population. A hybrid description is potentially reasonable in a situation where categorical diagnosis based on explicit operational criteria provides useful practical guidance for decisions regarding management of the condition, while a description in relation to a spectrum might enhance understanding of the nature of the problem and encourage a degree of flexibility in approaches to clinical management.

In both ICD-11 and DSM-5, the special status for first-rank symptoms or other bizarre delusions was removed. In previous editions, only one such symptom was required for a diagnosis of schizophrenia; in the current editions, two or more from the specified set of characteristic symptoms must be present. Subtypes of schizophrenia have been replaced by 'symptom specifiers' in ICD-11 and 'dimensional assessments' in DSM-5. Catatonia is no longer a subtype of schizophrenia but is a specifier applicable to psychotic disorders, mood disorders and general medical disorders.

DSM-5 Schizophrenia

In outline, DSM-5 criteria demand the presence of two or more from a set of five characteristic symptoms, impaired social/occupational function, a duration of continuous disturbance for six months including one month of active characteristic symptoms, the exclusion of schizoaffective disorder and major mood disorder, and the exclusion of the direct physiological effects of a drug or a general medical condition.

In more detail, the criteria are[2]:

A. *Characteristic symptoms*: two (or more) of the following symptoms, each present for a significant portion of time during a one-month period (or less, if successfully treated):
   i. Delusions
   ii. Hallucinations
   iii. Disorganised speech (e.g. frequent derailment or incoherence)
   iv. Grossly disorganised or catatonic behaviour
   v. Negative symptoms (e.g. affective flattening, poverty of speech or avolition)

B. *Social/occupational dysfunction*: dysfunction is present for a significant portion of the time since the onset. Occupational function, interpersonal relations or self care has been markedly below the level prior to the onset (or in cases with onset in childhood or adolescence, expected level of interpersonal, academic or occupational function has not been achieved).

C. *Duration*: there have been continuous signs of disturbance for at least six months, including the characteristic symptoms specified in section A (i.e. active-phase symptoms) for at least one month (or less, if successfully treated). At other times in the six months, prodromal or residual symptoms are present, such as negative symptoms or attenuated forms of two or more of the other symptoms listed in section A.

D. *Schizoaffective and mood disorder exclusion*: schizoaffective disorder and mood disorder with psychotic features can be ruled out, either because no major depressive, manic, or mixed episodes have occurred concurrently with the active-phase symptoms or – if mood episodes have occurred – their total duration has been brief relative to the duration of the active and residual periods.

E. *Substance/general medical condition exclusion*: the disturbance cannot be attributed to the direct physiological effects of a substance (e.g. a drug of abuse, medication) or a general medical condition.

F. *Relationship to a pervasive developmental disorder*: if there is a history of autistic disorder or another pervasive developmental disorder, the additional diagnosis of schizophrenia is made only if delusions or hallucinations are prominent for at least a month (or less, if successfully treated).

Although subtypes of schizophrenia are not defined in DSM-5, particular clinical features can be specified as dimensional assessments. The dimensional assessments are hallucinations, delusions, disorganised course, abnormal psychomotor behaviour, negative symptoms, cognitive impairment, depression, and mania.

The course of illness can be specified as first episode, multi-episode or continuous, with a modifying designation as currently symptomatic, in partial remission or in full remission.

ICD-11 Schizophrenia

For schizophrenia, symptoms from at least two of the following seven symptom categories must be present for most of the time during a period of at least one month or longer. At least one of the symptoms must be from the one of the four categories of core symptoms (i-iv)[1]:

i. Persistent delusions of any kind
ii. Persistent hallucinations in any modality
iii. Thought disorder (disorganisation, such as tangentiality or loose associations), resulting in severe cases of incoherence or irrelevant speech, or neologisms
iv. Distortions of self-experience (e.g. thoughts are not generated by the subject but by an external force, up to the point of passivity, such as thought insertion or thought withdrawal)
v. Negative symptoms such as apathy and anhedonia, paucity of speech, and blunting of emotional expressions (not due to depression or to medication)

vi. Disorganised behaviour, including odd, eccentric, aimless and agitated activity
vii. Psychomotor disorders (e.g. excitement, posturing, waxy flexibility, negativism, mutism, stupor)

Disorders attributed to the direct physiological effects of drug toxicity or a general medical condition, and cases in which affective symptoms predominate, are excluded.

The one-month duration criterion specified in ICD-10 was retained in ICD-11, in contrast to the requirement of continuous disturbance extending for a period of six months specified in DSM-5. The WHO Working Group based their recommendation for retaining the one-month criterion on the evidence of the high stability of the ICD-10 diagnosis over time compared to the diagnosis based on the DSM criteria. Furthermore, in contrast to the DSM criteria, there is no requirement for the impairment of social or occupational function in ICD-11.

In ICD-11, symptom specifiers – corresponding to dimensional assessments in DSM-5 – can be added to provide further clinical detail. The symptom specifiers are positive symptoms, negative symptoms, depressive symptoms, manic symptoms, psychomotor symptoms and cognitive impairments.

The possibility of depressive and manic symptom specifiers allows for the observation that these mood symptoms are observed commonly in schizophrenia. However, if depressive or manic symptoms are predominant, a mood disorder diagnosis should be made. If the symptom criteria for schizophrenia and a mood disorder of at least moderate severity are met simultaneously or within a few days of each other for a period of one month, the diagnosis should be schizoaffective disorder.

As in DSM-5, the course of illness can be specified as first episode, multi-episode or continuous, with a modifying designation as currently symptomatic, in partial remission or in full remission.

The Phenomena of Schizophrenia

The Schneiderian First-Rank Symptoms

In his attempt to define a set of symptoms that might provide a reliable basis for the diagnosis of schizophrenia, Kurt Schneider identified a group of experiences that have become known as 'first-rank symptoms'.[17] Schneider was careful to emphasise that schizophrenia involves not merely first-rank symptoms but also more widespread changes in mental function: 'A psychotic phenomenon is not like a defective stone in an otherwise perfect mosaic' (p.95). First-rank symptoms are not unique to schizophrenia: they are reported in approximately 10–15% of patients with manic-depressive psychosis and in patients with overt organic brain conditions.

Because these symptoms do not have either high specificity for schizophrenia nor high value in predicting long-term outcome, they are not assigned special diagnostic significance in either the DSM-5 or ICD-11. Nonetheless, first-rank symptoms appear to reflect a disturbance of ownership of one's own thoughts, feeling and behaviour, which are crucial elements of a sense of self. They therefore warrant attention in an attempt to understand the nature of schizophrenia.

Schneider did not give explicit definitions of the first-rank symptoms, and clinicians have subsequently employed various definitions that differ in detail. Mellor formulated a set of strict definitions and reported that 72 per cent of people with schizophrenia exhibit at least one such symptom.[18] The following descriptions of first-rank symptoms are based on Mellor's definitions,[18] although illustrations from Schneider's account[17] are also given where possible.

Voices Commenting

This symptom describes patients hearing a voice describing their actions as they occur. The actions are often quite mundane; although, in some instances, a special significance might be suspected. Schneider (p.97) describes a woman with schizophrenia who heard a voice say, whenever she wanted to eat: 'Now she is eating; here she is munching again.'

Voices Discussing or Arguing

Patients experience hallucinations of voices that discuss them or argue about them, referring to them in the third person. Schneider (p.97) refers to a patient who experienced auditory hallucinations night and day, 'like a dialogue, one voice always arguing against the other'.

Audible Thoughts (Gedankenlautwerden; écho de la pensée)

This is the experience of hearing one's own thoughts aloud. One of Schneider's patients reported: 'I hear my own thoughts. I can hear them when everything is quiet.' Another complained: 'When I try to think, my head gets full of noise; it's as if my own brain were in an uproar with my thoughts' (p.97).

Thought Insertion

This is the experience that thoughts that are not one's own have been inserted into one's mind. It is not merely a matter of being influenced to think a particular thought: the essence of the symptom includes the experience that the thought is not one's own.

> A skilled shirt-maker knew how large the collars should be but when she proceeded to make them there were times when she could not calculate at all. This was not ordinary forgetting, she had to think thoughts she did not want to think, evil thoughts. She attributed all this to being hypnotised by a priest. (Schneider, p.101)

Thought Withdrawal

This is the experience that thoughts are removed by an alien influence. Schneider (p.100) gives as an example:

> A schizophrenic man stated that his thoughts were 'taken from me years ago by the parish council'. They had constantly robbed him of all his thoughts.

The experience that one's thinking has stopped, leaving a state in which all thought is absent (thought blocking), is less specific to schizophrenia and is not regarded as a first-rank symptom.

Thought Broadcast

This is the experience that one's thoughts are broadcast so that others might share them. Schneider (p.101) describes a female patient who was so convinced that the doctor knew exactly what she was thinking that she suggested that she would stop talking and he could just listen. The belief that others can read one's thoughts is not in itself a first-rank symptom: the essential feature is the experience that one's thoughts are in the public domain.

Made Will

The patient has an impulsion to act that is experienced as arising from an alien source. The impulse is usually so strong that it is acted upon. The execution of the action itself is not experienced as alien. Mellor (p.17) gives as an example of the account of a patient who had emptied a urine bottle over the dinner trolley: 'The sudden impulse came over me that I must do it. It was not my feeling; it came into me from the X-ray department.' Schneider (p.119) describes a patient who was unable to respond to suggestions because 'thousands and thousands of wills act against me'.

Made Acts

This is the experience of one's actions being executed by an external influence, such that one is a passive observer of one's own actions. Mellor (p.17) reports a patient who described his fingers moving to pick up objects:

> but I don't control them . . . I sit there watching them move, and they are quite independent, what they do is nothing to do with me. I am just a puppet . . . I am just a puppet who is manipulated by cosmic strings.

Made Affect

Here, affects are experienced as imposed by an alien influence. A young woman described by Mellor (p.17) complained:

> I cry, tears roll down my cheeks and I look unhappy, but inside I have a cold anger because they are using me in this way, and it is not me who is unhappy, but they are projecting unhappiness into my brain.

Somatic Passivity

This is the experience of alien influence over bodily functions. Mellor (p.18) specifies that there two essential components: a somatic experience – which is usually, but not always, hallucinatory – combined with a delusional belief in the alien origin of that experience. The experience is most commonly one of visceral function. He gives the example of a young man's experience:

> X-rays [enter] the back of my neck, where the skin tingles and feels warm; they pass down the back in a hot tingling strip about six inches wide to the waist. Then they disappear into the pelvis which feels numb and cold and solid like a block of ice. They stop me from getting an erection.

Delusional Perception

This describes the attribution of abnormal significance, usually with self-reference, to a genuine perception without any comprehensible rational or emotional justification. Delusional perception is sometimes preceded by a delusional atmosphere, a sense of oddness or strangeness. Mellor (p.18) describes a young Irishman who felt a sense of unease while at breakfast with a fellow lodger, as if something frightening was about to happen. When the lodger pushed the salt cellar towards him, he perceived the event and understood his companion's intentions correctly. However, he suddenly knew he must return home to greet the pope, who was visiting Ireland to see the young man's family and reward them 'because Our Lord is going to be born again of one of the women . . . and because of this they are all born with their private parts back to front'.

Hallucinations and Illusions

Hallucinations in any of the sensory modalities occur in schizophrenia, although auditory hallucinations are the most common. Most characteristic are the three types of auditory hallucination identified as Schneiderian first-rank symptoms: voices commenting, voices discussing or arguing, and hearing one's own thoughts aloud. Second-person auditory hallucinations are also common. In the International Pilot Study of Schizophrenia (IPSS), conducted by the World Health Organization,[19] hallucinations involving voices speaking to the patient were recorded in 65 per cent of cases of acute schizophrenia.

Often, the voices are harsh, critical or frightening, although occasionally they are a source of comfort. In contrast to the situation in affective psychosis, hallucinations in schizophrenia are often mood incongruent insofar as their content cannot readily be understood as a consequence of the patient's mood.

Sometimes, the patient assumes it is the voice of a neighbour. Such a belief can become incorporated into a more extensive system of delusional beliefs of persecution by the neighbour, together with hallucinations in other sensory modalities. A patient who attributed the voices to neighbours also reported smelling gas, which they believed the neighbours had piped into his house. Other patients attribute the hallucinatory voice to God or to organisations such as state intelligence services. The perceived source can be located within the patient's own body. Patients sometimes attribute their experience to a transmitter embedded in their brain, or in some other organ. For example, a young man maintained that a transmitter had been implanted in his teeth.

Behaviour such as whispering or looking around as if seeking the source of the voice can provide a clue to the presence of hallucinations. An elderly man repeatedly denied hearing voices but was observed at times to suffer distraction and then to engage in whispering. When asked about the content of his whispered conversations, he described a dialogue with strangers.

The strictest definition of a hallucination is the experience of a sensory perception not based on a sensory stimulus. While the hallucinations of schizophrenia usually satisfy this strict definition, some patients report hearing voices that are triggered by a sensory stimulus. For example, a sound, such as the noise of a distant car engine, can trigger the voices. A patient who was frequently observed to sit hunched with his head to one side, so that his right ear was buried in the shoulder pad of his jacket, admitted that this posture diminished the voices. In contrast, others obtain relief by focusing attention on their surroundings and actively processing environmental information.

When patients with schizophrenia relate their experiences of hearing voices during acute episodes of the illness, they usually describe the perceptions as having the same sensory quality as voices arising from real sources in the external world and heard through the ears. At this stage of the illness, it is not uncommon for patients to act on commands issued by the voices. In contrast, in the chronic stage of the illness, it is quite common for patients to describe voices that are recognised as arising from within their own minds. These experiences resemble pseudo-hallucinations, which are sensory perceptions in the absence of external stimuli that patients clearly recognise as morbid products of their own mind. However, usually patients with chronic schizophrenia who describe the voices as arising in their own mind nonetheless remain ambivalent about their source. Such hallucinations should be afforded less weight in the process of diagnosis, but they can be very intrusive into the patient's mental activities and should not be ignored in assessing the impact of the patient's condition on his or her life.

Olfactory hallucinations occur, as do other olfactory disorders, including disturbances of the affective connotations of smells. Sometimes patients become convinced that they themselves are giving off an unpleasant odour. Somatic hallucinations are common and are often associated with delusional interpretations. A man who experienced a strange sensation in his bowels was convinced that a snake had entered through his anus. Another described the experience of being cut with a knife by his parents. While this statement might well have been understood as an expression of his tense relationship with his parents, he was adamant that the experience was real, not merely a metaphor.

Although visual hallucinations are usually regarded as evidence of an overtly organic psychosis, such hallucinations are not uncommon in schizophrenia. Sometimes, the patients experience them as personal – intended only for themselves – yet they believe in their reality. A patient described the appearance of King George V and Queen Mary regularly at the ward entrance. Both were dressed in full coronation regalia. When asked why others could not see them, she replied, 'Because they have come to see me.'

Rarely, visual hallucinations occur at the onset of an acute episode of illness as a feature of a dream-like (oneiroid) state in which the patient is detached from reality. In this altered state of consciousness, complex vivid visual hallucinations can occur, as can visual illusions, in which perceptions of real stimuli are distorted. Objects can be surrounded by an aura, have either an unnatural intensity of colour or be muted and grey, be changed in shape, be reduced in size (micropsia) or be enlarged (macropsia). The patient might report the experience that the scene has been encountered before (déjà vu). These specific distortions of reality are not characteristic of schizophrenia, and unless they are accompanied by other clinical features more typical of schizophrenia, some other organic disorder of the brain should be suspected.

Delusions

Virtually all patients with schizophrenia suffer from delusions at some time in their illness, and a wide variety of types of delusions can occur. Delusions of persecution and of reference have little diagnostic specificity but are nonetheless common in schizophrenia. In the IPSS, ideas of reference were reported in 70 per cent of cases and suspiciousness in 66 per cent.[19] Patients commonly report that television programmes make special reference to them. Delusions of grandiose identity or grandiose ability also occur in schizophrenia, although they are more typical of mania. In contrast to the situation in mania, where grandiose thinking is associated with elated mood, grandiose delusions in schizophrenia are usually not congruent with mood. Similarly, nihilistic delusions, which entail a belief that a part or all of one's own body is non-functioning or even absent – which are characteristic of depressive psychosis – can occur as mood-incongruent delusions in schizophrenia. For example, a middle-aged man suffering from schizophrenia stated that his head was absent, but apart from accompanying agitation, his concurrent mental state betrayed no underlying feelings or thoughts that might account for this nihilistic delusion.

In schizophrenia, delusional beliefs are sometimes beyond understanding insofar as they arise suddenly and without any foundation in preceding mental processes or because they refer to fantastic events or circumstances that could not possibly occur. For example, a young woman suddenly knew, with total conviction, that she was a cat. She jumped from a high window and broke her back. It was not possible to elicit any mental precursor to this notion. Another young woman woke one morning filled with a sense of cosmic strangeness and power as if she could ride a bicycle (which she had never previously done). She then stabbed herself in the abdomen with a bread knife. However, after her recovery, she could give no explanation of why she had done this.

Delusions can be either fragmentary or part of a system of linked, relatively self-consistent delusions. The man who claimed his head was absent also reported that there was blood all over his face and showed no awareness of the contradiction implied by these statements. Another patient repeatedly referred to the fact that an axe had split his head but could give no explanation of how this had happened or what consequences it had produced. In contrast, a middle-aged woman, who had been experiencing auditory hallucinations and thought insertion for several months before a real burglary at her house, subsequently developed a relatively self-consistent persecutory delusional system based on the premise that the intelligence services were keeping her under surveillance and placing pressure on her by transmitting messages to her.

Patients with schizophrenia sometimes have delusional memories. These are accounts of fictitious events or circumstances that the patient is convinced he or she has experienced in the past. For example, a young man was convinced that, several years previously, he had had an operation in which his abdominal organs had been removed. He held tenaciously to this belief despite the absence of a surgical scar.

In acute episodes, patients often act in accordance with their delusions. In the more chronic phase of the illness, however, it is common to encounter 'double orientation', in which there is a dissociation of affect and behaviour from the implications of the delusion. A man who maintained he was the Duke of Hamilton – and from time to time referred casually to a family member named Liz (Queen Elizabeth II) – nonetheless accepted without demur his humble accommodation.

Disorders of the Form and Flow of Thought

Form of Thought

Despite many attempts to define and classify the disorders of the form of thought that occur in schizophrenia since Bleuler introduced the apt term 'loosening of associations' more than 100 years ago,[5] these disorders remain perhaps the most enigmatic of all schizophrenic phenomena. One of the problems lies in the sheer variety of manifestations of disordered form of thought, and it is difficult to tease out the essential elements. There are at least three distinguishable classes of formal thought disorder in schizophrenia, which tend to differ with regard to the phase of illness in which they are most prominent (see Table 5.1.1 for definitions of the various phenomena).

i. There are phenomena such as tangentiality, derailment, perseveration and distractibility, which appear to reflect instability of goal in thinking. This class of disorders is most prominent during acute exacerbations of the illness.

Case Example

A 48-year-old woman who suffered from a sustained florid schizophrenic illness reported having a telephone in her head. When she was asked what she heard on the telephone, she replied: 'Well, it's like meeting people and I [pause] have a jug of hot tea and relax therapy, relaxation, and I can speak to the sinus arrhythmia doctor.' Her reply begins in a slightly tangential manner and then becomes derailed. At times, she has difficulty in finding words. The term 'sinus arrhythmia doctor' appears to be an idiosyncratic use of words to describe a psychiatrist. At another point in the interview, in an attempt to delineate suspected ideas of reference, the interviewer asked: 'Has there been anything about you on the TV?' She replied: 'There's been the union jack and the hospital fire alarm and plastic surgery.' Interviewer: 'Did those things have anything to do with you?' Patient: 'The Boer war.' These replies illustrate marked tangentiality and derailment.

ii. There are idiosyncrasies of thought and language. These include idiosyncratic use of words, idiosyncratic ideas and

Table 5.1.1 Disorders of the form of thought (synonyms or variants in parentheses)

Category	Symptom	Definition
Unstable goal	Tangentiality	Responses that are off the point
	Derailment	Inappropriate shift to a loosely related or unrelated idea during flow of speech (asyndetic thought)
	Distractibility	Shift to an irrelevant idea triggered by an external stimulus
Idiosyncratic thought and language	Idiosyncratic word use	Normal words used in an inappropriate context (word approximations, metonyms) or non-words (neologisms)
	Idiosyncratic ideas	Unusual ideas that appear to reflect peculiar, personal concepts, or ideas expressed in an unusual manner that impedes comprehension
	Idiosyncratic logic	Reasoning that does not follow normal rules of logic
	Incoherence	Incomprehensible speech, apparently reflecting absent or idiosyncratic connections between words ('word salad')
Weakening of goal	Empty speech	Utterances lacking an identifiable goal and composed mainly of vacuous phrases of the type normally used merely to maintain flow of speech (poverty of content of speech)
	Generalisation	Speech lacks specificity and conveys little information because of over-generalisation
	Unelaborated ideas	Ideas lack normal development; speech contains few adjectives, adverbs or modifying clauses
	Perseveration	Unwarranted repetition of a previously expressed word or idea

idiosyncratic logic. The idiosyncrasies of logic do not usually involve a failure of strict, syllogistic logic. Rather, they appear to reflect unusual lines of thought that, at least in some instances, appear to reflect a private logic that ignores the common knowledge of the world that guides normal thinking. For example, the woman who was asked why only she could see King George and Queen Mary at the doorway and replied 'because they have come to see me' appeared to be following an internally consistent line of thought but ignoring common knowledge of the world. In the past, clinicians might have described this as autistic logic, but it is preferable to avoid that term because this type of thinking is not identical to that characteristic of childhood autism. Idiosyncrasies of thought and language can occur at any phase of the illness. In particular, these disorders are sometimes prominent among the residual symptoms that persist after the resolution of the acute phase of illness. They also occur relatively frequently in some first-degree relatives, which suggests that these disorders may be a marker for a schizophrenic trait.

Case Examples

When asked about a scene depicting a boat tied to a tree, a patient with persisting stable symptoms replied: 'I'd like to get in the boat, put in on the canal and row it away, 'cos there's a waistline there. The tree here is er . . . somebody . . . a man or a woman will come there . . . they'll sit down because that's there . . . they'll feel uneasy and they'll take it and burn it.' His reason for wanting to get in the boat reveals both idiosyncratic logic and idiosyncratic use of the word 'waistline'. The subsequent sentence exhibits derailment. When asked whether he meant that they would burn the boat he said: 'Yes, only for a person in the mind . . . you put that up there so it's a Van Gogh, you know, Christ knows. What the hell is the boat doing there, you know you give five million quid for it, he'd change his mind.' The reply begins tangentially and becomes derailed. As a result of the derailment, it is unclear to whom the pronoun 'he' refers. The phrase 'only for a person in the mind' is an idiosyncratically expressed idea whose meaning is difficult to discern.

The idiosyncrasy of thought and language can be quite subtle. When asked about his daily activities, a 37-year-old man with only slight evidence of residual schizophrenic symptoms replied: 'I look at walls and windows and that bothers my life.' In poetry, such a sentence might be accepted as legitimate. Indeed, his reply might be regarded as a poignant description of the impoverishment of life faced by many patients. However, when idiosyncrasy in everyday speech impedes communication substantially, it indicates pathological thought.

iii. There are disorders that appear to reflect weakening of the goal of thinking, such as empty speech, un-informative generalisations and lack of elaboration of ideas. Empty speech is characterised by utterances that begin without any identifiable goal and is dominated by vacuous phrases, of the type that are used from time to time in normal speech to maintain flow (e.g. 'you know').

Patients do not seem to be sure of what they are saying, thinking or perceiving. Empty speech is similar in concept to poverty of content of speech, in which the amount of information is relatively low in proportion to the number of words uttered. It is noteworthy that in a comparison of formal thought disorders in acute mania and schizophrenia, after adjusting for differences in cognitive scores, a greater level of poverty of content of speech in schizophrenia was the only aspect of formal thought that differed between the two diagnostic groups.[20] Weakening of goal may also give rise to perseveration, although it is probable that several different pathological processes can contribute to perseveration.

There are also some disorders that appear to reflect the co-incidence of two different classes of phenomena. For example, the combination of markedly unstable goal with idiosyncratic use of language generates incoherence and, in extreme cases, 'word salad' (verbigeration).

Of these three classes of formal thought disorder, idiosyncrasy of thought and language is perhaps the most specific to schizophrenia, although instances occur occasionally in manic speech. In contrast, instability of goal is commonly encountered in mania. Weakening of goal is not a feature of mania, but it can be a prominent feature of speech in a variety of chronic brain disorders other than schizophrenia. The co-existence of all three types of thought disorder is rarely encountered in any condition other than schizophrenia. It should, however, be noted that occasional instances of all three classes of formal thought disorder occur in the speech of normal individuals; it is the frequency of occurrence and degree of disorder that distinguishes the thought of people with schizophrenia.

Flow of Thought

There are also a variety of disorders of the flow of thought (see Table 5.1.2). During acute phases, the flow of thought can be accelerated, generating pressure of speech. When this is combined with unstable goal, the pattern of speech closely resembles that seen in mania. During any phase of schizophrenic illness – but especially in chronic illness – there can be an impoverishment or slowing of thought, leading to poverty of speech, which is manifest as lack of spontaneous speech and brevity of replies. Poverty of speech is illustrated in the

Table 5.1.2 Disorders of the flow of thought

Symptom	Definition
Poverty of speech	Decreased amount of speech: brief replies, lack of spontaneous speech
Pressure of speech	Excessive rate of speech
Blocking	Transient interruptions of speech during which the subject experiences absence of thought

following response of a chronic patient to an invitation to describe a depiction of an active dock-side scene with a gang of workmen unloading a barge, several buildings and a pensive lady looking over the parapet of a bridge at the water below, all illuminated by a bright sun: 'Reminds me of some ... um ... er ... sun ... er ... clouds and sun ... [long pause].... That's all.'

Poverty of speech, which refers to the flow of speech averaged over a period of several minutes or more, differs from the phenomenon of blocking, which is manifest as brief interruptions of speech during which the patient has the experience of having no thoughts at all. It is possible that this phenomenon is closely related to the experience of thought withdrawal, but it lacks the delusional attribution of alien influence.

Positive and Negative Thought Disorder

The various disorders of form and flow of thought can be grouped into two major divisions: positive thought disorder, comprising unstable goal, idiosyncrasy and pressure of speech, and negative thought disorder, comprising weakening of goal and poverty of speech.

Such a dichotomy is consistent with the overlap in the nature of unstable goal and idiosyncrasy insofar as both involve a tendency to make connections between words or ideas on the basis of incidental features. However, it scarcely does justice to the variety and temporal course of thought disorders in schizophrenia.

Assessment of Formal Thought Disorder

The clinical assessment of thought disorder is difficult because the expression of these disorders depends on the extent to which the patient is given the opportunity to exhibit spontaneity and to direct the flow of conversation. Thought disorder can be more overt when the patient is faced with an intellectually challenging task or when explaining delusional beliefs.

There are several useful rating scales for thought disorder, but none is fully satisfactory. Andreasen developed a widely used scale for disorders of thought, language and communication (the TLC scale),[21] that provides definitions of 23 items that can be rated with reasonable reliability in a clinical interview. However, the TLC scale is not sensitive to relatively subtle idiosyncratic uses of language. Holzman and colleagues constructed the Thought Disorder Index (TDI), which is more sensitive to these subtle idiosyncrasies of schizophrenic thought, and reported that these idiosyncrasies are more characteristic of schizophrenia.[22] However, the procedure devised by Holzman for assigning TDI scores involves assessment of thinking during the completion of both the Rorschach test and the verbal subtests of the Wechsler Adult Intelligence Scale, which makes it too cumbersome for use in the setting of a clinical interview. Kircher and colleagues developed the 30-item Thought and Language Disorder (TALD) scale, capturing the full variety of formal thought disorders, including both observable aspects of speech and subjective experiences.[23]

Several studies have demonstrated that features detected by the computerised assessment of speech samples in the early phase of psychotic illness can predict subsequent evolution of the illness. Mota and colleagues used an automated analysis based on graph theory to demonstrate that disorganisation in speech samples collected during the first clinical contact predicted severity of negative symptoms and a diagnosis of schizophrenia six months later.[24] Bedi and colleagues used the automated analysis of transcripts of interviews of young people exhibiting clinical features indicative of risk of psychosis to identify semantic and syntactic features predicting later psychosis onset.[25] They found that a reduction of semantic coherence and two syntactic markers of speech complexity predicted later psychosis development with 100 per cent accuracy, outperforming prediction based on clinical interviews.

Disorders of Affect

Although disorders of thinking and perception are the most distinctive features of schizophrenia, disorders of affect are also a major component of the condition. Affect can be blunted, incongruous, unstable, irritable, depressed or elevated. Blunted and incongruous affect are characteristic of schizophrenia. Depressed affect is nonetheless common.

Blunted Affect

Blunted affect has long been regarded as a cardinal feature of chronic schizophrenia, but it is also prevalent in acute schizophrenia. For example, in the IPSS, it was reported in 66 per cent of cases of acute schizophrenia.[19] It is manifest as a failure to express feelings either verbally or non-verbally, even when talking about issues that would normally be expected to engage the emotions. Expressive gestures are rare, and there is little animation in facial expression or in vocal inflection.

In some cases, objective evidence of affective blunting is accompanied by subjective awareness of loss of the ability to experience emotion. More commonly, the patient is unaware of having blunted emotions. However, friends and relatives often find the difficulty in establishing emotional contact with the patient a source of frustration and distress.

Incongruous Affect

The expression of affect can be markedly inconsistent with the circumstances. A patient may laugh in a hollow and meaningless way for no understandable reason. A shallow, fatuous affect similar to that arising from damage to the frontal lobes of the brain is more common.

Depression

Depression can occur during various phases of schizophrenia. Dysphoric mood is very common in the prodromal phases preceding a psychotic episode. Overt depression is often present during acute psychotic episodes. Knights and Hirsch found a wide range of depressive features in 65 per cent of a sample of patients with acute schizophrenia.[26] In general, this overt depression shows some evidence of diminution as the psychotic episode resolves, but it is also common to find depression persisting or becoming apparent in the months following an acute episode. Depression also occurs in the chronic, stable phase of the illness. The point prevalence in this phase lies between 15 and 25 per cent.

In both the acute and stable phases of the illness, depressed mood usually occurs as part of a syndrome of depression similar to that occurring in primary depressive illness. In particular, the depressed mood is likely to be accompanied by anhedonia and negative cognitions, such as low self-esteem, pessimism and hopelessness, as well as suicidal ideation. Suicide itself is not rare. However, in some instances, suicide in schizophrenia occurs when there is no significant evidence of depression, which suggests that factors such as delusional ideation, hallucinatory voices, idiosyncratic judgement and reduced impulse control can play a part. Biological features of depression such as disturbance of sleep and appetite also occur in association with depressed mood.

The observation that depression is a feature of virtually all phases of schizophrenia has prompted various proposals regarding the relationship between depression and schizophrenia. Some of the evidence suggests that a liability to depression is simply one aspect of the diathesis to schizophrenia. A psychological response to the implications of having schizophrenia may also be a factor in the pathogenesis of depression.

Anhedonia

Anhedonia, which is a loss of the ability to experience pleasure, can be a feature of depression in schizophrenia. It also occurs independently of depression, especially in the chronic phase of the illness, when it tends to be associated with flattened affect, poverty of thought and decreased volition. When it occurs as part of a depressive syndrome, it often comprises loss of the ability to experience satisfaction in achievement and also loss of consummatory pleasure. When associated with flattened affect, anhedonia usually entails loss of the pleasures of the hunt rather than of the feast.

Disorders of Volition

In schizophrenia, volition can be either weakened or disjointed.

Weakened Volition

Weakened volition is manifest as a lack of spontaneous motor activity; it is often accompanied by a lack of spontaneity in speech and affect. The patient is inclined to sit inertly in an armchair or to remain in bed throughout much of the day.

Case Example

A 63-year-old woman, who lived alone in a flat provided by the local authority after her discharge from the mental hospital several years previously, lay in bed throughout the day, despite attempts by the community nurse, occupational therapist and doctor to engage her in activity. Left to her own devices, she would eat only candy bars bought for her by a friend. Her flat became increasingly squalid, and her physical health was at risk. She was readmitted to the hospital compulsorily, and after a month of treatment, showed some marginal improvement in her level of activity. However, her cooperation was limited by resentment concerning her compulsory admission. After discharge, she returned to her former state.

Disjointed Volition

The patient can be overactive in an ill-directed manner. There is a reduced ability to withstand impulses to act.

Case Example

An intelligent and artistic young woman, who had been unable to re-establish either stable social relationships or regular occupation after her psychotic symptoms abated, lived alone in a poorly furnished rented room. One day, she felt cold, so she gathered together a pile of paper and lit a fire on the carpet beside her bed. Fortunately, she managed to extinguish it before serious damage was done, but the carpet was ruined. She understood the probable consequences of lighting the fire. It appeared that she had been unable to suppress the impulse to act despite the ability to appreciate the likely consequences.

Catatonia

Catatonia is a disturbance of voluntary motor activity and hence overlaps with the disorders of volition described earlier. Catatonia is reflected in abnormalities of the form of motor activity and in the amount of activity (either underactivity or overactivity). It should be noted that both ICD-11 and DSM-5 emphasise that catatonia occurs in a variety of mental disorders, including mood disorders and disorders arising from overt brain trauma.

At times, an apparently normal motor act is arrested in mid-flight. For example, a patient might become frozen in the act of reaching out for the door handle to open a door and stand with an arm extended for many minutes. Catatonic phenomena described in the early years of the twentieth century were often more dramatic in character. Patients were more commonly reported to exhibit flexibilitas cereus (waxy flexibility), a condition in which the patient adopted a posture that could be adjusted by an examiner, as if the patient were a passively deformable wax model. Catatonic underactivity can be manifest as an apparently stuporous state, but one in which consciousness is usually maintained.

A catatonic act can appear to reflect abnormal compliance with or resistance to cues for action, resulting in a movement or posture that is inappropriate to the circumstances. For example, the patient might mimic a movement made by the examiner (echopraxia). At times, it is as if the patient is continually changing his or her mind about whether or not to execute a socially appropriate action such as shaking hands on meeting, alternating between extending and withdrawing a hand. Such ambivalence when exhibited in the sphere of motor actions is known as ambitendence. Catatonic acts can also be negativistic, such as withdrawing the hand when the interviewer appropriately proffers a hand.

Case Example

The wife of a 42-year-old man who had a 14-year history of schizophrenia summoned an ambulance to the house because her husband had collapsed. The ambulance men found him inert on the floor, mute but with his eyes open. In an attempt to establish his level of consciousness, they first rubbed the skin over his sternum and then twisted a handful of the trapezius muscle. He did not respond. Several days later in hospital, when he had resumed a normal level of activity, he reported being fully aware of the ambulance men's attempts to elicit a response and was angry at the way they had treated him. He could not account for his failure to respond.

Catatonic overactivity takes the form of apparently pointless activity that is usually repetitive, such as walking rapidly around and around a table for a period of a half an hour or more. In at least some cases, an abrupt switch from a state of underactivity to overactivity can occur.

In the pre-treatment era, a primary catatonic presentation of schizophrenia was relatively common, occurring in up to 20 per cent of new cases. Today, a primary catatonic schizophrenic illness is relatively rare, whereas the syndrome of catatonia is not uncommon. Catatonia has a spectrum of symptoms, ranging from the classical features (e.g. stupor, automatic obedience, echo phenomena, ambitendency and mutism) to a variety of lesser-known symptoms, such as whispered or robotic speech, unexplained foreign accents, tip-toe walking, hopping, rituals and mannerisms.

Catatonia has a multiplicity of causes. Classically, it was linked to schizophrenia. In more recent series, though, up to 25 per cent of cases are associated with mania, and catatonic attacks can also occur during a depressive episode. Catatonia may also be a presenting feature of a wide variety of metabolic and neurological disorders, including tumours, and hence a new case of catatonia always merits a comprehensive medical, psychiatric and neurological assessment, including a brain scan.

Violent Behaviour

Violent behaviour is usually the product of an interaction between an individual and his or her surroundings. The type and frequency of violent behaviour in schizophrenia are strongly dependent on social circumstances. Occasionally, patients do perpetrate serious violence against others. Violence against the self, such as self mutilation or suicide, is more common. Minor physical violence against people or property and verbal aggression are common. Describing such violence as if it were purely a manifestation of schizophrenia is potentially misleading.

There are several aspects of the mental disturbances in schizophrenia that can contribute to violence. Delusional misinterpretations can generate fear or anger. Hallucinatory voices sometimes instruct the patient to carry out a violent act. Irritability can arise as a consequence of persistent, intrusive and unpleasant psychotic experiences or as a direct consequence of the disease process on the level of cerebral arousal. Disturbance of volition can diminish control over impulses that are recognised to be inappropriate. Lack of judgement can result in a faulty evaluation of the consequences of an act or of its ethical implications.

Aggression can be directed against members of the patient's family, against mental health professionals and occasionally against members of the general public. The family of those patients living at home and the nursing staff caring for patients in hospital are quite commonly the target of verbal aggression and minor physical violence. Serious violence driven by delusions or hallucinations, though much rarer, sometimes has a fatal outcome. Again, family and professionals are at greatest risk. Even matricide, an extremely rare crime, can occur in schizophrenia. Therefore, careful assessment of the risk of violence is an important aspect of the assessment of acutely disturbed patients.

Case Example

A patient who was, in general, considerate and gentle towards others developed grandiose and persecutory delusions, becoming irritable and aggressive. The police were summoned; when a policeman appeared at his front door, the patient shot him with a bolt from a crossbow. After conviction in court, he was detained in a secure unit for treatment under the Mental Health Act. The episode of acute disturbance settled, and he was eventually transferred to an unlocked ward. He once again resumed his characteristic gentle and considerate manner in most matters, but he continued to maintain that the policeman deserved to be shot and that he had been right to do it. In light of this evidence of limited insight and lack of judgement, he was very closely supervised following discharge to a group home under a Home Office restriction order. After he had been living in the group home for about a year, the community nurse noted that he was again becoming agitated. When the community nurse returned a few days later, the patient was suspicious and angry. An urgent psychiatric assessment confirmed that he was harbouring the delusional belief that the community nurse was part of a conspiracy against him. He was compelled to return to hospital immediately under the terms of the restriction order. The manager of the group home subsequently found a partially assembled crossbow in the patient's room.

Cognitive Impairment

Patients with schizophrenia often perform poorly in formal tests of cognitive function, although the patterns of impaired performance vary between cases. Cognitive impairment is of clinical importance because its severity is an indicator of social and occupational outcome. Both ICD-11 and DSM-5 allow the formulation of the diagnosis to include a symptom specifier denoting cognitive impairment.

Virtually all aspects of cognitive function have been reported to show impairment in at least some people with schizophrenia. The diversity of cognitive impairments that can occur suggests that some may arise from non-specific abnormalities of brain structure or function that have increased the person's susceptibility to schizophrenia but that are only incidentally related to the core pathophysiological processes. On the other hand, certain cognitive impairments are especially prevalent, raising the possibility that these have a more specific link to the core processes, as considered later. Impairments of executive functions (characteristic of the role of the frontal lobes), of memory functions (associated with both the frontal and temporal lobes) and of various aspects of attention are common.

Executive Function

Failure of executive functions is illustrated by the deficit in performance in word-generation tasks, in which the patient is asked to generate as many words as possible in a given category in a specified time. Some patients with schizophrenia, like those with Alzheimer's disease, tend to produce few words. However, unlike the situation in Alzheimer's disease, if the patient is asked to perform the same task on numerous occasions, many different words are generated in total, indicating that the store of words is intact: the problem lies in employing strategies to obtain access to the store.

Ability to change strategies in response to changing task demands is another aspect of executive function commonly impaired in schizophrenia. This can be demonstrated by tasks such as the Wisconsin Card Sorting Test, in which the participant is required to discover a rule governing the sorting of cards according to specific features and, when the rule is changed, to discover the new rule. People with schizophrenia, like individuals with frontal lobe lesions, tend to make incorrect perseverative responses.

Memory

Many aspects of memory function can be impaired, especially declarative memories (e.g. recall of events or stories, paired associate learning, visual recall of designs). In the verbal domain, it is typical to find a disproportionate impairment of recall compared with recognition. At least in cases that are not too chronic, the deficit in recall can be overcome by preparing the patients with strategies for organising the material to be recalled. This suggests that, even in the case of memory, some of the deficit lies in the domain of developing strategies for the task.

Attention

Among the attentional impairments observed in schizophrenia are impairment of both selective attention and the ability to sustain attention.

Selective attention involves the ability to attend to a specific aspect of a situation in the face of competition from other features that tend to intrude. The Stroop task, in which the participant is presented with colour names printed in inks that are not congruent with those colour names and required to name the colour of the ink, tests selective attention and also the ability to select a response. People with schizophrenia, especially those suffering disorganisation of thought, are generally less able to suppress the influence of the irrelevant colour name.

The ability to sustain attention (vigilance) is commonly assessed using the continuous performance test (CPT). In this test, the participant is presented with a long series of varying stimuli, including irrelevant stimuli and designated target stimuli, and is required to respond whenever a target stimulus appears. Again, people with schizophrenia, along with a substantial number of their first-degree relatives, perform poorly.

The Origin and Time Course of Cognitive Impairment

In studies of twins discordant for schizophrenia, the twin with the illness usually does worse on such tests than the unaffected twin, even though the affected twin's performance may be within the normal range.[27] This suggests that, even in cases where there is no marked cognitive impairment, the illness obstructs the realisation of potential cognitive ability. Furthermore, the cognitive impairments are associated with development of overt illness, not merely with the genetic predisposition to the illness. Nonetheless, there is evidence of some impairment – most notably in episodic memory – in the non-affected twins relative to healthy controls, implying that genes play some role.[27] Longitudinal studies of large cohorts reveal that cognitive impairments can be discerned from early childhood in individuals who subsequently develop schizophrenia.[28]

The evidence regarding the evolution of cognitive impairment once the illness is established is complex. In a minority of cases, there is progressive decline over many years, but in many cases, cognitive performance stabilises and may even improve. Nonetheless, cognitive impairments are usually more persistent than psychotic symptoms. Indeed, the persistence of cognitive impairments raises the possibility that these impairments reflect the core pathophysiological processes underlying the clinical features of the illness.[13]

At least minor degrees of cognitive impairment are common in schizophrenia and indeed appear to be associated with a predisposition to a diverse range of mental disorders.[11,12] However, studies employing cluster analysis identify a distinct group of cases of schizophrenia characterised by more marked cognitive impairment.[29] It is possible that this distinguishable group of cases correspond to cases of classical schizophrenia, characterised by impoverished and/or disorganised mental activity,[13] which we will discuss further in the section on subtypes of illness.

Neurological Signs

Abnormal Involuntary Movements

Kraepelin in the nineteenth century described 'spasmodic phenomena' affecting the face and other parts of the body in his patients with a clear account of various involuntary movement disorders.

In 1926, several decades before the development of antipsychotic medication, Farran-Ridge also described a range of abnormal involuntary movements – which he attributed to basal ganglion disorder – in patients with schizophrenia. The movements include tics, twitches and grimaces. After the introduction of anti-dopaminergic antipsychotic medication in the mid-1950s, abnormal involuntary movements became more prevalent, although the onset of abnormal movements related to treatment is usually seen only after prolonged administration. Furthermore, the movements can be exacerbated by the withdrawal of antipsychotic medication and often persist long after cessation of treatment. Hence, these medication-related dyskinetic movements are called tardive dyskinesia.

Dyskinetic movements in schizophrenia fall into two groups: orofacial dyskinesia and trunk and limb dyskinesia. While the former is more characteristic of drug-induced dyskinesia, it is probable that aspects of the disease process itself contribute to both types. In particular, core negative symptoms such as poverty of speech and flat affect are associated with both. Orofacial dyskinesia is rare in young patients but increases rapidly in late middle age. The age range in which this increase in prevalence occurs is about a decade earlier in patients with marked negative symptoms in comparison with those without negative symptoms, which suggests that a pathological process underlying negative symptoms interacts with age-related neuronal degeneration in a way that hastens the onset of orofacial dyskinesia.[30]

Cortical Signs

Both dyspraxia and agnosia are common, at least among chronic patients. Typically, patients are clumsy or hesitant in performing motor sequences, or they have impairments of integration of sensory information such as dysgraphaesthesia or impaired two-point discrimination. These neurological signs have limited localising power, but they are probably indicative of impaired function of association cortex. They are related to core negative symptoms and, to a lesser extent, to disorganisation of mental activity.[31]

Abnormal Eye Movements

Saccadic intrusions in smooth pursuit eye movements are reported in 50–85% of patients and 40–50% of first-degree relatives. The familial pattern prompted Holzman and colleagues to propose the existence of a heritable neurological characteristic (a latent trait) that can be manifest as either schizophrenia or as an abnormality of smooth pursuit or both disorders.[32] In addition to saccadic intrusions in smooth pursuit, other abnormalities of eye movement occur. For example, some patients fail to suppress an automatic saccade towards a stimulus in the periphery when instructed to perform a saccadic movement away from the side of the stimulus (an antisaccade).

Insight

While some impairment of insight is implicit in the classification of schizophrenia as a psychotic illness, the degree to which unrealistic thinking interferes with the patient's understanding of the nature of the illness is quite variable, both over the course of the illness in an individual case and between cases. At its most severe level, impaired insight may lead patients to deny that they are suffering from an illness at all. It is difficult to engage them in any therapeutic programme. At less severe levels, patients may accept that they have an illness but deny that it is a mental illness. More commonly, patients do accept – at least implicitly – that they have a mental illness, but they have unrealistic ideas that diminish their ability to evaluate issues regarding treatment or to comprehend the impact of the illness on their lives. Assessment of the level of insight is especially important where there is a risk of dangerous behaviour.

Case Example

A 22-year-old man who had suffered a schizophrenic episode one year previously developed a delusional belief that he belonged to the Knights Templar, and he had to defend the temple against enemies. He assembled a collection of weapons, including guns and swords. His parents informed his general practitioner, but the 22-year-old man maintained he was not ill and was unwilling to accept medical assessment. When a social worker and psychiatrist came to his house to assess him with a view to compulsory admission to hospital under the Mental Health Act, he threatened them with a shotgun. The police were called and, in the ensuing gun battle, the patient and two police officers were injured. The patient was admitted to hospital compulsorily and treated with haloperidol. In the following weeks, he accepted that he required treatment with antipsychotic medication in hospital. Nonetheless, he continued to believe that he was besieged by enemies. In particular, he regarded his parents as enemies, possibly because of their attempts to seek medical help for him. Thus, despite an increase in the level of his insight during treatment, he developed only a partial appreciation of the nature of his condition and remained potentially dangerous.

Dimensions of Psychopathology in Schizophrenia

Kraepelin had created the concept of the illness that was subsequently named schizophrenia by bringing together three previously distinct illnesses – hebephrenia, catatonia and dementia paranoides – into a single disease entity. Diem had added dementia simplex in 1903. The amalgamation of these distinct illnesses was justified because, over the course of their illness, most individuals satisfying criteria for schizophrenia show features of more than one of the previously distinct disorders that had been brought together in the single illness category.

Nonetheless, schizophrenia is very heterogeneous in clinical profile. Attempts to identify discrete subtypes of schizophrenia during the twentieth century had limited success. Neither DSM-5 nor ICD-11 recognise the subtypes identified in previous editions. Nonetheless, the heterogeneity suggests that various distinguishable pathological processes can occur within schizophrenia. This leads to the proposal that schizophrenia is a disease in which there are a number of dimensions of psychopathology, reflecting distinguishable but related neuropathological processes, which might or might not occur together in a single case.

The Type 1/Type 2 Dichotomy

In an influential attempt to account for the heterogeneity of schizophrenia, Crow proposed that there were two independent dimensions, which he designated type 1 and type 2.[33] Type 1 schizophrenia was characterised by positive symptoms, which tend to be acute. Positive symptoms entail the presence of an abnormal mental process, including delusions, hallucinations and formal thought disorder. Crow proposed that type 1 schizophrenia reflected a biochemical imbalance, such as dopaminergic hyperactivity. Type 2 schizophrenia was characterised by negative symptoms that tend to be chronic. Negative symptoms reflect the absence of a mental function present in normal individuals, including poverty of speech and blunted affect. Crow proposed that type 2 schizophrenia arose from a structural abnormality of the brain. It should be noted that, despite the use of the labels 'type 1' and 'type 2', Crow did not consider that these types were distinct illnesses. He recognised that they reflected dimensions that often occurred together within a single illness.

As predicted by Crow's hypothesis, much evidence indicates that negative symptoms are more strongly associated with various indices of brain abnormality than are positive symptoms. However, the structural abnormalities revealed by X-ray computed tomography and magnetic resonance imaging are not associated exclusively with negative symptoms. Although the type 1/type 2 proposal now appears to be an oversimplification of the relationship between symptoms, it was perhaps the first credible attempt to link the symptoms of schizophrenia with underlying neuropathology in a way that accounted for the occurrence episodes of acute disturbance superimposed upon a background of enduring deficits. In particular, it provided a major stimulus to the investigation of the enduring deficits.

Three Syndromes of Characteristic Schizophrenic Symptoms

Most detailed analyses of the pattern of correlations between symptoms characteristic of schizophrenia – including factor analysis of studies limited to patients with persistent, stable symptoms – have revealed at least three distinguishable groups of symptoms:[34]

i. Psychomotor poverty (the core negative symptoms: poverty of speech, blunted affect, decreased spontaneous movement)
ii. Disorganisation (disorders of the form of thought, inappropriate affect)
iii. Reality distortion (the core positive symptoms: delusions, hallucinations)

In many ways, these three syndromes resemble the three principal psychotic illnesses that Kraepelin had amalgamated to form dementia praecox: reality distortion comprises symptoms that were a feature of dementia paranoides; disorganisation is similar to hebephrenia; and psychomotor poverty, which reflects diminished spontaneous activity, resembles the hypoactive phase of catatonia. It is important to emphasise that the syndromes can co-exist within an individual patient and hence reflect distinguishable dimensions of psychopathology within a single illness.

Each of the three syndromes is associated with a distinct pattern of impairment in neuropsychological tests, which suggests that there are three different patterns of underlying brain function. The evidence indicates that psychomotor poverty, disorganisation and reality distortion are, respectively, associated with impairment of the supervisory mental functions responsible for initiation, selection and monitoring of self-generated mental activity. A study of regional cerebral blood flow (rCBF) using positron emission tomography confirmed that each syndrome is associated with a particular pattern of cerebral activity.[35] For each syndrome, the associated pattern of rCBF embraces anatomically connected regions of association cortex and related subcortical nuclei. Furthermore, for each syndrome, the cerebral regions involved include those areas of cortex implicated in the corresponding supervisory mental function in normal individuals. Thus, the evidence suggests that there are several distinct patterns of brain malfunction in schizophrenia.

Many other studies have reported a similar segregation of schizophrenic symptoms, even in groups of patients who were more heterogeneous with regard to chronicity of symptoms.

Subsequent studies have provided support for these patterns, but not all of the data are consistent. One noteworthy inconsistency is that, in very early-phase cases, features of disorganisation and psychomotor poverty frequently co-exist. Factor analysis indicates that they share a relationship with a single underlying latent variable.[36]

Five Dimensions of Psychopathology in Schizophrenia

The three characteristic schizophrenic syndromes that emerge from the exploration of the relationships between persistent symptoms do not embrace the entire gamut of symptoms in schizophrenia. In particular, there are two additional syndromes that are usually transient: depression, characterised by low mood and depressive cognitions such as low self-esteem and pessimism, and psychomotor excitation, characterised by motor overactivity and excited, labile affect, which appears to be the polar opposite of psychomotor poverty and resembles the excited phase of catatonia.

Factor analyses of the symptoms assessed using the Positive and Negative Syndrome Scale (PANSS),[37] which covers the symptoms of schizophrenia in a comprehensive manner, reveal a complex pattern with five main factors:[38]

i. Core negative symptoms (including social withdrawal, lack of spontaneity, poor flow of conversation, blunted affect, motor retardation)
ii. Core positive symptoms (including delusions and hallucinations)
iii. Excitement (including poor impulse control, tension, hostility)
iv. Depressive symptoms (including anxiety, guilty feelings, depression, somatic concern)
v. Cognitive disorders (including difficulty in abstract thinking, disorientation and conceptual disorganisation)

The group of cognitive disorders resembles the disorganisation syndrome. Unfortunately, PANSS ratings do not provide a clear delineation of the disorganisation syndrome because several PANSS symptom items are defined in a manner that includes features of both disorganised and impoverished mental activity. For example, the blunted affect item includes inappropriate affect. Furthermore, it is noteworthy that in meta-analyses of factor analyses of PANSS symptoms,[39] the PANSS 'cognitive factor' receives loading for items such as mannerisms and posturing suggesting that cognitive disorganisation is related to disorganisation of behaviour as indicated in Liddle's three syndrome model.[34]

Thus, factor analysis of PANSS ratings confirms that virtually the entire gamut of schizophrenic symptoms can be accounted for by five principal dimensions of psychopathology. These dimensions apparently reflect five major pathological processes that generate five distinguishable syndromes. Although these five syndromes are distinguishable insofar as they can occur separately, evidence of more than one syndrome is detectable in the majority of patients. Furthermore, the probability of observing a particular combination of syndromes depends on the phase of illness, which suggests that there are various shared features linking these distinguishable syndromes. Overall, there appears to be a constellation of symptoms, all of which are related, but some of the relationships are closer than others, with the symptoms clustering into five major groups. Box 5.1.1 presents the five major groups of symptoms with item composition based on a synthesis of the consistent results of factor analyses using various symptom rating scales.

Box 5.1.1 Dimensions of psychopathology in schizophrenia

Reality distortion
- Delusions
- Hallucinations

Disorganisation
- (Positive) formal thought disorder
- Inappropriate affect
- Disjointed volition

Psychomotor poverty
- Poverty of speech
- Flat affect
- Motor underactivity

Psychomotor excitation
- Pressure of speech
- Irritability
- Motor overactivity

Depression
- Depressed mood
- Pessimism/hopelessness
- Low self-esteem/guilt
- Anhedonia

Non-specific psychopathology
- Attentional impairment
- Disorientation
- Anxiety
- Sleep disturbance
- Somatic complaints

Subtypes of Schizophrenia

Attempts to divide schizophrenia into distinct subtypes based purely on cross-sectional symptom profile have hitherto not been successful. However, division into subtypes that take account of the tendency of symptoms to persist or of the association between symptoms and impairments of cognition and role function show greater promise of identifying cases at greater risk of poor outcome.

Deficit versus Non-deficit Schizophrenia

Carpenter and colleagues introduced the concept of deficit schizophrenia to described cases exhibiting enduring primary negative symptoms.[40] Primary negative symptoms are not attributable to processes such as psychological reaction to positive symptoms, social circumstances or medication. The criteria for deficit schizophrenia require that these symptoms have been present for a least a year. The proposal that deficit schizophrenia constitutes a disease separate from non-deficit forms of schizophrenia is supported by a substantial body of evidence indicating distinct aetiological factors and distinguishable brain abnormalities.[41] Although there are inconsistencies, the balance of evidence also indicates greater cognitive impairment in deficit schizophrenia compared with non-deficit cases. [42]

Classical Schizophrenia versus Integrated Psychosis

There is substantial evidence that both the disorganisation syndrome and the psychomotor poverty syndrome are associated with impaired role function and cognitive impairment in established schizophrenia.[34,43] Furthermore, systematic review confirms that formal thought disorder is associated with impaired cognition and role functioning in the early stages of psychosis.[44] Longitudinal studies of the early phase of illness indicate that disorganisation and impoverishment predict both onset of overt psychosis and functional outcome over a period of several years.[45,46]

Taken together, these observations raise the possibility that disorganisation and impoverishment of mental activity, together with cognitive impairment, are the defining characteristics of a form of schizophrenia that is associated with an appreciable risk of poor long-term outcome.[13] In light of the resemblance of these clinical features to the characteristics of the illness described in the classical accounts by Kraepelin and Bleuler, this form of schizophrenia might reasonably be described as classical schizophrenia. Cases of non-affective psychosis that do not exhibit these features might be described as cases of integrated psychosis insofar as they exhibit psychotic symptoms with minimal disorganisation of mental activity and cognitive impairment. Although cases of non-affective integrated psychosis might satisfy current ICD and DSM criteria for schizophrenia, the concept of a continuous psychotic spectrum suggests that such cases are further from the 'schizophrenia pole' of the continuum.

Factor analysis of the relationships between clinical features in the stable phases of illness reveals a latent variable that accounts for the observed correlations between disorganisation, psychomotor poverty, cognitive impairment and poor occupational and social function,[47] supporting the proposal that these clinical features reflect a core process underlying classical schizophrenia. However, observation that disorganisation[45,46] and impoverishment[45] predict the onset of overt psychosis indicates that the pathophysiological process underlying classical schizophrenia can also lead to episodes of reality distortion.

Factor analysis identifies groups of clinical features that tend to occur together within a case. When the aim is to identify categories of patients that share relevant clinical features, the appropriate mathematical procedure is cluster analysis. Applying cluster analysis to a sample of cases with well-established schizophrenia, Farmer and colleagues identified two distinct groups: the larger group was characterised by later onset, good premorbid adjustment and well-organised delusions; the other group exhibited poor premorbid adjustment, early onset, a family history of schizophrenia, bizarre behaviour, incoherent speech and blunted affect.[48] The two groups identified by Farmer resemble the proposed categories of integrated psychosis and classical schizophrenia. The stability of this sub-typology of schizophrenia was confirmed using multivariate statistical techniques on a large independent data set.[49]

Because a very diverse range of genetic and environmental factors contribute to the aetiology of psychotic illnesses, as discussed in the introduction to this chapter, it is likely that there will be heterogeneity within any distinguishable categories. It is also likely that the boundaries between such categories will not be entirely clear-cut. Nonetheless, the pressing need to increase our understanding of the processes that lead to poor functional outcome in schizophrenia justifies a concerted effort to further clarify the clinical features of putative classical schizophrenia and to identify social, psychological and neurological processes that might contribute to this condition.

There is substantial overlap between the concepts of classical vs integrated schizophrenia and deficit vs non-deficit schizophrenia. Core negative symptoms (psychomotor poverty) are characteristic of both deficit and classical schizophrenia. The most noteworthy difference is the role of disorganisation in classical schizophrenia. In light of the evidence that disorganisation predicts risk of poor outcome in the early-phase cases[46] and is associated with impaired cognition and role function in established illness,[34,43] disorganisation should not be ignored in seeking to identify cases at risk of poor outcome.

A key question is whether or not the concept of classical schizophrenia merely brings together two distinguishable groups of cases or, alternatively, that there is an intrinsic relationship between the underlying processes leading to disorganisation and impoverishment of mental activity. Examination of disorganisation and impoverishment of speech suggests that there is an intrinsic relationship. Allen and colleagues demonstrated that diminished verbal fluency (assessed by quantifying the number of words in a particular category generated in a limited time) can reflect either difficulty in organising the search for words or premature abandonment of the search for words.[50] Allen reported that the occurrence of both difficulties is associated with impoverishment of speech together with the other cardinal aspects of psychomotor poverty: blunted affect and diminished spontaneous motor activity. The difficult in organising the search can also lead to the generation of task-inappropriate words. It is plausible that abandoning the search for words prematurely reflects an inhibitory process that defends against a tendency to produce inappropriate words.

More generally, these observations suggest that restricted expressions of mental activity ('negative symptoms') are an inhibitory defence against the ongoing tendency to produce inappropriate speech, affect or behaviour. This speculation is consistent with the observation that disorganisation plays a cardinal role in predicting poor outcome in the early phase of illness,[46] while psychomotor poverty becomes more marked in well-established illness.[51]

The Course and Prognosis of Schizophrenia

Despite the fact that Kraepelin distinguished dementia praecox (schizophrenia) from affective psychosis largely on the basis of time course – with dementia praecox typically beginning in adolescence and persisting throughout adult life – the course of schizophrenia as identified by current diagnostic criteria for schizophrenia shows substantial variability. There is variability in the mode of onset, in the degree of persistence of symptoms through the mid-stage of the illness, and in the long-term outcome. It is possible that at least in part, the diversity of illness course and outcome arises because the concept of schizophrenia has been extended to embrace disorders that were not part of the classical concept, and renewed focus on the pathophysiological processes that give rise to the classical picture might lead to improved approaches to treatment addressing these processes.[13] Conversely, it might be argued that undue focus on the classical concept of schizophrenia has impeded understanding of the large number of cases of non-affective psychosis that do not fit the classical concept.[3] These two viewpoints are not necessarily mutually exclusive. These viewpoints might be reconciled by a better understanding of heterogeneity and of the processes that shape outcome. In this section, we will review course and prognosis in a manner that acknowledges the heterogeneity of outcome while drawing attention to features that point towards identifying processes that shape outcome.

The Prodrome and Onset

At one extreme, the onset can be insidious, with subtle evidence of abnormality beginning in childhood, or even in infancy. In some cases, the patient's mother declares that, even in the first year of life, the patient differed from siblings in responsiveness. At school, one of several different patterns of behaviour may emerge: in some cases, the child is shy and socially awkward; in others cases, the child is hostile and disruptive in class. During adolescence, these patterns develop further. The shy, awkward child becomes introspective and socially isolated. The more disruptive child may, as an adolescent, become quite erratic in behaviour. In either case, the developing young adult finds it difficult to form stable, intimate relationships or to establish a consistent work record. Sooner or later, perhaps while still at school, a decline in performance becomes noticeable. In a minority, in unfavourable circumstances, there may be a drift into a vagrant lifestyle, with marked neglect of personal hygiene. In most cases, the illness eventually declares itself with delusions and hallucinations.

At the other extreme, the onset can be quite abrupt. In such cases, patients become unsettled over the course of a few weeks. They may experience dysphoric mood or irritability and a puzzled sense that something odd is happening. They often appear preoccupied. In some instances, obsessional thoughts intrude. Concentration deteriorates, and sleep is disturbed. From this unsettled state, delusions or hallucinations emerge, and behaviour is likely to become disruptive, even aggressive. There is a rapid deterioration in occupational performance and social activity. Such an onset often follows a stressful experience.

However, the majority of cases lie between these two extremes. The onset of florid symptoms occurs after a prodromal phase lasting many months, which begins with a subtle alteration of behaviour and may progress through a phase of preoccupation and social withdrawal before agitation becomes prominent and overt psychosis appears. Not uncommonly, onset occurs during the first year of a university or college course. The young person may be living away from home for the first time, and as pressures build up – perhaps as first-year examinations approach – the breakdown occurs.

Subtle disturbances in language can be discerned prior to the onset of the first episode using computer-based natural language processing analyses. For example, Bedi and colleagues demonstrated that in young people judged to be at risk on the grounds of prodromal features, reduction in the flow of meaning in speech (semantic coherence) and in syntactic complexity could predict subsequent psychosis onset with high accuracy.[25]

It is also noteworthy that drug-induced psychosis can be a precursor of a transition to schizophrenia. [52]

The distribution of age of onset of overt symptoms is one of the most characteristic features of schizophrenia. In males, the frequency of onset rises rapidly through adolescence to a peak at about age 22, followed by a steady decrease, such that onset after 40 is rare. In females, the frequency of onset rises through adolescence, but the peak is later, the distribution is somewhat broader and an appreciable risk of onset persists into middle age.

Outcome of the First Episode

In a major study conducted at Hillside Hospital, New York, of the course of illness in a cohort of patients who satisfied research diagnostic criteria for schizophrenia or schizoaffective disorder of predominantly schizophrenic type, Robinson and colleagues found that 87% achieved remission within the first year.[53] The median time to achieve remission was nine weeks.

The Medium-Term Evolution of the Illness

In a minority of cases, there is complete recovery after the first episode. In a systematic five-year follow-up study of a comprehensive, representative cohort of patients from a defined catchment area in Buckinghamshire, a relatively affluent rural English county, 16% of patients had only one episode and showed no residual impairment.[54] The patients had been selected according to present state examination diagnostic criteria, which place emphasis on the presence of Schneiderian first-rank symptoms and do not require appreciable persistence of symptoms. A similar proportion of recoveries were observed in the first-episode study conducted at Hillside Hospital, New York, in which patients were diagnosed according to research diagnostic criteria, which require a minimum of two weeks duration to minimise overlap with acute transient psychosis. Follow-up of the 87% of patients who had responded to treatment in the first year revealed that 18% did not have any relapses in the following five years.[55] Thus, approximately 16% of patients recover after a single episode, provided the diagnostic criteria do not demand substantial persistence.

A meta-analysis of longitudinal studies of remission and recovery of cases with episode psychosis, with an average follow-up period of seven years, found that 30% of cases with a diagnosis of schizophrenia had recovered.[56] There was however substantial variability between studies in the proportion reported to have recovered. Recovery rates were higher in North America than in Europe.

Longitudinal studies indicate that 20–30% of cases run an episodic course with relatively minor disability between episodes.[57] Even in such relatively good-outcome cases, it is common to find that the patient experiences brief periods of mild dysphoric symptoms and attentional difficulties several times a year. Some of these episodes of mild disturbance prove to be the prodromal phase of florid psychotic relapse.

In the middle range of the severity of illness are cases with appreciable degree of disability persisting between episodes of florid symptoms. Between episodes, the patient typically exhibits abnormal sensitivity to stress and some oddities of behaviour or lack of initiative but is able to sustain some relationships and may be able to work, albeit at lower level than might have been otherwise expected. The middle range also includes patients who have persisting delusions or hallucinations that interfere minimally with daily life so that occupational and social activities suffer only mild disruption. Some patients who initially exhibit an illness of medium severity appear to suffer a stepwise deterioration after successive episodes, and the rate of remission in later episodes is lower than in first episodes.[55]

Towards the severe end of the spectrum of illness, about 20–25% of patients achieve at best partial remission of symptoms and suffer from substantial persisting disability. The most severe cases, amounting to perhaps 5–10% of all cases, show severe persistent symptoms and behavioural disorder that seriously disrupts all aspects of life.

Long-Term Outcome

In contrast to the implication of Kraepelin's original choice of the name 'dementia praecox', there is a tendency for schizophrenia to resolve eventually in many cases, though the time scale of improvement can be several decades. The major studies that have followed patients for more than 20 years show that more than 50% of cases show either recovery or significant improvement over several decades.[57] Improvement was not confined only to those with mild illness. For example, Harding and colleagues studied 118 patients who satisfied DSM–III criteria for schizophrenia who had been representative of the most impaired third of the Vermont State Hospital inpatient population prior to a programme of active rehabilitation in the mid-1950s.[58] They were resettled in the community. Three decades later, 68% were judged either to have recovered or to have improved significantly.

Factors Predicting Outcome

There are no reliable guidelines for predicting outcome in an individual case. However, there are constitutional factors as well as features of the onset of illness that indicate an increased likelihood of better outcome.

Female gender, good premorbid social adjustment and a family history of affective disorder are associated with better outcome. Abrupt onset associated with major precipitants, onset at a later age and the presence of marked mood disturbance at onset are indicators of a relatively good prognosis. Family history of schizophrenia and poor premorbid adjustment predict poor outcome (Box 5.1.2).

As mentioned in the discussion of the concept of classical schizophrenia, psychomotor poverty and disorganisation preceding the illness not only predict likely onset of overt psychosis but also long-term poor outcome. In a 10-year follow-up study of adolescents, Dominguez and colleagues found that interpersonal deficits ('negative' features) and disorganisation predicted subsequent conversion to overt psychosis and secondary functional impairment.[45] A six-year follow-up of 41 adolescents at ultra-high risk found that disorganised symptoms were highly predictive of poor functional outcome.[46]

Some studies have found that long duration of untreated psychosis (DUP) is a predictor of poor outcome, although other studies have cast doubt upon this finding. In a comprehensive meta-analysis, Penttilä and colleagues found no significant correlation between DUP and occupational function.[59] However, they found statistically significant but weak correlation between DUP and social function. There was marked heterogeneity between studies. Overall, the evidence indicates only a weak relationship between DUP and long-term impairment of function.

Among neurobiological features, the extent of the structural abnormality of the brain is perhaps the one most consistently observed to be associated with poor outcome,

Box 5.1.2 Prognostic factors

Factors indicating poor prognosis

- Family history of schizophrenia
- Poor premorbid adjustment
- Insidious onset
- Impoverished/disorganised mental activity
- Onset in adolescence
- Marked cognitive impairment

Factors indicating good prognosis

- Evidence of schizoaffective features
- Marked mood disturbance at onset
- Family history of affective illness
- Female gender

although some studies have not confirmed this association. A follow-up investigation of cases presenting with clinical features of the 'at-risk state' reported that decreased grey matter volume in the frontal cortex at baseline predicted poor functional outcome after seven years irrespective of whether the individuals developed overt psychosis.[60]

One important debate that remains unresolved is whether or not long-term treatment with antipsychotic medication leads to greater impairment of cognition and role function in at least some cases.[61]

Other Primary Psychotic Disorders

Brief Psychotic Disorders

In ICD-11, acute and transient psychotic disorder (ATPD) is characterised by abrupt onset of positive psychotic symptoms that fluctuate rapidly in theme and intensity and persist no longer than three months. The symptoms include delusions, hallucinations, incomprehensible or incoherent speech, or any combination of these. In many cases, premorbid psychological and physiological stressors can be identified. Drug toxicity or conditions attributable to a general medical condition are excluded. The ICD-11 description focuses on the varied and fluctuating (polymorphic) nature of the symptoms.

A duration up to three months is specified for ATPD because the WHO Working Group on the Classification of Psychotic Disorders concluded that the modal duration of remitting psychoses with acute onset is two to four months. If the symptoms are not polymorphic but fit the description of the symptoms characteristic of schizophrenia and the duration is less than one month, a diagnosis of 'other specified primary psychotic disorder' should be made, whereas if the duration exceeds one month, the diagnosis should be schizophrenia provided all diagnostic requirements are met.

The diversity of the character of acute and transient psychotic disorders have led in the past to the assignment of various different names. These disorders have variously been described as cycloid psychosis, bouffée délirante and reactive psychosis.

In DSM-5, brief psychotic disorder is defined as the occurrence of one or more psychotic symptoms with a sudden onset and full remission within one month. The list of symptoms is the same as that of the symptoms characteristic of schizophrenia, apart from lack of negative symptoms. Unlike ICD-11, DSM-5 does not emphasise the polymorphic nature of the symptoms. If the disturbance persists for one to six months, the diagnosis of schizophreniform disorder should be made, provided all diagnostic requirements are met. Unlike the criteria for schizophrenia, the criteria for schizophreniform disorder do not specify a deterioration of function.

Schizophreniform Disorder

Schizophrenifom disorder is a condition within the schizophrenia spectrum described in DSM-5, with a symptom profile similar to schizophrenia but having a duration from one to six months. Because brief psychosis can last up to one month – and schizophrenia itself can only be diagnosed after six months – the diagnosis of schizophreniform disorder is used for illnesses lasting between one and six months. If the patient's disorder exceeds six months, schizophrenia should be diagnosed instead.

According to DSM-5, the patient should have at least two out of five key symptoms of schizophrenia: (i) delusions, (ii) hallucinations, (iii) disorganised speech, (iv) grossly disorganised or catatonic behaviour or (v) negative symptoms. At least one of these symptoms should be either (i), (ii) or (iii). Impaired occupational and social functioning may or may not be present, but in contrast to schizophrenia, it is not a diagnostic requirement.

DSM-5 schizophreniform disorder has two specifiers: firstly, the specifier 'with good prognosis' for cases with (i) confusion or perplexity, (ii) good premorbid social and occupational functioning, (iii) the absence of blunted affect; secondly, the specifier 'with poor prognosis' for cases with none of these features.

There are very few studies of the outcome of DSM-5 schizophreniform disorder, but there are studies based on DSM-IV, which has similar criteria for schizophreniform disorder as DSM-5. In a large study of 500 entrants to the Mclean-Harvard 1st episode project,[62] 19 (3.8%) subjects were assigned an initial diagnosis of DSM-IV schizophreniform disorder. At follow-up two years later, 17 out of the 19 (90%) had changed diagnosis mainly to schizoaffective disorder or schizophrenia, suggesting that – in most cases – schizophreniform disorder represents an early phase in the development of subsequent schizophrenia or schizoaffective disorder. On account of this, the category of schizophreniform disorder is not defined in ICD-11. The ICD-11 criteria for schizophrenia do not specify a minimum duration of six months to minimise the need for change in diagnosis as the illness progresses. Conditions that might be diagnosed as DSM-5 schizophreniform disorder would usually be diagnosed as schizophrenia or schizoaffective disorder according to ICD-11 criteria.

Schizoaffective Disorder

Schizoaffective disorder is characterised by symptoms of schizophrenia and affective disorder occurring in the same episode of a patient's illness. Kasanin used the term 'schizoaffective psychosis' to describe nine patients who exhibited a mixture of schizophrenic and affective symptoms.[6] Although the patients had been diagnosed as having dementia praecox, the outcome was better than expected. They were young, had good premorbid personalities and had been severely stressed before becoming ill.

In both DSM-5 and ICD-11, the criteria for schizoaffective disorder have been specified in a manner intended to minimise uncertainty about the assignment of a diagnosis. In both manuals, the criteria clearly describe schizoaffective disorder as a disorder with substantial contributions from symptoms characteristic of schizophrenia as well as symptoms of mood disorder. However, the nature of the required overlap between psychotic and mood symptoms differs between the two diagnostic manuals.

ICD-11 requires that symptom criteria for schizophrenia (e.g. delusions, hallucinations) and mood disorder (depressive or manic episode) of at least moderate severity must be met simultaneously or within a few days of each other for four weeks.

In DSM-5, the operational criteria for schizoaffective disorder are complex. The criteria specify a continuous period of illness during which there is a major mood episode (manic or depressive) in addition to two or more of the five characteristic symptoms of schizophrenia (as defined in section A of the criteria for schizophrenia). Hallucinations and delusions must be present for two or more weeks in the absence of a major mood episode (manic or depressive) during the entire lifetime duration of the illness. Symptoms that meet the criteria for a major mood episode are present for most of the total duration of both the active and residual portions of the illness. A major depressive episode must include depressed mood. The disturbance is not the result of the effects of a substance (e.g. a drug of misuse or a medication) or another underlying medical condition.

According to DSM-5, patients who only experience psychotic symptoms during mood episodes should receive a diagnosis of major depression or bipolar affective disorder with psychotic features. In contrast, schizoaffective disorder requires at least two weeks in which psychotic symptoms (delusions and hallucinations) occur without mood symptoms, in addition to symptoms of a major mood episode (depression or mania) being present for the majority of the total duration of the illness. If delusions and hallucinations are the dominant features for the majority of the duration of illness, a diagnosis of schizophrenia should be made.

In light of the fact that the operational diagnostic criteria of schizoaffective disorder have changed over the years, there is a paucity of informative studies reporting long-term outcome. Nonetheless, the available evidence indicates that the outcome of schizoaffective disorder is intermediate between bipolar mood disorder and schizophrenia, as in the cases originally described by Kasanin.[6] Tests of neuropsychological functions have demonstrated a close resemblance between schizoaffective disorder and schizophrenia.[63]

The difference between ICD-11 and DSM-5 in the specific diagnostic criteria for schizoaffective disorder – and the complex nature of the criteria adopted in DSM-5 – suggest that the boundaries of schizoaffectve illness reflect pragmatic operational diagnostic criteria rather than the naturally defined boundaries of a distinct disorder. Nonetheless, the observation that there are individuals who exhibit substantial symptoms characteristic of schizophrenia and also symptoms of mood disorder does reflect current understanding of aetiology and has important implications for treatment. The evidence that multiple genetic variations and multiple psychosocial factors contribute to the risk of psychotic illness, as outlined in the introduction to this chapter, suggests that an appreciable number of cases might be expected to exhibit approximately equal genetic predisposition to schizophrenia and bipolar disorder.

The finding that factor analyses of a comprehensive range of the symptoms occurring in schizophrenia yield five factors[39] and that two of these (depression and excitation) have the character of the two major types of mood episodes (major depression and mania) indicates that the pathological processes underlying mood disorders can also occur in schizophrenia. The evidence that pre-synaptic dopaminergic overactivity contributes to acute psychotic symptoms in both schizophrenia and bipolar disorder is consistent with the efficacy of dopamine-blocking medication in acute psychotic episodes in both disorders.[10]

Delusional Disorder

Delusional disorders are chronic psychotic conditions that have delusions as the predominant symptom. In particular, there are one or more persistent delusions without appreciable impoverishment or disorganisation of mental activity. Hallucinations, if present, are not prominent. DSM-5 requires that they are related to the delusional theme. Most aspects of social function are relatively well preserved. Nonetheless, an important aspect of assessment is the potential danger that the patient might pose to those who feature in their delusions.

DSM-5 requires the presence of one (or more) delusions with a duration of one month or longer, whereas ICD-11 specifies that delusions must be present for at least three months. DSM-5 specifies seven types of delusional disorder.

1. Erotomania (also known as de Clérambault's syndrome) – this syndrome is characterised by delusions in which the patient believes a particular person is in love with them. In many instances, though not invariably, this person may be a superior at work, a public figure or a celebrity. If this 'lover' denies feelings for the patient, further delusional elaborations might arise to explain why the 'lover' cannot publicly acknowledge this love and must communicate through secret messages and signs. Mellor[64] gives the example of a patient who believed that a rock star was in love with her and knew that the sequence of songs he performed had a secret message meant only for her. While erotomania is more common in women, it is more likely to lead to serious forensic problems in men. Feelings of love may become mixed with hostile and jealous feelings, posing a significant risk to the 'lover' and those close to him or her.
2. Grandiose type – the central theme of the delusion is the conviction of having some great (but unrecognised) talent or insight or having made some important discovery, often with a religious theme. Sometimes, the patient believes they have a special relationship with a famous person or

that they themselves are the famous person, whilst the actual famous person is deemed to be an imposter.

3. Jealous type (also known as the Othello syndrome) – the patient believes that his or her spouse or lover is unfaithful. The lack of rationality underlying the patient's belief is a crucial aspect of diagnosis. Establishing the reality of the partner's behaviour is not relevant. Treatment with antipsychotics seldom works. The condition creates a significant risk of homicide. 'Morbid jealousy' is a general term for pathological jealousy, occurring in delusional disorder or as a symptom in diverse psychiatric conditions, such as alcoholism. Mowat[65] found that 12 per cent of the male admissions to Broadmoor Hospital over two decades were the result of a homicide due to morbid jealousy. Examining the case records of these individuals revealed that their dangerousness and untreatability had been manifest on numerous occasions prior to the final denouement. Mowat recommended permanent geographical separation as the only viable management option for these couples.
4. Persecutory type – the patient believes that he or she is being conspired against, spied on, followed, poisoned or drugged, maliciously maligned or obstructed in the pursuit of goals. The patient might take legal action. A few become vexatious litigants.
5. Somatic type – the central delusional theme for this type involves bodily functions or sensations. The patient may believe that they are giving off a powerful odour. Other somatic delusions include the belief that the patient's skin is infested with parasites (delusional parasitosis, also known as Ekbom's syndrome) or that parts of their body are misshapen or not functioning.
6. Mixed – these are cases in which no one delusional theme predominates.
7. Unspecified – the dominant delusional belief cannot be clearly discerned or is not one of the above five specific types.

In some instances, the delusions are psychologically understandable. The case of the mass murderer Ernst Wagner, described in detail by Robert Gaupp,[66] illustrates the manner in which a delusion of reference progressed from oversensitive ruminations to devastating violent behaviour. Gaupp acquired a detailed understanding of this progression though meetings with Wagner on multiple occasions over the years following the murders in 1913.

Case Example

Wagner was a sensitive, intelligent, self-critical man. In his youth, he ruminated on the moral and physical implications of his masturbation. At times, he had suicidal ideas. He nonetheless did well academically and trained to be a school teacher. In his mid-thirties, while a schoolmaster in the village of Mühlhausen, he engaged in bestiality. He became convinced that the villagers were aware of this crime and mocked him. After completing his training as a teacher, he was transferred to a teaching position in another village. He married and had children but continued to ruminate on ideas related to the bestiality. He made two attempts at suicide. Over the next seven years, he plotted the destruction of the Mühlhausen villagers. After a further four years, he acted. He first killed his wife and children. He then travelled to Mühlhausen, set fire to the village and shot the villagers as they fled, killing nine and seriously wounding 12 others. During pre-trial examination, he was judged to be mentally ill and was committed to an insane asylum, where he spent the remaining 25 years of his life. During this time, he continued to engage in intellectual and cultural activities, including writing two plays.

In other cases, the formation of a delusion is not psychologically understandable, though the content might be related to the patient's personality and life experience. Theories underlying the treatment of delusions using cognitive therapy postulate that delusional thinking is an abnormality of cogni tive functioning that can be modified using cognitive-behavioural methods.[67] These cognitive abnormalities may be traits predisposing to the development of delusions, or states associated with the presence of delusions.

There are several types of delusional syndrome that involve misidentification. The Capgras syndrome is characterised by the delusion that a familiar person, or persons, have been replaced by an exact double. In the Frégolie syndrome, an unfamiliar person, or persons, is believed to be someone very familiar (usually a persecutor), even though their physical appearance is not the same. The content of these delusions appears to reflect dysfunction of specific brain circuits specialised for the recognition of others in relation to oneself. These delusional syndromes typically occur in the setting of degenerative conditions such as Alzheimer's disease, though they can occur in schizophrenia. The diagnosis and recommendations for treatment are determined not only by the occurrence of the relevant delusion but also by the associated clinical features.

Folie à deux is a condition in which the delusional belief is transferred from one person, the primary patient, to another, the secondary patient. Usually, the primary patient is more intelligent, older and dominant, while the secondary patient is less intelligent, sensitive and dependent. Folie à deux was known as 'shared psychotic disorder' in DSM-IV and 'induced psychotic disorder' in ICD-10. These categories were dropped from DSM- 5 and ICD-11 respectively. The condition should receive the diagnosis appropriate to the clinical features they present per the respective guidelines. The most frequently diagnosed psychiatric illness in the primary case is delusional disorder or schizophrenia. The secondary patient is commonly classified as suffering from delusional disorder, but in some instances, the clinical features might warrant diagnosis of another psychotic disorder.

Case example (from Mellor[64]):

A patient with schizophrenia believed that he should go into space so that he might destroy a satellite that was transmitting thought waves into his mind. His wife, who had a dependent personality and borderline intelligence but was otherwise normal, believed in his mission and his capabilities as a 'rocket scientist'. Sometime after his discharge from the hospital, both were apprehended by the police as they attempted to launch a plywood and aluminium foil 'spaceship' three metres high. He was sitting in this structure, which she was attempting to ignite.

Schizotypal Disorder

Schizotypal disorder is characterised by eccentric behaviour, thinking and affect. Although the symptoms appear to be attenuated forms of the symptoms occurring in schizophrenia, neither clear-cut delusions nor hallucinations occur. Instead, magical thinking, depersonalisation and derealisation, visual and somatic illusions, transient auditory hallucinations and stilted or over-elaborate speech are more typical. Factor analysis of the symptoms reveals three groups of symptoms resembling reality distortion (in attenuated form), disorganisation and psychomotor poverty – characteristic of schizophrenia.[68]

Schizotypal disorder is more common in individuals with a relative with schizophrenia. It emerges gradually during adolescent development and follows a chronic course with some fluctuation in intensity of symptoms but without clearly defined acute episodes or periods of remission. It does occasionally progress to schizophrenia.

Psychosis Associated with Substance Use or with General Medical Conditions

In DSM-5, psychosis associated with substance use or medical conditions is included in the chapter with schizophrenia spectrum disorders. In ICD-11, there is a separate section for mental disorders due to substance abuse or medical conditions. Nonetheless, the cross-linked framework for recording diagnosis in ICD-11 does allow psychosis due to substance abuse or a general medical condition to also be recorded in the section for schizophrenia spectrum disorders.

Irrespective of the formal system for recording these disorders, the observation that drug toxicity and a diverse range of medical conditions can present with psychotic symptoms has important implications not only on account of demonstrating the importance of general medical assessment as part of the investigation of a first-episode psychosis but also because of how psychotic responses to demonstrable disruption of brain structure and function shed light on the possible mechanisms of psychotic symptoms.

Toxicity with any of a very wide range of drugs of abuse or prescribed medications can produce psychotic symptoms. Drugs of abuse that produce an increase in dopaminergic neuro-transmission (e.g. cocaine, amphetamine) are especially prone to produce acute psychotic symptoms. Classic hallucinogens include LSD and psilocybin. Dissociative hallucinogens such as phencyclidine produce a diverse range of symptoms characteristic of schizophrenia, in addition to dissociative symptoms such as the experience of feeling disconnected from the surroundings or from one's own body. The mechanism of action of these drugs entails blockade of the NMDA class of glutamate receptors.

Tetrahydrocannabinol (THC), which is the constituent that confers high potency on cannabis, is psychotogenic. THC toxicity can be manifest as acute psychosis with both positive and negative symptoms.[69] The association of cannabis use with subsequent psychosis months or years later is also noteworthy. In a large multi-site, multinational study comparing cases of first-episode psychosis with controls representative of the local populations, Di Forte and colleagues found that daily cannabis use was associated with increased odds of psychotic disorder compared with users who had never used cannabis.[70] There were almost five-fold increased odds for daily use of high-potency types of cannabis. When the psychosis is not attributable to current drug toxicity, the psychotic disorder would be classified as schizophrenia provided the other relevant criteria for a diagnosis of schizophrenia are fulfilled.

Psychosis can be a manifestation of a diverse range of general metabolic conditions, including various endocrine disturbances. Hypothyroidism, elevated cortisol and hyperparathyroidism can present with acute psychosis. Psychosis can also arise from central nervous system infections. In the case of herpes simplex encephalitis, it appears the mechanism involves an autoimmune inhibition of NMDA receptors in the hippocampus.

In cases of psychosis arising from either degeneration or traumatic injury to the brain, the nature of the mental symptoms typically reflects disruption of the normal function of the damaged brain circuits. Frontal lobe damage produces two characteristic syndromes: pseudo-depression is similar in nature to the psychomotor poverty observed in schizophrenia, while pseudo-psychopathy is similar to the disorganisation symptom of schizophrenia. In frontotemporal dementia, which produces extensive and progressive damage to frontal and temporal lobes, disorganised mental activity is often prominent in the early phase, while impoverished mental activity is typical of the later phase.

Focal neural damage to areas such as the supplementary motor area or the temporoparietal junction produces symptoms such as the alien hand sign, which closely resemble the Schneiderian first-rank symptom, 'made acts'. However, patients with the relevant focal neural damage usually retain insight into the origin of the symptom. This observation supports the proposal that the symptom of 'made acts' arises in schizophrenia when there is damage to a specific brain system engaged in the sense of ownership of one's own acts, within the context of a more diffuse dysfunction of the brain.

In general, the observation that symptoms similar to those occurring in schizophrenia spectrum disorders can be produced by disruptions of identifiable brain systems supports the proposal that the form and content of mental symptoms typically reflects dysfunction in the brain system or networks normally engaged during the relevant aspect of mental activity. However, the time course is likely to depend on the molecular or cellular mechanism underlying the disruption.

Conclusion

The evidence we have reviewed indicates that psychotic disorders overlap in clinical features, aetiology and associated brain abnormalities. While each patient's psychosis is unique, patients share common features that transcend traditional categorical diagnostic boundaries. This should not surprise us: we face a constellation of overlapping disorders within which distinct categories have been imposed by operational diagnostic criteria devised on the basis of clinical experience and scientific evidence.

The defining characteristic of all of these disorders is reality distortion. However, there is marked heterogeneity in severity, time course and outcome. At the less severe end of the spectrum of severity is schizotypal disorder, in which reality distortion is attenuated. The features of schizotypal disorder are prominent expressions of characteristics that can be discerned in the non-clinical general population, indicating that the continuum of severity extends to levels that do not warrant description as a disorder. At the severe end of the spectrum lies schizophrenia. The tendency to conflate the term 'psychosis' with schizophrenia is potentially harmful, risking therapeutic pessimism in the minds of patients, clinicians and society at large. Particularly in the early stages, when reliable prediction of long-term outcome is unreliable, it is usually preferable to use the term 'psychosis' rather than 'schizophrenia'.

However, failure to identify the features of psychotic illness that indicate risk of a bad outcome for the sake of avoiding therapeutic pessimism is not sensible. The evidence that even severe cases of schizophrenia tend to recover over a period of decades[57,58] suggests that there is substantial scope for treatment that improves long-term outcome. Increased understanding of the features that predict poor outcome is a rational approach to developing such treatments.

The question of whether or not the relationships between shared clinical features of psychotic disorders are best described by dimensions that vary in severity in a continuous manner across cases or, alternately, fit best with the allocation of cases into discrete groups is unlikely to have a definitive answer that serves all purposes. The evidence regarding the existence of a general psychopathological factor, the p factor, occurring across virtually all known types of mental disorders – together with the evidence that the severity of the p factor is correlated with both severity of cognitive impairment and with the thinning of the cerebral cortex – suggest that some features reflecting prognosis are distributed on a continuum.[12]

On the other hand, the evidence from cluster analysis that cases of schizophrenia can be divided into two distinguishable groups on the basis of features associated with poor pre-illness adjustment and poor long-term outcome[48,49] supports the proposal that, for the purpose of optimising treatment, it might be potentially useful to distinguish classical from non-classical schizophrenia.[13] The non-classical cases satisfying contemporary ICD-11 or DSM-5 criteria for schizophrenia might reasonably be labelled 'integrated psychotic disorder'.

The growing evidence that the features of classical schizophrenia are associated with impaired function in identifiable distributed brain networks,[13] together with the evidence that the adult human brain exhibits plasticity, raises the possibility that neuromodulation therapies directed at modifying the function of specific brain circuits might provide effective treatment for the symptom of classical schizophrenia. Pessimism regarding treatment of the core features of classical schizophrenia is unwarranted.

Nonetheless, as clinicians we should bear in mind that despite the possible practical utility of making a categorical diagnosis to facilitate decisions about management, ultimately each patient is an individual. The art of good clinical practice includes recognising features specific to the individual while drawing on guidance derived from recognition of features that overlap with other cases. The evidence we have reviewed indicates that this is especially true of psychotic disorders.

References

1. World Health Organization. *ICD-11*. icd.who.int/en.
2. American Psychiatric Association. *Diagnostic and Statistical Manual of Mental Disorders (DSM-5)*. Washington, DC: American Psychiatric Publications; 2013.
3. Guloksuz S, van Os J. The slow death of the concept of schizophrenia and the painful birth of the psychosis spectrum. *Psychological Medicine* 2018;48 (2):229–44.
4. Kraepelin E. *Dementia Praecox and Paraphrenia* (trans. M Barclay). Edinburgh: Livingstone; 1919.
5. Bleuler E. *Dementia Praecox or the Group of Schizophrenias* (trans. J Zinkin 1951). London: Allen & Unwin; 1911.
6. Kasanin J. The acute schizoaffective psychoses. *American Journal of Psychiatry* 1933;90:97–126.
7. Linscott RJ, van Os J. An updated and conservative systematic review and meta-analysis of epidemiological evidence on psychotic experiences in children and adults: on the pathway from proneness to persistence to dimensional expression across mental disorders. *Psychological Medicine* 2013;43(6):1133–49.
8. Nieman DH, McGorry PD. Detection and treatment of at-risk mental state for developing a first psychosis: making up the balance. *The Lancet Psychiatry* 2015;2(9):825–34.
9. Craddock N, Owen MJ. The Kraepelinian dichotomy – going, going . . . but still not gone. *The British Journal of Psychiatry* 2010;196(2):92–5.
10. Jauhar S, Nour MM, Veronese M, et al. A test of the transdiagnostic dopamine hypothesis of psychosis using positron emission tomographic imaging in bipolar affective disorder and schizophrenia. *JAMA Psychiatry* 2017;74(12):1206–13.
11. Caspi A, Houts RM, Belsky DW, et al. The p factor: one general psychopathology factor in the structure

of psychiatric disorders? *Clinical Psychological Science* 2014;2(2):119–37.

12. Romer AL, Elliott ML, Knodt AR, et al. Pervasively thinner neocortex as a transdiagnostic feature of general psychopathology. *American Journal of Psychiatry* 2021;178(2):174–82.
13. Liddle PF. The core deficit of classical schizophrenia: implications for predicting the functional outcome of psychotic illness and developing effective treatments. *Canadian Journal of Psychiatry* 2019;64(10):680–5.
14. Berrios GE, Beer D. The notion of a unitary psychosis: a conceptual history. *History of Psychiatry* 1994;5(17):13–36.
15. Berrios GE, Rogelio L, Villagrán JM. Schizophrenia: a conceptual history. *International Journal of Psychology and Psychological Therapy* 2003;3(2):111–40.
16. Kraepelin E. *Die Erscheinungsformen des Irresciens* (*Patterns of Mental Disorder*, trans. H Marshal). In: Hirsch S, Shepherd M (eds.) *Themes and Variations in European Psychiatry*. Chichester: Wright; 1974: 7–30.
17. Schneider K. *Klinische Psychopathologie (Clinical Psychopathology)*, 5th ed. (trans. MW Hamilton). New York: Grune & Stratton; 1959.
18. Mellor CS. First rank symptoms of schizophrenia: I. the frequency in schizophrenics on admission to hospital. II. differences between individual first rank symptoms. *The British Journal of Psychiatry* 1970;117 (536):15–23.
19. World Health Organization. *The International Pilot Study of Schizophrenia*. Geneva: World Health Organization; 1973.
20. Kircher T, Stein F, Nagels A. Differences in single positive formal thought disorder symptoms between closely matched acute patients with schizophrenia and mania. *European Archives of Psychiatry and Clinical Neuroscience* 2021;272:395–401.
21. Andreasen NC. Thought, language, and communication disorders. I. clinical assessment, definition of terms, and evaluation of their reliability. *Archives of General Psychiatry* 1979;36 (12):1315–21.
22. Solovay MR, Shenton ME, Holzman PS. Comparative studies of thought disorders. I. Mania and schizophrenia. *Archives of General Psychiatry* 1987;44 (1):13–20.
23. Kircher T, Krug A, Stratmann M, et al. A rating scale for the assessment of objective and subjective formal Thought and Language Disorder (TALD). *Schizophrenia Research* 2014;160(1–3):216–21.
24. Mota NB, Copelli M, Ribeiro S. Thought disorder measured as random speech structure classifies negative symptoms and schizophrenia diagnosis 6 months in advance. *NPJ Schizophrenia* 2017;3:18.
25. Bedi G, Carrillo F, Cecchi GA, et al. Automated analysis of free speech predicts psychosis onset in high-risk youths. *NPJ Schizophrenia* 2015;1:15030.
26. Knights A, Hirsch SR. 'Revealed' depression and drug treatment for schizophrenia. *Archives of General Psychiatry* 1981;38(7):806–11.
27. Goldberg TE, Torrey EF, Gold JM, et al. Learning and memory in monozygotic twins discordant for schizophrenia. *Psychological Medicine* 1993;23 (1):71–85.
28. Jones P, Rodgers B, Murray R, et al. Child development risk factors for adult schizophrenia in the British 1946 birth cohort. *Lancet* 1994;344 (8934):1398–402.
29. Wenzel J, Haas SS, Dwyer DB, et al. Cognitive subtypes in recent onset psychosis: distinct neurobiological fingerprints? *Neuropsychopharmacology* 2021;46(8):1475–83. DOI:10.1038/s41386-021-00963-1.
30. Liddle PF, Barnes TRE, Speller J, et al. Negative symptoms as a risk factor for tardive dyskinesia in schizophrenia. *The British Journal of Psychiatry* 1993;163:776–80.
31. Liddle PF, Haque S, Morris DL, et al. Dyspraxia and agnosia in schizophrenia. *Behavioural Neurology* 1993;6(1):49–54.
32. Holzman PS, Kringlen E, Matthysse S, et al. A single dominant gene can account for eye tracking dysfunctions and schizophrenia in offspring of discordant twins. *Archives of General Psychiatry* 1988;45(7):641–7.
33. Crow TJ. Molecular pathology of schizophrenia: more than one disease process? *British Medical Journal* 1980;280(6207):66–8.
34. Liddle PF. The symptoms of chronic schizophrenia. A re-examination of the positive-negative dichotomy. *British Journal of Psychiatry* 1987;151: 145–51.
35. Liddle PF, Friston KJ, Frith CD, et al. Patterns of cerebral blood flow in schizophrenia. *British Journal of Psychiatry* 1992;160:179–86.
36. McGorry PD, Bell RC, Dudgeon PL, et al. The dimensional structure of first episode psychosis: an exploratory factor analysis. *Psychological Medicine* 1998;28 (4):935–47.
37. Kay SR. *Positive and Negative Syndromes in Schizophrenia*. New York: Brunner/Mazel; 1991.
38. Bell MD, Lysaker PH, Beam-Goulet JL, et al. Five-component model of schizophrenia: assessing the factorial invariance of the positive and negative syndrome scale. *Psychiatry Research* 1994;52(3):295–303.
39. Shafer A, Dazzi F. Meta-analysis of the positive and negative syndrome scale (PANSS) factor structure. *Journal of Psychiatric Research* 2019;115:113–20.
40. Carpenter WT, Heinrichs DW, Wagman AM. Deficit and nondeficit forms of schizophrenia: the concept. *American Journal of Psychiatry* 1988;145(5):578–83.
41. Kirkpatrick B, Galderisi S. Deficit schizophrenia: an update. *World Psychiatry* 2008;7(3):143–7.
42. Bora E, Binnur Akdede B, Alptekin K. Neurocognitive impairment in deficit and non-deficit schizophrenia: a meta-analysis. *Psychological Medicine* 2017;47 (14):2401–13.
43. Liddle PF. Schizophrenic syndromes, cognitive performance and neurological dysfunction. *Psychological Medicine* 1987;17(1):49–57.
44. Oeztuerk OF, Pigoni A, Antonucci LA, et al. Association between formal thought disorders, neurocognition and functioning in the early stages of psychosis: a systematic review of the last half-century studies. *European Archives of Psychiatry and Clinical Neuroscience* 2022;272(3):381–93.
45. Dominguez M-G, Saka MC, Lieb R, et al. Early expression of negative/disorganized symptoms predicting psychotic experiences and subsequent clinical psychosis: a 10-year study. *American Journal of Psychiatry* 2010;167(9):1075–82.
46. Ziermans T, de Wit S, Schothorst P, et al. Neurocognitive and clinical predictors of long-term outcome in

adolescents at ultra-high risk for psychosis: a 6-year follow-up. *PLoS ONE* 2014;9(4):e93994.

47. Rathnaiah M, Liddle EB, Gascoyne L, et al. Quantifying the core deficit in classical schizophrenia. *Schizophrenia Bulletin Open* 2020;1(1):sgaa031.
48. Farmer AE, McGuffin P, Spitznagel EL. Heterogeneity in schizophrenia: a cluster-analytic approach. *Psychiatry Research* 1983;8(1):1–12.
49. Williams J, Farmer AE, Wessely S, et al. Heterogeneity in schizophrenia: an extended replication of the hebephrenic-like and paranoid-like subtypes. *Psychiatry Research* 1993;49 (3):199–210.
50. Allen HA, Liddle PF, Frith CD. Negative features, retrieval processes and verbal fluency in schizophrenia. *British Journal of Psychiatry* 1993;163:769–75.
51. Pfohl B, Winokur G. The evolution of symptoms in institutionalized hebephrenic/catatonic schizophrenics. *British Journal of Psychiatry* 1982;141:567–72.
52. Murrie B, Lappin J, Large M, et al. Transition of substance-induced, brief, and atypical psychoses to schizophrenia: a systematic review and meta-analysis. *Schizophrenia Bulletin* 2020;46 (3):505–16.
53. Robinson DG, Woerner MG, Alvir JM, et al. Predictors of treatment response from a first episode of schizophrenia or schizoaffective disorder. *American Journal of Psychiatry* 1999;156(4): 544–9.
54. Watt DC, Katz K, Shepherd M. The natural history of schizophrenia: a 5-year prospective follow-up of a representative sample of schizophrenics by means of a standardized clinical and social assessment. *Psychological Medicine* 1983;13(3):663–70.
55. Robinson D, Woerner MG, Alvir JM, et al. Predictors of relapse following response from a first episode of schizophrenia or schizoaffective disorder. *Archives of General Psychiatry* 1999;56(3):241–7.
56. Lally J, Ajnakina O, Stubbs B, et al. Remission and recovery from first-episode psychosis in adults: systematic review and meta-analysis of long-term outcome studies. *British Journal of Psychiatry* 2017;211(6):350–8.
57. Ciompi L. Catamnestic long-term study on the course of life and aging of schizophrenics. *Schizophrenia Bulletin* 1980;6(4):606–18.
58. Harding CM, Brooks GW, Ashikaga T, et al. The Vermont longitudinal study of persons with severe mental illness, I: Methodology, study sample, and overall status 32 years later. *American Journal of Psychiatry* 1987;144(6):718–26.
59. Penttilä M, Jääskeläinen E, Hirvonen N, et al. Duration of untreated psychosis as predictor of long-term outcome in schizophrenia: systematic review and meta-analysis. *British Journal of Psychiatry* 2014;205(2):88–94.
60. Reniers RLEP, Lin A, Yung AR, et al. Neuroanatomical predictors of functional outcome in individuals at ultra-high risk for psychosis. *Schizophrenia Bulletin* 2017;43 (2):449–58.
61. Harrow M, Jobe TH. Long-term antipsychotic treatment of schizophrenia: does it help or hurt over a 20-year period? *World Psychiatry* 2018;17(2): 162–3.
62. Salvatore P, Baldessarini RJ, Tohen M, et al. McLean-Harvard International First-Episode Project: two-year stability of DSM-IV diagnoses in 500 first-episode psychotic disorder patients. *Journal of Clinical Psychiatry* 2009;70 (4):458–66.
63. Evans JD, Heaton RK, Paulsen JS, et al. Schizoaffective disorder: a form of schizophrenia or affective disorder? *Journal of Clinical Psychiatry* 1999;60 (12):874–82.
64. Mellor C. Schizoaffective, paranoid and other psychoses. In: Stein G, Wilkinson G. *Seminars in General Adult Psychiatry*, 2nd ed. Gaskell: London; 2007: 187–201.
65. Mowat RR. *Jealousy and Murder.* Tavistock: London; 1966.
66. Gaupp R. The scientific significance of the case of Ernst Wagner. In: Hirsch SR, Shepherd M (eds.) *Themes and Variations in European Pyschiatry.* Chichester: Wright; 1974: 121–33.
67. Garety PA, Freeman D. Cognitive approaches to delusions: a critical review of theories and evidence. *British Journal of Clinical Psychology* 1999;38 (2):113–54.
68. Wuthrich VM, Bates TC. Confirmatory factor analysis of the three-factor structure of the schizotypal personality questionnaire and Chapman schizotypy scales. *Journal of Personality Assessment* 2006;87(3):292–304.
69. Hindley G, Beck K, Borgan F, et al. Psychiatric symptoms caused by cannabis constituents: a systematic review and meta-analysis. *Lancet Psychiatry* 2020;7(4):344–53.
70. Di Forti M, Quattrone D, Freeman TP, et al. The contribution of cannabis use to variation in the incidence of psychotic disorder across Europe (EU-GEI): a multicentre case-control study. *Lancet Psychiatry* 2019;6(5): 427–36.

Causes and Outcome of Psychosis

Cecilia Casetta, Adrianna P. Kępińska, Simona A. Stilo and Robin M. Murray

Psychosis is characterised by distortions in thinking (e.g. fixed, false beliefs), perception (e.g. hearing voices or, less commonly, seeing things that are not there), emotions, language, sense of self and behaviour. Although it used to be thought that schizophrenia was a discrete entity, much recent evidence has shown that this is not so; schizophrenia does not have clear boundaries. Rather, it merges into schizoaffective disorder and bipolar disorder on the one hand and into schizotypal and paranoid personality on the other. It is best considered as the severe form of psychosis. The different psychotic disorders share some of the same risk factors and are sometimes associated with cognitive impairments, co-existing mental health conditions, substance misuse and physical health problems; the latter often develop over the course of the illness.

In the first part of this chapter, we will review genetic and then environmental risk factors for psychosis. Much knowledge has accumulated regarding both in the last two decades. We now know that the aetiology of psychosis is multifactorial. Genetic and environmental factors occasionally act alone but usually in combination, as well as operate at a number of levels and over time to influence an individual's likelihood to develop psychotic symptoms. Later, we will discuss the course and outcome of psychosis. Finally, we will discuss the relationship of the causes, and course, of illness to molecular and structural imaging abnormalities.

Genetic Risk Factors

Classic Genetic Studies

Interest in a genetic contribution to schizophrenia-like psychoses stretches back to Emil Kraepelin's Psychiatry Department at the University of Munich in the first part of the twentieth century. There, Kraepelin's collaborator Ernst Rüdin completed large studies showing that schizophrenia tended to run in families. However, Rüdin and many of his group became compromised by their collaboration with the Nazis. As a result, following World War II, research on psychiatric genetics became stigmatised and ground to a halt.

However, a few centres continued genetic studies. For example, at the Maudsley Hospital in London, Gottesman and Shields[1] showed a much higher concordance rate in monozygotic (MZ, identical) twins than in dizygotic (DZ, fraternal) twins. Other twin studies followed, again demonstrating differences in concordance rates – for example, Cardno et al.[2] reported 41% for MZ twins and 5% for DZ twins. The difference was attributed to the greater genetic identity of the former type. Researchers used twin studies to calculate the heritability (the proportion of the phenotype that can be attributed to genetic variation) of psychosis, with estimates up to 85%.

In the 1970s, the focus moved to adoption studies. Here, the Danish-American studies showed that the adopted-away children of mothers with schizophrenia still had a greatly increased risk of the disorder. Studies doing the opposite, following back the relatives of adoptees with schizophrenia, found the disorder to be more common in the biological relatives than the adoptive relatives (reviewed by Ingraham and Kety[3]).

Technological progress has dramatically changed our knowledge about the genetics of schizophrenia and indeed has reshaped the way we think about *nature and nurture.* Early theories assumed that schizophrenia might be the result of one or two major genes, or some unknown environmental factor. However, it subsequently became clear that transmission of one or two major genes could not explain the family inheritance of schizophrenia. On the basis of their twin study, Gottesman and Shields[1,4] argued that multiple genes contributed to liability to schizophrenia. As we shall see later, this was subsequently shown to be true.

Linkage and Candidate Gene Studies

In the 1980s, technologies for locating specific genes advanced rapidly. Initially, research focused on family linkage and candidate gene studies – studies searching for specific single genes that might contribute to psychiatric disorders. There was particular interest in genes that were postulated to be involved in the dopaminergic pathogenesis of schizophrenia such as *COMT, AKT1* and the dopamine D2 receptor gene, *DRD2.* Such studies continued for some 20 years but mostly failed to replicate,[5] with careful researchers failing to confirm the claims of their more cavalier colleagues. Reasons for this failure were small sample sizes with low statistical power, no accounting for population structure and different ancestries (which may have different patterns and frequencies of genes contributing to the disorder), too-liberal thresholds for statistical significance and, finally, publication bias towards positive results. The only gene consistently found to be implicated in schizophrenia was the dopamine D2 receptor *DRD2* gene.

GWAS Studies

In the 2000s, genotyping costs came crashing down, enabling large increases in genotyping and sample size.[5] Genome-wide association studies (GWAS) arrived, which analyse thousands of common genetic variants (single nucleotide polymorphisms, SNPs) without predefined hypotheses on which variants are related to a phenotype (e.g. disorder status). GWAS involved huge collaborative efforts that examined hundreds of thousands of people, not only for psychiatric and physical illnesses, but also for behavioural traits such as IQ and personality, or physical traits such as height. GWAS studies have shown that psychotic disorders are largely polygenic, with contributions from many genes and not a single gene of large effect.[6] Most gene variants make only a small contribution per variant to the risk of disorder. To detect this statistical signal, large samples are required. For this reason, research consortia now collect large-scale genetic and phenotypic data (e.g. the Psychiatric Genomics Consortium, or PGC).[7] For schizophrenia, GWAS samples shot up from 479 cases in 2008 to 69,369 cases and 236,642 controls in the most recent PGC study from 2022.[8]

In the landmark meta-analysis GWAS of schizophrenia from 2014,[9] 108 schizophrenia-associated loci were identified; by 2022, the number had increased to over 250.[8] Genes implicated in schizophrenia are involved in neurodevelopment, synaptic organisation, dopamine signalling (*DRD2*), calcium channel regulation (*CACNA1C*, *CLCN3*) and gamma-aminobutyric acid and glutamate neuro-transmission (e.g. *GRM3*, *GRIN2A*).[10]

An association has also been found with the major histocompatibility complex (MHC), on the short arm of chromosome 6, which is involved in immunity.[8] Complement component 4 (C4) genes within the MHC locus account in part for that MHC association signal. This is interesting because compliment genes are also involved in synaptic pruning, compatible with the theory that an abnormality in such pruning in adolescence may underlie the onset of schizophrenia in some cases.

Polygenic Risk Scores: As individual contributions of common SNPs to phenotypes are small,[11] researchers have combined information about multiple SNPs into a summary measure, called a polygenic risk score (PRS). This is a single aggregate score of an individual's genetic predisposition to a disorder (or other phenotype of interest). A PRS is calculated for an individual by summarising all those SNPs that were found associated with disorder status, with SNPs weighted by effect size from GWAS, multiplied by the allele count of each of those genetic variants.

PRS for schizophrenia (PRS-Sz) calculated from the latest PGC data explains about 7% of the variance of schizophrenia in case-control studies.[8] This is not, of course, powerful enough to be useful for screening for psychosis in the general population.

However, researchers have used PRS-Sz to test different hypotheses in targeted populations. For example, PRS-Sz was found to be able to differentiate schizophrenia from other psychosis,[12] while other studies have related the PRS-Sz to so-called endophenotypes (specific quantitative heritable biological traits) in relatives, such as magnetic resonance imaging (MRI) abnormalities or event-related potentials. PRS-Sz has also been applied to predicting the outcome of psychosis, but the effect is only modest. In general, the effect of PRS-Sz is not powerful enough to be of clinical use by itself at present; however, it could be used in conjunction with other clinical measures to triage people into screening for the disorder or be an additional measure where a diagnosis is unclear.[13]

Interestingly, in terms of the cognitive impairment seen in schizophrenia, it seems that premorbid IQ in schizophrenia is influenced by the same PRS for IQ that determines IQ in the rest of the population, while current IQ – after the onset of schizophrenia – is influenced additionally by the PRS-Sz.[14] Researchers have also examined the correlates of the PRS-Sz in unaffected individuals in the general population. Thus, Socrates et al.[15] showed that higher PRS-Sz was associated with negative traits, such as lower friendship and poorer family satisfaction and greater feelings of guilt and anxiety.

Overlap across Disorders: Analyses have shown a genetic overlap between major psychiatric disorders, or that specific genetic variants are causally associated with more than one disorder. For example, there is significant overlap of polygenic risk across schizophrenia, bipolar disorder (approximately two-thirds overlap), major depressive disorder, obsessive-compulsive disorder and, to a lesser extent, with ADHD, autism spectrum disorder and substance use disorders.[10]

Genetic overlap between schizophrenia and bipolar disorder is particularly important. Bipolar disorder PRS are significantly correlated with mania in schizophrenia[16] and psychosis in bipolar disorder.[17] On the other hand, schizophrenia PRS are significantly related to psychosis in bipolar disorder and negative symptoms in schizophrenia.[17] This research suggests that polygenic scores differentiate between psychosis symptom dimensions rather than disease status.[18]

The SNP-based heritability estimate in schizophrenia – the proportion of the variance explained by common genetic variants – is approximately 24%.[8] Obviously, this is much lower than the heritability estimates (up to 80%) derived from family and twin studies. The disparity is termed 'missing heritability' and is a continuing puzzle; it may in part be explained by current GWASs not being statistically powerful enough to detect all relevant variants but may also be explained by gene-gene interactions, gene-environment interactions or, importantly, rare genetic variation.

Rare Variants

Although by far the biggest component of the genetic contribution to schizophrenia is polygenic, in a small minority of cases (probably about 2%), rare variation is responsible. Rare variants have a frequency of less than 1% but generally carry a greater impact on risk for the disorder. Rare variants range from single nucleotide variants (SNVs), which alter only one or a small number of bases, to larger variants, which may involve thousands of bases. In terms of the former, an important report showed a significant association between *SETD1A* loss of function variants, which are likely to result in the loss of protein-coding function, and schizophrenia.[19]

Large variants may involve either deletions or duplications of genetic material and are called copy-number variations (CNVs) because they show differences in the numbers of repeats in the genome. Recent studies have implicated 12 rare copy-number variants.[20] The most common is the deletion on chromosome 22q11.2, which is responsible for the velocardiofacial syndrome (VCFS). Up to one-quarter of those with the VCFS deletion will develop a psychotic disorder. Most interestingly, non-psychotic carriers of the deletion show increased striatal dopamine synthesis, a well-established finding in schizophrenia.[21]

Most of the CNVs that have been implicated in schizophrenia are also associated with other neurodevelopmental disorders such as learning disabilities and autism; they are associated with poorer cognitive function in patients with schizophrenia than in those patients without a CNV[22] and are also a contributing factor to impairment in cognitive domains such as memory and perceptual reasoning in non-ill individuals who carry the CNV.[23] The penetrance of CNVs in schizophrenia seems to be additionally influenced by the burden of common risk alleles, with the clinical picture resulting from an additive joint effect between the two classes of risk variants.[24]

Ancestry

Ancestry differences are very important in gene discovery. Almost all the findings we have discussed hitherto have been reported for populations of European descent. This lack of diversity is still a major issue. Studies on the genetics of schizophrenia in East Asian populations have been published,[8,25] but the majority of GWAS data still come from populations of European descent.[26] As yet, there have been insufficient studies in large-scale samples of African and Latin origin to generalise the findings to diverse populations.

Epigenetics

Epigenetics in psychiatric disorders is a relatively new but burgeoning field (see Alameda et al.[27] for review). It refers to functional changes in DNA structural packaging or associated proteins (without any change in the DNA sequence itself) and which therefore influence where, when and how much genes are expressed. Epigenetic factors may account for some of the unexplained variance in psychiatric genetic studies and possibly mediate the interactions between genotype and known environmental risk factors. A significant proportion of the significant SNPs reported in the latest schizophrenia GWAS are in genetic regions regulating epigenetic processes. The main epigenetic processes in humans are histone modification regulating chromatin structure and DNA methylation; the latter has been the most researched.

As with gene hunting, epigenetic research in psychiatry started using a candidate gene approach but then progressed to epigenome-wide association studies (EWAS). DNA methylation changes, including those following environmental exposure, are tissue specific; therefore, it is not clear how relevant they can be to psychiatric clinical studies that only have access to peripheral tissues such as blood or saliva rather than brain.

However, there are certain situations in which methylation studied in peripheral tissues can be valuable. A robust association has been between tobacco smoking and DNA methylation changes detected in peripheral blood cells; indeed, the so-called tobacco methylation signature provides an accurate estimate of how much an individual has smoked in their lifetime as well as when and if they have stopped.[28] The effects of tobacco on methylation are an important confounder of studies of psychosis since patients often smoke much more heavily and frequently than controls.[28] Reports have been made of the effects on methylation of alcohol, tobacco and psychiatric medications so it is important to consider that some of the changes in DNA pathways found in psychotic patients may be led by such factors rather than the illness itself.

In an early study, Dempster et al.[28] performed a genome-wide analysis of DNA methylation on peripheral blood DNA samples obtained from MZ twin pairs discordant for major psychosis. The researchers found DNA methylation differences between twins discordant for schizophrenia and bipolar disorder, with epigenetic changes present especially in biological networks and pathways related to psychiatric disorder and neurodevelopment. More recently, Hannon et al.[29] meta-analysed EWAS results from seven psychosis and schizophrenia cohorts, identifying numerous DNA methylation differences between cases and controls with some evidence of overlap with genetic regions already implicated by GWAS. Some of the differences were only present in patients with treatment-resistant schizophrenia, possibly reflecting chronic exposure to antipsychotics or clozapine. Of the various environmental exposures thought to increase risk of psychosis, child abuse has been the most studied. However, these studies are at too early of a stage to have definitive findings.

Summary of Genetics

Family, adoption and twin studies have long suggested that schizophrenia has a genetic component. However, until the advent of molecular genetics, there was no definitive proof of this, and the field could not directly contradict those who denied that there was a genetic component. Then, molecular genetics arrived and showed that psychosis – like other psychiatric disorders – is polygenic, associated with thousands of genetic markers. In this way, there was a paradigm shift from seeking associations between psychosis and single genes (candidate genes) to seeking associations between psychosis and multiple genes, summarised as, for example, polygenic scores.

So far, advances in molecular genetics have not had a major impact in clinical practice. As Murray, GK and colleagues state,[13] 'On their own, PRS will never be able to establish or definitively predict a diagnosis of common complex conditions (e.g. mental health disorders), because genetic factors only contribute part of the risk and PRS will only ever capture part of the genetic contribution.' However, research advances at a considerable pace, and it may be that polygenic scores will be useful along with other information in certain circumstances – for example, assessing prodromal cases for risk of transition to full-blown psychosis.

On the other hand, it is useful to know if a patient carries a pathogenic CNV. One should particularly suspect this if the individual has a low IQ and other stigmata of neurodevelopmental impairment (e.g. minor physical anomalies or soft neurological signs). At present, there is no treatment for the effects of such CNVs, and the outcome tends to be worse than in most cases of psychosis. However, the knowledge of why their child has developed schizophrenia can be helpful to parents.

Environmental Risk Factors

Pregnancy and Birth Complications

Prenatal and perinatal complications, often collectively termed obstetric complications, have been implicated in the aetiology of psychosis since the 1930s. They are among the best replicated environmental risk factors for psychosis, and they have assumed particular importance in the genesis of the neurodevelopmental hypothesis of schizophrenia.[30]

Two major meta-analyses[31,32] have been carried out. Cannon's meta-analysis of prospective population-based studies found that three groups of complications were significantly associated with later schizophrenia: (1) complications of pregnancy (bleeding, diabetes, Rh incompatibility, pre-eclampsia), (2) abnormal foetal growth and development (low birthweight, congenital malformations, reduced head circumference) and (3) complications of delivery (uterine atony, asphyxia, emergency caesarean section).[31] However, estimates of effect sizes were generally less than two.

The more recent meta-analysis by Davies et al. (2020)[32] included a larger number of studies (n=152) and replicated most of Cannon's findings. Both meta-analyses concluded that foetal hypoxia and anoxia-related factors, where the developing brain is deprived of oxygen, are among those most consistently implicated. Recent studies have related asphyxia-related obstetric complications to smaller brain volumes[33] and lower cognitive abilities.[34]

Late winter or spring birth has often been reported as a risk factor for schizophrenia. However, it has a very small effect, and whether it is secondary to maternal infection or nutritional deficiency remains unclear. Some epidemiologic studies have associated exposure to viruses – particularly influenza infection[35] but also to rubella, varicella zoster virus, herpes simplex virus and toxoplasma gondii, as well as infections of the genital tract – with the offspring's risk for schizophrenia.

Furthermore, during maternal infection, inflammatory cytokine levels are elevated. Interestingly, mothers of patients with schizophrenia are reported to show elevated levels of maternal C-reactive protein and interleukin-8.[35] It is possible that the vaginal microbiome may play a role in this relationship. The microbiome is postulated to be altered by maternal infections, potentially leading to increased production of inflammatory products as well as to disrupted seeding of the neonatal microbiome at birth.

If a psychotic patient has a history of a major obstetric event, then what relevance does this have? It may have none, as the vast majority of babies exposed to such events develop entirely normally; the psychosis may be coincidental. However, the event is particularly likely to be significant if the patient has shown minor neurological signs or development problems in childhood (e.g. late milestones, lower IQ than siblings, behavioural problems). Should any of these be noted, then further investigation is warranted. In particular, structural MRI may establish if there is any evidence suggestive of early brain damage: irregular large ventricles, small hippocampi or cortical thinning. Neuropsychological testing may also be useful to elucidate overall intellectual functioning or any specific deficits.

Advanced Paternal Age

Advanced paternal age has long been reported in people with schizophrenia or psychosis. The meta-analysis of Davies and colleagues discussed earlier implicated parental age from age 34 and upwards. In relation to mothers, the situation is more complex with increased risk for psychosis in children of older mothers but also with maternal age younger than 20 years.[32] The main two explanatory theories regarding paternal age are (1) age-associated increase in sporadic de novo mutations in male germ cells[36] and (2) personality attributes of fathers making them more likely to enter marriage and reproduction late.[37]

Social Adversities and Trauma

Childhood Adversity: Social adversities and traumatic life events, either during childhood or adulthood, have been robustly associated with later psychosis. In a comprehensive review and meta-analysis of case-control, prospective and cross-sectional cohort studies, Varese et al. reported strong evidence that childhood adversity (defined as sexual abuse, physical abuse, emotional/psychological abuse, neglect, parental death and bullying) was associated with increased risk for psychosis in adulthood (overall OR=2.78).[38] Furthermore, there are now a number of reports of a relationship between childhood trauma and the severity of psychotic symptom presentation, particularly positive symptoms.[39]

The mechanisms that explain the association between childhood traumatic experience and psychotic disorders are likely to be complex and include biological mechanisms such as dysregulation of the hypothalamic-pituitary-adrenal axis[40] and psychological mechanisms such as changes to cognitive schema.[39] In relation to the latter, Alameda and colleagues[41] carried out a meta-analysis of possible mediators between child abuse and psychosis. The results showed solid evidence of mediation between child abuse and psychosis by negative cognitive schemas about the self and by post-traumatic stress symptoms, with possible evidence concerning depression.

Adverse Life Events: Life events more proximal to the onset of illness have also been investigated, though surprisingly less thoroughly. A review and meta-analysis by Beards et al. showed a three-fold increased odds of life events in the period prior to psychosis onset (with the time period under consideration ranging between 3 months and 3.6 years).[42] First-episode psychosis patients are also more likely to live alone, be single or unemployed, live in a rented accommodation, live in overcrowded conditions and receive an income below official poverty level, not only at first contact with psychiatric services but up to five years prior to the onset of psychosis.[43]

Social Geography

Social Class: Low social class at birth, usually measured by paternal occupation, has been reported to be associated with psychosis[44] though findings have not always been consistent.[45] There was an argument as to whether individuals 'drift' into the lower social classes because of the illness or its precursors or whether the lower social class itself is a risk factor for developing psychosis. However, most studies support the latter view.

Migration: There is a large body of research reporting high rates of psychotic disorders among migrant and minority ethnic groups.[46,47] Especially high rates have been reported for Black Caribbean and Black African populations in the UK[48] and Moroccan and Surinamese populations in the Netherlands.[49] Trends appear less clear in the global South. Risk seems to be higher among refugees compared to non-refugee migrants (i.e. IRR of 2.9 for refugees vs 1.7 for other migrants),[50] to persist into the second-generation migrants[46] and to change over time[51] with incidence rates that vary by region of origin, region of destination and their combination.

Several putative causal factors have been investigated in considering why there are variations in the occurrence of psychotic disorders in migrants. Higher incidence rates in the country of origin, selective migration or misdiagnosis of mood disorders all do not seem to be an explanation. One of the most striking findings in the literature is that rates of psychosis are higher among minority ethnic groups where they form a smaller proportion of the local population.[52] One possibility is that those living in areas of low ethnic density may suffer increased risk because of exposure to more discrimination and social adversity. Results from the large EU-GEI study, concerning 1,130 cases with a first-episode psychosis and 1,497 controls from sites in six countries (England, the Netherlands, Spain, France, Italy and Brazil) suggest that social adversity exposures at all stages of the migration process (before, during and after) are associated with increased odds of psychosis in migrants, independently of ethnicity or length of stay in the country of arrival.[53] Selten et al.[54] have suggested that the long-term experience of being excluded from the majority group (causing social defeat) increases risk via effects on the mesolimbic dopamine system, and Morgan et al. hypothesised a socio-developmental pathway in which exposure to adversity and trauma interacts with underlying genetic risk and impacts on neurobiological development (in particular, the stress response and dopamine systems) to create an enduring liability to psychosis.[55]

Urbanicity: Epidemiological studies have frequently associated birth, growing up and living in an urban environment with an increased risk of schizophrenia or psychosis in general. A meta-analysis, including a total of 47,087 cases with psychosis, found that the pooled OR for psychosis in urban environment compared with the rural environment was 2.39 (95% CI 1.62–3.51);[56] the more years a child spends in an urban area, the greater is the risk.

Numerous biological, social and economic mechanisms have been suggested to account for urbanicity effects such as exposure to prenatal and childhood infections like prenatal influenza and toxoplasma gondii infection, maternal obstetrical complications, cannabis use, social deprivation, income inequality, social fragmentation or greater exposure to stress, pollution or crime, but none of them has been consistently replicated.

Interestingly, a Danish register study showed a dose-response association between living near a green area during childhood (at age 10) and the risk of later development of schizophrenia. Risk decreased in the greenest areas.[57] Indeed, patients with psychotic disorders tend to reside in less-green neighbourhoods than the general population. Whether this is a result of the calming effect of nature or is confounded by social class is unknown.

Cannabis and Other Substance Use

There is good evidence that psycho-stimulants (such as amphetamines and cocaine)[58] can induce psychosis; methamphetamine psychosis has become a major problem in the Far East, Australia, South Africa and parts of USA. Psychosis can also occur – though less commonly – in association with the misuse of inhalants, nitrous oxide and steroids. A meta-analysis has also recently raised the question of whether tobacco use could be a risk factor for psychosis.[59]

However, most important is the large amount of evidence that points to an aetiological role for cannabis use. Prospective and case-control epidemiological studies consistently show a relationship between cannabis use and the development of psychosis with an estimated two- to three-fold increased risk.[60] The association is stronger for starting use at a lower age, with the use of high-potency cannabis with higher Δ9-tetrahydrocannabinol (THC) (the main psychoactive component of cannabis) and lower cannabidiol (CBD) concentrations, and in those individuals who used cannabis more frequently (especially daily use).[61] Meta-analyses have demonstrated a clear dose-response relationship between the level of use and the risk for psychosis.[62]

Indeed, current evidence shows that transient psychotic-like experiences can be inducted to healthy individuals by the administration of Δ9-tetrahydrocannabinol (THC) (Sherif et al. 2016 for a review[63]), and the EU-GEI study has found that if high-potency cannabis were no longer available, around 12% of first-episode psychosis cases across 11 Europe-wide sites could be prevented, rising to 30% in London and 50% in Amsterdam.[64]

Furthermore, continued cannabis use by those with psychosis is associated with increased risk of medication non-response and medication non-adherence as well as higher rates of recurrence of psychosis symptoms and rehospitalisations.[65]

Cumulative Effect of Environmental Risk Factors

None of the risk factors discussed earlier, by itself, is either necessary or sufficient for the development of psychosis. Most show a modest effect, and none seem specific for schizophrenia. A number of studies have now started examining the cumulative effect of multiple environmental factors on risk of psychosis as an aggregate index of the total number of risk factors or weighted sum. For example, Cougnard et al. reported an additive interaction between exposure to three risk factors—cannabis use, childhood trauma and urbanicity—and baseline psychotic experiences in predicting persistent psychotic symptoms three years later in the general population.[66] Stepniak et al. found that individuals who had been exposed to four or more environmental risk factors had a significantly lower age of onset than those exposed to three factors.[67]

Psychotic Symptoms in the General Population: We now know that subclinical psychosis is continuously distributed in the general population.[68] Psychotic-like symptoms may be experienced by up to 10 per cent of adults who do not fulfil the criteria for psychotic disorders. The evidence that clinical psychosis is an extreme end of a continuum reaching into the general population has facilitated research into the aetiological associations of minor psychotic symptoms; generally speaking, the risk factors for these minor symptoms are the same as those for clinical psychosis.

Gene-Environment Interplay

Any convincing model of the developmental cascade towards schizophrenia needs to include not only environment-environment interplay but also gene-environment interplay (GXE). The polygenic risk score for schizophrenia (PRS-Sz), which we discussed earlier, can be used to study the interplay of genes and environment. First, it can be used to examine whether environmental risk factors for psychosis are genuinely independent or are themselves subject to genetic influence. For example, it appears that genetic liability to schizophrenia, as measured by the PRS-Sz, has an effect (though small) in determining whether an individual is exposed to a risk factor (e.g. cannabis or urbanicity).[15] One can also address the question of how genes and environment act together to produce disease. It could be that the effects of the two simply add up to increase risk of psychosis or that some individuals are genetically susceptible to the effect of the environmental factor. Evidence so far tends to favour simple additive models, but much larger samples will be needed to examine this question properly.

The largest and most recently published study to date analysing the associations of polygenic risk score for schizophrenia and environmental exposures in 1,699 patients and 1,542 unrelated controls shows an additive interaction between polygenic risk score, lifetime regular cannabis use and exposure to early life adversities (sexual abuse, emotional abuse, emotional neglect and bullying) but not with the presence of other exposures such as hearing impairment, winter birth, physical abuse or physical neglect, confirming the need for future confirmatory studies.[69]

Conclusion Regarding Environmental Factors: Epidemiological studies have consistently shown a pattern of association between environmental risk factors and later onset of psychosis, which is suggestive of a causal relationship. However, there are a number of reasons why the association between environmental risk factors and psychotic outcomes may be overestimated or underestimated – such as bias (where incorrect estimates are due to measurements or sample selection), chance, confounding (a third explanation for the association) and reverse causation (where psychosis increases risk of an environmental exposure) – which should be taken in consideration when causality is inferred. Studying gene-environment interaction and gene-environment correlation (rGE) (genetic effects on environment exposure) may clarify the position.

In medicine, universal primary prevention has been shown to be more cost effective than developing 'high-tech' treatments for those with established disease. Persuading the general public not to smoke tobacco has saved many more lives than operating on those with lung cancer or thrombotic coronary arteries. Do we have equivalent opportunities to prevent mental disorder by diminishing population exposure to risk-increasing factors? The evidence concerning the high rates of mental disorder among the poor in inner cities raises the question of whether more equitable societies might reduce the frequency of serious mental illness. Although urban planning is beyond the expertise of mental health professionals, we can encourage policy makers – by presenting the evidence – that there is an urgent need to re-engineer our cities to improve public mental health. Improved perinatal care, supporting positive parenting and reducing poverty and income inequality can pay dividends for future generations.[70,71] Most importantly, the worldwide trend towards the increasing use of cannabis, especially of high-potency varieties, cries out for a preventive approach by bringing information about the risks of the daily consumption of high-potency cannabis to the general population.[71]

Course and Outcome

Onset

Psychotic disorders are rare in childhood but become more frequent with the onset of adolescence. Onset reaches a peak in males in the twenties and thereafter declines steadily.[47] The early peak in females is not as high as in males, but risk remains higher in older women than men; some studies suggest a second smaller peak between 45 and 55 years for women. Two reasons for these differences have been proposed. Firstly, all neurodevelopmental disorders are commoner in males (e.g. autism, ADHD) and, of course, schizophrenia is thought to be partly neurodevelopmental.[30] This could account for the greater early peak in males but not the second later peak in females. One possibility arises from evidence that oestrogen has a weak antidopaminergic effect; this might protect women in their reproductive years, but this effect would be lost with the menopause.

Outcome

Psychotic disorders are characterised by great heterogeneity in clinical and functional outcomes. Historically, the distinguishing feature of schizophrenia according to the Kraepelinian description of *dementia praecox* was its supposed progressively deteriorating course, which contrasted with the episodic and non-declining nature of mood disorders. However, more recent literature challenges this view, and there is an increasing recognition that many people diagnosed with schizophrenia can and will experience substantial symptomatic improvement and regain a degree of social and occupational functioning over time.

One reason why the pessimistic Neo-Kraepelian view was so widely accepted was that most follow-up studies were of patients with established psychosis. However, such studies are biased towards poor outcome by the fact that those who have already recovered are not included. To get a more balanced idea of the outcome, it is essential to follow-up patients from their first episode of psychosis. Morgan et al.[72] summarised the main findings from 13 such studies. They concluded that there was huge heterogeneity in reported outcomes and noted that 'estimates of proportions in remission or recovered (variously defined) at follow-up ranged from 20% to 78%, and the proportions in paid work at follow-up ranged from 19% to around 40%'.

Remission and Recovery: It dawned on investigators that one of the main reasons for inconsistencies in research findings was the lack of standardised measures of remission and recovery. In 2005, the Remission in Schizophrenia Working Group (RSWG) introduced a consensus definition of *symptomatic remission* and developed specific operational criteria for its assessment. The RSWG criteria involve *both*:

A. An improvement in symptoms, (e.g. PANSS item scores of 3, or SAPS and SANS item scores of 2)
B. A duration criterion of ⩾ 6 months for persistence of mild or absent symptoms. This is a longer period than previous definitions, in which the requisite duration was typically set at 8 to 12 weeks

These remission criteria can be further categorised as 'broad' or 'narrow'. 'Narrow' criteria comprise either symptom severity (mild or absent) and duration (mild or absent symptoms for ⩾ 6 months) or remission defined as patients being asymptomatic and attaining premorbid functioning sustained for ⩾ 6 months. 'Broad' criteria fulfil symptomatic remission but not duration criteria.[2]

In contrast to symptomatic remission, there is still a lack of consensus on definitions of both functional remission and recovery. Real-world indices of global functioning, involving social functioning (defined as involvement in social interactions and social activities) and maintaining satisfying relationships and occupation, are now recognised as key outcome measures for determining the success or otherwise of treatment.

'Recovery' is a multidimensional concept that incorporates symptomatic and functional improvement in social, occupational and educational domains, with a necessary duration component, which is usually considered ⩾ 2 years. Some studies use 'narrow' recovery criteria, meaning that both clinical and functioning dimensions are operationally assessed, along with a duration of sustained improvement for ⩾ 2 years. Recovery criteria can be defined as 'broad', if both clinical and level of functioning dimensions are assessed but with a duration for sustained improvement of ⩾ 1 year, or if either one or none of the symptom improvement and functioning dimensions are used or with an insufficient duration criterion.

Long-Term Outcome of Psychosis: In the last decade, the results have appeared from big cohorts of first episode of psychosis (FEP) patients who have been systematically followed up. We will now discuss these.

The *ÆSOP-10 study*[72] is a 10-year follow-up study of individuals with a FEP in South-East London and Nottingham (UK). Among the 387 FEP patients followed-up for a decade, most cases (77%) experienced at least one period of sustained remission, and at 10 years, 46% had been symptom free for ⩾ 2 years, meeting the criteria for recovery. On the other hand, 23% of cases did not experience a remission of psychotic symptoms of ⩾ 6 months at any point, whilst 44% formed an intermediate group that had had at least one remission and at least one episode. 12% (9% for non-affective) of all FEP recovered within six months and had no subsequent episode, 20% (14% for non-affective) never had an episode lasting more than six months, and around 50% (40% for non-affective) had not experienced symptoms in the two years prior to follow-up at 10 years. Taken together, the evidence showed that sustained periods of remission are not uncommon in FEP patients, and almost half of them recover. Among the diagnostic categories, schizophrenia was associated with a longer time to remission but, in accord with the growing consensus that a categorical diagnostic approach should be combined with symptom dimensions for a more accurate stratification of the patients, the best prediction of outcome was based on a model that combined the baseline categorical diagnosis and dimensional measures of psychopathology.[74]

The *GAP study*, in many ways the daughter of the ÆSOP study,[75] is a case-control study from South London. 410 FEP psychotic patients and 370 controls were followed up for up to five years from first contact with mental health services.[76] The remission rate during the first four years of illness was 59 per cent, with an average time to first remission of 18 weeks.

The *Suffolk County Mental Health Project*, a 20-year follow-up study of 373 first-admission psychotic patients (175 with a diagnosis of schizophrenia or schizoaffective disorder) from inpatient units in New York, reported much worse results.[77] The patients showed a substantial decline; their mean GAF score decreased from 49 at the six-month assessment down to 36 at the 20-year follow-up. These exceptionally poor long-term outcomes might be explained by the inadequate mental health care provided in Suffolk County. Some of the results from the study itself support this hypothesis, with indications that minor improvements in care could have resulted in better outcomes. For example, the frequency of medication visits was significantly associated with reductions of psychotic symptoms, probably due to improved adherence. Velthorst et al.[78] concluded that their findings support the importance of early intervention services for high-risk and FEP individuals.

Three other important long-term cohort studies have also been reported:

A. The OPUS study from Denmark[79] followed up with 374 FEP patients from a clinical trial of early intervention vs treatment as usual for 10 years.
B. Orygen – one of the first, and most famous, early psychosis intervention services in Melbourne, Australia – has resulted in a number of research programmes dealing with specific issues, including relapse prevention and promotion of psychosocial recovery.[80]
C. Harrow and colleagues[81] collected prospective 20-year data on 139 young FEP patients enrolled at the acute phase of hospitalisation as part of the Chicago Follow-up Study – a prospectively designed, longitudinal, follow-up programme. The study was remarkable for six re-assessments in the years after onset.

Systematic Review and Meta-Analysis: Lally et al.[73] put these and other data together and analysed 79 longitudinal studies representing 19,072 patients with FEP with at least one-year follow-up. They concluded that remission and recovery rates in FEP are more favourable than previously thought. The rate of remission among 12,301 individuals with FEP (mean follow-up of 5.5 years) was 58%. As expected, those with a diagnosis of affective psychosis had significantly higher remission and recovery rates compared with the schizophrenia group. The prevalence of recovery was 38% (mean follow-up 7.2 years), higher than the previously reported rates of 11–33% in multi-episode schizophrenia. However, when only studies using the 'narrow' recovery criteria were included in the analysis, the recovery rate went down to 25.2%. Recovery rates remained stable after the first two years, suggesting that a declining course of illness is not typical. This finding echoes the results of the famous study of Manfred Bleuler (1972), son of Eugene, who was one of the first to challenge the notion of the inevitable progressive decline in schizophrenia. Interestingly, although remission rates have improved over time, recovery rates have not.

Life Expectancy: People with psychotic disorders die younger than the rest of the population, with a 10-to-15-year reduction in life expectancy. Studies from many countries show that the trend of mortality rates in people with psychosis has not followed the same downward course as that of the general population, resulting in a growing disparity.[82]

Suicide accounts for only part of the excess mortality. Unhealthy lifestyle such as illicit drug use, poor diet and lack of exercise are implicated, with the most obvious remediable cause being the excessive use of tobacco compared to the general population (two to three times greater rates); some studies suggest that this may account for up to 70% of the excess deaths.[83] Long-term antipsychotic use also contributes to the high burden of metabolic side effects. Most second-generation antipsychotics confer a higher cardiometabolic risk than first-generation antipsychotics, leading to increased incidence of insulin resistance and diabetes, dyslipidaemia, weight gain and cardiac problems.

The five-year follow-up of the GAP study reported 2% of deaths among the patients enrolled at baseline. In the ÆSOP-10 study, 7% of patients had died during the 10-year follow-up, which is alarming, especially given the young age of the cohort. An even higher death rate was reported in the Suffolk County Mental Health Project, where 32% of the FEP patients died in the course of the 20 years follow-up.

The most worrying figures have come from a recent prospective observational analysis of a population-based cohort of individuals with a psychotic disorder in the USA. The 12-month mortality after the index psychosis diagnosis was approximately 24 times greater than that of the general USA population of the same age (2% vs <0.1% mortality rate). 61% of the cohort analysed were not on any antipsychotic medication at follow-up.[84]

A recent meta-analysis that estimates years of potential life lost and life expectancy in schizophrenia described an average of 14.5 years of potential life lost, which was higher for men than women (15.9 vs 13.6 years).[82] The overall weighted average life expectancy was estimated as 64.7 years, and it was lower for men than women (59.9 vs 67.6 years). As expected, lower life expectancy was found in Asia and Africa compared to Western countries.

Suicide: Suicide accounts for part of the excess mortality in psychosis, particulary in early years. Previous depression and suicide attempts, drug misuse, agitation or motor restlessness, living alone, fear of mental disintegration and poor medication compliance are the most relevant suicide risk factors in schizophrenia.[85] Suicide risk is higher in young patients, a finding that was replicated in both the ÆSOP-10 and GAP studies.

The follow-up of these two cohorts also showed that previous suicide attempts (HR=2.75 and 5.17, respectively) and depression (HR=1.55 and 1.16, respectively) were associated with an increased risk of suicidal behaviour in early psychosis, suggesting that early psychosis patients require particularly close monitoring. In terms of psychopathology, in the ÆSOP-10 cohort only, depression was associated with previous suicide attempts (scores medians in attempters vs non-attempters: 5.0 vs 0.0), whilst no direct association with insight scores were found.

Hospitalisation: Hospitalisation is an indicator of poor outcome in FEP, as it reflects the severity of illness and represents a significant portion of the public health burden. A meta-analysis[86] investigated the hospitalisation rate and length of stay in 81 longitudinal studies encompassing 23,280 FEP patients, with an average follow-up of seven years. Results showed that 55% had been hospitalised at least once during follow-up with an average length of stay of 116 days; the risk did not differ significantly depending on the length of follow-up. As hospitalisation is dependent on the nature and extent of local health care rather than being a global representative of illness severity, the authors investigated the proportion of patients hospitalised in different countries; it was highest in Australia and New Zealand (78.4%) compared to Europe (58.1%) and North America (48.0%) and lowest in Asia (32.5%).

Being in a stable relationship at the time of the first contact with mental health services was associated with reduced hospitalisation during follow-up, suggesting that social integration and strong social networks may improve outcomes of psychosis. Older age at illness onset was also associated with reduced hospitalisation rates during follow-up. Less-severe psychotic symptoms at onset were associated with a shorter length of hospitalisation, whilst longer duration of untreated psychosis (DUP) was associated with a longer length of stay.

Antipsychotic Medication

Many randomised-controlled trials have shown that antipsychotics have a prophylactic value in preventing psychotic relapses, based on the reduced relapse rate in those who continued treatment with antipsychotics. Leucht et al.[87] conducted a meta-analysis of 65 trials and found that antipsychotic maintenance treatment substantially reduces relapse risk in all patients with schizophrenia for up to two years of follow-up. More recently, a systematic review on very long-term outcome of schizophrenia investigated studies with follow-up periods of five years or more and found that the average proportion of patients with symptomatic remission at follow-up ranged between 16.4% in never-treated patients to 37.5% in patients who were systematically treated with antipsychotics.[88] The authors concluded that the long-term outcome of schizophrenia is highly variable, depending on access to mental health care, early detection of psychosis and pharmacological treatment. Their evidence supported the effectiveness of low-dose antipsychotic treatment for long-term maintenance in some patients.

However, some doubts have been raised about the universal long-term prophylactic use of standard doses of antipsychotics; most of the trials had follow-ups which usually lasted less than one year, and no solid evidence exists on whether the longer-term use (over three years) of antipsychotic is superior to a placebo while balancing the potential burden of side effects in the long-term.[89] The effect of most antipsychotics in inducing metabolic changes, obesity and diabetes, and ultimately cardiovascular problems, is well-known.

Data from Swedish and Finnish nationwide registers show a lower mortality in patients with chronic schizophrenia receiving long-term antipsychotics than in those with a similar duration of illness but no or little antipsychotic exposure.[90] However, this claim is disputed, and methodological concerns have been raised.[91]

Several long-term studies have claimed that a considerable number of patients diagnosed with schizophrenia who are not on antipsychotics have as good if not better outcome than those receiving treatment.[72,81] The main potential confounder in these studies is the lack of randomisation, with a lower intrinsic severity of disease in patients whose treatment was discontinued compared to those who continued. One of the few studies that tried to overcome this bias is a seven-year follow-up of a two-year open RCT comparing maintenance treatment and dose reduction in a group of FEP patients who had been initially treated successfully with antipsychotics. After six months of remission, patients were randomised for 18 months to either an approach encouraging antipsychotic dose reduction or discontinuation, or alternatively standard maintenance treatment. After the trial, treatment was at the discretion of the clinician. 18 months later, as expected, relapse rates were double in the reduction/discontinuation group compared to the maintenance group. However, after seven years, the group originally assigned to dose reduction experienced twice the recovery rate of the maintenance treatment group (40% vs 18%),[92] whilst no significant difference was found in symptom remission rate (69% vs 67%) between the groups. However, this was a small study, and it is important to emphasise that at seven years, only 21% of patients in the dose reduction/discontinuation group had actually stopped their antipsychotics, while a similar proportion had taken a mean daily dose of less than 1 mg of haloperidol for the previous two years. Furthermore, this trial was an open-label trial where the patient was considered a key-player in the discontinuation/dose reduction process, and successful discontinuation might be influenced by patient involvement and control, which might at least partially explain the positive results. The results of ongoing studies trying to replicate the findings of this trial will hopefully resolve this important issue.

Effects of Early Intervention: The OPUS trial, which investigated the long-term effect of a two-year specialised treatment for FEP vs treatment as usual, showed significant positive effects of assertive treatment on positive and negative symptoms, substance abuse, treatment adherence, lower dosage of antipsychotic medication, higher satisfaction with treatment and reduced burden to the family. However, many of these positive effects were not confirmed at five years – three years after the experimental treatment ended – although more patients who received OPUS treatment were able to live independently. Wils et al.[93] followed up with 496 patients diagnosed with a schizophrenia spectrum disorder originally included in the OPUS trial and found that 30 per cent of them had remission of psychotic symptoms at the time of the 10-year follow-up with no current use of antipsychotic medication. A similar pattern was found in the five-year follow-up study of the Lambeth Early Onset trial[94] and ÆSOP-10. These combined results suggest that a minority of patients with psychosis may be able to gradually reduce and eventually discontinue antipsychotics; this group may be between 20 per cent and 40 per cent.

Risk and Mediating Factors

Growing research have focused on factors that might influence outcome of psychosis. Young age at onset, male gender, black ethnicity, urbanicity, migration, history of trauma and poor social networks are among the most commonly reported risk factors for poorer outcome of psychosis. A brief description of the main findings will be discussed in the following sections.

Diagnosis: Worse outcomes are more common among patients diagnosed with non-affective compared to affective psychosis. In the ÆSOP-10 study, Morgan et al.[72] found that for those who achieved a good outcome, 30% had an acute onset and an undulating course, 35% had insidious onset and undulating course, 1% had acute onset and continuous course, and 1% had insidious onset and continuous course. Of note, the estimate that approximately 23% of all FEP (rising to 30% for non-affective psychoses) experienced a continuous course of illness is notably lower than the 33% noted by the WHO International Study of Schizophrenia (for all psychoses at 15 years).

Migration and Social Circumstances: Ethnic minority status and migration are important factors in the incidence but also the outcome of psychosis. In the ÆSOP and GAP studies, Black ethnicity was found – as in other UK studies – to be associated with more compulsory admissions and increased instances of police involvement compared with patients of White British ethnicity. These findings warrant action in mental health care and social policy to challenge and reduce this disparity.

On the other hand, supportive environment and positive social circumstances have been proposed as mitigating factors of psychosis outcome. Better social integration and strong social networks were shown to be associated with improved outcomes in FEP, and being in a stable relationship at the time of the first contact with FEP has been found to predict a reduced proportion of hospitalisation during follow-up.[86]

Childhood Adversities: Adverse experiences in childhood such as sexual abuse, physical abuse, emotional/psychological abuse, neglect, parental death and bullying are strongly associated with both the risk of psychosis and its outcome. In the GAP cohort, exposure to at least one type of childhood adversity was significantly associated with a lower likelihood of achieving symptomatic remission, as well as longer inpatient stays and compulsory admission over the five-year follow-up.[76] Childhood adversity predicted a poorer long-term outcome, with childhood physical abuse found associated with almost three-fold increased odds of not being in a relationship at one-year after onset compared to non-abused patients.

Duration of Untreated Psychosis: The critical phase theory is based on evidence that patients with FEP tend to have more fluctuating symptoms and level of functioning in the first years after onset and that these usually stabilise with time. Early intervention services are based on the idea that good care at this phase will have long-term benefits. Many early intervention researchers focused on the impact of duration of untreated psychosis and initiatives to reduce the time from onset of illness to initiation of treatment. The DUP is an important predictor of clinical and functional outcomes in schizophrenia, with longer DUP associated with poor prognosis.[83] A recent systematic review highlighted that greater DUP is also significantly associated with longer length of hospital admissions following FEP.[86]

However, a large systematic review involving 79 longitudinal studies on FEP failed to identify longer DUP as a moderator of remission or recovery rates,[73] questioning its role of marker or determinant of outcome. Due to its strong association with several other predictors of outcome, it has been hypothesised that the DUP might represent a marker of onset mode rather than an independent predictor of outcome.

Recreational Drug Use: Cannabis is the most commonly used illicit substance in patients with psychosis, with an extremely high prevalence among patients presenting with FEP in Western Europe and North America. As noted earlier, there is convincing evidence that cannabis is a major contributory factor for the emergence of psychotic disorders. A meta-analysis[95] confirmed that continued cannabis use after FEP has also been consistently shown to have a detrimental effect on outcome.

In the GAP cohort, patients who stopped using cannabis had the most favourable course of illness in the two years after illness onset.[96] In contrast, those who continued using high-potency cannabis daily showed an increased risk for a subsequent relapse, more relapses, less time until a relapse occurred and greater symptomatic severity. Continued use of cannabis was also associated with poorer adherence to prescribed antipsychotic medications, and high-frequency use of potent forms of cannabis adversely affected long-term outcome even in treatment-adherent patients, possibly by reducing the effectiveness of antipsychotic treatment.

As change in cannabis use after the onset of psychosis is a major determinant for clinical and functional outcome, specific intervention strategies aimed at helping patients to stop cannabis use should be routinely offered after FEP.

Treatment Resistance

Over 75 per cent of patients with first-episode psychosis respond to the first treatment with an antipsychotic medication.[97] However, in patients who do not improve with the first antipsychotic medication, response rates to subsequent non-clozapine antipsychotics are much lower. Recent data from a multicentric three-phase switching study (OPTiMiSE) confirm that, if remission is not achieved with the first antipsychotic medication, there is no benefit from switching antipsychotic medication instead of continuing on the same one and waiting to see whether remission can be achieved at a later stage.[98] Up to a third of patients with a diagnosis of schizophrenia show little to no symptomatic improvement despite treatment with multiple different antipsychotics. These people are considered treatment-resistant (TRS), which is defined as a failure to respond to adequate trials of two subsequent non-clozapine antipsychotics.[99]

The three crucial elements that define the concept of TRS are a validated diagnosis of schizophrenia as defined by diagnostic guidelines, adequate pharmacological treatment and persistence of symptoms despite adequate treatment, specifically failure of at least two adequate pharmacological trials with different antipsychotic drugs, meeting the following criteria:

a. Duration: oral antipsychotics for at least six weeks, or long-acting injectable antipsychotics (LAI) for at least six weeks after having reached steady state (may be up to four months after commencing treatment). A trial with a LAI is suggested in order to establish treatment resistance in case of suspected non-adherence.
b. Dose: total daily dose equivalent to 600 mg of chlorpromazine per day. If a trial has to be aborted due to intolerability prior to reaching criteria for an adequate therapeutic dose maintained for at least six weeks, it should not count as a failed trial.
c. No satisfactory symptom remission despite adequate treatment (minimum of 12 weeks duration of symptoms is required, defined as:
   1. Symptom improvement <20 per cent on a validated scale for symptom severity, such as the PANSS, the BPRS, the SANS or the SAPS
   2. Less than 'minimally improved' on the overall change in the Clinical Global Impression-Schizophrenia Scale (CGI-S)
   3. Score of <60 on SOFAS

The observed stability of recovery rates after the first two years from illness onset suggests that a progressive deterioration course of illness is not typical and that most patients with bad outcomes are apparent from the earlier stages of illness. This is supported by evidence indicating that although it can manifest at all stages of the disease, the vast majority of TRS patients (>70 per cent) are treatment resistant from illness onset.[100,101] A study using the 10-year outcome data from the ÆSOP-10 study suggested that there are two types of TRS. Seventy per cent of patients did not respond to an antipsychotic from their first contact with mental health services, whilst the other 30 per cent of TRS patients initially responded to antipsychotics before becoming resistant.[101] A replication from the GAP study largely confirmed these findings.[100] These results fit with the idea that there may be a distinctive poor outcome subgroup of FEP patients who show no striatal dopaminergic excess but rather have suffered neurodevelopmental damage with predominantly glutamatergic abnormalities who therefore fail to respond to traditional antidopaminergic medication.[101] In contrast, the loss of response in these patients who originally responded could be due to the emergence of dopamine receptor supersensitivity. Early identification of patients who require clozapine treatment has the potential to improve clinical outcomes and minimise the social and functional disability that results from prolonged untreated psychosis.

With respect to predictors of treatment resistance, data are still scarce, and it's not currently possible to accurately predict who will or will not respond to antipsychotic medication with certainty. The following sociodemographic and clinical predictors of TRS have been proposed:[101,102]

- Early onset
- Male gender
- Less education
- Poor premorbid social adjustment
- Lower premorbid IQ
- Comorbid personality disorder
- Recreational drug use

Biological Mechanisms Underlying Onset and Outcome of Psychosis

Abnormal Dopamine: The predominant biological theory of schizophrenia highlights the role of the excess pre-synaptic synthesis of DA in the striatum in the onset of positive symptoms. Consistent with this view, the diathesis–stress model suggests that the hypothalamus–pituitary–adrenal (HPA) axis may trigger a cascade of events resulting in neural circuit dysfunction, including alterations in DA signalling. Mizrahi et al.,[102] investigating the DA release in response to a psychosocial stress challenge in psychosis-related disorders, found that the largest stress-induced change in salivary cortisol was present in the schizophrenia group, followed by the clinical high-risk (prodromal) group, with an association between the per cent change in the cortisol response and the stress-induced DA release in the associative striatum.

Data provide intriguing evidence of an association between migration, hearing impairment, childhood abuse, low parental care and elevation in striatal dopamine synthesis. Acute administration of THC, the active ingredient of cannabis, has been reported to increase dopamine release. However, paradoxically, chronic cannabis use and also difficult premature birth are associated with decreased striatal dopamine. Perhaps, the individuals more vulnerable for psychosis have abnormalities within the hypothalamic–pituitary–adrenal (HPA) axis that contribute to dopaminergic and glutamatergic abnormalities that underlie psychotic symptoms.

Currently available antipsychotics do not target the primary pre-synaptic locus of excessive striatal dopamine but rather have their beneficial effects by blocking the post-synaptic effects on the D2 dopamine receptor of the (continuing) increased dopamine synthesis. One issue that is not yet resolved is the question of whether or not long-term use of antipsychotics upregulates D2 and D3 receptors, potentially leading to reduced effectiveness and increased risk of relapse at discontinuation of medication (antipsychotic-induced dopamine receptor supersensitivity).[89]

Whilst the dopamine hypothesis can account for certain aspects of the psychopathology of schizophrenia – especially positive symptoms (e.g. delusions, hallucinations, disorganised behaviour) – some studies suggest that the glutamatergic dysregulation, mainly through its interactions with other neurotransmitters like dopamine and gamma-aminobutyric acid, may account for cognitive and negative symptoms of schizophrenia.

Molecular neuroimaging studies have demonstrated a significant association between both striatal synaptic dopamine level and striatal D2 occupancy and short-term clinical response to antipsychotic treatment. However, TRS patients tend to not show the usual increase in pre-synaptic striatal dopamine synthesis capacity; it is not surprising that such patients do not respond to dopamine blockage since they do not show excess striatal dopamine. Some studies show elevated anterior cingulate cortex glutamate level in patients who do not show improvement despite antipsychotics. This could be due to distinct neurodevelopmental glutamatergic abnormalities in the subgroup of patients who failed to respond to conventional antipsychotic agents.

Patients with a family history of psychosis are more likely to respond poorly to antipsychotic drugs, suggesting a genetic influence in the development of TRS. However, evidence for genetic differences in TRS patients has been difficult to find.[103] Those with an abnormal MRI structural scan or poorer cognitive function are also more likely to be treatment resistant.

Brain Structural Abnormalities: The huge ENIGMA consortium studies have confirmed that people with schizophrenia show on average increased ventricular volumes and reductions in cortical thickness and surface area.[104] Indeed, subtle brain abnormalities are present at, and even before, onset of illness, especially in those who have suffered obstetric complications or those carrying CNVs. Two neurodevelopmental periods have been suggested as critical for the development of these abnormalities: a foetal/early infancy period, when early damage to the developing brain occurs,[30] and an adolescence/young adult period, during which excessive pruning may occur.[105]

It has become evident that brain abnormalities tend to worsen with the course of illness. Some such as Stone et al.[106] take this to represent a neurodegenerative process. However, longitudinal studies of patients show that long-term use of high-dose first-generation antipsychotics carries a risk of decreasing cortical volume and increasing ventricular volume; low-dose antipsychotics and second-generation antipsychotics have a smaller effect.[89] Animal studies show that similar abnormalities can be produced in monkeys and rats that are given antipsychotics.

There are other reasons why people with schizophrenia should show brain deterioration and cognitive imparment. They are more likely to develop metabolic syndrome, cardiovascular and cerebrovascular disorder, and diabetes, which are known to be associated with brain ageing and cognitive impairment in people with schizophrenia. Tobacco and cannabis smoking are other detrimental factors. In short, the changes in the brain as people with schizophrenia age could be due to lifestyle and factors associated with their illness rather than any intrinsic neurodegenerative process.[107]

Low- and Middle-Income Countries

The notion that people with schizophrenia in low- and middle-income countries (LMICs) experience more favourable outcomes than those in better-resourced settings was reported by a series of multicentre studies conducted by the WHO.[108] This apparently superior outcome has been hypothesised to arise from better social support.[109] However, recent research has challenged the notion of a more supportive family environment in LMICs and argued against the generalisability of the reported superior outcomes of schizophrenia in LMICs, highlighting the high mortality rates and the highly variable outcomes among different LMIC settings.[110] Furthermore, in LMICs, significantly higher multimorbidity was observed in people with self-reported psychosis than those with no psychotic symptoms.[111]

Cultural and social settings significantly shape the understanding of psychotic symptoms, and recent literature highlights how supernatural explanations of schizophrenia tend to be associated with greater self stigma and public stigma.[112] The severe shortage of mental health specialists in LMICs means that two-thirds of people with schizophrenia in LMICs do not access any evidence-based care,[113] and this care is usually sought only after seeing traditional healers. For example, in South Africa, it was found that nearly half of the people with psychosis had never accessed biomedical care whilst having sought the help of a traditional healer.[114] The use of traditional health practitioners as the first point of contact in LMICs has been found to be associated with longer DUP,[115] which is a well-established risk factor for poorer outcome in schizophrenia, so it's important that psychiatrists develop a good relationship with traditional healers so that these healers will rapidly refer those patients they cannot help.

Due to the limited coverage of community-based services, psychiatric hospitals remain the epicentre of biomedical care for most people with schizophrenia in LMICs, which leads to difficulties in the logistics of their long-term follow-up. Moreover, erratic antipsychotic medication supplies and difficulties paying for medication due to poverty often complicate care in LMICs. A recent review investigated the efficacy of psychosocial interventions for people with mental health conditions in LMICs[116] and found that community-based psychosocial interventions might have a strong effect on symptom severity and functioning in schizophrenia.

References

1. Gottesman II, Shields J. *Schizophrenia and Genetics: A Twin Study Vantage Point.* New York, NY: Academic Press; 1972.
2. Cardno AG, Marshall EJ, Coid B, et al. Heritability estimates for psychotic disorders: the Maudsley twin psychosis series. *Archives of General Psychiatry* 1999;56(2):162–8.
3. Ingraham LJ, Kety SS. Adoption studies of schizophrenia. *American Journal of Medical Genetics* 2000;97(1):18–22.
4. Gottesman, II, Shields J. A polygenic theory of schizophrenia. *Proceedings of the National Academy of Sciences of the United States of America* 1967;58 (1):199–205.
5. Duncan LE, Ostacher M, Ballon J. How genome-wide association studies (GWAS) made traditional candidate gene studies obsolete. *Neuropsychopharmacology* 2019;44 (9):1518–23.
6. Horwitz T, Lam K, Chen Y, et al. A decade in psychiatric GWAS research. *Molecular Psychiatry* 2019;24 (3):378–89.
7. Watson HJ, Yilmaz Z, Sullivan PF. The Psychiatric Genomics Consortium: history, development, and the future. In: Baune BT (ed.) *Personalized Psychiatry.* London, San Diego, CA, Cambridge, MA, Oxford: Academic Press; 2020:91–101.
8. Ripke S, Walters JT, O'Donovan MC. Mapping genomic loci prioritises genes and implicates synaptic biology in schizophrenia. *medRxiv* 2020. DOI: 2020.09.12.20192922.
9. Schizophrenia Working Group of the Psychiatric Genomics Consortium. Biological insights from 108 schizophrenia-associated genetic loci. *Nature* 2014;511:421–7.
10. Legge SE, Santoro ML, Periyasamy S, et al. Genetic architecture of schizophrenia: a review of major advancements. *Psychological Medicine* 2021;51(13):1–10.
11. Visscher PM, Wray NR, Zhang Q, et al. 10 years of GWAS discovery: biology, function, and translation. *American Journal of Human Genetics* 2017;101 (1):5–22.
12. Vassos E, Di Forti M, Coleman J, et al. An examination of polygenic score risk prediction in individuals with first-episode psychosis. *Biological Psychiatry* 2017;81(6):470–7.
13. Murray GK, Lin T, Austin J, et al. Could polygenic risk scores be useful in psychiatry? A review. *JAMA Psychiatry* 2021;78(2):210–9.
14. Legge SE, Cardno AG, Allardyce J, et al. Associations between schizophrenia polygenic liability, symptom dimensions, and cognitive ability in schizophrenia. *JAMA Psychiatry* 2021;78(2021):1143–51.
15. Socrates A, Maxwell J, Glanville KP, et al. Investigating the effects of genetic risk of schizophrenia on behavioural traits. *NPJ Schizophrenia* 2021;7(1):2.
16. Ruderfer DM, Fanous AH, Ripke S, et al. Polygenic dissection of diagnosis and clinical dimensions of bipolar disorder and schizophrenia. *Molecular Psychiatry* 2014;19:1017–24.
17. Bipolar Disorder and Schizophrenia Working Group of the Psychiatric Genomics Consortium. Genomic dissection of bipolar disorder and schizophrenia, including 28 subphenotypes. *Cell* 2018;173(7):1705–15.e16.
18. Quattrone D, Reininghaus U, Richards AL, et al. The continuity of effect of schizophrenia polygenic risk score and patterns of cannabis use on transdiagnostic symptom dimensions at first-episode psychosis: findings from the EU-GEI study. *Translational Psychiatry* 2021;11(1):423.
19. Singh T, Kurki MI, Curtis D, et al. Rare loss-of-function variants in SETD1A are associated with schizophrenia and developmental disorders. *Nature Neuroscience* 2016;19(4):571–7.
20. Rees E, Kirov G. Copy number variation and neuropsychiatric illness. *Current Opinion in Genetics & Development* 2021;68:57–63.
21. Rogdaki M, Gudbrandsen M, Daly E, et al. 142. State or trait? Investigation of dopamine function in individuals with 22q11 deletion. *Schizophrenia Bulletin* 2017;43:S75.
22. Hubbard L, Rees E, Morris DW, et al. Rare copy number variants are associated with poorer cognition in schizophrenia. *Biological Psychiatry* 2021;90(1):28–34.
23. Kendall KM, Bracher-Smith M, Fitzpatrick H, et al. Cognitive performance and functional outcomes of carriers of pathogenic copy number variants: analysis of the UK Biobank. *British Journal of Psychiatry* 2019;214 (5):297–304.
24. Bergen SE, Ploner A, Howrigan D, et al. Joint contributions of rare copy number variants and common SNPs to risk for schizophrenia. *American Journal of Psychiatry* 2019;176(1):29–35.
25. Lam M, Chen CY, Li Z, et al. Comparative genetic architectures of

schizophrenia in East Asian and European populations. *Nature Genetics* 2019;51(12):1670–8.

26. Mills MC, Rahal C. A scientometric review of genome-wide association studies. *Communications Biology* 2019;2:9.
27. Alameda L, Trotta G, Quigley H, et al. Can epigenetics shine a light on the biological pathways underlying major mental disorders? *Psychological Medicine* 2022;52(9):1645–65.
28. Dempster EL, Pidsley R, Schalkwyk LC, et al. Disease-associated epigenetic changes in monozygotic twins discordant for schizophrenia and bipolar disorder. *Human Molecular Genetics* 2011;20(24):4786–96.
29. Hannon E, Dempster EL, Mansell G, et al. DNA methylation meta-analysis reveals cellular alterations in psychosis and markers of treatment-resistant schizophrenia. *eLife* 2021;10:e58430.
30. Murray RM, Lewis SW. Is schizophrenia a neurodevelopmental disorder? *British Medical Journal (Clinical research ed.)* 1987;295 (6600):681–2.
31. Cannon M, Jones PB, Murray RM. Obstetric complications and schizophrenia: historical and meta-analytic review. *American Journal of Psychiatry* 2002;159(7):1080–92.
32. Davies C, Segre G, Estradé A, et al. Prenatal and perinatal risk and protective factors for psychosis: a systematic review and meta-analysis. *The lancet. Psychiatry* 2020;7 (5):399–410.
33. Wortinger LA, Engen K, Barth C, et al. Asphyxia at birth affects brain structure in patients on the schizophrenia-bipolar disorder spectrum and healthy participants. *Psychological Medicine* 2022;52(6):1050–59.
34. Wortinger LA, Engen K, Barth C, et al. Obstetric complications and intelligence in patients on the schizophrenia-bipolar spectrum and healthy participants. *Psychological Medicine* 2020;50 (11):1914–22.
35. Brown AS, Derkits EJ. Prenatal infection and schizophrenia: a review of epidemiologic and translational studies. *American Journal of Psychiatry* 2010 167 (3):261–80.
36. Malaspina D, Corcoran C, Fahim C, et al. Paternal age and sporadic schizophrenia: evidence for de novo mutations. *American Journal of Medical Genetics* 2002;114(3):299–303.
37. Petersen L, Mortensen PB, Pedersen CB. Paternal age at birth of first child and risk of schizophrenia. *American Journal of Psychiatry* 2011;168(1):82–8.
38. Varese F, Smeets F, Drukker M, et al. Childhood adversities increase the risk of psychosis: a meta-analysis of patient-control, prospective- and cross-sectional cohort studies. *Schizophrenia Bulletin* 2012;38(4),661–71.
39. Bentall RP, de Sousa P, Varese F, et al. From adversity to psychosis: pathways and mechanisms from specific adversities to specific symptoms. *Social Psychiatry and Psychiatric Epidemiology* 2014;49(7):1011–22.
40. Cullen AE, Fisher HL, Gullet N, et al. Cortisol levels in childhood associated with emergence of attenuated psychotic symptoms in early adulthood. *Biological Psychiatry* 2022;91(2):226–35.
41. Alameda L, Rodriguez V, Carr E, et al. A systematic review on mediators between adversity and psychosis: potential targets for treatment. *Psychological Medicine* 2020;50 (12):1966–76.
42. Beards S, Gayer-Anderson C, Borges S, et al. Life events and psychosis: a review and meta-analysis. *Schizophrenia Bulletin* 2013;39(4):740–47.
43. Stilo SA, Gayer-Anderson C, Beards S, et al. Further evidence of a cumulative effect of social disadvantage on risk of psychosis. *Psychological Medicine* 2017;47(5):913–24.
44. Castle DJ, Scott K, Wessely S, et al. Does social deprivation during gestation and early life predispose to later schizophrenia? *Social Psychiatry and Psychiatric Epidemiology* 1993;28 (1):1–4.
45. Morgan C, Kirkbride J, Leff J, et al. Parental separation, loss and psychosis in different ethnic groups: a case-control study. *Psychological Medicine* 2007;37(4):495–503.
46. Bourque F, van der Ven E, Malla A. A meta-analysis of the risk for psychotic disorders among first- and second-generation immigrants. *Psychological Medicine* 2011;41(5):897–910.
47. Jongsma HE, Turner C, Kirkbride JB, et al. International incidence of psychotic disorders, 2002–17: a systematic review and meta-analysis. *The Lancet. Public health* 2019;4(5): e229–e244.
48. Tortelli A, Errazuriz A, Croudace T, et al. Schizophrenia and other psychotic disorders in Caribbean-born migrants and their descendants in England: systematic review and meta-analysis of incidence rates, 1950–2013. *Social Psychiatry and Psychiatric Epidemiology* 2015;50(7):1039–55.
49. Selten JP, Veen N, Feller W, et al. Incidence of psychotic disorders in immigrant groups to The Netherlands. *British Journal of Psychiatry: The Journal of Mental Science* 2001;178:367–72.
50. Hollander AC, Dal H, Lewis G, et al. Refugee migration and risk of schizophrenia and other non-affective psychoses: cohort study of 1.3 million people in Sweden. *BMJ (Clinical research ed.)* 2016;352:i1030.
51. Oduola S, Das-Munshi J, Bourque F, et al. Change in incidence rates for psychosis in different ethnic groups in south London: findings from the Clinical Record Interactive Search-First Episode Psychosis (CRIS-FEP) study. *Psychological Medicine* 2021;51 (2):300–9.
52. Boydell J, van Os J, McKenzie K, et al. Incidence of schizophrenia in ethnic minorities in London: ecological study into interactions with environment. *BMJ (Clinical research ed.)* 2001;323 (7325):1336–8.
53. Tarricone I, D'Andrea G, Jongsma HE, et al. Migration history and risk of psychosis: results from the multinational EU-GEI study. *Psychological Medicine* 2022;52 (14):1–13.
54. Selten JP, van Os J, Cantor-Graae E. The social defeat hypothesis of schizophrenia: issues of measurement and reverse causality. *World Psychiatry: Official Journal of the World Psychiatric Association (WPA)* 2016;15 (3):294–5.
55. Morgan C, Charalambides M, Hutchinson G, et al. Migration, ethnicity, and psychosis: toward a sociodevelopmental model. *Schizophrenia Bulletin* 2010;36 (4):655–64.
56. Vassos E, Pedersen CB, Murray RM, et al. Meta-analysis of the association of urbanicity with schizophrenia.

Schizophrenia Bulletin 2012;38 (6):1118–23.

57. Engemann K, Pedersen CB, Arge L, et al. Childhood exposure to green space – A novel risk-decreasing mechanism for schizophrenia? *Schizophrenia Research* 2018;199:142–8.
58. Sara GE, Large MM, Matheson SL, et al. Stimulant use disorders in people with psychosis: a meta-analysis of rate and factors affecting variation. *Australian and New Zealand Journal of Psychiatry* 2015;49(2):106–17.
59. Gurillo P, Jauhar S, Murray RM, et al. Does tobacco use cause psychosis? Systematic review and meta-analysis. *The lancet. Psychiatry* 2015;2(8):718–25.
60. Di Forti M, Marconi A, Carra E, et al. Proportion of patients in south London with first-episode psychosis attributable to use of high potency cannabis: a case-control study. *The lancet. Psychiatry* 2015;2(3):233–8.
61. Di Forti M, Morgan C, Dazzan P, et al. High-potency cannabis and the risk of psychosis. *British Journal of Psychiatry: The Journal of Mental Science* 2009;195 (6):488–91.
62. Marconi A, Di Forti M, Lewis CM, et al. Meta-analysis of the association between the level of cannabis use and risk of psychosis. *Schizophrenia Bulletin* 2016;42(5):1262–9.
63. Sherif M, Radhakrishnan R, D'Souza DC, et al. Human laboratory studies on cannabinoids and psychosis. *Biological Psychiatry* 2016;79(7):526–38.
64. Di Forti M, Quattrone D, Freeman TP, et al. The contribution of cannabis use to variation in the incidence of psychotic disorder across Europe (EU-GEI): a multicentre case-control study. *The lancet. Psychiatry* 2019;6(5):427–36.
65. Schoeler T, Monk A, Sami MB, et al. Continued versus discontinued cannabis use in patients with psychosis: a systematic review and meta-analysis. *The lancet. Psychiatry* 2016;3(3):215–25.
66. Cougnard A, Marcelis M, Myin-Germeys I, et al. Does normal developmental expression of psychosis combine with environmental risk to cause persistence of psychosis? A psychosis proneness-persistence model. *Psychological Medicine* 2007;37 (4):513–27.
67. Stepniak B, Papiol S, Hammer C, et al. Accumulated environmental risk determining age at schizophrenia onset: a deep phenotyping-based study. *The lancet. Psychiatry* 2014;1(6):444–53.
68. Verdoux H, van Os J. Psychotic symptoms in non-clinical populations and the continuum of psychosis. *Schizophrenia Research* 2002; 54(1–2):59–65.
69. Vassos E, Sham P, Kempton M, et al. The Maudsley environmental risk score for psychosis. *Psychological Medicine* 2020;50(13):2213–20.
70. Murray RM, Ajnakina O, David A. Prevention of psychosis: moving on from the at-risk mental state to universal primary prevention. *Psychological Medicine* 2020;51(2):1–5
71. Murray RM, Cannon M. Public health psychiatry: an idea whose time has come. *World Psychiatry: Official Journal of the World Psychiatric Association (WPA)* 2021;20(2):222–3.
72. Morgan C, Lappin J, Heslin M, et al. Reappraising the long-term course and outcome of psychotic disorders: the AESOP-10 study. *Psychological Medicine* 2014;44(13):2713–26. DOI: 10.1017/S0033291714000282. Erratum in: *Psychological Medicine* 2014;44(13):2727.
73. Lally J, Ajnakina O, Stubbs B, et al. Remission and recovery from first-episode psychosis in adults: systematic review and meta-analysis of long-term outcome studies. *British Journal of Psychiatry* 2017;211(6):350–8. DOI: 10.1192/bjp.bp.117.201475.
74. Demjaha A, Morgan K, Morgan C, et al. Combining dimensional and categorical representation of psychosis: the way forward for DSM-V and ICD-11? *Psychological Medicine* 2009;39 (12):1943–55. DOI: 10.1017/S0033291709990651.
75. Murray RM, Mondelli V, Stilo SA, et al. The influence of risk factors on the onset and outcome of psychosis: What we learned from the GAP study. *Schizophrenia Research* 2020;225:63–8. DOI: 10.1016/j.schres.2020.01.011.
76. Ajnakina O, Lally J, Di Forti M, et al. Utilising symptom dimensions with diagnostic categories improves prediction of time to first remission in first-episode psychosis. *Schizophrenia Research* 2018;193:391–8. DOI: 10.1016/j.schres.2017.07.042.
77. Kotov R, Fochtmann L, Li K, et al. Declining clinical course of psychotic disorders over the two decades following first hospitalization: evidence from the Suffolk County Mental Health Project. *American Journal of Psychiatry* 2017;174(11):1064–74. DOI: 10.1176/appi.ajp.2017.16101191.
78. Velthorst E, Fett AJ, Reichenberg A, et al. The 20-year longitudinal trajectories of social functioning in individuals with psychotic disorders. *American Journal of Psychiatry* 2017;174(11):1075–85. DOI: 10.1176/appi.ajp.2016.15111419.
79. Melau M, Jeppesen P, Thorup A, et al. The effect of five years versus two years of specialised assertive intervention for first episode psychosis – OPUS II: study protocol for a randomized controlled trial. *Trials* 2011;12:72. DOI: 10.1186/1745-6215-12-72.
80. Cotton SM, Filia KM, Ratheesh A, et al. Early psychosis research at Orygen, The National Centre of Excellence in Youth Mental Health. *Social Psychiatry and Psychiatric Epidemiology* 2016;51 (1):1–13. DOI: 10.1007/s00127-015-1140-0.
81. Harrow M, Jobe TH, Faull RN. Does treatment of schizophrenia with antipsychotic medications eliminate or reduce psychosis? A 20-year multifollow-up study. *Psychological Medicine* 2014;44:3007–16.
82. Hjorthøj C, Stürup AE, McGrath JJ, et al. Years of potential life lost and life expectancy in schizophrenia: a systematic review and meta-analysis. *Lancet Psychiatry* 2017;4(4):295–301
83. Caponnetto P, Polosa R, Robson D, et al. Tobacco smoking, related harm and motivation to quit smoking in people with schizophrenia spectrum disorders. *Health Psychological Research* 2020;8(1):9042. DOI:10.4081/hpr.2020.9042
84. Schoenbaum M, Sutherland JM, Chappel A, et al. Twelve-month health care use and mortality in commercially insured young people with incident psychosis in the United States. *Schizophrenia Bulletin* 2017;43(6):1262–72. DOI: 10.1093/schbul/sbx009.
85. Challis S, Nielssen O, Harris A, et al. Systematic meta-analysis of the risk factors for deliberate self-harm before and after treatment for first-episode psychosis. *Acta Psychiatrica Scandinavica* 2013;127(6):442–54. DOI: 10.1111/acps.12074.

86. Ajnakina O, Stubbs B, Francis E, et al. Hospitalisation and length of hospital stay following first-episode psychosis: systematic review and meta-analysis of longitudinal studies. *Psychological Medicine* 2020;50(6):991–1001. DOI: 10.1017/S0033291719000904.

87. Leucht S, Tardy M, Komossa K, et al. Antipsychotic drugs versus placebo for relapse prevention in schizophrenia: a systematic review and meta-analysis. *Lancet* 2012;379(9831):2063–71. DOI: 10.1016/S0140-6736(12)60239-6.

88. Volavka J, Vevera J. Very long-term outcome of schizophrenia. *International Journal of Clinical Practice* 2018;72(7): e13094. DOI: 10.1111/ijcp.13094.

89. Murray RM, Quattrone D, Natesan S, et al. Should psychiatrists be more cautious about the long-term prophylactic use of antipsychotics? *British Journal of Psychiatry* 2016;209(5):361–5. DOI: 10.1192/bjp.bp.116.182683.

90. Taipale H, Tanskanen A, Mehtälä J, et al. 20-year follow-up study of physical morbidity and mortality in relationship to antipsychotic treatment in a nationwide cohort of 62,250 patients with schizophrenia (FIN20). *World Psychiatry* 2020;19(1):61–8. DOI: 10.1002/wps.20699.

91. Whitaker R. Viewpoint: do antipsychotics protect against early death? A critical view. *Psychological Medicine* 2020,50(16):2643–52. DOI: 10.1017/S003329172000358X.

92. Wunderink L, Nieboer RM, Wiersma D, et al. Recovery in remitted first-episode psychosis at 7 years of follow-up of an early dose reduction/ discontinuation or maintenance treatment strategy: long-term follow-up of a 2-year randomized clinical trial. *JAMA Psychiatry* 2013;70(9):913–20.

93. Wils RS, Gotfredsen DR, Hjorthøj C, et al. Antipsychotic medication and remission of psychotic symptoms 10years after a first-episode psychosis. *Schizophrenia Research* 2017;182:42–8. DOI: 10.1016/j.schres.2016.10.030.

94. Gafoor R, Nitsch D, McCrone P, et al. Effect of early intervention on 5-year outcome in non-affective psychosis. *British Journal of Psychiatry* 2010;196(5):372–6. DOI:10.1192/bjp.bp.109.066050

95. Schoeler T, Monk A, Sami MB, et al. Continued versus discontinued cannabis use in patients with psychosis: a systematic review and meta-analysis. *Lancet Psychiatry* 2016;3(3):215–25. DOI: 10.1016/S2215-0366(15)00363-6.

96. Schoeler T, Petros N, Di Forti M, et al. Association between continued cannabis use and risk of relapse in first-episode psychosis: a quasi-experimental investigation within an observational study. *JAMA Psychiatry* 2016;73 (11):1173–79. DOI: 10.1001/ jamapsychiatry.2016.2427.

97. Agid O, Arenovich T, Sajeev G, et al. An algorithm-based approach to first-episode schizophrenia: response rates over 3 prospective antipsychotic trials with a retrospective data analysis. *Journal of Clinical Psychiatry* 2011;72 (11):1439–44. DOI: 10.4088/ JCP.09m05785yel.

98. Kahn RS, Winter van Rossum I, Leucht S, et al. Amisulpride and olanzapine followed by open-label treatment with clozapine in first-episode schizophrenia and schizophreniform disorder (OPTiMiSE): a three-phase switching study. *Lancet Psychiatry* 2018;5 (10):797–807. DOI: 10.1016/S2215-0366 (18)30252-9.

99. Howes OD, McCutcheon R, Agid O, et al. Treatment-resistant schizophrenia: Treatment Response and Resistance in Psychosis (TRRIP) working group consensus guidelines on diagnosis and terminology. *American Journal of Psychiatry* 2017;174(3):216–29.

100. Lally J, Tully J, Robertson D, et al. Augmentation of clozapine with electroconvulsive therapy in treatment resistant schizophrenia: a systematic review and meta-analysis. *Schizophrenia Research* 2016;171(1–3):215–24. DOI: 10.1016/j.schres.2016.01.024.

101. Demjaha A, Lappin JM, Stahl D, et al. Antipsychotic treatment resistance in first-episode psychosis: prevalence, subtypes and predictors. *Psychological Medicine* 2017;47(11):1981–9. DOI: 10.1017/S0033291717000435.

102. Mizrahi R, Addington J, Rusjan PM, et al. Increased stress-induced dopamine release in psychosis. *Biological Psychiatry* 2012;71(6): 561–67.

103. Legge SE, Dennison CA, Pardiñas AF, et al. Clinical indicators of treatment-resistant psychosis. *British Journal of Psychiatry* 2020;216(5):259–66. DOI: 10.1192/bjp.2019.120.

104. van Erp TGM, Walton E, Hibar DP, et al. Cortical brain abnormalities in 4474 indviduals with schizophrenia and 5098 control subjects via the enhancing neuro imaging genetics through meta analysis (ENIGMA) consortium. *Biological Psychiatry* 2018;84(9): 644–54.

105. Keshavan MS, Anderson S, Pettegrew M. Is schizophrenia due to excessive synaptic pruning in the prefrontal cortex? The Feinberg hypothesis revisited. *Journal of Psychiatric Research* 1994;28(3):239–65.

106. Stone WS, Phillip MR, Yang LH, et al. Neurodegenerative model of schizophrenia: growing evidence to support a revisit. *Schizophrenia Research* 2022;243:154–62

107. Murray RM, Bora E, Modinos E, et al. Schizophrenia: a developmental disorder with risk of non-specific and avoidable decline. *Schizophrenia Research* 2022;243:181–6.

108. Jablensky A, Sartorius N, Ernberg G, et al. Schizophrenia: manifestations, incidence and course in different cultures. A World Health Organization ten-country study. *Psychological Medicine. Monograph Supplement* 1992;20:1–97.

109. Asher L, Fekadu A, Hanlon C. Global mental health and schizophrenia. *Current Opinion in Psychiatry* 2018;31 (3):193–9.

110. Cohen A, Patel V, Thara R, et al. Questioning an axiom: better prognosis for schizophrenia in the developing world? *Schizophrenia Bulletin* 2008;34 (2):229–44.

111. Stubbs B, Koyanagi A, Veronese N, et al. Physical multimorbidity and psychosis: comprehensive cross sectional analysis including 242,952 people across 48 low- and middle-income countries. *BMC Medicine* 2016;14(1):189.

112. Angermeyer MC, Carta MG, Matschinger H, et al. Cultural differences in stigma surrounding schizophrenia: comparison between Central Europe and North Africa. *British Journal of Psychiatry* 2016;208 (4):389–97.

113. Lora A, Kohn R, Levav I, et al. Service availability and utilization and treatment gap for schizophrenic disorders: a survey in 50 low- and middle-income countries. *Bulletin of the*

World Health Organization 2012;90 (1):47–54, 54a-54b.

114. Labys CA, Susser E, Burns JK. Psychosis and help-seeking behavior in rural KwaZulu Natal: unearthing local insights. *International Journal of Mental Health Systems* 2016;10:57.

115. Lilford P, Wickramaseckara Rajapakshe OB, Singh SP. A systematic review of care pathways for psychosis in low-and middle-income countries. *Asian Journal of Psychiatry* 2020;54:102237. DOI: 10.1016/j.ajp.2020.102237.

116. Barbui C, Purgato M, Abdulmalik J, et al. Efficacy of psychosocial interventions for mental health outcomes in low-income and middle-income countries: an umbrella review. *Lancet Psychiatry* 2020;7(2):162–72. DOI: 10.1016/S2215-0366(19)30511-5.

Drug Treatment of the Psychoses

Jonathan Rogers, Edward Chesney, Paul Morrison and Fiona Gaughran

History

Prior to the development of 'neuroleptic' or 'antipsychotic' drugs, the prospect for individuals with schizophrenia-like illnesses was bleak. Electroconvulsive therapy, developed in Italy in the late 1930s, provided relief for a few, while frontal lobotomy had a tranquilising effect but impaired numerous other cortical functions. Medications such as barbiturates merely provided sedation. However, the discovery of penicillin in 1928 led to the treatment of neurosyphilis, raising hopes by the middle of the twentieth century that a specific medical therapy might be possible for schizophrenia.[1]

The roots of modern psychopharmacology are found in the Ayurvedic medicine from the plant *Rauwolfia serpentina*, which had been used in India since around 1000 BCE for insanity. It was brought to the attention of Western medicine by Indian psychiatrists Bose and Sen, who described its effect on reducing blood pressure and violence in 1931. Reserpine, the active ingredient of the herb, acts by inhibiting the sequestering of monoamines into pre-synaptic vesicles. It was briefly popular as an antipsychotic in the 1950s until its ability to cause depression was noted.

Phenothiazine compounds were being used as early as the late 1800s by the German aniline dye industry, and they were found to function pharmacologically as antihistamine medications. In 1949, the French naval surgeon Henri-Marie Laborit, working in Tunisia, was investigating the potential of these antihistamines to reduce surgical shock. On his return to France, Laborit worked with Simone Courvoisier and Paul Charpentier at the Specia Laboratories of Rhone-Poulenc near Paris to refine the compounds, one of which was chlorpromazine, which was chosen as it was the least sedative. Laborit observed that patients who received chlorpromazine were less anxious and had a better mood, so he suggested its use to his psychiatric colleagues at the Val-de-Grace Hospital. It was noted to be effective in a patient with mania, but it was administered in combination, so it was difficult to ascertain what its specific effect would be, and it was soon abandoned in favour of electroconvulsive therapy (ECT).[2] However, Jean Delay and Pierre Deniker at the Saint-Anne hospital, also in Paris, heard about the experiment and published extensively on their own positive results with chlorpromazine in mania and psychosis in 1952. For further details of this history, see Ban (2007).[3]

The advent of chlorpromazine had an extraordinary effect on psychiatric practice. In France, patients were released from mechanical restraints and locked wards.[2] In the USA, there was a reported reduction of 90–95% in the incidence of violence and number of days in seclusion.[1] There was a subsequent rush to develop similar drugs, some of which (such as fluphenazine and thioridazine) were also antipsychotics, but one (imipramine) started the era of tricyclic antidepressants. However, the limitations of what were then termed 'neuroleptic' drugs quickly became apparent. Extrapyramidal side effects (EPSEs) and tardive dyskinesia were described as early as 1957.[4] It was also noted that these medications were not very effective for what would now be termed negative symptoms.[1]

Like many advances in psychiatry, the clinical progress with antipsychotic pharmacology predated the neurobiological understanding. It was not until 1963 that Carlsson and Lindqvist showed evidence for the blockade of monoamine receptors. It was only in 1975, having explored many other possibilities, that Seeman and colleagues demonstrated that antipsychotic activity was dependent on the antagonism of post-synaptic dopamine receptors.

Terminology evolved over time as well. One of the earlier descriptors for this class of drug was 'tranquilisers' and, later, 'major tranquilisers' to distinguish them from the benzodiazepines. This term, however, merely implies a calming effect, and thus Delay and Deniker preferred 'neuroleptic' on the basis of the extrapyramidal side effects – perpetuating the idea that these adverse effects were essential to the activity of the medications. The most commonly used term today is 'antipsychotic', but this term is also not without critics, who contend that it is insufficiently mechanistic and conflates symptoms with mental disorders.

The most significant development in antipsychotics since the advent of chlorpromazine has been the use of clozapine. Clozapine was discovered in 1959 and was the first antipsychotic drug to demonstrate an 'atypical' profile in that it did not induce extrapyramidal side effects – challenging the dogma that this was necessary for antipsychotic effect. It was introduced to widespread clinical practice in the 1970s, but its use was short-lived after a report of the death of eight patients in Finland with agranulocytosis. Despite the initial suggestion from the manufacturers that the monitoring of leukocyte count was necessary, it was almost completely withdrawn from use globally. It was only after convincing evidence for the superiority of clozapine compared to chlorpromazine for treatment-resistance schizophrenia was produced that the US Food and Drug Administration (FDA) approved it again.

'Atypical' antipsychotics other than clozapine started to come to market in the 1990s with the advent of drugs including olanzapine, risperidone and quetiapine. However, the concept of atypicality and whether these newer drugs have any superiority to older ones is controversial and discussed later. The other notable advance has been the development of long-acting injectable antipsychotic medications, which now exist for several typical and atypical antipsychotic medications.

New antipsychotics continue to come to market with the more recent advent of the partial agonists aripiprazole, brexpiprazole and cariprazine, but there is still a reliance on the modulation of post-synaptic dopamine receptors. Current identification of potential antipsychotics relies on the ability of drugs to suppress various motor and behavioural phenomena in the mouse or rat, which are limited models for schizophrenia itself.

Mechanisms

Molecules such as chlorpromazine, haloperidol, risperidone and so forth are effective against the core symptoms of psychosis. Chlorpromazine was discovered by serendipity; haloperidol and risperidone were discovered as antagonists of amphetamine and lysergic acid diethylamide (LSD) respectively. They are effective against delusional thinking, hallucinations, breakdown of ego boundaries and the agitation that is commonly associated with psychosis. They do not achieve this effect by a general sedative or major-tranquilising function. By the time of their introduction, a whole host of sedatives – including opiates – had already been tried for schizophrenia and had no impact whatsoever. The antipsychotics were different, but how they achieved their effect would remain a mystery for the best part of 20 years. This is not unknown in medicine. For instance, aspirin had been used for centuries, but the basis of the analgesic effect – inhibition of prostaglandin synthesis – was only discovered in the 1970s.

Of course, it is now readily appreciated that the (majority of) antipsychotics work on dopamine signalling in the brain. In particular, the antipsychotics dampen signalling at the dopamine D_2 receptor.[5] Generally, they function as *antagonists,* blocking the action of dopamine at the receptor. The antipsychotic drugs were in clinical use before dopamine was even recognised as a neurotransmitter. Acetylcholine and noradrenaline were the bona fide neurotransmitters – dopamine, which is an intermediate in the synthesis of noradrenaline, was regarded as no more than that, a mere precursor. The work of Nobel prize winner Arvid Carlsson and others in the 1960s and 1970s showed that dopamine was a neurotransmitter in its own right. That era of neurophysiology had two major themes: the characterisation of receptors for the various neurotransmitters as well as the elucidation of neurotransmitter release from nerve varicosities. Both research efforts made extensive use of radiolabelled molecules, either transmitters or drugs, to 'visualise' and quantify the fundamental component processes of synaptic signalling.

Dopamine receptors were initially classed as D_1 and D_2 on the basis of whether they stimulate (D_1) or inhibit (D_2) the production of an important signalling molecule inside neurons called cAMP (via G-proteins). Numerous antipsychotics were available for researchers, having been discovered using a highly predictive behavioural assay in rodents known as conditioned avoidance.[6] Pivotal experiments in the 1970s established that the affinity of a series of antipsychotic drugs for the dopamine D_2 receptor was linearly related to their dose range in clinical practice.[7] Antipsychotics such as sulpiride, which required clinical doses approaching 1000 mg/d to be effective, were found to have a low affinity for the dopamine D_2 receptor. At the other end of the scale, antipsychotics such as haloperidol, which were effective at doses below 5 mg/d, were found to have a very high affinity for the dopamine D_2 receptor.

Affinity: Affinity describes the strength of the chemical attraction between a drug and a receptor and can be quantified as a K_D value. Formally, the K_D value is the concentration of drug required to occupy 50 per cent of the available receptor population. High-affinity drugs have a low K_D value and vice versa.

By the 1990s, molecular biology had discovered and characterised five dopamine receptors in total, D_1–D_5. There was hope that this more detailed and accurate picture would present opportunities for a more refined clinical pharmacology. There was the idea of targeting one of the newly found subtypes, particularly D_4, in the hope of better efficacy and a better side-effect profile. Unfortunately, that effort led to a blind alley[8] – and this would turn out to be the case for several other approaches – which were nevertheless attractive on paper.

However, there were successes. One of the undoubted triumphs was the separation of the antipsychotic effect from the motor side effects: rigidity, tremor, bradykinesia and akathisia. High-affinity dopamine D_2 antagonists such as haloperidol are particularly prone to cause motor side effects. At one stage, it was even thought that motor side effects were an inevitable part of antipsychotic efficacy and that it was impossible to disentangle the two. Clozapine showed this not to be the case.

Following its introduction, it became apparent that clozapine does not cause motor side effects. Furthermore, it was also recognised – and ultimately demonstrated in clinical trials – that clozapine could be highly effective for patients with a stubbornly resistant and disabling psychotic illness, for whom other antipsychotics had failed. The unique clinical pharmacology of clozapine triggered an effort which, as yet, hasn't fully materialised: what is the mechanism responsible for clozapine's superior efficacy? One thing was certain, however, which was that clozapine had very weak affinity for the dopamine D_2 receptor, indirectly challenging the increasingly quite simplistic but never quite disproved notion that excess dopamine was at the roots of schizophrenia.

By the mid 1990s, the new methods in human psychopharmacology, such as positron emission tomography (PET) and single photon emission tomography (SPET), had demonstrated that an effective antipsychotic effect depended on the drug binding to roughly 65–80% of the total dopamine D_2 receptor pool in the basal ganglia.[9] (Higher binding increased the chances of motor disorder; lower binding could jeopardise the antipsychotic effect.) Clozapine behaved very differently though. Lyn Pilowsky and colleagues at the Institute of Psychiatry in London found that clozapine was effective in patients with schizophrenia despite very low D_2 binding in the basal ganglia. The low affinity of clozapine for the dopamine D_2 receptor could explain the absence of motor side effects in the clinic. This is also true of the otherwise unremarkable and relatively weak antipsychotic molecule quetiapine, which behaves similarly to clozapine in having fast dissociation from the D_2 receptor. If not via D_2, though, by which mechanism did clozapine have antipsychotic efficacy then? Indeed, it had an efficacy that went beyond merely addressing stubborn, hitherto treatment-resistant positive psychotic symptoms, but that also encompassed the so-called negative symptoms, the loss of drive, the diminution of the personality, the defining features of schizophrenia typically unresponsive to the other antipsychotics. The full benefits of clozapine could also be delayed by at least six months – another distinguishing feature – which has never been explained or attracted much speculation.

The field was initially attracted to the idea that clozapine's superior efficacy could be accounted for by the antagonism of a specific type of serotonin receptor. Earlier generations of pharmacologists had identified three serotonin receptor subtypes. The molecular biologists expanded this number to fourteen.[10] The receptor of interest in the case of clozapine was the $5HT_{2A}$ subtype.

Serotonin $5HT_{2A}$ receptor pharmacology was already of importance. The serotonin $5HT_{2A}$ receptor is the target for the psychedelic compounds psilocybin and LSD, which function as *agonists*, activating the receptor. Psychedelics can certainly transform the experience of lived reality in a fundamental manner whilst impairing insight.[11] As such, they can be said to elicit a psychotic experience, although perhaps with very little similarity – at least in phenomenological terms – to a typical, paranoid psychosis, the most common endogenous form of schizophrenia. The idea that LSD antagonists could be effective against endogenous psychosis led to the discovery of risperidone, a high-affinity $5HT_{2A}$ antagonist. However, risperidone is also a high-affinity dopamine D_2 receptor antagonist, confusing the picture. In time, the emerging class – of which risperidone was the prototype – became known as dual $D_2/5HT_{2A}$ receptor blockers, with the binding to the $5HT_{2A}$ being emphasised. Other members of the class include – at least on paper – olanzapine, ziprasidone, lurasidone, asenapine, iloperidone, lumateperone and clozapine. For a period, dual $D_2/5HT_{2A}$ receptor antagonism was heralded as a desirable quality in an antipsychotic molecule, especially given the apparent relationship with clozapine.

However, it soon became apparent that the other members of the $D_2/5HT_{2A}$ class fell short of clozapine in terms of efficacy.[12] Antagonism of the serotonin $5HT_{2A}$ receptor did not seem to confer additional benefit over and above D_2 blockade and could hardly be regarded as the special, unique feature of clozapine. Additionally, pure $5HT_{2A}$ receptor blockers are generally ineffective antipsychotics.[13] Overall, $5HT_{2A}$ appears to have been another blind alley for drug discovery in schizophrenia, although efficacy in Parkinson's psychosis was demonstrated for the inverse agonist pimavanserin, which might also have some benefits in schizophrenia, giving a last-gasp lifeline for serotonin-based antipsychotics.

Inverse agonist: Receptor systems have constitutive activity. Even in the absence of an agonist, a small proportion of the receptors will exist briefly in a conformation that activates an intracellular signalling cascade, say the synthesis of cAMP. An agonist binds and stabilises the active conformation of the receptor amplifying the magnitude of the signal. An inverse agonist binds and stabilises the inactive conformation of the receptor reducing baseline signalling. For completion, an antagonist, has equal preference for both the active and inactive conformations and has no impact upon the magnitude of baseline signalling, but it will compete with and block the effects of both an agonist and an inverse agonist at the receptor.

Somewhat unexpectedly, there is a case for re-incorporating the so-called typical or first-generation antipsychotics (such as trifluoperazine) into clinical practice again. Large trials in the USA and Europe have demonstrated that – clozapine aside – there is no difference in efficacy between the antipsychotics, regardless of when they were discovered or introduced into practice.[14,15] The differences between the various antipsychotics are increasingly seen, not in terms of efficacy but in terms of side effects, attributable to actions at other components (e.g. the histamine H1 receptor – sedation and weight gain, the hERG channel – long QTc) and certainly do not obey any imposed typical/atypical or first-generation/second-generation categorisation. Indeed, there is little rationale for such categorisation on either molecular or clinical grounds.[16] The SPET and PET studies from the 1990s brought some rationale to antipsychotic dosing and put paid to the former practice of exceptionally high-dosing, which brought very little except for risk. High-affinity dopamine D_2 receptor antagonists such as trifluoperazine and haloperidol can still be useful in the clinic, assuming there is prudence with the dosing and care to avoid motor side effects. However, the same is also true of risperidone and some of the other so-called dual $D_2/5HT_{2A}$ blockers.[16]

The basis of the superior efficacy of clozapine remains unknown. Aside from being the most efficacious molecule for schizophrenia, clozapine also probably heads the list for side effects.[17] Identification of the key molecular mechanisms underlying clozapine's antipsychotic effect could lead to the development of less-toxic related drugs. This remains an unaddressed priority for the field. Currently the most appealing candidate is partial agonist activity at a receptor for acetylcholine, termed M_4, which is enriched in the basal ganglia. The actions of clozapine at acetylcholine receptors are not shared by any other antipsychotic, typical or atypical, and stand out as a unique feature. There are five acetylcholine receptors in this class, and developing drugs with specificity has been a challenge but is important given the presence of the M_2 receptor in the heart.[16] Some encouraging signs suggest that specific partial agonist activity at cholinergic M_4 receptors could be a fruitful approach for drug discovery in schizophrenia.[18]

Another more immediate success has been the development of *partial agonists* for the dopamine D_2 receptor.[19] The prototype molecule is aripiprazole. Newer members of the class are brexpiprazole and cariprazine. This class appear to confer benefits in terms of a more favourable side-effect profile compared to the D_2 antagonists, namely an absence of high prolactin, sexual dysfunction, excessive sedation or weight gain. Dose-related akathisia is the only apparent downside of this class.

Partial agonist: At the receptor level, agonists stimulate a response – for example, enhanced cAMP production inside the neuron. Increasing the dose of agonist increases the magnitude of the response, but this soon reaches a plateau, the maximal response that the tissue can deliver. A full agonist stimulates the system at 100 per cent of its capacity. For a partial agonist, the plateau is much lower, say 30 per cent of the maximal response.

Aripiprazole, brexpiprazole and cariprazine are high-affinity, partial agonists at the dopamine D_2 receptor. They outcompete dopamine for the D_2 receptor and, on paper, offer protection against over-stimulation whilst not completely suppressing tissue systems. The partial agonists appear to have particular utility in first-episode psychosis, given their relatively benign side-effect profile, as well as for bipolarity.[16] They are less effective in more stubbornly ingrained psychoses. Aside from clozapine, however, this could be said of all the other antipsychotics.

For a brief period, glutamate pharmacology promised a new era of antipsychotic treatment.[20] The starting point was the psychopharmacology of ketamine. Akin to LSD/psilocybin, ketamine can completely transform the experience of lived reality and impair insight. It was argued that ketamine recreated not just the positive symptoms of schizophrenia but also the negative symptoms. As such, a drug which could antagonise ketamine might be effective against the whole spectrum of schizophrenic phenomena, not just the hallucinations, delusions and ipseity (sense of identity) disturbance but also the lack of drive, emotional flattening and poverty of thought that are predictive of social disability. Pre-clinical work led to the development of bitopertin (a glycine re-uptake inhibitor) and LY-2140023 (a metabotropic glutamate receptor group II agonist). Both molecules inhibit the effects of ketamine in animal models and were taken forward for human studies. The initial clinical trials were highly encouraging. However, both molecules floundered in larger, definitive studies, proclaiming glutamate – at least for the time being – as another blind alley for drug development in schizophrenia.[21,22] Unexpectedly, ketamine would re-appear as a treatment for stubborn, resistant depressive illness, and the clinical trials data have been supportive this time.

The endocannabinoid system has come to prominence in neuroscience. Endocannabinoids are important modulators of synaptic plasticity. In the basal ganglia, dopamine D_2 receptor activation gives rise to the synthesis of an endocannabinoid known as 2-Arachodonylglycerol (2-AG). Numerous studies have shown that 2-AG dampens cortical input to basal ganglia neurons.[23] At the same time, psychiatric practice was beginning to recognise that THC, the active ingredient of cannabis was psychotogenic and could even predispose to schizophrenia, if delivered in the absence of cannabidiol (CBD), another ingredient of the cannabis plant that had been bred-out of modern forms.[24]

Cannabinoid agonists – such as THC – stimulate CB_1 receptors, which are typically found on the terminals of glutamate and GABA neurons throughout the brain and especially enriched in structures such as the hippocampus, cerebellum, basal ganglia and cortex where circuit modification/learning occurs.[25] THC is a partial agonist at CB_1 receptors and, as such, delivers a sub-maximal response. A series of full agonists at the CB_1 receptors, the so-called synthetic cannabinoids, elicit a very florid, extreme psychotic reaction in users.

Similar to the case with LSD, ketamine and amphetamine, antagonists of THC represent candidates for the treatment of endogenous psychosis. Cannabidiol, the precise mechanisms of which remain unknown, has been shown to harbour antipsychotic properties,[26] although confirmation of efficacy against schizophrenia requires larger, definitive studies.

Phases of Treatment

At-Risk Mental State (ARMS)

The Psychosis Prodrome

Psychosis does not normally appear out of the blue. Two-thirds of patients who have experienced a psychotic episode are able to describe a prodromal period over the preceding months and years.[27] The symptoms are often non-specific; the most common are anxiety, low mood, social withdrawal and impaired concentration. A persistent decline in social and occupational function is common. Positive psychotic symptoms – while key from a diagnostic perspective – are not always present, often emerging at a later stage and are either fleeting or present in an attenuated form. Suspiciousness and unusual thought content are reported most frequently, while more extraordinary symptoms such as delusions, hallucinations and passivity phenomena are relatively rare.

In the past, the psychosis prodrome was only recognised retrospectively. However, there has been considerable effort to identify prodromal cases before they 'transition to psychosis'. Identifying individuals at this early stage presents a unique opportunity to alter the course or even prevent the development of psychotic disorders. There are several terms for the psychosis prodrome, including the 'clinical high-risk state' (CHR), the 'at-risk mental state' (ARMS) and the 'ultra-high-risk state' (UHR). Structured assessments to identify those most at risk of developing psychosis include the Structured Interview for Prodromal Syndromes (SIPS) and the Comprehensive Assessment of At Risk Mental States (CAARMS). The SIPS and CAARMS assess subjects according to the criteria for three distinct syndromes, which are described in Table 5.3.1.

An alternative approach is the 'basic symptoms' model. Rather than focusing on positive psychotic symptoms more generally, it aims to capture the specific subjective disturbances in thinking, language and attention that best predict the development of psychosis.[29] The Cognitive Disturbances (COGDIS) and Cognitive-Perceptive Basic Symptoms (COPER) criteria can be used to assess potential cases.[30] The COGDIS criteria are provided in Figure 5.3.1.

Prospective studies of CHR individuals have found that around 22 per cent develop a first episode of psychosis within three years.[31] While the majority do not develop psychosis, many continue to experience symptomatic and functional impairments. Sub-threshold psychotic symptoms may persist in some, while others are diagnosed with mood and anxiety disorders.

Clinical services for people at CHR offer psychoeducation, case management and clinical monitoring. UK NICE guidelines also recommend offering individual CBT with or without family interventions to all patients. Unfortunately, clinical trials examining the benefits of specific interventions have shown limited success. The most recent analyses suggest that no interventions, including cognitive behavioural therapy, family therapy, antipsychotics or omega-3 fatty acids, are more effective than case management alone at either reducing transition to psychosis or reducing attenuated positive psychotic symptoms.[32] Clinicians may still recommend specific pharmacological interventions to treat comorbid depression or anxiety disorders and, as a result, antidepressant, hypnotic and anxiolytic medications are often prescribed (see Chapters 3.3 and 6.1). Interventions to reduce substance misuse are also important (see Chapter 14); around a third of patients with psychoses smoke tobacco or use cannabis.[31] Antipsychotics are rarely prescribed as it is generally accepted that their benefits are unlikely to outweigh their harms. If antipsychotics are used, only very low doses should be prescribed on a trial basis with the aim of relieving symptoms and distress. Any prescription would be 'off-label'.

The overall value of the clinical services for CHR is controversial. The benefits of intervention at this early stage appear to be limited. Moreover, CHR services only identify a very small proportion (4–12.5%) of those who ever experience psychosis.[33] Other, more fundamental, criticisms of the field's foundations have also been made.[34] Even so, supporters of the CHR model highlight the potential benefits of engaging these help-seeking individuals at an early stage and providing interventions that may reduce their distress.

Presence of ≥2 of the following 9 basic symptoms with a SPI-A* score of ≥ 3 within the last 3 months:

- Inability to divide attention
- Thought interference
- Thought pressure
- Thought blockages
- Disturbance of receptive speech
- Disturbance of expressive speech
- Unstable ideas of reference
- Disturbances of abstract thinking
- Captivation of attention by details of the visual field

* Schizophrenia proneness instrument – adult version (204)

Figure 5.3.1 COGDIS criteria.

Table 5.3.1 Three types of psychosis prodrome

	CAARMS criteria	Proportion of total[1]	Psychosis at 6 months[1]	Psychosis at 24 months[1]
Attenuated psychotic symptoms	Symptoms below threshold levels for psychosis (either sub-threshold intensity or frequency) + Decline in social and occupational functioning	79–90%	10% (95% CI: 8–13%)	19%[15,16,18,20-25] (95% CI: 15–23%)
Brief limited intermittent psychotic symptoms	A recent history of frank psychotic symptoms that resolved spontaneously (without antipsychotic medication) within one week + Decline in social and occupational functioning	6–14%	10% (95% CI: 2–20%)	39% (95% CI: 7–51%)
Genetic risk and deterioration syndrome	Family history of psychosis in first-degree relative or schizotypal personality disorder + Decline in social and occupational functioning	3–7%	0% (95% CI: 0–1%)	3% (95% CI: 0–8%)

[1] Data from the meta-analysis by Fusar-Poli et al. 2016[28]

First Episode and Acute Psychosis

Treatment of Acute and First-Episode Psychosis

Expectant Management

Unless a patient is highly disturbed, antipsychotic medication does not need to be started immediately. For patients presenting with a first episode of psychosis or those presenting with novel symptoms, a period of assessment is often valuable to clarify a patient's diagnosis and formulation before its natural history is obscured by the effects of treatment. If psychotic symptoms have only been present for a few days, treatment with antipsychotics may not be necessary as the symptoms may spontaneously resolve without treatment. For those with a psychosis secondary to substance use, a period of abstinence may also be sufficient. However, if symptoms persist, it is important to initiate pharmacological treatment as a period of untreated psychosis of more than four weeks predicts 20 per cent more severe symptoms at follow-up compared to those whose psychosis is untreated for a week or less.[35]

Benzodiazepines, Antihistamines and Other Sedatives

In the first instance, distress, anxiety and agitation should be managed non-pharmacologically. However, if such symptoms are severe, sedative medication can be considered. Benzodiazepines are often prescribed regularly to manage agitation and aggression, though clinicians may be surprised how little evidence there is from randomised controlled trials supporting their effectiveness.[36] Diazepam and clonazepam are two of the most popular agents as their longer half-lives (~20–50 hours) should reduce the risk of rebound symptoms. However, this also means that they will slowly accumulate over time, risking oversedation if the patient is not reviewed regularly. Clonazepam has the additional advantage that it has a slower onset of action and may be less liable to be abused for recreational purposes. Antihistamines, such as promethazine, can also be prescribed regularly and may be less likely to lead to dependence. In emergency situations where there is severe distress or agitation, rapid tranquilisation may be required (see later).

For insomnia, a benzodiazepine with a shorter half-life (to avoid a hangover effect the following morning) is normally preferred. Zopiclone, zolpidem and other 'z-drugs' can also be used, though there is little to distinguish them from benzodiazepines from a pharmacological perspective as both are positive allosteric modulators of the $GABA_A$ receptor. As a result, NICE guidelines recommend that the choice should be based on cost alone.[37] An alternative to GABA-ergic agents is a melatonin receptor agonist. Ramelteon and melatonin are well tolerated and present no risk of dependency. There is also emerging evidence from several small clinical trials that suggest they may counteract the adverse metabolic effects of certain antipsychotics.[38]

Antipsychotics

Antipsychotics are the first-line treatment for psychosis. They have proven efficacy[39] and established safety, and their use is associated with reduced mortality over the long-term.[40] Every licensed antipsychotic reduces the activity of dopamine D_2 receptors, either by acting as antagonists or partial agonists. All antipsychotics also have activity at serotonin, histamine, adrenergic, muscarinic and other receptors.

Classification of Antipsychotics -- Antipsychotics have been classified according to their chemical structure (e.g. butyrophenones, benzisoxazoles, thioxanthenes), their propensity to cause extrapyramidal side effects (typical/atypical) and how recently they were developed (first-generation/second-generation). None of these categories is ideal as they either lack scientific validity or clinical value. In the last decade, there has been a drive to use a more scientifically based terminology: Neuroscience-based-Nomenclature (NbN).[41] NbN is an evidence-based system that aims to describe the pharmacology for all psychopharmacologically active agents. It is supported internationally and is based on each medication's pharmacological activity. An approved and easy-to-use app to support this (NBN2) is available online.

Discussing Antipsychotic Medication with Patients and Their Carers -- NICE guidelines recommend that patients should take an active role in discussions regarding antipsychotic medication. Failure to discuss medication changes can contribute to feelings of isolation and loss of control and may exacerbate paranoia or mistrust of mental health services. Patients should be supported to understand the expected benefits and adverse effects of treatment and be educated on how to seek help when adverse effects occur. The complexity of the discussion should reflect their level of understanding, and if possible, their family and carers should be involved. Clear explanation of adverse effects – particularly sensitive issues such as erectile dysfunction, amenorrhea and weight gain – may make it more likely for a patient to seek help at an early stage, reducing the likelihood of subsequent non-adherence.

Efficacy -- The latest meta-analyses report that the overall efficacy of antipsychotic medication is of a moderate size (Standardised mean difference – SMD 0.38) when compared to placebo treatment.[39] Antipsychotics have the greatest effect on positive symptoms (SMD 0.45), though their efficacy for treating negative symptoms (SMD 0.35), quality of life (SMD 0.35) and function (SMD 0.34) is not much lower. Between antipsychotics, the differences in efficacy are small but may be clinically significant when comparing the most and least effective agents. Clozapine excluded, the two most effective agents for overall symptoms appear to be amisulpride (0.73; 95% CrI 0.58–0.89) and olanzapine (0.56; 95% CrI 0.50–0.62).[42] Three of the least efficacious but commonly prescribed antipsychotics are lurasidone (0.36; 95% CrI 0.24–0.48), aripiprazole (0.41; 95% CrI 0.32–0.50) and quetiapine (0.42; 95% CrI 0.32–0.50), all of which possess licences for use in affective disorders in at least one jurisdiction.

Tolerability -- Arguably the most important feature of an antipsychotic is its tolerability. All antipsychotics have adverse effects – many of them unpleasant – so it is important to use the lowest effective dose. In practice, it can take a number of trials of different medications before a patient settles on a preferred agent. Important adverse effects to consider and discuss include:

- Extrapyramidal (dystonia, akathisia, tremor)
- Metabolic (weight gain, diabetes)
- Cardiovascular (prolonged QT and sudden cardiac death)
- Hormonal and sexual (erectile dysfunction, amenorrhoea, loss of libido)
- Mental (sedation, cognitive impairment, emotional flattening)

At a molecular level, adverse effects are largely determined by each agent's receptor binding profile, the prominence of which is driven by the concentration of the compound in an individual and determined by factors such as dose, genetics and drug interactions. Antagonism of histamine H_1 receptors causes sedation and weight gain. Akathisia is particularly common with D_2 receptor partial agonists. Blockade of $5HT_{2C}$ receptors can lead to weight gain[43] (which can be offset by adjunctive aripiprazole, a partial agonist at the receptor; see later). The section on side effects provides in-depth information on the assessment and management of adverse effects.

Evidence from Pragmatic Trials

Ideally, all clinical interventions should be supported by evidence from randomised controlled trials (RCTs). Randomisation of subjects and blinding of participants and researchers to allocated treatments minimise the biases present in observational research. However, most RCTs have major limitations. First, they have a tendency to recruit volunteers who are not representative of the wider patient population: they are less likely to have a severe illness or struggle to adhere to prescribed treatments. Further, many trials are often short, typically lasting for just a few weeks. Some of the most distressing adverse effects such as diabetes, tardive dyskinesia and gynaecomastia may take months to materialise and will not be accurately measured by short-term studies. Some of these limitations can be overcome with pragmatic trial designs. Pragmatic trials are often single-blind or open-label, have less proscriptive inclusion criteria, fewer outcome measures and may allow clinicians more flexibility to adjust medication dose. As a result, they are often able to recruit larger and more representative samples and are able to monitor response to treatment over a longer period. In the following section, we describe some of the most influential pragmatic trials and consider their implications.

One of the most influential studies was the CATIE trial.[44] It randomised 1,492 patients with schizophrenia to either olanzapine, perphenazine, quetiapine or risperidone for up to 18 months. While there were no differences between the different medications with regard to symptomatic improvement, there were meaningful differences in discontinuation rates. Olanzapine had the best result, with a discontinuation rate of 64%. Quetiapine had the worst, a discontinuation rate of 82%. The EUFEST trial randomised 498 patients with first-episode schizophrenia to amisulpride, olanzapine, ziprasidone, quetiapine and haloperidol for 12 months.[45] The best results, in terms of both treatment response and tolerability, were with amisulpride and olanzapine. Both achieved a greater than 50% reduction in symptoms for 67% of patients, compared to 37–56% for other agents. Discontinuation rates were 33% for olanzapine, 40% for amisulpride, 43% for ziprasidone, 53% for quetiapine and 72% for haloperidol. The third-largest study was the PAFIP-3 trial, which recruited 376 drug-naïve patients with first-episode psychosis and followed them up for three years.[46] The time until discontinuation varied considerably: from 855 days with olanzapine, 786 days with risperidone, 452 days with aripiprazole, 295 days with haloperidol and 251 days with ziprasidone, down to just 60 days with quetiapine. Participants in the quetiapine arm were considerably more likely to discontinue treatment due to lack of efficacy (50% for quetiapine vs 22% for other agents). Together, these studies highlight the most efficacious agents: olanzapine, amisulpride and perhaps risperidone too.

Olanzapine has high affinity for histamine H_1 receptors and is therefore a potent sedative. As a result, it is often considered in situations where there is significant agitation or aggression. Since olanzapine can have a considerable and rapid effect on weight and other metabolic outcomes, it is often worth considering switching to an alternative agent at an early stage, and indeed, some national guidelines recommend that olanzapine is not used as a first-line drug in first-episode psychosis.[47]

What Dose?

Studies using PET studies suggest that occupancy of 65–85% of D_2 receptors is associated with clinical response.[48] D_2 receptor occupancy is highly correlated with plasma antipsychotic levels (Pearson's $r = 0.77$, $P < 0.0001$).[49] However, due to large variation in pharmacokinetics between patients, antipsychotic dose is a poor predictor of action at the receptor and therefore of clinical response. Nevertheless, in many patients, antipsychotics achieve substantial occupancy (>65%) at relatively low daily doses (risperidone 3 mg, haloperidol 2 mg, olanzapine 7.5 mg and amisulpride 450 mg). Even at maximal doses, however, quetiapine struggles to achieve 50 per cent occupancy, perhaps underlying its uncertain efficacy.[50]

In first-episode psychosis, the dose of antipsychotic required is usually much lower than in established illness. High doses increase the risk of side effects and may not achieve substantial clinical benefit. Common antipsychotic medications used in first-episode psychosis and established schizophrenia, along with their most common side effects, are described later.

Maintenance

Maintenance Treatment and Relapse Prevention

Psychotic relapses are highly disruptive. Risks include self injury, suicide and violence to others, damage to personal relationships and societal stigma, unemployment and neglect of physical health. Maintenance treatment with antipsychotic medication is the most effective intervention to reduce these risks. In clinical trials of patients with schizophrenia – compared to placebo treatment, where 64% of patients will relapse within a year – only 27% on antipsychotic medication relapse (risk ratio [RR] 0.40, 95% CI: 0.33–0.49).[51] For patients with first-episode psychosis, antipsychotics reduce the risk of subsequent relapse by about 50%.[52] The number needed to treat is just three. Maintenance treatment is also associated with a large reduction in violent acts (2% vs 12%; RR 0.27, 95% CI: 0.15–0.52) and improved quality of life (standardised mean difference - 0.62, 95% CI: 1.15–0.09).[51]

Switching Medications and Optimum Dosing

Adverse effects are unpredictable and significant inter- and intra-individual variation in pharmacokinetics can make predicting the ideal dose of a new medication difficult. A variety of methods have been used to estimate equivalent doses, though there is no gold standard.[53] Results from a meta-analysis of placebo-controlled dose-finding trials are presented in Table 5.3.2.[54]

Most antipsychotics display a hyperbolic dose-response curve, so that at higher doses, any subsequent increase may only have a limited effect. The doses at which 95% of total efficacy are achieved (at a population level) are presented in Table 5.3.2. While trials of high and very high doses may be worthwhile in some individual cases, overall they risk increasing the burden of adverse effects without having a major impact on efficacy. Patients prescribed high doses should be closely monitored for adverse effects, and any trial should have clear objectives and be time limited.

Ideally, cross-titrating between antipsychotics should be done slowly and cautiously, bearing in mind that a change in presentation on switching may be due to withdrawal of an adverse effect of a previous drug, such as sedation.

Table 5.3.2 Doses at which 95% of total efficacy are achieved[4]

	Dose equivalent to risperidone 1 mg (mg/day)	95% effective dose (mg/day)
Amisulpride	86	537
Aripiprazole	1.8	11.5
Asenapine	2.4	15
Brexpiprazole	0.54	3.4
Haloperidol	1	6.3
Iloperidone	3.2	20.1
Lurasidone	23.5	147
Olanzapine	2.4	15.2
Paliperidone	2.1	13.4
Quetiapine	77	482
Risperidone	1	6.3
Sertindole	3.6	22.5
Ziprasidone	30	185

Antipsychotic Polypharmacy

Most guidelines are unenthusiastic about antipsychotic polypharmacy. The main concern is that combination antipsychotics increase the risk of adverse effects, QTc prolongation and drug-drug interactions without much evidence that they improve efficacy. The only clinical trials that support the practice are either open-label or low-quality; high-quality studies find no effect.[55] Thus far, the literature is heterogenous but suggests mortality risk is comparable between antipsychotic polypharmacy and monotherapy,[56] while switching from polypharmacy to monotherapy may risk relapse.[57] Despite guidelines and audits, antipsychotic polypharmacy is relatively common in clinical practice (~20 per cent).

If there is an exception to this rule, it is for aripiprazole, which is sometimes co-prescribed to improve tolerance rather than effect. Aripiprazole augmentation can help mitigate hyperprolactinaemia and weight gain caused by other antipsychotics and may even be an effective adjunct for treating negative symptoms.

Adherence

For most medical conditions, only about 50% of patients take their medication as prescribed. Adherence in patients with schizophrenia isn't any better: in a large study of US veterans, 39% had consistently good adherence to their antipsychotics, 43% had inconsistent adherence and 18% were poorly adherent.[58] Many factors may affect adherence, including lack of insight, poor motivation and memory impairment. Friends and family are also important and can have both a positive and negative impact; societal and self-stigma can also have a role. To aid adherence, clinicians can work with patients to select a medication that provides the ideal balance between efficacy and adverse effects to suit their individual needs. Long-acting injectable formulations are effective and can be offered early.

Promoting adherence is a collaborative process. An ideal approach is shared decision-making, where clinicians and patients work together to ensure that the patient is at the centre of decisions regarding their treatment. Shared decision-making has been shown to improve patients' perception of the therapeutic alliance, treatment satisfaction and self-rated medication compliance.[59] Many patients will, understandably, have a fundamental desire to try and manage their illness without the need for psychotropic medication; a non-dogmatic approach, where dose reduction and medication discontinuation are managed and supported, may be more effective in the long-term.

Unfortunately, there is little evidence to support specific psychological or behavioural interventions to improve adherence. Technological interventions, such as smart pill containers and digital text reminders, and interventions that engage family and carers are perhaps the most evidence-based.[60] Adherence therapy – a brief psychological intervention based on psychoeducation – motivational interviewing and CBT has been tested in six clinical trials.[61] In a meta-analysis, it was shown to be associated with symptomatic improvement despite having no impact on adherence. Tellingly, the only trial with an active control intervention (psychoeducation) demonstrated no benefit of treatment; the results of the other trials may simply be an artefact of increased therapeutic input.[62]

Long-Acting Injectable Formulations

Long-acting injectable (LAI) antipsychotics are more effective than oral formulations, and discussions on LAIs as an option may be valuable to have early in the course of the illness. This assertion is supported by evidence from across study designs.[63] They have been shown to reduce the risk of relapse in RCTs (relative risk [RR] 0.88, 95% CI: 0.79–0.99), cohort studies (RR 0.92, 95% CI: 0.88–0.98) and pre-post studies (RR 0.44 95% CI: 0.39–0.51). Study design is particularly relevant here. Patients recruited to RCTs are more likely to adhere to medication, minimising the potential benefit of an LAI. In cohort studies, selection bias has a major effect, as clinicians prescribe them for patients with more severe illness. In pre-post studies, where the same patients are examined before and after prescription of an LAI, regression to the mean is the main issue, which, unlike the biases in the other studies, will accentuate the benefits of LAI treatment. In summary, the real-world efficacy of LAIs is likely to be somewhere inbetween the estimates presented earlier. Arguably, more important than relapse is psychosocial function, which is also improved with LAI treatment relative to oral medication.[64]

Breakthrough Symptoms and 'Dopamine Supersensitivity'

Even when adherent to medication, many patients with psychosis relapse. Psychotic disorders are inherently dynamic, and symptoms fluctuate from week to week. A meta-analysis of clinical trials for LAI antipsychotics estimated that the average relapse rate is about 23 relapses per 100 participant-years, despite adherence being established.[65] The factor with the largest impact on the risk of relapse was the presence of tardive dyskinesia (HR = 2.4, 95% CI: 1.1–5.4, p = 0.038), which was even larger than diagnosis of a comorbid substance use disorder (HR = 1.6, 95% CI: 1.2–2.1, p = 0.0037).[65] From a neurobiological perspective, this is an intriguing finding as it supports the 'dopamine supersensitivity' hypothesis, which proposes that chronic D2 receptor blockade – as is achieved by almost all antipsychotic medications apart from partial agonists – will lead to a compensatory upregulation of D_2 receptors, as well as an increase in their sensitivity to dopamine. As a result, over time, the efficacy of antipsychotic treatment may wane, and higher and higher doses will be required to control symptoms. The treatment of choice for both tardive dyskinesia and emerging treatment resistance in such circumstances is clozapine.

Dose Reduction and Discontinuation

Recently, the recommendation that individuals with schizophrenia receive maintenance treatment with antipsychotics has been challenged. The main concerns include 'dopamine supersensitivity', the long-term effects of antipsychotics on brain volume, negative effects on physical health and long-term functional outcomes. As described earlier, there is some evidence to suggest that dopamine sensitisation may be an issue for some patients, though the size of the problem is not clear. Changes to brain volume are very concerning but are complicated by the fact that these changes are also seen in clinical high-risk subjects before treatment has even been started[66] and, in patients with established illness, these changes are also confounded by illness severity.[67] With regard to physical health, while antipsychotics may increase the risk of certain health problems, particularly cardiovascular disease, there is a large body of evidence to show that antipsychotics reduce overall mortality in the long-term.

Good long-term data on how antipsychotic treatment affects functional outcomes is in short supply. Clinical trials that last for years are unfeasible, and any observational research is vulnerable to confounding. One of the most prominent studies in this area was by Wunderink and colleagues.[68] It was a clinical trial that randomised 128 patients with remitted first-episode psychosis to either maintenance treatment with antipsychotics or a dose reduction/discontinuation regime over 18 months. In keeping with other studies, Wunderink and colleagues observed a higher relapse rate (43% vs 21%) in the discontinuation group. Of the 65 participants assigned to the dose reduction regime, discontinuation was achieved in 35 (46%) and maintained in 14 (22%) without relapse. However, after a subsequent five-year naturalistic follow-up, there was no difference in relapse rates (62% vs 69%) or symptomatic remission (69% vs 67%), and functional remission was much more common in the discontinuation group (46% vs 20%). Part of the observed effect may be because the groups were unbalanced, as the maintenance treatment group had more participants with a diagnosis of schizophrenia and fewer participants in employment at baseline. Hui and colleagues described a similar study where they randomised 178 patients with first-episode psychosis who had achieved full positive symptom remission to either maintenance treatment with quetiapine 400 mg or early treatment discontinuation for 12 months.[69] At 10 years, a poor clinical outcome was observed in more patients in the discontinuation group (39%) than the maintenance treatment group (21%), while functional outcome and rates of employment were similar. More research in this area is clearly required.

Whatever the evidence, many patients with psychosis, particularly those who have only experienced a single episode of illness, will want to try and manage their illness without medication. For a significant minority, this is a reasonable aim: in follow-up data from the OPUS study, a randomised trial of a specialised early intervention for patients with first-episode psychosis found that 30 per cent were not taking antipsychotics and had no symptoms 10 years later.[70] The factors that are associated with successful antipsychotic discontinuation are all markers for less severe illness: fewer symptoms, better social functioning, fewer previous relapses, shorter duration of untreated psychosis, older age at the onset of illness and lower antipsychotic dose before discontinuation.

It is often assumed that abruptly stopping medication presents the greatest risk of relapse, and it has been suggested that the dose of antipsychotic should be reduced in a hyperbolic manner – for example, by one-quarter every few months.[71] The theory behind this method is supported by data from dose-response studies[54] as well as neuroimaging research.[72] However, a meta-analysis of placebo-controlled clinical trials that required participants to stop their current antipsychotic before entering the trial found no difference in relapse rates between studies that required abrupt discontinuation with those that allowed more gradual discontinuation.[51] If antipsychotic withdrawal does lead to a rebound of psychosis, you would expect to observe a magnification of the effect size for antipsychotic treatment in the subsequent trial, an effect that is not observed.

Treatment-Resistant Schizophrenia (TRS)

Establishing Treatment Resistance

In first-episode schizophrenia, a trial of a single antipsychotic should lead to an adequate response (50 per cent or more reduction in psychotic symptoms) in about half of patients, with remission of symptoms achieved in about one-quarter, although higher response rates to a first antipsychotic of 76 per cent have been reported. If a patient's illness has not responded to an adequate dose of at least two antipsychotics (one of which should be a second-generation antipsychotic according to NICE guidelines), a diagnosis of treatment-resistant schizophrenia must be considered. As well as being evident from early on in a patient's illness course, treatment resistance can also emerge at a later stage.[73] Before treatment resistance is established, alternative explanations for non-response must be considered. These include:

- Incorrect diagnosis or over-looked comorbidity (especially affective, substance use and personality disorders as well as physical health conditions)
- Social and psychological factors
- Non-adherence to medication
- Inadequate dose or rapid metabolism of medication

In one study of 36 patients referred to a specialist service to support initiation of clozapine, only 56 per cent had a therapeutic level and 19 per cent had no detectable drug in their plasma.[74]

The OPTiMiSE Study

OPTiMiSE was a clinical trial that recruited patients within the first two years of a psychotic illness. The trial had three phases. In the first, all patients were treated with amisulpride, up to 800 mg/day. Those who did not meet criteria for symptomatic remission after four weeks were then randomly assigned, under double-blind conditions, to either continue amisulpride or switch to olanzapine – up to 20 mg/day – for a further six weeks. In the final phase, remaining volunteers started clozapine. Out of 446 patients who entered the trial, 56 per cent achieved remission after the first phase. 72 patients went on to complete the second phase comparing amisulpride with olanzapine. At the end of six weeks, there was no difference in remission between those who remained on amisulpride (15/33 [45%]) and those switched to olanzapine (17/39 [44%]) ($p = 0.87$). The findings suggest that there is little difference between non-clozapine antipsychotics when treating treatment-responsive schizophrenia. If the study is replicated, perhaps treatment resistance can be established and clozapine started after treatment with a single antipsychotic.

Clozapine

In the 1970s, clozapine was withdrawn from use after a series of deaths due to agranulocytosis were observed in Finland. Eventually, it was established that clozapine can be prescribed safely, as long as the white cell count is monitored regularly. This change in practice enabled the first trial, published in 1988, to demonstrate clozapine's unique effectiveness in treatment-resistance schizophrenia,[75] where it is now accepted as the gold-standard treatment.

The mechanism of action that underlies clozapine's effectiveness in treatment resistance has not been established. Clozapine has considerable activity at receptor targets other than dopamine. It also appears to have different activity at dopamine receptors, where it rapidly dissociates after binding to them, and at clinically effective doses, it has relatively low striatal dopamine D_2 receptor occupancy, around 40 per cent.[76]

Clozapine must be titrated slowly (in daily increments of 12.5–25 mg). Otherwise, side effects, such as postural hypotension and sedation, may be intolerable and potentially dangerous. Adverse effects tend to be the most severe early on in therapy but should lessen over time. Compared to other antipsychotics, clozapine perhaps has the widest range of adverse effects. Despite this, it is well tolerated, with a relative risk of all-cause discontinuation rates of about 76 per cent that of placebo in clinical trials.[42] During titration, the patient's pulse, temperature and blood pressure are measured both before and after each dose. Jurisdictions differ but, in the UK, white cell counts must be completed weekly for the first 18 weeks, fortnightly until week 52, and thereafter monthly.

Plasma Clozapine Levels

If clozapine is to be used well, it should be optimised, and therapeutic plasma levels can be very helpful in this process.

Women, non-smokers, people of Asian heritage and the elderly will achieve especially high clozapine levels at a given dose of clozapine. A plasma clozapine level of 350 μg/L is often cited as the target, though many patients will require much lower or higher levels to manage their illness. The sensitivity of the 350 μg/L cut-off for response is just 64 per cent, and for non-response, the specificity is 78 per cent.[77] Levels are at least useful for assessing compliance with treatment and the risk of seizures; if levels are above 600 μg/L, prophylaxis with an antiepileptic agent is recommended. In general, the best approach is to prescribe the lowest effective dose and level to minimise adverse effects.

The clozapine/norclozapine ratio has been used as an indicator of medication adherence though recent research has questioned its usefulness. Metabolism of clozapine to norclozapine is through cytochrome p450 1A2. This pathway is heavily influenced by the hydrocarbons in cigarette smoke and by inflammation. If someone on clozapine stops smoking tobacco, then their clozapine levels may double, with a concomitant increase in side effects; the same effect may occur during systemic infections.

Withdrawing Clozapine

Of patients who discontinue clozapine, around half stop due to adverse effects, 30 per cent due to non-compliance and 20 per cent due to lack of efficacy.[78] Ideally, clozapine should be withdrawn gradually, not only because of the risk of relapse, but also due to a cholinergic rebound effect that can cause severe nausea, vomiting, diarrhoea, sweating, headache, acute dystonia, dyskinesias and even catatonia.

If clozapine is discontinued in a patient with established treatment resistance, it is not clear what the best alternative medication might be. A large observational study (n = 2,250) of patients who had discontinued clozapine after at least one year of treatment examined outcomes according to the subsequent treatment choice.[79] Compared to treatment without antipsychotic medication, the risk of readmission was lowest for restarting of clozapine (adjusted hazard ratio, or aHR: 0.49), followed by oral olanzapine (aHR: 0.58) and antipsychotic polypharmacy (aHR: 0.62). Risk of treatment failure (defined as readmission, change of medication or death) was lowest for aripiprazole long-acting injectable (aHR: 0.42), reinitiation of clozapine (aHR: 0.49) and oral olanzapine (aHR: 0.69).

Clozapine-resistant Psychosis

Clozapine Resistance

In randomised controlled trials, only 40 per cent of treatment-resistant patients show an adequate response to clozapine.[80] In practice, higher rates of response may be achieved after prolonged treatment (up to 6 months) or by a trial of higher clozapine levels.[81] If response to clozapine remains limited, several aspects of a patient's presentation should be re-examined. Substance use, affective and other comorbidities should be reviewed and actively managed, adverse effects should be systematically reassessed as they may be impacting treatment tolerance or adherence (see later), and additional psychological and social interventions should be considered (see later). Once clozapine resistance is established, several treatment options have been reported, though the evidence base for each is very limited. Numerous meta-analyses have attempted to summarise the evidence from trials for different strategies but have found conflicting results.[82] Unfortunately, the field until recently has been complicated by variable definitions of treatment resistance and the presence of numerous small and low-quality trials.

Alternatives to Clozapine

Even in treatment-resistant patients, clozapine may not always be the best option. As well as clozapine resistance, patients may not be able to tolerate its adverse effects, may develop serious physical health problems such as agranulocytosis or myocarditis, or may simply be unable or unwilling to adhere to oral treatment. There is limited evidence to guide patients and clinicians on how to proceed in this unenviable situation. There is some evidence that high-dose olanzapine can reduce severity of psychosis to a similar degree as clozapine, but it was inferior to clozapine in relation to function and carried a higher metabolic burden.[83]

Augmentation Strategies

Adding a Second Antipsychotic

A meta-analysis of 12 randomised trials found limited benefits from augmenting clozapine treatment with an additional second-generation antipsychotic.[84] The effect on positive psychotic symptoms was not statistically significant (SMD = −0.21, 95% CI: −0.51 to 0.09, p = 0.170) although small-medium effects were demonstrated for negative symptoms (SMD = −0.38; 95% CI: −0.65 to −0.11, p = 0.005) and depressive symptoms (SMD = −0.35, 95% CI: −0.58 to −0.12, p = 0.003). The evidence for individual antipsychotics is much more limited, though aripiprazole may have a medium effect on overall symptoms (SMD = −0.57, 95% CI: −1.02 to −0.13, p = 0.01).[85] Administering the second antipsychotic as a long-acting injectable formulation is supported by several small mirror-image studies, but there needs to be further examination of safety and effectiveness, given that the rationale for choosing clozapine is that non-clozapine antipsychotics have been ineffective.

Adding an Antidepressant

There is some evidence that antidepressants may be beneficial in the management of schizophrenia. The majority of trials have examined fluoxetine, which - after meta-analysis - had a moderate-large effect on overall symptoms (SMD = −0.73, 95% CI: −0.97 to −0.50, $p<0.05$).[85] Of note, fluoxetine raises clozapine levels slightly. However, larger and higher-quality trials of antidepressant augmentation that include all schizophrenia patients (i.e. also including non-treatment-resistant individuals) find much smaller effects on overall, depressive,

Table 5.3.3 Promising antipsychotic treatment candidates

Agent	Mechanism of Action	Number of RCTs	Total Number of Participants	Comment	Ref
Anti-inflammatory agents	Various immune system targets	70	4,104	High likelihood of publication bias makes interpretation of results difficult	91
Memantine	A non-competitive NMDA receptor antagonist	11	570	Possible efficacy for negative symptoms SMD: 0.60, 95% CI: 0.08–1.12)	92
Sarcosine	Type 1 glycine transporter inhibitor	7	326	A meta-analysis found that sarcosine was associated with a significant positive effect on overall clinical symptoms (SMD: 0.51, 95% CI: 0.26–0.76)	93
Ondansetron	Serotonin 5-HT_3 receptor antagonist	5	304	Meta-analysis found improvements in negative (n=209; SMD: 0.96, 95% CI: 0.22–1.71) and general symptoms (n=171; SMD: 0.97, 95% CI: 0.02–1.91). No effect on positive symptoms	94
SEP-363856	Agonist at trace amine–associated receptors 1 serotonin 5-HT_{1A} receptors	1	245	Total PANSS score least-squares mean difference −7.5 points; 95% CI: −11.9 to −3.0) with SEP-363856 treatment	95
Xanomeline/ Trospium	Xanomeline: muscarinic (M1 and M4 receptors) agonist Trospium: peripheral acting muscarinic receptor antagonist	1	182	At week 5, PANSS total score demonstrated an 11.6-point improvement compared to placebo at p<0.0001	96
Cannabidiol	Inhibition of endocannabinoid metabolism (not established)	3	171	Encouraging results from two out of three trials	97 26 98

and negative symptoms (overall symptoms, SMD= −0.24, 95% CI:−0.39 to −0.09).[86]

Adding a Mood Stabiliser

There is little evidence that sodium valproate is effective in schizophrenia as most trials are low-quality. Trials including non-treatment-resistant patients do not support its efficacy. Only one low-quality trial has examined lithium add-on treatment,[82] and studies including non-treatment-resistant schizophrenia patients do not support its role, with the effectiveness of lithium disappearing when schizoaffective patients are excluded,[87] suggesting that lithium is effective for mood symptoms but not for schizophrenia.

Non-pharmacological Options

Out of the non-pharmacological augmentation strategies, electroconvulsive therapy (ECT) is the one with the most supporting evidence, though this is still very limited.[88] Out of 18 trials, none have compared ECT treatment with sham ECT, and only one managed to blind the assessors to treatment arm. Evidence for transcranial direct current stimulation (tDCS) and transcranial magnetic stimulation (TMS) is limited, with a recent meta-analysis showing no significant effect on auditory hallucinations from either tDCS or TMS.[89] However, a meta-analysis looking at cognitive symptoms suggests that tDCS may have promise.[90]

Novel Treatments

At present, all licensed treatments for psychosis are antagonists or partial agonists at the dopamine D_2 receptor. This is not because there has been a lack of effort to identify novel agents: the list of failed candidates is not a short one. Table 5.3.3 describes a selection of some of the more promising runners and riders. Each will require replication in large-scale high-quality clinical trials before they are licensed as treatments for schizophrenia.

Schizoaffective Disorder and Affective Comorbidities of Psychosis

The diagnosis of schizoaffective disorder has been defined in various ways and has been brought into question by some. It is certainly a heterogeneous disorder, and individuals are frequently switched between a diagnosis of schizoaffective disorder and affective or schizophrenia diagnoses, which has some implications for treatment. Unfortunately, schizoaffective disorder has not been subject to a large number of high-quality studies, meaning that practice guidance is often extrapolated from trials of schizophrenia or bipolar disorder or derived from studies with mixed populations including those with schizoaffective disorder. Moreover, caution should be exercised when extrapolating from studies with other disorders because there is some evidence that antipsychotic tolerability varies according to the underlying disorder.

Therefore, a pragmatic approach often consists of the principles in Table 5.3.4, though the evidence for this is weak. It is likely that the approach to a bipolar course of schizoaffective disorder is very different from a unipolar depressive course.

Table 5.3.4 Principles of pharmacotherapy in schizoaffective disorder

1.	Treat affective components of illness as comorbidities according to treatment guidelines for affective illnesses.
2.	Initial treatment should generally be with antipsychotics but consider a trial of a mood stabiliser if manic symptoms persist.
3.	It is unlikely that one size fits all, so personalise treatment to target an individual's symptoms.
4.	More than one agent is often appropriate, as there is rarely one drug that addresses all aspects of the illness.

The mainstay of treatment for schizoaffective disorder remains antipsychotic drugs, and it is predominantly patients at the manic pole who have been studied, although many trials do not specify the intercurrent polarity. A systematic review of randomised double-blind placebo-controlled trials in schizoaffective disorder found only three stand-alone trials and three post-hoc analyses, most of which examined individuals in the acute phase of illness.[99] Aripiprazole, ziprasidone and paliperidone (extended-release tablet) were each superior to placebo in single trials.[100–102] Interestingly, in the paliperidone trial, only the higher dose of 12 mg/day was effective.[102] Both olanzapine and risperidone were compared to haloperidol: olanzapine showed greater improvement in the PANSS, BPRS and MADRS totals compared to haloperidol, with greater difference in the PANSS negative subscale than the PANSS positive subscale;[103] a smaller trial of risperidone did not show any differences from haloperidol.[104] Two studies reported benefits of long-acting injectable formulations of risperidone and paliperidone in schizoaffective disorder.[105,106] There is some evidence for clozapine in individuals with schizoaffective disorder, both for affective and psychotic, either in the acute or maintenance phases.[107] One recent large-scale Scandinavian observational study found that clozapine, long-acting injectable antipsychotics and combination therapy with mood stabilisers were associated with the best outcomes.[108] The BAP guidelines note the poor evidence available on treatment of schizoaffective disorder and recommend treating schizomania first line with an antipsychotic based on individual patient characteristics.

In terms of mood stabilisers, there is even less evidence. Unlike antipsychotics, which have evidence in both schizophrenia and bipolar disorder, mood stabilisers do not have good evidence in schizophrenia. Observational data suggest that mood stabilisers as an adjunct to antipsychotic therapy reduce risk of hospitalisation for schizoaffective disorder compared to antipsychotic monotherapy.[108] Interestingly, a Cochrane review of lithium for antipsychotic augmentation in schizophrenia and schizoaffective disorder found that response rates were higher in the lithium augmentation group, but the effect became non-significant once patients with schizoaffective disorder were excluded.[109] In two retrospective studies, valproate seemed to be effective in schizoaffective disorder,[110,111] but the evidence is poor. There may be some role for valproate in targeting specific symptoms such as excitement and aggression. The addition of topiramate was not superior to placebo in one trial.[112] There is no evidence for the use of carbamazepine, which also risks interactions with other medications. The BAP recommend that a mood stabiliser should only be considered after an adequate trial of an antipsychotic, and it should be discontinued if it is not effective.

Depression is common in schizophrenia, with 40 per cent of individuals meeting criteria at any one time and up to 80 per cent when followed up longitudinally.[113] It may, however, be hard to distinguish from negative symptoms of schizophrenia. Depression is a poor prognostic indicator in schizophrenia and is a significant factor in suicides.[113,114] There is, however, little research into its treatment. Because depressive symptoms may be secondary to the psychosis, there was clinical consensus that treatment of depression should not begin until psychosis has been adequately treated. However, in practice, complete elimination of psychosis is not always possible, so both aspects of the illness may need to be treated concurrently, and trial evidence is limited. Some atypical antipsychotics have evidence for treatment-resistant depression, so they might be expected to be effective for depression in schizophrenia. In one study of haloperidol versus quetiapine, quetiapine resulted in a greater reduction in depressive symptoms.[115] Additionally, some of the newer antipsychotics – lurasidone and cariprazine – have demonstrated effectiveness in bipolar depression.[116] More specifically, both clozapine and lithium have been associated with a reduction in suicide rates in people with schizophrenia and bipolar disorder respectively.

The NICE psychosis guidelines recommend treating comorbid depression in line with isolated major depressive disorder. A meta-analysis of treatments for depression in schizophrenia found that antidepressants were effective with a number needed to treat of five.[117] A Cochrane review on the topic concluded that antidepressants might help, but the quality of the evidence was low and might reflect publication bias.[118] Importantly, however, there is no evidence that antidepressants cause a worsening of psychosis, although they are associated with a greater incidence of abdominal pain, constipation, dizziness and dry mouth. Overall, the BAP guidance advises that a therapeutic trial of antidepressants for depression in schizophrenia is justifiable. However, there are diagnostic and practical considerations to be considered before prescribing. In terms of diagnosis, negative symptoms, extrapyramidal side effects of antipsychotics and depression can be difficult to distinguish. Tricyclic antidepressants have anticholinergic activity, so they can reduce extrapyramidal side effects independent of any antidepressant activity, though they do not necessarily improve the negative symptoms of schizophrenia. Even in subsyndromal depression in schizophrenia, one trial of citalopram showed an improvement in depressive symptoms and quality of life,[119] though in unselected patients with schizophrenia, citalopram was not associated with a change in the PANSS score.[120] There is also the risk of precipitating a manic switch in bipolar schizoaffective disorder, so it is recommended that unopposed antidepressants are avoided in this group. Some practical considerations are illustrated in Table 5.3.5.

Table 5.3.5 Practical issues in prescribing antidepressants in schizophrenia

1.	Pharmacokinetic interactions between antipsychotics and antidepressants may occur, potentially increasing plasma concentrations of both drugs.
2.	Citalopram and escitalopram can prolong the QTc interval, so the MHRA states that concurrent prescription with QTc-prolonging antipsychotics is contraindicated.
3.	Antidepressant use in schizophrenia is not associated with increased mortality but, in fact, is associated with a reduced risk of overall mortality.
4.	High doses of benzodiazepines in schizophrenia are associated with higher rates of suicide and overall deaths.

Benzodiazepines should be avoided as treatment for anxiety. The BAP recommends an individual risk assessment before prescribing an antidepressant, taking into account the role of high-dose or combined antipsychotic prescriptions and the place of electrocardiogram (ECG) monitoring.

Specific Treatment Targets

Negative Symptoms

Negative symptoms consist of five highly inter-correlated domains: affective flattening, alogia (a reduction in speech output), avolition, anhedonia and attentional impairment. They are present at onset, often outlast an acute psychotic episode, predict a poor outcome and have a substantial impact on function. For some individuals, negative symptoms are the predominant feature of their illness, and it has been suggested this represents a distinct disease for which different pharmacotherapy may be required. Negative symptoms tend to respond poorly to current therapeutic modalities.

One helpful conceptual distinction is between primary negative symptoms – idiopathic features of the psychotic disorder – and secondary negative symptoms – those with another identifiable cause, many of which are reversible. Secondary negative symptoms may be due to positive symptoms (for instance, avolition due to paranoia), depression, extrapyramidal side effects, apathy due to obstructive sleep apnoea or medication-related sedation, prolonged institutionalisation and lack of stimulation or substance misuse. In practice, it can be difficult to distinguish these, but it is generally helpful when considering an individual with negative symptoms to identify any possible aetiology for secondary negative symptoms as an initial strategy.

The largest systematic review and meta-analysis of negative symptoms found that second-generation antipsychotics (SGAs), antidepressants, combinations of pharmacological agents and glutamatergic medications (N-acetyl cysteine, D-cycloserine, glycine, D-serine, ampakine, LY404039, sarcosine, memantine and D-alanine) had evidence for efficacy, while first-generation antipsychotics (FGAs) and neurostimulation did not.[121] However, although there may be some reduction in symptom scores, the clinical significance is doubtful. BAP guidelines therefore avoid recommending any particular treatment and suggest that, if a medication trial is undertaken for negative symptoms, there should be careful monitoring with a symptom scale designed specifically for negative symptoms, and treatment should be stopped if there is no clinically meaningful response. SIGN guidelines suggest augmentation with an antidepressant, lamotrigine or sulpiride.

Table 5.3.6 Antipsychotic medications that may be more effective in negative symptoms[123,124]

Amisulpride
Cariprazine
Aripiprazole (when used in augmentation)
Clozapine

In terms of antipsychotic use, their effect on negative symptoms appears to be modest, and it is possible that they act indirectly by improving positive symptoms rather than having intrinsic efficacy against negative symptoms. Four antipsychotic drugs may be more effective for negative symptoms (see Table 5.3.6), though the reasons for this are unclear. It is possible that clozapine appears better than some antipsychotics because of its favourable EPSE profile. One meta-analysis compared antipsychotic augmentation against monotherapy and found that negative symptoms improved more with augmentation – but only when augmenting with aripiprazole – and it was not clear how this compared to aripiprazole monotherapy.[55] It is interesting that two of the agents in Table 5.3.6 (aripiprazole and cariprazine) are partial agonists at the D_2 receptor. Cariprazine has been specifically marketed for predominant negative symptoms based on a trial comparing it to risperidone, but the difference between treatments was very small (1.5 points on the PANSS factor score for negative symptoms).[122]

Regarding antidepressant use, a Cochrane systematic review found five randomised controlled trials and concluded that there was some evidence for a greater clinical response but that it was weak.[125] Negative symptom domains implicated were affective flattening, alogia and avolition. Higher-quality studies tend not to show smaller effect sizes.

In terms of other approaches, psychostimulants can be used safely in stable patients with schizophrenia without worsening psychosis, and it is possible that they improve negative symptoms, but more evidence is required. Modafinil and armodafinil are also thought to be safe and well tolerated, but their effect on negative symptoms is very small.[126] Glutamatergic agents have proved disappointing with meta-analytic evidence that they are not superior to a placebo.[127] Anticonvulsants and 5-HT_3 antagonists only have preliminary evidence. Recent RCTs of promising treatments for negative symptoms included minocycline (a tetracycline antibiotic with immunomodulatory properties and supposed effects on glutamate-mediated excitotoxicity), bitopertin (a glycine reuptake inhibitor) and rTMS to the dorsolateral and prefrontal cortex, all of which failed to show any difference from placebo.

In view of the poor evidence for treatment, we propose a pragmatic approach as outlined in Table 5.3.7.

Table 5.3.7 Pragmatic approach to negative symptoms

1.	Assess for presence of secondary negative symptoms and address causative factors (e.g. physical illness, EPSEs, depression, lack of stimulation and substance misuse)
2.	Optimise existing antipsychotic regimen: a. Ensure positive symptoms are adequately treated b. Use the lowest effective dose
3.	Trial of one of the following approaches, carefully monitoring response and discontinuing if no clinical benefit: a. Switch to an antipsychotic with more evidence in negative symptoms b. Augment with an antidepressant (usually an SSRI) c. Augment with aripiprazole

Table 5.3.8 Approach to cognitive deficits

1.	Consider comorbidity with delirium, dementia or other disorder known to impair cognitive performance (e.g. obstructive sleep apnoea, Addison's disease, hypothyroidism, B12/folate deficiency)
2.	Consider impact of recreational drugs, especially opioids and benzodiazepines
3.	Reduce burden from prescribed medications, especially anticholinergics, opioids and benzodiazepines (see medichec.com)
4.	Treat positive symptoms with an antipsychotic
5.	Reduce antipsychotic to the minimum effective dose
6.	Consider an atypical antipsychotic

Cognition

Cognitive impairment in the psychoses has been recognised at least as far back as Kraepelin's term 'dementia praecox'. Full-scale IQ tends to be impaired in schizophrenia, but even in studies where there is matching for IQ, individuals tend to show impairments in specific domains, notably executive function, working memory, attention, processing speed, verbal fluency and verbal memory, albeit with a high degree of inter-individual variability. Unlike positive symptoms, cognitive impairment tends to be stable throughout the illness course rather than showing episodic relapses. In fact, lower IQ in adolescence is associated with an increased risk of schizophrenia, and cognitive impairment likely predates overt psychotic symptoms.[128] In addition to this intrinsic cognitive impairment, meta-analysis has found that individuals with schizophrenia are at higher risk of incident dementia (RR 2.29; 95% CI: 1.35–3.88).[129]

Cognitive impairment is an important treatment target because – despite advances in treatment of positive symptoms – functional improvement in schizophrenia has been limited. Both poorer baseline cognitive function and subsequent cognitive decline are associated with greater functional decline. Cognition has often been found to be the best predictor of functional status.[130]

There are currently no approved treatments for cognitive impairment in the psychoses. Reducing the cognitive burden from other medications is one approach (see Table 5.3.8). Benzodiazepine and opioid use have been associated with cognitive deficits in other disorders, so this is likely to compound any impairments.

Antipsychotics have been shown to have a small positive effect on multiple cognitive domains, but there is no correlation with dose. One small study found that reducing the dose of patients treated with high doses of antipsychotics has been associated with cognitive improvement.[131] In terms of which antipsychotic to use, there is some weak evidence suggesting that atypical antipsychotics are overall more beneficial for cognition and, certainly, the requirement for anticholinergic treatments for EPSEs from FGAs is likely to be deleterious. Unlike in positive symptom domains, it does not seem to be the case that clozapine is superior to other antipsychotics, and one RCT suggested it may even be worse.[132] A meta-analysis of cognitive effects of clozapine, olanzapine and risperidone found that different drugs had been associated with improvements in different symptom domains,[133] but the studies were generally small and open-label, and the overall findings may have been a product of which outcomes were chosen in studies of different pharmacological agents. If there are differences between antipsychotics, they are likely to be very small, as the large CATIE trial found overall modest improvements with antipsychotics but no significant differences between drugs.[134]

In terms of other pharmacological treatment options, data on antidepressants are sparse and conflicting.[135] Limited data on the use of electroconvulsive therapy (ECT) in the psychoses suggest that it is not associated with cognitive decline.[136]

Rapid Tranquilisation

Indications

There is a spectrum of agitated presentations for which rapid tranquilisation (RT) may be indicated. These range from agitation to 'acute behavioural disturbance', a severe form of sudden onset aggression with autonomic dysfunction, which can be a form of catatonia (see later) that the Royal College of Emergency Medicine recognises as a medical emergency.[137] There is often, but not always, aggression and sometimes violence. The aim of rapid tranquilisation is to induce a state of calmness and to curtail excessive motor activity, not to bring about sedation or sleep, although these do sometimes occur. The specific objectives of rapid tranquilisation are to prevent injury to others, prevent self harm, to prevent accidental injury to the person, to protect the clinical environment and to reduce distress.

General Principles

These objectives must be carefully balanced against the risks of rapid tranquilisation itself. The degree of restriction should be proportional to the severity of the risks, taking into account the current law and codes of practice.[138] Severe agitation itself (especially in the context of drug intoxication) can be associated with arrhythmia and hyperthermia.[137] On the other hand, physical restraint should also be minimised because this is associated with injuries and has contributed to deaths in health care and forensic settings.[137]

Practice in rapid tranquilisation is driven as much by theory and expert consensus as it is by robust evidence, as difficulties in obtaining consent for trials of rapid tranquilisation has led to limited evidence.

In terms of terminology, rapid tranquilisation is generally used to refer only to the use of parenteral medications. However, rapid tranquilisation should be considered as the end of a process after failure of other non-pharmacological and pharmacological interventions.

The final general principle is that, as with other syndromal presentations such as delirium, the primary management of agitation is addressing the underlying cause.[138] Even in patients with established schizophrenia, agitation that is unusual for their illness may herald a delirium, drug intoxication or drug withdrawal. More commonly in a psychiatric ward, there are issues related to personal autonomy, loss of contact with relatives, concerns about family and welfare, and difficult relationships with staff or other patients that can be resolved directly. There is RCT evidence for nicotine replacement therapy in reducing agitation in hospitalised inpatients with schizophrenia.

De-escalation

Prevention and reduction of agitation require the work of a multi-disciplinary team that is able to intervene at the levels of interpersonal relationships, environmental modifications, activities, psychological interventions and pharmacological interventions. Many patients who become agitated have a history of prior agitation so, for these people, an individualised de-escalation plan should be generated,[138] based on general principles, patient preferences and past experiences.

Although this requires the work of several professionals, in a situation of acute agitation, communication with the distressed person should primarily be conducted by a single member of the staff[139] to reduce over-stimulation and keep messaging simple and consistent. There are several distinct strategies to good de-escalation, which the BAP/NAPICU guidelines on rapid tranquilisation identify: continual risk assessment, self-control techniques, avoidance of provocation, respecting patient space, management of environment, passive intervention and watchful waiting, empathy, reassurance, respect and avoidance of shame, appropriate use of humour, identification of patient needs, distraction, negotiation, reframing events for patient, and non-confrontational limit setting.[138] This de-escalation should precede rapid tranquilisation and, where rapid tranquilisation does have to occur, de-escalation should continue.

More restrictive non-pharmacological strategies are often required alongside the rapid tranquilisation described later. For example, manual restraint is often required to safely administer intramuscular medications or to perform cannulation. Rapid tranquilisation may also be used alongside strategies such as segregation and seclusion.

Routes of Administration

Some medications, such as quetiapine or risperidone, only offer a single route. Many offer more than one option, and this is a significant factor in choice of agent.

When comparing different routes of administration, often the key question is time to onset of clinical effect. This is difficult to quantify and varies between individuals. A surrogate measure is often the time to peak plasma levels (T_{max}), which is used in Table 5.3.9, but this is probably an over-estimate of time to clinical effect. As a general rule, administration via the intravenous or inhaled routes is faster than administration via the intramuscular or buccal routes, which is faster than the oral route.

Other factors are also important though. Intramuscular injections can be painful and considered demeaning. Side effects may generally be less common with oral medications, or at least have a slower onset, allowing interventions to avert the side effects to be more effective. When comparing parenteral routes, intravenous administration provides more predictable plasma concentrations than intramuscular injection and may be more humane in settings such as a general hospital where a cannula may already be in situ. One study comparing the introduction of a structured intramuscular protocol to previous clinician-guided intravenous tranquilisation found that the duration of behavioural disturbance actually fell,[140] although this may be more a reflection on the use of a structured protocol than on the change in route. Treatment setting is likely to be an important factor, with inhaled loxapine more likely to be available in psychiatric intensive care units, psychiatric nurses being skilled in administering intramuscular injections under restraint, patients in general hospital wards more likely to be cannulated and patients in medical intensive care units having the availability of staff trained in advanced airways.

Bioavailability for different agents sometimes varies across routes, but this is not consistent between drugs. For instance, oral lorazepam has practically 100 per cent bioavailability, whereas for haloperidol, dose adjustment is necessary because oral bioavailability is only 60–70%. However, this is not always reflected in licensed doses. For example, the licensed oral doses of lorazepam and promethazine are both lower than their respective parenteral doses. Contrary to popular belief, orodispersible formulations of antipsychotics are not absorbed any more quickly than regular tablets; their advantage lies in their assistance in monitoring compliance.[138]

Medication Selection

A medication plan should be made in anticipation of agitation by a multi-disciplinary team including a psychiatrist and specialist pharmacist.[139] If rapid tranquilisation is used, a senior doctor should review all the patient's medications at least once daily.[139] There are several factors to consider when choosing the appropriate medication; these include patient preference, past response (both efficacy and side effects), medical comorbidity, pregnancy, intoxication and potential for interaction with other prescribed or non-prescribed medications.[138,139] Part of an individualised medication plan may include PRN medications, but these should not be prescribed routinely for all patients on admission.[139]

A few specific causes of agitation specifically guide choice of drug for rapid tranquilisation. The World Federation of Societies

Table 5.3.9 Medications commonly used in rapid tranquilisation. Adapted from Patel et al. (2018)[138]

Drug	Route	Formulations	Bioavailability	T_{max}
Clonazepam	PO	Tablet, liquid	90%	1–4 hr
	IM	Injection	93%	3 hr
Diazepam	PO	Tablet, liquid	76%	30–90 min
	IM	Injection	76%	30–90 min
	IV	Injection (emulsion, Diazemuls)	100%	≤15 min
Lorazepam	PO	Tablet	100%	2 hr
	IM	Injection	100%	1–1.5 hr
	IV	Injection	100%	Seconds–minutes
Midazolam	Buccal	Solution	75%	30 min
	IM	Injection	>90%	30 min
	IV	Injection	100%	Seconds–minutes
Aripiprazole	PO	Tablet, orodispersible, liquid	87%	3–5 hr
	IM	Injection	100%	1 hr
Haloperidol	PO	Tablet, liquid	60–70%	2–6 hr
	IM	Injection	100%	20–40 min
	IV	Injection	100%	Seconds–minutes
Olanzapine	PO	Tablet, orodispersible	Not known	5–8 hr
	IM	Injection	Not known	15–45 min
	IV	Injection	100%	Seconds–minutes
Quetiapine	PO	Tablet	Not known	1.5 hr
Risperidone	PO	Tablet, orodispersible, liquid	67–70%	1–2 hr
Loxapine	INH	Vapour	91%	2 min
Promethazine	PO	Tablet, liquid	25%	1.5–4 hr
	IM	Injection	100%	2–3 hr

of Biological Psychiatry recommends using benzodiazepines if agitation is due to alcohol withdrawal and using antipsychotics if agitation is due to alcohol intoxication.[141] Promethazine can be useful in benzodiazepine-tolerant patients.[138] It is common practice to administer an antipsychotic if agitation is caused by psychosis, but concomitant use of more than one antipsychotic should be avoided.[123] If a patient is antipsychotic-naïve or there is insufficient information to guide medication choice, NICE recommends using IM lorazepam.[139]

In terms of dosing, an observational study found that high doses of rapid tranquilisation (defined as more than 10 mg of midazolam, droperidol or haloperidol) were associated with a similar time to sedation but more adverse effects than more moderate dosing. If the BNF maximum dose is to be exceeded, this should only be done as part of a plan for an agreed therapeutic goal and directed by a senior doctor.[139]

Benzodiazepines

Benzodiazepines are contraindicated in respiratory depression, severe respiratory disease or sleep apnoea. They are also cautioned in porphyria, and the potential for abuse should be considered in individuals requesting prescriptions. Their side effects include oversedation, respiratory depression, ataxia, hypotension, falls, amnesia and, rarely, paradoxical excitement. There is more evidence for lorazepam in rapid tranquilisation than for any other agent.[138] Intramuscular midazolam has a faster action than many other intramuscular agents, but it also wears off more quickly, which can necessitate further injections.[138] Midazolam is also associated with more frequent oxygen desaturation and airway obstruction, occasionally requiring active airway management.[138] Diazepam has a long and variable half-life, so it can accumulate. If diazepam is administrated intravenously, it should be given in the emulsified form (Diazemuls) and administered slowly at 1 mL solution/minute.[138]

Antipsychotics

Antipsychotics are contraindicated where there is known QTc prolongation or risk factors for ventricular arrhythmias (such as prior ventricular arrhythmia, low serum potassium or recent myocardial infarction). They should also be avoided in 7individuals with Parkinson's disease or related alpha-synucleinopathies. Inhaled loxapine is contraindicated in respiratory distress or active airways disease (e.g. COPD or asthma). Side effects are often dose-dependent and are considered in-depth later in this chapter; of particular relevance for rapid tranquilisation are extrapyramidal side effects. Akathisia can mimic agitation, erroneously resulting in further antipsychotic administration. Acute dystonia can be life-threatening, intensely painful and must be treated immediately. Concomitant use of two or more antipsychotic drugs should be avoided.[123] Recent evidence shows that, for rapid tranquilisation, there is no difference in efficacy between first- and second-generation antipsychotics. However, side effects between agents can differ substantially. Acute dystonia occurs in approximately 5 per cent of those treated with intramuscular haloperidol and, for this reason, it should be avoided as monotherapy.[138] However, promethazine has anticholinergic properties, so the combination of haloperidol and promethazine is reasonable.[138]

Zuclopenthixol acetate (often known by its tradename Clopixol Acuphase) is not a rapid tranquilisation agent. Its T_{max} is 36 hours, and its effects last for several days. Its use is limited to obviating repeated intramuscular injections of antipsychotic drugs for rapid tranquilisation. An ECG should be performed before use.[138]

Medication Combinations

Some specific medication combinations have a synergistic effect; others are dangerous. As mentioned earlier, adding intramuscular promethazine to intramuscular haloperidol attenuates extrapyramidal side effects. Adding haloperidol to lorazepam is more sedative, but the effect disappears in the medium term.[138] Intramuscular benzodiazepines and intramuscular promethazine are commonly combined, but there is a lack of studies to support this strategy. Parenteral olanzapine should never be combined with parenteral benzodiazepines due to an increased risk of hypotension, bradycardia and respiratory depression.[141]

Monitoring

Monitoring recommendations rely on expert consensus. Prior to treatment initiation, an ECG is recommended for haloperidol, although NICE recognises that this may not always be possible, and there may be a balance of risks.[139] The approach advocated by the BAP is as follows:

- Following pre-RT medications (see Table 5.3.10): NEWS (National Early Warning Score) every hour for at least 1 hour
- Post-IM RT: NEWS every 15 minutes for at least 1 hour
- Post-IM RT in those who are oversedated, asleep or physically unwell: NEWS every 15 min for at least 1 hour + pulse oximetry until Pt ambulatory

Table 5.3.10 Summary of rapid tranquilisation algorithms

	BAP/NAPICU	NICE	Maudsley Prescribing Guidelines	RCEM
De-escalation	Various de-escalation techniques			
Oral, inhaled or buccal treatment	• Inhaled loxapine • Buccal midazolam • PO lorazepam • PO promethazine • PO aripiprazole • PO haloperidol • PO olanzapine • PO quetiapine • PO risperidone	-	If already taking an antipsychotic: • PO lorazepam • PO promethazine • Buccal midazolam If not already taking an antipsychotic: • PO olanzapine • PO risperidone • PO quetiapine • PO haloperidol • Inhaled loxapine *May repeat this step once*	-
1st-line RT	• IM lorazepam • IM promethazine • IM aripiprazole • IM droperidol • IM olanzapine	• IM lorazepam • IM haloperidol + IM promethazine	• IM lorazepam • IM promethazine • IM olanzapine • IM aripiprazole • IM haloperidol (least preferred)	Give IM or IV depending on risks of cannulation: • Benzodiazepines • Ketamine • Antipsychotics
2nd-line RT	• IM promethazine + IM haloperidol • IM lorazepam + haloperidol	• If partial response to 1st-line agent, consider further dose of that 1st-line agent. • If no response to 1st-line agent, consider dose of other 1st-line agent	• Repeat of 1st-line RT agent • Haloperidol + lorazepam • Haloperidol + promethazine	-
3rd-line RT	• IV lorazepam • IV midazolam • IV droperidol • IV olanzapine	-	• IV diazepam	-
Additional options	• IM zuclopenthixol acetate • ECT	-	• Repeat 3rd-line RT up to three times	-

- Post-IV RT, Pts who are unconscious (unrousable) and severely physically unwell: continuous monitoring with resuscitation facilities available

This monitoring may be very difficult in patients who remain aggressive and those in seclusion. However, even for patients who cannot be approached, the respiratory rate, consciousness level, pallor, dystonia, akathisia and signs of dehydration can be ascertained.[138] Patients in seclusion should therefore remain under direct eyesight observation.[138]

Intravenous options must be used only in settings where resuscitation equipment and clinicians trained to manage medical emergencies are present.[138] If administering intravenous diazepam, the patient should be kept supine for at least one hour. There should be immediate access to flumazenil whenever parenteral benzodiazepines are used; it should be administered if respiratory rate falls below 10 breaths/minute or SpO2 falls below 90 per cent.[138] Flumazenil can induce seizures, so it is contraindicated in those who are benzodiazepine-dependent, have a history of epilepsy or who are suspected to have taken an overdose of proconvulsant medications. If administering inhaled loxapine, a salbutamol inhaler should be available in case of bronchospasm, and its use requires some degree of patient cooperation.[142]

Algorithms

There is considerable overlap in the approaches advocated by different professional bodies, although some differences remain, partly due to the intended audiences of the guidelines. We summarise the major UK algorithms in Table 5.3.10.

Within each box, several options are provided – it is not suggested that these should be administered concurrently, unless this is explicitly mentioned. No preference is implied by the order of agents.

Catatonia

Definition

Catatonia is a psychomotor syndrome that occurs in a range of psychiatric, neurological and general medical conditions. It can occur in the psychoses, but the presence of catatonia does not necessarily suggest a diagnosis of schizophrenia; in fact, catatonia is probably more common in mood disorders. ICD-11 and DSM-5 both define catatonia as at least three of the following clinical features: catalepsy, waxy flexibility, stupor, agitation, mutism, negativism, posturing, mannerisms, stereotypies, grimacing, echolalia and echopraxia. The most commonly used catatonia rating scale, the Bush-Francis Catatonia Rating Scale, incorporates these features and is useful for gauging severity and treatment response.[143,144] The pathophysiology of catatonia remains poorly understood, but several lines of evidence suggest that there is GABA-ergic hypofunction in motor areas.

Lorazepam Challenge Test

The first pharmacological intervention for catatonia should usually be the lorazepam challenge. It has three distinct roles: to support a diagnosis of catatonia, to predict subsequent effectiveness of further benzodiazepines and to elucidate underlying psychopathology. The procedure is outlined in Table 5.3.11.

Table 5.3.11 Lorazepam challenge instructions

1.	Perform a baseline assessment of catatonic features, e.g. using the Bush-Francis Catatonia Rating Scale
2.	Administer a dose of lorazepam. Usually, 2 mg is optimal, but 1 mg may be considered in children, the elderly or those with respiratory disease. Lorazepam may be given IV, IM or PO.
3.	Re-assess catatonic features after 5 minutes (IV), 15 minutes (IM) or 30 minutes (PO). A positive test result is considered a 50% reduction in catatonic signs.
4.	If the test is initially negative, one further dose of lorazepam can be given at this point.
5.	Re-assess after 5, 15 or 30 minutes, as in step 3.

Overall Management Strategy

There are several goals for catatonia treatment, which must be considered concurrently:

1. Treat the catatonia itself, usually with benzodiazepines or ECT
2. Treat the underlying disorder
3. Prevent and treat any complications of catatonia

Treatment of the underlying disorder may involve restarting a medication, withdrawal of which has precipitated catatonia. This may occur for benzodiazepines and is a particular problem in the sudden cessation of clozapine, after which catatonia can rapidly develop within days.[145]

Benzodiazepines for Catatonia

For most patients, benzodiazepines are the mainstay of treatment for catatonia. There is most evidence for lorazepam, though diazepam and clonazepam have also been used. Reports suggest that other agents that increase signalling at the $GABA_A$ receptor, such as barbiturates and z-drugs are also effective. After a lorazepam challenge, a total daily dose of 4 mg should be started. Thereafter, the total daily dose (usually spread over four doses) should be increased daily by 2–4 mg until either (a) catatonia is lysed or (b) sedation or respiratory depression limit treatment. Doses of up to 20–30 mg of lorazepam have been required in some reports. Treatment with benzodiazepines has been found in a systematic review to be associated with response rates of between 66 per cent and 100 per cent.[146] However, in observational studies, responders have tended to have much shorter durations of catatonia than non-responders, suggesting that there may be a critical window for starting lorazepam treatment.

Electroconvulsive Therapy

Electroconvulsive therapy (ECT) is generally considered the definitive treatment for catatonia.[147] It may be used as an emergency treatment or where treatment with benzodiazepines has failed. There is double-blind sham-controlled RCT evidence for ECT in catatonia, which produced an approximately 90 per cent response rate, which was significantly superior to treatment with risperidone.[148]

There are some practical considerations when giving ECT for catatonia. Traditionally, bilateral ECT is used, but right unilateral ECT may also be effective.[149] One problem is that high doses of benzodiazepines can raise the seizure threshold. The simplest solution to this is to increase the dose of ECT. The rapid withdrawal of benzodiazepines before ECT can risk the appearance of ECT worsening catatonia.[149]

Role of Antipsychotics

The role of antipsychotics in catatonia treatment is controversial. On the one hand, there is the need to treat underlying psychosis or to restart an antipsychotic, the withdrawal of which has precipitated catatonia. On the other hand, catatonia is a strong risk factor for the development of neuroleptic malignant syndrome.[150,151] A pragmatic approach to this issue is to use antipsychotics where necessary with caution, using D_2 partial agonists or agents with weaker D_2 antagonism whilst giving benzodiazepine cover.

Other Treatments

The anticonvulsants valproate, carbamazepine and topiramate all have a few reports showing benefit in patients with catatonia, but the evidence is very limited.[146,152] There is growing evidence for the NMDA negative allosteric modulators memantine and amantadine.[153] These glutamatergic agents have few side effects, although their effect on catatonia can take several days (unlike the often immediate effect of benzodiazepines). There is likely to be substantial reporting bias in the case reports of all these alternative treatments, so it is unclear how effective they are.

Prevention and Treatment of Complications of Catatonia

Major complications of catatonia include dehydration, malnutrition, pressure sores, muscle contractures, venous thromboembolism, aspiration and urinary retention.[154] Much of the prevention of these relies on good nursing care, which ensures regular hydration as well as frequent repositioning and movement of limbs. There are, however, several prescribing considerations. Most prosaically, prescribing oral or intravenous fluids is often necessary. Food intake can be enhanced by prescribing doses of benzodiazepines to fall 30–60 minutes prior to mealtimes. Pharmacological venous thromboembolism prophylaxis in cases of prolonged immobility is indicated.

Organic Psychotic Disorders

General Principles

In this chapter, we predominantly discuss primary, or idiopathic, psychosis, such as in schizophrenia and related disorders. However, it is worth also considering the treatments available for secondary, or 'organic', psychotic disorders. The list of possible neurological and medical conditions that can cause psychosis is extremely long, but we list some of the most important in Table 5.3.12. We do not cover dementia and Parkinson's disease in this chapter, as they are major topics in their own right in old age psychiatry and neuropsychiatry. We refer readers to the Neuropsychiatric Disorders chapter of this volume. Organic psychotic disorders, which occur in clear consciousness, should be distinguished from delirium, which may feature delusions and hallucinations, although there is some overlap in the causes of these states.

Table 5.3.12 Important neurological and medical causes of psychosis

Epilepsy
Huntington's disease
Stroke
Drugs (prescribed and recreational)
Autoimmune encephalitis
Other inflammatory disorders
Thyroid disorders
CNS infections
Traumatic brain injury
Dementia
Parkinson's disease

Regardless of the aetiology of the psychosis, treatment of the underlying disorder is paramount. However, it is commonly the case that this cannot be further optimised or that, in the interim, psychiatric management is necessary. Psychopharmacological agents are often only needed temporarily, however, in contrast to common practice in schizophrenia. It is likely that the same pathophysiology of dysregulated dopamine signalling underlies organic psychosis as in primary psychotic disorders. Thus, antipsychotics are commonly used in a similar way, although there is little evidence for this approach. However, there are some important differences because onset of organic psychosis is generally later in life in patients with medical comorbidities and often more frailty. Therefore, lower doses may be required with greater regard to side effects and drug-drug interactions. Given the polypharmacy that many of these patients have, simple dosing regimens are preferred.

Epilepsy

Psychosis in epilepsy is a complex area with several possible aetiologies, as shown in Table 5.3.13.

Where psychosis is related to individual seizures, the primary management is the reduction of seizure frequency, usually by optimising antiepileptic drugs. For post-ictal psychosis, short-term treatment with either benzodiazepines (particularly in the early stages) or antipsychotics have been suggested.[155] Where use of an antiepileptic drug has been associated with psychosis – either directly or in alternative psychosis – dose reduction and careful retitration can be attempted with close monitoring.[155] Wherever psychotropic medications are used, care should be taken not to lower the seizure threshold.

Table 5.3.13 Possible aetiologies of psychosis in epilepsy

Psychosis aetiology	Description
Ictal psychosis	Complex partial seizures, usually involving the temporal lobe, feature psychotic symptoms that terminate with the seizure
Post-ictal psychosis	Following seizures, there is a lucid interval of at least several hours, after which psychosis develops, generally lasting several days
Interictal psychosis	Patients with epilepsy are at increased risk of a schizophrenia-like chronic psychosis that is not significantly temporally related to individual seizures. There tends to be several years from onset of epilepsy to onset of psychosis
Alternative psychosis	The phenomenon of psychosis emerging as seizure frequency drops, usually in concert with antiepileptic treatment. The EEG correlate of this is termed 'forced normalisation'
Antiepileptic drug-related psychosis	Numerous antiepileptic drugs have been associated with the onset of psychosis, most classically levetiracetam, topiramate and zonisamide. Withdrawal of vigabatrin has also been associated with psychosis

Huntington's Disease

Psychosis in Huntington's disease can be effectively treated with antipsychotic medications. In fact, antipsychotics are also sometimes used to treat chorea as well, so there may be beneficial side effects. However, the danger is that antipsychotics can worsen Parkinsonism and dystonia. For this reason, SGAs at low doses are preferred. Olanzapine and risperidone are most frequently used. Clozapine has been effective in some cases.

Stroke

Psychosis is an uncommon feature of stroke but can arise in the days, weeks or months following the event. As oedema and inflammation reduce, symptoms sometimes subside spontaneously. Thus, often watchful waiting can be the optimal strategy. If antipsychotics are required, it is often just on a temporary basis.[156] However, where possible, antipsychotics should be avoided due to the increased risk of stroke that they pose, which raises the possibility that they may increase the risk of further stroke. If they are used, there should be careful consideration of risks and benefits.

Drug-Induced

Psychosis can be caused by prescribed and recreational drugs. In both cases, cessation of the offending agent is advised, although this is often not straightforward. Clinical guidance on the treatment of psychosis related to recreational drugs is available from the Novel Psychoactive Treatment: UK Network (NEPTUNE, neptune-clinical-guidance.co.uk/). Corticosteroids are one of the most common culprits for medication-induced psychosis in clinical practice. Most patients can be managed with either a tapering of the steroid or antipsychotic treatment, but a minority require both to obtain resolution of symptoms. Lithium has also been used. Resolution is generally within a few days.

Autoimmune Encephalitis

Autoimmune encephalitis, and particularly NMDA receptor encephalitis, commonly features psychosis. Management often requires immunotherapy and, in cases of paraneoplastic syndromes, removal of the offending tumour. In cases of psychosis, antipsychotics are usually required as well, but their use can precipitate autonomic instability and extrapyramidal side effects. They should therefore be cautiously titrated.[157] Catatonia is common and occurs in as many as 88 per cent of individuals with NMDA receptor encephalitis.[158] It should generally be treated with benzodiazepines, although ECT has also been used with rapid effect.[157]

Inflammatory

Multiple sclerosis occasionally features psychotic symptoms and may even present with these prior to neurological diagnosis. If it is suspected that psychotic symptoms herald a relapse of multiple sclerosis, steroids may be administered, but antipsychotic medications are more commonly used with a preference for those at lower risk of inducing extrapyramidal symptoms.

Psychosis in systemic lupus erythematosus (SLE) often poses a treatment dilemma because it may either be due to neuropsychiatric involvement of SLE or to steroid treatment. For patients in whom steroids are thought to be blamed, tapering of steroids and replacement with other immunosuppression is recommended. In other cases, corticosteroids may be required, usually in combination with antipsychotics, to treat neuropsychiatric SLE.

CNS Infections

HIV and the opportunistic infections that may accompany it have numerous CNS manifestations, so diagnosis takes some care. Antipsychotics are usually used for management of psychotic symptoms. Antiretroviral medications are notorious for pharmacokinetic interactions, which may be checked using the Liverpool HIV Drugs Interaction Checker (www.hiv-druginteractions.org/). Equally important are pharmacodynamic interactions. For instance, NRTIs and protease inhibitors cause lipodystrophy, while protease inhibitors are associated with impaired glucose tolerance, both of which can compound the metabolic side effects of SGAs.[159] Moreover, tenofovir is associated with a reduction in bone mineral density, which is problematic in the context of antipsychotic-induced hyperprolactinaemia. The leukopenia produced by clozapine also requires careful monitoring given the immunosuppression in HIV and the tendency of some ARVs to cause bone marrow suppression.

Syphilis is a classic cause of psychosis and is currently undergoing a resurgence in certain populations. Primary treatment for neurosyphilis is with parenteral penicillin.

Thyroid Disorders

Hyper- and occasionally hypothyroidism have been associated with psychotic symptoms, sometimes as a presenting feature. Treatment consists of correcting the thyroid hormone balance, although antipsychotic use has also been required in some cases.

Traumatic Brain Injury

Psychosis in traumatic brain injury tends to develop months to years following the injury and is more common following damage to the temporal lobe. One recommended approach is to discontinue other medications that may worsen psychosis, to provide education to the patient and family, and to cautiously use SGAs.[160]

Side Effects

It is now clear that, although the most immediately apparent side effects of antipsychotic drugs were extrapyramidal, antipsychotics cause side effects across endocrine, neurological, cardiac, metabolic, haematological, ophthalmological and gastrointestinal systems. Occasionally, these side effects can be useful in addressing comorbid symptoms, but generally they are unpleasant and a significant cause of medication discontinuation. In rare cases, side effects can be life-threatening. However, despite this, there are now robust observational data demonstrating that, among individuals with schizophrenia, mortality is actually lower in those individuals on moderate doses of antipsychotics.[161] Moreover, there are potential gains of six to seven years of life expectancy to be enjoyed by implementing existing interventions to target modifiable risk factors for mortality in those with schizophrenia or schizoaffective disorder.[162]

Somnolence and Sedation

Somnolence and sedation are related issues in drug treatment. Sleep abnormalities are common in schizophrenia, with a reduction in slow-wave sleep reported. Medications can add additional problems, and sedation has been associated with difficulties in occupational and social function. In addition, it may contribute to falls in the elderly and weight gain. It can impair patients' ability to engage in rehabilitation programmes. Sedation, where present, is also likely to be a significant contributor to negative symptoms, but this may not be immediately obvious – for example, in the patient who does not get out of bed in the morning, where apathy may be thought to be responsible.

It is now recognised that sedation is not necessary for successfully treating psychosis. However, there are situations where it can be advantageous, and assisting with the initiation of sleep is often a benefit that patients will appreciate. Sedative properties of antipsychotics are particularly used in the setting of acute agitated psychosis for reducing arousal and helping to reset a sleep-wake cycle.

The mechanism of sedation is likely to include antagonism at α_1-adrenergic, H_1-histaminergic and M_1-cholinergic receptors. It is often more common at the start of treatment and may resolve spontaneously. The most sedative antipsychotics are clozapine, chlorpromazine and promazine, but loxapine, olanzapine, pipotiazine, quetiapine and zuclopenthixol also have significant sedative properties.[123]

Identification of medication-induced sedation or somnolence requires careful consideration of the timing over which symptoms have developed and of alternative hypotheses (for example, hypothyroidism, if there is insidious onset). If sedation has occurred shortly after drug initiation or an increase in dose, the best management may be patient education and watchful waiting in anticipation that side effects may ease. It always worth reviewing other medications for agents that may be contributing; benzodiazepines are often used on admission for agitation, but need for them tends to wane as a patient recovers, and these should be stopped in preference to antipsychotics. In all cases, patients prescribed medications with the potential to cause sedation should be warned not to drive if they feel sedated.

If sedation occurs during medication titration (for instance, with clozapine) slowing the titration schedule will often help. If the treatment dose has already been reached, reduction to the lowest effective dose is recommended. In cases where sedation seems disproportionately high compared to the antipsychotic dose, examination of plasma levels – particularly for clozapine – can be helpful, as sedation could be a sign of slow metabolism or a drug interaction.

If there is little scope to reduce the dose, the most useful strategy is often to change the timing of the antipsychotic. An awareness of drug half-lives can help here. Moving as much of the medication dose to the night-time as possible is recommended. If this results in 'hangover' drowsiness the next morning, bringing the dose forward to the early evening is another strategy.

In some cases, switching medications is the best option. The antipsychotics with the lowest propensity for sedation are amisulpiride, aripiprazole, brexpiprazole, cariprazine, risperidone and sulpiride, followed by haloperidol, trifluoperazine and ziprasidone.[123]

The final option is to add a medication to promote alertness. Modafinil, bupropion and stimulants have been tried, but the evidence is controversial.[163,164] A systematic review of modafinil use found that it showed a significant benefit in only one of four studies, and the authors stated that small sample sizes and contradictory results limit conclusions.[165] One strategy that may be worth trying is encouraging caffeinated drinks in the morning, but this can contribute to tachycardia and inhibits CYP1A2, which can increase plasma concentrations of clozapine and olanzapine. One observational study found that reducing the clozapine dose and augmenting with aripiprazole were each associated with a reduction in the number of hours of sleep, but they were only effective in about 40 per cent of individuals.[166]

Hyperprolactinaemia and Sexual Dysfunction

Sexual dysfunction is common and can comprise difficulties in attaining arousal, erection or orgasm. Numerous factors can contribute, many of which are more common in psychotic illnesses, including psychological stress, diabetes mellitus and medications (including prolactin-raising antipsychotic, serotonergic antidepressants and mood stabilisers that lower testosterone).[167]

Hyperprolactinaemia is one cause of sexual dysfunction (specifically, loss of libido, erectile dysfunction and impaired ability to orgasm) that is commonly related to antipsychotic drugs. It results from antagonism of the dopaminergic tuberoinfundibular pathway from the hypothalamus to the anterior pituitary, which normally results in tonic inhibition of prolactin release. Hyperprolactinaemia may be asymptomatic, but clinical features can include gynaecomastia, galactorrhoea, osteoporosis and subfertility. In addition, it may increase the risk of breast cancer in women. It may also occur in the presence of pituitary adenomas, hypothyroidism, chronic kidney disease and polycystic ovarian syndrome, as well as being raised physiologically in pregnancy and breast feeding. There are two forms of prolactin in the blood: free prolactin and macroprolactin, only the former of which is clinically relevant. The reference range also varies slightly between men and women, so local laboratory ranges should be checked. Prolactin-raising agents are said to be the typical antipsychotics in addition to risperidone, paliperidone and amisulpride, while other SGAs are described as prolactin-sparing. Prolactin can rise within hours of antipsychotic initiation and generally falls within a few days of discontinuation.

In routine assessment of patients prescribed antipsychotics, it is important to sensitively enquire about sexual dysfunction, as embarrassment often means that patients are reluctant to volunteer the information. Symptoms of hyperprolactinaemia should also be sought, including any history of fractures. Timing of symptoms is important, as a rapid onset of symptoms is more likely to be medication-related whereas an insidious progression might suggest another physical cause that requires investigation.[167] In terms of investigations, basic screening should include blood pressure and measurement of HbA1c and prolactin. Prolactin should be measured at baseline prior to starting an antipsychotic, once an adequate dose has been reached, and annually thereafter.[167] Prolactin can be raised by stress, waking and eating, so take the sample at least two hours after waking and one hour after a meal.

If prolactin is raised, macroprolactin levels should be requested to ascertain if this may be pseudohyperprolactinaemia. In a woman of childbearing potential, pregnancy should be ruled out. In the case of raised free prolactin, there should be enquiry about headache and visual impairment while screening for a bitemporal hemianopia as part of an assessment for a pituitary adenoma. Strategies for treating antipsychotic-induced hyperprolactinaemia include reducing the dose, switching the antipsychotic, adding aripiprazole (usually at 5 mg) or adding a dopamine agonist, although care needs to be taken around the worsening of psychosis.[168] If prolactin is greater than 2500 mIU/L, there should be a discussion with endocrinology, as antipsychotics tend not to generate a prolactin this high.

In terms of sexual dysfunction more generally, once hyperprolactinaemia has been ruled out, lifestyle changes – including a Mediterranean diet, weight loss, exercise and smoking cessation – may be effective.[167] Using a less sedative antipsychotic may also help. For erectile dysfunction, sildenafil can be useful and is mostly safe, although it can prolong the QTc interval and may increase the risk of hypotension.[167]

Motor Side Effects

Traditionally, the various motor side effects of antipsychotic drugs are often grouped together as extrapyramidal side effects. These are Parkinsonism, dystonia (both acute and tardive), akathisia, tardive dyskinesia and neuroleptic malignant syndrome. Antipsychotic-induced catatonia may also occur, and the reader is directed to the section on catatonia in this chapter. These separate disorders may be comorbid, and acute EPSEs are a risk factor for tardive dyskinesia. However, while there are similarities, the epidemiology and treatment of the specific motor side effects of antipsychotics show marked differences, so we consider them separately here. They are all thought to arise from antagonism of D_2 receptors in the nigrostriatal pathway. This is an area where understanding of the neurobiology through neuroimaging has had a profound effect on clinical practice: we now know from PET studies that the D_2 occupancy required for EPSEs is higher than the occupancy required for antipsychotic response.[169]

It had been thought with the advent of SGAs, that EPSEs would become a minor issue in antipsychotic treatment. However, the CATIE trial demonstrated that most of the supposed benefit of SGAs was lost when FGAs were prescribed at lower, more appropriate doses.[170] Likewise, the CUtLASS RCT showed no advantage in terms of quality of life, symptoms or care costs for non-clozapine SGA over FGA.[171] It is also sometimes unhelpful to conflate all FGAs and SGAs, and individual drugs have different propensities for EPSEs. Unfortunately, EPSEs have remained a serious problem with antipsychotics in the twenty-first century and may have a considerable contribution to the poor quality of life and stigma often attached to psychotic illnesses. They are also a factor in medication adherence.

There are some broad principles that apply to management of all EPSEs. Firstly, these disorders are not always obvious and may not be volunteered, so careful clinical examination and enquiry about symptoms are necessary. Rating scales, such as the Simpson-Angus Scale or the Abnormal Involuntary Movement Scale (AIMS) may be useful. As is generally the case, prevention is better than treatment, and these disorders are a reminder to only use antipsychotics where necessary and to keep minimise exposure where possible.

Parkinsonism

Parkinsonism is classically defined as a triad of tremor, rigidity and bradykinesia. In drug-induced Parkinsonism, the tremor is generally at 3–6 Hz and present at rest, though there may also be a postural tremor. Non-motor Parkinsonian symptoms, such as hypomimia, cognitive and emotional changes may also occur. For a formal diagnosis of drug-induced Parkinsonism, there should have been an absence of Parkinsonism prior to drug initiation, and the presence of Parkinsonism develops during drug use. It generally appears within a few weeks of starting an antipsychotic, increasing the dose or reducing the dose of a medication used to treat EPSEs. However, it has been reported to persist, or even progress, after discontinuation of an antipsychotic.[172]

In terms of the epidemiology, Parkinsonism has become less common in recent decades, although it may still occur in as many as 20–35% of those treated with antipsychotics.[173] FGAs do not seem to be any worse than SGAs if used at appropriate doses, but there is evidence for the following risk factors: older age, female sex, prior EPSEs, family history of Parkinson's disease, cognitive impairment and HIV infection.[173] In terms of treatment factors, Parkinsonism is clearly dose-dependent and is worsened by other drugs that reduce dopaminergic signalling, including metoclopramide, reserpine, tetrabenazine and calcium channel blockers. There is also some evidence that SSRIs, valproate, phenytoin and lithium may contribute,[172] although careful clinical examination is required, as lithium and valproate can cause other forms of tremor.

In terms of differential diagnosis, the affective blunting of Parkinsonism can resemble primary negative symptoms of schizophrenia. Other causes of Parkinsonism are also important to consider, most commonly idiopathic Parkinson's disease and vascular Parkinsonism. Although Parkinson's disease is a disorder of dopaminergic neurons whereas drug-induced Parkinsonism is due to antagonism of the post-synaptic receptors, there is an interesting relationship between these disorders. Antipsychotics can cause severe EPSEs in individuals with Parkinson's, and it seems that antipsychotic drugs can unmask presymptomatic Parkinson's. It is also possible that drug-induced Parkinsonism increases the risk of subsequent Parkinson's disease. In practice, a careful history and examination are important to distinguish these conditions, although the classic distinction between idiopathic Parkinson's being asymmetrical with secondary Parkinsonism (including drug-induced) being symmetrical is not specific enough to be diagnostically useful. Where there is doubt, a DAT (dopamine active transporter) scan can distinguish Parkinson's disease from idiopathic Parkinsonism.

In terms of treatment, the simplest option is often to reduce the antipsychotic to a dose that is just below the threshold for induction of EPSEs. This can be difficult, however, particularly with drugs that have a narrow of antipsychotic effect bounded by EPSEs at the upper end. It is also worth evaluating the continued need for an antipsychotic. The role of other contributing medications should also be considered. Switching to a drug with a lower risk of EPSEs is sometimes helpful and, in those very sensitive to Parkinsonism, clozapine can be considered. Antimuscarinic agents – such as benztropine, trihexyphenidyl and procyclidine – lack a solid evidence base, but they are generally effective in clinical practice and are recommended treatments. However, antimuscarinic agents can cause cognitive impairment (with a possible increase in dementia risk), worsen tardive dyskinesia and contribute to dry mouth (with a subsequent increase in dental problems), angle-closure glaucoma, constipation, tachycardia, urinary retention and impaired thermoregulation. This patient group is also often exposed to other medications with anticholinergic properties – including antipsychotics themselves – which can compound these effects. Therefore, use of antimuscarinic agents should be minimised, generally restricted to short-term use. There is occasionally an indication to prescribe a prophylactic antimuscarinic, but this should be reserved for individuals who are very sensitive to Parkinsonism. Regarding other agents, one RCT found amantadine to be similarly effective to anticholinergics,[174] and it may be used as an alternative. Dopamine agonists should be avoided due to the theoretical risk of worsening psychosis.

Dystonia

Dystonia is the abnormal and sustained contraction of a muscle group. It can affect the oculomotor muscles (oculogyric crisis), eyelids (blepharospasm), neck (torticollis or retrocollis), trunk (opisthotonos) or jaw (trismus). When it affects the larynx, it can obstruct the airway and be life-threatening. In its acute form, with a sudden onset, it tends to be painful and frightening. It can easily be confused with catatonic posturing or psychogenic movement disorders. There is also a tardive dystonia.

Dystonia appears to be less common than in early studies of FGAs, in which approximately 10 per cent of patients were affected. Recent studies suggest it occurs in up to 2 per cent of those on SGAs.[124,175] Risk factors are male sex, young age, cocaine use, high doses and parenteral administration.

Immediate management of acute dystonia requires securing the airway, where necessary. Antimuscarinics should be administered – PO, IM or IV – depending on urgency and availability.[124] After resolution, an oral antimuscarinic may be required to prevent recurrence, and dose adjustment of the antipsychotic is likely to be required.[175]

In tardive dystonia, there is little evidence, but use of anticholinergics, botulinum toxin injections, beta blockers and deep brain stimulation may be considered.[175]

Akathisia

Akathisia is the combination of a subjective sense of restlessness with objective constant voluntary movement in an attempt to ease this sensation. The movement often takes the form of pacing, rocking or fidgeting. It generally occurs within a few weeks of starting or increasing an antipsychotic, although it may occur in a chronic or tardive form. Akathisia may be distressing and can contribute to suicidal behaviour. Studies suggest it occurs in 20–30% of individuals prescribed FGAs and 5–15% in those on SGAs, but there is a lack of comparative studies.[124]

The crucial step in management of akathisia is to recognise it as a drug-induced extrapyramidal syndrome, rather than assuming that it is psychotic agitation, which can compound the problem with increasing antipsychotic doses. Dose reduction or switching are initial considerations. There is weak evidence for anticholinergics, propranolol, clonidine, gabapentin, mianserin, mirtazapine, trazodone and benzodiazepines.[124,175] Propranolol at 30–120 mg daily in divided doses may be tried in those without airway disease with monitoring of blood pressure.[175] Mirtazapine at 15 mg is another option.[123]

Tardive Dyskinesia

Tardive dyskinesia describes involuntary repetitive movements, excluding tremor, which are often the delayed effect of antipsychotic use. It can involve any body part, although occurs around the mouth or face in about 80 per cent of cases. Movements are complex and can be choreiform, athetotic or stereotypic. Similar movements sometimes occur in the elderly and have been reported in antipsychotic-naïve individuals with schizophrenia. They may be worsened by stress and have been linked to social withdrawal. Dyskinesia may also appear on antipsychotic withdrawal. Assessment of severity of symptoms (for example, using the AIMS) is helpful, but consideration of the functional impact is possibly more important. Dopamine receptor hypersensitivity is the leading pathophysiological theory.

The prevalence of tardive dyskinesia seems to differ dramatically across populations, ranging from 6.7% to 60% among patients with chronic schizophrenia. It is not clear whether FGAs confer a greater risk for tardive dyskinesia; at any rate, any difference is modest. The major factor in the aetiology of tardive dyskinesia is the duration of antipsychotic exposure, as risk increases by 4–5% per year of treatment. Other risk factors are older age, female sex, mood disorder, intellectual disability, substance misuse, diabetes, HIV, drug-free intervals, lithium use and early EPSEs.

If an individual is displaying marked dyskinesia, the first step is to consider whether this is a hallmark of a primary neurological disorder, which may also be responsible for the psychosis. Assessment should include a careful history of the symptoms, a review of neurological symptoms and a neurological examination, alongside blood tests for full blood count (FBC), liver function, thyroid function, bone profile and antiphospholipid antibodies. There may also need to be specific investigations where there is suspicion of disorders such as Wilson's disease, Huntington's disease or neuroacanthocytosis.

In terms of treatment, stopping anticholinergic therapy may result in an improvement. It is unclear whether stopping or switching antipsychotics is effective, but a switch to clozapine can be helpful, albeit with rather delayed results.[124] If tardive dyskinesia emerges on dose reduction, observation may be preferred, as this can resolve over several months. The use of benzodiazepines or increasing the antipsychotic dose may help in the short term, but long-term benzodiazepine use is fraught with problems, and greater antipsychotic exposure is ultimately likely to worsen the situation although it may have a role in life-threatening situations – for example, constant gagging.[175] There is some weak evidence for amantadine, botulinum toxin injections and ginkgo biloba. There are, however, promising treatments on the horizon. Tetrabenazine is a VMAT-2 (vesicular monoamine transporter 2) inhibitor that has been used for many years for tardive dyskinesia, but it has a substantial side-effect burden including depression, suicidal ideation, Parkinsonism, falls and QTc prolongation; if tardive dyskinesia is disabling, it is an option to consider.[124] The FDA has now licensed two similar drugs, deutetrabenazine and valbenazine, which have improved tolerability and are recommended for tardive dyskinesia, although they are not yet available in the UK.[175]

Neuroleptic Malignant Syndrome

Presentation

Neuroleptic malignant syndrome (NMS) is a rare neurological emergency that occurs as an idiosyncratic reaction to initiation or dose increase of dopamine antagonists or, in the closely related neuroleptic malignant-like syndrome, withdrawal of prodopaminergic drugs. There are consensus criteria for NMS – which have been validated – which lists the following criteria in descending order of priority: exposure to a dopamine antagonist or withdrawal of a dopamine agonist within 72 hours, oral temperature $\geq$ 38.0°C on two or more occasions, rigidity, mental status alteration, creatine kinase four or more times the upper limit of normal, sympathetic nervous system lability ($\geq$ 2 of raised blood pressure, blood pressure fluctuation, diaphoresis and urinary incontinence), hypermetabolism (heart rate $\geq$ 25% above baseline and respiratory rate $\geq$ 50% above baseline) and negative work-up for infectious, toxic, metabolic and neurological causes.[176,177] A very high temperature is particularly important, as it is more specific to NMS and confers a poorer outcome. A raised creatine kinase is non-specific, as it can be caused by agitation or IM injections. Although, in NMS, the creatine kinase is often very high. Other laboratory findings common in NMS are leucocytosis and myoglobinuria (suggested by haemolysed blood on urinalysis). In terms of timing, mental state changes (such as confusion) are often the first sign, followed by rigidity, then hyperthermia and autonomic dysfunction.[124] Unlike serotonin syndrome, NMS is not a common feature of antipsychotic overdose but rather an unpredictable reaction, usually within 3–9 days of starting an antipsychotic, although it can occur much later.

Frequency of NMS has declined from 1–3% in the 1980s to 0.02–0.03% in recent literature, which probably reflects changing prescribing practice more generally as well as a shift towards SGAs.[124] Risk factors are male sex, younger age, pre-existing neurological disorder, prior NMS, dehydration, high doses, rapid titration, IV antipsychotics and high ambient temperature.[124]

The differential diagnosis for NMS includes other medication-induced disorders (malignant hyperthermia, anticholinergic syndrome, serotonin syndrome, stimulant use), malignant catatonia, withdrawal of CNS depressants, sepsis, CNS infections, autoimmune encephalitis, vasculitis, heat stroke, benign increase in creatine kinase and fever due to clozapine withdrawal.

Regarding treatment, early recognition is critical. There is no trial data, so there is a reliance on (sometimes conflicting) expert opinion. The first step consists of immediately stopping the antipsychotic or restarting the pro-dopaminergic medication.[124] Once this has been done, NMS is generally a self-limiting illness, although recovery can be prolonged in individuals who have been using long-acting injectable antipsychotics.[175] However, extensive supportive treatment is required prior to recovery, often necessitating ICU admission. Rehydration, electrolyte correction, external cooling and correction of metabolic acidosis are often required. Intravenous fluids are used to prevent renal damage in the context of rhabdomyolysis. Antimuscarinics should be avoided, as they further impair thermoregulation.[124] When administering medications, the IM route should be avoided, as it may cause a further rise in the creatine kinase. Parenteral benzodiazepines can be used to reduce agitation and as myorelaxants. If the condition is more severe, bromocriptine, amantadine or dantrolene may be used.[124] ECT has also been effective in a few refractory cases.[124] After recovery, cautious antipsychotic re-challenge may be considered, but this should generally take place after at least two weeks with a less potent antipsychotic.[124]

Cardiac Side Effects

Cardiovascular disease is the single largest cause of death in schizophrenia.[178] In particular, patients with schizophrenia have a higher risk of both cardiac arrest and ventricular arrhythmias than the general population, although sudden cardiac death only accounts for approximately 5 per cent of deaths in psychiatric wards. The reasons for this cardiovascular mortality likely include a high prevalence of smoking, substance misuse, poor diet and lack of exercise in addition to the metabolic side effects and increased risk of type 2 diabetes from many antipsychotics. However, antipsychotic drugs do seem to confer a more direct risk for cardiac death via ventricular arrhythmias. Deaths tend not to be predictable and are rarely related to situations involved in rapid tranquilisation; where they are, they often result from asphyxia due to restraint rather than from a medication effect. Therefore, preventing cardiac death is as much about identifying and modifying risk factors as it is early identification and treatment of cardiac presentations. In considering cardiac side effects, we discuss a general approach before looking at the specific issues of QT prolongation, tachycardia and orthostatic hypotension.

General Assessment

When a patient on an antipsychotic is presenting with cardiac symptoms or signs, a thorough assessment is required. This should include a history of cardiac symptoms (chest pain, breathlessness, orthopnoea, paroxysmal nocturnal dyspnoea, syncope, ankle swelling and palpitations) as well as consideration of precipitants for symptoms (such as alcohol, drugs and exercise) and enquiry about a family history of sudden cardiac death. A cardiac examination should be performed, alongside a lying-standing blood pressure where there is any history of syncope. An ECG is necessary, and blood tests – in addition to routine haematology and chemistry – may include thyroid function, troponin, D-dimer, brain natriuretic peptide, HbA1c and blood glucose. A urine drug screen and urinalysis can be useful. A chest X-ray is often indicated. More specialist investigations may include an echocardiogram, a 24-hour ECG or an event recorder.[167]

QT Prolongation

The QT interval is measured in lead II of an ECG from the start of the Q-wave to the end of the T-wave. The QT interval, however, varies physiologically with the heart rate, so correction is required. To account for this, the Fridericia formula may be used, which has been shown to be superior to the older Bazett formula: $QTc = QT/\sqrt[3]{RR}$, where RR is the R–R interval and all timings are expressed in milliseconds.[179] Various online and app calculators are available, including mdcalc.com. The normal QTc is <440 ms for males and <470 ms for females.

A QTc greater than 500 ms is associated with an increased risk of the ventricular tachyarrhythmia torsade de pointes, which is fatal in approximately 10 per cent of cases.[178] The risk seems to be particularly increased in those with pre-existing cardiovascular disease. Lengthening of the QTc in sequential ECGs is a warning sign. Sertindole, pimozide, thioridazine, droperidol, intravenous antipsychotics and a high antipsychotic dose are risk factors for QTc prolongation. On average, droperidol, sertindole and ziprasidone increase the QTc by 15–35 ms, whereas quetiapine, haloperidol and olanzapine increase it by 5–15 ms, but there is inter-individual variation.

The other consideration is the impact of other conditions on the QT interval. A congenital long QT syndrome is present in approximately 1 in 4,000 people. In addition, low calcium, magnesium or potassium as well as other arrhythmias, thyroid disease, diabetes and anorexia nervosa are risk factors. Other drugs may contribute to a prolonged QT interval by pharmacokinetic interactions (increasing the plasma concentration of the antipsychotic, see later section on drug interactions) or by pharmacodynamic interactions (independently having a QT-prolonging effect). Other drugs known to prolong the QTc independently include macrolide antibiotics, ciprofloxacin, sotalol, amiodarone, quinidine and ondansetron. The effect of individual psychotropic and non-psychotropic medications can be checked at crediblemeds.org.

In terms of clinical practice, NICE recommends an ECG prior to antipsychotic initiation if it is specified in the summary of product characteristics (SPC), if there is pre-existing cardiovascular disease or cardiovascular risk factors, or if an individual is an inpatient. An already prolonged QTc contraindicates further QT-prolonging drugs. The ECG should be repeated once the steady state of an antipsychotic has been reached.[167] If the QTc is raised in a patient on an antipsychotic but it is no greater than 500 ms, consider a dose reduction, a switch to another antipsychotic, addressing other risk factors and a repeat ECG in one to two weeks; cardiology should be consulted if there are unexplained cardiac symptoms or if it is not possible to alter the antipsychotic. If the QTc is greater than 500 ms or there is an increase of more than 60 ms, the antipsychotic should be stopped immediately, and there should be a consultation with cardiology.[167]

Tachycardia

There are several important causes of tachycardia to be aware of: sinus tachycardia, supraventricular tachycardia, atrial fibrillation and ventricular tachycardia. These should be distinguished from a reflex tachycardia, which may accompany orthostatic hypotension. Antipsychotics, and particularly clozapine, can cause tachycardia via anticholinergic activity and possibly via antagonism of α_2-adrenergic receptors. Ventricular tachycardia is a medical emergency and, in the polymorphic form (torsade de pointes), is associated with QT prolongation. Sinus tachycardia has a broad differential diagnosis and is common in psychotic agitation, but it can also be a feature of many medical illnesses and sympathomimetic or anticholinergic drugs. Clozapine causes a sinus tachycardia in about a quarter of patients, which generally resolves after four weeks. However, if the sinus tachycardia is persistent and untreated, it may be a risk factor for cardiomyopathy. Often slowing the clozapine titration helps, but if symptomatic, tachycardia may be treated with bisoprolol 1.25–2.5 mg OD, with ivabradine as an option if a beta-blocker is not appropriate.[180]

Orthostatic Hypotension

Orthostatic hypotension is defined as a fall of 20 mmHg systolic or 10 mmHg diastolic blood pressure two to five minutes after five minutes of lying flat. It is common in older age, but it can also be a sign of volume depletion, autonomic nervous system dysfunction and cardiac disease. It may occur in up to 40 per cent of antipsychotic-treated patients, although there have been much lower estimates in some recent studies. It results from the antagonism of α_1-adrenergic receptors. It can result in falls and is particularly problematic when an individual wakes up at night. It is often more of an issue early in treatment and can be mitigated by slower titration. The contribution of other medications should also be assessed. Non-pharmacological interventions, such as sitting up slowly, hydration, salt intake, thromboembolism deterrent stockings and exercise can help.[167] If these fail, fludrocortisone or midodrine can be used.

Anticholinergic Side Effects

Anticholinergic, more specifically antimuscarinic, side effects of antipsychotics form an important burden of illness, particularly in the elderly. Even in a general adult population, they can be problematic. Nonetheless, there is some evidence that antipsychotics with greater anticholinergic side effects exhibit fewer extrapyramidal side effects.

Peripheral anticholinergic side effects tend to reduce secretions, causing dry mouth (which may be manifested by a patient needed to lick their lips before speaking and can result in dental caries and mouth ulcers), dry eyes, reduced bronchial secretions (risking mucous plugs in pre-existing airways disease) and impaired sweating (risking hyperthermia). In addition, constipation (even bowel obstruction), dilated pupils, blurred vision and tachycardia can result. In the longer term, these can be associated with glaucoma and an increased risk of acute coronary syndrome.

Central anticholinergic side effects are mostly related to cognitive impairment, which can affect concentration, attention and memory. This can contribute to delirium and may exacerbate pre-existing cognitive deficits in schizophrenia. These side effects have also been associated with an increased risk of falls. In the longer term, there is evidence that a high anticholinergic burden is a risk factor for dementia.

Finally, the anticholinergic syndrome can result from an overdose of anticholinergic medications, either intentionally or from a cumulative effect of multiple medications. This is a medical emergency and consists of a hyperactive delirium with tachycardia, dilated pupils, dry mucous membranes, reduced bowel sounds, hot skin and urinary retention. Seizures occasionally occur.

In terms of medications, some SGAs – and most especially clozapine – are worse than FGAs. Many of the drugs used to manage EPSEs are anticholinergic, but other common medications that are not prescribed for their anticholinergic properties have an intense anticholinergic burden notwithstanding.

The Medichec tool (medichec.com) can be used to check the anticholinergic burden of one or more medications, as well as the likelihood of dizziness and sedation.

In terms of prevention, an effort should be made to avoid polypharmacy and particularly multiple anticholinergic medications. Anticholinergic drugs should be avoided in those with closed-angle glaucoma or prostatic hypertrophy, as they risk worsening symptoms.[19] Where any new symptoms appear, the prescriber should consider whether these may be the result of anticholinergic side effects. There should also be a high index of suspicion for problems like dental caries and glaucoma.

Where the anticholinergic syndrome is suspected, an ABCDE resuscitation approach is necessary. An ECG should be performed, and fluid resuscitation is often required. Consider cooling techniques for hyperthermia and catheterisation if urinary retention has developed. Physostigmine, a cholinesterase inhibitor, has also been used. Most cases are much milder and more insidious. In this situation, it is important to identify the culprit(s) and to consider reducing the dose or switching to a less anticholinergic agent. Practical measures include dipping water regularly or sugarless gum for dry mouth or artificial tears for dry eyes. Constipation is considered in more detail under 'Clozapine-Specific Side Effects'.

Where there has been a high anticholinergic burden, the cessation or switching of the offending medication(s) can cause a withdrawal syndrome, which can be mistaken for side effects of the new drug. It may be a particular problem when discontinuing clozapine. Cholinergic rebound consists of diarrhoea, vomiting, rhinorrhoea, sweating, agitation and insomnia. In addition, movement disorders such as akathisia and Parkinsonism can emerge.

Diabetes and Impaired Glucose Tolerance

Diabetes mellitus can be diagnosed in various ways, most commonly with a random plasma glucose $\geq$11.1 mmol/L, a fasting plasma glucose $\geq$ 7.0 mmol/L or an HbA1c $\geq$ 48 mmol/mol. If the HbA1c is $\geq$ 48 mmol/mol in the absence of symptoms of diabetes, it should be repeated prior to a diagnosis being made. There is a particularly high risk of type 2 diabetes in antipsychotic treatment. Of those individuals with both schizophrenia and diabetes, a third of natural deaths are attributed to diabetes,[182] and diabetes is associated with a two-fold increase in mortality among these individuals.[183] Acute presentations of diabetes (including fatal episodes of diabetic ketoacidosis) have occurred in individuals on antipsychotics without a prior diagnosis of diabetes. Moreover, it is associated with complications in the form of both macrovascular and microvascular disease.

There are numerous factors that contribute to this risk of diabetes. It is partially mediated by obesity, but there is growing evidence for glucose dysregulation and insulin resistance even in non-obese people treated with antipsychotics.[184] Individuals with schizophrenia are more likely to have a poor diet and do insufficient exercise.[184] They also suffer from difficulties in accessing care.[184] In terms of pharmacological factors, clozapine and olanzapine are particularly high-risk for the development of diabetes, while aripiprazole and lurasidone are more benign. Even FGAs seem to contribute though. In addition, these patients may be on other medications, such as valproate and lithium, which can predispose to weight gain or glucose intolerance. Once diabetes is established, positive symptoms, such as agitation and paranoia, as well as negative symptoms, including apathy, can contribute to poor compliance with pharmacological and non-pharmacological treatment plans.[184]

In terms of prevention, from treatment initiation there should be discussion of the risk of diabetes on antipsychotics and the importance of lifestyle in addressing this. NICE states that HbA1c and fasting plasma glucose should be checked at baseline prior to starting an antipsychotic, 12 weeks after initiation, at one year and annually thereafter. If the HbA1c is 42–47 mmol/mol, the person should be offered an intensive structured lifestyle programme.[184] If this is unsuccessful, even in those individuals who remain pre-diabetic, metformin may be considered.[184]

Treatment is similar to the treatment of type 2 diabetes outside of the context of antipsychotic use with a strategy that progresses from diet to oral medications to insulin. Consideration should of course be given to switching the antipsychotic to one with a lower risk, but it is acknowledged that effective treatment of psychosis is important for self-management of diabetes.

Obesity

Obesity is a growing problem in Western society and is occurring at a younger age. It is associated with an increased risk of type 2 diabetes, osteoarthritis, hypertension, dyslipidaemia, ischaemic heart disease, heart failure, stroke, cancer, obstructive sleep apnoea, asthma, infections of various sorts, non-alcoholic fatty liver disease, gallstones, pancreatitis, chronic kidney disease, subfertility and polycystic ovarian syndrome. Those treated with antipsychotics are at substantially greater risk for obesity. As a minimum, therefore, the body mass index (BMI) should be measured at baseline, weekly for the first four to six weeks after starting an antipsychotic, every two to four weeks up to 12 weeks, at 6 months and annually thereafter.[184] See Lester and other tools as discussed in Chapter 16.

There is meta-analytic evidence for individual lifestyle counselling, followed by exercise interventions, psychoeducation, aripiprazole augmentation, topiramate, D-fenfluramine and metformin in weight reduction. Aripiprazole augmentation, topiramate and dietary interventions have evidence for reducing waist circumference.[185]

Lifestyle interventions should always be a component of 1st-line management of obesity and should generally be continued alongside other interventions.[184] Lifestyle interventions tend to result in a loss of 3 kg in weight or one point in BMI, a statistically significantly reduction in BMI on meta-analysis, although the effect is clinically insignificant[186] so prevention of weight gain is paramount. In first-episode psychosis, lifestyle interventions attenuate weight gain after antipsychotic initiation.[184] When giving dietary advice to patients, it helps to set small, realistic goals, such as losing 5–10% of body weight at a rate of 0.5 kg per week.[167] This can be achieved by eating three balanced meals a day, increasing fruit and vegetable intake, eating at the table without distractions (such as television) and waiting for 15–20 minutes for delayed satiety before considering second portions.[167] In more difficult cases, consider involving a dietician.

In terms of pharmacological interventions, a switch to an antipsychotic with a lower propensity for weight gain (such as aripiprazole, brexpiprazole, cariprazine, lurasidone or ziprasidone) should be considered.[184] Where a patient is gaining weight on olanzapine or clozapine, the addition of aripiprazole may be considered.[184] Where other pharmacological and non-pharmacological strategies have been considered, metformin may be used (even in the absence of T2DM) to promote weight loss, though it is less effective than intensive lifestyle intervention.[184] Bariatric surgery may be considered in severe cases.[167]

Dyslipidaemia

Dyslipidaemia may consist of raised total cholesterol, raised LDL cholesterol, lowered HDL cholesterol or raised triglycerides. Raised LDL cholesterol is a strong risk factor for cardiovascular disease and is associated with antipsychotic drug use. The BAP therefore recommends checking lipid profile (ideally fasting lipids, but otherwise random lipids suffice) at 12 weeks, six months and annually thereafter.[184] There is meta-analytic evidence for addressing disordered cholesterol with lifestyle interventions, topiramate, metformin and aripiprazole.[185] However, first-line management should consist of reducing alcohol intake, promoting smoking cessation, optimising control of any comorbid diabetes and advising on a diet low in saturated fats. The QRISK-3 calculator takes into account serious mental illness and antipsychotic use: it may be used to calculate 10-year cardiovascular risk. If risk is greater than 10 per cent, a statin should be initiated.[167]

In terms of triglycerides, there is evidence that topiramate, lifestyle interventions and metformin all reduce triglyceride levels,[185] but there is currently insufficient evidence that this lowers cardiovascular risk.[167]

Other Side Effects

There is a wide range of haematological side effects of antipsychotics. These include excesses of cell types (leukocytosis and eosinophilia) as well as cytopenias (leukopenia, neutropenia, thrombocytopenia and pancytopenia). Agranulocytosis, while most common in clozapine use (see later) can also occur with other antipsychotics. Most of these reactions occur within six weeks of starting the drug, so vigilance for symptoms that might result from a haematological abnormality is necessary during these early weeks.

Hepatic side effects may also occur and were a problem with chlorpromazine use, which was associated with cholestasis in 1–2% of patients. There is also the insidious increased risk of non-alcoholic fatty liver disease due to the metabolic side effects of SGAs. SGAs are sometimes considered to be safer, but they can occasionally cause a severe idiosyncratic acute liver injury.[187] There is no consensus on whether liver function tests should be routinely monitored.[187] An elevation in transaminases in individuals on an antipsychotic is common and is often due to non-alcoholic fatty liver disease. Where there is a raised alkaline phosphatase – or ALT and bilirubin are raised – consideration should be given to discontinuing the antipsychotic.

Adverse skin reactions occur in approximately 5 per cent of those on antipsychotics, most of which are fairly benign. Chlorpromazine, in particular, is associated with photosensitivity and skin hyperpigmentation, so patients should be warned to avoid direct sunlight and wear sunscreen. Allergic reactions to antipsychotics may also occur and may consist of erythema multiforme, a maculopapular rash, generalised urticaria, angioedema or exfoliative dermatitis. Usually this necessitates a switch to a structurally unrelated antipsychotic, but if the reaction is mild and the therapeutic benefit outweighs the risk, it may be possible to continue the antipsychotic.

Pneumonia is more common in patients treated with antipsychotics, with a relative risk of 1.83 (1.60–2.10), spanning both FGAs and SGAs.[188] Vigilance – especially in those with additional risk factors like old age, airways disease and smoking – is required.

The increased risk of venous thromboembolism on antipsychotics has also been confirmed in large-scale observational studies.[189] The risk is dose-dependent and is highest on clozapine, olanzapine and low-potency FGAs.[189] There is no evidence for any active interventions, so vigilance is suggested.[124]

Hypertension is often considered part of the metabolic syndrome and frequently occurs in those treated with antipsychotics alongside obesity, T2DM and dyslipidaemia. Existing NICE guidelines for the general population should be followed.

Clozapine-Specific Side Effects

Clozapine occupies a unique position in the management of treatment-resistant schizophrenia. Clozapine also has the broadest side-effect profile of the antipsychotics, although its value appears greatest in terms of its beneficial effect on life expectancy in people with schizophrenia. It is therefore important that people prescribed clozapine have every help to make it easy to tolerate. Active and regular enquiry about side effects is essential. The Glasgow antipsychotic side-effect scale for clozapine (GASS-C[190]) can be useful. Alternatively, if people are on a number of different medications, the original GASS[191] supplemented by the Bristol Stool Chart[192] can be used. In any case, it is important to enquire about side effects at every consultation, as clozapine levels vary depending on individual metabolic pathways, smoking habits, systemic inflammation and co-prescribed medications, and differences in levels will result in changes in tolerance.

The most high-profile side effect of clozapine is agranulocytosis, which – when the link was made – resulted in clozapine's withdrawal from the market in most countries. However, in countries where it continued to be prescribed, clozapine's relative benefit became apparent and was later confirmed by well-constructed clinical trials. Overall, the estimated cumulative risks of neutropaenia and agranulocytosis on clozapine are 3% and 0.8% respectively.[193] Meta-analytic data shows that the incidence of neutropaenia-related deaths on clozapine is 0.013%, while 2.1% of people who experienced severe neutropenia died.[194]

The re-licensing of clozapine in many countries was therefore conditional on regular neutrophil counts. The current threshold for discontinuing clozapine in the UK is 1.5×10^9/l, (unless there is a diagnosis of benign ethnic neutropaenia, when it drops to 1.0×10^9/l). The exact neutrophil thresholds for continuing clozapine prescription however vary from country to country. The FDA recently lowered the neutrophil threshold at which clozapine is stopped, meaning that it is less likely to be stopped inappropriately; discontinuing clozapine unnecessarily can result in a deterioration in mental state that can be damaging functionally and socially.

There are many other possible causes of neutropaenia, so a full risk-benefit assessment of a clozapine re-challenge needs to take these into account. However, a true clozapine-related agranulocytosis is likely to recur and difficult to prevent, so re-challenge is not advised. People are more likely to develop an initial agranulocytosis during the early weeks of clozapine use. Having developed an agranulocytosis as a direct reaction to clozapine, re-exposure to the drug risks a further drop in neutrophil count, which tends to be faster, reach a lower neutrophil nadir and take longer to resolve.

The monitoring of neutrophil count on clozapine has meant that if people develop clinically significant neutropenia, this is detected and managed early. The same cannot be said for the high risk of constipation on clozapine, which happens three times more often than on other antipsychotics, with reports of life-threatening and indeed fatal consequences. Schizophrenia itself is associated with constipation because of obesity, poor diet and sedentary behaviour. In addition, the anticholinergic effect of antipsychotics will reduce bowel motility, but for people on clozapine, bowel motility is further compromised by potent agonist activity at δ opioid receptors from clozapine's main metabolite, norclozapine. It is recommended that people monitor their bowel movements from the time they start clozapine – ideally using a tool such as the Bristol Stool Chart – and that regular enquiry is made, as people may not volunteer the information. There is also a case to be made for routine or early co-prescription with laxatives. Should people experience constipation early, continued use of gut motility agents may be indicated.[167] Bulk-forming laxatives should be avoided as the underlying cause is hypomotility.

Clozapine reduces the seizure threshold at higher doses or levels above the therapeutic range. Should a trial of treatment above the therapeutic range be indicated, prophylactic use of antiepileptic agents is required. The most common antiepileptic agents used are lamotrigine and, in keeping with safety guidelines (see later), sodium valproate. Lamotrigine also has some evidence for effectiveness in bipolar depression, which can occur comorbid with schizoaffective disorder. Therapeutic drug levels are important in people prescribed lamotrigine as levels are greatly affected by co-prescribed medications.

Additionally, some experience myoclonic jerks on clozapine, which should be considered if people report spillages or falls. An increasing frequency of myoclonic jerks can indicate a raised risk of a generalised seizure so should be assessed thoroughly. It is helpful to reduce the dose of clozapine if clinically appropriate. The most effective antiepileptic medication for myoclonic jerks is sodium valproate, with clonazepam also being effective. Lamotrigine is not effective in this context. However, sodium valproate can reduce neutrophil counts, which may complicate clozapine monitoring. Extremely importantly, sodium valproate is highly teratogenic and is not appropriate for use in women of childbearing potential unless in the presence of an extremely robust contraception plan.[195]

Hypersalivation can be troublesome on clozapine. It tends to be worse at night-time and is most marked in the early stages of treatment. It is socially embarrassing, affecting quality of life and has been suggested as being a contributory factor in the development of aspiration pneumonia on clozapine. The first step is to prescribe at the lowest effective dose as hypersalivation is associated with higher plasma levels. Strategies such as using chewing gum, using more more pillows at night-time and placing a towel on the pillow to prevent soaking overnight can be helpful. There are no medicines licensed for hypersalivation, but first-line treatments often include anticholinergic agents – most notably hyoscine, which has one double-blind RCT supporting its use.[196] However, anti-cholinergics can increase the risk of constipation so need to be managed carefully (see medichec.com). Many other drugs have been trialled in this area, including amisulpride and metoclopramide, with case reports of success with botulinum toxin.[123]

Sedation (see the section on 'Somnolence and Sedation' in this chapter) is prominent with clozapine especially early on in treatment. Using the lowest effective dose, skewing the dose towards bedtime and gradually making changes to best suit the lifestyle of the patient is helpful. Trials of targeted adjunctive medications have not identified a clear pharmacological strategy; negative trialled medications include modafinil.[197]

Weight gain and diabetes are addressed earlier but are likewise especially common on clozapine, so dietary and activity advice before treatment starts is essential. Notably, the emergence of glucose dysregulation can be rapid, with one study showing that 55 per cent of people developed an abnormal glucose tolerance test within three months of starting clozapine, independent of weight gain.[198]

Nocturnal enuresis is surprisingly common on many antipsychotics but especially so on clozapine, and specific enquiry may be needed to reveal its existence. A reasonable first approach is to reduce the level of nocturnal sedation by changing dosing times and distribution, although this may then have effects on daytime sedation. Avoiding fluids before bedtime can be helpful as well as setting alarms to wake up to urinate at night. In more challenging cases, desmopressin has been used, although sodium needs to be monitored.[123]

Gastro-oesophageal reflux disease is often observed in people taking clozapine. It is usually managed with proton pump inhibitors although some of these, such as omeprazole, can induce CYP1A2, which can affect the levels of clozapine.

Clozapine is associated with a risk of infections, including pneumonia. It is thought that this may result from the aspiration of saliva. Further, immunoglobulins levels appear to be lower in people taking clozapine,[199] with more prescriptions of antibiotics. It has been suggested that people receiving clozapine could be considered for a pneumococcus vaccination.[199] Many will be eligible for annual influenza vaccinations, while all patients with a serious mental illness should receive vaccination against Covid-19. Inflammation, in general, reduces CYP1A2 activity, so getting pneumonia or an infection can increase clozapine levels quite dramatically, and the clozapine dose should be reviewed.

Initiation of clozapine requires careful observation for at least the first four weeks. The dose starts low to prevent emerging side effects and is gradually titrated up. Blood pressure, pulse and temperature are monitored at least daily in the first four weeks as a sudden rise in clozapine dose can cause hypotension. Hypertension has also been observed in the first four weeks of clozapine use.

Clozapine itself induces an inflammatory response so fever can be observed in the first four weeks. If so, it is important to check that the neutrophil count has not dropped and to reduce the rate of titration. Should fever occur in the presence of other systemic indicators, it is important to look for underlying acute disorders such as myocarditis, neuroleptic malignant syndrome and pneumonia.

Nausea is most common during the first weeks of treatment. Anti-emetics can ameliorate, but some may be problematic in a given individual – for example, if there is known sensitivity to dopamine antagonists. Ondansetron is an effective anti-emetic but can worsen constipation, while domperidone should be avoided if there is any underlying cardiac risk or QT prolongation.

Tachycardia is quite common in the first four weeks of clozapine use and may be dose related. It is usually benign, but if it persists at rest and co-occurs with alterations in blood pressure, with chest pain or with fever, this may suggest myocarditis, necessitating urgent assessment, referral to cardiology and suspension or – if confirmed – discontinuation of clozapine. A benign isolated tachycardia can be treated with cardio-selective beta blockers or, if necessary, ivabradine, a negative chronotropic agent that acts on the funny channels of the heart.[180]

The dose at which one should first measure clozapine levels varies by sex, smoking habit and ethnicity – with females, non-smokers and people of Asian heritage more likely to have higher levels of clozapine at a given dosage.[200]

Clozapine has been associated with both myocarditis and cardiomyopathy. Clozapine-related myocarditis is likely a hypersensitivity response, which has a significant variation in reported incidence between 0.2 and 3%.[201] This variation may relate to differences in screening protocols, but the speed of titration may also be relevant, as may concurrent sodium valproate prescription. The risk for myocarditis is highest in the first two months after starting clozapine but has been reported later in treatment. Symptoms suggestive of myocarditis include hypotension, tachycardia, fever, flu-like symptoms, fatigue and dyspnoea, along with chest pain. An echocardiograph at baseline is helpful. Suggested screening for cardiac myocarditis includes vital signs (pulse, blood pressure, temperature and respiratory rate) taken daily for four weeks, alongside systematic questions about chest pain, fever, cough, shortness of breath and exercise capacity. Weekly c-reactive protein (CRP), troponin, FBC and ECG tests should be taken for the first four weeks. If the CRP goes above 100 mg per litre or troponin is more than twice the upper limit of normal, then clozapine should be stopped and the echocardiograph repeated.[123]

Cardiomyopathy is a later complication and can present with signs of heart failure. However, early cardiomyopathy may be asymptomatic, so any symptoms of palpitations, chest pain, syncope, sweating, reduced exercise capacity or breathing difficulties should be investigated, including with echocardiography. It is less frequent – about 1 out of 1,000 patients – although, again, there is a wide range.[123,201]

Drug Interactions

Drug Interactions and Pharmacogenomics

There is large inter-individual variation in drug response. This can be due to differences in both pharmacokinetics (drug absorption, distribution, metabolism and elimination) and pharmacodynamics (effects at the drug's biological targets). Together, these factors determine the efficacy, adverse effects and withdrawal symptoms that an individual experiences from each drug at different doses. In certain scenarios, the dose should be pre-emptively adjusted to reduce the risk of either failed treatment or intolerable adverse effects.

Absorption and the Food Effect

The timing of meals can have a significant effect on the bioavailability of antipsychotics. Ziprasidone's absorption doubles when taken with food. Larger meals have more consistent absorption, so it is recommended that ziprasidone is administered with a meal containing at least 500 calories. A similar effect is observed with lurasidone, which has a two to three times increase in absorption with food. A slightly smaller meal (350 kcals) is advised.

CYP Enzymes and Pharmacogenomics

The cytochrome P450 (CYP) enzymes are found in the liver but also in the gut, brain[202] and other tissues. There are over 50 different genes encoding CYP enzyme genes that are grouped in 18 families (*CYP1, CYP2, CYP3*). Just five enzymes account for the majority of drug metabolism: CYP1A2, CYP2C9, CYP2C19, CYP2D6 and CYP3A4. The three enzymes most relevant to antipsychotic metabolism are CYP1A2, CYP2D6 and CYP3A4.

As well as being substrates for CYP enzymes, some drugs and compounds will also induce or inhibit their activity, leading to knock-on effects on the metabolism of other medications (Table 5.3.14). Carbamazepine, for example, induces both CYP2D6 and CYP3A4 and can reduce the plasma concentrations of clozapine, risperidone, olanzapine and quetiapine by about 50 per cent. Fluoxetine inhibits several enzymes and may increase plasma levels of clozapine and risperidone by about 50 per cent and 75 per cent respectively.

Cigarette Smoking

Tobacco smoke contains aromatic hydrocarbons that induce cytochrome P450 enzymes, especially CYP1A2.[203] This can affect the metabolism of antipsychotics such as clozapine, haloperidol and olanzapine, reducing their plasma levels by 50 per cent. Abrupt cessation of smoking, as occurs when patients are admitted to hospital, can lead to rapid increases in plasma concentrations, thereby risking severe toxicity. Another common stimulant that induces CYP1A2 is caffeine. Systemic inflammation can reduce CYP1A2 activity, resulting in elevated plasma drug concentrations.

Grapefruit Juice

Grapefruit juice is a potent inhibitor of CYP3A4,[204] which is caused by a flavonoid compound known as naringin. It can increase the bioavailability of some medications – quetiapine, for example – by up to three times.

Pharmacogenomics: The Example of CYP2D6 and Risperidone

CYP enzyme activity depends on the set of alleles that each individual has. There are four categories of metaboliser: poor, intermediate, normal and ultrarapid. The enzyme with the greatest phenotypic variation is CYP2D6. One of its substrates is risperidone, which is metabolised by CYP2D6 to its active metabolite 9-OH-risperidone. Compared to normal metabolisers, poor and intermediate metabolisers have risperidone plasma concentrations that are about 1.4x and 1.6x higher and may, therefore, be more likely to experience adverse effects.[205] High CYP2D6 activity, on the other hand, reduces active drug exposure and may impact on treatment response. As a result, those who are both poor and ultrarapid metabolisers are more likely to switch medications within one year (odds ratios: 1.9 [95% CI: 1.1–3.1, p = 0.015] and 2.9 [95% CI: 1.4–6.0. p = 0.003] respectively).[205] It is recommended that poor metabolisers are prescribed doses about 30 per cent lower than usual. Some experts have suggested that patients should be genotyped before they start treatment in order to facilitate a more precise titration of dose.[205] The issue is particularly relevant in certain populations: 70 per cent of East Asians, for example, are poor or intermediate metabolisers compared to only 25 per cent of White Americans.

Pharmacodynamic Interactions

Pharmacodynamic interactions are where multiple drugs contribute to the same end effect. For example, alcohol, antihistamines and opiates – if taken together – risk dangerous oversedation. These interactions are listed in Table 5.3.15.

Table 5.3.14 CYP enzymes and selected interactions with antipsychotics

CYP Enzyme	Inhibitors	Inducers	Antipsychotic Substrates
CYP1A2	Fluvoxamine, ciprofloxacin, verapamil, erythromycin, caffeine	Tobacco, modafinil, phenytoin, omeprazole, rifampicin, carbamazepine	Asenapine, brexpiprazole, clozapine, chlorpromazine, olanzapine
CYP2D6	Fluoxetine, paroxetine, bupropion, duloxetine, promethazine, quinidine, ritonavir	Carbamazepine, rifampicin	Aripiprazole, brexpiprazole, cariprazine, chlorpromazine, haloperidol, iloperidone, olanzapine, risperidone, zuclopenthixol
CYP3A4	Fluoxetine, paroxetine, erythromycin, clarithromycin, ketoconazole, itraconazole, ritonavir, grapefruit juice	Carbamazepine, phenytoin, St. John's wort, modafinil	Aripiprazole, cariprazine, haloperidol, iloperidone, lurasidone, olanzapine, quetiapine, ziprasidone, zuclopenthixol

Data from electronic medicines compendium (EMC). www.medicines.org.uk/emc/

Table 5.3.15 Pharmacodynamic interactions

Risk	Antipsychotics	Other Agents
Anticholinergic excess (Blurred vision, constipation, dry mouth, urinary retention, confusion)	Clozapine, chlorpromazine, trifluoperazine	Hyoscine, atropine
Neutropaenia, agranulocytosis	Clozapine	Carbamazepine, cytotoxics, ciprofloxacin, erythromycin, metronidazole
Weight gain, metabolic syndrome, cardiovascular risk	Chlorpromazine, clozapine, olanzapine, quetiapine	Tricyclic antidepressants, mirtazapine, lithium, sodium valproate; also cigarette smoking and older age
Sedation	Chlorpromazine, clozapine, olanzapine, quetiapine	Alcohol, antihistamines, benzodiazapines, z-drugs, gabapentinoids, mirtazapine, opioids, trazodone, tricyclic antidepressants
Seizures	Clozapine, chlorpromazine	Alcohol and benzodiazepine withdrawal, buproprion, tricyclic antidepressants, trazodone
Orthostatic hypotension	Asenapine, clozapine, quetiapine, olanzapine, risperidone	Alcohol, antihypertensives, tricyclic antidepressants
Cardiorespiratory depression	Intramuscular olanzapine	Intramuscular lorazepam
Sexual dysfunction (erectile dysfunction)	All except aripiprazole, brexpiprazole and cariprazine (D_2 receptor partial agonists)	
QT prolongation	Haloperidol, pimozide, ziprasidone	Several antibiotics, antifungals,tricyclic antidepressants, citalopram, escitlopram, cyclosporine, methadone, tamoxifen

References

1. Carpenter WT, Davis JM. Another view of the history of antipsychotic drug discovery and development. *Molecular Psychiatry* 2012;17(12):1168–73. www.nature.com/articles/mp2012121 (accessed 9 September 2020).
2. Sneader W. *Drug Discovery: A History.* Chichester: Wiley; 2006. books.google.co.uk/books/about/Drug_Discovery.html?id=jglFsz5EJR8C (accessed 9 September 2020).
3. Ban TA. Fifty years chlorpromazine: A historical perspective. *Neuropsychiatric Disease and Treatment* 2007;3(4):495–500. www.ncbi.nlm.nih.gov/pubmed/19300578 (accessed 10 September 2020).
4. Schonecker M. Paroxysmal dyskinesia as the effect of megaphen. *Nervenarzt* 1957;28(12):550–3. www.ncbi.nlm.nih.gov/pubmed/13517450 (accessed 10 September 2020).
5. Kapur S, Remington G. Dopamine D(2) receptors and their role in atypical antipsychotic action: still necessary and may even be sufficient. *Biological Psychiatry* 2001;50(11):873–83.
6. Wadenberg M-LG. Conditioned avoidance response in the development of new antipsychotics. *Current Pharmaceutical Design* 2009;16 (3):358–70.
7. Seeman P, Lee T, Chau-Wong M, et al. Antipsychotic drug doses and neuroleptic/dopamine receptors. *Nature* 1976;261(5562):717–9. www.nature.com/articles/261717a0 (accessed 2 December 2021).
8. Tarazi FI, Zhang K, Baldessarini RJ. Dopamine D_4 receptors: beyond schizophrenia. *Journal of Receptors and Signal Transduction* 2004;24(3):131–47. www.tandfonline.com/doi/abs/10.1081/RRS-200032076 (accessed 2 December 2021).
9. Pani L, Pira L, Marchese G. Antipsychotic efficacy: relationship to optimal D2-receptor occupancy. *European Psychiatry* 2007;22(5):267–75. www.cambridge.org/core/journals/european-psychiatry/article/abs/antipsychotic-efficacy-relationship-to-optimal-d2receptor-occupancy/CA4F00CB4847264A20F18475396 7634F (accessed 2 December 2021)
10. Green AR. Neuropharmacology of 5-hydroxytryptamine. *British Journal of Pharmacology* 2006;147(S1):S145–52. onlinelibrary.wiley.com/doi/full/10.1038/sj.bjp.0706427 (accessed 2 December 2021).
11. Morrison PD, Murray RM. The antipsychotic landscape: dopamine and beyond. *Therapeutic Advances in Psychopharmacology* 2018;8(4):127–35. journals.sagepub.com/doi/full/10.1177/2045125317752915 (accessed 2 December 2021).
12. Leucht S, Cipriani A, Spineli L, et al. Comparative efficacy and tolerability of 15 antipsychotic drugs in schizophrenia: a multiple-treatments meta-analysis. *Lancet.* 2013;382 (9896):951–62.
13. Ebdrup BH, Rasmussen H, Arnt J, et al. Serotonin 2A receptor antagonists for treatment of schizophrenia. *Expert Opinion on Investigational Drugs* 2011;20(9):1211–23. www.tandfonline.com/doi/abs/10.1517/13543784.2011.601738 (accessed 2 December 2021).
14. William T. Carpenter MD, Robert W. et al. Special section on implications of CATIE: lessons to take home from CATIE. *Psychiatric Services* 2008;59 (5):523–5. ps.psychiatryonline.org/doi/abs/10.1176/ps.2008.59.5.523 (accessed 2 December 2021).
15. Naber D, Lambert M. The CATIE and CUtLASS studies in schizophrenia. *CNS Drugs*. 2012;23(8):649–59. link.springer.com/article/10.2165/00023210-200923080-00002 (accessed 2 December 2021).
16. Morrison P, Taylor DM, McGuire P. *The Maudsley Guidelines on Advanced Prescribing in Psychosis.* Hoboken, NJ: Wiley-Blackwell; 2020.
17. Legge SE, Hamshere M, Hayes RD, et al. Reasons for discontinuing clozapine: a cohort study of patients commencing treatment. *Schizophrenia Research* 2016;174(1–3):113–9.
18. Watt ML, Kehn L, Shaw DB, et al. The muscarinic acetylcholine receptor agonist BuTAC mediates antipsychotic-like

effects via the M4 subtype. *Neuropsychopharmacology* 2013;38 (13):2717–26. www.nature.com/articles/npp2013186 (accessed 2 December 2021).

19. Lieberman JA, III. Managing anticholinergic side effects. *Primary Care Companion of the Journal of Clinical Psychiatry* 2004;6(Suppl 2):20–3. www.ncbi.nlm.nih.gov/pubmed/16001097 (accessed 18 May 2021).
20. Stone JM, Morrison PD, Pilowsky LS. Glutamate and dopamine dysregulation in schizophrenia – a synthesis and selective review. *Journal of Psychopharmacology* 2007;21(4):440–52. journals.sagepub.com/doi/abs/10.1177/0269881106073126?casa_token=ynxkGb8 (accessed 2 December 2021).
21. Singer P, Dubroqua S, Yee B. Inhibition of glycine transporter 1: the yellow brick road to new schizophrenia therapy? *Current Pharmaceutical Design* 2015;21 (26):3771–87.
22. Li ML, Hu XQ, Li F, et al. Perspectives on the mGluR2/3 agonists as a therapeutic target for schizophrenia: still promising or a dead end? *Progress in Neuro-Psychopharmacology & Biological Psychiatry* 2015;60:66–76.
23. Xu H, Perez S, Cornil A, et al. Dopamine–endocannabinoid interactions mediate spike-timing-dependent potentiation in the striatum. *Nature Communications* 2018;9 (1):1–18. www.nature.com/articles/s41467-018-06409-5 (accessed 2 December 2021).
24. Di Forti M, Marconi A, Carra E, et al. Proportion of patients in south London with first-episode psychosis attributable to use of high potency cannabis: a case-control study. *The Lancet Psychiatry* 2015;2(3):233–8.
25. Katona I, Freund TF. Multiple functions of endocannabinoid signaling in the brain. *Annual Review of Neuroscience* 2012;35:529–58. www.annualreviews.org/doi/abs/10.1146/annurev-neuro-062111-150420 (accessed 2 December 2021).
26. McGuire P, Robson P, Cubala WJ, et al. Cannabidiol (CBD) as an adjunctive therapy in schizophrenia: a multicenter randomized controlled trial. *American Journal of Psychiatry* 2018;175 (3):225–31. ajp.psychiatryonline.org/doi/abs/10.1176/appi.ajp.2017.17030325 (accessed 2 December 2021).
27. Shah JL, Crawford A, Mustafa SS, et al. Is the clinical high-risk state a valid concept? Retrospective examination in a first-episode psychosis sample. *Psychiatric Services* 2017;68 (10):1046–52.
28. Fusar-Poli P, Cappucciati M, Borgwardt S, et al. Heterogeneity of psychosis risk within individuals at clinical high risk: a meta-analytical stratification. *JAMA Psychiatry* 2016;73(2):113–20.
29. Klosterkötter J, Hellmich M, Steinmeyer EM, et al. Diagnosing schizophrenia in the initial prodromal phase. *Archives of General Psychiatry* 2001;58(2):158–64.
30. Schultze-Lutter F, Michel C, Schmidt SJ, et al. EPA guidance on the early detection of clinical high risk states of psychoses. *European Psychiatry* 2015;30 (3):405–16.
31. Fusar-Poli P, Salazar De Pablo G, Correll CU, et al. Prevention of psychosis: advances in detection, prognosis, and intervention. *JAMA Psychiatry* 2020;77(7):755–65.
32. Davies C, Radua J, Cipriani A, et al. Efficacy and acceptability of interventions for attenuated positive psychotic symptoms in individuals at clinical high risk of psychosis: a network meta-analysis. *Frontiers in Psychiatry* 2018;9:187.
33. McGorry PD, Hartmann JA, Spooner R, et al. Beyond the "at risk mental state" concept: transitioning to transdiagnostic psychiatry. *World Psychiatry* 2018;17(2):133–42.
34. van Os J, Guloksuz S. A critique of the "ultra-high risk" and "transition" paradigm. *World Psychiatry* 2017;16 (2):200–6.
35. Howes OD, Whitehurst T, Shatalina E, et al. The clinical significance of duration of untreated psychosis: an umbrella review and random-effects meta-analysis. *World Psychiatry* 2021;20 (1):75–95.
36. Gillies D, Sampson S, Beck A, et al. Benzodiazepines for psychosis-induced aggression or agitation. *Cochrane Database of Systematic Reviews* 2013;4: CD003079.
37. National Institute for Clinical Excellence. *Guidance on the Use of Zaleplon, Zolpidem and Zopiclone for the Short-term Management of Insomnia.* 2004. www.nice.org.uk/guidance/ta77.
38. Igwe SC, Brigo F. Does melatonin and melatonin agonists improve the metabolic side effects of atypical antipsychotics?: a systematic review and meta-analysis of randomized controlled trials. *Clinical Psychopharmacology and Neuroscience* 2018;16(3):235.
39. Leucht S, Leucht C, Huhn M, et al. Sixty years of placebo-controlled antipsychotic drug trials in acute schizophrenia: systematic review, Bayesian meta-analysis, and meta-regression of efficacy predictors. *American Journal of Psychiatry* 2017;174(1):927–42.
40. Tiihonen J, Lönnqvist J, Wahlbeck K, et al. 11-year follow-up of mortality in patients with schizophrenia: a population-based cohort study (FIN11 study). *Lancet.* 2009;374(9690):620–7.
41. Zohar J, Stahl S, Moller H-J, et al. A review of the current nomenclature for psychotropic agents and an introduction to the neuroscience-based nomenclature. *European Neuropsychopharmacology* 2015;25 (12):2318–25.
42. Huhn M, Nikolakopoulou A, Schneider-Thoma J, et al. Comparative efficacy and tolerability of 32 oral antipsychotics for the acute treatment of adults with multi-episode schizophrenia: a systematic review and network meta-analysis. *Lancet* 2019;394 (10202):939–51.
43. Nguyen CT, Rosen JA, Bota RG. Aripiprazole partial agonism at 5-HT2C: a comparison of weight gain associated with aripiprazole adjunctive to antidepressants with high versus low serotonergic activities. *The Primary Care Companion for CNS Disorders* 2012;14(5):26654.
44. Lieberman JA, Stroup TS, McEvoy JP, et al. Effectiveness of antipsychotic drugs in patients with chronic schizophrenia. *New England Journal of Medicine* 2005;353(12):1209–23.
45. Kahn RS, Fleischhacker WW, Boter H, et al. Effectiveness of antipsychotic drugs in first-episode schizophrenia and schizophreniform disorder: an open randomised clinical trial. *Lancet.* 2008;371(9618):1085–97.
46. Gómez-Revuelta M, Pelayo-Terán JM, Juncal-Ruiz M, et al. Antipsychotic treatment effectiveness in first episode of psychosis: PAFIP 3-year follow-up randomized clinical trials comparing

haloperidol, olanzapine, risperidone, aripiprazole, quetiapine, and ziprasidone. *International Journal of Neuropsychopharmacology* 2020;23 (4):217–29.

47. Kreyenbuhl J, Buchanan RW, Dickerson FB, et al. The schizophrenia patient outcomes research team (PORT): updated treatment recommendations 2009. *Schizophrenia Bulletin* 2010;36(1):94–103.

48. Uchida H, Takeuchi H, Graff-Guerrero A, et al. Dopamine D2 receptor occupancy and clinical effects: a systematic review and pooled analysis. *Journal of Clinical Psychopharmacology* 2011;31(4):497–502.

49. Uchida H, Takeuchi H, Graff-Guerrero A, et al. Predicting dopamine D2 receptor occupancy from plasma levels of antipsychotic drugs: a systematic review and pooled analysis. *Journal of Clinical Psychopharmacology* 2011;31 (3):318–25.

50. Lako IM, van den Heuvel ER, Knegtering H, et al. Estimating dopamine D2 receptor occupancy for doses of 8 antipsychotics: a meta-analysis. *Journal of Clinical Psychopharmacology* 2013;33(5):675–81.

51. Leucht S, Tardy M, Komossa K, et al. Antipsychotic drugs versus placebo for relapse prevention in schizophrenia: a systematic review and meta-analysis. *Lancet* 2012;379(9831):2063–71.

52. Kishi T, Ikuta T, Matsui Y, et al. Effect of discontinuation v. maintenance of antipsychotic medication on relapse rates in patients with remitted/stable first-episode psychosis: a meta-analysis. *Psychological Medicine* 2019;49 (5):772–9.

53. Patel MX, Arista IA, Taylor M, et al. How to compare doses of different antipsychotics: a systematic review of methods. *Schizophrenia Research* 2013;149(1–3):141–8.

54. Leucht S, Crippa A, Siafis S, et al. Dose-response meta-analysis of antipsychotic drugs for acute schizophrenia. *American Journal of Psychiatry* 2020;177(4):342–53.

55. Galling B, Roldán A, Hagi K, et al. Antipsychotic augmentation vs. monotherapy in schizophrenia: systematic review, meta-analysis and meta-regression analysis. *World Psychiatry* 2017;16(1):77–89. doi.wiley .com/10.1002/wps.20387 (accessed 15 January 2021).

56. Buhagiar K, Templeton G, Blyth H, et al. Mortality risk from long-term treatment with antipsychotic polypharmacy vs monotherapy among adults with serious mental illness: A systematic review and meta-analysis of observational studies. *Schizophrenia Research* 2020;223:18–28.

57. Matsui K, Tokumasu T, Takekita Y, et al. Switching to antipsychotic monotherapy vs. staying on antipsychotic polypharmacy in schizophrenia: A systematic review and meta-analysis. *Schizophrenia Research* 2019;209:50–7.

58. Valenstein M, Ganoczy D, McCarthy JF, et al. Antipsychotic adherence over time among patients receiving treatment for schizophrenia: A retrospective review. *Journal of Clinical Psychiatry* 2006;67 (10):1542–50.

59. Hamann J, Holzhüter F, Blakaj S, et al. Implementing shared decision-making on acute psychiatric wards: a cluster-randomized trial with inpatients suffering from schizophrenia (SDM-PLUS). *Epidemiology and Psychiatric Sciences* 2020;29:e137.

60. Hartung D, Low A, Jindai K, et al. Interventions to improve pharmacological adherence among adults with psychotic spectrum disorders and bipolar disorder: a systematic review. *Psychosomatics* 2017;58(2):101–12.

61. Gray R, Bressington D, Ivanecka A, et al. Is adherence therapy an effective adjunct treatment for patients with schizophrenia spectrum disorders? A systematic review and meta-analysis. *BMC Psychiatry* 2016;16 (1):1–12.

62. Gray R, Leese M, Bindman J, et al. Adherence therapy for people with schizophrenia: European multicentre randomised controlled trial. *British Journal of Psychiatry* 2006;189 (6):508–14.

63. Kishimoto T, Hagi K, Kurokawa S, et al. Long-acting injectable versus oral antipsychotics for the maintenance treatment of schizophrenia: a systematic review and comparative meta-analysis of randomised, cohort, and pre–post studies. *The Lancet Psychiatry* 2021;8 (5):387–404.

64. Olagunju AT, Clark SR, Baune BT. Long-acting atypical antipsychotics in schizophrenia: a systematic review and meta-analyses of effects on functional outcome. *Australian and New Zealand Journal of Psychiatry* 2019;53(6):509–27.

65. Rubio JM, Schoretsanitis G, John M, et al. Psychosis relapse during treatment with long-acting injectable antipsychotics in individuals with schizophrenia-spectrum disorders: an individual participant data meta-analysis. *The Lancet Psychiatry* 2020;7 (9):749–61. linkinghub.elsevier.com/retrieve/pii/S2215036620302649

66. Mcintosh AM, Owens DC, Moorhead WJ, et al. Longitudinal volume reductions in people at high genetic risk of schizophrenia as they develop psychosis. *Biological Psychiatry* 2011;69 (10):953–8.

67. Haijma S V, Van Haren N, Cahn W, et al. Brain volumes in schizophrenia: A meta-analysis in over 18 000 subjects. *Schizophrenia Bulletin* 2013;39 (5):1129–38.

68. Wunderink L, Nieboer RM, Wiersma D, et al. Recovery in remitted first-episode psychosis at 7 years of follow-up of an early dose reduction/discontinuation or maintenance treatment strategy long-term follow-up of a 2-year randomized clinical trial. *JAMA Psychiatry* 2013;70(9):913–20.

69. Hui CLM, Honer WG, Lee EHM, et al. Long-term effects of discontinuation from antipsychotic maintenance following first-episode schizophrenia and related disorders: a 10 year follow-up of a randomised, double-blind trial. *The Lancet Psychiatry.* 2018;5 (5):432–42.

70. Wils RS, Gotfredsen DR, Hjorthøj C, et al. Antipsychotic medication and remission of psychotic symptoms 10 years after a first-episode psychosis. *Schizophrenia Research* 2017;182:42–8.

71. Horowitz MA, Jauhar S, Natesan S, et al. A method for tapering antipsychotic treatment that may minimize the risk of relapse. *Schizophrenia Bulletin* 2021;47 (4):1116–29.

72. Kapur S, Zipursky RB, Remington G, et al. 5-HT2 and D2 receptor occupancy of olanzapine in schizophrenia: a PET investigation. *American Journal of Psychiatry* 1998;155(7):921–8.

73. Emsley R, Nuamah I, Hough D, et al. Treatment response after relapse in a placebo-controlled maintenance trial in schizophrenia. *Schizophrenia Research* 2012;138(1):29–34.

74. McCutcheon R, Beck K, Bloomfield MAP, et al. Treatment resistant or resistant to treatment? Antipsychotic plasma levels in patients with poorly controlled psychotic symptoms. *Journal of Psychopharmacology* 2015;29 (8):892–7.

75. Kane J, Honigfeld G, Singer J, et al. Clozapine for the treatment-resistant schizophrenic: a double-blind comparison with chlorpromazine. *Archives of General Psychiatry.* 1988;45 (9):789–96.

76. Kapur S, Zipursky RB, Remington G. Clinical and theoretical implications of 5-HT2 and D2 receptor occupancy of clozapine, risperidone, and olanzapine in schizophrenia. *American Journal of Psychiatry* 1999;156(2):286–93.

77. Perry PJ, Miller DD, Arndt S V, et al. Clozapine and norclozapine plasma concentrations and clinical response of treatment-refractory schizophrenic patients. *American Journal of Psychiatry* 1991;148(2):231–5.

78. Ucok A, Yağcıoğlu EA, Yıldız M, et al. Reasons for clozapine discontinuation in patients with treatment-resistant schizophrenia. *Psychiatry Research* 2019;275:149–54.

79. Luykx JJ, Stam N, Tanskanen A, et al. In the aftermath of clozapine discontinuation: comparative effectiveness and safety of antipsychotics in patients with schizophrenia who discontinue clozapine. *British Journal of Psychiatry* 2020;217(3):498–505.

80. Siskind D, Siskind V, Kisely S. Clozapine response rates among people with treatment-resistant schizophrenia: data from a systematic review and meta-analysis. *Canadian Journal of Psychiatry* 2017;62(11):772–7.

81. Krivoy A, Joyce D, Tracy D, et al. Real-world outcomes in the management of refractory psychosis. *Journal of Clinical Psychiatry* 2019;80(5):18m12716.

82. Wagner E, Löhrs L, Siskind D, et al. Clozapine augmentation strategies – a systematic meta-review of available evidence. Treatment options for clozapine resistance. *Journal of Psychopharmacology* 2019;33(4):423–35.

83. Meltzer HY, Bobo W V, Roy A, et al. A randomized, double-blind comparison of clozapine and high-dose olanzapine in treatment-resistant patients with schizophrenia. *Journal of Clinical Psychiatry* 2008;69(2):274–85.

84. Bartoli F, Crocamo C, Di Brita C, et al. Adjunctive second-generation antipsychotics for specific symptom domains of schizophrenia resistant to clozapine: a meta-analysis. *Journal of Psychiatric Research* 2019;108:24–33.

85. Siskind DJ, Lee M, Ravindran A, et al. Augmentation strategies for clozapine refractory schizophrenia: a systematic review and meta-analysis. *Australian and New Zealand Journal of Psychiatry* 2018;52(8):751–67.

86. Helfer B, Samara MT, Huhn M, et al. Efficacy and safety of antidepressants added to antipsychotics for schizophrenia: a systematic review and meta-analysis. *American Journal of Psychiatry* 2016;173(9):876–86.

87. Leucht S, Helfer B, Dold M, et al. Lithium for schizophrenia. *Cochrane Database of Systematic Reviews* 2015;2015(10):CD003834.

88. Wang G, Zheng W, Li X-B, et al. ECT augmentation of clozapine for clozapine-resistant schizophrenia: a meta-analysis of randomized controlled trials. *Journal of Psychiatric Research* 2018;105:23–32.

89. Guttesen LL, Albert N, Nordentoft M, et al. Repetitive transcranial magnetic stimulation and transcranial direct current stimulation for auditory hallucinations in schizophrenia: systematic review and meta-analysis. *Journal of Psychiatric Research* 2021;143:163–75. pubmed.ncbi.nlm.nih .gov/34500345/ (accessed 2 December 2021).

90. Sun C-H, Jiang W-L, Cai D-B, et al. Adjunctive multi-session transcranial direct current stimulation for neurocognitive dysfunction in schizophrenia: a meta-analysis. *Asian Journal of Psychiatry* 2021;66:102887.

91. Jeppesen R, Christensen RHB, Pedersen EMJ, et al. Efficacy and safety of anti-inflammatory agents in treatment of psychotic disorders – a comprehensive systematic review and meta-analysis. *Brain, Behavior, and Immunity* 2020;90:364–80.

92. Vayisoğlu S, Karahan S, Yağcioğlu AEA. Augmentation of antipsychotic treatment with memantine in patients with schizophrenia: a systematic review and meta-analysis. *Turk Psikiyatr Dergisi* 2019;30(4):253–9.

93. Chang C-H, Lin C-H, Liu C-Y, et al. Efficacy and cognitive effect of sarcosine (N-methylglycine) in patients with schizophrenia: a systematic review and meta-analysis of double-blind randomised controlled trials. *Journal of Psychopharmacology* 2020;34 (5):495–505.

94. Zheng W, Cai D-B, Zhang Q-E, et al. Adjunctive ondansetron for schizophrenia: a systematic review and meta-analysis of randomized controlled trials. *Journal of Psychiatric Research* 2019;113:27–33.

95. Koblan KS, Kent J, Hopkins SC, et al. A Non-D2-receptor-binding drug for the treatment of schizophrenia. *New England Journal of Medicine* 2020;382 (16):1497–506.

96. Brannan SK, Sawchak S, Miller AC, et al. Muscarinic cholinergic receptor agonist and peripheral antagonist for schizophrenia. *New England Journal of Medicine* 2021;384(8):717–26. www.nejm .org/doi/full/10.1056/NEJMoa2017015 (accessed 2 December 2021).

97. Leweke FM, Hellmich M, Kranaster L, et al. Cannabidiol as a new type of an antipsychotic: results from a placebo-controlled clinical trial. *Biological Psychiatry* 2012;71(8):63S.

98. Boggs DL, Surti T, Gupta A, et al. The effects of cannabidiol (CBD) on cognition and symptoms in outpatients with chronic schizophrenia a randomized placebo controlled trial. *Psychopharmacology* 2018;235 (7):1923–32.

99. Murru A, Pacchiarotti I, Nivoli AMA, et al. What we know and what we don't know about the treatment of schizoaffective disorder. *European Neuropsychopharmacology* 2011;21 (9):680–90. www.sciencedirect.com/ science/article/pii/S0924977X1100040X (accessed 7 October 2020).

100. Glick ID, Mankoski R, Eudicone JM, et al. The efficacy, safety, and tolerability of aripiprazole for the treatment of schizoaffective disorder: Results from a pooled analysis of a sub-population of subjects from two randomized, double-blind, placebo-controlled, pivotal trials. *Journal of Affective Disorders* 2009;115 (1–2):18–26. www.sciencedirect.com/

science/article/pii/S0165032708005107 (accessed 7 October 2020).

101. Keck PE, Reeves KR, Harrigan EP, et all. Ziprasidone in the short-term treatment of patients with schizoaffective disorder: results from two double-blind, placebo-controlled, multicenter studies. *Journal of Clinical Psychopharmacology* 2001;21 (1):27–35. www.ncbi.nlm.nih.gov/pubmed/11199944 (accessed 7 October 2020).

102. Canuso CM, Lindenmayer J-P, Kosik-Gonzalez C, et al. A randomized, double-blind, placebo-controlled study of 2 dose ranges of paliperidone extended-release in the treatment of subjects with schizoaffective disorder. *Journal of Clinical Psychiatry* 2010;71 (05):587–98. article.psychiatrist.com/?ContentType=START&ID=10006877 (accessed 7 October 2020).

103. Tran PV, Tollefson GD, Sanger TM, et al. Olanzapine versus haloperidol in the treatment of schizoaffective disorder. *British Journal of Psychiatry* 1999;174(1):15–22. www.ncbi.nlm.nih.gov/pubmed/10211146 (accessed 7 October 2020).

104. Janicak PG, Keck PE, Dams JM, et al. A double-blind, randomized, prospective evaluation of the efficacy and safety of risperidone versus haloperidol in the treatment of schizoaffective disorder. *Journal of Clinical Psychopharmacology* 1981;21 (4):360–8. pascal-francis.inist.fr/vibad/index.php?action=getRecordDetail&idt=1061231 (accessed 7 October 2020).

105. Fu D-J, Turkoz I, Simonson RB, et al. Paliperidone palmitate once-monthly reduces risk of relapse of psychotic, depressive, and manic symptoms and maintains functioning in a double-blind, randomized study of schizoaffective disorder. *Journal of Clinical Psychiatry* 2015;76(03):253–62. www.psychiatrist.com/jcp/article/pages/2015/v76n03/v76n0303.aspx (accessed 6 October 2020).

106. Peuskens J, Olivares JM, Pecenak J, et al. Treatment retention with risperidone long-acting injection: 24-month results from the Electronic Schizophrenia Treatment Adherence Registry (e-STAR) in six countries. *Current Medical Research and Opinion* 2010;26(3):501–9. www.tandfonline.com/doi/full/10.1185/03007990903488670 (accessed 6 October 2020).

107. Rey Souto D, Pinzón Espinosa J, Vieta E, et al. Clozapine in patients with schizoaffective disorder: a systematic review. *Revista de Psiquiatria y Salud Mental* 2020;14(3):148–56. pubmed.ncbi.nlm.nih.gov/34400122/ (accessed 6 October 2020).

108. Lintunen J, Taipale H, Tanskanen A, et al. Long-term real-world effectiveness of pharmacotherapies for schizoaffective disorder. *Schizophrenia Bulletin* 2021;47(4):1099–107. academic.oup.com/schizophreniabulletin/advance-article/doi/10.1093/schbul/sbab004/6127087 (accessed 18 February 2021).

109. Leucht S, Kissling W, McGrath J. Lithium for schizophrenia. *Cochrane Database of Systematic Reviews* 2007;(3):CD003834. www.ncbi.nlm.nih.gov/pubmed/17636738 (accessed 7 October 2020).

110. McElroy SL, Keck PE, Pope HG. Sodium valproate: its use in primary psychiatric disorders. *Journal of Clinical Psychopharmacology* 1987;7(1):16–24. www.ncbi.nlm.nih.gov/pubmed/3102563 (accessed 22 October 2020).

111. Bogan AM, Brown ES, Suppes T. Efficacy of divalproex therapy for schizoaffective disorder. *Journal of Clinical Psychopharmacology* 2000;20 (5):520–2. www.ncbi.nlm.nih.gov/pubmed/11001235 (accessed 22 October 2020).

112. Roy Chengappa K, Kupfer DJ, Parepally H, et al. A placebo-controlled, random-assignment, parallel-group pilot study of adjunctive topiramate for patients with schizoaffective disorder, bipolar type. *Bipolar Disorders* 2007;9 (6):609–17. doi.wiley.com/10.1111/j.1399-5618.2007.00506.x (accessed 7 October 2020).

113. Upthegrove R, Marwaha S, Birchwood M. Depression and schizophrenia: cause, consequence or trans-diagnostic issue? *Schizophrenia Bulletin* 2016;43 (2):sbw097. academic.oup.com/schizophreniabulletin/article-lookup/doi/10.1093/schbul/sbw097 (accessed 22 October 2020).

114. McGinty J, Upthegrove R. Depressive symptoms during first episode psychosis and functional outcome: a systematic review and meta-analysis. *Schizophrenia Research* 2020;218:14–27. www.sciencedirect.com/science/article/pii/S092099641930581X?via%3Dihub (accessed 22 October 2020).

115. Emsley RA, Buckley P, Jones AM, et al. Differential effect of quetiapine on depressive symptoms in patients with partially responsive schizophrenia. *Journal of Psychopharmacology* 2003;17 (2):210–5. journals.sagepub.com/doi/10.1177/0269881103017002010 (accessed 22 October 2020).

116. Citrome L, Tocco M, Zeni C, et al. Assessing the benefit-risk ratio of approved treatments for bipolar depression using likelihood to be helped or harmed (LHH) analyses. *CNS Spectrums* 2021;26(2):146.

117. Gregory A, Mallikarjun P, Upthegrove R. Treatment of depression in schizophrenia: systematic review and meta-analysis. *British Journal of Psychiatry* 2017;211(4):198–204. www.cambridge.org/core/product/identifier/S0007125000280379/type/journal_article (accessed 22 October 2020).

118. Whitehead C, Moss S, Cardno A, et al. Antidepressants for people with both schizophrenia and depression. *Cochrane Database of Systematic Reviews* 2002;2002(2):CD002305. www.ncbi.nlm.nih.gov/pubmed/12076447 (accessed 7 October 2020).

119. Zisook S, Kasckow JW, Golshan S, et al. Citalopram augmentation for subsyndromal symptoms of depression in middle-aged and older outpatients with schizophrenia and schizoaffective disorder. *Journal of Clinical Psychiatry* 2009;70(4):562–71. www.psychiatrist.com/jcp/schizophrenia/citalopram-augmentation-subsyndromal-symptoms-depression/(accessed 22 October 2020).

120. Salokangas RKR, Saarijärvi S, Taiminen T, et al. Citalopram as an adjuvant in chronic schizophrenia: a double-blind placebo-controlled study. *Acta Psychiatrica Scandinavica* 1996;94 (3):175–80. doi.wiley.com/10.1111/j.1600-0447.1996.tb09844.x (accessed 22 October 2020).

121. Fusar-Poli P, Papanastasiou E, Stahl D, et al. Treatments of negative symptoms in schizophrenia: meta-analysis of 168 randomized placebo-controlled trials. *Schizophrenia Bulletin* 2015;41 (4):892–9. academic.oup.com/schizophreniabulletin/article/41/4/892/2338040 (accessed 12 November 2020).

122. Németh G, Laszlovszky I, Czobor P, et al. Cariprazine versus risperidone monotherapy for treatment of predominant negative symptoms in patients with schizophrenia: a randomised, double-blind, controlled trial. *Lancet* 2017;389(10074):1103–13. www.sciencedirect.com/science/article/pii/S0140673617300600 (accessed 14 January 2021).

123. Taylor D, Barnes TRER, Young AH. *The Maudsley Prescribing Guidelines in Psychiatry*, 14th ed. London: Wiley-Blackwell; 2021.

124. Barnes TR, Drake R, Paton C, et al. Evidence-based guidelines for the pharmacological treatment of schizophrenia: updated recommendations from the British Association for Psychopharmacology. *Journal of Psychopharmacology* 2020;34(1):3–78. www.ncbi.nlm.nih.gov/pubmed/31829775 (accessed 22 October 2020).

125. Rummel-C, Kissling W, Leucht S. Antidepressants for the negative symptoms of schizophrenia. *Cochrane Database of Systematic Reviews* 2006;(3):CD005581. www.ncbi.nlm.nih.gov/pubmed/16856105 (accessed 5 November 2020).

126. Andrade C, Kisely S, Monteiro I, et al. Antipsychotic augmentation with modafinil or armodafinil for negative symptoms of schizophrenia: systematic review and meta-analysis of randomized controlled trials. *Journal of Psychiatric Research* 2015;60:14–21. www.sciencedirect.com/science/article/pii/S0022395614002805 (accessed 12 November 2020).

127. Kishi T, Iwata N. NMDA receptor antagonists interventions in schizophrenia: meta-analysis of randomized, placebo-controlled trials. *Journal of Psychiatric Research* 2013;47(9):1143–9. www.sciencedirect.com/science/article/pii/S0022395613001398 (accessed 12 November 2020).

128. David AS, Malmberg A, Brandt L, et al. IQ and risk for schizophrenia: a population-based cohort study. *Psychological Medicine* 1997;27(6):1311–23. www.ncbi.nlm.nih.gov/pubmed/9403903 (accessed 31 March 2021).

129. Cai L, Huang J. Schizophrenia and risk of dementia: a meta-analysis study. *Neuropsychiatric Disease and Treatment* 2018;14:2047–55. www.ncbi.nlm.nih.gov/pubmed/30147318 (accessed 31 March 2021).

130. Bowie CR, Harvey PD. Cognitive deficits and functional outcome in schizophrenia. *Neuropsychiatric Disease and Treatment* 2006;2(4):531–6. www.ncbi.nlm.nih.gov/pubmed/19412501 (accessed 18 February 2021).

131. Kawai N, Yamakawa Y, Baba A, et al. High-dose of multiple antipsychotics and cognitive function in schizophrenia: the effect of dose-reduction. *Progress in Neuro-Psychopharmacology and Biological Psychiatry* 2006;30(6):1009–14. www.sciencedirect.com/science/article/pii/S0278584606000911 (accessed 18 February 2021).

132. Bilder RM, Goldman RS, Volavka J, et al. Neurocognitive effects of clozapine, olanzapine, risperidone, and haloperidol in patients with chronic schizophrenia or schizoaffective disorder. *American Journal of Psychiatry* 2002;159(6):1018–28. psychiatryonline.org/doi/abs/10.1176/appi.ajp.159.6.1018 (accessed 18 February 2021).

133. Meltzer HY, McGurk SR. The effects of clozapine, risperidone, and olanzapine on cognitive function in schizophrenia. *Schizophrenia Bulletin* 1999;25(2):233–56. academic.oup.com/schizophreniabulletin/article-lookup/doi/10.1093/oxfordjournals.schbul.a033376 (accessed 31 March 2021).

134. Keefe RSE, Bilder RM, Davis SM, et al. Neurocognitive effects of antipsychotic medications in patients with chronic schizophrenia in the CATIE Trial. *Archives of General Psychiatry* 2007;64(6):633–47. www.ncbi.nlm.nih.gov/pubmed/17548746 (accessed 31 March 2021).

135. Nielsen RE. Cognition in schizophrenia – a systematic review. *Drug Discovery Today: Therapeutic Strategies* 2011;8(1–2):43–8. www.sciencedirect.com/science/article/pii/S1740677311000337

136. Nielsen PR, Benros ME, Mortensen PB. Hospital contacts with infection and risk of schizophrenia: a population-based cohort study with linkage of Danish national registers. *Schizophrenia Bulletin* 2014;40(6):1526–32. www.ncbi.nlm.nih.gov/pubmed/24379444 (accessed 29 January 2020).

137. The Royal College of Emergency Medicine. *Guidelines for the Management of Excited Delirium / Acute Behavioural Disturbance (ABD)*. London: The Royal College of Emergency Medicine; 2016.

138. Patel MX, Sethi FN, Barnes TR, et al. Joint BAP NAPICU evidence-based consensus guidelines for the clinical management of acute disturbance: de-escalation and rapid tranquillisation. *Journal of Psychopharmacology* 2018;32(6):601–40. journals.sagepub.com/doi/10.1177/0269881118776738 (accessed 4 May 2021).

139. NICE. *Violence and Aggression: Short-Term Management in Mental Health, Health and Community Settings*. 2020. www.nice.org.uk/guidance/ng10.

140. Calver LA, Downes MA, Page CB, et al. The impact of a standardised intramuscular sedation protocol for acute behavioural disturbance in the emergency department. *BMC Emergency Medicine* 2010;10(1):14. bmcemergmed.biomedcentral.com/articles/10.1186/1471-227X-10-14 (accessed 4 May 2021).

141. Garriga M, Pacchiarotti I, Kasper S, et al. Assessment and management of agitation in psychiatry: expert consensus. *World Journal of Biological Psychiatry* 2016;17(2):86–128. www.tandfonline.com/doi/full/10.3109/15622975.2015.1132007 (accessed 4 May 2021).

142. Faden J, Citrome L. Examining the safety, efficacy, and patient acceptability of inhaled loxapine for the acute treatment of agitation associated with schizophrenia or bipolar I disorder in adults. *Neuropsychiatric Disease and Treatment* 2019;15:2273. www.tandfonline.com/doi/pdf/10.2147/NDT.S173567 (accessed 2 December 2021).

143. Bush G, Fink M, Petrides G, et al. Catatonia. I. Rating scale and standardized examination. *Acta Psychiatrica Scandinavica* 1996;93(2):129–36. www.ncbi.nlm.nih.gov/pubmed/8686483 (accessed 18 April 2018).

144. Bush G, Fink M, Petrides G, et al. Catatonia. II. Treatment with lorazepam and electroconvulsive therapy. *Acta Psychiatrica Scandinavica* 1996;93(2):137–43. doi.wiley.com/10.1111/j.1600-0447.1996.tb09815.x (accessed 24 August 2018).

145. Lander M, Bastiampillai T, Sareen J. Review of withdrawal catatonia: what does this reveal about clozapine? *Translational Psychiatry* 2018;8:139. www.nature.com/articles/s41398-018-0192-9 (accessed 22 January 2019).

146. Pelzer AC, van der Heijden FM, den Boer E. Systematic review of catatonia treatment. *Neuropsychiatric Disease and Treatment* 2018;14:317–26. www.ncbi.nlm.nih.gov/pubmed/29398916 (accessed 5 March 2018).

147. Fink M, Taylor MA. *Catatonia: A Clinician's Guide to Diagnosis and Treatment*. Cambridge: Cambridge University Press; 2006.

148. Girish K, Gill NS. Electroconvulsive therapy in lorazepam non-responsive catatonia. *Indian Journal of Psychiatry* 2003;45(1):21–5. www.ncbi.nlm.nih.gov/pubmed/21206808 (accessed 31 January 2020).

149. Denysenko L, Sica N, Penders TM, et al. Catatonia in the medically ill: etiology, diagnosis, and treatment. The Academy of Consultation-Liaison Psychiatry Evidence-Based Medicine Subcommittee monograph. *Annals of Clinical Psychiatry* 2018;30(2):140–55. www.ncbi.nlm.nih.gov/pubmed/29697715 (accessed 28 January 2021).

150. Rasmussen SA, Mazurek MF, Rosebush PI. Catatonia: our current understanding of its diagnosis, treatment and pathophysiology. *World Journal of Psychiatry* 2016;6(4):391. www.ncbi.nlm.nih.gov/pubmed/28078203 (accessed 18 August 2017).

151. Funayama M, Takata T, Koreki A, et al. Catatonic stupor in schizophrenic disorders and subsequent medical complications and mortality. *Psychosomatic Medicines* 2018;80(4):370–6. www.ncbi.nlm.nih.gov/pubmed/29521882 (accessed 9 May 2018).

152. Beach SR, Gomez-Bernal F, Huffman JC, et al. Alternative treatment strategies for catatonia: a systematic review. *General Hospital Psychiatry* 2017;48:1–19. www.sciencedirect.com/science/article/pii/S0163834317301378 (accessed 6 June 2018).

153. Carroll BT, Goforth HW, Thomas C, et al. Review of adjunctive glutamate antagonist therapy in the treatment of catatonic syndromes. *Journal of Neuropsychiatry and Clinical Neurosciences* 2007;19(4):406–12. psychiatryonline.org/doi/abs/10.1176/jnp.2007.19.4.406 (accessed 8 November 2017).

154. Clinebell K, Azzam PN, Gopalan P, et al. Guidelines for preventing common medical complications of catatonia: case report and literature review. *Journal of Clinical Psychiatry* 2014;75(6):644–51. www.ncbi.nlm.nih.gov/pubmed/25004188 (accessed 11 June 2018).

155. Trimble M, Schmitz B (eds.) *The Neuropsychiatry of Epilepsy*. Cambridge: Cambridge University Press; 2002. www.cambridge.org/core/product/identifier/9780511544354/type/book (accessed 6 May 2021).

156. Joyce EM. Organic psychosis: the pathobiology and treatment of delusions. *CNS Neuroscience & Therapeutics* 2018;24(7):598–603. www.ncbi.nlm.nih.gov/pubmed/29766653 (accessed 6 May 2021).

157. Pollak TA, Lennox BR, Müller S, et al. Autoimmune psychosis: an international consensus on an approach to the diagnosis and management of psychosis of suspected autoimmune origin. *The Lancet Psychiatry* 2020;7(1):93–108. www.sciencedirect.com/science/article/pii/S2215036619302901 (accessed 6 May 2021).

158. Rogers JP, Pollak TA, Blackman G, et al. Catatonia and the immune system: a review *The Lancet* 2019;6(7):620–30. www.sciencedirect.com/science/article/pii/S2215036619301907?via%3Dihub (accessed 22 August 2019).

159. Hill L, Lee KC. Pharmacotherapy considerations in patients with HIV and psychiatric disorders: focus on antidepressants and antipsychotics. *Annals of Pharmacotherapy* 2013;47(1):75–89. journals.sagepub.com/doi/10.1345/aph.1R343 (accessed 6 May 2021).

160. Arciniegas DB, Harris SN, Brousseau KM. Psychosis following traumatic brain injury. *International Review of Psychiatry* 2003;15(4):328–40. www.tandfonline.com/doi/full/10.1080/09540260310001606719 (accessed 6 May 2021).

161. Torniainen M, Mittendorfer-Rutz E, Tanskanen A, et al. Antipsychotic treatment and mortality in schizophrenia. *Schizophrenia Bulletin* 2015;41(3):656–63. academic.oup.com/schizophreniabulletin/article-lookup/doi/10.1093/schbul/sbu164 (accessed 7 May 2021).

162. Dregan A, McNeill A, Gaughran F, et al. Potential gains in life expectancy from reducing amenable mortality among people diagnosed with serious mental illness in the United Kingdom. *PLoS ONE* 2020;15(3):e0230674. dx.plos.org/10.1371/journal.pone.0230674 (accessed 7 May 2021).

163. Kane JM, Sharif ZA. Atypical antipsychotics: sedation versus efficacy. *Journal of Clinical Psychiatry* 2008;69(Suppl 1):18–31. www.ncbi.nlm.nih.gov/pubmed/18484805 (accessed 7 May 2021).

164. Miller DD. Atypical antipsychotics: sleep, sedation, and efficacy. *Primary Care Companion to the Journal of Clinical Psychiatry* 2004;6(Suppl 2):3–7. www.ncbi.nlm.nih.gov/pubmed/16001094 (accessed 7 May 2021).

165. Saavedra-Velez C, Yusim A, Anbarasan D, et al. Modafinil as an adjunctive treatment of sedation, negative symptoms, and cognition in schizophrenia. *Journal of Clinical Psychiatry* 2009;70(1):104–12 www.psychiatrist.com/JCP/article/Pages/modafinil-adjunctive-treatment-sedation-negative-symptoms.aspx (accessed 7 May 2021).

166. Ramos Perdigués S, Sauras Quecuti R, Mané A, et al. An observational study of clozapine induced sedation and its pharmacological management. *European Neuropsychopharmacology* 2016;26(1):156–61. www.ncbi.nlm.nih.gov/pubmed/26613638 (accessed 7 May 2021).

167. Taylor D, Gaughran F, Pillinger T. *The Maudsley Practice Guidelines for Physical Health Conditions in Psychiatry*. Hoboken, NJ: Wiley-Blackwell; 2020. www.wiley.com/en-gb/The+Maudsley+Practice+Guidelines+for+Physical+Health+Conditions+in+Psychiatry-p-9781119554202 (accessed 7 May 2021).

168. Gupta S, Lakshmanan DAM, Khastgir U, et al. Management of antipsychotic-induced hyperprolactinaemia. *BJPsych Advances* 2017;23(4):278–86. www.cambridge.org/core/product/identifier/S2056467800002668/type/journal_article (accessed 7 May 2021).

169. Kapur S. Relationship between dopamine D_2 occupancy, clinical response, and side effects: a double-

blind PET study of first-episode schizophrenia. *American Journal of Psychiatry* 2000;157(4):514–20. ajp.psychiatryonline.org/article.aspx?articleID=174052 (accessed 12 May 2021).

170. Caroff SN, Hurford I, Lybrand J, et al. Movement disorders induced by antipsychotic drugs: implications of the CATIE schizophrenia trial. *Neurologic Clinics* 2011;29(1):127–48. www.ncbi.nlm.nih.gov/pubmed/21172575 (accessed 18 June 2018).
171. Jones PB, Barnes TRE, Davies L, et al. Randomized controlled trial of the effect on quality of life of second- vs first-generation antipsychotic drugs in schizophrenia: cost utility of the latest antipsychotic drugs in schizophrenia study (CUtLASS 1). *Archives of General Psychiatry.* 2006;63(10):1079–87.
172. Shin H-W, Chung SJ. Drug-induced parkinsonism. *Journal of Clinical Neurology* 2012;8(1):15–21. www.ncbi.nlm.nih.gov/pubmed/22523509 (accessed 11 May 2021).
173. Ward KM, Citrome L. Antipsychotic-related movement disorders: drug-induced parkinsonism vs. tardive dyskinesia – key differences in pathophysiology and clinical management. *Neurology and Therapy* 2018;7(2):233–48. link.springer.com/10.1007/s40120-018-0105-0 (accessed 8 May 2021).
174. DiMascio A, Bernardo DL, Greenblatt DJ, et al. A controlled trial of amantadine in drug-induced extrapyramidal disorders. *Archives of General Psychiatry* 1976;33(5):599–602. www.ncbi.nlm.nih.gov/pubmed/5066 (accessed 11 May 2021).
175. American Psychiatric Association. *The American Psychiatric Association Practice Guideline for The Treatment of Patients with Schizophrenia,* 3rd ed. Washington DC: American Psychiatric Association Publishing; 2021. psychiatryonline.org/doi/full/10.5555/appi.books.9780890424841.Schizophrenia00pre.
176. Gurrera RJ, Caroff SN, Cohen A, et al. An international consensus study of neuroleptic malignant syndrome diagnostic criteria using the delphi method. *Journal of Clinical Psychiatry* 2011;72(09):1222–8. article.psychiatrist.com/?ContentType=START&ID=10007472 (accessed 12 May 2021).
177. Gurrera RJ, Mortillaro G, Velamoor V, et al. A validation study of the international consensus diagnostic criteria for neuroleptic malignant syndrome. *Journal of Clinical Psychopharmacology* 2017;37(1):67–71. journals.lww.com/00004714-201702000-00014 (accessed 12 May 2021).
178. Abdelmawla N, Mitchell AJ. Sudden cardiac death and antipsychotics. Part 1: Risk factors and mechanisms. *Advances in Psychiatric Treatment* 2006;12(1):35–44. www.cambridge.org/core/product/identifier/S1355514600002753/type/journal_article (accessed 13 May 2021).
179. Vandenberk B, Vandael E, Robyns T, et al. Which QT correction formulae to use for QT monitoring? *Journal of the American Heart Association* 2016;5(6):e003264. www.ncbi.nlm.nih.gov/pubmed/27317349 (accessed 13 May 2021).
180. Lally J, Brook J, Dixon T, et al. Ivabradine, a novel treatment for clozapine-induced sinus tachycardia: a case series. *Therapeutic Advances in Psychopharmacology* 2014;4(3):117–22.
181. Ribe AR, Laursen TM, Sandbaek A, et al. Long-term mortality of persons with severe mental illness and diabetes: a population-based cohort study in Denmark. *Psychological Medicine* 2014;44(14):3097–107. www.ncbi.nlm.nih.gov/pubmed/25065292 (accessed 19 May 2021).
182. Schoepf D, Potluri R, Uppal H, et al. Type-2 diabetes mellitus in schizophrenia: increased prevalence and major risk factor of excess mortality in a naturalistic 7-year follow-up. *European Psychiatry* 2012;27(1):33–42. www.cambridge.org/core/product/identifier/S0924933800069224/type/journal_article (accessed 19 May 2021).
183. Cooper SJ, Reynolds GP, Barnes T, et al. BAP guidelines on the management of weight gain, metabolic disturbances and cardiovascular risk associated with psychosis and antipsychotic drug treatment. *Journal of Psychopharmacology* 2016;30(8):717–48. www.ncbi.nlm.nih.gov/pubmed/27147592 (accessed 19 May 2021).
184. Vancampfort D, Firth J, Correll CU, et al. The impact of pharmacological and non-pharmacological interventions to improve physical health outcomes in people with schizophrenia: a meta-review of meta-analyses of randomized controlled trials. *World Psychiatry* 2019;18(1):53–66. onlinelibrary.wiley.com/doi/abs/10.1002/wps.20614 (accessed 20 May 2021).
185. Speyer H, Jakobsen AS, Westergaard C, et al. Lifestyle interventions for weight management in people with serious mental illness: a systematic review with meta-analysis, trial sequential analysis, and meta-regression analysis exploring the mediators and moderators of treatment effects. *Psychotherapy and Psychosomatics* 2019;88(6):350–62.
186. Slim M, Medina-Caliz I, Gonzalez-Jimenez A, et al. Hepatic safety of atypical antipsychotics: current evidence and future directions. *Drug Safety* 2016;39(10):925–43. link.springer.com/10.1007/s40264-016-0436-7 (accessed 21 May 2021).
187. Dzahini O, Singh N, Taylor D, et al. Antipsychotic drug use and pneumonia: systematic review and meta-analysis. *Journal of Psychopharmacology* 2018;32(11):1167–81. journals.sagepub.com/doi/10.1177/0269881118795333 (accessed 21 May 2021).
188. Jönsson AK, Spigset O, Hägg S. Venous thromboembolism in recipients of antipsychotics. *CNS Drugs* 2012;26(8):649–62. link.springer.com/10.2165/11633920-000000000-00000 (accessed 21 May 2021).
189. Hynes C, Keating D, McWilliams S, et al. Glasgow antipsychotic side-effects scale for clozapine – development and validation of a clozapine-specific side-effects scale. *Schizophrenia Research* 2015;168(1–2):505–13.
190. Waddell L, Taylor M. A new self-rating scale for detecting atypical or second-generation antipsychotic side effects. *Journal of Psychopharmacology* 2008;22(3):238–43. journals.sagepub.com/doi/abs/10.1177/0269881107087976 (accessed 2 December 2021).
191. Lewis SJ, Heaton KW. Stool form scale as a useful guide to intestinal transit time. *Scandinavian Journal of Gastoenterology* 2009;32(9):920–4. www.tandfonline.com/doi/abs/10.3109/00365529709011203 (accessed 2 December 2021).
192. Alvir JMJ, Lieberman JA, Safferman AZ, et al. Clozapine-induced agranulocytosis – incidence and risk factors in the United States. *New England Journal of Medicine* 1993;329(3):162–7. www.nejm.org/doi/full/10

.1056/Nejm199307153290303 (accessed 2 December 2021).

193. Myles N, Myles H, Xia S, et al. Meta-analysis examining the epidemiology of clozapine-associated neutropenia. *Acta Psychiatrica Scandinavica* 2018;138 (2):101–9. onlinelibrary.wiley.com/doi/full/10.1111/acps.12898 (accessed 2 December 2021).

194. David Baldwin AW. Withdrawal of, and alternatives to, valproate-containing medicines in girls and women of childbearing potential who have a psychiatric illness. Royal College of Psychiatrists; 2018.

195. Segev A, Evans A, Hodsoll J, et al. Hyoscine for clozapine-induced hypersalivation: a double-blind, randomized, placebo-controlled cross-over trial. *International Clinical Psychopharmacology* 2019;34(2): 101–7.

196. Freudenreich O, Henderson DC, Macklin EA, et al. Modafinil for clozapine-treated schizophrenia patients: a double-blind, placebo-controlled pilot trial. *Journal of Clinical Psychiatry.* 2009;70(12):1674–80.

197. Howes OD, Bhatnagar A, Gaughran FP, et al. A prospective study of impairment in glucose control caused by clozapine without changes in insulin resistance. *American Journal of Psychiatry* 2004;161(2):361–3. ajp.psychiatryonline.org/doi/abs/10.1176/appi.ajp.161.2.361 (accessed 2 December 2021).

198. Ponsford M, Castle D, Tahir T, et al. *Clozapine is associated with secondary antibody deficiency. British Journal of Psychiatry* 2019;214(2):83–9. www.cambridge.org/core/journals/the-british-journal-of-psychiatry/article/clozapine-is-associated-with-secondary-antibody-deficiency/59687F02595E18C19E0BC59374572995 (accessed 2 December 2021).

199. de Leon J, Schoretsanitis G, Kane JM, et al. Using therapeutic drug monitoring to personalize clozapine dosing in Asians. *Asia-Pacific Psychiatry* 2020;12(2):e12384. onlinelibrary.wiley.com/doi/full/10.1111/appy.12384 (accessed 2 December 2021).

200. Patel RK, Moore AM, Piper S, et al. Clozapine and cardiotoxicity – a guide for psychiatrists written by cardiologists. *Psychiatry Research* 2019;282:112491.

201. Ghosh C, Hossain M, Solanki J, et al. Pathophysiological implications of neurovascular P450 in brain disorders. *Drug Discovery Today* 2016;21 (10):1609–19.

202. Spina E, De Leon J. Metabolic drug interactions with newer antipsychotics: a comparative review. *Basic & Clinical Pharmacology & Toxicology* 2007;100 (1):4–22.

203. Ameer B, Weintraub RA. Drug interactions with grapefruit juice. *Clinical Pharmacokinetics* 1997;33(2):103–21.

204. Jukic MM, Smith RL, Haslemo T, et al. Effect of CYP2D6 genotype on exposure and efficacy of risperidone and aripiprazole: a retrospective, cohort study. *The Lancet Psychiatry* 2019;6 (5):418–26.

205. Schultze-Lutter F, Addington J, Ruhrmann S, et al. *Schizophrenia Proneness Instrument, Adult Version (SPI-A).* Rome: Giovanni Fioriti. 2007.

Chapter

5.4 Psychosocial Management of Psychosis

David Kingdon

Evidence-based interventions include psychological and social treatments and modes of service delivery such as early intervention for psychosis teams. Family work and individual cognitive behaviour therapy are the psychological approaches that have been best researched but remain limited in availability: assessment, engagement, case conceptualisation and specific work with hallucinations, delusions and negative symptoms have been adapted for clinical practice. The goal is self-determined recovery that will take into account key physical and mental health and social concerns, such as accommodation, employment and relationships.

Psychosis and schizophrenia are major mental disorders that can seriously disrupt individuals' lives, causing considerable distress and disruption and affecting their families and social circles. This results in substantial costs to society generally and particularly to mental health services (contributing to more than a half of inpatient costs) and physical health services as well as lost opportunities in education, relationships and employment. Yet, psychosis and schizophrenia are readily treatable with psychological and social interventions supplementing medications.[1] However, in contrast to severe physical illnesses, these interventions are rarely available or used effectively.

The terms 'psychosis' and 'schizophrenia' have become virtually interchangeable in clinical practice, although 'psychotic symptoms' can be present in organic, depressive, manic and personality disorders. Schizophrenia is being used less and less due to its very negative and inappropriate associations with inevitable and permanent deterioration and violence. In fact, most patients make full recoveries from their initial episodes; relapse is, however, common and a focus for early intervention. Very few patients require long-term residential care but the return to and maintenance of employment remains a major concern, with under 10 per cent of those in contact with services achieving this. Suicide is a higher risk than for the general population, but violence to others is less common than violence towards those with psychosis. 'Severe (and enduring) mental illness' is a broad concept that can include affective disorders such as bipolar disorder and severe depression as well as the group of schizophrenias.

As described in previous chapters of this book, psychosis exists on a continuum with normality, and whilst extremes of both are clearly identifiable, people may move in and out of psychosis with variations occurring in insight. Even where insight into being 'ill' is absent, often acceptance of assistance – even therapy and medication – can still be possible. Management will also take into account other associated conditions – for example, depression may be the predominant emotion, or anxiety, elation, disinhibition or physical illness may be causing delirium. Personality disorder has been particularly controversial (see Chapter 7.1), as individuals frequently describe psychotic symptoms such as hearing voices or paranoia, and the overlap with psychosis can cause debate and disagreement: people can experience and need support for both conditions.[2]

Eugen Blueler described a 'group of schizophrenias' in 1911, and it remains the case that presentations of psychosis can be variable. ICD-11 includes quite diverse presentations – for example, delusional disorder (systematised beliefs based on inaccurate conclusions), substance abuse precipitation, as well as psychotic conditions when neither are factors. It is also becoming increasingly clear that severe childhood trauma is a major factor in many presentations of psychosis as well as borderline personality disorder.[2,3] Complex post-traumatic stress disorder is a new and potentially very helpful and destigmatising category introduced in ICD-11. These differing presentations are important in relation to psychological and social approaches alongside case conceptualisation and the specific symptoms experienced that are the focus of intervention. The goal, however, is always the type of recovery chosen by the patient.

There are a range of causes of psychosis or 'the group of psychoses', and there is now a very well-developed body of work that has identified associations with epidemiological factors, life experiences and psychological predispositions.[4,5] Persecutory delusions are conceptualised as unfounded threat beliefs, developed in the context of genetic and environmental risk, and maintained by a number of psychological processes, including excessive worry, low self-confidence, poor sleep, anomalous experiences, reasoning biases and safety-seeking behaviours.[6] Voices in psychosis may be related to hypervigilance; autobiographical memory is especially related to trauma and drug misuse, inner speech and isolation/sensory or sleep deprivation.[7] Negative symptoms may result from dysfunctional attitudes, demoralisation, neglect (through institutionalisation) or isolation, or they may have a protective function in the avoidance of anxiety[8–10] and the precipitation of positive symptoms (e.g. voices and paranoia).

Psychological Treatment

Approaches to psychosis involve psychological, social and biological interventions. Cognitive behaviour therapy is now established as the psychological treatment of choice advocated by international treatment guidelines. Social approaches include employment and supportive initiatives as well as developments in service delivery including early intervention and case management. There is also evidence that social skills training can be effective, especially for negative symptoms.[11] There are widely available manuals[12] that describe teaching core abilities, individually and in groups – listening, requesting, expressing positive and negative feelings using conversation, having assertiveness, and using conflict management and broader relationship skills.

Psychological approaches to psychosis have a long history, but it is only in the past couple of decades that experimental studies have shown that specific ways of working can be effective. Previously, psychotherapeutic techniques were considered to be harmful in psychosis: there were pioneering approaches, but early controlled studies either found no effect or more benefit from a comparison of non-specific therapeutic approaches. There was also a justified concern that some approaches were primarily criticisms of society, especially family structures and services. Nevertheless, detailed clinical descriptions[13,14] were influential with many psychiatrists even where explanations were more controversial.

So there has always been, and to some extent remains, a degree of scepticism about how such approaches can effectively reduce distress from hallucinations or improve insight into delusions. By their very nature, delusions have been traditionally described as not being amenable to reason, so reasoning approaches seem inherently doomed to failure. There is also the more general perspective that psychosis has been shown to be associated with biological changes, and therefore, the implication can be drawn that biological methods are needed to rectify these problems.

Perhaps the latter issue is most straightforward to address. A disorder that has demonstrable biological origins (e.g. stroke) can still benefit from psychosocial methods in adaptation, motivation and rehabilitation – treatment of depression, occupational and physiotherapies – and these may, in the long term, play a major part in moving, as far as possible, towards recovery. The postulated non-amenability of delusions to reason may be key to the Jasperian definition in relation to an assessment, but such definitions don't specify that this need be a permanent state nor that more refined and newly developed methods of reasoning might not benefit the individual – just as medication can have beneficial effects. Again, it may well be that the person can also benefit in the short term and, particularly, the long term from being able to manage and live with the delusion and its consequences or implications and, similarly, with the hallucinations. It may still be possible to regain a more meaningful and less distressing and disabling existence.

Evidence for Psychological Interventions

There is now abundant evidence that family intervention[15] and cognitive behaviour therapy for psychosis (CBTP) adds value to medication. In one specific, yet to be replicated, study, family intervention and CBTP has had beneficial effects when medication is refused.[16] There has been debate about the CBTP studies involved, in particular when these have been meta-analysed. McKenna, Leucht and colleagues[17] have recently clarified the issues regarding outcomes and inclusion criteria, and their conclusion was unequivocal – CBT is effective against positive symptoms. Meta-analysis for negative symptoms also suggest effects where these are targeted.[18] Thus, for patients with such persistent symptoms, CBT has a beneficial effect over and above medication, and given the potential severity of the illness, it is now recommended by international guidelines including those from the American Psychiatric Association,[19] PORT[20] and the National Institute of Health and Clinical Excellence[21] in the UK.

Most studies have used CBT courses of 16 to 20 sessions with a dedicated trained therapist. There have also been successful studies that have been longer – for example, up to 50 sessions for patients with predominantly negative symptoms[22] – and shorter – 6 to 10 sessions, where mental health staff have had trained to supplement their clinical skills.[23] Brief targeted interventions have also been used: mindfulness groups for voices[24] and the use of an intervention for paranoia targeted at worry[25] are examples. Mindfulness has been widely researched and is quite widely available; it seeks to reconnect individuals with what is happening within and around them and can let then them stand back and observe what is happening. The worry intervention involves understanding the positives and negatives about worry – specifically, worry about others (as in paranoia) – problem-solve the causes and also be able to detach through the use of 'worry' periods.

This latter has been further developed into a modular 'Feeling Safe' intervention, which has been highly successful versus a non-specific therapy ('befriending') control.[26] The intervention focuses on the maintenance factors of persecutory delusions: worry, negative self-beliefs, anomalous experiences, sleep dysfunction, reasoning biases and safety behaviours. The SlowMo app, with clinical support, is targeted at reasoning techniques (e.g. countering the tendency to 'jump to conclusions') and has given promising results in paranoia.[27] Virtual reality (VR) is also now proving a very successful addition to CBTP, with automated VR cognitive therapy (gameChange) that can treat avoidance – especially severe agoraphobia and distress in patients with psychosis – with significant reductions in anxious avoidance of, and distress in, everyday situations.[28]

Psychosis is a term covering a very broad group of presentations, and specific problems can be challenging. Substance misuse is a common example, and there has been limited work using CBT. The one major study of CBTP with motivational interviewing did not show a positive result,[29] although it recruited very well and seemed very acceptable to patients. Interestingly, an earlier pilot, which incorporated family work as well as individual work, did have benefits. Moreover, it does seem that lower levels of substance misuse do not reduce likelihood of successful outcomes.[30] Childhood and later trauma is also frequently a major issue in psychosis. Trauma-focused CBT, eye movement desensitisation and reprocessing (EMDR – a psychotherapy that utilises eye movements), and prolonged exposure have been used in the treatment of such trauma and have recently been found to also be effective where psychosis is present.[31]

CBTP has also been used by case management[32] and UK early intervention teams,[33] and some of the techniques were included in the US RAISE early intervention study.[34] A brief needs assessment instrument (DIALOG) has been evaluated with community mental health teams, which systematically elicits individuals' satisfaction with domains in their life and then uses a solution-focused approach (DIALOG+) to address issues. It has also been shown to improve quality of life, to be cost effective and to have other benefits.[35] Training in improving communication with people with psychosis (TEMPO) using, in part, CBTP has improved the therapeutic relationship as experienced by the psychiatrists receiving the training and the individuals with whom they work.[36] This matters because the quality of the therapeutic relationship has been shown to be the most important indicator of collaboration/compliance.[37] CBTP can also directly improve attitudes to medication.[38,39] The description of CBTP provided in this chapter synthesises the elements of that training for use in clinical practice.

However, compliance therapy directed towards medication usage rather than a broader holistic approach does not seem to be successful.[40]

Finally, CBTP has been developed and seems most effective with broader service approaches – integrated with community, rehabilitation and recovery approaches and potentially the Open Dialogue(OD) approach[41] with its emphasis on the therapeutic relationship (currently, OD is being evaluated in a randomised controlled trial). OD is described thus:

> Working with families and social networks, as much as possible in their own homes, Open Dialogue teams work to help those involved in a crisis situation to be together and to engage in dialogue. It has been their experience that if the family/team can bear the extreme emotion in a crisis situation, and tolerate the uncertainty, in time, shared meaning usually emerges, and healing/recovery is possible.

Assessment

Cognitive behaviour therapy for psychosis builds on general clinical skills.[10,42] A good mental health assessment helps the individual and clinician understand how specific symptoms have developed. It provides good background information that can lead to an understanding of how and why specific beliefs or perceptions have arisen. The process of exploration and the 'guided discovery' of developing an inquiring dialogue is a key part of the approach to unravelling issues that may have occurred many years ago but can still affect current beliefs about the world and those around the individual. Understandability of paranoia, for example, can become clear where trust has been seriously damaged. Voices that originate from specific individuals or circumstances can also begin to make sense. Negative symptoms can become understandable as ways of avoiding uncomfortable situations that repeatedly cause distress and fear, resulting in avoidance and demoralisation or 'self-defeating' beliefs.[8] The CBT component of the assessment involves drawing out links between thoughts, feelings and behaviour, including specific patterns of such connections and, as interaction progresses, underlying beliefs that have a general pervasive effect.

Gathering information together is essential to moving forward but does need to be made sense of and formulated. Understanding predisposing, precipitating, perpetuating and protective factors initially can then be linked to current and underlying concerns, physical issues and the cognitive triad – thoughts, emotions and behaviours. Diagrams can be helpful where the interactions are complex and to clarify connections, but being able to summarise some brief, specific collaborative conclusions may be sufficient. For example, unless there is a specific reason, recognising that someone shouting or laughing out loud is usually a reaction to their own thoughts and circumstances rather to you (personalisation).

The amount of detail discovered during a full assessment can be overwhelming, and the process can lead to confusion about which area to focus on. Developing a collaborative formulation/case conceptualisation and thence a therapeutic plan for a broad approach, including social and physical treatments, can take you forward. Usually the specific concerns that the individual themselves have will need addressing first – voices may be causing considerable distress and interfering with daily living, or there may be social issues that interfere with progress.

Although studies have tended to focus on individual work, there have been a small number that have included families and shown very clearly that this can enhance recovery. Even small numbers of joint (or, if necessary, separate) sessions can allow collaborative development and the sharing of the formulation and development of individual coping strategies. Group work on specific topics – understanding voices or paranoia or improving motivation – can be useful, but the nature of psychotic symptoms is such that some individual work always seems to be necessary.

Case Conceptualisation

Case conceptualisation for individuals with psychosis is based on standard cognitive-behavioural approaches.[43] It needs to address key current and past events, thoughts, feelings and behaviours but also social circumstances and physical health issues. Positive symptoms will be included, but negative symptoms also need to be considered, as cognitive insights need to be converted into behavioural change (actions) for recovery to be a reasonable consideration. Individual symptoms, therefore, will need to be formulated to ensure that understanding is developed, and overall conceptualisation can then draw the different factors together. Key events are linked to emotions, behaviour and thoughts to enable a shared understanding of how these interact. It can then be possible to develop treatment strategies.

Clinical insight is an integral component of psychosis, and identifying areas of misunderstanding and their development collaboratively can enable alternative explanations to be explored. Acceptance of illness may not be crucial and even acceptance that paranoid or hallucinatory beliefs are mistaken may not matter if behaviour change (e.g. acting on the beliefs) can occur in order to improve relationships and functioning. For example, a patient may be convinced they are being persecuted by the government. The approach is to be accepting – not confrontational or to appear sceptical. Ask straightforward questions about how this persecution started and developed: Why did they believe the government was responsible? Which part of the government? Was it a particular individual? Why were they targeted? What had they done about it? What could they do about it? What did their family think? This allows the person to make a detailed examination of the belief and, in the process, to examine the reasoning behind it – and where doubts exist. It also may produce grievances that are warranted and actions that are reasonable to take. Most of all, the individual feels listened to, a formulation can be drawn up and a therapeutic relationship can be established even when, inevitably, there are differences of opinion.

Engagement

Engagement is key to any therapeutic interaction, although it has often been thought to be challenging with people with psychosis. Frequently, the problem is that the person will say that they have not felt that their concerns are understood or taken seriously. Therefore, simply listening by using a normalising perspective – assuming that reasons exist for things said and done – and addressing issues regarding the voices or delusions in a direct and open way can lead, paradoxically, to excellent engagement. If the person feels their paranoia is being investigated and their safety taken seriously, they're much more likely to work together with a clinician. It may well be that, after assessment, the beliefs that they have are not supported by evidence, but understanding why they feel the way they do can enhance the therapeutic relationship – and in most instances, there is some logic in the beliefs themselves. It becomes possible to understand why they believe what they do.

In some circumstances, symptoms may have been minimised in previous clinical interactions. Commonly, voices may have been described as 'pseudo-hallucinations', not 'real voices', or 'just thoughts' or dissociation, particularly where there is comorbid borderline personality disorder.[2] However, these experiences – voices as perceived by the individual – can be very distressing and the insight variable. Working with them can reduce that distress, help coping and be very engaging. Normalising symptoms in a way that helps them become understandable – for example, discussing how voices can occur with sleep deprivation, trauma or bereavement – can aid the person to recognise that the approach being taken is one that is accepting and non-judgemental.

Engagement is a continuous process that may fluctuate and need monitoring. Difficult periods can develop when discussing traumatic events or when the therapist is challenged by the individual (e.g. as to whether the therapist believes the person). It is sometimes necessary to 'agree to differ', which is a tactic that can work very well in defusing tension and allowing a refocusing on the impacts of beliefs. For example, 'I get what you are saying and that you are convinced about these issues, but I'm not so sure myself – maybe we can work on the effects it is having on you and keep you safe'. This type of engagement doesn't involve collusion or confrontation and respects the individual's perspective whilst not agreeing with it.

Working with Voices

It is very important to get a good understanding of how the voices heard by the individual are affecting them by considering their frequency, volume, pattern and level as well as the amount of distressing content, the actual content and the beliefs about the experiences. (Psychosis rating scales[44] provide a brief, useful and systematic way of assessing these processes.) Alongside this understanding of the phenomena, it is necessary to gain an understanding of who the patient thinks is speaking, whether they are identifiable and what are they saying. Sometimes, what is being said is so unpleasant and personal that the individual finds it very difficult to convey. In those circumstances, it can be sufficient and advisable to simply suggest that it may be too unpleasant to disclose material but that you recognise this, that it is very negative, and you can nevertheless do meaningful work on the associated effects – and beliefs. Voices can also be positive as well as negative and can be quite supportive, but – where these exist – it is their negative effects that usually need addressing.

Clarifying with the person that you recognise that what they're experiencing is in the form of speech, 'just like me speaking to you now, or perhaps louder' helps. The difference from ordinary speech is that the originator of the speech can't usually be seen. There may be different explanations for this that need to be explored: it may be that the sounds heard are coming through the walls from neighbours or are from God or the devil or other supernatural sources, or there is sometimes a technological reason whereby speech is projected to the individual only. Securing these explanations is very important, if they exist – but sometimes, indeed often, the individual is uncertain themselves about the origin of the voices. Sometimes, it is worth appraising why the individual thinks that other people, including the practitioner, can't hear their voices. It may be the case that the individual has doubts about their explanation, and it can be worth testing in session. Asking them to let the clinician know when they're hearing voices can allow assessment of what is happening at the time. Sometimes, there may be an explanation in terms of the distortion of sounds that they're hearing. Sometimes, recording the voice experiences on a phone can allow identification of misinterpretation or confirm recognition that the voices are not being heard in conventional ways – clarifying that this is not normal speech but something different.

Developing explanations is then the way to understand the experience. Any explanation that they have come to themselves can be explored, understood and discussed. They may well have already reached an understanding that the voices are something unique to themselves that relates to their past experiences and to the mental health problems that they have. Sometimes, the beliefs are delusional and paranoid, relating to persecution by people or agencies that they will specify, and it will be important to work with these as you would with delusional belief (see later in this chapter). Often, there is the opportunity to explain what is known about hallucinations. For example, when people hear voices, the area of the brain that is involved in speech (Broca's area) is active, so there is, in a very literal sense, inner speech occurring – what 'sounds' external is occurring in the brain. It can also be very helpful to describe situations in which hallucinations occur in the absence of psychosis – for example, sleep deprivation, bereavement, delirium and even when going off to or waking up from sleep. An explanation that many patients find helpful is related to sleep. When we are asleep, we hear speech; we just think of this speech as dreams, and when we wake up, they generally stop. Hallucinations have been described many times, including by Freud, as 'dreaming awake' or even a 'waking nightmare'. The fact that the person is hearing someone else's voice does not mean that it's not from their own mind – maybe memories – especially where the originating experience has been a particularly emotional and disturbing one. Memories of experiences like a car crash or a wedding are much more vivid, and these experiences can be recalled much more easily than everyday experiences. Hallucinations similarly are often related to emotional experiences.

However, this is not always the case, as sometimes the voices can present as muddled, jumbled thoughts that seem to have no particular meaning and may not be distressing but are puzzling. Explanation of the process of the generation of automatic thoughts can be helpful as the experience being described is often one of externalising such thoughts and the failure to recognise them as the individual's own.

Having clarified the nature of the voices, it is usually important to address the content. If this is neutral or positive, it may well be that the content is unimportant or may be a support for the individual. Although it can still be helpful to agree on an explanation for the phenomena, the voices may be listed as allies rather than a problem to deal with. Where the content is negative, each statement from the voice often takes the form of negative comments about the person – for example: 'you're useless' (or usually more venomous and vulgar) – and work with these statements can be managed in a very similar way to that which is used in cognitive therapy for depression. The evidence for and against the statements can be weighed and, importantly, some conclusion established that is often along the lines of 'I'm not that bad' or 'I'm trying my best'. Sometimes, it's important to understand the origin of the statements, which may have come from relationships in childhood. There may be particular phrases used by key individuals or related to specific instances of childhood trauma or bullying.

Key issues about the power relationship with the voices can be addressed by weighing up whether the statements made should be believed. This may mean questioning the authority of the originator of them. It may be part of the therapeutic work that addresses the specific issues related to trauma or relationships. Specific phrases can sometimes be valuable – often using those that have come from the conclusions drawn – so again, 'I'm doing my best' might be an example. Sometimes qualifying these phrases, with a short list of the reasons why we believe this, can be helpful. Thinking of them, or even saying it aloud when in an appropriate setting, to the voice can sometimes be a useful approach.

It is always worth exploring the ways that the individual has already developed in addressing voices. In general, heightened emotion, including anger, tends to lead to exacerbation, but this can be an individual response. Some people do find that cursing and swearing at the voice reinforces their power over it, but most find that this just leads to greater aggravation. Using different approaches to explore what works best can produce better coping. This can be in concert with approaches such as mindfulness or socialisation. Again, it is important to establish and reinforce those approaches that help.

Working with Delusions

Delusional beliefs may present as very accessible to discussion as they are usually the major concern that the individual has. In some circumstances, though, time and patience may be needed to elicit the concerns. This may be because they involve paranoid beliefs, which are essentially about lack of trust, and it may take time to build up sufficient trust for the individual to feel that the practitioner is not part of the conspiracy or at least that they can be trusted to listen to them, even if they don't believe the individual can help. Frequently, the individual has expressed their beliefs and not felt believed by practitioners or, more specifically, not felt that their beliefs are taken seriously. Assessing frequency, volume, pattern, degree of conviction and the level of distress gives a dimensional understanding that can be helpful, as with voices.[44]

Delusional beliefs have origins, and understanding how they began, what was happening in the period leading up to the belief presenting and what has happened to reinforce it since can be a very helpful process to the practitioner. It can also allow the individual to systematically examine their explanation of the beliefs themselves. It would be very unusual for someone to go through this process and then concur that they may have got it wrong, but it is quite frequent for this process to begin to sow internal doubts. This can mean that the process of exploring the delusion takes time: for most, this is a question of minutes, but just occasionally, especially with systematised delusions, it takes longer – although the exploration can be linked over a few sessions. Exploring the circumstances from start to finish can provide a continuity that enables the individual to feel they are listened to and accepted and also feel prepared to consider alternative approaches to their problems, even if not alternative explanations.

Fully exploring these issues can lead to specific plans and problem solving, which provides for an action – this might involve a letter or a written complaint to the police or a government official. This enables them to assemble and inevitably review the evidence for their belief and, frequently, then allows the person to move their life forwards. They are agreeing to differ with the practitioner but also accepting that there are limits to what they can do about the situation and that its domination of their life may be counter-productive. Sometimes, an inference-chaining approach – for example, 'What is it about people believing that you are the inventor of the internet that is important to you?' or 'Why would being an Admiral in the Navy matter?' or 'Why would being a great surgeon matter?' – can elicit material that can be worked on directly, such as about self-esteem or influence ('I could have saved my son from dying'), that can move the therapeutic relationship forward.

An alternative, or complementary, approach has recently been subject to specific evaluation; after initially establishing the relationship and assessing symptomatology, a 'worry intervention' can be offered – similar to that used in CBT for generalised anxiety disorder – on the basis that spending all day ruminating about the belief may not be helpful. Although the worry involved can have positive value in problem solving and possibly maintaining safety, it is leaving them little time in their life to do anything else. The belief itself is therefore not challenged, but it is suggested that using a 'worry period' regularly once or twice a day may be a way of concentrating on that concern for a set period but then leaving time free to do the normal day-to-day activities of life. The evidence is that this can then allow the individual to take control of the worry – manifested as their paranoia – and have a positive demonstrable benefit on the worry, the quality of life and indeed the delusional conviction.[25]

The aim of each of these approaches is not to convince the individual that they are wrong. It is to understand why they believe what they believe and what the impacts are on their and others lives and then to assist them to manage these beliefs more productively and with less associated distress.

Negative Symptoms

Although many CBTP studies have focused on positive symptoms, some have been broader in scope and successfully so.[22,45,46] Essentially, the cognitive-behavioural conceptualisation of negative symptoms considers possible individual psychosocial explanations – blunted affect can be a response to trauma or institutionalisation, low motivation can be due to demoralisation or self-defeating beliefs, poverty of speech can come from isolation. Generally, these explanations involve protection – by the avoidance of stressful circumstances, which can cause social and general anxiety and worsen ideas of reference and hallucinations. Engaging people experiencing negative symptoms can be challenging because they may feel much safer avoiding stress than becoming involved in anything that stimulates it, so identifying things that do motivate – for example, one patient revealed an obsession with the TV programme 'Star Trek' – could be used to develop conversation and actions to follow up on their interest. Addressing symptoms through CBT approaches needs to take into account an anticipated worsening of positive symptoms and develop management of stress and behavioural activation using mastery and pleasure diaries (rating specific activities according to the actual completion of them and positive response) with graded target setting. These can be effective over time, where CBT specifically targets negative symptoms,[22,47,48] in putting the gains made through understanding into improved quality of life and moving towards recovery. Social skills training and employment initiatives also have a major role to play.

Relapse Prevention and Medication Management

Developing lasting change and recovery (see further discussion in Chapter 20) can occur through understanding, anticipation and resilience. Recognising the emergence of anxiety and positive symptoms as possible signs of stress is important so they can be used as signals that social and psychological issues need to be addressed – often by problem solving and sometimes by enlisting support with family encouragement. An understanding can be developed that the use of medication is a coping strategy, which can assist with this resilience and reduce chances of relapse and which can be adapted to circumstances. This does not necessitate an acceptance of illness or even that the hallucinations and delusions are 'not real', just that the medication – for whatever reason, such as effects on sleep or stress – can be helpful. Studies have inevitably been relatively short term (one to two years) with one positive exception,[47] yet we know that psychosis can relapse. Clinicians, CMHTs and carers can provide booster sessions using the interventions described to maintain gains and minimise relapse.

Novel CBT Interventions

New directions have tended to be transdiagnostic (e.g. voices or paranoia) rather than developed for specific mental disorders. These include acceptance and commitment therapy (ACT), mindfulness training, positive psychology interventions, dialectical behaviour therapy, imagery modification, compassion focussed therapy (CFT) and metacognitive therapy (see Wright et al.[49] for further details). These 'third wave' interventions, following behaviour therapy and then cognitive behaviour therapy, have a less robust evidence base for implementation in the treatment of psychosis, but they all have found their place within the current psychosocial repertoire.

Mindfulness training for people with psychosis in a group format has been described and evaluated[24] as being both safe and therapeutic. It, however, seems likely that prolonged periods of mindfulness are not indicated. Instead, mindfulness techniques – such as the mindful breath, mindful walking and mindful eating – might be useful.[49] In particular, the body scan might unlock somatic memories of trauma that need specific therapy.

Imagery modification has been used for voice hearing as part of an avatar approach, where a therapist works to modify negative beliefs through a computer construction of a representation of the physical entity – as identified by the patient – of the 'voice'[50] with a construction of its sound and content. The therapist interacts with the patient through the image to reduce its power. Imagery is also part of a positive memory training approach,[51] which identifies the main emotion linked to distressing voice hearing (e.g. sadness) and then activates an image linked to the opposite emotional state (e.g. the euphoria of scoring a goal for your local soccer team) and then practicing with the image and linked emotion. Images linked to voice hearing triggered by unprocessed traumatic memories can also be modified during the process of CBT.

CBT for psychosis has now established itself as an evidence-based treatment alongside medication and other interventions (e.g. employment and case management) to the extent that clinical guidelines endorse it. It is continuing to develop, and research needs to keep pace with the newer third-wave approaches. However, availability of evidence-based CBT for psychosis remains a problem internationally.[52] Full training is available now in many countries, and services do need to consider how to access this training to provide the expertise for application, teaching and supervision. The techniques described can be used in psychiatric practice with supervision or peer support and by using the teaching materials available.[10,36,53] Most sessional therapy is likely to be provided by clinical psychologists or other trained therapists. Self-help and caregiver support materials are also available.[53–57]

Carer Support and Intervention

Work with families, couples and other caregivers – including those employed to work in supportive accommodation – varies from caregiver psychoeducation and social support to more structured involvement with individual families and groups of families. The evidence for the effectiveness of family work is strong and long established,[58,59] yet it remains unavailable to many.

This can be due to a lack of trained staff, inflexibility in meeting the needs of families (e.g. around working hours and location), the availability of families, the reluctance of individual patients to engage, and the lack of recognition of the importance of such work by clinical services. There are a number of questionnaires available that can help in assessing knowledge of schizophrenia and psychosis, as well as relative assessment and outcomes (e.g. burden of care).[60]

Approaches involve work with individual or groups of families, including couples. This should involve the individual experiencing psychotic symptoms if that is practical and agreed. There may be circumstances in which the family or individual wish to meet alone initially, and there may be occasions when the individual refuses access to the family. Families themselves do have the right to express their views, but individuals also have rights to confidentiality if such contacts occur. Overcoming these issues is often crucial to progress, and often, a way of negotiating can be found about what is said to the families or spouse and what is not. Practitioners can always listen to families, although this may need to be explained to the individual concerned so that trust is maintained. It may then be possible to give general advice even if specific information about the individual's care cannot be disclosed. General elements of support have been described in the Triangle of Care:[61]

1. Carers and the essential role they play are identified at first contact or as soon as possible thereafter.
2. Staff are 'carer aware' and trained in carer engagement strategies.
3. Policy and practice protocols regarding confidentiality and sharing information are in place.
4. Defined post(s) responsible for carers are in place.
5. A carer introduction to the service and staff is available, with a relevant range of information across the acute care pathway.
6. A range of carer support services is available.

Caregiver support and psychoeducation can be made available over a small number of sessions, which may be sufficient for the family's needs and circumstances.[46] Generally, however, family intervention will involve offering more sessions – at least 10 planned sessions over a period of between three months and a year.[62] It is important to take account of the relationship between the main carer and others in the family and the individual concerned. Usually, the process involves a clinical assessment, which gathers information about the composition of the household, their current life issues, their levels of distress, their coping strategies and areas of strength the family have. It will usually be helpful to allow the family to tell their story about how problems developed and led to the presentation of one individual to mental health services. This can help in developing the formulation of the individual's needs and of the family situation and dynamics. Developing and sharing this can be invaluable in reaching a common understanding on which future plans and expectations can be built. The work with the family will usually involve problem solving of general issues that they may have and specific issues in relation to the individual's distress, disability and behaviour. Coping strategies can be enhanced or developed, which help overcome difficult situations. There are often issues around medication and compliance that can be understood and worked through – generally, an educational rather than coercive approach is more likely to be successful and less stressful. Similarly, approaches in relation to the use of illicit drugs and alcohol may need careful consideration. How should families respond to hallucinatory or delusional behaviour (e.g. speech about being a super-hero or fabulously wealthy)? Collusion or confrontation tend not to be helpful whereas enquiry and discussion may be more helpful – often a pattern of response that is most helpful and least confrontational can be developed. Distress from voices may be supported through reference to coping strategies previously developed – for example, going to a quiet place or playing music or a computer game. Interference with others may need management, such as playing music through headphones rather than speakers or trying to speak inwardly rather than outwardly to voices. There may also be self-help groups available locally and nationally (e.g. RETHINK Mental Illness, Hearing Voices groups and MIND), which can support and provide advice.

Communication can be difficult, and this can be due to the nature of the problem that the individual has and their ability to articulate their concerns. It can also be due to styles of interaction within the family that can confusion to the individual. Supporting the family can involve helping them speak directly to each other, to listen to each other without interrupting, to avoid overgeneralising but also enable them to speak about specific instances where there have been difficulties and then looking at ways of managing these issues in the future. Problem solving involves identifying their individual problems, brainstorming some possible solutions, choosing one of them, doing it and then reviewing how well it worked. Setting some goals for the future can be helpful in relation to behaviours that have been problematic and tasks that need to be allocated and completed. This can then be put into a family care plan to complement the individual care plan that is drawn up during the individual work that's proceeding. Where issues are present between partners, a similar approach can be successful. For families and spouses, the issue of staying or separating can arise. For the latter, RELATE or Improving Access to Psychological Therapy (IAPT) services offering couple work and similar organisations may have a role.

Management therefore has specific, supportive, educational and treatment functions and includes negotiated problem solving or crisis management work. It is very important that the family are aware of where mental health care can be obtained and how, including through local councils and the voluntary sector. They can understandably become increasingly frustrated when they feel that they are not being listened to and necessary support isn't being made available. Clinicians have a key role in assessment, psychoeducation and management of families, even where they cannot be involved directly in scheduled family work.

Some of the original family work looked at issues specifically related to relapse. These identified criticism and over-protectiveness, described as 'high expressed emotion' (EE), as predictors of increased relapse.[63] This led to an initial series of studies on family work to identify those with high EE and also with high levels of face-to-face contact. Researchers developed interventions to modify these factors,[64] which have over time expanded to involve broader approaches to family work. It remains important to note that these factors may need communication management, although more general practical supports are often at least as important. Unfortunately, there has been a widespread interpretation – particularly in the USA – that this work implied criticism of the carers themselves with echoes of early psychodynamic descriptions of the *schizophrenogenic family*. As carers frequently may feel inappropriate guilt at the development of psychosis in their offspring, this can be an important issue to counter immediately where it appears to be arising – as it can detrimentally affect the carers themselves and their collaboration in treatment plans and family support.

There are also cultural circumstances were high expressed emotion may actually have positive benefits. Criticism likewise may have derived from a lack of appropriate support and consequent frustration. Dealing with these key issues will often be more important and engaging than focusing directly on critical behaviour or over-protectiveness. Paradoxically, many families have felt, and indeed been, criticised by professionals despite there being no evidence to support any approach by which families might make it less likely for psychosis to develop. However, what has been clear is that families often feel very under-supported by services, and this is particularly at times of crisis when they need advice guidance and direct support. Providing information about local crisis services is important as well as responses from those services when required.

Summary

Psychosis and schizophrenia are relatively common and cause distress and disability to many with major effects on individual, caregivers and society. Much is now understood about the causes, especially childhood trauma, drug misuse and psychological predispositions. Diagnosis is based on presenting symptoms – positive and negative – and whilst psychosis is on a continuum with normality and other mental disorders, it is usually distinguishable such that case conceptualisation and intervention can be applied. Psychosocial interventions now have a strong evidence base (e.g. CBT, family work, social skills training, supported employment and early intervention) but are frequently not available in the UK and, even more so, internationally or provided to evidence-based standards.[52] Clinicians can use psychosocial techniques, support colleagues (e.g. CMHTs and clinical psychologists) and advocate their use to patients, carers and service managers.

References

1. Maj M, van Os J, De Hert M, et al. The clinical characterization of the patient with primary psychosis aimed at personalization of management. *World Psychiatry* 2021;20(1):4–33.
2. Kingdon DG, Ashcroft K, Bhandari B, et al. Schizophrenia and borderline personality disorder: similarities and differences in the experience of auditory hallucinations, paranoia, and childhood trauma. *Journal of Nervous and Mental Disease* 2010;198(6):399–403.
3. Varese F, Smeets F, Drukker M, et al. Childhood adversities increase the risk of psychosis: a meta-analysis of patient-control, prospective- and cross-sectional cohort studies. *Schizophrenia Bulletin* 2012;38(4):661–71.
4. Radua J, Ramella-Cravaro V, Ioannidis JPA, et al. What causes psychosis? An umbrella review of risk and protective factors. *World Psychiatry* 2018;17(1):49–66.
5. Beck AT, Rector NA, Stolar N, et al. *Schizophrenia: Cognitive Theory, Research, and Therapy*. New York: Guilford Publications; 2011.
6. Freeman D. Persecutory delusions: a cognitive perspective on understanding and treatment. *Lancet Psychiatry* 2016;3 (7):685–92.
7. McCarthy-Jones S, Thomas N, Strauss C, et al. Better than mermaids and stray dogs? Subtyping auditory verbal hallucinations and its implications for research and practice. *Schizophrenia Bulletin* 2014;40(Suppl 4):S275–84.
8. Beck AT, Grant PM, Huh GA, et al. Dysfunctional attitudes and expectancies in deficit syndrome schizophrenia. *Schizophrenia Bulletin* 2013;39(1):43–51.
9. Kingdon D. Cognitive-behavioural therapy for psychosis. *British Journal of Psychiatry* 2004;184:85–6.
10. Kingdon D, Turkington D. *Cognitive Therapy of Schizophrenia*. New York: Guilford; 2004.
11. Turner DT, McGlanaghy E, Cuijpers P, et al. A meta-analysis of social skills training and related interventions for psychosis. *Schizophrenia Bulletin* 2018;44(3):475–91.
12. Bellack AS, Mueser KT, Gingerich S, et al. *Social Skills Training for Schizophrenia: A Step-By-Step Guide*. New York: Guilford Publications; 2013.
13. Laing RD, Esterson A. *Sanity, Madness and the Family. Vol. 1, Families of Schizophrenics*. London: Tavistock Publications; 1964.
14. Arieti S. *Interpretation of Schizophrenia*. New York: Basic Books Inc.; 1974.
15. Rodolico A, Bighelli I, Avanzato C, et al. Family interventions for relapse prevention in schizophrenia: a systematic review and network meta-analysis. *Lancet Psychiatry* 2022;9 (3):211–21.
16. Morrison AP, Turkington D, Pyle M, et al. Cognitive therapy for people with schizophrenia spectrum disorders not taking antipsychotic drugs: a single-blind randomised controlled trial. *Lancet* 2014;383(9926):1395–403.
17. McKenna P, Leucht S, Jauhar S, et al. The controversy about cognitive behavioural therapy for schizophrenia. *World Psychiatry* 2019;18(2):235–36.
18. Lutgens D, Gariepy G, Malla A. Psychological and psychosocial interventions for negative symptoms in psychosis: systematic review and meta-analysis. *British Journal of Psychiatry* 2017;210(5):324–32.
19. Keepers GA, Fochtmann LJ, Anzia JM, et al. The American Psychiatric Association practice guideline for the treatment of patients with schizophrenia. *American Journal of Psychiatry* 2020;177(9):868–72.
20. Kreyenbuhl J, Buchanan RW, Dickerson FB, et al. The schizophrenia patient outcomes research team (PORT): updated treatment recommendations 2009. *Schizophrenia Bulletin* 2010;36(1):94–103.
21. National Institute for Health and Care Excellence. *Psychosis and Schizophrenia in Adults: Prevention and Management*. London: NICE; 2014.
22. Grant PM, Huh GA, Perivoliotis D, et al. Randomized trial to evaluate the efficacy of cognitive therapy for low-functioning patients with schizophrenia. *Archives of General Psychiatry* 2012;69(2):121–7.
23. Turkington D, Kingdon DG, Rathod S, et al. Outcomes of an effectiveness trial of cognitive-behavioural intervention by mental health nurses in schizophrenia. *British Journal of Psychiatry* 2006;189:36–40.
24. Chadwick P, Strauss C, Jones AM, et al. Group mindfulness-based intervention for distressing voices: a pragmatic randomised controlled trial. *Schizophrenia Research* 2016;175(1–3):168–73.
25. Freeman D, Dunn G, Startup H, et al. Effects of cognitive behaviour therapy for worry on persecutory delusions in patients with psychosis (WIT): a parallel, single-blind, randomised controlled trial with a mediation analysis. *Lancet Psychiatry* 2015;2 (4):305–13.
26. Freeman D, Emsley R, Diamond R, et al. Comparison of a theoretically driven cognitive therapy (the Feeling Safe Programme) with befriending for the treatment of persistent persecutory delusions: a parallel, single-blind, randomised controlled trial. *Lancet Psychiatry* 2021;8(8):696–707.
27. Garety P, Ward T, Emsley R, et al. Effects of SlowMo, a blended digital therapy targeting reasoning, on paranoia among people with psychosis: a randomized clinical trial. *JAMA Psychiatry* 2021;78(7):714–25.
28. Freeman D, Lambe S, Kabir T, et al. Automated virtual reality therapy to treat agoraphobic avoidance and distress in patients with psychosis (gameChange): a multicentre, parallel-group, single-blind, randomised, controlled trial in England with mediation and moderation analyses. *Lancet Psychiatry* 2022;9 (5):375–88.
29. Barrowclough C, Haddock G, Wykes T, et al. Integrated motivational interviewing and cognitive behavioural therapy for people with psychosis and comorbid substance misuse:

randomised controlled trial. *BMJ* 2010;341:c6325.

30. Naeem F, Kingdon D, Turkington D. Cognitive behavior therapy for schizophrenia in patients with mild to moderate substance misuse problems. *Cognitive Behaviour Therapy* 2005;34 (4):207–15.
31. van den Berg DP, de Bont PA, van der Vleugel BM, et al. Prolonged exposure vs eye movement desensitization and reprocessing vs waiting list for posttraumatic stress disorder in patients with a psychotic disorder: a randomized clinical trial. *JAMA Psychiatry* 2015;72 (3):259–67.
32. Turkington D, Munetz M, Pelton J, et al. High-yield cognitive behavioral techniques for psychosis delivered by case managers to their clients with persistent psychotic symptoms: an exploratory trial. *Journal of Nervous and Mental Disease* 2014;202(1):30–4.
33. Morrison AP, French P, Stewart SL, et al. Early detection and intervention evaluation for people at risk of psychosis: multisite randomised controlled trial. *BMJ* 2012;344:e2233.
34. Kane JM, Robinson DG, Schooler NR, et al. Comprehensive versus usual community care for first-episode psychosis: 2-year outcomes from the NIMH RAISE early treatment program. *American Journal of Psychiatry* 2016;173(4):362–72.
35. Priebe S, Kelley L, Omer S, et al. The effectiveness of a patient-centred assessment with a solution-focused approach (DIALOG+) for patients with psychosis: a pragmatic cluster-randomised controlled trial in community care. *Psychotherapy and Psychosomatics* 2015;84(5):304–13.
36. McCabe R, John P, Dooley J, et al. Training to enhance psychiatrist communication with patients with psychosis (TEMPO): cluster randomised controlled trial. *British Journal of Psychiatry* 2016;209 (6):517–24.
37. Day JC, Bentall RP, Roberts C, et al. Attitudes toward antipsychotic medication: the impact of clinical variables and relationships with health professionals. *Archives of General Psychiatry* 2005;62(7):717–24.
38. Kemp R, Kirov G, Everitt B, et al. Randomised controlled trial of compliance therapy. 18-month follow-up. *British Journal of Psychiatry* 1998;172:413–9.
39. Rathod S, Kingdon D, Smith P, et al. Insight into schizophrenia: the effects of cognitive behavioural therapy on the components of insight and association with sociodemographics – data on a previously published randomised controlled trial. *Schizophrenia Research* 2005;74(2–3):211–9.
40. McIntosh AM, Conlon L, Lawrie SM, et al. Compliance therapy for schizophrenia. *Cochrane Database of Systematic Reviews* 2006;2006(3): CD003442.
41. Freeman AM, Tribe RH, Stott JC, et al. Open dialogue: a review of the evidence. *Psychiatric Services* 2019;70(1):46–59.
42. Wright JH, Turkington D, Kingdon DG, et al. *Cognitive-Behavior Therapy for Severe Mental Illness: An Illustrated Guide*. Arlington: American Psychiatric Publications; 2009.
43. Persons JB. *The Case Formulation Approach to Cognitive-Behavior Therapy*. New York: Guilford Press; 2012.
44. Haddock G, McCarron J, Tarrier N, et al. Scales to measure dimensions of hallucinations and delusions: the psychotic symptom rating scales (PSYRATS). *Psychological Medicine* 1999;29(4):879–89.
45. Sensky T, Turkington D, Kingdon D, et al. A randomized controlled trial of cognitive-behavioral therapy for persistent symptoms in schizophrenia resistant to medication. *Archives of General Psychiatry* 2000;57(2):165–72.
46. Turkington D, Kingdon D, Rathod S, et al. Outcomes of an effectiveness trial of cognitive-behavioural intervention by mental health nurses in schizophrenia. *The British Journal of Psychiatry* 2006;189(1):36–40.
47. Turkington D, Sensky T, Scott J, et al. A randomized controlled trial of cognitive-behavior therapy for persistent symptoms in schizophrenia: a five-year follow-up. *Schizophrenia Research* 2008;98(1–3):1–7.
48. Turkington D, Kingdon D, Turner T, et al. Effectiveness of a brief cognitive-behavioural therapy intervention in the treatment of schizophrenia. *British Journal of Psychiatry* 2002;180:523–7.
49. Wright N, Turkington D, Kelly O, et al. *Treating Psychosis: A Clinician's Guide to Integrating Acceptance and Commitment Therapy, Compassion-Focused Therapy, and Mindfulness Approaches within the Cognitive Behavioral Therapy Tradition*. Oakland: New Harbinger Publications; 2014.
50. Craig TK, Rus-Calafell M, Ward T, et al. AVATAR therapy for auditory verbal hallucinations in people with psychosis: a single-blind, randomised controlled trial. *Lancet Psychiatry* 2018;5(1): 31–40.
51. Steel C, Korrelboom K, Fazil Baksh M, et al. Positive memory training for the treatment of depression in schizophrenia: a randomised controlled trial. *Behaviour Research and Therapy* 2020;135:103734.
52. Kopelovich SL, Nutting E, Blank J, et al. Preliminary point prevalence of Cognitive Behavioral Therapy for psychosis (CBTp) training in the US and Canada. *Psychosis* 2022;14 (4):344–54.
53. Hazell C, Hayward M, Strauss C, et al. *An Introduction to Self-Help for Distressing Voices*. London: Robinson; 2018.
54. Freeman D, Freeman J, Garety P. *Overcoming Paranoid and suspicious Thoughts: A Self-Help Guide Using Cognitive Behavioural Techniques*. London: Robinson; 2016.
55. Turkington D, Kingdon D, Rathod S, et al. *Back to Life, Back to Normality. Vol. 1: Cognitive Therapy, Recovery and Psychosis*. Cambridge: Cambridge University Press; 2009.
56. Turkington D, Spencer HM. *Back to Life, Back to Normality. Vol. 2: CBT Informed Recovery for Families with Relatives with Schizophrenia and Other Psychoses*. Cambridge: Cambridge University Press; 2018.
57. Morrison AP, Renton J, French P, et al. *Think You're Crazy? Think Again: A Resource Book for Cognitive Therapy for Psychosis*. Abingdon: Routledge; 2014.
58. Ma CF, Chan SKW, Chien WT, et al. Cognitive behavioural family intervention for people diagnosed with severe mental illness and their families: a systematic review and meta-analysis of randomized controlled trials. *Journal of Psychiatric and Mental Health Nursins* 2020;27(2):128–39.
59. Pharoah F, Mari J, Rathbone J, et al. Family intervention for schizophrenia.

Cochrane Database of Systematic Reviews 2010(12):CD000088.

60. Barrowclough C, Tarrier N. *Families of Schizophrenic Patients: Cognitive Behavioural Intervention*. Cheltenham: Nelson Thornes; 1992.

61. Worthington A, Rooney P, Hannan R. *The Triangle of Care: Carers Included: A Guide to Best Practice in Mental Health Care in England*. London: Carers Trust; 2013. carers.org/downloads/resources-pdfs/triangle-of-care-england/the-triangle-of-care-carers-included-second-edition.pdf.

62. Lobban F, Barrowclough C. *A Casebook of Family Interventions for Psychosis*. Chichester: John Wiley & Sons; 2009.

63. Brown GW, Birley JLT, Wing JK. Influence of family life on the course of schizophrenic disorders: a replication. *British Journal of Psychiatry* 1972;121 (562):241–58.

64. Leff J, Berkowitz R, Shavit N, et al. A trial of family therapy v. a relatives group for schizophrenia. *British Journal of Psychiatry* 1989;154:58–66.

Anxiety Disorders

David S. Baldwin, Bethan Impey and Vasilios Masdrakis

Anxiety symptoms and anxiety disorders are common in community settings and primary and secondary medical care.[1] Anxiety symptoms are often mild and only transient, but many people are troubled by severe symptoms that cause both considerable personal distress and a marked impairment in social and occupational function. The principal anxiety disorders are currently considered to comprise panic disorder, generalised anxiety disorder, social anxiety disorder, agoraphobia, specific phobias, separation anxiety disorder and selective mutism. Additional conditions (not considered further here) include substance/medication-induced anxiety disorder, anxiety disorder due to another medical condition, other specified anxiety disorder and unspecified anxiety disorder.[2] Post-traumatic disorder and obsessive-compulsive disorder are now classified away from the anxiety disorders, so are considered elsewhere (see Chapters 6.2 and 6.4). Specific phobias are mainly considered elsewhere (see Chapter 6.3), and because selective mutism is most typically seen during childhood, it is outside the scope of this book. Together, anxiety disorders constitute the most frequent mental disorders, with an estimated 12-month prevalence of approximately 10–14% of the population, and they have a substantial associated socioeconomic burden[1]. According to the World Health Organization (WHO), anxiety disorders rank sixth among all disorders regarding the 'years lived with disability': mainly because they often have a prolonged debilitating course with a high proportion of only intermittent recovery (32.1%) or chronicity (8.6%) at nine-year follow-up.[3]

Although the societal impact of anxiety disorders is substantial, many of those who could benefit from psychological or pharmacological treatment are neither recognised nor treated. Recognition relies on maintaining a keen awareness of the psychological and physical symptoms of anxiety disorders, and accurate diagnosis rests on identifying the pathognomonic features of specific conditions. Decisions on the need for treatment should be determined by the severity and persistence of symptoms, the degree of associated psychological distress, the level of impact on everyday life, the presence of co-existing depressive symptoms, and other features such as history of a good response to or the poor tolerability of previous treatments. The choice of treatment is influenced greatly by patient characteristics and preferences, as well as by clinical experience. There is much overlap between the different anxiety disorders in effective and acceptable evidence-based therapies ('first-line' treatments include prescription of a selective serotonin re-uptake inhibitor [SSRI] or a course of cognitive behavioural therapy [CBT]), but there are important differences between anxiety disorders, which should influence some treatment decisions. It therefore helps to remain familiar with the characteristic features and evidence base for the treatment of each disorder.

Diagnosis and Differential Diagnosis

Generalised anxiety disorder (GAD). This is characterised by excessive and largely uncontrollable worrying that has lasted at least six months and is not restricted to particular circumstances (for example, only when attending a social gathering). The worries often centre on possible physical ill-health, affecting either themselves or family members, and patients can repeatedly present with 'medically unexplained' physical symptoms, often craving reassurance and sometimes requesting inappropriate medical investigations. Common features include apprehension, tension, difficulty in concentrating and heightened autonomic symptoms, such as dry mouth, palpitations and abdominal discomfort. GAD is one of the more frequent mental disorders in primary medical care but is often not recognised, possibly because only a minority present with the characteristic psychological symptoms.

Panic disorder. Accurate diagnosis depends on establishing the presence of recurrent unexpected surges of severe anxiety usually designated as 'panic attacks', which typically reach their peak within 10 minutes and last around 30–45 minutes. The severity of physiological symptoms (e.g. chest pain, racing heart) can cause some patients to believe they are in imminent danger of death, and the associated psychological distress may make some patients fear they might lose control or 'go mad'. Between panic attacks, patients typically experience relative freedom from anxiety (at least initially), although most are apprehensive about the possibility of experiencing further panic attacks (anticipatory anxiety). Panic disorder can occur with or without agoraphobia (with marked anxiety in feared situations from which escape might prove difficult or embarrassing), and agoraphobia can either precede, or more typically follow, the development of panic attacks. Patients with comorbid depression are typically more severely unwell and disabled by symptoms, tend to make greater use of health services, and generally have a worse prognosis.

Adult separation anxiety disorder (ASAD). Although it was traditionally regarded as a disorder in childhood, separation anxiety disorder is now also recognised as a condition affecting adults, either by continuing into or having an onset during adult life. As such, it is now grouped with other anxiety disorders within the current editions of the International Classifications of Disease (ICD-11)[4] and *Diagnostic and Statistical Manual of Mental Disorders* (DSM-5).[2] ASAD is characterised by the presence of anxiety and fear (which is atypical for the patient's age and development level) over separation from people and places to which the patient has a strong attachment. It is associated with clinically significant levels of psychological distress or an impairment in social, academic, occupational and other areas of functioning that is not explained by another disorder. The distinction of ASAD from conditions such as panic disorder (with or without agoraphobia), GAD and dependent personality disorder can sometimes be troublesome.

Social anxiety disorder (also known as social phobia). This is characterised by an intense and persistent fear of being scrutinised or negatively evaluated by others. Affected individuals generally anticipate ridicule or personal humiliation, avoiding many social situations or enduring them with great psychological distress. Common physical symptoms include blushing, dry mouth and a fear of inappropriate micturition. Some individuals experience panic attacks, although social anxiety disorder can usually be distinguished from panic disorder fairly easily because, in social anxiety disorder, the attacks occur expectedly in feared social or performance situations. Furthermore, in panic disorder, the presence of a friend typically provides at least some reassurance, whereas in social phobia, this often makes little difference. A significant proportion of those (approximately one-third) with social anxiety disorder develop secondary major depression, and distinguishing between the disorders can sometimes be difficult; however, in social anxiety disorder, the capacity to enjoy oneself usually remains, and energy levels are not significantly impaired. Many patients with social anxiety disorder consume excessive quantities of alcohol-containing drinks or use cannabis or other drugs, believing this may help quell anxiety before a social encounter.

Specific (also termed simple, or isolated) phobias. Specific fears of certain objects, animals or situations are very common, although only a minority of affected people present for treatment – this often being at a time of changing domestic or career responsibilities. The impairment associated with a specific phobia is usually quite limited, but the presence of a comorbid specific phobia can increase the disability associated with other anxiety disorders or depression. Specific phobias are considered in detail elsewhere (see Chapter 6.3).

Differential diagnosis of anxiety disorders. Some conditions can be confused with anxiety disorders (Table 6.1.1). Co-existing depressive symptoms often accompany anxiety disorders (and approximately one-third of people with anxiety

Table 6.1.1 Important differential diagnoses in patients with anxiety disorders

Condition	Differentiation from anxiety disorder
Depressive episode	Early morning waking, feeling worse in the morning, loss of capacity for pleasure, constipation, guilty thoughts and marked suicidal thoughts all suggest depression rather than anxiety. Depressive symptoms in anxiety disorders tend to develop after the psychological and somatic symptoms of the anxiety disorder (e.g. anticipation of embarrassment, anxiety and avoidance in social phobia).
OCD	Anxiety symptoms are usually present and may be severe, and whilst excessive worrying can have a ruminative quality, the predominant symptoms are obsessive ruminations (and images, doubts and impulses) and compulsive mental and physical rituals. Compulsive rituals rarely predominate in patients with anxiety disorders.
PTSD	Anxiety symptoms are usually present, and hypervigilance-related symptoms may be severe. Re-experiencing symptoms (such as flashbacks) and 'numbing' are not common features in patients with anxiety disorders.
Psychotic illness	Anxiety can be part of the prodrome before the onset of psychotic illness, but delusions, hallucinations and thought disorder are not seen in patients with primary anxiety disorders. Some patients with severe social anxiety disorder have marked interpersonal sensitivity in feared social or performance situations that can sometimes appear almost persecutory in nature, but the typical onset of anxiety symptoms in mid-adolescence and absence of interpersonal sensitivity outside of feared social situations helps to clarify diagnosis.
Psychostimulant use	Excess consumption of caffeine-containing drinks and drugs can result in physical and psychological symptoms of anxiety. Use of amphetamines, Ecstasy, cocaine, ketamine and hallucinogens can sometimes result in agitation and severe anxiety, including panic attacks and depersonalisation-derealisation experiences. Primacy of drug-seeking behaviour and physical signs of intoxication (e.g. stereotypic movements with amphetamine use) support the diagnosis of drug dependency. Many novel psychoactive substances (e.g. mephedrone) can cause anxiety, but their full side effect profiles are not yet fully established.
Drug withdrawal	Abrupt withdrawal of alcohol, barbiturates, benzodiazepines, gabapentinoids, opiates and some antidepressant drugs can result in agitation, tremor, dizziness, gastrointestinal upset and insomnia. Anxiety disorders are not associated with acute confusional states or marked autonomic instability. Characteristic physical signs are seen after withdrawal from certain drug classes; for example, pupillary dilatation in people withdrawing from opiates.
Illness anxiety disorder	Also known as 'hypochondriasis' and characterised by the unrealistic fear of having or being at risk of a serious medical condition, often with misinterpretation of typical bodily functions as being signs of illness. Sometimes difficult to distinguish from GAD and OCD, but in the former, hypochondriacal concerns are usually just one of many worries, and in the latter, ruminations are typically widespread and ritualistic behaviours more pronounced.
Physical illness	Anxiety symptoms are common in many physical health problems and can be the presenting feature – for example, in hyperthyroidism, hypoglycaemia, complex partial seizures, paroxysmal tachycardia and phaeochromocytoma.

disorders also meet syndromal criteria for major depression, this usually being described as 'comorbid'). Depressive symptoms in patients with anxiety disorders can include suicidal thoughts, may increase the associated impairment and can affect the prognosis adversely. Treatment of depression usually reduces the intensity of anxiety symptoms when depression is the primary diagnosis. However, when depression is comorbid or follows an anxiety disorder, each condition usually requires separate consideration and often separate targeted treatment. It is also important to ask about features of obsessive-compulsive disorder (OCD) and post-traumatic stress disorder (PTSD) when taking an anxiety history, as anxiety symptoms are common in these conditions, which are considered in detail elsewhere (see Chapter 6.2 and 6.4). Finally, it is worth remembering that anxiety symptoms can be so intense and worrisome thoughts so preoccupying as to appear almost delusional in nature (i.e. fixed, with inability to see alternate explanations), and in this presentation, psychosis should be considered within the differential diagnosis.

Epidemiology of Anxiety Disorders

Generalised anxiety disorder. GAD is one of the most common mental disorders in community and clinical settings. Epidemiological studies of nationally representative samples in the United States report a past-year prevalence of between 2.7–3.1% and a lifetime prevalence of GAD of between 5.1–11.9%. A review of epidemiological studies in Europe found a past-year prevalence of between 1.7–3.4% and a lifetime prevalence of between 4.3–5.9%. Worldwide estimates of the lifetime and 12-month prevalance are 3.7% and 1.8%, respectively.[5] The disorder is approximately twice as common in females as it is in males.

Comorbidity with major depression or other anxiety disorders is very frequent. In a nationally representative survey of United States adults, 66% of individuals with current GAD had at least one concurrent psychiatric disorder, and 90% of individuals with lifetime GAD had at least one comorbid psychiatric disorder. Worldwide, lifetime comorbidity has been estimated as 81.9%, and mood disorders have an estimated lifetime comorbidity of 63.0%.[5] Major depressive disorder is the most common comorbid condition, being reported in 39% of individuals with current GAD and 62% of individuals with lifetime GAD. Other common comorbid conditions in individuals with GAD (rates over the previous 30 days and lifetime) include social anxiety disorder (23% and 34%, respectively), specific phobia (25% and 35%) and panic disorder (23% and 24%). GAD may also be associated with increased rates of alcohol and other substance use disorders, PTSD and OCD. It is also common among patients with 'medically unexplained' chronic pain or chronic physical illness.[6]

Panic disorder and agoraphobia. Epidemiological studies estimate the lifetime prevalence of *panic attacks* to lie between 13.2–22% and the lifetime prevalence of *panic disorder* (with or without agoraphobia) to be between 1.7–4.7%.[7,8] Agoraphobia is included within DSM-5 as a 'stand-alone' condition, separate from panic disorder. Although the two conditions commonly co-occur, agoraphobia without panic attacks can be reliably characterised and differs from panic disorder with agoraphobia based on its incidence, gender distribution and treatment approaches. Panic disorder is approximately twice as frequent in women as in men. The median age of onset is 24 years, but approximately half of adults with the condition report significant anxiety-related problems during childhood. Panic disorder is found in all ethnic groups, but varying cultures may experience and report psychological distress through differing idioms – for example, it has been reported that White Americans report more trembling and shaking, whereas Hispanic Americans report more choking sensations. Risk factors for the development of panic disorder include younger age (less than 60 years), single status, socioeconomic disadvantage, lower educational attainment, unemployment, and birth in a different country to current national residence.

Panic disorder is associated with substantial functional impairment – for example, when compared to non-anxious individuals, quality of life is markedly reduced and impairments are similar to those experienced by patients with chronic medical illnesses such as diabetes mellitus. Panic disorder is typically accompanied by severe impairments in home, occupational and social functioning; reduced productivity at work; and financial decrements.[9] Although patients with panic disorder are frequent users of primary and secondary care medical services and although comorbidity with physical illness is common, the underlying anxiety disorder is often over-looked or misdiagnosed. There is frequent comorbidity with other anxiety disorders, major depression and alcohol or substance use disorders: approximately two-thirds of individuals with panic disorder meet criteria for another anxiety disorder, the lifetime comorbidity of major depression is estimated as 38%, and approximately 34% of adults with panic disorder with agoraphobia meet criteria for at least one lifetime substance use disorder. Treatment-seeking patients with bipolar disorder have a lifetime rate of panic of between 14–18%. Psychiatric comorbidity in panic disorder is associated with increased risk of suicide attempts, and panic disorder is probably associated with increased rates of cardiac dysfunction and disease, as well as cardiac death.[10]

Social anxiety disorder (SAD). Epidemiological studies suggest SAD is one of the more common mental disorders: the lifetime prevalence in the United States has been estimated as lying between 2.4–13.0% (the wide range probably being due to differences in the required level of functional impairment). The worldwide lifetime prevalence has been estimated as 4.0%: although the age of onset is early across the globe, there are substantial variations in the level of functional impairment and degree of comorbidity.[11] Risk factors for developing SAD include female sex, single status, unemployment and socioeconomic disadvantage. Cultural factors may affect the expression of social anxiety symptoms – for example, *taijin kyofusho* in Japan involves the fear of offending others by embarrassing them or making them feel uncomfortable. The typical longitudinal course of SAD is not fully established, although a chronic unremitting course is not uncommon.

Even in the absence of comorbidity, SAD is associated with reduced educational achievement, impairment at and absence from paid employment, weakened social support networks, increased use of health services and lowered quality of life. Most individuals with SAD have one or more comorbid conditions, the most frequent being major depression, other anxiety disorders, substance use disorders, eating disorders and sexual dysfunction. SAD may act as a predisposing factor for these subsequent comorbid conditions. There is an increased risk of attempted suicide and death by suicide. SAD has been found to be associated with obesity, stuttering, cardiac disease, autoimmune conditions and Parkinson's disease.

Separation anxiety disorder. Separation anxiety *symptoms* are not infrequent across the lifespan – for example, a prospective study involving adolescents and young adults (aged 14–24 years) found a 7.8% 'lifetime prevalence' of such symptoms. However, having symptoms of separation anxiety does not necessarily indicate the presence of separation anxiety *disorder*, as its diagnosis also rests on evaluating the degree of personal distress and level of impairment. In the US National Comorbidity Survey Replication (NCS-R) epidemiological study, the estimated lifetime prevalence of the disorder was 6.6%: the prevalence was higher in females than in males, especially in the subgroup in whom separation anxiety started in childhood.[12] Data from WHO World Mental Health Surveys involving 18 countries suggest an average lifetime prevalence of separation anxiety disorder in the general population of 4.8%.[13] Risk factors for lifetime separation anxiety disorder included female gender, reported childhood adversities and lifetime traumatic events, and these factors predicted separation anxiety disorder onsets in differing countries, as well as in childhood, adolescence and adulthood.

Epidemiological studies attest to the possibility of developing separation anxiety disorder for the first time during adult life (i.e. aged 18 years or older). In the NCS-R study, although 36.1% of 'cases' with an onset of separation anxiety in childhood experienced symptoms that persisted into adult life, the majority (77.5%) of 'cases' in adults had an onset during adulthood, and the WHO surveys found that 43.1% of lifetime onsets occurred in adulthood. A recent meta-analysis indicates that 72.4% and 75% of patients had an onset of illness by 14 and 18 years, respectively.[14] The typical duration of untreated illness in adult patients with separation anxiety disorder is uncertain, but the condition impairs social and work functioning markedly. In the NCS-R study, more than 40% had severe impairment in at least one life domain (most commonly in domains of social and personal life), this impairment being more marked in those with comorbidity, which was present in more than half the cases.[12]

Causes of Anxiety Disorders

The macro-circuitry (linked anatomical regions, see Figure 6.1.1) underlying both normal and pathological anxiety is probably similar: sensory stimuli enter the brain, processing starts in the thalamus, interpretation and evaluation occurs within the limbic system and medial prefrontal cortex, and – once a stimulus is evaluated as anxiety-provoking – the hypothalamus and brainstem trigger a physiological response to anxiety. In pathological anxiety, probable changes at the level of the micro-circuit (i.e. connections between neurons and associated interactions with glial cells, the blood vessel endothelium and surrounding specialised extracellular matrix ['perineuronal net'], within the individual anatomical regions) cause an imbalance in excitatory and inhibitory neurotransmitters (glutamate, g-aminobutyric acid). Serotonin acts in the brainstem (periaqueductal grey matter) to reduce the physiological response to anxiety and modulates anxiety processing in the limbic system. Opioids and neuropeptides (orexin, oxytocin, cholecystokinin) are also implicated in anxiety disorders.

Generalised Anxiety Disorder

Although data from twin studies are inconsistent, genetic factors may predispose individuals to developing GAD.[15] GAD may share a common heritability with major depression and with the personality trait of 'neuroticism' (an enduring tendency to worry and feel anxious, sad or guilty). Variations in the subtype of the glutamic acid decarboxylase gene may increase susceptibility to GAD, and increased frequency of the serotonin transporter gene-linked polymorphic region SS genotype has been reported. Findings from gene-environment studies indicate the importance of early developmental trauma and recent stressful life events – and their interaction with genetic markers – in developing GAD and anxiety sensitivity.[15]

GAD is more likely to occur in individuals with 'behavioural inhibition', (the tendency to be timid and shy in novel situations) than without this trait. GAD in adults is associated with a higher-than-average number of traumatic experiences and other undesirable life events in childhood, when compared to individuals without GAD,[16] and childhood maltreatment confers an increased risk of developing GAD following stressful experiences.[17]

Many explanations of the origin and persistence of the excessive and pervasive worrying that characterises GAD have been proposed.[18] These include constantly scanning the environment for cues of threat, the use of worrying as a strategy for solving problems or as a mechanism to avoid the fear response, the intolerance of uncertainty or ambiguity, and the worry about the uncontrollability and presumed dangerous consequences of worrying. Individuals with GAD show a bias towards generating negative interpretations of ambiguous material and tend be vigilant to threatening stimuli, often detecting 'threats' rapidly, particularly when the threat is

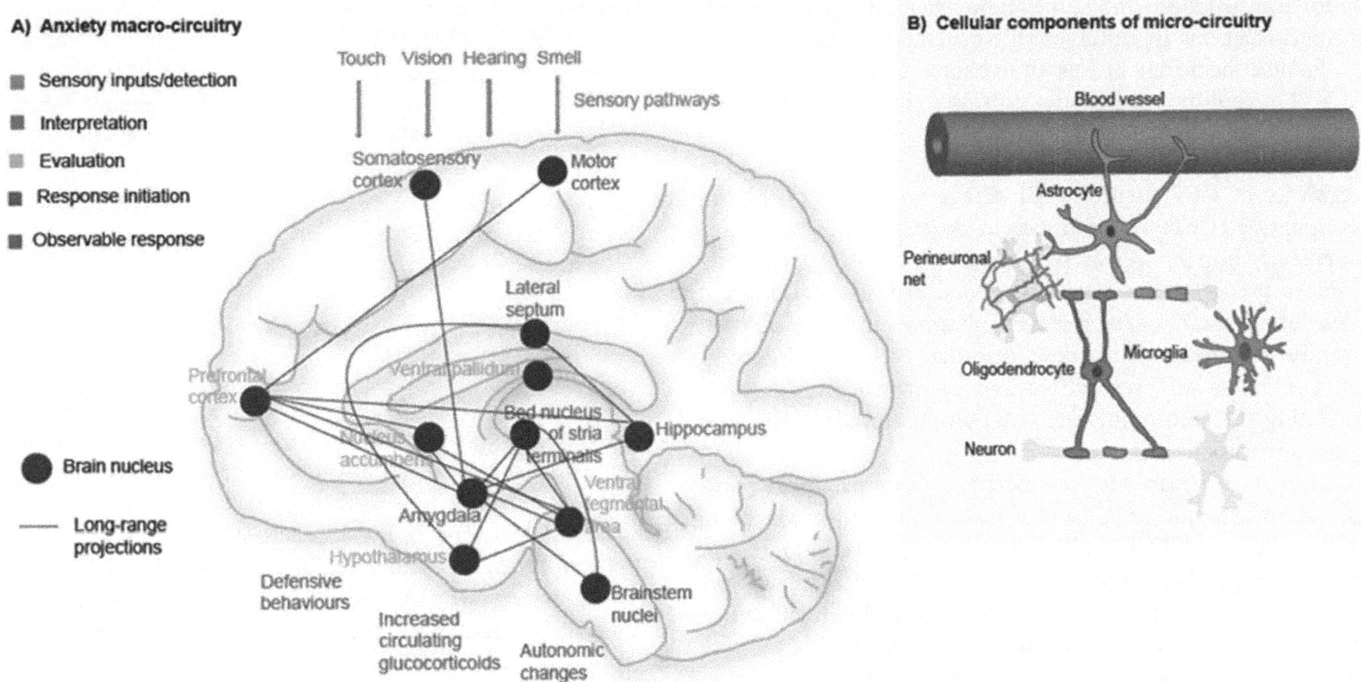

Figure 6.1.1 Macro-circuitry and micro-circuitry of anxiety. Part A illustrates brain nuclei that are linked via long-range projections to form the anxiety macro-circuit. These projections are inhibitory, excitatory or modulatory. These projections mean that the brain nuclei interact with and influence each other's function. The brain nuclei names (and other elements of sensory pathways) are shaded to indicate their role in anxiety processing. Part B illustrates the cellular components of micro-circuitry, which are found in each brain nucleus (except the perineuronal net, which is only found in certain regions).

presented in verbal-linguistic format (i.e. words) rather than pictorial form.[19] These biases appear to diminish with successful treatment, with CBT or an SSRI.

Investigations of neurotransmitters and other biomarkers in GAD tend to have been small or not replicated.[20] Evidence for possible neurotransmitter disturbances includes two case-control studies (with a total of 60 individuals) that found elevated levels of the norepinephrine metabolites 3-methoxy-4-hydroxyphenylgycol and vanillylmandelic acid, a case-control study that found a blunted growth hormone in response to clonidine (which suggests decreased post-synaptic alpha-2 adrenergic receptor sensitivity), and an observational study which found that elevated urinary levels of the serotonin metabolite 5-hydroxyindoleacetic acid were associated with greater somatic but not psychic anxiety symptoms. Other data suggest a possible role of acid-sensing ion channels in the amygdala[21] and elevated levels of C reactive protein and other proinflammatory cytokines.[22]

Neuroimaging studies suggest GAD might be associated with morphological and metabolic differences to controls, but studies tend to be small and to generate inconsistent findings.[23] Magnetic resonance imaging (MRI) has suggested reduced white matter volume in the dorsolateral prefrontal cortex, anterior limb of the internal capsule, and midbrain, while positron emission tomography (PET) demonstrated a relative increase in glucose metabolism in parts of the occipital, right posterior temporal lobe, inferior gyrus, cerebellum and right frontal gyrus as well as an absolute decrease in the basal ganglia in GAD patients when compared to a control group. A functional MRI study indicated greater anticipatory activity in the bilateral dorsal amygdala (both to aversive and neutral pictures), suggesting an enhanced anticipatory emotional responsiveness in GAD. A systematic review of neuroimaging studies indicates GAD is associated with difficulties in engaging the prefrontal cortex and anterior cingulate cortex during emotional regulation tasks.[24]

Panic Disorder

Awareness of both the often-extreme nature of a panic attack and the seemingly preferential response of patients with panic disorder to tricyclic antidepressants rather than benzodiazepine anxiolytics together encouraged the development of biological models for the aetiology of the condition, although psychological explanations have also been persuasive. Potential noradrenergic dysfunction has been suggested, based on the induction of panic attacks with yohimbine (an α2-adrenergic receptor antagonist) and the blunting of the growth hormone response to clonidine (an α2-agonist). Disturbances in serotonergic neuro-transmission have been suggested, as tryptophan depletion can alter respiratory ventilation, and SSRIs are often effective in the condition.[25] Altered $GABA_A$ receptor activity in brain regions associated with panic (including the orbitofrontal cortex, amygdala and insular cortex) suggests possible disturbances in GABAergic neuro-transmission, and some studies suggest a potential role for perturbations in glutamatergic neuro-transmission.[25]

Panic attacks may be related to cholecystokinin (CCK) and CCK-2 receptors, which are expressed in almost all brain regions. The centromedial nuclei of the amygdala – heavily implicated in panic neurobiology – are particularly rich in networks of CCK neurons. Challenge with cholecystokinin tetrapeptide (CCK-4) – a fragment of CCK – has been used extensively in panic research: it reliably and dose-dependently induces panic attacks after intravenous administration, and these attacks can be blocked by pharmacotherapy, both in healthy volunteers and panic disorder patients. Moreover, CCK interacts with several panic-relevant neurotransmitters, including the serotoninergic, GABAergic, noradrenergic and endocannabinoid systems.[26,27]

Hyperventilation and hypocapnia were originally considered to be a *cause* of panic attacks, and techniques to increase carbon dioxide (CO_2) levels during panic (breathing into and out of a paper bag) were used widely. However, subsequent studies demonstrated that CO_2 inhalation in high concentrations (35%) reliably *induces* panic attacks, primarily by acting on brainstem respiratory centres located in the reticular substance of the medulla oblongata and the pons. Currently, CO_2 hypersensitivity is considered a *risk factor* for panic vulnerability. A biological-evolutionary model proposed by Donald Klein posits that mechanisms underlying panic involve a hypersensitive 'suffocation monitor', which misfires a 'false suffocation alarm' (FSA) even when exteroceptive/interoceptive cues (including CO_2 levels) do not truly signal threat: hyperventilation serving to protect from panic by lowering CO_2 levels.[28] Klein later modified his FSA theory, proposing a physiological link between episodic functional endogenous opioid system malfunction and panic-like suffocation sensitivity, leading to the proposal of a 'respiratory subtype' of panic disorder. More recently, researchers have theorised that recurrent episodes of hyperactive amygdala-driven apnoea may contribute significantly to panic pathogenesis.[29]

Panic and fear are different phenomena, the former probably not being related to HPA-axis activity in contrast to fear/stress reactions. However, a 'neuroanatomical hypothesis' of panic disorder posits that fear and panic responses both emerge from a 'fear-circuit', centred in the amygdala with projections to other structures including the medial prefrontal cortex, hippocampus, hypothalamus, HPA-axis, brainstem, anterior cingulate cortex and insula. Disturbances in the coordination between cortical and brainstem functions may underly panic attacks, which explains how both pharmacotherapy and psychotherapy can reduce panic symptoms.[30]

A still-developing conceptualisation based on neural network theory encompasses altered function in three main networks: a central executive control network, the salience network and the default mode network.[31] The default mode network is active during internal thought, and increased connectivity has been associated with rumination, which may be relevant to GAD. However, in panic disorder, default mode network activity is decreased (Table 6.1.2). Supporting but not wholly consistent evidence includes aberrant dorsolateral prefrontal cortex activation to threat stimuli and emotion regulation tasks (executive network); hyperactivation of the dorsal anterior cingulate cortex and insula to external threat, as well as the fear of cardiovascular symptoms induced by CO_2 challenge (salience network); and altered hippocampal and ventromedial prefrontal cortex function in extinction and emotion regulation processes (default mode network).

Table 6.1.2 Triple network model of panic disorder: differences and similarities between patients and controls

	Central executive network	Salience network	Default mode network
Volume	Decreased	Decreased	Decreased
Activation	Inconsistent findings	Increased	Inconsistent findings
Within-network connectivity	No difference	Increased	Decreased

Psychological factors are also important. Panic attacks and disorder can emerge apparently spontaneously, but most affected individuals can identify a relevant life stressor in the year prior to the onset of panic-related symptoms.[32] It is unclear whether there is a true excess of undesirable life events or whether individuals who develop the condition are more sensitive to the aversive effects of bad experiences. Models based on fear learning have intuitive value. Panic attacks are associated with multiple interoceptive cues (for example, awareness of a racing heart) and exteroceptive cues (for example, a feared shopping mall), and these cues can be conceptualised as conditioned stimuli, capable of provoking fear and defensive responses (including autonomic and behavioural changes). Maintenance of the condition may occur through the generalisation of defensive responses to perceptually or conceptually similar stimuli (as examples, breathlessness or a cinema), leading to a broadening of feared situations (see Lissek et al.[33] for an expanded discussion). Patients with panic disorder show an increased fear-potentiated startle response to both unpredictable threats and images of safety cues. CBT for panic disorder involves the extinction of threat and fear responses by identifying and challenging cognitive distortions (including 'catastrophic' misinterpretations of symptoms) and by 'unpairing' conditioned stimuli from the unconditioned panic attack through progressive exposure.

Social Anxiety Disorder

As with other anxiety disorders, there is much uncertainty about the aetiology of social anxiety disorder.[34] Family and twin studies have indicated that social anxiety disorder has a genetic component, and the first genome-wide association study suggested potential genetic risk variants on chromosomes 1 and 6.[35] Epigenetic studies suggest a potential

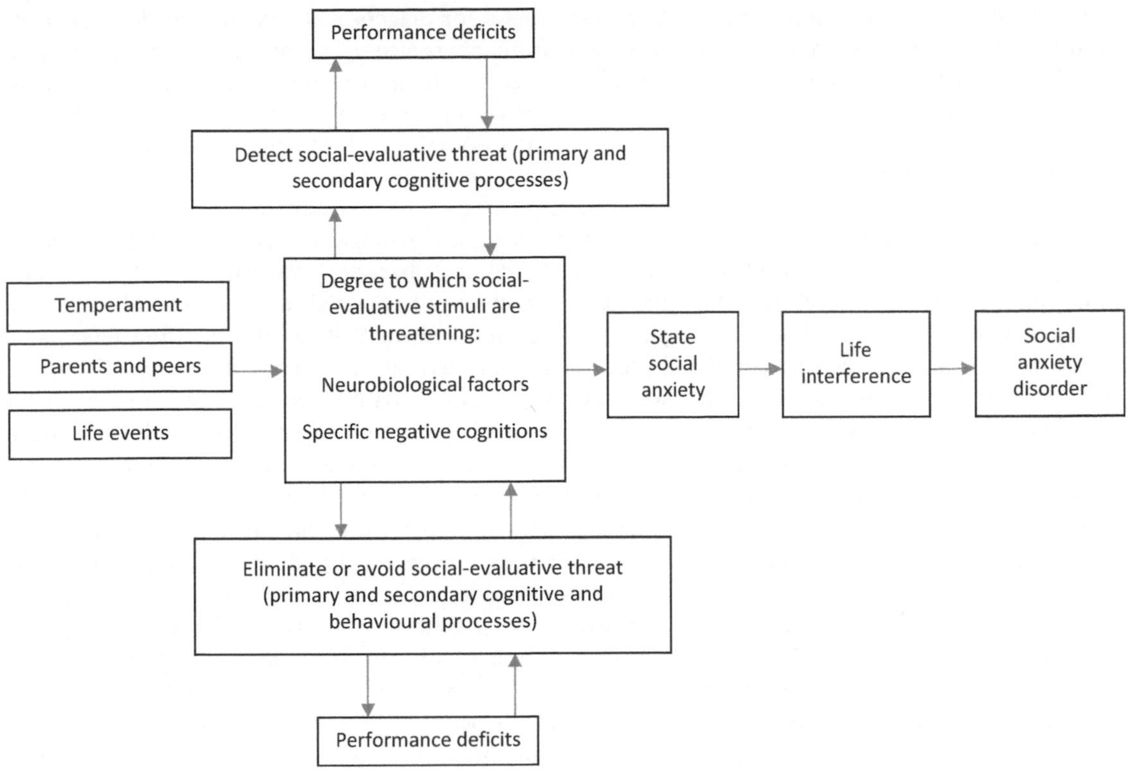

Figure 6.1.2 Integrated aetiological and maintenance model of social anxiety disorder.[39]

association between social anxiety traits and variations in the functioning of oxytocin – a hypothalamic neuropeptide known to be involved in establishing trust – in reducing distress, in helping 'read' the mental and emotional states of others and in facilitating prosocial behaviour. Oxytocin administration in patients with social anxiety disorder can alter amygdala-prefrontal connectivity and attenuate amygdala reactivity to fearful faces.[36] Investigations of heart rate variability provide some evidence for parasympathetic underactivity, and studies involving the Trier Social Stress Test suggest an increased cortisol response to stressful situations, particularly in men[34]. A series of small studies have suggested a possible role for disturbance in serotonergic neurotransmission, but findings relating to dopaminergic, GABAergic and noradrenergic neuro-transmission have been inconsistent.[37] Structural MRI studies have been inconclusive, but meta-analysis of functional MRI studies involving anxiety-provoking stimuli suggest social anxiety disorder is associated with increased brain activation in the amygdala, insula and prefrontal cortex as well as with altered function in subcortical networks involved in social cognition and self-reflection.[38]

Psychosocial factors likely to be important in the development and maintenance of social anxiety disorder include childhood temperament (with behavioural inhibition, considered in more detail later); parental psychopathology; neuroticism; peer criticism, heightened self-awareness and increased self-evaluation; biases in the processing of emotional information; and persistently negative expectations of social situations (see further details in Chapter 3.4). Many of these factors are integrated into the model of social anxiety disorder proposed by Wong and Rapee[39] (Figure 6.1.2).

Separation Anxiety Disorder

The aetiology of separation anxiety disorder in adults has not been explored extensively, and the potential roles of environmental and genetic factors and the ways in which they might interact is unclear.[40] Insights from studies of 'attachment' in anxious children may not necessarily be relevant to separation anxiety disorder in adults. Anxiety and the fear of abandonment are driving forces behind attachment formation, and attachment theory suggests 'securely attached' children should exhibit less anxious behaviour towards attachment figures, whereas 'insecurely attached' children could display symptoms of separation anxiety when an interpersonal relationship is threatened or an attachment figure is not consistently and reliably available.

Adult attachment style has two primary dimensions: attachment anxiety and attachment avoidance (which concerns the degree to which a person feels uncomfortable depending on and being emotionally close to others). Attachment anxiety, with apprehension over rejection and abandonment, has been associated with increased rates of psychopathology. Possible explanations for the observed association between *attachment anxiety* and depression include negative models of the 'self', low self-esteem, self-criticism and dysfunctional attributions to partners' behaviour.[41] By contrast, people high in *attachment avoidance* tend to invest less in interpersonal relationships, are less upset when those relationships end and are relatively low in commitment and relationship satisfaction.[42] Anxious attachment and separation anxiety appear highly correlated in patients with separation anxiety disorder, but not all individuals with separation anxiety disorder have an insecure attachment style.[43]

'Behavioural inhibition' is an early but persistent temperamental trait characterised by shyness, withdrawal, avoidance and fears of the unfamiliar, and it may be a developmental endophenotype for subsequent development of anxiety disorders. Separation anxiety symptoms are significantly correlated with recollections of difficulties associated with behavioural inhibition among adult patients with a primary diagnosis of affective disorders.[44] Separation anxiety disorder is also associated with the temperament and character dimensions of high 'harm avoidance' and low 'self-directedness' but is not especially linked to the dimension of 'intolerance of uncertainty'.[45]

Peripheral-type benzodiazepine binding site receptors, which have a role in the biosynthesis of steroids during stress and anxiety states, may have a significantly lower density in the subgroup of panic disorder patients in whom co-existing separation anxiety is prominent. Like panic disorder, separation anxiety disorder appears associated with hypersensitivity to inhaled CO_2.[46] Childhood separation anxiety disorder, adult panic disorder and hypersensitivity to 35% carbon dioxide challenge may all share a common latent intervening variable.[47] However, not all evidence accords with this hypothesis, as children with separation anxiety disorder do not react with panic or increased anxiety symptoms after hyperventilation challenge when compared to controls with panic or other anxiety disorders.

Oxytocin has an important role in mother-infant interactions, so it might be expected that oxytocin is altered in individuals with disordered attachment. Peripheral oxytocin levels are potential biological markers of the dynamics of social relationships,[48] and children with separation anxiety disorder may have significantly lower salivary oxytocin levels when compared to children with other anxiety-related conditions.[49] However, mutation analysis of the oxytocin gene reveals no consistent disturbance in patients with adult separation anxiety disorder, although single nucleotide and intron 2 molecular variants have been detected.[50] Attachment anxiety is linked to higher plasma cortisol levels, and further clarification of potential links between cortisol and oxytocin in mechanisms underlying the stress response is needed.[51]

General Considerations in the Pharmacological Treatment of Anxiety Disorders

The persistence of symptoms and associated impairment in functioning means that most patients who exceed the threshold criteria for diagnosis of anxiety disorders are likely to benefit from pharmacological or psychological interventions.[52] The need for treatment should be judged by ascertaining the severity and duration of symptoms, the impact on daily living, the presence and intensity of co-existing depressive symptoms, and other features such as a previous good response to medication or psychotherapy. The choice of treatment modality (pharmacological or psychological) should be influenced by clinical characteristics, patient preferences and the ready availability of potential interventions. Most clinical guidelines recommend an SSRI as the first-line pharmacological treatment across the range of anxiety disorders, whereas other antidepressant classes tend to be reserved for patients who do not respond to an SSRI or who tolerate it poorly (antidepressant drugs are considered elsewhere, see Chapter 3.3). There is no 'ideal' anxiolytic drug (Table 6.1.3): response rates to initial treatment are often disappointing, many patients experience unwanted side effects (such as drowsiness with benzodiazepines or pregabalin and sexual dysfunction with SSRIs), others will have a relapse of symptoms despite continuing with treatment, and some patients will be affected by troublesome discontinuation symptoms.

The overall efficacy of psychological and pharmacological approaches in the acute phase of treatment of anxiety disorders has been regarded as broadly similar, although this assumption has been questioned.[53] There is much overlap between the anxiety disorders for evidence-based effective therapies – such as prescription of an SSRI or a course of individual or group CBT – but there are some important differences between disorders in evidence-based treatments, such as the lack of evidence of efficacy for benzodiazepine anxiolytics in patients with OCD (Table 6.1.4). Depressive symptoms often accompany anxiety disorders: around one-third of people with anxiety disorders also meet diagnostic criteria for a depressive episode. Treatment of depression will

Table 6.1.3 Properties of the 'ideal' anxiolytic drug

Effectiveness considerations	*Acceptability considerations*
Effective across the full range of anxiety disorders	Once-daily dosage
Effective across the spectrum of symptom severity	Minimal adverse effects
Effective across age range	Minimal interference with everyday life
Effective in achieving remission in acute treatment	No development of tolerance
Effective in preventing relapse of symptoms	Safe in overdose
Rapid onset of action	Suitable in physically ill patients
Effective in treating co-existing depression	Free from interactions
Cost-effective	No discontinuation symptoms

Table 6.1.4 Pharmacokinetic parameters and prescribing correlates for some benzodiazepines

Compound	Bioavailability	Time to peak level (hrs)	Biological half-life (hrs)	Dosage and use(s)	Onset of effect
Midazolam	96% (IM route)	1.5–2.5	1.5–2.5	Single dose, sedation prior to anaesthesia	Very fast
Temazepam	96%	2–3	8–20	Night-time sleep induction	Fast
Flunitrazepam	64–77%	1–2	18–26	Night-time sleep induction	Fast
Lorazepam	85%	2	10–20	As required, panic attack	Fast
Alprazolam	80–90%	1–2	4–6 (IR) 10–16 (XR)	3 times daily, anxiolysis	Intermediate
Diazepam	76%	0.5–1.5	20–100	Twice daily, anxiolysis, management of alcohol withdrawal	Intermediate
Oxazepam	95%	1.5–3.0	6–9	3–4 times daily, anxiolysis	Intermediate–slow
Chlordiazepoxide	~100%	~4	5–30	3 times daily, anxiolysis, management of alcohol withdrawal	Slow
Clonazepam	90%	1–8	19–60	Once daily, anxiolysis, anticonvulsant	Intermediate–slow, but sustained

usually reduce anxiety symptoms when depression is the primary diagnosis. However, if an anxiety disorder is comorbid with (secondary) depression, each condition requires separate consideration and treatment – for example, a benzodiazepine anxiolytic prescribed for a patient with GAD may not relieve accompanying depressive symptoms, and CBT targeted against panic attacks and agoraphobic avoidance may not improve low mood.[52]

The strongest evidence for acute treatment of patients with anxiety disorders is for judicious prescription of an SSRI or by undertaking manualised CBT delivered by trained, supervised staff; in some disorders, it is uncertain whether combining these approaches is associated with greater improvement than with either treatment when given alone. SSRIs are considered in more detail elsewhere (Chapter 3.3). Continuation treatment that follows a satisfactory response to acute treatment (ideally resulting in remission of symptoms) is recommended for all patients with anxiety disorders, to consolidate the response and reduce the likelihood of relapse. It has been argued that psychological treatments may be more effective than pharmacological treatments in keeping patients well, but there is clear evidence that 'antidepressants' are highly effective in preventing relapse of symptoms in long-term treatment of patients with anxiety disorders.[54]

Current recommendations for pharmacological treatment are derived mainly from the findings of randomised double-blind placebo-controlled trials, which demonstrate robust efficacy and reasonable tolerability for many interventions, both in acute treatment and in preventing relapse. However, patients who participate in randomised controlled trials may have a better prognosis than patients treated in 'real-world' clinical settings, where the effects of treatment can often be disappointing. It is not currently possible to predict the likelihood of response for a given patient with great accuracy, and there are uncertainties about next steps in further management after non-response to first-line treatment approaches. Attempts to optimise clinical outcomes rest on making best use of available treatments, but there is much room for improvement. Improved outcomes could result from additional anxiolytic medications with novel mechanisms of action, leading to greater efficacy and improved acceptability in all patient groups; alternatively, novel treatments might lead to enhanced effectiveness and acceptability in specific patient subgroups, when combined with the use of reliable biomarkers for identifying which individuals are most likely to benefit.[55]

Benzodiazepine Anxiolytics

Benzodiazepines can be grouped according to chemical structure and pharmacokinetic properties, but they all share a common mechanism of action and produce a range of similar effects. Beneficial effects include the reduction of anxiety, the induction and maintenance of sleep, the relaxation of muscles, and the treatment and prevention of epileptic seizures. These properties are shared by most benzodiazepines to varying degrees, depending on their potency and pharmacokinetic profile. They also have a range of untoward adverse effects that may outweigh benefits in many patients, limiting their use in clinical practice. The balance of risk and benefit remains disputed and undergoes periodic reconsideration.[56,57]

Benzodiazepines enhance the effects of the major inhibitory neurotransmitter γ-aminobutyric acid (GABA), the endogenous ligand at $GABA_A$ receptors (ligand-gated chloride and bicarbonate ion channel complexes, comprising five transmembrane glycoprotein sub-units arranged around a central transmembrane channel) and at $GABA_B$ receptors (G-protein-coupled metabotropic receptors that stimulate the opening of inward-rectifying potassium channels). Benzodiazepines act as 'positive allosteric modulators' at $GABA_A$ receptors, resulting in anticonvulsant, anxiolytic, hypnotic and myorelaxant effects, but they have no effects on $GABA_B$ receptors, where baclofen and gamma hydroxybutyrate (GHB) are agonists. Each $GABA_A$ receptor contains two α sub-units, two ß sub-units and either a γ or δ sub-unit – differing sub-units are combined to produce a variety of receptor subtypes, with distinct distributions and specific pharmacological properties. Binding of a benzodiazepine to its site increases the affinity of the receptor for GABA, increasing the likelihood of the receptor 'opening' to allow the passage of chloride ions through the membrane; this influx normally results in neuronal hyperpolarisation and reduced 'excitability' of the target cell. Anxiolytic effects of benzodiazepines are thought to be mediated through α2 and α3 sub-units, sedative effects through the α1 sub-unit, and amnestic effects through the α5 sub-unit, which suggests α2/α3 subtype selective ligands might have beneficial anxiolytic effects whilst avoiding the problems of non-selective agents.

Benzodiazepines differ in potency, time to effect and duration of action, as well as the degree of lipophilicity and volume of distribution; some need repeated daily dosing, but others only need once-daily dosing to achieve desired effects (see Table 6.1.4). Many benzodiazepines (for example, diazepam) have long-lasting active metabolites, which can accumulate with repeated dosing – especially in elderly patients and those with liver disease, or in those with genetic variants leading to low or absent activity of relevant cytochrome P450 enzymes. With the exception of the 3-hydroxy-substituted benzodiazepines (lorazepam, oxazepam and temazepam) – which are conjugated with glucuronic acid) – all benzodiazepines undergo extensive hepatic metabolism, so medications that act as either inducers or inhibitors of hepatic enzymes can cause potentially clinically significant changes in plasma levels. For example, the SSRIs fluoxetine and fluvoxamine can impair the elimination of alprazolam and diazepam, presumably through inhibition of metabolism via CYP2C19 (diazepam) and CYP3A4 (both).[58]

Randomised controlled trials demonstrate efficacy of some benzodiazepines in some anxiety disorders, usually in acute treatment for reducing anxiety symptom severity and sometimes in long-term treatment for preventing relapse. There is good evidence for efficacy in the acute treatment of GAD, social anxiety disorder and panic disorder, but there is limited evidence for efficacy in OCD and PTSD.[52] There have been few direct comparisons of benzodiazepines with other medications, but benzodiazepines may have marginally superior efficacy in acute treatment in GAD, when compared to SSRIs and SNRIs.[59] Because of tolerability concerns (see later), most guidance suggests that alternatives should be preferred over benzodiazepines, which are generally reserved for patients who do not respond to a series of other treatments. Benzodiazepines have limited antidepressant effects, which is troublesome in anxious patients who are often also markedly depressed.

Benzodiazepine administration can result in dose-dependent sedation and drowsiness, mental slowing and anterograde amnesia (difficulty in forming new memories); somnolence typically becomes less prominent with continued use, though memory problems tend to persist. Stopping treatment with benzodiazepines is often associated with some improvement in cognitive performance.[60] Benzodiazepine administration can also cause a dose-dependent impairment in driving performance, which potentiates detriments due to alcohol consumption. Epidemiological studies suggest benzodiazepine use is associated with increased risk of road traffic accidents, above that seen with untreated mental disorders. Elderly patients are more vulnerable to adverse cognitive and psychomotor effects and eliminate drugs slower than younger patients, so an increased risk of falls should be considered before benzodiazepines are prescribed.

Tolerance to the effects of benzodiazepines can occur and is probably more pronounced for the anticonvulsant and hypnotic-sedative effects than for the anxiolytic effects; it is unusual for patients with anxiety disorders to incrementally increase their daily consumption. Tolerance may arise through multiple poorly understood mechanisms, including $GABA_A$ receptor uncoupling (whereby benzodiazepines exhibit decreased ability to facilitate GABA-induced ion flux), modifications in $GABA_A$ sub-unit expression, and compensatory glutamatergic, monoaminergic and neurosteroidal influences.[61] Dependence on benzodiazepines is usually recognised following the emergence of withdrawal symptoms on either abruptly stopping or rapidly reducing long-term treatment. The neural basis of habit-forming properties of benzodiazepines is not fully understood, but they increase the firing of dopaminergic neurones in the ventral tegmental area through effects on α1 sub-unit-containing $GABA_A$ receptors on nearby interneurons; this triggers the drug-evoked synaptic plasticity in excitatory afferents onto dopaminergic neurones and underlies drug reinforcement. Mechanisms underlying the experience of withdrawal symptoms are also not fully established, although down-regulation of benzodiazepine binding sites as well as increased calcium ion flux and serotonergic activity may be relevant.[61]

A broad range of physical and psychological withdrawal symptoms has been described (see Table 6.1.5); these are sometimes hard to distinguish from symptoms of underlying anxiety disorders, but perceptual disturbances (such as the sensation of 'tilting') are infrequent in untreated patients with anxiety disorders. Differential diagnoses reflect the presented clinical features, so they can include alcohol and drug intoxication or withdrawal, hypoglycaemia, cerebrovascular events and epilepsy. Withdrawal phenomena are usually short-lived (lasting less than four weeks) although their duration is influenced by individual pharmacokinetic factors, and some people describe markedly distressing symptoms long after stopping benzodiazepines.[62]

Possible risk factors for the development of benzodiazepine dependence include starting benzodiazepines at a younger age, lower length of education, minority ethnic group status, higher levels of anxiety and depressive symptoms, a history of alcohol or drug dependence, higher daily dosage, longer

Table 6.1.5 Clinical features reported or observed after benzodiazepine withdrawal[61]

Psychological symptoms	Physical symptoms	Complications
Increased anxiety	Trembling	Increased risk of seizures
Nervousness	Sweating	Poor motor coordination
Sleep disorders	Nausea and vomiting	Cognitive impairment
Inner restlessness	Motor agitation	Impairment of memory
Depressive symptoms	Dyspnoea	Perceptual impairments
Irritability	Increased heart rate	Hyperacusis
Psychosis-like conditions	Elevated blood pressure	Photophobia
Depersonalisation, derealisation	Headaches	Hypersomnia
Confusion	Muscle tension	Dysaesthesia and dyskinesia

Table 6.1.6 Principles of clinical management in benzodiazepine dependence and withdrawal[61]

1 Prevention
- *Primary*: avoidance of benzodiazepines, identification and treatment of psychological illness, awareness of at-risk patient groups, sensitivity to patient concerns about medication, restriction of benzodiazepine prescriptions to short-term treatment
- *Secondary*: restriction on automatic renewal of benzodiazepine prescriptions, practice-based clinical audits focused on prescribing practice, implementation of practice-based alerting systems to prompt discussion between prescribers and dispensers
- *Tertiary*: familiarity with and implementation of treatment withdrawal protocols, support of patients before, during and after withdrawal

2. Medication consolidation and gradual dose reduction
- Conversion of benzodiazepine polypharmacy to monotherapy, inpatient admission for very high dose users, dosage tapering at mutually agreed rate, avoidance of very prolonged reductions, avoidance of simultaneous withdrawal from benzodiazepines and opioids

3. Accompanying psychological interventions
- Techniques based on psychoeducation, motivational interviewing and instillation of confidence and optimism, CBT to support withdrawal and maintain abstinence as well as psychological treatment of underlying conditions

4. Concomitant psychotropic drug prescriptions
- Pharmacological treatment of underlying conditions such as major depressive disorder and generalised anxiety disorder, medication for facilitating abstinence in alcohol use disorder, occasional use of short-term administration to facilitate withdrawal, rare use of flumazenil in specialist services

5. Relapse prevention
- Approaches to managing persistent insomnia, continued treatment of underlying conditions, support in reducing alcohol consumption, attempts to address risk factors such as interpersonal discord, precarious employment and housing problems

duration of benzodiazepine use, shorter drug half-life, participation in self-help groups for medication dependence, and concomitant prescription of other psychotropic drugs. Other features such as a perceived 'reliance' on benzodiazepines to perform daily activities, continued use beyond the original treatment indication, taking of extra tablets before anticipated stressful events, 'doctor shopping', private prescriptions and reports of lost prescriptions may also be relevant. Problems with benzodiazepines may be perpetuated by a lack of knowledge of side effects and absence of psychosocial support, but they could be ameliorated by education about medication, an increased range of alternative forms of care, and targeted extended dialogue between patients and clinicians.[63]

Key aspects of clinical management of benzodiazepine dependence are summarised in Table 6.1.6.[61] *Primary prevention* emphasises limiting benzodiazepine anxiolytic or hypnotic prescriptions to short-term treatment and exercising considerable caution when considering prescriptions for older patients. Physicians may underestimate the importance of factors that can be helpful in avoiding inappropriate prescribing, such as patients' concerns about potential side effects and dislike of taking multiple medications. *Secondary prevention* includes systemic approaches to reducing the renewal of prescriptions, regular practice-based auditing and implementation of alerting systems to prompt discussions between prescribing physicians and dispensing pharmacists. *Tertiary prevention* focuses on tapering approaches and support of patients before, during and after withdrawal.

In patients with established dependence, benzodiazepines should be withdrawn gradually to minimise withdrawal symptoms – ideally, at a rate based on the ability of the patient to tolerate emerging symptoms. Recommendations on the pace of dosage reduction range widely, from reducing the initial benzodiazepine dose by 50 per cent approximately every week to reducing the daily dose by between 10 and 25 per cent every two weeks.[61] Brief psychological interventions may enhance the efficacy of gradual dose reduction. It is uncertain whether switching from a shorter-acting drug (such as lorazepam) to a longer-acting drug (such as diazepam or clonazepam) is advantageous, though patients who are taking multiple benzodiazepines should whenever possible be 'converted' to taking a single drug first. Approximate dosage equivalents are available (Table 6.1.7), but there is much variation between individuals in drug metabolism. Inpatient admission may be needed for the initial stages of withdrawal in patients taking very high doses (equivalent to 100 mg/day of diazepam, or greater).

Certain medications have been evaluated to ascertain whether they exert beneficial effects in easing benzodiazepine withdrawal, but the evidence of benefit is limited. Substitute pharmacotherapies given alone appear inferior to gradual dose reduction and, in combination, probably do not enhance its efficacy.[64] Subcutaneous or slow intravenous infusion of the $GABA_A$ receptor antagonist/partial agonist flumazenil has been found helpful in some patients, although its use can precipitate panic-like symptoms, seizures and psychosis-like

Table 6.1.7 Approximate dosages of common benzodiazepines and Z-drugs equivalent to 5 mg of diazepam

Drug	Dose
Chlordiazepoxide	12.5–15 mg
Clonazepam	0.25–1.0 mg
Loprazolam	0.5–1.0 mg
Lorazepam	0.5 mg
Lormetazepam	0.5–1.0 mg
Nitrazepam	5 mg
Oxazepam	10–15 mg
Temazepam	10 mg
Zaleplon	10 mg
Zopiclone	7.5 mg
Zolpidem	10 mg

experiences.[65] Psychological interventions are aimed at facilitating withdrawal, supporting subsequent abstinence and addressing any underlying disorders. CBT is used widely, although supporting evidence appears rather limited. Simple brief interventions (such as providing advice and information leaflets) can facilitate an initial reduction in benzodiazepine use but should probably be accompanied by other psychosocial interventions.[66]

Gabapentinoids

Gabapentinoids are medications used in a range of neurological or psychiatric conditions – some (gabapentin, pregabalin) have widespread clinical use. Gabapentin and pregabalin have analgesic, anticonvulsant and anxiolytic effects, but only pregabalin has a licence for treating patients with GAD. In the United Kingdom, at least half of all gabapentinoid prescriptions may be 'off-label', and concerns regarding widespread non-prescribed use has led to the reclassification of gabapentin and pregabalin as Class C controlled substances with accompanying regulations regarding prescriptions in April 2019.

The gabapentinoids are substituted derivatives of GABA and share the property of blocking α2δ-sub-unit-containing voltage-gated calcium channels within the CNS, most prominently after prolonged administration[67] – their molecular pharmacological mechanisms are complex.[68] Although gabapentin is a structural analogue of GABA, it does not bind to GABA receptors, convert into GABA or another GABA receptor agonist, or modulate GABA transport or metabolism. Furthermore, it is not a direct calcium channel blocker; it disrupts the regulatory functions of α2δ sub-units and their interactions with other proteins. Pregabalin shows high affinity binding to Type 1 and Type 2 proteins of the α2δ sub-unit of P/Q type voltage-gated calcium channels; it does not bind directly to $GABA_A$ or $GABA_B$ receptors or to sites allosterically linked to GABA but increases the density of GABA transporter proteins and extracellular GABA through a dose-dependent increase in L-glutamic acid decarboxylase activity. Through effects on calcium channels, pregabalin reduces glutamate release and may reduce synthesis of excitatory synapses and block 'trafficking' of new voltage-gated calcium channels to the cell surface. After oral administration, gabapentin exhibits non-linear kinetics, due to a saturatable transport mechanism in intestinal absorption, with decreased bioavailability at higher dosages. By contrast, pregabalin absorption is dependent upon active transport and is linear, with proportional increases in plasma levels across the dose range, maximal levels occurring within 60 minutes. Pharmacokinetic interactions with gabapentin and pregabalin are unlikely as they are not bound to plasma proteins and undergo negligible metabolism, approximately 98 per cent of the drugs being excreted unchanged in urine.

Gabapentin is often prescribed to patients with anxiety symptoms but appears to have only limited benefits in small studies involving patients with social anxiety disorder or panic disorder.[69,70] Pregabalin can be effective in patients with GAD, with similar effects in reducing psychological and physical symptoms of anxiety and reductions in the severity of sleep disturbance and co-existing depressive symptoms. However, adverse effects are common during short-term and long-term treatment.[71] Augmentation with pregabalin can be beneficial in reducing anxiety symptoms after an initial partial response of patients with GAD to SSRIs or SNRIs, and pregabalin monotherapy has been found efficacious in acute treatment and relapse prevention in social anxiety disorder.[52] It can reduce withdrawal symptoms from benzodiazepines and zolpidem and facilitate abstinence in previously alcohol-dependent patients.[72]

The most frequent adverse effects of gabapentin treatment are dizziness and drowsiness; fatigue, unsteadiness, nystagmus and peripheral oedema also occur commonly, and respiratory depression can occur when gabapentin is taken with opioids or benzodiazepines, or when used in patients with underlying respiratory illness. The most commonly reported adverse effects with pregabalin are dizziness and drowsiness (both occurring in approximately 30 per cent of patients with GAD); less common side effects including visual disturbances, unsteadiness and clumsiness.[71] Weight gain occurs in approximately 4 per cent of patients undergoing long-term treatment, and peripheral oedema is also reported (in up to 3 per cent of treated patients) but does not appear to be associated with hypertension, congestive heart failure or declining renal or hepatic function. There are potential pharmacodynamic interactions with other CNS depressants, and pregabalin overdose can be hazardous when combined with alcohol, benzodiazepines or opioids.

Gabapentin and pregabalin have addictive potential and the risk of misuse.[73] A systematic review indicates gabapentin can be taken for recreation, 'self-medication' or intentional self harm; patients with current or previous opioid misuse are at particular risk.[74] For pregabalin, the findings of pre-clinical

Table 6.1.8 Principles of clinical management of non-prescribed use of gabapentinoids

• Remember that gabapentinoid medicines have the potential for non-prescribed use
• Maintain awareness of clinical risk factors associated with potential hazards including non-prescribed use
• Avoid prescribing gabapentinoids to patients with current or previous alcohol or substance use disorders
• Warn patients about potential hazards before and during gabapentinoid treatment
• Follow local regulations about limiting treatment periods and stipulating the dosage of prescriptions
• Review patients regularly to determine whether there is a persistent need for continued treatment
• Monitor patients carefully but sensitively for signs of dependence and indicators of non-prescribed use
• Support patients who develop problems whilst reducing and withdrawing treatment
• Refer to colleagues with greater expertise in management of non-prescribed use if initial approaches prove unhelpful

investigations are inconsistent. It may have direct and indirect effects on the reward system and so possess the potential for abuse. However, it also attenuates opiate withdrawal symptoms, reduces alcohol consumption in animal models of opiate and alcohol dependence, and has been found helpful in facilitating withdrawal from alcohol, benzodiazepines, nicotine and zolpidem. 'Euphoria' (which was described in ~5 per cent of participants in early clinical trials with pregabalin for epilepsy) appears dose-dependent and seen across indications and has an uncertain course. Supra-therapeutic doses of pregabalin can result in a sense of contentment, enhanced empathy, increased sociability, dissociation and disinhibited behaviour, and non-prescribed use is reported, particularly in patients with a history of substance use disorders or after high dosages are prescribed.[75]

Non-prescribed use of gabapentin is associated with increased risks of all-cause and drug-related hospitalisation, particularly if combined with opioids, and pregabalin prescriptions in patients undergoing opioid maintenance therapy increase all-cause mortality. The increased risk of death may result from greater respiratory depression, prolonged gastrointestinal transit increasing gabapentin concentration, and delayed onset of effect of gabapentinoids when compared to injected opioids. Non-prescribed use may also be associated with withdrawal syndromes, including anxiety, depression, headache, joint and muscle pains, lethargy, shivering and sweating. There are also reports of agitation, disorientation, irritability and seizures.[73] The principles of clinical management of non-prescribed use of gabapentinoids are intuitive[76] and summarised in Table 6.1.8.

Buspirone and Related Azapirone Medications

The azapirones include buspirone (an anxiolytic), gepirone (which may have efficacy in depression and certain forms of sexual dysfunction), ipsapirone (an investigational drug), perospirone (an antipsychotic, used in Japan) and tandospirone (used in China and Japan for anxiolytic and antidepressant effects). Only buspirone has entered widespread clinical use in multiple countries: it is licensed for short-term treatment of anxiety in the United Kingdom and short- and long-term treatment of anxiety disorders in the United States. Mainly used in the treatment of GAD, it may be most beneficial when patients have not previously been treated with benzodiazepines.[77] It can augment the response to antidepressants in patients with social phobia and reduce symptoms of sexual dysfunction associated with SSRI treatment. The onset of effect is slower than with benzodiazepines, and buspirone is not helpful in reducing symptoms associated with withdrawal from alcohol, barbiturates or benzodiazepines.

The principal effects of buspirone probably derive from its 5-HT_{1A} agonist properties.[78] It is a high affinity full agonist at pre-synaptic 5-HT_{1A} inhibitory auto-receptors and a partial agonist at post-synaptic 5-HT_{1A} receptors. At low dosage, it blocks pre-synaptic D2 auto-receptors and enhances dopaminergic neurotransmission in the nigrostriatal pathway, but at higher dosage, it blocks post-synaptic D2 receptors. It also has high affinity as an antagonist at D3 and D4 receptors. It does not interact with the $GABA_A$ receptor complex, but some actions may be mediated by oxytocin release secondary to 5-HT_{1A} agonist effects. A metabolite [1-(2-pyrimidinyl)piperazine] is a potent terminal α2-adrenergic auto-receptor antagonist and may enhance noradrenergic activity and increase anxiety.

Extensive first-pass hepatic metabolism results in low bioavailability. Peak plasma levels occur within 90 minutes, but the elimination half-life is probably less than 11 hours. It should not be prescribed with monoamine oxidase inhibitors (MAOIs) or in patients with liver or kidney disease. Its metabolism (hydroxylation and methylation) is primarily through cytochrome CYP3A4, so plasma levels are increased by concomitant haloperidol prescription or by drinking grapefruit juice (both of which are CYP3A4 inhibitors) but are decreased by the CYP3A4 inducer carbamazepine.[58]

Although generally well tolerated, common problems include dizziness, headache, nausea and nervousness. Unlike benzodiazepines, buspirone does not cause sedation or psychomotor impairment. It appears to be safe in overdose, when taken alone. It does not cause euphoria, and there is no evidence of the development of tolerance or dependence. Studies in healthy volunteers indicate that buspirone lowers body temperature (through effects at 5-HT_{1A} pre-synaptic receptors) and increases plasma prolactin and growth hormone levels.

Beta Blockers (ß-blockers)

Although best known as 'cardiac drugs' for managing hypertension, correcting dysrhythmias and secondary prevention of myocardial malfunction, certain beta blockers (atenolol, propranolol) are still frequently used to reduce the severity of physical symptoms of anxiety, following the early discovery of their beneficial effects in reducing anxiety symptoms associated with hyperthyroidism.[79] However, despite traditional use of propranolol in reducing *physical* symptoms of anxiety, there is limited evidence of its efficacy in reducing *psychological* symptoms in patients with anxiety disorders.[80]

Beta blockers are competitive antagonists for epinephrine (adrenaline) and norepinephrine (noradrenaline) at three types of β-adrenergic receptors: β1 receptors are located mainly in the heart and kidneys; β2 receptors are mainly in the lungs, gastrointestinal tract, liver, uterus, vascular smooth muscle and skeletal muscle; and β3 receptors are in adipocytes. Some beta blockers block all types of receptors, whereas others are selective for certain receptors – the blockade of β-adrenergic receptors within the sympathetic branch of the autonomic nervous system reduces physical symptoms associated with the 'fight-or-flight' response. Some beta blockers (for example, oxprenolol) have intrinsic sympathomimetic activity (acting as partial agonists), which renders them unhelpful in managing patients with anxiety symptoms.

Propranolol (a non-selective β1- and β2- adrenergic receptor antagonist) is rapidly and completely absorbed, with peak plasma levels occurring within three hours of ingestion. Taking it with food increases its bioavailability, which is variable because of extensive first-pass hepatic metabolism. Being highly lipophilic, propranolol crosses the blood-brain barrier and can occur in high concentrations in the brain. Propranolol biotransformation is mediated mainly by CYP1A2 and CYP2C19, and co-administration of inhibitors of CYP2D6 (fluoxetine, paroxetine) can result in severe adverse events (severe bradycardia and atrioventricular block).[58] The main metabolite 4-hydroxypropranolol has a longer half-life (up to 7.5 hours) than the parent compound (3–4 hours) and is pharmacologically active. Atenolol (a selective β1-adrenergic receptor antagonist) is hydrophilic and so does not cross the blood-brain barrier. Pindolol (non-selective β1- and β2- antagonist, with intrinsic sympathomimetic activity) undergoes less first-pass metabolism but elimination is reduced in patients with renal disease; because of an additional antagonist effect at 5-HT_{1A} auto-receptors, it may advance the onset of action of some antidepressants.

Adverse effects of beta blockers include bronchospasm, dyspnoea, cold extremities, bradycardia, hypotension, heart failure, heart block and sexual dysfunction. Lipophilic compounds are more likely than hydrophilic compounds to cause insomnia and vivid dreams. Adverse effects associated with β2 receptor antagonist activity (bronchospasm, peripheral vasoconstriction, altered glucose and lipid metabolism) are less common with β1-selective agents. Hypoglycaemia can occur, as β2-adrenoceptors stimulate glycogen breakdown and pancreatic release of glucagon.

Generalised Anxiety Disorder

For all conditions, a summary of evidence for pharmacological and psychological interventions – with accompanying recommendations for treatment – has been provided by a consensus group from the World Federation of Societies of Biological Psychiatry; please refer to this for additional information, if required.[81]

Short-term pharmacological treatment (also known as 'acute phase pharmacotherapy'). First-line medications include some SSRIs (escitalopram, paroxetine and sertraline) and SNRIs (duloxetine, venlafaxine). Citalopram has been evaluated in a single study in elderly patients, where it was superior to placebo. The TCA imipramine is also effective but is probably less well tolerated than SSRIs and SNRIs. Trazodone has been found superior to placebo and similarly effective as imipramine and diazepam in a single RCT, but long-term studies have not been published. Pregabalin is efficacious in acute treatment studies, across patient subgroups, and reduces the likelihood of relapse[82] but is recommended as a second-line approach, due to its abuse potential. Some benzodiazepines (alprazolam, bromazepam, diazepam) are efficacious and, in meta-analysis, may have somewhat greater efficacy than SSRIs and SNRIs.[59] However, they are not recommended for routine use, due to tolerability and other concerns, and should probably be reserved for patients who have not responded to multiple previous treatments.[56]

Although efficacious in acute treatment (and in a relapse prevention study), the melatonin agonist/5-HT_{2C} antagonist agomelatine is only licensed for the treatment of depression. The 5-HT_{1A} agonist buspirone was found superior to placebo in six studies, although it was not significantly different to placebo in three studies; it appears less effective when compared to more established anxiolytics, and long-term studies have not been published. The multi-modal drug vortioxetine – which acts as a serotonin transporter (SERT) inhibitor, 5-HT_{1B} partial agonist, 5-HT_{1A} full agonist, and 5-HT_3 and 5-HT_7 antagonist – has been found efficacious in relapse prevention, but it has uncertain efficacy in acute treatment so is not currently recommended for routine use. The serotonin re-uptake inhibitor and 5-HT_{1A} partial agonist vilazodone – which is licensed for the treatment of major depression in Canada and the USA – has been found efficacious in three studies, but there are no published comparisons with reference drugs or long-term studies.

The antihistamine hydroxyzine has been found efficacious (although long-term studies have not been published), but daytime sedation can be troublesome. The second-generation antipsychotic quetiapine has also been found efficacious and is licensed for treatment of GAD in some countries, but tolerability problems such as weight gain and metabolic syndrome should make it reserved for patients who have not responded to other approaches. Other treatments that have been found efficacious in at least one acute treatment study include opipramol (a tricyclic anxiolytic, used widely in some European countries), the anticonvulsant valproate (which should not be used in women of reproductive potential)[83] and a lavender oil extract.

Long-term pharmacological treatment. GAD is generally regarded as a long-term condition that waxes and wanes in severity and typically requires long-term treatment. Guidelines recommend that after symptom remission, treatment should continue for at least six months in order to reduce the risk of relapse. In relapse prevention studies, escitalopram, paroxetine, venlafaxine, duloxetine, agomelatine, vortioxetine and pregabalin have all been found efficacious in preventing and delaying relapses. Benzodiazepines should only be used for long-term treatment when a series of other evidence-based approaches have not been found beneficial.

Medications after non-response. There have been rather few studies of further treatment after initial non-response, and only the addition of olanzapine or pregabalin to an SSRI have been found effective.

Psychological interventions. Whereas depression tends to relate to experiences of loss (see Chapter 3.3), anxiety symptoms usually relate to perceived threat to the self. Physical sensations, such as breathlessness or abdominal pain, may lead to negative thoughts – for example, worrying about or fear of serious illness, madness or even death. Life events, such as the death of a relative or the loss of a job, can be linked with negative thoughts of illness or poverty and to dysfunctional behaviour (e.g. reclusive isolation, excessive anger, alcohol consumption). CBT for GAD is quite practical and involves:[84,85]

- Collaborative education about anxiety and addressing misunderstandings about symptoms such as breathlessness, pain or palpitations
- Using techniques to deal with unhelpful thoughts (e.g. panic or excessive worry)
- Finding ways to tackle problems (e.g. paying bills, going to work or avoidance of social situations)

There may also be some underlying maladaptive assumptions that interfere with progress (e.g. low self-esteem or feelings of powerlessness), and these may need to be elicited, explored, understood and managed.

CBT has been found superior to being placed on a waiting list (as a control) but not consistently superior to active control treatment (i.e. comparisons other than waiting list); meta-analysis of studies with active controls indicates only a trend for a significant difference between CBT and control treatments, and a second meta-analysis found that whilst CBT exerted greater effects than being placed on a waiting list, it was not superior to psychological placebo.[86] Internet interventions based on CBT (iCBT) has also been found superior to placement on a waiting list, and an under-powered study found iCBT and face-to-face CBT to have broadly similar efficacy. Applied relaxation appears to have similar efficacy to being placed on a waiting list and to be less effective than CBT. Psychodynamic psychotherapy has unproven efficacy in GAD.

Only two studies have compared the combination of CBT with pharmacological treatment against either one given as monotherapy. One study found that combining CBT with diazepam was more effective than diazepam alone but not more effective than CBT alone; the other study found that combining CBT with venlafaxine was similar to venlafaxine monotherapy.

Exercise. A small study compared two forms of exercise (weight-lifting and cycling) to being placed on a waiting list in women undergoing pharmacological treatment, and it found that there were no significant differences between either the exercise condition and the waiting list control.[87]

Panic Disorder

Short-term pharmacological treatment. There is no evidence that psychotropic drugs are beneficial in reducing the duration and severity of a mild and short-lived panic attack, but short-acting benzodiazepines may sometimes be beneficial in patients experiencing longer-lasting and more severe panic attacks. SSRIs and the SNRI venlafaxine are first-line pharmacological treatments for panic disorder. The TCAs clomipramine and imipramine are probably as effective as SSRIs/SNRIs, but the frequency of adverse events is higher for TCAs, and only one placebo-controlled trial has been published for desipramine and lofepramine. The MAOI phenelzine has been evaluated in a single placebo-controlled trial, but because of potential severe interactions with dietary components or other medications, phenelzine should be reserved for patients who have not responded to other treatments. Studies with the reversible inhibitor of monoamine oxidase A (RIMA) moclobemide have produced inconsistent findings: two double-blind placebo-controlled studies found that it was not superior, but two adequately powered comparator-controlled studies found it to have similar beneficial effects to those with standard treatments. Trazodone, buspirone and propranolol do not appear effective, and only one under-powered comparison trial with mirtazapine has been published; however, the SNRI reboxetine was found efficacious in a small placebo-controlled study.[88]

TCAs and SSRIs do not appear to differ in their efficacy, although the rarely used tetracyclic maprotiline (a primarily noradrenergic antidepressant) proved inferior to the SSRI fluvoxamine. However, the adverse effect profile of TCAs and SSRIs differs; and in most comparisons, SSRIs are marginally better tolerated than TCAs. A study involving patients with comorbid panic disorder and major depressive disorder found that sertraline and imipramine were similarly effective, but sertraline was better tolerated and more acceptable. Comparisons among SSRIs do not reveal marked differences in efficacy, although escitalopram was superior to citalopram on some symptom domains in a placebo-controlled study.[89]

Benzodiazepine anxiolytics are effective but potentially addictive. The combination of benzodiazepines with an antidepressant (SSRIs, SNRIs or TCAs) can result in an earlier reduction in symptom severity, when compared to antidepressant monotherapy, but not with a greater likelihood of overall treatment response. In a study examining this combination, patients were treated with paroxetine and clonazepam or with paroxetine and placebo. Combined treatment with paroxetine and clonazepam resulted in more rapid response than with the SSRI alone, but there was no differential benefit beyond the initial few weeks of therapy.

Alprazolam has been compared to imipramine in a number of studies, and no differences were found in global improvement. There are no direct double-blind comparisons of SSRIs and benzodiazepines in panic disorder. An open comparison found that clonazepam had an earlier onset of effect and greater overall benefit than paroxetine, and clonazepam was better tolerated. A meta-analysis found that SSRIs were associated with more adverse effects than benzodiazepines in short-term treatment of panic disorder,[90] and a network meta-analysis (including 87 studies, 12 drug classes, and 12,800 participants) indicated that the balance of remission and adverse events is probably best with SSRIs. Among the SSRIs, escitalopram or sertraline may be preferable.[91]

Long-term pharmacological treatment. Panic disorder tends to persist for many years, with a fluctuating course. Treatment should continue for several months after symptom remission to reduce the likelihood of relapse. Double-blind placebo-controlled relapse prevention studies have shown that certain SSRIs (citalopram, fluoxetine, paroxetine, sertraline), venlafaxine, clomipramine, imipramine and the benzodiazepine alprazolam are all efficacious in reducing relapse (both the proportion of relapses and the time to relapse). Such studies also indicate that, after symptom remission with acute treatment, a further 6–12 months of treatment course is warranted. For SSRIs, the daily dosage in maintenance treatment should probably be the same as in short-term treatment, although an open study of maintenance treatment with imipramine suggests that halving the daily dosage does not increase the likelihood of relapse.[92]

Medications after non-response. If initial treatment proves ineffective after medication has been prescribed at the maximum tolerated daily dosage, patients can be advised to switch to another first-line treatment (for example, from an SSRI to an SNRI, or between SSRIs). If this approach also proves ineffective, second-line approaches can be considered. Lastly, drugs or drug combinations that were effective in open studies and case reports may be an option.[93]

Psychological interventions. CBT for panic disorder typically comprises exposure-based techniques to reduce agoraphobic avoidance as well as cognitive techniques including interoceptive exposure to counter anticipatory anxiety and panic attacks. CBT is the psychological intervention with the most substantial evidence but has been mainly compared against waiting list controls. When compared to active controls (including psychological placebo, pill placebo, relaxation and self-exposure), supporting evidence is less striking: meta-analysis indicates a significant but small effect.[81] A previous meta-analysis had indicated CBT had an average pre-post effect size similar to that of a pill placebo.[53] Despite concerns regarding methodology (including variable blinding), CBT-based interventions delivered remotely (iCBT) appear superior to waiting list controls and more effective than active control (relaxation) in one study, as well as similarly effective as individual CBT.[94] In meta-analysis of pre-to-post effect sizes, iCBT was marginally less effective than face-to-face CBT and less effective than medication.[94] The evidence for psychodynamic psychotherapy is limited and not encouraging. In one study, it was less effective than relaxation, and in most comparisons with CBT, psychodynamic psychotherapy was inferior. Applied relaxation (AR) appears superior to progressive muscle relaxation, but studies comparing AR with CBT or psychodynamic psychotherapy are inconclusive. Eye movement desensitisation and reprocessing (EMDR) does not appear effective in patients with panic disorder.

In most direct comparisons, CBT and medication have similar efficacy. However, some comparisons are underpowered and potentially unreliable. Most studies that compared psychotherapy (mostly CBT) and various medications found no significant difference between interventions. However, in five studies, medication was superior, and in two studies, CBT was superior. In investigations of combination treatment, most studies found that the combination of psychotherapy with medication was superior to psychotherapy alone. In studies without a control condition, patients with residual symptoms whilst on medication improved after CBT was introduced.

It is often stated that gains from CBT are maintained after treatment is stopped, whereas patients treated with medication have a relapse of symptoms after treatment is withdrawn. However, follow-up studies that compared the durability of effect of CBT or drug therapy do not show a clear advantage for CBT; in two studies, CBT had an advantage, one study found that medication was superior, and three studies found no significant differences between interventions. In a meta-analysis based on pre-to-post effect size differences in studies in which patients were followed up after treatment was ended, gains with CBT and other psychotherapies were maintained for up to 24 months, but medications (and placebo) also demonstrated enduring effects[95].

Several studies have examined whether D-cycloserine, which is a partial N-methyl-D-aspartate (NMDA) receptor agonist, might facilitate fear extinction and enhance exposure therapy (presumably by either enhancing NMDA receptor function during extinction or by reducing NMDA receptor function during fear memory consolidation). These studies have generated inconsistent findings, with the majority of studies finding no advantage for the combination.

Exercise. Two placebo-controlled studies have examined the value of exercise. The first compared running, clomipramine or a placebo and found exercise and clomipramine to be superior to placebo, although exercise was less effective than clomipramine. In the second, participants received either paroxetine or a placebo, combined with either exercise or relaxation training; paroxetine was superior to the placebo, but exercise was not superior to relaxation. These studies suggest exercise has some beneficial effects in panic disorder, but it should not be the sole treatment approach and should be combined with standard treatments (medication or CBT).

Separation Anxiety Disorder

Because of limited evidence, few recommendations can be made for adults with separation anxiety disorder. In children with the condition, two studies have found that CBT is superior to being placed on a waiting list, but comparisons with active controls are lacking. A double-blind placebo-controlled study in children who had not responded to CBT found that both the TCA imipramine and placebo lead to improvements, with no significant difference between groups. In adults with the condition, a small double-blind placebo-controlled trial found that vilazodone (which has both SSRI and 5-HT_{1A} agonist properties) was not superior to placebo.[96]

Social Anxiety Disorder

Short-term pharmacological treatment. The SSRIs escitalopram, fluvoxamine, paroxetine and sertraline are potential first-line medications. For citalopram, only one double-blind placebo-controlled study has been published, and the evidence for fluoxetine is inconclusive. The SNRI venlafaxine is another potential first-line medication, but the related compound desvenlafaxine was not found superior to placebo in one study. The calcium channel modulator pregabalin was found to be effective in two studies, but evidence for efficacy for gabapentin is limited to a single study.

The MAOI phenelzine can be effective in some patients. However, due to its adverse effect profile and interaction liability, it should probably be reserved for treating patients who have not responded to other interventions.[97] Findings with the RIMA moclobemide are inconsistent, as it was superior to placebo in some studies but did not separate from placebo in others; a meta-analysis of placebo-controlled studies of moclobemide found it to be significantly superior to placebo but with a small effect size.

The benzodiazepines bromazepam and clonazepam were each found effective in a single placebo-controlled study, but due to possible tolerability and safety concerns, they should only be used in carefully selected patients. The antidepressant mirtazapine was efficacious in one placebo-controlled study, as was the NMDA receptor antagonist ketamine (given intravenously) in a double-blind placebo-controlled study, but buspirone was not efficacious in a single double-blind placebo-controlled study, and the beta blocker atenolol was not superior to placebo in two such studies. For additional details, see Bandelow et al.[81]

Long-term pharmacological treatment. SAD is usually a long-lasting condition that typically requires prolonged treatment. Double-blind placebo-controlled relapse prevention studies have found escitalopram, paroxetine, sertraline, venlafaxine, phenelzine, pregabalin and moclobemide to all be more effective than placebo.[81]

Medications after non-response. In a double-blind placebo-controlled study, patients who had not responded to sertraline were randomised to continue with sertraline (plus placebo) or sertraline plus clonazepam or venlafaxine; there was a numerical advantage for clonazepam augmentation, when compared to continuing sertraline (plus placebo) or switching to venlafaxine, but the difference between clonazepam and placebo augmentation was not statistically significant, nor was the difference between sertraline plus placebo versus venlafaxine.[98]

Psychological interventions. Treatment with CBT is more effective than being placed on a waiting list, but in 14 comparisons with active control conditions, only two found a significant advantage for CBT. A meta-analysis of studies with active controls indicates a significant though small difference between CBT and active controls. Internet psychotherapeutic interventions based on CBT (iCBT) have been found superior to being placed on a waiting list in most studies and to be as effective as face-to-face CBT and more effective than relaxation. Virtual reality exposure therapy was found superior to being placed on a waiting list in some but not all studies; when compared to *in vivo* exposure in under-powered studies, findings have been inconsistent. Psychodynamic psychotherapy cannot be recommended as it was not found superior when compared to an active control and was inferior to CBT. CBT was found to be less effective than pharmacological treatment in one study, but data on combining CBT with pharmacological treatments are inconclusive. Some data arise from comparisons with drugs that are not first-line medications (e.g. phenelzine, moclobemide or clonazepam), although the combination of CBT with sertraline was not superior to either treatment, given as monotherapy. Adding psychodynamic psychotherapy to clonazepam was not superior to monotherapy with clonazepam. Evaluations of the potential of D-cycloserine for enhancing the effects of exposure therapy or CBT have produced inconsistent findings. For additional details, see Bandelow et al.[81]

Potential Developments in Anxiolytic Drugs

Existing pharmacological and psychological treatments for patients with anxiety disorders are not ideal, and a wide range of novel targets for potential anxiolytics is being explored.[99] Given the accumulating evidence that affective disorders are associated with peripheral and neuroinflammation, there appears to be some scope for 'repurposing' existing anti-inflammatory agents, possibly as monotherapy or more probably as an augmentation approach whilst patients continue other treatments. The anxiety response to CO_2 challenge appears at least partly mediated by complex chemosensory systems involving pH-sensitive ion channels, known as 'acid-sensing ion channels' (ASICs), and one particular receptor (ASIC1a) is involved in cued and contextual fear conditioning and may help to prevent suffocation by inducing active defence responses.[21,100,101] This suggests that ASIC-1A receptor antagonists could have anxiolytic potential.[101] Orexin receptor antagonists can attenuate anxiety-like behaviour in animals,[102] and increasing availability of drugs with this pharmacological property for clinical use opens the possibility for exploring their anxiolytic effects in experimental medicine models of anxiety.[103] Selective ligands targeted at specific $GABA_A$ sub-units (the α-2 and α-3 sub-units) may prove to have anxiolytic effects, with a lower liability for sedation, tolerance and dependence.[104] Finally, there is much interest in the potential anxiety-reducing effects of cannabinoid and psychedelic agents – based on rather limited evidence[105,106] – but more robust evidence of efficacy, tolerability and safety from large-scale randomised placebo-controlled trials is needed before such compounds could be incorporated into routine clinical practice.

References

1. Penninx BW, Pine DS, Holmes EA, Reif A. Anxiety disorders. *Lancet* 2021;397: 914–27.
2. American Psychiatric Association. *Diagnostic and Statistical Manual of Mental Disorders*, 5th ed. Arlington, VA: APA; 2013.
3. Solis EC, van Hemert AM, Carlier IVE, et al. The 9-year clinical course of depressive and anxiety disorders: new NESDA findings. *Journal of Affective Disorders* 2021;295: 1269–79.
4. World Health Organization. *ICD-11: International Classification of Diseases*, 11th revision. Geneva: World Health Organization, 2019.
5. Ruscio AM, Hallion LS, Lim CCW, et al. Cross-sectional comparison of the epidemiology of DSM-5 generalized anxiety disorder across the globe. *JAMA Psychiatry* 2017;74(5):465–75.
6. Culpepper L. Generalized anxiety disorder and medical illness. *Journal of Clinical Psychiatry* 2009;70(Suppl 2):20–4.
7. Kessler RC, Chiu WT, Jin R, et al. The epidemiology of panic attacks, panic disorder, and agoraphobia in the National Comorbidity Survey Replication. *Archives of General Psychiatry* 2006;63(4):415–24.
8. de Jonge P, Roest AM, Lim CC, et al. Cross-national epidemiology of panic disorder and panic attacks in the world mental health surveys. *Depression and Anxiety* 2016;33(12):1155–77.
9. Alonso J, Mortier P, Auerbach RP, et al. Severe role impairment associated with mental disorders: results of the WHO World Mental Health Surveys International College Student Project. *Depression and Anxiety* 2018;35 (9):802–14.
10. Albert CM, Chae CU, Rexrode KM, et al. Phobic anxiety and risk of coronary heart disease and sudden cardiac death among women. *Circulation* 2005;111(4):480–7.
11. Stein DJ, Lim CCW, Roest AM, et al. The cross-national epidemiology of social anxiety disorder: data from the World Mental Health Survey Initiative. *BMC Medicine* 2017;15(1):143.
12. Shear K, Jin R, Ruscio AM, et al. Prevalence and correlates of estimated DSM-IV child and adult separation anxiety disorder in the National Comorbidity Survey Replication. *American Journal of Psychiatry* 2006;163(6):1074–83.
13. Silove D, Alonso J, Bromet E, et al. Pediatric-onset and adult-onset separation anxiety disorder across countries in the World Mental Health Survey. *American Journal of Psychiatry* 2015;172(7):647–56.
14. Solmi M, Radua J, Olivola M, et al. Age at onset of mental disorders worldwide: large-scale meta-analysis of 192 epidemiological studies. *Molecular Psychiatry* 2022;27(1):281–95.
15. Gottschalk MG, Domschke K. Genetics of generalized anxiety disorder and related traits. *Dialogues in Clinical Neuroscience* 2017;19(2):159–68.
16. Safren SA, Gershuny BS, Marzol P, et al. History of childhood abuse in panic disorder, social phobia, and generalized anxiety disorder. *Journal of Nervous and Mental Disease* 2002;190 (7):453–6.
17. Bandoli G, Campbell-Sills L, Kessler RC, et al. Childhood adversity, adult stress, and the risk of major depression or generalized anxiety disorder in US soldiers: a test of the stress sensitization hypothesis. *Psychological Medicine* 2017;47(13):2379–92.
18. Koerner K, McEvoy P, et al. Cognitive-behavioral models of generalized anxiety disorder (GAD): towards a synthesis. In: Gerlach AL, Gloster AT (eds.) *Generalized Anxiety Disorder and Worrying: A Comprehensive Handbook for Clinicians and Researchers.* Hoboken, NJ: John Wiley & Sons; 2021: 117–50.
19. Goodwin H, Yiend J, Hirsch CR. Generalized anxiety disorder, worry and attention to threat: a systematic review. *Clinical Psychology Review* 2017;54:107–22.
20. Sutherland-Stolting A, Liao B, Kraus K, et al. Pathogenesis of generalized anxiety disorder. In: Simon NM, Hollander E, Rothbaum BO, Stein DJ (eds) *Textbook of Anxiety, Trauma and OCD-Related Disorders* (third edition). Washington, D.C.: American Psychiatric Association Publishing; 2020:181–96.
21. Wemmie JA, Taugher RJ, Kreple CJ. Acid-sensing ion channels in pain and disease. *Nature Reviews. Neuroscience* 2013;14(7):461–71.
22. Costello H, Gould RL, Abrol E, et al. Systematic review and meta-analysis of the association between peripheral inflammatory cytokines and generalised anxiety disorder. *BMJ Open* 2019;9(7): e027925.
23. Schienle A, Wabnegger A. Structural and functional neuroanatomy of generalized anxiety disorder. In: Gerlach AL, Gloster AT (eds.) *Generalized Anxiety Disorder and Worrying: A Comprehensive Handbook for Clinicians and Researchers.* Hoboken, NJ: John Wiley & Sons; 2021: 151–71.
24. Goossen B, van der Starre J, van der Heiden C. A review of neuroimaging studies in generalized anxiety disorder: "So where do we stand?". *Journal of Neural Transmission (Vienna)* 2019;126 (9):1203–16.
25. Webler RD, Coplan JD. Pathogenesis of panic disorder. In: Simon NM, Hollander E, Rothbaum BO, et al. (eds.) *Textbook of Anxiety, Trauma and OCD-Related Disorders*, 3rd ed. Washington, DC: American Psychiatric Association Publishing; 2020:373–84.
26. Zwanzger P, Domschke K, Bradwejn J. Neuronal network of panic disorder: the role of the neuropeptide cholecystokinin. *Depression and Anxiety* 2012;29(9):762–74.
27. Rehfeld JF. Cholecystokinin and panic disorder: reflections on the history and

some unsolved questions. *Molecules* 2021;26(18):5657.

28. Klein DF. False suffocation alarms, spontaneous panics, and related conditions. *An integrative hypothesis. Archives of General Psychiatry* 1993;50 (4):306–17.
29. Feinstein JS, Gould D, Khalsa SS. Amygdala-driven apnea and the chemoreceptive origin of anxiety. *Biological Psychology* 2022;170:108305.
30. Dresler T, Guhn A, Tupak SV, et al. Revise the revised? New dimensions of the neuroanatomical hypothesis of panic disorder. *Journal of Neural Transmission (Vienna)* 2013;120 (1):3–29.
31. Menon V. Large-scale brain networks and psychopathology: a unifying triple network model. *Trends in Cognitive Sciences* 2011;15(10):483–506.
32. Manfro GG, Otto MW, McArdle ET, et al. Relationship of antecedent stressful life events to childhood and family history of anxiety and the course of panic disorder. *Journal of Affective Disorders* 1996;41(2):135–9.
33. Lissek S. Toward an account of clinical anxiety predicated on basic, neurally mapped mechanisms of Pavlovian fear-learning: the case for conditioned overgeneralization. *Depression and Anxiety* 2012;29(4):257–63.
34. Bas-Hoogendam J, Roelofs E, Westenberg P, et al. Pathogenesis of social anxiety disorder. In: Simon N, Hollander E, Rothbaum BO, et al. (eds.) *Textbook of Anxiety, Trauma, and OCD-related Disorders*. Washington, DC: The American Psychiatric Association Publishing; 2020: 429–44.
35. Scaini S, Belotti R, Ogliari A. Genetic and environmental contributions to social anxiety across different ages: a meta-analytic approach to twin data. *Journal of Anxiety Disorders* 2014;28 (7):650–6.
36. Neumann ID, Slattery DA. Oxytocin in general anxiety and social fear: a translational approach. *Biological Psychiatry* 2016;79(3):213–21.
37. Bandelow B, Baldwin D, Abelli M, et al. Biological markers for anxiety disorders, OCD and PTSD: a consensus statement. Part II: Neurochemistry, neurophysiology and neurocognition. *The World Journal of Biological Psychiatry* 2017;18(3):162–214.
38. Bruehl AB, Delsignore A, Komossa K, et al. Neuroimaging in social anxiety disorder – a meta-analytic review resulting in a new neurofunctional model. *Neuroscience & Biobehavioral Reviews* 2014;47:260–80.
39. Wong QJJ, Rapee RM. The aetiology and maintenance of social anxiety disorder: a synthesis of complimentary theoretical models and formulation of a new integrated model. *Journal of Affective Disorders* 2016;203: 84–100.
40. Scaini S, Ogliari A, Eley TC, et al. Genetic and environmental contributions to separation anxiety: a meta-analytic approach to twin data. *Depression and Anxiety* 2012;29 (9):754–61.
41. Bartholomew K, Horowitz LM. Attachment styles among young adults: a test of a four-category model. *Journal of Personality and Social Psychology* 1991;61(2):226–44.
42. Greenberg MT. Attachment and psychopathology in childhood. In: Cassidy J, Shaver PR (eds.) *Handbook of Attachment: Theory, Research, and Clinical Applications*. New York: Guilford Press; 1999: 469–96.
43. Pini S, Abelli M, Troisi A, et al. The relationships among separation anxiety disorder, adult attachment style and agoraphobia in patients with panic disorder. *Journal of Anxiety Disorders* 2014;28(8):741–6.
44. Pini S, Abelli M, Costa B, et al. Relationship of behavioral inhibition to separation anxiety in a sample (N = 377) of adult individuals with mood and anxiety disorders. *Comprehensive Psychiatry* 2022;116:152326.
45. Boelen PA, Reijntjes A, Carleton RN. Intolerance of uncertainty and adult separation anxiety. *Cognitive Behaviour Therapy* 2014;43(2):133–44.
46. Atlı O, Bayın M, Alkın T. Hypersensitivity to 35% carbon dioxide in patients with adult separation anxiety disorder. *Journal of Affective Disorders* 2012;141(2–3):315–23.
47. Roberson-Nay R, Eaves LJ, Hettema JM, et al. Childhood separation anxiety disorder and adult onset panic attacks share a common genetic diathesis. *Depression and Anxiety* 2012;29 (4):320–7.
48. Crockford C, Deschner T, Ziegler TE, et al. Endogenous peripheral oxytocin measures can give insight into the dynamics of social relationships: a review. *Frontiers in Behavioural Neuroscience* 2014;8:68.
49. Lebowitz ER, Leckman JF, Feldman R, et al. Salivary oxytocin in clinically anxious youth: associations with separation anxiety and family accommodation. *Psychoneuroendocrinology* 2016;65:35–43.
50. Costa B, Pini S, Martini C, et al. Mutation analysis of oxytocin gene in individuals with adult separation anxiety. *Psychiatry Research* 2009;168 (2):87–93.
51. Gordon I, Zagoory-Sharon O, Schneiderman I, et al. Oxytocin and cortisol in romantically unattached young adults: associations with bonding and psychological distress. *Psychophysiology* 2008;45(3):349–52.
52. Baldwin DS, Anderson IM, Nutt DJ, et al. Evidence-based pharmacological treatment of anxiety disorders, post-traumatic stress disorder and obsessive-compulsive disorder: a revision of the 2005 guidelines from the British Association for Psychopharmacology. *Journal of Psychopharmacology* 2014;28 (5):403–39.
53. Bandelow B, Reitt M, Röver C, et al. Efficacy of treatments for anxiety disorders: a meta-analysis. *International Clinical Psychopharmacology* 2015;30 (4):183–92.
54. Batelaan NM, Bosman RC, Muntingh A, et al. Risk of relapse after antidepressant discontinuation in anxiety disorders, obsessive-compulsive disorder, and post-traumatic stress disorder: systematic review and meta-analysis of relapse prevention trials. *BMJ* 2017;358:j3927.
55. Stein DJ, Craske MG, Rothbaum BO, et al. The clinical characterization of the adult patient with an anxiety or related disorder aimed at personalization of management. *World Psychiatry* 2021;20 (3):336–56.
56. Baldwin DS, Aitchison K, Bateson A, et al. Benzodiazepines: risks and benefits. A reconsideration. *Journal of Psychopharmacology* 2013;27 (11):967–71.
57. Silberman E, Balon R, Starcevic V, et al. Benzodiazepines: it's time to return to the evidence. *British Journal of Psychiatry* 2021;218(3):125–27.

58. Muscatello MR, Spina E, Bandelow B, et al. Clinically relevant drug interactions in anxiety disorders. *Human Psychopharmacology* 2012;27(3):239–53.

59. Gomez AF, Barthel AL, Hofmann SG. Comparing the efficacy of benzodiazepines and serotonergic anti-depressants for adults with generalized anxiety disorder: a meta-analytic review. *Expert Opinion on Pharmacotherapy* 2018;19(8):883–94.

60. Barker MJ, Greenwood KM, Jackson M, et al. Persistence of cognitive effects after withdrawal from long-term benzodiazepine use: a meta-analysis. *Archives of Clinical Neuropsychology* 2004;19(3):437–54.

61. Baldwin DS. Clinical management of withdrawal from benzodiazepine anxiolytic and hypnotic medications. *Addiction* 2022;117(5):1472–82.

62. Taylor S, Annand F, Burkinshaw P, et al. *Dependence and Withdrawal Associated with Some Prescribed Medicines*. London: Public Health England; 2019.

63. Sirdifield C, Chipchase SY, Owen S, et al. A systematic review and meta-synthesis of patients' experiences and perceptions of seeking and using benzodiazepines and Z-drugs: towards safer prescribing. *Patient* 2017;10(1):1–15.

64. Parr JM, Kavanagh DJ, Cahill L, et al. Effectiveness of current treatment approaches for benzodiazepine discontinuation: a meta-analysis. *Addiction* 2009;104(1):13–24.

65. Gallo AT, Hulse G. Pharmacological uses of flumazenil in benzodiazepine use disorders: a systematic review of limited data. *Journal of Psychopharmacology* 2021;35(3):211–20.

66. Mugunthan K, McGuire T, Glasziou P. Minimal interventions to decrease long-term use of benzodiazepines in primary care: a systematic review and meta-analysis. *British Journal of General Practice* 2011;61(590):e573–8.

67. Dolphin AC. Voltage-gated calcium channels and their auxiliary subunits: physiology and pathophysiology and pharmacology. *Journal of Physiology* 2016;594(19):5369–90.

68. Calandre EP, Rico-Villademoros F, Slim M. Alpha$_2$delta ligands, gabapentin, pregabalin and mirogabalin: a review of their clinical pharmacology and therapeutic use. *Expert Review of Neurotherapeutics* 2016;16(11): 1263–77.

69. Berlin RK, Butler PM, Perloff MD. Gabapentin therapy in psychiatric disorders: a systematic review. *Primary Care Companion for CNS Disorders* 2015;17(5).

70. Ahmed S, Bachu R, Kotapati P, et al. Use of gabapentin in the treatment of substance use and psychiatric disorders: a systematic review. *Frontiers in Psychiatry* 2019;10:228.

71. Baldwin DS, den Boer JA, Lyndon G, et al. Efficacy and safety of pregabalin in generalised anxiety disorder: a critical review of the literature. *Journal of Psychopharmacology* 2015;29 (10):1047–60.

72. Freynhagen R, Backonja M, Schug S, et al. Pregabalin for the treatment of drug and alcohol withdrawal symptoms: a comprehensive review. *CNS Drugs* 2016;30(12):1191–200.

73. Evoy KE, Sadrameli S, Contreras J, et al. Abuse and misuse of pregabalin and gabapentin: a systematic review Update. *Drugs* 2021;81(1):125–56.

74. Smith RV, Havens JR, Walsh SL. Gabapentin misuse, abuse and diversion: a systematic review. *Addiction* 2016;111(7): 1160–74.

75. Hägg S, Jönsson AK, Ahlner J. Current evidence on abuse and misuse of gabapentinoids. *Drug Safety* 2020;43 (12):1235–54.

76. Baldwin DS, Masdrakis V. Non-prescribed use of gabapentinoids: mechanisms, predisposing factors, associated hazards and clinical management. *European Neuropsychopharmacology: The Journal of the European College of Neuropsychopharmacology* 2022;63:6–8.

77. Chessick CA, Allen MH, Thase M, et al. Azapirones for generalized anxiety disorder. *Cochrane Database of Systematic Reviews* 2006;2006(3):CD006115.

78. Loane C, Politis M. Buspirone: what is it all about? *Brain Research* 2012;1461:111–8.

79. Turner P, Granville-Grossman KL. Effect of adrenergic receptor blockade of the tachycardia of thyrotoxicosis and anxiety state. *Lancet* 1965;2 (7426):1316–8.

80. Steenen SA, van Wijk AJ, van der Heijden GJ, et al. Propranolol for the treatment of anxiety disorders: systematic review and meta-analysis. *Journal of Psychopharmacology* 2016;30 (2):128–39.

81. Bandelow B, Allgulander C, Baldwin DS, et al. World Federation of Societies of Biological Psychiatry (WFSBP) guidelines for treatment of anxiety, obsessive-compulsive and posttraumatic stress disorders – Version 3. Part I: Anxiety disorders. *The World Journal of Biological Psychiatry* 2023;24 (2):79–117.

82. Feltner D, Wittchen HU, Kavoussi R, et al. Long-term efficacy of pregabalin in generalized anxiety disorder. *Internation Clinical Psychopharmacology* 2008;23(1):18–28.

83. Baldwin DS, Amaro HJF. Prescription of valproate-containing medicines in women of childbearing potential who have psychiatric disorders: is it worth the risk? *CNS Drugs* 2020;34(2):163–69.

84. Kennerley H. *Overcoming Anxiety: A Self-Help Guide Using Cognitive Behavioural Techniques*. London: Robinson; 2014.

85. Willson R, Branch R. *Cognitive Behavioural Therapy for Dummies*. Chichester: John Wiley & Sons; 2019.

86. Chen TR, Huang HC, Hsu JH, et al. Pharmacological and psychological interventions for generalized anxiety disorder in adults: a network meta-analysis. *Journal of Psychiatric Research* 2019;118:73–83.

87. Herring MP, Jacob ML, Suveg C, et al. Feasibility of exercise training for the short-term treatment of generalized anxiety disorder: a randomized controlled trial. *Psychotherapy and Psychosomatics* 2012;81(1):21–8.

88. Versiani M, Cassano G, Perugi G, et al. Reboxetine, a selective norepinephrine reuptake inhibitor, is an effective and well-tolerated treatment for panic disorder. *Journal of Clinical Psychiatry* 2002;63(1):31–7.

89. Bandelow B, Stein DJ, Dolberg OT, et al. Improvement of quality of life in panic disorder with escitalopram, citalopram, or placebo. *Pharmacopsychiatry* 2007;40(4):152–6.

90. Quagliato LA, Cosci F, Shader RI, et al. Selective serotonin reuptake inhibitors and benzodiazepines in panic disorder: a meta-analysis of common side effects in acute treatment. *Journal of*

Psychopharmacology 2019;33 (11):1340–51.

91. Chawla N, Anothaisintawee T, Charoenrungrueangchai K, et al. Drug treatment for panic disorder with or without agoraphobia: systematic review and network meta-analysis of randomised controlled trials. *BMJ* 2022;376:e066084.
92. Mavissakalian M, Perel JM. Clinical experiments in maintenance and discontinuation of imipramine therapy in panic disorder with agoraphobia. *Archives of General Psychiatry* 1992;49 (4):318–23.
93. Chen MH, Tsai SJ. Treatment-resistant panic disorder: clinical significance, concept and management. *Progress in Neuro-Psychopharmacology and Biological Psychiatry* 2016;70:219–26.
94. Bandelow B, Wedekind D. Internet psychotherapeutic interventions for anxiety disorders – a critical evaluation. *BMC Psychiatry* 2022;22(1):441.
95. Bandelow B, Sagebiel A, Belz M, et al. Enduring effects of psychological treatments for anxiety disorders: meta-analysis of follow-up studies. *British Journal of Psychiatry* 2018;212 (6):333–38.
96. Schneier FR, Moskow DM, Choo TH, et al. A randomized controlled pilot trial of vilazodone for adult separation anxiety disorder. *Depression and Anxiety* 2017;34 (12):1085–95.
97. Chamberlain SR, Baldwin DS. Monoamine oxidase inhibitors (MAOIs) in psychiatric practice: how to use them safely and effectively. *CNS Drugs* 2021;35(7):703–16.
98. Pollack MH, Van Ameringen M, Simon NM, et al. A double-blind randomized controlled trial of augmentation and switch strategies for refractory social anxiety disorder. *American Journal of Psychiatry* 2014;171(1):44–53.
99. Sartori SB, Singewald N. Novel pharmacological targets in drug development for the treatment of anxiety and anxiety-related disorders. *Pharmacology & Therapeutics* 2019;204:107402.
100. Vollmer LL, Strawn JR, Sah R. Acid-base dysregulation and chemosensory mechanisms in panic disorder: a translational update. *Transl Psychiatry* 2015;5(5):e572.
101. Vullo S, Kellenberger S. A molecular view of the function and pharmacology of acid-sensing ion channels. *Pharmacol Res* 2020;154:104166.
102. Salvadore G, Bonaventure P, Shekhar A, et al. Translational evaluation of novel selective orexin-1 receptor antagonist JNJ-61393215 in an experimental model for panic in rodents and humans. *Translational Psychiatry* 2020;10(1):308.
103. Fagan HA, Huneke NTM, Domschke K, Baldwin DS. The role of the orexin system in the neurobiology of anxiety disorders: potential for a novel treatment target. *Neuroscience Applied* 2024;3:103922.
104. Maramai S, Benchekroun M, Ward SE, et al. Subtype selective γ-aminobutyric acid type A receptor (GABA. *Journal of Medicinal Chemistry* 2020;63(7):3425–46.
105. Black N, Stockings E, Campbell G, et al. Cannabinoids for the treatment of mental disorders and symptoms of mental disorders: a systematic review and meta-analysis. *Lancet Psychiatry* 2019;6(12):995–1010.
106. Weston NM, Gibbs D, Bird CIV, et al. Historic psychedelic drug trials and the treatment of anxiety disorders. *Depression and Anxiety* 2020;37 (12):1261–79.

Post-traumatic Stress Disorder

Jonathan I. Bisson

Diagnosis and Classification

Although the characteristic symptoms of post-traumatic stress disorder (PTSD) have been recognised for many centuries, it was first included as a diagnosis in 1980 in the third edition of the *Diagnostic and Statistical Manual of Mental Disorders* (DSM).[1] Since then, the diagnostic criteria have undergone several changes, and it is now included as a trauma and stressor related disorder in DSM-5[2] and as a disorder specifically associated with stress in ICD-11.[3] Increasing recognition of the heterogeneity of presentations covered by the PTSD diagnosis – and a desire for increased clinical utility – led the World Health Organization to include the sibling condition of complex PTSD (CPTSD) in ICD-11.

The Traumatic Event

PTSD is one of the few psychiatric conditions that requires exposure to a specific type of event before diagnosis can be made. The exact nature of qualifying traumatic events has been much debated, with some people arguing that this requirement should be dropped and – like the majority of psychiatric conditions – the diagnosis be made purely on the nature of the symptom presentation. After some deliberation, both DSM-5 and ICD-11 have retained the specific traumatic event requirement; a key argument for this has been to prevent overdiagnosis, although it is important to acknowledge that some people will present with the characteristic symptoms of PTSD to non-qualifying traumatic events. Indeed, a study of 4,558 adults living in South Wales found that 47 per cent reported having experienced a traumatic event, and just under half of these were non-qualifying traumatic events.[4] The commonest non-qualifying event reported was the death of a parent, and there was little difference in prevalence of PTSD symptoms described in those who experienced a qualifying traumatic event and those who did not.

The DSM-5 definition of a qualifying traumatic event is that it should involve actual or threatened death, serious injury or sexual violence. There are, however, important caveats to this. For example, if an event is learnt about, it only counts as a qualifying event if it occurred to a close family member or close friend, and the nature of the trauma must have been violent or accidental. So, in theory, learning about a close relative having a severe heart attack would not be sufficient to cause PTSD, but witnessing it could be. The ICD-11 definition of 'extremely threatening or horrific event or series of events' allows a greater degree of interpretation but, nevertheless, the event has to be objectively very severe to qualify. According to both the DSM-5 and ICD-11 classification systems, a wide variety of events that can be very traumatic to individuals would not qualify – for example, parental separation, divorce and verbal bullying.

The Symptoms

Table 6.2.1 provides a summary of the main symptom clusters of PTSD according to DSM-5 and ICD-11 and of CPTSD according to ICD-11. There are now major differences in the diagnostic criteria for PTSD between the main classification systems, and they have effectively diverged – rather than converged – over time.[5] DSM-5 has kept the single diagnosis of PTSD but broadened the definition to include more features

Table 6.2.1 *The main symptom clusters of PTSD and CPTSD*

	DSM-5 PTSD	ICD-11 PTSD	ICD-11 CPTSD
Exposure to a severe traumatic event(s)	X	X	X
Re-experiencing symptoms	X	X	X
Avoidance symptoms	X	X	X
Hyperarousal symptoms	X	X	X
Negatively distorted cognitions and mood related to the traumatic event	X		
Emotional dysregulation			X
Interpersonal relationship difficulties			X
Negative self-concept			X

typically associated with more complex presentations. ICD-11 has narrowed the definition of PTSD, aiming to make it more clinically useful, and included the separate diagnosis of CPTSD to recognise a distinct constellation of symptoms experienced by some people following traumatic events. The result is that DSM-5 PTSD is a more complicated diagnosis than ICD-11 PTSD and includes people with more shame-based and guilt-based difficulties rather than fear-based difficulties alone. In contrast, the core symptoms of ICD-11 PTSD are very much based on fear, but people with additional disturbances in self-organisation (including more shame- and guilt-based phenomena) are included in the CPTSD diagnosis.

DSM-5 Symptom Criteria

DSM-5 PTSD has 20 symptom criteria that are divided into four separate clusters. The first cluster comprises intrusion symptoms, including nightmares, dissociative reactions (e.g. flashbacks) and psychological distress at exposure to reminders; the presence of one or more of these is required for the diagnosis. The second cluster concerns persistent avoidance (e.g. of memories, thoughts and external reminders); one or more forms of avoidance is required for the diagnosis. The third cluster covers negative alterations in cognitions and mood associated with the traumatic event(s) and is a new cluster, although some of the symptoms included (e.g. markedly diminished interest) were present in the DSM-IV definition of PTSD. New symptoms in this cluster include distorted cognitions around blame; persistent feelings such as shame, guilt or fear; and persistent negative beliefs or expectations about oneself, others or the world; at least two symptoms from this cluster are required. The final cluster also requires two or more symptoms to be present and concerns increased reactivity and arousal related to the traumatic event, including irritability, hypervigilance and sleep disturbance.

In addition to satisfying the traumatic event and symptom criteria, a duration of at least a month as well as significant distress or functional impairment are also required for a PTSD diagnosis. The presence of depersonalisation or derealisation leads to a 'with dissociative symptoms' specification, and a delay in the criteria being met for at least six months after the traumatic event leads to a 'with delayed expression' specification.

ICD-11 Symptom Criteria

ICD-11 PTSD has six symptom criteria across three clusters, which overlap with three of the DSM-5 ones. At least one symptom from each cluster is required for the diagnosis. The re-experiencing cluster requires vivid intrusive memories, flashbacks or nightmares, and it is widely accepted as having a higher threshold than for the DSM-5 intrusion cluster. The avoidance cluster covers the same symptoms as those included in DSM-5, and the persistent perceptions of heightened current threat cluster only includes hypervigilance and an enhanced startle reaction. For a diagnosis to be made, symptom duration has to be 'for at least several weeks', and the symptoms must cause significant impairment in important areas of functioning. It is noteworthy that the ICD-11 classification has avoided including criteria that are less specific and less likely to discriminate between different conditions, such as diminished interest, concentration difficulties and sleep disturbance.

ICD-11 CPTSD requires the criteria for a diagnosis of ICD-11 PTSD to be met along with '*severe and persistent (1) problems in affect regulation; (2) beliefs about oneself as diminished, defeated or worthless, accompanied by feelings of shame, guilt or failure related to the traumatic event; and (3) difficulties in sustaining relationships and in feeling close to others*'. These symptoms should also cause significant impairment in important areas of functioning. Although not a requirement for the CPTSD diagnosis, it is recognised that CPTSD is more commonly associated with exposure to more complex traumatic events, multiple traumatic events and more prolonged traumatic events than with exposure to single traumatic events of short duration.

A key example of the type of trauma exposure associated with CPTSD is childhood abuse and, although rejected by ICD-11, it has been argued that CPTSD should be considered a developmental disorder. Others have argued that it is synonymous with borderline personality disorder but, although the conditions can co-occur and both are associated with a history of childhood abuse, there are clear differences that can be used to help differentiate between these diagnoses.[6] The CPTSD diagnosis focuses on the effects of trauma, PTSD symptoms are a core element, and there is a stable negative self-concept and avoidance of relationships. For borderline personality disorder, suicide attempts and self-injurious behaviour are key features along with lack of a stable self-concept and fears of abandonment.

Prevalence

Sadly, qualifying traumatic events for PTSD are not uncommon, and it has been reported that the majority of the global population will experience at least one qualifying traumatic event at some point during their lives.[7] Most epidemiological work to date has focused on DSM (mainly DSM-IV) defined PTSD. In the last Adult Psychiatric Morbidity Survey in the United Kingdom,[8] 31.4% of respondents people reported exposure to a likely PTSD qualifying traumatic event, and 4.4% screened positive for DSM-IV PTSD in the past month. Rates of exposure and PTSD were similar in women and men, but screening positive for PTSD in the past month was particularly high in women aged 16 to 24 (12.6%).

68,894 people from 24 countries completed the World Health Organization's (WHO) mental health survey assessment of DSM-IV PTSD.[7] 70.4% reported having experienced a trauma in their lifetime, and the conditional risk of PTSD after exposure was 4%. A more recent survey of a representative sample of 1,051 adults in the UK exposed to a qualifying traumatic event considered the prevalence of screening positive for ICD-11 PTSD and CPTSD.[9] Of those surveyed, 5.3% met the criteria for PTSD and 12.9% for CPTSD, with the latter being associated with younger age and interpersonal trauma.

It is well recognised that individuals exposed to more extreme forms of trauma are more likely to develop PTSD. The WHO study described earlier found a wide range of conditional risks associated with different types of traumatic events; the highest was for rape (19%). In common with other types of traumatic event, rates of PTSD in those affected by disasters varies according to a person's proximity to the event and their role in it. A review of the epidemiology of PTSD after disasters estimated rates at 30–40% among direct victims of disasters, 10–20% among rescue workers and 5–10% in the general population.[10]

COVID-19 Pandemic

The Covid-19 pandemic was very traumatic to many people, and a proportion of people will have developed or will develop PTSD due to the traumatic nature of their experiences during the pandemic. Several research studies have now considered traumatic stress symptoms in samples representative of the UK population. For example, a study of 2,025 adults living in the United Kingdom between 23 and 28 March 2020 found that 16% reported symptoms compatible with an ICD-11 diagnosis of PTSD.[11] A systematic review and meta-analysis of studies that considered common mental disorder prevalence during the pandemic found a mean prevalence of PTSD of 21.94%,[12] but interpretation of the results is limited by the heterogeneous methods employed by the included studies, unknown baseline prevalence levels, and the lack of determination of the nature of traumatic events reported.

Frontline health care workers are recognised as a group that has been exposed to multiple qualifying traumatic events through their work during the pandemic. A recent systematic review found 14 studies of health care workers completed during the pandemic;[13] rates of significant post-traumatic stress symptoms ranged between 2.1% and 73.4%. A survey completed between October and November 2020 by just over 2,000 people with lived experience of mental illness explored how traumatic they had found the Covid-19 pandemic.[14] Of those surveyed, 39% reported finding at least one element traumatic, meaning that the majority did not identify their experience as a traumatic one. Respondents were asked to identify the experience that troubled them most, and the vast majority would not have fulfilled the traumatic event criterion for a diagnosis of PTSD. The most-reported 'most troubling experience', reported by around 27%, was 'generalised worry', with 'lockdown and restrictions' being the next most-reported one. Clear PTSD qualifying events such as exposure to death accounted for less than 7% of responses. Other 'most troubling experiences' included exposure to Covid-19, other people not following the rules, the government's response, having to wear face coverings, coverage in the news media and finances. Just over 13% of all participants reported symptoms sufficient to qualify for a diagnosis of ICD-11 PTSD to a Covid-19 event, but this reduced to 1.1% when the traumatic event criterion was included.

Outcome

As indicated earlier, the majority of people exposed to a qualifying traumatic event do not go on to develop PTSD or CPTSD, but a significant minority do. The natural course of PTSD varies between different people. A six-year follow-up study of people admitted to a general hospital in Australia for at least 24 hours due to physical injury following a traumatic event allowed five distinct trajectories of PTSD symptoms to be modelled (see Figure 6.2.1).[15] By far, the commonest trajectory (seen in 73 per cent of this sample) was a 'resilient' one, whereby the individual never experienced distressing mental health symptoms for a sustained period.

External factors associated with a more marked and possibly pathological mental health response following exposure to a traumatic event include greater proximity to the event and its direct effects. Internal factors are likely to be equally important in determining mental health response and include past mental health difficulty, family psychiatric difficulty, immediate reaction to stressors, coping style and perception of social support.[16]

Neurobiology

Although far from being fully understood, knowledge about the neurobiology of PTSD has increased significantly over the last decade, not least around the involvement of neurotransmitters, neuropeptides and glucocorticoids in the processing of traumatic memories and the development and maintenance of PTSD. These include catecholamines, opioids, gamma-aminobutyric acid (GABA), glutamate, serotonin, oxytocin and cortisol. There is also considerable evidence that overactivity of the amygdala, driven by overactivity of the noradrenergic system, plays a significant role and that attenuation of this should be beneficial in preventing and treating PTSD.[17] More recently, increasing attention has been paid to the role of consolidation and reconsolidation of traumatic memories due to increasing evidence that memories are more amenable to being retrieved and changed than originally thought.[18]

Psychological Theories

Several psychological theories have been developed to explain the development and maintenance of PTSD.[19] Perhaps the best known are fear conditioning theories that underpin the use of exposure therapies for the treatment of PTSD through the mechanism of habituation. It is argued that PTSD develops when a traumatic event (the unconditioned stimulus) becomes associated with a conditioned stimulus (e.g. walking through a park for people with PTSD following an assault that occurred

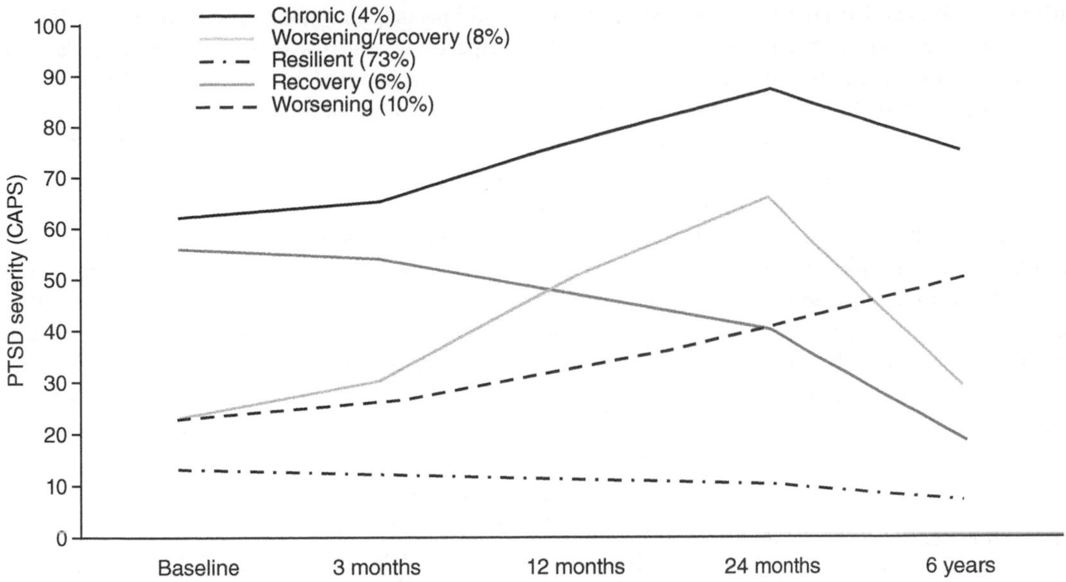

Figure 6.2.1 Symptom trajectories following traumatic events over six years.[15]

in a park), and reinforcement of this link occurs through exposure to the conditioned stimulus, causing further distress, leading to avoidance and a vicious circle. A widely cited expansion of this theory to better explain the phenomenology of PTSD is emotional processing theory, which argues that fear is activated through associative networks. Other commonly cited theories of PTSD argue for a greater cognitive contribution. The dual representation theory proposes that PTSD involves two different memory systems, situationally accessible and verbally accessible – the former giving rise to symptoms such as nightmares and flashbacks, and the latter to the distorted cognitions characteristic of PTSD. The cognitive theory of PTSD argues that it arises from excessive negative appraisals producing a sense of current threat, and this has underpinned the development of cognitive therapy for PTSD.

Prevention

The fact that PTSD requires exposure to a particular type of traumatic event provides more possibilities for prevention than for most psychiatric disorders. This extends to intervention before predicted exposure to traumatic events occurs (e.g. in the military and emergency services). A recent systematic review[20] concluded that there was insufficient evidence to recommend any pre-incident intervention, although attention bias modification training was noted to show some signs of being beneficial, and further work in this area is clearly warranted. More attention has been paid to universal (prevention delivered to everyone exposed to a traumatic event) and indicated (targeted at certain groups of individuals exposed to a traumatic event) interventions.

There has been a lot of interest in a universal intervention commonly referred to as psychological debriefing (PD), in which people exposed to traumatic events are provided with a single session that aims to reduce the risk of mental health sequelae. This was first described as critical incident stress debriefing for groups of ambulance personnel following traumatic events but was subsequently adapted for use with individuals and labelled psychological debriefing. A series of randomised controlled trials (RCTs) and systematic reviews have led to the conclusion that psychological debriefing is ineffective and may cause harm to some people.[21] This has culminated in recommendations against its use, including by the National Institute for Health and Care Excellence (NICE) in the UK.[22]

More recent systematic reviews of single-session preventative interventions have continued to find an absence of evidence for individual psychological debriefing.[20] A few studies with longer-term follow-up have suggested the potential for harm, but meta-analysis of primary – three to six months post-trauma – endpoints reveal neutral impact.[20] There clearly remains insufficient evidence to recommend individual PD, and the same is true for group debriefing, although no clear signal of potential harm has been found for this approach. Interestingly, an adapted form of group PD – that included some cohesion training – delivered to army personnel in China dealing with the aftermath of an earthquake found it to be more effective than standard group PD.[23] It would be premature to recommend any form of debriefing, but this adapted form of group PD seems worthy of further research and has met the criteria required to be recognised as an intervention with emerging evidence in the latest International Society for Traumatic Stress Studies (ISTSS) prevention and treatment guidelines.[24]

The best evidence for prevention comes from studies that have identified individuals with symptoms of PTSD and then provided a more formal trauma-focused intervention – similar, albeit often briefer, to those interventions provided for the treatment of PTSD.[20] Cognitive behavioural therapy with a trauma focus (CBT-TF) has the best evidence, but there is emerging evidence for eye movement desensitisation and reprocessing (EMDR). The evidence for such interventions gets better when restricted to individuals who satisfy the criteria for acute stress disorder in the first month following exposure to a traumatic event or the criteria for PTSD within three months of a traumatic event.[25] There is more limited evidence for the preventative value of pharmacological approaches.[26] Hydrocortisone is the only drug that has some emerging evidence of preventing the development of PTSD, but the main studies to date have all been with participants who are severely physically unwell, raising major questions around the generalisability of the findings.

Treatment

The evidence is much better for the treatment of PTSD than for the prevention of it. There is now strong and robust evidence for the use of various psychological interventions and pharmacological interventions, although the effect size associated with pharmacological interventions is lower than that for psychological interventions. That said, effect sizes are usually calculated for psychological interventions when compared to wait list or usual care controls whereas, for pharmacological interventions, the comparison is against placebo, which represents a higher bar.[27]

Psychological Treatment

Psychological treatments for PTSD can broadly be divided into those with a trauma focus and those without a trauma focus. The former include cognitive behavioural therapies with a trauma focus such as prolonged exposure therapy,[28] cognitive therapy for PTSD[29] and more eclectic forms of therapy that combine both cognitive and exposure work. Eye movement desensitisation and reprocessing is the other established form of trauma-focused psychological treatment. Less-established, but emerging, trauma-focused therapies are those that are purported to work through the mechanism of reconsolidation, with reconsolidation of traumatic memories being the best researched to date.[30] The best-evidenced psychological treatments for PTSD are considered individually below.

Cognitive Behavioural Therapy with a Trauma Focus (CBT-TF)

CBT-TF aims to treat PTSD by addressing thoughts, beliefs or behaviour. CBT-TF usually involves homework and covers a range of components, the prominence of which vary according to the type of CBT-TF delivered. Key components include psychoeducation, exposure work, cognitive work and more general relaxation/stress management. CBT-TF has the best efficacy/effectiveness evidence of all treatment options for PTSD. A recent systematic review and meta-analysis included 51 RCTs with 1,380 participants and found a large effect size of around 1.32 compared to wait list or usual care controls. The review also found increasing evidence that some CBT-TFs may be better than others, with prolonged exposure therapy,[28] cognitive therapy for PTSD,[29] cognitive processing therapy[31] and eclectic, non-specific forms of CBT-TF faring best. This led to these interventions being recommended more strongly in recent guidelines that differentiated between different treatments.[24,32]

Cognitive therapy for PTSD[29] focuses on the identification and modification of negative appraisals and behaviours that lead the person with PTSD to over-estimate current threat. It also involves the modification of beliefs related to other aspects of the experience and how the individual interprets their behaviour during the trauma (e.g. issues concerning guilt and shame). Cognitive processing therapy[31] focuses on the evaluation and modification of problematic thoughts that have developed following the traumatic experience(s). For example, using cognitive techniques to challenge typical thoughts of PTSD – that the individual is to blame for their trauma or that the world is now unsafe. An optional component of CPT is the development of a detailed, written narrative account of the trauma. Prolonged exposure therapy[28] involves using a verbal narrative technique with a detailed recounting of the traumatic experience that is then recorded and listened to on a repeated basis with the goal of habituation. In addition, real-life repeated exposure to avoided and fear-evoking situations – that are now safe but associated with the trauma – is undertaken, again with the aim of habituation.

Increasing attention is also being given to alternative forms of delivery of CBT-TF, designed to increase access and improve cost-effectiveness without reducing clinical effectiveness. Internet-based CBT-TF uses internet-based programmes to treat people with PTSD sufferers using CBT-TF approaches. The best evidence for such approaches is when self-help using an internet-based programme is guided by a therapist who has less contact with the patient than in traditional face-to-face CBT-TF. There is now good evidence that such approaches are effective,[33] with a recent RCT demonstrating non-inferiority of one guided self-help programme against face-to-face CBT-TF.[34] Although less well evidenced overall, some alternative forms of CBT-TF have been developed for particular groups of people with PTSD – for example, narrative exposure therapy for refugees and asylum seekers with a focus on helping recipients to develop a coherent, chronological, autobiographical narrative of their life that includes their traumatic experiences (a testimony) with the therapist facilitating emotional processing with cognitive-behavioural techniques.

Eye Movement Desensitisation and Reprocessing (EMDR)

EMDR is a standardised, eight-phase, trauma-focused therapy involving the use of bilateral physical stimulation (eye movements, taps or tones). Targeted traumatic memories are considered in terms of an image, the associated cognition, the associated affect and body sensation. These four components are then focused on as bilateral physical stimulation occurs. It is hypothesised that EMDR stimulates the individual's own information processing in order to help integrate the targeted memory as an adaptive contextualised memory. Processing targets involve past events, present triggers and adaptive future functioning. EMDR, at times, uses restricted questioning related to cognitive processes paired with bilateral stimulation to unblock processing.

EMDR has become a very popular treatment with many people now trained to deliver it. It has a robust evidence base, and a recent systematic review and meta-analysis[30] included 11 trials with 415 participants and an effect size of 1.23. This and the absence of difference between EMDR and CBT-TF in meta-analyses of head-to-head trials makes it difficult to choose between them, and EMDR is strongly recommended as a treatment of PTSD by several guidelines. A sensitivity analysis performed for the latest NICE guidelines for PTSD,[22] however, found an absence of evidence for EMDR in the treatment of combat-related PTSD in military veterans. The four RCTs that have considered EMDR in the treatment of combat-related PTSD in military veterans only included 92 participants; two studies were positive, and two were neutral.[35] Risk of bias was identified in all studies along with significant clinical and statistical heterogeneity, reducing confidence in the reliability of the finding and making interpretation of it difficult and highlighting the need for more research in this area. The finding did, however, result in NICE not recommending the use of EMDR for combat-related PTSD.

Reconsolidation of Traumatic Memories (RTM)

RTM involves the activation of a traumatic memory and then a procedure that includes imagining a black-and-white movie of the event – dissociated from its content – and re-winding it when fully associated over two seconds. This is designed to change the perspective from which the memory is recalled. There has been increasing interest both in terms of prevention and treatment of PTSD through the mechanism of reconsolidation to facilitate improvement in symptoms of PTSD. The idea is that when a memory is laid down, there is a short period – perhaps up to six hours – where the memory is unstable and more malleable to change. It has also been found that traumatic memories can be mobilised and made more malleable, even many years after a traumatic event. Two positive RCTs of RTM have been published with further RCTs of RTM and related interventions underway. Advocates of this approach point to advantages over CBT-TF in terms of number of sessions and the level of exposure to traumatic events required being less than techniques designed to work through the mechanism of habituation – for example, prolonged exposure therapy.

Psychological Treatments without a Trauma Focus

For many years, trauma-focused psychological treatments have been recommended as the treatments of choice by various guidelines and rightly so, given their superior evidence. However, this can underplay the fact that non-trauma-focused psychological treatments can help reduce symptoms of PTSD. This is particularly true for CBT without a trauma focus. A recent meta-analysis included seven studies with 318 participants and found an effect size of 1.06. This is slightly inferior to the effect sizes described earlier but an effect that would likely be felt very positively by someone with PTSD. CBT without a trauma focus includes a heterogeneous group of therapies that use a variety of non-trauma-focused techniques commonly used in generic CBT, including but not limited to stress management, emotional stabilisation, relaxation training, breathing retraining, positive thinking and self-talk, assertiveness training, thought stopping and stress inoculation training. It is clearly a valid treatment option for people who do not tolerate trauma-focused approaches, are not in a position to engage with them, or make an informed choice not to engage with them.

Present-centred therapy is another evidence-based non-trauma-focused approach to treat people with PTSD. Designed to target daily challenges that people with PTSD encounter because of their symptoms, it includes psychoeducation about the impact of PTSD symptoms, the development of effective strategies to deal with day-to-day challenges and homework to practice newly developed skills.

Pharmacological Treatments

Given our knowledge of the neurobiology of PTSD, there is good reason to believe that pharmacological treatment approaches should be beneficial. Considerable evidence exists, for example, from animal research on fear conditioning and from clinical research on PTSD to suggest that the overactivity of the noradrenergic system is a fundamental element of PTSD, and attenuation should be beneficial.[36] There are various ways to do this, either directly through drugs that work through their effects on adrenergic receptors (e.g. propranolol and prazosin) or indirectly (e.g. hydrocortisone to reduce noradrenaline release).

There is now strong evidence that some pharmacological treatments are effective for the treatment of PTSD.[37] The best evidenced are the selective serotonin re-uptake inhibitors fluoxetine, paroxetine and sertraline as well as the serotonin and noradrenaline re-uptake inhibitor venlafaxine. There is robust evidence for the efficacy of all of these drugs compared to placebo, but the effect sizes are small (0.3–0.4) leading the ISTSS guidelines to recommend them as 'interventions with low effect'.[24] As stated earlier, it is important to note that effect sizes generated in comparison with a placebo control are likely to be smaller than those generated for trials using a wait list or usual care control as is the case for psychological treatments for PTSD. There is limited work comparing psychological and pharmacological treatments directly for the treatment of PTSD, and until such work is available, their true relative efficacies will not be known. At present, their purported relative efficacies are influenced by assumptions regarding the comparability of effect sizes calculated in two different ways.[38]

Current guidelines, including NICE[22], ISTSS[24] and the Australian National guidelines,[32] have effectively concluded that trauma-focused psychological treatments are superior to pharmacological treatments, but all the guidelines do recommend the use of pharmacological treatments for PTSD. It is likely that many people with PTSD who are prescribed drugs will experience clinically significant improvement; many of the pharmacological RCTs report over 50 per cent improvements in PTSD symptoms at baseline for those taking drugs. Pharmacological treatments should form part of the treatment arsenal to deliver an evidence-based approach to the treatment of people with PTSD. Even though they should be considered as second line to trauma-focused psychological treatments, there are several reasons medication is prescribed, over and above failure to tolerate or respond to trauma-focused therapy. These include informed personal choice, long waits for therapy, lack of stability and other factors that prevent trauma-focused psychological treatment being delivered safely and effectively.

In addition to pharmacological monotherapy, there is good RCT evidence that some drugs can augment the effects of monotherapy.[37] Prazosin and risperidone are the best-evidenced drugs for augmentation, but there is also some evidence for quetiapine in the treatment of PTSD, and this is preferred by some to risperidone due to its side effect profile. Another approach that has attracted a lot of interest in recent years is that of pharmacologically assisted psychotherapy. The drug with the best evidence in this regard is MDMA; RCTs have shown that its use in combination with a particular form of psychotherapy can reduce symptoms of PTSD,[39] although more work is needed before it can be routinely recommended.

Most guidelines recommend the prescription of specific drugs without detailed guidance on how to prescribe them. It is clear from the RCT evidence available that people with PTSD often require a higher dose than the starting dose for most of the recommended drugs; indeed, for all the recommended drugs, the mean dose administered in RCTs was closer to the maximum dose than the starting dose.[38] A team in Cardiff has synthesised the available evidence around prescribing to produce a prescribing algorithm.[38] This provides advice on how to prescribe in a stepped manner and also includes evidence-informed approaches to managing marked insomnia and agitation, along with recommending other drugs with more limited evidence – but some evidence of effect (amitriptyline, mirtazapine and phenelzine) – for people who do not respond or tolerate other drugs. This algorithm has been adopted by the Australian guidelines for the treatment of PTSD,[32] and the main summary of it is shown in Figure 6.2.2.

Non-psychological and Non-pharmacological Treatments

A range of other interventions also have some evidence of effectiveness for the treatment of PTSD, although it would be premature to recommend the routine use of any of them. Such approaches have been recommended as interventions with emerging evidence by the latest ISTSS guidelines[24] and include acupuncture, neurofeedback, transcranial magnetic stimulation and yoga.

Treatment of CPTSD

It is well recognised that CPTSD is often more challenging to treat than PTSD, and as a relatively new diagnosis, there is an absence of RCT evidence to determine the best approach to take. Several of the RCTs that underpin the evidence base for PTSD have, however, included people with more complex presentations, and many participants would have been likely to have satisfied the criteria for CPTSD if this had been assessed. It, therefore, seems reasonable for treatment approaches for CPTSD to be informed by the evidence base for PTSD.

Two recent systematic reviews and meta-analyses have attempted to use evidence that predates the CPTSD diagnosis to inform treatment approaches. One meta-analysis[40] included 51 RCTs of psychological interventions for PTSD in which clinically significant disturbances in self-organisation symptoms were assessed. Cognitive behavioural therapy, exposure alone and EMDR were superior to the usual care for PTSD symptoms – negative self-concept and disturbed relationships – but few RCTs reported effects on affect dysregulation. The second meta-analysis[41] considered interventions following exposure to complex trauma defined as sustained, repeated or multiple forms of traumatic exposure. Ninety-four RCTs with 6,158 participants were included; the majority were of populations diagnosed with PTSD. Phased modular psychological interventions that included skills-based and trauma-focused strategies were the most promising interventions for emotional dysregulation and interpersonal problems. These reviews appear to support a phased, multicomponent approach, and there is already good evidence for the use of at least one such approach – skills training in affective and interpersonal regulation coupled with narrative exposure work for the treatment of PTSD. This approach has now been enhanced to include a module on self-concept[42] – thereby covering all the symptom clusters of CPTSD – and is currently being evaluated.

Until better evidence emerges, it seems appropriate to consider a phased approach coupled with a trauma-focused one for CPTSD, although it is noteworthy that there has been a debate in the field regarding the need for phasing, and this may well be determined by personal factors and specific

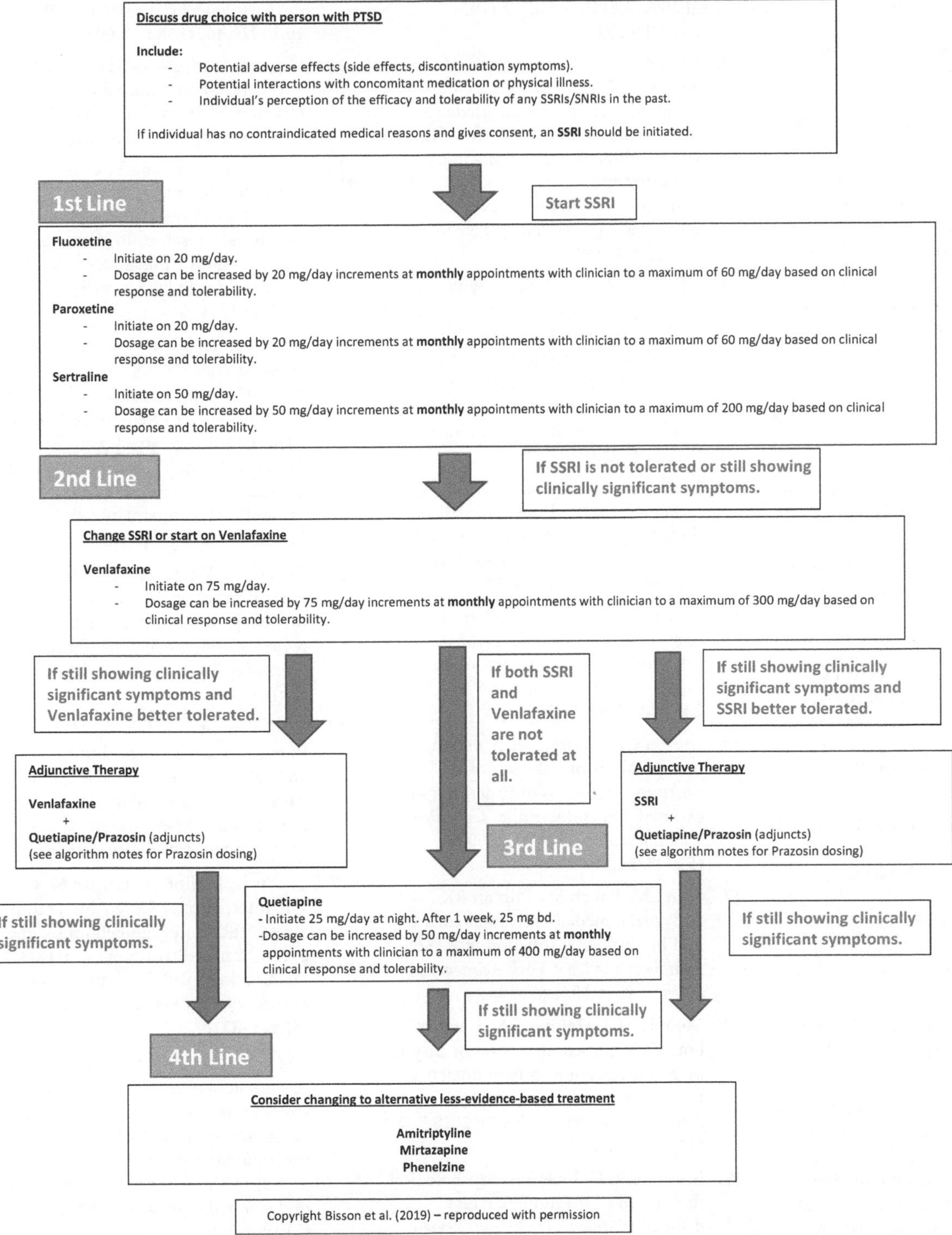

Figure 6.2.2 PTSD pharmacological prescribing algorithm.

symptoms rather than an individual diagnosis per se. Research and clinical experience suggest that many people with CPTSD do find it difficult to engage with trauma-focused work without a period of stabilisation work. It is to be hoped that treatment for PTSD and CPTSD moves towards a more personalised approach with interventions being tailored to meet the specific needs of people with these conditions.

Concluding Remarks

PTSD and CPTSD cause significant distress to people affected by them. Despite the limited evidence for effective preventative interventions, there is strong evidence for effective psychological and pharmacological treatments. Early detection and treatment are vital to reduce the individual and societal impact of these common mental disorders.

References

1. American Psychiatric Association. *Diagnostic and Statistical Manual of Mental Disorders*, 3rd ed. Washington, DC: American Psychiatric Publishing, 2000.
2. World Health Organization. (2018). *International Classification of Diseases for Mortality and Morbidity Statistics*, 11th Rev. icd.who.int/browse11/l-m/en
3. American Psychiatric Association. *Diagnostic and Statistical Manual of Mental Disorders*, 5th ed. Washington, DC: American Psychiatric Publishing, 2013.
4. White J, Pearce J, Morrison S, et al. Risk of post traumatic stress disorder following traumatic events in a community sample. *Epidemiology and Psychiatric Sciences* 2015;24(3):249–57.
5. Bisson JI. What happened to harmonisation of the PTSD diagnosis?: the divergence of ICD11 and DSM5. *Epidemiology and Psychiatric Sciences* 2013;22(3):205–7.
6. Cloitre M, Garvert DW, Brewin CR, et al. Evidence for proposed ICD-11 PTSD and complex PTSD: a latent profile analysis. *European Journal of Psychotraumatology* 2013;4. DOI: 10.3402/ejpt.v4i0.20706.
7. Kessler RC, Aguilar-Gaxiola S, Alonso J, et al. Trauma and PTSD in the WHO World Mental Health Surveys. *European Journal of Psychotraumatology* 2017;8 (sup5):1353383.
8. McManus S, Bebbington P, Jenkins R, et al. (eds.) *Mental Health and Wellbeing in England: Adult Psychiatric Morbidity Survey 2014*. Leeds: NHS Digital; 2016.
9. Karatzias T, Hyland P, Bradley A, et al. Risk-factors and comorbidity of ICD-11 PTSD and Complex PTSD: findings from a trauma-exposed population based sample of adults in the United Kingdom. *Depression and Anxiety*, 2019;36(9):887–94.
10. Galea S, Nandi A, Vlahov D. The epidemiology of post-traumatic stress disorder after disasters. *Epidemiologic Reviews* 2005;27:78–91.
11. Shevlin M, McBride O, Murphy J, et al. Anxiety, depression, traumatic stress and COVID-19-related anxiety in the UK general population during the COVID-19 pandemic. *BJPsych Open* 2020;6(6):e125. DOI: 10.1192/bjo.2020.109.
12. C′enat JM, Blais-Rochette C, Kokou-Kpolou CK, et al. Prevalence of symptoms of depression, anxiety, insomnia, posttraumatic stress disorder, and psychological distress among populations affected by the COVID-19 pandemic: a systematic review and meta-analysis. *Psychiatry Research* 2021;295:113599.
13. d'Ettorre G, Ceccarelli G, Santinelli L, et al. Post-traumatic stress symptoms in healthcare workers dealing with the COVID-19 pandemic: a systematic review. *International Journal of Environmental Research and Public Health* 2021;18(2):601. DOI: 10.3390/ijerph18020601
14. Lewis C, Lewis K, Roberts A, et al. COVID-19-related posttraumatic stress disorder in adults with lived experience of psychiatric disorder. *Depression and Anxiety* 2022;39(7):564–72.
15. Bryant RA, Nickerson A, Creamer M, et al. Trajectory of post-traumatic stress following traumatic injury: 6-year follow-up. *British Journal of Psychiatry* 2015;206(5):417–23.
16. Brewin CR, Andrews B, Valentine JD. Meta-analysis of risk factors for posttraumatic stress disorder in trauma-exposed adults. *Journal of Consulting and Clinical Psychology* 2000;68 (5):748–66.
17. Shin LM, Rauch SL, Pitman RK. Amygdala, medial prefrontal cortex, and hippocampal function in PTSD. *Annals of the New York Academy of Sciences* 2006;1071:67–79.
18. Monfils MH, Holmes EA. Memory boundaries: opening a window inspired by reconsolidation to treat anxiety, trauma-related, and addiction disorders. *Lancet Psychiatry* 2018;5 (12):1032–42.
19. Brewin CR, Holmes EA. Psychological theories of posttraumatic stress disorder. *Clinical Psychology Review* 2003;23(3):339–76.
20. Bisson JI, Astill Wright L, Jones KA, et al. Preventing the onset of post traumatic stress disorder. *Clinical Psychology Review* 2021;86: 102004.
21. Rose A, Bisson J, Churchill R, et al. Psychological debriefing for preventing post traumatic stress disorder (PTSD). *Cochrane Database of Systematic Reviews* 2002;2:CD000560. DOI: 10.1002/14651858.CD000560.
22. National Institute for Health and Care Excellence. *Post-Traumatic Stress Disorder NICE guideline [NG116]*. 2018. www.nice.org.uk/guidance/ng116.
23. Wu S, Zhu X, Zhang Y, et al. A new psychological intervention: '512 Psychological Intervention Model' used for military rescuers in Wenchuan Earthquake in China. *Social Psychiatry and Psychiatric Epidemiology* 2012;47:1111–9.
24. International Society for Traumatic Stress Studies (ISTSS). *ISTSS PTSD Prevention and Treatment Guidelines: Methodology and Recommendations*. 2018. istss.org/getattachment/Treating-Trauma/New-ISTSS-Prevention-and-Treatment-Guidelines/ISTSS_PreventionTreatmentGuidelines_FNL-March-19-2019.pdf.aspx.
25. Roberts N, Kitchiner N, Kenardy J, et al. Early psychological intervention following recent trauma: a systematic review and meta-analysis. *European Journal of Psychotraumatology* 2019;10 (1):1695486.
26. Astill Wright L, Sijbrandij M, Sinnerton R, et al. Pharmacological prevention and early treatment of post-traumatic stress disorder and acute stress disorder: a systematic review and meta-analysis. *Translational Psychiatry* 2019;9(1):334.
27. Bisson JI, Berliner L, Cloitre M, et al. The International Society for Traumatic Stress Studies new guidelines for the prevention and treatment of PTSD: methodology and development process. *Journal of Traumatic Stress* 2019;32 (4):475–83.
28. Foa E, Dancu CV, Hembree EA, et al. A comparison of exposure therapy, stress inoculation training, and their combination for reducing posttraumatic stress disorder in female assault victims. *Journal of Consulting and Clinical Psychology* 1999;67 (2):194–200.
29. Ehlers A, Clark DM, Hackmann A, et al. Cognitive therapy for post-traumatic stress disorder: development and evaluation. *Behaviour Research and Therapy* 2005;43(3):413–31.
30. Lewis C, Roberts NP, Andrew M, et al. Psychological therapies for post-traumatic stress disorder in adults: systematic review and meta-analysis. *European Journal of*

Psychotraumatology, 2020;11 (1):1729633.

31. Resick P, Nishith P, Weaver TL, et al. A comparison of cognitive-processing therapy with prolonged exposure and a waiting condition for the treatment of chronic posttraumatic stress disorder in female rape victims. *Journal of Consulting and Clinical Psychology* 2002;70(4):867–79.
32. Phoenix Australia. *The Australian Guidelines for the Prevention and Treatment of Acute Stress Disorder (ASD), Posttraumatic Stress Disorder (PTSD) and Complex PTSD.* 2020. www.phoenixaustralia.org/australian-guidelines-for-ptsd/
33. Simon N, Robertson L, Lewis C, et al. Internet-based cognitive and behavioural therapies for post-traumatic stress disorder (PTSD) in adults. *Cochrane Database of Systematic Reviews* 2021;5(5): CD011710.
34. Bisson JI, Ariti C, Cullen K, et al. Guided, internet based, cognitive behavioural therapy for post-traumatic stress disorder: pragmatic, multicentre, randomised controlled non-inferiority trial (RAPID). *BMJ* 2022;377.
35. Kitchiner N, Lewis C, Roberts N, et al. Active duty and ex-serving military personnel with post-traumatic stress disorder treated with psychological therapies: systematic review and meta-analysis. *European Journal of Psychotraumatology* 2019;10(1): 1684226
36. Southwick SM, Bremner JD, Rasmusson A, et al. Role of norepinephrine in the pathophysiology and treatment of posttraumatic stress disorder. *Biological Psychiatry* 1999;46(9):1192–204.
37. Hoskins MD, Bridges J, Sinnerton R, et al. Pharmacological therapy for post-traumatic stress disorder: a systematic review and meta-analysis of monotherapy, augmentation and head-to-head approaches. *European Journal of Psychotraumatology* 2021;12 (1):1802920.
38. Bisson JI, Baker A, Dekker W, et al. Evidence-based prescribing for post-traumatic stress disorder. *British Journal of Psychiatry* 2020;216 (3):125–26.
39. Hoskins MD, Sinnerton R, Nakamura A, et al. Pharmacological-assisted psychotherapy for post-traumatic stress disorder: a systematic review and meta-analysis. *European Journal of Psychotraumatology* 2021;12(1):1853379.
40. Karatzias T, Murphy P, Cloitre M, et al. Psychological interventions for ICD-11 Complex PTSD symptoms: systematic review and meta-analysis. *Psychological Medicine* 2019;49(11):1761–75.
41. Coventry PA, Meader N, Melton H, et al. Psychological and pharmacological interventions for posttraumatic stress disorder and comorbid mental health problems following complex traumatic events: systematic review and component network meta-analysis. *PLOS Medicine* 2020. doi.org/10.1371/journal.pmed.1003262.
42. Cloitre M, Karatzias T, McGlanachy E. *Enhanced STAIR Narrative Therapy for CPTSD. Treatment Manual.* Unpublished Manuscript. 2019. Further details: classic.clinicaltrials.gov/ct2/show/NCT04752072 (accessed 14 September 2023).

Specific Phobias

Julius Burkauskas, Naomi A. Fineberg, Arun Enara, Giovanna Cirnigliaro and Lynne M. Drummond

Specific phobia is a condition characterised by an intense reaction of fear and avoidance to a situation or an object perceived as dangerous. Individuals might rationally understand the situation is not in reality dangerous, but often even the thought of the specific situation or object evokes intense anxiety. Various studies have reported on the lifetime prevalence of specific phobia, which ranges from 3 to 15 per cent, with incidence predominantly occurring during adolescence. This disorder often leads to a reduction in the quality of life and can cause significant functional impairment. Various theories from genetic to psychological, including those drawing inferences from psychodynamic and cognitive behavioural therapies, offer explanations about the aetiology of specific phobia. Exposure therapy and SSRIs are recognised treatment options for individuals with specific phobias.

Background

Fear is a universal and essential emotion. Without it, the human race would have fallen over cliffs and failed to run from sabre-toothed tigers. Thus, from an evolutionary perspective, fear is crucial for survival. Individuals differ in their baseline level of fear (trait anxiety) and the situations that provoke fear (state anxiety). However, not all fear is rational and based on a threat to survival.

We all might have fears that are irrational but unstoppable. These fears are often embarrassing but do not make us change our lifestyle. They lie on a continuum with phobic disorders.

Phobias have been defined as morbid fears that are involuntary, cannot be reasoned away and lead to avoidance of the feared object or situation.[1] Clearly, they overlap with morbid fears. Most individuals with phobic disorder, however, have made major adjustments to their lifestyle to avoid the phobic stimulus.[2]

Case Example

A twenty-five-year-old woman has developed a specific phobia of spiders. She is afraid that a spider might enter her ear while she is asleep and, this way, reach and damage her brain. Rationally, she knows this is impossible, but this does not decrease her fear, and she has very high anxiety any time a spider might be somewhere nearby. She is on a constant lookout for spiders wherever she goes. Her quality of life has been affected heavily in recent years, as she bought a country house by the lake for weekends and holidays. What was initially planned as a perfect place for friends and family gatherings is now considered a fear zone as she finds it almost impossible to go there because of her fear of spiders. Once, she saw a tiny spider on her pillow in the evening there. As she was not able to touch the spider and it ran away, her friend that was staying with her had to keep searching for the spider for almost three hours, as she refused to go to sleep before the spider was caught. After this incident, she became reluctant to go to the country house and is often upset this place no longer gives her happiness. She often asked her family members to check a room that she was about to enter – in case there might be some spiders there – and often refused to go to family gatherings or to visit friends if they lived outside of the city. As her life was getting more and more restricted, the woman decided to seek professional help.

Working definitions of the most commonly seen types of phobic disorder are given in Table 6.3.1, along with their relative prevalence, age at onset and sex incidence.

Diagnosis

The *Diagnostic and Statistical Manual (5th ed.)*, DSM-5,[4] defines specific phobia as an excessive fear triggered by a particular object or situation. The extent of the fear is disproportional to the actual danger of the object or situation, and this fear occurs almost immediately when the individual with phobia is in contact with the feared stimulus.

Unlike in DSM-IV,[5] in DSM-5, there is no requirement for the individual to know that their fear is disproportionate to the reality. This criterion was changed as it was realised that many children did not meet this criterion. The individual either goes to lengths to avoid the feared object or situation or tolerates it only with extreme distress. The phobia significantly impacts the individual's school, work or personal life. The symptoms should have been in existence for at least six months. The patient must not have another disorder that could explain the symptoms before diagnosing specific phobia.

Many anxiety disorders have similar symptoms. Therefore, the therapist must rule out other disorders before diagnosing a specific phobia.

In the International Statistical Classification of Diseases and Related Health Problems (11th ed.), ICD-11,[3] specific phobia falls under the anxiety or fear-related disorders group,

Table 6.3.1 Types of phobias*

Disorder	Prevalence	Onset	Sex incidence	Feared situation	Comments
Agoraphobia	One of the commonest and most handicapping phobias in psychiatric practice	Early adult life	Females more frequently affected than males	Fear of crowded places, travelling by public transport, supermarkets, enclosed spaces	Can present with or without panic disorder
Social anxiety disorder	The next most common phobia seen in psychiatric clinics after agoraphobia	Adolescence	Equal	Can be generally fearful of all social situations or specific (e.g. eating, drinking, blushing, vomiting)	Psychological therapy will depend on whether it is general or specific. This phobia is the most studied from the psychopharmacological standpoint
Specific animal phobia	Rarely seen in psychiatric practice and more likely in general practice	Early childhood (usually before the age of seven years)	More common in adult women but equal sex incidence in childhood	Dogs, cats, spiders, insects and so on	Specificity to the animal. Self-help packages are popular with these patients
Miscellaneous specific phobias	May present in a variety of ways	Varies	Overall equal	Heights, enclosed places, flying, thunder and so on	
Blood and injury phobia	Possibly more common than is ever recorded as these individuals tend to avoid all clinical situations	Often starts in adolescence and may improve in middle age	Equal	Medical or dental procedures, blood	Parasympathetically mediated fainting response rather than sympathetically mediated fight, flight or freeze reaction

* Please note that social anxiety disorder and agoraphobia are discussed in Chapter 6.1.

characterised by extreme fear and anxiety resulting in behavioural disturbances to the extent of impairing an individual's personal, family, social, educational, occupational or other important areas of functioning. Subcategories of anxiety or fear-related disorders defined in ICD-11 are generalised anxiety disorder, panic disorder, agoraphobia, specific phobia, social anxiety disorder, separation anxiety disorder and selective mutism.

The diagnosis of phobic disorder depends on a history of the fear being provoked by specific objects or situations. The anticipation of fear often leads to avoidance of these stimuli, or the stimuli is endured with dread. However, the ICD-11 differs a little from previous versions of ICD as it states that avoidance is not a prerequisite for the diagnosis. Panic may occur, and in such cases, the phobia is given diagnostic precedence over the panic symptoms.

Areas of Controversy

The relative importance of panic in the classification of phobic disorders is controversial. Panic may be viewed as very high levels of anxiety. During exposure to fear-provoking situations, some individuals suffer from incapacitating panic. This panic may also result from the anticipation of a future fear-provoking event. Thus, panic can be seen as a secondary reaction to the feared situation.

However, other workers have argued that the panic attack is the primary event, with the phobic anxiety developing as a secondary phenomenon. According to this view, panic has a separate biological basis to its genesis and should take precedence over the phobic anxiety in terms of classification and treatment. This controversy is demonstrated by the difference in the ICD and DSM views on classification.

In recent years, the debate has focused on the nosological position of panic disorder and its links to agoraphobia. While some psychiatrists have been inclined to accept that the apprehension of going out causes the panic, others have viewed the experience of panic as the core problem, which causes the fear of going out and having a panic attack away from the security of the home.

There are persuasive arguments in favour of both positions, and it is possible that the explanation lies in an intermediate model, one with interconnecting biological and environmental factors that act through the hypersensitivity of the autonomic nervous system.[4]

In clinical samples, almost all individuals presenting with symptoms of agoraphobia also have a history of panic disorder. In contrast, agoraphobia without a history of panic disorder is consistently reported in community samples, although the rates may have been exaggerated, and the disorder lacks strong support as a separate entity.[5] Some 35–50% of those with panic disorder in community settings also suffer from agoraphobia.[6] Individuals with panic and agoraphobia report more comorbid disorders and are more disabled than those with uncomplicated agoraphobia.

Specific Phobias: Differential Diagnosis and Comorbidity

As with the other anxiety disorders, the problem of comorbidity often confounds the diagnostician. Approximately

80 per cent of individuals with phobia also fulfil criteria for other anxiety disorders, to the extent that it can be impossible to determine a single, primary source of anxiety.[7] The presence of comorbidity has increased the burden of the disorder. In recent years, most studies of phobic anxiety have concentrated on social anxiety disorder, generalised anxiety and panic, all of which are frequently comorbid with agoraphobia and specific phobias. For example, suicidality increases from an estimated rate of 1 per cent for uncomplicated social phobia to 16 per cent for comorbid disease.

Obsessive-Compulsive Disorder

Obsessive-compulsive disorder can be easily mistaken for phobic disorder. There are important similarities and differences between the two conditions. These are highlighted in Table 6.4.1 in Chapter 6.4 on 'Obsessive-Compulsive and Related Disorders'.

Generalised Anxiety Disorder

Generalised anxiety disorder (GAD) is manifested as symptoms of worry and anxiety that occur in a generalised and persistent manner and are not related to specific cues. Results from community surveys suggest that the onset of phobic disorders, such as agoraphobia and specific phobias, may predict the later onset of GAD.[8]

In comorbid cases, it may be hard to distinguish the phobia, in which case a behavioural test – where the therapist observes the patient in a variety of situations – can be diagnostic.

Panic Disorder

This condition has already been discussed in relation to agoraphobia. The essential features of panic disorder are recurrent attacks of severe anxiety that are not restricted to any specific situation and, therefore, occur unpredictably.

Depression

Individuals with depression often experience symptoms of anxiety. In more severe cases, anxiety combined with inertia can lead to symptoms almost identical to agoraphobia or social anxiety disorder.

On the other hand, the restricted life of the individual with agoraphobia or social anxiety disorder can lead to depression. Indeed, depression occurs in roughly 50 per cent of individuals with panic, agoraphobia or social anxiety. A study by Batinic et al.[9] emphasised that depression and agoraphobia/generalised anxiety and panic disorder often go hand in hand. Suicidal behaviours are particularly seen in those with high anxiety complicated by a depressive disorder during their lifetime, and there is considerable cross-sectional and longitudinal comorbidity with dysthymia.[9] Often, the phobia precedes the onset of depression, which may be considered as a secondary reaction associated with the demoralising effect of chronic anxiety.[10]

In cases of doubt, it is usually advisable to treat the depression first and then to examine the residual symptoms.

Post-traumatic Stress Disorder (PTSD)

This condition can mimic phobic disorder and, therefore, can overlap the diagnoses. A few individuals develop phobia after a traumatic event, which leads to heightened arousal and other symptoms of PTSD.

Anxious/Avoidant Personality Disorder

This is a controversial diagnosis, characterised by severe social avoidance, low self-esteem, sensitivity to rejection and avoidance of risks starting from an early age. It appears to respond to treatments that are effective for social anxiety disorder and may, therefore, be regarded as a pervasive form of social anxiety disorder rather than as a true disorder of personality.[11,12]

Substance Misuse

A study by Arias et al.[13] showed that, when individuals with substance misuse were examined, those with a dual diagnosis fared worse than those with pure dependence. Bipolar, agoraphobia and generalised anxiety were the most frequent comorbidities in substance use disorder and resulted in higher rates of suicide.[13] The associated problems of tolerance and dependence also confounded the clinical picture. The experience of a 'hangover' after an alcoholic binge with symptoms of dry mouth, palpitation, headache and nausea are all very similar to those of high anxiety.

Physical Disorders

Physical conditions such as pheochromocytoma,[14] imbalance of thyroid hormones,[15] hypoglycaemia,[16] mitral valve regurgitation,[17] Parkinson's disease,[18,19] variant Creutzfeldt–Jakob disease[20] and AIDS[21] can all present with features similar to anxiety and panic and may be mistaken for phobic anxiety disorder. Physical disorders can be excluded by careful history taking followed by relevant physical examination.

Compared with individuals with or without other forms of psychiatric illness, those with agoraphobia and panic disorder show an increased risk of medically unexplained symptoms, are associated with a high use of medical services, and experience increased mortality from both cardiovascular and cerebrovascular disease.[6] A survey of 86 individuals with asthma revealed a high prevalence of phobic anxiety disorders, with agoraphobia, panic disorder with or without agoraphobia and social anxiety disorder occurring in 26.8%, 13.9% and 9.3% of those surveyed, respectively.[22]

Another possible confusion is postural orthostatic tachycardia syndrome (PoTS), where individuals experience extremely high pulse rates and dizziness or fainting due to low blood pressure.[23,24] Individuals may be fearful of going out with this condition for fear of fainting. This disorder has only recently been examined and fully described.[23] It is known to frequently co-exist in individuals with Ehlers-Danlos Syndrome,[25] who in the past have been described as having high levels of anxiety. A German study found that, once the symptoms attributable to the autonomic dysfunction were removed, individuals with PoTS did not experience more anxiety disorders than the general population.[26]

Epidemiology

Prevalence

Agras et al.[27] found a total prevalence of phobic disorder in the general population of Vermont, USA, to be 77 people per 1,000. However, severely disabling phobias were found in only 2.2 per 1,000 of the population, and only one person per 1,000 was actively receiving treatment.[27]

Half the clinical cases involved agoraphobia, but less than 10 per cent of the total phobic population had the condition.[27] This early study showed that clinical populations are not a good sample to understand the prevalence of a condition in the community.

One of the many problems in epidemiological research involves deciding where the cut-off between annoying, minor personal difficulty and clinically relevant phobic anxiety should be.

It is generally acknowledged that phobic disorders are extremely common. The US National Comorbidity Survey[7] examined a range of demographic parameters in 8,098 non-institutionalised respondents, aged 15–54 years. DSM-III-R diagnoses were established, and the results showed lifetime (and 30-day) prevalence rates of 13.3% (4.5%) for social phobia, 11.3% (5.5%) for specific phobia and 6.7% (2.3%) for agoraphobia.[7] Other studies in America and Europe (e.g. Wardenaar, et al.,[28] Lépine and Lellouch[29]) support high frequencies of disorder. Interestingly, although individuals with agoraphobia perceived themselves to be less impaired, a higher proportion of this group sought professional help than those with social anxiety disorder or specific phobia.[7]

Gender

Women appear to suffer from anxiety disorders approximately twice as often as men. This includes phobic disorders and agoraphobia, as well as generalised anxiety disorders, panic disorder and specific phobia.[28,30,31]

Onset and Course of Phobic Disorders

Specific phobias usually start early in childhood, as early as eight years old,[28] and although many phobias continue into adolescence, the majority improve over time. However, a review found that the peak population prevalence of specific phobic disorder occurs in middle or old age.[32]

Agoraphobia usually occurs in the late teens or early twenties and is rarely seen in childhood. It is also observed to run a chronic, enduring course and is responsible for considerable impairment.[5,33,34]

Future directions of studies analysing specific phobia should include specific neuroimaging studies and the integration of imaging and genetic data to gain a better understanding.[35]

Aetiology

Although genetic, behavioural and cognitive theories of aetiology have been proposed, much of the research has concentrated on social phobia and panic disorder with little emphasis on agoraphobia and specific phobias.

Genetic Theories

The genetic epidemiology of phobias – investigating the interrelationship of agoraphobia, social anxiety disorder, animal phobias and situational phobias – has been examined separately in females and males in two large twin studies.[36,37] The results for females showed that agoraphobia had the highest rates of comorbidity. Greater concordance in the monozygotic twins than in the dizygotic twins supported the importance of genetic mechanisms. A statistical analysis indicated that a third of the variance in liability to phobias was attributable to genetic factors, whereas the remainder was linked to environmental influences, such as parental attitudes and issues around upbringing. Model fitting suggested that for all except animal phobias, familial aggregation was better explained by genetic rather than specific environmental factors.[36] In the second study – which looked at male twins – agoraphobia, social anxiety disorder, animal phobias, situational phobias and blood/injection/injury phobias were all found to aggregate within twin pairs. The aggregation was again thought largely to result from genetic factors, with the heritability ranging from 25 to 37 per cent. Multi- variate analysis revealed a genetic factor common to all phobias tested, as well as other genetic factors specific to each phobia and a common familial-environmental factor.[37] The authors concluded that genetic risk factors are partially common to all phobias and partially specific to particular subtypes, and these factors also play a moderate role in the aetiology of phobias. Family environment also plays a role in the origin of social and agoraphobia.[36,37]

Neurotransmitters

In children, there is evidence that both selective serotonin reuptake inhibiting drugs and also selective serotonin norepinephrine inhibitors are helpful in all types of anxiety disorder, including specific phobias. This implies that these drugs dampen the fear response.[38]

Similarly, the same authors reported the apparent efficacy of benzodiazepines in reducing fear in children and adolescents, suggesting that the inhibitory neurotransmitter gamma-aminobutyric acid (GABA) may be inherent in the phobic anxiety response. However, the authors point out the limited number of studies performed in this age group that demonstrates this.

Psychological Theories

Psychoanalytic Theories

The original and classic account of a child with phobic disorder is Freud's description of a young boy with a specific fear of horses. The boy, Hans, became frightened of horses after he witnessed an accident involving a horse while he was out walking with his father. Freud believed that this fear of horses was a substitute for his unconscious hatred and fear of his father. Thus, phobias were viewed by Freud as resulting from unresolved Oedipal complex.

More modern psychoanalytic views of phobic disorder still tend to concentrate on the theory that anxiety is displaced from one feared object to an associated one – that is, from an unconscious feared object or situation to a conscious, and therefore avoidable, object or situation.[39]

In a recent review of various aspects of anxiety disorders, Goodwin[40] suggests that anxiety, depression and obsessive-compulsive syndromes may all be due to similar mechanisms that present in various ways due to various influencing factors.

Behavioural Theories

The reproduction of phobic-like reactions in the laboratory led to the popularity of conditioning theories for the development of phobias. In their famous case of 'Albert', Watson and Rayner[41] demonstrated that an 11-month-old child with a positive interest in furry animals developed a fear of rats after a steel bar was struck, making a loud noise, whenever he put out his hand towards a white rat. This case was not replicated, however, and the theory of a straightforward relationship between the genesis of phobias and classical conditioning was modified by other workers, who commented on individual differences in the susceptibility to aversive stimuli.[42] Eysenck[43] suggested that individuals who condition easily are more likely to develop phobias. Other workers emphasised that the intensity and amount of reinforcement following any action also has an effect on the degree of conditioning that takes place.[44]

Early in the development of behavioural treatments for phobias, Mowrer's[45] view of fear acquisition was widely accepted as the model for the development of clinical phobias. According to this view, classically conditioned fear leads to avoidance behaviour. Avoidance leads to a reduction of fear, and thus the avoidance behaviour is reinforced by a reduction in anxiety.

This model, however, was soon challenged. First, it was acknowledged that individuals with phobia are often unable to recall traumatic experiences relating to the onset of their phobia.[46,47] Second, several workers had failed to replicate Watson and Rayner's[41] experiment.[48,49] Third, the model did not fit with the gradual onset of phobias usually seen in clinical practice.[50] Finally, it did not explain the common stereotyped patterns of fear-provoking objects and situations.

In a series of laboratory-based experiments with adult volunteers, Ohman et al.[51,52] demonstrated that humans are much more likely to be aversively conditioned to phylogenetically old, fear-relevant stimuli (e.g. snakes and spiders) than to neutral stimuli (e.g. flowers and mushrooms).

In 1965, Marks[1] proposed the concept of 'prepotency', which is the tendency for a particular species to attend preferentially to certain stimuli of evolutionary importance rather than to other, evolutionary unimportant stimuli, even when these stimuli are encountered for the first time. Seligman's concept of preparedness extended this evolutionary model further.[53] Preparedness refers to the idea that certain stimuli are more likely to be associated with each other and with certain responses.

Is Blood/Injection/Injury Phobia Separate from Other Phobias?

Blood/injection/injury phobia is one of the most interesting phobias. Not only is it difficult to judge the prevalence of the condition (as people who have it tend, by definition, to avoid medical personnel), but the autonomic response to the phobic stimulus is different from that in other phobias. Whereas many individuals with phobia fear that they may faint in their phobic situation, this actually rarely happens as the sympathetic response and increased cardiac output prevents fainting. In blood/injection/injury phobia, however, the vaso-vagal reaction frequently does cause fainting.[54] Presumably, this makes sense in evolutionary terms because – whereas with most threatening situations a fight-or-flight reaction is necessary for survival – once injury is realised, or at least inevitable, a reduction in cardiac output is more likely to be life-saving. Individuals with blood/injection/injury phobia demonstrate this response in an exaggerated form. It is therefore important to ensure that any individual with this condition is exposed to phobic stimuli only when lying down; otherwise, injury from falling could occur.

Behavioural Overview

Overall, the behavioural view of the genesis of phobic disorder is that individuals vary in trait anxiety and susceptibility to conditioning. Phobias are an almost-universal experience in childhood but generally pass with age. In some individuals, these fears persist. Many sufferers have a family history of phobic disorder, and genetic factors as well as modelling by close family members may be implicated in the development of the phobia. Once a phobia has developed, the patient will tend to escape from the fear-provoking situation. This escape causes the anxiety to abate. Because high anxiety is extremely unpleasant, the reduction in anxiety resulting from escape is like a reward and reinforces the escape behaviour. Thus, every episode of short-lived exposure followed by escape serves to strengthen the phobic escape and avoidance behaviour. In the case of social anxiety disorder, if children are unduly restricted (e.g. by anxious parents) and are not given the opportunity to engage in social interactions, they may not acquire the necessary skills for later life. Thus, family attitudes may reinforce avoidant behaviours and make the disorder worse.[55]

Cognitive Theories

In the cognitive model of phobic anxiety developed by Aaron T. Beck in the USA, it is not the stimulus or the situation that causes the anxiety but the individual's expectations and interpretation of the situation.[56] Clark[57] developed this model further with the cognitive model of panic. In this model, once an individual feels anxious, they may focus on specific physical symptoms of anxiety. If these symptoms are interpreted as evidence of a bad event, the anxiety is further increased. This, in turn, leads to exacerbation of the anxiety symptoms.

Case Example

A 50-year-old man had a fear that he might drop dead from a myocardial infarction. While standing in a supermarket queue, he noticed that his pulse was rapid. He viewed this as evidence that something was wrong with his heart and that he may experience a myocardial infarction at any moment. Unsurprisingly, this thought led to heightened anxiety and an even faster pulse, and thus a vicious circle of anxiety was established. It is easy to see how this unpleasant experience led to the man fleeing homeward and subsequently avoiding situations linked to the anxiety.

Sociological Theories

The nature versus nurture debate depends on whether it is believed that children inherit their phobias from a parent or whether the phobias are learned. There are no adoption studies of parents with phobic disorder to answer this question. However, many clinicians working with individuals with phobia believe that the trait anxiety levels and ease of conditioning are inherited. The type and the extent of the fear are probably linked directly to environmental factors.

Treatment of Phobias

Behavioural Psychotherapy

The behavioural treatment of phobic disorders is a prolonged, graduated exposure in real life to the feared situation. It is based on the understanding that individuals with phobias have learned to escape or avoid fear-provoking phobic situations. This avoidance and escape behaviour strengthen the association between the stimulus and anxiety. In therapeutic exposure, the individual is asked to stay in a previously agreed fear-provoking situation until the anxiety engendered by the stimulus reduces by at least half. This process takes approximately 1 hour, and the reduction in anxiety is called habituation.

Most individuals with handicapping phobias are not willing or able to engage immediately with the most feared object or situation. For this reason, the patient and the therapist need to work out a hierarchy of different exposure situations. For example, a woman with a severe spider phobia may find that sitting in a room with a spider would cause maximal anxiety scoring 8 on a 0–8 scale of anxiety. Saying the word 'spider' may be given an anxiety rating of 2 on the same scale. A drawing of a spider may be rated a 4, a photograph of a spider rated a 5, a moving film image of a spider rated a 6 and a spider in an enclosed jar rated a 7. Once this has been established, the patient and therapist need to agree on an initial exposure task that will cause the patient to experience anxiety but at a level that he or she feels able to tolerate.

Once the patient has performed the first exposure task and experienced habituation of the anxiety, the same task needs to be repeated regularly by the patient as self-exposure homework. This should ideally be performed three times a day but at least daily. The patient should find that, on repeated exposure, the anxiety is progressively lessened and that it also lasts for progressively shorter periods. Once the first stage has been conquered, the patient is moved on to the next task in the hierarchy.

The most effective exposure has been shown to be:

- Prolonged rather than of short duration[58]
- In real life rather than in fantasy[59]
- Regularly practised, with self-exposure homework tasks[60]

Although exposure treatment sounds time-consuming, it can be cost efficient as patients perform much of the therapy themselves. In a study of the treatment of agoraphobia by Mathews et al.,[61] the total therapist time used was only seven hours.

Many individuals with mild to moderate phobias can treat themselves using self-exposure and regular monitoring by either a therapist or even a specially written computer program.[62] However, it was shown that therapist-directed exposure during one session (maximum three hours) was significantly better in reducing phobia (post-treatment and one year later) than self-directed exposure via a manual (during a two-week period).[63] Examples of self-help manuals include the time-tested *Living with Fear*.[64]

Therapists can easily learn the skills required to administer an exposure programme or to advise patients on self-exposure by reading one of the practical guides to therapy.[65] and by obtaining supervision from a registered behavioural psychotherapist.

Cognitive Therapy

Exposure therapy is successful for most individuals with anxiety disorders. However, cognitive therapy may have a place in treating those patients who have failed to respond to exposure therapy or who cannot or are unwilling to enter exposure situations because of their extreme fear.

Cognitive therapy requires more therapist training than exposure therapy. The type of cognitive therapy that has been described for use with individuals with phobia is that developed by Beck and Emery.[56] Faulty negative automatic thoughts that cause the individual to feel anxious are identified and challenged by the patient and therapist working collaboratively. Some individuals with agoraphobia develop safety behaviours to reduce their anxiety. These behaviours can interrupt the success of a behavioural programme, and it may be necessary to use cognitive techniques to encourage an individual to abandon safety behaviours.[66]

Exposure treatment has been shown to be effective in 66 per cent of individuals with agoraphobia[67] and highly effective for individuals with a variety of specific and social phobias.[68] A naturalistic study of patients with agoraphobia failed to show any benefit of cognitive sessions in addition to exposure therapy.[69] A recent systematic review of nine studies comparing virtual reality versus *in vivo* exposure therapy found no difference in efficacy between the two approaches for specific phobia and agoraphobia.[70] As an emerging technology, it is expected that virtual reality will soon become an innovative clinical tool for individuals with specific phobia.[71,72] Findings of a recent meta-analysis also suggest that cognitive behavioural therapy for specific phobia is associated with improved outcomes compared with control conditions for up to12 months after treatment completion but not beyond.[73]

Recent reviews have summarised the best evidence for factors resulting in positive therapy effects for exposure treatments. These include low trait anxiety, high motivation and high self-efficacy prior to exposure therapy, high cortisol levels and heart rate variation, the evocation of disgust in addition to anxiety, the avoidance of relaxation (as this technique might hinder results), a focus on cognitive changes, context variation, sleep and memory-enhancing drugs (d-Cycloserine) during exposure therapy.[74] Modifiable risk factors without professional intervention include social support, coping and physical activity, while risk factors making exposure less likely to work include addiction (especially cigarette smoking for agoraphobia) and avoidance.[75]

Targeted cognitive techniques probably have a role in overcoming specific problems for some individuals. For example, cognitive therapy can be used to alter faulty beliefs and self-judgement in social anxiety.[76,77] Clark's[57] model of panic and treatment using hyperventilation and cognitive therapy can be used for some individuals with agoraphobia and panic.

Nowadays, few psychoanalytically trained therapists would advocate their form of treatment for individuals with a phobia. There are therefore no outcome studies on this type of intervention.

A population-based cross-sectional WHO World Mental Health survey including participants from 24 countries (n = 112,507) assessed lifetime specific phobia treatment outcomes.[78] Individuals with specific phobia were asked whether during their lifetime they spoke to a professional about their specific phobia and whether they ever received treatment that they considered helpful. A summary of participants' reports showed that specific phobia treatment was helpful for 23.0% of individuals for the first professional seen, but this proportion rises to 85.7% with persistent help-seeking, indicating that specific phobia is highly treatable.[79]

A Cochrane database study examined the use of psychological therapies in individuals with panic disorder both with and without agoraphobia. These included behavioural, cognitive and third wave approaches using mindfulness, as well as psychodynamic approaches and even supportive psychotherapy. Overall, this review concluded that it was difficult to show any meaningful differences between all different psychological therapies.[80]

Pharmacological Treatments

Exposure-based therapies constitute the most effective treatment for specific phobia. However, pharmacotherapies can still be considered for patients suffering from specific phobias in case they were non-adherent or resistant to exposure-based therapies or where such therapies were innaccessible.

The considerable literature on the drug treatment of the phobic disorders is almost exclusively confined to the treatment of panic disorder, general anxiety disorder and social phobia presented in Chapter 6.1. This is because the symptoms of specific phobia are adequately reduced with the drug therapy indicated for other anxiety disorders, mainly SSRIs, SNRIs and benzodiazepines. Moreover, specific phobia is less disabling and common compared to the other anxiety disorders.[81]

Benzodiazepines such as diazepam, alprazolam and midazolam are useful in the short-term reduction of subjective self-reported fear during the exposure to the feared object or situation but be aware of the risks of dependency. Anaesthetic drugs for the treatment of dental phobia are ineffective unless conducted with the inhalation of anaesthetic nitrous oxide, which seems to work both in the short term and the long term. Cognitive enhancers such as D-cycloserine, glucocorticoids and yohimbine hydrochloride seem to be more effective than placebo, at least in the short term, in treating specific phobia symptoms. Beta-adrenergic antagonists have been examined but with inconsistent results. The author of this review concluded that pharmacotherapies for specific phobias focusses on drugs that enhance the efficacy of exposure-based therapies sessions by reducing anticipating phobia-related fear or by enhancing cognition during these sessions.[82]

Combination Treatment for Phobic Disorders

Both psychological and pharmacological treatments have their benefits and drawbacks. Psychotherapy may be more challenging for the patient and more difficult to come by; its effects may develop more slowly but are likely to endure, and there are no major safety concerns. On the other hand, pharmacotherapy is easily obtained, acts quickly and, in the case of the newer drugs, is also safe and well tolerated, but the drugs probably need to be taken long term to ensure sustained effectiveness.[83]

In general, patients and therapists find that combining treatments works best in clinical practice, although formal examination of the outcome of this approach is only just being undertaken. Key elements in the psychological approach – including explanation, education and engagement of the patient in the therapeutic alliance – are prerequisites for optimising the clinical effect of drug treatment.

References

1. Marks IM. *Fears and Phobias*. London: Heinemann Medical Books; 1969.
2. Craske MG, Stein MB. Anxiety. *The Lancet*. 2016;388(10063):3048–59.
3. WHO. (World Health Organization). *ICD-11 for Mortality and Morbidity Statistics. Mental, Behavioural or Neurodevelopmental Disorders*. icd.who.int/browse11/l-m/en. (accessed 1 June 2019).
4. Faravelli C, Paionni A. Panic disorder: clinical course, etiology and prognosis. In: Nutt DJ, Ballenger JC, Lépine J-P (eds.) *Panic Disorder: Clinical Diagnosis, Management and Mechanisms*. London: Martin Dunitz; 1999:25–44.
5. Andrews G, Slade T. Agoraphobia without a history of panic disorder may be part of the panic disorder syndrome. *The Journal of Nervous and Mental Disease* 2002;190(9):624–30.
6. Baldwin DS, Birtwistle J. The side effect burden associated with drug treatment of panic disorder. *Journal of Clinical Psychiatry* 1998;59(Suppl. 8):39–44.
7. Magee WJ, Eaton WW, Wittchen H-U, et al. Agoraphobia, simple phobia, and social phobia in the National Comorbidity Survey. *Archives of General Psychiatry* 1996;53(2):159–68.
8. Kessler RC, Wittchen H-U. Patterns and correlates of generalized anxiety disorder in community samples. *Journal of Clinical Psychiatry* 2002;63:4–10.
9. Batinic B, Opacic G, Ignjatov T, et al. Comorbidity and suicidality in patients diagnosed with panic disorder/agoraphobia and major depression. *Psychiatria Danubina* 2017;29(2):186–94.
10. Goodwin RD. Anxiety disorders and the onset of depression among adults in the community. *Psychological Medicine* 2002;32(6):1121–4.
11. Frandsen FW, Simonsen S, Poulsen S, et al. Social anxiety disorder and avoidant personality disorder from an interpersonal perspective. *Psychology and Psychotherapy: Theory, Research and Practice* 2020;93(1):88–104.
12. Ballenger JC, Davidson JR, Lecrubier Y, et al. Consensus statement on social anxiety disorder from the International Consensus Group on Depression and Anxiety. *Journal of Clinical Psychiatry* 1998;59(17):54.
13. Francisco A, Nestor S, Pablo V, et al. Madrid study on the prevalence and characteristics of outpatients with dual pathology in community mental health and substance misuse services. *Adicciones* 2013;25(2):118–27.
14. Kogan CS, Stein DJ, Maj M, et al. The classification of anxiety and fear-related disorders in the ICD-11. *Depression and Anxiety* 2016;33(12):1141–54.
15. Burkauskas J, Pranckeviciene A, Bunevicius A. Thyroid Hormones, Brain, and Heart. In: Iervasi G, Pingitore A, Gerdes AM (eds.) *Thyroid and Heart: A Comprehensive Translational Essay*. London: Springer International Publishing; 2020: 339–60.
16. Bispham JA, Hughes AS, Driscoll KA, et al. Novel challenges in aging with type 1 diabetes. *Current Diabetes Reports* 2020;20(5):1–9.
17. Willits I, Keltie K, de Belder M, et al. Safety, effectiveness and costs of percutaneous mitral valve repair: a real-world prospective study. *PLoS ONE*. 2021;16(5):e0251463.
18. Forbes EJ, Byrne GJ, O'Sullivan JD, et al. Defining atypical anxiety in Parkinson's disease. *Movement Disorders Clinical Practice* 2021;8(4):571–81.
19. Lintel H, Corpuz T, Paracha S-u-R, et al. Mood disorders and anxiety in Parkinson's disease: current concepts. *Journal of Geriatric Psychiatry and Neurology* 2021;34(4):280–8.
20. Brandel J-P, Knight R. Variant Creutzfeldt–Jakob disease. *Handbook of Clinical Neurology* 2018;153:191–205.
21. Brandt C, Zvolensky MJ, Woods SP, et al. Anxiety symptoms and disorders among adults living with HIV and AIDS: a critical review and integrative synthesis of the empirical literature. *Clinical Psychology Review* 2017;51:164–84.
22. Nascimento I, Nardi AE, Valença AM, et al. Psychiatric disorders in asthmatic outpatients. *Psychiatry Research* 2002;110(1):73–80.
23. Raj SR, Guzman JC, Harvey P, et al. Canadian cardiovascular society position statement on postural orthostatic tachycardia syndrome (POTS) and related disorders of chronic orthostatic intolerance. *Canadian Journal of Cardiology* 2020;36(3):357–72.
24. Safavi-Naeini P, Razavi M. Postural orthostatic tachycardia syndrome. *Texas Heart Institute Journal* 2020;47(1):57–9.
25. Miller AJ, Stiles LE, Sheehan T, et al. Prevalence of hypermobile Ehlers-Danlos syndrome in postural orthostatic tachycardia syndrome. *Autonomic Neuroscience* 2020;224:102637.
26. Wagner C, Isenmann S, Ringendahl H, et al. Anxiety in patients with postural tachycardia syndrome (PoTS). *Fortschritte der Neurologie-psychiatrie* 2012;80(8):458–62.
27. Agras S, Sylvester D, Oliveau D. The epidemiology of common fears and phobia. *Comprehensive Psychiatry* 1969;10(2):151–6.
28. Wardenaar KJ, Lim CC, Al-Hamzawi AO, et al. The cross-national epidemiology of specific phobia in the World Mental Health Surveys. *Psychological Medicine* 2017;47(10):1744–60.
29. Lépine J-P, Lellouch J. Classification and epidemiology of social phobia. *European Archives of Psychiatry and Clinical Neuroscience* 1995;244(6):290–6.

30. Bandelow B, Michaelis S. Epidemiology of anxiety disorders in the 21st century. *Dialogues in Clinical Neuroscience* 2015;17(3):327.
31. McLenon J, Rogers MAM. The fear of needles: a systematic review and meta-analysis. *Journal of Advanced Nursing* 2019;75(1):30–42.
32. Eaton WW, Bienvenu OJ, Miloyan B. Specific phobias. *The Lancet Psychiatry* 2018;5(8):678–86.
33. Noyes R, Reich J, Christiansen J, et al. Outcome of panic disorder: relationship to diagnostic subtypes and comorbidity. *Archives of General Psychiatry* 1990;47 (9):809–18.
34. Batelaan NM, Rhebergen D, Spinhoven P, et al. Two-year course trajectories of anxiety disorders: do DSM classifications matter? *Journal of Clinical Psychiatry* 2014;75(9):985–93.
35. Bas-Hoogendam JM, Groenewold NA, Aghajani M, et al. ENIGMA-anxiety working group: rationale for and organization of large-scale neuroimaging studies of anxiety disorders. *Human Brain Mapping* 2022;43(1):83–112.
36. Kendler KS, Neale MC, Kessler RC, et al. The genetic epidemiology of phobias in women: the interrelationship of agoraphobia, social phobia, situational phobia, and simple phobia. *Archives of General Psychiatry* 1992;49 (4):273–81.
37. Kendler KS, Myers J, Prescott CA, et al. The genetic epidemiology of irrational fears and phobias in men. *Archives of General Psychiatry* 2001;58(3):257–65.
38. Wehry AM, Beesdo-Baum K, Hennelly MM, et al. Assessment and treatment of anxiety disorders in children and adolescents. *Current Psychiatry Reports* 2015;17(7):52.
39. Hughes P. *Dynamic Psychotherapy Explained.* Abingdon: Radcliffe Medical Press; 1999.
40. Goodwin GM. The overlap between anxiety, depression, and obsessive-compulsive disorder. *Dialogues in Clinical Neuroscience* 2015;17(3):249.
41. Watson JB, Rayner R. Conditioned emotional reactions. *Journal of Experimental Psychology* 1920;3(1):1.
42. Pavlov IP. *Conditioned Reflexes; an Investigation of the Physiological Activity of the Cerebral Cortex.* London: Oxford University Press; 1927.
43. Eysenck HJ. *The Dynamics of Anxiety and Hysteria: an Experimental Application of Modern Learning Theory to Psychiatry.* London: Routledge & Kegan Paul; 1957.
44. Spence K, Haggard D, Ross L. Intrasubject conditioning as a function of the intensity of the unconditioned stimulus. *Science.* 1958;128 (3327):774–5.
45. Mowrer OH. *Learning Theory and Personality Dynamics.* New York: The Ronald Press Company; 1950.
46. Buglass D, Clarke J, Henderson A, et al. A study of agoraphobic housewives. *Psychological Medicine* 1977;7(1):73–86.
47. Goldstein AJ, Chambless DL. A reanalysis of agoraphobia. *Behavior Therapy* 1978;9(1):47–59.
48. English HB. Three cases of the 'conditioned fear response'. *The Journal of Abnormal and Social Psychology* 1929;24(2):221.
49. Thorndike EL. *The Psychology of Wants, Interests and Attitudes.* New York: Appleton-Century; 1935.
50. Emmelkamp PM. Anxiety and fear. In: Emmelkamp PM, Bellack AS, Hersen M, et al. (eds.) *International Handbook of Behavior Modification and Therapy.* Boston: Springer; 1982: 349–95.
51. Öhman A. Face the beast and fear the face: animal and social fears as prototypes for evolutionary analyses of emotion. *Psychophysiology* 1986;23 (2):123–45.
52. Öhman A, Fredrikson M, Hugdahl K, et al. The premise of equipotentiality in human classical conditioning: conditioned electrodermal responses to potentially phobic stimuli. *Journal of Experimental Psychology: General* 1976;105(4):313.
53. Seligman ME. Phobias and preparedness. *Behavior Therapy* 1971;2 (3):307–20.
54. Bienvenu OJ, Eaton WW. The epidemiology of blood-injection-injury phobia. *Psychological Medicine* 1998;28 (5):1129–36.
55. Beidel DC. Social anxiety disorder: etiology and early clinical presentation. *The Journal of Clinical Psychiatry* 1998;59(Suppl 17):27–32.
56. Beck AT, Emery G. *Anxiety Disorders and Phobias: a Cognitive Perspective.* New York: Basic Books; 1985.
57. Clark DM. A Cognitive Model of Panic Attacks. In: Rachman S, Maser JD (eds.) *Panic: Psychological Perspectives.* Hillsdale, NJ: L. Erlbaum Associates; 1988: 71–89.
58. Stern R, Marks I. Brief and prolonged flooding: a comparison in agoraphobic patients. *Archives of General Psychiatry* 1973;28(2):270–6.
59. Emmelkamp PM, Wessels H. Flooding in imagination vs flooding in vivo: a comparison with agoraphobics. *Behaviour Research and Therapy* 1975;13(1):7–15.
60. McDonald R, Sartory G, Grey S, et al. The effects of self-exposure instructions on agoraphobic outpatients. *Behaviour Research and Therapy* 1979;17(1):83–5.
61. Matthews AM, Gelder MG, Johnston DW. *Agoraphobia: Nature and Treatment.* Abingdon: Routledge; 1981.
62. Ghosh A, Marks IM, Carr A. Therapist contact and outcome of self-exposure treatment for phobias: a controlled study. *The British Journal of Psychiatry.* 1988;152(2):234–8.
63. Öst L-G, Salkovskis PM, Hellström K. One-session therapist-directed exposure vs. self-exposure in the treatment of spider phobia. *Behavior Therapy* 1991;22(3):407–22.
64. Marks IM. *Living with Fear: Understanding and Coping With Anxiety.* New York: McGraw-Hill; 1978.
65. Stern RS, Drummond LM. *The Practice of Behavioural and Cognitive Psychotherapy.* Cambridge: Cambridge University Press; 1991.
66. Wells A, Papageorgiou C. Worry and the incubation of intrusive images following stress. *Behaviour Research and Therapy* 1995;33(5):579–83.
67. Mathews AM, Gelder MG, Johnston DW, et al. *Agoraphobia: Nature and Treatment.* London: Tavistock; 1981.
68. Marks IM. *Cure and Care of Neuroses: Theory and Practice of Behavioral Psychotherapy.* Chichester: John Wiley & Sons; 1981.
69. Burke M, Drummond LM, Johnston DW. Treatment choice for agoraphobic women: exposure or cognitive-behaviour therapy? *British Journal of Clinical Psychology* 1997;36(3):409–20.
70. Wechsler TF, Kümpers F, Mühlberger A. Inferiority or even superiority of virtual reality exposure therapy in phobias? – A systematic review and

quantitative meta-analysis on randomized controlled trials specifically comparing the efficacy of virtual reality exposure to gold standard in vivo exposure in agoraphobia, specific phobia, and social phobia. *Frontiers in Psychology* 2019;10:1758.

71. Park MJ, Kim DJ, Lee U, et al. A literature overview of virtual reality (VR) in treatment of psychiatric disorders: recent advances and limitations. *Frontiers in Psychiatry* 2019;10:505.
72. Oing T, Prescott J. Implementations of virtual reality for anxiety-related disorders: systematic review. *JMIR Serious Games* 2018;6(4):e10965.
73. van Dis EAM, van Veen SC, Hagenaars MA, et al. Long-term outcomes of cognitive behavioral therapy for anxiety-related disorders: a systematic review and meta-analysis. *JAMA Psychiatry* 2020;77(3):265–73.
74. Böhnlein J, Altegoer L, Muck NK, et al. Factors influencing the success of exposure therapy for specific phobia: a systematic review. *Neuroscience & Biobehavioral Reviews* 2020;108:796–820.
75. Zimmermann M, Chong AK, Vechiu C, et al. Modifiable risk and protective factors for anxiety disorders among adults: a systematic review. *Psychiatry Research* 2020;285:112705.
76. Marks IM. Advances in behavioral-cognitive therapy of social phobia. *Journal of Clinical Psychiatry* 1995;56 (Suppl 5):25–31.
77. Coupland NJ. Social phobia: etiology, neurobiology, and treatment. *Journal of Clinical Psychiatry* 2001;62:25–35.
78. de Vries YA, Harris MG, Vigo D, et al. Perceived helpfulness of treatment for specific phobia: findings from the World Mental Health Surveys. *Journal of Affective Disorders* 2021;288:199–209.
79. de Roos NM, de Vries JH, Katan MB. Serum lithium as a compliance marker for food and supplement intake. *American Journal of Clinical Nutrition* 2001;73(1):75–9.
80. Pompoli A, Furukawa TA, Imai H, et al. Psychological therapies for panic disorder with or without agoraphobia in adults: a network meta-analysis. *Cochrane Database of Systematic Reviews* 2016;4(4): CD011004.
81. Williams T, Hattingh CJ, Kariuki CM, et al. Pharmacotherapy for social anxiety disorder (SAnD). *Cochrane Database of Systematic Reviews* 2017;10 (10):CD001206.
82. Khali RB. Non-antidepressant psychopharmacologic treatment of specific phobias. *Current Clinical Pharmacology* 2015;10(2):131–138.
83. Nutt D, Baldwin D, Beaumont G, et al. Guidelines for the management of social phobia/social anxiety disorder. *Primary Care Psychiatry.* 1999;5 (4):147–55.

Further Reading

Drummond LM. *CBT for Adults.* Cambridge: Cambridge University Press/ Royal College of Psychiatrists; 2018.

Chapter

6.4

Obsessive-Compulsive and Related Disorders

Lynne M. Drummond, Arun Enara, Giovanna Cirnigliaro, Julius Burkauskas and Naomi A. Fineberg

Introduction

Obsessive-compulsive disorder (OCD) is a chronic and debilitating illness. It has a specific natural history and treatment response that merits separate attention. This chapter provides a comprehensive update on the origins, aetiology and treatment of OCD. We also touch upon advances in the understanding of a group of less–well researched disorders related to and currently classified together with OCD, termed the 'obsessive-compulsive and related disorders' (OCRDs). However, the main focus of this chapter will be on OCD.

Historical Perspective

Our understanding of obsessive-compulsive disorder (OCD) has changed over time. Notwithstanding, obsessions and compulsions have consistently remained the core symptoms for establishing the diagnosis. In the early twentieth century, there was an effort to understand and treat many mental conditions using psychoanalysis. According to Freud, OCD was linked to an 'anal phase' of infant development. However, this theory did not result in successful treatment and management of the condition. Thereafter, OCD has gained the reputation of being an extremely chronic condition, frequently unresponsive to available interventions.

One of the first full descriptive accounts of OCD in the British medical literature was by Professor Sir Aubrey Lewis, in which he emphasised the importance of unwanted thoughts (obsessions) that came into the patient's mind but were actively resisted by the patient.[1]

In the 1960s and 70s, two major breakthroughs led to the discovery that people living with OCD could be helped. It was found that clomipramine, a tricyclic drug that has an action on the serotonin system, had a 'direct anti-obsessive action', and this finding led to the controlled trials of its usage published in the 1980s.[2] Almost simultaneously, the application of learning theory to understand OCD led to the development of the psychological treatment of graded exposure with response prevention.[3] We now know that OCD is a common condition that can be treated with some success. However, many patients fail to receive the help and treatment they require, and a substantial proportion continue to remain symptomatic in spite of accessing adequate treatment.

Diagnosis and Classification

Obsessive-Compulsive Disorder (OCD)

The diagnosis of OCD is based on a characteristic symptom profile, of which obsessions and compulsions represent core features.

Obsessions are intrusive and unwanted thoughts, images or impulses that cause anxiety or distress and which the patient tries, at least in the early stages of the illness, to resist. These emotionally charged thoughts are recognised as being a product of the patient's own mind but are seen as contrary to his or her wishes or personality (i.e. they are 'ego dystonic'). Examples include a parent thinking of harming a loved child or a religious person having blasphemous thoughts. The sufferer may try very hard not to have the obsessive thought. This in itself can lead to an increased frequency and intensity of the thought. The reader can try this out by carrying out a simple experiment of self-observation: put this book down and try to think about anything at all *except* a pink hippopotamus. Most people will immediately have the visual image of a pink hippopotamus when attempting this exercise, illustrating how hard it is to dismiss a 'forbidden' thought. Obsessional thoughts have a much greater persistency and are thus much more difficult to dismiss.

Compulsions may be either overt actions or covert 'neutralising' thoughts. These are activities designed to reduce the anxiety caused by the obsessional thought or to 'put the thought right' in some way. For example, a person with an obsession that he or she has been contaminated by a dreaded disease may compulsively wash to 'undo' the contamination; a minister plagued by blasphemous obsessions may have to repeat a stereotyped prayer to 'undo' or neutralise the obsession. These activities, however, are either not linked with the fear in reality (e.g. a spinster with thoughts of having sex with strangers in a shop may have the compulsion to wash her hands repeatedly) or they are clearly excessive. For example, a man with the obsession that his home may be burgled may check that he has locked the front door 25 times.

The *Diagnostic and Statistical Manual, 5th edition* (DSM-5),[4] and the International Classification of Diseases, 11th revision (ICD-11),[5] provide standardised diagnostic criteria for OCD. Although there are clear similarities between the two systems, a few minor but important differences exist (Table 6.4.1). Both DSM-5 and ICD-11 rely on the presence of time-consuming

Table 6.4.1 Differences in ICD-10, DSM-5 and ICD-11 classification of OCD

	ICD-10	DSM-5	ICD-11
Classifications	Neurotic, stress related and somatoform disorders	Obsessive-compulsive and related disorder	Obsessive-compulsive and related disorder
Duration criteria	2 weeks	No duration criteria	No duration criteria
Qualifiers	• Predominant obsessions • Predominant compulsions • Mixed obsessions and compulsions	• Insight – Good–fair, poor, absent–delusional • Tic-related	• Insight – Fair to good and poor to absent
Insight	Recognised as individual's own thoughts	Insight can vary from good to poor	Insight can vary from good to poor
Affect	No description	Obsessions cause 'marked anxiety or distress'. Associated features include a range of affects	Obsessions commonly cause anxiety. Under additional features, a range of affects is described
Compulsions	Mental compulsions not recognised	Mental compulsions recognised	Mental compulsions recognised
Comorbid diagnosis	In the presence of prominent symptoms of depression or antedating symptoms of depression, a diagnosis of depression is made. Obsessive-compulsive disorder diagnosis discouraged in the presence of schizophrenia or Tourette's syndrome	Can be diagnosed along with other disorders	Can make a diagnosis of obsessive-compulsive disorder in the presence of other disorders like Tourette's syndrome, schizophrenia or depression
Associated disorders		Includes body dysmorphic disorder, hoarding disorder, trichotillomania (hair pulling disorder), excoriation (skin picking) disorder.	Includes body dysmorphic disorder, hypochondriasis, olfactory reference disorder, hoarding disorder, skin picking disorder, trichotillomania

obsessions or compulsions that result in significant distress or significant impairment in personal, family, social, educational, occupational or other important areas of functioning. Compulsions may be mental or physical. The individual attempts to ignore or suppress the obsessions or neutralise them by performing compulsions. It was recognised both in the DSM-5 and ICD-11 that insight into the irrationality of the obsessions or compulsions in OCD can be highly variable, fluctuating within an individual at different times and under varying circumstances. Thus, a measure of insight is adopted as a specifier and ranges between good to fair and poor to absent. In the DSM-5, the presence of a tic – which may affect treatment outcomes – was also included as another specifier.

The major differences in the two contemporary classificatory systems, along with the ICD-10, are summarised in Table 6.4.1.

The DSM-5 represented a major shift in the classification of OCD, as a new and separate category of obsessive-compulsive and related disorders (OCRDs; also called obsessive-compulsive spectrum disorders in the psychiatric literature) was created (Table 6.4.2). These disorders were grouped together due to their frequent comorbidity and similar symptomatology. Previously, OCD had been classified as an anxiety disorder. Body dysmorphic disorder had been classified as a somatoform disorder, and trichotillomania had previously been categorised as an impulse-control disorder. It was recognised that OCD often co-exists with anxiety symptoms and many anxiety disorders, but it was thought justifiable to create a subgroup of the disorders.

ICD-11[5] also adopted an obsessive-compulsive and related disorders (OCRD) grouping, comprising a similar but not identical list of disorders (Table 6.4.2). A field trial recently found that – compared to the ICD-10 – the ICD-11 criteria had greater clinical utility in diagnosing OCD and the other OCRDs, suggesting that this new method of grouping disorders was beneficial.[6]

Table 6.4.2 Obsessive-compulsive and related disorders in the DSM-5 and ICD-11

DSM-5	ICD-11
Obsessive-compulsive disorder (OCD)	**Obsessive-compulsive disorder (OCD)**
Body dysmorphic disorder	**Body dysmorphic disorder**
Hoarding disorder	**Hoarding disorder**
Trichotillomania (hair-pulling disorder)	**Trichotillomania (hair-pulling disorder)**
Excoriation (skin-picking) disorder	**Excoriation (skin-picking) disorder**
Substance/medication-induced obsessive-compulsive and related disorder	**Hypochondriasis**
Obsessive-compulsive and related disorder due to another medical condition	**Olfactory reference disorder**
Other specified obsessive-compulsive and related disorder	**Other specified obsessive-compulsive or related disorders**
Unspecified obsessive-compulsive and related disorder	**Obsessive-compulsive or related disorders, unspecified**

Body Dysmorphic Disorder (BDD)

Body dysmorphic disorder (BDD) involves obsessive thoughts about irregularities or abnormalities in appearance. They are usually related to imagined or perceived minor defects, which are exaggerated, and occur together with related compulsive acts including checking one's appearance (e.g. in the mirror or other reflective surfaces), comparing one's appearance with others and attempts at camouflage (e.g. with make-up or even cosmetic surgery). Unlike OCD, the obsessions and compulsions of BDD are restricted to specific appearance-related themes. People with severe BDD may attempt to remediate their perceived disfigurement with cosmetic surgery, but they do not usually obtain satisfaction from this. Some people with BDD even attempt 'do it yourself' surgery, and this can end up with dangerous consequences. As with OCD, levels of insight in BDD may be impaired – to the extent that the individual with BDD may believe they actually are disfigured.

Hoarding Disorder

Hoarding disorder is a pattern of behaviour characterised by compulsive and excessive acquisition, often along with the inability or unwillingness to discard large quantities of objects that would seemingly qualify as useless or without value, resulting in a cluttered and congested environment. This can become a serious health or wellbeing hazard. Hoarding disorder is another OCRD that is commonly associated with impaired insight, and it is sometimes the family members or affected neighbours who raise the alarm. In such cases, concerted efforts to engage the individual may be needed in order to fully evaluate and manage the problem.

Trichotillomania

Trichotillomania (hair-pulling disorder) is often a debilitating condition characterised by compulsive pulling out of one's own body hair (e.g. head, eyebrows, lashes, pubic hair), leading to hair loss, scarring, distress and marked functional impairment. People with this disorder are frequently ashamed and do their utmost to hide their symptoms (e.g. with hair pieces, make-up or scarves), even from their doctors. Vigilance for trichotillomania is recommended in anyone presenting with unusual headwear, especially if there is a known history of another OCRD.

Excoriation Disorder

Skin-picking disorder (excoriation disorder) is characterised by compulsive, disfiguring picking of the skin (e.g. around fingernails, lips) leading to skin lesions. It may be associated with severe nail biting. As in trichotillomania, the disorder is associated with significant distress or functional impairment.

Hypochondriasis

Hypochondriasis involves the obsessive preoccupation with fears of having a serious disease that persists despite adequate medical reassurance to the contrary. Somatic symptoms do not need to be present and, if they are present, are usually mild. The individual may however be hypervigilant for signs of illness and catastrophically mistake normal bodily sensations as malign. The hypochondriacal ruminations are accompanied by compulsive 'neutralising' behaviours that usually involve checking for bodily symptoms, requesting investigations and checking of health-related information to seek reassurance. Nowadays, this form of medical checking frequently takes place on the internet (termed cyberchondria). This checking or reassurance seeking only serves to increase anxiety.

Olfactory Reference Syndrome

Olfactory reference syndrome involves obsessive ruminations about the fear that one emits a foul or unpleasant body odour that causes extreme offence to others. The disorder is also characterised by compulsive neutralising behaviours such as frequent showering or excessive deodorant use to camouflage the imagined odour or by social avoidance and isolation. As with BDD, in some cases, insight may be impaired, and the individual believes he or she really does smell. Interpersonal interactions are avoided or endured with significant distress, shame and embarrassment.

Apart from OCD, the OCRDS tend to be a relatively poorly recognised group of disorders with limited research of evidence related to epidemiology, course and treatment. It is to be expected that the new classification will improve our understanding of these disorders. Therefore, the following sections of this chapter will focus on OCD and make reference to the other disorders where appropriate.

Common Symptoms of OCD

Most patients with OCD experience a mixture of different obsessions and compulsions. Excessive or unrealistic fears about contamination are consistently reported as the commonest form of obsession and are usually accompanied by washing or cleaning compulsions or avoidance of situations that might lead to contamination. These individuals may, for example, find it difficult to visit the hospital or outpatient clinic. Other common obsessions include the irrational fear that harm will befall on themselves or their loved ones, obsessions relating to aspects of the body being diseased or disfigured, and pathological doubts. These obsessions are commonly linked to repetitive checking behaviours, which can extend to asking family members or doctors for help or reassurance. An overwhelming need for orderliness or symmetry is another common symptom that links itself to tidying and arranging compulsions. Unwelcome or perverse sexual obsessions can be particularly distressing and embarrassing, to the extent that sufferers may be reluctant to divulge these symptoms for fear of being labelled as a sexual deviant. Other themes include abnormal assessment of risk, excessive doubt and the need for completeness.

Obsessions without compulsions can also occur, but careful examination in most cases identifies some form of mental compulsion. Usually the extremely distressing intrusive thought is followed by the individual searching for evidence that they have not performed their worst fear or seeking reassurance from others.

Case Example

A 40-year-old man presented with a 20-year history of incapacitating ruminations concerning homosexuality. He spent roughly 10 hours a day ruminating and had been unable to work or socialise because of his problem. Although initially reluctant to discuss his ruminations, he eventually admitted that he had worries that he might have touched men's bottoms. This had led him to worry that he was homosexual, despite the fact that he had been married for 15 years and had no homosexual fantasies or experience. Whenever he was near another man, he would think that he might have touched the man on the bottom. This made him feel anxious. He would then have the urge to try to relive in his mind every movement he had made since first seeing the man to check that he had not touched the man's bottom. Although this checking reduced his anxiety a little, he would soon doubt his recall and repeat the checking activity several times. From this example, it can be seen that the obsessional thought was 'I have touched his bottom', which was followed by repeated covert checking compulsions. Since these compulsions took the form of mentally visualising his own actions, they could easily have been over-looked if the patient had not been asked to report exactly what went through his mind. Some obsessions take the form of obsessional images. In the previous example, another man might have the mental image of himself actually touching another man's bottom.

Compulsions without obsessions have also been described. Many of these patients have suffered from OCD for several decades, and it appears that the original obsession – or reason for performing the compulsion – has been lost over time. The compulsions, therefore, seem to persist as a form of habit. Patients with obsessional slowness appear to have pure compulsive activity without a history of obsession.[6] These patients take several hours to get up, get dressed or have a bath. They deny any clear obsessional thoughts that lead to this extreme difficulty.

Case Example

A 24-year-old man had a 10-year history of slowness. Washing and shaving in the morning took between two and five hours to complete, so that he felt unable even to attempt to get up and dressed. Initially, he would spend an hour going over in his mind the activities he was going to perform. Following this, he set out all the objects he was going to use in advance. He would put his razor on the shelf and then stand and stare at it for several minutes before picking it up and putting it down again. This placing of objects and repetition could continue for as much as an hour. Once this was completed, the actual actions of shaving and washing were similarly methodically performed, with each action being followed by close scrutiny, prolonged periods of thought and repetition.

Although patients with obsessional slowness deny obsessional thoughts, the motivation for their slowness is usually an effort to ensure that everything they do is performed perfectly, thus driving a need to break down actions into components and mentally check each one. By aiming at perfection, they constantly fail and thus have to try harder, which takes increasingly longer. A frequent experience is that of obsessional doubt. This is the subjective feeling of doubt that an action has been performed, or performed 'properly', even though the person knows that he or she has done it.

Case Example

A man had obsessions that his house might burn down. On leaving the house, he would check all the electrical switches and gas taps. Immediately after the compulsive checking, he had doubts that he had checked everything properly and therefore repeated the checks many times. On one level, he knew that he had checked everything, but he felt he could not trust his memory. Such repetition can be understood in terms of the temporary anxiety-reducing effect of compulsive rituals.

OCD with Poor Insight

Most patients with OCD show insight into the irrationality of their symptoms – at least in some circumstances (e.g. while sitting in a relaxed state without immediate compelling obsessive fears) – but show poorer insight in other circumstances (e.g. whilst experiencing troubling intrusions). Some patients may have more limited insight throughout the full course of the illness.[7] Some individuals with very poor insight are extremely difficult to engage in therapy and appear deluded. Matsunaga et al.[8] examined a group of individuals with OCD with poor insight. They compared patients with OCD and poor insight with those with good insight. Overall treatment with clomipramine and cognitive behavioural therapy (CBT) resulted in improvement in insight as well as OCD symptoms for those with poor insight. However, a more recent study that compared people with OCD with poor insight against those with good insight found that those with poor insight were more difficult to treat – for example, they were likely to have been untreated for longer, to have been prescribed antipsychotics, to have sensory phenomena (e.g. sense of unpleasant smell) or to have hoarding symptoms.[9] In another study, a comparison with those diagnosed with schizophrenia plus OCD symptoms, found that patients with poor insight OCD had similar functional impairment at the start of treatment but fared much better after six months on treatment.[10]

OCD: Differential Diagnosis and Comorbidity

Boundary with Normality

Mild forms of obsessions, such as repetitive behaviour checking or superstitious acts, are common in everyday life. In popular culture, for example, people may refer to someone having an 'obsession' as someone who intensely enjoys a sport such as football. Alternatively, many of us might have had horrible, frightening or abhorrent intrusive thoughts on occasions (e.g. standing on the station platform and suddenly thinking you may jump in front of the train), which causes you to step back and be temporarily anxious. These are automatic thoughts and can occur in everyone. In OCD, it is the repetitive nature of the thoughts that is the key. This often leads to these thoughts dominating the individual's life and causes significant functional impairment.

In order to diagnose OCD, an individual needs to have obsessions or compulsions as their core symptoms, and the diagnosis should only be made if the symptoms are time-consuming or associated with impairment or distress. Indeed, some mild obsessive behaviours may have a benefit to the individual in terms of achieving their life goals. In OCD, however, the behaviours have become an end in themselves, which interferes with the attainment of life goals and happiness.

The obsessions and the urge to perform compulsions are, by definition, unpleasant and cause the individual distress. Indeed, obsessions are often abhorrent and frightening. Compulsions usually reduce the distress caused by the obsession to some extent, but the relief is short-lived. Sometimes, neither obsessions nor compulsions are obvious and may need further exploration to be revealed. Some people describe their obsessions as being a 'voice', but further questioning reveals that this is, in reality, an intrusive thought and that it can be recognised as such.

Recurrent intrusive thoughts, impulses or images also occur in other OCRDs. For example, the preoccupation with bodily appearance in BDD, the preoccupation with illness in hypochondriasis or the preoccupation with hair pulling in trichotillomania. Other more rewarding preoccupations – such as with sex, shopping, eating or gambling – are not OCD but are examples of increased impulsive behaviours or behavioural addiction and should not be diagnosed as OCD. The overlap between compulsivity and impulsivity is currently an area being widely researched as it is increasingly recognised that there is overlap between the psychobiological mechanisms underpinning both types of symptoms.[9]

Depression

An association between OCD and depression has been noted for many years.[11,12] A diagnosis of OCD can be made in the presence of comorbid depression, as long as the ruminations are not exclusively restricted to depressive themes. In the large US Epidemiologic Catchment Area studies,[13,14] one-third of adults with OCD also met DSM criteria for major depression at the time of interview, and three-quarters reported a history of depression at some time during their illness. Moreover, 12 per cent of individuals diagnosed with depression also had a history of OCD. A study of childhood OCD showed that the depression was equally likely to pre-date as to follow the obsessional illness.[15] The link between OCD and depression remains poorly understood, and some symptoms usually associated with depression – such as anxiety, lack of pleasure, concentration difficulties and lack of drive – may also be part of OCD. It is thought that some individuals have a vulnerability to both disorders.

Given that OCD can be severely disabling, it is not surprising that sufferers become dysphoric, often leading to developing depression. In such cases, treatment of the underlying OCD leads to an improvement of both conditions. Further, many patients are secretive about their OCD and cope for years despite severe obsessional symptoms. They choose to present to their doctor for treatment only when depression supervenes, and it significantly impacts their functioning. In these cases, it is important to not miss the OCD, since the depression is likely to respond fully only if the underlying OCD is treated adequately.

OCD and Phobic Disorders

Phobic disorders can easily be confused with OCD. Important similarities and differences between the two conditions are highlighted in Table 6.4.3.

Spider phobia is an example of a specific animal phobia where the fear is purely related to the presence of spiders in the vicinity. Contrast this with the following case of OCD.

Case Example

Eleanor had a 10-year history of fear of contamination by household dirt with the concern that she might catch diseases, which could then be passed on to others and would result in her feeling responsible for this plague. She viewed spiders as evidence that a place was dusty and 'unclean'. This made her avoid any situations where she had seen spiders in the past. Even if she saw a spider in her garden through the window, she would feel anxious and resort to cleaning rituals, which consisted of stripping off all her clothes – which she considered contaminated – and repeatedly washing them in multiples of four, which she considered a good number.

A spider phobic has an extreme fear of spiders and will avoid any situation that causes him or her to think about spiders. Eleanor's problem is different. Her fear is not of the spiders themselves but of the *consequences* that may result from contact with spiders and dust. The development of *elaborate belief systems* in people with OCD is also demonstrated in Eleanor's case, where she performed her stereotyped washing rituals in multiples of four.

Table 6.4.3 Comparison of obsessive-compulsive disorder (OCD) and phobias

Similarities	Differences
Fear is a core feature	Unlike in phobias, in OCD, the fear is not of the situation itself but of its consequences
Avoidance of situations that provoke thoughts, anxiety or rituals	Unlike in phobias, in OCD, elaborate belief systems develop around the rituals

Tourette Syndrome

Tourette syndrome (TS) commonly presents with symptoms of OCD, estimates ranging from 35 to 50%.[16] Furthermore, the families of TS sufferers have a raised incidence of OCD (as well as of TS, tics and agoraphobia[17]). The incidence of TS in OCD is lower (5–7%), although tics are reported in 20–30% of individuals with OCD. It can sometimes be difficult to distinguish between compulsive rituals and tics. Close questioning about the reasons why movements are performed is often required. Compulsions are performed to reduce the anxiety associated with an obsessional idea, whereas tics are performed to reduce discomfort or tension, which is often worsened by stress and anxiety. Patients with TS often turn out to be more resistant to conventional treatments. Tic-related OCD is recognised as a specific subgroup in the DSM-5, and patients with this comorbidity may particularly benefit from treatment with SSRI and adjunctive dopamine antagonist drugs.[18]

Obsessive-Compulsive (Anankastic) and Other Personality Disorders

Obsessive-compulsive personality disorder (OCPD) is marked by long-standing 'egosyntonic' attitudinal traits and behaviours involving an excessive need for orderliness, control and rigid perfectionism. These traits and behaviours are usually present by the time a person reaches adulthood and are visible in a variety of situations. They may include stubbornness, frugality and hoarding and can be extremely debilitating. ICD-11 has taken a novel, dimensional approach to diagnosing personality disorders. A recent review found evidence that the category of anakastia in ICD-11 is diagnostically valid, clinically useful and overlaps with the DSM-5 OCPD criteria. The clinical utility of this new approach has to be further determined through more studies in diverse clinical and cultural groups.[19]

OCPD is one of the commonest personality disorders, and mild degrees of this may offer an advantage to the individual.[20] It was traditionally thought that OCD tended to develop in those with pre-existing obsessional personalities. Systematic studies, however, have identified OCPD in only a minority of cases of OCD, with other forms of personality disorders occurring more commonly. Up to 5 per cent of individuals with OCD have a schizotypal personality disorder, which tends to confer a poor prognosis characterised by inadequate social function, poor treatment compliance and poor insight.

Emotionally unstable personality disorder (EUPD) is also sometimes seen in patients with OCD. Indeed, it may be that childhood trauma has resulted in both OCD and EUPD. A small study by Ramos-Barbera and Drummond (2018), presented at the ECNP congress, found that OCD patients with EUPD were less likely to significantly improve with intensive treatments when compared with patients with comorbid OCPD or autism.

Schizophrenia and Other Psychoses

Schizophrenia is more common in patients with OCD. In a study based on Danish registers, prior diagnosis of OCD was associated with an increased risk of developing schizophrenia and schizophrenia spectrum disorders later in life.[21] In addition, patients with OCD and their relatives are more likely to be diagnosed with bipolar disorder, schizoaffective disorder and schizophrenia compared with the general population.[22]

Some atypical antipsychotic medicines that act on the glutamatergic system, most markedly clozapine, can precipitate OCD-like symptoms in patients with schizophrenia.[23] Preliminary evidence suggests that the comorbid obsessive-compulsive syndrome needs specific treatment, since antipsychotic medications used on their own are generally ineffective.

Case Example

A young, male long-stay inpatient with a diagnosis of schizophrenia made himself exceedingly unpopular on his ward because of his compulsion to use excessive amounts of toilet paper, which continually blocked the toilets.

Autism

Autism is a developmental disorder that can present in people with a range of intellectual abilities. Traditionally, it was thought to be much more common in men, but recent studies suggest that the condition is often under-diagnosed in women, who are often better at hiding their social interaction difficulties, and large studies have suggested that the male to female ratio for autism may be 3–4:1.[24] There is increasing evidence suggesting a high prevalence of previously undiagnosed ASD in patients presenting for treatment for OCD.[25] ASD traits are associated with greater OCD symptom severity and poor insight.

Anorexia Nervosa and Bulimia Nervosa

The link between obsessive-compulsive symptoms and eating disorders has been recognised for well over 50 years.[26] Of course, intrusive thoughts and forced behaviours relating specifically to weight, body size and food intake are integral to the eating disorder and do not constitute OCD as such. However, many individuals may also have obsessions and compulsions unrelated to food. Thiel et al.,[27] using standardised rating instruments, showed that 37 per cent of a cohort of 93 anorexic or bulimic females concurrently fulfilled DSM criteria for OCD. OCD comorbidity correlated positively with the severity of the eating disorder. Other studies looking at people with OCD have reported a high lifetime prevalence of anorexia nervosa and bulimia nervosa, reaching 6–12%.[27]

Increased rates of eating disorders are also described in people with autism spectrum disorder.[28] Conversely, people diagnosed with anorexia nervosa were found to score higher than average on a scale measuring autistic symptoms.[29]

Stammering and Stuttering

Some individuals with OCD have to perform compulsive rituals that results in a lack of clarity in spoken speech. Common examples are patients who need to check that every word they say is totally accurate or patients who may count the number of words in their sentence or letters in their words before uttering them. Careful assessment may be needed to reveal the problem, and patients with speech abnormalities should be screened for obsessional psychopathology.

Recently, stammering and stuttering has been linked to a prior history of streptococcal infection.[30] Some workers have reported the finding that some children who present with rapid onset of neurological symptoms and OCD have had recent streptococcal or other infections.[31]

Epidemiology of OCD

Large-scale epidemiological surveys have shown a relatively high prevalence of OCD. Worldwide, a six-month prevalence of between 1.3%[32] and 2%[13] and a lifetime prevalence of 1.9% to 3.3% has been reported.[33] These rates of disorder could be related to the fact that many people with OCD do not seek medical help but battle alone in the community. Alternatively, the relatively high rates seen in community surveys may result from the inclusion of people with mild obsessional symptoms without functional impairment.

Community prevalence studies also identify a female to male ratio of around 1.5:1. Women commonly suffer from compulsive washing and avoidance, whereas men more frequently have checking rituals or ruminations.[34,35] Males predominate in surveys of OCD referrals – reflecting, perhaps, a greater illness severity in males. A study of patients with refractory OCD treated in the community[36] showed a predominance of men (around 56 per cent) in the most profoundly ill group requiring inpatient treatment.[37]

The mean age at onset of OCD is earlier than that of depression, occurring at around 20 years of age. Males tend to develop the illness earlier, with incidence rates peaking in the early teens, compared to the early twenties for females.[38] OCD was once thought to be rare in children, but we now know that it is in fact one of the commonest mental disorders, affecting 1–5% of children and adolescents in community samples.[39] The clinical pattern mirrors that in adults, and boys tend to develop symptoms earlier than girls.

The course of OCD can vary from a relatively benign form – in which the sufferer experiences occasional, discrete episodes interspersed between symptom-free periods – to a malignant form with unremitting symptoms and substantial social impairment. A remarkable 40-year follow-up study looked at a cohort of 144 individuals who had been treated in the hospital for OCD by the investigators. Treatment started before the development of more-effective treatments that are available today.[40] The study found that 60% showed signs of improvement within the first 10 years of hospital admission, rising to 80% by the end of the study, but only 20% achieved full remission; another 60% continued to experience significant symptoms, 10% showed no improvement whatsoever and 10% had deteriorated. In 60% of cases, the type of symptoms had changed over the course of the illness, and 20% of those whose symptoms initially improved subsequently relapsed, sometimes after as long as 20 years of being free of symptoms (and hence, early recovery does not appear to rule out the possibility of relapse).

In spite of the early onset and chronic, unremitting course of the untreated illness, people with OCD do not usually present for treatment until many years have elapsed, often until they are in their early middle age. Poor recognition of the disorder and stigma are likely reasons. As a result, the duration of untreated illness in OCD counts as one of the longest for any mental disorder and is thought to contribute to poor outcomes.[41,42] Therefore, incentives for improving recognition and timely treatment are encouraged.[43,44]

Approximately half of all OCD patients who present for treatment are single.[34] This probably reflects the pervasive effect of OCD on sustaining relationships as a result of which many people with OCD are living alone and relatively unsupported by family members. In the most profound refractory groups, only 19.2% of patients requiring inpatient treatment were married or cohabiting.[37]

OCD is seen in cultures as diverse as India[45] and Hong Kong,[46] as well as the Western countries. Recent studies have noted, however, that OCD is likely to be under-diagnosed in African Americans in the USA.[47] Religion is thought to play a part in the genesis of some cases; studies have suggested that the disorder is more common in people who have had a strict religious upbringing, although it does not appear to be related to any particular denomination.[48,49] A recent review by Nicolini et al.[50] concluded that religion and religiosity impacted on the content of obsessions but that culture and religion did not alter the prevalence of OCD.

Aetiology

There are many theories for the aetiology of OCD. Most of these are not mutually exclusive, and a multifactorial aetiology is likely.

Genetics

A genetic component to OCD has been recognised from the earliest descriptions of the disorder. A recent review demonstrated the complexity of the genetics of OCD and presented some of the latest evidence regarding the networks of genes involved in synaptic transmission, neurodevelopment, and the immune and inflammatory changes associated with this disorder.[51]

Animal models have implicated various genes in the development of OCD. These include genes coding for scaffolding proteins within cellular membranes – including SLC6A4, which codes for the serotonin transporter protein, as well as SAPAP3 and SCL1A1, which are intimately involved in the structure of the glutamate receptor.[52,53] However, large-scale population-based studies designed to search for consistent genetic abnormalities within OCD samples, such as the recent Genome Wide Association Studies (GWAS), have not so far conclusively demonstrated any single gene abnormality in OCD, possibly owing to methodological issues.[54,55]

Early work exploring the heritability of OCD focused on family and twin studies, but more recent work has used other models.

Family Studies

A number of family studies have been performed regarding OCD,[56] and their results demonstrate that OCD runs closely in families. However, there is also a high rate of other psychiatric illnesses in the relatives of probands.[57] OCD itself occurs in roughly 10% of the first-degree relatives of patients, compared with 1.9% in controls.[58] A recent large study of familial aggregation demonstrated that the risk of OCD in full siblings of patients with tic-related OCD and patients with non-tic-related OCD was estimated at 10.63 and 4.52%, respectively, suggesting that tic-related OCD is a more familial form and may have a different aetiology.[59] This form of information can be helpful in discussions between clinicians and patients, including those planning a family.

Twin Studies

Familial aggregation of a disorder is a prerequisite for genetic transmission, but it does not prove genetic transmission because the family unit also transmits environmental and cultural influences that shape human development. Twin studies, to some extent, control for the cultural effects of shared sibling-ship and may therefore give a better indication of heritability.

The twin method involves comparing the rate of concordance for OCD among monozygotic twins with that among dizygotic twins. If the concordance among monozygotic twins is higher, it is taken as robust evidence of a genetic contribution to the expression of the disorder. Several twin studies have looked at anxiety and 'neuroticism'. They showed a strong likelihood of heritability. Few studies, however, have looked specifically at OCD. Historically, Carey and Gottesman[60] carefully examined 15 pairs of monozygotic and dizygotic twins with OCD and found that 87% of the monozygotic and 47% of the dizygotic twins were concordant for obsessive symptoms or traits, supporting the view that genetic components are implicated. A more recent, larger study of 220 pairs of non-clinical twins suggested that the heritability of obsessive-compulsive traits was 74%.[61,62]

Other Methods of Studying Heritability

Other techniques, such as segregation analysis, may be used to refine our understanding of heritability. Three such studies have been applied to OCD.[63-65] The results showed that if you take the OCD population all together, inheritance patterns are hard to model and do not fit any simple Mendelian rule. However, if you select out those families who have many members affected (i.e. that are clearly familial), a pattern of 'mixed model' transmission emerges. This mixed model implies a gene of major effect combined with a multigenic background. Thus, it is likely that there are several genes involved in OCD, and individuals may be more or less affected by a variety of different genetic mechanisms.

It is clear that the genetic model of OCD is far from straightforward. For example, it has recently been reported in a study examining expression of synaptic genes in post-mortem human brain samples that patients with OCD have reduced expression of genes related to excitatory glutamatergic synapses in the lateral and frontal regions of the orbitofrontal cortex.[66] Other studies have looked at gene methylation, which may control the expression of genes related to OCD, and its impact on the expression of the illness.

Neurotransmitters

OCD and the Serotonin Hypothesis

The evidence for an abnormality in serotonin neurotransmission in patients with OCD rests mainly on the results of drug treatment studies, which have consistently shown that drugs with potent inhibitory effects on the neuronal re-uptake of serotonin (5-HT) – and thereby increase serotonin availability at the level of the synapse – are effective treatments, while anxiolytic and antidepressant agents acting predominantly on other neurotransmitter systems are not.

Clomipramine is a tricyclic antidepressant that acts predominantly by reducing the re-uptake of serotonin into the presynaptic neurons following its release into the synaptic cleft. It has only weak actions on noradrenergic transmission, although one of its metabolites has noradrenergic effects. Many trials have compared clomipramine with placebo as well as other tricyclic drugs, which have consistently shown superiority for clomipramine. For example, clomipramine has been shown to be more effective in OCD than the predominantly noradrenergic antidepressants desipramine[67] and nortriptyline.[68]

Since the discovery of clomipramine's efficacy, more highly selective serotonin re-uptake inhibitors (SSRIs) – such as fluvoxamine, fluoxetine, paroxetine, sertraline and citalopram – have been extensively investigated and also found to be effective in OCD. Recent studies also suggest that higher doses of SSRI are more efficacious and that the effect develops over time and is lost when treatment is discontinued (for clinical information on dosing, please see later).[43,69,70] People with OCD tend to react slowly to clomipramine or SSRIs, with benefits often not apparent until the patient has been on a full dose of medication for up to three months. Thereafter, benefits can continue to accrue for at least two years.[43]

While these findings point to serotonin being important for recovery and provide a rationale for further investigation of serotonergic neuro-transmission in OCD, we need to be cautious about extrapolating too far from these data. In spite of extensive investigation, the 'serotonin hypothesis' for OCD – which proposes that OCD results from a specific dysfunction in the 5-HT system – remains speculative, and the mechanism by which clomipramine and SSRIs exert their effects in OCD remains unknown.[71]

Platelet Studies

The area of biological markers for OCD has recently been reviewed by Bandelow et al.[72] Platelets have been used as an accessible model of intracerebral neurons *vis-à-vis* re-uptake of serotonin, since they possess very similar serotonin transporter and re-uptake machinery. Several studies have investigated the platelet serotonin transporter using a variety of radiolabelled ligands. A reduction in the number of transporter sites in OCD patients compared with controls has been found, which appears to be state dependent and may be reversed after successful treatment with SSRIs.[73] While we cannot necessarily infer that the same process is occurring in the brain, these findings provide further support for a link between OCD and serotonin neuro-transmission.

Pharmacological Responses

More than 17 subtypes of serotonin receptor have been identified, and the question of which receptors might be most implicated in OCD has been raised. Besides blocking the serotonin transporter, clomipramine enhances the responsiveness of the post-synaptic 5-HT1A receptor and desensitises the 5-HT2C receptor, whereas SSRIs reduce somato-dendritic and terminal auto-receptor responsiveness.[74] These changes are associated with gradually increasing serotonergic neurotransmission across the synapse. The effects are particularly marked in the orbitofrontal cortex,[75] an area strongly implicated in OCD from neuroimaging studies (see later). The anti-obsessional effect of SSRIs has been linked to increasing activation of 5-HT2 pathways.[76]

The use of neurochemical probes to explore the sensitivity of various 5-HT receptor subtypes provided some further suggestive information about the role of serotonin in OCD. m-Chlorophenylpyperazine (m-CPP), an agonist at 5-HT1A, 5-HT1D and 5-HT2C receptors and which also blocks 5-HT3 receptors, was found in a series of experiments to exacerbate OCD symptoms.[77] mCPP-induced symptoms were reversed by co-administration of 5-HT antagonists such as metergoline and ritanserin.[69,70,78] These findings suggested that OCD may be associated with hypersensitivity of these 5-HT receptors in brain regions involved in the production of OC symptoms, such as the orbitofrontal and anterior cingulate cortices or the caudate nucleus.[77] However, these largely historical findings have not so far translated into viable theories. Although we cannot rule out the involvement of other subtypes, future studies of these receptors with modern neuroimaging modalities like MRS would clarify our understanding.

Other Neurotransmitters and OCD

Based on the existing evidence, it seems unlikely that OCD results exclusively from a dysregulation of serotonin. For example, roughly one-third of clinical cases fail to respond to treatment with SSRIs.[79,80] McDougle and Goodman,[81] for example, have argued that OCD is mediated by serotonin neurons in most cases, but for some patients, there is additional pathology in the dopamine system. They cite evidence from studies of combination drug treatments as well as recent neuroimaging studies (see later). A small amount of supportive neurochemical data links OCD with dysfunction in the noradrenaline systems and certain neuropeptides such as arginine, vasopressin and oxytocin.[82]

In recent years, there has been increased interest in the role of glutamate in the development and treatment of OCD. Glutamate is the most abundant neuroexcitatory chemical in the brain and has a function in learning, cognition and memory. Neuroimaging and studies of cerebrospinal fluid (CSF) in OCD patients suggest abnormalities in intracerebral glutamate transmission in OCD.[83] Some atypical antipsychotics, particularly clozapine, are thought to either precipitate or worsen OCD symptoms in some patients. It is possible that this effect results from actions on glutamatergic systems.[84,85] Other agents working on the glutamatergic system (ketamine, topiramate, memantine, N-acetyl cysteine, riluzole) have been found to have a beneficial effect on OCD in small-scale clinical trials (Table 6.4.4).

Neuroimaging

Structural Imaging and OCD

Neuroimaging in OCD has been performed since the late 1980s. Cortico-striatal circuits control a variety of neurobiological functions, including motor control, reward and cognition. The orbitofrontal cortex is connected to the corpus striatum, globus pallidus and thalamus in a functional loop that supports switching between behaviours.[86] The involvement of cortico-striatal circuitry, particularly orbitofrontal cortex and ventral striatum, in OCD is supported by imaging data from several studies that have explored anatomical aspects (brain volume, shape, density) of cortical and subcortical nodes in this circuitry.[87] Recent meta-analyses illustrate additional involvement of other brain regions – in particular, the parietal cortex, limbic areas and cerebellum.[88,89] The latest large-scale meta-analyses from the Enhancing Neuroimaging Genetics through Meta-Analysis (ENIGMA) consortium show greater pallidum volume, smaller hippocampus volume and parietal cortical thinning in OCD patients.[90,91] These abnormalities appear to be subtle and varying. Moreover, the extent to which they are unique to OCD or common to other psychiatric disorders remains unclear, as insufficient comparative and longitudinal studies are currently available.[87]

Functional Imaging in OCD

In the last 20 years, functional magnetic resonance imaging (fMRI) has been used to investigate brain dynamic alterations

Table 6.4.4 Other pharmacological agents in treatment-resistant OCD

Used as monotherapy	Study	Design	Outcome
D-amphetamine (single dose)	Insel et al. 1983 Joffe et al. 1991	Double-blind RCT Double-blind RCT	D-amphet > placebo D-amphet > placebo; Methylphenidate = placebo
Morphine	Koran et al. 2005	Double-blind RCT	Morphine > placebo
Ketamine (IV) (single dose)	Bloch et al. 2012 Rodriguez et al. 2013	Open-label Double-blind RCT	No responders at 3d Ketamine > placebo at 7d
Mirtazapine	Koran et al. 2005	Double-blind discontinuation	MIR > placebo
Used in combination with serotonin re-uptake inhibitors	**Study**	**Design**	**Outcome**
Lamotrigine	Bruno et al. 2012 Khalkhali et al. 2016	Double-blind RCT Double-blind RCT	Lamotrigine > placebo Lamotrigine > placebo
Topiramate	Berlin et al. 2010 Mowla et al. 2010 Afshar et al. 2014	Double-blind RCT Double-blind RCT Double-blind RCT	Compulsions sig, Total Y-BOCS NS Topiramate > placebo NS
Memantine	Haghigi et al. 2013 Ghaleiha et al. 2013 Modaresi et al. 2017	Double-blind RCT Double-blind RCT Double-blind RCT	Memantine > placebo Memantine > placebo Memantine > placebo
N-acetyl cysteine	Afshar et al. 2012 Sarris et al. 2015 Paydari et al. 2016 Costa et al. 2017	Double-blind RCT Double-blind RCT Double-blind RCT Double-blind RCT	N-AC > placebo NS N-AC > placebo NS
L-carnosine	Arabzadeh et al. 2017	Double-blind RCT	L-carnosine > placebo
Granisetron	Askari et al. 2012	Double-blind RCT	Granisetron > placebo

in OCD. Early studies focused on assessing regional brain differences between patients with OCD and healthy controls in task-based fMRI, focusing on tasks of executive functioning and emotional processing. Later studies have investigated interregional connectivity. Other fMRI approaches have been used to predict clinical outcomes across various treatment modalities. Results from these studies suggest the existence of functional changes in the different nodes of the cortico-striatal-thalamo-cortical circuits. However, it has not yet been possible to build a fully coherent framework from the available findings.[92]

Magnetic resonance spectroscopy (MRS) is another technique for examining localised brain activity in OCD.[93] It has been hypothesised that OCD symptoms may result from an imbalance in the concentration of different neurotransmitters within the cortico-striatal circuitry, but the available MRS studies – which have focused on measuring local concentrations of glutamate, glutamine and gamma-amino-butyric acid – report inconsistent results, probably due to methodological limitations.[94-97] However, changes in the concentration of N-acetylaspartate, a marker of neuronal density, in dorsal and rostral anterior cingulate cortex has been relatively consistently revealed and found to normalise after successful clinical treatment.[98,99] Another relatively consistent MRS finding in OCD patients is a higher level of thalamic choline, a marker of cell membrane turnover.[100]

Positron emission tomography (PET) affords precise measurement of brain neurotransmitters and their receptors, complementing MRS methodology. A few PET studies have been performed in OCD and have reported abnormal receptor binding across different neurotransmitters including 5-HT, dopamine and glutamate.[83,101] However, once again, these results remain inconclusive.[93]

Electroencephalography (EEG) and OCD

EEG monitoring provides good temporal resolution but relatively less good anatomical resolution for changes in intracerebral neuronal activity. One of the most widely used tools in this area is the event-related potential (ERP), which is an electrical signal registered in response to a specific sensory, motor or cognitive stimulus. A component of the ERP, called error-related negativity (ERN), is generated after the commission of an error.[102] Enhanced ERN amplitudes are found in patients with OCD and their healthy relatives, implicating the enhanced ERN as an electrophysiological trait marker of vulnerability to the disorder.[103,104] Other different ERP components are currently under investigation, while high-density electroencephalography has recently emerged as a more precise technique for future research applications.[105]

Immunological Processes and OCD

Similarities between OCD and obsessions occurring in children with Sydenham's chorea led to the investigation of immunological processes in childhood OCD. Sydenham's chorea is a manifestation of rheumatic fever caused by infection with group A beta-haemolytic streptococci. Antibodies directed at the bacteria react with neurons in the basal ganglia and cause damage to neuronal structures, leading to characteristic movement disorders and, in over 80 per cent of cases, obsessions and compulsions. Moreover, one-third of children with early-onset OCD also show signs of choreiform movements. This has led to the hypothesis that infection with group A beta-haemolytic streptococci can produce conditions grouped together under the acronym PANDAS (paediatric autoimmune neuropsychiatric disorders associated with streptococci), including subgroups of paediatric OCD and tics. Patients with rheumatic fever show high levels of circulating anti-caudate antibodies and a specific B-lymphocyte antigen, labelled D8/17. This antigen also appears to be over-represented in children with OCD, Tourette's syndrome and chronic tic disorder and has been proposed as an immunological marker of susceptibility to rheumatic fever or motor consequences of infection.

Following on from these findings, it was discovered that other agents that cause common childhood infections could also result in a similar pattern of neurological symptoms and OCD. It has therefore been suggested that the syndrome be relabelled as paediatric autoimmune neurological syndrome (PANS) or childhood autoimmune neurological syndrome (CANS).[30] A study that examined adult patients with profound, chronic, refractory OCD found that these patients did not have high levels of anti-streptococcal antibodies but almost one-fifth of the sample had high levels of anti-nuclear antibodies, and these were higher than in a control group of patients treated in a psychiatric ward for conditions other than OCD.[106]

Novel brain imaging using PET has demonstrated evidence of glial cell activation in cortico-striatal circuitry, further suggesting an inflammatory or immunological aetiology for OCD and pointing to the importance of investigating other biological methods for treatment, such as medications targeting gliosis or immune modulation.[107]

Another novel area of exploration is in the microflora of the gut and the impact this may have on the development of various psychiatric syndromes. If the gut does not have a healthy range of bacteria, the theory is that the walls become 'leaky', and this leads to potential autoimmune conditions such as asthma. There has been some speculation that this may lead to some cases of OCD. A study by Turna et al. showed that patients with OCD had a limited range of gut bacteria when compared with controls.[108]

Psychological Theories

Psychoanalytic Theories

Sigmund Freud proposed that the symptoms of OCD arise as a compromise between conflicting forces in the mind.[109] For Freud, at the heart of obsessional neurosis are unconscious, aggressive instincts. Unacceptable urges – particularly, hostile urges – are admitted into awareness because of incomplete repression, necessitating defensive responses in the form of compulsive rituals to reduce guilt and anxiety. Due to the limited evidence available in regard to these theories and its usefulness in resolving OCD symptoms, it will not be discussed further.

Behavioural

Obsessions can be viewed as learned responses to specific situations.

Case Example

A 42-year-old man gave a 5-year history of blasphemous thoughts, which were provoked by the sight of churches, crosses or religious personnel. These obsessions started after the death of his mother. It could be postulated that her death caused an agitated and aroused state. At this time, previously neutral stimuli, such as churches, produced aversive blasphemous thoughts. Instead of ignoring these thoughts, which would have allowed his anxiety to habituate, he made efforts to suppress the thoughts and avoid situations that might provoke them. Because anxiety is an aversive experience, anything that reduces anxiety can be viewed as a positive reinforcer. Thus, the man's behaviour in avoiding situations and trying to suppress his anxiety-provoking thoughts was reinforced. This reinforcement served to strengthen the association between the previously neutral stimuli – the thoughts and his avoidance behaviour.

Compulsive behaviours or rituals are inefficient ways of reducing anxiety, as they cause only a small amount of relief and their effect is short-lived before anxiety increases again, which leads to a repetition of the ritual.

Case Example

A 30-year-old secretary had a 10-year history of fear that she might contaminate her children with toxoplasma from dog faeces. Upon returning to her house, she would strip off all her clothes and engage in washing rituals, in a set routine from the head downwards. This activity reduced her anxiety and was thus reinforced. Every time she performed washing rituals, the association between the thoughts and the washing rituals was strengthened. However, once she had finished washing, she would be plagued by doubt that she had performed the ritual totally correctly and so would start the washing ritual again. This sequence of anxiety followed by the washing ritual was repeated 20–30 times before she gave up in a state of exhaustion and continued anxiety. It can be seen that she spent most of her time with high levels of anxiety, with only partial and temporary relief from her rituals. These rituals themselves served to increase the problem by not allowing her anxiety to habituate naturally.

It seems difficult to understand why the individual does not habituate to an obsessional thought after hours spent every day thinking about it. Careful analysis of the content of the thought will generally reveal that there is an anxiety-provoking obsession followed by an anxiety-reducing ritualistic thought, which acts in the same way as covert rituals in temporarily reducing the anxiety and reinforcing the process.

Most people with OCD also use reassurance as an attempt to reduce the anxiety associated with their obsessional thoughts.[110]

Case Example

A man with a fear that he might cause a fire by leaving the gas on would perform repeated checking rituals. After this, he would repeatedly seek reassurance from his wife that everything had been switched off. This reassurance seeking resembled a ritual, as it temporarily reduced his anxiety, but the effect was short-lived and then further reassurance was required.

One reason why compulsive behaviour does not habituate or may even increase in the course of OCD is that, through repetition, they turn into maladaptive habits (i.e. stimulus response behaviours that are cued by specific environmental stimuli). In fact, many patients with chronic OCD report that they do not understand why they continue to perform compulsions and suggest that this form of behaviour may have become habitual. Evidence from neuroscience showing a bias towards responding in a habitual way both in rewarding and aversive situations lends support to this hypothesis.[111]

Evolutionary/Behavioural Theories

The question arises as to why the themes of obsessions are so remarkably similar. Obsessions can be divided into one of the following categories:

- Fear of contamination with harm to self
- Fear of contamination with harm to others
- Acts of omission with harm to self
- Acts of omission with harm to others
- Acts of commission with harm to self
- Acts of commission with harm to others
- Loss of objects
- Perfectionism

A limited degree of perfectionism can be an advantage in life – for example, over hygiene. In unprecedented situations, where risk is heightened – such as during the 2020–2021 coronavirus pandemic – social avoidance and repetitive washing and checking behaviours are considered vital for public health. Thus, obsessional-type symptoms can be viewed as being potentially advantageous and may thus have been selectively preserved within our genetic make-up. Members of a species are likely to respond more to stimuli with evolutionary significance.[112] In other words, it is easy for a child to learn fear of spiders, whereas fear of trees rarely occurs and would be expected to be preceded by an aversive event associated with a tree. It does seem that most obsessional fears are of situations that might be evolutionarily inherent to our species.[113]

Disgust Sensitivity

Behavioural immune theory suggests that disgust makes an individual avoid contact with substances that are evolutionarily likely to carry pathogens or contaminants. It is theorised that contamination fears in OCD may be a result of heightened disgust sensitivity, which is an evolutionarily valid emotion. A few empirical studies[114, 115] have recorded a positive association between OCD symptoms and disgust propensity, which is a self-reported tendency to be disgusted by verbally presented, hypothetical disgusting situations, such as 'stepping on dog poop' or 'seeing a rat run across my path in a park'. After the development of the disgust scale, a few studies[116,117] observed a modestly sized relationship between neuroticism and disgust sensitivity. Disgust sensitivity in such cases may also be mediated by parental modelling.

Cognitive Theories

Cognitive theories of OCD are compatible with the behavioural theories proposed earlier. In fact, they can be viewed as an elaboration or extension of behavioural theory. Cognitive theories stem from the idea that faulty thinking patterns are learned as a result of early childhood experiences. These maladaptive patterns or schemes may lie hidden for many years until activated by a later traumatic event or experience. A review by Rachman[118] examined the various cognitive theories of OCD and suggested that both an overinflated sense of personal responsibility as well as overestimation of danger may have a role to play, at least in compulsive checkers.[118] Wells' metacognitive model of OCD proposes that it is about the importance and meaning of thoughts for the individual that leads to the need to control thoughts and the need to perform rituals to prevent the feared consequences. The metacognitions that he believed are specific to OCD are thought fusion beliefs (i.e. 'If I think something, it is important'), beliefs about rituals and stop signals – or, in other words, the inability to feel satisfied and stop repeating thoughts or actions.[119] A recent study from Finland examined the metacognitions of people with OCD and concluded that a need to control thoughts contributed to checking, cleaning and rumination symptoms; cognitive self-consciousness contributed to symptoms of slowness; uncontrollability and danger contributed to doubt symptoms; and positive beliefs contributed to checking symptoms.[120]

Patients with OCD show impairments on a range of cognitive functions, in particular when tested on inhibition and cognitive flexibility. They show difficulty inhibiting habitual or behavioural responses when signalled to do so or when the behaviour no longer confers an advantage, and they show inflexibility in the use of environmental cues to adaptively modify behaviour according to changing contingencies. Cognitive disinhibition may explain why patients with OCD are unable to stop repeating their obsessional thoughts and compulsive behaviours. Cognitive inflexibility may explain why the obsessions and compulsions follow such rigid and stereotyped behavioural patterns. Deficits in inhibition and cognitive flexibility can also be seen in other OCRDs such as trichotillomania, body dysmorphic disorder and hoarding disorder. These deficits are also found in the healthy first-degree relatives of OCD patients, suggesting that they represent a marker of the vulnerability to neurobiological abnormality shared among members of OCD families.[121,122]

Sociological Theories

There are obvious problems in separating the effects of genetics and environment. It is perhaps surprising that the majority of children who have a parent with OCD do not show signs of the disorder. However, a minority do exhibit obsessive-compulsive symptoms, which may be similar to or completely different from those of the parent. Most experts believe that the influence of genetics outweighs that of social learning (or modelling, to use a behavioural term), although more research in this area is needed.

Although the onset of OCD can be insidious or sudden, studies have shown that people with the condition have more life events in the year preceding onset than do matched controls.[123] Life events varied from losses – such as bereavement, redundancy and head injury – to those that would on the surface appear more positive. This finding links behavioural theories with neuro-biological hypotheses.[62] Life events causing increased arousal, if aversive, could be linked to a previously neutral stimulus (e.g. electrical plugs). According to classical conditioning theory, the patient may become conditioned to respond with fear and high arousal, constantly checking for the danger of electrical plugs and ensuring they are safe.

Treatment

Prior to the 1960s, OCD was considered untreatable. In the following decades, a relatively narrow range of psychotherapies and pharmacotherapies have been found to be effective. Cognitive behavioural therapies involving exposure and response prevention (ERP) and pharmacotherapy with a serotonin re-uptake inhibitor (SRI) or clomipramine represent well-established treatments. Substantial improvement can be achieved in many patients following standard treatment, and early intervention is likely to improve outcomes further,[44] though a substantial proportion of patients fail to respond or go on to relapse.

According to the National Institute for Health and Clinical Excellence[118, 124] guidelines on the treatment of OCD (published in 2005, updated in 2013, checked in 2019 and now listed for updating), the current standard of care in the United Kingdom is to offer either behavioural psychotherapy or medication as first-line treatment for adults with OCD. In the case of children or adolescents, behavioural psychotherapy is usually offered first. Medication is offered if psychotherapy is declined or they are unable to engage or benefit from therapy, with arrangements for adverse event monitoring. Established psychological and pharmacological treatments appear to be equally effective, and it is not clear whether a combination of both is superior to psychological or pharmacological monotherapy.[125]

The evidence-based treatment of OCD depended upon the introduction of methods for the standardised assessment of the disorder. The Yale-Brown Obsessive Compulsive Scale (Y-BOCS)[126] is a widely accepted and validated quantitative measure of obsessive-compulsive symptom severity that can also be helpful in clinical practice. It is divided into two parts (1. symptom checklist, 2. ten severity questions), and the score is independent of the type or number of obsessions or compulsions. Each item rates from 0 (no symptoms) to 4 (extreme symptoms), with a total range of 0 to 40. The total score classifies severity into subclinical, mild, moderate, severe and extremely severe. A 25 per cent improvement in the baseline Y-BOCS represents a clinically relevant change equivalent to a minimal partial response. Similarly, a five-point worsening of the remission Y-BOCS can be used to represent a clinical relapse.[127]

If an adequate response to treatment with an SSRI alone or CBT alone or their combination does not occur, second-line strategies include high-dose treatment with SRIs, switching/combining SRIs and augmentation with antipsychotics. Failure to respond to these therapeutic options may indicate refractoriness to treatment. Thus, if the symptoms remain severe and debilitating, it may be necessary to consult with specialist services for consideration of somatic treatments such as neurostimulation or neurosurgery (see later).

Psychological Treatment

Exposure and Response Prevention (ERP)

Exposure and response prevention (ERP) is the psychological treatment of choice for patients with obsessions and compulsions. It consists of prolonged, graded exposure in real life to the feared situation together with self-imposed response prevention. In order to perform this treatment, the patient needs to be educated about OCD and how the temporary reduction in anxiety produced by the performance of compulsive rituals actually serves to strengthen the association between obsessive thought and compulsive ritual, thus worsening the condition.

Exposure works on the observation that a patient who has an intense fear of a situation, when confronted with the situation will either escape or perform activities (compulsions or rituals) to reduce or prevent the harm he or she fears will result. High anxiety is extremely unpleasant. Escape and compulsive behaviours reduce anxiety. Therefore, the escape behaviours are reinforced by the reduction of the anxiety. Consequently, the conditions are worsened by each episode of brief exposure and escape. In exposure treatment, the aim is to produce prolonged periods of contact with the feared situation until the anxiety naturally reduces (habituation). Compulsions reduce anxiety, and this serves to reinforce the ritual. However, the reduction in anxiety produced by a compulsive ritual tends to be small and the effect temporary. Instead, rituals prevent therapeutic exposure and increase the tendency to ritualise further.

With treatment, patients are asked to expose themselves to the fear-provoking situation and remain in that situation until the anxiety has substantially reduced. This usually takes between 60 and 90 minutes. Although this is a simple technique, the skill lies in the therapist accurately assessing the correct fear-provoking cues, educating the patient about the therapy and helping the patient to agree on a level of exposure that will cause a degree of anxiety that can be tolerated.

Although exposure is the cornerstone of the treatment of OCD, it needs to be combined with response prevention – that is, with encouragement not to perform compulsions, either physical or mental. This can usually be achieved by demonstrating to the patient how they interfere with exposure. The same exposure tasks are then repeated by the patient at least daily (preferably three times a day) until there is little anxiety even at the commencement of the exposure. A more anxiety-provoking situation can then be tackled until the patient has completed the tasks on the 'anxiety hierarchy' devised with the therapist.

Graduated exposure and response prevention is a quick and cost-efficient treatment that can be easily applied in many general practice and hospital settings, but it is often unavailable outside specialist services. Although some basic training is required, this can easily be obtained by reading about clinical techniques[128,129] and by obtaining supervision from a trained behavioural psychotherapist. It has been found that instruction in self-exposure techniques may be all that is required for many patients. For more intransigent cases, individual therapist exposure rarely involves more than 10–15 hours of therapist time. Moreover, ERP can most usefully be applied in the patient's home-setting, where the symptoms are usually maximal.[36]

Over the years, the most effective exposure has been shown to be (1) prolonged rather than of short duration, (2) in real life rather than in fantasy and (3) regularly practiced, with self-exposure homework tasks. In addition, the efficacy of self-exposure has been demonstrated in individual, group and online delivery.[130, 131] Patients with pure obsessional ruminations have always been considered difficult to treat. This may partly have been because therapists have not identified the associated covert, anxiety-reducing compulsions (as discussed earlier). The cornerstone of treatment for obsessions is exposure to the anxiety-provoking thought and resistance to the covert mental ritual.

One way of maintaining exposure to the anxiety-provoking thoughts involves the use of a personal recording. The aim is to use this recording to prolong exposure without allowing the patient time to perform mental rituals. Originally, this technique involved using a cassette tape but can now be easily achieved on a mobile phone recording.

Cognitive Behavioural Therapy (CBT)

Although cognitive behavioural therapy has been advocated for OCD, there is no clear evidence that, in general, it produces any better results than simple exposure and response prevention.[132] There is more evidence in favour of using targeted cognitive techniques to overcome specific problems in exposure therapy. For example, cognitive therapy may be helpful in reducing the strength of belief in irrational obsessions or the erroneous sense of responsibility that may characterise some patients with OCD. Descriptions of current thinking about optimal psychological treatments for OCD have been published recently.[43] The outcome of treatment is fully discussed in the next section. In recent years, there has been an increased interest in using what have become known as third-wave or third-generation CBT interventions (first wave being behavioural, second wave being cognitive and behavioural). With respect to OCD, these are loosely based on Eastern concepts and meditation. Patients are taught to focus the mind away from the danger-related intrusive thoughts and onto benign, non-threatening stimuli.[133]

Outcome of ERP and CBT

The treatment of OCD using straightforward graduated exposure and self-imposed response prevention has been shown, by controlled trials, to be effective in the majority of patients who complete the treatment. Despite these good results, many patients fail to engage in exposure treatments, while others relapse and require booster sessions. It is advisable to follow-up with patients to ensure that their gains are maintained and that if signs of relapse develop, they can be dealt with promptly before the patient has reverted to pre-treatment levels of disability. The usual practice is to see patients 1, 3, 6 and 12 months after treatment. Even in previously treatment-refractory samples, an over 30 per cent reduction in Y-BOCS scores can be achieved using CBT.[36] Recent studies have tended to include patients with predominantly obsessions and few overt compulsions in overall outcome results.[134] Many recent studies have tended to favour using ERP combined with some cognitive reattribution. There have been many studies comparing ERP with CBT using such methods. Most have tended to show equivalence with very little advantage generally shown for the addition of more sophisticated techniques.

Although there have been multiple studies and many previous meta-analyses examining the relative merits of ERP, CBT and other psychological interventions, a recent meta-analysis by Reid et al. demonstrated many problems in psychological therapy outcome research.[135] The authors conclude that although a large effect size was found for CBT with ERP in reducing the symptoms of OCD, this is dependent on the control group chosen. For example, the advantage of CBT over treatment with SRIs was found to be null when adequate dosages of SRIs were prescribed. There were also concerns about methodological consistency and the fact that the efficacy was strongly linked to researcher commitment in many studies. Moreover, studies of ERP or CBT in OCD have often been small in scale, without adequate control groups, and lack consistency in the active components of treatment.

Poorly applied cognitive therapy may make some patients with OCD worse. This is because the process of looking for evidence to confirm or refute the obsessions can become incorporated into rituals. Lastly, cognitive therapy may not be cost-efficient, as it requires specialist training and supervision for the therapist, and therapy can be of relatively long duration.

Psychodynamic Psychotherapy

Although some psychoanalysts do still recommend psychodynamic psychotherapy for patients with OCD, most would agree with Cawley's view that 'there is no evidence to support or refute the proposition that formal psychotherapy helps patients with obsessional disorders'.[136]

Pharmacotherapy

Which Drugs Are Effective in OCD?

The selectivity of pharmacological response to drugs that act as inhibitors of the synaptic re-uptake of serotonin (serotonin re-uptake inhibitors, SRIs), such as clomipramine and the SSRIs, distinguishes OCD from the other anxiety disorders and from depression, in which both noradrenergic and serotonergic medications appear effective.

The discovery that clomipramine is an effective treatment for OCD was an important breakthrough. It is well established that the anti-obsessional actions of clomipramine do not depend on an antidepressant effect – since the seminal study by Montgomery that specifically excluded patients with comorbid depression – and demonstrated efficacy against placebo at a relatively modest daily dose of 75 mg.[137] On the other hand, clomipramine is associated with unpleasant and potentially dangerous side effects, such as convulsions, cardiotoxicity and cognitive impairment. Sexual dysfunction has been reported in up to 80 per cent of patients on clomipramine, compared with 30 per cent of those on SSRIs, and drop-out rates due to side effects are considerably lower for SSRIs than for clomipramine. A few head-to-head comparator studies of adequate statistical power indicated equivalent efficacy for SSRIs and clomipramine but superior tolerability for SSRIs.[2]

Skapinakis et al. performed a meta-analysis that demonstrated efficacy for SSRIs as a whole compared to placebo; individual SSRIs produced similar effect sizes, and there was no evidence to suggest superiority of any individual drug.[125] As a result of their improved tolerability, SSRIs are now recommended as the first-line and clomipramine as the second-line treatment for OCD. Among the SSRIs, fluvoxamine, fluoxetine, paroxetine, sertraline, citalopram and escitalopram have been found to be effective in large-scale randomised controlled trials.[2] In the face of equivalent efficacy, the choice of SSRI depends on a balance between patient preference, the side-effect profile and the potential for drug-drug interaction. In circumstances where patients are taking other medications, consideration of pharmacokinetic effects – in particular, at the level of the hepatic cytochrome P450 metabolising enzymes – is relevant. Sertraline, citalopram or escitalopram may be preferred because they are relatively weak enzyme inhibitors. However, as citalopram and escitalopram are shown to prolong the QTc interval in a dose-dependent manner and as OCD often requires the maximum licensed SSRI dosage to produce optimal benefits, careful consideration is required before these agents are prescribed. Fluoxetine and its active metabolite have long half-lives, resulting in fewer withdrawal reactions and advantages for patients who frequently forget their medication.

In conclusion, improved safety and tolerability indicate that SSRIs should be used as the first choice treatment, with clomipramine reserved for those who cannot tolerate SSRIs or who are a non-responder to them.[124] OCD is a chronic illness, so treatment need to be effective over the longer term. There is limited long-term follow-up data, but studies of SSRI treatment responders suggest that treatment-related improvements are maintained without tolerance developing for at least two years.[136,138]

What Is the Most Effective Dose and How Long Does It Take?

The treatment response in OCD is slow. Incremental improvement occurs over weeks and months, and improvement can continue for up to two years if treatment is continued. In a meta-analysis, SSRIs as a group versus placebo produced a statistical difference in Y-BOCS only after 6–13 weeks of treatment.[139] Thus, it is important to encourage patients to continue the treatment in the early stages, if progress seems slow.

Fixed-dose studies have been performed with paroxetine, fluoxetine, sertraline and citalopram. The results have on the whole shown an advantage for the higher doses, though there has been some inconsistency.[2] The British Association for Psychopharmacology treatment guideline suggests starting with the lowest efficacious daily dosage of SSRIs, which may subsequently be increased in case of insufficient response.[140] However, slow up-titration could be challenging for severely ill patients, for whom a prompt response is desired. The APA guidelines recommend up-titration of SSRI to maximum approved doses within four to six weeks and waiting for an additional six weeks to assess effectiveness.[141] (Please note that clomipramine, citalopram and escitalopram have dose-dependent side effects that limit their use at high-dose levels – see 'Treatment of SRI-refractory OCD'.)

For How Long Should Pharmacotherapy Continue?

Clinical evidence shows that drug discontinuation is associated with a gradual worsening of OCD, which is improbable to represent a temporary withdrawal effect. A meta-analysis of several placebo-referenced randomised controlled trials investigating stable treatment responders demonstrated that continuing SSRI treatment significantly reduced relapse rates.[69] These findings indicate that treatment should be continued to protect against relapse.

Treatment of SRI-refractory OCD

Most studies have defined treatment response as a 25–35% improvement in baseline Y-BOCS scores. A substantial minority of patients fail to respond, and around 40% of patients maintain residual symptoms in spite of continued treatment.[69] Patients experiencing a less than 25% reduction of their baseline Y-BOCS score after three months of SRI treatment, of which at least six weeks was at maximal tolerated dose, may be considered SRI-refractory.[141] Results from various evidence-based studies have identified four main pharmacological approaches for these patients.

1. *A higher dose of SSRI.* Whereas clomipramine should not usually be prescribed above the maximum recommended dose due to the risk of potentially dangerous side effects (see later), in the case of SSRIs, it is possible to gain a better response by gradually increasing the dosage to levels exceeding the licensed maximum (e.g. up to 400 mg for sertraline).[142,143] SSRIs in high dose appear relatively well tolerated by patients with OCD. For example, in a double-blind study, 66 OCD treatment-resistant patients were randomised to sertraline in doses of 200 mg/day or 250–400 mg/day; significantly greater improvements were seen in the high-dose group, while both groups showed similar levels of adverse events.[144] Other open-label studies have tested off-label doses of escitalopram reaching 50 mg/day with some success.[145] The American Psychiatric Association OCD Guideline provides a list of the upper doses of SSRI that are not licensed but are occasionally prescribed for patients who have failed to respond to conventional doses.[141] The Royal College of Psychiatrists has issued clinical guidance on the safe prescribing of medications outside their licensed indications.[146] Consideration of high-dose treatment should be reserved for patients who are not experiencing unwarranted adverse effects, and full consent needs to be obtained. Citalopram and escitalopram require particular caution because of dose-dependent effects on cardiac conduction, and if used in supramaximal doses, additional ECG monitoring is needed.

Owing to the increased risk of convulsions and cardiotoxicity, the use of higher doses of clomipramine cannot be recommended without additional safeguards such as the monitoring of plasma drug levels or the use of electrocardiography.

2. *Intravenous administration of SRI.* This has been hypothesised to be more effective than oral SRI, owing to improved bioavailability, and some patients have benefited from this route of administration. According to a few open-label studies, intravenous clomipramine[147] or citalopram[80] could be of short-term advantage for severe OCD patients for whom a fast treatment response is wanted.
3. *Drug combination strategies.* There is increasing evidence that adding low doses of antipsychotic agents may be helpful in case of treatment-resistant OCD. Dopamine-receptor blocking drugs do not appear effective as monotherapy in OCD, although they are the treatment of choice for Tourette's syndrome. However, the conventional antipsychotic haloperidol and the atypical antipsychotics risperidone, olanzapine, quetiapine and aripiprazole have each been found to be effective when added to ongoing SSRI treatment in placebo-controlled studies investigating SRI-refractory cases. A recent meta-analysis of 12 double-blind, randomised, placebo-controlled trials indicated that significantly more patients responded to augmentation with an antipsychotic than placebo.[148] Atypical antipsychotics are associated with lower rates of extrapyramidal side effects and are therefore recommended to be used before haloperidol.
4. *Novel pharmacological strategies.* A range of diverse drug treatments, such as memantine, riluzole, ketamine and D-amphetamine, are currently undergoing investigation as 're-purposed' treatments for OCD. They have not yet been sufficiently tested for their use to be fully recommended. A list of pharmacological agents with at least preliminary evidence of efficacy in OCD is shown in Table 6.4.4.

Neurosurgery and Neuromodulation

Refractoriness to psychological and pharmacological treatment may indicate a role for somatic treatments such as neuromodulation or neurosurgery, especially when symptoms are severe, chronic and debilitating.

Although extensively used in the middle of the twentieth century, nowadays, neurosurgery in the UK is strictly reserved for those patients with OCD with the most profound, intractable illness under statutory safeguards to ensure the grounds for surgery can be fully justified. The most common procedures involve capsulotomy and anterior cingulotomy, targeting areas in the internal capsule and the anterior cingulate cortex respectively. The procedures serve to disconnect areas of the frontal cortex from subcortical structures by creating lesions made either using standard surgical procedure, radioactive elements, radiofrequency or a gamma knife. Today, ablative procedures are mostly performed using stereotactic methods, targeted using neuroimaging guidance in carefully selected patients.[149]

In a recent systematic review by Pepper et al.[150] studying the response rate of anterior capsulotomy for OCD, the consolidated estimate of response rates (35% drop in Y-BOCS score) was reported to be 73%, with 24% achieving remission (Y-BOCS score < 8). Within the older literature (mostly radiofrequency thermal lesions with a few gamma knife surgeries), using a bespoke grading scheme, 90% were rated as having 'responded', with 39% 'symptom free'. A recent meta-analysis suggest that among the available procedures, capsulotomy seemed to be the most effective.[151]

Deep brain stimulation (DBS) is emerging as a promising alternative procedure for severe intractable OCD. In this procedure, electrodes carrying electrical pulses from a battery inserted under the pectoral muscles are placed in sites within subcortical brain areas, including the anterior limb of the internal capsule, the ventral capsule, the nucleus accumbens or the ventral caudate nucleus, the subthalamic nucleus, or the inferior thalamic peduncle.[152] DBS has been found to change neuronal activity in cortico-striatal brain circuits. Evidence suggests that different electrode localisations target specific networks leading to different clinical effects. A recent mechanism of effect study by Tyagi et al. compared DBS to the ventral capsule and the subthalamic nucleus. All six previously highly refractory patients in this study showed improvements in OCD symptoms alongside, in the case of subthalamic nucleus DBS, improvement in cognitive inflexibility and, in the case of ventral capsule DBS, improvement in depressed mood.[153] A recent metanalysis of 14 studies of DBS estimated an overall 76 per cent response rate in treatment-refractory OCD patients, with 57 per cent being full responders.[152]

While DBS involves surgery and is a highly invasive procedure, less invasive methods of neurostimulation not requiring surgery that target the more superficial cortical nodes involved in similar neural pathways have been investigated. Repetitive transcranial magnetic stimulation (rTMS) and deep transcranial magnetic stimulation (dTMS), mainly targeting the dorsolateral prefrontal cortex and orbitofrontal cortex, are the techniques most commonly applied in OCD. A recent meta-analysis of several individual, mostly small studies – most of which showed positive findings – concluded that rTMS showed inconclusive evidence of short-term efficacy in OCD and recommended that a definitive study be conducted.[161] A recent multicentre double-blind controlled trial of dTMS showed evidence that this technique is well tolerated and efficacious.[134] Other non-invasive strategies that offer the potential for self-application, and therefore may be more suitable for treating OCD 'at scale', such as transcranial direct current stimulation (tDCS) and transcranial alternating current stimulation (tACS) are also currently under investigation.[43]

Obsessive-Compulsive Related Disorders (OCRDS)

Apart from OCD, the OCRDS tend to be a relatively poorly recognised group of disorders with limited research of evidence related to epidemiology, course and treatment. It is to be expected that the new classification will improve our understanding of these disorders. Therefore, the following sections of this chapter will focus on OCD and make reference to the other disorders where appropriate.

Body Dysmorphic Disorder (BDD)

Body dysmorphic disorder (BDD) involves obsessive thoughts about irregularities or abnormalities in appearance. They are usually related to imagined or perceived minor defects, which are exaggerated, and occur together with related compulsive acts including checking one's appearance (e.g. in the mirror or other reflective surfaces), comparing one's appearance with others and attempts at camouflage (e.g. with make-up or even cosmetic surgery). Unlike OCD, the obsessions and compulsions of BDD are restricted to specific appearance-related themes. People with severe BDD may attempt to remediate their perceived disfigurement with cosmetic surgery but do not usually obtain satisfaction from this. Some people with BDD even attempt 'do it yourself' surgery, and this can end up with dangerous consequences. As with OCD, levels of insight in BDD may be impaired, to the extent that the individual with BDD may believe they are disfigured.

BDD often can occur in an individual who has other obsessive-compulsive disorders including OCD, skin picking and trichotillomania, although depression and social anxiety disorder are the most common comorbid conditions. One of the main differential diagnoses for BDD is to distinguish it from anorexia nervosa. Indeed, both conditions do appear very similar with preoccupation about bodily appearance and attempts to rectify perceived bodily 'flaws' by taking drastic remedial action. Whereas BDD and anorexia can co-exist, the differentiating feature is that, in BDD, weight loss is not the central theme. Suicidal ideation and self harm are extremely common in BDD.[154]

Whereas insight into the truth of the intrusive thoughts in OCD vary between individuals and in the individual over time and depending on circumstance, people with BDD usually have little insight and truly believe they are disfigured, repulsive and ugly despite evidence to the contrary.[155]

Treatment of BDD

Poor insight is common in BDD and means that most patients do not present to clinicians seeking help, or if they do, they frequently ask for help with depression or following an episode of self harm. These patients tend to seek 'remedies' for their perceived bodily flaws and thus seek referral to cosmetic surgeons, aesthetic medicine specialists, orthodontists, dermatologists and others who they feel may 'correct' their 'abnormalities'. For this reason, there would undoubtedly be a benefit if all patients trying to access cosmetic treatments were screened. Clearly, this would be impossible to implement, and some screening questionnaires present a simpler alternative with referral for psychological assessment for those who cause concern. It should be borne in mind, however, that some patients with BDD will seek to perform 'corrective' self-surgery once their desire for surgery is thwarted and – together with the high suicidal behaviours – this makes this group of patients particularly at risk of self harm. The treatment of BDD has recently been reviewed by an international group of experts.[156]

Psychopharmacology

There have been few randomised controlled trials of drug treatment in BDD. To date, those that have taken place have shown benefit for clomipramine, fluoxetine and escitalopram, with little benefit shown from SNRIs.[156] Open trials have also shown benefit across the SSRIs. It has however also been noted that higher doses of SSRIs are often necessary, and benefit accrues over a prolonged time (similar to OCD). Maximum doses for the various SSRIs are sertraline 400 mg/day, fluoxetine 120 mg/day, citalopram 40 mg/day, escitalopram 60 mg/day (with an ECG recommended at doses exceeding 20 mg/day), fluvoxamine 450 mg/day and paroxetine 100 mg/day.[156] These doses are above the maximum dosages recommended by most countries' regulatory agencies, and patients need to be made aware of this and the pros and cons discussed with them.

Unlike in OCD, there is scant evidence to suggest that the addition of a low-dose antipsychotic to the SRI treatment is of benefit. This remains due to a lack of studies rather than definitive evidence.

Psychological Treatment

The studies of BDD have generally shown treatment with CBT incorporating some ERP. There have however been wide variations in additional treatments that have been applied. For example, a study by Wilhelm et al.[157] included advanced cognitive therapy, whereas others have been more ERP based.[158]

An example of treatment using mainly ERP based therapy for BDD is given here.

> Extract from *Everything You Need to Know About OCD* by LM Drummond. Cambridge: Cambridge University Press; 2022.[159]
>
> Ryan, a 41-year-old man, was referred to the clinic by his general practitioner (GP), who was reluctant to refer Ryan for more surgery without a psychiatric opinion. Since his teens, Ryan has been convinced that his nose is too big. At age 35, he underwent a surgical operation to reduce the size of his nose (rhinoplasty). Initially, he felt better and gained more confidence, but then he began to worry that his nose was still rather large. He returned to the surgeon, who told Ryan that he could not recommend further operations. Ryan then went to see several doctors, all of whom told him there was nothing wrong with his nose. Due to this, Ryan became convinced that if he could afford to visit a cosmetic surgeon privately, he could obtain the 'perfect' nose. However, he had asked the GP to send him for one final opinion before he used his life's savings to have surgery. The GP refused to refer him unless Ryan agreed to a psychiatric assessment.
>
> When he arrived for the appointment, Ryan was very unenthusiastic and did not want to engage with the therapist at all. He kept saying, 'If I just have the surgery, I'll be OK'. The therapist suggested to him that he was unlikely to get further surgery, and there was no evidence that the last surgery had helped. Cosmetic surgery is an imprecise science. One person's idea of a 'perfect' nose may differ greatly from another person's idea. Anyone seeking a 'perfect' nose is likely to be disappointed. Ryan believed this was wrong and that he definitely needed surgery (Figure 6.4.1). The therapist suggested two possible explanations for the way he was feeling:
>
> - He had an extremely large nose which was ugly as he believed and was the cause of comment for everyone who saw him. The only way to rectify this situation would be for Ryan to have surgery.
> - It was the way Ryan felt about his nose which caused the problem, and this fed into a vicious cycle.
>
> Ryan listened to the therapist's theory but said he still believed that the first explanation was correct and that only surgery would correct it. He did, however, agree to have five sessions of CBT 'if only to convince my doctor that I really do need surgery'. The therapist agreed to this. Ryan appeared depressed and miserable, and the therapist was

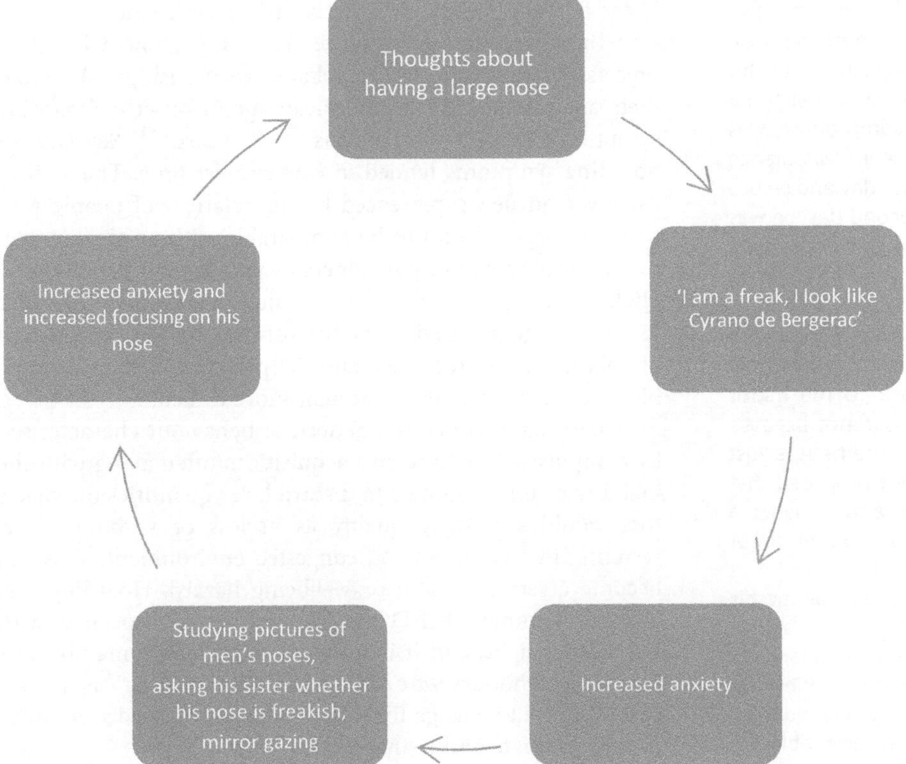

Figure 6.4.1 Cognitive behavioural model for Ryan's concerns regarding his nose.

concerned about his low mood. Ryan admitted his mood had been low recently, but he believed this was purely since he had not received surgery. Although he admitted to suicidal thoughts, he denied any plans but felt he might commit suicide if he did not ultimately get the surgery that he believed he needed. The therapist suggested that his symptoms of depression may be helped by treatment with an SSRI, but Ryan was adamant that he did not need this. Ryan was asked to make a list of other men with large noses and bring it to the next session. The following week, Ryan arrived with a list of people with large noses, including the French film actor Gerard Depardieu and other successful politicians and actors. The therapist asked Ryan what he noticed about these men. He replied, 'I know what you are going to say, yes, they all have big noses and yes, they have all had successful careers and success with women but that is different to me as my nose is much worse!' The therapist asked Ryan to bring some photographs of men he believed were attractive to the next session. For the remainder of this session, Ryan agreed to walk along the High Street with the therapist to observe how many people stared at Ryan's nose. The result of this was that contrary to Ryan's prediction, no one stared at his nose.

The next week, the therapist measured the length and breadth of Ryan's nose and also the length and breadth of his face. Ryan agreed that the nose should be in proportion with the face. From these figures was calculated the width and length ratio for his nose. Similar measurements were taken from the photographs that Ryan had brought. It was soon discovered that Ryan's nose was average in both length and width. Ryan dismissed this by saying that 'mine still looks much larger'. For homework this week, the therapist asked Ryan not to look in the mirror for more than five minutes three times a day and only to check his hair. In addition, he was asked to not telephone his sister for reassurance about his nose. Ryan did not believe that either of these requests was reasonable. A compromise was therefore reached whereby he would seek reassurance and mirror gaze as much as he liked on one day and record his anxiety throughout the day. On the second day, he was to carry out the programme as suggested by the therapist and record his anxiety. For the rest of the week, he could do whichever he believed was the most useful.

When Ryan returned the next week, his records showed that he felt better when he did not mirror gaze or seek reassurance. However, he had gone back to the mirror gazing and telephoning his sister for reassurance because he believed that by following the programme he was 'just trying to forget my problem'. The therapist proposed that Ryan walk around the hospital grounds and conduct a survey of people asking them what they thought about his nose. Ryan was fairly shy about this to begin with but did agree. Most people were complimentary about his nose, which was described as 'chiselled' and 'a fine Roman nose', and others were neither complimentary nor critical and said 'just looks normal'. After completing the survey, the therapist asked Ryan what he concluded from this exercise, and he said, 'It does seem that the problem is more the thoughts about my nose rather than my nose'. From this point onwards, Ryan worked well in therapy, but he still did not wish to continue beyond five sessions. He agreed to reduce the time he spent in front of the mirror and to stop asking his sister for reassurance about his nose. He has decided to put his request to see a cosmetic surgeon 'on hold' for a while but says that although he is willing to try to 'live with my nose' for the next few months, he will seek surgery if his preoccupation with his nose increased again.

Outcome of BDD Treatment

As stated earlier, there have been few trials conducted on BDD, and they favour pharmacological treatment with SSRIs at higher dosages than those used for depression and continued for a long time to accrue maximum benefit.[156] Studies of psychological treatment of BDD have the problem of generally small numbers, at risk of researcher bias and a lack of uniformity in the approaches. An additional issue is that many studies use waiting list controls, which tend to inflate the efficacy of the active treatment.[156] A pragmatic approach however would suggest that a combination of treatment with an SSRI and CBT involving ERP appears to offer the best treatment for these patients.

Hoarding Disorder

Hoarding is a common condition, affecting approximately 2–6% of the adult population in Western countries. Hoarding occurs in both women and men at similar rates. People with hoarding disorder tend to live alone and are less likely to have family or friends visit their home. Hoarders sometimes report a preference for being alone with their objects, as they give more reliable relationships. A recent meta-analysis found that the mean age of onset of hoarding symptoms across studies was 16.7 years.[160] Severity of hoarding symptoms tended to worsen over time. The level of caregiver burden experienced by the relatives of people who hoard has been found to be comparable with or greater than that reported by family members of people with dementia.[161] High comorbidity rates of major depressive disorder (50–52%), generalised anxiety disorder (24%) and social phobia (23%) are reported, and the presence of these comorbid disorders can make treatment more difficult.

Hoarding disorder is a pattern of behaviour characterised by compulsive and excessive acquisition, often along with the inability or unwillingness to discard large quantities of objects that would seemingly qualify as useless or without value, resulting in a cluttered and congested environment. This can become a serious health or wellbeing hazard. Hoarding disorder is another OCRD that is commonly associated with impaired insight, and it is sometimes the family members or affected neighbours who raise the alarm. In such cases, concerted efforts to engage the individual may be needed in order to fully evaluate and manage the problem.

An excellent recent review on the topic is given in Bratiotis et al.[162] from which the later account is taken. Hoarding disorder is characterised by difficulty parting with possessions because of strong urges to save the items. Difficulty discarding usually includes items thought to be of little value and results in an accumulation of a large number of possessions that clutter up the home. As early as 1947, Erich Fromm described a 'hoarding orientation' in which a person's security depended on collecting and saving objects. In 1962, the Scandinavian psychiatrist Jens Jansen referenced 'collector's mania' to describe older adults who filled their rooms with an overabundance of objects.

Hoarding disorder has only recently been recognised as a significant psychiatric disorder, appearing for the first time in official glossaries as recently as DSM-5[4] and ICD-11,[5] without any mention in DSM-IV[163] or ICD-10.[164] It is now classed within the obsessive-compulsive group, and DSM-5 has six criteria:

- Persistent difficulty discarding or parting with possessions, regardless of their actual value.
- This difficulty is due to a perceived need to save the items and to the distress associated with discarding them.
- The difficulty discarding possessions results in the accumulation of possessions that congest and clutter active living areas and substantially compromises their intended use. If living areas are uncluttered, it is only because of the interventions of third parties (e.g. family members, cleaners or the authorities).
- The hoarding causes clinically significant distress or impairment of functioning (including maintaining a safe environment for oneself or others).
- The hoarding is not attributable to another medical condition (e.g. brain injury, cerebrovascular disease, Prader–Willi syndrome).
- The hoarding is not better explained by the symptoms of another mental disorder (e.g. obsessions in obsessive-compulsive disorder, decreased energy in major depressive disorder, delusions in schizophrenia or another psychotic disorder, cognitive defects in major neurocognitive disorder, restricted interests in autism spectrum disorder).

Specify if with excessive acquisition: the majority of cases (80 per cent) are in this group. The assessor should also comment on whether it is with good insight or poor insight, absent insight or delusional beliefs

In contrast to OCD, people with hoarding disorder are sometimes not distressed by their hoarding behaviours, whereas those with OCD are usually very distressed by their symptoms. People with hoarding disorder also often fail to appreciate the negative effect of their hoarding on either themselves or others such as family members and neighbours. On an individual level, accumulated possessions can result in difficulty in completing basic human functions, such as socialising, preparing food, bathing and mobilising when rooms and hallways are stuffed full of clutter. This applies especially to older hoarders. Severe hoarding behaviour can ultimately result in the degradation of the home, with the neglect of routine maintenance and homes becoming squalid, mouldy, pest-infected or structurally unsound because of excessive weight of clutter or water damage. Severely cluttered family environments are associated with increased childhood distress, reduced social interaction and greater family conflict. A common presentation is through child social services as a result of a child neglect investigation. Specifically, problems associated with hoarding behaviour provoke health and safety concerns for both the occupant of the home and for those who live nearby, such as neighbours with shared walls. For example, the risk of fire increases when combustibles are stored near heat sources or electrical wiring, and blocked exits create safety hazards for residents and emergency responders. A study by Lucini et al.[165] found that 60 per cent of hoarding-related fires spread beyond its source, in contrast with only 10 per cent of non-hoarding fires. Other legal ramifications can include the involvement of child welfare services, older adult and guardianship services and animal welfare organisations.

Diagnosis is usually obvious on entering the subject's home, but specialised assessment tools are helpful in defining treatment goals, and these include the HOMES Multidisciplinary Risk Assessment or the Cleanliness and Clutter Scale, whilst the phenomenon of squalor is measured with the Homes Environment Index. References for these scales and many others are given in Lucini et al.[165]

The neurobiology of hoarding behaviours is still unclear, and MRI and fMRI studies of hoarding behaviours are in their infancy and involve only small numbers of subjects, but they suggest the involvement of the anterior cingulate gyrus and the insula. Hoarding, as well as hoarding symptoms, showed heritability ranging from 45% to 71%, just below that of OCD, which is around 74%. In a community-based paediatric sample, study findings indicated that the L_G+S variant of 5-HTTLPR was significantly associated with hoarding in men, whereas a trend was shown for variation downstream of HTR1B to be linked with hoarding in women.

Management

At a superficial level, it appears that the obvious treatment is to simply hire a service to clean out the home and, if there is obstruction, then to forcibly remove the hoarder from his home to accomplish this. However, this does not work because of the resentment at forcible removal and high rates of recidivism. Empirically, it has been found that a joint therapist-client harm reduction approach works best with the goal of reducing the harms associated with the hoarding. Treatment is usually as a weekly CBT programme and often includes components of decision-making training, sorting and discarding exercises, organisation training, exposure to non-acquiring cognitive restructuring and motivational interviewing.[166] CBT has been found to be particularly effective at addressing the difficulty in discarding, reducing clutter volume and decreasing acquiring behaviours. Regular home visits by the therapist are strongly recommended. There is increasing interest in group CBT over individual CBT because of the general advantages of group-based therapies, including greater social interaction and involvement as well as expected higher cost-efficiency.[167] Peer-facilitated CBT for hoarding is an alternative group treatment that has been found to be as effective as psychologist-led group CBT. The 'Buried in Treasures workshop' is a manualised, peer-facilitated CBT composed of 15 structured sessions that provide psychoeducation regarding hoarding disorder, motivation enhancement, cognitive restructuring and discarding exercises.[168] There is also an increased interest in VR-based therapies.

Severe hoarding behaviour commonly results in diverse public health and safety concerns, which in turn, necessitate community interventions. Medication sometimes helps, and there are small RCT trials showing benefits for paroxetine, venlaflaxine SR at a high dosage of 225 mg, and atomoxetine (an ADHD medication). Medication appears to be useful for 'difficulties in discarding' but not for overall hoarding behaviours, and presently there is no data on whether it can be usefully combined with CBT.[162]

Trichotillomania

Trichotillomania (hair-pulling disorder) is often a debilitating condition characterised by the compulsive pulling out of one's own body hair (e.g. head, eyebrows, lashes, pubic hair), leading to hair loss, scarring, distress and marked functional impairment. People with this disorder are frequently ashamed and do their utmost to hide their symptoms (e.g. with hair pieces, make-up or scarves), even from their doctors. Vigilance for trichotillomania is recommended in anyone presenting with unusual headwear, especially if there is a known history of another OCRD.

Francois Hallopeau, a French dermatologist, introduced the term trichotillomania to denote an irresistible urge to pull one's hair.[169] This is often associated with subsequent rituals, such as mouthing the hair afterwards or even ingesting it (trichophagia). Most sufferers report a state of tension before pulling their hair out, with some relief and gratification afterwards. DSM- 5 criteria include recurrent pulling out of one's hair resulting in noticeable hair loss and repeated attempts to decrease or stop hair pulling. The hair pulling is not due to another dermatological or psychiatric disorder.

The hair pulling is not described as painful; rather, individuals report tingling and pruritis in the affected areas. Afterwards, there may be a sense of gratification and tension release. As well as the scalp, the eyebrows, eyelashes, beard and pubic hair may be involved. Hair pulling tends to occur during states of relaxation – while sitting down watching television, reading or studying – but it is usually done in secret. Around 20 per cent of subjects report eating their hair. Amongst children (usually aged one to five years) who swallow their hair, a few may develop a tracheo-bezoar (a hair ball in the stomach) and present with epigastric pain, vomiting and a palpable mass, a condition sometimes leading to surgery and occasionally having a fatal outcome.

Many patients feel ashamed of their habit, which therefore may be undeclared. A study of associated psychiatric comorbidity showed an increased lifetime prevalence for major depression, simple phobia, generalised anxiety disorder and possibly also for alcohol and substance misuse.[170] Rates of co-occurring OCD are significantly higher in individuals with trichotillomania (13–27%) than those found in the community (1–3%), and rates of trichotillomania among individuals with OCD have ranged from 4.9% to 6.9%, which is greater than the rate of 0.5%–2.0% found in the community. The repetitive motor symptoms of hair pulling share some similarity with the repetitive compulsive rituals of OCD, and these parallels suggest that similar neurobiological processes are involved and have led to the reclassification of the disorder as being in the OCD family rather than it being an impulse disorder.

Patients may spend one to three hours a day in hair pulling, which leads eventually to severe baldness. Sometimes, areas of complete alopecia appear, but a thinning of the hair is more common with a predilection for the thinning to occur in the crown or parietal regions of the scalp. Sometimes, eyebrows and eyelashes may be completely absent. Hair-pullers commonly also engage in nail biting, thumb sucking, head banging, gnawing and other types of self-mutilation. The course is usually chronic but with relapses and remissions.

The main differential diagnosis is with alopecia areata. Both disorders present with bald patches; however, in trichotillomania, the short, broken strands of hair will appear alongside normal hairs, while in alopecia, all the hairs are short. In addition, when the hair regrows, there is no change in pigmentation in trichotillomania, whereas this can occur in alopecia areata. Among those who deny the habit of hair pulling, a scalp biopsy will demonstrate the traumatic nature of the disorder with categen hairs, absence of inflammation and scarring, and dilated follicula infundibula. Hair follicle changes, known as tricomalacia, are said to be characteristic and differentiate the disorder from alopecia. Occasionally, other causes of hair loss such as hypothyroidism, tinea capitis and syphilis may also need to be excluded,

Epidemiology

A recent large general population survey of trichotillomania found an overall prevalence rate of 1.7% with no differences between the sexes. Presentation is usually within general practice or dermatology clinics, and onset is typically in childhood and adolescence, with females having a younger age of onset at a mean age of 14 years as compared to a male mean age at 19 years The most common co-occurring disorders were 'any anxiety' disorder (53%), depression (45%), ADHD (29%), PTSD (29%) and OCD (29%).

Management

The disorder often starts in childhood and has a prolonged course, and behavioural strategies appear to be the most useful. Behavioural interventions for trichotillomania have generally included three core elements: first, awareness training, wherein techniques such as self-monitoring are implemented to improve the patient's awareness of their pulling and increase the patient's awareness of the urges that precedes pulling; second, stimulus control, which includes a variety of methods that serve as 'speed bumps' to reduce the likelihood that pulling behaviour begins; and third, competing response training, where patients are taught at the earliest sign of pulling, or of the urge to pull, to engage in a behaviour that is physically incompatible with hair pulling for a brief period of time until the urge subsides. This is known as habit reversal. The latter technique involves asking the patient to practise some alternative motor response, such as grasping or clenching the hands for three minutes, that competes with the urge to pull hair. Behavioural regimes rely on identifying situations where the habit takes place – for example, while reading or watching television – and response prevention is attempted in these situations. Pulling can be both automatic (i.e. outside awareness) and focused (i.e. in response to identifiable affective triggers) within each individual. Relaxation therapy is sometimes also helpful. Another component of the behavioural regime is 'overcorrection' or positive attention, which requires patients to brush or comb their hair or repair eye make-up (for eyelash pullers) after each episode of hair pulling.

Facial screening by covering the patient's scalp with a soft cloth is sometimes helpful. Patients will often deliberately cover affected areas out of feelings of shame but also to protect these areas from further damage.

There is some RCT evidence for the efficacy of certain drugs: the opioid antagonist naltrexone, the glutamate modulator *N*-acetylcysteine, and the atypical neuroleptic olanzapine. An earlier study found evidence for clomipramine in women with trichotillomania, which suggests a possible link with obsessive-compulsive disorder. However, a controlled trial showed no significant benefit from fluoxetine (60 mg daily) when compared with waiting list controls, although the same trial demonstrated significant benefits for behavioural therapy. Hypnotherapy has been reported as helpful in individual cases and so may be worth trying. While both behaviour therapy and drug treatment may offer some relief in the short term, little is known about relapse rates, prevention or long-term outcome.[171, 172]

Skin-Picking Disorder (Excoriation Disorder)

Skin-picking disorder (excoriation disorder) is characterised by the compulsive, disfiguring picking of the skin (e.g. around fingernails, lips) leading to skin lesions. It may be associated with severe nail biting. As in trichotillomania, the disorder is associated with significant distress or functional impairment.

DSM-5 also includes 'Excoriation' (skin-picking disorder) within its chapter on 'Obsessive Compulsive and Related Disorders', but some authors consider it to be a behavioural addiction. The main features of this condition are recurrent picking of the skin, usually the face, arms and hands, but it can be from any site or multiple sites. It may result in skin lesions, which can become infected, but for the most part, results in low self-esteem, guilt and shame, and subjects try and cover affected areas. Most individuals use their fingernails, but some will use tweezers, scissors or pins, and they may spend many hours a day engaged in this activity. It is usually done when the subject is alone and in secret except occasionally in the presence of close family members. The condition does not often present for treatment but may be observed in general practice settings or dermatology clinics but rarely in psychiatric clinics. Individuals often try and stop the habit but find this difficult or impossible to do. A general population study of skin-picking disorder found a point prevalence of 1.4% – with a small female excess – and other mental health comorbidities were common, with generalised anxiety disorder (63.4%), depression (53.1%) and panic disorder (27.7%) being the most frequently endorsed. It can occur amongst those with learning difficulties and is a feature of the Prader–Willi syndrome. The preceding affect is often one of anxiety or boredom and, once started, the skin picking offers tension relief. The differential diagnosis includes psychotic disorders such as delusional parasitosis, formication as in the DTs, non-suicidal self harm, cocaine addiction and other dermatological disorders – most commonly, scabies. Treatments are with CBT strategies similar to those described for trichotillomania, as described earlier.[173]

Hypochondriasis

The term hypochondriasis refers to the obsessive preoccupation that the individual is suffering from a serious medical condition despite having received medical reassurance that this is not the case. Any physical symptoms or complaints that occur appear minor compared to the patient's distressed and anxious state. In addition, many of these patients are hypervigilant towards normal bodily sensations. The intrusive thoughts about disease are accompanied by 'neutralising' behaviours such as repeatedly checking for symptoms, seeking medical tests and reassurance as well as repeatedly checking the internet for information (cyberchondria). This checking or reassurance seeking only serves to increase anxiety. As well as the considerable cost to the wellbeing and health of the individual, there is an additional cost in terms of the usage of medical facilities and unnecessary investigations to a health service.[174]

Hypochondriasis is a relatively common condition estimated to be found in 0.04–4.5% of the general population, 0.3–8.5% in GP surgeries and 12–20% in specialty hospital clinics.[175] It is thought that hypochondriasis affects men and women in equal numbers and often starts in adolescence or early adult life.[176]

Table 6.4.5 Location of hypochondriasis in the major classification systems (DSM and ICD)

DSM-IV-TR: Somatoform Disorders	DSM-5: Somatic Symptom Disorders and Related Disorders	ICD-10: Somatoform Disorders	ICD-11: Obsessive Compulsive and Related Disorders
Somatisation Disorder	**Somatic Symptom Disorder**	Somatisation Disorder	Obsessive-Compulsive Disorder
Undifferentiated Somatoform Disorder		Undifferentiated Somatoform Disorder	Body Dysmorphic Disorder
Pain Disorder	Conversion Disorder	Dissociative (Conversion) Disorder	Olfactory Reference Disorder
Hypochondriasis	**Illness Anxiety Disorder**	Persistent Somatoform Pain Disorder	**Hypochondriasis**
Conversion Disorder	Factitious Disorder	**Hypochondriacal Disorder**	Hoarding Disorder
Somatoform Disorder Not Otherwise Specified	Other Specified Somatic Symptom and Related Disorder	Somatoform Autonomic Dysfunction	Body-Focused Repetitive Behaviour Disorders
Body Dysmorphic Disorder	Unspecified Somatic Symptom and Related Disorder	Other Somatoform Disorders	Substance-Induced Obsessive-Compulsive or Related Disorders
		Somatoform Disorder, Unspecified	Secondary Obsessive-Compulsive or Related Syndrome
			Other Specified Obsessive-Compulsive or Related Disorders
			Obsessive-Compulsive or Related Disorders, Unspecified

In some individuals, hypochondriasis is a brief, self-limiting problem that may be precipitated by life events and stressors. In approximately 5 per cent, it can go on to be a serious and life-changing condition.[177]

When hypochondriasis interferes with functioning, it can have devastating effects on the individual. There is an increased risk of suicide[178] as well as interference with social, occupational and family functioning and a possible neglect of general physical health, which are seen as unrelated to their main fear.[179]

Classification of Hypochondriasis

Hypochondriasis was included as a mental disorder in the DSM classification system from the third edition in 1980 onwards and originally grouped along with somatisation disorder in the somatoform disorders. The main difference between the two disorders is that, in the former, the excessive concern regarding health arises from a fear of having a serious illness as opposed to having to deal with physical symptoms – which are usually absent or very mild – while in the latter, the distress is caused by the presence of the physical symptoms themselves (see also the discussion of hypochondriasis in Chapter 6.6 on 'Bodily Distress'). In the DSM-5,[4] hypochondriasis was renamed as illness anxiety disorder, and the family was renamed as somatic symptom disorders and related disorders. This classification has caused some controversy, as somatic symptoms do not seem to be a primary feature of illness anxiety disorder (hypochondriasis).

In contrast, in the ICD-11 redaction,[5] the term hypochondriasis was retained, and the disorder was moved from the ICD-10 'Somatoform Disorders' to join the 'Obsessive Compulsive Disorder and Related Disorders' owing to recognition of the prominence of obsessive and compulsive symptomatology (Table 6.4.5).

Treatment of Hypochondriasis

By definition, people with hypochondriasis worry that they may have a serious physical condition requiring medical intervention. Such patients are not likely to easily agree to see a psychiatrist, for fear that any real health-related concerns will be over-looked. However, medical interventions tend to reinforce and strengthen hypochondriacal beliefs. For example, if a man has abdominal pain and believes he has stomach cancer, any physician he attends will most likely order a number of tests to look at possible diagnoses. Once those tests are negative, the physician will reassure the patient. As with OCD, this reassurance will improve his anxiety, and he feels relief. However, this relief may be short-lived as he thinks that the problems that he is describing could be serious – hence the need for investigation – or there is a possibility that the doctor could be wrong or that the tests have missed some vital sign. He therefore returns to the doctor again. Many patients with hypochondriasis therefore end up seeking medical opinions from multiple places and having many medical investigations, all of which fails to resolve the anxiety and distress.

Psychopharmacology

Considering how much of a problem hypochondriasis presents within the health systems, there are surprisingly few studies examining medication and treatment. Overall, treatment with SSRIs is recommended for the treatment of hypochondriasis.[180] As with OCD and BDD, it would be expected that doses at the upper limits of prescribing would be advised, and findings from at least one study suggests this is the case, but more work is needed to confirm this for hypochondriasis.[181]

Psychological Treatment -- CBT appears effective in the acute treatment of hypochondriasis.[181] Treatment involves first engaging the patient. In the case of patients expressing unwillingness to take psychotropic medication (as they believe they have a physical condition), psychotherapy can be an effective initial step. Treatment starts by asking the patient to try a new way of behaving for a few weeks in which they do not engage in seeking medical reassurance. The case history here demonstrates this.

Extract from *Everything You Need to Know About OCD* by LM Drummond. Cambridge: Cambridge University Press; 2022.[159]

Ash is a 25-year-old man who was referred for assessment by the gastro-enterology team. He was extremely reluctant to see a psychiatrist but was eventually persuaded by being told that many patients benefit from seeing the psychiatrist irrespective of their diagnosis as any emotion can have an effect of the bowel.

The history showed that Ash is the only child of quite elderly parents and had been a much-wanted child as it had taken his parents many attempts at in-vitro fertilisation to conceive him. Consequently, he had been quite 'molly-coddled' as a young child and was always described as 'sickly', requiring considerable time away from school although no serious pathology had ever been found.

At the age of 18 years, Ash had moved away from home to attend university. He developed some abdominal pains and went to the student health centre. They told him that this was most likely due to his poor diet since leaving home. Ash, however, was not happy with this and started searching the internet. He convinced himself that he suffered from a form of ulcerative colitis and that he would die from the complication of carcinoma unless this was dealt with. After several visits to the health centre, they eventually sent him to the hospital to see a gastro-enterologist. The consultant at the clinic performed a sigmoidoscopy on Ash and reassured him there was nothing wrong. Initially, Ash was relieved but over the next few days he was plagued by thoughts such as:

- 'Doctors can get things wrong . . . what if he missed the pathological area.'
- 'I only had sigmoidoscopy and that can only examine the lower bowel. Maybe the upper bowel is affected.'
- 'Maybe he's only telling me there's nothing wrong because he thinks I'm really ill and the prognosis is hopeless.'

These thoughts meant that Ash asked for an urgent return visit to the clinic and eventually was given a colonoscopy. Each new test reduced his anxiety for a while, but then the catastrophic thoughts would creep back in. Eventually, the local clinic refused to see him. By this time, Ash was so crippled by his anxieties that he was no longer attending to his studies. He returned home where his parents were very concerned about his weight loss. Ash had started to restrict his diet to that advised for people with ulcerative colitis and thus was avoiding most sources of insoluble fibre (e.g. bran, whole foods and sweet corn) and also any dairy produce including milk, cheese and cream. As well as trying to avoid physical activity in case it upset his bowel, Ash took a variety of tablets from health food shops consisting of a range of vitamin and mineral supplements and also Chinese medicines supposed to act on the bowel. Over the next few years, Ash ended up having more and more investigations and going to see a multiplicity of NHS and private gastro-enterologists. Every time he was discharged from a clinic, his anxiety would rocket, and he would seek out another physician and surgeon. At the time of referral to the psychiatric clinic, Ash had a BMI of only 16 and spent most of his days lying in bed. He was pale and unwell and spent his time searching for a cure for his 'ulcerative colitis'. His parents were extremely anxious and really did believe Ash had a serious medical condition. His mother said, 'Look at the state of him, he's undernourished and can barely get out of bed . . . there must be something seriously wrong with him that the doctors haven't found.' The family had spent over £10, 000, which they could barely afford, to try and get a diagnosis for Ash.

The case history of Ash demonstrates how medical practitioners unwittingly exacerbate the symptoms of health anxiety. Most patients will attend their GP or hospital clinic and happily accept the outcome of relevant tests. However, medicine is not an exact science, and there are hardly any situations when a doctor can honestly say he or she is 100 per cent certain. If a patient returns and becomes insistent, then the doctor – mindful of the potential for medico-legal allegations and negligence claims if a diagnosis is over-looked – will often concede to the patient's demands and order further tests. As can be seen from Ash's history, this can form a vicious cycle with a downward spiral of the patient.

In treating patients with health anxiety, the first thing the psychiatrist needs to do is to establish with the patient that there will be no more medical tests or seeking of reassurance for the duration of psychological treatment. This is easier said than done. Patients with health anxiety really believe they have a serious physical illness that may threaten their lives and so it will seem as if the therapist is asking them to take a big risk. One way of approaching this is to present two scenarios to the patient. This can be demonstrated in the story of the treatment of Ash.

Ash was very unwilling at first to agree to stop consulting doctors about his bowels. He felt this would be 'dangerous' and that his symptoms may progress and worsen. The therapist said:

> 'I understand your concern about your bowels, but if we look at this, you have been seeking a diagnosis for over seven years now. I am asking you to agree to no further investigations for the next four

months whilst we start to look at alternative answers. I am going to propose to you that there are two possible explanations for your situation.'

'Firstly, your current belief is that you have a serious bowel condition such as ulcerative colitis and that this will result in a life-threatening situation. All the doctors and specialists who have seen you have managed to miss this diagnosis but that if you keep on seeing more specialists and having more tests, you will eventually obtain a diagnosis of inflammatory bowel disease.'

'My theory is that you do indeed suffer from a variety of bowel symptoms. These symptoms may well have been precipitated originally by a poor diet when you left home. However, once you became anxious that you had a serious bowel disease, your anxiety increased. Chronic and high anxiety can cause various symptoms which you describe such as colicky pain, intermittent diarrhoea and constipation and a feeling of nausea. Every time you go and see a specialist, you feel better for a day or two and then start to worry they may have over-looked the diagnosis, and your anxiety and symptoms get worse. In addition, your restricted diet has made you severely underweight. This diet may well be contributing to your bowel symptoms, and also being malnourished means you will have low energy, lack of drive and a feeling of malaise. This in turn leads you to spend increasing time in bed. Remaining in bed makes you weaker and also has a deleterious effect on your physical symptoms.'

Ash did not agree with the therapist's theory but, persuaded by his parents, agreed to give it a try and agreed that initially he would not consult any bowel specialists for the next six weeks. The therapist gave him the following chart (Figure 6.4.2) to take away. Ash also agreed to stop the Chinese medicine but decided to remain on the vitamin supplements.

In therapy, the first thing was to try to modify some of Ash's beliefs about his symptoms. He was asked to search the internet and to discover some of the symptoms caused by anxiety and to see if any of these symptoms matched the ones he had. Over the next few sessions, the emphasis was placed on examining Ash's symptoms and thoughts and, by working jointly with Ash, trying to discover if there were any alternative explanations other than serious bowel disease for his symptoms. At the end of several sessions, Ash conceded that his belief that his symptoms were caused by anxiety had increased from 0 to 40 per cent. He was asked if he would be willing to try expanding the repertoire of his diet. After a long discussion, Ash agreed to include dairy produce in his diet for a week to see if this caused his symptoms to improve or deteriorate.

Ash managed to incorporate dairy produce without ill effect and was successfully challenging many of his thoughts concerning serious bowel disease. He was already spending less time in bed, but the therapist worked with him to look at introducing graded exercise to gradually increase his physical activity. He found that as he grew stronger and was eating a better diet, his symptoms were less prominent. After several weeks, he agreed to eat wholemeal and foods rich in fibre. Once a full and varied diet was established, he agreed to stop his vitamin and mineral supplements.

Ash started some more detailed work with the therapist examining some of his thoughts and the deeper beliefs that he held about his health and fitness. Many of these were successfully challenged, and he stopped seeing himself as weak and sickly and began to understand that he could, indeed, be a strong and healthy man. Following on from this, Ash decided to try to take up judo. He enrolled in a local class and, to his surprise, not only enjoyed the sport but was reasonably good at it.

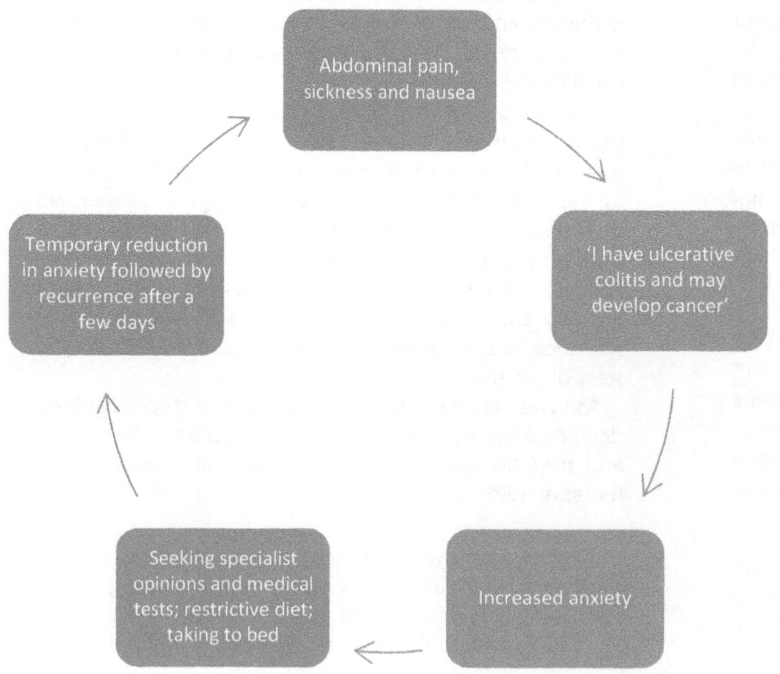

Figure 6.4.2 Therapy chart.

Currently, Ash looks like a strong, fit, healthy and happy young man. He no longer restricts his diet, although he does try to maintain a healthy diet, which he believes helps him perform better in judo competitions.

Outcome of Hypochondriasis Treatment

There have been studies examining treatment with CBT as well as SSRIs. Overall, large effect sizes have often been reported with CBT for hypochondriasis. A recent meta-analysis of this subject found that the type of CBT used varied in type and efficacy. A high chance of researcher bias was found in the CBT studies.[181]

Olfactory Reference Syndrome

Olfactory reference syndrome involves obsessive ruminations about the fear that one emits a foul or unpleasant body odour that causes extreme offence to others. The disorder is also characterised by compulsive neutralising behaviours, such as frequent showering or excessive deodorant use, to camouflage the imagined odour or by social avoidance and isolation. As with BDD, in some cases, insight may be impaired, and the individual believes he or she really does smell. Interpersonal interactions are avoided or endured with significant distress, shame and embarrassment. At this time, there is no evidence base for treatment separate from other conditions.

Conclusion

Our understanding of OCD and the related disorders has increased dramatically since the early days. Despite this, they still remain poorly understood and often over-looked by mental health services. This is despite OCD having a considerable mortality and high economic burden. The OCD-related disorders of skin picking and hoarding disorder have only been described since the updating of DSM in 2013, and so, it is unsurprising that the research is often patchy and inconclusive in these areas. It is hoped that better understanding and research will help to refine treatments and increase the availability of treatment and support.

References

1. Lewis A. *Inquiries in Psychiatry: Clinical and Social Investigations.* London: Routledge and Kegan Paul; 1967. www.ocdhistory.net/20thcentury/lewis.html. (accessed 19 July 2021).
2. Fineberg NA, Gale TM. Evidence-based pharmacotherapy of obsessive-compulsive disorder. *International Journal of Neuropsychopharmacology* 2005;8(1):107–29. DOI: 10.1017/s1461145704004675.
3. Foa EB. Cognitive behavioral therapy of obsessive-compulsive disorder. *Dialogues in Clinical Neuroscience.* 2010;12(2):199–207. DOI: 10.31887/DCNS.2010.12.2/efoa.
4. American Psychiatric Association. *Diagnostic and Statistical Manual of Mental Disorders: DSM-5.* 5th ed. Washington, DC: American Psychiatric Publishing, Inc; 2013.
5. World Health Organization. *ICD-11 Mortality and Morbidity Statistics. Mental, Behavioural or Neurodevelopmental Disorders.* icd.who.int/browse11/l-m/en (accessed 1 June 2019).
6. Kogan CS, Stein DJ, Rebello TJ, et al. Accuracy of diagnostic judgments using ICD-11 vs. ICD-10 diagnostic guidelines for obsessive-compulsive and related disorders. *Journal of Affective Disorders* 2020;273:328–40. DOI: 10.1016/j.jad.2020.03.103.
7. Foa EB. Failure in treating obsessive-compulsives. *Behavior Research and Therapy* 1979;17(3):169–76. DOI: 10.1016/0005-7967(79)90031-7.
8. Matsunaga H. [Clinical features, treatments and outcome of obsessive-compulsive disorder (OCD) focusing on the assessment and characteristics of patients with treatment-refractory OCD]. Seishin Shinkeigaku Zasshi. 2013;115(9):967–74.
9. Fineberg NA, Potenza MN, Chamberlain SR, et al. Probing compulsive and impulsive behaviors, from animal models to endophenotypes: a narrative review. Neuropsychopharmacology. 2010;35(3):591–604. DOI: 10.1038/npp.2009.185.
10. Matsunaga H, Kiriike N, Matsui T, et al. Obsessive-compulsive disorder with poor insight. *Comprehensive Psychiatry* 2002;43(2):150–7. DOI: 10.1053/comp.2002.30798.
11. Lewis AJ. Melancholia: a clinical survey of depressive states. *Journal of Mental Science.* 1934;80(329):277–378.
12. Kendell RE, Discipio WJ. Obsessional symptoms and obsessional personality traits in patients with depressive illnesses. *Psychological Medicine* 1970;1(1):65–72. DOI: 10.1017/s0033291700040022.
13. Myers JK, Weissman MM, Tischler GL, et al. Six-month prevalence of psychiatric disorders in three communities 1980 to 1982. *Archives of General Psychiatry* 1984;41(10):959–67. DOI: 10.1001/archpsyc.1984.01790210041006.
14. Robins LN, Helzer JE, Weissman MM, et al. Lifetime prevalence of specific psychiatric disorders in three sites. *Archives of General Psychiatry* 1984;41(10):949–58. DOI: 10.1001/archpsyc.1984.01790210031005.
15. Swedo SE, Rapoport JL, Leonard H, et al. Obsessive-compulsive disorder in children and adolescents. Clinical phenomenology of 70 consecutive cases. *Archives of General Psychiatry* 1989;46(4):335–41. DOI: 10.1001/archpsyc.1989.01810040041007.
16. Montgomery MA, Clayton PJ, Friedhoff AJ. Psychiatric illness in Tourette syndrome patients and first-degree relatives. *Advances in Neurology* 1982;35:335–9.
17. Eapen V, Robertson MM, Alsobrook JP, et al. Obsessive compulsive symptoms in Gilles de la Tourette syndrome and obsessive compulsive disorder: differences by diagnosis and family history. *American Journal of Medical Genetics* 1997;74(4):432–8. DOI: 10.1002/(sici)1096-8628(19970725)74:4<432::aid-ajmg15>3.0.co;2-j.
18. Bloch MH, Landeros-Weisenberger A, Kelmendi B, et al. A systematic review: antipsychotic augmentation with

treatment refractory obsessive-compulsive disorder. *Molecular Psychiatry* 2006;11(7):622–32. DOI: 10.1038/sj.mp.4001823.

19. Gecaite-Stonciene J, Lochner C, Marincowitz C, et al. Obsessive-compulsive (anankastic) personality disorder in the ICD-11: a scoping review. *Frontiers in Psychiatry* 2021;12:646030. DOI: 10.3389/fpsyt.2021.646030.
20. Fineberg NA, Reghunandanan S, Kolli S, Atmaca M. Obsessive-compulsive (anankastic) personality disorder: toward the ICD-11 classification. *Brazilian Journal of Psychiatry* 2014;36 (Suppl 1):40–50. DOI: 10.1590/1516-4446-2013-1282.
21. Meier SM, Petersen L, Pedersen MG, et al. Obsessive-compulsive disorder as a risk factor for schizophrenia: a nationwide study. *JAMA Psychiatry* 2014;71(11):1215–21. DOI: 10.1001/jamapsychiatry.2014.1011.
22. Cederlöf M, Lichtenstein P, Larsson H, et al. Obsessive-compulsive disorder, psychosis, and bipolarity: a longitudinal cohort and multigenerational family study. *Schizophrenia Bulletin* 2015;41 (5):1076–83. DOI: 10.1093/schbul/sbu169.
23. Fernandez-Egea E, Worbe Y, Bernardo M, et al. Distinct risk factors for obsessive and compulsive symptoms in chronic schizophrenia. *Psychological Medicine* 2018;48(16):2668–75. DOI: 10.1017/s003329171800017x.
24. Loomes R, Hull L, Mandy WPL. What is the male-to-female ratio in autism spectrum disorder? A systematic review and meta-analysis. *Journal of the American Academy of Child and Adolescent Psychiatry* 2017;56 (6):466–74. DOI: 10.1016/j.jaac.2017.03.013.
25. Wikramanayake WNM, Mandy W, Shahper S, et al. Autism spectrum disorders in adult outpatients with obsessive compulsive disorder in the UK. *International Journal of Psychiatry in Clinical Practice* 2018;22(1):54–62. DOI: 10.1080/13651501.2017.1354029.
26. Du BF. Compulsion neurosis with cachexia (anorexia nervosa). *American Journal of Psychiatry* 1949;106 (2):107–15. DOI: 10.1176/ajp.106.2.107.
27. Thiel A, Broocks A, Ohlmeier M, et al. Obsessive-compulsive disorder among patients with anorexia nervosa and bulimia nervosa. *American Journal of Psychiatry* 1995;152(1):72–5. DOI: 10.1176/ajp.152.1.72.
28. Cashin A, Buckley T, Trollor JN, et al. A scoping review of what is known of the physical health of adults with autism spectrum disorder. *Journal of Intellectual Disabilities* 2018;22 (1):96–108. DOI: 10.1177/1744629516665242.
29. Tchanturia K, Smith E, Weineck F, et al. Exploring autistic traits in anorexia: a clinical study. *Molecular Autism* 2013;4(1):44. DOI: 10.1186/2040-2392-4-44.
30. Alm PA. Streptococcal infection as a major historical cause of stuttering: data, mechanisms, and current importance. Frontiers in Human Neuroscience. 2020;14:569519. DOI: 10.3389/fnhum.2020.569519.
31. Swedo SE, Frankovich J, Murphy TK. Overview of treatment of pediatric acute-onset neuropsychiatric syndrome. *Journal of Child and Adolescent Psychopharmacology* 2017;27(7):562–5. DOI: 10.1089/cap.2017.0042.
32. Weissman MM, Bland RC, Canino GJ, et al. The cross national epidemiology of obsessive compulsive disorder. The Cross National Collaborative Group. *Journal of Clinical Psychiatry* 1994;55 (Suppl):5–10.
33. Karno M, Golding JM, Sorenson SB, et al. The epidemiology of obsessive-compulsive disorder in five US communities. *Archives of General Psychiatry* 1988;45(12):1094–9. DOI: 10.1001/archpsyc.1988.01800360042006.
34. Noshirvani HF, Kasvikis Y, Marks IM, et al. Gender-divergent aetiological factors in obsessive-compulsive disorder. *British Journal of Psychiatry* 1991;158:260–3. DOI: 10.1192/bjp.158.2.260.
35. Drummond LM. The treatment of severe, chronic, resistant obsessive-compulsive disorder. An evaluation of an in-patient programme using behavioural psychotherapy in combination with other treatments. *British Journal of Psychiatry* 1993;163:223–9. DOI: 10.1192/bjp.163.2.223.
36. Boschen MJ, Drummond LM. Community treatment of severe, refractory obsessive-compulsive disorder. *Behaviour Research and Therapy* 2012;50(3):203–9. DOI: 10.1016/j.brat.2012.01.002.
37. Boschen MJ, Drummond LM, Pillay A, et al. Predicting outcome of treatment for severe, treatment resistant OCD in inpatient and community settings. *Journal of Behavior Therapy and Experimental Psychiatry* 2010;41 (2):90–5. DOI: 10.1016/j.jbtep.2009.10.006.
38. Rasmussen SA, Eisen JL. Epidemiology of obsessive compulsive disorder. *Journal of Clinical Psychiatry* 1990;51 (Suppl):10–3; discussion 4.
39. Flament MF, Cohen D. Child and adolescent obsessive-compulsive disorder: a review. *Obsessive-Compulsive Disorder* 2000;4:147–201.
40. Skoog G, Skoog I. A 40-year follow-up of patients with obsessive-compulsive disorder [see comments]. *Archives of General Psychiatry* 1999;56(2):121–7. DOI: 10.1001/archpsyc.56.2.121.
41. Albert U, Barbaro F, Bramante S, et al. Duration of untreated illness and response to SRI treatment in obsessive-compulsive disorder. *European Psychiatry* 2019;58:19–26. DOI: 10.1016/j.eurpsy.2019.01.017.
42. Dell'Osso B, Benatti B, Grancini B, et al. Investigating duration of illness and duration of untreated illness in obsessive compulsive disorder reveals patients remain at length pharmacologically untreated. *International Journal of Psychiatry in Clinical Practice* 2019;23(4):311–3. DOI: 10.1080/13651501.2019.1621348.
43. Fineberg NA, Hollander E, Pallanti S, et al. Clinical advances in obsessive-compulsive disorder: a position statement by the International College of Obsessive-Compulsive Spectrum Disorders. *International Clinical Psychopharmacology* 2020;35(4):173–93. DOI: 10.1097/yic.0000000000000314.
44. Fineberg NA, Dell'Osso B, Albert U, et al. Early intervention for obsessive compulsive disorder: an expert consensus statement. *European Neuropsychopharmacology* 2019;29 (4):549–65. DOI: 10.1016/j.euroneuro.2019.02.002.
45. Khanna S, Kaliaperumal V, Channabasavanna S. Reactive factors in obsessive compulsive neurosis. *Indian Journal of Psychological Medicine* 1986;9 (2):68–73.

46. Lo WH. A follow-up study of obsessional neurotics in Hong Kong Chinese. *British Journal of Psychiatry* 1967;113(501):823–32. DOI: 10.1192/bjp.113.501.823.

47. Chasson GS, Williams MT, Davis DM, et al. Missed diagnoses in African Americans with obsessive-compulsive disorder: the structured clinical interview for DSM-IV Axis I disorders (SCID-I). *BMC Psychiatry* 2017;17(1):258. DOI: 10.1186/s12888-017-1422-z.

48. Raphael FJ, Rani S, Bale R, et al. Religion, ethnicity and obsessive-compulsive disorder. *International Journal of Social Psychiatry* 1996;42 (1):38–44. DOI: 10.1177/002076409604200105.

49. Rasmussen SA, Tsuang MT. Clinical characteristics and family history in DSM-III obsessive-compulsive disorder. *American Journal of Psychiatry* 1986;143(3):317–22. DOI: 10.1176/ajp.143.3.317.

50. Nicolini H, Salin-Pascual R, Cabrera B, et al. Influence of culture in obsessive-compulsive disorder and its treatment. *Current Psychiatry Reviews* 2017;13 (4):285–92. DOI: 10.2174/2211556007666180 115105935.

51. Saraiva LC, Cappi C, Simpson HB, et al. Cutting-edge genetics in obsessive-compulsive disorder. *Faculty Reviews* 2020;9:30. DOI: 10.12703/r/9-30.

52. Ahmari SE, Dougherty DD. Diessecting OCD circuits: from animal models to targeted treatments. *Depression and Anxiety* 2015;32(8):550–62. DOI: 10.1002/da.22367.

53. Chamberlain BL, Ahmari SE. Animal models for OCD research. In: Fineberg NA, Robbins TW (eds.) *The Neurobiology and Treatment of OCD: Accelerating Progress.* Berlin/Heidelberg: Springer; 2021: 55–96.

54. Purty A, Nestadt G, Samuels JF, et al. Genetics of obsessive-compulsive disorder. *Indian Journal of Psychiatry* 2019;61(Suppl 1):S37–S42. DOI: 10.4103/psychiatry.IndianJPsychiatry_518_18.

55. Strom NI, Soda T, Mathews CA, et al. A dimensional perspective on the genetics of obsessive-compulsive disorder. *Translational Psychiatry* 2021;11(1):401. DOI: 10.1038/s41398-021-01519-z.

56. Pauls L, Fineberg P, Marazziti D, et al. The role of genetic factors in OCD. In: Fineberg N, Marazziti D, Stein DJ (eds.) *Obsessive Compulsive Disorder: A Practical Guide.* London: Taylor & Francis. 2001: 61–77.

57. McGuffin P, Reich T. Psychopathology and genetics. In: Lesse S. (ed.) *Comprehensive Handbook of Psychopathology.* Washington, DC: American Psychiatric Association Publishing; 1984: 47–75.

58. Pauls DL, Alsobrook II JP, Goodman W, et al. A family study of obsessive-compulsive disorder. *American Journal of Psychiatry* 1995;152(1):76–84. DOI: 10.1176/ajp.152.1.76.

59. Brander G, Kuja-Halkola R, Rosenqvist MA, et al. A population-based family clustering study of tic-related obsessive-compulsive disorder. *Molecular Psychiatry* 2021;26(4):1224–33. DOI: 10.1038/s41380-019-0532-z.

60. Carey G. Twin and family studies of anxiety, phobic and obsessive disorders. In: Klein DF, Rabkin JG (eds.) *Anxiety: New Research and Changing Concepts.* New York: Raven Press; 1981: 117–36C.

61. Burton CL, Park LS, Corfield EC, et al. Heritability of obsessive-compulsive trait dimensions in youth from the general population. *Translational Psychiatry* 2018;8(1):191.

62. Mataix-Cols D, Boman M, Monzani B, et al. Population-based, multigenerational family clustering study of obsessive-compulsive disorder. *JAMA Psychiatry* 2013;70(7):709–17.

63. Nicolini H, Hanna G, Baxter L, et al. Segregation analysis of obsessive compulsive disorders. *Preliminary results. Ursus Medicus* 1991;1:25–8.

64. Cavallini MC, Di Bella D, Pasquale L, et al. 5HT2C CYS23/SER23 polymorphism is not associated with obsessive–compulsive disorder. *Psychiatry Research* 1998;77(2):97–104.

65. Alsobrook II JP, Leckman JF, Goodman WK, et al. Segregation analysis of obsessive-compulsive disorder using symptom-based factor scores. *American Journal of Medical Genetics* 1999;88 (6):669–75.

66. Piantadosi SC, Chamberlain BL, Glausier JR, et al. Lower excitatory synaptic gene expression in orbitofrontal cortex and striatum in an initial study of subjects with obsessive compulsive disorder. *Molecular Psychiatry* 2021;26(3):986–98.

67. Zohar J, Insel TR. Obsessive-compulsive disorder: psychobiological approaches to diagnosis, treatment, and pathophysiology. *Biological Psychiatry* 1987;22(6):667–87.

68. Thorén P, Åsberg M, Cronholm B, et al. Clomipramine treatment of obsessive-compulsive disorder: I. A controlled clinical trial. *Archives of General Psychiatry* 1980;37(11):1281–5.

69. Fineberg NA, Pampaloni I, Pallanti S, et al. Sustained response versus relapse: the pharmacotherapeutic goal for obsessive–compulsive disorder. *International Clinical Psychopharmacology* 2007;22(6):313–22.

70. Bloch MH, McGuire J, Landeros-Weisenberger A, et al. Meta-analysis of the dose-response relationship of SSRI in obsessive-compulsive disorder. *Molecular Psychiatry* 2010;15(8):850–5.

71. Blier P, Abbott FV. Putative mechanisms of action of antidepressant drugs in affective and anxiety disorders and pain. *Journal of Psychiatry and Neuroscience* 2001;26(1):37.

72. Bandelow B, Baldwin D, Abelli M, et al. Biological markers for anxiety disorders, OCD and PTSD: a consensus statement. Part II: Neurochemistry, neurophysiology and neurocognition. *The World Journal of Biological Psychiatry* 2017;18(3):162–214.

73. Marazziti D, Conti L, Pfanner C, et al. No correlation between aggression and platelet 3H-paroxetine binding in obsessive-compulsive disorder patients. *Neuropsychobiology* 2001;43(3):117–22.

74. Hjorth S, Bengtsson H, Kullberg A, et al. Serotonin autoreceptor function and antidepressant drug action. *Journal of Psychopharmacology* 2000;14(2):177–85.

75. Maia TV, Cooney RE, Peterson BS. The neural bases of obsessive-compulsive disorder in children and adults. *Development and Psychopathology* 2008;20(4):1251–83.

76. El Mansari M, Blier P. Responsiveness of 5-HT1A and 5-HT2 receptors in the rat orbitofrontal cortex after long-term serotonin reuptake inhibition. *Journal of Psychiatry and Neuroscience* 2005;30 (4):268–74.

77. Aouizerate B, Guehl D, Cuny E, et al. Updated overview of the putative role of the serotoninergic system in obsessive-compulsive disorder. *Neuropsychiatric Disease and Treatment* 2005;1 (3):231–43.

78. Hollander E, Fay M, Cohen B, et al. Serotonergic and noradrenergic sensitivity in obsessive-compulsive disorder: behavioral findings. *The American Journal of Psychiatry* 1988;145(8):1015–7.

79. Erzegovesi S, Cavallini MC, Cavedini P, et al. Clinical predictors of drug response in obsessive-compulsive disorder. *Journal of Clinical Psychopharmacology* 2001;21 (5):488–92.

80. Pallanti S, Hollander E, Bienstock C, et al. Treatment non-response in OCD: methodological issues and operational definitions. *International Journal of Neuropsychopharmacology* 2002;5 (2):181–91.

81. McDougle CJ, Goodman WK. Obsessive-compulsive disorder: pharmacotherapy and pathophysiology. *Current Opinion in Psychiatry* 1991;4:267–72.

82. Leckman JF, Goodman WK, North WG, et al. Elevated cerebrospinal fluid levels of oxytocin in obsessive-compulsive disorder: comparison with Tourette's syndrome and healthy controls. *Archives of General Psychiatry* 1994;51(10):782–92.

83. Karthik S, Sharma LP, Narayanaswamy JC. Investigating the role of glutamate in obsessive-compulsive disorder: current perspectives. *Neuropsychiatric Disease and Treatment* 2020;16:1003–13.

84. Marinova Z, Chuang D-M, Fineberg N. Glutamate-modulating drugs as a potential therapeutic strategy in obsessive-compulsive disorder. *Current Neuropharmacology* 2017;15(7):977–95.

85. Sharma LP, Reddy YJ. Obsessive-compulsive disorder comorbid with schizophrenia and bipolar disorder. *Indian Journal of Psychiatry* 2019;61 (Suppl 1):S140.

86. Alexander GE, Crutcher MD, DeLong MR. Basal ganglia-thalamocortical circuits: parallel substrates for motor, oculomotor, 'prefrontal' and 'limbic' functions. *Progress in Brain Research* 1991;85:119–46.

87. Veltman D. Structural imaging in OCD. In: Fineberg N, Robbins TW (eds.) *The Neurobiology and Treatment of OCD: Accelerating Progress*. Berlin: Springer; 2021: 201–29.

88. Eng GK, Sim K, Chen S-HA. Meta-analytic investigations of structural grey matter, executive domain-related functional activations, and white matter diffusivity in obsessive compulsive disorder: an integrative review. *Neuroscience & Biobehavioral Reviews* 2015;52:233–57.

89. Hazari N, Narayanaswamy JC, Venkatasubramanian G. Neuroimaging findings in obsessive-compulsive disorder: a narrative review to elucidate neurobiological underpinnings. *Indian Journal of Psychiatry* 2019;61(Suppl 1):S9.

90. Boedhoe PS, Schmaal L, Abe Y, et al. Distinct subcortical volume alterations in pediatric and adult OCD: a worldwide meta-and mega-analysis. *American Journal of Psychiatry* 2017;174(1):60–9.

91. Boedhoe PSW, Schmaal L, Abe Y, et al. Cortical abnormalities associated with pediatric and adult obsessive-compulsive disorder: findings from the ENIGMA Obsessive-Compulsive Disorder Working Group. *American Journal of Psychiatry* 2018;175 (5):453–62. DOI: 10.1176/appi.ajp.2017.17050485.

92. Soriano-Mas C. Functional brain imaging and OCD. In: Fineberg N, Robbins TW (eds.) *The Neurobiology and Treatment of OCD: Accelerating Progress*. Berlin: Springer; 2021: 269–300.

93. Biria M, Cantonas L-M, Banca P. Magnetic resonance spectroscopy (MRS) and positron emission tomography (PET) imaging in obsessive-compulsive disorder. In: Fineberg N, Robbins TW (eds.) *The Neurobiology and Treatment of OCD: Accelerating Progress*. Berlin: Springer; 2021: 231–68.

94. Zhang Z, Fan Q, Bai Y, et al. Brain gamma-aminobutyric acid (GABA) concentration of the prefrontal lobe in unmedicated patients with obsessive-compulsive disorder: a research of magnetic resonance spectroscopy. *Shanghai Archives of Psychiatry* 2016;28(5):263.

95. Zheng H, Yang W, Zhang B, et al. Reduced anterior cingulate glutamate of comorbid skin-picking disorder in adults with obsessive-compulsive disorder. *Journal of Affective Disorders* 2020;265:193–9.

96. Fan S, Cath DC, van den Heuvel OA, et al. Abnormalities in metabolite concentrations in Tourette's disorder and obsessive-compulsive disorder – A proton magnetic resonance spectroscopy study. *Psychoneuroendocrinology* 2017;77:211–7.

97. Li Y, Zhang CC, Weidacker K, et al. Investigation of anterior cingulate cortex gamma-aminobutyric acid and glutamate-glutamine levels in obsessive-compulsive disorder using magnetic resonance spectroscopy. *BMC Psychiatry* 2019;19(1):1–9.

98. Yalçin Ö, Şener Ş, Boyunağa ÖLK, et al. Comparing brain magnetic resonance spectroscopy findings of pediatric treatment-naive obsessive-compulsive disorder patients with healthy controls. *Turkish Journal of Psychiatry* 2011;22 (4):222–9.

99. Yücel M, Harrison BJ, Wood SJ, et al. Functional and biochemical alterations of the medial frontal cortex in obsessive-compulsive disorder. *Archives of General Psychiatry* 2007;64 (8):946–55.

100. Parmar A, Sharan P, Khandelwal SK, et al. Brain neurochemistry in unmedicated obsessive-compulsive disorder patients and effects of 12-week escitalopram treatment: 1H-magnetic resonance spectroscopy study. *Psychiatry and Clinical Neurosciences* 2019;73(7):386–93.

101. Escobar AP, Wendland JR, Chávez AE, et al. The neuronal glutamate transporter EAAT3 in obsessive-compulsive disorder. *Frontiers in Pharmacology* 2019;10:1362.

102. Weinberg A, Dieterich R, Riesel A. Error-related brain activity in the age of RDoC: a review of the literature. *International Journal of Psychophysiology* 2015;98(2):276–99.

103. Riesel A. The erring brain: error-related negativity as an endophenotype for OCD – A review and meta-analysis. *Psychophysiology* 2019;56(4):e13348.

104. Perera MPN, Bailey NW, Herring SE, et al. Electrophysiology of obsessive compulsive disorder: a systematic review of the electroencephalographic literature. *Journal of Anxiety Disorders* 2019;62:1–14. DOI: 10.1016/j.janxdis.2018.11.001.

105. Fineberg N, Robbins TW. *The Neurobiology and Treatment of OCD: Accelerating Progress*. Berlin: Springer; 2021.

106. Nicholson TR, Ferdinando S, Krishnaiah RB, et al. Prevalence of anti-basal ganglia antibodies in adult obsessive-compulsive disorder: cross-

sectional study. *The British Journal of Psychiatry* 2012;200(5):381–6.

107. Meyer J. Inflammation, obsessive-compulsive disorder, and related disorders. In: Fineberg N, Robbins TW (eds.) *The Neurobiology and Treatment of OCD: Accelerating Progress*. Berlin: Springer; 2021: 31–53.

108. Turna J, Grosman Kaplan K, Anglin R, et al. The gut microbiome and inflammation in obsessive-compulsive disorder patients compared to age-and sex-matched controls: a pilot study. *Acta Psychiatrica Scandinavica* 2020;142 (4):337–47.

109. Freud S. *The Standard Edition of the Complete Psychological Works of Sigmund Freud* (trans. JE Strachey). London: Hogarth Press; 1964.

110. Warwick HM, Salkovskis PM. Reassurance. *British Medical Journal (Clinical Research Edition)* 1985;290 (6474):1028. DOI: 10.1136/ bmj.290.6474.1028.

111. Gillan CM, Robbins TW, Sahakian BJ, et al. The role of habit in compulsivity. *European Neuropsychopharmacology* 2016;26(5):828–40.

112. Eisenstein E, Eisenstein D, Smith JC. The evolutionary significance of habituation and sensitization across phylogeny: a behavioral homeostasis model. *Integrative Physiological & Behavioral Science* 2001;36:251–65.

113. Stein DJ, Hermesh H, Eilam D, et al. Human compulsivity: a perspective from evolutionary medicine. *European Neuropsychopharmacology* 2016;26 (5):869–76.

114. Tybur JM, Lieberman D, Griskevicius V. Microbes, mating, and morality: individual differences in three functional domains of disgust. *Journal of Personality and Social Psychology* 2009;97(1):103.

115. Haidt J, McCauley C, Rozin P. Individual differences in sensitivity to disgust: a scale sampling seven domains of disgust elicitors. *Personality and Individual Differences* 1994;16 (5):701–13.

116. Olatunji BO, Haidt J, McKay D, et al. Core, animal reminder, and contamination disgust: three kinds of disgust with distinct personality, behavioral, physiological, and clinical correlates. *Journal of Research in Personality* 2008;42(5):1243–59.

117. Druschel B, Sherman MF. Disgust sensitivity as a function of the Big Five and gender. *Personality and Individual Differences* 1999;26(4):739–48.

118. Rachman S. A cognitive theory of compulsive checking. *Behaviour Research and Therapy* 2002;40 (6):625–39.

119. Wells A, Papageorgiou C. Relationships between worry, obsessive-compulsive symptoms and meta-cognitive beliefs. *Behaviour Research and Therapy* 1998;36(9):899–913.

120. Tümkaya S, Karadağ F, Yenigün EH, et al. Metacognitive beliefs and their relation with symptoms in obsessive-compulsive disorder. *Archives of Neuropsychiatry* 2018;55(4):358.

121. Robbins TW, Vaghi MM, Banca P. Obsessive-compulsive disorder: puzzles and prospects. *Neuron* 2019;102 (1):27–47.

122. Fineberg NA, Apergis-Schoute AM, Vaghi MM, et al. Mapping compulsivity in the DSM-5 obsessive compulsive and related disorders: cognitive domains, neural circuitry, and treatment. *International Journal of Neuropsychopharmacology* 2018;21 (1):42–58.

123. Mckeon J, Roa B, Mann A. Life events and personality traits in obsessive-compulsive neurosis. *The British Journal of Psychiatry* 1984;144 (2):185–9.

124. National Institute for Health and Care Excellence. *Obsessive-Compulsive Disorder and Body Dysmorphic Disorder: Treatment. Clinical Guideline [CG31]*. London: National Intitute of Clinical Excellence; 2005.

125. Skapinakis P, Caldwell DM, Hollingworth W, et al. Pharmacological and psychotherapeutic interventions for management of obsessive-compulsive disorder in adults: a systematic review and network meta-analysis. *The Lancet Psychiatry* 2016;3(8):730–9.

126. Goodman WK, Price LH, Rasmussen SA, et al. The Yale-Brown obsessive compulsive scale: I. Development, use, and reliability. *Archives of General Psychiatry* 1989;46(11):1006–11.

127. Hollander E, Stein DJ, Fineberg NA, et al. Quality of life outcomes in patients with obsessive-compulsive disorder: relationship to treatment response and symptom relapse. *Journal of Clinical Psychiatry* 2010;71 (6):784–92. DOI: 10.4088/ JCP.09m05911blu.

128. Drummond LM, Edwards LJ. *Obsessive Compulsive Disorder: All You Want to Know About OCD for People Living With OCD, Carers, and Clinicians*. Cambridge: Cambridge University Press; 2018.

129. Dennington L. *CBT for Adults: a practical guide for clinicians*. L.M. Drummond London: Royal College of Psychiatrists, 2014. pp. 284, £ 28.50 (pb). ISBN: 978-1-909-72627-7. *Behavioural and Cognitive Psychotherapy* 2015;43(6):767–8.

130. Wootton BM. Remote cognitive–behavior therapy for obsessive–compulsive symptoms: A meta-analysis. *Clinical Psychology Review* 2016;43:103–13.

131. Rogers MA, Lemmen K, Kramer R, et al. Internet-delivered health interventions that work: systematic review of meta-analyses and evaluation of website availability. *Journal of Medical Internet Research* 2017;19(3): e90.

132. McLean PD, Whittal ML, Thordarson DS, et al. Cognitive versus behavior therapy in the group treatment of obsessive-compulsive disorder. *Journal of Consulting and Clinical Psychology* 2001;69(2):205.

133. Külz AK, Landmann S, Cludius B, et al. Mindfulness-based cognitive therapy (MBCT) in patients with obsessive-compulsive disorder (OCD) and residual symptoms after cognitive behavioral therapy (CBT): a randomized controlled trial. *European Archives of Psychiatry and Clinical Neuroscience* 2019;269:223–33.

134. Simpson HB, Maher MJ, Wang Y, et al. Patient adherence predicts outcome from cognitive behavioral therapy in obsessive-compulsive disorder. *Journal of Consulting and Clinical Psychology* 2011;79(2):247.

135. Reid JE, Laws KR, Drummond L, et al. Cognitive behavioural therapy with exposure and response prevention in the treatment of obsessive-compulsive disorder: a systematic review and meta-analysis of randomised controlled trials. *Comprehensive Psychiatry* 2021;106:152223.

136. Cawley R. Psychotherapy and obsessional disorders. In: Beech HR (ed.) *Obsessional States*. London: Methuen; 1974: 259–89.

137. Montgomery S. Clomipramine in obsessional neurosis: a placebo-

controlled trial. *Pharmaceutical Medicine* 1980;1:189–92.

138. Fineberg NA, Reghunandanan S, Brown A, et al. Pharmacotherapy of obsessive-compulsive disorder: evidence-based treatment and beyond. *Australian & New Zealand Journal of Psychiatry* 2013;47(2):121–41.

139. Soomro GM, Altman DG, Rajagopal S, et al. Selective serotonin re-uptake inhibitors (SSRIs) versus placebo for obsessive compulsive disorder (OCD). *Cochrane Database of Systematic Reviews* 2008;2008(1):CD001765.

140. Baldwin DS, Anderson IM, Nutt DJ, et al. Evidence-based pharmacological treatment of anxiety disorders, post-traumatic stress disorder and obsessive-compulsive disorder: a revision of the 2005 guidelines from the British Association for Psychopharmacology. *Journal of Psychopharmacology* 2014;28 (5):403–39.

141. American Psychiatric Association, Koran LM, Hanna GL, et al. Practice guideline for the treatment of patients with obsessive-compulsive disorder. *American Journal of Psychiatry* 2007;164(7 Suppl):5–53.

142. Pampaloni I, Sivakumaran T, Hawley C, et al. High-dose selective serotonin reuptake inhibitors in OCD: a systematic retrospective case notes survey. *Journal of Psychopharmacology* 2010;24(10):1439–45.

143. Vaughan R, O'Donnell C, Drummond LM. Blood levels of treatment resistant obsessive-compulsive disorder patients prescribed supra-normal dosages of sertraline. *European Neuropsychopharmacology* 2018;28 (6):767–8.

144. Ninan PT, Koran LM, Kiev A, et al. High-dose sertraline strategy for nonresponders to acute treatment for obsessive-compulsive disorder: a multicenter double-blind trial. *Journal of Clinical Psychiatry* 2006;67(1):15–22.

145. Dougherty DD, Jameson M, Deckersbach T, et al. Open-label study of high (30 mg) and moderate (20 mg) dose escitalopram for the treatment of obsessive-compulsive disorder. *International Clinical Psychopharmacology* 2009;24(6):306–11.

146. Aitchinson KJ, Baldwin DS, Barnes TR, et al. Use of licensed medicines for unlicensed applications in psychiatric practice. 2017.

147. Karameh WK, Khani M. Intravenous clomipramine for treatment-resistant obsessive-compulsive disorder. *International Journal of Neuropsychopharmacology* 2016;19(2): pyv084.

148. Dold M, Aigner M, Lanzenberger R, et al.Antipsychotic augmentation of serotonin reuptake inhibitors in treatment-resistant obsessive-compulsive disorder: an update meta-analysis of double-blind, randomized, placebo-controlled trials. *International Journal of Neuropsychopharmacology* 2015;18(9):pyv047.

149. Etherington L-A, Matthews K, Akram H. New directions for surgical ablation treatment of obsessive compulsive disorder. In: Fineberg N, Robbins TW (eds.) *The Neurobiology and Treatment of OCD: Accelerating Progress*. Springer; 2021: 437–60.

150. Pepper J, Zrinzo L, Hariz M. Anterior capsulotomy for obsessive-compulsive disorder: a review of old and new literature. *Journal of Neurosurgery* 2019;133(5):1595–604.

151. Lai Y, Wang T, Zhang C, et al. Effectiveness and safety of neuroablation for severe and treatment-resistant obsessive–compulsive disorder: a systematic review and meta-analysis. *Journal of Psychiatry and Neuroscience* 2020;45(5):356–69.

152. Bergfeld IO, Dijkstra E, Graat I, et al. Invasive and non-invasive neurostimulation for OCD. *Current Topics in Behavioral Neuroscience* 2021;49:399–436. DOI: 10.1007/7854_2020_206.

153. Tyagi H, Apergis-Schoute AM, Akram H, et al. A randomized trial directly comparing ventral capsule and anteromedial subthalamic nucleus stimulation in obsessive-compulsive disorder: clinical and imaging evidence for dissociable effects. *Biological Psychiatry* 2019;85 (9):726–34.

154. Angelakis I, Gooding PA, Panagioti M. Suicidality in body dysmorphic disorder (BDD): a systematic review with meta-analysis. *Clinical Psychology Review* 2016;49:55–66.

155. Rosen JC, Reiter J, Orosan P. Cognitive-behavioral body image therapy for body dysmorphic disorder. *Journal of Consulting and Clinical Psychology* 1995;63(2):263.

156. Castle D, Beilharz F, Phillips KA, et al. Body dysmorphic disorder: a treatment synthesis and consensus on behalf of the International College of Obsessive-Compulsive Spectrum Disorders and the Obsessive Compulsive and Related Disorders Network of the European College of Neuropsychopharmacology. *International Clinical Psychopharmacology* 2021;36(2):61.

157. Wilhelm S, Phillips KA, Didie E, et al. Modular cognitive-behavioral therapy for body dysmorphic disorder: a randomized controlled trial. *Behavior Therapy* 2014;45(3):314–27.

158. McKay D, Todaro J, Neziroglu F, et al. Body dysmorphic disorder: a preliminary evaluation of treatment and maintenance using exposure with response prevention. *Behaviour Research and Therapy* 1997;35 (1):67–70.

159. Drummond LM, Edwards LJ. *Everything You Need to Know about OCD*. Cambridge: Cambridge University Press; 2022.

160. Zaboski BA, Merritt OA, Schrack AP, et al. Hoarding: a meta-analysis of age of onset. *Depression and Anxiety* 2019;36(6):552–64.

161. Drury H, Ajmi S. Fernández de la Cruz L, et al. Caregiver burden, family accommodation, health, and well-being in relatives of individuals with hoarding disorder. *Journal of Affective Disorders* 2014;159:7–14.

162. Bratiotis C, Muroff J, Lin NXY. Hoarding disorder: development in conceptualization, intervention, and evaluation. *Focus (American Psychiatric Publishing)* 2021;19 (4):392–404. DOI: 10.1176/appi.focus.20210016.

163. American Psychiatric Association. *Diagnostic Criteria From DSM-IV*. Washington, DC: American Psychiatric Association; 1994.

164. World Health Organization. *The ICD-10 Classification of Mental and Behavioural Disorders: Clinical Descriptions and Diagnostic Guidelines*. Geneva: World Health Organization; 1992.

165. Lucini G, Monk I, Szlatenyi C. *An Analysis of Fire Incidents Involving Hoarding Households*. Melbourne, Australia: Worcester Polytechnic Institute; 2009.

166. Steketee G, Frost RO. *Compulsive Hoarding and Acquiring.* Oxford: Oxford University Press; 2006.

167. Bodryzlova Y, Audet JS, Bergeron K, et al. Group cognitive-behavioural therapy for hoarding disorder: systematic review and meta-analysis. *Health & Social Care in the Community* 2019;27(3):517–30.

168. Linkovski O, Zwerling J, Cordell E, et al. Augmenting Buried in Treasures with in-home uncluttering practice: pilot study in hoarding disorder. *Journal of Psychiatric Research* 2018;107:145–50.

169. Chamberlain SR, Odlaug BL, Boulougouris V, et al. Trichotillomania: neurobiology and treatment. *Neuroscience & Biobehavioral Reviews* 2009;33(6):831–42.

170. Christenson GA, Mackenzie TB, Mitchell JE. Characteristics of 60 adult hair pullers. *The American Journal of Psychiatry* 1991;148(3):365–70.

171. Grant JE, Chamberlain SR. Trichotillomania. *American Journal of Psychiatry* 2016;173(9):868–74.

172. van Minnen A, Hoogduin KA, Keijsers GP, et al. Treatment of trichotillomania with behavioral therapy or fluoxetine: a randomized, waiting-list controlled study. *Archives of General Psychiatry* 2003;60(5):517–22.

173. Grant JE, Chamberlain SR. Prevalence of skin picking (excoriation) disorder. *Journal of Psychiatric Research* 2020;130:57–60.

174. Starcevic V. Hypochondriasis and health anxiety: conceptual challenges. *The British Journal of Psychiatry* 2013;202(1):7–8.

175. Tyrer P, Cooper S, Tyrer H, et al. Increase in the prevalence of health anxiety in medical clinics: possible cyberchondria. *International Journal of Social Psychiatry* 2019;65(7–8):566–9.

176. Meng J, Gao C, Tang C, et al. Prevalence of hypochondriac symptoms among health science students in China: a systematic review and meta-analysis. PloS one. 2019;14(9):e0222663.

177. Newby JM, Hobbs MJ, Mahoney AE, et al. DSM-5 illness anxiety disorder and somatic symptom disorder: comorbidity, correlates, and overlap with DSM-IV hypochondriasis. *Journal of Psychosomatic Research* 2017;101:31–7.

178. Tyrer P, Tyrer H. Health anxiety: detection and treatment. *BJPsych Advances* 2018;24(1):66–72.

179. Gustavsson A, Svensson M, Jacobi F, et al. Cost of disorders of the brain in Europe 2010. *European Neuropsychopharmacology* 2011;21 (10):718–79.

180. Somashekar B, Jainer A, Wuntakal B. Psychopharmacotherapy of somatic symptoms disorders. *International Review of Psychiatry* 2013;25 (1):107–15.

181. Fineberg NA, Pellegrini L, Clarke A, et al. Meta-analysis of cognitive behaviour therapy and selective serotonin reuptake inhibitors for the treatment of hypochondriasis: implications for trial design. *Comprehensive Psychiatry* 2022: 152334.

Chapter

6.5

Functional Neurological Disorder

Matt Butler and Timothy R. Nicholson

Introduction

This chapter gives an overview and update on functional neurological disorder (FND), also known as dissociative neurological symptom disorder and previously known as conversion disorder. FND is the presence of neurological symptoms that are not explained or explainable by a neurological disorder. FND is no longer a diagnosis of exclusion. Instead, wherever possible, it is ruled-in by distinct features of history and examination – the latter known as positive clinical signs. FND encompasses multiple subtypes, from seizures to motor disorders to sensory abnormalities. Symptoms often co-occur, sometimes in a striking fashion.

FND is a prototypical neuropsychiatric disorder, lying in the artificial gaps between neurology and psychiatry. This is to the detriment of patients, whose care can be over-looked as clinicians struggle to determine which service is best placed to manage the complex disorder. FND has been called medicine's 'silent epidemic', a 'crisis in neurology', and 'psychiatry's blind spot'.[1] In the media, stories of complex presentations of functional neurological disorder are often portrayed as 'medical mysteries', indicating a lack of presence and understanding of the disorder in public as well as medical discourse,[2] leading to missed diagnoses and treatment opportunities.

Historically, FND has been assumed to be a purely stress-related psychiatric disorder, but over recent decades, this simplistic conception has been supplanted by more nuanced models of symptom generation. Undoubtedly, FND remains incompletely understood; however, significant advances in the understanding of the disorder have been made in the past two decades. Gone is the strict Freudian emphasis on the 'conversion' of repressed psychic pain or trauma into somatic symptoms. Instead, whilst keeping in mind the potential aetiological relevance of stressors and trauma, clinicians diagnosing and managing FND are now encouraged to elicit positive clinical signs, which reliably distinguish FND from other neurological disorders.

The history of FND is compelling, not least as an exemplar of how brain disorders have been conceptualised over time. Throughout the history of Western medicine, symptoms resembling FND have been referred to in myriad ways: from hysteria to conversion disorder to medically unexplained symptoms (not to mention many of the more derogatory epithets). Most in the field have now settled on FND, an aetiologically neutral term preferred by most patients.[3]

FND challenges the questionable dichotomies of brain versus mind, mind versus body, conscious versus subconscious and individual versus society. This chapter strives to avoid these dualisms wherever possible. In FND, the biological, psychological, sociological – and everything in between – may be relevant to the patients in front of us.

History

The first written accounts of something resembling FND can be found in the texts of the Old Babylonian Empire period (second millennium BCE).[4,5] Whilst to trained modern eyes these texts do suggest functional neurological symptoms, there is no convincing evidence that early civilisations had any sense of what the brain was or did. Their vignettes are descriptive, not explanatory, and apart from the fact that functional disorders are as old as history, there is not too much else we can learn.[6]

Hysteria, the old – and now pejorative – term for FND-like symptoms, originated in classical Greek medicine, with some mention of uterine causes for symptoms in the Hippocratic Corpus. Nevertheless, the extent to which the Greeks believed in a wandering womb (hystera) – and how much this influenced their medical practice – is debated. We know with more certainty that the Greeks did believe in physical causes to most illnesses, including neuropsychiatric disorders like epilepsy.[6]

As with much of their culture, Greek medical thought was absorbed by the Romans, who took the idea of the wandering womb more seriously. Physicians of the Roman Empire, such as Galen (129–216 CE), promoted variations on uterine theories. These Romanised versions of Greek thought were, throughout most of the Middle Ages, the only accessible source of knowledge on medical practice; so the uterine theory persisted, such that the disorder was seen as one exclusively affecting women through and beyond antiquity.[6] As well as the recycled writings of classical philosophers and physicians, physicians in the European Middle Ages were influenced by religious beliefs, and during this period, functional symptoms were probably often thought to have spiritual or supernatural causes.[7]

Following the famous anatomist Thomas Willis (1621–1675) – who had identified the brain as the source of thoughts and emotion and who had described convulsive hysteria – Thomas Sydenham (1624–1689), another pioneering English physician, was perhaps the first to repopularise the notion of a physical basis of hysteria. Sydenham presciently noted that hysteria was the second commonest presentation in his patients and wrote of how significant stressors can cause the 'animal spirits [to] run into disorderly motions', leading to physical symptoms.[8] Sydenham and his contemporaries were harbingers of an era of thought that has lasted ever since: brain disorders have natural rather than supernatural causes. In tandem with Robert Burton's seminal work *The Anatomy of Melancholy*, the reciprocal relationship between mind and body was also beginning to be taken seriously.[9]

Jean-Martin Charcot (1825–1893) is widely held as one of the most influential figures in the history of FND as well as the father of neurology. He was the superintendent of the large Salpêtrière Hospital in Paris, at the time an asylum for women. Charcot was renowned for his diligent clinical examinations, and he was driven by a desire to categorise hysteria and to find pathological correlates for the protean symptoms he saw in his female patients via clinico-pathological correlation. For most of his career, he was convinced that there were dynamic lesions in the brain responsible for the symptoms. Although he worked primarily with women, Charcot stressed that hysteria was not a solely female disease and that many of the male railroad workers he examined also had the disorder.

Charcot argued that hysteria was a hereditary disorder (in keeping with the general view in medicine and society at the time) but accepted that environmental factors were relevant: he linked precipitating psychological or physical trauma or stress with the development of hysteria. Along with his co-workers, he produced an album of hundreds of photographs for his published *Iconography*, in which he unsuccessfully attempted to document the hypothesised predictable progression of hysterical symptoms. Nevertheless, he successfully demonstrated that functional neurological symptoms represented the patient's own ideas of illness, rather than that which is fully compatible with established anatomical and physiological knowledge.[10] Charcot also popularised the use of hypnosis in the disorder, both as a means to investigate symptoms formation and as well as a treatment modality.

There is a direct, if tantalisingly brief, link between Charcot and another figure who looms large in the world of hysteria in the nineteenth century. Sigmund Freud (1856–1939), then a neurologist and neuroscientist and yet to develop his psychoanalytic theory, visited Paris in the winter of 1884–1885 to study under Charcot. He watched the professor demonstrate the progression of hysteria at the latter's famous 'Leçons du mardi' and mingled with Charcot and his associates. Although Freud's interest in hysteria likely stemmed from this period in his early career, it is less clear how much Charcot's ideas on the disorder directly influenced Freud.[10]

Freud developed his theory of conversion in his work with (often wealthy and female) Viennese clients. In his book *The Neuro-Psychoses of Defence* (1894), which was a published a year before his seminal *Studies in Hysteria*, Freud suggested that conversion symptoms arose when an 'incompatible idea is rendered innocuous by the sum of excitation being transformed into something somatic'[11] (p. 49). This involved two processes: the repression of intolerable thoughts or feelings and then the conversion of these into physical symptoms. Freud's concept of conversion would come to be one of the preferred terms for FND throughout the twentieth century and has only very recently been replaced as the official primary term for the disorder in DSM-5-TR (the 2022 update of DSM-5) and ICD-11.

Another contemporary of Freud, Pierre Janet (1859–1947), has a less well-known but still vital place in the history of FND. Janet studied hysteria (his doctoral thesis was supervised by Charcot) and, like Freud, conceptualised the disorder as one which stemmed from psychological processes. Unlike Freud, Janet argued that functional disorders arose via the mechanism of dissociation (discussed later, and ICD-11's preferred term over functional), with patients suffering from symptoms due to difficulties in integrating motor or sensory function with conscious attentional processes.

Psychological processes had thus risen to become the generally accepted explanations for FND, even after Freud quietly ceased his writings on conversion (for reasons still not entirely understood). Nevertheless, the period around the turn of the century was one in which FND – still mostly known then as hysteria – continued to garner interest from physicians in the United Kingdom as well as France, with prominent neurologists such as William Gowers and Hughlings Jackson treating and writing about the disorder.

The arrival of the First World War (1914–1918) suddenly reanimated interest in functional symptoms on a large scale, as healthy young men returned from the abject horrors of the trenches with multiple neurological disorders. Soldiers displayed myriad symptoms including speech pathologies, dystonia, tremor and gait disorders. These initially defied clear explanation, but rapidly escalating cases created an emerging crisis for the army and a rapid prioritisation for understanding the cause. At first, blast-related neuropathology was posited; however, later the conception moved closer to psychological aetiology akin to the contemporary understanding of FND. These cases were eventually conceived as 'shell shock', a term that was initially encouraged and then banned by the British Army. For all its horrors, the presence of shell shock provided indisputable empirical evidence that healthy young men were perfectly capable of developing functional neurological symptoms.[12]

Following the cessation of the First World War and the precipitous drop in shell shock cases, the twentieth century became a relative dark age for FND. Descriptive accounts of hysteria (as it was still mostly known) were removed from medical textbooks, probably due to a combination of factors such as the Home Office inquiry into shell shock, the rise of the clinicopathological method (i.e. correlating clinical signs to laboratory findings), and increasing interest in Freudian conceptions of conversion, which were of little interest to neurologists at the time.[13] This loss of curiosity about FND arose at a time when neurology and psychiatry bifurcated into artificially separate disciplines, in a small part due to the misinterpreted evangelising of Freud's ideas and work. Interest in FND would only re-emerge in earnest at the beginning of the twenty-first century.

FND in the Modern World

Over the past two decades, there has been a significant resurgence of research and clinical interest in FND. As we have seen, terminology has now largely settled on 'functional' as an aetiologically neutral term preferred by patients.[3,14] Other terms have baggage. 'Psychogenic' is a familiar term, but and as with 'conversion disorder', it relies too heavily on unevidenced psychological and Freudian concepts. 'Non-organic', another commonly used term, implicitly suggests an unhelpful substance dualism, and as with 'medically unexplained symptoms', only serves to define symptoms by what they are not. Hysteria and 'pseudo' (neurological symptoms) incorrectly suggest a deliberate or performative aspect.

Modern advances in our understanding of FND, led by Edinburgh neurologist Jon Stone and neuropsychiatrist Alan Carson, began with work establishing how common and robust FND diagnoses are; converging evidence has clearly shown that FND is no more likely to be later reversed as a diagnosis than any other neurological disorder (see later). Following this, research and clinical interest turned to the re-emergence of positive clinical signs as a reliable means to distinguish FND from other neurological disorders. This allowed patients with FND to be given an explanation to what might be happening to them, rather than simply being told that there is nothing wrong. There have been concurrent advances in the biological understanding of FND (discussed in detail later), exemplified by functional neuroimaging studies that have indicated that FND can be distinguished from, for example, feigned symptoms mimicking the disorder.

Despite these advances, many people with FND continue to have a poor quality of life.[15,16] The complexity of the disorder, as well as enduring stigma and a pervasive implication that symptoms are feigned or malingered, has generally led to the rejection of people with FND from both neurological and psychiatric services.[17,18] Patients are sometimes left behind, and it is not uncommon for years to pass before a clinician offers a diagnosis. Much of this substandard care likely arises due to the lack of training on recognising and managing FND, as well as the scarcity of funding for appropriate services for this common disorder. We still have much more work to do in understanding FND, particularly working out who might be at risk of developing symptoms and how we might treat them once they have been diagnosed.

Clinical Features

The clinical phenotypes of FND vary widely: any aspect of neurological function that can normally be consciously accessed can be affected by FND. Nevertheless, the disorder is commonly grouped into subtypes which broadly describe similar symptom profiles. Although individualised formulations are invariably more important and useful, these classifications are not only important in a descriptive sense, but it also help direct clinicians to specific treatment options. The subtypes generally include motor FND, functional seizures, sensory FND and increasingly functional cognitive syndrome.

DSM-5-TR and ICD-10 Classification

As above, with the text revision of the DSM-5 (DSM-5-TR), functional neurological symptom disorder is now the primary category, which lies under the chapter 'Somatic Symptoms and Related Disorders'. In the ICD-11, FND is classified as dissociative neurological symptom disorder (a term less commonly used in the FND literature). A positive step in this iteration of the manual has been the inclusion of the cognitive subtype of FND, which is increasingly recognised as a key symptom and a common reason to present to memory clinics (see later). Summaries of the current classifications are in Table 6.5.1. There have been calls for the incorporation of pain and

Table 6.5.1 Classifying FND in the DSM-5 and ICD-11. Subtypes with corresponding classifiers in both manuals are bold

	DSM-5 (2013) and DSM-5-TR (2022)	ICD-11 (2019)
Chapter	Somatic symptom and related disorders	06 Mental, behavioural or neurodevelopmental disorders
Classification	F44.X Functional neurological symptom disorder	6B60 Dissociative neurological symptom disorder
Subtypes	F44.4: With motor symptoms (**weakness or paralysis**, **abnormal movement**, swallowing, **speech**) F44.5: **With attacks or seizures** F44.6: With sensory symptoms (anaesthesia or **sensory loss**, **visual**/olfactory/**hearing disturbance**) F44.7: With mixed symptoms Specify if: - Acute (<6 months) or persistent (>6 months) - With or without psychological stressor	6B60.0 **Visual** 6B60.1 **Auditory** 6B60.2 Vertigo or dizziness 6B60.3 **Sensory** 6B60.4 **Non-epileptic seizures** 6B60.5 **Speech** 6B60.6 **Paresis or weakness** 6B60.7 Gait 6B60.8 **Movement** 6B60.9 Cognitive 8A00.3 Functional Parkinsonism 8A02.3 Functional dystonia or spasms 8A04.4 Functional tremor

somatic symptom subtypes of FND into future classifications of the disorder.[19]

In the ICD-11, some FND subtypes (functional Parkinsonism, dystonia and tremor) have appropriately appeared for the first time in the neurological chapters. This chapter-straddling, as with other neuropsychiatric conditions such as the dementias, suggests it is time to consider the merging of these chapters into a unifying brain disorders category, which would remove the need to perpetuate false dualisms.

Epidemiology

FND most commonly arises in young adults,[20] and women are over-represented with a ratio of roughly 3:1.[21] Conservative estimates suggest there are 8,000 new diagnoses of FND per year in the United Kingdom, with up to 100,000 living with the disorder.[21] These rates are roughly equivalent to, for example, multiple sclerosis.[22] Even so, FND is probably more common than is assumed, in part due to the limited education of medical professionals on the disorder, heterogenous diagnostic codes in diagnostic manuals and hospitals,[23] and poor coding in health care systems when diagnosed by clinicians.[24]

It is commonly stated that FND is the second most common disorder in neurology outpatient clinics, echoing the prescient observations of Sydenham, although this may only be strictly true when a broad view of functional symptoms is taken.[25,26] FND is certainly common in emergency departments, particularly when presenting in similar fashion to acute stroke, cauda equina syndrome or epileptic seizure.[27] There are some estimates that suggest that 1 in 10 acute neurology admissions are for FND.[28] Despite these often acute presentations, it is not infrequent for patients to wait several years after the onset of their symptoms to receive a diagnosis of FND.[20]

Making the Diagnosis

In general, FND is best characterised as any neurological symptom that is neither explained nor explainable by recognised neurological disease. To extrapolate, this means that symptoms deviate from those expected in any other neurological condition, either by discrepancy with the anatomical or physiological understanding of what occurs when nervous structures or systems are damaged, or by virtue of distinct patterns of variability (e.g. distractibility). Positive clinical signs can be used to actively discriminate from other neurological disorders.

Consensus opinion remains that a formal diagnosis of FND should be undertaken by someone who is experienced in neurology or neuropsychiatry, but initial assessment and management can appropriately take place in primary or non-specialist secondary care settings.[29] Once a diagnosis of FND has been made, the stability is no different to other disorders, with a misdiagnosis rate of 1–4%; in fact FND is far more commonly incorrectly labelled as another neurological disorder than vice versa.[1]

Taking a History

It is crucial to get a good sense of the patient's journey that led to you before you begin any assessment, and it is worth exploring what understanding and concerns they may have about seeing you as a psychiatrist. Patients with functional symptoms have often been dismissed, disbelieved, accused of not having real symptoms or told they are being 'crazy or mad'. Time spent proactively dispelling such misconceptions and reassuring the patient that you know their symptoms and sufferings are very real is often required.

Patients with FND commonly have a number of core and associated symptoms. When taking a history, it is worth focusing on each symptom in turn and eliciting the exact form of the symptom, when it arises and what makes it better or worse. Directly ask about common comorbidities such as fatigue, pain, sleep disturbance, anxiety, panic attacks (which often occur at symptom onset), depression and other common potential functional symptoms such as memory or cognitive problems, dizziness or balance issues, and gastrointestinal, urinary and bowel symptoms.

Ask about how functionally impaired the person is, both as a result of their FND symptoms but also from comorbidities. Asking about good and bad days can help to determine the degree of symptom variability. Clarify if there was an initial precipitating event (physical or psychological injury or stressor) which led to the symptoms and whether there have been any acute or chronic stressors. It is worth checking in with the patient's illness beliefs early on and sensitively introducing the notion of FND if it is a differential.

If there is a link to symptom worsening when stressed, this can be very helpful later when explaining and justifying the diagnosis. However, it is worth asking about this carefully and sensitively at an appropriate juncture (often asking indirectly or obliquely). The same approach should be taken when asking about past stress and trauma. These explorations may be left to subsequent appointments if it doesn't feel like the right time to enquire or if the patient is clearly resistant to any such enquiry.

Investigations

As well as keeping relevant differential diagnoses for any symptoms in mind, it is important to always remember that FND often develops from and therefore often co-exists with other neurological disorders; be prepared to make two concurrent diagnoses, if required. Although FND is not a diagnosis of exclusion, appropriate investigations (e.g. blood tests, neuroimaging, neurophysiology) should certainly still be considered where necessary, particularly when there is suspicion of co-occurring or alternative differential diagnoses.[1]

Nevertheless, be mindful that ordering investigations is not always a benign process. In a minority of patients, even seemingly innocuous inappropriate investigations can lead to direct and indirect harm, not only in terms of adverse events and economic costs but also by fuelling anxiety and symptom monitoring. This is especially the case if positive or borderline results of unclear relevance are found, a situation which becomes increasingly likely with the increasing number of tests performed.[30]

Positive Clinical Signs

Positive clinical signs allow for active diagnosis and differentiation from other neurological presentations with a high degree of accuracy and stability.[31] There are numerous positive clinical signs, many of which have excellent sensitivity and specificity (discussed in turn later).[1] Positive clinical signs for diagnosing FND have been known about for at least a century.[32] Nevertheless, emphasis only began to be placed on their diagnostic use over the past two decades or so.

The movement towards the use of positive clinical signs has been a large part of the recent improvements in recognising and treating patients with functional neurological symptoms. These changes have been reflected in diagnostic manuals; since the publication of the DSM-5 in 2013, FND is no longer seen as a diagnosis of exclusion. This movement towards a 'rule-in' neurological diagnosis was also accompanied by the removal of the need to identify a relevant psychological stressor – a legacy from Freudian conceptions of the disorder – which was an essential diagnostic criterion in DSM-IV but is now a subspecifier (Table 6.5.1).

Demonstrating positive clinical signs to the patient and using them as a method to explain the symptoms can also be an effective means of helping patients understand this complex disorder. Positive clinical signs often illustrate a specific mechanism distinct to other disorders and show the reversibility of symptoms, even if transiently. It is also certainly more reassuring for the person to hear that they are being diagnosed on the basis of something other than 'your tests all came back normal'.[1] Despite the utility of positive clinical signs, FND should rarely be diagnosed solely on the presence of a single clinical sign.

Associated Symptoms

Many patients with FND have associated symptoms, which are often disabling but are not part of either the core FND diagnosis or a comorbidity. These symptoms include (chronic) pain, headache, fatigue and bowel and bladder dysfunction. Some associated symptoms are almost as common in FND as the 'core' neurological symptoms themselves and may have more of a negative effect on quality of life.[20] Population-level data has indicated that these associated symptoms are much more common than comorbid psychiatric disorders. The presence of associated symptoms such as pain and fatigue may help contribute to positively discriminating FND from other causes of neurological symptoms.[33]

Comorbidities

FND is commonly comorbid with other neurological conditions.[34] Motor FND is particularly common in disorders such as Parkinson's disease and multiple sclerosis, and the co-occurrence of functional seizures and epilepsy is often seen. Patients with FND may have comorbid psychiatric disorders such as anxiety and post-traumatic stress disorder (PTSD) and other dissociative symptoms such as depersonalisation and derealisation, although there is a large proportion of patients for whom this is not the case.[20,35,36]

Although there are certainly indications that stress and psychiatric conditions worsen FND symptoms (as they would any physical disorder), the indications are equally as strong that the relatively high presence of psychiatric syndromes emerges from the challenges of living with a debilitating and challenging disorder.[37] It is worth emphasising to patients (and colleagues) that FND is not 'caused' by psychiatric disorders.

Subtypes

Although FND may be grouped into subtypes depending on the presenting or main feature, co-occurrence of multiple neurological symptoms is extremely common.[20] Subtypes are discussed in turn later.

Motor FND

Weakness and Paralysis

Functional paralysis can affect any combination of muscles, but it often affects one or several limbs or the face unilaterally or bilaterally. Patients with functional paralysis may be able to continue with the usual tasks of daily living, but in the more severe cases – such as tetraplegia or bilateral leg weakness – patients may be wheelchair or even bed bound.

Leg Weakness/Paralysis

Leg weakness may emerge in the context of an acute presentation, such as hemiparesis mimicking a stroke. In the case of unilateral functional leg weakness, the patient may drag their leg behind them (rather than circumduct it), a form of gait that is specific to the diagnosis of functional leg weakness and reflects a mental model of how a leg would move if paralysed rather than the reality of nerve damage affecting the leg muscles.[38] Other aspects of gait may point towards a functional cause, such as excessive hesitation and effort, knee buckling, or falling towards support (i.e. a sudden loss of tone at each step).[1]

On the examination chair, functional paralysis in the limbs may be associated with 'give-way' weakness: initial demonstration of strength followed by a loss of strength. Perhaps the most sensitive and most validated sign in FND is Hoover's sign, in which patients are unable to extend their affected hip into the examination bed; however, the examiner will be able to feel downward pressure (hip extension) when the contralateral limb is raised (flexed at the hip), due to the presence of stabilising spinal reflexes.[39] Hoover's sign is positive when involuntary extension is stronger than voluntary extension. A similar concept exists for hip abduction, which is weak in affected legs on voluntary movement, but strength normalises when the contralateral hip is abducted against resistance.[29]

Arm Weakness

As with leg weakness, functional arm weakness can be demonstrated via give-way weakness, drift without pronation (when arms are extended with palms facing downwards). The 'flex-ext' sign is the upper limb version of Hoover's sign: it is positive when the involuntary flexion of the affected arm at the elbow when extending the healthy elbow against resistance is stronger than the voluntary flexion at the elbow. However, it is less well validated than Hoover's sign and generally not found to be clinically useful.

Facial Weakness

Hemifacial weakness may be associated with visible contraction of the platysma muscle and lack of a positive 'other Babinski sign' (positive when the ipsilateral eyebrow is raised in hemifacial spasm).

Tremor

Functional tremor tends to affect the upper limbs but can affect any part of the body, including the head and trunk. A small study showed patients with functional tremor significantly over-estimate the proportion of the day they spend with tremor (although patients with organic tremor also over-estimated to a lesser extent).[40] This is likely a reflection of the fact that FND is an attentionally mediated disorder, with distraction leading to improvement in symptoms.

Eliciting positive clinical signs in functional tremor depends on this tendency for symptoms to improve with distraction. Over a period of time during an assessment, if the tremor varies in amplitude, frequency or direction, this is suggestive of a functional cause. Functional tremor is further suggested if immobilisation of the tremulous limb leads to the tremor emerging in another part of the body.[1] 'Entrainment' of an upper limb tremor can also aid the diagnosis of a functional cause. To demonstrate this, patients with unilateral tremors are asked to make movements of their unaffected corresponding limb (e.g. pinch their unaffected forefinger and thumb together) at a different frequency to that of the tremor, ideally set by the examining clinician rather than the patient. If the tremor ceases or is entrained (i.e. takes on the same rhythm as the pinching), or if the patient is unable to copy the movement, this strongly suggests functional tremor.[29]

Myoclonus

Functional myoclonus is the occurrence of rapid intermittent muscular contractions in the affected body part. Truncal or axial myoclonus is over-represented in functional cases in comparison to other causes, although limbs may be affected too. Functional myoclonus will often be described by patients as 'shocks', or 'jerks'. The positive clinical signs for functional myoclonus rest on the same principles as functional tremor (see earlier), with variability and distractibility pointing towards a functional diagnosis.

There has been some suggestion that EEG evidence of motor planning in the form of a *Bereitschaftspotential* ('readiness potential' in German) in the motor and supplementary motor cortices prior to the myoclonic activity may aid diagnosis of functional myoclonus. Nevertheless, current evidence suggests that this is neither sensitive nor specific enough to reliably distinguish functional myoclonus from other causes.[41]

Dystonia

Functional dystonia occurs when there is a fixed flexion of a limb, commonly of the distal portion. The symptoms are typically unilateral and, if affecting the arm, usually feature a tightly closed fist and, in the leg, an inverted and dorsiflexed foot. There are no positive clinical signs associated with the disorder, but the co-occurrence of prominent pain or anaesthesia (often affecting the whole limb in a non-dermatomal distribution) and rapid onset is suggestive of FND. Physical injury, often relatively mild, is a common precipitating event in functional dystonia.

Tics

Functional tics can take the form of any rapid movement (including vocalisation). Distinguishing functional tic-like disorders from tic disorders of other aetiology (e.g. Tourette's syndrome) is challenging, even for movement disorders specialists. It should be emphasised – as with all other FND – that functional tics may co-exist with their non-functional counterparts, and the presence of one does not exclude the other. Functional tic-like symptoms are suggested by the rapid onset of symptoms (often at an older age than is usual for other tic disorders), a high frequency of upper limb or trunk movements, and poor response to conventional treatments for tic disorders.[42]

Functional Parkinsonism

Functional Parkinsonism presents with many of the motor signs seen in, for example, Parkinson's disease. The disorder often develops in those who have had contact with someone with Parkinson's disease. On examination, patients will display variability in their motor symptoms (for example, bradycardia during assessment but not on complex movements such as tying laces), entrainment of tremor, and variable resistance to passive movements in the absence of cogwheel rigidity. Other suggestive signs include preservation of pincer movement and absence of decrement during finger tapping. Ancillary signs usually seen in Parkinson's, such as migrographia, anosmia and hypersalivation, are usually absent.

Patients should not have neuroimaging to rule-out the disorder if there is sufficient clinical suspicion. Nevertheless, should clinical examination be equivocal, a dopamine transporter–single-photon emission computed tomography (DAT-SPECT) scan will be normal in patients with functional Parkinsonism, in contrast to Parkinson's. Management is as with other functional motor disorders, and levodopa challenges should be discouraged due to strong placebo effects. Chronic disability is common, even when functional Parkinsonism is correctly recognised.[43]

Sensory FND

Somatosensory Dysfunction

Functional hypo-aesthesia, anaesthesia and other sensory abnormalities commonly accompany other functional symptoms but may also exist independently. Sensory abnormalities in FND can range from feelings of numbness to paraesthesia ('pins and needles') to complete sensory loss (anaesthesia). Often, the symptoms of functional sensory loss are associated with other functional symptoms (e.g. paralysis or dystonia).

Sensory loss or changes that do not follow dermatomal distribution – for example, hemisensory loss from the midline or loss of sensation distally from the shoulder or hip joint encompassing the whole limb – are strongly indicative of a functional cause. These patterns reflect an internal representation of how a sensory deficit would manifest rather than the impact of direct disruption of afferent inputs. Confirmation of intact sensory pathways can be obtained using somatosensory evoked potentials, which characterise nervous impulses from the periphery to the somatosensory cortex.[44]

Visual Dysfunction

Patients with functional blindness may present with loss of their entire visual field or incomplete visual loss such as 'tubular blindness'. Similarly, visual blurring which stops short of blindness may also feature. In a patient with tubular visual loss, a functional cause can be clinched by demonstrating that the visual loss is the same at, say, 50 cm as it is at 150 cm. In peripheral visual loss of other causes, the field of vision would expand at further distances, which is in keeping with the knowledge of physics and optics.[29]

Although controversial, there is putative overlap between functional visual disorders and 'visual snow syndrome', a debilitating disorder in which patients experience continuous visual disturbance that resembles a poorly tuned analogue television. This has been conceptualised as a brain network disorder characterised by attentional modulation of visual processing and top-down predictive errors leading to distorted visual experience.[45]

Auditory Disorders

There are a number of auditory symptom syndromes that can have functional aetiologies, ranging from hearing loss to auditory processing disorders to positive phenomena such as tinnitus. Functional hearing loss can be investigated with physiological hearing tests such as auditory evoked potentials and otoacoustic emission testing, which can be used to demonstrate intact auditory pathways. Further suggestive signs include normal voice volume in the presence of bilateral hearing loss or a positive Stenger test (see reference) in unilateral hearing loss.[46] A subset of functional auditory disorders is 'acoustic shock', which presents in some people who are exposed to a sudden unexpected sound; the resulting syndrome includes tinnitus, hyperacusis, balance disturbance, hypervigilance and sleep disturbance.

Functional auditory disorders present to psychiatric services relatively uncommonly, and it is relatively less well characterised than other functional symptoms. Unfortunately, the audiological literature has tended to conflate functional hearing loss with malingering, which is only likely relevant in a subset of cases. It is recognised that more research into these symptoms and their treatments is required.[47]

Functional Seizures

Patients with functional seizures, often also known as 'attacks', present with a wide range of symptoms or seizure types, from transient episodes of unresponsiveness to prolonged fits involving significant whole-body movements. Many report a feeling of detachment or dissociation prior to the onset of the seizures, although this may not be remembered and is indicative rather than diagnostic.[29]

Diagnosis is complicated by the fact that the co-occurrence of epileptic and functional seizures is common – almost one-quarter of patients with a diagnosis of functional seizures also have epilepsy – and the presence of either does not preclude the other.[48] People with functional seizures may have a worse quality of life than those diagnosed with epileptic seizures.[21] Consequently, it becomes very important to ask about how many types of seizure a patient has – both from them and carers that witness the events – and take a good history of the clinical features, ideally accompanied by video footage taken by carers.

Functional seizures generally last longer than their epileptic counterparts, and a seizure duration of over two minutes is considered highly specific for functional seizures. Up to a third of patients intubated in critical or intensive care for status epilepticus have in fact had a prolonged functional seizure, meaning there is a serious risk of iatrogenic harm if functional seizures are not correctly recognised.[49] Similarly, a significant minority of patients admitted for investigation of treatment-refractory epilepsy eventually receive a diagnosis of functional seizures, meaning a proportion of patients are incorrectly medicated, sometimes for years.[48]

Video telemetry recordings of seizure activity with no associated abnormal discharges on electroencephalogram (EEG) is the gold-standard for diagnosis of functional seizures. In some patients, the probability of a seizure during an EEG investigation can be increased through non-invasive methods such as hyperventilation-photic stimulation with suggestion that this might induce a seizure. This non-deceptive method, which is commonly used in 'activation clinics', quickly and safely induces a response in most patients. This can reduce the need for prolonged telemetry, with major cost and time benefits for both health care systems and the patients themselves.[50]

Of course, this is not always possible, but thankfully, there are also a number of semiological features that point towards a functional cause, which according to the International League Against Epilepsy criteria, can be sufficient for a diagnosis of 'possible' or 'probable' functional seizures.[51] As stated earlier, video recordings of the seizures – for example, on smartphones – can be helpful if the seizures do not occur during medical reviews.

Irregularity and variability to the seizure pattern, including evolution of the movements, are suggestive of a functional cause. During functional seizures, patients may have their eyes shut (in contrast to tonic-clonic and other epileptic seizures), show side-to-side head movements, asynchronous arm movements, an arching back ('*arc de cercle*') and pelvic thrusting.[1] In contrast to the period of post-ictal confusion following tonic-clonic epileptic seizures, patients with functional seizures may come round quickly, and crying post-seizure is common in functional seizures.[29]

Urinary incontinence and ictal injury can occur in both epileptic and functional seizures and is thus limited as a discriminatory marker, although severe injuries in FND are rare, such as deep tongue lacerations from biting and major head or musculoskeletal injuries from falls. Prolactin may be useful specifically to distinguish between functional seizures and tonic-clonic epilepsy (raised 20 minutes post-seizure in the latter), although its use is limited by the fact that other forms of epilepsy are seldom associated with raised prolactin, and therefore negative prolactin is not useful as a predictor of functional seizures.[52]

Panic disorder is an important differential, and diagnosis is complicated by the fact that functional seizures may be triggered by panic attacks, although the subjective experience of panic can be relatively hidden to the point that it has been suggested many FND seizures are perhaps best described as a 'panic attack without panic'.[53]

Functional Cognitive Disorders

Functional cognitive symptoms may present independently or as part of an FND with other primary symptoms. It is increasingly recognised as a distinct disorder (e.g. inclusion in ICD-11, see Table 6.5.1) as well as a common co-occurring symptom alongside other forms of FND.[20] In either case, it is often responsible for significant disability and distress.

Functional cognitive disorder is a key differential in dementia, with up to a quarter of those visiting a memory clinic meeting criteria.[54] As such, it has been referred to as 'dementia's blind spot'.[55] There is an overlap with state and trait anxiety, as well as depression; however, functional cognitive disorder is a separate entity to cognitive disorders that result from psychiatric illnesses.

Symptoms are those which suggest attentional diversion, such as losing concentration in conversation or when reading, mild word-finding difficulties, or forgetting why one came into a room. Patients may feel that cognition is effortful and may struggle to remember specific 'overlearned' information such as PIN numbers or passwords. Subjective cognitive concerns are not necessarily a precursor to mild cognitive impairment and dementia.[54]

Standard neurocognitive tests may be poor discriminators of functional cognitive disorders in comparison to progressive neurodegenerative disorders. Nevertheless, in comparison to those who end up with a diagnosis of dementia, patients with functional cognitive syndromes are more likely to attend clinic alone, more likely to be concerned about their symptoms, and are more likely to be able to give rich and specific accounts of instances of memory loss.[56] Internal inconsistency (i.e. with observed behaviour or between situations) within the memory symptoms is strongly suggestive of a functional cause. Table 6.5.2 demonstrates some examples of clinical features at interview that would suggest functional memory problems as compared to dementia.

Research into functional cognitive syndrome is burgeoning, but there remain limited evidence-based treatments for the disorder. Expert opinion suggests that a cognitive behavioural approach to symptoms may be helpful, as well as attempting to reassure concerned patients that cognitive lapses are normal in healthy adults and that cognitive aids or safety strategies (such as making reminder notes) are often counterproductive.[57]

Functional Amnesia

Distinct from functional cognitive disorders is functional (or dissociative) amnesia, which refers to difficulties in conscious recall, particularly of autobiographical events. Anterograde amnesia may or may not be present in varying degrees.[58]

The literature is heterogenous; however, functional amnesia may be:

- Global: a sudden complete loss of autobiographical memories
- Focal: amnesia for specific autobiographical details or time periods
- Fugue state: a loss of personal identity associated with aimless wandering, often of a few days' duration

As with many functional disorders, predisposing factors include a severe precipitating stressor, childhood adversity and a current or previous neurological disorder (including head injury and previous neurological amnesia). The key to differentiating functional from other neurological causes of amnesia is in the loss of personal identity, which does not occur in other neurological causes, and the presence of other neurological symptoms, which always occur in other neurological causes.[59]

Functional amnesia cases can be distinguished from transient global amnesia by the fact that the latter does not feature a loss of personal identity, is better characterised by sudden

Table 6.5.2 Features of the memory clinic interview that would suggest dementia versus functional cognitive symptoms. Adapted from Reuber et al.[56]

Diagnostic feature	More suggestive of dementia	More suggestive of functional memory problems
Who attends the memory clinic?		
Is the patient accompanied?	Yes (Accompanied persons (AP) include family or friends)	No
Responding to neurologists' specific questions about memory problems		
'Who is most concerned about the memory problems?'	No reply from patient, 'I don't know', or AP states they are most concerned	The patient
'Can you give me an example of the last time your memory let you down?'	No response, partial or incomplete answer, or the patient offers a routine common problem ('it's daily')	Provides detailed specific example
Working and episodic memory exhibited within the present consultation		
Ability to recall a recent episodic memory during interaction	Not demonstrated	Repetitions marked by phrases such as 'like I said' or 'as I said'
Responding to compound questions	Unable to attend to different parts of compound questions	Can attend to different parts of compound questions
How patients respond to neurologists' questions		
Prevalence of verbal 'I don't know' responses	Frequent	Infrequent, related to new issues not previously considered
Patients' elaborations and length of turns at talk	Short, literal answers	Long responses, sharing of additional, unsolicited details
Repetition	More frequent repetition of own and others' utterances	Less frequent, marked as repetitions
Production of talk	Struggle to reply to questions, communication difficulties	Able to reply when questioned

anterograde memory dysfunction (which tends to recover after a period of up to 24 hours), and tends to feature prominent perseveration or repeated questioning.[60]

Treatment of functional amnesia is challenging, and approaches may involve psychological therapy.[61] Historically, there has been some success with abreaction therapy[62] and hypnosis[58] in cases of persistent functional amnesia. Both are used less commonly in contemporary medical practice but may still have a place in severe cases. Treating any mental disorders which (not uncommonly) co-occur, as well as addressing ongoing psychosocial stressors, may also prove useful.[59]

Other Functional Syndromes

Dizziness or Unsteadiness (Persistent Postural-Perceptual Dizziness)

Persistent postural-perceptual dizziness (PPPD or 'triple PD') – not to be confused with benign paroxysmal positional vertigo (BPPV) – constitutes one or more symptoms of dizziness, unsteadiness or non-spinning vertigo that occurs on most days for at least three months. The symptoms are episodic (i.e. periods without symptoms are compatible with diagnosis) and may vary in severity but tend to last for hours at a time.

Often, the disorder is triggered by an event that unsettles balance and perception, such as acute vestibular syndrome or a panic attack. Trait anxiety and excessive vigilance towards symptoms are risk factors for PPPD emerging from such events. Symptoms are commonly exacerbated by situations such as walking, eating in a busy restaurant and being in complex visual environments, such as with intricately patterned carpets.[63]

The Bárány Society criteria for persistent postural-perceptual dizziness (Table 6.5.3) can be used to guide diagnosis, and they rest on features of the history as detailed earlier.[64] As with all FND, PPPD is not a diagnosis of exclusion, and clinicians can avoid requesting investigations if the history meets the diagnostic criteria, although it is sensible to order investigations relevant to any differential diagnoses. A minority of patients may develop a secondary functional gait disorder, which arises in the context of cautious and deliberate movements induced by the vertiginous experience.

Treatment for PPPD takes a rehabilitative approach, with patients guided to slowly retrain their abnormal reflexive responses to movement and visual stimuli. PPPD may also be one of the few functional disorders in which medication such as selective serotonin re-uptake inhibitors may be directly effective, although strong evidence for this is lacking. Similarly, cognitive behavioural therapy (CBT) has some, albeit inconsistent, evidence for efficacy in PPPD.[63]

Speech

Functional speech disorders can take any form, but they manifest most often as relatively distinct subtypes of dysphonia, stuttering or prosodic abnormalities. Foreign accent syndrome is felt to be a functional subset of the latter in many cases. Nevertheless, in some cases, a structural cause has been suggested; for a full discussion of possible discriminatory factors between the two, see McWhirter et al.[65] As with any

Table 6.5.3 The Bárány Society criteria for persistent postural-perceptual dizziness[64]

Criteria for the diagnosis of persistent postural-perceptual dizziness (PPPD)
All five criteria (A-E) must be fulfilled to make the diagnosis.
A. One or more symptoms of dizziness, unsteadiness or non-spinning vertigo are present on most days for three months or more. 1. Symptoms last for prolonged (hours-long) periods of time, but they may wax and wane in severity. 2. Symptoms need not be present continuously throughout the entire day.
B. Persistent symptoms occur without specific provocation, but they are exacerbated by three factors: 1. Upright posture 2. Active or passive motion without regard to direction or position 3. Exposure to moving visual stimuli or complex visual patterns
C. The disorder is precipitated by conditions that cause vertigo, unsteadiness, dizziness or problems with balance including acute, episodic or chronic vestibular syndromes, other neurologic or medical illnesses, or psychological distress. 1. When the precipitant is an acute or episodic condition, symptoms settle into the pattern of criterion A as the precipitant resolves, but they may occur intermittently at first and then consolidate into a persistent course. 2. When the precipitant is a chronic syndrome, symptoms may develop slowly at first and worsen gradually.
D. Symptoms cause significant distress or functional impairment.
E. Symptoms are not better accounted for by another disease or disorder.

FND, functional speech disorders may co-exist with other motor speech disorders of other aetiology. Patients may have associated functional orofacial signs, such as facial weakness or palsy, as described earlier.

Functional mutism (or aphonia) is a particular form of functional speech disorder. There may be a complete inability to vocalise, or the patient may mouth words with accurate but inaudible articulatory movements. The unconscious phenomenon of functional mutism should be contrasted with that of selective mutism, in which there is conscious reluctance to speak in certain situations, particularly in anxiety-provoking scenarios.[66] Functional mutism can be distinguished from neurogenic mutism via the absences of associated symptoms, including severe motor impairments elsewhere in the body, cognitive impairment or globally reduced consciousness. History taking in functional mutism may uncover recent verbal conflicts or difficulties in speaking out. Writing ability is often preserved in functional mutism, but the use of aids should be discouraged in order not to perpetuate symptoms.[66,67]

The diagnosis of functional speech disorders often requires the input of an expert in speech and language therapy, and there are positive clinical signs which suggest the diagnosis. Patients may show evident variability in their speech during examination, and the speech of someone with functional speech disorder may improve when they are distracted. Patients may also retain the ability to sing, particularly favourite old songs, which rely less on conscious speech production and more on implicit or procedural memory. In the absence of other signs suggesting myasthenia gravis, fatiguability of speech is suggestive of functional speech disorder. In most cases, treatment is directed towards speech therapy by a speech and language therapist with appropriate experience.[66]

Functional Coma

Functional stupor or coma is defined as a prolonged attack of unresponsiveness or significantly reduced responsiveness to external stimuli. It is relatively rare, although cases do present to emergency departments and general medical wards, and general anaesthesia (e.g. for surgical procedures) has been noted as a specific trigger. Patients with functional coma often have significant levels of unresponsiveness and anaesthesia, although they are physiologically awake. There are presumed, but not definite, cognitive and memory impairments during these states. There is an overlap between pervasive refusal syndrome and resignation syndrome (discussed later) in children.

Functional coma should be distinguished from other neuropsychiatric causes of coma-like syndromes, such as severe depression or catatonia. A full neurological assessment is required in every case, and investigations to probe differentials (blood tests, toxicology, neuroimaging, lumbar puncture, EEG) are often required. Given the extensive differentials and potential life-threatening nature of coma, the diagnostic net should be cast wide, even if functional coma is suspected.

On examination, resistance to eye opening as well as eyes deviating towards the floor may be useful in some cases, although having eyes open or undeviating is not incompatible with functional coma. The use of noxious stimuli (e.g. sternum or nail bed pressure) is not as helpful as might be intuited, as patients with functional coma often have significant anaesthesia; these tests are neither sensitive nor specific for functional coma. Similarly, there is conflicting evidence on the use of the 'hand drop' test, where patients' arms are lifted and dropped to their face. Instead, transient retention of tone when the arm is dropped towards the bed (not necessarily the face) may be a more useful test.[68]

Patients inevitably recover from functional coma without any specific treatment. Supportive medical interventions such as nasogastric feeding, intravenous fluids or catheterisation may be required, but of course, these are not without risk. There is some suggestion that talking to the patient to demonstrate wakefulness via the signs suggested above may be beneficial, as well as calm reassurance within earshot.

Functional Urological Syndromes

Although outside of the handbook classification, there is increasing recognition that patients with FND may have bladder symptoms, with one sample indicating a prevalence in almost half.[20] Urinary symptoms may be the main or sole presenting feature in some patients, and research is underway to delineate these syndromes. Broadly, patients may present in acute urinary retention, with presentations resembling cauda equina, or may have chronic issues in voiding urine.

It is well recognised that many patients presenting in acute urinary retention with lower limb signs or back pain do not have neuroradiological evidence of cauda equina nerve root compression. It is increasingly recognised that a proportion of these 'scan-negative' cases have a functional cauda equina syndrome, which may be triggered by acute pain or, conversely, analgesic medicines such as gabapentin or opioids.[69] Further risk factors include the presence of other FND symptoms and psychiatric comorbidity. Nevertheless, clinically distinguishing these cases from those of acute cord compression prior to spinal imaging is challenging, and a diagnosis of FND may only occur post-hoc.[70]

In contrast, some people (often women) may suffer with chronic urinary retention of uncertain cause, which is sometimes diagnosed as Fowler's syndrome. These cases often feature urinary sphincter abnormalities, which can be correlated with abnormal discharges on sphincter electromyography (EMG). It has been suggested that a proportion of these patients may have a form of chronic functional urinary retention, with similar risk factors to those for acute functional urinary retention. Treatment options lack a current evidence base, although bladder retraining and medication rationalisation are important principles.[71]

There are other related urological and gynaecological disorders, such as painful bladder syndrome and vaginismus, which may have overlap with functional urological syndromes. These represent important areas for clinical and research development.

Prognosis

There is some evidence to indicate that limiting time from onset of functional neurological symptoms to diagnosis and treatment has a positive effect on prognosis.[72] Nevertheless, for myriad reasons, clinical samples indicate that 40–50% of those with FND are no better at 7–10 year follow-up.[72–74] Such reasons include the fact that high-quality evidenced-based treatments in FND are currently lacking,[31] and optimal treatment programmes can be difficult to access for many. Nevertheless, there is some reason for optimism that the prognosis might be improving with increasing availability of FND-specific evidence-based treatments. It is also thought that the co-occurrence of significant comorbidities is a poor prognostic factor; specific examples include chronic pain, polypharmacy and complex psychiatric comorbidities such as PTSD and severe personality disorders, particularly those with a borderline pattern.

Inpatient health care costs of FND in the United States are estimated to be around $1.2 billion per year, equivalent to the most severe neurodegenerative disorders.[23] There are limited data on costs associated with FND in the UK; however, a 2009 analysis that classified FND amongst all somatisation disorders found a cost to the NHS of £3 billion/year, with an attendant £14 billion loss of productivity.[75] Patients with severe illness often require expensive inpatient treatment programmes.[76]

Outcome measurement in FND is tricky, in part because of the clinical heterogeneity of the disorder. Recent attempts at standardising outcome measures have been made, and this may help to better inform generalisable findings of granular outcomes in FND treatments.[77] Of course, outcomes in FND diagnosed and treated in secondary care is likely to be worse, by definition, than those seen in primary care or indeed not seen at all.

Aetiology and Risk Factors

Research on FND has led to a more nuanced understanding of longitudinal dimensional risk, most notably via the stress-diathesis model. This suggests that each person has a certain susceptibility to developing FND based on a combination of three factors. The first is the background biological risk, of which limited information is known. The second is predisposing factors, such as maltreatment in early childhood. The third is precipitating factors in adulthood. In those with FND, relative contributions of each of these three factors has been sufficient to move the person over the symptom threshold line.[78] In any case, we must keep in mind that a risk factor does not equal a cause.

Biological Risk

Although it is likely that genetic and neurodevelopmental factors are a factor in the risk of developing FND, there are currently very limited studies on this topic. As with most brain disorders, it is likely that any biological risk factors will involve the complex interplay of genes and environment. Indeed, there have been reports of FND showing familial clustering; whilst certainly not ruling out a gene-environment predisposition, given the capacity for transmission between close-knit groups (see later), this does not necessarily confirm a genetic element.[79] Other stress-related disorders have shown moderate degrees of heritability,[80] and studies have indicated that genetic and functional alterations in the hypothalamic-pituitary-adrenal axis interact with childhood abuse to increase the risk of developing disorders such as PTSD.[81]

A single epigenetic study has shown increased methylation of the oxytocin receptor gene (OXTR), which codes for a receptor associated with social behaviour and the stress response, in patients with FND.[82] In another case-control study, a polymorphism in catechol-O-methyltransferase (an enzyme that, amongst many functions, degrades catecholamine neurotransmitters) was not associated with FND.[83] Indirect evidence for the modulation of gene expression in FND patients has been found in studies that have shown decreased serum brain-derived neurotropic factor (BDNF) in FND versus controls; BDNF has been suggested to play a role in mediating trauma-related neuroplasticity in FND.[84] Research has identified myriad candidate genes for future exploration. Clearly, there is more work to be done in this area.

Predisposing Factors

Childhood Maltreatment

Childhood maltreatment is common across the whole of psychiatry but also across the rest of medicine and neurology. Negative experiences in childhood are associated not only with worse psychological outcomes, but they are also associated with poorer physical health, including evidence of persistent immune modulation and chronic inflammation.[85] Whilst our explanatory models of FND have moved beyond linear relationships between trauma and symptoms, it is still a role of psychiatrists to address these common risk factors where and when appropriate.

Early life maltreatment is one of the most robust risk factors for the development of FND. Nevertheless, a theme that runs through all the evidence supporting this assertion is that childhood adversity is not relevant to all those who develop the disorder. A meta-analysis of case-control studies (a mix of healthy, psychiatric and neurological control groups) found a prevalence of 49% for emotional abuse, 24% for sexual abuse and 30% for physical abuse. Odds ratios indicated these rates were much higher than healthy controls (OR 8.6) but less so in comparison to neurological controls (OR 2.5) or psychiatric controls (OR 2.0).[86]

We would advise those seeing FND patients not to persistently search for trauma when it is not there. Particularly on the first connection with a patient, it may be prudent not to zealously pry. Nonetheless, discussions around trauma should be invariably introduced at some point, in a balanced and non-judgemental way that does not inadvertently lead the patient to feel blamed for their symptoms. Discuss these issues confidently and compassionately but at the patient's own pace.

Biological Effects of Maltreatment

Systemic inflammation has been proposed to be a factor in the precipitation or perpetuation of functional neurological symptoms, which may be a modulated experience of childhood maltreatment (as earlier). Small, uncontrolled samples of FND patients have indicated that markers of inflammation are raised above normative ranges.[87,88] Other research has indicated that FND may be associated with hypothalamic-pituitary-adrenal axis dysfunction, with a flatter cortisol awakening response in FND patients versus controls, which may be mediated by emotional abuse in childhood.[89]

Precipitating Factors

Although a precipitating factor is not always identifiable, FND symptoms commonly arise during or following psychosocial stressors (which are as varied as life itself) or after physical insults or disorder. There may be a mix of the two. On occasion, clusters of FND symptoms may arise in multiple people contemporaneously.

Acute Psychosocial Stressors

The same meta-analysis detailed earlier found a moderate association between precipitating stressors in adulthood and the development of FND symptoms.[86] Clinical experience also suggests that identifiable stressors are relevant for a large subset of patients with FND. In one study, in the month before symptom onset, at least one severe life event was identified in 56% of patients with FND, which was significantly more than 21% of patients with depression. The majority of the stressors occurred within 24 hours prior to the development of symptoms. Roughly half of the stressors were rated as having a high 'escape' potential, which meant that the impact of a stressor was felt to be ameliorated by being ill with neurological symptoms.[90]

In the case of chronic FND, ongoing psychosocial stressors may be associated with interpersonal dynamics that 'trap' the patient into their illness, despite the often well-meaning efforts of those around them.

Evolution from Physical Insults or Injuries

FND symptoms may also arise or emerge from physical symptoms or injury (or, commonly, the pain that accompanies these).[91] Precipitating physical injury appears to be particularly common in functional dystonia, where it may be causally related in two-thirds of cases.[37] Functional weakness may arise acutely from episodes such as panic attacks, migraine or painful injury to the limb.[92] FND motor reactions to medical procedures such as vaccinations are not uncommon.[93,94]

Social Contact (Epidemic Functional Illness)

On some occasions, the development of functional symptoms may be mediated by close social contact – for example, within families or carers of those with neurological illness. The progression of similar symptoms in people in regular contact with each other is likely due to illness or symptom models being subconsciously imitated, which may be more likely to happen in times of high stress.

In other distinct cases, functional symptoms may spread in clusters between large groups of people. Here, we use the term 'epidemic functional illness' as an alternative to other terms such as the more pejorative 'mass hysteria' or less aetiologically neutral 'mass psychogenic or sociogenic illness' to describe this phenomenon.

These epidemics of functional illnesses have historical precedent. There are specific accounts of epidemics of symptoms from the Middle Ages that may have borne some relation to FND (although perhaps more akin to a dissociative or trance-state), which at the time were attributed to demonic possession. The most infamous were the 'dancing manias'; the most devastating affected up to 400 citizens of Strasbourg, who danced involuntarily for several weeks in 1518. The cases tended to follow extremely stressful social periods, such as outbreaks of the bubonic plague or serially poor harvests. In other cases, Galenic humoral imbalance was blamed, and similar epidemics in in Southern Italy were attributed to tarantula spider bites. This phenomenon lives on in the performances of Tarantella folk dances in the region.[95]

Epidemic functional illnesses are more likely to arise in close-knit communities (e.g. school, workplaces) and often occur in times of stress. Symptoms vary across time and place, but they often feature anxiety-related components such as dyspnoea and (pre)syncope, as well as more classical neurological symptoms of any form. The outbreaks often incorporate narratives about contemporary fears or social anxieties,[96] such as 'railway spine' during the nineteenth century locomotive boom, the twentieth and twenty-first century fears of terrorism and 'targeted acoustic attacks' by foreign agents,[7] and clusters of functional illnesses triggered by SARS-CoV-2 vaccinations.[94]

Epidemic functional illness clusters represent a group of individuals who have developed functional neurological symptoms in a related manner: it does not represent a distinct disorder. In these settings, social contagion is a particularly strong factor in the development of symptoms but is never the sole risk. The same predisposing and precipitating factors apply as with any other cases of FND.

Often, epidemics of functional illness are confined to a specific time and place, relying on culturally bound factors – such as geographically or culturally specific accepted means of displaying distress – which prevents their spread afar. As an example, resignation syndrome is a likely epidemic functional illness affecting children, which is characterised by an initial depressive withdrawal phase followed by a functional coma-like state, often for many months or years. The disorder solely affects children seeking refugee status in Sweden or other specific regions – such as some Pacific islands – and is typically seen in those who have a history of significant traumatic experience(s).[97]

Nevertheless, in the modern era, the interconnectivity of people across time and space – particularly on social media – is likely to mean that epidemic functional illnesses are no longer solely confined to specific regions or time periods. The capacity for functional neurological symptoms to spread via social media was noted during the Covid-19 pandemic, when an upsurge in functional tic presentations – mostly in young women viewing others with similar symptoms on the TikTok video-sharing app – was noted.[98]

Mechanistic Hypotheses

Historically, FND was conceptualised as entirely psychological or trauma related; however, more nuanced modern conceptions focus on the role of stress and genetic vulnerability.[78] This gene-environmental interplay has been typified by mechanistic theories that suggest that at least some features of FND may be explained by aberrant co-optation of evolutionarily conserved mechanisms, such as dissociation in the face of life-threatening and uncontrollable situations.[99] Neurobiological models of FND incorporate brain pathways such as the default mode network (DMN), and computational models implicate attentional biases and 'over-weighted priors', which refers to brain systems prioritising incorrect internally-generated models of the body over contradictory sensory input.[100]

As neuroscience and philosophy of mind have moved away from the idea of the brain as an isolated computing machine sitting independently in the environment, so too have ideas on FND. It is now generally accepted that human conscious (and unconscious) experience relies on an embodied brain that is dynamically interacting with its environment, constantly making predictions about the body and the environment which it uses to model experience and behaviour. In other words, the brain is a predictive organ. Stretched to a logical conclusion, human experience has been described as a 'controlled hallucination'.[101]

Models of FND have treaded in this furrow, with evidence-based findings supporting the conception that FND is a disorder of the brain's ability to dynamically form verifiable predictions about the reciprocal relationships between environment and body. For example, a patient with functional weakness may be unable to move their limb volitionally due to a mismatch between the model of what the limb can do and the competing sensory evidence arising from the limb.

Nevertheless, like all illnesses, FND is multiple realisable: it can be appropriately conceptualised from neuroreceptor alterations all the way to interpersonal and societal (and even global) relationships. No single form of conceptualising the disorder will ever be sufficient to fully understand what is going on in the patient in front of us.

Bayesian Brain

The dynamic brain introduces some concepts of Bayesian prediction modelling, which states that neural predictions are generated and continuously updated via the amalgamation of prior knowledge of conditions ('priors') with novel sensory information ('posteriors'). Bayesian ideas of FND, most eloquently argued by Edwards et al.,[100] posit that incorrect and abnormally strong preconscious ideas of bodily states (priors) are prioritised over sensory information. For example, strong predictions that one cannot move a limb is prioritised over the afferent sensory input indicating an intact and functioning leg. In the case of FND following a physical insult, it may be that the brain is prevented from updating its predictive model of the injury despite physical healing.

How the problems with predictive coding might arise is yet to be fully understood; however, it may be due to the diversion of resources towards regions of the brain implicated in emotional or threat response, such as the limbic system.[29,100] There have been attempts to unify predictive coding theories of FND symptom generation with emotional processing alterations,[102] which builds upon previous theories that highlighted the disruptive effects of aberrant emotional processing in FND.[103] The predictive coding model has been broadened from FND to incorporate other functional and somatic symptoms.[104]

Dissociation

'Dissociation' was a term first described by Pierre Janet, who described it as the mind compartmentalising certain processes in response to stress or trauma. He proposed that under a variety of conditions – including trauma – a rogue 'idea', such as that of a weak limb, could become fixed and separated from the consciousness that was too weak to exert control over it.[105] The term 'dissociation' has remained influential to this day and remains the preferred term for functional neurological symptoms in the ICD-11.

Since Janet, the term has acquired multiple fluid meanings, and in broad terms, can refer to either a sense of detachment from the world (e.g. depersonalisation or derealisation) or alternatively, a loss of conscious or voluntary control over a process that is otherwise intact. Although the former definition may be seen in some patients with FND, it is the latter that is more relevant mechanistically.

Functional limb paralysis, for example, may arise from the dissociation (compartmentalisation) of the ability to consciously control the function of movement of the limb. The underlying function is not impaired (and therefore the symptom is reversible); however, it is split off from volitional control. There are commonly experienced situations that healthy people have where functions are compartmentalised and occur outside of conscious awareness, such as having a conversation whilst driving. In FND, the ability to regain conscious access to the function is not present.[106]

People with FND have higher levels of dissociation as measured by clinical scales in comparison to healthy and neurological controls; those with a seizure subtype of FND appear to have greater levels of dissociation than other forms. The presence of identifiable dissociation is associated with more severe symptoms and worse quality of life.[107]

Neuroimaging

FND probably involves both structural and functional network alterations[108] and is a disorder which likely transcends aberrations in single brain networks. Despite the significant advances made in the field of FND functional neuroimaging, there remains a lack of large-scale and replicated findings. Given the heterogeneity of the disorder, a reliable imaging biomarker for FND remains (and may well remain) elusive.

Structural

Research data has indicated structural differences in FND patients, including reduced volumes in motor and limbic system regions (see Perez et al.[111] for references). Around a quarter of patients with functional seizures may have abnormal findings on structural neuroimaging, although the clinical significance of these is uncertain.[109] Large-scale collaborative international research is currently underway to combine research datasets to increase the power of structural analyses of brain morphology in FND.[110]

Functional

As well as structural alterations, FND features multi-network alterations as evidenced by functional disruptions within and across limbic, attentional, agency and sensorimotor networks.[111] FND can be reliably distinguished from simulated symptoms in research settings via functional neuroimaging.[112] A recent comprehensive review of studies[111] found that the limbic and paralimbic cortices (specifically cingulate cortex and amygdala) are overactive in FND, and heightened connections between the limbic and motor cortices are implicated in an attentional diversion model, in which altered connectivity leads to symptom generation. FND patients have shown increased connectivity in brain regions that comprise the default mode network, such as the medial prefrontal cortex and posterior cingulate cortex (PCC), both in resting-state and task-based paradigms.[113–119] The right temporoparietal junction, an area responsible for self and agency, has also been implicated.[111]

Treatments

Current treatment options for FND are limited, and many patients have severe long-term symptoms despite best-available treatment.[1,31] Nevertheless, there are simple, and sometimes effective, steps that clinicians can take to manage and treat patients.

General Principles

Professionals treating FND should engender a positive sense of recovery in the patient, which is best achieved using a collaborative manner whilst avoiding the simplistic 'all tests are negative, it's good news!' approach. Legitimise the patient's suffering, use the diagnosis confidently and compassionately, and demonstrate how recovery might be possible. A note of cautious optimism is often best, tailored to the individual factors that might make a good outcome more or less likely.

A recognition that patients may have been passed around by services – and perhaps dismissed by clinicians – may help the patient feel listened to. Theirs is a complex disorder that is still incompletely understood, and so it is no wonder that some may struggle to understand or accept the diagnosis, at least initially. Compassionate and patient repetition of key concepts from multiple members of the multi-disciplinary team is key.

Although there are some indications that clinicians have a conception that patients with FND favour physical explanations to their disorder at the expense of psychological contributions, this is not borne out by the data.[120] In fact, the average patient with functional neurological symptoms has a nuanced conception of their disorder and is able to incorporate both physical and psychological explanations.[20]

As much as possible, patients should be encouraged to limit or stop their reliance on external aids – for example, wheelchairs or walking aids in functional motor disorder or memory aids in functional cognitive disorder. Many patients might feel alone in their suffering, particularly if understanding is lacking, but fortunately, there are several helpful and supportive patient groups available (e.g. www.fndhope.org).

Psychoeducation

Explanation of FND should begin at first suspicion of the disorder; practical guides on how to inform patients of their diagnosis can be found in, for example, Carson, et al.[121] Emphasis should rest on the mind-body nature of the disorder, and patients should never be told that it is 'all in their mind' as this will be conflated with the disorder not being real or valid, or that it is somehow their fault. A compassionate and thorough explanation of FND symptoms can in itself help improve patient care and quality of life, and this could be the sole treatment required for a subset of patients,[122] although the longitudinal effect of this is yet to be confirmed by data.

Although the computer metaphor of the mind has significant limitations, it can be a useful means of framing symptoms to patients. FND can be described as a 'software' problem or glitch, which is occurring in a piece of hardware which is functioning without issue. Patients can be directed to an excellent online resource for explaining FND (neurosymptoms.org), and clinicians may also find this resource useful in terms of providing simple practical examples of useful explanatory phrases. FND patient groups and charities (e.g. FND Hope and FND Action) also provide information on the disorder, resources and both informal and formal support networks. Of course, patients should never be dismissed with just website addresses and instructions to do their own research.

Patients can be referred to psychoeducational groups that aim to further explore FND, how it arises and the effect on patients' lives. The evidence is limited for effects on core FND symptoms; however, evaluations of psychoeducation groups consistently show high levels of patient satisfaction and positive modifications to the way patients relate to their disorder.[1]

Physiotherapy and Other Rehabilitative Treatments

Physiotherapy can be an effective treatment for patients with motor forms of FND. As detailed in consensus recommendations, physiotherapy for FND rests on the general principles we've seen earlier, as well as specific principles of exercise such as encouraging early use of affected body parts and focusing on utilising automatic movements (for example, by employing distraction techniques).[123] A feasibility trial of 29 functional motor patients who received specialist physiotherapy showed 72% rated their symptoms as improved at six months compared to 18% in the control group.[124] The resulting large (n = 335) RCT is due to report soon after writing (www.physio4fmd.org).

Recent guidelines on FND-specific occupational therapy[125] and speech and language therapy[66] rest on similar principles and lay down a clear path for development of further evidence-based rehabilitative approaches to FND.

Psychological Therapy

Psychological therapy is a promising option for some forms of FND, particularly functional seizures where the evidence base is the most sophisticated and for which physiotherapy is not applicable. Cognitive behavioural therapy (CBT) has received the most interest and, as with any disorder, works best where there are targetable disordered cognitive or behavioural pathways. Full or partial acceptance that there may be a psychological component to their disorder is often necessary for psychological therapy to get off their ground.

Cognitive Behavioural Therapy (CBT)

There have been previous indicators that CBT is effective at reducing functional seizure frequency. However, the largest study on this to date (the CODES trial) did not find evidence to support this from a 12-session programme in comparison to standard medical care at 12 month follow-up. Nevertheless, almost all secondary outcomes such as quality of life and enhanced ability to manage symptoms were significantly improved in the intervention group.[126] There is also modest evidence that self-guided CBT may be helpful in other forms of FND.[127] The evidence is less strong for other subtypes. However, it is an appropriate option where services allow, and clinicians should strive to use CBT principles throughout management and treatment pathways.

Psychodynamic

Possibly as a result of the movement away from the Freudian conception of conversion as an explanatory model for FND, as well as the inherent difficulties that psychodynamic therapy has in fitting into structured trial methodology, there is limited modern evidence for the use of psychodynamic therapy in FND. The evidence to support its use is limited by this lack of case-control studies, although other forms of evidence have shown modest improvements, but these may be in other domains rather than primary symptoms.[128]

Nevertheless, psychodynamic therapy should not be neglected, and the emphasis on emotional and interpersonal conflicts may be beneficial to a subset of patients who have significant histories of childhood maltreatment or in whom chronic stressors (e.g. interpersonal conflicts) have a negative impact on FND symptoms, as they would in many disorders.

Psychodynamic interpersonal therapy has shown some promise but with limited evidence to date.[129]

Other Psychological Therapies

There are also promising, albeit very limited, data on the use of mindfulness-based therapy,[130] individually tailored psychological approaches[131] and dialectical behavioural therapy.[1]

Medication

Although many people with FND are often on several psychotropic medications, there is no specific evidence for medications to treat FND itself.[132] Nevertheless, it is often helpful to treat common comorbidities such as pain, headache, insomnia, depression, anxiety and PTSD, perhaps with a lower threshold than would be the case for these disorders in isolation. Clinicians making a diagnosis of FND should aim to collaboratively de-prescribe any psychopharmacological agent that is not treating an established comorbidity. A significant minority of patients may take non-prescribed medications or substances as a form of self-management of their symptoms.[133]

Despite this, there are specific cases in which the use of psychoactive medications on a day case basis may be effective. Therapeutic sedation with dissociative anaesthetics such as propofol (or rarely, ketamine), also known as abreaction, has a small but suggestive evidence base in cases of severe refractory FND, particularly functional coma and dystonia. The mechanisms by which this is suggested to work include demonstrating reversibility, interrupting attentional diversion, and a non-deceptive leveraging of suggestibility to encourage recovery.[134]

There have been suggestions that (es)ketamine[135,136] and psychedelics[137] could be used in a similar means to induce recovery in severe FND, although there is currently no firm evidence for either. A neuroimaging study of psilocybin (a psychedelic) with psychological support in FND (NCT05723276) and a randomised-controlled trial of psilocybin in conjunction with physiotherapy for motor FND are due to commence at the time of writing (ACTRN12621000578808).

Non-medical Treatments

A number of non-medical treatments have been trialled in FND, including hypnosis, botulinum toxin and non-invasive neurostimulation techniques such as transcranial magnetic stimulation (TMS).[1] It has been suggested that many of these treatments may leverage a placebo effect, which may be particularly effective given meta-analytic evidence that people with FND have heightened responsiveness to verbal suggestion.[138] The placebo effect may be particularly pronounced in response to botulinum toxin (in functional dystonia, for example), which can lead to immediate relief of symptoms despite the neuromuscular blocking actions taking around 72 hours to have an effect.[139] There is lively debate about whether utilising placebo and suggestibility should be seen as a problem or a valuable therapeutic option in FND.[140]

Electrical therapy – the use of electrical charges with a therapeutic aim – has a long history in the treatment of FND.[141] There has been recent renewed interest in the use of electrical stimulation in the form of TMS as a targeted and better-tolerated intervention. Although some results have been promising from case series and RCTs for motor and visual symptoms, the studies to date have been too small and methodologically heterogenous in terms of the stimulation targets, stimulation parameters and trial design (especially regarding control intervention) to allow robust conclusions regarding efficacy of this treatment modality.[142,143] It is also unclear what potential mechanism(s) of action may be relevant beyond placebo until definitive trials are completed.

Conclusions

FND incorporates a complex spectrum of common symptoms that lie between neurology and psychiatry. Patients can be left with highly disabling symptoms with limited treatment options, although in a good proportion, full recovery is possible with currently available treatment methods. FND is no longer a diagnosis of exclusion, and a flourishing of research in the twenty-first century has elucidated biological, psychological and social factors that are relevant to the disorder. FND is the prime example of a neuropsychiatric disorder, and its challenges and complexities make for a tough but rewarding condition to diagnose and treat.

There is no one-size-fits-all approach to diagnosing and treating a patient with FND. A personalised approach, considering the multiple aetiological mechanisms and potential management strategies that are sensitive to the patient's perspective and current understanding of the condition, are the key to a patient's engagement with optimal treatment options and improving outcomes.

It is hoped that the recent thrust of research into FND, the improvements of clinical services and equitable access, and the developing education of health care professionals and the wider public will continue. Those in the field of FND have much more work to do, particularly in identifying why certain people are vulnerable to developing the disorder, as well as how we might best treat those for whom conventional treatments have been unable to help.

References

1. Aybek S, Perez DL. Diagnosis and management of functional neurological disorder. *BMJ* 2022;376:o64.
2. Popkirov S, Nicholson TR, Bloem BR, et al. Hiding in plain sight: functional neurological disorders in the news. *Journal of Neuropsychiatry and Clinical Neurosciences* 2019;31(4):361–7.
3. Stone J, Wojcik W, Durrance D, et al. What should we say to patients with symptoms unexplained by disease? The 'number needed to offend'. *British Medical Journal* 2002;325(7378):1449–50.

4. Reynolds EH, Kinnier Wilson J V. Neurology and psychiatry in Babylon. *Brain* 2014;137(9):2611–9.
5. Wilson JVK, Reynolds EH. Translation and analysis of a cuneiform text forming part of a Babylonian treatise on epilepsy. *Medical History* 1990;34 (2):185–198.
6. Reynolds EH. Hysteria in ancient civilisations: a neurological review: possible significance for the modern disorder. *Journal of the Neurological Sciences* 2018;388:208–13.
7. Bartholomew RE, Baloh RW. Challenging the diagnosis of 'Havana Syndrome' as a novel clinical entity. *Journal of the Royal Society of Medicine* 2019;113(1):7–11.
8. Sydenham T. *Dr. Sydenham's Compleat Method of Curing Almost All Diseases, and Description of their Symptoms*. 6th ed. London: STET; 1724.
9. Trimble M, Reynolds EH. A brief history of hysteria: from the ancient to the modern. *Handbook of Clinical Neurology* 2016;139:3–10.
10. Goetz CG. Charcot, hysteria, and simulated disorders. *Handbook of Clinical Neurology* 2016;139:11–23.
11. Freud S. *The Neuro-Psychoses of Defence. Standard Edition*, Vol. 3. London: Hogarth Press; 1894.
12. Popkirov S, Wessely S, Nicholson TR, et al. Different shell, same shock. *BMJ* 2017;359:j5621.
13. Fend M, Williams L, Carson AJ, et al. The Arc de Siècle: functional neurological disorder during the 'forgotten' years of the 20th century. *Brain* 2020;143(4):1278–84.
14. Ding JM, Kanaan RAA. Conversion disorder: a systematic review of current terminology. *General Hospital Psychiatry* 2017;45:51–5.
15. Jones B, Reuber M, Norman P. Correlates of health-related quality of life in adults with psychogenic nonepileptic seizures: a systematic review. *Epilepsia* 2016;57(2):171–81.
16. Glass SP, Matin N, Williams B, et al. Neuropsychiatric factors linked to adherence and short-term outcome in a U.S. functional neurological disorders clinic: a retrospective cohort study. *Journal of Neuropsychiatry and Clinical Neurosciences* 2018;30(2):152–9.
17. MacDuffie KE, Grubbs L, Best T, et al. Stigma and FND: a research agenda targeting the clinical encounter. *CNS Spectrums* 2020;1–6.
18. Lidstone SC, Araújo R, Stone J, et al. Ten myths about functional neurological disorder. *European Journal of Neurology* 2020;27(11):e62–e64.
19. Maggio J, Alluri PR, Paredes-Echeverri S, et al. Briquet syndrome revisited: implications for functional neurological disorder. *Brain Communications* 2020;2 (2):fcaa156. DOI: 10.1093/braincomms/fcaa156.
20. Butler M, Shipston-Sharman O, Seynaeve M, et al. International online survey of 1048 individuals with functional neurological disorder. *European Journal of Neurology* 2021; 28 (11):3591–602. DOI: doi.org/10.1111/ene.15018.
21. Bennett K, Diamond C, Hoeritzauer I, et al. A practical review of functional neurological disorder (FND) for the general physician. *Clinical Medicine (Northfield Il)* 2021;21 (1):28–36.
22. MS Society. *MS in the UK*. www.mssociety.org.uk/what-we-do/our-work/our-evidence/ms-in-the-uk (accessed 7 December 2021).
23. Stephen CD, Fung V, Lungu CI, et al. Assessment of emergency department and inpatient use and costs in adult and pediatric functional neurological disorders. *JAMA Neurology* 2020;78 (1):88–101.
24. Herbert LD, Kim R, Hassan AAO, et al. When neurologists diagnose functional neurological disorder, why don't they code for it? *CNS Spectrums* 2021;26:664–74.
25. Stone J, Carson A, Duncan R, et al. Who is referred to neurology clinics? – the diagnoses made in 3781 new patients. *Clinical Neurology and Neurosurgery* 2010;112(9):747–51.
26. Carson A, Lehn A. Epidemiology. *Handbook of Clinical Neurology* 2016;139:47–60.
27. Finkelstein SA, Cortel-LeBlanc MA, Cortel-LeBlanc A, et al. Functional neurological disorder in the emergency department. *Academic Emergency Medicine* 2021;28:685–96.
28. Beharry J, Palmer D, Wu T, et al. Functional neurological disorders presenting as emergencies to secondary care. *European Journal of Neurology* 2021;28(5):1441–5.
29. Stone J, Burton C, Carson A. Recognising and explaining functional neurological disorder. *BMJ* 2020;371:m3745. DOI: 10.1136/bmj.m3745.
30. Butler M, Scott F, Stanton B, et al. Psychiatrists should investigate their patients less. *BJPsych Bulletin* 2021;46 (3):1–4.
31. Espay AJ, Aybek S, Carson A, et al. Current concepts in diagnosis and treatment of functional neurological disorders. *JAMA Neurology* 2018;75 (9):1132–41.
32. Head H. An address on the diagnosis of hysteria. *British Medical Journal* 1922;1 (3204):827–9.
33. Lagrand T, Tuitert I, Klamer M, et al. Functional or not functional; that's the question. *European Journal of Neurology* 2021;28(1):33–9.
34. Stone J, Carson A, Duncan R, et al. Which neurological diseases are most likely to be associated with 'symptoms unexplained by organic disease'. *Journal of Neurology* 2012;259 (1):33–8. DOI: 10.1007/s00415-011-6111-0.
35. Brown RJ, Reuber M. Psychological and psychiatric aspects of psychogenic non-epileptic seizures (PNES): a systematic review. *Clinical Psychological Review* 2016;45:157–82.
36. Matin N, Young SS, Williams B, et al. Neuropsychiatric associations with gender, illness duration, work disability, and motor subtype in a U.S. functional neurological disorders clinic population. *Journal of Neuropsychiatry and Clinical Neurosciences* 2017;29 (4):375–82.
37. Baizabal-Carvallo JF, Hallett M, Jankovic J. Pathogenesis and pathophysiology of functional (psychogenic) movement disorders. *Neurobiology of Disease* 2019;127:32–44.
38. Daum C, Hubschmid M, Aybek S. The value of 'positive' clinical signs for weakness, sensory and gait disorders in conversion disorder: a systematic and narrative review. *Journal of Neurology, Neurosurgery, and Psychiatry* 2014;85 (2):180–90.
39. Hoover CF. A new sign for the detection of malingering and functional paresis of the lower extremities. *Journal of the American Medical Association* 1908;LI(9):746–7.

40. Pareés I, Saifee TA, Kassavetis P, et al. Believing is perceiving: mismatch between self-report and actigraphy in psychogenic tremor. *Brain* 2012;135(Pt 1):117–23. DOI: 10.1093/brain/awr292.
41. Perez DL, Aybek S, Popkirov S, et al. A review and expert opinion on the neuropsychiatric assessment of motor functional neurological disorders. *Journal of Neuropsychiatry and Clinical Neurosciences* 2020;33(1):14–26.
42. Ganos C, Martino D, Espay AJ, et al. Tics and functional tic-like movements. *Neurology* 2019;93(17):750–8.
43. LaFaver K, Espay AJ. Diagnosis and treatment of functional (psychogenic) parkinsonism. *Seminars in Neurology* 2017;37(2):228–32.
44. Voon V, Cavanna AE, Coburn K, et al. Functional neuroanatomy and neurophysiology of functional neurological disorders (Conversion disorder). *Journal of Neuropsychiatry and Clinical Neurosciences* 2016;28 (3):168–90.
45. Klein A, Schankin CJ. Visual snow syndrome as a network disorder: a systematic review. *Frontiers in Neurology* 2021;12:724072. www.frontiersin.org/articles/10.3389/fneur.2021.724072.
46. Paul R. Kileny, Teresa A. Zwolan, Heidi K. Slage. Diagnostic audiology and electrophysiologic assessment of hearing. In: Hillman TA, Cummings W Jr, Haughey BH, et al. *Cummings Otolaryngology: Head and Neck Surgery*. St. Louis: Mosby; 2005: 2022.
47. Baguley D, Cope T, McFerran D. Functional auditory disorders. In: Hallett M, Stone J, Carson AJ (eds.) *Functional Neurologic Disorders*. Cambridge, MA: Academic Press; 2016: 367–78.
48. Kutlubaev MA, Xu Y, Hackett ML, et al. Dual diagnosis of epilepsy and psychogenic nonepileptic seizures: systematic review and meta-analysis of frequency, correlates, and outcomes. *Epilepsy & Behavior* 2018;89:70–78.
49. Walker MC, Howard RS, Smith SJ, et al. Diagnosis and treatment of status epilepticus on a neurological intensive care unit. *QJM* 1996;89(12):913–20.
50. Baslet G, Bajestan SN, Aybek S, et al. Evidence-based practice for the clinical assessment of psychogenic nonepileptic seizures: a report from the American Neuropsychiatric Association Committee on Research. *Journal of Neuropsychiatry and Clinical Neurosciences* 2021;33(1):27–42.
51. Lafrance WC, Baker GA, Duncan R, et al. Minimum requirements for the diagnosis of psychogenic nonepileptic seizures: a staged approach: a report from the International League Against Epilepsy Nonepileptic Seizures Task Force. *Epilepsia* 2013;54(11):2005–18.
52. Wang Y-Q, Wen Y, Wang M-M, et al. Prolactin levels as a criterion to differentiate between psychogenic non-epileptic seizures and epileptic seizures: A systematic review. *Epilepsy Research* 2021;169:106508.
53. Goldstein LH, Mellers JDC. Ictal symptoms of anxiety, avoidance behaviour, and dissociation in patients with dissociative seizures. *Journal of Neurology, Neurosurgery, and Psychiatry* 2006;77(5):616–21.
54. McWhirter L, Ritchie C, Stone J, et al. Functional cognitive disorders: a systematic review. *The Lancet Psychiatry* 2020;7(2):191–207.
55. Ball HA, McWhirter L, Ballard C, et al. Functional cognitive disorder: dementia's blind spot. *Brain* 2020;143 (10):2895–903.
56. Reuber M, Blackburn DJ, Elsey C, et al. An interactional profile to assist the differential diagnosis of neurodegenerative and functional memory disorders. *Alzheimer Disease and Associated Disorders* 2018;32 (3):197–206. journals.lww.com/alzheimerjournal/Fulltext/2018/07000/An_Interactional_Profile_to_Assist_the.5.aspx
57. McWhirter L, King L, McClure E, et al. The frequency and framing of cognitive lapses in healthy adults. *CNS Spectrums* 2022;27(3):331–8. DOI: 10.1017/S1092852920002096.
58. Staniloiu A, Markowitsch HJ. Dissociative amnesia. *The Lancet Psychiatry* 2014;1(3):226–41.
59. Harrison NA, Johnston K, Corno F, et al. Psychogenic amnesia: syndromes, outcome, and patterns of retrograde amnesia. *Brain* 2017;140(9):2498–510.
60. Arena JE, Rabinstein AA. Transient global amnesia. *Mayo Clinic Proceedings* 2015;90(2):264–72.
61. Cassel A, Humphreys K. Psychological therapy for psychogenic amnesia: successful treatment in a single case study. *Neuropsychological Rehabilitation* 2016;26(3):374–91.
62. Poole NA, Wuerz A, Agrawal N. Abreaction for conversion disorder: systematic review with meta-analysis. *British Journal of Psychiatry* 2010;197 (2):91–5. DOI: 10.1192/bjp.bp.109.066894.
63. Popkirov S, Staab JP, Stone J. Persistent postural-perceptual dizziness (PPPD): a common, characteristic and treatable cause of chronic dizziness. *Practical Neurology* 2018;18(1):5–13.
64. Staab JP, Eckhardt-Henn A, Horii A, et al. Diagnostic criteria for persistent postural-perceptual dizziness (PPPD): consensus document of the committee for the Classification of Vestibular Disorders of the Bárány Society. *Journal of Vestibular Research* 2017;27 (4):191–208.
65. McWhirter L, Miller N, Campbell C, et al. Understanding foreign accent syndrome. *Journal of Neurology, Neurosurgery, and Psychiatry* 2019;90 (11):1265–9.
66. Baker J, Barnett C, Cavalli L, et al. Management of functional communication, swallowing, cough and related disorders: consensus recommendations for speech and language therapy. *Journal of Neurology, Neurosurgery, and Psychiatry* 2021;92 (10):1112–25.
67. Maurer CW, Duffy JR. Functional speech and voice disorders. In: LaFaver K, Maurer CW, Nicholson TR, et al. (eds.) *Functional Movement Disorder: An Interdisciplinary Case-Based Approach*. New York: Springer International Publishing; 2022:157–67.
68. Ludwig L, McWhirter L, Williams S, et al. Chapter 28 – functional coma. In: Hallett M, Stone J, Carson AJ (eds.) *Functional Neurologic Disorders*. Amsterdam: Elsevier; 2016: 313–27.
69. Gibson LL, Harborow L, Nicholson T, et al. Is scan-negative cauda equina syndrome a functional neurological disorder? A pilot study. *European Journal of Neurology* 2020;27 (7):1336–42. DOI: 10.1111/ene.14182.
70. Hoeritzauer I, Pronin S, Carson A, et al. The clinical features and outcome of scan-negative and scan-positive cases in suspected cauda equina syndrome: a retrospective study of 276 patients. *Journal of Neurology* 2018;265 (12):2916–26.

71. Hoeritzauer I, Stone J, Fowler C, et al. Fowler's syndrome of urinary retention: a retrospective study of co-morbidity. *Neurourology and Urodynamics* 2016;35 (5):601–3.

72. Gelauff J, Stone J, Edwards M, et al. The prognosis of functional (psychogenic) motor symptoms: a systematic review. *Journal of Neurology, Neurosurgery, and Psychiatry* 2014;85(2):220–6.

73. Gelauff JM, Carson A, Ludwig L, et al. The prognosis of functional limb weakness: a 14-year case-control study. *Brain* 2019;142(7):2137–48.

74. Carson AJ, Best S, Postma K, et al. The outcome of neurology outpatients with medically unexplained symptoms: a prospective cohort study. *Journal of Neurology, Neurosurgery, and Psychiatry* 2003;74(7):897–900.

75. Bermingham SL, Cohen A, Hague J, et al. The cost of somatisation among the working-age population in England for the year 2008–2009. *Mental Health in Family Medicine* 2010;7(2):71–84.

76. Nicholson C, Francis J, Nielsen G, et al. Barriers and enablers to providing community-based occupational therapy to people with functional neurological disorder: An interview study with occupational therapists in the United Kingdom. *British Journal of Occupational Therapy* 2021;85 (4):262–73.

77. Pick S, Anderson DG, Asadi-Pooya AA, et al. Outcome measurement in functional neurological disorder: a systematic review and recommendations. *Journal of Neurology, Neurosurgery, and Psychiatry* 2020;91(6):638–49.

78. Keynejad RC, Frodl T, Kanaan R, et al. Stress and functional neurological disorders: mechanistic insights. *Journal of Neurology, Neurosurgery, and Psychiatry* 2019;90(7):813–21.

79. Stamelou M, Cossu G, Edwards MJ, et al. Familial psychogenic movement disorders. *Movement Disorders* 2013;28 (9):1295–1298.

80. Smoller JW. The genetics of stress-related disorders: PTSD, depression, and anxiety disorders. *Neuropsychopharmacology* 2016;41 (1):297–319.

81. Binder EB, Bradley RG, Liu W, et al. Association of FKBP5 polymorphisms and childhood abuse with risk of posttraumatic stress disorder symptoms in adults. *JAMA* 2008;299 (11):1291–305.

82. Apazoglou K, Adouan W, Aubry J-M, et al. Increased methylation of the oxytocin receptor gene in motor functional neurological disorder: a preliminary study. *Journal of Neurology, Neurosurgery, and Psychiatry* 2018;89 (5):552–4.

83. Armagan E, Almacıoglu ML, Yakut T, et al. Cathecol-O-methyl transferase Val158Met genotype is not a risk factor for conversion disorder. *Genetics and Molecular Research* 2013;12(1):852–8.

84. Diez I, Larson AG, Nakhate V, et al. Early-life trauma endophenotypes and brain circuit–gene expression relationships in functional neurological (conversion) disorder. *Molecular Psychiatry* 2021;26(8):3817–28.

85. Danese A, Pariante CM, Caspi A, et al. Childhood maltreatment predicts adult inflammation in a life-course study. *Proceedings of the National Academy of Sciences* 2007;104(4):1319–24.

86. Ludwig L, Pasman JA, Nicholson T, et al. Stressful life events and maltreatment in conversion (functional neurological) disorder: systematic review and meta-analysis of case-control studies. *The Lancet Psychiatry* 2018;5(4):307–20.

87. van der Feltz-Cornelis C, Brabyn S, Ratcliff J, et al. Assessment of cytokines, microRNA and patient related outcome measures in conversion disorder/ functional neurological disorder (CD/ FND): the CANDO clinical feasibility study. *Brain, Behavior, and Immunity - Health* 2021;13:100228.

88. Kozlowska K, Chung J, Cruickshank B, et al. Blood CRP levels are elevated in children and adolescents with functional neurological symptom disorder. *European Child & Adolescent Psychiatry* 2019;28(4):491–504.

89. Weber S, Bühler J, Vanini G, et al. Identification of biopsychological trait markers in functional neurological disorders. *Brain* 2022;146(6):2627–41.

90. Nicholson TR, Aybek S, Craig T, et al. Life events and escape in conversion disorder. *Psychological Medicine* 2016;46(12):2617–26. DOI: 10.1017/ S0033291716000714.

91. Stone J, Carson A, Aditya H, et al. The role of physical injury in motor and sensory conversion symptoms: a systematic and narrative review. *Journal of Psychosomatic Research* 2009;66 (5):383–90.

92. Stone J, Warlow C, Sharpe M. Functional weakness: clues to mechanism from the nature of onset. *Journal of Neurology, Neurosurgery, and Psychiatry* 2012;83(1):67–9.

93. Butler M, Coebergh J, Safavi F, et al. Functional neurological disorder after SARS-CoV-2 vaccines: two case reports and discussion of potential public health implications. *Journal of Neuropsychiatry and Clinical Neurosciences* 2021;33 (4):345–8.

94. Butler M, Tamborska A, Wood GK, et al. Considerations for causality assessment of neurological and neuropsychiatric complications of SARS-CoV-2 vaccines: from cerebral venous sinus thrombosis to functional neurological disorder. *Journal of Neurology, Neurosurgery, and Psychiatry* 2021;92(11):1144–51.

95. Waller J. *A Time to Dance, a Time to Die: The Extraordinary Story of the Dancing Plague of 1518*. Cambridge: Icon Books; 2008. books.google.co.uk/ books?id=n3ghAQAAMAAJ.

96. Bartholomew RE, Wessely S. Protean nature of mass sociogenic illness: from possessed nuns to chemical and biological terrorism fears. *British Journal of Psychiatry* 2002;180:300–6.

97. von Knorring AL, Hultcrantz E. Asylum-seeking children with resignation syndrome: catatonia or traumatic withdrawal syndrome? *European Child & Adolescent Psychiatry* 2020;29(8):1103–9.

98. Hull M, Parnes M. Tics and TikTok: functional tics spread through social media. *Movement Disorders Clinical Practice* 2021;8(8):1248–52.

99. Kozlowska K, Scher S, Helgeland H, et al. Asylum-seeking children in shutdown: Neurobiological models. *Developmental Child Welfare* 2021;3 (3):282–309.

100. Edwards MJ, Adams RA, Brown H, et al. A Bayesian account of 'hysteria'. *Brain* 2012;135(11):3495–512.

101. Seth A. Illuminating consciousness. *New Scientist* 2021;251(3350):44–8.

102. Jungilligens J, Paredes-Echeverri S, Popkirov S, et al. A new science of emotion: implications for functional neurological disorder. *Brain* 2022;145 (8):2648–63.

103. Pick S, Goldstein LH, Perez DL, et al. Emotional processing in functional neurological disorder: a review, biopsychosocial model and research agenda. *Journal of Neurology, Neurosurgery and Psychiatry* 2019;90 (6):704–11. DOI: 10.1136/jnnp-2018-319201.

104. Van den Bergh O, Witthöft M, Petersen S, et al. Symptoms and the body: taking the inferential leap. *Neuroscience and Biobehavioral Reviews* 2017;74(Part A):185–203. DOI: 10.1016/j.neubiorev.2017.01.015.

105. Janet P. *The Major Symptoms of Hysteria: Fifteen Lectures Given in the Medical School of Harvard University*. London: Macmillan; 1907.

106. Brown RJ. Dissociation and functional neurologic disorders. *Handbook of Clinical Neurology* 2016;139:85–94.

107. Campbell MC, Smakowski A, Rojas-Aguiluz M, et al. Dissociation and its biological and clinical associations in functional neurological disorder: systematic review and meta-analysis. *BJPsych Open* 2023;9(1):e2.

108. Begue I, Adams C, Stone J, et al. Structural alterations in functional neurological disorder and related conditions: a software and hardware problem? *NeuroImage. Clinical* 2019;22:101798.

109. Asadi-Pooya AA, Homayoun M. Structural brain abnormalities in patients with psychogenic nonepileptic seizures. *Neurological Sciences* 2020;41 (3):555–9.

110. Butler M. Functional neurological disorder mega-analysis. *OSF* 2022. osf.io/jdya7 (accessed 16 February 2023).

111. Perez DL, Nicholson TR, Asadi-Pooya AA, et al. Neuroimaging in functional neurological disorder: state of the field and research agenda. *NeuroImage, Clinical* 2021;30:102623.

112. Spence SA, Crimlisk HL, Cope H, et al. Discrete neurophysiological correlates in prefrontal cortex during hysterical and feigned disorder of movement. *Lancet* 2000;355(9211):1243–4.

113. Cojan Y, Waber L, Carruzzo A, et al. Motor inhibition in hysterical conversion paralysis. *NeuroImage* 2009;47(3):1026–37.

114. de Lange FP, Roelofs K, Toni I. Increased self-monitoring during imagined movements in conversion paralysis. *Neuropsychologia* 2007;45 (9):2051–8. DOI: 10.1016/j.neuropsychologia.2007.02.002.

115. de Lange FP, Toni I, Roelofs K. Altered connectivity between prefrontal and sensorimotor cortex in conversion paralysis. *Neuropsychologia* 2010;48 (6):1782–8. DOI: 10.1016/j.neuropsychologia.2010.02.029.

116. de Lange FP, Roelofs K, Toni I. Motor imagery: a window into the mechanisms and alterations of the motor system. *Cortex* 2008;44(5):494–506. DOI: 10.1016/j.cortex.2007.09.002.

117. Hassa T, de Jel E, Tuescher O, et al. Functional networks of motor inhibition in conversion disorder patients and feigning subjects. *NeuroImage. Clinical* 2016;11:719–27.

118. Czarnecki K, Jones DT, Burnett MS, et al. SPECT perfusion patterns distinguish psychogenic from essential tremor. *Parkinsonism & Related Disorders* 2011;17(5):328–32.

119. Nahab FB, Kundu P, Maurer C, et al. Impaired sense of agency in functional movement disorders: an fMRI study. *PLoS One* 2017;12(4):e0172502.

120. Lehn A, Bullock-Saxton J, Newcombe P, et al. Survey of the perceptions of health practitioners regarding functional neurological disorders in Australia. *Journal of Clinical Neuroscience* 2019;67:114–23.

121. Carson A, Lehn A, Ludwig L, et al. Explaining functional disorders in the neurology clinic: a photo story. *Practical Neurology* 2016;16(1):56–61.

122. Stone J, Carson A, Hallett M. Explanation as treatment for functional neurologic disorders. *Handbook of Clinical Neurology* 2016;139:543–53. DOI: 10.1016/B978-0-12-801772-2.00044-8.

123. Nielsen G, Stone J, Matthews A, et al. Physiotherapy for functional motor disorders: a consensus recommendation. *Journal of Neurology, Neurosurgery, and Psychiatry* 2015;86 (10):1113–9.

124. Nielsen G, Buszewicz M, Stevenson F, et al. Randomised feasibility study of physiotherapy for patients with functional motor symptoms. *Journal of Neurology, Neurosurgery, and Psychiatry* 2017;88:484–90.

125. Nicholson C, Edwards MJ, Carson AJ, et al. Occupational therapy consensus recommendations for functional neurological disorder. *Journal of Neurology, Neurosurgery, and Psychiatry* 2020;91(10):1037–45.

126. Goldstein LH, Robinson EJ, Mellers JDC, et al. Cognitive behavioural therapy for adults with dissociative seizures (CODES): a pragmatic, multicentre, randomised controlled trial. *The Lancet Psychiatry* 2020;7 (6):491–505.

127. Sharpe M, Walker J, Williams C, et al. Guided self-help for functional (psychogenic) symptoms. *Neurology* 2011;77(6):564–72.

128. Gutkin M, McLean L, Brown R, et al. Systematic review of psychotherapy for adults with functional neurological disorder. *Journal of Neurology, Neurosurgery, and Psychiatry* 2021;92:36–44.

129. Mayor R, Howlett S, Grünewald R, et al. Long-term outcome of brief augmented psychodynamic interpersonal therapy for psychogenic nonepileptic seizures: seizure control and health care utilization. *Epilepsia* 2010;51 (7):1169–76.

130. Baslet G, Dworetzky B, Perez DL, et al. Treatment of psychogenic nonepileptic seizures: updated review and findings from a mindfulness-based intervention case series. *Clinical EEG and Neuroscience* 2014;46(1):54–64.

131. Reuber M, Burness C, Howlett S, et al. Tailored psychotherapy for patients with functional neurological symptoms: a pilot study. *Journal of Psychosomatic Research* 2007;63(6):625–32.

132. O'Connell N, Nicholson T, Blackman G, et al. Medication prescriptions in 322 motor functional neurological disorder patients in a large UK mental health service: a case control study. *General Hospital Psychiatry* 2019;58:94–102.

133. Butler M, Seynaeve M, Bradley-Westguard A, et al. Views on using psychoactive substances to self-manage functional neurological disorder: online patient survey results. *Journal of Neuropsychiatry and Clinical Neurosciences* 2023;35(1):77–85. DOI: 10.1176/appi.neuropsych.21080213.

134. Stone J, Hoeritzauer I, Brown K, et al. Therapeutic sedation for functional (psychogenic) neurological symptoms. *Journal of Psychosomatic Research* 2014;76(2):165–8.

135. Vendrell-Serres J, Soto-Angona Ó, Rodríguez-Urrutia A, et al. Improvement of functional neurological disorder after administration of esketamine nasal spray: a case report. *Therapeutic Advances in Psychopharmacology* 2021;11:1–6. DOI:10.1177/20451253211022188.

136. Moccia L, Lanzotti P, Pepe M, et al. Remission of functional motor symptoms following esketamine administration in a patient with treatment-resistant depression: a single-case report. *International Clinical Psychopharmacology* 2022;37(1):21–4. journals.lww.com/intclinpsychopharm/Fulltext/2022/01000/Remission_of_functional_motor_symptoms_following.4.aspx.

137. Butler M, Seynaeve M, Nicholson TR, et al. Psychedelic treatment of functional neurological disorder: a systematic review. *Therapeutic Advances in Psychopharmacology* 2020;10:1–15. DOI:10.1177/204512532091212.

138. Wieder L, Brown R, Thompson T, et al. Suggestibility in functional neurological disorder: a meta-analysis. *Journal of Neurology, Neurosurgery, and Psychiatry* 2021;92(2):150–7.

139. Burke MJ, Lidstone SC. Placebo effects and functional neurological disorder: helpful or harmful? In: LaFaver K, Maurer CW, Nicholson TR, et al. (eds.) *Functional Movement Disorder: An Interdisciplinary Case-Based Approach.* New York: Springer International Publishing; 2022: 367–78.

140. Burke MJ, Faria V, Cappon D, et al. Leveraging the shared neurobiology of placebo effects and functional neurological disorder: a call for research. *Journal of Neuropsychiatry and Clinical Neurosciences* 2019;32(1):101–4.

141. McWhirter L, Carson A, Stone J. The body electric: a long view of electrical therapy for functional neurological disorders. *Brain* 2015;138(Part 4):1113–20.

142. Oriuwa C, Mollica A, Feinstein A, et al. Neuromodulation for the treatment of functional neurological disorder and somatic symptom disorder: a systematic review. *Journal of Neurology, Neurosurgery, and Psychiatry* 2022;93 (30):280–90.

143. Aniwattanapong D, Nicholson TR. Transcranial magnetic stimulation (TMS) as treatment for functional movement disorder. In: LaFaver K, Maurer CW, Nicholson TR, et al. (eds). *Functional Movement Disorder: An Interdisciplinary Case-Based Approach.* New York: Springer International Publishing; 2022: 379–99.

Chapter

6.6

Bodily Distress Disorder, Chronic Pain and Factitious Disorders*

David Kingdon

Pierre Briquet, the French physician and psychologist, published his *Treatise on Hysteria* in 1859 on 430 patients that provided the basis for today's bodily distress/somatisation/chronic primary pain disorder (Briquet syndrome) diagnosis.[1] Briquet wrote that hysteria was a 'neurosis of the brain in which the observed phenomena consist chiefly of a perturbation of vital activities, which serve as the manifestation of affective feeling'. While sensorimotor functional neurological symptoms were part of the original symptom complex, pain was a core symptom. Briquet wrote, 'There is not a single woman with this neurosis who does not have some muscle pain during the course of the illness.'

Bodily Distress Disorder

Bodily distress disorder has been introduced into ICD-11 for a group of symptoms (see Box 6.6.1) that have proved difficult to describe and for whom descriptive terms have proved controversial.[2] They present with physical symptoms, but medical examination fails to establish a link with any known physical disease. Patients may have developed a belief, variable in strength, that they have a physical disorder with a biological cause. Degrees of the disorder are described in ICD-11: mild, moderate and severe. At initial presentation, patients may be open to alternative hypotheses of causation (e.g. stress or life event or lifestyle-related explanations) and prepared to consider social and psychological approaches. Unfortunately, such explanations may not be made available, and the patient perceives that they are being told that 'there is nothing wrong with you'. Symptoms may be described as 'unexplained' when psychosocial explanations may be readily available and appropriate – although these explanations may be resisted if introduced insensitively. This, in turn, causes frustration, damages the relationship with health care professionals and strengthens beliefs in physical causes.

Classifying the disorders associated with somatic concerns has been a challenging exercise in psychiatric nosology.[2] Previous classifications of these conditions in ICD-10 and DSM-V did not fare much better than earlier attempts.[3] Even though not exactly identical, these classifications were broadly similar, and criticisms of either system are therefore generally applicable to both. Among the most salient criticisms are those relating to their utility in routine clinical practice. A central feature of the definition of these disorders – that the symptoms are not due to physical or medical causes – was criticised for being unreliable and for posing a fundamental nosological problem: defining a disorder on the basis of the

Box 6.6.1 ICD-11 Bodily distress disorder

Bodily distress disorder is characterised by the presence of bodily symptoms that are distressing to the individual and excessive attention directed towards the symptoms, which may be manifest by repeated contact with health care providers. If another health condition is causing or contributing to the symptoms, the degree of attention is clearly excessive in relation to its nature and progression. Excessive attention is not alleviated by appropriate clinical examination and investigations and appropriate reassurance. Bodily symptoms are persistent, being present on most days for at least several months. Typically, bodily distress disorder involves multiple bodily symptoms that may vary over time. Occasionally, there is a single symptom – usually pain or fatigue – that is associated with the other features of the disorder. The symptoms and associated distress and preoccupation have at least some impacts on the individual's functioning (e.g. strain in relationships, less effective academic or occupational functioning, abandonment of specific leisure activities).

Exclusions

- Tourette syndrome
- Hair pulling disorder
- Dissociative disorders
- Hypochondriasis
- Body dysmorphic disorder
- Excoriation disorder
- Gender incongruence
- Sexual dysfunctions
- Tic disorders
- Sexual pain-penetration disorder
- Postviral fatigue syndrome
- Chronic fatigue syndrome
- Myalgic encephalomyelitis

* Acknowledgements to Tom Brown and Harold Merskey for material adapted and utilised from their chapter in the 2nd edition of *Seminars in General Adult Psychiatry*.

absence of a feature rather than the presence of a problem. Some patients object to the term 'somatoform', which they think implies that their symptoms are of doubtful clinical importance and are 'in their heads' or not real. Furthermore, the notion that the symptoms are medically unexplained is often rejected by patients as essentially an issue of detection – essentially a medical failure.

ICD-10 used the term 'somatoform disorders', which included somatisation disorder and hypochondriasis, and the DSM-5 created a new grouping called 'Somatic Symptom and Related Disorders', in which the prototypic condition is somatic symptom disorder. Even though this diagnosis can be given to a condition with 'one or more somatic symptoms', it nevertheless requires that 'excessive thoughts, feelings or behaviours are related to the somatic symptoms or associated health concerns'. Specifically, for a diagnosis of somatic symptom disorder, at least one of three psychological criteria should be present: health anxiety, disproportionate and persistent concerns about the medical seriousness of the symptoms, and excessive time and energy devoted to the symptoms or health concerns. Only one symptom is required (e.g. pain or cough) for both DSM-5 and ICD-11.

Traditionally, there have been two approaches to the classification of patients with bodily distress (somatisation) symptoms. The first highlights a number of symptomatic medical syndromes, such as irritable bowel syndrome and chronic fatigue syndrome. The alternative approach has been to look for an underlying psychiatric disorder – for example, depression or anxiety, both of which commonly present somatically – or to assign a diagnosis of somatoform disorder. Both approaches have their limitations. First, it is common for patients with functional somatic syndromes to also have an underlying psychiatric disorder, usually depression or an anxiety disorder. It should, however, be noted that by no means do all patients with these somatic syndromes have underlying or co-existing psychiatric disorder. Second, there is increasing evidence that significant overlap exists between syndromes. Wessely et al.[4] postulated that the existence of distinct somatic syndromes is an artefact of medical specialisation. The particular syndrome(s) diagnosed depends on which type of medical specialist the patient sees. Their literature review revealed that diagnostic criteria for the 12 syndromes they reviewed overlap; patients who have one somatic syndrome also met criteria for one or more of the other syndromes. Sex incidence, prevalence of co-existing psychiatric disorder, treatment, prognosis and response to treatment are broadly similar.

The term 'bodily distress disorder' is neutral about causation, allows for diagnosis of medical illness where symptoms and signs emerge, and may be more acceptable to patients. Much bodily distress is related to physical symptoms arising from life circumstances and can be related to the effects of anxiety and depression. Stress on muscles or joints as well as headaches, abdominal discomfort or palpitations from activity or inactivity can all be described as bodily distress.

Bodily distress disorder is a broad and general term which on the face of it could be used to describe a variety of conditions that were not included in the classification. These are specified as exclusions (see Box 6.6.1). Some of these conditions are described elsewhere in this edition, such as dissociative disorders (under Functional Neurological Disorder – Chapter 6.5) and hypochondriasis and body dysmorphic disorder (under Obsessive-Compulsive and Related Disorders – Chapter 6.4). Hypochondriasis has been moved to OCD and related conditions in ICD-11 due to the occurrence of repetitive cognition and behaviours as well as task-related neural activation patterns on brain imaging[2] and because, unlike body distress disorders, hypochondriasis responds to some of the same treatments used for obsessive-compulsive and related disorders. It has however been suggested that hypochondriasis is better understood and described as health anxiety and grouped with other anxiety disorders.[3] There is indeed a case for all these conditions to be described and categorised similarly. A description of hypochondriasis is provided in Chapter 6.4, but due to its relationship to bodily distress disorder, information is also provided here. DSM-5 retains hypochondriasis under the section on 'Somatic Symptom and Related Disorders'.

Terminology has therefore historically been a major issue. Older terms such as hysteria and hypochondriasis are now unacceptable to patients although, as described, the latter is retained in current classifications. The term 'functional disorder' has been found, perhaps surprisingly, to be acceptable to most patients[5] and is used in the new category 'Functional Neurological Disorders' (see Chapter 6.5).

These conditions are particularly sensitive to external sociocultural factors, especially to prevailing notions of illness within both the medical profession and the wider community. The literature in this area of medicine often begins from a point of view that separates so-called mental illness from physical illness. This dichotomy can be useful for practical purposes (service provision) but is often unhelpful with the individual patient where the interaction is dynamic and continuous. Physical symptoms can arise from mental conditions, and the latter can contribute to physical illness. Medicine now fully accepts the notion of a biopsychosocial understanding and management of various disorders, whether it be anxiety, schizophrenia or chronic pain. This is held to be a monistic approach – that is, one that is unitary in terms of body-mind relationships and is reflected in considering each aspect in explanation and management.

ICD-11 BDD should not be confused with another new concept, the 'bodily distress syndrome' (BDS), included in the primary health care section of ICD-11, ICPC.[6] This diagnosis is based on twenty-five 'bothering somatic symptoms' grouped in four symptom clusters (cardiopulmonary, gastrointestinal, musculoskeletal and general) occurring within the past four weeks. To establish the diagnosis of BDS – either single-organ type (one or two systems) or multiorgan type (three or all four systems) – in a busy primary care clinic is, reportedly, less time-consuming than diagnosing BDD because the assessment of psychobehavioral criteria is not required. This is the major reason given for including an adapted but broader version of the BDD concept.

BDD Diagnostic Requirements

Features required for diagnosis include distressing bodily symptoms that typically, but not essentially, involve multiple bodily symptoms, which may vary over time. Attention is directed towards the symptoms, which may manifest in persistent preoccupation with the symptoms or their consequences despite appropriate clinical examination and investigations by repeated contacts with health care providers. Where they have an established medical condition, the degree of attention related to the symptoms is disproportionate. Related distress and preoccupation result in significant impairment in personal, family, social, educational, occupational or other important areas of functioning. The symptoms or the associated distress and preoccupation are not better accounted for by another mental disorder.

Severity of Bodily Distress Disorder

Severity is defined in terms of mild, moderate and severe bodily distress disorder:

- Mild: the individual spends only a limited amount of time focusing on symptoms (e.g. no more than one or two hours per day) and is able to focus on other unrelated topics with mild impairment in personal, family, social, educational, occupational or other important areas of functioning
- Moderate: persistent preoccupation with the distressing symptoms and their consequences, frequent medical visits and substantial time and energy focusing on the symptoms and their consequences (e.g. several hours per day) with moderate impairment
- Severe: pervasive and persistent preoccupation with severe impairment in personal, family, social, educational, occupational or other important areas of functioning (e.g. unable to work, alienation of friends and family, abandonment of nearly all social and leisure activities)

The most common bodily symptoms associated with bodily distress disorder include pain (e.g. musculoskeletal pain, backache, headaches), fatigue and gastrointestinal and respiratory symptoms, although patients may be preoccupied with any bodily symptom. The individual can generally provide a detailed description of the symptoms, but it may be difficult for clinicians to account for the symptoms in anatomical or physiological terms.

Over-interpretation or catastrophisation about their bodily symptoms – dwelling on the most extreme negative consequences – can occur, leading to avoidance of normal activities and severe distress, which may in turn lead to other symptoms associated with inactivity (e.g. stiffness and muscle weakness, muscle pain following minimal exertion).

Course Features

In about half of individuals diagnosed with bodily distress disorder seen in primary care, bodily symptoms resolve within 6 to 12 months.[7] Individuals with a severe disorder and those with multiple bodily symptoms tend to experience a more chronic and persistent course and are more likely, but more resistant, to being seen by mental health professionals, particularly liaison services. The presence of multiple bodily symptoms is commonly associated with greater impairment in functioning as well as with poorer treatment response for any co-occurring mental or medical conditions.[7] Older adults with bodily distress disorder are more likely than younger adults with the condition to have multiple bodily symptoms, and symptoms are more likely to be persistent. The diagnosis of bodily distress disorder in older adults can be challenging due to the higher likelihood of medical conditions that may account for symptoms or are comorbid with bodily distress disorder.[7]

Bodily distress (somatic) symptoms are common in all black and minority ethnic groups, especially among persons seeking health care (see Chapter 17). Differences in rates of bodily symptoms may be related to cultural reporting styles. Symptoms that are common in one cultural group may be less common in other groups – for example, whereas pain symptoms are common across cultures, symptoms such as heat in the body or in the head, crawling sensations, heaviness, or complaints of 'gas' or abdominal bloating are common in certain cultural group but not in others.[7] Culture may influence explanatory models, with symptoms variously attributed to forms of bodily energy, humours or other ethnophysiological concepts as well as religious, spiritual, personal, family or environmental stresses.

In the initial edition of this book, a number of disorders were separately described, and their treatment outlined. These included irritable bowel syndrome, functional chest pain and chronic fatigue syndrome. Since then, the concept of functional somatic symptoms and syndromes has been developed, and it now seems sensible to discuss these various syndromes together(see Wessely et al.,[4] discussed earlier). These syndromes constitute a huge clinical caseload both in primary care and in specialist hospital clinics. In contrast to 'real' illness, this group are often described as a 'burden', which perpetuates the denigration and then disregard of people who can be very distressed and disabled and for whom effective interventions should be made available. Every hospital specialty has its own syndrome (see Table 6.6.1), and patients with these syndromes account for 30–40% of new outpatient referrals in hospital clinics.

Concern about physical symptoms is the usual reason for patients to consult doctors. Doctors are trained to diagnose diseases and treat them; yet, in only a minority of cases do

Table 6.6.1 Somatic symptom/bodily distress disorders in hospital clinics

Specialty	Syndrome
Infectious diseases	Chronic fatigue syndrome
Gastroenterology	Irritable bowel syndrome
Cardiology	Atypical chest pain
Respiratory medicine	Hyperventilation syndrome
Rheumatology	Fibromyalgia
Neurology	Tension headache
Gynaecology	Chronic pelvic pain
Gynaecology	Premenstrual syndrome

doctors identify the disease that accounts for the patient's symptoms, at least in primary care.[8] Most symptoms therefore remain unexplained even after medical assessment. It is worth noting that ICD-11 lists 'functional syndromes' in individual systems categories (e.g. GI, GU and CVS), which effectively duplicates BDD categorisation; it may, however, be useful in discussion with individual patients and for medical specialties.

Typically, the patient with severe BDD (somatisation disorder) will present with a multiplicity of symptoms occurring over a long period of time in different body systems. The symptoms will be unaccounted for by underlying physical disorder, although they will continue to be attributed to medical problems by the patient. Most commonly, the symptoms are very subjective and thus difficult to objectively measure – for example, pain and fatigue. Occasionally, however, patients will present with more concrete symptoms more predictive of organic illness, such as melaena, and specimen examples can be requested. Typically, patients begin to present in their teens or 20s. Diagnosis has, however, frequently been delayed and considered, or at least management commenced, only after multiple referrals and multiple investigations, and sometimes even after surgical exploration or intervention. It has been common for these patients to have had numerous non-diseased organs removed before diagnosis is made, discussed with the individual and referral for psychiatric assessment considered. The most common organs removed have been the appendix, gall bladder and uterus.

There are numerous clues to the detection of the condition: patients often present with complex histories, having seen numerous specialists and having voluminous case notes. The early age of onset of unexplained symptoms should be apparent from searching the case notes and general practitioner's records and, indeed, presentation of a diagnosis of severe BDD is usual, though not inevitably, before age 40. Patients with severe BDD may deny or minimise emotional problems. Although, discussion of life circumstances – often most effectively within the context of a personal and social history – can improve detection and, approached sensitively, be accepted or at least entertained by the patient. Patients have high lifetime rates of depression and anxiety disorders, and self harm is common. A variety of personality traits have been associated with severe BDD[9] and may colour the way the patient presents. Bass[9] has indeed suggested that somatisation disorder is perhaps best seen as a personality disorder.

There is frequently difficulty or confusion about the overlap between BDD and both malingering and factitious disorder. In practice, this distinction can be difficult. Malingerers usually deliberately feign illness to avoid something difficult or unpleasant or to gain personal advantage. Patients with factitious disorder also intentionally feign symptoms to mimic disease or self-induce disease or injury. Although it has been stated that, in somatisation disorder, the motive is unconscious and that this distinguishes it from malingering, in clinical practice, the conscious/unconscious distinction is difficult to make (as discussed elsewhere in this chapter). It is likely, particularly with the passage of time, that both factitious and malingering symptoms may sometimes mix with BDD.

Epidemiology

Epidemiological studies suggest these syndromes as a group are common, and they are mainly encountered in primary care. Community studies carried out in the DSM–III era suggested a community prevalence of 0.4% for strictly defined somatisation disorder.[10] However, the prevalence of somatic symptom disorders in the general population is now estimated to be 5–7%.[11] Modifying the criteria by reducing the large number of symptoms required by ICD-10 and DSM-IV leads to the prevalence rising considerably. Bass and May[12] claimed that 4% of the general population and 9% of patients admitted to tertiary care have chronic multiple functional somatic symptoms. Prevalence of 35% has been reported in medical outpatient departments[11] and even higher in some specialist clinics, such as gastroenterology and neurology. About half the patients with a functional somatic syndrome (and more in specialist settings) have symptoms persisting for over a year. Lieb and colleagues[13] interviewed 3,021 adolescents and young adults using the Munich adaptation of the Composite International Diagnostic Interview (CIDI) – which included 46 somatosensory symptoms, all derived from DSM-IV. Interviewers cross-checked that a reported symptom was not part of an existing known condition or due to a drug or alcohol and that it was also clinically significant (e.g. involving a visit to the doctor, medication taken or some functional impairment). Just over half the population had a lifetime experience of at least one of these symptoms. The 12-month prevalence of these symptoms was also very high. Thus, 33% reported a pain symptom, including 11% headache, 9% abdominal pain, 4% back pain and 4% joint pain. A gastrointestinal symptom was reported by 13%, neurological symptoms by 9% and conversion symptoms by around 7%. Somatisation disorder is generally reported to be more common in women, with a sex ratio of 2:1. It is found across a range of cultures.[14]

In primary care settings, the use of different measures and different samples leads to considerable variation in prevalence rates, but most studies indicate an overall prevalence of 8–22%.[11] Persistent somatoform pain disorder is not considered separately from somatoform disorder as the epidemiology is similar.[15] A recent primary care study[6] found 17% of attenders fulfilled the bodily distress syndrome criteria (note above – this is broader than BDD); it is particularly common among patients aged 41–65 years, people with impaired mental and physical health status, and patients with limited socioeconomic resources. Patients with BDS had high comorbidity with depression and anxiety, although mental morbidity did not account for their poor health-related quality of life.

Prognosis

In a systematic review, Hartman[16] reported that approximately 50% to 75% of the patients with 'medically unexplained symptoms' (MUS) improved, whereas 10% to 30% deteriorated. In patients with hypochondriasis, recovery rates vary between 30% and 50%. In studies on MUS and hypochondriasis, the number and severity of somatic symptoms at baseline influenced the course of these conditions. Comorbid anxiety and depression did not seem to predict the course of hypochondriasis.

Aetiology

Its aetiology is multifactorial. An association with both physical and sexual abuse and an exposure to parents with complaints of poor physical health has been found. A history of unexplained (i.e. bodily distress) symptoms during childhood is also associated with an adult diagnosis of BDD. Numerous psychological theories have attempted to account for the origins of bodily distress symptoms. These vary from psychodynamic theories to cognitive theories. The role of biological function in BDD has been studied in some syndromes but inconclusively.

The role of doctors and the health care system in causing and perpetuating functional symptoms is significant. Inappropriate reassurance, over-investigation, spurious diagnoses and treatments, and reinforcing disability are all major contributions to chronicity in these syndromes. The patient's own knowledge and beliefs about symptoms and the behaviours engaged in when symptomatic are also highly relevant to the aetiology of these syndromes.

Management

Many patients with functional somatic symptoms do not present to doctors at all but deal with the symptoms themselves. Of those who present to doctors, most are treated in primary care. For some, symptoms are self-limiting, and a brief explanation and reassurance are all that is required. Some, usually those with more persistent or disabling symptoms, reach hospital clinics. In this section on management, we emphasise a tiered approach to care and outline a general approach to managing these patients in primary care settings, before describing the more specialist care that patients will require. NICE clinical guidelines[17] for anxiety, depression, chronic fatigue syndrome and irritable bowel syndrome may all be relevant. There is not a specific UK guideline for bodily distress disorder/somatisation, but the Danish College of General Practitioners have produced a very useful guideline for functional disorders.[18] A meta-analysis[19] has provided evidence for the efficacy of antidepressants even in the absence of clear-cut depression or anxiety. Antidepressants had a greater effect on physical symptoms than on psychological symptoms. The evidence was greater for tricyclic antidepressants than for SSRIs, although there was evidence of efficacy for both.

In medical practice, the following principles are widely held to be useful:[20]

1. One doctor, usually the general practitioner, should be identified as the patient's main medical carer, should coordinate the patient's care and, in particular, should communicate with any other health care professionals who become involved with the patient.
2. Time spent carrying out an initial comprehensive assessment is worthwhile. Patients need to be allowed to talk about their physical symptoms, including when they are seeing psychiatrists. Their views on the aetiology of their symptoms should be actively sought (but not initially actively challenged, especially during the engagement phase with the patient). Any concerns expressed about psychosocial factors should be encouraged, and the doctor and the patient should negotiate an agreed problem list to be tackled.
3. The validity of the patient's physical symptoms needs to be strongly acknowledged. Patients will often be anxious that doctors think their symptoms are 'all in my mind' or 'imaginary'. Accepting the symptoms as real and empathising with the patient's suffering is extremely helpful in engaging the patient in a collaborative management plan. Physical examination can be a useful part of this, although clear limits have to be set on investigations and referrals to specialists. Such referral without a clear clinical reason is usually unhelpful but may need careful explanation.
4. After the initial engagement phase, the doctor should attempt to broaden the agenda and facilitate discussion of relevant psychosocial problems. The goals of management should be clearly negotiated. Functional improvement and damage limitation rather than a cure should be the aim. The patients should be encouraged to think in terms of coping with symptoms rather than in terms of total symptom relief.
5. Primary care management of patients and their partners/families[21] involves giving simple advice, explanations and reassurance; detecting psychiatric disorders (e.g. anxiety and depression) with appropriate advice, prescribing and management; dealing with obvious cognitive and behavioural factors that exacerbate disability (e.g. disease

conviction, avoidance behaviours, checking behaviours); and providing care and referral for patients with persistent symptoms.

Development of appropriate interview skills for doctors attempting to manage patients with multiple bodily distress symptoms[22] includes attention to language used. Words associated with psychiatry (e.g. depression or anxiety) at the early stages of engagement may only confirm the patient's suspicion that the doctor thinks it is simply a psychiatric problem or that the patient is exaggerating symptoms. The explanation given to patients about their symptoms can be crucially important. The explanation should embrace physiological factors (e.g. hyperventilation or overactivity of the autonomic nervous system), behavioural factors (e.g. checking or selective attention to particular body parts) and emotional factors (e.g. relationship of physical symptoms to stress or fear). Examples where stress is recognised to cause physical symptoms – being 'sick' with fear before an interview or when in danger – or describing the positive benefits of hyperventilation and alertness when under threat – 'fear, fight or flight reaction' – can sometimes be relevant.

Patients with persistent symptoms are usually reluctant to engage with mental health services, although not invariably so – they can also be relieved when support is suggested, such as 'talking therapy' (previously known as IAPT), and can self-refer. Preparation of the patient for referral is crucial and should emphasise the need to learn to cope with persistent symptoms rather than merely representing an assessment for underlying psychiatric problems. Where counselling is rejected or fails, involvement of a psychiatrist can be successful with their ability to use their medical knowledge and skills to assess, explain and manage symptoms. Where the situation becomes protracted and fraught, joint consultations[23] involving combinations of a general practitioner, mental health practitioner/psychologist, physician and psychiatrist can be very useful at disentangling misunderstanding and helping the patient feel they are not merely being disregarded or 'dumped' on to mental health services.

Specialist Treatment

A minority of patients will require specialist psychiatric treatment. Patients in this group are more likely to have problems engaging with psychiatric services, and the principles outlined in relation to the management of somatisation disorder earlier are equally relevant here. Psychiatric services based in general hospitals or primary care are more acceptable to most of the patients than services based in psychiatric hospitals. Liaison psychiatrists have particular expertise and experience in organising and delivering these services (see Chapter 19). Although this is improving, unfortunately, these services are still not uniformly available in the UK, and even where they do exist, liaison services cannot provide a comprehensive service for all these patients. Part of the role of the liaison psychiatrist, therefore, is to help educate and advise colleagues in the appropriate management of such patients.

Psychological treatment is based on cognitive behavioural approaches. The Improving Access to Psychological Therapies ('talking treatments') programme in the UK offers open access for interventions for 'people with long-term conditions and medically unexplained symptoms' (i.e. including symptoms of bodily distress).[24] More complex presentations – for example, where personality disorder/complex trauma are factors – may require referral to psychologists based in mental health services with support from the community mental health team (CMHT). Systematic review of 15 studies of CBT[25] for 'somatoform disorders and medically unexplained physical symptoms' has demonstrated that it could alleviate and have a sustained benefit on somatic, anxiety and depressive symptoms and improve physical functioning but did not affect doctor visits or improve social functioning.

Treatment for health anxiety[26,27] builds on the model that underpins cognitive behavioural therapy (CBT, see Chapter 3.4), identifying dysfunctional beliefs that influence perceptions of critical incidents (e.g. onset of disturbing physical symptoms or illness/death of close relative) and negative automatic thoughts ('I've got cancer'). These lead to health anxiety and become complicated by avoidant behaviours and mood, as well as physical and cognitive changes. Avoidant behaviours may include social avoidance, bodily checking and reassurance seeking; cognitive factors include preoccupation, bodily focusing and selective attention on specific symptoms; physical maintaining factors include hyperventilation, abdominal discomfort or dizziness; these in turn can contribute to depression. Management focuses, as previously discussed, on engagement, self-monitoring and cognitive restructuring (e.g. generating alternative explanations). Behavioural tasks are especially important to positive outcomes – for example, exposure to daily living is supported to overcome avoidance and improve mood. As therapy progresses, identification and reattribution of core beliefs and assumptions may become possible.

Hypochondriasis

The word 'hypochondriasis' literally means 'below the cartilage' and was first used by Smollius in 1610.[28] It was applied to various mental states that were thought to be caused by changes in the organs of the hypochondrial region, particularly the liver and the spleen.[29] Burton (1651)[30] and James Boswell (1777–83)[31] used the word to describe a sub-division of melancholia or depression. Thomas Willis (1684)[32] is credited with being the first to make the distinction between hypochondriasis and hysteria. He regarded the latter as an organic brain disease and challenged the uterine view of hysteria, which had prevailed for many centuries.

George Cheyne (1733)[33] wrote an important treatise on hypochondriasis, hysteria and melancholy entitled *The English Malady*. He described his own depressive and hypochondriacal symptoms and wrote in the preface of the book that it was 'intended as a legacy and dying speech only to my fellow sufferers'. He attributed these disorders to the pressures of modern living (in the eighteenth century), by which he meant the influences of mechanisation, city dwelling and affluence. Robert Whytt recognised nervous disorders, hypochondriacal symptoms and hysterical ones. Some think that he was describing depression, hypochondriasis and hysteria. It seems rather that he recognised the occurrence of anxiety and depression and the somatic complaints related to them. At the beginning of his book,[34] he wrote 'physicians have bestowed the character of nervous on all those disorders, whose nature and causes they were ignorant of', a comment which remains apposite. He later wrote:

> To wipe off this reproach, and, at the same time to throw some light on nervous hypochondriac and hysteric complaints, is the design of the following observations.

At the end of his book he wrote about low spirits saying, 'Hypochondriac and hysteric patients are commonly affected with this complaint in a greater or less degree', and he later refers to 'low spirits or melancholy'.

His diagnostic concerns remain of interest, including his concern about diagnosis by exclusion. Whytt also gave sensible advice on management, which included the wise counsel not to promise a cure, plus the prescription of exercise, dietary change and, for severe cases, opium. The recent concept of hypochondriasis as a morbid preoccupation with health emerged only in the nineteenth century, when Falret (1822)[35] referred to abnormal beliefs about one's health as 'hypochondria'. The description of hypochondriasis by Gillespie (1928)[36] paved the way for the DSM-III and DSM-IV concepts of hypochondriasis as a syndrome with disease phobia and disease conviction at its heart.

Since the late 1970s, the dominant terminology in this field has been 'somatisation' (from the Greek word 'soma', for body). It was first used early in the twentieth century by Stekel, who described a group of neuroses that presented with physical symptoms.[36] In the latter half of the twentieth century, the term was championed by Lipowski,[37] who defined it as:

> a tendency to experience and communicate somatic distress and symptoms which are unaccounted for by pathological findings and to attribute them to physical illness and to seek medical help for them.

With specific reference to the term 'hypochondriasis', recent literature has preferred the more acceptable term 'health anxiety', which is much easier to use with patients, who see 'hypochondriasis' as an accusation rather than a diagnosis. Health anxiety[38] refers to attitudes, fears and beliefs about health, based on appraisals of bodily symptoms and signs. Some degree of health anxiety is virtually universal. It lies on a continuum from mild to severe and disabling. Severe clinically and socially significant health anxiety would meet DSM/ICD criteria for hypochondriasis.

Clinical Features

The ICD-11 criteria for hypochondriasis (see also Chapter 6.4) are outlined in Box 6.6.2.

The core features are disease phobia and disease conviction, as well as a preoccupation with disease that persists despite medical investigation and reassurance. Sufferers are often preoccupied with intrusive thoughts around the themes of having an actual disease or fear of developing an actual disease. Disturbing, frightening images and fear of death are also common. The thoughts have the quality of over-valued ideas, are held with some conviction and rarely respond to reassurance for any length of time. Misinterpretation of normal sensations is extremely common, as is a tendency to self-examine. These patients often engage in checking behaviours, such as monitoring pulse rate and blood pressure, or examining minor skin lesions and body parts (e.g. breasts or testes). Sometimes, checking behaviours can produce or exacerbate the very symptoms the patient fears; for example, patients with globus sensation ('globus hystericus') who fear cancer of the oesophagus or larynx often check by repeated swallowing, an action that itself leads to globus sensation. In contrast to patients with somatisation disorder, these patients often have a narrow symptom focus, being preoccupied with a specific organ or specific disease (although this preoccupation can change and move from system to system).

Any body area may be involved, although symptoms relating to the chest, abdomen, head and neck are particularly common.[29] Most patients are in some pain. Medical assessment and examination do not reveal any evidence of disease, despite which the patient's preoccupation and concerns persists. It is, of course, the case that physical and psychiatric disorder may co-exist, and inevitably patients with hypochondriasis will at some point develop physical disorders. This highlights one of the great difficulties in managing patients with hypochondriasis. In clinical practice, what usually happens is that, in the early stages of the patient's presentation, there is a phase of zealous over-investigation on the part of professionals in the hunt for organic disease. When none is

Box 6.6.2 ICD-11 hypochondriasis

Hypochondriasis is characterised by persistent preoccupation or fear about the possibility of having one or more serious, progressive or life-threatening illnesses. The preoccupation is accompanied by either (1) repetitive and excessive health-related behaviours, such as repeatedly checking of the body for evidence of illness, spending inordinate amounts of time searching for information about the feared illness, repeatedly seeking reassurance (e.g. arranging multiple medical consultations) or (2) maladaptive avoidance behaviour related to health (e.g. avoids medical appointments). The symptoms result in significant distress or significant impairment in personal, family, social, educational, occupational or other important areas of functioning.

found, there can follow a policy of under-investigation and non-investigation, even in the presence of ominous symptoms indicative of organic disorder. Development of disease and presentation of new conditions can then be missed and, even where this is not the case, patients frequently can relay experiences where family members, or others, have been misdiagnosed with serious consequences.

Epidemiology

Estimates of the prevalence of hypochondriasis have been fairly wide ranging. It is probably higher among medical patients than in the general population,[39] and particular medical specialties have even higher prevalence, with a figure as high as 10 per cent being described in an ear, nose and throat clinic.[40] The demographic risk factors for hypochondriasis are somewhat different from those for bodily distress disorders. The sex incidence appears to be equal (in contrast, bodily distress disorder has a female to male ratio of 2:1 – see earlier). No convincing relationships between age, education and occupational status have been found.[41]

Aetiology

There is considerable interest in the role of early childhood environment. For both bodily distress symptoms and hypochondriasis, a number of studies have shown that an adverse childhood environment can predispose to adult somatisation and hypochondriasis.[42] Some studies have also found – in contrast to neglect – over-protectiveness and over-concern on the part of parents can also lead to hypochondriasis.[43] Life events, including medical life events such as myocardial infarction, and cognitive factors involving problematic appraisals of body sensations[44] may also contribute. Higher levels of personality disorder (PD) in patients with hypochondriasis have been found than controls, but a more recent comparison has shown that PD is no more common than in two comparative anxiety disorders.[45]

Differential Diagnosis

The existence of a primary hypochondriasis syndrome has been disputed since hypochondriasis symptoms frequently accompany other psychiatric disorders, notably depression and anxiety disorder, including specific illness phobias, obsessive-compulsive disorder and panic disorder. Occasionally, hypochondriacal delusions are also a feature of schizophrenia. A small minority of patients do have missed physical illness, especially neurological and endocrine disorders. Indeed, Creed concluded that neither somatisation disorder and hypochondriasis can be regarded as definite psychiatric disorders distinct from anxiety and depression.

Classification systems have made it clear that a diagnosis of hypochondriasis and bodily distress disorder should not be made if one of the other psychiatric syndromes better accounts for the symptoms, but this diagnostic practice should not mean that important, distressing symptoms are not addressed. Clarification of the order of onset of symptoms and the longitudinal course of the disorder often resolves diagnostic doubt, and treatment of other syndromes may impact on the hypochondriacal or BD symptoms. However, this is not necessarily the case, and a holistic approach should always be employed.

Some patients with specific illness phobias fear illnesses that they have not yet even encountered – for example, HIV – in contrast to patients with hypochondriasis, who are preoccupied with diseases they believe they have. Similarly, patients with panic disorder present with symptoms such as fear of dying or having a heart attack, which can lead to confusion with hypochondriasis. The obsessional nature of intrusive thoughts and images in hypochondriasis can lead to confusion with obsessive-compulsive disorder (note its inclusion in the OCD section of ICD-11). Patients with the latter have obsessions and compulsions across a whole range of areas and not just disease and illness. Patients who present with hypochondriacal delusions in the context of psychosis will, in accordance with the diagnosis, have other features of a psychotic illness. However, in delusional disorder itself, a somatic delusion may be the only manifestation of the disorder, and differentiation from hypochondriasis may be based on the reasons given for the health belief rather than the degree of conviction, which is high in both.[46]

Finally, transient hypochondriacal symptoms can occur after serious medical disorders (e.g. cancer or ischaemic heart disease). Following such illnesses, some patients become preoccupied with any bodily symptom and interpret these symptoms as a sign, rightly or wrongly, of ongoing disease. Appropriate medical evaluation and then explanation and reassurance in these cases may help to resolve the symptoms. Family concern can also be an important factor to identify and manage.

Measurement of Hypochondriasis and Health Anxiety

Two scales generally used in both clinical practice and research to measure hypochondriasis are the Whiteley Index[47] (Box 6.6.3) and the Illness Attitude Test.[48] The scales attempt to measure three core elements of the DSM-IV concept of hypochondriasis: disease phobia, disease conviction and lack of response to medical reassurance. These scales have been criticised by Kirmayer and Robbins,[41] who claim they sample a limited range of patients' symptoms, mood and attitude and tell us little about behaviour. Lucock and Morley[49] have developed a self-report questionnaire known as a health anxiety questionnaire, dealing with health preoccupation, illness phobia, reassurance seeking and interference with day-to-day living.

Management

Many authors on hypochondriasis comment on the difficult nature of the doctor–patient relationship, and much of the

Box 6.6.3 The Whiteley Index

1. Do you often worry about the possibility that you have a serious illness?
2. Are you bothered by many pains and aches?
3. Do you find that you are often aware of various things happening in your body?
4. Do you worry a lot about your health?
5. Do you often have the symptoms of very serious illnesses?
6. If a disease is brought to your attention (through the radio, television, newspaper or someone you know) do you worry about getting it yourself?
7. If you feel ill and someone tells you that you are looking better, do you become annoyed?
8. Do you find that you are bothered by many different symptoms?
9. Is it easy for you to forget about yourself and think about all sorts of other things?
10. Is it hard for you to believe the doctor when he or she tells you there is nothing for you to worry about?
11. Do you get the feeling that people are not taking your illness seriously enough?
12. Do you think that you worry about your health more than most people?
13. Do you think there is something seriously wrong with your body?
14. Are you afraid of illness?

discussion earlier on severe bodily distress can be applied (see also the hypochondriasis section in Chapter 6.4).

One issue that often arises in the early stages of treatment is the role of reassurance. Explanation and reassurance given in the context of an adequate medical assessment for a patient with whom one has a good therapeutic relationship can constitute adequate treatment in themselves. However, Warwick and Salkovskis[50] draw attention to the dangers of providing reassurance at the wrong time and in the wrong way. They emphasise that reassurance can be taken to be dismissive and patronising whereas advise providing an explanation of the investigations undertaken and the nature and cause of bodily symptoms – both physical and arising from the effects of anxiety (e.g. hyperventilation), with resulting effects including paraesthesiae and breathlessness, abdominal discomfort or intercostal pain – can be more effective. They caution against repeatedly reassuring patients, especially if that involves simply ordering more and more tests or examining them too often. Such manoeuvres may reinforce abnormal illness behaviours in a manner similar to reinforcing rituals in obsessive-compulsive disorder: while it can lead to a short-term reduction in anxiety, the fear and anxiety will return, along with an increased urge to seek further reassurance. An approach that emphasises collaboration in exploring possible factors relating to the symptoms is more productive and potentially less confrontational. Reassurance should also not be given prematurely – that is, before the results of investigations and evaluations are known or before patients have had a good opportunity to ventilate adequately. Patients given the freedom to fully describe their physical complaints frequently move on to spontaneously talk about psychosocial issues sooner or later. Functional improvement and reduction in distress rather than total symptom relief will be the goal of care with agreement that the symptoms are not 'all in your head' or 'in your imagination', as they may report other health care staff have said to them previously – or they have assumed that that is what they think.

Warwick et al.[51] published a randomised controlled trial of CBT in patients with hypochondriasis. This study had a 16-session programme involving the use of both cognitive and behavioural procedures, and patients were compared with a waiting-list control group. The treatment group did considerably better than the control group. The trial established the efficacy of CBT in patients with hypochondriasis, and subsequent trials have confirmed this.[52] The basic components of CBT are as described for health anxiety generally, mentioned earlier.

There is evidence for pharmacological therapies, specifically fluoxetine, in hypochondriasis. Patients with secondary hypochondriacal symptoms will respond to drug treatment of the primary syndrome; a recent study has shown comparative effects with CBT, but most are effective with both. Fallon compared placebo, CBT, fluoxetine or joint treatment with both fluoxetine and CBT, and results were improvements in the joint treatment group, 47.2%; single active treatment group, 41.8%; and placebo group, 29.6%.[53]

Chronic Pain

Pain is understood as the unpleasant experience that we usually attribute to some physical event. The International Association for the Study of Pain adopted the following definition of pain in 1994:

> 'An unpleasant sensory and emotional experience associated with actual or potential tissue damage or described in terms of such damage.'[54]

The purpose of this definition is to direct attention away from the notion that we cannot define pain in somebody who does not have any physical problem (i.e. tissue damage is not necessary for pain). In the pain literature, a distinction is made between nociception and pain itself, to explain the highly variable and frequently unpredictable relationship between tissue damage and pain. Nociception refers to the activity in the central nervous system (CNS) produced by potentially tissue-damaging stimuli such as thermal, mechanical or chemical agents. Pain is the perception of nociception and is an entirely subjective experience. A wide variety of influences – including psychiatric disorder, cultural influences, childhood experiences and so on – may influence the degree of pain a person develops for a given nociceptive experience. The clinician may judge that the pain perceived by the patient is disproportionate to the extent of the tissue damage in the course of the clinical assessment, but this does not necessarily mean the pain is of psychogenic origin.

Non-nociceptive pain can still arise from a definite organic cause, such as trigeminal neuralgia, or from some organic cause yet to be identified, a psychological cause or some combination of these causes. It is also important to realise that the vast majority of non-nociceptive pains, including those thought to be psychological, are not factitious or due to malingering but are experienced as very real by the patient.

Jones et al.[55] have reviewed the mechanisms involved in nociception processing, which include some important findings from functional MRI (fMRI) and PET scan studies. It is now clear that the stimulus in terms of anticipation of pain is almost as important as the pain stimulus itself, and anticipation can activate most of the central nociceptive system, particularly areas like the medial prefrontal cortex and the anterior cingulate gyrus, with the only difference being the magnitude of the response. This anticipatory response can be blocked by benzodiazepines, which indicates the importance of anxiety as a mediator. Attention alone can also alter nociceptive responses, and the beneficial effects of distraction in pain control are well known. Bantick et al.[56] have shown that psychological distraction will diminish fMRI responses to painful stimuli, particularly in the orbitofrontal cortex, and selective attention probably plays some (as yet undefined) role in the somatic pain syndromes, where pain seems to be associated with very much heightened degrees of distress. Patients with chronic atypical facial pain also show changes on PET scanning. They show an enhanced response in the anterior cingulate cortex and other parts of the central pain systems to thermal stimulation in comparison with controls.[57] Ikkos[54] discusses the emerging understanding which highlights the importance of dopamine-expressing GABAergic neurons in the nucleus accumbens. They suggest that D1 expression is associated with a sense of pleasure and approach behaviour and D2 with a sense of punishment and behavioural inhibition. Regulation of these (i.e. D1 and D2 expression) may be mediated by nigrostriatal and medial frontal striatal pathways within the brain, increasingly understood as a 'predictive' organ. This is reinforced by the understanding that the expectations of patients shape pain (e.g. anxiety levels immediately after an accident and post-traumatic stress at four months can predict persistence), and the single best predictor of response to treatment through individualised pain management programmes was expectation of improvement – not the site, type, intensity, chronicity or other characteristic of the pain itself.[54]

Classification of Pain Disorders

Both DSM-IV and ICD-10 approached the difficult notion of psychological causation in different ways. ICD-10 came down rather more firmly in favour of psychogenic causation – and furthermore, holds out the hope that clinical examination can establish this. Thus, the text states:

> pain occurs in association with emotional conflict or psychosocial problems that are sufficient to allow the conclusion that they are the main causative influences.

DSM-IV was rather more reticent in this respect and does not use the word 'cause' but states:

> psychological factors are judged to have an important role in the onset, severity, exacerbation or maintenance of the pain.[58]

DSM-5 no longer includes a pain-specific mental disorder. DSM-5 somatic symptom disorder with predominant pain replaces DSM-IV pain disorder. It has been argued by Katz et al.[59] that this disorder is not recommended for people with chronic pain because it lacks validity and is overly inclusive and stigmatising. Instead, adjustment disorder remains the most appropriate, accurate and acceptable diagnosis for people who are overly concerned about their pain.

ICD-11 classifies chronic pain under 'Symptoms, signs or clinical findings, not elsewhere classified: Pain: Chronic Primary Pain' but now describes biopsychosocial factors:

> Chronic primary pain is chronic pain in one or more anatomical regions that is characterised by significant emotional distress (anxiety, anger/frustration or depressed mood) or functional disability (interference in daily life activities and reduced participation in social roles). Chronic primary pain is multifactorial: biological, psychological and social factors contribute to the pain syndrome. The diagnosis is appropriate independently of identified biological or psychological contributors unless another diagnosis would better account for the presenting symptoms.

Patients with pain disorders are certainly not a homogeneous group, and many do not have psychiatric illness. Conversion mechanisms are not found to be common in chronic pain syndromes.[60] ICD-11 gives examples of individual pain syndromes such as chronic primary pain, including fibromyalgia (chronic widespread pain), complex regional pain syndrome, chronic primary headache and orofacial pain, chronic primary visceral pain and chronic primary musculoskeletal pain (e.g. following whiplash injuries).

Some psychiatric illness can cause pain as part of the illness – for example, headaches with depression, and as the depression resolves, these headaches sometimes improve as well. Low back pain and neck pain, which are the commonest types of chronic pain, generally have a physical initiating event, and as information increases, these types of pains have more often been found to have continuing physical causes. Bizarre pains can sometimes occur in both depression and schizophrenia, and these may be intractable. They should not be classified as pain disorder but rather as a symptom of the primary psychiatric condition. In addition, those who suffer from a chronic physical illness associated with pain may be liable to develop secondary emotional changes – social withdrawal, situational disorders, reactive depressions and occasionally major depressive disorder.

Severity in ICD-11 is described as no, mild, moderate or severe pain, and distress or pain-related interference with pattern and onset are described as intermittent or persistent with/without overlaid attacks.

NICE[61] guidance for chronic pain describes pain that persists or recurs for more than three months and which is not secondary to an underlying condition that adequately accounts for the pain or its impact. In the UK, the prevalence of chronic pain is uncertain, but it appears to be common, affecting perhaps one-third to one-half of the population. It is not known what proportion of people with chronic pain either need or wish for treatment. The prevalence of chronic primary pain is unknown, but it is estimated to be between 1 per cent and 6 per cent in England.

According to NICE, the experience of pain is always influenced by social factors (including deprivation, isolation, lack of access to services), emotional factors (including anxiety, distress, previous trauma), expectations and beliefs, mental health (including depression and post-traumatic stress disorder) and biological factors.

Management of Pain Disorders

Management should be collaborative, supportive and with shared decision-making. Primary and secondary pain can co-exist. Pain management (at least for severe and persistent pain) is now mainly undertaken in multi-disciplinary pain clinics, including anaesthetists and psychologists. Support from psychiatrists varies, but they will be involved where they are already in contact with patients or on request. Commonly in complex cases, they can assist in the identification and management of comorbid anxiety or depression, personality disorder or bodily distress disorder.

Assessment should follow a standard psychiatric approach, including enquiry about specific items (see Box 6.6.4).

It is important to acknowledge the distress and disturbance that they experience and involve family and friends if possible.

Box 6.6.4 Specific assessment items[61]

- Lifestyle and day-to-day activities, including work and sleep disturbance
- Physical and psychological wellbeing
- Stressful life events, including previous or current physical or emotional trauma
- Current or past history of substance misuse
- Social interaction and relationships
- Difficulties with employment, housing, income and other social concerns
- Views on living well
- The skills that the individual has for managing their pain
- What helps when their pain is difficult to control
- Their understanding of the causes of their pain
- Their expectations of what might happen in the future in relation to their pain
- Their understanding of the outcome of possible treatments

Advice can be provided and a care and support plan developed, including advice on exercise programmes and physical activity for chronic primary pain, acceptance and commitment therapy (ACT), cognitive behavioural therapy (CBT) for pain, and acupuncture (see comprehensive evidence review in NICE guideline[61]). Psychological treatments[62] are informed by a biopsychosocial model of pain as well as psychological research that has identified the central role of the behavioural, cognitive and emotional factors that are believed to contribute to the perpetuation, if not the development, of chronic pain and pain-related disability and emotional distress.[63] ACT is based on the psychological flexibility model; it extends previous forms of CBT and integrates many CBT-related variables into six core therapeutic processes. ACT is a process-based therapy that fosters openness, awareness and engagement through a wide range of methods, including exposure-based and experiential methods, metaphors and values clarification.[64]

Pharmacological usage can be increased in response to the distress expressed by patients. Advice is offered, essentially, that evidence only exists for antidepressants, which can have an effect in absence of depression.

Factitious Disorders

Munchausen Syndrome

Munchausen syndrome was first characterised by Richard Asher[65] in 1951. He described patients who falsified illness and sought medical help in several different locations over long periods of time. Most of Asher's original cases resembled organic emergencies of several types: abdominal (*laparotomophilia migrans*), haemorrhagic (*haemorrhagica histrionica*) and neurological (*neurologica diabolica*). These accounts of illness, 'dramatic and untruthful', were compared to those of the 'Baron of Munchausen', a character created in 1785 by writer Rudolf Erich Raspe and based on German-born baron Hieronymus Karl Friedrich Freiherr von Münchhausen, who was prone to telling fanciful stories. The old eponymous name of Munchausen is still used as it is uniquely memorable, but in modern classifications, the term 'factitious disorders' is now preferred.

In factitious disorders, symptoms are intentionally induced or feigned so that the patient can assume the sick role. Factitious disorders are serious mental disorders in which a person deceives others by purposely getting sick or by inflicting a self injury. Both ICD-11 and DSM-5 have a similar classification:

I. Factitious disorder imposed on self
II. Factitious disorders imposed on another

Factitious Disorder Imposed on the Self

There are no sound epidemiological studies of the phenomenon because of the elusive nature of the subjects, and the vast bulk of the literature on the topic comprises of single case reports, but it is thought that around 1 per cent of admissions to general hospitals may have Munchausen's syndrome.

Although people with factitious disorder have some knowledge, they are usually unaware of why they are doing this, and their purpose is to assume a sick role. In the related syndrome of malingering, patients do have conscious knowledge as to why they are falsifying or exaggerating their symptoms, and this is with a purpose such as to obtain money or to simulate sickness to obtain a hospital bed for the night.

There are multiple types of clinical pictures that simulate known physical disorders, and the bulk of the medical literature on the problem takes the form of single case histories, but this is of little use in obtaining any understanding of the core features of the syndrome. However, Krahn et al.[66] collected 93 cases diagnosed over 21 years from the Mayo Clinic in Minnesota, a clinic renowned for its excellence and high diagnostic standards. Most of the 93 patients were women (72%), and just under half of these women (47%) were women with either a training in or practical experience of health work, and so they had both the knowledge and skill to simulate a physical illness. In most cases in Krahn's series, diagnosis was made through laboratory tests, which were inconsistent with the clinical story. Some examples include cases of recurrent hypoglycaemia, where exogenous insulin was identified; in non-healing wounds, mouthwash was found in the wound; in cases of recurrent haematuria, glass fragments were found in the urine; and in cases of diarrhoea and hypokalaemia, thiazide diuretics were detected in urine toxicology. There are innumerable other ingenious falsifications of known disease pictures in the literature. The diagnosis is rarely made at the initial presentation but rather comes to light later on as the pattern of deception manifests itself. Whether the condition presents to the general physician, psychiatrist or GP, the doctor needs to assume the mantle of a detective and search for inconsistencies, deception and dishonesty.

Hospital wandering (the 'hospital hopper') was more common among men, and the Munchausen subtype is said to consist of pathological wandering from one hospital to another, pathological lying and a presentation with dramatic complaints. Pain was present in 85 per cent of the patients and known substance misuse in around 30 per cent. The authors stressed that an important differential diagnosis is to work out whether the patient is only seeking analgesics or whether the main aim is to assume the sick role. Many of these subjects are prone to gross persistent lying. Bass[67] noted that this is probably the most reliable sign and is almost always associated with factitious disorders. He stated that the following features are associated with this pattern of gross lying, also known as *pseudologia phantastica:*

- It is not determined by situational factors, whereas in malingering, the lying is determined by situational factors
- There may be a kernel of truth
- It is often fantastic, with self-aggrandisement
- It may be compulsive and recurring (i.e. the patient cannot seem to stop lying)
- The underlying motive is attention seeking
- It may be very destructive

Box 6.6.5 Specific categories of evidence used to confirm the diagnosis of factitious disorders

1. Inexplicable laboratory results (e.g. foreign material in a biopsy sample or body fluid)
2. Obvious inconsistency between history and results of physical examinations and tests
3. Patient admission of self-induced illness
4. Records from other institutions showing similar evaluations or contradictory information
5. Criminal conviction for Munchausen by proxy
6. Observed tampering with wounds (e.g. removal of dressing, interfering with drips)
7. Surreptitious use of medications

Criteria used in the study by Krahn et al.[66]

Examination of the patient's case notes from several sources and the demonstration of inconsistencies between the patient's case notes from other hospitals and the current history usually provides the first clue of the pathological lying in a patient with a factitious disorder (see Box 6.6.5). Bass[67] suggests that subtle types of brain damage, particularly to the frontal lobes, may be important and quotes cases where lesions in the prefrontal cortex occurring during infancy resulted in chronic persistent motiveless lying later in life, but the aetiology remains unknown.

Munchausen by Proxy: Factitious Disorder Imposed on Another (FII)

This condition was first described by Meadow[68] in 1977. He reported on two cases: the first where a mother poisoned her child with salt and the second where the mother provoked extensive medical investigations of her child over time. He also observed how pleasant and cooperative the Munchausen mothers were in regard to their children's investigations in contrast to the more normal but highly anxious mothers of truly sick children. The Munchausen mothers seemed to enjoy the attention of the ward staff. Soon afterwards, there was a flood of case reports, and the syndrome was renamed by Bentovim[69] initially as 'induction illness syndrome'. The condition is now known 'factitious illness imposed on another (FII)' in both the ICD-11 and DSM-5.

It is usually diagnosed by paediatricians and is considered to be a form of child abuse; because there have been deaths (mainly through poisoning by salt), it is considered a highly dangerous form of abuse. Gray and Bentovim[69] in 1996 published one the first series of cases and classified them into four groups:

1. Failure to thrive through withholding of food
2. Children who were alleged to be 'highly allergic' to foodstuffs, and parents would shop around in search of doctors who would blame different foodstuffs for the child's condition so that eventually these children were getting insufficient food. Once hospitalised and given ordinary hospital food, these children gained weight, and it became clear the descriptions of food allergy were greatly exaggerated
3. Parents who described worrying symptoms such as fits, repeated cyanotic episodes, passing large amounts of urine or blood in the urine
4. Active administration of substances or active interference with the child's medical treatment (e.g. interfering with wound healing)

Numerous case reports have since appeared in the literature, but it is only in recent years that attempts to put these diverse single case studies together through meta-analysis, and there are two such studies in the literature.

The first of these, by Yates and Bass,[70] included 796 perpetrators – some single case studies and others small series – and the main results were that nearly all abusers were female (97.6%) and the victim's mother (95.6%), and most were married (75.8%). Mean caretaker age at the child's presentation was 27.6 years. Perpetrators were frequently reported to be in health care-related professions (45.6%), to have had obstetric complications (23.5%) or to have histories of childhood maltreatment (30.0%). The most common psychiatric diagnoses recorded were factitious disorder imposed on self (30.9%), personality disorder (18.6%) mainly Cluster B, and depression (14.2%).

The second series, by Abdurrachid,[71] covered 81 case reports with broadly similar results. Again, almost all perpetrators were female (91% female, 1% male and 7% unreported). Twenty-three cases (28%) had a perpetrator with psychiatric diagnosis: factitious disorder imposed on self (10%), depression (9%) and personality disorders (7%). In more than one-third of cases (36%), there was a history of a familial conflict or abuse. Fourteen cases (17%) had perpetrators working in health care. The most common type of falsification was induction (74%); however, 15% of cases had more than one type of falsification. The most common outcomes were separation (37%), no follow-up (22%), imprisonment (14%), death of victim (12%), treatment of the perpetrator (10%), continued living together (4%) and suicide of perpetrator (1%). Recurrence was present in more than three quarters of cases.

Factitious disorder imposed on others can also occur in health care settings whereby the perpetrator is a health care professional who induces signs of illness or kills patients under their care. In May 1993, Beverley Allitt, a state-enrolled nurse then aged 31, was found guilty of the murder of four young children, of the attempted murder of a further three children, and of causing grievous bodily harm with intent on a further six children. All of the victims had been in her care in the paediatric ward of the Grantham and Kesteven General Hospital. Issues around the diagnosis of 'Munchausen's syndrome by proxy' and its distinction from severe personality disorder were played out during her trial and in subsequent legal reviews of her sentencing.[72] In a similar case, in 2006, a nurse Benjamin Green[73] was convicted of two counts of murder and fifteen counts of grievous bodily harm involving injecting patients with drugs to induce respiratory arrests. The trial judge described the psychiatric reports in this latter case as 'not particularly illuminating'. However, having an awareness that these behavioural patterns occur is important for all health care professionals as the potential consequences are devastating.

Diagnosis

The initial diagnosis of the behavioural pattern is now usually made by paediatricians, and their training nowadays includes having knowledge and awareness of this syndrome. GPs and other health professionals are less aware of the condition, possibly because it is so uncommon. Once suspected, a multi-disciplinary approach should be adopted. The initial stage should be a detailed chronology of the case notes of the child incorporating all the previous medical records and a social history of the suspected perpetrator and the family. The medical history of siblings may reveal similar behaviours have occurred before. If suspicion remains high, risks to the child should be assessed. If present, the case should be referred to social service, and the child and perpetrator should be separated. Health care professionals should evaluate the persistence of signs and symptoms in the child in the absence of the caregiver. Psychiatric support should be sought, both for the victim and the perpetrator. In some cases that have been particularly difficult to pin down (e.g. recurrent cyanotic attacks in small children), covert surveillance in hospital has been used to observe the mother-child interaction, and occasionally, mothers have been shown to place a pillow over the baby's head. However, there have been ethical concerns about covert surveillance because of the absence of consent.

An essential criterion in the DSM-5 for the diagnosis of FII is identified deception, which is conscious, carefully planned and well concealed. Different types of falsification are shown in Box 6.6.6.

Box 6.6.6 Types of falsification in FII

False information given to doctor:

1. Withholding information: failing to provide critical information
2. Exaggeration: grossly exaggerating the child's symptoms so he appears to be more ill than he truly is
3. Simulation: altering biological specimens or procedures to yield abnormal results
4. Induction: directly creating symptoms or impairments
5. Coaching: manipulating another to give answers to the clinician that corroborates the claims of the abuser

The distinction between abuse in FII and other situations lies in the intention of the perpetrator. In FII, the falsification provides gains to the perpetrator, unconscious motivations that fulfil their psychological needs of solitude, attachment, family status or love. Whereas in malingering, the gains are more obviously material (e.g. money).

There is now good awareness of the condition amongst paediatricians, but there is less awareness amongst GPs and other health professionals, possibly because it is a relatively uncommon condition in the general population. There have not been any proper epidemiological published studies, but it is estimated to occur in around 0.5 out of 100,00 of the population, and based on published studies, a mortality of 10 per cent is sometimes cited.

Psychopathology

There is no single psychopathology underlying cases of FII, but many perpetrators have had deprived or abusive childhoods and have been victims themselves, and it is thought[74] that they are seeking to draw attention to their distressing inner world consequent on their own earlier trauma and deprivation. *Help seekers* use the factitious illness to communicate their own feelings of distress and usually readily accept psychotherapy. *Doctor addicts* are obsessed with the goal of obtaining medical treatment and are typically more suspicious, antagonistic and paranoid. *Active inducers* cause active and direct harm, are very resistant to therapeutic interventions and are clearly the most dangerous.

Diagnosis is difficult, especially distinguishing fabricated illness from real illness because both can occur together or distinguishing from the simple excessive anxiety in a mother with a sick child. However, the FII mother has a persistence for more and more investigation and diagnostic procedures and hospital admissions, so these ultimately become distressing to the victim. Psychotic or delusional mothers are excluded from FII in DSM-5.

At one time, it was thought that these mothers were criminal and should be dealt with in the criminal justice system. However, today, a therapeutic approach is usually adopted. The focus of therapy should be on the perpetrator taking accountability for their abuse. Psychological treatment such as narrative therapy, trauma-focused cognitive behaviour therapy, dialectical behaviour therapy and family therapy may all have their place. The parents should be involved in drawing up plans for the child and the wellbeing of the family. However, where there is non-engagement and repeated denial of the abuse, there may be little alternative but to proceed to separation, which may be for the long term.

Outcomes are variable. In one series from the Park hospital[75] in Oxford, 17 mothers were treated in the hospital, 10 were reunited with their children and 3 were discharged home without their children. This indicates that some mothers are treatable. In another series,[71] only 4 out of 81 mothers were reunited with their child and, even then, there were recurrences after being reunited, indicating a watchful eye needs to be kept after a successful reunification as a few cases can become chronic and relapsing.

Malingering

The essential feature of malingering is the intentional production of false or grossly exaggerated physical or mental symptoms. It is not included in either DSM-5 or ICD-11 as a mental disorder. In the previous DSM-IV, it was not in the main text, but malingering appeared in their appendix entitled 'conditions for further study', but presumably it did not make the grade because it is not included in the main text of the DSM-5. In the DSM-5, malingering gains mention only as a differential diagnosis to factitious disorder. In ICD -11, it is not classed as a mental disorder but can be found as one of 24 'reasons for contacting health services' and assigned a code QC30.

However, its absence from both official glossaries does not mean that the condition does not exist or that psychiatrists do not encounter it in their daily work. Far from it, malingering is common in a variety of settings. In civilian settings, this is most often to avoid work, obtain financial compensation or to obtain drugs. In forensic settings, this is to avoid the court or diminish a prison sentence, and in a military setting, it is to avoid military service.

Malingering needs to be distinguished from factitious disorder – where there is also simulation of illness to gain the sick role, but the patient is less aware of their motivation – whereas in malingering, it is deliberate and conscious. Because malingering can simulate almost any medical or psychological condition, a unitary description is not feasible, but the fraudulent presentation is usually apparent to specialists in that particular field. In a hysterical conversion state, the motivation is said to be entirely unconscious, and the gain is intra-psychic (e.g. relief from intolerable anxiety). Malingering can be superimposed on genuine illness as well, and this presents a difficult challenge to the physician. By far the most common presentation of feigned illness is in medico-legal practice, particularly in personal injury cases because large sums of money can be obtained through a false but successful claim. It is thought that somewhere between 7–15% of all claims may have a dishonest component.[76] Because it is impossible to sustain the picture of a false injury day and night for seven days a week, insurance companies arrange for 24-hour surveillance of such claims, which is often successful in revealing the obvious dishonesty. Exaggerated claims also occur most commonly in cases of PTSD, work-related stress and the cognitive symptoms of head injuries following road traffic accidents, but specialised psychometry can usually detect the difference from a feigned memory loss from a genuine one.

Conclusion

Patients with bodily distress, hypochondriasis and chronic pain experience symptoms that impair their functioning and cause them significant degrees of discomfort; they also represent a significant public health challenge. Problems in classification/nosology continue to bedevil this area, and these difficulties – along with the use of the language of psychiatric classification, which most patients find unacceptable – continue to lead to the DSM/ICD terms being little-used in day-to-day clinical practice, including liaison psychiatry. Biological, psychological and social factors are relevant to both the aetiology and the maintenance of these syndromes, as well as to their treatment. In recent years, a variety of effective biological and psychosocial approaches to treatment have been developed, and these patients can now be considered as a group for whom medical and psychological approaches should be offered.

References

1. Maggio J, Alluri PR, Paredes-Echeverri S, et al. Briquet syndrome revisited: implications for functional neurological disorder. *Brain Communications* 2020;2(2):fcaa156.
2. Gureje O, Reed GM. Bodily distress disorder in ICD-11: problems and prospects. *World Psychiatry* 2016;15(3):291–2.
3. Mayou R. Is the DSM-5 chapter on somatic symptom disorder any better than DSM-IV somatoform disorder? *British Journal of Psychiatry* 2014;204(6):418–9.
4. Wessely S, Nimnuan C, Sharpe M. Functional somatic syndromes: one or many? *Lancet* 1999;354(9182):936–9.
5. Stone J, Wojcik W, Durrance D, et al. What should we say to patients with symptoms unexplained by disease? The "number needed to offend". *BMJ* 2002;325(7378):1449–50.
6. Budtz-Lilly A, Vestergaard M, Fink P, et al. Patient characteristics and frequency of bodily distress syndrome in primary care: a cross-sectional study. *British Journal of General Practice* 2015;65(638):e617–e23.
7. World Health Organization. *ICD-11: International Classification of Diseases (11th revision).* Geneva: World Health Organization; 2019.
8. Kroenke K, Mangelsdorff AD. Common symptoms in ambulatory care: incidence, evaluation, therapy, and outcome. *American Journal of Medicine* 1989;86(3):262–6.
9. Bass C. Somatoform disorders: aspects of liaison psychiatry. *Current Opinion in Psychiatry* 1993;6(2):210–5.
10. Swartz M, Blazer D, George L, et al. Somatization disorder in a community population. *American Journal of Psychiatry* 1986;143(11):1403–8.
11. Creed F, Henningsen P, Fink P. *Medically Unexplained Symptoms, Somatisation and Bodily Distress: Developing Better Clinical Services.* Cambridge: Cambridge University Press; 2011.
12. Bass C, May S. Chronic multiple functional somatic symptoms. *BMJ* 2002;325(7359):323–6.
13. Lieb R, Pfister H, Mastaler M, et al. Somatoform syndromes and disorders in a representative population sample of adolescents and young adults: prevalence, comorbidity and impairments. *Acta Psychiatrica Scandinavica* 2000;101(3):194–208.
14. Simon G, Gater R, Kisely S, et al. Somatic symptoms of distress: an international primary care study. *Psychosomatic Medicine* 1996;58(5):481–8.
15. Fröhlich C, Jacobi F, Wittchen HU. DSM-IV pain disorder in the general population. *European Archives of Psychiatry and Clinical Neuroscience* 2006;256(3):187–96.
16. olde Hartman TC, Borghuis MS, Lucassen PL, et al. Medically unexplained symptoms, somatisation disorder and hypochondriasis: course and prognosis. A systematic review. *Journal of Psychosomatic Research* 2009;66(5):363–77.
17. National Institute of Health and Care Excellence. *Mental Health, Behavioural and Neurodevelopmental Conditions.* www.nice.org.uk/guidance/conditions-and-diseases/mental-health-behavioural-and-neurodevelopmental-conditions (accessed 2 September 2023).
18. Danish College of General Practitioners. *Clinical Guideline: Functional Disorders.* vejledninger.dsam.dk/media/files/10/clinical-guideline-functional-disorders-dsam-2013.pdf (accessed 24 February 2023).
19. O'Malley PG, Jackson JL, Santoro J, et al. Antidepressant therapy for unexplained symptoms and symptom syndromes. *Journal of Family Practice* 2009;48(12):980–90.
20. Mai F. Somatization disorder: a practical review. *Canadian Journal of Psychiatry* 2004;49(10):652–62.
21. Mayou R, Bass CS. *Treatment of Functional Somatic Symptoms*: Oxford University Press; 1995.
22. Salmon P, Peters S, Stanley I. Patients' perceptions of medical explanations for somatisation disorders: qualitative analysis. *British Medical Journal* 1999;318:372–76.
23. Sharpe M, Protheroe D, House A. Joint working with physicians and surgeons. In: Peveler R, Feldman E, Friedman T (eds.) *Liaison Psychiatry: Planning Services for Specialist Settings.* Berlin: Springer Science & Business; 2000: 195–206.
24. National Collaborating Centre for Mental Health. *The Improving Access to Psychological Therapies (IAPT) Pathway for People with Long-term Physical Health Conditions and Medically Unexplained Symptoms.* www.rcpsych.ac.uk/docs/default-source/improving-care/nccmh/iapt/nccmh-iapt-ltc-full-implementation-guidance.pdf?sfvrsn=de824ea4_4.
25. Liu J, Gill NS, Teodorczuk A, et al. The efficacy of cognitive behavioural therapy in somatoform disorders and medically unexplained physical symptoms: a meta-analysis of randomized controlled trials. *Journal of Affective Disorders* 2019;245:98–112.
26. Kent C, McMillan G. A CBT-based approach to medically unexplained symptoms. *Advances in Psychiatric Treatment* 2009;15(2):146–51.
27. Asmundson G, Taylor S, Cox B. *Health Anxiety: Clinical and Research Perspectives on Hypochondriasis and Related Conditions.* Hoboken, NJ: Wiley; 2001.
28. Veith I. *Hysteria: The History of a Disease.* Chicago: University of Chicago Press; 1965.
29. Kenyon FE. Hypochondriacal states. *British Journal of Psychiatry* 1976;129:1–14.
30. Burton R. *The Anatomy of Melancholy: What it Is, with All the Kinds, Causes, Symptons, Prognostics & Several Cures*

of It. New York: Empire State Book Company; 1924.

31. Boswell J. *On Hypochondria (1777–83).* London: William Kimber and Co; 1951.
32. Willis T. *An Essay of Pathology of the Brain and Nervous Shock in Which Convulsive Diseases Are Treated Of.* London: Dring Lee & Harper; 1684.
33. Cheyne G. *George Cheyne: The English Malady (1733).* Abingdon: Routledge; 1733.
34. Whytt R. Observations on the nature, causes and cure of those disorders which are commonly called nervous, hypochondriac, or hysteric: to which are prefixed some remarks on the sympathy of the nerves. London: Beckett & du Hondt; 1767.
35. Falret J-P. *De l'hypochondrie et du suicide: considérations sur les causes, sur le siège et le traitement de ces maladies, sur les moyens d'en arrêter les progrès et d'en prévenir le développement.* Paris: Croullebois; 1822.
36. Gillespie R. Hypochondria: its definition, nosology and psychopathology. *Guy's Hospital Reports* 1928;78:408–60.
37. Lipowski ZJ. Somatization: the concept and its clinical application. *American Journal of Psychiatry* 1988;145 (11):1358–68.
38. Asmundson G, Taylor S, Cox B. *Health Anxiety: Clinical and Research Perspectives on Hypochondriasis and Related Conditions.* West Sussex, UK: John Wiley & Sons Ltd; 2001.
39. Speckens AE, Spinhoven P, Sloekers PP, et al. A validation study of the Whitely Index, the Illness Attitude Scales, and the Somatosensory Amplification Scale in general medical and general practice patients. *Journal of Psychosomatic Research* 1996;40(1):95–104.
40. Schmidt A, Roosmalen Rv, Beek Jvd, et al. Hypochondriasis in ENT practice. *Clinical Otolaryngology & Allied Sciences* 1993;18(6):508–11.
41. Kirmayer LJ, Robbins JM. Three forms of somatization in primary care: prevalence, co-occurrence, and sociodemographic characteristics. *The Journal of Nervous and Mental Disease* 1991;179(11):647–55.
42. Barsky AJ, Wool C, Barnett MC, et al. Histories of childhood trauma in adult hypochondriacal patients. *The American Journal of Psychiatry* 1994;151(3):397–401.
43. Parker G, Lipscombe P. The relevance of early parental experiences to adult dependency, hypochondriasis and utilization of primary physicians. *British Journal of Medical Psychology* 1980;53(4):355–63.
44. Warwick HMC. Cognitive therapy in the treatment of hypochondriasis. *Advances in Psychiatric Treatment* 1998;4(5):285–91.
45. Fallon BA, Harper KM, Landa A, et al. Personality disorders in hypochondriasis: prevalence and comparison with two anxiety disorders. *Psychosomatics* 2012;53(6):566–74.
46. Kingdon D, Rathod S, Turkington D. Psychotic disorders with hypochondriacal features: delusions of the soma. In: Asmundson G, Taylor S, Cox B (eds.) *Health Anxiety: Clinical and Research Perspectives on Hypochondriasis and Related Conditions.* West Sussex, UK: John Wiley & Sons Ltd; 2001: 324–37.
47. Pilowsky I. Dimensions of hypochondriasis. *British Journal of Psychiatry* 1967;113(494):89–93.
48. Kellner R. *Somatization and Hypochondriasis.* Santa Barbara, CA: Greenwood; 1986.
49. Lucock MP, Morley S. The health anxiety questionnaire. *British Journal of Health Psychology* 1996;1(2):137–50.
50. Clark DM, Salkovskis PM, Hackmann A, et al. Two psychological treatments for hypochondriasis: a randomised controlled trial. *The British Journal of Psychiatry* 1998;173(3):218–25.
51. Warwick HM, Clark DM, Cobb AM, et al. A controlled trial of cognitive-behavioural treatment of hypochondriasis. *British Journal of Psychiatry* 1996;169(2):189–95.
52. Cooper K, Gregory JD, Walker I, et al. Cognitive behaviour therapy for health anxiety: a systematic review and meta-analysis. *Behavioural and Cognitive Psychotherapy* 2017;45(2):110–23.
53. Fallon BA, Ahern DK, Pavlicova M, et al. A randomized controlled trial of medication and cognitive-behavioral therapy for hypochondriasis. *American Journal of Psychiatry* 2017;174 (8):756–64.
54. Ikkos G, Ramanuj PP. Brain and pain: old assumptions and new science about chronic pain. *BJPsych Advances* 2020;26 (3):156–8.
55. Jones A, Kulkarni B, Derbyshire S. Pain mechanisms and their disorders: imaging in clinical neuroscience. *British Medical Bulletin* 2003;65(1):83–93.
56. Bantick SJ, Wise RG, Ploghaus A, et al. Imaging how attention modulates pain in humans using functional MRI. *Brain* 2002;125(2):310–9.
57. Derbyshire S, Jones A, Devani P, et al. Cerebral responses to pain in patients with atypical facial pain measured by positron emission tomography. *Journal of Neurology, Neurosurgery & Psychiatry* 1994;57(10):1166–72.
58. Klein J. Chronic pain, psychopathology, and DSM-5 somatic symptom disorder. *Canadian Journal of Psychiatry* 2015;60 (11):528.
59. Katz J, Rosenbloom BN, Fashler S. Chronic pain, psychopathology, and DSM-5 somatic symptom disorder. *The Canadian Journal of Psychiatry* 2015;60 (4):160–67.
60. Merskey H. Shellshock. In: Berrios GE, Freeman HL (eds.) *150 Years of British Psychiatry, 1841–1991.* London: Gaskell; 1991: 245.
61. National Institute for Health and Care Excellence. *Chronic Pain (Primary and Secondary) in Over 16s: Assessment of All Chronic Pain and Management of Chronic Primary Pain.* www.nice.org .uk/guidance/NG193 (accessed 7 February 2023).
62. Williams ACC, Fisher E, Hearn L, et al. Psychological therapies for the management of chronic pain (excluding headache) in adults. *Cochrane Database of Systematic Reviews* 2020;8:CD007407.
63. Kerns RD, Sellinger J, Goodin BR. Psychological treatment of chronic pain. *Annual Review of Clinical Psychology* 2011;7:411-34.
64. Feliu-Soler A, Montesinos F, Gutiérrez-Martínez O, et al. Current status of acceptance and commitment therapy for chronic pain: a narrative review. *Journal of Pain Research* 2018;11:2145–59.
65. Asher R. Münchhausen syndrome. *Lancet* 1951;1(6650):339–41.
66. Krahn LE, Li H, O'Connor MK. Patients who strive to be ill: factitious disorder with physical symptoms. *American Journal of Psychiatry* 2003;160(6):1163–8.

67. Bass C, Halligan PW. Illness related deception: social or psychiatric problem? *Journal of the Royal Society of Medicine* 2007;100(2):81–4.

68. Meadow R. Munchausen syndrome by proxy. The hinterland of child abuse. *The Lancet* 1977;310(8033):343–5.

69. Gray J, Bentovim A. Illness induction syndrome: paper I—a series of 41 children from 37 families identified at The Great Ormond Street Hospital for Children NHS Trust. *Child Abuse & Neglect* 1996;20(8):655–73.

70. Yates G, Bass C. The perpetrators of medical child abuse (Munchausen Syndrome by Proxy) – A systematic review of 796 cases. *Child Abuse & Neglect* 2017;72:45–53.

71. Abdurrachid N, Marques JG. Munchausen syndrome by proxy (MSBP): a review regarding perpetrators of factitious disorder imposed on another (FDIA). *CNS Spectrums* 2022;27(1): 16–26.

72. England and Wales High Court (Queen's Bench Division). *Decisions.* Allitt, Re [2007] EWHC 2845 (QB) (6 December 2007) www.bailii.org/ (accessed 23rd March 2023).

73. Oxford Mail. *Killer Nurse Jailed for at Least 30 Years.* www.oxfordmail.co.uk/news/757898.killer-nurse-jailed-least-30-years/ (accessed 7 March 2023).

74. Schreier HA, Libow JA. Munchausen syndrome by proxy: diagnosis and prevalence. *American Journal of Orthopsychiatry* 1993;63(2):318–21.

75. Berg B, Jones DP. Outcome of psychiatric intervention in factitious illness by proxy (Munchausen's syndrome by proxy). *Archives of Disease in Childhood* 1999;81 (6):465–72.

76. Rogers R, Sewell KW, Goldstein AM. Explanatory models of malingering: a prototypical analysis. *Law and Human Behavior* 1994;18(5):543–52.

Chapter

7.1 Clinical Features and Implications of New Classification of Personality Disorders

Peter Tyrer

Personality disorder represents a diagnosis very different from others in psychiatry. This is because it describes a long-standing integral part of a person, not just an affliction that has happened. Because of the sensitivity of ascribing a core part of a person's being to the impersonality of a diagnostic term, the subject has been widely stigmatised. However, the condition – however named – is very common and affects one-tenth of the population. In this chapter, the clinical features of personality disorder identified in the new ICD-11 severity classification are described and their value illustrated. A fuller description of the ICD-11 classification can be found in another publication.[1]

There are five levels of diagnosis of personality disorder – including the subsyndromal form, personality difficulty, which is by far the most common. The diagnosis of borderline personality disorder is the most used in practice, but it is a heterogeneous term that overlaps with almost every other disorder in psychiatry. All personality disorders have approximately equal genetic and environmental precursors, and the involvement of childhood adverse experiences and trauma is unfortunately true for this as for all psychiatric disorders.

The two core features of all personality disorders are persistent problems in interpersonal social functioning and distorted self-perception. These are relatively easy to identify but should be examined independently of any current mental state disorder, as temporary disturbance in personality functioning can occur in all mental illness.

Introduction

The term 'personality disorder' has become widely criticised and, to a large extent, stigmatised in recent years, and this impression has developed to a greater extent than other diagnoses. This is unfair because personality and personality disorder are all on the same spectrum, one that extends from having no personality problems at one extreme to severe personality disorder at the other. Everybody is on this spectrum somewhere. Those that have no personality problems at all and those at the opposite end with severe personality disorder are both by definition very rare.

In this chapter, I will give the essentials of the subject as it stands at present, but the reader must appreciate that a great deal of change is taking place, and I will try and minimise confusion as much as possible. Because there is a substantial minority of people who would like to abolish the diagnosis of personality disorder, I also include some sections at the end of the chapter to help the practitioner in dealing with criticisms of the use of the term, whether or not it is being used appropriately.

The Core Features of Personality Disorder

The assessment of personality disorder is considered quite a complex process, and most of the instruments that are used to assess it are longer than almost all other assessments in psychiatry. It has to be granted that it is virtually impossible to make a full assessment of someone's personality by any instrument known to man, and the best descriptions are found in novels rather than scientific tomes. There is also a tendency in assessments to examine each of the different areas of function in personality disorder as though they were completely separate from each other. This particularly applies to the present classification system (ICD-10, DSM-IV and DSM-5), where textbooks devote chapters to each of the categories of personality disorder as though they stand alone.[2, 3]

However, the two features that are common to every person manifesting the features of personality disorder are interpersonal social dysfunction and a lack of self-awareness, best expressed as a lack of mutual understanding. The second of these is difficult to define. Neither of these is difficult to detect. Here are some examples: the person who gratuitously picks an argument in order to indulge in profanity, the elderly man who abuses all his carers indiscriminately, the 'know all' who interrupts and talks over others, the one who persists in an argument by refusing to give way over a trivial tiny point, and the isolated relative who turns up at a funeral wearing a yellow shirt and jeans and does not realise this is not appropriate dress. These are not necessarily indicative of personality disorder but, in some cases, can be construed as a personality difficulty when they offend.

The definition of personality disorder in ICD-11 is not very different from that in ICD-10 and, as it is still going to be the defining language for diagnosis, it is worth looking at it more closely for the clues to its detection:

'Personality disorder is characterised by problems in functioning of aspects of the self (e.g. identity, self-worth, accuracy of self-view, self-direction), and/or interpersonal dysfunction (e.g. ability to develop and maintain close and mutually satisfying relationships, ability to understand others' perspectives and to manage conflict in relationships) that have persisted over an extended period of time (e.g. 2 years or more). The disturbance is manifest in patterns of cognition, emotional experience, emotional expression and behaviour that are maladaptive (e.g. inflexible or poorly regulated) and is manifest across a range of personal and social situations (i.e. is not limited to specific relationships or social roles). The patterns of behaviour characterising the disturbance are not developmentally appropriate and cannot be explained primarily by social or cultural factors, including socio-political conflict, in personal, family, social, educational, occupational or other important areas of functioning.'[4]

Examination of these core features has often been neglected in the past. The descriptions of the individual categories are so enticing, they are immediately noticed, and whether or not the core features are present is often over-looked.

Problems in Self-Function

In the definition earlier, jargon and confusion rule the first sentence. Identity disturbance is a complex concept; I am an identical twin and have always had it. It may be present in personality disorder but in only a minority, mainly in the group commonly described as borderline or emotionally unstable. However, many with highly obsessional, dissocial (psychopathic) and detached (schizoid) disorders have very firm ideas about their identities – not ones we would necessarily share but certainly not fluctuating.

Self-worth also varies among different people with personality disorder. For those with persistent negative thinking, it is a common feature but equally so in those with depression. It also fluctuates greatly with mood disturbance. Also, some with personality disorder are very impressed by their self-worth. Certain famous public figures come to mind in whom intimations of personality disorder have never been far away. 'Accuracy of self-view' is clumsily expressed, but it is a better and more general concept for the group that equates to some extent with mutual understanding. If you do not understand yourself, you do not understand others. However, lack of self-awareness with respect to personality is a better way of putting it. It is when you get a totally blank expression in response to explaining why somebody else is distressed by something that has been said or done that you realise that this valuable check on behaviour is wanting.

Absence of self-direction is often an important part of personality malfunction but, again, is found in many other conditions. It is frequent in common mood disorders and in the schizophreniform conditions, where it joins up with negative symptoms.

So, for the busy clinician, an in-depth analysis of self-function is not going to be possible in assessing those with personality disorder. It is the interpersonal dysfunction that is much more prominent. However, the inability of those with personality problems to understand others (often expressed as a 'failure to read other people') is part of the picture and links very closely with social dysfunction.

Interpersonal Dysfunction

The inability to make mutually satisfying relationships is really the core feature of all personality disorder. It is always a good idea in the first clinical interview to leave personality assessment to the end. By doing this, so many of the elements of interpersonal dysfunction will have become apparent in the history of the problem and the personal and family history. A chequered employment history with a failure to make full use of talents, a succession of partners in relationships ending in disaster, or an absence of any meaningful relationships at all, they all point towards a diagnosis of personality disorder. The descriptions from patients are often amplified by anger, paranoia and blaming of others, but it does not take much perspicacity to realise the prime mover in these episodes is the patient, not the other parties.

Maladaptive Patterns of Cognition, Emotional Experience, Emotional Expression and Behaviour

These are not easy elements to identify. The key word is 'maladaptive'; the expression of emotions – whether highly charged or under-played – can be highly appropriate and adaptive. If it is imposed into the wrong situation, it can create great distress and disturbance. Emotionally inappropriate behaviour – sometimes, rather unfairly, called emotional incontinence – is a prominent feature of the borderline personality disorder group. Because it is so focused on emotional reaction, emotionally inappropriate behaviour is sometimes felt to be external to the central personality disorder construct and should be looked at independently.[5]

Persistence over an Extended Period of Time (Two Years or More)

This is a key element in diagnosis, but it should not be taken too literally. In the past, definitions of personality disorder have usually added terms such as 'ingrained', 'pervasive' and 'persistent' that have led to the conclusion that personality disorder is immutable, contributing greatly to the stigma attached to the condition. Personality is more or less immutable, although it becomes more settled and stable with increasing age, but personality disorder is not. It is the least stable of all diagnoses in clinical practice, with less than 10 per cent of patients receiving a specific personality diagnosis on repeat admissions compared with 47 per cent for schizophrenia.[6] In cohort studies, personality disorder has been found to change greatly over time.[7,8]

You may find comments on social media, where the diagnosis of personality disorder continues to be assaulted as though it was stigma on stilts, along the lines of 'if personality is stable and personality disorder unstable, the diagnosis is nonsense?' The reason is simple; maladaptive behaviour in one setting may be adaptive in another, so while the personality persists, the disorder disappears, at least for a time.

There is also concern, particularly in child and adolescent psychiatry, that an early diagnosis of personality disorder may blot subsequent life chances and so create unnecessary hardship. Although the incidence ('incidence' chosen deliberately here instead of 'prevalence') of personality disorder in younger people is higher than in older people,[9] however, there is now good research showing that personality disorder can be reliably diagnosed and managed in adolescence.

It also has to be emphasised that many other psychiatric disorders persist for years and can masquerade as personality disorders, so persistence should not be relied upon too strongly in making the diagnosis. The key difference in the definition of personality disorder in ICD-11 compared with ICD-10 is the allowance to diagnose the condition at any age, provided the features have been present for at least two years. This is likely to lead to an increase in the prevalence of personality disorders, but it is still likely to be less than one or two per cent.[10]

Substantial Distress or Significant Impairment in Functioning

This is a necessary requirement to the diagnosis. It emphasises that even if you have all the other features of personality disorder and are highly successful – either as a consequence of your personality or independently of it – then the diagnosis should not be made. This may seem odd but, in practice, is rarely a problem in diagnosis. People can be highly successful but succeed because they exploit and diminish others, and so 'substantial distress' certainly applies in these instances.

It is also fair to say that, in clinical practice, psychiatrists will seldom come across patients in this world who are seeking treatment for their personality disorder, unless they are within the emotionally unstable group.

When Should Personality Disorder Be Diagnosed?

Isolated examples of maladaptive behaviour do not constitute personality disturbance, but if they are repeated often in similar form over a long period, then personality disorder should seriously be considered. At a psychiatric interview, many of these behaviours will become apparent, and irritation will tend to turn the interviewer towards the diagnosis. 'Personality disorder: the patients psychiatrists dislike', wrote Lewis and Appleby in 1988;[11] Chartonas et al.[12] repeated this conclusion 30 years later. People with personality disorder can be unlikeable; because they fail to tune into you, you cannot tune into them, and if they annoy you – irrespective of their true diagnosis – a diagnosis of personality disorder will satisfy your displeasure. So, the cycle is established: those with personality disorder feel misunderstood and wrongly conclude that abolishing the diagnosis will solve their problems.

Other Clinical Features of Personality Disorder: The Borderline Controversy

Presentation

Most of those diagnosed with personality disorder in current practice have emotionally unstable or borderline personality disorder. This condition only accounts for around 15 per cent of all personality disorders according to epidemiological data (see later). So why is this the condition most identified in clinical practice? It is because this group is the only one that seeks treatment, often urgently, whereas the others may attend for help with other conditions but do not ask to have their personality problems addressed. Personality disorders can be separated into Type R (treatment resisting) and Type S (treatment seeking) groups;[13] borderline is one of the few Type S disorders.[14]

So, even though borderline accounts for such a small proportion of identifiable personality disorders, it had led to more than 90 per cent of papers and books on treatment, and almost all the pathways for personality disorder are essentially focused on this group. You might say there is nothing wrong with this; services have to be sensitive to who presents; services cannot ignore them. However, if we ignore all the other personality disorders, we do their sufferers a disservice.

Is the Borderline Condition a Personality Disorder?

All diagnoses are temporary concepts, and so none can be regarded as immutable. However, there are important differences between borderline and all other personality disorders. Over the course of the last hundred years, it has become increasingly clear that personality depends on long-lasting traits that allow personality structures to remain constant over a long period. Many of these traits have been moulded by evolutionary necessity;[15] borderline symptoms have never had an evolutionary lift.

The symptoms – or operational criteria as DSM-5 has it – are a mixture of behaviours, moods and patterns, as well as also interpersonal dysfunction, but they are not traits.[4] What is more, the symptoms cover the whole of psychiatry (Table 7.1.1). If we accept that all personality disorders require both difficulties in interpersonal relationships and poor self-awareness, then borderline clearly does not apply, as those with the condition are usually all too well aware of their impact on others – often in retrospect – and suffer greatly as a consequence.

The defenders of the diagnosis can point to the following:

- The wide use of the diagnosis shows that practitioners recognise it frequently in the patients they see
- Most of the successful treatments of personality disorder are for the borderline condition
- A considerable amount of increased understanding has come about in neuropsychology and developmental psychology through study of borderline personality disorder

Table 7.1.1 The heterogeneity of borderline personality disorder

Borderline personality feature	Overlapping mental disorder(s)
Unstable relationships	The only one that is linked to personality disorder
Uncertain identity	Dissociative identity disorder
Rapid swings of mood	Bipolar disorder
Impulsive behaviour	Substance misuse
Fear of abandonment	Anxiety disorders
Frequent self harm	Depressive disorders
Chronic emptiness	Depressive disorders
Episodes of anger	Substance misuse, impulse control disorders
Transient dissociative symptoms	Dissociative disorders
Psychotic symptoms	Schizophrenia and related disorders

- When services have been set up in different countries of the world, they have almost all been concerned with the management of borderline personality disorder

You could say that this information is evidence-based, but it is not. If you carried out a similar review about the use of leeches in the eighteenth century, all four of these criteria would apply. At that time, there were even sophisticated texts about the relative success of different leeches in bloodletting.

If Borderline Is Not a Personality Disorder, Where Does It Belong?

Every careful study of borderline personality shows that emotional instability is a core part of the syndrome. Indeed, Marsha Linehan, the best-known researcher in the subject, has always felt it is best looked at as a disorder of emotional dysregulation. It is naturally unstable, and by being so, it should be denied inclusion among the personality disorders when it is present alone. However, because it is so heterogeneous, it overlaps with other personality disorders. A clinical diagnosis of borderline personality disorder can include any of the following: emotional dysregulation alone; emotional dysregulation with personality disorder (following the ICD-11 definition); emotional dysregulation with personality disorder and severe risk to self or others (possibly leading to compulsory detention); and emotional dysregulation with personality disorder and comorbid mood, substance misuse and eating disorders. This is not a satisfactory form of classification.

A good diagnosis has to be consistent in form and over time. Neither of these is true of the borderline condition. As well as being a potpourri of symptoms, feelings and behaviour, the clinical features show great variation in them over time. To take one example, Zanarini and her colleagues[16] found that, 10 years after an original diagnosis of borderline personality disorder, self harm and impulsive behaviour resolved quickly, feelings of emptiness and general depression persisted longer, and fear of abandonment and anxious mood hardly moved at all. It is perhaps not surprising, therefore, that the main positive effects of treatment discussed in the next chapter of this book are shown for self harm and impulsive behaviour.

Emotional dysregulation disorder could well be a diagnosis within the mood disorders, but this is outside the scope of this chapter and is not included in ICD-11 or DSM-5.

The Dangers of Borderline Personality Disorder

One of the other problems with borderline symptoms is that they are infectious. Readers will be aware of adolescents in online chat rooms developing suicide pacts and other self-harming strategies or of celebrities with inner turmoil and are then encouraged to disclose all their feelings. Those that have symptoms are also encouraged to write about their symptoms, and the pattern of their ups and downs becomes a morbidly fascinating subject. In other countries, where the more important preoccupations are to get enough food to support your family and deal with external threat, borderline personality disorder does not seem to exist.

An important subject for those who have emotional dysregulation is validation, first given emphasis by Marsha Linehan.[17] Validation of a person's feelings represents an acceptance that 'their responses make sense and are understandable' and that 'they are taken seriously and not discounted or trivialised'.[18] This is absolutely correct, but it must not be extended to apply to disagreements over care when a practitioner makes a recommendation that differs from that of the patient. Claiming in this circumstance that feelings have been invalidated is untrue, and there is no place for power politics in resolving it. Practitioners should follow the advice of Newton-Howes,[19] who advocates 'cautious paternalism' in resolving it.

Trauma and Personality Disorder

Many authorities now regard personality disorder as a condition that has been created by trauma and, therefore, invalidates the notion of personality disorder as a diagnosis. It is perfectly true that many patients with personality disorder have had major traumatic episodes in their lives, but a majority do not have significant adversities, particularly in early life which so many regard as the important stage of development for the negative effects of adversity. When careful reviews have been carried out into the incidence of trauma in patients with personality disorder, the results do not show that borderline personality disorder has a directly specific association with trauma. This is because many other psychiatric disorders have higher rates of past childhood trauma than those without psychiatric illness[20] and, across the world, childhood neglect and adversity accounts for nearly 30 per cent of all psychiatric disorders.[21] Personality disorder – particularly borderline – are increasingly treated within 'trauma-informed services', but these need to apply to all disorders when childhood neglect is identified.

The new ICD-11 classification has taken account of this issue in creating a new diagnosis of complex PTSD. For this diagnosis, individuals must fulfil the criteria for PTSD but also have symptoms of disturbances in self-organisation, which include emotional dysregulation, negative self-concept and interpersonal difficulties. The latter disturbances obviously have some overlap with borderline personality disorder – and this has been shown in studies[22,23] – but to some extent, they can be distinguished from borderline personality disorder.[23] This shows that the emergence of complex PTSD may have a reasonably distinct symptom profile.

Trauma-informed care is likely to be reserved for those with complex PTSD, whether or not they have personality disorder also.

Assessment of Personality Disorder by Self-Rating

For those who doubt their ability to assess personality disorder – or are concerned that the apparent personality disturbance is equivocal as it could be linked to mental state – the possibility of giving questionnaires can be considered. The simplest of these is the Standardised Assessment of Personality Abbreviated Scale (SAPAS),[24] which is readily available. A score of four on the scale suggests a person may have personality disorder. The evidence that interpersonal social dysfunction is probably the most important element of personality disorder is illustrated by the structure of a five-item scale derived from the Social Functioning Questionnaire[25] (see the end of the chapter). A score of four or more on the scale gives a strong indication that the person has a personality disorder. The advantage of the scale is it can be given without any mention of personality if the assessor is worried about bringing this term up in the course of an interview.

More recently there have been new instruments designed to assess ICD-11 personality disorder, both in terms of severity[26] and personality domains[27] (as described later). For those interested in the DSM-5 Alternative Model (see later), this is also examining personality disorder in terms of severity in an equivalent way.[28]

The Diagnosis of Personality Disorder

Until recently, the diagnosis of personality disorder was made in two ways. The first was introduced in DSM-III to give a separate axis to the classification of personality dysfunction, Axis II. One of the reasons for providing a second axis of classification was to give more attention to a group of conditions that might otherwise be forgotten. Once Axis II had been decided, a categorical diagnosis was made of 10–13 disorders (some, like passive-aggressive and masochistic) have been removed over the years.

However, a serious problem arose in the submission of the Task Force for the Revision of Personality Disorders in advance of DSM-5 in 2013. The American Psychiatric Association turned down a suggested 'hybrid model' of combined categorical and dimensional disorders and reverted to the previous descriptions in DSM-IV. However, the hybrid system kept going and became the Alternative Model for Personality Disorders (AMPD), and this is now used more often than DSM-IV, at least among the research community (see comparisons in Table 7.1.2).

In DSM-5, the separate axis for personality disorder (Axis II) was scrapped, and this led to some concern.[29] Personality disorders are not diagnosed very often, and there was a fear that they might be even less noticed. The ICD-11 revision group (2010–2017) recommended the removal of all categorical diagnoses in favour of a single dimension of severity with anchor points for different levels (Figure 7.1.1) with only one category, borderline, being added as a qualifying 'pattern descriptor'.[30]

Table 7.1.2 Current and immediate past classifications of personality disorder

DSM-IV-TR	ICD-10	AMPD	ICD-11
Borderline	Emotionally unstable, including borderline and impulsive	Borderline	No categories included – diagnosis made by severity of disorder with domain trait qualifiers (see Figure 7.1.1) but with the option of adding borderline as a pattern descriptor, if preferred
Antisocial	Dissocial	Antisocial	
Narcissistic	(Never included)	Narcissistic	
Histrionic	Histrionic		
Avoidant	Anxious	Avoidant	
Dependent	Dependent		
Schizoid	Schizoid	Schizotypal	
Schizotypal			
Obsessive-compulsive	Anankastic	Obsessive-compulsive	
No good equivalents in any classification			

DSM = Diagnostic and Statistical Manual of Mental Disorders. ICD = International Classification of Diseases. AMPD = Alternative Model for Personality Disorders.

	Personality difficulty	Mild personality disorder	Moderate personality disorder	Severe personality disorder
No evidence of dysfunction	Dysfunction in discrete settings	Persistent dysfunction but integrated life present	More severe problems with risk to self/others	Very severe breakdown of function

Figure 7.1.1 Spectrum of severity for personality disturbances.

Reasons for the ICD-11 Classification

Why has there been such a radical change in the classification of personality disorders? There are two main reasons. The first is the unsatisfactory nature of the existing classifications. The second is the development of greater stigma about these types of disorder, shown both by the general population and all health professionals, including psychiatrists. Personality disorder is avoided and so seldom diagnosed. National statistics suggest that personality disorder is diagnosed in only 1 to 3% of all psychiatric patients, but epidemiological data suggested 10% of the population[31] and 30 to 80% of all psychiatric patients (depending on the type of service) have this disorder.[14,32,33]

Although there are 10 different diagnostic categories in DSM-IV and ICD-10, only two of them are used in practice – antisocial (dissocial) and borderline personality (emotionally unstable) disorders. The consequence has been that personality disorder has been pushed further and further towards the edges of psychiatry and become the province of specialist workers in the field.

When the ICD-11 work group for the revision of personality disorders were set up by the World Health Organization, it was recognised that what was needed was a simple way of diagnosing personality disturbance that is socially inclusive rather than stigmatising, which could be used widely by all practitioners. This has been achieved by a single spectrum of severity (Figure 7.1.1).

The spectrum of personality disorder is shown in the figure. As mentioned earlier, most people have at least some degree of personality problems; it is difficult to attach stigma to something we all have. The epidemiological data has been collected in good faith – and without bias – so we have to accept these data as the best available, assuming we have the thresholds right. This has only recently been recognised in classification systems. One of the reasons why the unattractive labels such as histrionic, narcissistic, antisocial, borderline and emotionally unstable have become so stigmatised is that they place people into cardboard stereotypes. Very few people can pile all their personality characteristics into one diagnostic box; they overflow, except for the more extreme disorders. The diagnosis that has persisted more than any other is the borderline category, which has even squeezed into the ICD-11 classification as a 'pattern specifier' – but not as a diagnosis, as it is equivalent to a domain trait.[30] Many will wish to continue using the terms 'emotionally unstable' and 'borderline', and they are at liberty to do so, but the ICD-11 classifcation has a much better way of defining this group of disorders than the borderline specifier. Those with traits in the negative affective and dininhibited domains are very different from those in the negative affective and dissocial ones, and those with negative affective, dissocial and disinhibited features are probably more difficulty to treat than others. Giving all equivalence is not helpful.

These categories are going to disappear in the new classification of personality disorder (ICD-11), which was introduced formally in January 2022. Once ICD-11 is established, personality disorder will only be diagnosed according to the spectrum above. For clinical purposes, only mild, moderate and severe personality disorder will qualify as actual personality disorders. The condition called personality difficulty is much more common but is not a formal personality disorder.

The diagnosis of personality disorder is qualified by what are called trait domains. These are not diagnoses but descriptive additions to the level of personality disorder. There are five of them – negative affectivity (a complex set of syllables describing tendencies towards anxiety, depression and anger), detachment (the tendency to avoid close relationships), disinhibition (the tendency to act on impulse and regret it afterwards), dissociality (or antisocial in United States, describing aggression, lack of empathy and selfish behaviour) and anankastia (a word that will be unfamiliar to many but which describes excessive concern over detail and order, as well as perfectionism). One or more of these can be added to the severity of the personality disorder to explain the condition in more detail.

What Is the Difference between Personality Difficulty, Mild and More Severe Personality Disorders?

People with personality problems differ only in the severity of their symptoms and behaviour. The two core components of all personality disorders are difficulties in interpersonal relationships and a lack of self-understanding of why other people behave the way they do. In the case of personality difficulty, these are only shown in certain situations and do not apply to other ones. So, for example, a person who gets on with most people may be antagonistic towards others that are seen as authority figures. In interviews and other situations with dominant figures, they show this antagonism, but it is not present in other settings at all. This explains why personality difficulty is so common and why most people avoid the situations when these adverse personality features might be shown.

People who cross the threshold into full personality disorder differ in that those who have mild features can still maintain fairly good relationships with many people but are often held back in their social and occupational roles. In those with moderate personality disorder, these problems are more severe, only a few relationships are maintained, and occupational and social performance is impaired. As personality disorder gets more severe, there is an increasing risk of harm to self or others, and – in the case of very severe personality disorder – this risk is often sufficient to place people in institutional settings to protect others.

What Is the Cause of Personality Disorder and When Does It Develop?

Most research has established that the effects of genetics and those of environment are roughly equal in determining personality disorder,[34] including borderline personality disorder,[35] but of course, these can also interact. There are no specific genes associated with personality disorder, and exactly how it is transmitted is not known. More is known about environmental causes and triggers. Abuse in any form, physical aggression, sexual abuse and neglect are all potential triggers for subsequent personality disorder. Most of these occur early in life. Whether or not the cause is environmental or genetic, the features of personality disorder are often present in late childhood or early adolescence. These include truancy, refusal to comply with instructions (oppositional behaviour), impulsive behaviour, drug misuse and excessive nervousness. These, of course, overlap with other childhood disorders and should not automatically be regarded as personality problems. However, all parents and caregivers should be aware that these features could be the precursors of personality disturbance later in life. This is one of the points in favour of diagnosing personality disorder in youth.

Why Is It Important to Recognise Personality Disorder at All Levels of Severity?

If personality disorder has an impact on the outcome of other mental disorders, it is important for it to be recognised as early as possible. Unfortunately, this is not normally the case. One of the reasons why the term 'personality disorder' has been stigmatised is that the diagnosis is far too often made when a person has not responded to a treatment to which they, in the mind of the therapist, should have responded. It is certainly true that if a personality disorder is present at the same time as a mental disorder, there is generally a worse outcome,[36–39] but this may be because the personality aspects are seldom given attention. It is true that there are a number of studies that do not demonstrate this. Many of these studies are dependent on the method in which personality disorder has been assessed, but the results of the largest systematic reviews and meta-analyses are quite clear. There are obviously going to be exceptions; a recent one concerns cognitive behavioural therapy in health anxiety in which much better response was shown in those with personality disorder, particularly if the personality problems were more severe.[40]

What Is the Course of Personality Disorder?

One of the myths about personality disorder that contributes to stigma is that, once it has been diagnosed, it is a condition that will stay with you for life. This is completely untrue. Personality disorder changes dramatically over time irrespective of treatment, sometimes for the better, sometimes for the worse.[8,41,42] Because, until recently, there have been very few treatments available for personality problems, we do not know if successful treatment in the short term is extended to the long term. It used to be thought that personality disorder improved in older age – the word often used is mellowed – but this has not been confirmed. A great deal depends on whether the older person is adapted to the environment in which they are placed, and this will become an increasing issue as the population gets steadily older.

Criticisms of Personality Disorder

In the last part of this chapter, I would like to deal with various shibboleths that come up repeatedly when personality disorder is mentioned. Many of these arise from misconceptions that promulgate stigma. Some of these are held by some senior members of the profession, and their views might have been partly sustained by the unsatisfactory diagnostic system that has existed until the present.

Personality Disorder as a Diagnosis Is Redundant; I Never Use It

It is perfectly possible to practise as a good psychiatrist without ever using the term 'personality disorder'. However, this does not mean the term is not recognised. It is kept in the background of your mind as a samizdat subject that can only be talked about in code. Some term has to be used when you need to communicate with another health professional, and even then, the words 'personality difficulty' may leak out. Increasingly, the term 'complex emotional needs' is being used to avoid the words many of us would like to disappear. This is nonsense. We all have complex emotional needs and, unless these words are formally defined in a different way, they just become a form of fireside chat. These particular words are often used in those with emotionally unstable borderline personality disorder, but this ignores the much bigger proportion of those with personality disorders who do not recognise 'complex emotional needs' as anything more than psychobabble.

The big advantage of the ICD-11 is that by embracing the spectrum of personality disturbance, there is no reason to avoid the terminology. Even if you are completely put off by the term, personality disorder, you can still use wording such as 'to the right of the personality spectrum' when talking to those people who would be regarded as having a personality disorder.

Personality Disorder Is a Term Used to Express Your Dislike of a Patient

This is unfortunately still remarkably extant. The gap between Lewis and Appleby in 1988[11] and Chartonas et al.[12] in 2017 is nearly 30 years, but they express the same sentiment. This attitude is reflective of cognitive dissonance, the natural tendency to avoid conflicting beliefs. Psychiatrists are trained to help people with mental illness and receive a boost when praised or seemingly understood. When a patient does not respond in kind, or retaliates with fire and brimstone, it is easy to rationalise and conclude that they have a condition that is untreatable, and then the patient can be dismissed from care without any misgivings.

If all psychiatrists made an assessment of personality status at first interview, this particular trap could be avoided.

Personality Disorder Is Grossly Overdiagnosed; It Is Rare

When personality disorder is assessed using accepted instruments by epidemiological investigators who have no prior opinions or consistent bias, around one in ten of the population has a personality disorder, with a lower proportion in low-income countries.[43]

As Personality Disorder Is Untreatable, It Is Best Ignored

Although the next chapter in this book shows that this is not true, this shibboleth is widely followed. It is true that for milder degrees of personality dysfunction, we have very little data to go on as these conditions have been largely unrecognised. However, we do know some useful facts. In particular, other mental disorders have a different trajectory when personality disorder is also present, and this should influence treatment. The points relevant to the practising psychiatrist are:

Relapse of mood disorders is more frequent when significant personality disorder is present.[44,45]

Patients with personality disorder treated with anti-anxiety drugs are more likely to get withdrawal symptoms when they try to stop the drug, even if they withdraw slowly.[1,46,47]

The benefits of psychological treatment for mental state disorders are more likely to persist after treatment is concluded than if treated with drug therapies.[40,48,49]

Short Social Functioning Questionnaire (SSFQ)

Please look at the statements below and tick the reply that comes closest to how you have been generally:

Statement	Reply	Score
1. I complete my tasks at work and home satisfactorily.	Most of the time	0
	Quite often	1
	Sometimes	2
	Not at all	3
2. I find my tasks at work and at home very stressful.	Most of the time	3
	Quite often	2
	Sometimes	1
	Not at all	0
3. I have difficulties in getting and keeping close relationships.	Severe difficulties	3
	Some problems	2
	Occasional problems	1
	No problems at all	0
4. I feel lonely and isolated from other people.	Almost all the time	3
	Much of the time	2
	Not usually	1
	Not at all	0
5. I enjoy my spare time	Very much	0
	Sometimes	1
	Not often	2
	Not at all	3

References

1. Tyrer P, Mulder R. *Personality Disorder: From Evidence to Understanding.* Cambridge: Cambridge University Press; 2022.
2. Livesley WJ, Larstone R. *Handbook of Personality Disorders: Theory, Research, and Treatment.* New York: Guilford Publications; 2018.
3. Lejuez CW, Gratz KL. *The Cambridge Handbook of Personality Disorders.* Cambridge: Cambridge University Press; 2020.
4. World Health Organization. *ICD-11: International Classification of Diseases (11th revision).* Geneva: World Health Organization; 2019.
5. Tyrer P. Why borderline personality disorder is neither borderline nor a personality disorder. *Personality and Mental Health* 2009;3(2):86–95.
6. Baca-Garcia E, Perez-Rodriguez MM, Basurte-Villamor I, et al. Diagnostic stability of psychiatric disorders in clinical practice. *British Journal of Psychiatry* 2007;190:210–6.
7. Seivewright H, Tyrer P, Johnson T. Change in personality status in neurotic disorders. *Lancet* 2002;359(9325):2253–4.
8. Yang M, Tyrer H, Johnson T, et al. Personality change in the Nottingham Study of Neurotic Disorder: 30-year cohort study. *Australia and New Zealand Journal of Psychiatry* 2022;56 (3):260–9.

9. Sharp C. Bridging the gap: the assessment and treatment of adolescent personality disorder in routine clinical care. *Archives of Disease in Childhood* 2017;102(1):103–8.
10. Tyrer P, Crawford M, Sanatinia R, et al. Preliminary studies of the ICD-11 classification of personality disorder in practice. *Personality and Mental Health* 2014;8(4):254–63.
11. Lewis G, Appleby L. Personality disorder: the patients psychiatrists dislike. *British Journal of Psychiatry* 1988;153:44–9.
12. Chartonas D, Kyratsous M, Dracass S, et al. Personality disorder: still the patients psychiatrists dislike? *BJPsych Bulletin* 2017;41(1):12–7.
13. Tyrer P, Mitchard S, Methuen C, et al. Treatment rejecting and treatment seeking personality disorders: Type R and Type S. *Journal of Personaliy Disorders* 2003;17(3):263–8.
14. Ranger M, Methuen C, Rutter D, et al. Prevalence of personality disorder in the case-load of an inner-city assertive outreach team. *Psychiatric Bulletin* 2004;28(12):441–3.
15. Beck AT, Davis DD, Freeman A. *Cognitive Therapy of Personality Disorders*. New York: Guilford Publications; 2015.
16. Zanarini MC, Frankenburg FR, Reich DB, et al. The subsyndromal phenomenology of borderline personality disorder: a 10-year follow-up study. *American Journal of Psychiatry* 2007;164(6):929–35.
17. Linehan M. *Cognitive-Behavioral Treatment of Borderline Personality Disorder*. New York: Guilford Press; 1993.
18. Linehan M. *DBT Skills Training Manual*. New York: Guilford Publications; 2014.
19. Newton-Howes G. The case for cautious paternalism in the emergency management of patients with borderline personality disorder. *BJPsych Bulletin* 2021;45(2):86–9.
20. Werbeloff N, Hilge Thygesen J, Hayes JF, et al. Childhood sexual abuse in patients with severe mental illness: demographic, clinical and functional correlates. *Acta Psychiatrica Scandinavica* 2021;143(6):495–502.
21. Kessler RC, McLaughlin KA, Green JG, et al. Childhood adversities and adult psychopathology in the WHO World Mental Health Surveys. *British Journal of Psychiatry* 2010;197(5):378–85.
22. Frost R, Hyland P, Shevlin M, et al. Distinguishing complex PTSD from borderline personality disorder among individuals with a history of sexual trauma: a latent class analysis. *European Journal of Trauma & Dissociation* 2020;4(1):100080.
23. Jowett S, Karatzias T, Shevlin M, et al. Differentiating symptom profiles of ICD-11 PTSD, complex PTSD, and borderline personality disorder: a latent class analysis in a multiply traumatized sample. *Personality Disorders: Theory, Research, and Treatment* 2020;11(1):36.
24. Moran P, Leese M, Lee T, et al. Standardised Assessment of Personality–Abbreviated Scale (SAPAS): preliminary validation of a brief screen for personality disorder. *The British Journal of Psychiatry* 2003;183(3):228–32.
25. Tyrer P, Yang M, Tyrer H, et al. Is social function a good proxy measure of personality disorder? *Personality and Mental Health* 2021;15(4):261–72.
26. Bach B, Brown TA, Mulder RT, et al. Development and initial evaluation of the ICD-11 personality disorder severity scale: PDS-ICD-11. *Personality and Mental Health* 2021;15(3):223–36.
27. Kim YR, Tyrer P, Hwang ST. Personality Assessment Questionnaire for ICD-11 personality trait domains: development and testing. *Personality and Mental Health* 2021;15(1):58–71.
28. Weekers LC, Hutsebaut J, Kamphuis JH. The Level of Personality Functioning Scale-Brief Form 2.0: update of a brief instrument for assessing level of personality functioning. *Personality and Mental Health* 2019;13(1):3–14.
29. Newton-Howes G, Mulder R, Tyrer P. Diagnostic neglect: the potential impact of losing a separate axis for personality disorder. *British Journal of Psychiatry* 2015;206(5):355–6.
30. Tyrer P, Mulder R, Kim YR, et al. The development of the ICD-11 classification of personality disorders: an amalgam of science, pragmatism, and politics. *Annual Review of Clinical Psychology* 2019;15:481–502.
31. Winsper C, Bilgin A, Thompson A, et al. The prevalence of personality disorders in the community: a global systematic review and meta-analysis. *The British Journal of Psychiatry* 2020;216(2):69–78.
32. Keown P, Holloway F, Kuipers E. The prevalence of personality disorders, psychotic disorders and affective disorders amongst the patients seen by a community mental health team in London. *Social Psychiatry and Psychiatric Epidemiology* 2002;37:225–29.
33. Beckwith H, Moran PF, Reilly J. Personality disorder prevalence in psychiatric outpatients: a systematic literature review. *Personality and Mental Health* 2014;8(2):91–101.
34. Livesley WJ, Jang KL. The behavioral genetics of personality disorder. *Annual Review of Clinical Psychology* 2008;4:247–74.
35. Skoglund C, Tiger A, Rück C, et al. Familial risk and heritability of diagnosed borderline personality disorder: a register study of the Swedish population. *Molecular Psychiatry* 2021;26(3):999–1008.
36. Newton-Howes G, Tyrer P, Johnson T. Personality disorder and the outcome of depression: meta-analysis of published studies. *The British Journal of Psychiatry* 2006;188(1):13–20.
37. Newton-Howes G, Tyrer P, Johnson T, et al. Influence of personality on the outcome of treatment in depression: systematic review and meta-analysis. *Journal of Personality Disorders* 2014;28 (4):577–93.
38. Skodol AE, Grilo CM, Keyes KM, et al. Relationship of personality disorders to the course of major depressive disorder in a nationally representative sample. *American Journal of Psychiatry* 2011;168(3):257–64.
39. Skodol AE, Geier T, Grant BF, et al. Personality disorders and the persistence of anxiety disorders in a nationally representative sample. *Depression and Anxiety* 2014;31 (9):721–28.
40. Tyrer P, Wang D, Tyrer H, et al. Influence of apparently negative personality characteristics on the long-term outcome of health anxiety: secondary analysis of a randomized controlled trial. *Personality and Mental Health* 2021;15(1):72–86.
41. Zanarini MC, Frankenburg FR, Hennen J, et al. The longitudinal course of borderline psychopathology: 6-year

prospective follow-up of the phenomenology of borderline personality disorder. *American Journal of Psychiatry* 2003;160(2):274–83.

42. Gunderson JG, Stout RL, McGlashan TH, et al. Ten-year course of borderline personality disorder: psychopathology and function from the Collaborative Longitudinal Personality Disorders study. *Archives of General Psychiatry* 2011;68(8):827–37.

43. Winsper C, Bilgin A, Thompson A, et al. The prevalence of personality disorders in the community: a global systematic review and meta-analysis. *British Journal of Psychiatry* 2020;216 (2):69–78.

44. Goddard E, Wingrove J, Moran P. The impact of comorbid personality difficulties on response to IAPT treatment for depression and anxiety. *Behaviour Research and Therapy* 2015;73:1–7.

45. Tyrer P, Tyrer H, Yang M, et al. Long-term impact of temporary and persistent personality disorder on anxiety and depressive disorders. *Personality and Mental Health* 2016;10 (2):76–83.

46. Tyrer P, Owen R, Dawling S. Gradual withdrawal of diazepam after long-term therapy. *Lancet* 1983;1(8339):1402–6.

47. Schweizer E, Rickels K, De Martinis N, et al. The effect of personality on withdrawal severity and taper outcome in benzodiazepine dependent patients. *Psychological Medicine* 1998;28 (3):713–20.

48. Pomeroy JC, Ricketts B. Long-term attendance in the psychiatric outpatient department for non-psychotic illness. *The British Journal of Psychiatry* 1985;147(5):508–16.

49. Conradi HJ, de Jonge P, Kluiter H, et al. Enhanced treatment for depression in primary care: long-term outcomes of a psycho-educational prevention program alone and enriched with psychiatric consultation or cognitive behavioral therapy. *Psychological Medicine* 2007;37(6):849–62.

Chapter 7.2

Clinical Approaches to Personality Disorder (AKA Complex Emotional Needs)*

Oliver Dale and Andrew Howe

The meeting of two personalities is like the contact of two chemical substances: if there is any reaction, both are transformed
Modern Man in Search of a Soul – *Carl Jung*

Introduction

Our brief is to consider how to care for patients who meet the criteria for a diagnosis of personality disorder. We will do so by reflecting on the role of the psychiatrist in creating a resilient, honest and caring clinical environment delivering interventions in a considered and coherent manner. Central to this is the relationship between doctor and patient, which includes not only direct clinical care but also the orchestration of work across the multi-disciplinary team and other agencies through clinical leadership.

We approach personality disorders as a relational problem in which the patient experiences their difficulties through their relationships with themselves and the world around them. These difficulties often – though not exclusively – are a developmental consequence of adverse childhood experience, brought to life within the therapeutic relationship itself. This inevitably means the work is challenging, but it also means that the way we comport ourselves and lead becomes central to the therapeutic culture.

Much has been written on the challenges of working with people who are diagnosable with personality disorder, but perhaps less acknowledged is how these challenges represent not only the very material fundamental to our primary task but also the reason it is such rewarding work given the right circumstances.

This chapter is split into three parts: the first gives an overview of the relational scene, the second a pathophysiological description, and the final section a more detailed description of how care and interventions can be delivered. The focus is mainly on general adult psychiatry and inevitably leans towards the community; however, the principles outlined are relevant across health and social care.

* With thanks to Julia Blazdell and Keir Harding.

Setting the Scene

Personality Disorder: A Recent History

When the last version of this chapter was published in 2007, some 75 years after Stern's paper, a degree of therapeutic optimism and clinical imperative was emerging. Scientific evaluation, conceptual development and political pressure had brought personality disorder into the mainstream of mental health services. Some attribute the ensuing flurry as being brought about following the conviction of Michael Stone for the murder of Lin and Megan Russell. The perpetrator had been known to mental health services previously and had a diagnosis of personality disorder. The Royal College of Psychiatrists at the time articulated a concern that its members could not be held responsible for the consequences of patients with personality disorder if it had neither the legal framework nor the resources to manage the condition. Furthermore, there was a view in some quarters that such conditions were 'untreatable'.

Many psychiatrists at the time held a more nuanced view with regard to what was and was not treatable. What is clear is that some saw the diagnosis of personality disorder as a means to exclude difficult patients. The term was therefore often avoided, sometimes with the explicit agreement of the patient. There were, however, notable exceptions, and the Cassel and Henderson hospitals used the term with pragmatic ambivalence (see Box 7.2.1).

In 2003, The National Institute for Mental Health England published the seminal paper *Personality Disorder: No Longer a Diagnosis of Exclusion.*[1] This kickstarted the National Personality Disorder Programme, which was to run until 2011. At the time, only 17 per cent of English NHS mental health trusts reported having a dedicated service, and only 40 per cent reported having 'some level of service'. The report highlighted how diagnosis alone could determine whether the service provided longer-term care and treatment or whether the patient was offered occasional moments of crisis care, typically in A&E.

Box 7.2.1 Cassel and Henderson hospitals

The Henderson and Cassel hospitals established the practice of therapeutic communities. Both operated a psychosocial approach in which patients and staff shared the responsibility for the running of the hospital so that no group owned being 'entirely well' or 'entirely unwell'. Therapy was a part of the programme but was not seen as the principal intervention, simply part of a whole.

Tom Main, author of 'The Ailment', worked along Eileen Skellern – who coined the phrase 'your patients are your greatest resource'. Such thinking and approaches arguably gave rise to co-production.

The Henderson, which closed in 2008, famously had a saying that 'the diagnosis of personality disorder brought you to our door, and that is where you can leave it'.

The Cassel Hospital continues to treat adults through a residential and outreach programme. It is also the national host for the current iteration of the Knowledge & Understanding Framework.

Good practice examples were drawn into the programme, and a small group of pilot services were established to test out different approaches. The learning from these pilots was explored through a Delphi[2] and disseminated across health and social care as well as the criminal justice system. A final review of the programme was prepared in 2011.[3] It concluded the pilot services demonstrated the following assumptions reflecting the importance of:

- Human relationships
- The psychosocial environment
- Investment in the programme
- Leadership
- Effective teamwork
- The establishment of good networks and partnerships

These have been further developed into a quality network scheme run by the Royal College of Psychiatrists' Centre for Quality Improvement – Enabling Environments.[4] Enabling Environments provides a transdiagnostic approach to creating healthy social environments.

An assumption of the national programme was that personality disorder was 'everyone's business'. This meant delivering most of the care through mainstream mental health services alongside partner agencies. In addition, strategically placed, local specialist services would provide care at a local level for those with more complex needs. A key objective to support such an assumption was a training programme called the Knowledge and Understanding framework (KUF), providing a stepped model of training co-delivered by lived experience practitioners alongside 'experts by profession'. It – along with the community interest company, emergence (small e), that was led by service users – was to become the exemplar of co-production.

From the outset, the national programme understood lived experience practitioners could bring a skill-set that was as important, and sometimes more relevant, than that of a clinician. As such, fair remuneration ensured a balance of power which, in the case of KUF, created a vibrant training experience through the incorporation of a range of teaching methods alongside experiential learning. The KUF programme ceased to formally function in 2018 but has continued, and it is believed 100,000 people in health, social care and the criminal justice system have attended the three-day awareness training. In 2021, NHS England, HM Prison and Probation Service, and Health Education England commissioned a revamped KUF programme given its success in demonstrating an improvement in understanding[5] and reducing staff burnout.[6]

The national programme itself was closed following the 2008 financial crisis, although the criminal justice side continued. In the absence of a national strategy, it was left up to a hope that local services would continue the evolution, driven by local priorities. The British and Irish Group for the Study of Personality Disorder (BIGSPD) took on the task, albeit informally, of maintaining the programme's relationships and has evolved into an association of services as opposed to a purely scientific organisation.

The hands-off strategy meant a lack of a whole systems approach and an absence of institutional learning. A chaotic and piecemeal picture emerged. Whilst a 2015 survey of English mental health NHS trusts[7] found 84 per cent reported having a dedicated service with 100 per cent reported offering some level of service, there was a concerning level of heterogeneity. Furthermore, an increasing confusion between service and intervention emerged, meaning that patients required a good degree of engagement, motivation and psychosocial readiness to be helped, and the most vulnerable were the most poorly served with interventions still delivered in fits and starts through crisis contacts.

At the same time, the last two decades have seen a significant development of both epidemiological and interventional evidence. Evans'[8] review of the literature sets out the key findings from this period. Perhaps two of the most prominent ones are life expectancy, which is roughly 18 years less on average,[9] and the £12.3 billion cost to the public purse predicted by 2026.[10] Alongside the description of such economic and human burden, a raft of – largely psychological – interventions were developed and demonstrated to be both cost-effective and affordable. Representing such progress, NICE guidance for self harm,[11] borderline[12] and antisocial[13] personality disorders were developed.

There is no doubt that an enormous amount of progress has been made, and yet, personality disorder remains in the spotlight. The NHS Long Term Plan and its Community Mental Health Framework has made personality disorder a key priority. Behind such efforts is a recognition that – for many – progress has been at best limited, whilst others argue we have – if anything – gone backwards through an increasing entrenchment of diagnostically driven interventional approaches. All agree, however, that care could and should be improved, best summarised in the Consensus Statement on Personality Disorder.[14]

What or Who Are We Treating?

Putting aside the controversies around concept, classification and label – and despite the variety in presentation – the DSM-5 field trials demonstrate that psychiatrists have good inter-rater reliability when it comes to identifying borderline personality disorder.[15]

This is curious as patients typically present with comorbidities. For instance, a large-scale household survey found those with a cluster B diagnosis have considerable levels of anxiety or affective disorders[16] with an odds ratio of 20.3 (5.7–71.6). So, whilst a more superficial conceptual problem – say depression – might bring a patient to our attention, we pick up that there is *something underlying* the presentation. When the something is described as personality disorder, we are saying something occurred either in our relationship with the patient or elsewhere that leaves us wondering. This is an emerging awareness, and if we are truly to help, this means engaging with something uncertain and difficult to grasp hold of, partly because it is occurring in a reaction *between* patient and clinician.

We would argue that what the study by Regier et al.[15] is describing is as much an unconscious reaction than a purist application of diagnostic criteria. A key myth to dispel, however, is that unconscious is *not* synonymous with being unaware but is more accurately an affective or feeling-toned awareness. Being receptive to this awareness allows the psychiatrist and patient to go beyond 'treating' the depression with a simple transactional intervention. By being curious about what these depressed feelings mean, we help the patient create a curiosity about their internal world and, in turn, we help establish what we call the 'real therapeutic relationship'.

We all have our leanings, and our relationships are coloured by our own valences derived from our own history. This points to something fundamental; as a phenomenon of relationships, you the clinician are stepping into the patients' internal world with them and bringing your own traumas and idiosyncrasies into the mix. Whilst this is true of all caring and professional roles, it is most present in this field. This is deeply challenging as it means having to confront the fact that our thoughts, feelings and even actions inevitably fall short of the idealised professional. For these reasons, all of us find this challenging, but many also find it deeply rewarding.

Talion Law

Such intimate work demands trust. Some[17] conceptualise these difficulties as themselves having stemmed from a failure in epistemic trust – defined as the capacity to trust new knowledge gleaned from the social environment. Trust is imperative to learn, but it also gives an experience of belonging and so creates a safe environment.

Box 7.2.2 Talion Law

'An Eye For an Eye'

The Law of Retaliation (*lex talionis*) is an early legal system based on a principle that the punishment should be proportionate to the crime.

Some consider Talion Law to have been established to replace feuds and vendettas, which were extreme and threatening social disorder.

Psychoanalytic theories describe an 'internal' legal system governed by a superego, which punishes the patient through an internal critical force.

The critical patient, therefore, is likely to be illustrating a regime they have had to endure for much of their lives.

Whilst such a voice ultimately leaves the patient isolated, it is a defence, there to guard against the vulnerability that arises in trusting someone and expressing their true selves. It is a self-care system in over-drive.

It is common for patients to describe not being able to trust clinicians. Given the role of trauma and adversity in the patient's presentation, one might think that this gives us a simple explanation as to why. We will show later that there is much more to the conflicts that dominate the field that relate to impossible expectations placed upon patients and clinician alike.

This is the territory of the rescue fantasy, which is a form of therapeutic over-optimism (i.e. that if therapy is provided in the right way, it is certain to be helpful and pain free with immediate results). Related to this is the concept of 'relentless hope',[130] which protects us from facing the reality of the patient's past, present and future. Whilst denial protects us from grief, in its place, grievance stalks the treatment as patient and clinician clings to the hope of something transformative.

An indication of failure risks interpreting the clinician or 'system' as uncaring, or perhaps more importantly because of its role in iatrogenic harm, we see the patient as failing in their role and so blame them for the challenges of the work. Perilously, such powerful reactions can leave the patient considering themselves at fault; helpless or hopeless, ultimately, they are to blame. West[18] describes this phenomenon as a form of 'Talion Law' (see Box 7.2.2).

Therapeutic Nihilism

It is well known that a large group of patients fit frankly neither into the psychotic nor into the psychoneurotic group, and that this border line group of patients is extremely difficult to handle effectively by any psychotherapeutic method. . .. I had to stop treatment leaving them not much benefited
Stern, 1938

Some consider Stern to have coined the term 'borderline', and we have quoted him here to illustrate how the field has a long history of locating the problem in the patient. Furthermore, the quote describes what we might refer to as 'therapeutic nihilism' – the sense, to a varying degree, of hopelessness in the work that both patient and clinician carry. It is this combination of both blame and failure that is potentially so destructive and what we must understand.

To underline the point, these are *feelings* clinicians and patient might repeatedly experience. These are not necessarily *facts,* however, and keeping that in mind is a challenge because it is as much an unconscious, automatic experience as it is conscious observation. It is feeling-toned and, therefore, colours everything to the extent that it was only relatively recently accepted that treatment was beneficial through the cold light of randomised controlled trials.

Yet, whilst this nihilism has dogged the field, it is also telling us something about the patient's interpersonal relationships as well as their internal world. Stern's 'feeling' is illuminating because this transference observation is data that informs us of the patients' view of themselves and their life. At the centre of such nihilism is a deep sense of shame and an expectation of rejection, which not only form a drive behind the patient's destructive behaviours but also the iatrogenic harm we risk if we are not live up to such powerful forces.

Box 7.2.3 Common factor theory

Refers to the argument that the power of therapeutic intervention almost entirely comes from the therapeutic relationship.

Saul Rosenweig is credited for starting to describe this in an article in 1936. This has been developed further into different models.

The contextual model frames the impact of therapy occurring through:

1. The real relationship
2. Expectations
3. Specific ingredients.

A review by Wampold[22] places the impact of common factors as accounting for between 30 and 70 per cent of the effect size.

One might consider that the real relationship:

- Is private but not secret
- Allows disclosure of difficult material
- Seeks understanding not judgement
- Is valued by both parties
- Is intimate yet professional
- Is inquisitive and not overly directive

Borderline as a Relational Psychosis

For now, we will ask the reader to consider borderline as simply a state of mind that reflects an early stage of development in which our capacity to think and manage our experiences is underdeveloped. It is a state in which unconscious communication processes and affective content predominates. Sometimes referred to as mentalising, holding something in the mind requires an interaction between conscious and unconscious process – the conscious component of this and the relationship between the two being developed through the experience of being thought about, or that it requires a dependable mentalising environment in order to create a mentalising function for oneself.

We might consider that our task, therefore, is to help the patient understand their experiences by thinking about them, making sense of them and communicating an understanding in a way in which they can use. One might think of the clinical relationships as a highly emergent one – at the outset you don't know where 'it' will take you and your patient. It is also a process that is inherently dependent upon one another.

A predominance of unconscious process, however, makes this especially emergent and uncertain, so it can set up quite a conflicted, confusing and anxiety-provoking process. This is especially true when considering our patients' early experiences of care will have given rise to adaptations warding against dependence on others. Equally important though is to consider how health care systems often undermine the creation of 'dependency' and relationship – for instance, through the avoidance of continuity of care.

We will explore this later, but for now, it is worth stating that thinking and being thought about are not easy, nor necessarily benign. The confusion within the patient, clinician and the health care community around this patient has a defensive, protective function. Such confusion can be so significant and persistent that the authors view such an experience as a form of relational psychosis – a state of collective mind in which it is very difficult to think about and describe the experience.

As psychiatrists, we have a very important role in leading a culture of thoughtfulness and understanding. We do this through developing a collective formulation, ultimately aiming to create an experience for the patient that helps them explore and comprehend their internal world. This is a living, relational and to some degree unconscious process – it is as much a feeling-toned process as a cognitive one (see Box 7.2.3).

Care and Treatment

The scientific method has been key to our understanding, but the empirical approach is equally limited. Hinshelwood[19] described psychiatry as having two opposite attitudes, one emphasising the patient as a *scientific object*, the other emphasising the patient as a *suffering subject.* The word patient derives from 'the one who suffers', and Hinshelwood argued that we tend to retreat to scientific objectification when under pressure, and this leaves us potentially blind to suffering.

Medication lends itself to the scientific method, but equally, psychological interventions can be prescribed and given as an aliquot. With manualisation making them amenable to randomised controlled trials, discrete treatments are of preference as the agents of change and the suffering becomes side-lined.

Add in the recovery model, a laudable aim to minimise the presence of an institution in a patient's life, the caring relationship risks being seen as irrelevant, even harmful. Suddenly, we are left with a clinical leaning away from suffering and a system designed to intervene as opposed to care.

The evidence is before us though. For instance, a multicentre RCT exploring lamotrigine in borderline personality disorder[20] found that both the active and placebo group had a clinically and statistically significant improvement in the weeks after joining the study that was sustained throughout follow-up. A qualitative study by the same team[21] lent further credence to common factor theory[22] and the power of the relationship; however, in this case, it was with the trial team.

Palliative medicine well understands that those with serious illnesses not only live more comfortable but also longer lives if treatment appropriately shifts from curative intervention to symptom management.[23] A psychiatric version of this is to recognise that our job is as much to care for people as it is to treat them or eradicate risks. Therefore, our wish is to underline this distinction between care and treatment.

Relational Practice in the Service of Care and Treatment

By foregrounding relational practice patients, we can better choose and prepare for interventions tailored to form part of a considered and uniquely individual clinical strategy. It is from this therapeutic alliance that the patient is supported to explore interventions, providing them a space for reflection and consolidation. In doing so, we create a coherent, patient-centred approach that respects the challenges and so makes the most effective use of an intervention's efficacy.

Through clinical leadership, the psychiatrist brings the patient and different components of service and partner agencies together, with the psychiatrist negotiating with the patient and colleagues to consider what is realistic and operating within respective legal and policy frameworks that guide the management of risk.

Containment relates to not only the reliable application of these processes, but equally the management of the feeling experiences that such work generates. Coherent care is based on being able to think about the patient, but whilst thinking can manage anxieties, it can equally generate them. Perhaps the most famous work describing this is 'The Ailment' by Tom Main,[24] in which he explores how our desire to help and our need to be successful can undermine our capacity to care in the face of intractable problems. Isabel Menzies, investigating the nursing practice later, specified the social defences deployed within caring institutions to manage these anxieties[25] and the emotional challenges of caring.

Both papers describe unconscious processes present in caring that can drive us towards states of mind in which we are less able to think. Although part and parcel of everyday life, when ill or stressed, we are all drawn to these defences. The relationships between patient, carers and the institution become challenged, creating a social environment prone to fragmentation and conflict. Containment comes out of an understanding that caring for the patient, both their healthy and unhealthy aspects, means tending to the institutions' capacity for healthy and unhealthy behaviours.

As Hinshelwood describes, 'poorly organised institutions risk enhancing the internal disorganisation of their severely disorganised members'.[26] As such, the psychiatrist has a critical role in leading such a community through not only their direct relationship with the patient, but also through their relationships with the social system around the patient. In such a system, the psychiatrist is an authority figure, both in terms of the holistic clinical expertise that they bring but also the power invested in them by the state through legislation and the institution through the consultant role.

Psychopathological Description

Personality Disorder Classification

The two predominant classification systems (ICD and DSM) take different approaches to classification. The former uses a dimensional model – of which personality forms one dimension – and the latter takes a categorical approach, describing discrete disease or disorder entities.

Given this is a UK publication, our approach is weighted towards ICD. The 11th version is current and has redefined personality disorder diagnoses by introducing a matrix of severity sitting alongside a smaller number of descriptors representing dysfunction across the five personality traits (see Chapter 7.1). These changes have been controversial. The introduction of severity has been largely welcomed. However, the loss of the perhaps most widely used clinical descriptions of borderline and dependent have caused confusion. Whilst some clinicians consider the new framework able to capture such qualities, the backlash resulted in the retention of the borderline term; however, not within the structure itself.

ICD-11

Severity is described in Table 7.2.1. Note that personality difficulty is a subclinical description.

Tables 7.2.2 and 7.2.3 describe some of demographic characteristics that describe what we might see at different levels of severity.[27]

Having established the degree of severity, the five traits of personality within a personality disorder are considered. These are modelled from the 'Big 5 personality traits' (openness, conscientiousness, extraversion, agreeableness and neuroticism)

- **Negative Affectivity:** describes a broad range of negative emotions that are out of proportion to the situation, emotional lability, negative attitudes, poor self-esteem and mistrustfulness

- **Detachment**: describes both social and emotional detachment and perhaps could be considered as avoidant
- **Disinhibition**: relates to self-centredness and a lack of empathy
- **Dissociality:** includes impulsivity, distractibility, irresponsibility, recklessness and lack of planning
- **Anankastia:** includes perfectionism, rigid control over emotional expression and stubbornness

Through such a lens, the personality disorders of ICD-10 may therefore be described using several different traits above. Given the recent changes of ICD-11, our evidence base remains firmly organised around ICD-10. Some extrapolation and interpretation are required.

Prevalence

There are many estimates of prevalence, but we would suggest reading Coid et al.,[16] which provide an authoritative estimate of a 4.4% community prevalence. Of note, borderline is more common in men whilst the most common disorder overall is anankastic (see Table 7.2.4).

The prevalence within various settings is set out below:

- 24% of primary care attendees[28]
- 52% in psychiatric outpatients[29]
- 27% in inpatient services[30]
- Up to 80% prison population[31]
- As a primary diagnosis, personality disorder reduces the likelihood of admission to an acute psychiatric hospital by 0.4 (0.3–0.56)
- As a comorbid diagnosis, personality disorder with schizophrenia or bipolar affective disorder increases the likelihood of being in the top 10% of users of inpatient services – with an odds ratio of 2.2 (1.8–2.7) – and raises the odds of detention by 1.6 (1.4–1.9).[32]

This concept of comorbidity raises an important conceptual point taken up by the model of DSM, which is to ask what is it that we are treating in 'personality disorder'? Some argue that

Table 7.2.1 Severity of personality disorder

Personality difficulty	Personality difficulty (not a disorder), with personality dysfunction only in certain settings
Mild personality disorder	Personality dysfunction is persistent but does not prevent normal functioning
Moderate personality disorder	Persistent interpersonal and self pathology, with disruption in personal, social and occupational areas
Severe personality disorder	Severe personality disruption, with high risk of harm to self or others

Table 7.2.2 Demographic characteristics at different levels of severity

Impact on Employment Odds Ratio by personality disturbance level					
Employment status	**Personality difficulty**	**Simple disorder**	**Complex disorder**	**Severe disorder**	**x2 for overall comparison d.f = 3**
Part time	1.11 (0.96–1.28)	1.11 (0.68–1.06)	0.83 (0.68–1.06)	2.32 (1.58–3.41)	24.81*
Unemployed	1.23 (0.86–1.76)	1.61 (1.09–2.38)	2.15 (1.35–3.42)	6.42 (3.67–11.23)	42.77*
Economically inactive	1.38 (1.19–1.60)	1.38 (1.19–1.60)	1.36 (1.08–1.69)	5.09 (3.45–7.52)	77.08*

* P< 0.001

Table 7.2.3 Further demographic characteristics at different levels of severity

Odds Ratio of aetiological and forensic factors					
	Personality difficulty	**Simple disorder**	**Complex disorder**	**Severe disorder**	**x2 for overall comparison d.f = 3**
School expelled	1.00	1.26	1.65*	9.56**	119.0**
Run away	1.74**	2.76**	3.47**	19.3**	266.6**
Homeless	1.43**	1.72**	2.29**	8.83**	154.3**
Sexually abused	1.61**	2.31**	3.55**	5.60**	110.2**
Institutional care before 16	0.91	0.94	0.94	10.5**	151.4**
LA care before 16	1.04	0.89	1.32	8.13**	128.3**
Conduct disorder	1.49**	2.97**	3.19**	>20**	>400**
Ever convicted	1.22	1.67*	2.11**	10.6**	99.4**

*P<0.05 ** P<0.001

Table 7.2.4 Personality disorder prevalence (%)

	Male	Female	Total
Paranoid	1.2 (0.4–3.1)	0.3 (0.1–1.0)	0.7 (0.3–1.7)
Schizoid	0.9 (0.3–2.6)	0.8 (0.2–3.5)	0.8 (0.3–1.7)
Schizotypal	0.02 (0.0–0.1)	0.1 (0.03–0.3)	0.06 (0.02–0.2)
Antisocial	1.0 (0.5–2.1)	0.2 (0.05–0.7)	0.6 (0.3–1.1)
Borderline	1.0 (0.3–3.2)	0.4 (0.2–1.1)	0.7 (0.3–1.7)
Avoidant	1.0 (0.3–2.8)	0.7 (0.3–1.8)	0.8 (0.4–1.7)
Dependent	0.2 (0.04–1.0)	0.02 (0.0–0.2)	0.1 (0.03–0.5)
Anankastic	2.6 (1.0–6.6)	1.3 (0.3–5.6)	1.9 (0.9–4.3)
Total	**5.4 (3.2-9.1)**	**3.4 (1.7-6.7)**	**4.4 (2.9-6.7)**

Table 7.2.5 Prevalence of comorbidities[16]

	Cluster A	Cluster B	Cluster C
Mental disorder	**OR (95% CI)**	**OR (95% CI)**	**OR (95% CI)**
Functional psychosis	2.83 (0.59–13.6)	7.44 (2.20–25.2)**	2.52 (0.66–9.54)
Affective/anxiety disorder	2.70 (0.99–7.34)	20.3 (5.70–71.6)***	4.21 (1.93–8.80)*
Alcohol dependence	1.61 (0.45–5.71)	4.21 (1.69–10.5)*	0.46 (0.10–2.13)
Hazardous drinking	0.83 (0.29–2.42)	1.51 (0.65–3.48)	0.36 (0.13–0.99)*
Drug dependence	1.32 (0.22–7.76)	1.87 (0.57–6.11)	1.93 (0.53–7.07)

Weighted multilevel multivariate logistic regression: estimated odds ratio, models adjusted for gender, age, social class and marital status. Significance: * ($p \leq 0.05$), ** ($p \leq 0.01$) and *** ($p \leq 0.001$).

it is the comorbidities that drive the presentation – it is the depression, anxiety, impulse disorders (self harm, eating disorder, addictions) that motivate help-seeking behaviour. Others point out that it is not the personality that is disordered but several associated difficulties such as emotional regulation, distress tolerance, interpersonal effectiveness and dissociative experiences. This is sometimes conceptualised by the concept of Galenic syndrome[33] after the Greek physician who first described the relationship between personality and disease. For prevalence of comorbidities, see Table 7.2.5.

The prevalence of personality disorder amongst the following patient groups is:

- Up to 39% in eating disorders[34]
- 53% in substance misuse[35]
- 63% in somatisation disorder[36]

Complex Emotional Needs

Some maintain there are significant problems with the label and the concept behind it, suggesting that complex PTSD (cPTSD) offers an alternative with a 'benign face validity'.[37] Putting to one side that trauma's role is not the only determinant in personality disorder, self harm is not included in cPTSD criteria for ICD-11 either. The label of personality disorder appears to preference an idea that the caring relationship is complicated by an ongoing traumatic experience in the here and now and within the relationship itself, whilst PTSD and cPTSD imply a historic trauma outside of the immediate and current caring relationship.

What appears to be happening clinically is that the vagaries of patient, clinician and service mean it is common for different diagnoses to be used and personality disorder diagnosed with considerable idiosyncracy. Authoritative data is lacking. However, the level of clinical coding appears below what research suggests, and the role of personality disorder remains subsumed within a plethora of other labels. The Royal College of Psychiatrists titling the position paper 'Services for People *diagnosable with* Personality Disorder', is a pragmatic reflection of both the concerns around the label and its inconsistent application.

Furthermore, the concern about stigma is what led the NIHR Mental Health Policy Research Unit to adopt the term complex emotional needs (CEN) with its recent programme of research into personality disorder. CEN is not a diagnostic category nor does it have an epidemiological basis, but it does have a practical utility in the clinical setting, which seems to capture the old adage that a neurologist diagnoses what they can't treat, and a psychiatrist treats what they can't diagnose.

Outcomes

Impact on the Individual's Health

Life expectancy is 63.3 years for women and 59.1 years for men, 18.7 years and 17.7 years shorter than females and males respectively in the general population in England and Wales.[9]

The mechanism of action remains unclear; however, a separate study[38] demonstrated that after adjusting for age, sex, social class, hypertension, diabetes, smoking and alcohol consumption, the presence of a personality disorder diagnosis increased the risk of stroke (OR = 1.9, 95% CI, 1.0–3.5) and ischaemic hear disease (OR = 1.4, 95% CI, 1.0–1.9).

Impact on Self Harm and Suicide

- 9–10% of people with personality disorder die by suicide[39]
- Between 45–77% of people dying by suicide have personality disorder[40]
- 46% presenting to A&E with self harm have personality disorder[41]

Impact on Parenting

Parental personality disorder is associated with the following:

- Maternal personality disorder increases the risk of experiencing postnatal anxiety by 2.84 (95% CI, 1.31–6.15) and postnatal depression by 1.98 (95% CI, 0.81–4.81)[42]
- Maternal personality disorder increased risk of depression and self-harming behaviours in young people by 2.27 (1.45–3.54)[43]

- 50% of children with conduct disorder have a parent with personality disorder, and interventions for their parents produced improvements in a ratio of 8:1[44] as compared to those without interventions

Impact on Violence

Drawing on a large household survey, González et al.[45] made the following observations:

- Borderline personality disorder is only associated with intimate partner violence (IPV)
- For men and women, impulsivity was associated with violence
- For men, paranoid ideation is associated with violence. Additional associations with being male included repetitive incidents, along with incidents causing injury
- For women, relational instability was associated with violence, mostly towards intimate partners and causing no injury
- Violence causing injury and repetitive violence is more strongly associated with comorbid substance misuse, anxiety and dissocial personality disorder

Other studies report that gender does not moderate the effects of IPV, and increases in the number of types of borderline personality disorder symptoms correlates with the number of types of violent acts.[46]

Impact on Forensic Behaviours

From work on personality disorder and offending behaviour,[47] the following relationships have been found:

Multiple incidences of violence in forensic setting are:

- Five times more likely with borderline and eight times more likely with dissocial personality disorder compared to those with no personality disorders
- 25 times more likely with both, compared to none

Incidences of serious violence (causing injury) in forensic settings are:

- 3.5 times more likely with borderline and 10 times more likely with dissocial personality disorder when compared to none
- 20 times more likely with both, compared to no personality disorder

Aetiology

A clear pathophysiological understanding of personality disorder remains elusive. Whilst the prevailing thesis is that early environmental adversity is critical, it is unable to explain the variance. Many people with a trauma history do not develop mental disorder, whilst trauma can result in a range of different disorders. A mixture of genetics and environment seems relevant, but the scope of this chapter means only an indicative description is possible.

Biological Associations

The role of genetic phenotype presents a complex and uncertain picture. Overall, the inheritability of borderline personality disorder is considered to be around 40 per cent, but it may be as high as 60 per cent.[48]

There is interest in the functional polymorphism of the monoamine oxidase A metaboliser, which may moderate the effect of maltreatment.[49] Epigenetics have, however, become an interesting area, with some considering this could contribute to different presentations and outcomes within subgroups,[50] whilst others have found evidence to support observed gender differences in the development of personality disorder and make putative mechanisms through which childhood trauma modulates gene expression.[51]

Adverse Childhood Experiences

Adverse childhood experiences is a catch-all term for childhood neglect and trauma. This is a particularly subjective area as a person's narrative of early life events will only highlight the trauma that they feel they have experienced whilst acts of omission are subject to reporting bias.

A study funded by Public Health Wales[52] identified that 47% of the population had at least one ACE, whilst 14% experienced four or more. This cut off was more strongly associated with 'health-harming behaviours', defined as violence victimisation (OR: 14.2, 95% CI, 9.1–22.1), high-risk drinking (OR: 4.4, 3.1–6.4) and low mental wellbeing (OR: 4.7, 3.4–6.4).

A meta-analysis of 97 published studies[53] found people with borderline personality disorder are 13.91 (95% CI, 11.11–17.43) times more likely to report childhood adversity than non-clinical controls and 3.15 (95% CI, 2.62–3.79) times more likely than other psychiatric groups. Emotional abuse (OR: 38.11, 95% CI, 25.99–55.88) and neglect (OR: 17.73, 95% CI, 13.01–24.17) demonstrated the strongest correlations.

The role of early infantile neglect is very difficult to quantify and yet clearly relevant. Through the long-term follow-up of the adopted Romanian orphans following the collapse of the Soviet Union, researchers were able to define a dose-dependent exposure to parental neglect dependent on the amount of time spent within a Romanian orphanage as well as the distance the infant's cot was from the nursing station. The team[54] demonstrated the cognitive impact of neglect appeared reversible following adoption into a stable home. There remained, however, a dose-dependent relationship between neglect and the adult expression of autistic spectrum disorder, inattention and hyperactivity, disinhibited social engagement, and self and parent-reported emotional problems.

Social Associations

Social determinants are increasingly considered relevant and, in their editorial on trauma informed approaches, Sweeney and Taggart[55] – citing Hatch and Dohrenwend[56] as well as Paradies[57] – make the argument that inequalities of race, gender and poverty should be considered a form of trauma in their own right, whilst also exposing the individual to more frequent episodes of adversity. As such, there is considered an 'intersectionality' of adverse experience.

Developmental Psychopathology

Although we can be reasonably that certain genes and environment play a role in the development of personality disorder, a detailed psychopathological description of both the development and presentation can only be offered in the most tentative of ways. What is proposed here is how we have come to understand how this thing that we call personality disorder and why the nature of the work is the way it is.

Personality Disorder: A Gene-Environment Neurodevelopmental Disorder

We start from a position that the ego – the conscious and autobiographical sense of self, I – develops over time following birth and requires an attentive parental environment capable of thinking about the infant. Psychological development also requires a broader development of psyche grounded within the soma (body). All of this establishes a complex interrelationship between these various aspects of ourselves within a social and physical environment.

If the infant comes into a world that does not meet their physical and psychosocial needs, the development of these different aspects is impaired, their integration undermined, and the quality of these interrelationships affected. Furthermore, the limits of neuroplasticity mean these impacts have lifelong expression. We consider, therefore, personality disorder as a neurodevelopmental disorder arising out of an early gene and environment interaction.

Development of a Structured Psyche

Whilst a distinction between conscious and unconscious is not controversial, it was Carl Jung who described how the unconscious was one of two centres of 'awareness', the other centre being consciousness. He described how the Self (capital S) represented the unconscious mind and contained within it the ingredients for all psychic life (including the ego) as well as our drive towards individuation, which is equivalent to the term 'self-actualisation'. Individuation arises out of these two centres working together so the individual can transcend the challenges of living to achieve a grounded, ontologically coherent, sufficiently expressed life (see Table 7.2.6).

Using PET scanning, Damasio et al.[58] describes a close neuroanatomical relationship between emotion, feeling and homeostasis, supporting the idea of a multidimensional neural map with both coarse and refined neural pathways. They propose that some feelings are available to conscious thought and others are not, with a 'top-down' (conscious) modification from the orbitofrontal cortex and an 'as-if body loop mechanism' '*that drives activity in somatosensory maps from within the brain, independently of actual body signalling*'.

In a separate paper, Damasio[59] describes two centres of consciousness, divided into the 'core' and 'extended consciousness', with the ego equating to the extended consciousness and the core being the unconscious. Core consciousness is the immediate and psychosomatic experience of the moment, whilst the extended consciousness places the individual at a point in time and is aware of the past and future and the world around it. The extended consciousness is conscious and cognitive, it is 'I am who I am'; the unconscious is affective and psychosomatic. Damasio situates extended consciousness only in humanity, but core consciousness is common amongst animals.

Unconscious, Primary Process and Psychotic Thinking

Both Jung and Freud considered the contents of the unconscious as being affective in nature. We might also argue that they both considered it to be psychotic. However, to maintain a distinction between what we clinically refer to as psychosis, the term 'primary process' has been adopted. One might more accurately consider what we refer to as psychosis as being a state in which our ego function becomes overwhelmed by unconscious material. Importantly, ego contact with our unconscious can impact our capacity to think (think of a dream). What borderline is describing is how ego function is partially impaired by this affective part of our mind. To borrow from dialectical behavioural therapy, we have an emotional mind and a logical one. A wise mind, which is not always the preferred state, is something of a collaboration between the two.

An analogy is that, in the depths of a hallucinogenic trip, there remains a rudimentary I, but it is dominated by affectivity, it knows no bounds, it is filled with awe and terror, and it is completely connected to the universe. It is omnipotent and omniscient. West, referencing Matte Blanco[60], describes these states as being 'an experience of infinite effect'.

To summarise:

- the unconscious is affective in nature, feeling-toned and psychosomatic and is involved in the homeostasis of both body and mind (as opposed to the ego, which is rational and cognitive)
- the term 'unconscious' is a misnomer as we are aware of it, and it might be thought of as the seat of sentience
- Our awareness of our affective (and bodily) world fluctuates dependent upon our mental state

We might summarise the structural mind as such:

Table 7.2.6 The structural mind summarised

Core	Extended
Unconscious	Ego
Sentience	Conscious
Affective	Cognitive
Psychotic, 'primary process': timeless, boundless, no dimensions	Non-psychotic thinking: boundaried, time, space, autobiographical

Primary Affects, Drives and Conscious Modification

Taking this further, Alcaro et al.[61] describe the 'first neuro-evolutional layer of the mind . . . the affective core of the self'. Reviewing neuroscientific literature, they explore the brain stem commonalities across the animal kingdom.

With the brain stem remaining critical for conscious thought, lesions often result in a complete loss of conscious functioning. In cases of hydranencephaly – where the cerebral cortex and higher limbic areas are absent, leaving subcortical brain stem functioning only – there are observable forms of consciousness based on positive and negative affective states. Hence why the terms 'core' and 'extended' appear apt as conscious thinking is *extended* out of a core.

This affective core self demonstrates three affective states:

- **Visceral affects:** are an awareness of internal bodily states perceived as moods or feelings; they also effect homeostatic mechanisms such as the endocrine system.
- **Instinctual affects:** refer to a disposal to act, avoiding or approaching certain situations. Examples include sexual and locomotor behaviours.
- **Sensorial affects:** give perceptual experiences an affective value – for example, the pleasure of warmth or the unpleasantness of a startling sound.

The contents of the affective core can be further categorised into systems shared amongst mammalian brains. These 'primary affects' are thought to have developed to move animals to action to promote survival. Such behaviours could be described as impulsive as they are governed by a here-and-now affect, not a conscious plan.

Systems within the affective core are defined as follows:

- **SEEKING system:** moves animal to look for resources
- **RAGE system:** moves animals to compete for or defend resources
- **FEAR system:** moves animals to avoid danger
- **LUST system:** moves animals to identify potential mates and reproduce

There are also three uniquely mammalian systems that promote social bonding[62]:

- **CARE system:** moves mammals to care for offspring
- **PANIC/GRIEF (separation distress) system:** promotes drive to social bonding
- **PLAY system:** moves mammals to physically play and build social bonds.

* Note that we have adhered to academic convention, first set out by Panksepp, by presenting these systems in capitals.

Demonstrated through brain stimulation studies,[61] the activation of certain brain stem areas modifies our subjective states and generates emotions. In this first primal layer of the brain, these emotional states drive behaviour. These affective states are a primary unconscious form of experience that pervade at birth and move to a mediating role between the cortical part of the brain and the brainstem through development. Such affective states, given their primal and later mediating role, are a key part of learning, brain development and social bonding.

Neuroscientific literature suggests personal experiences cluster around primal affective states. The capacity for higher cortical function (top-down) modification of primal affective states is dependent upon the level of arousal experienced and the level of development of higher cortical function. In other words, an intense personal experience – say, a trauma – clustered around an aroused affective state is harder to mediate or keep under ego control. Limited top-down modification and cortical access leaves the experience within the homeostatic, bodily realm, just as trauma is often described as *being stored in the body*.

Neglect, Self-Care Systems and Negative Affective Core

Drawing in the work of observation data, developmental psychologists Edward Tronick and Andrew Gianino[63] describe the generation of a 'negative affective core', setting out how mother and infant are in a state of flux between emotional match and mismatch. Typically, mismatch is followed by repair, which may be initiated by the infant attempting to engage the care givers' attention. If successful, they learn to regulate their distress through interactions with another and develop both a conscious sense of connection and agency. If unsuccessful, then this can present as a high-stress experience, and the infant gives up and focusses on an independent self-regulation to achieve affective homeostasis. This sets the foundation for a self-care system that does not rely on human social connection and is less influenced by top-down, conscious mechanisms using the orbitofrontal cortex.

Such a situation has obvious implications for interpersonal relationships, but there are more profound implications as this is mirrored by an *intrapersonal* impact. Not only is this milieu setting up something in which there is a detachment from those around the person, but they are also less connected within themselves. As West[64,65] suggests, people prone to borderline states of mind shift more readily from an extended to a *more* core conscious position. Such a position means thinking and feeling can become dominated around particular primal affective states. Clinically, patients present with emotional lability with a predominance of negative emotional reactions, sometimes to highly specific situations such that they are 'triggered' by touchpoints.

Core Consciousness, Psychotic Communication and Relational Psychosis

Another implication of this lack of cortical and social involvement in emotional regulation and thinking is that whilst this core is a sentient world, it is one of unconscious communication. Our conscious thought and communication are extended out of an ancient, primitive form of unconscious thought and communication that continues to operate.

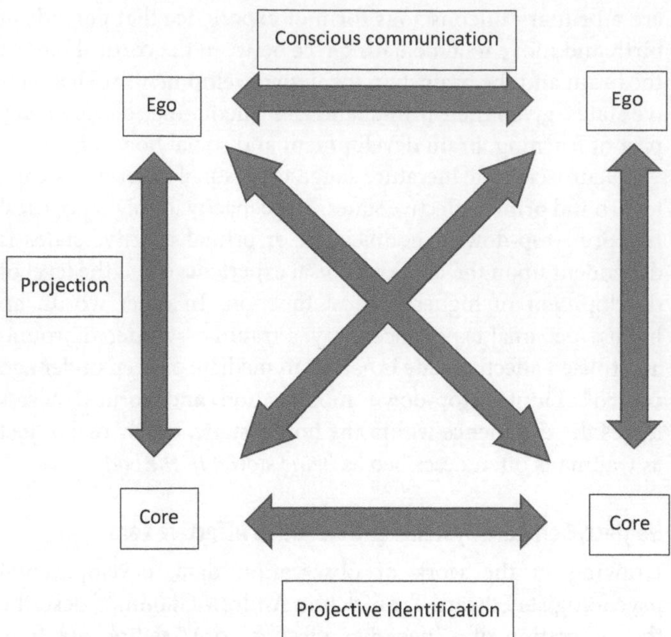

Figure 7.2.1 Explanatory diagram.

From an ego perspective, this can be experienced as bizarre – even magical – as these communications are ruled by primary process, and the transfer of information is to some degree 'underground' through unconscious interconnection. This is what we mean by projection and the completely unconscious phenomenon of projective identification, also known as participation mystique (see Figure 7.2.1).

This means that much of our communication between ourselves and our patients is occurring at this unconscious, feeling-toned level. There is always some degree of primary process connection between clinician and patient. However, given the challenges of the work as well as our own personal traumas, this becomes a relational psychosis in a pathological sense in places. This might explain what Main was referring to when he said that the staff did not own all the wellness and the patients not all the illness.

Personality Disorder or Disruption to the Expression of the Personality

Assuming creative life requires both core and extended consciousness working in balance, we might consider how adverse neurodevelopment may give rise to an imbalance with a greater risk of being overwhelmed by affective states – the consequences of being overwhelmed manifesting in distress plus a liability to impulsive action. Given the vicissitudes of life, such a situation can set up a chaotic, confused and traumatised autobiography, leaving the individual lacking in confidence with themselves in their environment and their capacity to live and learn. The problem of epistemic trust is, therefore, as much about lacking faith in themselves as opposed to others.

Such a conclusion might mean some form of retreat and detachment from the external world, through behaviour, grievance or addictions. The consequence of which is that the individual has a greater struggle to achieve individuation and a coherent identity. The problem is, however, compounded by the fact that at some level they 'see' their predicament very clearly in that – in some situations – they sense a life not lived.

From this perspective, the term 'personality disorder' contains within it a profound misunderstanding as the patient is clear about who they are, the personality is not disordered, it is the expression of their personality that is, such expression having been disrupted by chance events, early adverse experiences and increased exposures to traumas and challenges in later life.

A Clinicopathological Description

Drawing this together, we might consider how these concepts map on to the clinical experience.

Impairments of Mentalisation

Starting from the position of impairments of the early mentalising environment, the patient has a preference towards a self-care system. This means that the primary affective systems are less subject to both cortical modification and social bonding through attachments. This results in limitations in both a conscious awareness of their own psyche and soma as well as of those around them. Thinking – both something done within oneself (introverted thinking) and with others (extraverted thinking) – is impaired, and the extended conscious function is more susceptible to becoming overwhelmed.

Emotional Intensity and Impulse Disorders

Areas of unmodified primary affect systems leave the individual prone to becoming dysregulated through triggers. Triggers may relate to 'memories', particularly traumatic ones, which are stored in a more primary process manner. As such, a 'recollection' becomes extremely intense and vivid, giving rise to severe distress. Difficulties with cognitive and social modification present the individual with a preponderance of bodily or action-based mechanisms to regain homeostasis. This might result in behaviours such as self harm, violence, addictions or eating disorder amongst others. Such actions achieve homeostasis through somatosensory and neuroendocrine mechanisms but undermine attempts at social modification and a social-care system.

Dissociative Experiences

In severe distress, core consciousness predominates and gives rise to primary process thinking. This entails a breakdown in time and space alongside a confusion between psyche and soma, so that historical memory and current experience become blurred. The individual might have dissociative experiences, which include depersonalisation, derealisation, hallucinations and flashbacks. In flashbacks, 'memory' remnants encoded at a core consciousness level have a 'here and now' quality.

Borderline and Relational Psychosis

Borderline states predispose to primary process forms of communication. These are akin to psychotic processes but, in this context, take on a relational aspect. This means high levels of arousal and a corresponding drift towards core conscious processes is induced in those around the patient. In addition, our patient's use of earlier forms of 'thinking' draws us into corresponding in kind. Being with someone in great distress is distressing and likely gets in touch with our own primary affect systems.

Negative Affectivity

This relates to the development of a self-care system in which, instead of incorporating the emollient voice of a caregiver in creating affective homeostasis, the infant is left with an absence that is filled by other means. Clinically, patients report a negative 'voice' that wards against dependence and reliance upon others through a fundamental belief that they will be rejected. Such protection is maintained through a hostile and derogatory *intrapersonal* relationship creating a secret pact, maintaining a distance from those around and hiding one's true self. This is what psychoanalysts refer to as a critical superego, what some CBT therapists describe as the poisonous parrot, and dialectical behavioural therapy (DBT) therapists call judgement thoughts. Such *intrapersonal* difficulties are mirrored in *interpersonal* difficulties, as such judgement thoughts drive the Talion Law type view of the world.

Problems of Self-Actualisation

This conspires to create several interpersonal and intrapersonal difficulties, which to varying degrees fluctuate and differ between individuals. Whilst often temporary, crises occur at the moment of challenge and transition in life. Readers may be familiar with crisis occurring at the same time as car-coordinators change or a long-awaited therapy begins. Such difficulties can therefore become extremely disruptive to the individual's life course and hinder treatment.

Prognosis and Life Course

The definition of personality disorder includes the idea that the patients' difficulties are 'persistent and pervasive'. Clinicians have often considered the presence of lifelong difficulties, appearing in adolescence, as key to making a clinical diagnosis.

Such thinking is overly simplistic, however, as functional impairments may only arise at transitional points in people's lives, and later developmental stages might precipitate presentations. These are probably more subjective and idiosyncratic and go beyond a simplistic definition. As such, leaving higher education or training, settling into an intimate relationship, having children, the children leaving home, a parent dying, reaching retirement or developing an illness might be highly relevant and specific transitions, personally meaningful to an individual. Accordingly, personality disorder might manifest at later stages in life, with a seeming functional history preceding it.

Another misconception is the idea that a diagnosis of personality disorder confers an understanding that the patient will experience chronic difficulties. A recent meta-analysis[66] concerning the long-term course of BPD noted that between 50-70% of patients achieved remission in the long term. Depressive symptoms and functional impairment were also shown to improve as patients aged, whilst they quoted a mean rate for completed suicide at 4%.

This is in keeping with other reviews,[67] suggesting that the prognosis of borderline is more favourable than many other psychiatric conditions. Many of the symptoms, particularly the behavioural difficulties, become remitting in the first few years following diagnosis, and there is a generally favourable outcome with treatment. The prognosis of other personality disorders is not well described in the literature.

Management and Treatment of Personality Disorder

A Relational Approach to Personality Disorder

The relational nature of personality disorder presents both a challenge and an opportunity. The very thing that is found challenging is the very thing that mediates help. Every interaction with our colleagues and our communities becomes an opportunity for therapeutic intervention. In what systemic therapists call isomorphic process, even distant interactions can profoundly influence the care.

What we set out here is a relational approach, which draws upon the field's history and current policy framework. For a more detailed overview, we would point the reader to a *Qualitative Thematic Meta-synthesis* (in press), as well as qualitative evidence looking at both clinician[68] and service user experience[69] about what works.

Service Structures

At the time of writing, the Community Mental Health Framework (CMHF) is redeveloping mental health systems to integrate primary and secondary care at a primary care network level. The CMHF itself falls within a broader service landscape (see Chapter 20). A more detailed description can be found within the Royal College of Psychiatrists's Position Statement on Services for People Diagnosable with Personality Disorder.[70]

Whilst the traditional community health team model has continued to evolve, several personality disorder specific models and schema have been developed. Good psychiatric management,[71] structured clinical management (SCM, see Box 7.2.4)[72] and practical management of personality disorder[73] are widely adopted and adapted. No model shows an advantage over another,[74] and a one-size-fits-all approach will effectively exclude a considerable number of patients.

Box 7.2.4 Structured clinical management

This was originally designed as a control intervention to compare against MBT and found to be very effective.

Each patient is allocated a worker who may be a care coordinator.

Programme typically lasts 18 months.

Entails one group contact and one individual contact a week. There are three phases:

Introductory phase: setting short-term goals and creating a safety plan

Active phase: working on managing emotions and problem solving skills

Next steps: includes consolidating and plans for the future

Some call the group 'the emotional regulation group', and it is very similar to the DBT skills group or Systems Training for Emotional Predictability and Problem Solving (STEPPS). Many services co-produce this group with a lived experience practitioner.

Our approach outlined is a pragmatic one for the generalist working within an adult community mental health team. We assume appropriate personality disorder specific interventions and reflective practice are available within the service. Where they are not, practitioners can be trained in co-production, delivering skills-based approaches and also establishing case-based discussion groups. Even with quite limited resources, such an approach should be capable of meeting all but the most complex of needs with the advantage of containing the different models and approaches that are available in order to create a rich ecosystem with which to engage, care and treat. Such flexibility and generalism is key to respecting the Galenic nature of the work.

Furthermore, it can provide a framework to hold the long-term work that many – clinicians and patients included – consider key. It is also worth remembering that specialist services are only as effective as the local service that makes the referral as a partnership between the two is vital to ensure the patient's progress is grounded within their local community and that both specialist and general service develop through supporting one another.

Public Health Model Approach

Arguments about the role of specialist services is as protracted as the label. Some of this reflects a confusion between service and therapeutic modality.

Whilst some light can be found in this economic evaluation of community services,[74] public health models approach health and social needs, particularly those with variable severity and complexity, in a comprehensive way – for our purposes, the way the difficulties associated with personality disorder and the resources within a broadly defined local community interact to impact an individual's capacity to live their life. ICD-11 lends itself to this approach, and the Royal College of Psychiatrists's position statement and CMHF adopt a similar philosophy, accepting that personality disorder is 'everyone's business'.

We, therefore, advocate for a whole systems approach, which includes both mainstream and specialist – one which provides a rich tapestry of interventions, designed to prevent, intervene early, care for and treat those with a wide degree of difficulty and risk. Whilst bespoke personality disorder interventions should be widely available, only those with the most complex difficulties and the hard to reach would require a specialist service.

Key Principles

Trauma Informed Care (TIC)

TIC is a shift through foregrounding the role of trauma both as an antecedent to mental ill health as well as a consequence of any ensuing difficulties. TIC practice describes how we might create services that promote feelings of safety and control. A useful editorial by Sweeney and Taggart[55] sets out some of the thinking; alongside this and other guidance, we consider the following principles key:

- Explicitly acknowledge the links between trauma and mental health
- Recognise trauma takes many forms and include social determinants and 'intersectionality'
- Accept services run the risk of re-traumatising people through exclusion, fragmentation of care and the use of power to impose interventions
- Ensure staff are confident in making trauma enquiries and do so in the knowledge that they can provide continuity of care and that people move at their own speed
- Provide a range of interventions that address safety, promote prevention, teach skills, foster self-acceptance and create meaningful activity
- Empower through respecting that symptoms and behaviours serve a purpose and engage the patient as an active participant in their care as opposed to a passive recipient
- Promote a culture of hope and belonging through co-production

Containment and Boundaries

Such statements are difficult to deliver. Not only that, whilst they sound benign, achieving them is not. To understand why, we need to explore the terms 'containment' and 'boundary'.

Container-Contained -- Bion set out that to make sense of our emotional mind, we need a significant other and that our capacity for thinking is dependent upon a stable link with this other. This is what he meant by container-contained.

In health, we seek out and rely upon a range of relationships – formal, social and intimate – which allow us to explore our internal world and make sense of the environmental and the developmental challenges we face. This is a neverending process, and our approach to it is heavily influenced through the mechanisms set out earlier. Although there are exceptions to the rule, most of us require a sufficient experience of 'real' relationships within our social networks in which we can honestly explore and make sense of our lives. Without such help, we are unable to think and are left at the mercy of emotional dysregulation.

Our patients therefore present us with two tasks. The first is to give them the opportunity of a significant other with whom a stable link can be formed, and the second is to support them in the development of significant others outside of the clinic in the real world. Perhaps we might distinguish these as the creation of a real therapeutic relationships in the service of creating real relationships.

The Drama Triangle -- Real therapeutic relationships are, however, challenging for both patient and clinician. We might understand this through the concept of the drama triangle as described by Stephen Karpman in the 1960s. It describes how conflict in human relationships can be understood as having three different positions: victim, rescuer and persecutor. Relationships can get stuck in a coarse occupation of one position, but equally, people can move around the positions and even occupy different positions simultaneously.

This is an ancient and universal idea and probably fundamental to human psychological development. Hugh Gee[75] explores this in a paper using the painting of Saint George and the Dragon by Uccello, highlighting that throughout time and in every culture, we are drawn to such themes – just think of the modern hero films. The illustration we are using here may seem a little quaint to our eye, but when painted in 1470, to the average person this painting would have been an awesome, terrifying sight.

These are life and death anxieties, and so, what is being confronted can provoke retreat and retrenchment through complaint or disengagement, even self harm and suicide. If we are to help our patient achieve real relationships, then the real therapeutic relationship must be resilient enough to contain this threatening material.

Arguably, what is so threatening is mourning, both in terms of what has come to pass and a realisation of what can never be. The patient's request to be made 'normal' or to 'deal with' the trauma can have an aspect of a relentless unrealistic hope. Freud's classic paper 'Mourning and Melancholia' is an early exploration of what we might refer to now as the psychic retreat of melancholia warding us against loss that confronting reality brings. Here, the loss is the loss of an idealised version of ourselves and the injustice of adversity.

Grievance and Its Role in Avoiding Grieving -- What Adolph Stern appears to have described in his original paper is a sense of being stuck in a process of intractable conflict to avoid mourning. No one wants to mourn, but for some, resolution is necessarily avoided as it may be protecting the individual from a very serious breakdown. Remaining in conflict can be preferable, through its ability to maintain relationships as well as organising a sense of identity, purpose and meaning.

We might posit that different personality types deploy different approaches to lessen the emotional dysregulation that follows greater contact with these fundamental and universal challenges.

- **Negative affectivity:** withdrawal through hopelessness and helplessness
- **Detachment**: safety through distance and withdrawal
- **Disinhibition**: distraction and denial created through abandon
- **Dissociality**: safety created through control over another
- **Anankastia:** overcontrol, with a focus on detail at the expense of the bigger picture

These are largely unconscious processes and more structural than 'choice', but regardless, our patients are working to mourn the scars of adversity as it affects their life. The adversity also risks giving a profoundly held view that real relationships are dangerous as not only are others unreliable, but also that the monsters within themselves are so threatening and unattractive that rejection is inevitable.

Realistic hope, one of modest expectation and created through real relationships, is not only terrifying but can be the bitterest of pills to swallow. In its place, a relentless hope might take its place, described by Martha Stark as

> a defense to which the patient clings in order not to have to feel the pain of . . . disappointment in the object, the hope a defense ultimately against grieving.

The object in this case is the idealised version of our lives and selves. To go on living, false hope is – it seems – better than none.

The Rescue Phantasy and the Negative Therapeutic Reaction -- Returning to the drama triangle, the corresponding counterpart to the idealised version of the patient is an idealised version of the clinician. This is how we might understand why we are 'asked' to adopt the rescuer position. The patient's realisation, however, that there is no quick fix in the form of a pill, a new home, a type of therapy or whatever is not only disappointing, but unbelievable. Whilst there are times when staff display judgemental, uncaring and even incompetent behaviours, there is a pervading atmosphere that staff are experienced as uncaring or incompetent people.

Complaints can redouble following a 'contact' between patient and clinician in which the seriousness of the patient's dilemma is understood, shared and made real. A key challenge for the clinician is to disentangle when they need to do something different – or perhaps make an apology – from when they are simply in the midst of the therapeutic work. Clinician and patient may hold onto the contact, deepening the relationship and taking the path to healthy dependency. At other times, the contact is denied, grievance taken and dependent vulnerability avoided. Such dependency can be attacked – sometimes through violence – typically to the self but also potentially to others. More commonly, it is through a complaint and occasionally a request to change clinicians. This is what some call the negative therapeutic reaction.

Typically, a conflicted position is occupied in which the patient engages by moving in and out of acknowledging the contact and the importance of the relationship. Disavowal of the contact, whilst maintaining it, is a compromise to make the dependency less threatening whilst allowing engagement to deepen. Acknowledging even small indications of progress is critical, but it can be difficult as it might feel like patient can only 'hug you in the back'.

Boundaries of the Real Therapeutic Relationship -- For it to do its work, the real therapeutic relationship needs to be safe enough but not at the expense of avoiding meaningful, if difficult, exploration. This means it needs to be focused on both the therapeutic task and the needs of the patient as well as held within the confines of the institution, service and role of the practitioner. It also needs to tolerate being rubbished and accept that it is neither omnipotent nor powerless. Boundaries are a remarkably difficult thing to define; however, we would consider the following important.

The Relationship Provides 'Continuity of Care' -- There will be variations depending on different roles, but it means we minimise disruption as much as possible and allocate a lead clinician who stands as a reference point for thinking about the patient, decision-making and accountability. Assuming our ambition is to help the patient live in the community, the community mental health team remains central whether the patient is receiving specialist treatment elsewhere or is admitted to an acute ward.

For the community psychiatrist, whilst not working intensely with a patient, there is a commitment to being available to both the patient and colleagues in between planned contacts. This should also be maintained if the patient is discharged and referred back. This is the provision of the stable other, and a psychiatrist or a GP providing a longitudinal relationship over many years can provide something profoundly intimate. Such an intimacy has its challenges for both clinician and patient and can become highly claustrophobic at times. Working through these challenges can present profound opportunities, say in challenging a perception that they are unbearable, for instance.

Henri Rey's description of the 'brick mother' is a helpful reminder that an institution can also 'hold' a continuity of care,[76] so whilst perhaps less individually intense, it is worth considering when trying to understand the patient's experience.

The Relationship Is Private but Not Secret -- The relationship is dependent upon the safety of both clinician and patient. Appropriate information sharing plays a key role in the creation of safety. As such, data sharing should be on both a need-to-know basis with informed consent where possible. This might mean that when asked by the family or the patient to share information, even if it is with the patient's apparent consent, we uphold the private nature of the work. Modelling from the outset that unnecessary disclosure compromises the therapeutic space, we demonstrate how we consider that our job is to create a stable, personal, private link that can withstand the test of time and vicissitudes of life.

There are, however, limits. Whilst most of the time we can receive information and not transmit it, where there is a need to protect life and limb, we may have to act without consent. This practice is typically set out within information governance policies, overseen by a dedicated team and Caldicott Guardian. In practice, in an imminent crisis, safeguarding concern or for the prevention of serious crime, disclosure through appropriate channels is necessary. It is important to observe policy and process such as disclosure to the Nearest Relative only or directly to social services, the DVLA or the police. This is critical to creating a safe, real therapeutic relationship that is firmly grounded in a legal framework. It is important to not assume that people understand the intricacies of information governance, so being clear and explicit about the boundaries is important and, when in doubt, check and report back to the patient.

Both Parties Are Committed to the Relationship -- Perhaps the most challenging aspect for the clinician, patient and institution is a commitment to long-term therapeutic caring relationships as distinct from time-limited interventions.[69]

These are difficult relationships to maintain and are high risk. The longer they go on for, the greater the likelihood of an incident, say of self harm. As the realness of the relationship deepens, the greater the truth contained within them, and sometimes, this can prove very challenging. These are relationships that are needed and typically not wanted.

Complaints from the patient or others acting on their behalf are common, and yet in the face of such criticism, the clinician may need to quietly recognise the patient's need to furiously disavow their commitment and connection. Whilst the patient may need to disavow the commitment, for the clinician to do so would be catastrophic.

The Relationship Creates an Opportunity for Disclosure -- Our efforts are designed to create a space within which the disclosure and witnessing of difficult material can be safely achieved. In doing so in a way that does not judge and accepts what has been brought, the patient is given an experience of being accepted which, we hope, will help them begin to accept themselves. Therapeutic work can be seen as creating an accepting interpersonal relationship with the aim of creating an accepting intrapersonal relationship.

The Relationship Is Honest -- Disclosure is no use if it is negated or a blind eye turned to it; it may do more harm than good. Staying with the patient and what they bring means holding onto the narrative in a way that is respectful of the truth and acting accordingly as well. This can manifest in quite practical ways such as noting repeated requests for medication or therapy after multiple previous unhelpful attempts or the patient asking to do something that is patently unhelpful. Sometimes saying no is the hardest thing to do, but it might be the most important, but only if you are willing to 'stay with' the patient and the conflict subsequently.

Disclosure by clinicians is very complex. Whilst it is important to draw on personal experience, being explicit in clinical contacts has various pitfalls. Quite often, the urge to disclose something can be made use of in such a way that still respects the focus on meeting the patient's needs. Our advice is to make use of colleagues to consider any disclosure beforehand.

Group versus Individual and Education versus Therapy

Some therapeutic approaches are considered more educational than therapy, whilst therapies might be more cognitive and others more emergent and relational. There is a lack of evidence exploring the nature of these different components and who they work best for and when. However, if we use the drama triangle to consider this, there are certain things we can do to turn the heat of the interaction down.

Group work, especially if it is psychoeducational, is one way to do so. Having other people in the room lessens the intensity of interactions between individuals as members do not get so stuck in a particular position. This means that whilst there might be moments when one is in the thick of it, there are also opportunities to observe others when they are helped by others in the group who have the advantage of being less invested in and therefore dysregulated in a moment.

Dialectical behavioural therapy (DBT), Systems training for emotional predictability and problem solving (STEPPS) and emotional regulation groups (ERG) strictly focus on the material being learnt and avoid narrative to lessen dysregulation. As such, discussing events that might be very shameful, for instance, are avoided.

Whilst such approaches are helpful in engaging and managing harmful behaviours, sometimes there is a sense that they don't sufficiently give the experience of depth in connection. Many programmes therefore run group and individual contacts alongside one another to manage this. However, some models are more relational than others – schema, MBT and psychodynamic interventions being highly relational and emergent as opposed to CBT and DBT, for instance.

The greater the structure and presence of the therapy, the better it is at dealing with dysregulation in the present, but at the expense of therapeutic intimacy. This remains more art and opinion than science, but there seems a reasonable consensus that different people need different things at different times.

Assessment

Diagnosis

Standardised assessments tend to be used in research whilst most clinicians construct diagnosis through detailed history taking, clinical examination and exploring with the patient what makes sense to them and is helpful. It is worth stating that diagnosis will always be a limited construct, but it can be a helpful one to organise thinking and arrange for needs to be met. Formal psychometric testing is sometimes used in specialist services but principally for service evaluation.

One screening tool is the Standardised Assessment of Personality Abbreviated Scale (SAPAS). This is an eight-question, yes–no answer questionnaire in which a score of three or more gives a sensitivity of 0.94 and specificity of 0.85.[77]

Diagnostic Counselling

A World Café event exploring attitudes amongst clinicians and those with a lived experience found a range of contrasting views about the diagnostic label but described that such perspectives were influenced by the way the diagnosis was explained, alongside the availability of services and interventions.[78]

A small interpretive phenomenological analysis study noted five themes around receiving a diagnosis.[79] These were:

- Knowledge is power
- Uncertainty about what the diagnosis meant
- Diagnosis as rejection
- Diagnosis is about not fitting
- Hope and the possibility of change

These themes note both positive and negative experiences of diagnosis. The authors recommended that clinicians tailor the diagnostic counselling around them.

A qualitative study investigating the diagnosis of mood disorders, which included personality disorder,[80] focused on the potential mismatch between the clinicians' assumptions about receiving a diagnosis and the patient experience. Instilling hope through discussing available treatments and that symptoms improve over time can impact the experience of diagnosis.

A systematic review[81] highlights the importance of a considered and confident counselling in shaping attitudes and imparting hope to the patient. They found the following were likely to reinforce the perception of stigma and rejection:

- A lack of information about the diagnosis
- A reluctance by professionals to convey the diagnosis
- A withheld diagnosis

Positive interpretations of the diagnosis included:

- Efficacy in providing a clearer understanding of the self
- The diagnosis helping to make sense of their difficulties
- Connecting with others

Diagnostic counselling in the clinical encounter plays a crucial role in establishing trust, and many patients find the diagnosis of personality disorder a helpful construct. That said, it is often helpful to be open about the different experiences people describe, the stigma and that some find it patently unhelpful. Some consider complex post-traumatic stress disorder more accurate as well as validating, whilst others find depression and anxiety more fitting. We advocate a pragmatic approach that is more interested in engagement and exploration, whilst trying to uphold the need to be honest. Regardless of which diagnosis is used, our task is to inform the patient and ensure access to the most fitting care and treatment. What is explored in the session and what is placed on a clinic letter will allow for discretion, and service design needs to adopt a similarly pragmatic and flexible approach.

Recovery Colleges have a particularly important role in supplementing counselling, and an example of this synergy along with a pragmatic approach to diagnosis can be found in the evaluation of the course Learning About Thinking Emotions & Relationships (LATER).[82]

Formulation

Formulation is the process of understanding the meaning within the patient's presentation. As we get to know the patient, we understand what and why they are troubled. In the creation of a formulation, not only are we co-creating a plan driven by the patient's agenda, but we are also giving them an experience of being understood.

As is now clear to the reader, the creation of a formulation is a disturbing process. A review of formulations found that while they most often instilled hope and understanding, some found it upsetting.[83]

There are different approaches, and for simplicity, we will give two that are in common use.

The 'Five Ps' of Formulation

Perhaps the simplest structure and one that may more accurately be considered a history-gathering approach.

Presenting Problem -- Current difficulties and how they affect the person's life at that time. A TIC approach would frame this question as 'what has happened to you?' as opposed to 'what is wrong with you?'

Predisposing Factors -- Biological, psychological and social factors that pose a risk of developing a specific problem.

Precipitating Factors -- Real world events that preceded and influenced the onset of the problem. Examples are often social but could include trauma or changes in health.

Perpetuating Factors -- Factors that maintain the current difficulties and can be wide ranging – for example, substance use, staying in an abusive relationship or insomnia. Can also be internal, such as the personal templates people have developed for thinking about themselves, others and the world.

Protective Factors -- Include support, skill, interests or anything that results in a high change of reducing symptoms.

This might be considered a 'strengths-based' question, with some advocating this should be placed right at the beginning of an assessment. Again, these can also be personal templates of thinking, as well as behaviours that may have both helpful and unhelpful qualities.

Power Threat Meaning Framework

Published by the British Psychological Society, the power threat meaning framework (PTM)[84] is described as a structure for identifying patterns in emotional distress, unusual experiences and troubling behaviour. Although purported to be an alternative to psychiatric classification, it lacks an epidemiological underpinning and syndromic classification system. It is included here as a formulation tool.

The PTM identifies patterns of emotional distress in the following domains with subcategories:

Power: What Has Happened to You? -- Describe what it is that has affected you. In this context, this will likely be an act of omission or commission that has had a negative impact upon the person. It may include something from any of these areas

- Biological or embodied
- Coercive and restrictive
- Legal
- Economic and material
- Ideological
- Social, cultural and spiritual
- Interpersonal and relational, including moderation by available resources

Threat: How Did It Affect You? -- Describe how the above power operation has impacted upon you. This could include, for instance, emotional distress, effect on the sense of belonging, loss of self-expression, or a fear to life and limb.

Meaning: What Sense Did You Make Of It? -- Describe the experience of the meaning of the power problem and the way it threatened the individual. We are particularly interested in the threat responses. Explore with the patient what they did to survive. This might be automatic biological responses or more consciously selected ones with a range of behavioural consequences, such as self harm, addictions or remaining in abusive relationships.

The framework helps identify broad patterns of threat responses and the meaning encapsulated within them. The aim is that an individual narrative is developed as opposed to one defined externally by diagnosis and, in doing so, encourages the patient to develop a curiosity about their internal world. When the conversation begins to explore how the patient responded, strengths are inevitably exhibited, and the patient can begin to own their agency.

Risk Assessment and Management

The NICE Self Harm Guidance does not recommend the use of actuarial risk assessments – the categorisation of risk as high or low is likely to do more harm than good. In keeping with this and the adage that past behaviour is the best predictor of future behaviour, we recommend a succinct summary of risk behaviours.

Considering our legal duties and ethical framework enshrined in the Mental Health Act, we suggest organising descriptions of risk along the lines of the 3rd criterion for detention (i.e. risks to self, health and others).

For pragmatic reasons, we are going to focus briefly on risks to self. These can take many forms – most obviously self harm and suicide – but also include addictions, self-neglect and exposure to domestic violence and many others. When exploring risk of suicide, there are some key considerations:

- Although risk factors for completed suicide do change, they are more often static. These include being male, the presence of physical health problems and any history of deliberate self harm, mental disorder or substance misuse. A list of previous incidents is not required, simply the presence or absence of a factor.
- Understanding the lethality of a suicidal act includes exploring any preparations for death to manage personal affairs, the use of an apparent lethal means and an avoidance of discovery. Survival after such acts should make the clinician extremely cautious in constructing plans.

Approaches to risk management should hold in mind the importance of engagement around the specific problem. This is probably also true in considering the risks to others. The clinician is therefore often presented with the dilemma that the more they manage the risk for patients, the greater the longer-term risk to the patient. Crisis interventions, particularly those involving detention, tend to undermine developing ways of managing distress and dysregulation, especially if they are continued for any length of time. Restrictions and round-the-clock supervision might provide the patient and clinician with a sense of relief, but at the same time, they tend to harm the very things that make life worth living through disrupting meaningful social and occupational activity.

Documentation of risk should explore these factors and describe the risk dilemmas the clinicians and the patient are tussling with. Furthermore, whilst a plan might exclude a crisis intervention, other – more appropriate – interventions should be considered instead, such as a contact with a clinician they know. Regardless of the decision, scrutinising it through case discussion and sharing responsibility with colleagues is an important part of managing one's own anxiety and so help to create a more thoughtful response.

Tasks of Care and Treatment

We are going to describe treatment as having three tasks, which have both a fractal and circular nature to them in that they can describe each individual session as well as a treatment programme overall: stabilise, explore and consolidate (see Figure 7.2.2). Progress is not linear, and these distinctions are artificial in that we use them to help reflect on the work.

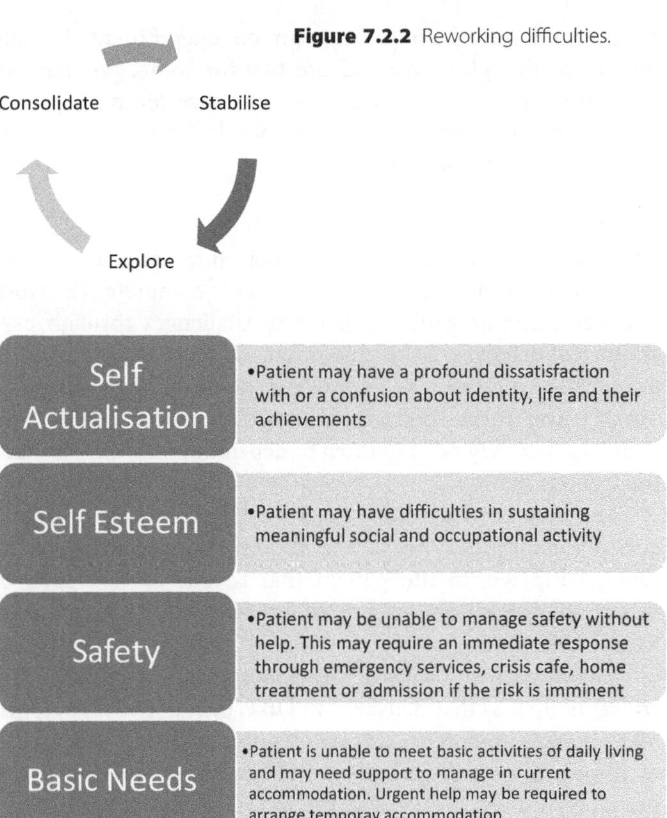

Figure 7.2.2 Reworking difficulties.

Figure 7.2.3 Initial task – to work out where you are.

It may also be helpful to consider that some roles have a greater emphasis on delivering treatments or interventions, such as psychologists, psychotherapists or occupational therapists, whilst others are more designed to organise and deliver longitudinal care, such as doctors, nurses, social workers and support workers. This is also a forced dichotomy, but a key consideration is to support colleagues to keep to the confines of their role and service.

Stabilise

Although many present in crisis, every single referral and every re-encounter will involve some degree of anxiety and a need to settle and re-establish the connection. For those with whom there is no previous contact or are amid a crisis, this is more obvious, but it is equally true of an encounter within an established relationship. The first task is to work out where you are.

This may require active enquiry, and Maslow's hierarchy of needs is a helpful aide memoire (see Figure 7.2.3). It is important to acknowledge that a patient's priority may not follow the hierarchy, yet we should still follow it, even as the salience of substance misuse or other harmful behaviours can sometimes over-ride this hierarchy. Without safety, nothing more significant can be achieved. This may mean that goal setting needs to be negotiated whilst avoiding power battles by accepting one's powerlessness. This can be sobering for the patient and may help focus them on engagement. Equally important though is to recognise that for some, problems of self-actualisation may become as life threatening as those arising out of failing to meet basic needs. The sense of a life not lived can provoke suicidality.

Explore

Engaging someone in exploring their internal and external world is not straightforward, nor is it ever complete. The work is uncertain, emergent and liable to challenges through psychological defences. Difficulties might arise out of confronting unrealistic expectations or out of the shame and guilt that arise out of being understood, or perhaps the fear that comes from realising that they need to learn to depend upon others to have their needs met.

The aim is to develop a culture of enquiry and stoke a curiosity about their mind and, in doing so, create an internal relationship within the patient that is able to take note of things in order develop a broader presence of mind, even when under stress.

Such a curiosity may be developed by learning skills and concepts such as that delivered in DBT, or it may be developed by learning to mentalise through being coached by a clinician, or it may be supported by simply being shown an interest in, perhaps all three. Either way the job is to help the patient sit more comfortably in their internal world and to exist more comfortably in the external one.

We are all conflicted about engaging in such a process as it means deepening a real therapeutic relationship through the exploration of truth. Although the clinician might not disclose the personal meaning, this is a mutual process and provokes our own personal, sometimes painful, reflections. For our patients, however, it is understandably more challenging as there is a power imbalance; the focus is on them, and they are kept out of the clinician's private life, so they don't get to explicitly see the meaning to the clinician.

Learning is a painful process, and ambivalence is integral even if it is disavowed. Exploration in a boundaried manner involves making connections and maintaining a presence focused on the therapeutic task, which can feel threatening – particularly as we are holding a narrative, which in some cases may stretch over many years. Holding such a story might mean grappling with demands that are either harmful or unhelpfully collusive, such as through the dismissal or denigration of another or through a request that seems unrealistic. Understanding what lies behind such requests and assertions can be experienced as a challenge, and the patient may be feel judged when a harmful or therapy-interfering behaviour is opened up.

Dealing with the aftermath of a meaningful contact can produce a movement away from it or a denial. This can occur in the moment, but equally it may arise out of contacts that are more apparently warm or easy. This is often later in the gap between sessions and might be understood that, whilst making sense of the past can bring relief, it can also bring sadness, anxiety, shame and guilt.

Some interventions are more focused on implicit exploration as opposed to more explicit enquiry. Occupational, vocational and social interventions can support the establishment of activities that powerfully challenge core beliefs, say through belonging to a group or perhaps through self-reflection through social activity and observation of others within their community. Here the patient is developing skills to manage their emotional world whilst also developing interpersonal skills and problem solving but through approaches which are used on a daily basis.

It is in these interventions where changes to the patient's social environment are made to develop activities of daily living as well as social and occupational activities – ultimately with the aim of broadening their relational field and creating real relationships alongside the real therapeutic relationships. Furthermore, such activities held within a wider therapeutic framework with a collection of different interventions can support each other synergistically.

Consolidate

Paying attention to the ingredients of the real therapeutic relationship, we aim to provide a safe, long-term space within which the emotional and cognitive experiences of these different areas of therapeutic activity can be understood and developed. One might consider the task is to create a secure attachment figure from which a safe base is established to explore the internal and external worlds. Accepting that exploration will incur destabilisation of that stable link, as described by Bion, is important to validate the experience and digest the emotional experience. The fewer the real relationships in the patient's life, the greater the reliance upon the real therapeutic relationships.

Some consolidation will occur within the interventions themselves, but sometimes a space outside of a therapy or intervention is helpful. This could come from the lead clinician or the care coordinator or perhaps a colleague in a crisis service, or this might mean the individual worker – often a psychiatrist – supporting a group intervention and vice versa in a way that gives the patient space to reflect on difficult encounters or the aftermath of dealing with a meaningful connection.

Such consolidation might be quite everyday and simply reflect a developing sense of reliability and relational permanence. Sometimes, it might be very significant and occur within ruptures within the therapeutic relationship. Such ruptures might become very severe and protracted and could precipitate a crisis. Ensuring that there is continuity of care is critical as a crisis managed within a relationship, even very early on and even one in which there is existing conflict, is far more likely to be resolved without escalation than by a stranger and often involves some form of repair to the therapeutic relationship.

A common example might be the period of mourning that occurs after a substantial therapy. During this phase, a range of complex experiences may arise, and having someone who is not there to replace the therapy but is there to accompany the patient through such a period is key. For some, this might mean drawing on years of experience of working with the patient and a continued commitment to the patient during this phase can have great meaning. The psychiatrist is perhaps uniquely placed for this work, and the long-term, open-ended nature of community work can mean a real therapeutic relationship that develops a particular intimacy as it spans the years. This is not too dissimilar for GPs, except the difference here is that we may have worked with people with more profound difficulties and with a greater intensity and for whom there are few real relationships.

As we get to know the patient, there is a therefore a circularity to the work, and a reworking of the difficulties presents itself. Hopefully, a movement is achieved so that the same path is not simply retrodden, and the circle becomes a spiral with a direction of travel. Recognising and making explicit small changes to this pattern are key to acknowledge the progress to both patient and colleagues, and such reflections then give a sense of real hope and help.

Interventions Delivering Care and Treatment

Most psychiatrists working in the community will lead the care of a small caseload of patients who are care coordinated and a larger group whose care they lead alone. There will also be a larger group of patients who are known to psychiatric service, but whose care is held by the GP. This larger group can be offered an institutional continuity of care and also given a sense of containment, much like Rey's 'brick mother'. There is, however, increasing evidence of the impact of continuity in predicting mortality, acute hospitalisation and out of hours care. This has been largely demonstrated in primary care,[85] but the lessons are equally relevant for us here.

What distinguishes who is offered what has as much to do with individual clinicians and services as it does the patient. However, severity is a poor predictor, and perhaps the most important question for the team to consider is what is the most helpful response and who is best placed to help?

The Organisation of Care

Assessment and allocation

Every patient, whether they have complex or low-level needs, requires a thorough and expert assessment with diagnostic counselling and an appraisal of options and access to psychological education and wellbeing interventions. This is especially true if there is the presence of self harm due to the risks associated with it.

If the patient is actively being cared for by the service, the patient needs to be informed who to approach if they have a question or a concern. This typically means being given an accountable clinician who has oversight of their care. Typically, this rests with a consultant psychiatrist but may on occasion be held with the GP if the intervention is well circumscribed.

In addition to the lead clinician, a range of colleagues from different backgrounds will be brought in at different times for particular tasks. Who, when, what and why depends on the careful and considered negotiation between lead clinician and patient with the overview of the MDT so that the care plan is appropriately scrutinised.

Management of Planned Contacts

Once allocated a lead clinician or care coordinator, establishing a transparent and predictable routine is fundamental; any deviation can be misinterpreted by the patient just as much as it can betray the clinician's disavowed antipathy towards the patient. The need to respect time boundaries cannot be overstated.

Much maligned, the psychiatric clinic can play a very powerful role in the provision of containment whilst delivering sustainable progress whilst acknowledging almost all, if not all, the progress will occur outside of the therapeutic setting. The following are key:

- Creating a predictable setting – keep the same room for each appointment, explain any variations, begin and end on time. Even if the patient turns up late, see the patient for the time that remains.
- Making the next appointment at the end of each appointment there and then is a powerful intervention. Not only does this respect the patient's everyday life and plans, but you know they have the date and time, and the patient knows you are committed to working with them, even if the appointment has just been 'difficult'.
- Ensuring the patient knows how to contact you between appointments gives an experience of presence and being held in mind and an availability whilst also placing you in position to manage any eventualities and underscoring the patient's agency in their treatment.

Management of Unplanned Contacts

Each clinical setting needs to establish protocols for managing contacts outside of appointments. This will need to include a plan for out of hours and establish clear lines of communication between crisis services and the lead clinician.

A common approach is to have established phone numbers and an escalation procedure with the first point of every clinical contact being the lead clinician or care coordinator and from there escalating up stepwise through to the emergency services, if necessary. Quite often the contact is straightforward, but sometimes, an urgent response is required. Agreement within the team about who does what and when is fundamental before you establish these protocols.

Reflecting on any unplanned contacts forms a key task in stabilisation, and any aberration from the agreed plan should be explored.

Interventions Preferencing Stabilisation

Crisis Planning

It is important to hold in mind that self-harming behaviours have a function and a value to the patient, even if they are motivated to change them. Exploring this duality with the patient is important at the outset before exploring alternatives to these self-harming behaviours and strategies for managing self harm events.

Crisis and contingency planning should form a part of every patient's care plan. It is far more effective to plan how to respond to a crisis when not in crisis. Some therapeutic approaches such as SCM and DBT will take the patient through detailed plans, which may include different techniques and skills to reduce and manage distress through behavioural and relational techniques.

Crisis plans should entail a personal escalation plan starting with actions for the individual, drawing on their own real relationships, and then incrementally setting out how professional help is recruited. For a response from a clinician, it should be agreed who responds outside of planned appointments. This is typically those providing the care as opposed to the interventions so as to keep those delivering the interventions on task. When more immediate support is required, it is inevitable some form of duty arrangement, preferably near the patient's team is required, before the inclusion of the crisis team, crisis cafes and 24-hour telephone helplines. Most would accept that A&E or emergency services should be considered as a final option.

Some advocate an acceptance that self-harming behaviours will persist, and harm minimisation strategies should be considered. A mixed methods analysis of patient records[86] classified such techniques as:

- **Substitution**: through use of rubber bands or ice
- **Simulation**: through drawing red lines on the skin
- **Defer or Avoid:** through use of an alternate and less harmful injury
- **Damage Limitation:** through use of aseptic techniques, for example

Crisis and Home Treatment Team

Crisis and Home Treatment Teams (CHTT) are suggested as alternatives to inpatient hospital admissions. A published review of those with an emotionally unstable personality disorder (EUPD) diagnosis treated by a CHTT[87] explores the care of 64 referrals received over a three-year period. In 34 per cent of cases, patients were subsequently admitted to hospital, as CHTT input was not able to help effectively. The study also noted significant polypharmacy, with 68 per cent of patients being prescribed three or more regular medications. Anecdotally, brief episodes of home treatment care well integrated with the community team can present a viable alternative to admission.

Admission

There is no clear empirical consensus for the benefit or adverse outcomes of admission for those diagnosed with personality disorder, but there is a perceived wisdom that acute psychiatric inpatient treatment can be unhelpful. There is a lack of objective evidence for this view, and admissions are common.

Concerns regarding the risk of iatrogenic harm seem to underlie this view, with several different factors involved including the ward environment itself being one that has high levels of emotional dysregulation, that admissions disrupt relationships in the community as well as social and occupational activities, and a perception that professionals assuming the responsibility for risk management creates a dynamic of doing to the patient as opposed to getting alongside them. Other factors worth considering are that impositions through the Mental Health Act and ward practices used to manage incidents risk re-traumatisation.

These concerns are especially true if repeated admission is becoming established as a pattern of crisis. In such circumstances, careful attention to understanding and planning for crisis through multi-agency and across-team case discussion is essential.

NICE guidance is a little more circumspect and can see a role for the management of acute crises and prevention of harm to self and others. Some literature describes unplanned hospital admissions having limited value and potential negative consequences that hinder long-term recovery.[88,89] More recently, the concept of the brief admission suggests it may prevent self harm and suicide in patients with BPD (see Table 7.2.7).[90] Patients described the nursing contact as being a critical factor.

A longitudinal naturalistic observational study[91] found that extended inpatient treatment can result in significant and clinically meaningful symptomatic and functional improvement in borderline personality disorder without iatrogenic effects; however, this appears to have been a hospital with a degree of specialisation.

Other studies have demonstrated well-structured specialist programmes, particularly those with voluntary and highly

Table 7.2.7 Agreed components of brief admissions (BA) from a Delphi Study[129]

• Absence of key community professionals can be a reason to request admission
• Patients can request BAs
• A BA can help patients persevere following therapy
• Plan should be agreed by patient, community and ward team
• Talking about self harm should not be taboo
• Patients can attend ward events on leave
• Nurse contact during a BA is important to decrease stress
• A BA can help patients better endure their daily lives
• Contacts with other patients can be of benefit
• Not all behaviours are to be accepted during the BA
• A stay with friends can be as effective as a BA
• A discharge letter should be sent to the community team
• A BA can only be offered in conjunction with community care

specialist treatment combining inpatient and step-down community phases, have shown a benefit; however, some evidence questions whether residential treatment confers an advantage.[92] Such studies though have considerable methodological flaws due to a lack of control groups, and they fail to adequately include risk and harm into their models of severity nor do they consider the role of engagement and containment, which may allow for these patients to engage in intensive rehabilitation that would have otherwise not been possible in the community.

Compulsion Through Mental Health Act

Although this principally refers to detention in hospital, in some circumstances, community treatment orders have been used for specific indications. There is a lack of empirical data on the use of compulsion in treatment in personality disorder. Where it may be useful is to take control of a crisis in which high levels of distress appear to pose an imminent threat to safety and make clear thinking and the ability to plan impossible. Civil compulsion for longitudinal treatment is, however, increasingly perceived to be more harmful than helpful, and a recent report by BIGSPD into the use of out-of-area placements highlights concerns and a lack of consensus about practice and viable alternatives.[93]

Accepting admission and compulsion have a harmful aspect means careful attention to the 4th criteria for detention is necessary; namely, whether detention is an appropriate (and effective) treatment. For some patients, the management of short-term risks often comes at a cost of increasing the longer-term risks and often for questionable therapeutic benefit. In considering such risk dilemmas, it is important that the clinician document how they have used colleagues and appropriate expertise to scrutinise such decisions so that a thoughtful plan is created, and responsibility is appropriately distributed within the institution.

Pharmacological Treatments

Use of medication is not recommended unless it is for comorbid conditions such as depression.[94] This guidance reflects a complete absence of any medications licensed for the treatment of personality disorder. NICE suggests that short-term use of sedative or antipsychotic medication for acute crises may be reasonable but limits this to a low number of weeks.

Although it is acknowledged that comorbidities can be treated with medication, it becomes quite questionable as to whether the emotional dysregulation and negative affectivity of borderline are being targeted as opposed to a putative anxiety or affective disorder.

Despite this advice, 92 per cent of patients with a diagnosis of personality disorder are prescribed medication, much of which is considered off-licence.[95] Internationally, similar results have been found.[96]

There is a dearth of effectively controlled, published research into the use of medications for personality disorder. A Cochrane review[97] for pharmacotherapy of BPD found limited evidence through small, short-term studies suggesting mood stabilisers (topiramate, sodium valproate and lamotrigine) and antipsychotics (aripiprazole, olanzapine and haloperidol) might be of use for affective dysregulation. Evidence for SSRIs in the treatment of borderline were lacking. Since the Cochrane paper, there has been a further systematic review,[98] which does not substantially alter this position. We can more emphatically say that the long-term use of lamotrigine has no advantage over placebo.[20]

On the matter of treating comorbidities, evidence suggests that comorbid personality disorder considerably reduces the effectiveness of medication in depression (or 2.18, 95% CI, 1.70–2.8).[99]

A review paper by Li,[100] exploring the psychodynamics of psychopharmacology, suggested that the taking of medication can be a 'form of organising experience' given its procedural nature. Li also postulates that medication, and the prescription, can be seen as a transitional object. Conversely, it has also been felt to be symptomatic of the need for a 'quick fix' of distressing symptoms, and clinicians should reflect that they are equally susceptible to this desire in reaching for a prescription.

A pragmatic and engaging approach is that this motivation could be worked with benefit to the therapeutic relationship.[101] An important aspect to highlight in the management of medication is that the data suggests that, once started on medication, the presence of a personality disorder diagnosis appears to adversely impact the monitoring and review arrangements indicative of best practice.[95]

It is likely that medication will be used. However, it is possible to ensure that the gaining of informed consent, along with the management and monitoring of medication, is conducted according to best practice. In such a way, we can give the patient an experience of a clinician who is able to tolerate uncertainty, who is supportive but ultimately caring in the way they shape the patient's use of medication. In such a way, harmful combinations or addictive medications may be avoided, or if they are used, their harm is moderated through pragmatic harm minimisation approaches.

Interventions Preferencing Exploration

Occupational Interventions

A recent article suggests occupational therapists should treat more patients with a diagnosis of personality disorder[102] due to the complex occupational work such difficulties bring. In a study by Potvin et al.,[103] participants with personality disorder viewed self-care tasks as painful, and some tasks that patients found beneficial to manage emotional dysregulation were disruptive to social activities.

One key area for occupational therapy is to support discharge from an inpatient admission. Birken and Harper[104] found that patients struggled to develop a routine, engage in social activities and manage their home environment after discharge. As such, occupational therapy (OT) is a key component of working with the patient and in planning discharge from inpatient admission.

Engagement in meaningful occupational activity can be beneficial for some through giving structure and access to social activity and helping to identify competencies. The relationship between chronic emptiness and days out of work is well known, but this can – even after significant psychological intervention – persist.[105] In others, unrealistic and ill-timed expectations can further deepen differences through exposure to social challenges leading to a greater sense of marginalisation. We suggest that just as any intervention can unwittingly be harmful, occupational progress cannot be assumed to be an independent benefit of therapy, nor can it be assumed to be beneficial for all at any time.

Such interventions are best targeted in the context of a broader care plan, which is sensitive to the patient's situation and developed through expert clinical direction.

Peer Support

Peer support has been found to improve relationships and a sense of self for patients[106] and is of benefit to mental health services for personality disorder.[107] A recent paper[108] described two models of peer support for personality disorder. In one form, peer support workers were part of mental health teams. In the other, they played a complementary role to treatment as usual. The paper also considered views of peer support workers, patients and other mental health care professionals. Overall peer support was felt to be beneficial by all the groups interviewed.

Psychological Treatments

This section will briefly explore the most common approaches. It is worth reflecting also on the nature of the interventions, which could be considered to fall across a spectrum with the most educational and behavioural at one end and the most relational and exploratory or emergent at the other.

Short-Term Psychological Interventions -- These are explicitly not recommended by NICE. However, we would caution against a simplistic interpretation of this guidance. Although robust empirical data remains lacking, brief focused interventions within a wider plan and relational framework can be useful. These typically take on a psychological educational approach. Observational data is beginning to report positively, including a 10-week Recovery College intervention,[82] and a 24-week programme also appeared favourable in an RCT feasibility trial.[109]

Systems Training for Emotional Predictability and Problem Solving (STEPPS) -- STEPPS is a once-weekly, twenty-week duration, group psychotherapy for patients with borderline personality disorder. Developed in the 1990s, it is based on CBT principles and teaches patients emotional regulation skills. STEPPS is designed for health care services where resources and personnel are limited. The Cochrane review into psychological therapies for BPD[110] found STEPPS reduced BPD symptom severity, psychosocial dysfunction, dissociation symptoms and interpersonal problems at the end of treatment. These benefits were not often maintained in follow-up. The STEPPS approach had no positive effects on impulsivity and affective symptoms. However, the noted benefits and low resource burden of STEPPS make it a useful approach and can form a part of a wider therapeutic ecosystem.

Cognitive Behavioural Therapy -- CBT refers to several different therapy techniques and has been adapted for a wide range of mental disorders. For the treatment of personality disorders, there are two prevailing adaptations that are most in practice in the UK – dialectical behavioural therapy and schema-focused therapy. We will describe them separately here. For a more extensive review, we refer you to the review by Matusiewicz and colleagues.[111]

Dialectical Behavioural Therapy (DBT) -- DBT is an evidence-based therapy for 'chronically parasuicidal' borderline patients steeped in cognitive behavioural therapy and mindfulness practice.[111] Designed by Marsha Linehan, who experienced the difficulties associated with borderline personality disorder herself, it is the most widely used and studied intervention globally. The goals of treatment are ordered in a hierarchy, with the most important being a reduction in parasuicidal behaviours, followed by therapy-interfering behaviours and finally working on behaviours that interfere with the quality of life.

Dialectical refers to the technique of holding two opposing views with a hope that a synthesis is reached, whilst the behavioural approaches focus on the application of a chain analysis to better understand target behaviours. Through a mixture of psychological education, practice in the real world supported by homework and diary keeping, and reinforcement through group process, alternative solutions are developed.

The full programme takes place over one year and combines once-weekly individual and group work. The group work is strictly focused onto learning skills and problem solving to make the most of the material learnt. It is a six-month programme, repeated to make a full year and structured around four modules:

- Mindfulness
- Distress tolerance
- Emotional regulation
- Interpersonal effectiveness

The individual sessions are directive and structured around the hierarchy of treatment goals, exploring the patient's behaviour in each area between sessions. Detailed chain analysis exploring behavioural and environmental events that proceeded a behaviour is made with alternative solutions explored. Another key concept worth mentioning is the consideration of the tendency to have critical thoughts directed towards the self and others, or 'judgement thoughts', often present within a crisis.

DBT is increasingly used as a stand-alone six-month group for people with less-serious suicidal behaviours, often as part of a wider programme of treatment and care. It is probably the most widely evidenced therapy programme.

Schema-Focused Therapy -- Developed by Jeffrey Young in 1994, schema therapy is an integrative therapy drawing on a range of CBT, gestalt and psychodynamic therapies. It draws on an understanding that pervasive, self-defeating patterns of thoughts, feelings and behaviours called early maladaptive schemas are present in us all, but early adversity can lead to a propensity to these developing due to the mismatch between the infants need and their environment. There are, so far, 18 schemas described.

In addition to these schemas, the therapy explores how these can combine to form 'modes'. An example might include the angry-protector or the abandoned-abused child mode. How the patient enters into these modes and their impact upon the patient in terms of having their needs met are explored. This is largely in individual therapy, but group variants have also been offered.

Evidence remains limited and is exclusively focused on borderline personality disorder. A helpful review can be found by Schneider Bakos and colleagues.[113]

Mentalisation-Based Therapy -- MBT is a manualised treatment approach designed specifically for borderline.[114] Its chief assumption is that individuals with BPD have disorganised attachment and lack the capacity to mentalise. Mentalisation concerns our ability to 'understand actions by both other and oneself in terms of thoughts, feelings, wishes, and desires'.[114]

Mentalisation is an imaginative activity key to self-determination and affect regulation. If our own mental states as children were understood and met by caring, attentive and non-threatening adults, then our ability to mentalise is developed accordingly. Everyone's capacity to mentalise is impaired by stress, and what demarcates borderline personality disorder is the propensity to enter non-mentalising states of mind, giving rise to emotional dysregulation, impulsivity and interpersonal difficulties.

The MBT focus of treatment (Chapter 5 of Bateman and Fonagy[114]) is on the mind of the patient, with encouragement to consider how they think and feel about themselves or others, how this affects responses to others and how this influences action. Prior to starting therapy sessions, patients are often given an introductory course to the concept of mentalising and the aims of therapy.

MBT is offered on an individual and group basis with a recommended duration of 18 months. Given it is a manualised treatment, it has less stringent criteria for applications to training (for example, there is no need for personal psychotherapy).

Psychodynamic Therapy -- The term psychodynamic refers to the mind being an ever-changing system consisting of conscious and unconscious elements.[115] It is based on the idea that there is unconscious mental activity that affects our conscious feelings, thoughts and behaviours.

The therapist in psychodynamic therapy seeks to understand the ways in which the patient is affected by thoughts and feelings that are unconscious. This information can come from a variety of sources, both from descriptions of external events or the relationship between patient and therapist. The therapist must decide if they disclose their interpretations or take a more supportive stance and allow awareness to develop over time.

Psychodynamic therapy is not a manualised treatment, which makes it difficult to empirically investigate. Other variables such as a therapist's particular therapeutic stance, number of sessions per week or durations of treatment complicate a standardised approach to therapy.

The term has become a bit of a catch-all and may include psychoanalytically orientated therapy, transference-focused therapy and simply psychodynamic counselling. The reader will also note the considerable overlap with other therapies.

Some have attempted to manualise psychodynamic therapy, and perhaps the most widely adopted version is transference-focused psychotherapy, which was developed specifically for borderline pathology. In an RCT comparison with mainstream psychotherapy, whilst both approaches demonstrated an improvement, TFP was more efficacious in changing borderline symptomatology, psychosocial functioning and personality organisation.[116]

The Tavistock Adult Depression Study is relevant to this area given its 'ecological' approach to the inclusion of patients. This RCT into treatment-resistant depression did not exclude patients with comorbid 'Axis II' difficulties and offered one group individual psychotherapy and the other group treatment as usual (TAU), which was effectively routine follow-up and possible referral for other interventions. There was no difference between the groups during treatment, with a modest rate of remissions, but post-treatment, there emerged a clear difference, with 44 per cent of the treatment group no longer meeting diagnostic criteria for major depressive disorder, compared with 10 per cent of those receiving TAU at 24 months follow-up.[117]

Group Psychotherapy -- Most therapeutic approaches employ groups, whether this is part of a formal therapy programme or simply part of delivering social or occupational interventions. Whatever their form, specialist and mainstream services use groups not only for their pragmatic advantages, but because they are in and of themselves clinically extremely important in providing a therapeutic experience.

Much has been written about the therapeutic and antitherapeutic processes operating within groups. The Institute of Group Analysis defines group analysis as 'a form of psychotherapy by the group, of the group, including its conductor...

[it] aims to achieve a healthier integration of the individual in his or her network of relationships'.

What is probably most relevant to our considerations here is that groups exploit two key processes in providing help. Set out by Pearce and Pickard,[118] 'belongingness', defined as a pervasive drive to form and maintain a minimum quantity of lasting significant relationships, and 'responsible agency', which is essential to behavioural change, are explored with respect to a therapeutic community. We would suggest that these are fundamental to the group process more generally.

Regardless of these more esoteric explorations, group psychotherapy itself has been widely studied as an intervention in the treatment of personality disorder. A recent meta-analysis concluded that group psychotherapy had a large effect on reduction of BPD symptoms ($g = 0.72$, 95% CI, 0.41–1.04, $p<0.001$) and a moderate effect on suicidality/parasuicidality symptoms ($g = 0.46$, 95% CI, 0.22–0.71, $p<0.001$) when compared with TAU.[117]

Art Therapy -- Art therapy is often used in specialist personality disorder services and wider mental health services. A recent meta-analysis[120] considered the use of art therapies in the treatment of borderline personality disorder. Only five studies qualified for inclusion, all of which had small sample sizes, were mostly pilot studies and lacked post-treatment follow-up. The approaches to art therapy were mostly psychodynamic, although they included mentalisation and DBT-based approaches. Patients reported benefits including a greater awareness of trauma, the development of relaxation and coping techniques, better interpersonal functioning as well as being more able to communicate their needs.

A small RCT of cluster B/C personality disorders[121] compared 10 weeks of once-weekly art therapy to waiting list controls. The study found art therapy reduced personality disorder psychopathology and maladaptive schema modes and increased positive measures of acceptance. Concerning the patients' views of art therapy in PD, a large (n=528) quantitative survey of PD patients who had participated in art therapy reported benefits, primarily in emotional and social functioning.[122]

These papers show that art therapy has the potential to benefit patients with personality disorder, both subjectively and objectively. Whilst art therapies might lack the evidence base of some of the more mainstream interventions, we would agree that art therapy should be universally available given its capacity to engage patients and its flexibility in working alongside other interventions and modalities.

The Therapeutic Community -- TC treatments are a group-based, participative approach to treating mental health problems. Haigh and Pearce[123] describe the development of these treatments from the Second World War at the Northfield Military Hospital to current practice, which is largely in the community, although the Cassel Hospital continues to run a modified residential programme for those with severe personality disorder. TC approaches are widely adopted in community-based residential placements, as well as rehabilitation placements for addictions and some prisons such as HM Grendon.

The therapeutic community model at the Henderson Hospital was extensively researched, and four 'themes' were identified operating within it: democratisation, permissiveness, reality confrontation and communalism. Contemporary theory emphasises the role of exploiting 'belonginess' and the 'culture of enquiry'.

The model promotes patient empowerment through flattened hierarchies and shared decision-making. It is the staff's responsibility to monitor destructive group processes and prevent them from taking over the community, but the patients take on the day-to-day activities within the community. The TC itself does not denote a modality of therapy, although it is particularly suited to group analysis,[123] and other therapies can become incorporated into programmes such as psychoanalytic, DBT and art therapies.

Chiesa et al.[124] compared three treatment programmes for PD. Two of the programmes studied had a TC component, and the third consisted of general psychiatric management. Participants in the TC model had better outcomes than the general psychiatric model at the end of treatment. In a further study at 72 months post-treatment, these outcomes were maintained.[125] One RCT comparing four TCs to treatment as usual for patients with a PD diagnosis showed significant improvements in satisfaction, aggression and self harm compared to treatment as usual.[126]

Nidotherapy -- Deriving from the Latin term for 'nest', nidotherapy describes the systematic manipulation of the environment to treat symptoms of mental illness. A core idea is finding the views, aspirations and understanding of the patient and then trying to realistically change the environment to fit these needs, even if the needs are seen as pathological. It focusses on function rather than symptoms and is heavily patient-centred. It is thought to be particularly suited to patients with personality disorder as it helps shift the focus away from the patient to the environment and is mostly an emotionally neutral process.[127] One small RCT of 12 sessions of nidotherapy found it significantly reduced inpatient bed use.[128]

Therapies Comparison -- Given the range of different therapies, it is very easy to slip into a 'what works best' type of mentality. For the general psychiatrist, this can seem like a very unhelpful competition, and we would advocate that a service develops a broad range of different therapeutic opportunities, given the broad range of patients we treat.

With that health warning in mind, a 2020 Cochrane review of psychological interventions considered 75 RCTs exploring 16 different types of therapy.[110] They made the following conclusions:

- Treatment ranged from one to 36 months
- DBT is the most investigated therapy, followed by MBT

- Pooled analysis showed that the therapies reduced BPD severity, improved psychosocial functioning and reduced depression
- There was no reduction in suicide as an outcome
- No specific therapies showed an advantage on reducing attrition
- DBT was more effective at reducing self harm and improving psychosocial function
- MBT was more effective at reducing suicidality and depression
- Comparisons between different therapies are of limited value due to poor data quality, however

It is worth noting that many patients will not receive structured therapy interventions and that, at any one time, only a small portion of people on a caseload are engaged in an active psychological or psychotherapeutic treatment intervention. Patients will move in and out of interventions and, quite often, not see them through to completion. It is advisable for the clinician to therefore not see therapy as the sine qua non of the task, but to understand therapy and these interventions as merely tools to create a thoughtful psychosocial environment for the patient that can stand the test of time and help the individual make the best of life in their local community.

Conclusion

There are few areas of psychiatry that present the clinician such a personal and potentially rewarding challenge as the field of personality disorder. What we have set out here is, we hope, a way of approaching the work. It is inevitably more focused on attitude and understanding than a list of instructions. Given the foundation in relationship, the individual clinician will do well to draw on understanding themselves – their strengths, wishes and weaknesses – so that they can meet the challenge with integrity. If they do, they will find this work deeply rewarding, even if only quietly so.

This is an area of political controversy though. With its foundations so deeply embedded in inequality and injustice, it requires leadership and engagement. Psychiatrists, with their broad training in biopsychosocial approaches, legal frameworks and leadership are well placed to meet those challenges and advocate for their patients.

References

1. National Institute for Mental Health in England. *Policy Implementation Guidance for the Development of Services for People with Personality Disorder; Personality Disorder; No Longer a Diagnosis of Exclusion.* 2003. www.candi.nhs.uk/sites/default/files/Documents/pd_no_longer_a_diagnosis_of_exclusion.pdf.
2. Crawford MJ, Price K, Rutter D, et al. Dedicated community-based services for adults with personality disorder. *Delphi Study* 2008;88:342–3.
3. Wilson L, Haigh R. *INNOVATION IN ACTION: Review of the Effectiveness of Centrally Commissioned Community Personality Disorder Services.* 2011. static1.squarespace.com/static/649eb5cc35e2d04d639bb189/t/64d0b49fed254708aff24d7e/1691399329191/2011+Innovation-in-Action.pdf.
4. Haigh R, Harrison T, Johnson R, et al. Psychologically informed environments and the 'Enabling Environments' initiative. *Housing, Care Support* 2012;15(1):34–42.
5. Lamph G, Latham C, Smith D, et al. Evaluating the impact of a nationally recognised training programme that aims to raise the awareness and challenge attitudes of personality disorder in multi-agency partners. *Journal of Mental Health Training, Education and Practice* 2014;9(2):89–100.
6. Finamore C, Rocca F, Parker J, et al. The impact of a co-produced personality disorder training on staff burnout, knowledge and attitudes. *Mental Health Review Journal* 2020;25(3):269–80.
7. Dale O, Sethi F, Stanton C, et al. Personality disorder services in England: findings from a national survey. *BJPsych Bulletin* 2017;41(5):247–53.
8. Evans S, Sethi F, Dale O, et al. Personality disorder service provision: a review of the recent literature. *Mental Health Review Journal* 2017;22(2):65–82.
9. Fok MLY, Hayes RD, Chang CK, et al. Life expectancy at birth and all-cause mortality among people with personality disorder. *Journal of Psychosomatic Research* 2012;73(2):104–7.
10. McCrone P, Dhanasiri S, Patel A, et al. Paying the price: the cost of mental health care in England to 2026. *British Journal of Psychiatry* 2008;184:386–92.
11. National Institute for Health and Care Excellence. *The Short-Term Physical and Psychological Management and Secondary Prevention of Self-Harm in Primary and Secondary Care.* London: NIHCE; 2004.
12. National Institute for Health and Care Excellence. *Borderline Personality Disorder: Treatment and Management.* London: NICE; 2008.
13. National Institute for Health and Care Excellence. *Antisocial Personality Disorder: Treatment, Management and Prevention.* 2010. www.ncbi.nlm.nih.gov/pubmed/21834198
14. Lamb N, Sibbald S, Stirzaker A. Shining lights in dark corners of people's lives: reaching consensus for people with complex mental health difficulties who are given a diagnosis of personality disorder. *Criminal Behaviour and Mental Health.* 2018;28(1):1–4.
15. Regier DA, Kuhl EA, Kupfer DJ. The DSM-5: classification and criteria changes. *World Psychiatry* 2013;12(2):92–8.
16. Coid J, Yang M, Tyrer P, et al. Prevalence and correlates of personality disorder in Great Britain. *British Journal of Psychiatry* 2006;188(May):423–31.
17. Orme W, Bowersox L, Vanwoerden S, et al. The relation between epistemic trust and borderline pathology in an adolescent inpatient sample. *Borderline Personality Disorder and Emotion Dysregulation* 2019;6(13).

18. West M. Self-disclosure, trauma and the pressures on the analyst. *Journal of Analytical Psychology* 2017;62 (4):585–601.
19. Hinshelwood RD. The difficult patient. *British Journal of Psychiatry* 1999;174 (3):187–90.
20. Crawford MJ, Sanatinia R, Barrett B, et al. The clinical effectiveness and cost-effectiveness of lamotrigine in borderline personality disorder: a randomized placebo-controlled trial. *American Journal of Psychiatry* 2018;175(8):756–64.
21. Sanatinia R, Afzal S, MacLaren T, et al. Improved mental health among LABILE study participants: a qualitative exploration. *Personal Mental Health* 2019;13(2):75–83.
22. Wampold BE. How important are the common factors in psychotherapy? An update. *World Psychiatry* 2015;14 (3):270–7.
23. Gwande A. *Being Mortal, Illness, Medicine and What Matters in the End.* London: Profile Books; 2015.
24. Main TF. The ailment*. *British Journal of Medical Psychology* 1957;30 (3):129–45.
25. Menzies IEP. A case-study in the functioning of social systems as a defence against anxiety. *Human Relations* 1960;13(2).
26. Hinshelwood R. Psychoanalytic origins and today's work: the Cassel heritage. In: Campling P, Haigh R (eds.) *Therapeutic Communities: Past, Present and Future.* London: Kingsley; 1999: 39–49.
27. Yang M, Coid J, Tyrer P. Personality pathology recorded by severity: national survey. British Journal of Psychiatry. 2010;197(3).
28. Moran P, Jenkins R, Tylee A, et al. The prevalence of personality disorder among UK primary care attenders. *Acta Psychiatrica Scandinavica* 2000;102 (1):52–7.
29. Keown P, Holloway F, Kuipers E. The prevalence of personality disorders, psychotic disorders and affective disorders amongst the patients seen by a community mental health team in London. *Social Psychiatry and Psychiatric Epidemiology* 2002;37 (5):225–9.
30. Lewis KL, Fanaian M, Kotze B, et al. Mental health presentations to acute psychiatric services: 3-year study of prevalence and readmission risk for personality disorders compared with psychotic, affective, substance or other disorders. *BJPsych Open* 2019;5(1):e1.
31. Slade K, Forrester A. Measuring IPDE-SQ personality disorder prevalence in pre-sentence and early-stage prison populations, with sub-type estimates. *International Journal of Law and Psychiatry* 2013;36(3–4):207–12.
32. Fok ML-Y, Stewart R, Hayes RD, et al. The impact of co-morbid personality disorder on use of psychiatric services and involuntary hospitalization in people with severe mental illness. *Social Psychiatry and Psychiatric Epidemiology* 2014;49(10):1631–40.
33. Tyrer P, Mulder R, Newton-Howes G, et al. Galenic syndromes: combinations of mental state and personality disorders too closely entwined to be separated. *British Journal of Psychiatry* 2022;1–2.
34. Herzog DB, Keller MB, Lavori PW, et al. The prevalence of personality disorders in 210 women with eating disorders. *Journal of Clinical Psychiatry* 1992;53(5):147–52. www.ncbi.nlm.nih.gov/pubmed/1592839
35. Bowden-Jones O, Iqbal MZ, Tyrer P, et al. Prevalence of personality disorder in alcohol and drug services and associated comorbidity. *Addiction* 2004;99(10):1306–14.
36. Garcia-Campayo J, Alda M, Sobradiel N, et al. Personality disorders in somatization disorder patients: A controlled study in Spain. *Journal of Psychosomatic Research* 2007;62 (6):675–80.
37. Watts J. Problems with the ICD-11 classification of personality disorder. *The Lancet Psychiatry* 2019;6(6):461–3
38. Moran P, Stewart R, Brugha T, et al. Personality disorder and cardiovascular disease. *Journal of Clinical Psychiatry* 2007;68(1):69–74.
39. Paris J. Chronic suicidality among patients with borderline personality disorder. *Psychiatric Services* 2002;53 (6):738–42.
40. Cheng ATA, Chen THH, Chen C-C, et al. Psychosocial and psychiatric risk factors for suicide. *British Journal of Psychiatry* 2000;177(4):360–5.
41. Haw C, Hawton K, Houston K, et al. Psychiatric and personality disorders in deliberate self-harm patients. *British Journal of Psychiatry* 2001;178(1):48–54.
42. Hudson C, Spry E, Borschmann R, et al. Preconception personality disorder and antenatal maternal mental health: a population-based cohort study. Journal of Affective Disorders. 2017;209:169–76.
43. Bonin E-M, Stevens M, Beecham J, et al. Costs and longer-term savings of parenting programmes for the prevention of persistent conduct disorder: a modelling study. *BMC Public Health* 2011;11(1):803.
44. Pearson RM, Campbell A, Howard LM, et al. Impact of dysfunctional maternal personality traits on risk of offspring depression, anxiety and self-harm at age 18 years: a population-based longitudinal study. *Psychological Medicine* 2018;48(1):50–60.
45. González RA, Igoumenou A, Kallis C, et al. Borderline personality disorder and violence in the UK population: categorical and dimensional trait assessment. *BMC Psychiatry* 2016;16 (1):180.
46. Hines DA. Borderline personality traits and intimate partner aggression: an international multisite, cross-gender analysis. *Psychology of Women Quarterly* 2008;32(3):290–302.
47. Freestone M, Howard R, Coid JW, et al. Adult antisocial syndrome co-morbid with borderline personality disorder is associated with severe conduct disorder, substance dependence and violent antisociality. *Personality and Mental Health* 2013;7(1):11–21.
48. Amad A, Ramoz N, Thomas P, et al. Genetics of borderline personality disorder: systematic review and proposal of an integrative model. *Neuroscience and Biobehavioral Reviews* 2014;40:6–19.
49. Caspi A. Role of genotype in the cycle of violence in maltreated children. *Science* 2002;297(5582):851–4.
50. Gescher DM, Kahl KG, Hillemacher T, et al. Epigenetics in personality disorders: today's insights. *Frontiers in Psychiatry* 2018;9:579.
51. Arranz MJ, Gallego-Fabrega C, Martín-Blanco A, et al. A genome-wide methylation study reveals X chromosome and childhood trauma methylation alterations associated with borderline personality disorder. *Translational Psychiatry* 2021;11(1):5.

52. Ashton K, Bellis M, Hughes K. Adverse childhood experiences and their association with health-harming behaviours and mental wellbeing in the Welsh adult population: a national cross-sectional survey. *Lancet* 2016;388: S21.

53. Porter C, Palmier-Claus J, Branitsky A, et al. Childhood adversity and borderline personality disorder: a meta-analysis. *Acta Psychiatrica Scandinavica* 2020;141(1):6–20.

54. Sonuga-Barke EJS, Kennedy M, Kumsta R, et al. Child-to-adult neurodevelopmental and mental health trajectories after early life deprivation: the young adult follow-up of the longitudinal English and Romanian Adoptees study. *Lancet* 2017;389 (10078):1539–48.

55. Sweeney A, Taggart D. (Mis) understanding trauma-informed approaches in mental health. *Journal of Mental Health* 2018;27(5):383–7.

56. Hatch SL, Dohrenwend BP. Distribution of traumatic and other stressful life events by race/ethnicity, gender, SES and age: a review of the research. *American Journal of Community Psychology* 2007;40(3–4):313–32.

57. Paradies Y. A systematic review of empirical research on self-reported racism and health. *International Journal of Epidemiology* 2006;35(4):888–901.

58. Damasio AR, Grabowski TJ, Bechara A, et al. Subcortical and cortical brain activity during the feeling of self-generated emotions. *Nature Neuroscience* 2000;3(10):1049–56.

59. Damasio A. *The Feeling of What Happens: Body and Emotion in the Making of Consciousness*. 1st ed. Boston: Houghton Mifflin Harcourt; 2000.

60. Matte BI. *The Unconscious as Infinite Sets*. London: Karnac; 1975.

61. Alcaro A, Carta S, Panksepp J. The affective core of the self: a neuro-archetypical perspective on the foundations of human (and animal) subjectivity. *Frontiers in Psychology* 2017;8(Sep):1424.

62. Panksepp J. Crossing the brain-mind rubicon: how might we scientifically understand basic human emotions and core affective feelings of other animals? *Neuropsychoanalysis* 2014;16(1):39–44.

63. Tronick E, Gianino A. Interactive mismatch and repair: challenges to the coping infant. *Zero Three* 1986;6(3): 1–6.

64. West M. The narrow use of the term ego in analytical psychology: the 'not-I' is also who I am. *Journal of Analytical Psychology* 2008;53(3):367–88.

65. West M. Identity, narcissism and the emotional core. *Journal of Analytical Psychology* 2004;49(4):521–51.

66. Álvarez-Tomás I, Ruiz J, Guilera G, et al. Long-term clinical and functional course of borderline personality disorder: a meta-analysis of prospective studies. *European Psychiatry* 2019;56 (1):75–83.

67. Biskin RS. The lifetime course of borderline personality disorder. *Canadian Journal of Psychiatry* 2015;60 (7):303–8.

68. Foye U, Stuart R, Trevillion K, et al. Clinician views on best practice community care for people with complex emotional needs and how it can be achieved: a qualitative study. *BMC Psychiatry* 2022;22(1):72.

69. Trevillion K, Stuart R, Ocloo J, et al. Service user perspectives of community mental health services for people with complex emotional needs: a co-produced qualitative interview study. *BMC Psychiatry* 2022;22(1):55.

70. Royal College of Psychiatrists. *Position Statement 01/2020, Services for People Diagnosed with Personality Disorder*, 2000.

71. Gunderson J, Masland S, Choi-Kain L. Good psychiatric management: a review. *Current Opinion in Psychology* 2018;21:127–31.

72. Bateman A, Fonagy P. Randomized controlled trial of outpatient mentalization-based treatment versus structured clinical management for borderline personality disorder. *American Journal of Psychiatry* 2009;166(12):1355–64.

73. Livesley J. *Practical Management of Personality Disorder*. 1st ed. New York: Guilford Press; 2003.

74. Botham J, Clark A, Steare T, et al. Community interventions for people with complex emotional needs that meet the criteria for personality disorder diagnoses: systematic review of economic evaluations and expert commentary. *BJPsych Open* 2021;7(6): e207.

75. Gee H. The archetypal themes in Uccello's painting: St George and the Dragon. *Harvest* 1995;41: 38–46.

76. International Journal of Psychoanalysis. Obituary: Henri Rey (1912–2000). *International Journal of Psychoanalysis* 2017;82(2):397–9.

77. Moran P, Leese M, Lee T, et al. Standardised Assessment of Personality – Abbreviated Scale (SAPAS): Preliminary validation of a brief screen for personality disorder. *British Journal of Psychiatry* 2003;183 (3):228–32.

78. Lamph G, Dorothy J, Jeynes T, et al. A qualitative study of the label of personality disorder from the perspectives of people with lived experience and occupational experience. *Mental Health Review Journal* 2022;27 (1):31–47.

79. Horn N, Johnstone L, Brooke S. Some service user perspectives on the diagnosis of Borderline Personality Disorder. *Journal of Mental Health* 2009;16(2):255–69. www.tandfonline .com/doi/full/10.1080/ 09638230601056371.

80. Bilderbeck AC, Saunders KEA, Price J, et al. Psychiatric assessment of mood instability: qualitative study of patient experience. *British Journal of Psychiatry* 2014;204(3):234–9.

81. Lester R, Prescott L, McCormack M, et al. Service users' experiences of receiving a diagnosis of borderline personality disorder: a systematic review. *Personality and Mental Health* 2020;14(3):263–83. onlinelibrary.wiley .com/doi/10.1002/pmh.1478

82. Rocca F, Finamore C, Stamp S, et al. Psychoeducation for borderline personality difficulties: a preliminary study. *Mental Health Review Journal* 2021;26(3):226–37.

83. Macneil CA, Hasty MK, Conus P, et al. Is diagnosis enough to guide interventions in mental health? Using case formulation in clinical practice. *BMC Medicine* 2012;10:111.

84. Johnstone L, Boyle M, Cromby J, et al. *The Power Threat Meaning Framework: Overview*. Leicester: British Psychological Society; 2018.

85. Sandvik H, Hetlevik Ø, Blinkenberg J, et al. Continuity in general practice as predictor of mortality, acute hospitalisation, and use of out-of-hours care: a registry-based observational study in Norway. *British Journal of*

General Practice 2022;72(715): e84–90.

86. Cliffe C, Pitman A, Sedgwick R, et al. Harm minimisation for the management of self-harm: a mixed-methods analysis of electronic health records in secondary mental healthcare. *BJPsych Open* 2021;7(4):e116.
87. Turhan S, Taylor M. The outcomes of home treatment for borderline personality disorder. *BJPsych Bulletin* 2016;40(6):306–9.
88. Krawitz R, Jackson W, Allen R, et al. Professionally indicated short-term risk-taking in the treatment of borderline personality disorder. *Australasian Psychiatry* 2004;12(1):11–7.
89. Paris J. Implications of long-term outcome research for the management of patients with borderline personality disorder. *Harvard Review of Psychiatry* 2002;10(6):315–23.
90. Helleman M, Goossens PJJ, Kaasenbrood A, et al. Evidence base and components of Brief Admission as an intervention for patients with borderline personality disorder: a review of the literature. *Perspectives in Psychiatric Care* 2014;50(1):65–75.
91. Fowler JC, Clapp JD, Madan A, et al. A naturalistic longitudinal study of extended inpatient treatment for adults with borderline personality disorder: an examination of treatment response, remission and deterioration. *Journal of Affective Disorders* 2018;235: 323–31.
92. Chiesa M, Cirasola A, Fonagy P. Four years comparative follow-up evaluation of community-based, step-down, and residential specialist psychodynamic programmes for personality disorders. *Clinical Psychology & Psychotherapy* 2017;24(6):1331–42.
93. Zimbron J, Harding K, Jones E, et al. *Out of Area Placements for people with a Personality Disorder Diagnosis in England*. 2022. The British and Irish Group for the Study of Personality Disorder. bigspd.org.uk/wp-content/uploads/2023/07/OOA-Report-A4-NEW-v2.pdf
94. National Institute for Health and Care Excellence. *Borderline Personality Disorder: Recognition and Management*. London: NIHCE; 2009. www.nice.org .uk/guidance/CG78.
95. Paton C, Crawford MJ, Bhatti SF, et al. The use of psychotropic medication in patients with emotionally unstable personality disorder under the care of UK Mental Health Services. *Journal of Clinical Psychiatry* 2015;76(4):e512–8.
96. Paolini E, Mezzetti FAF, Pierri F, et al. Pharmacological treatment of borderline personality disorder: a retrospective observational study at inpatient unit in Italy. *International Journal of Psychiatry in Clinical Practice* 2017;21(1):75–9.
97. Lieb K, Völlm B, Rücker G, et al. Pharmacotherapy for borderline personality disorder: Cochrane systematic review of randomised trials. *British Journal of Psychiatry* 2010;196(1):4–12.
98. Hancock-Johnson E, Griffiths C, Picchioni M. A focused systematic review of pharmacological treatment for borderline personality disorder. *CNS Drugs* 2017;31(5):345–56.
99. Newton-Howes G, Tyrer P, Johnson T. Personality disorder and the outcome of depression: meta-analysis of published studies. *British Journal of Psychiatry* 2006;188(1):13–20.
100. Li TCW. Psychodynamic aspects of psychopharmacology. *Journal of the American Academy of Psychoanalysis and Dynamic Psychiatry* 2010;38 (4):655–74.
101. Williams P. Discussion of Terry Owens' paper. *Journal of Infant, Child, and Adolescent Psychotherapy* 2013;12 (1):10–6.
102. Harding K. Enhancing the occupational therapy role around 'personality disorder' and self-harm. *British Journal of Occupational Therapy* 2020;83 (9):547–8. doi.org/10.1177/ 0308022620947642.
103. Potvin O, Vallée C, Larivière N. Experience of occupations among people living with a personality disorder. *Occupational Therapy International*. 2019; Article ID 9030897. https://doi.org/10.1155/2019/9030897
104. Birken M, Harper S. Experiences of people with a personality disorder or mood disorder regarding carrying out daily activities following discharge from hospital. *British Journal of Occupational Therapy* 2017;80(7):409–16. dx.doi.org/ 10.1177/0308022617697995.
105. Miller CE, Lewis KL, Huxley E, et al. A 1-year follow-up study of capacity to love and work: what components of borderline personality disorder most impair interpersonal and vocational functioning? *Personality and Mental Health* 2018;12(4):334–44.
106. Brightman B. Peer support and education in the comprehensive care of patients with borderline personality disorder. *Psychiatric Hospital* 1992;23 (2):55–9.
107. Ng F, Townsend ML, Jewell M, et al. Priorities for service improvement in personality disorder in Australia: perspectives of consumers, carers and clinicians. *Personality and Mental Health* 2020;14(4):350–60.
108. Barr KR, Townsend ML, Grenyer BFS. Using peer workers with lived experience to support the treatment of borderline personality disorder: a qualitative study of consumer, carer and clinician perspectives. *Borderline Personality Disorder and Emotion Dysregulation* 2020;7(1):1–14.
109. Crawford MJ, Thana L, Parker J, et al. Structured psychological support for people with personality disorder: feasibility randomised controlled trial of a low-intensity intervention. *BJPsych Open* 2020;6(2):e25.
110. Storebø OJ, Stoffers-Winterling JM, Völlm BA, et al. Psychological therapies for people with borderline personality disorder. *Cochrane Database of Systematic Reviews* 2020;2020(5).
111. Matusiewicz AK, Hopwood CJ, Banducci AN, et al. The effectiveness of cognitive behavioral therapy for personality disorders. *Psychiatric Clinics of North America* 2010;33(3):657–85.
112. Linehan MM, Armstrong HE, Suarez A, et al. Cognitive-behavioral treatment of chronically parasuicidal borderline patients. *Archives of General Psychiatry* 1991;48(12):1060–4.
113. Schneider Bakos D, Eduardo Gallo A, Wainer R. Systematic review of the clinical effectiveness of schema therapy. *Contemporary Behavioral Health Care* 2015;1(1):11–5.
114. Bateman A, Fonagy P. *Mentalisation-Based Treatment for Personality Disoders: A Practical Guide*. Oxford: Oxford University Press; 2016.
115. Cabaniss D, Cherry S, Douglas C. *Psychodynamic Psychotherapy*. 2nd ed. Hoboken, NJ: Wiley Blackwell; 2017.
116. Doering S, Hörz S, Rentrop M, et al. Transference-focused psychotherapy v. treatment by community psychotherapists for borderline

personality disorder: randomised controlled trial. *British Journal of Psychiatry* 2010;196(5):389–95.

117. Fonagy P, Rost F, Carlyle J, et al. Pragmatic randomized controlled trial of long-term psychoanalytic psychotherapy for treatment-resistant depression: the Tavistock Adult Depression Study (TADS). *World Psychiatry* 2015;14(3):312–21.
118. Pearce S, Pickard H. How therapeutic communities work: specific factors related to positive outcome. *International Journal of Social Psychiatry* 2013;59(7):636–45.
119. McLaughlin SPB, Barkowski S, Burlingame GM, et al. Group psychotherapy for borderline personality disorder: a meta-analysis of randomized-controlled trials. *Psychotherapy* 2019;56(2):260–73.
120. Van Lith T. Art therapy in mental health: a systematic review of approaches and practices. *Arts in Psychotherapy* 2016;47:9–22.
121. Haeyen S, van Hooren S, van der Veld W, et al. Efficacy of art therapy in individuals with personality disorders cluster B/C: a randomized controlled trial. *Journal of Personality Disorders* 2018;32(4):527–42. doi.org/10.1521/pedi_2017_31_312.
122. Haeyen S, Chakhssi F, Van Hooren S. Benefits of art therapy in people diagnosed with personality disorders: a quantitative survey. *Frontiers in Psychology* 2020;11:686.
123. Pearce S, Haigh Rex. *The Theory and Practice of Democratic Therapeutic Community Treatment*. London: Jessica Kingsley Publications; 2017.
124. Chiesa M, Fonagy P, Holmes J, et al. Residential versus community treatment of personality disorders: a comparative study of three treatment programs. *American Journal of Psychiatry* 2004;161(8):1463–70.
125. Chiesa M, Fonagy P, Holmes J. Six-year follow-up of three treatment programs to personality disorder. *Journal of Personality Disorders* 2006;20 (5):493–509.
126. Pearce S, Scott L, Attwood G, et al. Democratic therapeutic community treatment for personality disorder: randomised controlled trial. *The British Journal of Psychiatry* 2017;210 (2):149–156.
127. Tyrer P. Nidotherapy in the treatment of personality disorder. *Psychiatry* 2008;7(3):121–3.
128. Ranger M, Tyrer P, Miloseska K, et al. Cost-effectiveness of nidotherapy for comorbid personality disorder and severe mental illness: randomized controlled trial. *Epidemiology and Psychiatric Sciences* 2009;18(2): 128–36.
129. Helleman M, Goossens PJJ, van Achterberg T, et al. Components of Brief Admission as a crisis intervention for patients with a borderline personality disorder: results of a Delphi study. *Journal of the American Psychiatric Nurses Association* 2017;24 (4):314–26. doi.org/10.1177/1078390317728330.
130. Stark M. *Relentless Hope: The Refusal to Grieve*. Chicago: International Psychotherapy Institute; 2017.

Chapter

7.3 Antisocial and Other Personality Disorders, Impulse Control Disorders, and Non-substance Addictive Disorders

George Stein

The previous two chapters have covered the broad approach to personality disorders adopted by ICD-11 and has focused on the diagnosis and treatment of borderline personality disorder (DSM-5)/emotionally unstable personality disorder (ICD-11), which is the most common category of personality disorder presenting to the National Health Service (NHS) and with evidence of the effectiveness of treatment. It is the only trait category specifically named in the new ICD-11.

Other categories of personality disorders are encountered in clinical practice, and these are described and named in DSM-5. The most important of these individual categories is antisocial personality disorder.

There is also a category of conditions known as 'impulse disorders', where subjects experience an impulse to commit some action that may give them pleasure and are said to be ego-syntonic yet result in distress to the individual or harm to others, such as gambling and internet gaming disorder. Addictions to substances are discussed in Chapter 14.

Antisocial Personality Disorder (ASPD)

Antisocial personality disorder has been recognised since the earliest times. This may be because of the propensity of such individuals to commit serious crimes such as murder, which would be alarming in any society, and the earliest judicial systems would therefore have recorded these. Thus, as soon as societies such as those in Mesopotamia or ancient Israel acquired writing skills, they recorded the main features of ASPD. In ancient Israel, the condition is well described in the Old Testament in the book of Proverbs written between 800 and 400 BCE. The book of Proverbs is a series of aphorisms and lessons taught by fathers to their sons on how to lead a happy, successful and moral life.[1] In the original Hebrew version, there are several different character types mainly having different features of ASPD, but all these types are translated into the English Bible using the single word 'fool', which entails considerable loss of meaning. The most aggressive type is the *belial* (scoundrel) and is described in a short poem in Proverbs 6.[12-19] This character stirs up trouble, is manipulative and has several key psychopathic traits including arrogance, dishonesty, impulsivity, violence; he sheds blood and mistreats his family. The picture is of an aggressive psychopath, and he fulfils diagnostic criteria for DSM-5 antisocial personality disorder. Other character types described in the book of Proverbs are the *pethi,* who is a psychopath with learning difficulties; the *Kesil,* who also has ASPD; the *ewil,* who is a psychopath with normal intelligence; and the *les*, who is a narcissistic type who also has ASPD.

The modern era probably starts with Pinel,[2] who in 1806, wrote of a condition called '*manie sans delire*'. Among his cases he described was a non-psychotic but ill-tempered French nobleman who, in a fit of rage, pushed a woman down a well. In 1835, Prichard[3] described a condition called 'moral insanity', which comprised 'a morbid perversion of the natural feelings, tempers, moral dispositions and natural impulses without any defect in intellectual reason and functions or any insane delusions or hallucinations', and thus, he was probably the first to exclude cases of learning difficulties and insanity from the concept of 'moral insanity'. Back in France, Trélat[4] coined the term '*folie lucide*' to describe 'lucid madmen who in spite of their disturbed reason respond to all questions to the point and to the superficial observer looked quite normal', while impulsive behavioural states such as homicidal and suicidal monomanias were held to be cases of 'impulsive insanity' in the scheme of Dagonet.[5]

There are also many twentieth-century contributions to this subject. Henderson[6] described three psychopathic types – aggressive, inadequate and creative. The latter accounting for the high intelligence found among some deviant characters. Cleckley (1941) provided a series of detailed clinical descriptions of psychopathic individuals in his seminal book *The Mask of Sanity,*[7] and they included a minister of the church, a lawyer, a physician and even a psychiatrist!

Clinical Features of Antisocial Personality Disorder (DSM-5)/Dissocial Personality Disorder (ICD-10)

Individuals with this personality syndrome tend to take advantage of others, are 'out for number one' and have little investment in moral values. They tend to be deceitful, to lie or mislead and to engage in unlawful or criminal behaviour. They have little empathy, appear to experience no remorse for harm or injury caused to others, and may show reckless disregard for the rights, property or safety of others. They tend to act impulsively, without regard for consequences, and present as immune or invulnerable. They tend to be unreliable and irresponsible (e.g. they may fail to meet work obligations or honour financial commitments). People with this syndrome try to manipulate the emotions of others to get what they want. They tend to be angry or hostile, to seek power or influence over others and to be critical of others. They sometimes appear to gain pleasure or satisfaction by being sadistic or aggressive. They may abuse alcohol. They tend to be conflicted about authority and are prone to get into power struggles. They have little psychological insight into their motives and behaviour. They may have an exaggerated sense of self- importance.

Some severe cases are obviously callous and will have committed serious crimes. In social or family situations, there is a tendency to try to dominate or, at the very least, demean other people. Confrontation on some personal issue may provoke revenge, and among those with poor impulse control, this may rapidly escalate into violence.

Dissocial individuals usually have a clear intellectual grasp of the moral values of society and may even superficially acknowledge that they should change their behaviour. They repeatedly fail to learn from experience or fail to respond to conventional regimes of punishment such as prison. Some may be so grossly insensitive as to be genuinely unaware of the feelings of others, but most are all too keenly aware of the foibles and weaknesses of other people and take advantage of them. A sham apology, or expression of contrition, may sometimes be made, but there is little genuine guilt or remorse. In recent years, research psychologists have focused on the so called 'dark traits' as described by Paullus;[8] these comprise the three personality traits of Machiavellianism, narcissism and psychopathy. Machiavellianism refers to falseness or deceitfulness, externalisation of guilt, emotional coldness and manipulation of interpersonal relations for self-gain. Narcissism is characterised by exaggerated self-esteem and grandiosity, egoism, arrogance and exploitation of interpersonal relations, as well as seeing others as a means to bolster self-perception. These traits are said to reflect ethically, morally and socially questionable behaviour that lie at the core of psychopathic criminality.

Boredom and a low tolerance of frustration are common amongst antisocial individuals, and they are often unable to sustain the tedium of a job or the day-to-day responsibilities of a marriage. Some may resort to thrill-seeking behaviours, such as gambling, promiscuity or substance misuse. In spite of their almost total lack of respect for the rights of others, many have a superficial charm and a mask of civility, but eventually, the mask drops. While some people with the condition – especially when it is severe – may become criminals, it is important to note that the majority do not. Perhaps it is only the unsuccessful antisocial individuals who end up in prison. One study showed that serious felonies occurred only in around a fifth of those who fulfilled criteria for antisocial personality disorder. Rather more frequent are problems with aggression, work and promiscuity. Men tend to have more illegal occupations, traffic offences, arrests and greater promiscuity. Women with antisocial personality disorder are more often deserted, hit their spouses, manifest child neglect or abuse, or have failed to work steadily.

Two psychodynamic mechanisms are commonly employed by antisocial individuals – rationalisation and projection. Aggressive behaviour and unkind actions are rationalised by viewing them as 'hard but honest', whilst those with a more vivid imagination resort to lying. Projection and projective identification permit the individual to disown their own malevolent impulses and attribute them to others. Attacks on other people are then justified, as subjects view themselves as the persecuted victim. Millon[9] pointed out that there are many more people with milder psychopathic traits who are neither criminal nor sufficiently dysfunctional to satisfy current diagnostic criteria. The ruthless and conniving business person, the brutalising sergeant or the vindictive head teacher all discharge their hostile impulses under the guise of their respectable occupation.[10]

Psychopathy and the PCL-20

As noted earlier, Cleckley's book gave a vivid description of all the features of antisocial personality disorder. Hare[11] extracted 22 traits that he thought were central to the condition and provided the first checklist of the main features (PCL-22) of the psychopath; in 1990, he revised this list, bringing the list down to 20 items (PCL-R-20) after having eliminated two items: drug and alcohol misuse as well as a previous diagnosis of psychopathy. Both these items were behaviours rather than trait items, and the final list of the PCL-R is shown in Table 7.3.1. Each item scores either 0 = absent; 1 = present

Table 7.3.1 PCL-R items in Hare's checklist

PCL-R items
Glib and superficial charm*
Grandiose sense of self-worth*
Need for stimulation
Pathological lying*
Conning/manipulative*
Attack of remorse or guilt*
Shallow affect*
Callous/lack of empathy*
Parasitic lifestyle
Poor behavioural controls
Sexual promiscuity
Early behaviour problems
Lack of realistic long-term goals
Impulsivity
Irresponsibility
Failure to accept responsibility for own actions*
Many short-term marital relationships
Juvenile delinquency
Revocation of conditional release
Criminal versatility

Items with an * indicate interpersonal or affective items (Factor 1)

or 2 = present and severe, giving a maximum score of 40. Anyone scoring over 30 is considered a severe 'Cleckley psychopath'. The PCL-R is divided into two factors or clusters of features. Factor 1 corresponds to the interpersonal and affective aspects whereas Factor 2 represents the socially deviant lifestyle. Items on this scale has been widely used in research into ASPD, and it can be used in everyday clinical work to check if the client being assessed has any antisocial traits. In Canada, the PCL-20 is used by the parole board to assess the level of risk in granting parole, as a high score is a reasonable predictor of the risk for re-offending.

ICD-11 has jettisoned the specific character types and instead has a system of rating the severity of the overall personality disorder and then attaching this to one of five domains; for ASPD, this is the realm of *dissociality*. Both DSM-5 and ICD-11 emphasise that the primary disorder in these individuals is one of interpersonal relationships, and it is the severity of this dysfunction that is the key feature for attaching a diagnosis of personality disorder to this malfunction.

Epidemiology

There have been around eight major epidemiological studies on ASPD since the year 2000,[12] with prevalence's ranging from 0.7 per cent (in Scandinavia) through to 4.3 per cent (USA). Although these studies applied DSM criteria, there were methodological differences between them (see Howard and Duggan[12]). Rates were higher in American than European studies and greater in men than women in all studies. ASPD was strongly associated with being male, socially disadvantaged, poorly educated, financially poor and single, indicating there is a large social contribution to the disorder. High rates of ASPD were found in prisons. A recent large meta-analysis of studies of prison populations[13] found that around 47 per cent of prisoners fulfilled criteria for ASPD, with rates being higher for those on remand than for already sentenced population. Amongst prisoners, recidivism is more frequent among those with ASPD, but this is partially explained by higher rates of substance abuse in this group.

Comorbidity is common for all PDs, and ASPD is commonly associated with drug misuse and alcohol misuse, anxiety and depression, with rates varying between studies. The finding that a person could have more than one personality disorder was one of the main criticisms of the older system of subtyping and led the ICD-11 system of 'domains'. For ASPD, *dissociality* is particularly relevant. Both DSM-5 and ICD-11 emphasise the severity of interpersonal dysfunction as the key feature for diagnosing personality disorder in an individual.

Aetiology

As in most other disorders, causation appears to be multifactorial with a mixture of genetic and environmental factors. A meta-analysis[14] of 51 twin and family studies found a hereditability of 0.41 for antisocial behaviours, which is quite high but lower than for the psychoses. The environmental contribution was 0.59, and most of this was non-shared environment (0.43), indicating that individual factors were important, and the shared environment component was small at 0.16.

The most important of the biological factors appear to relate to the brain: an early EEG study[15] showed widespread increased theta activity in both the central and temporal regions of the brain (theta waves are slow waves on an EEG at 4–7 cycles per second) and are found in children and adolescents, but most people mature out of them. The most recent quantitive EEG studies in a population of volent offenders found an excess of both theta and delta activity and decreased alpha activity in the right frontotemporal and left temporo-parietal regions, and these changes were significantly greater amongst subjects fulfilling criteria for DSM-5 antisocial disorder. Using PCL-R criteria to define psychopathy, changes in fast beta activity in the fronto-tempero-limbic regions were greater in those diagnosed as psychopaths than amongst non-psychopaths.[16] MRI studies have found higher grey matter volume in the inferior parietal lobule and white matter volume in the precuneus. Fractional anisotropy studies have found reduced white matter integrity in a variety of brain regions.[17] Structural and functional aberrancies involving the limbic and paralimbic systems including reduced integrity of the uncinate fasciculus appear to be associated with core psychopathic features.

In keeping with these neuropsychiatric findings are the observations that head injuries, particularly in children, are associated with an earlier onset of ASPD. Traumatic brain injury in childhood appeared to predispose to adolescent drug and alcohol misuse,[18] and it was only in this group that criminality developed. Age also has a powerful influence on the prevalence of antisocial behaviours; there is, for example, a 10-fold increase in such behaviours during adolescence. This increase is most likely due to an environmental influence, because the meta-analysis showed that the heritability of juvenile delinquency was only 0.07 while, for more mature adults, the figure was 0.43. Moffitt[19] proposed that there are two groups of juvenile delinquents: (1) a smaller core group with childhood difficulties and juvenile delinquency who then develop adult antisocial personality disorder, and in this group, the condition is probably genetically determined, and (2) a much larger group of more normal adolescents, who transiently venture into delinquency only during their adolescence and who lack any significant degree of genetic loading.

Aggressive behaviour is also a key feature of anti-social personality disorder, and studies have shown that aggression is one of the most stable character traits over time – there is only gradual attenuation with increasing age. Aggression at the age of eight correlates highly with aggression at age of 30, as measured by spouse abuse, self-reported physical aggression and criminality. Among men, an early history of temper tantrums predicts later divorce, ill-tempered parenting behaviours and a poor work record.[20]

Birth complications may also play a small role, but they appear to interact with social factors. Obstetric data on a large birth cohort was collected[21] and combined with measures of maternal rejection in an objective way (e.g. mother seeking abortion or stating the child was not wanted, or the child was brought up in an institution). The study found that around 2% of children with rejecting mothers (thus defined) committed a violent crime as an adult. For those with only birth complications, the rate was just under 3%. However, for those infants who had the combination of both birth complications and early maternal rejection, the rate for violent crimes in adulthood was very much higher, at 9%. Although only 4.5% of the sample had the combination of both birth complications and maternal rejection, this subgroup accounted for around 18% of violent crime for the whole cohort. The study provides some support for the interactive bio-social model and shows how the accumulation of risk factors is probably more important any single risk factor.

Certain childhood psychiatric disorders such as ADHD, oppositional defiant disorder and conduct disorder are sometimes precursors of adult ASPD. Thus, a follow-up study of children aged 6–12 years with attention deficit disorder showed that 9% were later incarcerated, compared with only 1% of the control group.[22]

The early follow-up studies by Robins[23] demonstrated that all adults with ASPD had shown some antisocial behaviour during childhood. This led to the writers of the DSM-III (1980) criteria for antisocial personality disorder to include a history of antisocial behaviour before the age of 15 among its core diagnostic criteria, and this criterion was retained in both DSM-IV and DSM-5. A 26-year follow-up study[24] of young adults who spent time in care (an especially vulnerable group) found that 40% of the conduct-disordered group met the criteria for antisocial personality disorder, compared with only 4.3% of those with no conduct disorder. Farrington found the risk of a poor outcome for childhood conduct disorder amongst those from a criminogenic environment was increased in the presence of adverse family circumstances; these included parental mental illness, parental marital discord, divorce, inconsistent discipline and family chaos, foster placements, and physical or sexual abuse.

Moffitt[19] suggested a biopsychosocial model hypothesising that genetic and obstetric causes interact at a biological level and result in CNS abnormalities that predispose to the characteristic neuro-psychological deficits. Children with these deficits who are then reared in unfavourable environments may go on to develop conduct disorder and the more severe antisocial disorders of adult life, while such negative tendencies may be gradually extinguished for those reared in more favourable environments.

Treatment

The National Institute for Health and Social Care (NICE) has produced a guideline[25] that covers principles for working with people with antisocial personality disorder, including dealing with crises. Its intended aims are to help people with antisocial personality disorder manage feelings of anger, distress, anxiety and depression, as well as to reduce offending and antisocial behaviour. It is acknowledged that no treatment for ASPD based on RCTs exists but that, nevertheless, people with ASPD may present to services in distress, and the conditions that affect them such as anxiety, depression, self harm, substance misuse and psychosis may be treatable in their own right. The latest Cochrane review on ASPD[26] did not find any convincing evidence for any of the eight psychological approaches reviewed nor have any of the Cochrane reviews on pharmacotherapy found any positive treatment effects.[27] It is important to acknowledge this with patients, parents and referrers as well as in court reports, where there may be expectations that the ways of modifying the underlying condition (i.e. ASPD) are available. However, ways of coping with conditions associated with it are available and should be offered by mental health services.

DSM-5 Clusters A, B and C

As described in Chapter 7.1, ICD-11 has abandoned the categorical classification of personality disorder, replacing it with a two-dimensional classification system: one dimension describing severity and a second, which includes five separate domain types, corresponding to the previous trait system. By contrast, DSM-5 has retained the previous categories defined in DSM-IV, but in recognition of the unsatisfactory nature of this system, it has proposed an experimental alternative classification system named the 'DSM-5 alternative model'. This is not in the main text but given in a separate chapter near the end of the manual.[28] This model comprises a mixture of severity criteria and trait domains, although these domains are not the same as those in ICD-11.

Both DSM-IV and DSM-5 have retained the division of personality disorders into three clusters A, B and C (see discussion later), and the way this works is shown in Table 7.3.2.

Table 7.3.2 DSM-IV and DSM-5 Clusters A, B and C personality disorders (PD)

DSM-IV/DSM-5	Main features
Cluster A: Paranoid ('eccentric')	
Paranoid	Suspicious, feelings of perception
Schizoid	Cold, detached, isolated
Schizotypal	Isolated, eccentric ideas
Cluster B: Antisocial ('dramatic')	
Antisocial	Behaviour disorder, callous, antisocial actions
Borderline	Instability of mood, behaviour and relationships
Histrionic	Shallow, dramatic, egocentric
Narcissistic	Self-centred, grandiosity, entitlement
Cluster C: Avoidant ('fearful')	
Avoidant	Hypersensitive, timid, self-conscious
Dependent	Submissive, helpless
Obsessive-compulsive	Doubt, caution, obsessional

The most recent meta-analysis[29] based on global studies of personality disorders gave an overall prevalence of PD of 7.8% in populations, with global rates of cluster A comprising 3.8%, cluster B comprising 2.8% and cluster C comprising 5%. In terms of costs to the community (both financial and social), the externalising disorders of cluster B are by far the most costly and do the greatest harm to the self and others, with borderline personality disorder being dealt with mainly by health services and antisocial personality disorder by criminal justice systems. This global review found lower rates for PD in lower- and middle-income countries (4.6%) as compared to higher income predominantly Western countries (9.3%).

Cluster A Personality Disorders

Three types are in this group: paranoid, schizoid and schizotypal. These PDs may have some relationship to schizophrenia. Thus, in the DSM-IV and DSM-5, they are placed in the personality disorders chapter, but in the ICD-10 and ICD-11, schizotypal disorder is placed in the schizophrenia chapter. Paranoid personality disorder and schizoid personality disorder are neither described nor named, which is in line with the ICD-11 intention to eliminate the named subtypes.

The link with schizophrenia derives from earlier family and cross adoption studies investigating the genetics of schizophrenia. These studies showed that amongst the first-degree relatives of those with schizophrenia, there was a raised rate of people with personality disorders. Most often but not exclusively, these were cluster A types: paranoid schizoid and schizotypal, and these personality disorders were often quite severe.

Paranoid Personality Disorder

Kretschmer[30] described a condition he called *paranoia sensitiva*: an extraordinary sensitivity to rejection by others and a consequent tendency to resist social contacts because of difficulty in trusting others, suspiciousness and ease in taking offence. Sometimes, they may be insensitive to the feelings of others and fail to trust even those whom they should trust, such as parents or spouses, and they blame others instead for their behaviour. As a result of their mistrust of authority figures such as doctors, they rarely present for help. Because paranoid personalities also have a high degree of anxiety associated with almost any type of attachment, they tend to become isolated, resulting in a gradual impairment of reality testing. These subjects maintain their self-esteem by projecting their malevolence onto others, by denying any personal weakness, and by promoting self-aggrandisement through grandiose and persecutory fantasies. Morbid jealousy of a non-delusional type may sometimes occur. A small number may become *querulous litigants*, who may sue other people – often repeatedly – usually over trivial issues. Common forensic presentations include stalking, harassment and violence. An unusual complication of paranoid personality in old age is the so-called senile squalor or *Diogenes syndrome*. These people neglect themselves to such a severe extent that they end up living in extreme squalor. Macmillan and Shaw[31] found that while half their cases were psychotic, the remainder had lifelong premorbid severe personality traits of being independent, suspicious, unfriendly, obstinate, secretive and quarrelsome – a pattern suggestive of paranoid personality disorder.

Epidemiology and Aetiology

The median community prevalence rate is 1% in community surveys; in psychiatric clinics prevalence ranges from 2–10% and amongst psychiatric inpatients, 10–30%. The highest rates of 23% are found in prison populations. Aetiology, as with all personality disorders, is a mixture of genetic and environmental factors. Thus, 30% of family members of those with delusional disorder have paranoid personality disorder traits compared to 3% of family members of controls. Data based on the Norwegian twin register[32] found a heritability of 68%. Childhood abuse was also related to paranoid personality disorder, in a dose-response relationship, even when the paranoid symptoms were sub-threshold for the diagnosis.

Paranoid personality disorder in DSM-5 describes a pervasive distrust and suspiciousness of others such that the motives are interpreted as malevolent, beginning by early adulthood and presenting in a variety of contexts including suspicion without sufficient basis or that others are exploiting, harming or deceiving them; preoccupation with unjustified doubts about the loyalty or trustworthiness of friends or others; reluctance to confide in another because of unwarranted fear that the information will be used against them; hidden negative meanings read into innocent remarks or events; persistent bearing of grudges; misperception of attacks on his or her character or reputation; or recurrent unwarranted suspicions regarding the fidelity of a partner. In all nosologies, paranoid personality disorder excludes psychotic symptoms, including paranoid delusions and hallucinations as encountered in schizophrenia or delusional disorder. However, it is now generally accepted that delusional conviction and strongly held belief lie on a continuum, so this is a question of degree. Paranoia is also a common symptom in psychotic depression, bipolar disorder, delusional disorder and substance abuse, all of which will require a separate diagnosis and management.

Paranoid thoughts that are not severe enough to constitute a disorder are common in the community. Data from the Adult Psychiatric Morbidity Survey[33] found 18.6% reported mild, non-bizarre paranoia. A smaller percentage (1.8%) endorsed the feeling that there is a plot to cause them serious harm, indicating a more serious level of paranoia.

There is no known treatment for paranoid PD, although successful psychological treatments for paranoia do now exist (see Chapter 5.4). However, as many of those with PPD are not in contact with services or only fleetingly so (e.g. where family members seek help or they affect others by their behaviour), a sufficient number of subjects with PPD to conduct a controlled trial have not as yet been assembled. As has occurred with paranoia studies, trials could conceivably be constructed with individuals who will sometimes accept supportive approaches and family encouragement to enter into studies, even where highly suspicious of treatment and despite their central belief that there is nothing wrong with them. Nevertheless, it is important to acknowledge to relatives, referrers and others that there is no evidence currently that psychiatric intervention is effective, although it is likely to be beneficial – in a general sense – to form or maintain relationships with the individual; isolation is likely to only maintain or worsen the condition.

Schizoid Personality Disorder

Bleuler[34] first coined the term 'schizoidie' to describe a trait he believed was present in everyone, varying only in its degree of biological penetrance. He suggested in its full-blown form, it led to schizophrenia. In milder cases, however, he thought it resulted in a schizoid personality. The modern concept has at its core a profound lack of emotion, warmth or any concept of the normal give-and-take of human relationships. This prevents the patient from making or sustaining close relationships. Even in a mandatory situation such as work, communication tends to be formal or perfunctory. Jobs involving the expenditure of physical or mental energy are generally shunned, and activities such as reading or watching television are preferred by people with a schizoid personality disorder. They rarely present with symptomatic complaints and, to others, seem to be introspective and vague. Ruminating about philosophy, science and religion are commonplace and may become the sole concern.

Schizoid personality disorder is similar in definition to autistic spectrum disorder (ASD)(see Chapter 9), and many cases previously diagnosed as schizoid PD would nowadays probably be more appropriately diagnosed as ASD. A recent study using a rigorous personality interview found that around half the subjects diagnosed with ASD also fulfilled criteria for schizoid or avoidant PD.[35]

Schizotypal Personality Disorder

The term 'schizotypal' was first coined by the analyst Rado[36] as an abbreviation of the 'schizophrenic phenotype'. Today, the term 'schizotypy' refers to both people with schizotypal personality disorder (STPD) and healthy individuals in the general population with certain personality traits and a latent liability for psychosis. In ICD-11, this is not classified as a personality disorder but is instead included with the psychotic disorders, as befits its genetic association with schizophrenia. However, in the American DSM system, it is placed in the personality disorder chapter with the diagnostic criteria being unchanged between DSM-IV and DSM-5.

Clinical Features

The category came into being as a way of describing the many people who had symptoms suggestive of schizophrenia, sometimes with a family history of schizophrenia, but lacking the full-blown picture of schizophrenia. Like those with schizoid personalities, people with a schizotypal personality disorder are aloof and isolated, but their inner world is not as barren. There may be referential ideas, odd beliefs, magical thinking and suspiciousness, but these are not of delusional intensity. Unlike those with schizoid personalities, people with a schizotypal personality disorder have some degree of relatedness to others and a feeling of being part of the world. Nonetheless, sometimes individuals complain of feelings of estrangement and depersonalisation, and they may socially isolate themselves for long periods. During these phases, there may be inappropriate affect, paranoid ideation and communication in odd and circumstantial ways. DSM-5 criteria for schizotypal personality disorder is described later.

Schizotypal personality disorder is described in DSM-5 as a pervasive pattern of social and interpersonal deficits marked by acute discomfort and reduced capacity for close relationships as well as by cognitive and perceptual distortions beginning in early adulthood, including ideas of reference; social anxiety; strange behaviour, affect, speech, appearance, beliefs or magical thinking; and unusual perceptual experiences (e.g. illusions). They tend to lack close confidants – other than relatives – and view others with generalised suspiciousness. The symptoms should not be due to schizophrenia or pervasive developmental disorder. The ICD-11 text places the disorder amongst the schizophrenias but states its course resembles that of a personality disorder. It gives a roughly similar syndromal picture to that described as in DSM-5 and given earlier.

The condition needs to be distinguished from normal eccentricity where there is no impairment of function or from other psychotic disorders, especially delusional disorder, schizophrenia and bipolar disorder. The presence of persistent psychotic symptoms rules out schizotypal personality disorder. Neurodevelopmental disorders, especially milder forms of ASD, also need to be excluded, but they usually have a much earlier onset.

Prevalence is low, and the DSM-5 text gives a median prevalence of 1.9 per cent or less. Almost all family studies of schizophrenia have found an excess of both schizophrenia and schizotypal personality disorder among first-degree relatives.[37] Many of the modern neuropsychiatric investigations that have been applied to schizophrenia have also been applied to STP, and these often reveal brain abnormalities similar in type – though of lesser magnitude – to those found in schizophrenia. Modern MRI and fractional anisotropy studies have found brain abnormalities in schizotypal personality disorder. First, there appears to be about a 13 per cent reduction in caudate nucleus volumes in never-medicated subjects compared to those with STP. Secondly, SPD subjects exhibited reduced asymmetry in the middle temple gyrus and the inferior temporal gyrus, which are brain areas associated with language processing and executive functioning. These findings lend further weight to the view of schizotypy being a part of the schizophrenia spectrum of disorders. A heritability of 71 per cent for schizotypal personality disorder has been reported. The conversion rates from STPD to schizophrenia spectrum disorders vary between 20 and up to 40 per cent depending on the duration of the follow-up interval.[37] One of the aims of the modern early intervention services is to reduce this rate of conversion, and advocates of these services claim some success in doing this. There are a few treatment studies that suggest that risperidone and thiothixene have beneficial effects in controlled trials, but as with schizoid personality disorder, getting subjects to take any medication is very difficult so trial data is limited.

Histrionic Personality Disorder

Histrionic personalities turn to others for protection and the rewards of life, and they present with dramatic attention-seeking behaviours. The core features are self-dramatisation, lability of mood, sexual provocativeness, egocentricity and excessive demand for praise and approval. Initially, there is an appearance of openness and some social skill. However, the histrionic person is also shallow, flirtatious and manipulative. Hyperbolic speech and melodramatic descriptions are noticeable. The outside world is everything, and introspection is avoided. Early analysts[38] stressed fixation at an infantile level, with child-like behaviour and confusion between fantasy and reality. It is more frequently diagnosed in women than men, and one of the difficulties in the older concept is that it represents a caricature of femininity.[39] A meta-analysis gave a median prevalence of 1.3% based on six studies,[40] and a twin study[41] found the disorder had a high heritability, similar to other cluster B disorders, $h^2 = 0.67$.

Comorbid Disorders

Histrionic personalities are prone to anxiety, particularly at times of separation, and generalised anxiety disorder and agoraphobia may occur. It was once thought that conversion symptoms and other dissociative phenomena such as amnesia, fugues and multiple personality disorder were more common among histrionic types, but their frequency is probably no greater than in the other personality disorders.[39] Somatisation is sometimes associated, and the combination of multiple somatic complaints with a histrionic personality disorder is sometimes referred to as Briquet's syndrome. Short-lived histrionic features are sometimes observed among those with depressive episodes but, as the depression resolves, these also cease, and this should not be confused with more long-standing histrionic personality disorder.

The condition is not often diagnosed today – it is a term that can be used pejoratively – and, as it is often comorbid with borderline personality disorder (see previous Chapter 7.2), it is often diagnosed as borderline personality disorder.

Narcissistic Personality Disorder

In Greek mythology, Narcissus was a hunter from Thespiae in Boeotia who was known for his great beauty. According to Tzetzes, he rejected all romantic advances, eventually falling in love with his own reflection in a pool of water, staring at it for the remainder of his life. After he died, in his place sprouted a flower bearing his name. Most people are familiar with the trait of narcissism, and the category of narcissistic personality has been retained in DSM-5 (cluster B) mainly as a result of the influence of Freudian psychoanalysis in the USA. It is not included in ICD-10 or ICD-11, being a diagnosis that is rarely made outside the USA.

People with this disorder have a grandiose sense of self-importance. They may be preoccupied by fantasies of success, power, brilliance or ideal love. They believe it is their right to receive special treatment, and their self-esteem is usually based on a blind, naive assumption of personal worth. These feelings of superiority are fragile, and there may be an exhibitionistic need for constant attention and admiration from others. Depression sometimes arises from deep feelings of envy towards the people that they perceive to be more successful. Criticism or failure will sometimes trigger a personal collapse. Friendships are one way and develop only if they feel they will profit the individual. In romantic relationships, the partner is often treated as little more than an object to bolster self-esteem. Cognitively, they tend to be expansive, with a pervasive sense of well-being. They have little or no idea that their behaviour may be unempathic or objectionable, and others may describe them as arrogant. To call someone a narcissist today would be highly pejorative and so, not surprisingly, the diagnosis is little used in the UK. Using pooled data,[40] prevalence was found to be very low at 0.2% or less.

Avoidant Personality Disorder (AVPD)

Avoidant personality disorder (AVPD), in the DSM-5, is characterised by extensive avoidance of social interaction driven by fears of rejection and feelings of personal inadequacy.

As stated earlier, Kretschmer[30] identified two types of schizoid individual: the anaesthetic and hyperaesthetic type. The anaesthetic type corresponds to DSM-5 schizoid personality, and the hyperaesthetic corresponds to avoidant personality disorder. Avoidant people – in contrast to those with a schizoid personality disorder – will actively seek contact, yet at the same time they are so sensitive to rejection and feelings of humiliation that relationships rarely develop. ICD-10 used the term 'anxious personality', and in ICD-11, the two domains of negative affectivity and detachment are used to describe these individuals.

Those with AVPD are habitually self-conscious, persistently in a state of tension and express an overwhelming need for security. There is a tendency to exaggerate the negative aspects of everyday situations. They feel their loneliness and isolated experience deeply and may complain of it yet, at the same time, also have a strong yet unexpressed desire to be accepted. Avoidant personalities tend to be excessively introspective, unsure of their identity and self-worth. The central dynamic is the struggle between affection and mistrust. Their life is restricted and one of great psychic pain. Among the more artistically inclined, the need for affection and closeness may appear in poetry, or else become sublimated into intellectual pursuits such as music or art. Other people are actively sought out because to be alone with one's despised self may impose an even greater torment, yet other people are also avoided because of feelings of shame and humiliation. They have few friends, although they may wish for more. Relationships are unlikely to be sustained unless the partner provides a degree of uncritical acceptance. Generalised anxiety disorder is most frequently associated, but depression resulting from the miserable lives these people lead may also occur. Social phobias are such a pervasive part of the avoidant pattern that it is difficult to say where the social phobia ends and the personality disorder begins, but some authorities view AVPD essentially as a severe variant of social anxiety disorder. There are, though, several distinguishing features. First, in the avoidant personality, the pattern is much more pervasive, while in social phobia, individuals are usually capable of making some normal relationships, at least within the family. Second, individuals with social phobia are intensely phobic about meeting people in specific situations, such as going to a restaurant or meeting a large group at work, but they are rather less likely to be troubled by relationships in general.

Compared to controls, persons with AVPD are less likely to be married or cohabiting and to be in paid work; they are likely to be less well educated but more likely to be receiving a disability payment. Research suggests that the criteria for AVPD are distinct from schizoid PD, but it also points to a possible relationship with schizophrenia. Thus, an increased prevalence of AVPD in the relatives of probands with schizophrenia has been reported using the UCLA schizophrenia family study data,[42] leading some to class avoidant PD as a schizophrenia spectrum disorder. A median prevalence rate of 1.1% has been found based on 11 studies,[40] while the heritability was given as 0.66. There is very little data on treatment, which is the same as for social phobia, but it is unusual for the condition to improve or get better.

Dependent Personality Disorder

This group is characterised by excessive emotional dependence on others with an intense need for social approval and affection. They suppress their own needs to fit in with the wishes of others. They may be self-effacing, ever agreeable, docile or ingratiating, and this may be apparent in their manners and posture. They search for an all-powerful partner who will supply them with the necessary nurturance and affection and then cling on to them in a dependent relationship. Dependent personalities may make relationships with assertive partners that are ostensibly very close. Many fail to enter long-standing relationships in adult life, but rather choose to stay at home, dependent on their parents until middle age when their parents may pass on.

Freud[43] described oral dependent characters. The word 'inadequate' has since been used indiscriminately in association with personality disorders, but Sullivan[44] described an 'inadequate type' that corresponds to the DSM-5 dependent personality disorder. Beneath their affability, they are searching for attention and approval. Self-deprecation is often used to obtain reassurance or at the very least to avoid reprimand. Self-esteem is low, and they find decision-making difficult, which they leave to others. Other traits include self-doubt, excessive humility, submissiveness and a self-perception of incompetence. There are often expressions of loneliness. This is a state reflecting a person's subjective distress over limited opportunities for socialisation and difficulties in establishing close interpersonal relationships. Despite their strong reliance on others, people high in interpersonal dependency have difficulties establishing and maintaining close relationships, and they become vulnerable to depression when these relationships break down and feelings of isolation supervene. A transient state of dependency resembling dependent personality disorder can occur in normal people after a major loss, and recent losses should always be taken into account before diagnosing dependent personality disorder. Depression may also share a number of features of dependent personality disorder, and dependent traits such as indecisiveness or feelings of helplessness may become exaggerated during a depressive episode but will disappear as the depression resolves.

More severe dependent personality disorders are found among those with the somatoform disorders, particularly somatisation disorder and hypochondriasis. Here, there is a lifelong pattern of dependency, with constant seeking of reassurance in the context of a medical setting. Patients with long-standing psychiatric illness of any type may also develop a dependent pattern, but in these cases, the personality before the onset of the axis I disorder is generally normal. Mattia and Zimmerman (2001) – based on 10 studies – gave a median prevalence rate[40] of 1.9% for dependent personality disorder, with the disorder probably more frequent among women. An estimate[45] for its heritability of $h^2 = 0.66$ is given.

Obsessive-Compulsive Personality Disorder

This category in DSM-5 was previously also known as anankastic personality disorder, and the trait domain of anankastia has been retained in ICD-11. It is characterised by perfectionism, punctiliousness, indecisiveness, reluctance to take risks, rigidity and orderliness. People with an anankastic personality have difficulty with uncertainty and a great need to be in control. Chance has to be reduced to a minimum, and any unplanned situation is avoided. They like routine and may have a timetable for each day, which is not permitted to vary from week to week. They may be rigid in their views, lack spontaneity and – in extreme cases – insist on others adhering to their views and timetables, leading to disagreements and resentment by partners. Difficulties in discarding old objects can lead to hoarding behaviours, and severe hoarding can sometimes be traced to an underlying obsessive-compulsive personality disorder. With regard to money, they may be stingy or miserly and often live at a standard of life far below what they can afford because of a need to control expenditure because of their fear of some future catastrophe.

They present as neat, stiff and formal, although they are rarely referred for this reason alone since these traits, in a milder form, may be valued by society. Minor degrees of obsessionality are not only commonplace but may even be desirable when they underpin reliability and competence, a pattern that should not be classified as personality disorder. Thus, many successful academics who are highly organised and meticulous in their work owe some of their success to their obsessional traits.

Obsessional personalities may present with any axis I disorder. They are readily distinguished from obsessive-compulsive disorder as, in the latter, there are true obsessions and compulsions, and the premorbid personality is usually normal. However, in occasional subjects, the personality disorder and the obsessive-compulsive disorder occur together, in which case DSM-5 states both conditions should be diagnosed. Obsessive-compulsive personality disorder appears to be more common amongst those with Parkinson's disease and was found to be four times more frequent than in an age-matched non-Parkinsonian control group.[46]

Hereditary factors may be aetiologically relevant. Of all the categories of personality disorder studied by Torgersen,[41] obsessional personality disorder had the highest heritability at $h^2 = 0.78$.

Other Personality Disorders in DSM-5

DSM-5 also has a category of 'personality change due to a medical condition'. It is well-known that certain medical conditions such as head injury can result in permanent personality changes. To diagnose this category of personality disorder, there should be good evidence that the personality was normal before the onset of the medical condition and that the changes seem to be linked to the pathophysiology of the medical condition. Subtypes are described according to the dominant symptomatology, and these include a labile type as sometimes occurs in multiple sclerosis, a disinhibited type where there is poor impulse control resulting in sexual indiscretions, an apathetic type presenting with apathy and indifference, an aggressive type presenting with aggressive behaviours, and a paranoid type where the presentation is with suspiciousness and paranoid ideation. Combined types may present as any combinations of these subtypes, and this is common following head injury.

The DSM-5 manual also includes a category of 'other specified personality disorders', where the features suggest a personality disorder but do not meet the full criteria for any of the listed personality disorders and the clinician chooses to give the reason for not making the diagnosis (e.g. mixed personality features). A final category in DSM-5 is 'unspecified personality disorder', which is similar to the above, but the clinician chooses *not* to provide the reasons for not making the diagnosis of a personality disorder, and this might include reasons such as 'insufficient information'. In clinical practice, the presenting features of personality disorder are commonly of mixed types, or the attempt to fit the picture with one of the known categories does not work, and so these latter two groupings are sometimes used. The ICD-11 scheme is more flexible and better able to accommodate clinical pictures that do not seem to fit any known category.

Impulse Control Disorders

The earlier schemes of DSM-IV and ICD-10 both described a group of patients with impulsive behaviour disorders, characterised by failure to resist an impulse that is usually ego-syntonic but often harmful to the individual. The person experiences increasing tension before committing the impulsive act and a sense of pleasure or gratification once it has been completed. These conditions are not personality disorders and probably represent a residual category. They included five main disorders: kleptomania, pyromania, trichotillomania, intermittent explosive disorder and pathological gambling. Compulsive buying is sometimes also considered to be an impulse disorder but was not included as such in either the DSM-IV or ICD-10.

Major changes have occurred in DSM-5, where the corresponding chapter is entitled 'Disruptive, Impulse Control and Conduct Disorders' and included childhood as well as adult disorders. The childhood disorders covered in this DSM-5 chapter are oppositional defiant disorder and conduct disorder and will not be covered here. DSM-5 pathological gambling disorder has been renamed as 'gambling disorder' and has been reclassified as an addiction disorder. It is considered to be a 'non-substance addictive disorder' because of its resemblance to other addictive disorders. A new condition 'internet gaming disorder' is now included in ICD-11, but in the DSM-5, this has been added in as one of the 'conditions for further study' indicating that its status is presently unclear. Also, trichotillomania has been reclassified as an obsessive-compulsive disorder as has escoriation or skin picking disorder, and these are described therefore in Chapter 6.4.

Population base rates for these disorders are unknown, but rates may be increased among psychiatric patients. A specially devised instrument for diagnosing impulse disorders[47] was applied to inpatients who had been admitted for a variety of affective disorders. Impulse disorders were common amongst those suffering from affective disorders, occurring as comorbid conditions. The following rates were reported: kleptomania, 8%; pathological gambling, 7%; intermittent explosive disorder, 6.4%; pyromania, 3.4%; and trichotillomania, 3.4%.

Some patients had more than one impulse control disorder. A French study[48] that applied the same interview to a group of patients with major depression found that almost a third had an associated impulse control disorder. Those with depression who also had an impulse control disorder were more likely to be bipolar than those who did not have an impulse control problem (19% versus 1.3%).

Gambling

Gambling involves risking something of value in the hope of obtaining something of greater value. For the most part, it is a leisure activity, but for a few individuals who gamble to excess, it is far from a leisure activity and becomes a damaging addiction. Since the mid-1980s, there has been unprecedented growth in commercial gambling, and the annual global gambling industry in 2021 was estimated to total $261.8 billion[49] and is expected to grow. This growth is driven by increasing acceptance of legal gambling, the intersection of gambling and financial technologies, the impacts of internet and mobile devices, the spread of gambling to traditionally non-gambling settings and other globalisation forces. In the UK, gambling firms derived 40 per cent of their slots revenue[50] from just 1 per cent of their players, who each lost on average £10,491. Few individuals or families can bear financial losses of this magnitude without experiencing break-ups or a great deal of misery.

Australian and New Zealand studies found the burden of harm associated with gambling is similar in magnitude to major depressive disorder and alcohol misuse and dependence.[51] The gambling-related burden of harm was 2.5 times more than for diabetes and 3.0 times more than drug use disorder. This burden is primarily due to its financial impact, damage to relationships and health, emotional/psychological distress and adverse impacts on work and education. This burden is disproportionately carried by disadvantaged and marginalised sectors of the population and contributes to health and social disparities.

Pathological gambling used to be classified as an impulse control disorder in DSM-III, DSM-IV and ICD-10, but recent research has demonstrated many commonalities between serious gambling and substance abuse disorder, and so it is now classed as a 'non-substance addictive disorder' in both DSM-5 and ICD-11.

Addicted individuals gamble with high frequency, and even though they sustain losses, they return for more and will often seek to 'chase their losses' by increasing their stakes. Their thinking may become distorted, as they often deny their losses or are ignorant of the extent of these losses, recalling only their wins. They do not know when to stop. They sometimes experience withdrawal feelings when not actively engaged in gambling, and yielding to such impulses perpetuates the addictive process. Absenteeism from work as well as poor work or school performance due to their preoccupation with gambling can result in job loss or educational failure. They may lie to conceal their losses from friends and family. They may also engage in 'bailout behaviour', appealing to family and others to bail them out, and this can sometimes result in divorce and separations. Some will become involved with financial crime, including theft, embezzlement or fraud. The matter becomes serious when family relationships, jobs or education courses are damaged. Individuals with gambling disorder have poor general health and utilise medical services at higher rates than matched populations.

DSM-5 gambling disorder grades severity by the number of criteria met: 4–5 is classed as mild disorder, 5–7 as moderate severity and 8–9 as severe disorder. In addition to the change in classification to an addictive disorder, the diagnostic criteria for gambling disorder in the DSM-5 differ from those for pathological gambling (PG) in DSM-IV in two key aspects. Firstly, the critera of 'commission of gambling-related illegal acts' has been removed. Secondly, the total number of criteria required for a diagnosis of gambling disorder has been lowered to four (whereas five were required for a diagnosis of pathological gambling in DSM-IV).

Gambling disorder is described as persistent and recurrent problematic gambling behaviour leading to clinically significant impairment or distress with a need to gamble with increasing amounts of money in order to achieve the desired excitement. This leads to preoccupation with gambling – persistent thoughts of reliving experiences, planning the next time or how to get money – with restlessness or irritability when attempting to cut down or stop. Repeated unsuccessful attempts are made to manage the behaviour but, after failing to win, returns to recoup loses. They will try to conceal the extent of involvement with gambling – seriously jeopardising relationships, jobs, educational or career opportunities – and they may borrow or steal to fund their habit.

ICD-11 has separate categories for gambling disorder predominantly off-line or predominantly online in recognition that a huge amount of gambling is now conducted through the internet either on the computer or phone. The criteria for gambling disorder in ICD-11 are much simpler than the DSM-5, there being only three clauses:

i. Impaired control over the gambling (e.g. its frequency, duration and termination)
ii. Increasing priority given to the extent that gambling takes precedence over other areas of life
iii. Continued escalation of the gambling, despite negative consequences, including significant impairment of personal, family and occupational areas of function

Pathological gambling needs to be distinguished from non-disordered gambling, where severity, frequency and losses are far lower, and the experience is more pleasurable; from professional gambling, where risks are limited and strict discipline is observed; from gambling in a manic episode; and from personality disorders, particularly antisocial personality disorder where recklessness is a feature. Amongst subjects where both personality disorder and gambling are present, both conditions should be diagnosed. Amongst patients with Parkinson's disease, dopaminergic medications can sometimes trigger gambling behaviours.

Epidemiology

The DSM-5 gives figures of a lifetime prevalence for gambling disorder in males of 0.6% and for females of 0.2%. There are higher rates for African Americans at 0.9% compared to white groups, where the rate is about 0.4%. Similar ethnicity differences have also been found in one study in the UK. International comparisons show prevalence rates are generally low in Europe, high in Asia and intermediate in Australasia and North America. There is some interest in the milder forms of gambling (e.g. where only three or four of the DSM criteria are present). This group of 'at-risk gamblers' may be two to three times larger than those with pathological gambling. If prevention is going to succeed, it will be intervention in this group that will be critical. In the USA, 'at-risk gamblers' are more likely to be men, young people, divorced or single, and non-Western immigrants. Furthermore, 'at-risk gamblers' are more likely to have gambling problems in the family.

There is growing concern about gambling amongst adolescents of school age, and it is known to be associated with alcohol and drug use and depression.[52] At-risk problem gambling, in comparison to low-risk gambling, is linked to negative health correlates such as poor school performance, depression and use of substances – such as tobacco, alcohol, cannabis and other drugs – among adolescents.[53] A large multi-nation European country school-based survey found 12.5% of all adolescents had gambled either online or offline, and 3.6% displayed problem gambling. Excitement-seeking gambling is associated with more permissive gambling-related attitudes and riskier gambling behaviours. Adolescents may be prone to engage repetitively in behaviours that generate short-term rewards (e.g. substance use and gambling) at the expense of longer-term achievements, with some experiencing addictions and related negative consequences.

Aetiology is a mixture of genetics and social factors. Rates are higher amongst those with friends and family who gamble. A recent analysis of gambling data in a large American twin study[54] gave hereditability figures of h^2=45.8% for 'common gambling' and 35.6% for 'skill gambling'. At-risk gamblers are more likely to have other family members with problem gambling. Easy availability – such as the presence of casinos – is also a factor, and there is little doubt that the extensive advertising by the gambling industry is effective in increasing both ordinary as well as pathological gambling. The male sex has been consistently found to predominate in gambling over females, but in recent years – in parallel with other societal changes for equal pay and the like – this gap is narrowing.

Females have a later onset, but they progress more rapidly to states of severe pathological gambling. They more often gamble because of depression, boredom and isolation and more frequently use bingo, scratch cards and lotto, which provides a slower gambling experience and hence a more prolonged diversion from their boredom and depression. Depression is also more common in female gamblers. The male pattern is of an earlier onset with more 'exciting' types of gambling such as casinos, cards (especially blackjack), sports and horse racing betting and fruit machine gambling and is more often associated with traits of impulsivity and recklessness. Fixed odds betting machines offer a very intense experience where it is possible to lose a lot of money in a very short space of time.

People stop and start gambling behaviours frequently, and binge gambling may occur. Thus, for a given locality – although rates remain fairly stable over time – during a 12-month period, around half the subjects either cease gambling or move out of pathological gambling status, only to be replaced by an equal number of subjects who acquire this status, some of whom are relapsing from a previous gambling history.[51]

Comorbidity

There are strong links to other addictions, particularly to smoking and drinking behaviours. With regard to smoking, those who both smoke and gamble show higher rates of pathological gambling. There are also links to depression. Modern genomic studies have shown that links to substance abuse and depression relate mainly to a common genetic aetiology. Affective disorders are common, and around 20 per cent of pathological gamblers will have made at least one suicide attempt. Public Health England[55] have estimated that gambling has made a contribution in 409 suicides each year, around 8 per cent of all UK suicides, indicating that gambling disorder was a very significant hazard to health. A systematic review and meta-analysis in treatment-seeking patients found 75% had one or more comorbidities,[47] including nicotine dependence (56%), depression (30%) and alcohol abuse (18%) and dependence (15%). There are complex bi-directional relationships between such disorders. Antisocial personality disorder and ADHD may also sometimes be associated.

Treatment

When help-seeking occurs, it is typically 'crisis driven', often occurring after experiencing severe harm (e.g. suicide attempt). Only 10 per cent of pathological gamblers present for treatment, and there are only two designated clinical centres for treating gamblers in the UK: one in West London and the other in Leeds. However, given the harms gambling causes, there is clearly a need for many more gambling clinics. People who have gambling problems often experience cognitive distortions (faulty thinking), impulsiveness and poor decision-making. Challenging these cognitive distortions is an effective way to reduce gambling behaviour and stay in recovery. Research has shown that CBT reduces gambling behaviour[56] by helping the person identify the thoughts, attitudes and beliefs that lead them to gambling. Examples of cognitive distortions in problem gambling include believing that skills or knowledge can influence the likelihood of winning at cards or sports betting, that playing longer will allow them to recoup losses, and that a certain outcome – such as a rolling a '6' – is due to happen. Clients can be taught how to analyse their gambling-related decisions and motivations, as well as their adoptions of rituals, techniques or strategies that they believe will increase their likelihood of winning. The CBT objective then becomes an exercise in refuting these cognitive distortions by helping clients realise that there is no connection between their gambling beliefs and gambling outcomes.

The Inventory of Gambling Situations is an evidence-based tool that can be used to help identify the situations that lead people to gamble and create an effective plan for relapse prevention.[57] Thus, after identifying what leads a person to gamble, they can then develop strategies to help them change their thought processes, which ultimately can impact their decision-making.

CBT is effective not only in an in-person, one-on-one format but also when delivered in group settings or through self-directed online programmes with minimal therapist support. Motivational interviewing and cognitive remediation for which the target is the various cognitive deficits associated with gambling behaviours have also been explored as possible therapeutic interventions, but their role is yet to be determined.

There have been two double-blind, placebo-controlled studies of naltrexone and nalfemene treatment that suggest significant clinical efficacy over placebo in treating gambling disorder, particularly in treating individuals who are family-history positive for alcohol addiction. A large number of other psychotropics have been investigated, but none have been shown to be effective in placebo-controlled trials. Social approaches such as enabling partners to secure the control of family income sometimes help but are difficult to enforce. Maintenance of gambling abstinence can be assisted by attending 'Gamblers Anonymous', which operates in a similar manner to Alcoholics Anonymous and uses the 12-step approach.

Gambling has always been a morally and politically contentious issue. Some, especially the church, having witnessed and supported families that have been financially devasted by a member with a severe gambling disorder are fiercely opposed to gambling, gambling advertising and any activity that promotes gambling. Others adopt a more permissive attitude, regarding gambling as an innocent leisure activity. This is the line the gambling industry promotes. As a token acknowledgement of the dangers, in its advertising, the industry claims it always promotes 'responsible gambling' yet, at the same time, is fully aware that much of its profits derives from problem gamblers. Presently, gambling clinics are paid for by the NHS, although many have questioned whether the gambling industry itself – which makes huge profits – should not also finance these clinics.

The National UK Research Network for Behavioural Addictions (NUK-BA) was established to promote understanding, research and treatments for behavioural addictions including gambling disorder.[58] They have proposed to the government that they establish a levy on the profits of the gambling companies to (1) conduct independent longitudinal research on the prevalence of disordered gambling (gambling disorder and at-risk gambling), as well as gambling harms, including in vulnerable and minority groups; (2) select and refine the optimal pragmatic measurement tools; (3) identify predictors (vulnerability and resilience markers) of disordered gambling in people who gamble recreationally, including in vulnerable and minority groups, longitudinally; (4) conduct randomised controlled trials (RCTs) on psychological interventions and pharmacotherapy for gambling disorder; (5) optimise the understanding of the neurobiological basis of gambling disorder, including genetics, impulsivity and compulsivity, and biomarkers; and 6) develop clinical guidelines based upon the best possible contemporary research evidence to guide effective clinical interventions. They also highlight the need to consider what can be learnt from other countries' approaches towards mitigating gambling-related harms.

Gaming Disorder

Whilst many individuals get satisfaction from internet computer games, an increasing number of young people spend many hours a day playing them to the detriment of relationships and responsibilities. This is a new disorder appearing for the first time in ICD-11 as a behavioural addiction. DSM-5 includes a similar condition in its chapter on 'conditions for further study'. It is characterised as 'a pattern of persistent or recurrent (electronic) gaming behaviour characterised by impaired control over the behaviour, giving increasing priority to gaming to the extent that it takes precedence over other life interests and daily activities; and continuation or escalation of gaming despite negative consequences'.

For gaming disorder to be diagnosed, the following criteria concerning the online/offline gaming behaviour ('digital gaming' or 'video gaming') must be present for at least 12 months:

1. Impaired control over gaming
2. Increasing priority given to gaming over other activities
3. Continuation or escalation of gaming despite the occurrence of negative consequences

The latter comprises personal (psychological and physical well-being), social, educational, work and financial areas. Non-pathological gaming has little or no adverse consequences.

A recent meta-analysis[59] found an overall prevalence of around 3%. High rates of the problem are found in China and other South-East Asian countries, as well as prevalence rates of 2.1 to 2.6% of youth in North America, 0.2 to 4.4% in Oceania, and 0.2 to 12.3% of youth in Europe. In the child and adolescent population, prevalence of internet gaming disorder as high as 8% have been observed, and rates rose further during the recent Covid pandemic. In most studies, there was comorbidity with a wide variety of other disorders, with anxiety, depression and ADHD being most frequent, but other disorders also occurred. Fortunately, data is emerging that the disorder is treatable and has a reasonable response to pharmacotherapy (antidepressants, methylphenidate, bupropion) as well as to standard psychotherapies such as CBT. Best results were obtained in combined drug and psychotherapy programmes, especially when parents were involved the treatment programmes.[60] In China, there was some resistance to a conventional psychiatric approach as Chinese parents were reluctant to have their offspring tarnished with a psychiatric label, and so parents often opted for a bootcamp approach, which was of unknown efficacy.

Intermittent Explosive Disorder

Typically patients with this condition have recurrent outbursts of temper (tantrums, tirades, verbal arguments or fights), and episodes do not last more than 30 minutes. The degree of aggressiveness is out of proportion to any precipitating social stress, and it is usually triggered by minor conflict.

The episodes can occur independently of any other diagnosis. Individuals or their relatives usually describe the episodes as ‘spells’ or ‘attacks’. Associated with the violent outbursts are feelings of tension, relief after the episode, followed by remorse. Many describe racing thoughts and an energy surge during the episodes, followed by lowering of mood and decreased energy. Most subjects have a lifetime comorbidity with a mood disorder, especially bipolar disorder.

In general, onset is in adolescence, and men predominate by a 4:1 ratio, although some women describe similar symptoms pre-menstrually. The diagnosis is not commonly made in the UK but is popular in America and many other countries. There is some doubt as to whether a pure category really exists, as many individuals with intermittent explosive disorder are usually comorbid for some other condition such as personality disorder, substance misuse, a psychosis or an organic personality change. There is also a suggestion of a link to bipolar disorder, with the episodes representing micropsychotic episodes of very rapid onset.

Intermittent explosive disorder in DSM-5 and ICD-11 comprises recurrent behavioural outbursts due to a failure to control aggressive impulses. This can be verbal (e.g. tantrums or arguments) or physical aggression towards property, animals or individuals and may or may not cause damage or destruction of property or physical injury. The level of aggression is unpremeditated, not for specific gain and out of proportion to the provocation or any stressors. Marked distress occurs in the individual as well as possible impairment in occupational or interpersonal functioning or financial or legal consequences.

The disorder is sometimes sub-divided according to whether the episodes result only in verbal threats to people, in attacks on people, in attacks only onto property or in physical attacks onto both people and property. Attacks on people are obviously more serious than attacks on property alone.[61] A study of comorbidity based on a CIDI interview to a large American population found an overall prevalence rate of 0.8% at all ages, but amongst adolescents (13 years to 17 years), 7.8% met diagnostic criteria, indicating this is primarily a disorder of youth. The following odds ratios for comorbidity were observed: all anxiety disorders, 7.2; bipolar disorder, 6.8; alcohol use disorder, 6.8; any substance abuse, 7.5; and externalising disorders (e.g. conduct disorder), 9.0. Suicidality (suicidal thoughts) was present in 38% and suicidal behaviours in 26%. There were no differences in comorbidity[62] between the different subtypes. FMRI studies[63] have shown specifically elevated hostile attribution and an anger response to socially ambiguous stimuli, as well as an enhanced amygdala (AMYG) and reduced orbitofrontal cortex (OFC) responses to anger faces.

Management of Aggression

Psychological and pharmacological approaches have a place; traditionally, anti-epileptics have been the mainstay of the latter for impulsive aggressive behaviours. A recent review of the topic[64] identified five drugs with at least one RCT evidence for efficacy: phenytoin, carbamazepine, lithium, lamotrigine and valproate, although phenytoin is not licensed for this indication. There was no support for levetiracetam. Controlled trials for fluoxetine[65] show that it may also be effective even in the absence of depression, and these trials found that fluoxetine was associated with full remission of aggressive behaviours in 29% of patients and full or partial remission in 46% of patients, and there is one double-blind trial amongst aggressive prisoners showing a large beneficial effect for lithium.[66] Anti-psychotics such as olanzapine or quetiapine are sometimes helpful, although some patients find them too sedative to continue using them over the long term. The clinician should offer treatment for impulsive aggression, either when it occurs on its own or when it is part of another comorbid disorder as is often the case. Even if the drug fails to abolish the episodes altogether, it often ameliorates the severity or frequency of the outbursts. In practice, initial drug selection may be ‘hit and miss’, but starting with an antiepileptic is common, and then systematically working through the different options may yield a successful strategy. Some guidance can be garnered from the associated comorbidities – for example, if there is comorbid depression, then fluoxetine might be a good starting option.

Psychological management of aggressive behaviours is better known as anger management and is offered by some services in the criminal justice system, such as the probation or domestic violence services, but is not usually offered by NHS psychiatric services. Training in positive and safe management of violence and acute psychological distress is, however, a standard part of NHS mandatory training and is central to personalised relationship-based approaches. These have evolved over time to become an essential part of reducing the fear, confusion and distress that underpins conflict and aggression in mental health settings.

Kleptomania

Kleptomania, from the Greek for 'stealing madness' refers to the irresistible impulse to steal unneeded items, and the DSM-5 provides a useful description. It regards the essential feature of the condition as a recurrent failure to resist the impulse to steal items that are not needed for personal use or that have little personal value. The person concerned may experience a rising sense of tension before the theft and then experience pleasure, gratification and anxiety reduction afterwards. The objects stolen usually have little value, and the person sometimes offers to pay for them, gives them away or sometimes hoards them. It is usually diagnosed in pre-court evaluations for shoplifting, but even amongst shoplifters, it is rare. Thus, in one series,[67] only 13 of 338 shoplifters (3.8%) were diagnosed as having kleptomania.. The DSM-5 gives an estimate of around 5% of shoplifters having the disorder. The DSM-5 excludes recurrent stealing behaviours due to schizophrenia, mania or dementia from its category of kleptomania. Lifetime psychiatric comorbidity is frequent, mainly with other impulse control (20–46%), substance use (23–50%) and mood (45–100%) disorders. The urges to steal and the rewarding emotional aspects of stealing were associated with greater illness severity. Frequency of urges to steal, reporting a positive feeling from the act of stealing, and certain comorbidities (anorexia nervosa, bulimia nervosa and OCD) were significantly and positively associated with illness severity.[68] Individuals with kleptomania suffer significant impairment in their ability to function socially and occupationally. Kleptomania may respond to cognitive behavioural therapy, and there is one RCT showing a beneficial effect of naltrexone; there are also case reports that various pharmacotherapies (e.g. lithium, anti-epileptics and antidepressants) are sometimes helpful.

Shoplifting itself is not a psychiatric disorder and, in English law, it is classed as a type of theft, but it is briefly considered here because it may be the presenting feature for a wide variety of psychiatric disorders. An observational study[69] found that up to 2 per cent of customers who enter a store will shoplift. Most shoplifting is for financial gain, but in pre-court evaluations, different case series have found that somewhere between 5 and 15 per cent of those detained are suffering from psychiatric disorders. Most commonly, this is depression, especially amongst women with low self-esteem, but substance abusers may shoplift to fund their habit, and those with severe mental illness who have become destitute may also do so to help feed themselves. A psychiatric court report will often usefully help divert people away from the criminal justice system to the appropriate mental health service.

Pyromania

Pyromania is a rare disorder in adults and is characterised by multiple episodes of deliberate fire-setting. These individuals have a fascination with fire and may experience tension or affective arousal before setting a fire. They may be both curious and fascinated by fire and may go to watch fires in their neighbourhood or set off false alarms. They often derive pleasure from institutions, personnel and equipment associated with fire and may spend time trying to get affiliated with their local fire department or even become fire fighters.

Fire-setting of itself is not a disorder but a presenting symptom and may result in danger to others and serious property damage. It is more common among juveniles, where it usually presents as one feature of a more global conduct disorder, but it can occasionally also occur with ADHD, adjustment disorder and learning difficulties. Alongside enuresis and cruelty to animals, fire-setting is one of the three behaviours commonly referred as the McDonald triad for sociopathy, which can predict adult crime.[70] A recent large-scale epidemiological American study of fire setters in the general population[71] found an overall prevalence of around 1 per cent and strong associations with ASPD. Around half of the individuals will have used mental health services at some time in their lives, which has increasingly been recognised by fire services in developing their preventative strategies. Men were more likely than women (male to female ratio=4:1) to be involved in fire-setting. The odds ratios of comorbidities with other common psychiatric disorders were given as alcohol abuse disorder, 3.0; drug abuse, 7.8; major depression, 1.8; bipolar disorder, 4.7; any anxiety disorder, 2.8; and pathological gambling, 7.8. The latter figure highlights the association between the various impulse disorders.

Pyromania as defined in DSM–5 and ICD–11 excludes fire-setting as a consequence of mental illnesses such as depression, schizophrenia or alcoholism. Pyromania also needs to be distinguished from intentional fire-setting (arson), where the motivation may be for revenge, profit, sabotage, to attract attention or even to make a political statement. After these exclusions, 'pure' pyromania in adults is extremely rare. For example, in one series of 283 convicted arsonists, mental health problems were present in 90% (36% with a major mental disorder – either schizophrenia or bipolar disorder – and 64% with alcohol), but there were only three cases of pyromania (1%).[72] There are few longitudinal studies and so the relationship between adult pyromania and juvenile fire-setting is unclear, but presumably many adult cases will have had their onset in childhood. Children and adolescents with fire-setting behaviours are often both curious about and fascinated by fire, in contrast to adult arsonists, who rarely show such an interest.

Arson is a serious crime – usually carrying a hefty prison sentence – although if mental illness is present, a psychiatric disposal will be considered. In the nineteenth century, pyromania was classed as one of the 'monomanias', and there were vigorous debates between psychiatrists and Judges at the time whether an insanity defence could be applied. Today, an insanity defence cannot be used in ordinary uncomplicated pyromania.

References

1. Stein G. Proverbs and personality disorder: male types of anti-social personality disorder. In: Stein G (ed.) *The Hidden Psychiatry of the Old Testament.* Lanham, MD: Hamilton Books; 2018: 384–436.
2. Pinel P. *A Treatise on Insanity* (translated by DD Davis, 1962). New York, NY: Hafner; 1806.
3. Prichard JC. *A Treatise on Insanity, and Other Disorders Affecting the Mind.* London: Gilbert & Piper; 1835.
4. Trélat U. *La folie lucide, étudiée et considérée au point de vue de la famille et de la société.* Paris: Kraus Reprint; 1861.
5. Dagonet M. *Des impulsions dans la folie et de la folie impulsive.* Paris: Masson; 1870.
6. Henderson DK. *Psychopathic States.* London: Chapman & Hall; 1939.
7. Cleckley H. *The Mask of Sanity* (2nd ed.). St Louis, MO: Mosby; 1941.
8. Paullus DL. Towards a taxonomy of dark personalities. *Current Directions in Psychological Science* 2014;23(6):421–6.
9. Millon T. *Disorders of Personality: DSM–III Axis II.* New York: John Wiley & Sons; 1981.
10. Casey P. Clinical features of the personality disorders and impulse control disorders. In: Stein G, Wilkinson G (eds.) *Seminars in General Adult Psychiatry.* Gaskell: RCPsych Publications; 2007: 432–87.
11. Hare RD. *Manual for the Hare Psychopathy Checklist–Revised.* Toronto: Multi-Health Systems; 2003.
12. Howard R, Duggan C. *Antisocial Personality: Theory, Research, Treatment.* Cambridge: Cambridge University Press; 2022.
13. Fazel S, Danesh J. Serious mental disorder in 23000 prisoners: a systematic review of 62 surveys. *The Lancet* 2002;359(9306):545–50.
14. Rhee SH, Waldman ID. Genetic and environmental influences on antisocial behavior: a meta-analysis of twin and adoption studies. *Psychological Bulletin* 2002;128(3):490.
15. Hill D, Watterson D. Electroencephalographic studies of psychopathic personalities. *Journal of Neurological Psychiatry* 1942;5(1–2):47–65.
16. Calzada-Reyes A, Alvarez-Amador A, Galán-García L, et al. EEG abnormalities in psychopath and non-psychopath violent offenders. *Journal of Forensic and Legal Medicine* 2013;20 (1):19–26.
17. Jiang W, Shi F, Liu H, et al. Reduced white matter integrity in antisocial personality disorder: a diffusion tensor imaging study. *Scientific Reports* 2017;7:43002.
18. Weil ZM, Karelina K. Lifelong consequences of brain injuries during development: from risk to resilience. *Frontiers in Neuroendocrinology* 2019;55:100793.
19. Moffitt TE, Lynam DR, Silva PA. Neuropsychological tests predicting persistent male delinquency. *Criminology* 1994;32(2):277–300.
20. Coid J. Current concepts and classification of psychopathic disorder. In: Tyrer PJ, Stein G (eds.) *Personality Disorder Reviewed.* London: Gaskell; 1993: 113–64.
21. Raine A, Brennan P, Mednick SA. Birth complications combined with early maternal rejection at age 1 year predispose to violent crime at age 18 years. *Archives of General Psychiatry* 1994;51(12):984–8.
22. Mannuzza S, Klein RG, Konig PH, et al. Hyperactive boys almost grown up. IV. Criminality and its relationship to psychiatric status. *Archives of General Psychiatry* 1989;46(12):1073–9.
23. Robins L. Epidemiology of anti-social personality disorder. In: Michels R, Cavenar JO, Cooper AM, et al. (eds.) *Psychiatry.* Philadelphia: Lippincott; 1986: 1–14.
24. Zoccolillo M, Pickles A, Quinton D, et al. The outcome of childhood conduct disorder: implications for defining adult personality disorder and conduct disorder. *Psychological Medicine* 1992;22(4):971–86.
25. National Institute for Health and Clinical Excellence. *Antisocial Personality Disorder: Prevention and Management. NICE Guideline (CG77).* London, UK: National Institute for Health and Clinical Excellence; 2009.
26. Gibbon S, Khalifa NR, Cheung NH, et al. Psychological interventions for antisocial personality disorder. *Cochrane Database of Systematic Reviews* 2020;9(9):CD007668.
27. Khalifa NR, Gibbon S, Völlm BA, et al. Pharmacological interventions for antisocial personality disorder. *Cochrane Database of Systematic Reviews* 2020;9(9):CD007667.
28. American Psychiatric Association. *Diagnostic and Statistical Manual of Mental Disorders: DSM-5.* Washington, DC: American Psychiatric Association; 2013.
29. Winsper C, Bilgin A, Thompson A, et al. The prevalence of personality disorders in the community: a global systematic review and meta-analysis. *British Journal of Psychiatry* 2020;216 (2):69–78.
30. Kretschmer E. *Der sensitive Beziehungswahn: ein Beitrag zur Paranoiafrage und zur psychiatrischen Charakterlehre.* Berlin: Springer-Verlag; 1918.
31. Macmillan D, Shaw P. Senile breakdown in standards of personal and environmental cleanliness. *British Medical Journal* 1966;2(5521):1032–7.
32. Kendler KS, Aggen SH, Neale MC, et al. A longitudinal twin study of cluster A personality disorders. *Psychological Medicine* 2015;45(7):1531–8.
33. McManus S, Bebbington PE, Jenkins R, et al. *Mental Health and Wellbeing in England: The Adult Psychiatric Morbidity Survey 2014.* London: NHS Digital; 2016.
34. Bleuler E. Die probleme der schizoidie und der syntonie. *Zeitschrift für die gesamte Neurologie und Psychiatrie* 1922;78(1):373–99.
35. Ketelaars C, Horwitz E, Sytema S, et al. Brief report: adults with mild autism spectrum disorders (ASD): scores on the autism spectrum quotient (AQ) and comorbid psychopathology. *Journal of Autism and Developmental Disorders* 2008;38(1):176–80.
36. Rado SE. Schizotypal organization: preliminary report on a clinical study of schizophrenia. In: Rado SE, Daniels GE (eds.) *Changing Concepts of Psychoanalytic Medicine.* New York: Grune & Stratton; 1956: 225–36.
37. Kirchner SK, Roeh A, Nolden J, et al. Diagnosis and treatment of schizotypal personality disorder: evidence from a systematic review. *NPJ Schizophrenia* 2018;4(1):20.
38. Chodoff P, Lyons H. Hysteria, the hysterical personality and hysterical

conversion. *American Journal of Psychiatry* 1958;114(8):734–40.

39. Wittels F. The hysterical character. *Medical Review of Reviews* 1930;36:186.

40. Mattia JL, Zimmerman M. Epidemiology. In: Livesley WJ (ed.) *Handbook of Personality Disorders: Theory, Research, and Treatment.* New York: Guilford Press; 2001: 107–23.

41. Torgersen S, Lygren S, Oien PA, et al. A twin study of personality disorders. *Comprehensive Psychiatry* 2000;41 (6):416–25.

42. Fogelson DL, Nuechterlein KH, Asarnow RA, et al. Avoidant personality disorder is a separable schizophrenia-spectrum personality disorder even when controlling for the presence of paranoid and schizotypal personality disorders: The UCLA family study. *Schizophrenia Research* 2007;91(1–3):192–9.

43. Freud S. Three essays on sexuality. *The Complete Works of Sigmund Freud.* (trans. J Stachey et al.). London: Hogarth Press and the Institute of Psycho-Analysis; 1953.

44. Sullivan HS. *Conceptions of Modern Psychiatry.* New York: Norton; 1947.

45. Gjerde LC, Czajkowski N, Røysamb E, et al. The heritability of avoidant and dependent personality disorder assessed by personal interview and questionnaire. *Acta Psychiatrica Scandinavica* 2012;126(6):448–57.

46. Nicoletti A, Luca A, Raciti L, et al. Obsessive compulsive personality disorder and Parkinson's disease. *PLoS One* 2013;8(1):e54822.

47. Grant JE, Levine L, Kim D, et al. Impulse control disorders in adult psychiatric inpatients. *American Journal of Psychiatry* 2005;162(11):2184–8.

48. Lejoyeux M, Arbaretaz M, McLoughlin M, et al. Impulse control disorders and depression. *The Journal of Nervous and Mental Disease* 2002;190(5):310–14.

49. Ibisworld. *Market Size Statistics – Global.* www.ibisworld.com/global/market-size/.

50. The Guardian. *Gambling Losses in Online Gaming Very Skewed to Deprived Areas – UK study.* www.theguardian.com/society/2022/jun/09/gambling-losses-online-gaming-deprived-areas-uk-study (accessed 27 March 2023).

51. Browne M, Rawat V, Tulloch C, et al. The evolution of gambling-related harm measurement: lessons from the last decade. *International Journal of Environmental Research and Public Health* 2021;18(9):4395.

52. Weinberger AH, Franco CA, Hoff RA, et al. Gambling behaviors and attitudes in adolescent high-school students: relationships with problem-gambling severity and smoking status. *Journal of Psychiatric Research* 2015;65:131–8.

53. Rahman AS, Balodis IM, Pilver CE, et al. Adolescent alcohol-drinking frequency and problem-gambling severity: adolescent perceptions regarding problem-gambling prevention and parental/adult behaviors and attitudes. *Substance Abuse* 2014;35 (4):426–34.

54. Huggett SB, Winiger EA, Palmer RHC, et al. The structure and subtypes of gambling activities: genetic, psychiatric and behavioral etiologies of gambling frequency. *Addictive Behaviors* 2021;113:106662.

55. Public Health England. *Gambling-Related Harms: Evidence Review.* www.gov.uk/government/publications/gambling-related-harms-evidence-review (accessed 6 March 2023).

56. Cowlishaw S, Merkouris S, Dowling N, et al. Psychological therapies for pathological and problem gambling. *Cochrane Database of Systematic Reviews* 2012;11:CD008937.

57. Littman-Sharp N, Turner N, Toneatto T. *Inventory of Gambling Situations (IGS).* Toronto: Center for Addiction and Mental Health; 2009.

58. Bowden-Jones H, Hook RW, Grant JE, et al. Gambling disorder in the UK: key research priorities and the urgent need for independent research funding. *Lancet Psychiatry* 2022;9(4):321–29.

59. Stevens MW, Dorstyn D, Delfabbro PH, et al. Global prevalence of gaming disorder: a systematic review and meta-analysis. *Australia and New Zealand Journal of Psychiatry* 2021;55(6): 553–68.

60. Chang C-H, Chang Y-C, Yang L, et al. The comparative efficacy of treatments for children and young adults with internet addiction/internet gaming disorder: an updated meta-analysis. *International Journal of Environmental Research and Public Health* 2022;19 (5):2612.

61. McLaughlin KA, Green JG, Hwang I, et al. Intermittent explosive disorder in the National Comorbidity Survey Replication Adolescent Supplement. *Archives of General Psychiatry* 2012;69 (11):1131–9.

62. Scott KM, de Vries YA, Aguilar-Gaxiola S, et al. Intermittent explosive disorder subtypes in the general population: association with comorbidity, impairment and suicidality. *Epidemiology and Psychiatric Sciences* 2020;29:e138.

63. Coccaro EF, McCloskey MS, Fitzgerald DA, et al. Amygdala and orbitofrontal reactivity to social threat in individuals with impulsive aggression. *Biological Psychiatry* 2007;62(2):168–78.

64. Felthous AR, McCoy B, Nassif JB, et al. Pharmacotherapy of primary impulsive aggression in violent criminal offenders. *Frontiers in Psychology* 2021;12:744061.

65. Coccaro EF, Kavoussi RJ. Fluoxetine and impulsive aggressive behavior in personality-disordered subjects. *Archives of General Psychiatry* 1997;54 (12):1081–8.

66. Sheard MH, Marini JL, Bridges CI, et al. The effect of lithium on impulsive aggressive behavior in man. *American Journal of Psychiatry* 1976;133 (12):1409–13.

67. Arieff AJ, Bowie CG. Some psychiatric aspects of shoplifting. *Journal of Clinical and Experimental Psychopathology* 1947;8(3):565–76.

68. Grant JE, Chamberlain SR. Symptom severity and its clinical correlates in kleptomania. *Annals of Clinical Psychiatry* 2018;30(2):97–101.

69. Buckle A, Farrington DP. An observational study of shoplifting. *The British Journal of Criminology* 1984;24 (1):63–73.

70. Hellman DS, Blackman N. Enuresis, firesetting and cruelty to animals: a triad predictive of adult crime. *American Journal of Psychiatry* 1966;122 (12):1431–5.

71. Blanco C, Alegría AA, Petry NM, et al. Prevalence and correlates of fire-setting in the United States: results from the National Epidemiologic Survey on Alcohol and Related Conditions (NESARC). *Journal of Clinical Psychiatry* 2010;71(9):1218–25.

72. Ritchie EC, Huff TG. Psychiatric aspects of arsonists. *Journal of Forensic Sciences* 1999;44(4):733–40.

Chapter 8

Neuropsychiatric Disorders

Andrea E. Cavanna and Alan Carson

Neuropsychiatry has a long and fascinating history as a discipline at the interface between neurology and psychiatry that combines clinical observations with modern investigational techniques. Historically, organic psychiatry has focused on clinical syndromes with regional connections affecting the four cortical lobes and the corpus callosum. Behavioural neurology has developed from early observations of classical neurocognitive syndromes, including aphasia, alexia, apraxia, agnosia and Gerstmann syndrome. A number of common neurological conditions often present with specific psychiatric symptoms: traumatic brain injury, cerebrovascular disease, brain tumours, epilepsy, movement disorders, infectious diseases and autoimmune neurological disorders such as multiple sclerosis, systemic lupus erythematosus and autoimmune encephalopathies. The differential diagnosis between delirium, dementia and pseudodementia can pose significant challenges. Finally, several toxic, metabolic and endocrine disorders can have clinically relevant neuropsychiatric manifestations.

Introduction

Historical Overview

Neuropsychiatry is a clinical discipline concerned with conditions arising from disorders of brain structure and function. Neuropsychiatrists specialise in the diagnosis and treatment of the psychiatric symptoms of patients with neurological disorders and organic diseases that indirectly affect the brain. A comprehensive approach to neuropsychiatry requires the integration of biological factors with the personal, family and social context. Therefore, knowledge and application of concepts and techniques derived from psychiatry, neurology, neuropsychology, genetics, pharmacology and medicine are essential to clinical practice.

Neuropsychiatry is not simply the sum of neurology and psychiatry, but an independent discipline with a long tradition.[1,2] The core assumption of neuropsychiatry can be traced back to the words of Hippocrates in the fifth century BCE: 'Men ought to know that from nothing else but the brain come joys, delights, laughter and sports, and sorrows, griefs, despondency and lamentations. And by this, in an especial manner, we acquire wisdom and knowledge, and see and hear and know what are foul and what are fair, what are bad and what are good, what are sweet and what are unsavory [. . .] And by the same organ we become mad and delirious, and fears and terrors assail us [. . .] All these things we endure from the brain when it is not healthy [. . .] In these ways I am of the opinion that the brain exercises the greatest power in the man' (*On the Sacred Disease*, 400 BCE). Interestingly, the same approach was endorsed by British molecular biologist and Nobel Prize winner Francis Crick (1916–2004) two and half millennia after Hippocrates' writings: 'You, your joys and your sorrows, your memories and your ambitions, your sense of personal identity and free will, are in fact no more than the behaviour of a vast assembly of nerve cells and their associated molecules'.[3]

The origins of modern neuropsychiatry can be traced back to the work of German neuroanatomist Franz Gall (1758–1828) and his collaborator Johann Spurzheim (1776–1832). Gall first elaborated his theory of organology (developed as phrenology by Spurzheim) based on five principles: (1) the brain is the organ of the mind, (2) the mind can be analysed into independent faculties, (3) the mental faculties are innate and have their seat in the cerebral cortex, (4) the size of each brain structure is an indication of its functional capacity and (5) the correspondence between the shape of the skull and the cortex of the brain is such that the size of the cerebral organs and their potential role in the psychological make-up can be determined by inspection. Despite the limitations of a far-too-literal approach to brain-behaviour relationships, the phrenologists paved the way for the scientific exploration of brain-behaviour correlations.

Wilhelm Griesinger (1817–1868, Figure 8.1) expanded on his predecessors' work on the localisation of mental diseases and their symptoms and famously stated that 'psychological diseases are diseases of the brain'. More recently, his words were echoed by the words of one of the fathers of behavioural neurology, Norman Geschwind (1926–1984): 'it must be realized that every behaviour has an anatomy'.

Between Griesinger and Geschwind, there were important advances in the study of the localisation of brain functions. British neurologist John Hughlings Jackson (1835–1911) conducted studies in epilepsy that fostered the development of modern methods of clinical localisation of brain lesions and the investigation of localised brain functions. American psychologist Karl Lashley (1890–1958) shed light on the neurobiological basis for sensorimotor and memory representations in the brain.

Sigmund Freud (1856–1939) began his career as an experimental neurologist, as documented by his early attempts to construct an anatomical/physiological model of the mind.

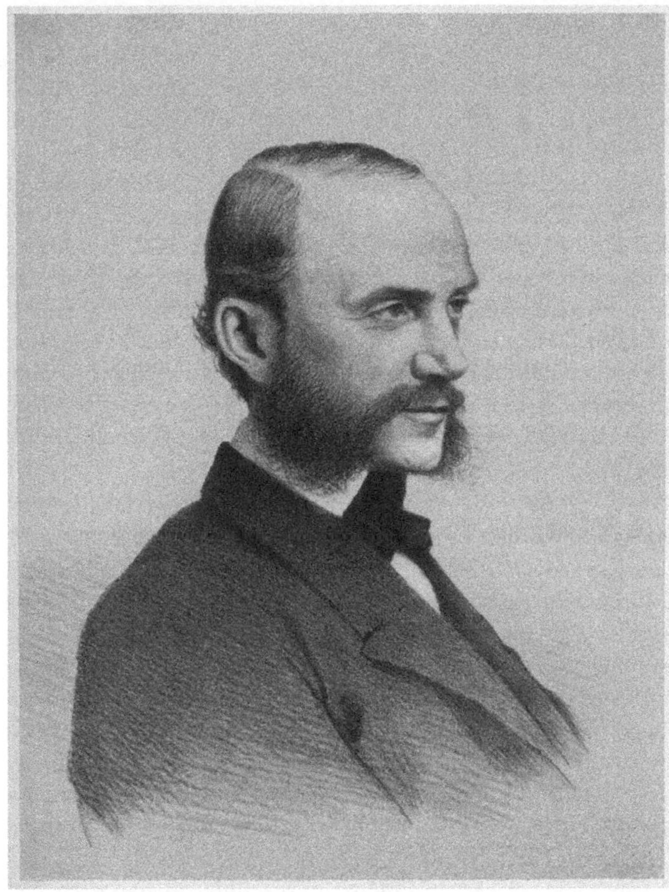

Figure 8.1 Wilhelm Griesinger (1817–1868).

Before abandoning his project, Freud argued that times would come when scientific methods would be sufficiently developed to allow for the construction of such a model. From a different perspective, with the description and classification of symptomatic psychoses in 1908, German neurologist Karl Bonhoeffer (1868–1948) laid the foundation for a categorisation into exogenous and endogenous psychiatric disorders. In the 1960s, Russian neuropsychologist Alexander Luria (1902–1977) provided an extensive description of the frontal lobe syndromes with original methods for their clinical evaluation, for which he is often credited as a father of modern neuropsychological assessment. Neuropsychiatry gradually progressed throughout the end of the twentieth century, culminating in the establishment of the British Neuropsychiatry Association in 1987 and the American Neuropsychiatric Association in 1988, and so inaugurated the contemporary era of clinical neuropsychiatry.

Investigations

Neuroimaging

Structural Neuroimaging

In addition to the lesion method, neuropsychiatrists have long investigation techniques to explore the brain bases of specific behavioural functions. In the mid-part of the twentieth century, new technologies became available to neuroscientists to identify and localise brain lesions, but these were mainly characterised by their invasive nature and poor resolution. It was not until the 1960s, when Sir Godfrey Hounsfield and Alan Cormack introduced brain computerised tomography (CT scanning), that the nature and localisation of a lesion could be identified and monitored in an essentially non-invasive manner. Brain CT scans can detect most cortical lesions, large vascular infarctions, demyelination and white matter changes (leucodystrophy), as well as hydrocephalus. Volumetric indices of brain atrophy may contribute to the diagnosis of neurodegenerative conditions.

Table 8.1 Structural neuroimaging techniques: computerised tomography (CT) and magnetic resonance imaging (MRI)

	CT	MRI
Development	1960s	1970s
Widespread use	From the 1970s	From the 1980s
Exposure to radiations	Yes	No
Major contraindications	Nil	Metal implants
Scanning time	Very short	Short
Spatial resolution	High	Very high

The phenomenon of nuclear magnetic resonance was discovered by Edward Purcell and Felix Bloch in the late 1970s. Brain magnetic resonance imaging (MRI) scans provide images in much finer detail than CT and have now largely supplanted CT as a structural diagnostic tool in neuropsychiatry. MRI takes advantage of the high prevalence of hydrogen in the body, especially within organs that are rich in water and fat, such as the brain. The MRI signal is generated by the magnetic properties of the hydrogen nucleus (consisting of a single positively charged proton) exposed to a strong oscillating magnetic field around the area to be imaged. MRI differentiates between grey and white matter, outlines major blood vessels and detects small lesions, particularly in the posterior fossa and pituitary regions, areas poorly visualised by CT. In addition to sensitively detecting lesions such as white matter changes and infarcts, MRI assists in the differential diagnosis of focal tissue pathology, as well as detects and allows quantitative estimations of cerebral atrophy. Important applications in neuropsychiatry include the assessment of the relationship between brain pathologies such as cerebrovascular disease or traumatic brain injury and psychiatric symptoms. More advanced MRI methods were developed and widely implemented during the 1990s, including voxel-based morphometry (VBM) for measuring grey matter volumes with greater accuracy as well as diffusion tensor imaging (DTI) for the detailed characterisation of white matter. The main characteristics of structural neuroimaging techniques, CT and MRI, are summarised in Table 8.1.

Functional Neuroimaging

A link between brain circulation and metabolism was first suggested by Charles Smart Roy (1854–1897) and Charles

Scott Sherrington (1857–1952) in 1890. In the same year, William James (1842–1910) – in his introduction of the concept of brain blood flow variations during mental activities – briefly reported the studies of the Italian physiologist Angelo Mosso (1846–1910, Figure 8.2). Mosso is credited with the first recordings of brain pulsations in patients with skull breaches and with the invention of the 'human circulation balance', which could non-invasively measure the redistribution of blood during emotional and intellectual activity.

The development of functional techniques in neuroimaging was spurred by Seymour Kety's initial investigations of brain blood flow in mental illness during the 1940s.[4] Functional neuroimaging techniques allow the visualisation of brain activity in vivo. Both single photon emission computed tomography (SPECT) and positron emission tomography (PET) assess cerebral function as a function of brain metabolism. Observations of regional differences in blood flow can be made following the introduction of radioactive tracers in the bloodstream, such as fludeoxyglucose in PET. This contains the short-lived radionuclide fluorine-18, which emits a positron that collides with an electron ('annihilation reaction') and produces gamma radiation, resulting in radiation safety issues associated within its use. Dopamine transporter SPECT imaging (DaTscan) is a sensitive method that employs ioflupane as a contrast agent to detect presynaptic dopamine neuronal dysfunction, a hallmark of idiopathic Parkinson's disease. Functional magnetic resonance imaging (fMRI) directly captures increases in blood oxygenation (blood oxygenation level-dependent contrast, BOLD) correlating with increased neuronal firing. Neuroimaging research in neuropsychiatry makes extensive use of fMRI protocols. Magnetic resonance spectroscopy (MRS) is a safe and non-invasive tool used to extract in vivo biochemical information from both grey and white matter, with potential diagnostic application in neuropsychiatric conditions. PET, fMRI and MRS are leading areas of research into brain function and mapping, with the potential to enhance clinical practice.[5]

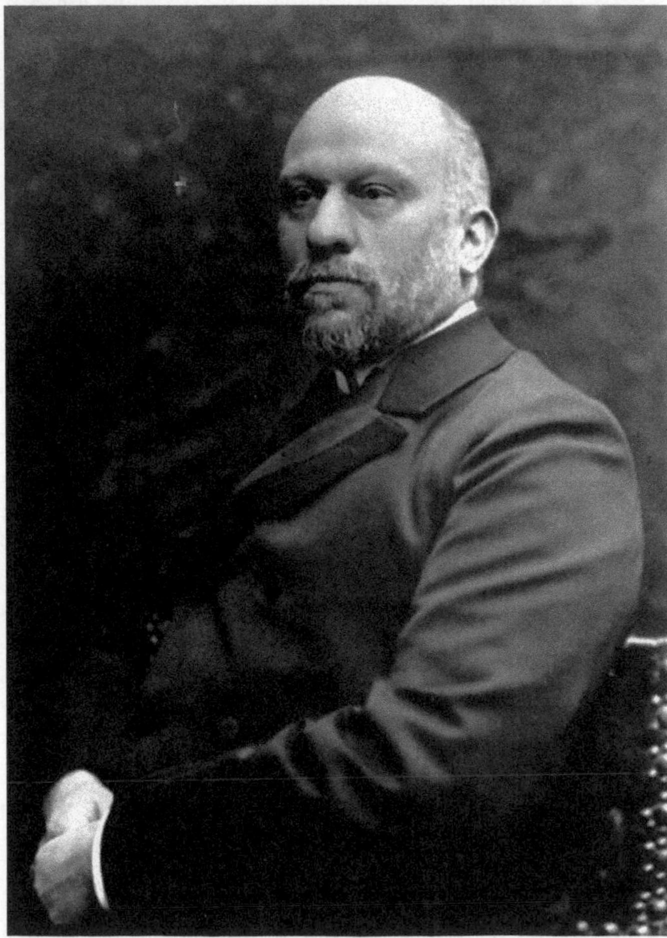

Figure 8.2 Angelo Mosso (1846–1910).

Neurophysiology

Electroencephalography (EEG) was first developed by German psychiatrist Hans Berger (1873–1941, Figure 8.3) for the assessment of cortical electrical activity in 1924. The EEG reading is classified into four characteristic waveforms according to frequency: delta rhythms (less than 4 Hz), theta (4–7 Hz), alpha (8–13 Hz) and beta (over 13 Hz). Prolonged EEG recordings, such as ambulatory EEG and video EEG, are often needed to capture paroxysmal spells of abnormal behaviours. Focal abnormalities are most consistent with localised disorders such as focal seizures, tumours, abscesses, subdural haematomas or cerebral infarctions; diffuse slowing occurs in generalised seizures, toxic and metabolic disorders, as well as advanced degenerative diseases. Developments in neurophysiological techniques include magnetoencephalography (MEG) and simultaneous EEG-fMRI recording, which allows for multimodal investigations combining the temporal resolution of EEG with the spatial resolution of MRI to improve diagnostic accuracy in epilepsy.[6]

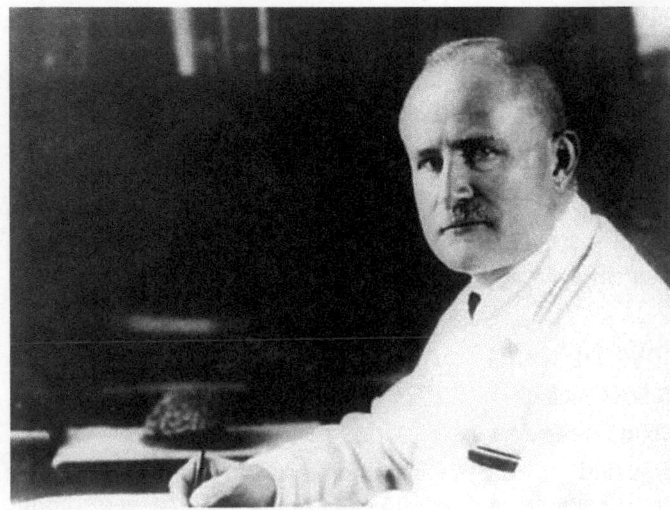

Figure 8.3 Hans Berger (1873–1941).

Neuropsychology

Formal neuropsychological measures can improve the reliability and validity of the clinical data in the assessment of the mental status of neuropsychiatric patients. The assessment of the cognitive state should be viewed as a 'screening' procedure and is certainly no substitute for proper neuropsychological assessment by a neuropsychologist. The most commonly used global measures of cognition include the Mini-Mental State Examination (MMSE), the Addenbrooke's Cognitive Examination (ACE) and the Montreal Cognitive Assessment (MoCA). The MMSE was developed by Folstein and colleagues in 1975 in order to differentiate 'organic' from 'functional' psychiatric patients and is currently a standard tool in screening for impairment of global cognitive function. The MMSE tests registration, attention and calculation, recall, language, ability to follow simple commands and orientation, within an administration time of 5–10 minutes. The ACE, later modified to ACE-III, is a short cognitive test for the detection of early dementia and the differentiation of dementia subtypes. The cognitive domains of the ACE-III correlate significantly with standardised neuropsychological tests used in the assessment of attention, language, verbal memory and visuospatial function. The MoCA is characterised by excellent sensitivity but poor specificity for the detection of mild neurocognitive disorders.

Individual measures addressing one or more aspects of cognition and behaviour should be carefully selected so that the neurocognitive assessment can be tailored to the individual patient.[7] When choosing a measure, clinician time, patient time and training requirements should be taken into consideration.

A simple way to test for general orientation is to ask patients for time and place, as well as age, date of birth and – if appropriate – time since last outpatient consultation.

Tests for attention mainly focus on the speed of information processing component, and they include the digit span test, the serial 7s test and the backwards spelling tests. In the digit span test, subjects are read a sequence of numbers and asked to repeat the same sequence back to the examiner in order (forward span) or in reverse order (backward span). The digit span test is also a measure of working memory. In the serial 7s test, subjects are asked to count down from one hundred by sevens. In addition to attention, this simple task tests the domains of memory and mental calculation. In the backwards spelling test, subjects are asked to spell words with complex spelling such as 'WORLD' backwards. This test is similar to the days/months backwards test, in which subjects are asked to name the days of the week or the months of the year in reverse order. Both tests tap into multiple domains, including concentration, working memory and executive function.

The Frontal Assessment Battery (FAB) is a useful tool for executive function testing. The FAB is a brief battery of six neuropsychological tasks probing frontal lobe function, designed to be completed in about 10 minutes. The similarities component assesses conceptualisation and abstract reasoning by asking subjects to explain in what way two objects such as a banana and an orange are alike. The lexical fluency component assesses mental flexibility by asking subjects to say as many words as they can beginning with a given alphabetical letter. The programming component assesses executive control through the Luria test: the examiner makes a fist, a slicing movement and a slapping movement with the hand, in sequence, to the words 'punch', 'cut' and 'slap', and then asks the patient to mimic with his own hand the series of fist–edge–palm. The conflicting instructions component assesses sensitivity or resistance to interference by asking the subject to tap twice when the examiner taps once and vice-versa. The Go–No Go component assesses inhibitory control by asking the subject to tap once when the examiner taps once, and to refrain from tapping when the experimenter taps twice. Finally, the prehension behaviour component assesses environmental autonomy by checking that the subject is not excessively dependent on environmental cues: the examiner brings his/her hands close to the subject's hands and touches the palms of both the patient's hands to see if the subject spontaneously takes them. The FAB is particularly helpful in the assessment of different types of dementias and traumatic brain injury affecting the frontal lobe.

Tests of language probe multiple aspects of verbal and non-verbal communication. In the confrontational naming tests, subjects are asked to name readily available items (e.g. 'pen') as well as more specific items (e.g. 'cufflinks'). In the comprehension test, subjects are asked to follow a single-stage instruction (e.g. 'Use your right hand to touch the tip of your nose') as well as multiple-staged instructions (e.g. 'Use your right hand to touch your left knee, left ear, right knee'). In the repetition (conduction) test, subjects are asked to repeat a difficult sentence (e.g. 'The rain in Spain falls mainly on the plain'). Subjects can be asked to read a short paragraph and write a brief sentence in order to assess their reading and writing skills. Finally, spontaneous verbal expression (phrase length, fluency and grammar), as well as possible alterations of form and content can be assessed during routine conversation with the patient.

Long-term memory and learning are best assessed by separately addressing their main components. Episodic memory refers to personally experienced events and comprises retrograde memory (for past events) and anterograde memory (for newly encountered information). Retrograde memory can be routinely tested during history taking; in addition, it is possible to ask patients about past personal events, such as facts and incidents ('autobiographical' memories). Anterograde memory can be assessed by testing the patient's recall of a given name after repetition by the examiner (immediate recall), as well as after five minutes (delayed recall). A second important memory system involves memory for word meaning and general knowledge (semantic memory); this component can be easily tested by asking patients for the description of recent news events.

The clock drawing test, which is commonly used to test visuospatial function, reflects frontal and temporoparietal functioning and is a valuable screening tool for dementia.

In the clock drawing test, the subject is instructed to draw a clock reading a specific time (generally 11:10). After the task is complete, the examiner draws a clock with the hands set at the same specific time and asks the subject to copy the image.

It is often advisable to complement the flexible use of tests that probe the individual domains of cognition with psychometric instruments developed to assess behavioural symptoms. The Neuropsychiatric Inventory assesses 10 classes of behavioural abnormalities in patients with dementia and other neuropsychiatric disorders domains of psychopathology. Behavioural testing can include measures of delirium or agitation (disinhibition, aggression and impulsivity), such as the Delirium Rating Scale (DRS), the Agitated Behaviour Scale (ABS), the Confusion Assessment Protocol (CAP) and the Pathologic Laughing and Crying Scale (PLACS). Other helpful behavioural scales encompass formal measures of affect and anxiety. These include the Patient Health Questionnaire (PHQ-9), the Quick Inventory for Depressive Symptomatology (QIDS), the Hamilton Depression Scale and the Beck Depression and Anxiety Inventories.

Syndromes with Regional Connections

Frontal Lobe

The frontal lobe occupies more than one-third of the brain's cortex and phylogenetically is the most recently evolved region of the brain. In consideration of its wide-ranging connections, it can be argued that the frontal lobe is involved in controlling virtually the entire repertoire of human behaviours. Posteriorly to anteriorly, within the frontal lobe are located the motor and pre-motor areas (responsible for the initiation of voluntary motor actions), Broca's area (speech production) and the prefrontal cortex (higher control functions).

Frontal lesions affecting the motor cortex lead to contralateral paresis, with initial muscle flaccidity and subsequent spasticity.

Lesions of Broca's area (inferior frontal gyrus) on the dominant side result in expressive aphasia (inability to produce speech), first described by French neurologist Paul Broca (1824–1880, Figure 8.4) in aphasic patients with left frontal lobe lesions. *Lesions to the corresponding area on the non-dominant hemisphere* can result in speech production lacking emotional tone (expressive aprosodia).

The key role played by the prefrontal region in neuropsychiatry is probably best exemplified by the celebrated case of Phineas Gage (1823–1860).[8] At the age of 25, while working as a railroad company foreman, Gage sustained a remarkable accident caused by an explosion at his construction site. A tamping rod was accidentally propelled at great velocity upwards through his left orbit and damaged his brain. Gage lost his left eye but survived the accident with a recovery that was described as remarkable, as there was no evidence of any sensory, motor or cognitive deficits. However, over the following years, his treating physician John Harlow was able to document puzzling changes in his behaviour and personality. Before the accident, Gage was described as 'the most efficient and capable foreman', whereas after the accident, Harlow wrote that Gage had become 'fitful, irreverent, indulging at times in the grossest profanity (which was not previously his custom), manifesting but little deference for his fellows, impatient of restraint or advice when it conflict with his own desires'. Harlow famously reported that Gage was 'no longer Gage'. The extent of the damage to Gage's left prefrontal cortex was determined in 1994 by Portuguese neurologist Antonio Damasio, who published the results of a computerised reconstruction of the trajectory of the tamping rod based on careful measurement of the damaged skull.[9]

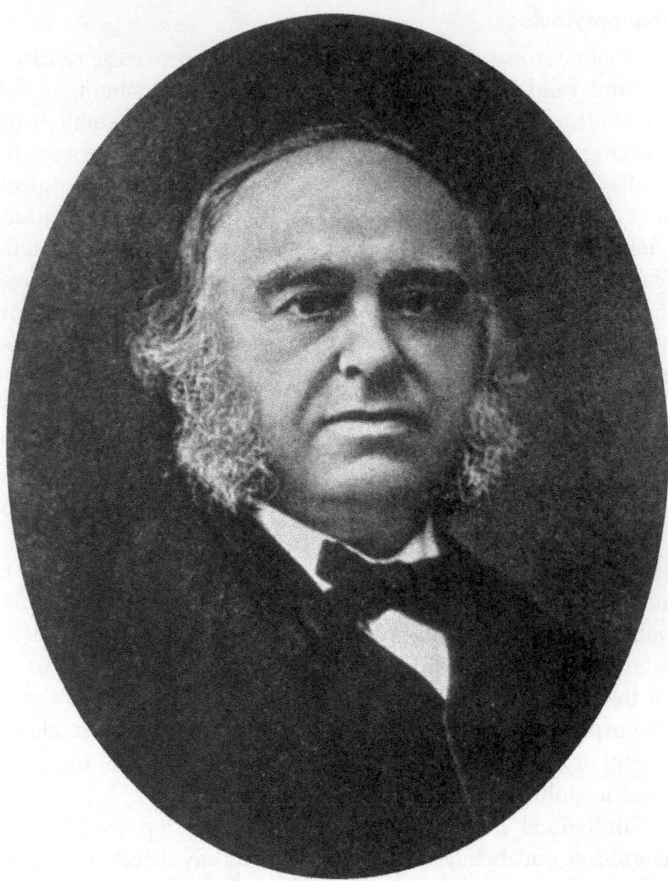

Figure 8.4 Paul Broca (1824–1880).

In 1949, Portuguese neurosurgeon Egas Moniz (1874–1955) received the Nobel Prize for his work in the field of psychosurgery after he had developed the surgical procedure of prefrontal leucotomy in the 1930s. Based on the known involvement of the frontal lobe in higher functions, personality and behaviour, Moniz hypothesised that intentionally damaging the neuronal tracts in the frontal lobe in patients with mental illnesses would lead to clinical improvement. A modified technique was adopted by American neurologist Walter Freeman (1895–1972), who was credited with performing several thousands of frontal lobotomies between the 1930s and the 1950s, after which this pioneering type of psychosurgery was gradually abandoned.

The prefrontal cortex has subcortical connections that include parallel cortico-striato-thalamo-cortical circuits, which originate from different portions of the prefrontal cortex and project to the striatum, globus pallidus and thalamus and back to the cortex again.[10] From a clinical perspective, it is possible to distinguish three major lesional syndromes based on prefrontal regions of primary involvement: the orbitofrontal syndrome, the ventromedial syndrome and the dorsolateral syndrome.

The orbitofrontal syndrome resembles Phineas Gage's clinical presentation and is predominantly characterised by disinhibition, with impaired social judgement, tactlessness, inappropriate sexual conduct and over-talkativeness. Pressure of speech can be related to childish excitement or silliness ('moria', described by Moritz Jastrowitz in 1888) and a tendency to tell inappropriate jokes, puns or pranks ('Witzelsucht', described by Hermann Oppenheim in 1890). Inappropriate affect can be accompanied by mood lability, often presenting with a shallow and fatuous euphoria. Lack of insight and impaired empathy can lead to gross errors of judgement with impulsiveness, irritability and aggressiveness. Some patients may no longer carry out the necessary activities of daily living and display poor self care.

The ventromedial syndrome, like the orbitofrontal syndrome, has prominent behavioural manifestations. It is characterised by abulia, apathy and emotional indifference, often associated with reduced psychomotor activity, impaired task maintenance and mutism. There can be loss of engagement with activities of daily living and incontinence, with or without distress.

The dorsolateral syndrome is mainly characterised by executive dysfunction. Patients typically have difficulties with planning, organisation, problem solving, abstract reasoning, creativity and generation of ideas. There can be significant inflexibility, perseveration and poor abstraction skills. Sequencing of behaviour, judgements of temporal order and performance on simultaneous tasks are often impaired. Concentration, attention and the ability to maintain a behavioural set without perseveration seem to be particularly affected in patients with dorsolateral prefrontal lesions. Moreover, stimulus-bound behaviours can be observed. Specifically, there may be evidence of an 'environmental dependency syndrome', also termed 'forced utilisation behaviour' and first described by Lhermitte in 1983 – patients feel compelled to reach out and purposefully use objects that are presented to them in an unintentional manner (e.g. a hammer and a nail).

Any pathological process affecting the prefrontal cortex can have far-reaching consequences in terms of neuropsychiatric presentations. The most common causes of prefrontal lobe syndromes include traumatic brain injury, hydrocephalus, neurodegenerative disorders, cerebrovascular diseases, infectious disorders, multiple sclerosis and excessive alcohol use.

Temporal Lobe

In addition to lateralisation (left hemisphere – usually the dominant one in terms of language function – versus right hemisphere), the temporal lobe can be functionally divided into its lateral aspect and medial aspect.

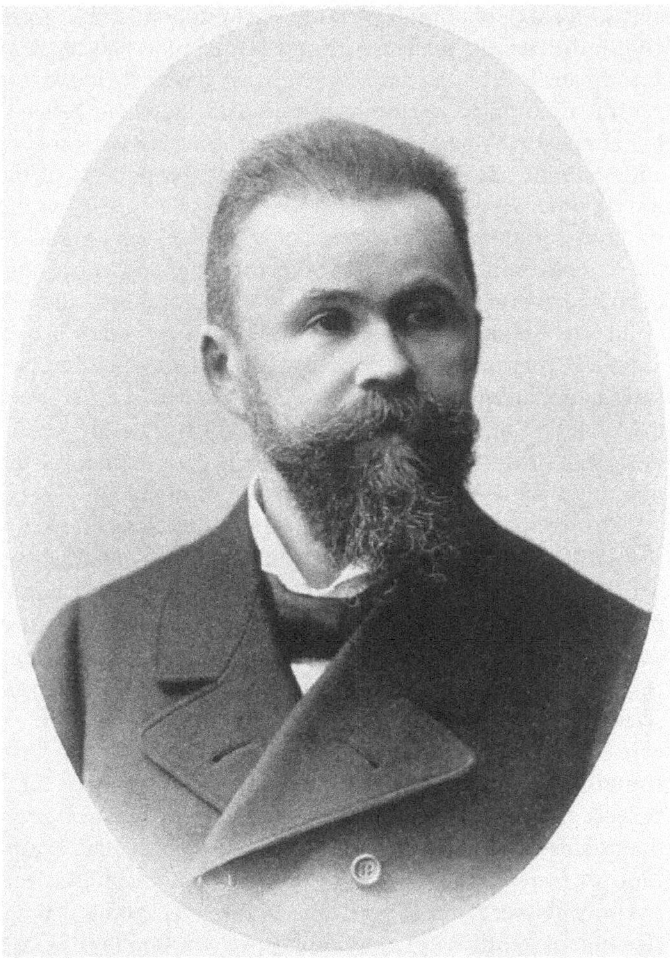

Figure 8.5 Carl Wernicke (1848–1905).

Lesions of the dominant temporal lobe may lead to language problems, including receptive aphasia or Wernicke's aphasia, first described by German psychiatrist Carl Wernicke (1848–1905, Figure 8.5) in 1874 and characterised by a severe comprehension deficit to spoken language. Speech production can be fluent but with nonsense words ('word salad').

Non-dominant temporal lesions may yield few symptoms, such as visuospatial difficulties or prosopagnosia. Lesions restricted to the temporal poles may also be silent. *Bilateral damage to the primary auditory cortex (Heschl's gyrus)* can result in cortical deafness, in which patients have difficulty with both verbal and non-verbal material.

The medial aspect of the temporal lobe contains major components of the limbic system and contributes to emotional regulation. The description of the limbic system was first published in 1878 by Paul Broca (1824–1880) and subsequently refined by James Papez (1883–1958) and Paul MacLean (1913–2007). The limbic system encompasses an interconnected set of cortical and subcortical structures, including the cingulate gyrus, hippocampus, parahippocampal gyrus, fornix, mammillary body, mammillothalamic tract, anterior thalamic nucleus, amygdala, septum and nucleus accumbens.[11] The nucleus accumbens, also referred to as ventral striatum, is currently viewed as a crossroad between the basal ganglia and the limbic system, or between 'motion' and 'emotion'. Histologically, the cortical components of the limbic system have three layers (allocortex), as opposed to the six layers of the neocortex. According to MacLean's model of the triune brain, the ability of processing and expressing primary emotions (e.g. fear, pleasure, pain, anger) allowed by the development of the limbic system in mammals played a central role in the development of interpersonal bonding skills and maternal care.[12] In MacLean's words, 'the history of the evolution of the limbic system is the history of the evolution of the mammals, and the history of the evolution of the mammals is the history of the evolution of the family'.

The central role played by the limbic system in the regulation of emotions is exemplified by the multifaceted behavioural and psychological manifestations of mesial temporal lobe epilepsy (temporo-limbic epilepsy), the most common type of focal epilepsy.[13] The underlying pathology is often mesial temporal lobe sclerosis or hippocampal sclerosis. *Mesial temporal seizures* typically present with an experiential aura; staring and oral automatisms are also common. The possible association with olfactory auras reflects the involvement of the olfactory cortex, located in the uncus and parahippocampal gyri. Experiential symptoms encompass a wide range of emotions, including fear, anxiety, pleasure and depression. Depersonalisation, déjà vu (feeling of familiarity) and jamais vu (unfamiliarity) can also be reported. Ictal fear has been associated with epileptiform discharges, primarily originated within the amygdala. Overall, dysfunction of the amygdala has been implicated in anxiety symptoms, including post-traumatic stress and panic attacks, which are driven by the experience of fear. Moreover, deep temporal structures have been targeted in psychosurgical procedures (stereotactic amygdalotomy, limbic leucotomy) mainly for the treatment of medically refractory aggressive behaviours.

Klüver-Bucy syndrome was first described in 1937, when Heinrich Klüver (1897–1979) and Paul Bucy (1904–1992) included bilateral temporal lobectomy in rhesus monkeys as part of their studies on animal models of behaviour. These procedures resulted in specific behavioural changes: loss of natural fear for dangerous stimuli, visual agnosia, placidity, environmental exploration, hypersexuality and hyperorality. Bilateral damage to the amygdala was thought to result in loss of fear. Elements of Klüver-Bucy syndrome can be observed in patients with acquired brain pathologies affecting both temporal lobes, including neurodegenerative disorders and herpes simplex encephalitis. The clinical picture encompasses excessive oral tendencies – including bulimia – and urges to touch objects in sight, placidity and loss of fear or anger, with apathy, altered sexual activity, visual agnosia and sometimes prosopagnosia.

Bilateral medial temporal lobe lesions, resulting in bilateral hippocampal damage, can produce a severe and selective amnesic syndrome (anterograde amnesia). The key role of the hippocampus for long-term memory storage is probably best exemplified by the striking case of the amnesic patient H.M. (Henry Molaison, 1926–2008).[14] At the age of 27, H.M. underwent a surgical procedure involving bilateral anterior temporal lobectomy for treatment-refractory epilepsy. The removal of both hippocampi resulted in the inability to form new declarative memories, with preserved procedural or implicit memory skills.

Amnesic syndromes can result from a variety of underlying pathologies: nutritional deficiency in association with alcohol misuse, malnutrition or malabsorption syndromes (Wernicke-Korsakoff syndrome, caused by thiamine deficiency), infection (e.g. herpes simplex encephalitis), head injury, anoxia, vascular lesions or deep midline tumours. *Patients with Wernicke-Korsakoff syndrome* typically try to compensate for their retrograde memory loss with confabulation: incorrect memories that the patient holds to be true, often consisting of real memories jumbled up and recalled inappropriately.

Parietal Lobe

Parietal lobe lesions affecting the primary sensory cortex can cause contralateral cortical sensory loss, which is marked by the loss of recognition of objects by palpation (astereognosia) and of figures written on the hand (agraphaesthesia), as well as impaired sensory localisation. In addition to neurological symptoms, parietal lobe lesions may produce a complex and florid variety of cognitive deficits, especially visuospatial difficulties.[15] Overall, the effects of parietal lesions vary depending on whether the dominant or non-dominant lobe is affected.

Non-dominant parietal lesions are classically associated with disturbed body image and an impaired sense of position in the environment. Neglect of the left side of the body and of the external space can occur. These deficits can present clinically with problems in multiple activities, including drawing, walking, driving and dressing. There may also be denial of the disability (anosognosia) or an attitude of indifference towards it (anosodiaphoria).

Dominant parietal lobe lesions are associated with dysphasia and agnosia. Anterior lesions may be associated with motor dysphasia, and posterior ones with sensory dysphasia. In addition to astereoagnosia and agraphaesthesia, patients can present with tactile agnosia (inability to name an object by touch alone) and autotopoagnosia (inability to identify own body parts).

Dominant parietal lobe lesions affecting its inferior portion can cause Gerstmann syndrome, a combination of finger agnosia (difficulty in naming fingers), dyscalculia (difficulty with numbers), dysgraphia (difficulty with writing) and right-left disorientation.

Bálint syndrome is a rare and poorly understood triad of severe neuropsychological deficits, including simultanagnosia (inability to perceive the visual field as a whole), oculomotor apraxia (difficulty in fixating the eyes) and optic ataxia (inability to move the hand to a specific object by using vision). The most common causes include bilateral infarction in the parieto-occipital region, neurodegenerative disorders and traumatic brain injury affecting the border of the parietal and occipital lobes.

Postero-medial parietal cortex lesions (precuneus and surrounding regions) are rare and can disrupt the 'default mode network', involved in maintaining consciousness during the resting state.[16]

Occipital Lobe

The occipital lobe is primarily concerned with higher order visual processing, as it contains the primary visual cortex (striate cortex, corresponding to Brodmann area 17) and the visual association cortex (prestriate cortex: Brodmann areas 18 and 19).

Focal lesions affecting the *primary visual cortex* lead to contralateral homonymous visual defects: blind spots (scotomas) and partial blind spots (amblyopias) in the contralateral visual field. Overall, trauma, migraine and epilepsy affecting the occipital lobe can cause elemental hallucinations (such as flashes of light) and distortion of vision. Cortical blindness presents with loss of vision – in the presence of normal optic fundi and preservation of pupillary light reflexes – and is often caused by extensive bilateral occipital cortex lesions. Blindsight, originally described by Lawrence Weiskrantz (1926–2018) and colleagues in the 1970s, is the ability of patients who are cortically blind due to lesions in their primary visual cortex to respond to visual stimuli that they do not consciously see.[17] *Anton syndrome* is rare and comprises full cortical blindness along with anosognosia and confabulation of visual experience. The most common cause of Anton syndrome is an ischaemic stroke involving bilateral occipital lobes due to the involvement of posterior cerebral arteries.

Bilateral damage to the visual association cortex results in visual agnosia, the inability to recognise the meaning of what is seen. Visual agnosia is most commonly caused by stroke, tumour, traumatic brain injury or degenerative disease. Bilateral lesions of the occipital cortex may also lead to Bálint syndrome, consisting of inability to perceive the visual field as a whole (simultanagnosia), difficulty in fixating the eyes (oculomotor apraxia) and inability to move the hand to a specific object by using vision (optic ataxia).

Corpus Callosum

Complete callosal damage may lead to different forms of apraxia and alexia, mainly caused by the non-dominant hemisphere's lack of access to speech centres in the dominant hemisphere (left hemisphere in most people). Left-sided neglect can develop as a result of underactivation of the non-dominant hemisphere following extensive callosal lesions. Complete transection of the corpus callosum (callosotomy) can be performed surgically for the treatment of refractory seizures. The *resulting disconnection syndrome ('split-brain' syndrome)* was first described in the 1960s by Roger Sperry (1913–1994), who was awarded the Nobel Prize in 1981. After surgical callosotomy, contralateral transfer of information can be significantly affected. For example, patients have been shown to become unable to verbalise the name of an object selectively presented to the non-dominant visual cortex in specific experimental protocols.

Anterior callosal lesions can lead to the alien hand sign, with loss of control over spontaneous and automatic movements of the non-dominant hand.

Posterior callosal lesions, associated with lesions of the left occipital lobe, can lead to pure word blindness (alexia without agraphia).

Neurocognitive Syndromes

Aphasia

Neurocognitive syndromes are characterised by brain pathologies associated with neuropsychological manifestations (Table 8.2).

Aphasias are a group of acquired disorders of language secondary to brain disease affecting the dominant hemisphere. The left hemisphere is the dominant hemisphere for language in the vast majority (95–99%) of right-handed people, as well as in the majority (60–70%) of left-handed people. Based on the early clinical and pathological reports of aphasic patients by Broca (1861) and Wernicke (1874), two different types of aphasia have been described.

Non-fluent or motor aphasia is associated with pathology anterior to the major central sulcus, in the dominant frontal lobe (Broca's aphasia). Primary motor aphasia is characterised by problems with speech expression; patients with Broca's aphasia have non-fluent spontaneous speech, with decreased output (fewer than 50 words and often fewer than 10 words per minute). There is evidence of increased effort to produce words, choice of wrong words, dysarthria leading to mispronunciation and disturbance of rhythm. Patients tend to use short sentences, often with single words, as well as telegraphic speech (utterance of meaningful nouns and verbs, with omission of prepositions and adjectives). Perseveration is commonly observed. Comprehension is relatively intact, whereas repetition, reading and writing are invariably affected. In over 80 per cent of cases, motor aphasia is accompanied by right-sided hemiplegia.

Fluent or sensory aphasia indicates pathology posterior to the major central sulcus, in the dominant temporal lobe (Wernicke's aphasia). Primary sensory aphasia is characterised

Table 8.2 Main groups of neurocognitive syndromes

Main groups of neurocognitive syndromes
Aphasia
Alexia
Apraxia
Agnosia
Gerstmann syndrome

by problems with speech comprehension; patients with Wernicke's aphasia have impaired auditory comprehension, often to the point that very little of what is heard can be understood (receptive aphasia). Patients with Wernicke's aphasia have fluent, paraphasic speech with defective repetition and impaired writing and reading. Speech production is effortless and without hesitation; however, its content is filled with empty phrases and circumlocutions, lacking meaningful nouns and verbs ('word salad'). The main types of errors include paraphasias (substitutions with similar sounding phonemes or words) and the use of meaningless nonsense words or neologisms. A lack of accompanying neurological signs can lead to misdiagnosis as psychosis or confusion.

Conduction aphasia is a third major aphasic syndrome and is caused by lesions of the arcuate fasciculus, which connects Wernicke's area with Broca's area. Patients with conduction aphasia display an impairment of repetition of speech out of proportion to all other deficits.

In *transcortical or borderzone aphasia*, the underlying pathology is located outside the peri-Sylvian region, in the vascular borderzone between the territory of the middle cerebral artery and that of the anterior or posterior cerebral arteries. Patients with transcortical or borderzone aphasia have intact or relatively good ability to repeat spoken language, despite serious aphasia.

In *anomic or nominal aphasia*, confrontation naming is affected more than any other language function, with low-frequency names or words being particularly affected.

Global aphasia is characterised by language deficits that encompass expressive, receptive, nominal and conductive components, with lesions including and extending beyond both Wernicke's and Broca's areas.

Alexia and Dyslexia

Alexia is an acquired inability to comprehend written language caused by brain damage. Based on the presence or absence of associated agraphia, there are two forms of alexia.

In alexia with agraphia (parietal-temporal alexia), disturbances of reading appear as letter word and numerical blindness, and all aspects of writing (from spontaneous to dictation) are affected.

In alexia without agraphia (occipital alexia), reading is impaired, whereas writing and spelling are intact. The hallmark of this condition is the paradoxical inability of patients to read the words they have just written. In contrast to parietal-temporal alexia, spelled words are usually recognised.

Developmental reading disorders are commonly referred to as *dyslexias*, a term also used to denote partial as opposed to complete loss of reading. The different types of acquired reading disorders are classified as letter-by-letter dyslexia, surface dyslexia and deep dyslexia.

Letter-by-letter dyslexia is characterised by pronounced slowness in reading and results from 'word blindness'.

Surface dyslexia consists in a pronounced difficulty in reading irregular words (as opposed to regular words), likely due to semantic memory deficits. This condition is usually accompanied by a naming deficit.

Deep dyslexia results from a deficit of the phonological system, responsible for the grapheme-phoneme conversion. Patients with deep dyslexia display particular difficulty in reading non-words – as well as impairments in reading abstract words – in working memory and in other aspects of language.

The percentage of people with dyslexia is unknown, but it is estimated to be between 5% and 15%, with figures varying across countries adopting different writing systems. Most cases of dyslexia are diagnosed in childhood by adopting a multi-component approach to assessment. Likewise, the management of dyslexia involves compensation strategies, therapy and educational support. Evidence from functional neuroimaging studies indicates that parts of the left hemisphere of the brain involved with reading – such as the inferior frontal gyrus, inferior parietal lobule and the middle and ventral temporal cortex – could be characterised by abnormal activity in patients with dyslexia. The cerebellar theory of dyslexia proposes that impairment of cerebellum-controlled muscle movement affects the formation of words and the automatisation of complex tasks, such as reading. Less common cases of adult-onset dyslexia usually occur as a result of brain injuries or neurodegenerative processes affecting left hemisphere structures and pathways involving the cerebellum.

In addition to disturbances in memory and perception, patients with posterior forms of dementia – such as Alzheimer's disease – can present with progressive language deficits. Initially, patients report anomia, resulting in semantic substitutions and circumlocutions, as well as impoverishment of spontaneous speech and vocabulary. These symptoms can be followed by simplified syntax, reliance on stock phrases, impaired comprehension and writing, verbal perseveration, vague and meaningless content and paraphasias. In the final stages of the disease, patients present with language incoherence and, occasionally, mutism.

Apraxia

Apraxias are a group of disorders affecting the spatial, temporal and force elements of learned, skilled purposeful movements. It is important to note that, the cognitive-motor problems reported by patients with apraxias are not attributable to weakness, akinesia, incoordination, sensory loss, intellectual deterioration, poor comprehension or uncooperativeness. There are several forms of apraxia, presenting with a variety of different errors under different conditions. In his original description in 1900, German neurologist Hugo Liepmann (1863–1925) recognised two main types of apraxia: ideational apraxia and ideomotor apraxia.

In ideational apraxia, there is an impaired ability to correctly perform a sequence or a series of actions as part of a multi-step task. Patients with ideational apraxia can fail to carry out coordinated sequences of actions such as folding a letter, inserting it into an envelope and stamping it. Forms of ideational apraxia can occur in patients with dementia and with lesions of the corpus callosum.

In ideomotor apraxia, there is failure to perform command actions that can usually be performed spontaneously, such as waving goodbye or stirring a cup of tea. Patients with ideomotor apraxia often retain the ability to spontaneously use tools, such as brushing one's hair in the morning without being instructed to do so. Ideomotor apraxia is typically associated with lesions of the dominant left hemisphere.

Orobuccal or buccofacial apraxia presents with difficulties in performing purposeful, skilled movements with the face, mouth, lips or tongue. Patients typically report problems when attempting to blow a kiss, blow out a match or suck on a straw. Orobuccal apraxia is often associated with lesions of the inferior frontal region and the insula. Patients with altered spatial organisation of actions, in the absence of any apraxia for individual movements, have constructional apraxia.

Constructional apraxia typically leads to difficulties in driving a car, using machinery and laying a table. Likewise, difficulties with the ability to draw or copy a figure or picture form the basis of many diagnostic tests.

Dressing apraxia is defined as an inability to correctly dress oneself. Patients with this condition can have difficulties relating the spatial form of garments to the body, such as orienting an arm to a sleeve, as well as doing up ties, zips, buttons and laces. Dressing apraxia is often associated with bilateral or right-sided parieto-occipital lesions.

Agnosia

Originally described by Heinrich Lissauer (1861–1891) in 1889, agnosia involves three distinct processing stages of visual object recognition: analysis of objects by their visual sensory properties (occipital lobe), formation of a percept or apperception (lateralised to the right parietal lobe) and association between the percept and its meaning (lateralised to the left occipitotemporal region). Agnosia is a disorder of object recognition, which cannot be attributed to sensory defects, mental deterioration, attentional disturbances, aphasic misnaming or unfamiliarity with the object. Patients with agnosia have intact primary sensory perception and intact ability to name the object once it has been recognised. The failure of recognition usually afflicts a single sensory modality: vision, hearing or touch. Patients with visual agnosia cannot name objects by sight, but they can identify them by other means, such as touch or hearing.

Prosopagnosia refers to the inability to recognise familiar faces and to learn new ones. Patients with severe forms of prosopagnosia cannot recognise their own face in a mirror. Prosopagnosia is typically caused by lesions affecting the occipito-temporal junction and resulting in the disconnection between the inferior visual association cortex and the temporal cortex. Prosopagnosia should be distinguished from Capgras syndrome, in which the patient believes that familiar persons have been replaced by physically identical doubles or impostors.

Gerstmann Syndrome

Gerstmann syndrome, described in 1924 by Austrian American neurologist Josef Gerstmann (1887–1969), results from parietal lobe lesions in the dominant hemisphere. The full syndrome includes four components, which often fail to cluster together: finger agnosia, right-left disorientation, dyscalculia and dysgraphia. Finger agnosia is characterised by the loss of ability to recognise, name, identify, indicate or select individual fingers, either on the patient's own body or on another person's body. Patients with right-left disorientation cannot carry out instructions that involve an appreciation of right and left. Patients with acquired dyscalculia associated with a left parietal lesion cannot do simple additions and subtractions, despite the absence of dementia or dysphasia. Finally, dysgraphia is a writing disorder presenting with impaired handwriting, orthographic coding and finger movement sequencing.

Neurological Disorders

Traumatic Brain Injury

Overview of Traumatic Brain Injury

Brain injury is one of the main causes of disability and mortality worldwide, particularly in younger men. Improvements in diagnostic techniques and care pathways, including better neurosurgical and intensive care management, have improved survival following brain injury. The long-term sequelae of brain injury, with both neuropsychiatric and neurocognitive problems, have become increasingly recognised, as they affect the functional outcomes and health-related quality of life, as well as add burden on carers. However, a substantial proportion of patients, including those with severe disabilities, do not present themselves to medical or psychiatric services and fail to receive neurorehabilitation treatment. This lack of referral to care, combined with the relatively common occurrence of brain injury, has led to the definition of brain injury as a 'silent epidemic'.

The concept of acquired brain injury encompasses traumatic brain injury and non-traumatic brain injury, such as hypoxic-ischaemic injury. Traumatic brain injury, in turn, can be subclassified into open (or penetrating) traumatic brain injury (with fracture of the skull and breach of the dura mater) and closed traumatic brain injury (without breach of the skull and dura mater). Common causes of closed traumatic brain injury are assaults, falls, road traffic accidents and blast injuries typically encountered in war veterans.

Multiple physical mechanisms can be involved in causing a traumatic brain injury. In addition to the direct impact on the skull or the brain itself, primary damage to the brain can occur as a result of either horizontal or rotational acceleration or deceleration injuries. Horizontal acceleration or deceleration injury typically cause brain contusion at the site of the injury ('coup') and on the opposite side of the brain ('contrecoup'). The rotational acceleration or deceleration can result in diffuse shearing of long central fibres and micro-haemorrhages at the level of the corpus callosum and rostral brainstem. Diffuse axonal injury and Wallerian degeneration of axons in the subcortical white matter and atrophic enlargement of ventricles can be the result of severe head injuries. Moreover, the rotational acceleration or deceleration can cause centrifugal pressure waves reaching the poles of the brain, which can undergo repeated buffeting against the skull and tentorium. The brain regions at higher risk of being damaged include the frontal poles, orbitofrontal cortex, temporal poles and medial temporal structures. The brainstem and midbrain may also be damaged after buffeting against the rim of the foramen magnum and the tentorial edge. Secondary injury to the brain can be the result of intracranial haemorrhage and increased intracranial pressure, among other factors.

A few standardised measures are currently available to assess the severity of traumatic brain injury. These include the Glasgow Coma Scale, an accumulative 15-point scale (15 = fully alert) based on responsiveness in the three areas of eye opening, gross motor activity and verbalisation. If accurately recorded, this measure can give an indication of outcome: a score as low as 3 at 24 hours after injury indicates an 80% chance of bad outcome (death, vegetative state or severe disability), whereas a score of 15 at 24 hours is associated with a bad outcome in only 6% of patients. Other early predictors of outcome include the length of post-traumatic amnesia and the duration of loss of consciousness. Post-traumatic amnesia refers to the duration of amnesia from the time of the injury to the restoration of normal continuous memory and is a good measure of diffuse axonal injury. A post-traumatic amnesia of 1–24 hours is regarded as moderate, while a post-traumatic amnesia of over 24 hours is regarded as severe and is more likely to be associated with some permanent disability. It has been suggested that a post-traumatic amnesia of less than one hour predicts return to work within a month, a post-traumatic amnesia of less than one week return to work within four months, and a post-traumatic amnesia of more than one week predicts invalidism for a year, as well as a 50–70% prevalence of severe psychiatric and intellectual disability at five-year follow-up. The Mayo Classification System for Traumatic Brain Injury Severity is also widely used by clinicians. The occurrence of neuropsychiatric sequelae of traumatic brain injury can be predicted by a number of factors, including the location, severity and extent of the brain damage. Contributing factors include, but are not limited to, premorbid personality, development of post-traumatic epilepsy and past or pre-existing psychiatric problems. With regard to the location of the brain lesion:

Frontal polar damage is associated with poor judgement and insight, apathy, and impaired problem solving

Orbitofrontal damage tends to result in impaired social judgement, impulsivity, excitability and childish behaviour

Temporal lobe damage causes memory loss and speech problems, as well as irritability and aggressiveness

Diffuse axonal injury characteristically leads to attentional problems, slowed thinking, poor concentration and other cognitive deficits

Traumatic brain injury can affect people of all ages. However, young children and adolescents are more likely to sustain a traumatic brain injury than persons in other age groups, with males being affected twice as frequently as females. Mortality rates depend on severity, but they are highest in those with severe injury and in the elderly. Children with pre-injury behavioural problems and psychiatric disorders appear to have a higher risk of sustaining a traumatic brain injury.

In younger children, traumatic brain injury is more commonly related to abuse, falls and pedestrian or bicycle accidents, whereas in older adolescents, it is more likely to be caused by road traffic accidents. Only a minority of traumatic brain injuries are severe; however, their consequences can be wide-ranging and long lasting. Children who suffered a severe traumatic brain injury typically develop a range of neuropsychiatric problems that can significantly affect schooling and alter educational achievements and subsequent occupational outcomes. Case management should involve additional school-based intervention for extra educational support and family interventions, in addition to a comprehensive neurorehabilitation package.

Acute Presentation of Traumatic Brain Injury

Acute post-traumatic amnesia and agitation are commonly reported immediately after traumatic brain injury.[18] Patients can present with confusion, disorientation, hyperactivity and inability to learn new information. The duration of these symptoms is variable and correlates with the severity of brain injury and functional outcomes. Agitation is characterised by psychomotor restlessness, automatisms, impulsivity, aggressiveness, emotional lability and impaired insight. These behavioural manifestations can be accompanied by transient alterations in the autonomic nervous system, including tachycardia and changes in temperature and clamminess. Patients with pre-existing psychiatric or neurological conditions (especially with frontal lobe and paralimbic pathology), as well as those with a history of alcoholor substance misuse are at higher risk of developing agitation after traumatic brain injury.

Acute agitation can predict the development of chronic neuropsychiatric problems, especially if it is prolonged, severe and associated with neuroimaging abnormalities. Prospective objective assessment of post-traumatic amnesia and detailed clinical assessment of an agitated patient after traumatic brain injury are recommended, as they contribute to the determination of the severity of traumatic brain injury and have both diagnostic and prognostic implications. Although post-traumatic amnesia and agitation have been associated with focal lesions and decreased cerebral perfusion within the frontal and temporal lobes, these symptoms can be reported by patients without any detectable structural lesions.

The treatment of agitated behaviour during post-traumatic amnesia requires careful management of the environment, with prioritisation of safety and minimisation of external stimulation. Pharmacotherapy can be useful in the management of patients with acute agitation or aggressiveness; however, the evidence base for any pharmacological class or individual agent is poor. Beta-blockers such as propranolol and pindolol could be effective in controlling post-traumatic brain injury agitation; however, their use needs to be carefully monitored due to their effects on blood pressure and the risk of falls resulting from postural hypotension. Second-generation antidopaminergic agents, such as risperidone, quetiapine and olanzapine, are commonly used for severe forms of acute agitation. The use of first-generation antidopaminergic agents such as haloperidol is limited by their tolerability profile, with concerns about extrapyramidal side effects and an increased risk of worsening of both motor and cognitive functions. The antiepileptic agents carbamazepine and valproate are used as mood stabilisers to treat agitation and aggressiveness after traumatic brain injury. The available evidence is weaker for other antiepileptic agents such as oxcarbazepine, lamotrigine or gabapentin, whereas the use of levetiracetam is contraindicated, as it can exacerbate agitation and aggressiveness, as well as causing irritability and affective symptoms. Benzodiazepines are sometimes used as sedatives in acute emergency settings; however, their regular use should be avoided as it can negatively affect neurocognition and paradoxically worsen aggressiveness. Other pharmacological agents that have been used for the treatment of agitation and aggressive behaviour following traumatic brain injury include methylphenidate, amantadine, buspirone and modafinil.

Neuropsychiatric Aspects of Traumatic Brain Injury

Mild Traumatic Brain Injury: Post-concussion Syndrome

The vast majority of traumatic brain injuries are rated as mild in severity. The clinical presentation of mild traumatic brain injury includes a combination of somatic symptoms (headache, dizziness, blurred vision), cognitive symptoms (problems with attention, concentration, memory) and neuropsychiatric symptoms (affective symptoms, anxiety, irritability, fatigue, sleep problems), collectively referred to as post-concussion syndrome.[19] Over 50 per cent of people after minor head injuries have symptoms (especially headache and dizziness) for up to two months, but only 12 per cent are symptomatic after one year. An individual's expectations of sequelae may have powerful effects.

The nosological status of post-concussion syndrome has been debated, as its multiple symptoms are non-specific in nature and show a considerable overlap with other psychiatric conditions, such as post-traumatic stress disorder and other anxiety disorders. The symptoms of post-concussion syndrome usually develop immediately or within the first one or two weeks after injury. The first symptoms to appear are often somatic and cognitive symptoms. Neuropsychiatric symptoms tend to develop slightly afterwards and may persist for weeks or months. The majority of people who sustained a mild traumatic brain injury and developed post-concussion syndrome show full recovery within days or weeks. However, a small proportion of patients continue to experience persisting symptoms, even after several months. A number of factors have been associated with more severe and persistent forms of post-concussion syndrome, including older age, female gender, previous history of mild traumatic brain injury, comorbid psychiatric disorders or substance misuse and compensation claims. Illness perceptions about the negative consequences of mild traumatic brain injury on physical, social and psychological wellbeing have also been shown to predict the development and persistence of post-concussion syndrome.

The management of patients with mild traumatic brain injury and post-concussion syndrome is symptomatic, and patients should be offered early advice and timely reassurance about outcome and return to work, as appropriate. Both non-pharmacological interventions and pharmacotherapy have been proposed for the treatment of post-concussion syndrome.[20] In addition to education and reassurance, psychological treatment approaches currently in use encompass cognitive rehabilitation, cognitive behavioural therapy and mindfulness-based intervention. More experimental treatment approaches include exercise-based rehabilitation, repetitive transcranial magnetic stimulation and hyperbaric oxygen therapy, but further studies are needed to prove their clinical effectiveness. The most commonly prescribed medications are antidepressants – particularly selective serotonin re-uptake inhibitors – targeting the main psychiatric comorbidities, such as anxiety and affective symptoms.

Severe Traumatic Brain Injury: Psychiatric Sequelae

Traumatic brain injuries that are classed as severe are a small minority of all cases, but they can lead to the development of chronic neuropsychiatric symptoms. The most common long-term neuropsychiatric consequences of severe traumatic brain injury are summarised in Table 8.3.

Following severe traumatic brain injury patients can develop affective symptoms, apathy, anxiety, psychotic symptoms and organic personality changes. There is evidence for an

Table 8.3 Most common neuropsychiatric sequelae of severe traumatic brain injury

Depression
Apathy
Anxiety
Delusional disorders
Schizophrenia-like psychosis
Personality change
Chronic traumatic encephalopathy

increased risk of developing dementia. Neurocognitive problems such as impaired attention, concentration and memory are also commonly reported. Early recognition and management of the neuropsychiatric sequelae of traumatic brain injury are important because of their significant impact on health-related quality of life and overall functioning.

Depression is the most commonly reported psychiatric problem following traumatic brain injury.[21] Beyond injury severity, psychosocial stressors and employment status have been noted to contribute to depressive symptoms and psychological distress. Depression after traumatic brain injury is associated with poorer cognitive functioning, increased anxiety, greater functional disability and decreased health-related quality of life. A number of cognitive and physical manifestations of depression – including difficulties with concentration, tiredness and changes in sleep and appetite – show a degree of overlap with the core features of brain injury. Consequently, the assessment of depression in patients who suffered traumatic brain injury can be challenging and requires a thorough neuropsychiatric assessment. Evidence suggests that antidepressants are effective in treating depression in neurological settings. Both cognitive behavioural interventions and pharmacotherapy with serotonergic agents (especially sertraline and citalopram) are used as evidence-based first-line treatments for depression after traumatic brain injury.[22]

Apathy, also described as amotivation and abulia, is commonly seen following traumatic brain injury. Symptoms of apathy encompass behavioural, cognitive and emotional dimensions: patients often report reduced goal-directed behaviour, lack of motivation, diminished initiative and lack of concern. It is important to conduct a thorough neuropsychiatric assessment, as apathy can be confused with depression, cognitive impairment and alterations of the level of consciousness. Apathy can be associated with poor outcomes, as it leads to poor engagement in neurorehabilitation and affects family, social and occupational functioning. Cognitive interventions and behavioural approaches, such as activity scheduling, are the most commonly used first-line management strategies. In more severe cases, these interventions can be combined with pharmacotherapy, including dopaminergic agents (selegiline), central nervous system stimulants (methylphenidate), cholinesterase inhibitors (donepezil) and other medications, such as selective serotonin re-uptake inhibitors and modafinil.

Anxiety is commonly reported by patients who sustained a traumatic brain injury. The clinical spectrum of anxiety disorders includes acute stress reaction, generalised anxiety disorder, panic disorder, specific phobic disorders and post-traumatic stress disorder. There is a considerable overlap between post-traumatic stress disorder and symptoms of traumatic brain injury, particularly post-concussion syndrome. The diagnostic process can be further complicated by the co-occurrence of other neuropsychiatric sequelae of traumatic brain injury – as well as increased alcohol consumption and substance abuse – because these conditions can alter the presentation of post-traumatic stress disorder. Anxiety management is often best delivered as part of a comprehensive neurorehabilitation programme, with a combination of cognitive behavioural therapy and pharmacotherapy (mainly serotonergic agents).

There is some evidence for an increased prevalence of psychotic symptoms following traumatic brain injury, with male gender, alcohol and substance abuse and pre-existing psychiatric conditions as the main risk factors.[23] Psychotic symptoms tend to correlate with frontal, temporal or hippocampal lesions, and cognitive deficits affecting memory and executive functions are commonly reported. Organic psychosis following traumatic brain injury usually presents as delusional disorders (Capgras syndrome, reduplicative paramnesia, Othello syndrome, Cotard syndrome, somatic delusions) and schizophrenia-like psychosis (auditory hallucinations and persecutory delusions). Long-term follow-studies of soldiers who received head injuries in the Second World War revealed a raised rate of the later development of chronic paranoid psychosis, often coming on 10–15 years after the original injury. Negative psychotic symptoms are not typically present. In addition to primary schizophrenia, the differential diagnosis includes secondary forms of psychosis, such as substance-induced psychosis or schizophrenia-like psychosis of epilepsy. The acute presentation of traumatic brain injury with agitation and behavioural problems associated with post-traumatic amnesia can be confused with psychosis. The treatment of traumatic brain injury-associated psychosis is similar to the treatment of psychotic symptoms in general, with special consideration to pharmacological interactions and tolerability in terms of impact on cognitive functions.

Organic personality change (persistent changes in behaviours and emotions after traumatic brain injury) is often reported by patients, carers and relatives as the most distressing long-term consequence of brain injury. The most common changes in personality and behaviour include irritability, frustration, anger, aggressiveness, impulsivity, emotional lability and disinhibition. Socially inappropriate behaviours and inappropriate expressions of affection can be the result of impaired judgement and lack of insight. A few manifestations of personality change can have a degree of overlap with affective symptoms and cognitive impairment. Both prefrontal lobe damage and anterior temporal lesions can result in severe clinical manifestations, associated with poor engagement with rehabilitative treatment, as well as poor emotional and occupational functioning. Patients with pre-existing psychiatric disorders, including personality disorders, appear to have a higher risk of developing organic personality changes. It is clear that people who suffer head injuries do not constitute a 'normal' population. It has been shown that as many as 50 per cent of patients admitted to one rehabilitation unit have evidence of premorbid specific learning disabilities. The neuropsychiatric assessment should include collateral history from family and carers and explore premorbid levels of function.

A comprehensive neuropsychological assessment helps in establishing the nature and severity of cognitive deficits that may have an impact on behaviour. The management of organic personality change involves a combination of targeted pharmacotherapy and behavioural programmes, to be delivered within neurorehabilitative services. Pharmacological options commonly used in clinical practice include serotonergic agents, mood stabilisers and atypical antipsychotics. Central nervous system stimulants and dopaminergic drugs can prove helpful, especially in patients with comorbid apathy symptoms.

Traumatic brain injury is considered to be the best-established environmental risk factor for the development of dementia. The risk seems to be higher with increased severity of injury, multiple traumatic brain injuries and increased age at injury. Both acceleration of brain atrophy and diminished cognitive reserve have been found to increase the impact of neurodegenerative changes in later life, thereby increasing the risk of dementia.

Chronic traumatic encephalopathy is characterised by chronic neuropsychiatric symptoms and cognitive problems. This condition is associated with typical neuropathological changes, resulting from repeated rotational traumatic brain injuries – for example, multiple sports-related concussions originally seen in professional boxers (dementia pugilistica or 'punch drunk' syndrome). The neuropathological appearance of CTE is different from other tauopathies, such as Alzheimer's disease. On a microscopic scale, the pathology includes neuronal loss and tau deposition, occurring as dense neurofibrillary tangles, neurites and glial tangles. Macroscopically, brain changes include cortical and cerebellar atrophy, as well as enlargement of the lateral ventricles and the third ventricle. Chronic traumatic encephalopathy is thought to be associated with a reduced cognitive reserve and increased chances of a neurodegenerative process becoming clinically apparent as a result of cerebellar, pyramidal and extrapyramidal damage. Neurological manifestations include dysarthria, reduced movement and facial immobility, followed by ataxia, tremor and spasticity. In addition to dementia, patients often present with apathy, irritability, disinhibition, as well as paranoid symptoms. Initially, the condition was thought to be exclusive to boxers, but in recent years, professional footballers who head the ball too vigorously and rugby players also seem to be at risk; there are presently debates about the management of such risks in school sports.

Cerebrovascular Disease

Stroke is a sudden, potentially fatal and disabling clinical syndrome characterised by an acute loss of focal cerebral function with symptoms lasting more than 24 hours and thought to be due to either spontaneous brain haemorrhage (haemorrhagic stroke) or inadequate cerebral blood supply to a part of the brain (ischaemic stroke). In turn, ischaemic stroke can be the result of insufficient blood flow, thrombosis or embolism associated with diseases of the blood vessels, heart or blood. A transient ischaemic attack, often referred to as a 'ministroke' is an acute loss of focal cerebral function or ocular function with symptoms lasting less than 24 hours and thought to be due to the same causative factors as stroke. Despite being characterised by temporary symptoms, transient ischaemic attack carries a high risk of stroke, especially in the first few days of its onset.

Stroke is one of the leading causes of death and disability, as a quarter of strokes are fatal within a year, and over a third of stroke survivors are left with severe disability, resulting in significant health and economic burden. Although cerebrovascular disease mainly affects older people, about one in four strokes occurs in those under the age of 65 years of age. The most common modifiable risk factors for stroke and transient ischaemic attack are hypertension, atrial fibrillation, carotid artery stenosis, diabetes and smoking.

Stroke syndromes result in a wide array of symptoms, which tend to occur abruptly and reach maximum severity shortly after onset. The nature of the sequelae of a stroke depends on the site of the vascular lesion (i.e. on the main cerebral artery occluded or the area of haemorrhage). Stroke syndromes are broadly classified into those arising from the anterior circulation (the carotid territory and its branches) and those arising from the posterior circulation (the vertebrobasilar territory). Patients with anterior circulation syndrome can present with a combination of contralateral motor weakness, homonymous visual field defect and higher cortical deficits (most commonly aphasia in strokes affecting the left hemisphere and neglect in strokes affecting the right hemisphere). Other types of ischaemic strokes affecting the anterior circulation are lacunar strokes: subcortical infarcts generally involving deep-seated structures, such as the basal ganglia. Posterior circulation stroke syndromes have varied presentations, depending on the location of the vascular lesion (e.g. cerebellar ataxia, visual field defects).

Approximately 85% of strokes are ischaemic, with the remaining 15% being haemorrhagic (10% intracerebral haemorrhage plus 5% subarachnoid haemorrhage). History taking and neurological examination are usually sufficient in making the diagnosis of a stroke. One of the main roles of structural neuroimaging in acute stroke presentations is the differential diagnosis between ischaemic and haemorrhage pathologies. The commonest pathophysiological mechanisms underlying ischaemic strokes are thromboembolism originating from atheromatous large vessels (such as the carotid arteries and aortic arch), cardio-embolism (usually related to atrial fibrillation or other cardiac pathologies) and small vessel disease related to hypertension and diabetes (often resulting in lacunar strokes). Primary intracerebral haemorrhage occurs mainly in patients with hypertension, followed by patients with underlying vascular abnormalities, including intracranial aneurysms, arteriovenous malformations, cavernomas or brain tumours. Subarachnoid haemorrhage affects a younger population than other types of strokes. The usual cause is a

Table 8.4 Most common neuropsychiatric manifestations of stroke

Depression
Fatigue
Apathy
Emotional lability
Phobic disorders
Generalised anxiety disorder
Psychosis

ruptured intracranial aneurysm, while vascular malformation such as angiomas are less frequent.

The acute management of stroke focuses on the delivery of evidence-based interventions to revascularise a blocked artery within the first few hours of onset of an ischaemic stroke. This can be achieved via intravenous thrombolysis with a tissue plasminogen activator, such as alteplase, or via mechanical thrombectomy (in a subset of acute ischaemic stroke patients with proximal anterior circulation large-vessel occlusion). Timely admission to an acute stroke unit is associated with a reduction in both mortality and disability after a stroke. Long-term secondary prevention approaches for both ischaemic strokes and transient ischaemic attacks include antiplatelet therapy, statins, antihypertensives, oral anticoagulants for atrial fibrillation, antidiabetic medications and lifestyle modifications, such as weight loss and smoking cessation.

The neuropsychiatric manifestations of stroke are common and can have an adverse impact on rehabilitation and functioning. The most common neuropsychiatric manifestations of stroke are summarised in Table 8.4.

Unfortunately, these symptoms are often underappreciated by stroke health professionals in clinical settings. In addition to cognitive impairment, patients can develop a range of post-stroke neuropsychiatric manifestations, including depression, apathy, fatigue, emotional lability, anxiety and psychosis. These neuropsychiatric sequelae of stroke are associated with a decreased likelihood of returning to work, poorer health-related quality of life and long-term disability, regardless of stroke severity.

Post-stroke depression occurs in around one-third of cases.[24] The main predictors of the development of depression after stroke are pre-existing affective disorders, higher stroke severity and physical disability. No consistent association has been found between post-stroke depression and age, gender, lesion location or cognitive impairment. The aetiology of post-stroke depression is likely to be multifactorial, and the assessment requires particular consideration for selected symptoms. For example, patients with anhedonia exhibit a genuine loss of interest or pleasure in activities, rather than the loss of ability to take part due to stroke-related physical limitations. The differential diagnosis of post-stroke depression includes the reasonable resignation in an elderly person, understandable distress at the disability, personality traits and cognitive impairment.

The somatic features of post-stroke depression include changes in sleeping pattern, loss of appetite and fatigue. Post-stroke fatigue is defined as the experience of significant fatigue, lack of energy or increased need to rest, leading to difficulty in taking part in everyday activities. Clinically significant apathy affects approximately a quarter of patients and appears to be related to disruption to fronto-subcortical circuits, resulting in reduced spontaneous action or speech production.[25] Emotional lability can develop weeks after a stroke and presents with sudden episodes of incontrollable crying or, less commonly, laughter that appear disproportionately intense to the provoking stimulus. Tearfulness typically occurs in response to emotionally congruent stimuli, with a significantly lowered threshold compared to the pre-stroke status. Psychoeducation, social interaction, exercise and other psychosocial interventions are recommended for the treatment of patients with mild depressive symptoms. Both serotonergic antidepressants and structured psychological therapy may be considered in more severe cases, as post-stroke depression can interfere with rehabilitation and result in increased mortality in the long term.

Anxiety disorders (mainly phobic disorders and generalised anxiety disorder) affect around a quarter of stroke survivors.[26] Anxiety after a stroke is predicted by pre-existing anxiety and affective disorders, whereas studies of association between anxiety and lesion location or stroke severity have yielded inconsistent findings.

Post-stroke anxiety can develop in the acute setting or during rehabilitation and become persistent; it has been shown to affect patients' health-related quality of life.

Phobia is defined as a disproportionate fear to the danger of well-defined situations or stimuli, and it clinically presents with unpleasant emotional states, ranging from mild nervousness and tension to autonomic symptoms such as palpitations, sweating and hyperventilation (full-blown panic attack).

Anticipatory anxiety and persistent avoidant behaviours may prevent patients with phobic anxiety from participating in usual activities.

Adaptive fear resulting from stroke-related physical impairments and maladaptive phobic fear may be considered on a continuum, with the differential diagnosis established by expert neuropsychiatric judgement, taking into account the individual patient's biological, psychological and social factors.

Generalised anxiety disorder developed after stroke is characterised by persistent and difficult-to-control worries about multiple daily life events. In addition, patients with generalised anxiety disorder can report feeling tension, fatigue, difficulty concentrating, irritability or sleep disturbance.

Panic attacks with autonomic symptoms can also occur occasionally in the context of generalised anxiety disorder. The treatment of anxiety disorders after stroke is based on a combination of cognitive behavioural therapy using exposure techniques (especially for agoraphobia and other specific phobias) and pharmacotherapy (selective serotonin re-uptake inhibitors and serotonin-noradrenaline re-uptake inhibitors).

New-onset schizophrenia-like psychotic disorders after a stroke are a less frequent occurrence. The most common cause of psychotic symptoms in the period immediately following a stroke is delirium, in which fleeting hallucinations and delusions usually present on a background of fluctuating consciousness. In addition to pre-existing psychosis, a psychosis after a stroke has occasionally been found to be associated with post-stroke epilepsy. Circumscribed delusions sometimes arise in patients who developed anosognosia after a stroke and are almost invariably associated with right hemisphere brain damage.

Peduncular hallucinosis is a rare psychotic syndrome characterised by complex visual hallucinations. This condition is typically associated with infarcts involving the pons and the midbrain and appears to occur with a slightly increased frequency as a complication of interventional neuroradiologic procedures.

Somatoparaphrenia, which can occur after stroke, refers to delusional beliefs that they do not own the limbs of the affected side of the body, which is usually the left side. In addition to unilateral spatial and body neglect, there can be both motor and somatosensory deficits. The denial of hemiparesis with confabulation can be accompanied by delusion of non-ownership, as patients often develop the belief that the limb is truly not their own or that it has been amputated and replaced by an artificial limb.

Brain Tumours

Brain tumours are a neoplastic pathology with important neuropsychiatric implications; of all types of tumours, brain tumours cause the highest rates of distress, depression and cognitive impairment.[27] The incidence of tumours of the central nervous system increases with advancing age, although there is an important peak in childhood (especially tumours primarily arising in the brainstem and cerebellum). Around 90 per cent of patients with brain tumours have neuropsychiatric symptoms, and in around 20 per cent, these are the presenting symptoms. The clinical presentations vary considerably across all ages, tumour sites and tumour types. The majority of brain tumours (about 85 per cent of cases) are metastases spreading from other tumour sites. There is relatively little research on the neuropsychiatry of cerebral metastases compared to primary brain tumours, particularly high-grade glioblastoma. Primary brain tumours arise within the central nervous system, with most tumours being of neuroepithelial origin.

The neuropsychiatric manifestations of brain tumours encompass general effects, local effects (arising from damage to the area of the brain affected by the tumour) and non-metastatic complications, which include the psychological effects on patients and their families. Brain tumours cause local tissue destruction or compression of surrounding structures. The general effects of brain tumours are mainly due to raised intracranial pressure and include headache (the most common initial presenting symptom in about half of the cases), drowsiness, confusion and apathy. The local effects depend on both the nature and the location of the brain tumour. Rapidly growing malignancies are associated with more severe neuropsychiatric symptoms, whereas slow-growing benign tumours – such as meningiomas – may present with subtle changes in mental state and personality. The association between tumour site and psychiatric presentation is often unreliable, and many neuropsychiatric presentations cannot be confidently linked with lesion location.[28]

With regard to the site of metastases:

Small cell carcinoma of the lung most commonly metastasises to the frontal lobe, cerebellum and parietal lobes

Large cell carcinoma of the lung often metastasises to the occipital lobe

Squamous cell carcinoma of the lung often metastasises to the cerebellum

Breast carcinoma secondaries often go to the cerebellum and basal ganglia

Malignant melanoma metastases tend to localise within the frontal and temporal lobes

A considerable proportion of patients with brain metastases have involvement of multiple sites, thus having complex presentations, especially confusion and cognitive impairment. Most primary brain tumours occur in the posterior fossa, frontal lobe and temporal lobe, with the parietal lobe, pituitary and occipital lobes being less often involved. Frontal and temporal lobe tumours are much more likely to present with psychiatric symptoms than parietal, occipital or infra-tentorial tumours. Focal seizures (with or without secondary generalisation) may be a presenting feature, especially with temporal and occipital tumours.

In addition to contralateral motor signs, frontal lobe tumours have been associated with three main neuropsychiatric presentations: orbitofrontal syndrome (especially disinhibition, irritability, emotional liability and personality changes), dorsolateral prefrontal syndrome (attention deficits and perseverative behaviours) and medial frontal syndrome (abulia, apathy, indifference, psychomotor retardation and, in severe cases, akinetic mutism). Temporal lobe tumours can cause a variety of neuropsychiatric complications, including memory deficits, affective symptoms and psychotic symptoms (complex visual, auditory, olfactory or gustatory hallucinations). Parietal lobe tumours present with alterations in contralateral cortical sensation. In addition to disturbances of body image, depression and personality changes have occasionally been reported. Gerstmann syndrome (agraphia, acalculia, finger agnosia and right-left disorientation) can be observed in patients with a brain tumour within the dominant parietal lobe. Occipital lobe tumours are typically associated with contralateral visual field deficits, simple visual hallucinations (flashes of lights of various shapes) and failure to recognise familiar faces (prosopagnosia).

Pituitary adenomas may cause headache and multiple endocrine disturbances, as well as mental slowing and apathy, and are occasionally associated with emotional lability and paranoid ideation.

Craniopharyngiomas and other neoplastic lesions of the hypothalamus can produce wide-ranging endocrine dysfunction, frontal apathy, subcortical slowing and somnolence. The combination of worsening intellectual deficit and hypersomnolence is suggestive of a diencephalic tumour.

Sensory or sensorimotor peripheral neuropathy, myopathy with bulbar palsy and subacute cerebellar degeneration are well-known non-metastatic neurological complications of brain tumours. The non-metastatic neuropsychiatric complications include encephalopathies. Specifically, limbic encephalopathy causes memory deficits associated with affective symptoms, anxiety and occasionally hallucinations. Finally, brain tumours cause considerable psychological complications, with a potentially significant impact on health-related quality of life, as well as a burden for caregivers. Moreover, a substantial proportion of patients with a brain tumour have unmet supportive care needs, and this is often felt in equal measure by their family members.

Epilepsy

Seizures and Epilepsy

Epileptic seizures are defined as the clinical manifestations of abnormal, excessive or synchronous brain activity, resulting in transient alterations of consciousness or motor control.[29] Epileptic seizures have two key elements: paroxysmal abnormalities of the electrical activity of the brain – which can be detected by electroencephalography or EEG – and associated abnormality of brain function (at the same time as the electrical discharge). Epilepsy is a disease characterised by an enduring predisposition to generate recurrent epileptic seizures, with neurobiological, cognitive, psychological and social consequences. Epilepsy is diagnosed when patients have either two unprovoked seizures occurring greater than 24 hours apart or one unprovoked seizure with a probability of further seizures similar to the general recurrence risk (at least 60 per cent) after two unprovoked seizures, occurring over the following 10 years.[30] Conversely, in patients who have been seizure-free for the preceding 10 years, without antiepileptic drugs for the preceding five years, the diagnosis of epilepsy is considered to be resolved. The lifetime prevalence of epileptic seizures in the general population is as high as 5 per cent, whereas the prevalence of epilepsy is considerably lower, up to 1 per cent.[31] The ages of seizure onset follow a bimodal distribution, with a peak in early life (developmental types of epilepsy) and a second peak during old age, when patients can present with symptomatic or lesional epilepsy.

Epileptic seizures can be either focal or generalised, depending on whether the onset of the seizure discharge is localised to part of the cerebral cortex or involves simultaneously both cerebral hemispheres.[32] Focal seizures are further divided into seizures with and without motor manifestations. The assessment of consciousness during an epileptic seizure (operationally defined as the patient's awareness of self and environment) allows the classification of focal seizures into 'focal impaired awareness seizures' (previously called 'complex partial seizures') and 'focal aware seizures' (previously referred to as 'simple partial seizures').

Generalised seizures are characterised by the involvement of both hemispheres from the onset of the seizure discharge and therefore invariably present with impaired awareness. Generalised seizures are primarily divided into motor and non-motor (absence) seizures. *Motor seizures* are further classified based on the type of their motor manifestations: tonic-clonic (classical convulsions or grand mal seizures) or other motor manifestations (e.g. clonic only, tonic only, myoclonic, atonic).

Non-motor seizures with focal onset can have autonomic, behavioural, cognitive, emotional or sensory manifestations, whereas non-motor seizures with generalised onset correspond to 'absence seizures'.

Absence seizures are characteristically associated with regular 3 Hz spike and slow-wave activity on electroencephalography.

Epileptic auras are subjective sensory or psychic phenomena due to focal seizures that can generalise.[33] The aura is, in itself, a focal aware seizure. The spread of the abnormal epileptic activity can result in a secondary generalisation, with loss of consciousness and bilateral convulsions, reflecting involvement of both cerebral hemispheres. The duration of the ictal phase varies between different seizure types, from a few seconds (e.g. absence seizures) to a few minutes (e.g. temporal lobe seizures).

Post-ictal mental state abnormalities typically involve confusion, tiredness and headache, and they may include paralysis of a limb (Todd's paresis).

Status epilepticus is defined as a seizure associated with at least five minutes of continuous clinical or electrographic epileptic activity, or recurrent epileptic activity without recovery between seizures.

The different types of epilepsies are classified according to syndromes.[34] Each epileptic syndrome can present with multiple seizure types. The terminology in use often reflects historical syndromic concepts – for example, psychomotor epilepsy (mesial temporal lobe epilepsy), nocturnal frontal lobe epilepsy, Janz syndrome (juvenile myoclonic epilepsy), Lennox-Gastaut syndrome and West syndrome.

The main line of management in epilepsy is with medications. There are over 20 antiepileptic drugs that are currently in use for the treatment of epilepsy. About half of them are currently licensed for use in monotherapy, whereas the available evidence for the remaining ones restricts their use to adjunctive (add-on) therapy only. Although there is no formula to choose which antiepileptic drug to use for a particular patient, effectiveness on specific seizure types combined with tolerability profiles can guide rational pharmacotherapy. Narrow-spectrum antiepileptic drugs include phenytoin, carbamazepine and oxcarbazepine, whereas examples of broad-spectrum antiepileptic drugs are valproate, levetiracetam, lamotrigine, topiramate and zonisamide. In general, narrow-spectrum antiepileptic drugs work for specific types of seizures (e.g. focal seizures, absence seizures, myoclonic seizures), whereas broad-spectrum antiepileptic drugs have additional effectiveness for a wider variety of seizures (e.g. focal seizures plus absence and myoclonic seizures). Among the most commonly prescribed agents, valproate is indicated for all seizure types, but it is contraindicated in women of childbearing potential or during pregnancy. Knowledge of the tolerabilty profiles of individual antiepileptic drugs is key to neuropsychiatry, as most agents have significant behavioural effects.[35] A few antiepileptic drugs have psychiatric indications, especially as anti-anxiety agents (e.g. pregabalin) or as mood stabilisers (e.g. valproate, carbamazepine, lamotrigine). Evidence on antiepileptic drug combinations (dual therapy or polytherapy) is virtually non-existent, and the final decision of combining specific antiepileptic drugs is based on the experience of the individual clinician. Up to a third of patients with epilepsy have refractory seizures that fail to respond to antiepileptic medications. Selected patients with refractory focal seizures can undergo resective epilepsy surgery (e.g. anterior temporal lobectomy), vagal nerve stimulation and other neurostimulation techniques that can often provide promising alternatives.

Besides the avoidance of known psychological precipitants of seizures (e.g. depression, anxiety and tiredness, especially if associated with sleep deprivation), a number of psychological and behavioural approaches may prove beneficial to some patients: cognitive behavioural therapy, biofeedback and conditioning procedures are among the most commonly indicated non-pharmacological strategies.

Behavioural symptoms are commonly reported in the context of epilepsy, especially in patients with refractory focal impaired awareness seizures. Psychiatric symptoms in epilepsy can be classified according to the temporal relationship with the epileptic seizure itself. Ictal and peri-ictal psychiatric symptoms are directly related to the seizure discharge and have an episodic pattern, whereas interictal disorders are unrelated in time to the seizure and tend to have a chronic course.

Ictal and Peri-ictal Phenomena

Both ictal and peri-ictal disorders are characterised by symptoms that are temporally related to the epileptic seizure.[36] The acute disruption of cerebral activity that occurs with the seizure discharge can present clinically with alterations in consciousness or acute changes in behaviour.

Preictal behavioural symptoms can herald a seizure and typically present as affect changes, dysphoria, anxiety, irritability, impulsivity and short attention span. The gap between preictal symptoms and clinical seizures can range from hours to up to three days. The behavioural manifestations tend to worsen during the 24 hours prior to the seizure and remit postictally, although persistence for a few days after the seizure can be seen.

Ictal psychiatric symptoms are the direct clinical expression of seizure activity and are often associated with temporal lobe seizures, which are the most common type of focal seizures. The deep mesial temporal structures – particularly the amygdala and hippocampus – can be highly epileptogenic, as in mesial temporal sclerosis. Most frontal lobe seizures involve motor activity. However, frontal seizures arising in the cingulate region may give rise to affective changes as well as complex automatisms, similarly to those seen in temporal lobe seizures. Moreover, frontal lobe seizures arising from the supplementary motor area can present with complex motor manifestations (e.g. bimanual/bipedal automatisms – such as clapping or stamping – and complex verbalisations like singing) and semi-purposive automatisms that can be mistaken for functional neurological symptoms. Parietal and occipital seizures are less common and less likely to be seen by neuropsychiatrists, although occasionally abnormal somatosensory and visual perceptions may also be misdiagnosed as functional neurological symptoms.

Ictal emotions are particularly common in patients with temporal lobe epilepsy, as seizure-induced alterations of the contents of consciousness are often the expression of epileptic auras of temporal lobe seizures.[37] The most common ictal affective symptoms are unpleasant emotions, especially fear, terror, anxiety, guilt, sadness, depression, anger and embarrassment. Ictal fear or panic is reported in around 60 per cent of experiential auras, followed by ictal depression (15 per cent). The differential diagnosis between ictal fear and panic attack disorder can be challenging. Ictal fear as a manifestation of an epileptic aura is typically brief (less than 30 seconds in duration) and stereotypical, occurs independently to stressful events, and may be followed by other ictal phenomena, such as motor automatisms, confusion and autonomic symptoms (especially salivation). The severity of the sensation of fear can range from mild to moderate. Conversely, panic attacks typically have longer duration (5–20 minutes, which at times may persist for several hours) and high intensity. Panic attacks are characteristically associated with significant autonomic symptoms, including tachycardia, diffuse diaphoresis and shortness of breath (but not excessive salivation). Contrary to panic attacks, ictal fear is not always recalled after a seizure; however, witnesses may report that the patient appeared terrified.

Ictal symptoms of depression are the second most frequent ictal psychiatric manifestations. Patients can suddenly report severe depression of mood, as well as feelings of anhedonia, guilt or suicidal ideation that typically are of short duration and stereotypical. Ictal affective changes occur out of context and tend to be associated with other ictal phenomena. More rarely, patients can experience positive or pleasant emotions, such as exhilaration, mirth, blissful happiness, euphoria, ecstasy or sexual excitement. Dreamy states are brief alterations of the contents of consciousness that can occur in a variety of psychological states and, in uncinate seizures, originating in the temporal lobe.

Ictal dissociative symptoms include derealisation and depersonalisation. Derealisation is the alteration in one's sense of external reality, whereas depersonalisation is the alteration in an individual's sense of personal reality and experience of self, occasionally accompanied by out-of-body experiences and autoscopy (seeing one's double). Both derealisation and depersonalisation may be difficult to distinguish from panic disorder, resulting in diagnostic confusion. During seizures (especially temporal lobe seizures), patients might recall past events or situations.

Ictal flashbacks tend to be more vivid and intrusive than commonplace recollections. In déjà vu (literally 'already seen') or déjà vécu ('already lived') experiences, feelings of recognition or familiarity can be inappropriately attached to the present. The opposite experiences can also occur and are referred to as jamais vu ('never seen') or jamais vécu ('never lived'). False recollections or paramnesias have also been reported.

Ictal violence most commonly occurs as the result of poor handling of a confused ictal or post-ictal patient. Violent behaviour as part of an automatism or post-ictal state is an extremely rare occurrence and is usually poorly directed, brief, purposeless, fragmentary, simple and repetitive. Occasionally, patients can display continuation of a behaviour instigated before the seizure began. Ictal violence is usually sudden, with paroxysmal onset, and results in behaviours that are grossly out of proportion to any stress, precipitant or provocation. There can be hazy recollection (or amnesia) for the ictal episode. Patients who recall performing a serious assault or destruction of property characteristically show genuine remorse. Overall, such uncontrollable storms of aggression are out of character, and between episodes, there is a lack of generalised aggressiveness.

Automatisms are part of the seizure associated with alterations of consciousness; patients experiencing an automatism usually show simple, repetitive movement or wandering with confusion and irritation, lasting less than five minutes in the majority of patients.

Epileptic psychoses temporally associated with epileptic seizures may be either ictal or post-ictal. Ictal psychosis is the result of ongoing paroxysmal brain discharges. The duration of ictal psychosis can be longer when associated with non-convulsive status epilepticus. Commonly reported ictal psychotic symptoms include organic perceptual abnormalities, with complex visual or auditory hallucinations and illusions with distortion of body image. After their seizures, patients might be able to recall seeing complex scenes or faces, or hearing voices or musical tunes. The contents of seizure-induced hallucinations are often described as familiar, although it is not always possible to identify them with precision. Associated symptoms can include altered speed of thoughts and forced thinking (inability to voluntarily control thoughts). EEG recording is an early and essential investigation in atypical confusional psychoses, as it can be diagnostic for ictal psychosis.

Post-ictal behavioural symptoms characteristically present after a symptom-free period ranging from several hours to one week after a seizure or, more frequently, a cluster of seizures. The average duration of the lucid interval is 24–48 hours. Post-ictal psychotic episodes can last from a few days to several weeks, but usually remit spontaneously after one to two weeks.

Post-ictal psychosis is typically reported by patients with refractory seizures for more than 10 years and is often associated with temporal lobe seizures and secondarily generalised tonic-clonic seizures. Affective features, erratic behaviours, hallucinations, confusion and amnesia have all been reported as part of this condition. Post-ictal psychosis characteristically presents with paranoid delusional beliefs (sometimes with religious themes) accompanied by affective changes. Fugues and twilight states are two common types of post-ictal psychosis.

Post-ictal fugues are prolonged dissociative episodes of wandering, altered behaviour and amnesia, which may last for hours or even days.

Twilight states are characterised by abnormal perceptual and affective experiences associated with cognitive impairment, perseveration and occasional paranoid hallucinatory disturbances. Other post-ictal behavioural symptoms include depression, anxiety and autonomic manifestations, which can last for 24 hours or more and can overlap with other psychiatric symptoms.

Both ictal and peri-ictal behavioural symptoms should initially be treated by optimising the antiepileptic pharmacotherapy, as complete control over seizure-related behavioural symptoms can only be achieved with remission of the underlying epilepsy.

Interictal Disorders

Anxiety and Affective Disorders

The link between epileptic seizures and behavioural disturbances has been recognised since Hippocrates' writings around 400 BCE. The behavioural symptoms reported by patients with epilepsy have often been shown to have a deeper impact on their health-related quality of life than the actual seizures. Epilepsy, behaviour and cognition have a complex relationship, with clinically relevant implications for the selection of the most appropriate antiepileptic drugs.[38] From a neuropsychiatric perspective, it is important that treatment interventions for patients with epilepsy are not restricted to the achievement of seizure freedom, but they incorporate the management of behavioural and cognitive manifestations.

Patients with epilepsy report a higher prevalence of psychiatric co-morbidity compared to the general population.[39] It has been estimated that interictal behavioural symptoms are relatively frequent in the epilepsy population, affecting between 30 and 50 per cent of patients (Table 8.5).

Table 8.5 Main epilepsy-associated interictal psychiatric disorders

Depression
Anxiety
Interictal dysphoric disorder
Schizophrenia-like psychosis of epilepsy
Alternative psychosis
Gastaut-Geschwind syndrome

Anxiety and affective disorders are the most frequent psychiatric comorbidities, with lifetime prevalence rates of up to 35 per cent. The prevalence rates of psychotic disorders are higher in patients with epilepsy than in the general population (7–10% versus 0.4–1%). Although psychotic disorders are reported less frequently than anxiety and affective disorders, these symptoms can be highly disabling. Specific personality traits have been associated with temporal lobe epilepsy (temporal lobe epilepsy personality disorder or Gastaut-Geschwind syndrome). Finally, a substantial proportion of patients with epilepsy present with comorbid functional neurological symptoms, especially psychogenic nonepileptic attacks, thus posing significant diagnostic challenges.

Interictal psychiatric disorders are thought to have a multifactorial aetiology, with the contribution of neurobiological, psychological and social factors, as well as behavioural adverse effects of antiepileptic drugs.[40] The early recognition and initial evaluation of interictal psychiatric disorders are important steps in the formulation of a comprehensive management plan that takes into account the complexities of the neuropsychiatric manifestations in the context of epilepsy. In addition to identifying the behavioural manifestations of epilepsy, neuropsychiatrists implement treatment interventions tailored to the individual patient with epilepsy and comorbid anxiety and affective symptoms, as well as psychotic disorders. Chronic psychiatric disorders appear to be more frequent in patients with refractory seizures and localisation-related epilepsy (especially temporal lobe epilepsy). Specifically, it has been suggested that both behavioural and personality changes may occur as a consequence of chronic temporo-limbic irritability.

Depression and anxiety are the most common interictal psychiatric disorders, occurring with a lifetime prevalence that is significantly higher in comparison with the general population.[41] The clinical presentation of interictal affective symptoms overlaps with that of primary psychiatric conditions seen in the wider community. Associated features include high anxiety and hostility, and there is a relationship with a long history of epilepsy. Female patients with epilepsy appear to have particularly higher risk of developing depression.[42] Moreover, patients with treatment-refractory epilepsy are more likely to develop specific types of phobias – such as fear of seizures, social phobia and agoraphobia – as a result of experiencing recurrent and unpredictable seizures. The fear of having an epileptic seizure in public, and of its possible consequences, can be linked with specific phobias and avoidance behaviours.

The aetiology of depression in epilepsy has a biological component as well as a psychosocial component. The former includes reduced monoaminergic activity, whereas the latter encompasses the experience of external locus of control and learned helplessness. Social stigma and limitations in selected life activities are likely to play a role as contributing factors.

Intermittent dysphoric symptoms are frequently reported by patients with chronic epilepsy; these include anergia, depressed mood, insomnia, atypical pains, anxiety, phobic symptoms, euphoric moods and paroxysmal irritability. The presence of at least three intermittent dysphoric symptoms with fluctuating clinical course and variable duration (from hours to days) prompts the diagnosis of interictal dysphoric disorder, a condition described by Swiss psychiatrist Dietrich Blumer.

Patients who have previously undergone epilepsy surgery (especially temporal lobe resection) have an increased risk of developing an affective disorder. Affective symptoms as behavioural complications of epilepsy surgery are more frequent in the first postsurgical year and can prove difficult to treat. A comprehensive neuropsychiatric assessment is recommended for the assessment and treatment of presurgical psychiatric comorbidities, and this may minimise the risk of postsurgical behavioural complications.

The first step in the treatment of affective symptoms and anxiety in the context of epilepsy is the optimisation of the pharmacotherapy of seizures.[43] The choice of the most appropriate antiepileptic agent(s) should be based on multiple factors, including the patient's demographic data and epilepsy data (seizure type, epileptic syndrome), the behavioural and cognitive profiles of individual antiepileptic drugs, their interaction profile and impact on reproductive functions, and the presence of other comorbidities. Based on the available data on the behavioural effects of antiepileptic drugs, a few selected antiepileptic drugs can prove beneficial in patients with comorbid anxiety (e.g. GABAergic agents such as gabapentin and pregabalin), whereas other drugs can be more indicated in patients with comorbid depression (e.g. lamotrigine).

Cognitive behavioural therapy has been shown to be helpful for the treatment of both affective symptoms and anxiety in patients with epilepsy. SSRIs should be considered as first-line pharmacological treatment options, based on their favourable tolerability profile and safety in terms of seizure threshold lowering effect. A few of the older antidepressants (notably monoaminoxidase inhibitors, tricyclic antidepressants and bupropion) are potentially epileptogenic, although most modern antidepressants are clearly effective and safe. Nearly all antidepressant medications will increase seizure frequency when taken in overdose; these medications must be started at low dosage, and increases must be slow. There can be clinically relevant interactions between antiepileptic drugs and antidepressants. A few antiepileptic drugs (e.g. phenobarbitone, phenytoin, carbamazepine) are liver-enzyme inducers and are therefore likely to reduce levels of antidepressants. Neuropsychiatrists also need to be aware of the possible enzyme-inhibiting effects of SSRIs such as fluoxetine and fluvoxamine, which may lead to increases in antiepileptic drug levels (especially phenytoin and carbamazepine). Although regular antiepileptic drug level monitoring in patients with epilepsy is not recommended as routine, where clinically indicated, optimisation of antiepileptic drug therapy can be guided by blood level monitoring in complex polypharmacy regimens.

Schizophrenia-like Psychosis of Epilepsy

Psychotic symptoms occur with a higher prevalence in patients with epilepsy, especially temporal lobe epilepsy.[44] The clinical picture of chronic schizophrenia in patients with epilepsy can be different to the presentation of primary schizophrenia and is often referred to as schizophreniform psychosis of epilepsy or schizophrenia-like psychosis of epilepsy. This condition is characterised by paranoid psychosis, often with positive symptoms such as hallucinations, and warm affect. Negative symptoms are rarely reported, and there is no increased family history of schizophrenia. Risk factors include seizures with a mesial temporal focus, ictal fear and onset of epilepsy in adolescence. The psychosis typically emerges 10–15 years after the onset of epilepsy, and there is usually a good premorbid function and less personality deterioration.

Delusions and hallucinations reported by patients with epilepsy have been described as 'more empathisable', because 'the patient remains in our world'. Overall, the schizophrenia-like psychosis of epilepsy is characterised by lesser severity and better response to therapy than primary schizophrenia, often resulting in a more favourable outcome. The pathophysiology of schizophrenia-like psychosis of epilepsy might be related to kindling mechanisms. It has been suggested that functional problems in the connections between the sensory cortex and limbic structures, resulting from chronic irritability of temporal lobe cortex, can eventually result in paranoid delusions about the significance of everyday sensory inputs. Caution should be used when treating psychotic symptoms in patients with epilepsy with antipsychotic medications because of the seizure threshold lowering effects of most antipsychotic medications. Atypical antipsychotics (with the exception of clozapine) are generally safer than first-generation antipsychotics; the first-generation antipsychotics with the lowest risk of seizure induction include haloperidol, fluphenazine, perphenazine and trifluoperazine.

Forced Normalisation

The relatively rare phenomenon of alternative psychosis is the development of acute psychotic (and sometimes anxiety/affective) symptoms when the seizures are brought under control. Conversely, remission of the behavioural symptoms can be reported upon recurrence of the epileptic seizures. This alternation of seizures and behavioural symptoms in a small group of patients with epilepsy was first noticed by Swiss chemist Heinrich Landolt. The improvement in behavioural problems is concomitant to EEG abnormalities, whereas seizure control is accompanied by normalisation of the EEG, a phenomenon referred to as forced normalisation or Landolt phenomenon. Albeit rare, this phenomenon can be of considerable clinical relevance, as the patients alternate between periods of clinically manifest seizures with normal behaviour and periods of seizure freedom accompanied by behavioural symptoms. Forced normalisation has been reported in association with the use of several antiepileptic drugs, as well as epilepsy surgery.

Gastaut-Geschwind Syndrome and Aggressive Behaviours

French epileptologist Henri Gastaut (1915–1995) and American behavioural neurologist Norman Geschwind (1926–1984) independently postulated that a specific type of personality disorder could arise from persistent temporal lobe seizure discharges. Temporal lobe epilepsy personality syndrome, also referred to as Gastaut-Geschwind syndrome, is a pattern of chronic behavioural changes (not necessarily maladaptive) described in patients with temporal lobe epilepsy. The Bear-Fedio questionnaire allows a systematic screening for 18 different personality traits that have been linked to temporal lobe epilepsy. The main features of temporal lobe epilepsy personality syndrome are hyperreligiosity, hypergraphia, hyposexuality and viscosity (an interictal language disturbance characterised by verbal stickiness). Humourless sobriety, dependence, irritability, circumstantiality, obsessionality, preoccupation with pseudo-philosophical concerns and ruminative intellectual tendencies are all features that have been associated with temporal lobe epilepsy personality syndrome.

There is evidence that violent or aggressive behaviour can be seen more commonly in people with epilepsy than in a normal control population. For example, the rate of criminal offences is higher in the epilepsy population than in the general population. Specifically, it has been suggested that patients with temporal lobe epilepsy could be at higher risk of developing interictal aggression and violence.

Cognitive Impairment

Both absence seizures and brief focal discharges may go unnoticed by the patient or those nearby and yet can significantly impair registration of memory. Post-ictal amnesia and partial amnesias may be misdiagnosed as a dementing process, especially if frequent seizures result in an almost continuous post-ictal state. There is no link between epilepsy and intellectual impairment, apart from cases of seizures associated as a secondary phenomenon with brain damage (congenital or otherwise). Interictal cognitive impairment and decline may be the result of sedative antiepileptic drugs, interrupted and poor education, parental attitudes and personal reactions to the illness. The cognitive profile of individual antiepileptic drugs should be taken into account in the neuropsychological assessment of patients with epilepsy. For example, topiramate has been associated – in a proportion of cases – with mental slowing and reduced verbal fluency (word-finding difficulties).

Non-convulsive status and possibly subclinical paroxysmal discharges, such as hippocampal spike activity, can also contribute to cognitive disturbances.

Specific memory and learning deficits can be associated with specific types of epilepsy – for example, verbal memory impairment with left temporal lobe epilepsy and impaired attention with generalised epilepsy. The aetiology of the epilepsy is the main determinant of cognitive impairment. Early onset, disease duration and seizure frequency are weakly related to cognitive impairment. Intellectual decline in patients with epilepsy is usually associated with severe personality deterioration and is more commonly seen in association with reduced reserves due to brain damage, resulting in early dementia.

Psychogenic Nonepileptic Attacks

Psychogenic nonepileptic attacks or dissociative seizures (previously referred to as pseudoseizures and hysterical seizures, among other terms) can pose significant diagnostic challenges even to experienced neurologists. Psychogenic nonepileptic attacks clinically resemble epileptic seizures. However, they are not accompanied by the characteristic changes in the brain's electrical activity. A substantial proportion of patients diagnosed with treatment-refractory epilepsy suffer from psychogenic nonepileptic attacks. Moreover, patients with epilepsy can present with a combination of epileptic seizures and psychogenic nonepileptic attacks. A pre-existing psychiatric disorder is more commonly found in patients with psychogenic nonepileptic attacks. With regard to the clinical phenomenology, these patients are more likely to present with eye closure and bizarre behaviours (such as screaming, head shaking and pelvic thrusting) than patients with epileptic seizures. Intermittent convulsions, active resistance to forceful eye opening, preserved consciousness with bilateral motor manifestations, and abrupt recovery following a prolonged episode are strong indicators of a psychogenic nonepileptic attack. Surface electroencephalography does not characteristically show any epileptiform abnormalities either during or after the clinical episode; however, this can also occur in certain epileptic seizures (e.g. seizures arising from the medial aspect of the frontal lobe). Moreover, occasional inter-ictal epileptiform discharges are not rare in healthy people. Therefore, simultaneous video and electroencephalographic recording of a typical clinical episode (ictal video EEG during videotelemetry) is currently considered the gold standard investigation for the differential diagnosis between psychogenic nonepileptic attacks and epileptic seizures. Serum prolactin levels measured immediately after the clinical episode are not particularly useful, as raised levels can be detected in both convulsive seizures and hypermotor psychogenic nonepileptic attacks (false positives). The management of psychogenic nonepileptic attacks starts at the moment of diagnosis communication, with reassurance and psychoeducation as cornerstones of the therapeutic process. If previously initiated, antiepileptic drugs can be gradually decreased until discontinuation, as appropriate. In such cases, cognitive and behavioural approaches should initially address the change in diagnosis, in addition to the psychotherapeutic exploration of the patient's past. There is evidence that patients with psychogenic nonepileptic attacks have a higher prevalence of previous traumatic experiences, especially a history of sexual abuse.

Movement Disorders

Parkinson's Disease

Both hyperkinetic and hypokinetic movement disorders can be associated with psychiatric symptoms (Table 8.6).

Parkinson's disease is a neurodegenerative condition consisting of both motor and non-motor features, with mean age at onset at around 60 years. Parkinson's disease is one of the most common neurological disorders of later life; its prevalence is around 1–2 per 1,000 in the general population, with higher figures in the elderly. Men are slightly more likely to be affected than women; however, the genetic risk is low. The key motor features of Parkinson's disease, first described in 1817 by James Parkinson (1755–1824), encompass the clinical triad of tremor, rigidity and bradykinesia.[45] Parkinsonian tremor may affect the hands (pronation/supination), jaw, tongue, head or lower limbs. It has a 'pill rolling' appearance, with high amplitude and low frequency (4–6 Hz), and is typically present at rest, but disappears during sleep. Rigidity has a 'lead pipe' quality and, on examination, it is possible to observe the 'cogwheel' phenomenon. Bradykinesia (or, in more severe cases, akinesia) presents with slowness of initiating movement and overall poverty of movement. Further clinical features of Parkinson's disease include postural instability, reduced arm swinging, freezing of gait, abnormal trunk posture ('camptocormia'), reduced facial mimicry ('poker face'), micrographia, oculomotor abnormalities, excessive salivation, seborrhoea, constipation, subjective sensory disturbance and fatigue.

The neuropathological hallmark of Parkinson's disease is the progressive loss of dopaminergic neurons within the pars compacta of the substantia nigra. Pathological intracellular accumulations of Lewy bodies can be observed, initially within the brainstem and olfactory structures, subsequently in the midbrain and, finally, across cortical areas (Braak staging).

Table 8.6 Most common movement disorders associated with psychiatric symptoms

Parkinson's disease
Tourette syndrome
Huntington's disease
Dystonia
Wilson's disease
Fahr's disease
Progressive supranuclear palsy
Sydenham's chorea

Rapid eye movement (REM) sleep behaviour disorder can precede the onset of obvious motor signs, possibly reflecting early-stage pathological involvement of brainstem structures.

The motor symptoms of Parkinson's disease can respond, at least for a few years, to pharmacotherapy. Dopamine replacement therapy encompasses levodopa (administered with COMT inhibitors, such as entacapone or opicapone, to reduce its peripheral metabolism) and dopamine receptor agonists (pramipexole, ropinirole, rotigotine and, in selected cases, apomorphine). MAO-B inhibitors can be useful to reduce oxidative damage, preserve cell membranes and enhance cell survival. Surgical therapies, especially deep brain stimulation targeting the subthalamic nucleus, can be an option for patients who no longer respond to pharmacotherapy or develop severe motor fluctuations (on-off phenomenon) and dyskinesias as adverse effects of dopamine replacement therapy.

The non-motor features of Parkinson's disease include a range of psychiatric symptoms and can affect patients' health-related quality of life to a greater extent than motor disability.[46] An association between depression and Parkinson's disease is well established; moreover, depression has been shown to potentially cause the greatest impairment in patients' well-being. Depression in the context of Parkinson's disease can be understood both as a reactive process to a serious disabling illness and as an integral part of the disease process itself, in consideration of the involvement of central monoamines. Patients with Parkinson's disease frequently report dysphoric mood – with sadness and feelings of hopelessness – whereas guilt and self-deprecation are relatively rare. The diagnosis of depression can be difficult because of the overlap between clinical features of classical depression and symptoms of Parkinson's disease, such as hypomimia (reduced facial mimicry resulting in 'facial masking' or 'poker face'), loss of concentration, cognitive slowing, sleep problems and weight loss. Pervasive low mood, severe anhedonia and diurnal variation in mood suggest a diagnosis of depression in patients with Parkinson's disease.

The full range of anxiety disorders, as well as apathy, are common in patients with Parkinson's disease – with or without comorbid depression – and should be distinguished from variations related to changes in motor state (end of dose effects). Affective symptoms in Parkinson's disease are best managed using standard treatment approaches for major depression, especially serotonergic agents. Co-administration of SSRIs and MAO-B inhibitors such as selegiline can result in increased risk for serotonergic syndrome. Likewise, caution is required when using SSRIs together with dopamine replacement therapies because of nausea as an emerging adverse effect. Among psychological interventions, cognitive behavioural therapy has been shown to be potentially useful for the treatment of depression in patients with Parkinson's disease.

The most common form of psychosis in patients with Parkinson's disease is associated with the use of dopaminergic agents.[47] The development of psychosis is the primary cause of family breakdown and nursing home placement in this patient population. Organic psychosis in the context of Parkinson's disease is characterised by a higher prevalence of visual hallucinations over auditory and olfactory hallucinations; these can take the form of people and animals, which are often perceived as non-threatening pareidolic illusions. Hallucinations often occur overnight, can be preceded by vivid dreams and nightmares, and can be accompanied by affective changes. Associated psychotic symptoms include pareidolic illusions, as well as persecutory and paranoid delusions, often of reference and infidelity (Othello syndrome).

About one-third of patients with Parkinson's disease treated with dopaminergic medications can develop impulse control disorders. Patients can present with a wide range of reward-seeking behaviours: compulsive eating, hypersexuality, pathological gambling and compulsive shopping are among the most frequently reported manifestations.[48] The term 'punding' describes pleasure-driven repetition of purposeless and stereotyped behaviours, such as assembling and disassembling complex machines and sorting out objects.

Overall, decreased and increased dopamine receptor stimulation are thought to exert opposite effects on the behavioural symptoms of patients with Parkinson's disease. Hypodopaminergic states have been associated with decreased motivational states, such as anhedonia, anxiety, apathy and depression. Hyperdopaminergic states have been linked to the development of impulse control disorders, punding and dopamine dysregulation syndrome (compulsive and excessive use of dopamine replacement therapy).[49]

Reduction of the dopamine replacement therapy is the first step in the treatment of psychotic symptoms and impulse control disorders, including punding. However, decreasing the dosage of antidopaminergic agents is often problematic, as it may lead to an exacerbation of the Parkinsonian symptoms. Discontinuation of anticholinergic medications can prove beneficial for patients with behavioural problems aggravated by cognitive symptoms. Antidopaminergic medications can be recommended in patients with persistent and severe behavioural symptoms. The highest level of evidence supports the use of clozapine, also in consideration of its relatively low rate of extrapyramidal adverse effects. Other atypical antipsychotic agents – such as quetiapine, risperidone and aripiprazole – can be considered as valuable alternative options. Pimavanserin, an atypical antipsychotic that targets serotonin neuro-transmission, has shown promise for the treatment of psychosis in patients with Parkinson's disease.

Cognitive behavioural therapy can be helpful in the pragmatic management of pathological reward-seeking behaviours. Patients treated with deep brain stimulation are often able to reduce the dosage of their dopamine replacement therapy, leading to a decrease in impulse control disorders. However, deep brain stimulation has occasionally been associated with the development of both affective symptoms and impulsivity.

Dementia in Parkinson's Disease

Cognitive disturbances are frequently reported by patients with Parkinson's disease. In addition to generalised global dementia, this patient population has an increased risk of developing focal and specific cognitive deficits, drug-induced confusional states and depression-related cognitive difficulties.

Age is the most important single determinant for the prevalence of dementia among people with Parkinson's disease. About 40 per cent of patients develop dementia, with significantly higher risk after the age of 70 years and 10–15 years after the diagnosis. Elderly patients with Parkinson's disease are also at higher risk of developing reversible confusional states associated with the use of antiparkinsonian medications. Patients with comorbid depression show a greater intellectual decline, with particular problems in frontal lobe tasks. The clinical presentation of dementia in patients with Parkinson's disease shows a considerable overlap with Lewy body dementia, suggesting the existence of a spectrum of neuropsychiatric disorders caused by accumulation of Lewy bodies within the cerebral cortex: problems with movement, widespread cognitive deficits, affective dysregulation and fluctuating consciousness. The results of treatment trials of acetylcholinesterase inhibitors have shown that the use of rivastigmine may be associated with improved cognition.

Tourette Syndrome

Tourette syndrome, first described in 1885 by Georges Gilles de la Tourette (1857–1904, Figure 8.6), is a tic disorder characterised by the presence of both motor and vocal tics.[50] Tics are defined as involuntary, sudden, rapid, recurrent, non-rhythmic movements or vocalisations. Tourette syndrome is a neurodevelopmental disorder, with onset in childhood and a chronic course. Other chronic tic disorders include persistent motor or vocal tic disorders, whereas the diagnostic category of provisional tic disorder is used for patients with tics that have been present for less than one year since onset.

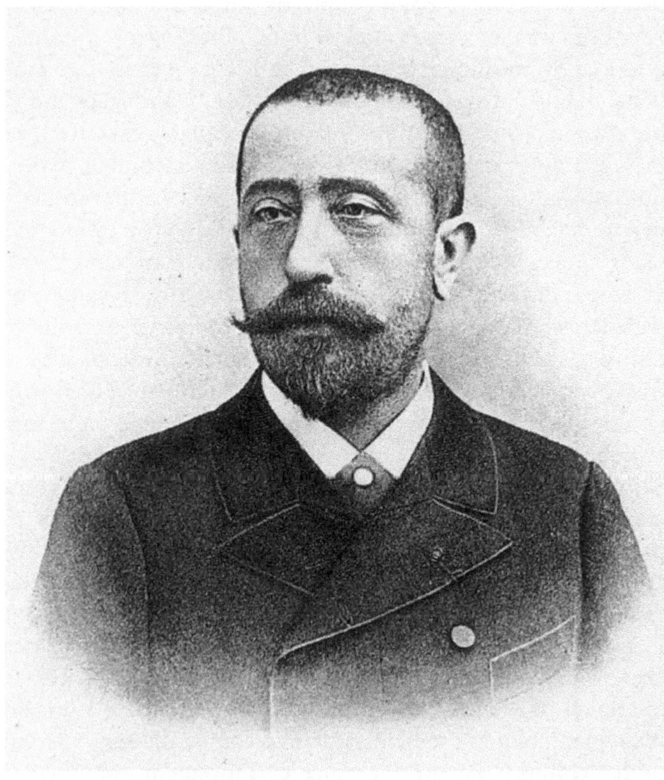

Figure 8.6 Georges Gilles de la Tourette (1857–1904).

Once thought to be a rarity, Tourette syndrome is no longer considered a rare medical condition: up to 1 per cent of school-age children fulfil current diagnostic criteria for this condition. It has been estimated that as many as 200,000–330,000 individuals in the United Kingdom have symptoms consistent with Tourette syndrome, with different degrees of severity.[51]

The average age at onset of tics is five to seven years, and tics are three to four times more common in boys than girls. The most frequent initial tics involve the eyes, especially blinking. Other simple motor tics include eye rolling, mouth opening, facial grimacing, neck stretching, shoulder shrugging, abdominal crunching, kicking or toe scratching. Complex motor tics involve multiple muscular districts, possibly resulting in whole body movements such as jumping, squatting, turning or hitting. Simple vocal tics (most commonly sniffing, grunting, throat clearing, coughing, snorting, humming) tend to develop after the motor tics. Complex vocal tics involve words and include echolalia (repeating others' words), palilalia (repeating own words) and coprolalia (involuntary swearing as a tic). Coprolalia is not included among current diagnostic criteria: it has been documented in up to 30 per cent of patients with Tourette syndrome in specialist clinics and in only about 10 per cent of patients in the wider community. A subset of patients can also report echopraxia (copying behaviours), palipraxia (repetition of voluntary actions, usually a set number of times or until the action feels 'just right'), copropraxia (inappropriate obscene gestures) and non-obscene socially inappropriate behaviours. Other complex tics, such as mental coprolalia and coprographia, may be revealed only on direct questioning.

Most patients with Tourette syndrome report that their tics are preceded by sensory symptoms: a subjective feeling of mounting inner tension, referred to as 'premonitory urge', that is temporarily relieved by tic expression.[52] Assessment of the premonitory urges is particularly useful for the differential diagnosis between tics and other repetitive behaviours, such as stereotypies and mannerisms.

The natural course of tics is characterised by a waxing and waning pattern, with significant changes in frequency, severity and body location throughout life. Tics typically peak in severity during early adolescence, and most patients report a variable degree of improvement by adulthood. Tics are characteristically exacerbated by environmental factors such as stress, anxiety, self-consciousness and excitement. Conversely, relaxation and engagement in non-stressful mental and physical tasks requiring active concentration, including playing sports and musical instruments, are often reported as tic-alleviating factors. The environment can modulate tic expression in multiple ways, including the perceived nature of social interactions.

The exact pathophysiology of Tourette syndrome is not fully understood. However, the available evidence points towards functional alterations at the level of the basal ganglia. Specifically, converging lines of evidence suggest dysfunction in striato-thalamo-cortical circuitries, with predominant involvement of dopaminergic pathways. Tourette syndrome is a genetically heterogeneous condition with multiple heritability patterns. The exact role of environmental factors (both immunological and perinatal factors) in the aetiology of the condition has not been fully clarified.

It has consistently been shown that in the majority of patients with Tourette syndrome (about 90 per cent), motor and vocal tics are associated with specific behavioural problems.[53] The most common psychiatric comorbidities are obsessive-compulsive disorder or sub-threshold obsessive-compulsive behaviours. The phenomenology of obsessive-compulsive symptoms often differs between patients with Tourette syndrome and patients with obsessive-compulsive disorder. Specifically, patients with Tourette syndrome report a significantly higher prevalence of tic-related obsessive-compulsive symptoms – such as concerns for symmetry, evening-up behaviours, arithmomania (counting), ordering, and 'just-right' perceptions – whereas patients with obsessive-compulsive disorder have a higher rate of concerns for contamination, cleaning and washing rituals. Tics are mainly driven by premonitory urges that are more physical in nature and are described as feelings of physical discomfort, pressure and need to release inner energy or tension, whereas compulsions are triggered by anxiety and intrusive thoughts. Moreover, compulsions tend to be more ritualistic and routine-like in nature.

Hyperactivity, distractibility and impulsivity are relatively common in patients with Tourette syndrome, especially in younger ones. The combination of Tourette syndrome and attention-deficit/hyperactivity disorder is common and adds greatly to the burden of both conditions on both patients and carers. In many cases, it can be difficult to disentangle hyperactivity associated with tic expression and attention deficits due to active tic suppression from the presence of comorbid attention-deficit/hyperactivity disorder. Collateral history from family members and teachers often plays a key role in the clinical assessment of attention-deficit/hyperactivity disorder in younger patients with Tourette syndrome. Impulsivity in the context of Tourette syndrome can be related to the expression of self-injurious behaviours and rage attacks. Other comorbid behavioural conditions include affective and anxiety disorders, with multifactorial origins. Moreover, patients with other neurodevelopmental disorders, such as autism spectrum disorders, have an increased risk of developing tics compared to the general population. Finally, there is preliminary evidence suggesting an increased prevalence of personality disorders. The findings of clinical studies dissecting the neuropsychiatric spectrum of tic disorders have suggested that Tourette syndrome could be seen as a gradient of disorders of increasing complexity, ranging from 'pure Tourette syndrome' (tics only) to 'Tourette syndrome plus' (tics plus comorbid behavioural symptoms).

The use of disease-specific health-related quality of life measures for both paediatric and adult patients with Tourette syndrome allows an accurate assessment of the differential impact of tics and behavioural comorbidities on patients' wellbeing.[54] In turn, knowledge about patients' perception of the determinants of their quality of life provides treating clinicians with useful indications for prioritising management strategies.

Psychoeducation is the first step in the management of Tourette syndrome. Information about tics and behavioural comorbidities should be shared with the patient's family, teachers, employers and other professionals involved. Pharmacotherapy is the mainstay of treatment for the motor and vocal tics, as well as for some of the associated behaviours.[55] The most commonly used medications are alpha-2 agonists, which modulate noradrenergic neuro-transmission and antidopaminergic drugs. Overall, alpha-2 agonists such as clonidine and guanfacine are well tolerated, as adverse effects including drowsiness, dry mouth, headache and postural hypertension tend to be dose-dependent. Alpha-2 agonists have proven particularly helpful in younger patients diagnosed with Tourette syndrome and attention-deficit/hyperactivity disorder. Among first-generation antidopaminergic drugs, the anti-tic effects of haloperidol, pimozide and fluphenazine have been widely documented, although these agents are characterised by poor tolerability profiles. Second-generation antidopaminergic drugs (such as risperidone) and substituted benzamides (such as sulpiride) can be equally effective, but they can be associated with adverse effects including hyperprolactinaemia, sedation and weight gain. Aripiprazole, a newer dopamine modulator with partial agonist properties, tends to be better tolerated. Augmentation strategies with antidopaminergic drugs can be particularly helpful for patients who present with tic-related obsessive-compulsive disorder, possibly based on the shared involvement of fronto-striatal dopaminergic pathways. Other potentially useful medications are pre-synaptic monoamine depletors (tetrabenazine) and antiepileptic drugs (topiramate). Serotonergic medications (SSRIs and the tricyclic agent clomipramine) have been found to be potentially useful in patients with comorbid obsessive-compulsive symptoms, affective symptoms and anxiety. In addition to distraction techniques, behavioural approaches for tic management include habit reversal training and exposure with response prevention. Habit reversal training is based on the patient's awareness of the premonitory urge occurring before a tic and the replacement of the tic itself with a competing response – a more comfortable or acceptable movement or sound. Exposure with response prevention is based on the habituation to the premonitory urge following prolonged voluntary suppression of all tics. Finally, the neurosurgical procedure of deep brain stimulation can be considered in carefully selected severe and treatment-refractory cases.[56] Based on the available evidence, the most promising brain targets are the thalamus and the globus pallidus. With the availability of improved treatment strategies, it has become possible to improve health-related quality of life for an increasing number of people with tics.

Huntington's Disease

Huntington's disease is a rare neurodegenerative movement disorder characterised by chorea. Choreic ('dance-like') movements are abrupt, irregular and purposeless. The hereditary nature of chorea was already noted in its first description by George Huntington (1850–1916, Figure 8.7) in 1872.

The prevalence of Huntington's disease has been estimated as 3–15 per 100,000 and appears to be on the rise in Western countries, as a result of improved case ascertainment, reduced stigma and increased longevity. Huntington's disease follows an autosomal dominant heritance model.[57] It is caused by a single genetic change: expansion of the CAG trinucleotide within the huntingtin gene on the short arm of chromosome 4 leads to protein misfolding and development of the huntingtin protein (Htt). The huntingtin protein tends to aggregate and is toxic to nervous system cells, particularly striatal neurons. The progressive accumulation of the huntingtin protein throughout life leads to symptoms that are usually obvious from middle age but can present at any age. There are no gender differences in either age of onset or clinical characteristics of Huntington's disease. However, inheritance from the paternal side is more likely among early-onset cases. At a population level, the age at onset of motor manifestations is inversely proportional to the length of CAG repeats, as higher numbers of repeats tend to correlate with earlier development of chorea. At the level of the individual patient, the number of CAG repeats is a poor predictor of the age at onset, as the speed and timing of progression have been shown to be modulated by multiple genes. CAG repeat lengths of 40 can be regarded as a 'positive genetic test'. CAG lengths between 36 and 39 are referred to as 'reduced penetrance alleles' and are often associated with later age of onset and prodromal behavioural changes, especially affective symptoms. Higher CAG lengths (for instance, 55 and over) tend to be associated with a juvenile form of Huntington's disease, historically referred to as the Westphal variant. The juvenile form is characterised by an earlier and faster progression than adult-onset Huntington's disease.

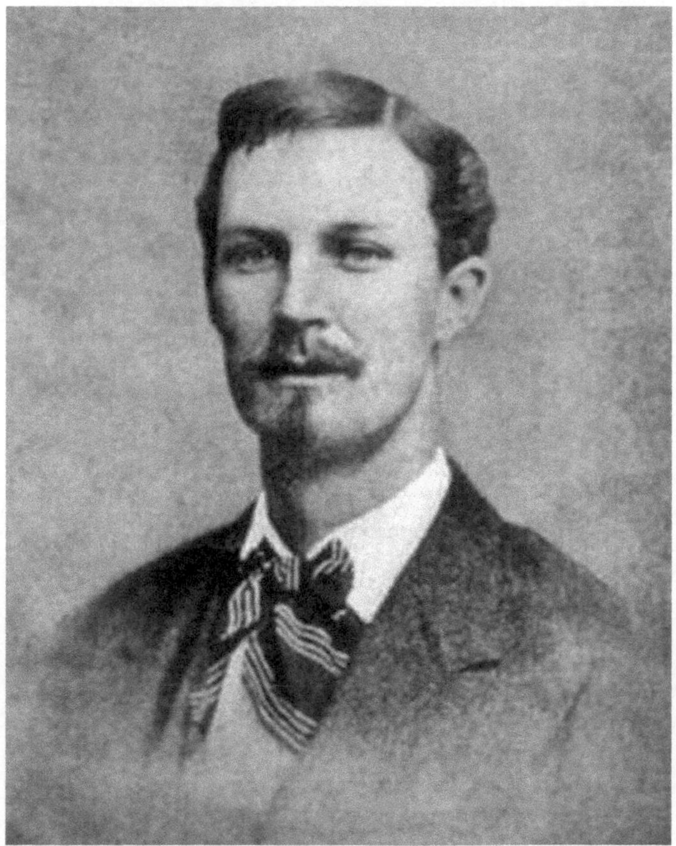

Figure 8.7 George Huntington (1850–1916).

Subtle brain changes (mainly affecting the striatum) can be detected prior to the onset of the motor symptoms. There is evidence that the brain adopts compensatory mechanisms to preserve its functions from an early stage. Likewise, specific non-motor symptoms including irritability, apathy and changes in social cognition can develop years prior to the motor manifestations. Moreover, rigidity, akinesia and cognitive changes – including executive function deficits – tend to be more pronounced in the juvenile variant of Huntington's disease, accompanied by psychiatric symptoms such as depression, anxiety, impulsivity and aggression. Prenatal testing and pre-implantation genetic diagnosis are among the reproductive strategies used to prevent the genetic change from being inherited. Specifically, in pre-implantation genetic diagnosis, the couple conceive in the same way as in vivo fertilisation. The new embyro is allowed to grow and a sample of cells from the embryo are tested for the Huntington's gene: if present, that embryo is not used for implantation. Only embryos free of disease are implanted, and the technique is being used for multiple untreatable genetic disorders. In affected individuals, genetic tests can have a diagnostic value or a predictive value (genetic counselling protocol).

The treatment for Huntington's disease is currently symptomatic, as disease-modifying treatments based on gene suppression therapy are currently only under development. Pharmacotherapy targeting dopaminergic neuro-transmission can improve chorea, often at the expense of worsening mental state (apathy and dysphoria) and cognition. In addition to the pre-synaptic depletor of monoamines tetrabenazine, antidopaminergic drugs such as risperidone, olanzapine, sulpiride and tiapride are often used to treat chorea. In consideration of its metabolic profile, olanzapine can be particularly useful in people who are liable to lose weight. Clonazepam can be helpful for the treatment of both dystonic and myoclonic features. Physical activity is also recommended, as it can improve general health in people with Huntington's disease, possibly delaying obvious onset.

Patients with Huntington's disease typically present with a range of motor, behavioural and cognitive disturbances.[58] Motor symptoms include chorea, athetosis and dystonia, in conjunction with Parkinsonian features as the disease develops. The most common behavioural symptoms are depression, anxiety, apathy, irritability and psychosis. Affective symptoms occur in about half of the patients with Huntington's disease and are often associated with anxiety.

The clinical manifestations of depression in Huntington's disease are relatively evenly distributed between male and female patients and can relapse and remit much more quickly than in major depression. Moreover, affective symptoms are most common in the pre-motor and early stages of the condition and tend to become less frequent as the disease progresses. The most commonly prescribed medications for depression, anxiety, apathy and irritability belong to the class of SSRIs, with the addition of mirtazapine as a second-line option, especially for patients with sleep disturbances.

A substantial minority of patients (5 to 15 per cent) develop psychosis. Delusional symptoms are more commonly reported as earlier manifestations, whereas organic hallucinations tend to occur in the later stages of the disease, as a direct consequence of the failing brain. Specific alterations in social cognition – including progressive deficits in theory of mind, with problems with empathy and understanding of irony – can be reported by family members and carers in early stages. The progressive deterioration that characterises Huntington's disease leads to problems with executive functions, problem solving, attention and multi-tasking. The diagnosis of dementia is commonly reported in the later stages of the disease.

Dystonia

Dystonia is a movement disorder characterised by sustained or intermittent muscle contractions that cause abnormal motor patterns or postures.[59] This condition was first described in 1911 by German neurologist Hermann Oppenheim (1858–1919, Figure 8.8), who termed it dystonia musculorum deformans. Dystonic movements are currently recognised as being typically patterned, twisting in nature and possibly tremulous. The abnormal movements are often initiated or worsened by voluntary action and are characteristically associated with overflow muscle activation. The exact pathophysiological mechanisms underlying the different forms of dystonia are only partially understood. Functional alterations in the basal ganglia (especially the striatum) and their connections with cortical areas (as well as cerebellum circuitries) point towards a shared defect in sensori-motor integration.

Dystonias encompass a heterogeneous group of clinical manifestations: some forms of dystonia are focal and affect isolated body parts, whereas others are generalised, impacting virtually every movement. Moreover, some forms of dystonia have onset in early childhood, whereas others become manifest later in life.

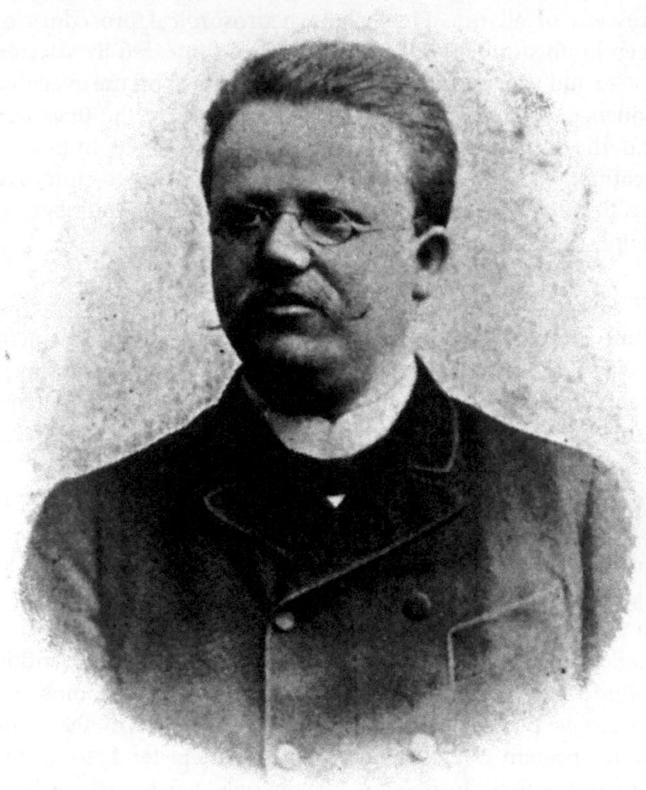

Figure 8.8 Hermann Oppenheim (1858–1919).

Focal dystonias, the most frequent forms of dystonia, usually present in middle age and are more common in women.

Spasmodic torticollis (idiopathic cervical dystonia) is caused by involuntary contractions of the neck muscles, which result in abnormal postures or involuntary movements of the head in any of the three possible planes of rotation. A minority of cases can be precipitated by neck injury and traumas. Relapses are common, and most patients develop a chronic disease.

Essential blepharospasm is a form of primary focal dystonia affecting eye closure. Unilateral blepharospasm is often associated with hemifacial spasm.

Oromandibular dystonia affects muscles of the lower face and jaw.

A few forms of primary focal dystonias were categorised as cramps and task-specific or occupational spasms (e.g. writer's cramp).

Writer's cramp is a focal dystonia characterised by postural cramps when the patient attempts to write. Associated symptoms often reported by patients include pain, postural and action tremor and abnormalities of hand grip. The increase in muscular tension and an atypical dystonic limb posture when writing is attempted characterises the so-called simple writer's cramp. If the abnormal postures also develop with any other activity, patients are diagnosed with dystonic writer's cramp.

Musician's focal dystonia is a task-specific dystonia characterised by the onset of involuntary muscle contractions and movements, which may appear in musicians after years of fine and repetitive movements during performances. It usually affects the most active muscles (typically of the hand) and therefore differs between instruments. Pathological trajectories in brain plasticity processes required to achieve advanced musical skills could play a central role in the development of musician's dystonia.

Generalised forms of primary dystonia typically start in childhood. *Segmental dystonia* affects more than one contiguous part of the body, whereas *hemidystonia* affects all the muscles in one-half of the body. Dystonias can also be symptomatic of underlying conditions, including stroke, cerebral palsy, neuroleptic drugs, Wilson's disease and Huntington's disease.

The treatment of dystonia is mainly symptomatic and largely depends on the distribution of motor symptoms. The most commonly prescribed medications for patients with dystonia include anticholinergic agents, baclofen and benzodiazepines. Intramuscular botulinum toxin injections and deep brain stimulation are more invasive treatment interventions. Physiotherapy is tailored to patients' individual needs and aims at optimising function and independence.

Levodopa-responsive dystonia (Segawa syndrome) is a rare genetic form of dystonia that usually presents in childhood, with leg-onset dystonia. In the majority of cases, there is marked diurnal variation, with worsening of symptoms throughout the day. Importantly, dopamine can restore almost-normal movement, suggesting that all children who develop dystonia should receive dopamine as a trial, even if they do not display diurnal variation.

Behavioural symptoms are commonly reported by patients with focal dystonia and can have a significant impact on their health-related quality of life.[60] Specifically, patients with cervical dystonia report a high prevalence of anxiety and affective symptoms. Likewise, patients with blepharospasm seem to have an increased risk of developing affective disorders than healthy controls. With regard to generalised forms of dystonia, increased rates of obsessive-compulsive disorder have been detected in patients with myoclonus dystonia, as well as recurrent depression in patients with genetic vulnerability to dystonia (DYT1 mutation). It has been suggested that behavioural changes can be an intrinsic component of the neuropsychiatric spectrum of dystonia. Preliminary findings indicate that anxiety and affective symptoms can precede the onset of the motor manifestations of dystonia. It has been suggested that dysfunction within cortico-limbic-striatal pathways could be a common pathophysiological substrate for the neuropsychiatric manifestations of dystonia. The treatment of behavioural symptoms in patients with dystonia is often empirical. Psychotherapy can address specific affective and anxiety symptoms, with positive implications for both mental and physical aspects of health-related quality of life in this patient population. Finally, the differential diagnosis with psychogenic dystonia can pose significant challenges, especially in patients with focal dystonic symptoms.

Other Movement Disorders

Wilson's Disease

Wilson's disease, or hepato-lenticular degeneration, was first described by American-born British neurologist Samuel Kinnier Wilson (1878–1937) in 1912. Wilson's disease is an uncommon genetic disorder of copper metabolism with an autosomal recessive pattern of inheritance. It is caused by mutations within the ATP7B gene, which codes for a copper carrier membrane protein, located on chromosome 13. Inheritance of the altered gene from both parents is required to develop Wilson's disease.

The pathophysiological process is an accumulation of copper deposits in the liver, brain, kidney, cornea and bone. Brain deposits affect the basal ganglia and lead to a number of neurological manifestations, primarily affecting motor function. Tremor and rigidity are common early signs, often associated with muscle rigidity and spasms. Dystonia is commonly present in patients with Wilson's disease, especially a dystonic facial expression known as risus sardonicus that creates a fixed and exaggerated smile. Dysarthria and dysphasia are occasionally reported. Most patients develop symptoms in the first two decades, and earlier onsets are associated with more aggressive course. The diagnosis is confirmed by low ceruloplasmin levels combined with low serum copper levels and increased 24-hour urinary copper excretion. In the eye, deposits in the cornea – particularly in Descemet's membrane – are responsible for the characteristic yellow to green to brown Kayser-Fleischer ring, which is almost invariably associated with neurological or psychiatric disorder. Ophthalmological examination using the slit lamp test reveal the presence of the characteristic Kayser-Fleischer rings and sunflower cataract in the eyes. Kayser-Fleischer rings are abnormal golden-brown discolorations in the eyes that are caused by deposits of excess copper. Kayser-Fleischer rings show up in about 97 per cent of people with Wilson's disease. Sunflower cataracts show up in one out of five people with Wilson's disease. These are characterised by a distinctive multicoloured centre with spokes that radiate outward. The build-up of copper in other organs can cause bluish discoloration in the nails, kidney stones, premature osteoporosis, lack of bone density, arthritis, menstrual irregularities and low blood pressure.

Hepatic involvement is present in about half of the patients, who can develop hepatitis and sclerosis. Treatment is lifelong as the mortality of those who discontinue it is high. In addition to the use of copper chelating agents, such as penicillamine, a diet that restricts foods high in copper (liver, cocoa, chocolate, mushrooms, shellfish, nuts, dried fruits and vegetables) is prescribed. If chelating agents and a low copper diet fail to work, then a liver transplant should be considered, as this is curative in 85 per cent of cases. Behavioural changes have been documented in a substantial proportion of patients with Wilson's disease, occasionally as presenting symptoms.[61] The psychiatric symptoms most frequently reported by patients are affective symptoms, with emotional lability, aggression and irritability. Anxiety, organic delusional states and catatonia have also been reported. Severe cognitive impairment is rare.

Fahr's Disease

Basal ganglia calcification documented by neuroimaging is often an incidental finding without clinical significance. In more severe cases, the changes may be associated with extrapyramidal symptoms and subcortical dementia in middle-aged people or occasionally with psychotic symptoms in younger people. Affective symptoms have also been reported. Basal ganglia calcification can be associated with a deficiency of parathyroid hormone. In a proportion of cases, patients have chronic renal failure or vascular, anoxic or infective cerebral lesions. However, many cases are idiopathic, and a few may be familial. Fahr's disease (familial basal ganglia calcification) is a rare autosomal dominant condition first noted in 1930 by German pathologist Karl Theodor Fahr (1877–1945). It begins in early adult life with progressive dementia, convulsions and rigidity. The diagnosis is based on idiopathic bilateral deposits of calcium in the strio-pallido-dentate area.

Progressive Supranuclear Palsy

Progressive supranuclear palsy, also referred to as Steele-Richardson-Olszewski syndrome, is a rare neurodegenerative disorder characterised by upgaze paralysis ('Mona Lisa stare'), pseudobulbar palsy, prominent dysarthria, rigidity of the neck and upper trunk and cognitive problems. The neuropsychological impairment is characteristic of subcortical dementia, with bradyphrenia, executive deficits, forgetfulness and visuospatial problems. Progressive supranuclear palsy belongs to a group of Parkinson's disease-related conditions, often referred to as 'Parkinson plus syndromes', as patients present with the core Parkinsonian features plus additional symptoms, which are often treatment-refractory. The Parkinsonian features resemble an akinetic rigid syndrome, whereas the behavioural changes are of the frontal lobe type, with inertia and stereotyped behaviours.

Sydenham's Chorea

Sydenham's chorea – historically referred to as St Vitus dance – is characterised by sudden, involuntary, irregular, jerky movements of the extremities, frequently associated with emotional instability and muscle weakness.[62] Sydenham's chorea is a possible consequence of rheumatic fever in children and is found in 10–30% of children with rheumatic fever, most commonly in prepubertal girls. It is rare in adulthood, although it can reappear in adult females as chorea gravidarum. The onset of the condition may be gradual, with children being described as clumsy. There can be complaints from teachers at school of poor attention and deteriorating handwriting, as well as stumbles and falls. Facial grimacing and a variety of speech disorders can be reported. Most of the choreiform movements subside during sleep and are exacerbated by emotions. Characteristically, if the patient is asked to extend the arms, hands and fingers, flexion of the wrists and hyperextension of the metacarpophalangeal joints are observed. Other motor signs include an inability to hold the tongue still when it is protruded and spasmodic contractions of the hands when the patient intentionally grips objects or the examiner's hands ('milk maid grip'). With regards to behavioural manifestations, obsessive-compulsive symptoms have been noted in the context of Sydenham's chorea.

Infectious Diseases

Human Immunodeficiency Virus

Infections with the human immunodeficiency virus (HIV) are seen worldwide, with the highest prevalence in sub-Saharan Africa and an increasingly significant impact in India, China and Eastern Europe. HIV enters the brain via infected macrophages and monocytes, and they can be found in the central nervous system in the early stages of the infection. Cerebral pathology is found in the vast majority of patients with HIV. Breakdown of the blood-brain barrier, loss of white matter density, neuronal loss and astrocyte and oligodendrocyte injury are responsible for the neuropsychiatric manifestations of HIV infection. Cerebrospinal fluid analysis has two main roles: to exclude the presence of opportunistic infection and to measure viral load. This latter has been shown to reliably correlate with the psychiatric and cognitive manifestations of HIV. Neuroimaging is most useful in excluding other conditions and central nervous system complications, such as other infections, progressive multifocal leukoencephalopathy and lymphoma. The prognosis of HIV infection has considerably improved since the beginning of the epidemic due to the widespread availability of combination antiretroviral therapy.

Psychiatric disorders are more common in populations with HIV, especially in the advanced stages of the disease. Psychiatric symptoms can negatively impact outcomes of people living with chronic HIV infection. For example, adequate treatment of depression can lead to improved psychosocial functioning and health-related quality of life.

HIV-positive individuals are twice as likely to be diagnosed with depression than HIV-negative individuals.[63] The risk of developing depression appears to be higher in patients with advanced HIV at presentation or a previous history of psychiatric disease. Moreover, depression has been associated with HIV disease progression and higher rates of mortality. The somatic features of depression – such as fatigue, insomnia, malaise and loss of appetite – overlap with symptoms that are commonly seen in the advanced stages of HIV infection. Anhedonia and cyclical mood variations are due to depression, whereas HIV-related lethargy is characterised by apathy, tiredness and lack of emotional engagement. Depression has been shown to have a negative impact on the ability of patients with HIV to cope with their condition and to comply with antiretroviral medication. Early recognition and treatment of depression in patients with HIV are important for reducing morbidity and mortality. However, there is no consensus on the most effective class of antidepressant agents.

HIV-positive individuals have a higher prevalence of mania compared to the general population. The rate of mania increases with the progression of HIV and correlates with the neurocognitive degeneration that is associated with advanced disease. HIV-related mania is characterised by key features of irritability and agitation, rather than feelings of elation and euphoria.

Anxiety symptoms and obsessive-compulsive disorder tend to be related to issues around the illness and its stigma. Patients can report repeatedly checking for progression of the illness, as well as obsessive thoughts about previous sexual partners.

Psychotic symptoms (delusions, hallucinations, formal thought disorder) are less common than affective disorders in the context of HIV and are typically associated with advanced stages of the disease. Patients with a past history of psychiatric illness and patients with poor cognitive performance have a higher risk for the development of new-onset psychosis, especially if they take no treatment for HIV.

Both psychiatric disorders and epileptic seizures may also occur in the later stages of HIV because of secondary pathologies, such as fungal infections, toxoplasmosis or central nervous system lymphoma. New-onset psychosis can be reported by patients taking antiretrovirals. The onset of an episode of psychoses in patients diagnosed as having HIV can be particularly alarming, as both referrers and sufferers demand immediate attention. Overall, a number of neuropsychiatric symptoms – including anxiety, dizziness, insomnia, nightmares, amnesia and agitation – have been reported as adverse effects of antiretroviral therapy.

Psychopharmacology plays an important role in patients with HIV, as untreated psychiatric disease in HIV is associated with increased morbidity and mortality. When prescribing pharmacological agents acting on the central nervous system, it is important to consider possible interactions with antiretroviral therapy. These could be particularly relevant with serotonergic agents and benzodiazepines. Specifically, there is the potential for increased levels of selective serotonin reuptake inhibitors such as fluoxetine when used in combination with antiretrovirals, which are known to act as inhibitors of the cytochrome P450 enzymes. Likewise, the benzodiazepines alprazolam, midazolam and triazolam are dependent on the isoform 3A4 of the cytochrome P450 for metabolism; potent inhibitors of this CYP isoform, such as the antiretroviral ritonavir, can decrease clearance of these medications and result in oversedation.

The relationship between HIV and psychiatric disorders is bidirectional: patients with psychiatric symptoms are at an increased risk of HIV infection because of their multiple, often illness-related, risk behaviours. Patients with psychiatric conditions who misuse substances (dual diagnosis group) have higher rates of HIV infections. Intravenous drug users, patients with a deteriorated chronic psychosis and those with severe personality disorders who engage in high-risk behaviours are clinical populations in which there should be increased suspicion of HIV infection.

In most cases, there are no early neuropsychological deficits in otherwise-asymptomatic HIV infections, as significant cognitive decline tends to be confined to late stages of the disorder. Moreover, the prevalence of *HIV-associated dementia* decreased considerably with the introduction of antiretroviral therapy[64] In developed countries, HIV-associated dementia has become relatively rare, and it is usually associated with treatment failure, late diagnosis or undiagnosed advanced disease. HIV-associated dementia is significantly more common and continues to be a clinically relevant issue in the developing world due to poor access to antiretroviral therapy. HIV-associated dementia is a subcortical type of dementia characterised by marked cognitive impairment that produces severe interference with activities of daily living.[65] Commonly reported brain imaging findings are white matter hyperintensity and cortical atrophy with ventricular dilatation. Key cognitive and behavioural manifestations include attentional deficits, concentration problems, forgetfulness, psychomotor retardation, apathy, social withdrawal and increased irritability. Problems with memory and concentration are among the most common early symptoms. Moreover, the early stages of HIV-associated dementia can present with a clinical picture resembling depression. HIV testing might be indicated in selected patients presenting with purely somatic symptoms of depression, such as weight loss and anorexia. HIV-associated dementia is a progressively disabling condition because of the variable degree of motor involvement; motor abnormalities tend to increase with disease progression, especially ataxia, bradykinesia, hyperreflexia, spasticity and pyramidal signs. Patients often complain of slowing and impairment of fine movements, as well as gait disturbances associated with tremor and lower limb weakness. Late-stage symptoms may also include seizures, incontinence and peripheral neuropathic pain. Although advanced cognitive deficits such as HIV-associated dementia are considerably less common than in the past, milder forms of cognitive impairment persist despite effective antiretroviral therapy.

Mild cognitive impairment in HIV can be subtle, and the diagnosis can be achieved through detailed neuropsychometric testing by an experienced neuropsychologist. Access to estimates of premorbid status via collateral history from third parties is often required for the specialist assessment. Brain imaging can show hazy white matter hyperintensity, with or without diffuse atrophy, or can be normal. Prevalence estimates vary considerably, depending on the definitions and methods used for the assessment. Mild cognitive impairment has a different phenotype compared to HIV-associated dementia: it is characterised by cortical deficits in learning, memory and executive functions, as opposed to a subcortical dementing process. The causes of mild cognitive impairment in patients with HIV are often multifactorial, and the direct impact of HIV on cognition can be difficult to determine. Contributing factors to be considered in clinical practice include antiretroviral therapy neurotoxicity, alcohol and substance abuse, cerebrovascular disease, hepatitis C co-infection and comorbid psychiatric disorders.

HIV infection is a preventable and treatable cause of cognitive impairment.[66] Antiretroviral therapy is indicated in patients with cognitive problems in the context of HIV. In patients taking antiretroviral therapy, first consideration must be given to whether HIV is adequately controlled in the blood and whether there is any need to adjust the dose of antiretroviral therapy. The presence of any comorbid conditions or drug toxicities that could be contributing to cognitive problems should be explored. Since HIV-associated dementia is associated with advanced infection, prognosis can be poor. A degree of improvement in cognitive function can be seen following initiation of effective antiretroviral therapy. Long-term survival can be achieved with adequate restoration of the immunological profile. Milder forms of cognitive impairment in people receiving antiretroviral therapy are characterised by a considerably better prognosis, although cognitive and behavioural problems can affect compliance to HIV treatment.

Syphilis

Neurosyphilis was first described in the late nineteenth century and identified as an organic cause of dementia and psychosis. Syphilis was common in Europe during the eighteenth and nineteenth centuries. It declined rapidly throughout the twentieth century, with the widespread use of antibiotics. In developed countries, rates of admissions to psychiatric institutions due to syphilis have decreased significantly since the pre-antibiotic era. However, infections can still be seen, especially in selected populations such as homosexual men and patients with HIV. In addition to persistently high rates in sub-Saharan Africa, recent increases in the prevalence of syphilis have been reported in the United Kingdom and the rest of the Western world, primarily due to unsafe sexual practices. The index of suspicion should be kept high in individuals with unusual psychiatric presentations.

Syphilis is caused by Treponema pallidum, one of the pathogenic bacteria referred to as spirochaetes. The diagnosis of symptomatic neurosyphilis is based on clinical features, supported by lumbar puncture and serological testing for systemic syphilis. Detection of cerebrospinal fluid abnormalities can result in the diagnosis of asymptomatic neurosyphilis. Patients with asymptomatic neurosyphilis have serological or clinical evidence of systemic syphilis, combined with abnormal cerebrospinal fluid findings, in the absence of neurological symptoms or signs. Neuroimaging abnormalities including cerebral infarction, arteritis and non-specific white matter lesions can have a supporting value in the diagnostic process. Serological tests can be divided into non-treponemal tests (such as the Venereal Disease Research Laboratory, or VDRL) and treponemal tests (such as Fluorescent Treponemal Antibody Absorption, or FTA-Abs), to be used in combination. Moreover, all patients diagnosed with neurosyphilis should be tested for other sexually transmitted infections – particularly HIV – in consideration of the high rates of co-infection.

Syphilis is classically divided into four stages: the localised primary lesion, secondary meningitis, tertiary meningovascular stage and central nervous system involvement (tabes dorsalis and general paresis of the insane). In terms of pathological changes, all stages are characterised by specific inflammatory responses. Once considered a late manifestation of syphilis, central nervous system involvement is currently recognised as a phenomenon that may happen at any stage of infection. In addition, congenital syphilis may affect newborns, although the condition may not be diagnosed until later.

Following the development of the primary lesion, patients generally present with secondary meningitis within a year of infection. Syphilitic meningitis may present with signs of meningism, headache, lethargy, forgetfulness, irritability, malaise, papilloedema, nausea and vomiting. Occasionally, patients can develop an acute confusional state or convulsions. Associated cranial nerve phenomena include ophthalmoplegias and the so-called Argyll Robertson pupil (small, irregular pupils that accommodate but do not react to light).

Tertiary meningovascular syphilis presents, on average, seven years after the primary infection. Patients can display a wide range of focal neurological symptoms, from mild headache to stupor, cranial nerve involvement, aphasia, seizures, progressive dementia and hemiplegia. The protean manifestations of this condition are due to endarteritis of small, medium and large blood vessels, potentially resulting in ischaemia, thrombosis or infarction.

Tabes dorsalis (degeneration of the different fibres of the dorsal roots) develops, on average, 21 years following the primary infection, as a result of the degeneration of the posterior roots and columns of the spinal cord. In addition to pupillary abnormalities, dorsal column sensory dysfunction and ataxia, patients typically complain of stabbing severe pains in the legs.

If untreated, a minority of patients can develop the so-called general paresis of the insane, approximately 10–24 years after the primary infection.[67] The general paresis is a neuropsychiatric disorder associated with cerebral atrophy in the anterior two-thirds of the cerebral hemispheres. Different forms of paresis have been described based on the observed changes in mental state. The neuropsychiatric manifestations of neurosyphilis usually begin with changes in personality and temperament, such as shallow affect (apathy or mild euphoria), irritability, reduced emotional control and other frontal lobe personality changes, often resulting in out-of-character behaviours or socially disinhibited actions that bring the patient to the attention of medical professionals. Delusions are a prominent feature of the psychiatric symptoms seen in neurosyphilis.[68] Fleeting persecutory delusions and grandiose delusions that revolve around power, money and social superiority are often reported. As the disease progresses, the delusions can be replaced by feelings of apathy and generalised disinterest. Patients can present with depressive symptoms, including low mood, melancholic delusions and suicidal thoughts – often against a background of a dementing process caused by the progressive disease.

Dementia in the context of syphilis is characterised by forgetfulness, poor concentration, slowed thinking, loss of insight and deterioration in cognitive abilities such as calculation and recall. Confusion can be exacerbated by recurrent episodes of impaired consciousness. Dementia can be complicated by persecutory delusions and can be interspersed by episodes of euphoria, depression or delirium. In addition to the most frequent neurological findings – including pupillary abnormalities, tremor, dysarthria, brisk reflexes and incoordination – patients can develop focal seizures and, more rarely, transient cerebrovascular episodes.

Historically, mercury was a long-standing treatment for syphilis. Another common treatment approach for syphilis was fever therapy – by infecting the patient with malaria, then treating the malaria with quinine. Nowadays, early treatment with high-dose penicillin remains the cornerstone of the management for neurosyphilis, as it prevents the subsequent development of general paresis. Antipsychotic drugs are indicated for both psychotic symptoms and agitation, whereas antidepressants can be used for affective symptoms. The extent of symptom resolution varies, depending on the clinical stage of neurosyphilis reached by patient before treatment. In the pre-antibiotic era, prognosis was considerably poorer, as patients diagnosed with severe neurocognitive dysfunction as a result of general paresis only had an average survival of a few years.

Syphilis can be transmitted during pregnancy or during birth (congenital syphilis). One-third of syphilitic infants present with symptoms; of these, about one in five develops neurosyphilis over the first couple of years of life. Infection with syphilis during pregnancy can also be associated with miscarriage. In certain world regions (such as sub-Saharan Africa) and specific populations (such as drug users and HIV-positive individuals), syphilis contributes to a substantial proportion of perinatal deaths.

Meningitis

Although bacterial and viral meningitis are not classically associated with neuropsychiatric presentations or the development of subsequent psychiatric disease, subtle cognitive deficits after acute infection have occasionally been reported. Tuberculous meningitis is a treatable but insidious condition caused by Mycobacterium tuberculosis and characterised by neuropsychiatric features, often without meningism[69] Rates of tuberculous meningitis are considerably higher in immunocompromised patients, especially in HIV-positive individuals.

The early stage of tuberculous meningitis is defined by subtle personality or gradual behavioural changes (e.g. apathy, irritability, low mood) that are often first noticed by those closest to the patient. Patients can also report psychotic symptoms, such as hallucination and delusions. The confusional state can resemble clinical pictures seen with alcohol-related encephalopathies, as it often includes amnesia. Overall, the psychiatric features in patients with tuberculous meningitis have a non-specific presentation, which is not always typical of a central nervous system infection. Specifically, subtle changes in consciousness and personality may be apparent to relatives but not easily captured during clinical assessments. At times, patients can present with euphoria despite their extreme memory difficulties. Neurosyphilis is an important differential diagnosis in patients with tuberculous meningitis who display neuropsychiatric features.

Anti-tuberculous treatment should be started as soon as the diagnosis is confirmed, as untreated tuberculous meningitis can lead to hydrocephalus and possibly coma. Even after treatment completion, recovery can be slow, and memory can take some time to return to baseline function.

Encephalitis

Most cases of infectious encephalitis have a viral aetiology. The most common cause of encephalitis in the United Kingdom is the herpes simplex virus type 1, which is responsible for a severe form of sporadic encephalitis. Other forms of encephalitis can have a geographically restricted endemic cause, such as the Japanese encephalitis virus. In a substantial proportion of cases, the cause of encephalitis remains unknown, as no aetiological agent can be identified with certainty.

Patients with encephalitis usually present with severe, progressive headache, vomiting, papilloedema, fever and altered mental status, following a prodromal flu-like illness. Fever can be mild, inconsistent or fluctuating. Alterations of both consciousness and mental state can manifest as mild somnolence, delirium, disorientation, psychotic symptoms, catatonia or, in severe cases, coma. The presence of seizures or other focal neurological deficits reflects parenchymal inflammation and is more supportive of a diagnosis of encephalitis, as opposed to meningitis. The psychiatric symptoms depend on the area of the brain affected and often precede classical features of parenchymal inflammation, such as seizures or other focal neurological signs.[70] Dysphasia, auditory hallucinations, memory loss, emotional lability, behavioural changes and other psychiatric symptoms or focal neurological signs indicative of temporal lobe dysfunction are usually suggestive of herpes simplex involvement. Patients can present with features of aggression and socially inappropriate behaviours in the case of frontal lobe involvement. The combination of acute confusion and hallucinations increases the risk of a misdiagnosis of delirium tremens or a metabolic encephalopathy.

Neurological assessment and lumbar puncture for cerebrospinal fluid analysis are essential diagnostic steps. In herpes simplex virus encephalitis, brain imaging findings may be normal early in the disease, but they can subsequently reveal specific changes in the temporal lobes, especially with magnetic resonance imaging. Electroencephalography in the acute stage of herpes simplex encephalitis can show a variety of abnormalities and can be useful for the diagnostic process.

A timely diagnosis is vital since delayed therapy is associated with poor prognosis. Initially, the patient should be stabilised, and antiepileptic drugs can be useful to provide seizure control. Early treatment with the antiviral agent aciclovir has a significant effect on reducing mortality and morbidity. It is widely recognised that both psychiatric symptoms and neuropsychological sequelae can persist long after treatment and can be debilitating. Specifically, patients can be left with quite significant post-encephalitic neuropsychiatric disorders, encompassing personality change, disturbed behaviours and social disinhibition. Other psychiatric symptoms that are commonly reported after encephalitis include anxiety and affective symptoms. With regards to cognitive dysfunction, the most debilitating feature can be severe anterograde amnesia, as well as less severe retrograde memory impairment.

Other Central Nervous System Infections

Subacute Sclerosing Panencephalitis

A number of other central nervous system infections have been found to be associated with psychiatric symptoms (Table 8.7).

Subacute sclerosing panencephalitis is a severe, rare condition that presents several years after an acute measles infection. Subacute sclerosing panencephalitis is thought to be caused by a slow measles virus (paramyxovirus). Slow viruses may stay dormant in humans for extended periods of time, then for reasons yet unknown may become reactivated. The initial symptoms include subtle cognitive deterioration and affective symptoms, typically in childhood or adolescence. Poor academic performance is often the result of gradual intellectual decline, associated with personality and behavioural change. Seizures and motor features can present at any time and typically include myoclonic jerking of the head, trunk and limbs. In the more advanced stages of the disease, patients can develop various degrees of visual impairment and significant neurological dysfunction, including paresis and eventually coma. Characteristic electroencephalographic patterns indicative of subacute sclerosing panencephalitis show stereotyped bilateral (asymmetrical) synchronous and periodic complexes. Raised antibody titres for measles virus and raised gamma-globulin can be found in the cerebrospinal fluid following lumbar puncture. Brain imaging can show white matter lesions and eventual atrophy at the level of the brainstem and other structures. In most cases, subacute sclerosing panencephalitis is a highly devastating and progressive central nervous system infection with a fatal course. In patients who survive, cognitive dysfunction often persists long after the acute phase of the illness.

Table 8.7 Rarer central nervous system infectious disorders associated with psychiatric symptoms

Subacute sclerosing panencephalitis
Cysticercosis
Whipple disease
Lyme disease
Trypanosomiasis
Typhus
Toxoplasmosis
Malaria

Cysticercosis

Cysticercosis is caused by infection with Taenia solium, a cestode parasite. Humans act as hosts for the cysticercus, the larval form of the parasite that is typically found in the faecal matter of pigs. The highest rates of infection are found in areas of Latin America, Asia and Africa that have poor sanitation and free-ranging pigs that have access to human faeces. It is rare in Western Europe. Central nervous system involvement occurs in the majority of cases, with the formation of multiple cysts within the brain (in addition to the muscle, skin and various organs). Most clinical features manifest themselves when the larvae die. The resulting inflammatory process leads to the classical presentation of isolated seizures, which can subsequently progress to epilepsy with calcification of the cysts. Raised intracranial pressure and a variety of focal neurological symptoms may also occur, depending on the site of the cysts. Meningitis has been reported with localisation of the cysts to the meninges. Psychiatric and cognitive symptoms develop as a consequence of the general deterioration in more severe cases or are due to the associated epilepsy. Neurocysticercosis has been associated with affective and psychotic symptoms, both in the acute phase and as a longer-term complication of infection.[71] The diagnostic process is based on a combination of clinical assessment, serological testing and brain imaging demonstrating the cysts. Treatment is based on the use of antiparasitic agents such as albendazole and praziquantel, and management involves antiepileptic drugs, anti-inflammatory agents and surgery in the rare case of significant hydrocephalus.

Whipple Disease

Whipple disease is a rare, multisystem disease caused by the bacterium Tropheryma whipplei. Although the main feature is malabsorption due to involvement of the gastrointestinal system, the brain can also be affected. Whipple disease is diagnosed more commonly among men over the age of 50, with weight loss due to malabsorption, arthralgia and lymphadenopathy. Central nervous system involvement is reported in approximately half of cases, with cognitive changes being the most common symptoms. A slowly progressive dementia occurs in some of the reported cases. Psychiatric features include affective symptoms, anxiety and psychosis. Ocular abnormalities, especially vertical supranuclear gaze palsy, are frequently reported. Oculomasticatory myorhythmia is a pathognomonic sign of Whipple disease involving the central nervous system. Oculomasticatory myorhythmia is characterised by continuous, smooth, pendular convergent and divergent oscillations of the eyes and concurrent synchronous contraction of masticatory muscles. The diagnosis is mainly based on duodenal biopsies. Prolonged antibiotic therapy may be required for the management of the systemic disease.

Lyme Disease

Lyme disease is caused by the spirochaete Borrelia burgdorferi, a bacterium that is transmitted to humans via tick bites. The condition is particularly prevalent in North America. The characteristic erythema migrans rash develops a few days or weeks following a tick bite. Accompanying symptoms include headache, myalgia and fever. Lyme disease involving the central nervous system is referred to as neuroborreliosis and is characterised by neurological symptoms, such as subacute meningitis, painful radiculitis and transverse myelitis. More rarely, neuroborreliosis can present with acute anxiety and affective changes. The neuropsychiatric presentation encompasses difficulty with concentration and recall, as well as chronic fatigue syndrome.[72] Depression as a late complication of neuroborreliosis is relatively common. Diagnosis is made with antibody testing of the cerebrospinal fluid and serum, with focus on the ratio of cerebrospinal fluid antibody level to serum antibody level. However, antibody tests in the first few weeks of infection may be negative, as the antibody response takes several weeks to reach a detectable level. Oral antibiotics are indicated for the management of Lyme disease; neurological complications require longer treatment.

Trypanosomiasis

African Trypanosomiasis, or sleeping sickness, is due to the protozoans Trypanosoma brucei gambiense and Trypanosoma brucei rhodesiense and is transmitted by the tsetse fly. An initial febrile illness associated with the fly bite progresses into the sleeping sickness stage. Central nervous system involvement is characterised by an insidious development of a variety of neurological symptoms in the form of tremors, incoordination, seizures, paralysis, confusion, headaches, apathy and daytime somnolence with restlessness at night. Both speech problems and extrapyramidal signs (including choreiform movements, tremor and other Parkinsonian features) have been observed. Psychiatric features are reported by the majority of patients, who can present with personality change, psychosis, affective disorder and cognitive decline. In the final phase of Trypanosoma brucei gambiense infection, progressive neurological involvement results in coma and death, usually occurs within weeks to months. Symptoms of Trypanosoma brucei rhodesiense infection are more slowly progressive, and the prognosis is more favourable with adequate treatment. Central nervous system involvement is less common with the South American variety of trypanosomiasis (Chagas disease), caused by Trypanosoma cruzi.

Typhus

The most common cause of typhus is the parasite Rickettsia prowazekii, which is transmitted by the body louse. In recent history, typhus was the big killer in the concentration camps of World War II, claiming Anne Frank as one of its victims. It is thought that there is direct central nervous system infection, with microscopic nodules in vessel walls and thrombosis resulting in neuropsychiatric symptoms as a prominent feature of the condition. Typhus fever presents with fever, headache, cough, myalgia, rash, insomnia and delirium. Both cerebellar and peripheral neurological symptoms may occur, and survivors often show persistent cortical damage. Psychotic symptoms are the most commonly reported psychiatric features, and central nervous system involvement becomes more severe towards the later stages of the febrile period. Treatment of the acute infection is with antibiotics, usually doxycycline.

Toxoplasmosis

Both congenital toxoplasmosis (a possible cause of learning disability) and adult toxoplasmosis are caused by the protozoan Toxoplasma gondii. The most common form of transmission is via ingestion of poorly cooked meat, and water contaminated with oocysts from cat excreta may also cause infection. In the 2011 United Kingdom National Screening Committee (UK NSC) review, congenital toxoplasmosis was estimated to affect 1 out of 10,000 live births, of which less than 5% would have severe neurological impairment and 20–30% would have intracranial or ocular lesions by three years old. The infection is often latent or subclinical. Infection during pregnancy is of particular concern because the organism may be transmitted through the placenta. First trimester infection is associated with a 10–15% risk of foetal infection, second trimester exposure is associated with a 25% risk and, for the third trimester, the risk of foetal exposure is 75%.

Congenital toxoplasmosis can be a severe condition if the infection occurs early in the first trimester, but most infected infants are asymptomatic at birth. The symptoms of congenital toxoplasmosis may become apparent after the first few days of life, and the clinical presentation encompasses seizures, microcephaly, spasticity, opisthotonos, chorioretinitis, microphthalmus, optic atrophy and other eye lesions, as well as internal hydrocephalus. Cerebral calcified nodules may be present on neuroimaging, and there can be liver and spleen involvement. Symptoms of the infantile form are similar to the congenital form but do not show calcification in the brain. Learning disability, which may be severe, is a later manifestation. All affected infants should be treated to prevent subclinical infection and later reoccurrences of infection, and women should be offered treatment as soon as the infection is diagnosed during pregnancy. Spiramycin reduces the risk of transmission from mother to baby and is not active against the parasite. It is offered routinely to women in France who are infected. If the baby is found to be infected, a combination of pyrimethamine and sulphadiazine can be taken, although this combination may have haematological adverse effects.

Malaria

Malaria is a protozoan disease transmitted by the bite of the Anopheles mosquito. Most cases of cerebral malaria and fatalities are due to infection by the protozoan Plasmodium falciparum, which remains common in tropical Africa, South America and parts of South-East Asia. Cerebral malaria occurs in a small proportion of affected individuals. Sporules of the parasite cause thrombosis in the brain capillaries, with haemorrhage and oedema, resulting in a diffuse encephalopathy. Generalised seizures occur in approximately half of adult cases, with higher proportions in children. Cerebral malaria can present with a range of neuropsychiatric syndromes: disturbances of consciousness, stupor and coma or acute delirium; acute psychosis or personality change; movement disorders with tremors; a stroke-like syndrome with focal neurological disorders; depression or apathy without fever. Neurological deficits appear to be associated with childhood cases of cerebral malaria. Malaria not only kills many people, but in endemic areas, leaves many individuals with lasting mild to moderate cognitive deficits. Malarial infections have been found to be major predictors of children's performance in the key subjects of language and mathematics. Moreover, subtle cognitive deficits of executive function and information processing have been reported, especially if the original illness is associated with reduced levels of consciousness. Travellers returning from endemic areas who have not taken antimalarial agents are at risk, and they may present to primary care or acute care services with fever and a neurological presentation. The diagnosis is straightforward – but only if the assessing physician considers the possibility and requests examination of the blood slide, where the parasites are obvious.

Creutzfeldt-Jacob Disease

Creutzfeldt-Jacob disease (CJD) is a prion disease, also referred to as transmissible spongiform encephalopathy. The eponym was introduced by German neuropathologist Walther Spielmeyer (1879–1935) in 1922, after the German neurologists Hans Gerhard Creutzfeldt (1885–1964) and Alfons Maria Jakob (1884–1931). In prion disease, the prion protein (PrPc) – a normal cellular brain protein – undergoes conformational change into an insoluble form termed PrPSc (prion protein, scrapie). Unlike other infectious diseases, prion disease is both heritable and transmissible, since the conformational change from PrPc to PrPSc can occur in three ways: spontaneously (accounting for at least 85 per cent of cases of CJD), genetically (comprising about 10 per cent of CJD cases and all the inherited forms, such as Gerstmann-Straussler syndrome) and transmissibly by exposure to a 'seed' of PrPSc. There are two main clinical syndromes associated with prion disease in humans: CJD and variant CJD (vCJD). Additionally, cases of iatrogenic CJD (exposure via pituitary-derived hormones, tissue grafts or neurosurgery) and prion diseases inherited via autosomal dominant transmission have been reported. A wide range of point mutations and insertions in the PRNP gene on chromosome 20 causes inheritable prion disease. People homozygous for a methionine-valine polymorphism at codon 129 of PrPc have been shown to be at increased risk for sporadic (methionine) and iatrogenic (valine) CJD. In the mid-twentieth century, an epidemic of a different transmissible spongiform encephalopathy called kuru devastated the Fore tribe in the Eastern Highlands of Papua New Guinea. The epidemic likely started when a villager developed sporadic Creutzfeldt-Jakob disease and died. The infection was passed on at mortuary feasts, where villagers consumed their deceased relatives as a mark of respect and mourning; when villagers ate the brain, they contracted the disease, and it was then spread to other villagers who ate their infected brains. Lessons from the kuru epidemic in Papua New Guinea suggested long incubation periods of human prions of 10–15 years in humans after exposure, with a range of 4–40 years.

Sporadic CJD classically presents with the clinical triad of dementia, myoclonus and ataxia. The mean age at onset is 60 years (range 45 to 75 years). The clinical picture progresses to akinetic mutism and death within a median of four months, with approximately 70 per cent of sufferers dying within six months. Patients frequently present with additional neurological features, including extrapyramidal and pyramidal signs, cerebellar ataxia and cortical blindness. Sporadic CJD is also characterised by the neuropathological triad of vacuolar (spongiform) change, astrocytosis and neuronal loss. The neuropathological aspect of vCJD is different and involves diffuse vacuolation and PrP-containing amyloid plaques surrounded by petals of spongiosis (florid or 'daisy' plaques). From the clinical perspective, vCJD has a median age of onset of 26 years (range 12–74 years), with a median length of illness of 13 months (range 6–39 months). Two-thirds of patients with vCJD present with psychiatric manifestations (anxiety and affective symptoms, irritability, insomnia, loss of interest and withdrawal), which are reported by approximately one-third of patients with sporadic CJD. Patients with vCJD typically develop disorientation and memory problems, alongside aggressiveness, hallucinations and neurological features, starting with altered sensation or pain in the limbs or face. In the 1980s and 1990s, a bovine form of transmissible spongiform encephalopathy spread in cattle in an epidemic fashion because of the previous habit of feeding cattle with the processed remains of other cattle. In turn, consumption by humans of bovine-derived foodstuff that contained prion-contaminated tissues resulted in an outbreak of vCJD in the 1990s and 2000s.

The diagnosis of CJD and vCJD can be challenging. It may initially be suspected in a person with rapidly progressing dementia, particularly when involuntary movements, coordination/balance problems and visual disturbances are reported. Further testing supports the diagnosis and may include electroencephalography (generalised periodic sharp wave pattern, particularly in the later stages), lumbar puncture (cerebrospinal fluid analysis for elevated levels of 14-3-3 protein) and neuroimaging (cortical and subcortical MRI abnormalities). There is currently no effective cure for CJD; therefore, treatment aims to relieve symptoms. Medications such as antidepressants can help with anxiety and depression, and painkillers are used to relieve pain.

Long Covid

While the Covid-19 pandemic was caused by a respiratory coronavirus, there have been clinically relevant implications for neuropsychiatry, especially with regard to the long-term effects of coronavirus ('long covid'). It has been reported that most people who contract Covid-19 feel better in a few days and make a full recovery within 12 weeks. However, for some people, symptoms can last longer, regardless of the severity of their initial clinical presentation. The most commonly reported symptoms in the context of post-Covid-19 syndrome include fatigue, shortness of breath, chest pain, cough, palpitations, joint pain, gastrointestinal symptoms and dermatological rashes. Neurologically, patients often report headache, dizziness, tinnitus, paraesthesia, changes to sense of smell or taste and insomnia. These symptoms can be accompanied by anxiety and affective symptoms. Finally, with regard to cognition, patients often report problems with memory and concentration ('brain fog'). Little is known about the pathophysiology and long-term course of the neuropsychiatric sequelae of Covid-19. However, there is likely to be ongoing need for psychiatric input into this global patient population.

Autoimmune Neurological Disorders

Multiple Sclerosis

Multiple sclerosis, together with systemic lupus erythematosus and the more recently identified autoimmune encephalopathies, is an autoimmune neurological disorder of central relevance to neuropsychiatry (Table 8.8).

Multiple sclerosis is a demyelinating disorder of the central nervous system that accounts for the most common cause of chronic neurological disability in young adults. The French neurologist and psychiatrist Jean-Martin Charcot (1825–1893, Figure 8.9) was the first person to use the clinic-pathological method to recognise multiple sclerosis as a distinct disease in 1868. The neuropsychiatric manifestations of multiple sclerosis include both psychiatric and cognitive symptoms and often impact significantly on morbidity.[73] Patients with multiple sclerosis can present with psychiatric symptoms that occur at any stage of the disease (depression, bipolar affective disorder and psychosis). Another group of psychiatric symptoms are more common at later stages of the disease, usually in association with cognitive impairment (euphoria, pseudobulbar affect and personality changes).

Affective symptoms are common and occur throughout the natural history of disease.[74] Both the degree of disability and disease duration have been related to depression in patients with multiple sclerosis. Moreover, their neurovegetative symptoms (e.g. fatigue and sleep problems) can confuse the diagnosis. Suicide risk in patients with multiple sclerosis is twice that of the general population, with severity of affective symptoms, alcohol abuse and isolation as the main risk factors for suicidal ideation. The biology of depression in multiple sclerosis encompasses both psychosocial determinants and specific lesion locations (especially prefrontal and temporal cortex). The efficacy of antidepressant medications and cognitive behavioural therapy has been assessed in a few studies on patients with multiple sclerosis.

Table 8.8 Main autoimmune neurological disorders associated with psychiatric symptoms

Multiple sclerosis
Systemic lupus erythematosus
Autoimmune encephalopathies

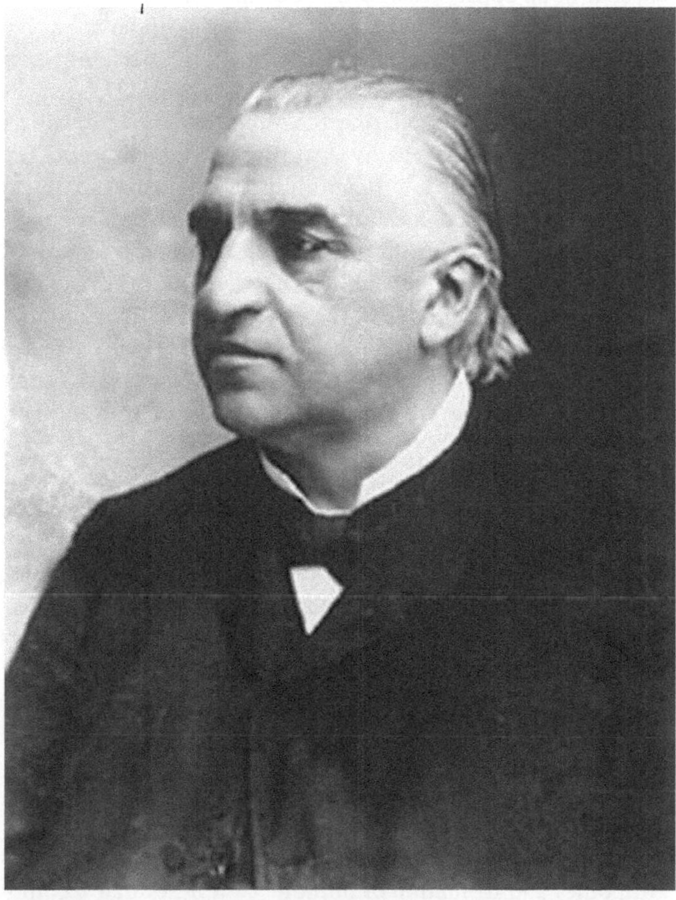

Figure 8.9 Jean-Martin Charcot (1825–1893).

Patients with multiple sclerosis have an increased risk of developing bipolar affective disorder, possibly due to biological inflammatory mechanisms. There does not seem to be a significant role for emotional distress due to diagnosis or disability, as bipolar affective symptoms at disease onset are not uncommon. There is relatively little research on the treatment of bipolar affective disorder in patients with multiple sclerosis. Both mood stabilisers (e.g. lithium, valproate) and sedative agents (benzodiazepines) are used in routine clinical practice.

Patients with multiple sclerosis have also been found to have an increased risk of developing psychotic episodes during the course of their disease. Little is known about the biological basis of psychosis in multiple sclerosis, and treatment is often empirical, with atypical antipsychotics being preferred because of the lower risk of extrapyramidal adverse effects.

Specific affective and behavioural symptoms can develop in more advanced stages of the disease, correlating with higher disability, cognitive dysfunction and heavier total lesion load on neuroimaging. Euphoria, elation, lack of insight and denial of disability can be reported, even in the presence of marked physical morbidity, potentially causing significant distress to the caregivers. Patients with pseudobulbar affect display affective states that are not representative of the underlying emotion: uncontrollable laughing or crying episodes, often in the absence of an appropriate stimulus or the corresponding emotion. The biological mechanisms are poorly understood, but they appear to involve pontine, brainstem and periventricular lesions. First-line therapy for this distressing condition usually involves serotonergic pharmacotherapy. Personality changes involving irritability, apathy and disinhibition are also frequently observed in late-stage multiple sclerosis and might correlate with lesion location. The most common cognitive symptoms in patients with multiple sclerosis involve memory, attention and abstracting ability. The severity of the cognitive impairment correlates with the overall extent of pathology seen in neuroimaging. Cognitive deficits are often over-looked but can add considerably to the patient's distress; cognitive rehabilitation, supportive psychotherapy and family support can be helpful.

Finally, the psychiatric effects of treatment interventions for multiple sclerosis should also be taken into consideration. Specifically, the use of corticosteroids can be associated with affective disorders, particularly mania and rarely psychotic symptoms. The possible link between treatment with interferon and development of affective symptoms in patients with multiple sclerosis is more controversial.

Systemic Lupus Erythematosus

Systemic lupus erythematosus is a chronic inflammatory disorder characterised by a relapsing-remitting course. The aetiology is autoimmune, and the pathophysiological mechanisms include loss of immune tolerance, production of autoantibodies and formation of immune complexes that accumulate in tissues, leading to systemic inflammation. Systemic lupus erythematosus with involvement of the central nervous system (neurolupus) presents with a wide spectrum of neurological and psychiatric symptoms, encompassing focal neurological manifestations (especially seizures), cognitive deficits and behavioural problems.[75]

Neuropsychiatric systemic lupus erythematosus develops slowly and fluctuates in severity. The diagnosis is clinical, as the relationship with pathological brain changes (inflammatory changes to small blood vessels) and systemic disease activity is inconsistent. The onset of cognitive and behavioural symptoms of neuropsychiatric systemic lupus erythematosus tends to occur in the later stages of the disease, often in episodes lasting for a few weeks. Multiple neuropsychiatric symptoms may be present at the same time or sequentially. The most frequent psychiatric manifestations are psychosis, affective and anxiety symptoms, cognitive dysfunction and acute confusional state.

Psychosis is a rare but serious presentation of neuropsychiatric systemic lupus erythematosus that is usually reported in the context of other manifestations of disease activity. The clinical manifestations resemble those of a psychotic episode in patients with schizophrenia. Pharmacotherapy involves antipsychotic agents; if there is evidence of generalised systemic lupus erythematosus activity, steroids and immunosuppressive therapy are warranted. The vast majority of patients show complete remission early on in the course of treatment.

Affective and anxiety symptoms are common manifestations of neuropsychiatric systemic lupus erythematosus. The aetiology is likely to be multifactorial, with contributions from the pathological activity and reactive processes to a severe, debilitating chronic condition. The spectrum of symptoms encompasses major depression; affective disorders with depressive, manic or mixed features; generalised anxiety; specific phobias; panic disorder or obsessive-compulsive disorder. In addition to antidepressant medications, biofeedback-assisted cognitive behavioural therapy has been shown to be potentially beneficial. Immunosuppressive pharmacotherapy aimed at controlling generalised pathological activity might also lead to improvement of affective symptoms.

Mild to moderate cognitive dysfunction is relatively common in patients with systemic lupus erythematosus, whereas severe cognitive dysfunction can affect a minority of patients. Risk factors for progressive cognitive problems include generalised systemic lupus erythematosus activity, neuroimaging evidence of central nervous system pathology (cortical atrophy or focal lesions), positive antiphospholipid antibodies and hypertension. The most commonly affected cognitive domains encompass attention, visual and verbal memory, executive function and psychomotor speed. Management strategies aim at treating exacerbating causes and controlling neurovascular risk factors.

Finally, brief acute confusional state – characterised by fluctuating level of consciousness and decreased attention – can be a neuropsychiatric complication of a minority of patients with systemic lupus erythematosus. Once other possible underlying causes such as infections or metabolic problems have been ruled out, treatment with a combination of steroids and immunosuppressive agents can be administered.

Corticosteroid-induced psychiatric disease occurs in a minority of patients treated with steroids and presents primarily as an affective disorder, rather than as psychosis. In this subgroup of patients with systemic lupus erythematosus, immunosuppressive pharmacotherapy aiming at controlling a primary psychiatric dysfunction might worsen the condition; symptoms typically resolve with discontinuation of corticosteroid treatment.

Autoimmune Encephalopathies

The discovery of encephalopathy syndromes associated with antibodies targeting neuronal surface antibodies heralded the modern era of autoimmune encephalitis. Up until the end of the previous century, limbic encephalitis had largely been recognised as a paraneoplastic phenomenon. The diagnosis of autoimmune encephalitis is of importance to the neuropsychiatrist, as patients often respond to immunotherapies and can recover from most psychiatric and cognitive problems.

Autoimmune encephalitis commonly presents with neuropsychiatric symptoms. Clinical red flags for the possibility of autoimmune encephalitis in patients presenting with psychiatric symptoms encompass the subacute onset of seizures, alterations of consciousness, dysarthria, headache, catatonia, motor symptoms, cognitive impairment and autonomic symptoms.[76] Supportive findings from neurological investigations include medial temporal lobe pathological changes and atrophy on structural neuroimaging, regional hypermetabolism on functional neuroimaging, electroencephalographic abnormalities and lymphocytic pleocytosis in the cerebrospinal fluid. The different antibody-associated forms of autoimmune encephalitis are classified according to the antigenic target, which is typically a neurotransmitter receptor or an associated protein.

NMDAR-antibody encephalitis is the most common form of autoimmune encephalitis. First described in 2007 in young women with ovarian teratoma presenting with psychosis, seizures and catatonia, NMDAR-antibody encephalitis has subsequently been clinically characterised as a severe multistage disorder with symptomatic progression in the majority of cases. Viral or viral-like prodromes occur in approximately 20 per cent of patients, followed by progression to significant behavioural disturbances, cognitive deficits and seizures. Psychiatric presentations include psychotic symptoms (delusions, visual and auditory hallucinations) and aggression.[77] The psychotic clinical picture is polymorphic, with predominant affective components. In addition to psychosis, NMDAR-antibody encephalitis appears to have a particularly close association with catatonia. In later stages of the disease, patients can develop motor manifestations (including catatonia), dysautonomia and coma.

NMDAR-antibody encephalitis affects mainly children and younger adult females, and the diagnosis is based on the presence of cerebrospinal fluid or serum NMDAR antibodies. There is epidemiological evidence that prevalence rates may be higher than those of herpes simplex encephalitis and approximate to 1–2 per million per year. Around 80 per cent of patients initially present to psychiatry services, although this proportion has reduced with time and increasing awareness of the disorder among physicians. Cases of NMDAR-antibody encephalitis presenting with isolated psychiatric symptoms (mainly psychosis) are relatively rare. Overall, the differential diagnosis between autoimmune encephalitis presenting with isolated psychiatric symptoms and a primary psychiatric disorder associated with neuronal auto-antibodies can be challenging.

Encephalitis associated with antibodies to voltage-gated potassium channel (VGKC) was first described in 2001. The most common symptoms are memory deficits, disorientation and temporal lobe seizures, although psychiatric features – including psychosis, anxiety and affective symptoms – have also been reported. VGKC-antibody encephalitis tends to present in later life, with a male to female ratio of approximately 3:2. The antibodies mostly bind specific proteins that are tightly connected to the VGKC, namely LGI1 and CASPR2.

LGI1 antibodies are predominantly associated with classical limbic encephalitis, usually of non-paraneoplastic origin. The clinical presentation at onset includes facio-brachial dystonic seizures: brief dystonic posturing of one arm and the ipsilateral side of the face.

Limbic encephalitis associated with CASPR2 antibodies more typically presents with insomnia, confusion and psychotic symptoms (hallucinations), as well as autonomic dysfunction and peripheral nervous system hyperexcitability, resulting in muscle fasciculations and cramps. This rare clinical picture, referred to as Morvan syndrome, can be misdiagnosed as a primary psychiatric disease if the peripheral and systemic features are neglected.

Other antibodies associated with an autoimmune form of limbic encephalitis are directed against the AMP-A receptor or the GABA-B receptor. These conditions are typically associated with tumours (especially affecting the breast, lung and thymus) but – like non-paraneoplastic limbic encephalitis – often respond to immunotherapies, which can provide at least a degree of symptom relief. Newly described forms of autoimmune encephalitis involve dopamine D2 receptor antibodies, which have been described in paediatric dyskinetic encephalitis lethargica, and IgLON5 antibodies, which have been associated with an encephalopathy syndrome featuring prominent parasomnias with breathing dysfunction and gait disorder.

Delirium and Dementia

Delirium

Delirium is an acute neuropsychiatric syndrome characterised by a complex constellation of cognitive impairments and behavioural disturbances that reflect underlying global

Table 8.9 Key clinical features of delirium

Criterion	Description
Disturbance in attention*	Reduced ability to direct, focus, sustain and shift attention
Disturbance in awareness*	Reduced orientation to the environment
Disturbance in cognition	Memory deficit, disorientation, impairment in language, impairment in visuospatial ability or perception

*The disturbance in attention and awareness develops over a short period of time (usually hours to a few days), represents a change from baseline and tends to fluctuate in severity during the course of a day.

impairment of brain function. This condition is sometimes referred to as acute confusional state, toxic confusional state, acute organic reaction, acute brain failure, toxic encephalopathy or acute organic psychosis, although some of the previous names are no longer in widespread use. Delirium is currently defined as an acute neurocognitive disorder characterised by prominent disturbance of consciousness, attention and other cognitive and perceptual functions. The clinical picture is summarised by the current diagnostic criteria, which require an acute/subacute disturbance in attention and awareness, plus an additional disturbance in at least one cognitive domain (Table 8.9).

Delirium tends to fluctuate and has temporal links to physical illness, trauma or drug toxicity, especially in the elderly. There is evidence from the history, physical examination or laboratory findings that the clinical presentation of delirium is caused by another medical condition, substance intoxication or withdrawal (either a drug of abuse or a medication), exposure to a toxin or is due to multiple aetiologies. The possible causes of delirium encompass a wide range of pathological processes (Table 8.10).

Delirium is usually due to a widespread disturbance of cerebral metabolism and requires urgent attention, as it is potentially reversible. The concept of subsyndromal delirium is used for patients who present with an attenuated delirium syndrome and do not meet full diagnostic criteria. Subsyndromal delirium often occurs during the evolution or resolution of a delirious episode, and it is characterised by a better outcome compared to full syndromal delirium.

Delirium is relatively common in clinical settings, with approximately one in five patients developing delirium at some time during hospitalisation. Rates are higher among patients in medical intensive care units and palliative care settings. Outside general hospital settings, it is estimated that 5 to 10 per cent of long-term residents of care homes typically have delirium at any time. Overall, elderly people are at higher risk because of changes that occur in the brain with ageing that increases their vulnerability to delirium. Patients with dementia are particularly vulnerable to developing delirium. Delirium has a considerable impact on patient outcomes and health care costs. Patients with delirium experience more prolonged hospitalisations, a higher number of complications (possibly including dementia), greater health care costs, reduced functional independence and increased mortality. Delirium can go unrecognised in a considerable proportion of cases because of its fluctuating nature, complex clinical presentation, overlap with dementia, lack of formal cognitive assessment, and underestimation of its potentially serious clinical consequences.

Table 8.10 Most common causes of delirium

Cause	Main examples
Degenerative disease	Dementias complicated by acute or subacute
Space-occupying lesions	Cerebral tumour, subdural haematoma, cerebral abscess
Trauma	Concussion, intracranial haematoma
Infections	Meningitis and encephalitis, focal infections, septicaemia
Vascular pathologies	Cerebrovascular accidents, hypertensive encephalopathy, vasculitis
Epilepsy	Psychomotor seizures, petit mal status, post-ictal states
Metabolic abnormalities	Uraemia, liver disorder, electrolyte disturbances, acidosis, alkalosis, hypercapnia, porphyria
Endocrine disorders	Diabetes, hyperthyroidism, hypothyroidism, parathyroid disorders, adrenal disorders, hypopituitarism
Intoxications	Drug and alcohol intoxication, drug withdrawal, chemical toxins, neuroleptic malignant syndrome
Anoxia	Lung disease, heart disease, anaemia, carbon monoxide poisoning
Vitamin deficiency	Wernicke encephalopathy, pellagra, B12 and folic acid deficiency
Other causes	Surgical procedures, pain, hypothermia, heat stroke

The main clinical features of delirium include a wide range of cognitive and psychiatric disturbances that impact upon consciousness, awareness of the immediate environment, generalised impairment of cognitive abilities, mental state and psychomotor behaviour. Consciousness can be affected both qualitatively (alterations of the subjective contents of consciousness) as well as quantitatively (alterations in the general level of wakefulness or arousal), with either reduced arousal or hyperaroused states. Disturbances to attention are considered the cardinal cognitive disturbance of delirium and present with impairment of the ability to direct, focus, sustain and shift attention. Reduced attentiveness can range from mild distractibility, losing the thread of conversations and failing to grasp complex details, to reduced interaction, lack of spontaneous speech production and inability to orient to salient stimuli, including bodily needs.

Early cognitive symptoms encompass minor forgetfulness and disorientation for time and place. Patients with delirium can have loss of topographical memory, resulting in them losing their way when wandering from home or driving to work. The memory deficit is often patchy, so that defective recall of remote events and partially correct information may be incorporated into confabulatory answers. Impaired new learning typically is an associated key feature. Other cognitive abilities potentially affected include executive functions and visuospatial abilities. Speech is often slurred or hesitant, with simple, poorly organised and often repetitious sentences. There can be circumlocutions, slips of the tongue, substitutions of words (paraphasias) and nominal dysphasias.

Other core features of delirium include psychiatric symptoms encompassing disturbances of thoughts and emotions. Perceptual abnormalities and other psychotic features most commonly present in the form of visual or tactile hallucinations, as well as illusions (distortions of shape, size and position of the patient's body and surroundings). Misperceptions are commonly reported, especially at night. Associated features include dissociative symptoms (both depersonalisation and derealisation) and delusions. Ideas of reference and paranoid delusions tend to be simple, fleeting, changeable, readily elicited by the environment and interpreted as hostile and persecutory. In general, thinking is incoherent, illogical, fragmented, undirected and characterised by impoverished content, with intrusive images lending a dream-like quality. Emotional lability is common in patients with delirium. Irritability, anger, anxiety, depression and unpredictable shifts in mood are often observed in varying combinations. Sustained lowering of affect can be mistaken for depressive illness. Variations in emotional arousal can range from panic to apathy, with the possibility of shifting between the two. Autonomic arousal can be present, with tachycardia, sweating, dilated pupils and hypertension.

Patients with delirium vary considerably with regard to their patterns of psychomotor activity. Two main 'hyperactive' and 'hypoactive' presentations have long been recognised, with an additional 'mixed' category for patients who experience alternations of increased and decreased motor activity within short time frames. In the majority of patients, spontaneous motor activity is reduced, but others present with a contrasting pattern characterised by hyperactivity, restlessness and excessive reactions to environmental stimuli. The most important example of the hyperactive variant is delirium tremens, observed in the context of alcohol withdrawal. In this condition, hyperkinetic manifestations often include a flapping tremor of the hands called asterixis. Other perseverative or repetitive stereotyped motor behaviours can also occur. Most commonly, shifts occur between states of lethargy and marked excitement (mixed subtype). In terms of underlying aetiology, hyperactive presentations are more common in younger patients and substance-related delirium, and they are linked to a better prognosis.

The temporal course of a delirium episode characteristically involves an acute onset that may be rapid (over hours) or more gradual (over a few days). As delirium worsens, patients become increasingly distractible, with either drowsiness or hyper-alertness and excitement. Diurnal fluctuation of symptoms is a common feature of delirium – for example, reduced responsiveness may shift unpredictably to outbursts of excitement. Often, the clinical picture is reported to worsen at night and improve in the morning, when patients may calm down and ask coherent, pointed questions. Overall, lucid intervals – or brief irregular episodes of improved thinking and behaviour – are characteristic of delirium and occur more often during daylight hours. Conversely, confusion is often more marked at night, and as a result, the sleep-wake cycle is frequently disrupted or reversed.

The outcome of delirium is highly variable, ranging from a brief transient episode characterised by full recovery to a more persistent illness associated with longer-term cognitive problems and functional impairment. Patients with delirium are prone to serious complications including feeding problems, dehydration, pneumonia, urinary incontinence and falls. Delirium is also independently associated with adverse outcomes. In addition to an increased risk of dementia, delirium is associated with subsequent development of post traumatic stress disorder and depression. Poor outcomes tend to correlate with the severity and duration of delirium.

It is estimated that about half of the cases of delirium are missed, misdiagnosed or diagnosed late in clinical practice. Lower detection rates are associated with a number of factors, including hypoactive presentations, comorbid dementia, previous psychiatric history and prominent pain symptoms. Routine systematic cognitive testing coupled with formal screening for delirium in high-risk cases is an assessment strategy that can improve detection rates.[78]

Since delirium is characterised by a prominent disturbance of attention, bedside tests that focus upon the ability to sustain attention can be useful screening tools. In most cases, delirium testing begins with assessing the level of arousal. Patients who respond to the clinician's presence but cannot cooperate with testing should be classed as having severe inattention consistent with delirium. The second phase of assessment for delirium focuses upon diagnosis and can be assisted by a variety of diagnostic approaches. In addition to laboratory tests, consideration of neurophysiological and imaging studies is often indicated.

The differential diagnosis of delirium is broad, as it can be easily mistaken for other neurocognitive and neuropsychiatric disorders such as dementia, depression or functional psychoses. Specifically, distinguishing the 3 D's of delirium, depression and dementia requires careful history taking, with collateral source where possible, as well as thorough examination and investigation for acute medical conditions. The presence of diffuse slowing on electroencephalography is more indicative of delirium.

The occurrence of delirium reflects a dynamic interplay between predisposing and precipitating factors. The most consistent predictors for delirium are older age, cognitive impairment or dementia, severe comorbid illness, functional impairment and exposure to psychoactive medications. The most common causes of delirium vary with patient age, but adolescents and young adults frequently report drug and alcohol intoxication and withdrawal syndromes, whereas in the elderly, infections and polytherapy are often identified. Systemic causes of delirium are usually characterised by the absence of focal neurological signs.

Delirium is a syndrome of generalised disturbance to brain function, reflecting widespread disturbance of neural networks. The aetiological heterogeneity of delirium suggests that delirium has many potential underlying mechanisms.[79] The pathogenesis of delirium is thought to involve two components: direct brain insults and aberrant stress responses. Direct brain insults can be the results of hypoxia, hypercapnia, hypoglycaemia, hyponatraemia, drugs, stroke and trauma, which directly disrupt cerebral functioning. Aberrant stress responses are thought to be mediated by cytokines and result in dysregulation of the hypothalamic-pituitary-adrenal axis and glucocorticoid levels, vagal transmission, and communication between the brain and the periphery. The main neurochemical disturbances associated with delirium involve reduced cholinergic function and hyperdopaminergic states. Anticholinergic agents can precipitate delirium, whereas antidopaminergic medications are the most commonly used pharmacotherapy for delirium. The spectrum of clinical symptoms reported by patients with delirium – ranging from disturbances of attention, arousal and thought to cognitive problems and disruption of the sleep-wake cycle – reflects widespread involvement of both cortical and subcortical structures.

The management of delirium has two main components, symptomatic and aetiological. In addition to the implementation of risk-reduction strategies addressing patient, illness and treatment factors, strategies of pharmacological prophylaxis (especially antidopaminergic agents) have been explored. The treatment of the underlying cause of delirium presupposes an accurate diagnosis, as well as careful consideration of aetiological processes and aggravating environmental factors. Both non-pharmacological and pharmacological strategies should be part of a care plan tailored to the individual needs of each patient.[80] Prudent use of antidopaminergic medications has long been the gold standard short-term pharmacotherapy for delirium.[81] The most commonly used agents include risperidone, olanzapine, quetiapine and haloperidol, whereas benzodiazepines have a limited role in delirium management. Treatment interventions should also address post-delirium care in order to minimise functional loss, address any psychological sequelae and reduce the risk of further episodes.

Dementia

Overview of Dementia

The term 'dementia' encompasses a range of progressive conditions mainly characterised by variable changes in cognition and behaviour.[82] Overall, dementia is common and is the major cause of long-term disability in old age, since age is the most significant risk factor for its development. From an epidemiological point of view, the prevalence of dementia is about 5 per cent in those over the age of 65 years and 15 per cent in those over 80 years. In high-income countries, it is expected that the number of individuals diagnosed with dementia will increase significantly over the next decades, due to the ageing of the population and advances in treating other age-related pathologies. In younger patients, the most common causes of dementia are Huntington's disease and Creutzfeldt-Jakob disease; older patients present most commonly with Alzheimer's disease (previously referred to as posterior type of dementia), frontotemporal dementia (previously referred to as anterior type of dementia), dementia with Lewy bodies, vascular dementia, alcoholic dementia and prion disease (Table 8.11). There is a relative excess of dementia of Alzheimer type among women and of vascular dementia among men.

Table 8.11 Main dementia syndromes

Neurodegenerative dementias	Alzheimer's disease
	Dementia with Lewy bodies
	Frontotemporal dementia
Non-neurodegenerative dementias	Vascular dementia
	Hydrocephalus
	Dementia caused by infective agents

Two main patterns of intellectual impairment have been described in patients with dementia. The more common pattern reflects cortical dysfunction, whereas the less common pattern is subcortical dementia. The cortical pattern of intellectual decline is characterised by deficits in language, learning, perception, calculation and praxis skills. The subcortical pattern presents more often with disordered motivation, affect, attention and arousal. There is, however, a considerable overlap in both clinical and neuropsychological presentations, and mixed cortical/subcortical patterns are frequently observed, especially in patients with focal or multifocal pathology.

From an aetiological perspective, it is possible to differentiate neurodegenerative and non-neurodegenerative dementias, depending on whether the underlying cause is primary neuronal loss. The most common neurodegenerative types of dementia are Alzheimer's disease, frontotemporal dementia, dementia with Lewy bodies and other forms of dementia associated with motor disorders. The heterogeneous group of non-neurodegenerative dementias includes vascular dementia, hydrocephalus and dementia caused by infective agents, as well as a number of other potentially reversible types of dementia. The differential diagnosis of dementia encompasses delirium, focal neurological or organic syndromes, psychiatric disorders (pseudodementia), mild cognitive impairment and age-associated memory impairment (benign senescent forgetfulness).[83]

Pseudodementia is a relatively common condition characterised by memory impairments secondary to a psychiatric syndrome that mimics dementia. Although the intellectual changes resemble those caused by degenerative dementias, cognitive deficits in pseudodementia are potentially reversible. The patient has a primary psychiatric disorder but no identifiable neurological disease that can account for the mental changes. Functional psychiatric disorder masquerading as dementia is most often associated with clinical depression, anxiety and transient stress, as well as – less frequently – schizophrenia, hypochondriasis, factitious and dissociative disorders. Ganser syndrome is a rare dissociative disorder (previously classified as factitious disorder) characterised by nonsensical or wrong answers to questions and often associated with other dissociative symptoms. The syndrome has also been called hysterical pseudodementia or prison psychosis – because the syndrome occurs most frequently in prison inmates, where it may be seen as an attempt to gain leniency from prison or court officials.

Clinical diagnostic criteria for dementia increasingly emphasise the need for supporting evidence from biomarkers, including both neuroimaging and laboratory tests, which may improve diagnostic accuracy in early stages. The neuropsychological assessment in the context of suspected dementia includes different tasks designed to probe a set of independent, but overlapping, domains of cognition: attention, learning and memory, visuospatial and constructional skills, language, executive functions and social cognition. In addition to the more comprehensive neuropsychological batteries, brief cognitive screening instruments have been developed and validated to provide an estimate of overall cognitive function and assist in the identification of patients who require a detailed cognitive evaluation. The Mini-Mental State Examination (MMSE), the Montreal Cognitive Assessment (MoCA) and the Addenbrooke's Cognitive Examination-III (ACE-III) are among the most commonly used general screening instruments. In addition, the occurrence and severity of behavioural symptoms can be assessed using the Neuropsychiatric Inventory (NPI) or the Cambridge Behavioural Inventory (CBI).

The treatment of primary dementia is still limited in both scope and efficacy. Acetylcholinesterase inhibitors (donepezil, galantamine and rivastigmine) are currently indicated for the cognitive symptoms. The NMDA antagonist memantine indirectly facilitates dopaminergic function, thereby exerting positive effects on attention, information processing and executive functions.

Mild Neurocognitive Disorder

Changes in cognitive functioning are prevalent in ageing populations, and there appears to be a continuum between normal and abnormal mental function in those individuals who will ultimately develop dementia. The commonly used notion of 'benign senescent forgetfulness' implies that age-related changes in memory functions are part of 'normal' ageing and not associated with central nervous system pathology. In addition to 'major neurocognitive disorder' (that replaced the previous diagnostic label of 'dementia or other debilitating conditions'), the DSM-5 introduced in 2013 the concept of mild neurocognitive disorder, defined by a noticeable decrement in cognitive functioning that goes beyond normal changes seen in ageing. Patients with mild neurocognitive disorder show evidence of modest cognitive decline from a previous level of performance in one or more cognitive domains (complex attention, executive function, learning and memory, language, perceptual motor or social cognition). Such evidence is based on two elements: concern (of the individual, a knowledgeable informant or the clinician) that there has been a mild decline in cognitive function as well as modest impairment in cognitive performance (preferably documented by standardised neuropsychological testing). The cognitive deficits documented in patients with mild neurocognitive disorder do not interfere with capacity for independence in everyday activities. Importantly, mild neurocognitive disorder does not necessarily progress to dementia. The current understanding of this condition is derived from research on mild cognitive impairment. Although there is currently no clear treatment for mild neurocognitive disorder, a clear need for experimental therapies focusing upon secondary prevention (decreasing the risk of progression to major neurocognitive disorder) has been identified.

Neurodegenerative Dementias

Alzheimer's Disease

Alzheimer's disease is a neurodegenerative type of dementia first described by German psychiatrist and neuropathologist Alois Alzheimer (1864–1915, Figure 8.10) in 1901. Patients

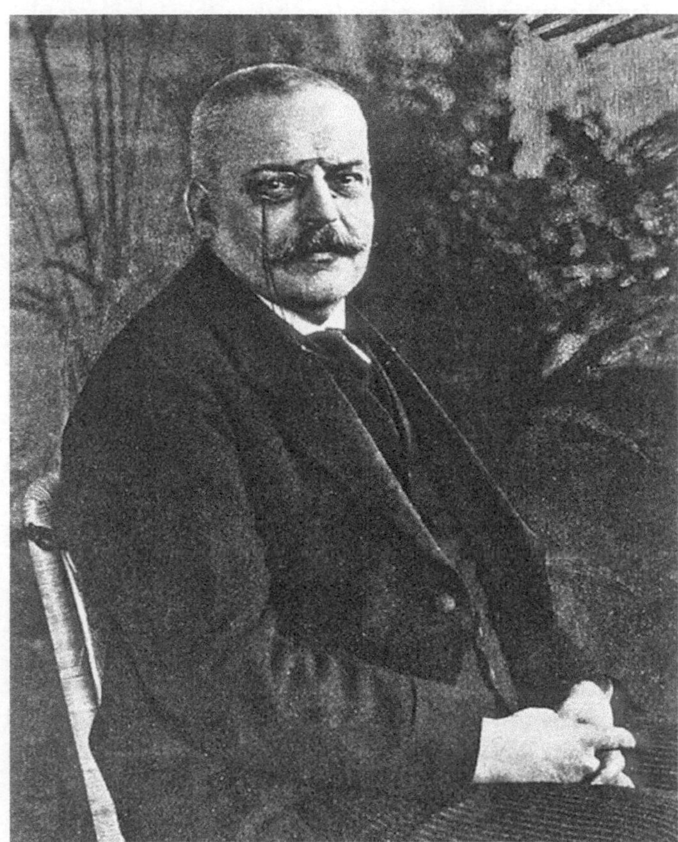

Figure 8.10 Alois Alzheimer (1864–1915).

with Alzheimer's disease characteristically present with deficits in episodic memory (both verbal and visual components), as well as variable alterations in attention and visuospatial skills.[84] In the initial stages of the disease, social cognition, language and behaviour are relatively intact, although a proportion of patients can present with early executive deficits. Overall, complaints about memory – occasionally accompanied by subtle memory deficits on cognitive testing – become increasingly common with ageing. Importantly, only a minority of subjects reporting memory problems will develop Alzheimer's disease, and it remains difficult to predict with certainty the outcome in any individual. The specific pattern of memory deficits with impaired encoding of information, together with impaired recall and recognition, tends to be associated with the early hippocampal pathology seen in Alzheimer's disease.[85]

According to the current classification, neurocognitive disorder due to Alzheimer's disease is subdivided into major and mild disorders, which exist along a continuum. At the mild neurocognitive disorder level, simple tasks such as remembering a shopping list, keeping track of a TV programme or planning a meal are described as being more difficult or requiring extra time but still achievable, whereas at the level of major neurocognitive disorder, such tasks can only be achieved with assistance of others or are abandoned altogether. If psychometry is performed, patients with major neurocognitive disorders score at two or more standard deviations below cultural norms (i.e. below the 3rd percentile), whereas the performance of patients with mild neurocognitive disorders lies in the one to two standard deviation range (i.e. between the 3rd and 16th percentiles). For major neurocognitive disorder, probable Alzheimer's disease is diagnosed if there is clear evidence of decline in memory and learning and at least one other cognitive domain, steadily progressive and gradual decline in cognition, and no evidence of mixed aetiology (e.g. cerebrovascular disease or other condition likely contributing to cognitive decline). Probable Alzheimer's disease is also diagnosed if there is evidence of a causative Alzheimer's disease genetic mutation from family history or genetic testing; otherwise, possible Alzheimer's disease should be diagnosed. For mild neurocognitive disorder, probable Alzheimer's disease is diagnosed if there is evidence of a causative Alzheimer's disease genetic mutation from either genetic testing or family history. Possible Alzheimer's disease is diagnosed if there is no such evidence, but there is clear evidence of decline in memory and learning and at least one other cognitive domain, steadily progressive and gradual decline in cognition, and no evidence of mixed aetiology.

Behavioural and psychological symptoms are reported by the majority of patients with Alzheimer's disease in residential care and are a cause of particular concern to carers. The most common behavioural changes include apathy and agitation. Affective symptoms, organic delusions (particularly delusions of theft and misidentifications), hallucinations, anxiety, irritability and restlessness are frequently reported. Behavioural and psychological symptoms, together with initial language impairment and a younger age of onset, have been associated with a more rapid decline.

The clinical course varies across individual patients; however, a pattern consisting of three consecutive phases is often described. The most common complaints during the earliest stages (1–3 years) include forgetfulness, as well as naming and word-finding difficulties. Possible alterations of visuospatial skills might cause problems in driving and drawing. Affective symptoms developing at this stage tend to be reactive to the underlying cognitive impairment, and performance anxiety may be considerable. The progressive decline in memory and other cognitive functions (thinking, reasoning, information processing) has an insidious onset and bears an increasingly more significant impact on activities of daily living. During the second stage (2–10 years), cognitive impairments become more severe and are accompanied by a constellation of focal deficits, encompassing apraxia, agnosia, comprehension difficulties and problems with mental calculation. Anosognosia is commonly reported, and disorganisation in both household tasks and financial affairs is increasingly more pronounced. The terminal stages of Alzheimer's disease (about 8–12 years) are characterised by global dementia, mutism, stupor and double incontinence. The loss of the unitary and coherent sense of personal identity becomes complete.

The aetiology of Alzheimer's disease remains a topic of intense research interest, focusing on the role of both genetic and non-genetic factors. In addition to increasing age, having a first-degree relative with Alzheimer's disease increases the risk of developing the condition. The cardinal neuropathological features of Alzheimer's disease are the presence of extracellular neuritic plaques and intracellular neurofibrillary tangles (aggregates of microtubule-associated protein tau). These findings allow the confirmation of the diagnosis at post-mortem or cortical biopsy. Both neuropathological changes can occur in normal ageing, with neurofibrillary tangles being most commonly confined to the hippocampi. However, they become significantly more widespread and prevalent in dementia. Other neuropathological features associated with Alzheimer's disease include hippocampal granulovacuolar degeneration, aluminium and amyloid deposition, hyaline degeneration and loss of both neurons and synaptic connections, resulting in alterations of acetylcholine, noradrenaline and serotonin neuro-transmission. The degree of neuronal loss and cholinergic depletion correlates with measures of cognitive and behavioural function better than other pathological markers.

The finding of various neurotransmitter depletions has led to efforts at replacement therapy, in particular with regard to cholinergic pathways. Three different acetylcholinesterase inhibitors (donepezil, rivastigmine and galantamine) are currently in use, with moderate efficacy on the cognitive symptoms but less clear benefit on disease severity, disability and health-related quality of life. The modest benefit of acetylcholinesterase inhibitors could be related to the complexity of neuro-transmission breakdown in Alzheimer's disease, which affects multiple chemical systems. The rationale for the use of NMDA antagonist memantine is the role played by the glutamatergic system in neurodegeneration across multiple types of dementia. The efficacy of other pharmacological options – such as cyclo-oxygenase 2 inhibitors, hormone replacement therapy and antioxidants – is yet unproven.

Dementia with Lewy Bodies and Extrapyramidal Syndromes

Dementia with Lewy bodies is a neurodegenerative type of dementia that presents clinically in a disease continuum with idiopathic Parkinson's disease.[86] The symptoms of dementia with Lewy bodies include both cognitive deficits and motor impairment. Lewy bodies, first identified in 1910 by German-born American neurologist Fritz Heinrich Lewy (1885–1950), are characteristically found in the substantia nigra of patients with Parkinson's disease, as well as in the hippocampus, limbic system and neocortex of patients with dementia with Lewy bodies. From a histological perspective, Lewy bodies are eosinophilic intraneuronal inclusions, composed of abnormally phosphorylated, neurofilament proteins aggregated with ubiquitin and alpha-synuclein. Dementia with Lewy bodies shares clinical and pathological features with both Alzheimer's disease and Parkinson's disease as a consequence of the depletion of acetylcholine and dopamine. Likewise, the neuropathological changes of dementia with Lewy bodies are mixed, with features of both Alzheimer's disease (amyloid plaques and, less frequently, tau neurofibrillary tangles) and Parkinson's disease (alpha-synuclein).

Dementia with Lewy bodies is relatively common in old age, accounting for 15–20% of cases in hospital series. The clinical presentation is characterised by impaired concentration, with fluctuating levels of attention throughout the day and visual hallucinations. Such fluctuations may pose significant challenges to the neuropsychological assessment. Memory deficits, similar to those seen in patients with Alzheimer's disease, are also common. The differential diagnosis of dementia with Lewy bodies includes Alzheimer's disease and other types of dementia, as well as Parkinson's disease, delirium and late-onset affective and delusional disorders.

Cognitive dysfunction – as well as psychosis, apathy and agitation – can respond to pharmacotherapy with acetylcholinesterase inhibitors. There is some evidence that acetylcholinesterase inhibitors may be more effective in dementia with Lewy bodies than in Alzheimer's disease, especially in mild disease. Specifically, treatment with rivastigmine may reduce psychotic symptoms such as visual hallucinations and may benefit activities of daily living. The most commonly reported adverse effects include diarrhoea, muscle cramps, dizziness, insomnia, nausea and vomiting.

A number of extrapyramidal syndromes can be associated with dementia. About a quarter of patients with late-stage idiopathic Parkinson's disease can develop dementia (Parkinson's disease dementia). Atypical Parkinsonian disorders can present with variable cognitive deficits.[87] Corticobasal degeneration is associated with a wide range of cognitive deficits, including impairment in memory, language and visuospatial skills. In particular, visuospatial impairment is often closely related to limb apraxia. Moreover, patients with corticobasal degeneration may develop a non-fluent type of aphasia, which can resemble the clinical presentation of early-stage progressive non-fluent aphasia. Progressive supranuclear palsy is associated with subtle executive deficits, as well as reduced verbal production. Huntington's disease, Wilson's disease and rarer disorders can present with a subcortical type of dementia. In addition to movement disorders, the main clinical features include memory problems, dysarthria, psychomotor retardation, affective symptoms and impaired insight and problem-solving.

Frontotemporal Dementia

Frontotemporal dementia is the most common cause of dementia in younger patients after Alzheimer's disease and presents with a range of behavioural and cognitive deficits. The average age at onset of frontotemporal dementia is between 35 and 65 years, with a variable illness duration and an equal sex distribution.[88]

About half of patients with frontotemporal dementia present with the behavioural variant of frontotemporal dementia, which is characterised by marked changes in personality, behaviour (e.g. disinhibition or apathy) and interpersonal conduct. Performance on cognitive testing may appear intact initially, although detailed testing usually demonstrates evidence of executive dysfunction and disinhibition. Deficits in language and memory may become increasingly prominent as the disease progresses. Overall, the breakdown in personality and social conduct occurs in the context of relative preservation of the instrumental functions of perception, spatial skills, praxis and memory. Specifically, patients with the behavioural variant of frontotemporal dementia present with an insidious onset and gradual progression of disinhibition, tactlessness and other alterations in social (interpersonal) conduct, including loss of empathy. The accompanying features encompass dysregulation of personal conduct (apathy, inertia, perseverative and compulsive behaviours, including hyperorality, humming, foot tapping and other stereotyped behaviours), loss of insight, emotional blunting, alterations in speech production (echolalia, mutism) and dysexecutive neuropsychological profile. Based on the individual clinical picture, the behavioural variant of frontotemporal dementia is sometimes subdivided into disinhibited, apathetic and stereotypic presentations.

The diagnosis of the behavioural variant of frontotemporal dementia is based on the presence of marked and progressive behavioural disturbances. The key distinguishing features from Alzheimer's disease are the prominent alterations in social cognition (loss of social awareness), hyperorality, stereotyped and perseverative behaviour, reduced speech production and relatively preserved memory and spatial orientation. With regard to investigations, electroencephalography is typically normal. Structural changes consistent with bilateral frontotemporal atrophy are revealed by magnetic resonance imaging, whereas functional neuroimaging shows anterior abnormalities (hypometabolism).

The behavioural variant of frontotemporal dementia was previously known as Pick disease, as it was first described by Arnold Pick in 1892. Pick reported the classic behavioural changes of indifference, poor judgement and insight, diminished creativity, careless dressing and antisocial behaviour, as well as aphasia. The neuropathology reveals bilateral atrophy of the frontal and temporal lobes and degeneration of the striatum, whereas the histology shows the presence of Pick bodies: spherical inclusion bodies found in the cytoplasm of affected cells and consisting of tau fibrils as a major component together with a number of other protein products, including ubiquitin.

A considerable proportion of cases of frontotemporal dementia are familial, mainly with autosomal dominant transmission. Mutations in the tau gene were first found in frontotemporal dementia with Parkinsonism linked to chromosome 17 (FTDP-17). An important cause of familial and apparently sporadic frontotemporal dementia is the C9orf72 (chromosome 9 open reading frame 72) repeat expansion, associated with an atypical or slowly progressive phenotype of the behavioural variant of frontotemporal dementia. The C9orf72 repeat expansion has been found to be common across the disease spectrum of frontotemporal dementia and motor neuron disease.[89]

Less common phenotypes of frontotemporal dementia are the temporal lobe variants, collectively referred to as primary progressive aphasia: a fluent type called semantic dementia and a non-fluent type called progressive non-fluent aphasia.

In the semantic dementia phenotype, there is progressive loss of word meaning and object or face identity, as well as behavioural disturbances, whereas orientation and episodic memory are spared. The neuroimaging presentation is that of asymmetric anterior temporal lobe atrophy, usually more prominent on the left hemisphere. From the pathological point of view, semantic dementia is tightly associated with the 43-kDa transactivation-responsive DNA-binding protein (TDP43)-positive intraneuronal inclusions.

In contrast, *progressive non-fluent aphasia* is characterised by motor speech errors (speech apraxia) and grammatical errors (agrammatism). Histologically, this variant is more commonly associated with underlying tau positive pathology. Neuroimaging findings show focal atrophy involving the inferior frontal cortex and anterior insular cortex of the left hemisphere. A third variant of primary progressive aphasia, logopenic progressive aphasia, is an atypical form of Alzheimer's disease characterised by marked word-finding difficulties, impaired sentence repetition (despite relatively preserved single word repetition) and minor phonological or grammatical errors in spontaneous speech. The underlying pathology shows brain atrophy involving more posterior (parietal) left hemispheric regions. The differential diagnosis between the aphasia syndromes in the context of dementia can be challenging, especially in non-fluent cases.

Other Types of Dementias

Vascular Dementia

Vascular dementia, also referred to as vascular cognitive impairment, is the most common type of non-neurodegenerative dementia. At a clinical level, the differential diagnosis between vascular dementia and Alzheimer's disease is based on the common involvement of subcortical and frontal functions in vascular dementia and the predominance of memory decline in Alzheimer's disease. Moreover, patients with vascular dementia have a history of multiple strokes and focal signs on neurological examination, marked white matter signal change on magnetic resonance imaging, and subtle differences on cognitive examination. Vascular dementia of acute onset usually follows a succession of strokes or a strategically placed single large infarction. The term 'multi-infarct dementia' was coined by Canadian neurologist Vladimir Hachinski in 1974. Following abrupt episodes of hemiparesis, sensory changes, dysphasia and other focal syndromes resulting from strokes, patients present with a fluctuating course and a stepwise deterioration in cognitive functions, culminating in dementia. The most important characteristics of multi-infarct dementia are acute onset with stepwise deterioration, evidence of cerebrovascular disease and focal neurology. Specifically, patients often present with episodes of nocturnal confusion, depression, pseudobulbar palsy (emotional incontinence with dysarthria and dysphagia), somatic complaints, ataxia and small-stepped gait, in the context of relative preservation of personality. Although the main predisposing factor is hypertension, multi-infarct dementia can also result from multiple, widespread cerebral emboli from extracranial sources. The Hachinski ischaemic score is a simple clinical tool used for differentiating the main types of dementia, such as primary degenerative dementia, multi-infarct dementia and mixed type dementia. The scale items include history of hypertension and stroke, as well as symptoms suggesting cerebral vascular events; high Hachinski ischaemic scores are closely related with cerebrovascular disease and its vascular factors.

The pathology of subcortical vascular dementia is characterised by lacunar infarcts, resulting from the occlusion of a single small perforating artery supplying the subcortical areas of the brain, and leukoaraiosis, resulting from more diffuse subcortical arteriosclerotic ischaemia of deep white matter. The lacunar state was first described by Pierre Marie in 1901, whereas diffuse leukoaraiosis was described by Otto Binswanger in 1894 and called Binswanger disease by Alois Alzheimer in 1902. The cerebral cortex is usually preserved, and patients with chronic hypertension often present with a more insidious cognitive deterioration. The clinical presentation encompasses pseudobulbar palsy with emotional lability, abulia, bradyphrenia, problems with concentration and memory, extrapyramidal signs and incontinence. Subcortical white matter ischaemia may be a more frequent and important cause of vascular dementia than multiple cortical infarcts. Finally, cortical infarcts and leukoaraiosis are commonly seen in patients with Alzheimer's disease and contribute to the decline of their cognitive performance. There is evidence from autopsy studies that a considerable proportion of patients over the age of 65 years show mixed pathology, with both a vascular component and a neurodegenerative component. In cerebrovascular disease, subcortical cholinergic pathways can be damaged by stroke or white matter disease, and acetylcholinesterase inhibitors have a modest effect in vascular cognitive impairment.

Hydrocephalus

Normal pressure hydrocephalus, also referred to as Hakims-Adams syndrome, was first described in 1965. The most common causes of hydrocephalus are brain tumours, particularly in the posterior fossa, obstructing the cerebral aqueduct and thereby the flow of cerebrospinal fluid. In most cases, the diagnosis is confirmed by structural neuroimaging. However, the differential diagnosis between hydrocephalus due to abnormal cerebrospinal fluid dynamics from hydrocephalus ex vacuo secondary to cerebral atrophy can be challenging, especially in the elderly.

The syndrome of normal pressure hydrocephalus is characterised by Hakim's triad of symptoms (dementia, gait disorder and urinary incontinence), in the absence of routine evidence of raised intracranial pressure. In most cases, there is no antecedent cause. However, this condition may develop years after meningitis, severe head injury with bleeding, or subarachnoid haemorrhage. Normal pressure hydrocephalus may respond to ventricular drainage.

In communicating hydrocephalus, the obstruction to cerebrospinal fluid is in the subarachnoid space (usually around the basal cisterns) rather than within the ventricular system. Patients with communicating hydrocephalus present with a treatable form of subacute progressive dementia. Accompanying features include headache, ataxia and gait disturbance, possibly in the absence of signs of raised intracranial pressure.

Dementia Caused by Infective Agents

Chronic infections are important possible causes of treatable dementia, accompanied by systemic manifestations, meningeal involvement, cerebrospinal fluid and brain imaging abnormalities. In addition to HIV-associated dementia (a subcortical type of dementia) and Creutzfeldt-Jacob disease (subacute spongiform encephalopathy or neurocognitive disorder due to prion disease), significant cognitive impairment has been observed in patients affected by a range of slow virus infections, as well as bacterial encephalitis and chronic meningitis. Of particular interest is neuroborreliosis or Lyme disease; Lyme encephalopathy is a chronic mild delirium, which potentially associates with both dementia and psychosis.

Toxic, Metabolic and Endocrine Disorders

Alcohol-Related Brain Damage

Epidemiology and Pathophysiology

Alcohol (ethyl alcohol or ethanol) is a psychoactive substance contained in alcoholic beverages.

Acute alcoholic poisoning results in drunkenness, but its dangerousness rises with increasing blood alcohol levels. After one or two drinks, a non-tolerant occasional drinker will display mild changes in affect, behaviour, cognition and motor control. If more is consumed and the blood alcohol level rises above 100 mg/100 ml, emotional lability and disinhibited behaviour – accompanied by impairment of judgement, memory and attention; slurring of speech; and incoordination – will be manifested. Similar symptoms may occur after head injury, post-ictally and as a result of hypoglycaemia. Beyond 200 mg/100 ml, these changes become marked. At around 300 mg/100 ml, depression of medullary function occurs, with the attendant risk of cardiorespiratory failure and coma. High blood alcohol levels inhibit gluconeogenesis and may induce severe hypoglycaemia, especially in malnourished individuals, children and adolescents; the usual signs may be missed if the individual is comatose and hypothermic. Hypovolaemia, lactic acidosis and acute renal failure are additional risks. The median lethal blood alcohol level is 400–500 mg/100 ml.

Intoxicated patients require careful assessment and management. The margin between narcosis and dangerous respiratory depression is narrower than with other central nervous system depressants such as anaesthetic agents. There is *great* danger attached to the practice of leaving a severely intoxicated person to 'sleep it off'. Coma due to alcohol is a medical emergency, as death may occur through aspiration or respiratory depression. Careful consideration should be given to alternative explanations of coma in a patient who misuses alcohol, particularly stroke, head injury, drug overdose, subdural haematoma, hypoglycaemia, liver failure, circulatory failure and hypothermia. Similar risks exist in the custody cells in police stations, where a significant proportion of deaths are due to alcohol poisoning.

Long-term alcohol misuse has detrimental effects on both the liver and the brain. Wernicke-Korsakoff syndrome is arguably the best-known manifestation of alcohol-related brain damage, a term that encompasses the wide spectrum of neuropsychiatric and cognitive symptoms that may develop as a consequence of direct alcohol toxicity and the indirect effects of thiamine deprivation.

Alcohol-related brain damage clinically presents with the acute, subacute and chronic effects of both alcohol and thiamine deficiency on the neurophysiology of the brain (Table 8.12).[90]

Table 8.12 Main neuropsychiatric manifestations of alcohol intoxication

Acute	Wernicke encephalopathy
Subacute	Dysexecutive syndrome and memory problems
Chronic	Korsakoff syndrome

It has been estimated that up to 1.5% of the general population have alcohol-related brain changes at post-mortem. However, the prevalence may be as high as 30–50% in socioeconomically deprived populations and high-risk communities, such as people attending alcohol treatment services. The presentation of alcohol-related brain damage is typically between the ages of 50 and 60 years. Women tend to present with a shorter drinking history and at a younger age than men.

The term Wernicke-Korsakoff syndrome captures both the acute (Wernicke encephalopathy) and the chronic (Korsakoff syndrome) manifestations of thiamine deficiency. Wernicke encephalopathy is a disorder of abrupt onset characterised by the classical clinical triad of ophthalmoplegia/nystagmus, delirium and ataxia – first described in 1881 by Carl Wernicke (1848–1905) in Germany. In 1887, Russian psychiatrist Sergei Korsakoff (1854–1900, Figure 8.11) described an illness characterised by pronounced impairment of recent and retrograde memory ('cerebropathia psychica toxaemica').

Korsakoff 'psychosis' was subsequently linked to Wernicke encephalopathy, as a proportion of patients with acute Wernicke disease proceed to Korsakoff syndrome. Thiamine deficiency does play a significant role in the aetiology of alcohol-related brain damage. Reduced dietary intake, as well as the direct effects of chronic alcohol abuse on the storage and utilisation of thiamine, can result in thiamine deficiency. The mammillary bodies and thalamic radiation appear to be particularly vulnerable to thiamine deficiency. Moreover, excessive alcohol ingestion can result in both enhancement of inhibitory GABAergic neuro-transmission and reduction of long-term potentiation at the level of NMDA receptors (a key process for learning and memory). The documented alterations in both GABAergic and glutamatergic pathways, combined with the evidence that the frontal lobes are particularly vulnerable to alcohol misuse, have been liked with alcoholic blackouts and amnesia associated with acute or binge drinking. The combined effects of thiamine deficiency and alcohol toxicity has been linked to widespread alterations to cortex and subcortical structures through neuronal depletion and white matter changes. The generalised cortical reduction results in ventricular enlargement and cortical atrophy.

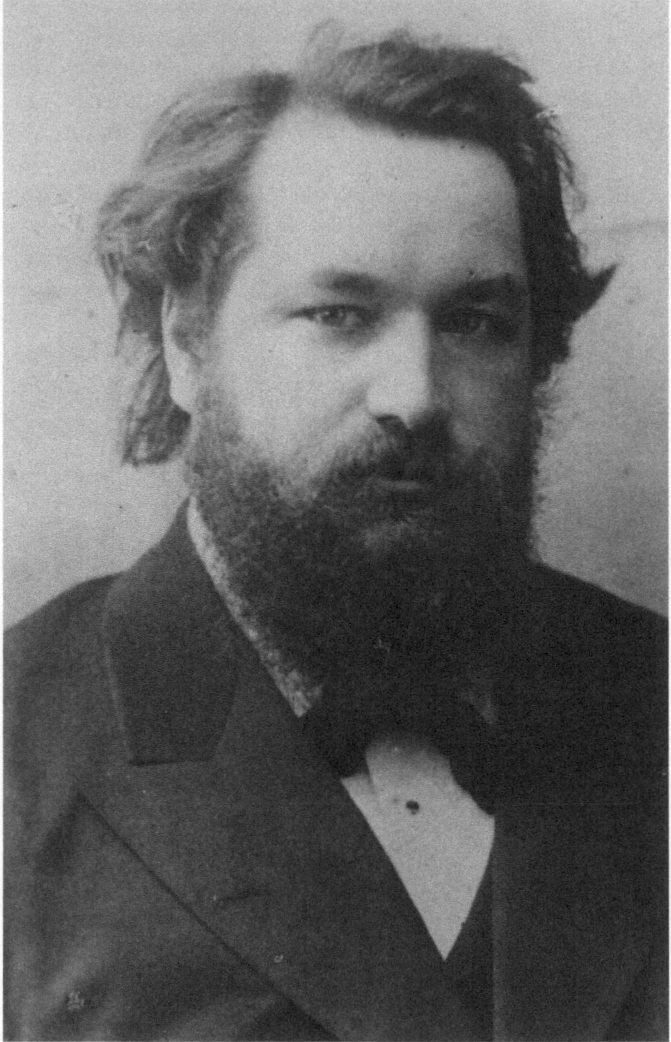

Figure 8.11 Sergei Korsakoff (1854–1900).

Acute Manifestations

Alcohol-induced amnesia is the loss of memory for actions and events occurring when intoxicated with alcohol. These 'memory blackouts' are commonly reported by dependent drinkers, as well as by occasional drinkers quite early in their drinking history. The memory gaps usually last for a few hours, although they can be longer. En-bloc memory loss is typically induced by large amounts of alcohol; it has a discrete onset and terminates with a sense of lost time and apprehension. Fragmentary memory loss is characterised by partial loss of memory, in which islets of recollection persist and often coalesce to produce a somewhat imperfect record of the lost events.

Memory blackouts should be distinguished from the memory impairment of thiamine deficiency resulting in Wernicke encephalopathy. The acute presentation of Wernicke encephalopathy is characterised by a classical triad of neurological signs: oculomotor abnormalities, cerebellar dysfunction and altered mental state. The acute clinical presentation may not be confined to the symptoms of Wernicke syndrome and may include features of limbic system, fronto-cerebellar-pontine and general cortical involvement. Moreover, up to a fourth of patients presenting in acute hospital settings also have a history of head injury or cerebrovascular disease, which can compromise cognitive performance. The differential diagnosis encompasses other frequently encountered conditions, such as hepatic encephalopathy and other causes of delirium. Red flags include malnutrition, neglect, history of frequent hospital admissions and physical problems, such as liver failure, pancreatitis and neuropathies.

Wernicke encephalopathy may co-exist with other vitamin deficiency disorders. Niacin deficiency is commonly found among people who misuse alcohol and usually presents with the triad of skin lesions, gastrointestinal disorders and mental changes (delirium, hallucinations, insomnia, anxiety and depression).

Wernicke encephalopathy is an acute emergency and warrants prompt intervention and physical stabilisation. Neuroimaging investigations can show the typical pattern of symmetrical thalamic lesions, as well as lesions in mammillary bodies, tectal plate and periaqueductal areas. However, more widespread lesions can also be reported, and negative findings do not rule out Wernicke encephalopathy, highlighting the importance of a detailed neuropsychiatric and cognitive assessment. Intravenous thiamine is the mainstay of treatment in the acute setting; other vitamin deficiencies have to be appropriately assessed and treated. Although the key features of Wernicke encephalopathy (ophthalmoplegia, ataxia and delirium) usually resolve within a few days after starting treatment, nystagmus can persist as a marker of the episode. Incomplete recovery of memory is relatively common.

Subacute Manifestations

The subacute manifestations of alcohol-related brain damage can be difficult to recognise, more insidious in onset and consequently rarely treated. Specifically, the presentation of dysexecutive syndrome is more insidious than the acute presentation of Wernicke encephalopathy and cognitive problems. Most patients present with various degrees of dysexecutive syndrome as a result of frontal cortex disturbance. These features – including problems in reasoning and processing complex information, understanding of risk, abstracting and manipulating memory, as well as acquiring novel information – can pose significant challenges to educational and therapeutic programmes targeting alcohol addiction.

Patients can develop increasing difficulties in social awareness, higher order reasoning and complex decision management. Over time, memory problems can become more evident, affecting the level of functioning and health-related quality of life in both family and work environments. With increasing cognitive impairment and long-standing intellectual damage, patients are at risk of social disengagement, domestic isolation and malnutrition.

Assessment of the less-obvious cognitive dysfunction that characterises the subacute manifestations of alcohol-related brain damage should focus on the dysexecutive syndrome and varying memory problems. This is particularly relevant to community settings and alcohol treatment services. The different degrees of subacute cognitive dysfunction across differing intellectual domains are thought to be a consequence of both the direct effects of alcohol and the indirect effects of thiamine deficiency. Treatment with thiamine should be offered to patients at risk of thiamine deficiency, who may present with a variety of symptoms including dizziness, diplopia, nausea, apathy, fatigue, insomnia and lack of concentration. These symptoms often co-occur with a history of poor nutrition, recurrent episodes of vomiting, weight loss and other nutritionally related conditions.

Chronic Manifestations

In the absence of thiamine treatment, Wernicke encephalopathy tends to progress to wider involvement of diencephalic and hippocampal networks, resulting in the chronic presentation of Korsakoff syndrome.[91] However, in a few cases, Korsakoff syndrome can present without an explicit history of Wernicke encephalopathy. Although the preceding episode of Wernicke encephalopathy may have occurred unnoticed, this condition is not an absolute prerequisite for the development of Korsakoff syndrome and related, more permanent, cognitive disorders.

Korsakoff syndrome is characterised by alterations of the mental state in which memory and learning are affected to a significantly greater extent than other cognitive functions in an otherwise alert and responsive patient. Both working memory (the ability of immediate recall of small amounts of information) and implicit memory (including procedural memory) are usually preserved. Semantic memory can be variably affected, whereas long-term episodic memory – including autobiographical memory – is frequently compromised, resulting in retrograde amnesia that may span several years.

The cognitive problems are typically complicated by false memories or confabulations. Complex, spontaneous confabulations are often characterised by the juxtapositioning of events in the person's life and are associated with orbitofrontal and ventromedial frontal pathology. Momentary confabulations are fleeting intrusion errors or distortions resulting from a challenge to the memory.

Chronic alcoholic hallucinosis can be accompanied by changes in mental state, personality and behaviour resembling those seen in patients with schizophrenia. There is evidence that cortical atrophy, especially frontal atrophy, occurs in patients with Wernicke-Korsakoff syndrome. However, it is often difficult to distinguish a primary alcoholic dementia from the effects of thiamine deficiency.

Marchiafava-Bignami disease is characterised by demyelination of parts of the corpus callosum, the anterior commissure and other areas of the brain, most often described in patients with chronic alcoholism. Nutritional factors (especially thiamine deficiency) are implicated in the pathophysiology. Marchiafava-Bignami disease may present clinically as a frontal lobe syndrome or as a progressive dementia evolving over a few years. The diagnosis can be challenging because of the variability of the clinical picture, with the complications of alcoholism potentially obscuring the presentation. Neurological signs such as dysarthria, dysphasia, dyspraxia, ataxia and hemiparesis are typically accompanied by physical deterioration leading to stupor and coma. This condition is associated with a poor prognosis, with residual severe disability in survivors.

Hepatic encephalopathy is the organic reaction of the brain to liver disease. Hepatocerebral disturbance in people who misuse alcohol occurs as a consequence of the development of a shunt between the portal and systemic circulation; as a consequence of this, toxins from the portal system enter the cerebral circulation unchanged by the liver. The neuropsychiatric manifestations include personality changes, irritability, altered mood, restlessness, psychotic symptoms and nocturnal wakefulness with daytime hypersomnia.[92] With regard to cognitive impairment, patients can report attention deficits, memory problems and confabulation. Progression leads to the onset of delirium, catatonia, stupor or coma. As patients deteriorate, they can develop a variety of neurological signs, including pyramidal, extrapyramidal and cerebellar signs. With time, flapping tremor ('asterixis'), dysarthria and muscle rigidity become noticeable. So-called liver breath ('foetor hepaticus') is often reported.

Hypoglycaemia, electrolyte imbalance, renal failure, infection and cerebral oedema may all contribute to the alterations of the mental state in patients with hepatic failure.

Alcohol-induced hypoglycaemia is an often-over-looked cause of morbidity in chronic, dependent drinkers who are malnourished. The cause is thought to be a reduced hepatic output of glucose, due to reduced hepatic stores of glycogen and suppression of gluconeogenesis during alcohol metabolism. In addition to autonomic symptoms, hypoglycaemia may induce generalised seizures. Alcohol-related electrolyte and acid-base disturbance in people who misuse alcohol include hyponatraemia, hypokalaemia, hypophosphataemia and hypomagnesaemia.

Early diagnosis and administration of thiamine for the acute presenting syndrome can prevent longer-lasting damage in people with alcohol-related brain damage. Although this is recognised as a potentially severe and incapacitating condition, resulting in significant morbidity and service utilisation, a considerable proportion of patients are likely to improve naturally if nutritionally stable, alcohol-free and supported in their recovery.

Longer-term psychosocial management is based on interventions targeting specific cognitive and behavioural domains.[93] Specifically, there is evidence that structured, specialised and purposeful psychosocial interventions may be associated with relatively good outcomes, reducing morbidity, alcohol misuse and service utilisation.[94]

Alcohol Withdrawal Syndromes

Alcohol withdrawal syndromes encompass the range of physical and mental changes experienced by dependent drinkers who withdraw from alcohol. Three major overlapping syndromes have been described: simple alcohol withdrawal, acute alcoholic hallucinosis and alcohol withdrawal delirium. Both complete and partial cessation of alcohol intake can result in withdrawal features, and the severity of symptoms is linked to the quantity and duration of alcohol consumption, as well as the drinking pattern.

In *simple withdrawal*, between 3 and 12 hours after drinking cessation, a dependent drinker can experience the symptoms of the withdrawal, including tremulousness and a range of physical and mental changes. Tremulousness is most apparent at the upper limbs and presents with different degrees of severity. The simple withdrawal features tend to subside one to two days into the withdrawal period, although neuropsychiatric symptoms such as insomnia, anxiety and depression can persist for a few weeks. About 12–18 hours into withdrawal, generalised epileptic seizures ('rum fits') can complicate this otherwise benign syndrome, especially in people who have a pre-existing history of epilepsy. Hypoglycaemia, hyponatraemia and hypomagnesaemia should be excluded as possible causes of seizures in the drinker.

Alcoholic hallucinosis is an important neuropsychiatric manifestation. Alcohol is the most common cause of hallucinosis in the general population. Perceptual disturbances are a common accompaniment of complete or partial alcohol withdrawal in dependent drinkers, and they can occur where drinking has recommenced but the features of withdrawal (including withdrawal delirium) are incompletely suppressed. Alcohol hallucinosis can be a consequence of nutritional, traumatic, toxic, metabolic or biochemical disturbances. The hallucinations are usually fleeting in nature, occur 12–48 hours into withdrawal, and are most pronounced during the first night. Most patients report visual hallucinations – as well as illusions, vivid dreams and other misperceptions – which can affect mood and become chronic in a minority of cases as described earlier.

Alcohol withdrawal delirium, historically referred to as delirium tremens (also known as the DTs), usually occurs within 18–36 hours of abstaining from alcohol. Patients characteristically present with clouding of consciousness and confusion; hallucinations and illusions affecting any sensory modality; and marked tremor. Visual hallucinations are typically experienced as vivid, as well as usually accompanied by auditory and tactile hallucinations. In contrast to alcoholic hallucinosis, there is usually a degree of cognitive impairment. Patients can also report secondary delusions, agitation, tremulousness, affective changes, insomnia or sleep-cycle reversal, as well as autonomic nervous system overactivity. Autonomic changes are usually striking and can include tachycardia, sweating, changes in blood pressure and pupil dilation. Approximately a third of patients develop epileptic seizures, which often precede the onset of delirium. Most episodes end abruptly with sleep within 72 hours or less, but there is a risk of relapses after apparent recovery. Memory for the preceding events is usually either incomplete or absent. The combination of hyperthermia and dehydration can precipitate circulatory collapse and contribute to mortality, especially when dependent drinkers with delirium tremens are alone at home.

The severity of alcohol withdrawal states appears to be linked to both the amount and the duration of recent drinking. Physical examination should be part of the comprehensive assessment, including autonomic arousal (temperature, pulse, blood pressure, sweating), tremor, agitation, signs of liver disease, infection and dehydration. Mental state examination should assess anxiety and affective symptoms, abnormal perceptions and thoughts, cognition (especially orientation and memory), as well as the degree of insight.[95] Simple withdrawal features of a mild degree or with uncomplicated alcohol withdrawal hallucinosis can be managed as outpatients, with the short-term use of benzodiazepines and vitamin supplements. Prophylactic treatment with antiepileptic drugs may be warranted in patients with a history of recurring withdrawal seizures.

Delirium tremens requires a more intensive care package within an inpatient setting, especially if the patients have significant autonomic overactivity, severe agitation, physical complications, a history of poor compliance with outpatient detoxification regimens, or poor home support.

Central pontine myelinolysis is a rare, but potentially fatal, acute osmotic demyelination syndrome selectively affecting the central basis of the pons. This condition was first described in 1959 as a disease affecting alcoholics and the malnourished, developing pseudobulbar palsy, quadriplegia, confusion and coma over a period of days. The involvement of electrolyte disturbances in the pathophysiology of central pontine myelinolysis is in line with the observations that rapid correction of hyponatraemia may lead to its development.

Pathological intoxication, also called alcohol idiosyncratic intoxication, has been defined as an acute brain syndrome manifested by marked behavioural changes (aggressiveness or psychotic reaction) after minimal alcohol intake in people with no pre-existing mental disorder. This condition was said to occur predominantly in persons with low tolerance to alcohol, but it was omitted from the DSM-IV because its existence was deemed to be controversial.

Drug Use

Stimulants

A number of recreational drugs have been associated with neuropsychiatric manifestations (Table 8.13).

Central nervous system stimulant drugs of abuse, including amphetamines and cocaine, can have clinically significant effects from a neuropsychiatric point of view. The acute effects of stimulants typically encompass euphoric mood, increased energy, improved concentration and thinking speed. The most common behavioural correlates are restlessness, agitation, hyperarousal and insomnia. However, depression is also frequently associated with stimulant misuse, since discontinuation of the drug leads to a 'crash' period characterised by decreased levels of energy, hypersomnia, anxiety and impaired concentration and cognition. During the first few days of the 'crash' phase, stimulant users often report prominent affective symptoms, which might contribute to the difficulty in assessing depression. Symptoms of abstinence, including reduction in mood, can persist for days or weeks depending on the specific drug of abuse. For example, affective symptoms can be reported for a few days following ecstasy (3,4-methylenedioxymethamphetamine, or MDMA) use; these manifestations are often described as the 'midweek blues' after MDMA use at the weekend. It has been estimated that about one-third of individuals with stimulant dependence develop depression in their lifetime. The overlapping presentations of depression and withdrawal in substance use are likely to be related to their shared neurobiological mechanisms, including alterations in dopaminergic and serotonergic pathways as well as dysregulated endogenous opioid function. Additionally, stimulant substance misuse can be associated with depression and anxiety indirectly by influencing adverse life events, via its negative impact on education and overall level of functioning. Individuals with substance misuse problems should be regularly assessed for the possible development of affective symptoms, with a view to implement treatment strategies for depression in a timely fashion. Stimulant substance misuse disorder should be treated alongside any comorbid psychiatric disorder. In addition to psychosocial interventions, serotonergic agents are among the most commonly prescribed pharmacotherapeutic options.

The association between stimulant abuse and psychosis is not rare and is likely to be caused by the increase in dopaminergic neuro-transmission. Psychotic symptoms associated with amphetamine use are similar to those reported by patients with paranoid schizophrenia: delusions, auditory hallucinations and ideas of reference. In most cases, psychotic symptoms resolve within hours or days of amphetamine use. A history of previous episodes of amphetamine-induced psychosis and a comorbid diagnosis of schizophrenia are associated with an increased risk of developing a psychotic episode in people who use amphetamines.

Likewise, cocaine use can induce a range of psychotic symptoms, especially transient paranoid delusions and auditory hallucinations.[96] Catatonic signs have also been documented in the context of cocaine use.[97] Male gender, greater addiction severity, agitation and aggressive behaviours have all been found to be associated with cocaine-induced psychosis. Stimulant-induced psychotic symptoms are usually self-limiting and resolve within a few days after cessation of use.[98] Pharmacotherapy is based on the use of dopamine

Table 8.13 Most common classes of recreational drugs associated with neuropsychiatric adverse effects

Cocaine, amphetamines and other central nervous system stimulants
Cannabis
Opiates
Hallucinogens

receptor antagonists, as well as benzodiazepines for the acute treatment of associated agitation.

Caffeine – as well as other xanthines such as theobromine and theophylline – are found in coffee, tea, soft drinks and chocolate and have stimulant effects on the central nervous system. The clinical symptoms of intoxication include restlessness, agitation, insomnia, diuresis, gastrointestinal disturbances, tachycardia, muscular contractions and alterations of thought and speech. Prolonged caffeine use can lead to physical tolerance and dependence. Individual susceptibility to intoxication is variable, and withdrawal symptoms include headache, irritability, poor concentration, anxiety and hypersomnia.

Cannabis

Cannabis is one of the most frequently used drugs of abuse worldwide. Cannabis use can lead to acute transient psychotic episodes during intoxication, as well as persistent psychosis after acute intoxication.[99] Specifically, cannabis intoxication has been associated with transient paranoid ideation. The increased risk of developing psychotic disorders following regular or heavy cannabis use persists beyond the half-life of cannabinoids. Cannabis containing higher tetrahydrocannabinol to cannabidiol ratios results in a higher risk of psychotic outcomes. In addition to cannabis, a number of synthetic compounds acting as cannabinoid receptor agonists increase the risk of developing psychosis and agitation during intoxication.[100] Dopamine receptor antagonists are widely used for the treatment of cannabis-induced psychotic symptoms. Regular cannabis use has been reported to be associated with an increased risk of depression and, to a lesser extent, anxiety. Moreover, patients with a diagnosis of bipolar affective disorder have increased rates of cannabis use, and there is evidence of cannabis use inducing and exacerbating manic symptoms.[101] Effective management of affective disorders with standard pharmacological and non-pharmacological treatments may lead to a reduction in cannabis use. The development of catatonic states after chronic, persistent high-dose synthetic cannabinoid use has been reported in patients without a previous diagnosis of psychosis. Catatonic symptoms can be reversed with abstinence and benzodiazepine treatment.

Opiates

Affective disorders – including depression and bipolar disorder, as well as anxiety – are commonly comorbid with opioid substance misuse and dependence.[102] Individuals with opiate misuse also have an increased prevalence of bipolar affective disorder. It has been suggested that the positive mood effects of opiates may contribute to the precipitation of manic episodes. The management of individuals with opiate dependence and associated affective disorders involves supporting them to stop or reduce their drug use through validated psychological approaches. In opioid dependence, engagement and stabilisation with opioid substitution treatment have been shown to result in improved affective symptoms. Serotonergic pharmacotherapy might also be helpful in order to optimise the management of comorbid anxiety disorders. Opiate-induced psychosis is rare, and opiate withdrawal psychosis clinically presents with auditory hallucinations and paranoid delusions.[103]

Hallucinogens

Drugs of abuse containing several plant intoxicants such as psilocybin ('magic mushrooms') can cause hallucinations and other acute psychotic symptoms. Hallucinogen persisting perception disorder occurs following cessation of use of a hallucinogen. Individuals can also re-experience perceptual symptoms that were experienced while intoxicated. Hallucinogen persisting perception disorder occurs most frequently after lysergic acid diethylamide (LSD) use. Flashbacks associated with hallucinogen use may also include psychosis with visual hallucinations, affective changes, panic attacks and dissociative symptoms. The mechanisms underpinning hallucinogen-induced psychosis and hallucinogen persisting perception disorder appear to be related to excitotoxic alterations of serotonergic and GABAergic neuro-transmission. Finally, ketamine – a drug used in anaesthesia – is also a substance of misuse known to potentially cause hallucinations as well as excitability, dissociative symptoms and delirium.

Neuropsychiatric Adverse Effects of Neuropharmacology

Cerebral intoxication with neuropharmacology can be an unrecognised cause of neuropsychiatric morbidity because of poor knowledge of the adverse effects of a medication as well as patients' denial or understatement about their usage (Table 8.14).

The potential adverse effects of medications used in neurology should always be considered in the clinical approach to behavioural and cognitive impairment. Cognitive adverse effects have been more commonly reported with the use of sedating antiepileptic drugs, including barbiturates and benzodiazepines.[104] Topiramate use has been associated with cognitive problems affecting attention, memory and executive function, as well as verbal fluency (word-finding difficulties). The behavioural profiles of antiepileptic drugs show a wide variability, depending on the individual agent, its dosage and the clinical characteristics of the patient.[105] A few antiepileptic drugs have been associated with the development of worsening of psychiatric symptoms, such as

Table 8.14 Most common neuropharmacological classes associated with neuropsychiatric adverse effects

Antiepileptic drugs
Dopaminergic drugs
Anticholinergic drugs
Ephedrine and other over-the-counter drugs

irritability and aggressiveness in patients with epilepsy treated with levetiracetam. Conversely, lamotrigine appears to be a safer option for patients with epilepsy and comorbid affective or psychotic symptoms. Pharmacological interactions between antiepileptic drugs and psychiatric drugs can have clinically relevant implications and should be taken into account in order to optimise pharmacotherapy in patients with epilepsy. Interactions can result in increased levels of either the antiepileptic drug or the psychiatric medication (with consequent risk of toxicity) or in reduced levels of either agent (with consequent risk of poor seizure control or ineffective treatment of psychiatric symptoms). A few antiepileptic drugs (e.g. levetiracetam) and psychiatric medications (e.g. citalopram) carry lower chances of causing clinically significant pharmacological interactions.

Organic psychosis with visual hallucinations, as well as a range of impulse control disorders, can be among the effects of dopamine replacement therapy in patients with Parkinson's disease. Dopamine agonists use has been associated with neuropsychiatric symptoms, especially when patients with Parkinson's disease are prescribed medications that are administered in a pulsatile mode.

Anticholinergic medicines can contribute to the development of psychosis in patients with Parkinson's disease. Overall, several medications used in neurology practice have anticholinergic effects that can cause adverse cognitive effects. Anticholinergic medications, especially in the elderly, can exhaust cognitive reserve and exacerbate the clinical presentation of neurodegenerative dementia. Both tricyclic antidepressants, such as amitriptyline and nortriptyline, and selective serotonin re-uptake inhibitors, especially paroxetine, are known to have anticholinergic effects. These medications should be used with caution in the elderly and in patients with a diagnosis of dementia or delirium.

The symptoms of anticholinergic intoxication are essentially those of atropine intoxication, caused by the antimuscarinic agent found in the plant atropa belladonna. These include dry mouth, reduced bronchial secretions, decreased sweating, fever, impairment in pupillary accommodation (with pupil dilation) resulting in blurred vision, tachycardia, difficulty passing urine and reduced bowel sounds. Neuropsychiatric symptoms can also be reported: fatigue, headache, ataxia, restlessness and excitement. Without effective intervention, ensuing delirium and hallucinations can be followed by coma. Memory problems can be a prominent feature. The differential diagnosis of anticholinergic intoxication includes the neuroleptic malignant syndrome, in which the dilated pupils are absent. Tricyclic antidepressants and clozapine can have prominent anticholinergic properties, whereas anticholinergic drug intoxication can be managed with an anticholinesterase agent such as physostigmine.

Psychosis, delirium, chronic affective symptoms and personality changes can be the consequences of intoxication, dependence or withdrawal from over-the-counter drugs. Intoxication has also been reported from medicinal substances administered topically, including eye drops and nasal compounds. Dependence does not always begin accidentally, as some compounds – such as ephedrine – have long been regarded as convenient amphetamine substitutes. Ephedrine was introduced into Western medicine as a bronchodilator and has a similar structure to amphetamines. Ephedrine and derivatives are among the most widely used over-the-counter medications, as they are key ingredients of remedies for the common cold. Their toxic effects include paranoid psychosis – with ideas of reference, delusions of persecution and hallucinations – almost invariably in a setting of clear consciousness. This clinical presentation can achieve significance when considering the differential diagnosis of schizophrenia. Depression and somnolence have been reported during withdrawal.

Environmental Elements and Other Chemical Substances

The most common poisons and brain intoxicants of environmental origin associated with neuropsychiatric symptoms are summarised in Table 8.15.

Aluminium intoxication can occur as a result of dialysis, from industrial exposure, from parenteral nutrition or from ingestion. Occupational exposure to aluminium has been associated with cognitive and behavioural symptoms – ranging from memory impairment to actual dementia – as well as a range of neurological disturbances.

Arsenic is found in compounds employed as herbicides and insecticides, as well as within the metal, paint and dye industries. Natural geological contamination of ground water occurs in some parts of Bangladesh and can induce chronic arsenic poisoning. The clinical presentation reflects the dose received and includes headache, nausea and other gastrointestinal symptoms, paraesthesias, seizures, delirium and coma. Neuropsychiatric presentations most commonly reflect

Table 8.15 Most common poisons and brain intoxicants of environmental origin associated with neuropsychiatric symptoms

Metals	Solvents	Pesticides	Gases
Aluminium	Carbon disulphide	Carbamates	Carbon monoxide
Arsenic	Carbon tetrachloride	Organochlorines	Ethane
Lead	Ethylene glycol	Organophosphates	Methane
Manganese	Isopropanol		Nitrous oxide
Mercury	Methanol		
Thallium	Methyl bromide		
	Methylene chloride		
	Toluene		
	Trichloroethane		
	Trichloroethylene		

subacute intoxication, with fatigue, weakness, muscular pain and anorexia. Psychiatric symptoms resemble schizophrenia, whereas cognitive impairment encompasses problems with learning and memory. Arsenic intoxication can be detected in urine, hair and nails.

Lead poisoning, also known as plumbism and saturnism, is a relatively common form of intoxication and is due to the accumulation of lead. This is still an occupational hazard – particularly for printers, painters and workers manufacturing batteries – despite efforts to remove lead from our environment. The main systemic features of lead poisoning include gastrointestinal symptoms, mild anaemia, weakness and fatigue. Acute brain intoxication results in irritability, insomnia, headache, hallucinations, memory problems, delirium and coma. Reported complications include seizures and raised intracranial pressure. Accidental exposure to lead can result in insidious accumulation, presenting with ataxia, peripheral neuropathy, anorexia, fatigue, irritability, insomnia and memory problems. Chronic organic lead intoxication presents with neuropsychiatric symptoms that overlap with both schizophrenia and hypomania. The diagnosis can be confirmed by the presence of high lead levels in blood and urine, associated with hypochromic anaemia. Recovery after severe lead poisoning is often incomplete; the neuropsychiatric sequelae include cognitive symptoms, seizures and other neurological deficits. The effects of lead on children and the developing brain may be more serious, as decreased cognition has been found to be associated with increased blood levels of lead.

Manganese miners, battery and steel plant workers, welders and glass workers have an increased risk of developing manganese intoxication. A neuropsychiatric presentation referred to as 'manganese madness' characterises the first few months after exposure. The most frequently reported symptoms include hallucinations, mania, ataxia, dysarthria, fatigue, anorexia, insomnia and memory problems. The clinical picture subsequently evolves to include more prominent neurological symptoms. In the later stages of chronic intoxication, patients can develop progressive Parkinsonism, personality changes and dementia ('manganism').

Mercury intoxication can result from exposure to the elemental liquid or vapour and is associated with pathological changes in the brain. The systemic features of chronic poisoning include gingivitis and dental problems, excessive salivation, anorexia, renal damage, anaemia, hypertension, tremor, peripheral neuropathy and ataxia. Historically, hat makers used mercury to help make the wool more pliable, unaware of the toxic effects of inhaled mercury vapour. The resulting psychotic presentation was immortalised as 'the Mad Hatter' in Lewis Carroll's *Alice's Adventures in Wonderland*. The most commonly reported psychiatric features are also referred to as 'erethism', and they include fatigue, depression, irritability, insomnia, apathy, shyness, nervousness and social anxiety. More extreme cases with prolonged exposure to mercury vapours can present with personality changes, memory problems and delirium. Minamata disease was a severe outbreak of mercury poisoning first discovered in the Japanese city of Minamata in 1956. It was caused by the release of methylmercury in the industrial wastewater from a local chemical factory; this highly toxic chemical accumulated in seafood, which – when eaten by the local population – resulted in mercury poisoning.

Thallium salts are odourless, colourless and tasteless and are used in the manufacture of optical lenses, semiconductors, fireworks and jewellery, as well as catalysts in several chemical processes. Acute thallium poisoning presents with prominent neuromuscular and gastrointestinal symptoms. Neuropsychiatric features may develop after a few days and include paraesthesias, headache, ptosis, optic atrophy, myopathy, seizures, psychosis, delirium and dementia. Cardiac arrhythmias can result in sudden death. Hair loss, parotid enlargement and skin lesions are the main systemic manifestations that develop in the more chronic stages of thallium poisoning.

Organic solvents have toxic effects on the central nervous system, in addition to other major organs. A number of products such as lighter fuels, adhesives, dry cleaning fluids, aerosols and nail-polish removers often contain more than one solvent, whose effects can be additive or synergistic with one another.

Carbon disulphide (an organic solvent used in the manufacture of rubber and plastics) exposure can cause include fatigue, depression, irritability, insomnia, mania and delirium. Chronic behavioural, motor and cognitive changes can also develop over time.

Carbon tetrachloride is a highly toxic halogenated hydrocarbon solvent. Transient exposure can cause irritation to the eyes, nose and throat; nausea; dizziness; drowsiness; diplopia and headache can result from transient exposure. A more severe clinical picture can be the consequence of continued higher-level exposure: delirium, seizures, coma and potentially death. Severe delayed systemic effects affect the hepatic, renal and gastrointestinal systems.

Ethylene glycol is employed as a solvent and in antifreeze, but it may be taken as an alcohol substitute. Inebriation can be followed by central nervous system depression, sedation, coma and death. Systemic complications can include severe metabolic acidosis and acute renal failure. The effects of diethylene glycol and propylene glycol resemble those of ethylene glycol.

Isopropanol vapour, either ingested or exposure, can lead to intoxication. The clinical picture overlaps with the one caused by ethanol intoxication, although symptoms tend to be more delayed and prolonged. In addition to neuropsychiatric disturbances, gastrointestinal symptoms can be particularly severe. Muscle spasms can be a useful pointer to the diagnosis.

Methanol poisoning can be caused by the adulteration of alcoholic beverages. The initial state of intoxication resembles that with ethanol intoxication. The products of methanol metabolism in the body can lead to severe metabolic acidosis and retinal ganglion cell damage, resulting in scotomata and blindness. The onset of neuropsychiatric symptoms – including visual changes, fatigue, delirium and coma – can be delayed for a few days. Impoverished alcoholics in the United Kingdom would sometimes resort to drinking 'meths' to satisfy their cravings, whereas criminal gangs continue to sell methanol as alcohol with resulting clusters of deaths and blindness in the Indian subcontinent.

Methyl bromide is an insecticide, and intoxication has been reported to induce persistent neuropsychiatric sequelae, encompassing hallucinations, memory problems, aphasia and incoordination.

Methylene chloride is both a solvent and a refrigerant and is metabolised to carbon monoxide, a toxic gas with narcotic and hypoxic effects on the brain.

Toluene is a solvent and a central nervous system depressant. Its inhalation causes an initial excitatory effect, followed by a depressive phase that may result in alterations of consciousness. During the excitatory phase, individuals can typically report euphoria, disinhibition, excitement, tinnitus, dizziness, diplopia, respiratory and gastrointestinal disturbances. Associated neuropsychiatric features include seizures, paraesthesias, psychotic symptoms, delirium and coma. Regular use can lead to dependency, tolerance and withdrawal phenomena. Solvent misuse is often associated with behavioural changes (especially social withdrawal and anorexia). Acute intoxication with the aromatic hydrocarbon benzene produces symptoms that are similar to those caused by toluene. Dyspnoea and impaired gait may persist for weeks, and chronic exposure has been associated with the development of haematological disorders.

Trichloroethane is an aerosol propellant and industrial degreasing solvent, and acute low-level exposure has mild behavioural effects, whereas massive exposure has been linked to permanent neurological sequelae, presumably as a result of cerebral hypoxia.

Trichloroethylene can cause cranial neuropathies, mainly affecting the trigeminal nerve. At higher levels of exposure, the clinical features resemble those of acute solvent intoxication, with the possibility of effect potentiation in case of concomitant alcohol abuse.

In the United Kingdom, the majority of solvent misusers now employ butane; previously, adhesives containing toluene and acetone were most widely used. Fluorinated hydrocarbons (freons) and butane appear to be disproportionately associated with fatalities, possibly due to their cardiotoxicity. Intoxicated individuals can become sensitised to the effects of endogenous and exogenous catecholamines. Solvent misuse should be suspected in the presence of an odour on the breath, freeze marks on the face, a peri-oral rash, glue on the hands or garments and possession of solvent containers. Behavioural changes include social withdrawal and anorexia, as well as those of intoxication. Laboratory detection is difficult; blood levels of solvents are detectable for 12 hours to five days, depending on the type of solvent.

A number of pesticide compounds have been shown to potentially cause neuropsychiatric symptoms. *Chlorinated pesticide compounds* cause central nervous system stimulation. Poisoning symptoms can include facial paralysis, dizziness, ataxia, tremor, seizures and delirium. Epileptic seizures have been particularly associated with chlorinated cyclodienes such as aldrin, dieldrin, heptachlor and chlordane. Chronic inhalation of the once commonly used herbicide *paraquat* has been associated with diffuse parenchymal lung disease ('paraquat lung').

Both *carbamates* (e.g. *carbyl*) and *organophosphate compounds* exert their neurotoxicity by acting as inhibitors of the acetylcholinesterase enzyme. *Organophosphate compounds* are known to be used as both pesticides and chemical weapons. For example, *O-isopropyl methylphosphonofluoridate (Sarin)* is a colourless and odourless gas that was extensively used by the Syrian government on its own people during the Syrian civil war. Likewise, *malathion*, *diazinon* and *parathion* act as irreversible acetyl-cholinesterase inhibitors, often resulting in fatal overdoses. The acute phase of intoxication is characterised by a number of features, including headache, vomiting, gastrointestinal symptoms, sweating, excess salivation and lacrimation, muscle weakness, cramps, fasciculations, wheezing, miosis and blurred vision, as well as memory problems and delirium. After a few days, patients can develop weakness or paralysis affecting their proximal limb, neck and respiratory muscles. Transient cranial neuropathies, fatigue and irritability have also been reported. Finally, possible delayed effects include distal sensorimotor neuropathy and corticospinal damage. From a neuropsychiatric perspective, lasting anxiety and affective symptoms have been described in individuals exposed to organophosphate pesticides, with endocrine disruption as a possible contributing factor.

It has been estimated that pesticide self-poisoning accounts for 14–20% of suicides worldwide.[106] In Western or industrialised countries, both illicit drugs (mainly opioids) and psychiatric drugs (mainly anxiolytics and antidepressants) are used for suicide purposes. In contrast, in low-income countries, such as India, or developed countries with significant agricultural areas, such as China, most suicides by poisoning occur through ingestion of pesticides. This has been linked to the observation that both carbamates and organophosphates are more easily available in predominantly agricultural countries.[107] *Dichloro-diphenyl-trichloroethane (DDT)* has major restrictions on its use because, being highly fat soluble, it is biomagnified in the food chain of animals. Further bans on highly hazardous pesticides, such as *paraquat* and *parathion*, have proven effective in reducing rates of suicide due to pesticide ingestion across most developing countries.

Nitrous oxide has been misused as a euphoriant for a long time. Acute exposure can cause delirium, whereas prolonged exposure has been associated with degeneration of the posterior and lateral columns of the spinal cord.

Carbon monoxide is a colourless and odourless gas formed by the incomplete combustion of organic material.

Inadequately maintained gas appliances are a notorious cause of carbon monoxide poisoning. Moreover, carbon monoxide poisoning in exhaust-filled cars has occasionally been reported as a means of suicide. Carbon monoxide reduces the oxygen-carrying capacity of blood and causes hypoxia. Likewise, small straight-chain aliphatic hydrocarbons such as methane and ethane are thought to have a toxic effect by inducing hypoxia.

Hypoxic or *anoxic brain injury* is primarily due to reduced oxygen supply to the brain, whereas hypoxic-ischaemic injury is the result of reduced cerebral blood flow (e.g. after a cardiac arrest), reduced oxygen supply or both.

In psychiatric settings, in addition to suicide attempts from exhaust fume inhalation resulting in carbon monoxide poisoning, hypoxic brain injury can occur after suicidal attempts by hanging. Certain specific central nervous system structures are particularly vulnerable to hypoxic brain injury: the arterial boundary zones and watershed areas of the cerebral cortex, Ammon's horns of the hippocampus, basal ganglia, thalamus and cerebellum. In addition to gait abnormality and involuntary movements, the clinical presentation of hypoxic brain injury includes a range of cognitive and neuropsychiatric problems. Cognitive symptoms include impairments in memory, executive function, attention and visuospatial functions. Changes in personality and behaviour include emotional lability, impulsivity, irritability, disinhibition, poor judgement and lack of insight. Alterations of consciousness can present as part of lethargy, mental slowing and delirium.

Altitude-related hypoxia can cause acute changes in the mental status as described earlier, usually becoming apparent above 4,000 m.

Carbon monoxide exposure to high levels can result in a syndrome of delayed neurotoxicity. Permanent sequelae of anoxic brain injury can include motor deficits, affective and personality disturbance, amnesic syndrome and dementia.

Metabolic, Endocrine and Mitochondrial Disorders

Metabolic Disorders

The most common metabolic disorders associated with neuropsychiatric symptoms are summarised in Table 8.16.

Table 8.16 Most common metabolic disorders associated with neuropsychiatric symptoms

Acute intermittent porphyria
Adrenoleukodystrophy
Alpha mannosidosis
Cerebrotendinous xanthomatosis
Fabry disease
Homocystinurias
Maple syrup urine disease
Metachromatic leukodystrophy
Niemann-Pick disease type C
Phenylketonuria
Tay-Sachs disease

Acute intermittent porphyria is an inherited metabolic disorder associated with heme biosynthesis defects and leading to excess urinary porphyrin and precursor secretion. The resulting metabolic abnormalities are reflected in alterations to GABAergic and serotonergic transmission. Acute intermittent porphyria most commonly presents in younger women with abdominal pain, peripheral neuropathy and neuropsychiatric symptoms. The most commonly reported psychiatric symptoms include psychosis, depression, anxiety, agitation and delirium.

Adrenoleukodystrophy is an X-linked recessive metabolic disorder due to mutations to a peroxisomal protein that oxidises very long-chain fatty acids, resulting in their accumulation in oligodendrocytes and adrenocortical cells. Although males are predominantly affected, female carriers may show a clinical phenotype due to inactivation of the normal allele. Phenotypes in adulthood include a predominantly spinal form (affecting the dorsal columns and corticospinal tract) and a cerebral form (characterised by inflammatory demyelination with a posterior predilection, in addition to the thalamus, corpus callosum and brainstem). With regard to the psychiatric presentation, patients most commonly report affective and psychotic symptoms, which may precede motor changes by a number of years.

Alpha mannosidosis is a recessive lysosomal storage disorder caused by mutations on the gene that encodes the enzyme alpha-mannosidase, which catabolises oligosaccharides. The resulting accumulation of oligosaccharides at the level of both glial cells and neurones initially affects the myelination process and subsequently neuronal structures. The childhood-onset form is usually characterised by moderate learning difficulties, hearing problems and immunodeficiency, whereas the indolent form with onset in adulthood may present with schizophrenia-like psychosis, followed by the development of ataxia, hearing loss and subcortical cognitive decline.

Cerebrotendinous xanthomatosis is a recessive metabolic disorder of cholestanol metabolism due to mutations in the gene coding for the enzyme sterol-27-hydroxylase. Cholestanol and its precursors accumulate in the extensors, neck and Achilles tendons, as well as in the brain (both grey and white matter), resulting in severe white matter and cerebellar nuclei pathology. Characteristic neurological symptoms include ataxia, pyramidal signs, seizures and peripheral neuropathy. Cognitive symptoms can also be prominent, with the development of dementia. Patients with cerebrotendinous xanthomatosis can often present with a range of psychiatric symptoms, encompassing psychosis, personality change, agitation and occasionally depression. Younger patients characteristically present with behavioural and personality disturbances associated with learning disabilities, whereas older patients typically present with affective and psychotic symptoms associated with frontal-subcortical dementia.

Fabry disease is an X-linked recessive disorder of glycolipid metabolism caused by mutations to the gene encoding the alpha-galactosidase enzyme. The gene defect results in accumulation of globotriaosylceramide in blood vessels and other tissues. Males are predominantly affected, whereas female carriers vary in the degree of presentation due to variable inactivation of the X chromosome. Disrupted vascular endothelium leads to the development of cutaneous angiokeratomas, hypohydrosis and corneal opacities. Patients typically present with episodes of peripheral pain and acroparaesthesia, precipitated by exercise or metabolic demand and potentially resulting in a chronic pain syndrome in adulthood. Vascular disease also affects the kidney, the heart and the brain. Patients often present with affective symptoms, which are likely to be multifactorial in origin, in line with the burden of pain and disease more generally.

A number of inherited metabolic disorders lead to elevated serum and urinary homocystine. *Defects in cystathione synthase* result in elevated levels of sulfur-containing aminoacids, which in turn can alter glutamatergic neuro-transmission and monoamine release. Disrupted collagen metabolism can result in dermatological and ophthalmological problems, arachnodactyly and scoliosis, as well as dystonia, seizures, learning disabilities and arteriovenous thromboembolism. The most frequent neuropsychiatric symptoms are aggressiveness, anxiety and affective symptoms, followed by psychotic features.

The *homocystinurias* are caused by defects involving the methionine synthetase and methylenetetrahydrofolate reductase enzymes. The resulting high levels of homocysteine can lead to a range of neuropsychiatric symptoms, including mental retardation, seizures, hypotonia and learning disabilities, as well as increased risk of developing psychosis.

Maple syrup urine disease is a recessive metabolic disorder caused by mutations in the genes that regulate branched chain amino acid catabolism. The resulting alterations affect synaptic and glial function and myelination, as well as inducing neuronal apoptosis. Monoaminergic, glutamatergic and GABAergic neuro-transmission are also affected. The name of the disorder derives from the sweet-smelling bodily fluids that have been detected in patients diagnosed with this condition. The clinical presentation can include ataxia and pyramidal features. Dietary restriction allows patients to survive into adulthood. However, they often develop motor signs and subtle executive deficits and attentional problems. Children may present with attentional deficits, whereas adults typically develop anxiety and affective symptoms.[108]

Metachromatic leukodystrophy is an autosomal recessive disorder linked to deficiency of the enzyme aryl-sulfatase A, which results in sulfatide accumulation in myelinated structures, as well as the kidney and gallbladder. On neuroimaging, leukodystrophy is characterised by periventricular white matter changes with an anterior preponderance, sparing subcortical fibres. In addition to the pyramidal and cerebellar motor signs, patients can present with psychotic symptoms, executive impairment, reduced speed of processing and attentional dysfunction. The cognitive symptoms can ultimately progress into dementia, with a clinical presentation that overlaps with that of frontotemporal dementia.

Niemann-Pick disease type C is a hereditary progressive disorder of cholesterol metabolism that causes intracellular cholesterol accumulation, particularly in neurones. Affected children present with hepatosplenomegaly and cholestasis, associated with seizures and learning disability. The form with onset in adolescents or adults frequently presents with neuropsychiatric symptoms (especially psychosis) prior to the development of neurological signs, as well as less clinically significant visceral symptoms. The most common genetic defect results in the accumulation of toxic GM2 and GM3 gangliosides, neurofibrillary tangles and neuroaxonal dystrophy that affects white matter diffusely and subcortical grey matter more focally within the cerebellum, thalamus, basal ganglia and hippocampus. Clinically, the most common manifestations are ataxia, dystonia, memory impairment and executive deficits. Moreover, brainstem changes can result in a characteristic vertical supranuclear gaze palsy.

Phenylketonuria is an autosomal recessive disorder caused by mutations in the gene for phenylalanine hydroxylase, which converts phenylalanine into tyrosine, the precursor for monoamines. This leads to the depletion of serotonin and dopamine within the central nervous system, which is associated with severe disruption of normal development. The resulting hyperphenylalaninemia affects cholesterol and protein synthesis, which in turn alters synaptic structure and myelination. Untreated phenylketonuria results in learning disability, seizures and death in childhood. Treatment is by dietary restriction of phenylalanine and supplementation of tyrosine. Despite treatment, patients often report high levels of anxiety and affective symptoms, reflecting monoaminergic depletion. Patients often have subtle executive and attentional deficits, which – like phenylketonuria-associated neuropsychiatric symptoms – tend to worsen when dietary control is poor and phenylalanine levels increase.

Tay-Sachs disease is an autosomal recessive sphingolipid storage disorder caused by impairment in the beta-hexosaminidase A enzyme, which results in accumulation of GM2 gangliosides within neuronal lysosomes. The resulting damage to neuronal cells affects mainly the cerebellum, thalamus, brainstem and substantia nigra. Children with Tay-Sachs disease can develop paresis, seizures, cerebellar signs and rapid degeneration; the disease is fatal. A later-onset form has been described, presenting with concomitant neuropsychiatric symptoms in early adulthood: dysarthria, ataxia, tremor, as well as psychotic and affective symptoms. Although cognitive function may be normal, patients often report subtle deficits in memory and executive function. Ashkenazi Jews have a relatively high incidence of Tay-Sachs and other lipid storage diseases. It has been estimated that in the United States, about 1 in 27 to 1 in 30 Ashkenazi Jews is a recessive carrier (in the general population, the incidence of carriers as heterozygotes is about 1 in 300). It is now possible to test for carrier status for Tay-Sachs, and it is customary for orthodox Jews in America – who usually have arranged marriages – to cross check their prospective partner for this.

Endocrine Disorders

The most common endocrine disorders associated with neuropsychiatric symptoms are summarised in Table 8.17.

Hyperthyroidism is a hypermetabolic state resulting from excessive activity of thyroid hormones. The most common causes of hyperthyroidism are diffuse toxic hyperplasia (thyroid-stimulating antibodies in Graves' disease), single functioning adenoma (toxic solitary goitre) and toxic multinodular goitre. Hyperthyroidism can also be due to exogenous thyroxine or iodine administration, thyroid carcinoma or other tumours. The development of clinical symptoms of hyperthyroidism is typically of insidious onset. In addition to chorea, periodic paralysis, myopathy and myasthenia, patients can present with psychiatric symptoms – particularly affective symptoms, anxiety and irritability. Affective symptoms are the most common neuropsychiatric features of hyperthyroidism – occurring in up to one-third of patients – and often developing prior to the physical manifestations.[109] In addition to mood disturbances, patients can report insomnia, reduced libido, weight loss and fatigue. Contrary to major depressive disorder, appetite is invariably increased in the context of hyperthyroidism. Although the severity of depression does not appear to be related to the extent of the biochemical hyperthyroidism, affective symptoms typically respond to measures that restore the euthyroid state. A mixture of affective and psychotic disturbances can be detected in the context of mild global impairment of cognition. Moreover, affective symptoms are often comorbid with generalised anxiety and agitation. Anxiety symptoms tend to correlate with the severity of the thyrotoxic features. The differential diagnosis between anxiety and hyperthyroidism can be difficult. Distinctive eye signs (exophthalmos) and later age at anxiety onset typically point towards the diagnosis of Graves' disease. Psychotic symptoms, including paranoid delusions and auditory hallucinations, have been reported in a minority of patients. Cognitive dysfunction is less common than in hypothyroidism and can include attentional deficits, short-term memory problems, slow reasoning and thought processing speed, as well as frank delirium. Fulminant episodes of delirium occur in a small percentage of patients with hyperthyroidism and are usually accompanied by high fever, tachycardia, hypotension, vomiting and diarrhoea. This acute presentation has been referred to as 'thyroid crisis' or 'thyroid storm'. A minority of patients with thyrotoxicosis, more usually older ones, present with apathetic detachment in the absence of psychomotor agitation. This presentation, termed 'apathetic' hyperthyroidism, is of slower onset and is associated with poor appetite and weight loss. Moreover, these patients have an increased risk of developing cardiovascular complications.

Table 8.17 Most common endocrine disorders associated with neuropsychiatric symptoms

Hyperthyroidism
Hypothyroidism
Cushing syndrome
Addison's disease
Hyperparathyroidism
Hypoparathyroidism
Acromegaly
Hypopituitarism
Diabetes mellitus
Insulinoma
Phaeochromocytoma

Hypothyroidism is a hypometabolic state resulting from inadequate thyroidal secretion of T3 and T4. *Endemic or sporadic hypothyroidism* present from birth is usually associated with learning disability and has traditionally been referred to as 'cretinism'. *Myxoedema* is the term applied to hypothyroidism in the child or adult. This endocrine disorder is significantly more common in women and is most frequently a disorder of middle life. The most common cause of hypothyroidism in adults is primary autoimmune hypothyroidism related to antithyroid antibodies. Less common causes include end-stage chronic thyroiditis or multinodular goitre, as well as adverse effects of drugs that affect thyroid function (e.g. lithium, carbamazepine and phenytoin). In particular, lithium treatment has been shown to affect the thyroid gland directly by inhibiting release of iodine, T3 and T4 as well as indirectly by inducing thyroid auto-antibodies. The clinical presentation of hypothyroidism includes characteristic physical features such as fatigue, poor appetite, constipation, cold intolerance and pain symptoms. In addition to physical and mental slowing, hypothyroidism can be associated with a variety of neuropsychiatric symptoms.[110] Affective symptoms, fatigue, anhedonia and hypersomnolence are commonly reported in patients with hypothyroidism and typically respond to treatment of the hypothyroid state. Depression is often associated with generalised anxiety symptoms. Hypothyroidism may also be a risk factor for the development of bipolar affective disorder. A range of psychotic symptoms – including paranoid delusions, misidentification, hallucinations, and thought disorder – can emerge after the onset of physical symptoms and have been described as 'myxoedematous madness'. Cognitive symptoms are commonly reported, occurring in about half of the cases. The spectrum of neuropsychological deficits ranges from reduced psychomotor speed, short-term memory problems, impaired visual-perceptual skills, executive dysfunction and difficulties with concentration to states of frank dementia.

Hyperadrenalism or Cushing's syndrome, first described in 1932 by American neurosurgeon Harvey Cushing

(1869–1939), is mainly due to overproduction of adrenocorticotrophic hormone from the anterior pituitary secondary to a pituitary adenoma. Less common causes include adrenal tumours and adrenocorticotrophic hormone-secreting tumours such as oat cell carcinoma of the lung. Cushing's syndrome is significantly more common in women and usually presents in mid-adulthood, but it can occur at any age. The characteristic features of Cushing's syndrome include hypertension, muscle weakness, fatigue, osteoporosis and dermatological changes. Truncal obesity involves the upper face ('moon face'), back ('buffalo hump') and trunk ('pot belly'). Female patients may experience hirsutism, acne and amenorrhoea, whereas men can report decreased libido and impotence. Psychiatric symptoms are reported by the majority of patients with Cushing's syndrome.[111] The most common psychiatric symptom is depression, often presenting with comorbid anxiety. Affective symptoms may present prior to physical symptoms and typically respond to treatment of the underlying cause. Elevated mood and manic symptoms have been rarely reported. Apathy, fatigue, agitation and – rarely – psychotic symptoms have also been reported. Cognitive impairment occurs in about half of the patients, presenting as deficits in verbal memory, attention and visuomotor/visuospatial skills. Frank delirium is relatively uncommon and is usually associated with high cortisol levels, advanced disease, older age and physical complications secondary to the disorder (especially supervening infection or other metabolic disorder such as metabolic alkalosis). *Exogenous steroid administration* – in contrast to idiopathic Cushing's syndrome – are more often characterised by mood elation. Neuropsychiatric symptoms can include emotional lability, manic symptoms, euphoria, agitation, pressured speech, hallucinations, delusions, anxiety, distractibility, insomnia, depression, perplexity and apathy. These manifestations tend to be dose-dependent, and milder reactions respond well to a gradual reduction in steroid dosage.

Addison's disease or primary adrenocortical insufficiency, first described in 1855 by British physician Thomas Addison (1793–1860), is due to autoimmune disease and is more common in women. Other inflammatory or destructive processes, dysfunction of the hypothalamic-pituitary axis, withdrawal of exogenous steroid treatment, or inborn failure of enzyme function can also lead to hypofunction of the adrenocortical system. The onset of systemic symptoms is insidious, with progressive fatigue, weakness, anorexia, weight loss, nausea, abdominal pain, hypotension and dermatological changes. The most commonly reported neuropsychiatric symptoms include depression, apathy, anxiety and irritability. Psychotic symptoms and alterations of consciousness are relatively rare, but they may herald an acute adrenal crisis ('Addisonian crisis'), with frank delirium, seizures and coma. Cognitive deficits, such as memory impairment, are often present, especially in patients with electrolyte abnormalities. The parathyroid glands maintain calcium homeostasis through the release of parathyroid hormone. The parathyroid hormone, in turn, increases serum calcium via stimulating bone osteoclasts to release calcium and through increasing its absorption in the gut and kidneys.

Hyperparathyroidism is usually diagnosed after an incidental finding of hypercalcaemia, with increased parathyroid hormone release being usually caused by a single functioning adenoma. More rarely, multiple adenomas may occur as part of a multiple endocrine neoplasia syndrome. The systemic symptoms of hypercalcaemia include fatigue, weakness, general malaise, thirst, polyuria, renal colic, gastrointestinal symptoms and abdominal pain. A number of neuropsychiatric symptoms have been described in patients with hyperparathyroidism. Affective symptoms and anxiety are the most commonly reported psychiatric manifestations. Psychotic symptoms – including hallucinations and persecutory or paranoid delusions – are less frequent. Hypercalcaemia due to primary hyperparathyroidism is also an important cause of attentional deficits, short-term memory dysfunction and acute confusional states. Delirium, referred to as 'parathyroid crisis', is associated with higher calcium levels. Overall, more severe hypercalcaemia leads to more severe neuropsychiatric disturbance, and symptoms generally respond to appropriate treatment such as parathyroidectomy.

Hypoparathyroidism is most commonly secondary to inadvertent removal of the parathyroid glands, usually as a consequence of thyroid surgery. More rarely, patients can have primary parathyroid disease or end-organ unresponsiveness to circulating parathyroid hormone (pseudohypoparathyroidism). Impaired parathyroid hormone production leads to hypocalcaemia, which clinically presents with symptoms of neuromuscular excitability – such as paraesthesia, muscle cramps, facial grimacing and convulsions. Secondary hypoparathyroidism often presents with more acute neuropsychiatric manifestations, including affective symptoms, irritability, psychotic symptoms and delirium. The neuropsychiatric manifestations of primary hypoparathyroidism can have a more insidious onset with emotional lability, impaired concentration and cognitive impairment. There is typically a correlation between the severity of neuropsychiatric symptoms and the degree of hypocalcaemia, and appropriate normalisation results in symptom resolution.

Acromegaly results from hypersecretion of growth hormone after puberty and is usually caused by a pituitary adenoma. Patients present with characteristic overgrowth of the head and extremities, often accompanied by headache, hypertension and glucose intolerance. Patients often present with psychiatric manifestations, including apathy, indifference, lack of spontaneity, inappropriate emotions, mood swings, reduced libido and, more rarely, psychotic symptoms. Psychiatric changes are thought to be multifactorial in origin. In the absence of raised intracranial pressure, cognitive deficits are not usually reported.

Hypopituitarism is most commonly due to a pituitary adenoma with a prolonged onset, and it can present with a number of systemic and neuropsychiatric manifestations.

Impaired libido and impotence can be early symptoms. Most patients with hypopituitarism develop psychiatric features, such as affective symptoms, apathy, inertia and, more rarely, schizophreniform psychosis. Memory impairment may be present. Delirium usually reflects impending or actual metabolic derangement, with increased risk of coma. A few manifestations of hypopituitarism, including impaired appetite, weight loss and scanty axillary and pubic hair can resemble the clinical picture of anorexia nervosa. The psychiatric symptoms of hypopituitarism typically respond well to hormone replacement.

Diabetes mellitus is a common endocrine disorder characterised by hyperglycaemia due to absolute or relative insulin deficiency. The vast majority of patients have type 2 diabetes mellitus (i.e. the non-insulin dependent form) that can be caused by insulin resistance linked to obesity, excess growth hormone, thyroxine, cortisol, adrenalin, pregnancy, medications and liver disease. Poor diabetic control is associated with affective symptoms. Changes in cognition, profound dehydration, polydipsia and polyuria, shallow respiration, hyperthermia, hypotension and tachycardia can all herald alterations of consciousness and diabetic coma.

In addition to misuse of hypoglycaemic medications, hypoglycaemia may be the result of different pathological processes, most commonly insulinomas. *Insulinomas* are tumours of the beta-cells located in the islets of the pancreas, which result in unregulated insulin secretion. This leads to fasting hypoglycaemia (relieved by glucose ingestion) and weight gain. Hypoglycaemia is characterised by hunger, weakness, restlessness, sweating, palpitations, faintness, headache, flushing and ataxia but may also include malaise, anxiety and dissociative symptoms. Inappropriate and aggressive behaviours have been reported, whereas seizures occur in a minority of patients. The triad of hypoglycaemia, central nervous system symptoms and prompt relief after intravenous administration glucose (Whipple's triad) forms the basis of diagnosis. For conditions of extreme starvation, hypoglycaemia may also induce permanent damage, as the central nervous system has a single source of energy – glucose – and the reserves of glycogen and glucose are small. The damage tends to occur in a rostro-caudal fashion: the middle layers of the cerebral cortex and the hippocampus are most affected, followed by the basal ganglia and the anterior thalamus. The effects of an insulinoma usually unfold insidiously, and in subacute hypoglycaemia, the symptoms of excess sympathetic activity are usually absent. Patients can present with affective symptoms, sleep problems, seizures, behavioural changes ranging from apathy to disinhibition, and cognitive deficits mainly affecting memory. In chronic hypoglycaemia, personality changes can occur, and memory is often affected, possibly resulting in global and irreversible cognitive deficits, including dementia.

Phaeochromocytomas are catecholamine-secreting tumours that originate most commonly in the chromaffin cells of the adrenal medulla, followed by similar cells located in sympathetic ganglia. The excessive secretion of catecholamines may be continuous or sporadic, resulting in the characteristic triad of palpitations, headache and profuse sweating. The variability of the presentation is partly due to the variation in the nature and quantity of catecholamines released. Paroxysmal symptoms occur in a substantial proportion of patients with phaeochromocytoma and may resemble anxiety symptoms, particularly panic attacks. The systemic manifestations encompass hypertension (and postural hypotension), pallor, perspiration, headache, tachycardia, tremor, nausea, abdominal and chest pain, as well as cardiac pathology. These clinical features may occur spontaneously or may be precipitated by exercise, postural changes, raised intra-abdominal pressure, acute psychological stress or emotional excitement. In addition to seizures, neuropsychiatric features can include intense anxiety, overarousal, affective symptoms and delirium.[112]

Mitochondrial Disorders

Mitochondrial disorders are multisystem disorders that can present with a wide range of neuropsychiatric symptoms.[113] These disorders can result from either mitochondrial or nuclear DNA mutations, and they are characterised by complex genetic patterns. The clinical suspicion of a mitochondrial disorder should be increased in patients with atypical psychiatric presentations, accompanied by signs of neurological, endocrine and cardiac dysfunction. The multisystem involvement is typically combined with a maternal history and a progressive course of the disease. The most common mitochondrial disorders associated with neuropsychiatric symptoms are mitochondrial encephalomyopathy, lactic acidosis, stroke-like episodes syndrome (MELAS) and Wolfram disease.

Mitochondrial encephalomyopathy, lactic acidosis, and stroke-like episodes syndrome (MELAS) is the most common mitochondrial disorder and presents before early adulthood after a period of normal development. The vast majority of cases of MELAS are due to a mutation in MT-TL1, an RNA transfer gene. The characteristic features of MELAS are stroke-like episodes that typically occur within the cortex (temporo-parieto-occipital regions), the basal ganglia, the cerebellum and the brainstem. Clinically, patients can develop hemiparesis, hemianopia and cortical blindness, often associated with migraines and vomiting. Elevated levels of lactic acid have been correlated with the range and severity of neurological manifestations, including strokes, deafness, retinopathy and seizures, as well as diabetes and cardiac abnormalities. Both affective and psychotic symptoms have been reported in association with MELAS. The diagnosis of MELAS is based on the clinical syndrome (neurological signs or symptoms, cognitive decline and evidence of strokes on imaging), elevated serum lactic acid levels and muscle biopsy showing ragged red fibres (expression of mitochondrial proliferation in response to mitochondrial failure).

Wolfram disease is a rare autosomal recessive mitochondrial disorder caused by a mutation in the WFS1 gene encoding an endoplasmic reticulum transmembrane protein.[114] Wolfram disease, also known as DIDMOAD (diabetes insipidus, diabetes mellitus, optic atrophy, deafness) is a multisystem disorder most commonly presenting with diabetes in childhood. Visual problems and optic atrophy, diabetes insipidus and sensorineural deafness typically develop at a later stage. Psychiatric manifestations, including psychotic symptoms, are relatively common. The diagnosis of Wolfram disease is based on clinical suspicion and confirmed by genetic analysis.

Nutrients

Vitamins

The most common vitamin deficiencies associated with neuropsychiatric symptoms are summarised in Table 8.18.

Vitamin B1 (thiamine) is an essential factor for several coenzymes involved in respiration. Thiamine deficiency is most commonly seen in the context of alcohol dependence, as alcohol can compromise the absorption and utilisation of thiamine.[115] Less common causes of thiamine deficiency are anorexia nervosa, hyperemesis gravidarum, severe renal disease requiring dialysis, and malabsorption syndromes associated with gastrointestinal malignancies and other pathologies, as well as bariatric surgery for obesity. Historically, thiamine deficiency has been associated with a number of systemic symptoms, collectively known as beriberi. In 'wet beriberi', oedema due to cardiac failure is prominent, whereas *in 'dry beriberi'*, the neurological features predominate over the cardiovascular manifestations. Specifically, in addition to weakness and myalgia, there is extensive peripheral nerve damage, leading to widespread sensorimotor deficits and muscle wasting. Fatigue and emotional disturbances are also common in beriberi. Acute neuropsychiatric manifestations of thiamine deficiency are observed in Wernicke encephalopathy (classically described as the triad of confusion, cerebellar ataxia and ophthalmoplegia). Since the vast majority of patients progress to develop Korsakoff syndrome, the two conditions are often grouped together as Wernicke-Korsakoff syndrome. Thiamine is poorly absorbed when given orally, especially in alcoholics or those with malabsorption syndromes. Therefore, patients with acute neuropsychiatric presentations suggestive of Wernicke encephalopathy are administered parenteral high-dose thiamine, whereas patients at risk of developing Wernicke-Korsakoff syndrome receive oral thiamine. The most consistent neuropathological findings in Wernicke-Korsakoff syndrome are atrophy of the mammillary bodies. However, oedema and micro-haemorrhages may also be seen in periventricular, midbrain and brainstem structures. Damage to the anterior thalamic nuclei seems to be critical in the development of the chronic amnestic symptoms reported by patients with Korsakoff syndrome.

Table 8.18 Most common vitamin deficiencies associated with neuropsychiatric symptoms

Vitamin B1 (thiamine)
Vitamin B3 (niacin)
Vitamin B6 (pyridoxine)
Vitamin B9 (folate)
Vitamin B12 (cobalamin)
Vitamin A (retinol)
Vitamin C (ascorbic acid)
Vitamin D

Vitamin B3 (niacin) is an essential co-factor in multiple reactions involved in the metabolism of carbohydrates and proteins, as well as in the chemical processes leading to cell assembly. Deficiency of vitamin B3 leads to the development of pellagra – a multisystem condition characterised by dermatitis, diarrhoea and dementia (the 'three Ds'). If untreated, the condition invariably results in death (the 'fourth D'). Pellagra is currently considered a rare condition in the Western world, although the diagnosis can still occasionally be made in chronic alcoholics and others at risk of malnourishment. The diagnosis of pellagra can be challenging because niacin deficiency in alcoholics can be under-recognised, photosensitive dermatitis can be absent, and the neuropsychiatric features can be variable and non-specific. The most commonly reported neuropsychiatry symptoms range from subacute fatigue and dysphoria to acute confusion, abnormal behaviours and memory impairment, occasionally accompanied by psychotic symptoms.[116] Clinical presentations similar to those caused by pellagra may occur in conditions affecting tryptophan metabolism, since tryptophan is a precursor of niacin. For example, pellagra-like features are observed in patients with Hartnup disease, a rare autosomal recessive condition associated with an abnormality of the tryptophan transporter gene.

Isolated deficiency of vitamin B6 (pyridoxine) is currently rare, but it may occur in alcoholism, chronic renal failure and other serious metabolic conditions. Patients taking isoniazid or penicillamine also have an increased risk of vitamin B6 deficiency. Vitamin B6 deficiency can be associated with treatment-refractory epilepsy, as well as polyneuropathy, although the latter tends to occur in the presence of multiple micronutrient deficiencies.[117]

Vitamin B9 (folate) deficiency during pregnancy is associated with neural tube defects in the developing foetus, and this led to a widespread public health recommendation about providing folate supplementation to pregnant women. However, folate deficiency is more common in the elderly and might be associated with depression. It is thought that a subset of folate-deficient patients can develop neuropsychiatric symptoms.[118] Moreover, genetic variables influencing the mechanisms by which folate is transported and utilised in the central nervous system might confer susceptibility to specific neuropsychiatric conditions. For example, folate deficiency is common in dementia, especially Alzheimer's disease, and is thought to increase the vulnerability to neurodegeneration. Individuals with cerebral folate deficiency have an abnormally low folate level in the central nervous system – despite normal serum levels – due to problems in the active transport of folate across the blood-brain barrier. Cerebral folate deficiency in early life may result from autoimmunity to folate receptors within the central nervous system, and it has been suggested that this can lead to the development of neuropsychiatric symptoms (e.g. autistic, spastic-ataxic, epileptic and schizophrenic syndromes).

Since *vitamin B12 (cobalamin)* acts in concert with vitamin B9 (folate) in several metabolic processes, there is considerable overlap in the clinical features of their deficiencies. However, cobalamin deficiency is characterised by higher prevalence and more severe neurological features than folate deficiency. Specifically, both vitamins are crucial in the conversion of homocysteine to methionine, which is essential for the production of myelin. Vitamin B12 is also required for the biochemical pathways that lead to purine synthesis; its deficiency leads to impaired erythrocyte production, resulting in megaloblastic anaemia (pernicious anaemia). *Vitamin B12 deficiency* is relatively common and results primarily from a lack of dietary intake, although gastrointestinal disorders can also play a role, as gut intrinsic factor is required for cobalamin absorption. Pernicious anaemia has been associated with a wide range of neuropsychiatric features. In infants, vitamin B12 deficiency may result in failure to thrive, hepatosplenomegaly and altered central nervous system development, with subsequent weakness, hypotonia and cognitive deficits. In adults, particularly the elderly, pernicious anaemia is often associated with both atherosclerosis and neurological disturbances. Early loss of vibration sense and peripheral sensory changes are commonly reported. Progressive degeneration of the dorsal and lateral columns of the spinal cord is a severe neurological complication, resulting in numbness, paraesthesia and weakness. If untreated with vitamin B12 replacement, neurological symptoms can progress to spasticity, paraplegia and severe ataxia. Low vitamin B12 has been associated with affective and psychotic symptoms, as well as subtle cognitive impairments, which tend to improve with vitamin supplementation. Chronic use (and abuse) of the nitrous oxide gas leads to low serum levels of vitamin B12 and clinical manifestations of its deficiency, including subacute spinal cord degeneration.

Vitamin A (retinol) is considered a prohormone, as it is oxidised intracellularly to the active metabolite retinoic acid. Retinoic acid is important in the embryological development of the central nervous system. In particular, it has a crucial role in the development and maintenance of the structures of the eye; vitamin A deficiency is the most common cause of nutritional blindness. Abnormal vitamin A levels, or anomalies in its functions, have also been linked to neuropsychiatric disorders. It seems likely that vitamin A deficiency might confer an increased vulnerability to dementia, as low levels of this vitamin are commonly found in patients with Alzheimer's disease and mild cognitive impairment. A possible link between vitamin A and other neuropsychiatric conditions, such as autism and schizophrenia, has been proposed. Likewise, it has been proposed that patients taking isotretinoin (an isomer of retinoic acid) for acne might have an increased risk of developing depression.[119] Fatigue has also been reported as a relatively common adverse effect of isotretinoin, whereas psychosis and aggressiveness have been described more rarely. Vitamin A – like vitamins D, E and K – can accumulate in the body. *Excessive ingestion of exogenous vitamin A ('hypervitaminosis A')* can lead to neuropsychiatric manifestations, including affective symptoms, sleep changes, headache, irritability and confusion.

Deficiency of vitamin C (ascorbic acid) leads to scurvy, a condition of historical relevance that – in the developed world – is currently encountered only in the context of severe physical or mental illness, such as advanced self-neglect associated with dementia.[120] There are also isolated case reports of scurvy occurring in patients with anorexia nervosa and schizophrenia. It cannot be ruled out that vitamin C deficiency is underdiagnosed in high-risk groups, although it can be difficult to attribute specific symptoms to nutritional deficits. Scurvy is characterised by connective tissue degeneration, leading to hyperkeratosis, severe joint and muscle pain, dental avulsion, oedema and spontaneous haemorrhage. According to historical reports, fatigue and irritability are the most common neuropsychiatric symptoms, especially in the early stages of the disorder. In addition to the classic acute presentations of scurvy, there could be a more insidious subacute neuropsychiatric form of the condition, characterised by fatigue, weakness and extrapyramidal symptoms.[121]

Lack of vitamin D is the most common vitamin deficiency worldwide, particularly where there is little exposure to sunlight, which is required for dermal vitamin D synthesis. Vitamin D deficiency has been associated with a wide range of neuropsychiatric disorders, including Parkinson's disease, dementia and schizophrenia. However, the exact relevance of vitamin D to these conditions remains unclear. Since vitamin D deficiency causes hypocalcaemia, it is likely that the central nervous system effects of the nutritional deficiency are due at least in part to low calcium levels.

Electrolytes and Minerals

The most common electrolyte and mineral imbalances associated with neuropsychiatric symptoms are summarised in Table 8.19.

Table 8.19 Most common electrolyte and mineral imbalances associated with neuropsychiatric symptoms

Calcium
Iodine
Iron
Magnesium
Phosphorus
Potassium
Selenium
Sodium
Zinc

In addition to hypoparathyroidism, *calcium deficiency* can arise from poor dietary intake. The classic neurological presentation of hypocalcaemia is a state of neuromuscular hyperexcitability characterised by paraesthesia, muscle cramps, facial grimacing and convulsions. The most commonly reported psychiatric features including affective symptoms, irritability, psychotic symptoms and delirium. Cognitive symptoms can also be reported. *Hypercalcaemia* can also present with neuropsychiatric symptoms, as well as systemic features. Depression and anxiety are the most commonly reported psychiatric manifestations, followed by psychotic symptoms and cognitive deficits, including acute confusional states.

Nutritional iodine deficiency can be present where diet depends largely on crops grown in low-iodine soils. Iodine is essential for normal thyroid function, and iodine deficiency typically presents as hypothyroidism with goitre. Iodine deficiency during pregnancy is known to be associated with severe impairment of central nervous system development in the foetus. Prenatal and infant iodine deficiency is an important cause of preventable learning disabilities and disrupted motor development. Severe maternal deficiency of iodine leads to a characteristic syndrome in the child (historically referred to as 'cretinism'), which includes short stature, spasticity, deafness, mutism, learning disability and often hypothyroidism.[122]

Iron deficiency has a high prevalence, arguably being the most common micronutrient deficiency worldwide. Reported neuropsychiatric symptoms are related to microcytic anaemia and include weakness, fatigue and dysphoria. It has also been suggested that iron deficiency might be associated with affective symptoms and neurodevelopmental conditions, although the possible role played by iron in these disorders is unclear, as the direction of the causal relationship between the psychiatric disorder and the poor nutritional intake is uncertain.

Magnesium is involved in different metabolic processes and has a key role in regulating the function of cell membrane ion channels within the central nervous system. The symptoms of *hypomagnesaemia* mimic those of hypocalcaemia. Specifically, the neuropsychiatric manifestations of magnesium deficiency include affective symptoms, anxiety, agitation, disorientation, personality changes, apathy, seizures, hallucinations and delirium. *Hypermagnesaemia* is usually an uncommon consequence of chronic kidney disease, rather than being the result of excess nutritional intake. In addition to malaise, nausea and vomiting, hypermagnesaemia can cause neuropsychiatric symptoms – including a severe acute encephalopathy, with areflexia, flaccid paralysis, dysarthria, ataxia and alterations of consciousness.

Hypophosphataemia, together with co-existing metabolic derangements including hypokalaemia, hypomagnesaemia and deficit of thiamine, can be encountered in the so-called refeeding syndrome. This condition has been described in malnourished individuals, especially homeless people admitted for assessment of psychosis, chronic alcohol misusers undergoing detoxification, patients with eating disorders and subjects with extreme degrees of self-neglect. Upon starting to feed, a shift from fat to carbohydrate metabolism occurs, triggering insulin secretion. This, in turn, stimulates a massive cellular uptake of phosphate, which can precipitate clinically significant hypophosphataemia. As phosphate concentrations drop, patients can report rhabdomyolysis, leucocyte dysfunction, hypotension, arrhythmias, respiratory and cardiac failure, seizures, delirium, coma and sudden death.

Hyperkalaemia can be caused by decreased renal excretion of potassium, due to either reduced glomerular filtration rate (e.g. chronic renal failure or acute oliguric renal failure) or reduced tubular secretion (e.g. Addison's disease or pharmacotherapy with potassium-sparing diuretics). Other possible causes of hyperkalaemia are transcellular potassium shifts, occurring with acidosis, cell destruction (induced by trauma, burns, rhabdomyolysis and haemolysis), diabetic hyperglycaemia and hyperkalaemic periodic paralysis.

Hyperkalaemic periodic paralysis is an autosomal dominant condition characterised by intermittent episodes of paralysis that can occur spontaneously, after exercise or following excessive dietary intake of potassium. Hyperkalaemia causes an organic brain syndrome characterised by a range of neuromuscular symptoms and other manifestations that can be mistaken for functional neurological symptoms: dysarthria, weakness, and, in more severe cases, flaccid paralysis and delirium.

Hypokalaemia can result from inadequate intake of potassium, excessive renal loss, vomiting and diarrhoea. Other causes of hypokalaemia include potassium shifts into the intracellular compartment as a result of alkalosis, insulin therapy or periodic hypokalaemic paralysis. *Periodic hypokalaemic paralysis* is a rare, autosomal dominant condition characterised by episodic weakness or paralysis triggered by the ingestion of a high load of carbohydrate. The intermittent neuromuscular manifestations of hypokalaemia can be mistaken for functional neurological symptoms.

Hypernatraemia can be caused by excessive water loss (e.g. pyrexia, burns, hypercatabolism, and diabetes insipidus), water loss exceeding sodium loss (e.g. sweating, vomiting, diarrhoea, osmotic diuresis), inadequate fluid intake (e.g. patients with alterations of consciousness) and excessive administration of sodium (e.g. salt poisoning). The systemic symptoms of dehydration include tachycardia, low-amplitude pulse, decreased jugular venous pressure, reduced skin turgor and postural hypotension. Hypernatraemia causes brain shrinkage, associated in extreme cases with subdural, subarachnoid or intracerebral haemorrhages. Commonly reported neuropsychiatric symptoms include weakness, irritability, psychotic symptoms, drowsiness, delirium and coma.

Hyponatraemia is caused by depletion or dilution of sodium reserves. Iatrogenic hyponatraemia can be due to incorrect intravenous infusion regimens or diuretic treatments, as well as a number of pharmacological agents, including amitriptyline, carbamazepine, haloperidol and lithium. Hyponatraemia can also be induced through excessive beer drinking ('beer potomania'). Patients with renal disorders, hepatic cirrhosis, congestive heart failure and Addison's disease are at risk of developing hyponatraemia. Finally, the syndrome of *inappropriate antidiuretic hormone secretion (SIADH)* is identified by the presence of a low serum sodium concentration in the presence of relatively concentrated urine. The neuropsychiatric symptoms of acute hyponatraemia are due to brain swelling, and they overlap with the manifestations of water intoxication (polydipsia). These include headache, blurred vision, tremor, ataxia, muscle cramps, seizures, delirium and coma. Chronic hyponatraemia may present with muscle weakness, drowsiness and hypersomnia. Rapid correction of hyponatraemia may lead to the development of central pontine myelinolysis.

Water intoxication associated with polydipsia and polyuria is quite common in psychiatric patients, particularly those with schizophrenia. Primary polydipsia is often accompanied by the sensation of dry mouth, and it is an important source of morbidity and mortality. In addition to polyuria, the early features of water intoxication include vomiting, headache, blurred vision, tremor and exacerbation of psychosis. Muscle cramps, ataxia and stupor have also been reported. This condition can go unnoticed until generalised seizures delirium or coma occur. In symptomatic patients, the diagnosis of water intoxication is confirmed by a plasma sodium level of less than 120 mmol/l. If the patient presents with overhydration due to acute hyponatraemia, management involves administration of intravenous hypertonic saline until the serum sodium levels stabilise to within a normal range. In addition to fluid restriction, behavioural treatments may involve the use of a token economy to provide positive reinforcement to desirable behaviour. Different pharmaceutical agents may be used in an attempt to achieve control over the polydipsia. These include atypical antipsychotics and the tetracycline antibiotic demeclocycline, which can induce nephrogenic diabetes insipidus. A number of emerging pharmacological options for the treatment of psychogenic polydipsia require further investigation.

Central pontine myelinolysis is a rare but potentially fatal acute disorder first described in people who are dependent on alcohol as well as undernourished individuals. This condition typically occurs in conjunction with life-threatening illnesses, which can be unrelated to alcohol use. Central pontine myelinolysis clinically presents with pseudobulbar palsy, quadriplegia, delirium and coma. The diagnosis is often confirmed after death, with characteristic histological findings (circumscribed areas of demyelination within the pons and, less commonly, in extrapontine sites; the term 'osmotic demyelination syndrome' encompasses all presentations).

Selenium deficiency often co-occurs with iodine deficiency, contributing to the hypothyroid symptoms. Moreover, low selenium may be associated with anxiety and affective symptoms, and it has been suggested that selenium deficiency could be a risk factor for the development of dementia.

Zinc deficiency resembles the symptoms of scurvy, as the metabolism of zinc is closely related to that of vitamin C. The main systemic features include skin lesions, poor wound healing and increased susceptibility to infectious. Lack of zinc in infancy is associated with growth retardation, hypogonadism and delayed motor development. Specific neuropsychiatric symptoms related to zinc deficiency include abnormalities of taste and olfaction, associated with anorexia and weight loss. In prolonged zinc deficiency, other neuropsychiatric features occur, such as cerebellar ataxia, fatigue, affective symptoms, paranoid delusions and hallucinations. A possible association between zinc deficiency and the development of anxiety disorders, memory impairment and progressive dementia has also been suggested.

References

1. Trimble MR. *The Intentional Brain: Motion, Emotion, and the Development of Modern Neuropsychiatry*. Baltimore, MD: Johns Hopkins University Press; 2016.
2. Trimble MR. The intentional brain: a short history of neuropsychiatry. *CNS Spectrums* 2016;21(3):223–9.
3. Crick F. *The Astonishing Hypothesis: The Scientific Search for the Soul*. London: Simon & Schuster; 1994.
4. Lagopoulos J. Evolution of brain imaging in neuropsychiatry: past, present and future. *Acta Neuropsychiatrica* 2010;22(3):152–4.
5. Worbe Y. Neuroimaging signature of neuropsychiatric disorders. *Current Opinion in Neurology* 2015; 28(4):358–64.
6. Shelley BP, Trimble MR, Boutros NN. Electroencephalographic cerebral dysrhythmic abnormalities in the trinity of nonepileptic general population, neuropsychiatric, and neurobehavioral disorders. *Journal of Neuropsychiatry and Clinical Neurosciences* 2008;20 (1):7–22.
7. Daffner KR, Gale SA, Barrett Am, et al. Improving clinical cognitive testing: report of the AAN Behavioral Neurology Section Workgroup. *Neurology* 2015;85(10):910–8.
8. Thiebaut de Schotten M, Dell'Acqua F, Ratiu P, et al. From Phineas Gage and Monsieur Leborgne to H.M.: revisiting disconnection syndromes. *Cerebral Cortex* 2015;25(12):4812–27.
9. Damasio H, Grabowski T, Frank R, et al. The return of Phineas Gage: clues about the brain from the skull of a famous patient. *Science* 1994;264 (5162):1102–5.
10. Alexander GE, DeLong MR, Strick PL. Parallel organization of functionally segregated circuits linking basal ganglia and cortex. *Annual Review of Neuroscience* 1986;9:357–81.
11. Catani M, Dell'Acqua F, Thiebaut de Schotten M. A revised limbic system model for memory, emotion and behaviour. *Neuroscience and Biobehavioral Reviews* 2013;37(8):1724–7.
12. MacLean P. *The Triune Brain*. New York: Plenum; 1990.
13. Cavanna AE, Rickards H, Ali F. What makes a simple partial seizure complex? *Epilepsy & Behavior* 2011;22(4):651–8.
14. Squire LR. The legacy of patient H.M. for neuroscience. *Neuron* 2009;61 (1):6–9.

15. Critchley M. *The Parietal Lobes.* Baltimore: Williams and Wilkins; 1953.
16. Cavanna AE, Trimble MR. The precuneus: a review of its functional anatomy and behavioural correlates. *Brain* 2006;129(Pt 3):564–83.
17. Weiskrantz L. *Blindsight: A Case Study and Implications*. Oxford: Oxford University Press; 1986.
18. Marshman LA, Jakabek D, Hennessy M, et al. Post-traumatic amnesia. *Journal of Clinical Neuroscience* 2013;20 (11):1475–81.
19. Marshall S, Bayley M, McCullagh S, et al. Updated clinical practice guidelines for concussion/mild traumatic brain injury and persistent symptoms. *Brain Injury* 2015;29 (6):688–700.
20. Hadanny A, Efrati S. Treatment of persistent postconcussion syndrome due to mild traumatic brain injury: current status and future directions. *Expert Review of Neurotherapeutics* 2016;16(8):875–87.
21. Osborn AJ, Mathias JL, Fairweather-Schmidt AK. Depression following adult, non- penetrating traumatic brain injury: a meta-analysis examining methodological variables and sample characteristics. *Neuroscience and Biobehavioral Reviews* 2014;47:1–15.
22. Bhatnagar S, Iaccarino MA, Zafonte R. Pharmacotherapy in rehabilitation of post-acute traumatic brain injury. *Brain Research* 2016;1640(Pt A):164–79.
23. Batty RA, Rossell SL, Francis AJ, et al. Psychosis following traumatic brain injury. *Brain Impairment* 2013;14 (1):21–41.
24. Bartoli F, Lillia N, Lax A, et al. Depression after stroke and risk of mortality: A systematic review and meta-analysis. *Stroke Research and Treatment* 2013: 862978.
25. van Dalen JW, Moll van Charante EP, Nederkoorn PJ, et al. Poststroke apathy. *Stroke* 2013;44(3):851–60.
26. Campbell Burton CA, Murray J, Holmes J, et al. Frequency of anxiety after stroke: a systematic review and meta- analysis of observational studies. *International Journal of Stroke* 2013;8 (7):545–59.
27. Krebber AM, Buffart LM, Kleijn G, et al. Prevalence of depression in cancer patients: a metaanalysis of diagnostic interviews and self-report instruments. *Psychooncology* 2014;23(2):121–30.
28. Madhusoodanan S, Opler MG, Moise D, et al. Brain tumor location and psychiatric symptoms: is there any association? A metaanalysis of published case studies. *Expert Review of Neurotherapetics* 2010;10(10):1529–36.
29. Cavanna AE, Ali F. Epilepsy: the quintessential pathology of consciousness. *Behavioural Neurology* 2011;24(1):3–10.
30. Fisher RS, Acevedo C, Arzimanoglou A, et al. ILAE official report: a practical clinical definition of epilepsy. *Epilepsia* 2014;55(4):475–82.
31. Fiest KM, Sauro KM, Wiebe S, et al. Prevalence and incidence of epilepsy: a systematic review and meta-analysis of international studies. *Neurology* 2017;88 (3):296–303.
32. Fisher RS, Cross JH, French JA, et al. Operational classification of seizure types by the International League Against Epilepsy: position paper of the ILAE Commission for Classification and Terminology. *Epilepsia* 2017;58 (4):522–30.
33. Monaco F, Mula M, Cavanna AE. Consciousness, epilepsy, and emotional qualia. *Epilepsy & Behavior* 2005;7 (2):150–60.
34. Scheffer IE, Berkovic S, Capovilla G, et al. ILAE classification of the epilepsies: position paper of the ILAE Commission for Classification and Terminology. *Epilepsia* 2017;58 (4):512–21.
35. Cavanna AE. *Behavioural Neurology of Antiepileptic Drugs: A Practical Guide.* Oxford: Oxford University Press; 2018.
36. Mula M. Epilepsy-induced behavioral changes during the ictal phase. *Epilepsy & Behavior* 2014;30:14–6.
37. Ali F, Rickards H, Cavanna AE. The assessment of consciousness during partial seizures. *Epilepsy & Behavior* 2012;23(2):98–102.
38. Kerr MP, Mensah S, Besag F, et al. International consensus clinical practice statements for the treatment of neuropsychiatric conditions associated with epilepsy. *Epilepsia* 2011;52 (11):2133–8.
39. Jones R, Rickards H, Cavanna AE. The prevalence of psychiatric disorders in epilepsy: a critical review of the evidence. *Functional Neurology* 2010;25 (4):191–4.
40. Berg AT, Altalib HH, Devinsky O. Psychiatric and behavioral comorbidities in epilepsy: a critical reappraisal. *Epilepsia* 2017;58 (7):1123–30.
41. Elger CE, Johnston SA, Hoppe C. Diagnosing and treating depression in epilepsy. *Seizure* 2017;44:184–93.
42. Bangar S, Shastri A, El-Sayeh H, Cavanna AE. Women with epilepsy: clinically relevant issues. *Functional Neurology* 2016;31(3):127–34.
43. Kanner AM. Management of psychiatric and neurological comorbidities in epilepsy. *Nature Reviews. Neurology* 2016;12(2):106–16.
44. Kanner AM, Rivas-Grajales AM. Psychosis of epilepsy: a multifaceted neuropsychiatric disorder. *CNS Spectrums* 2016;21(3):247–57.
45. Poewe W, Seppi K, Tanner CM, et al. Parkinson disease. *Nature Reviews. Disease Primers* 2017;3:17013.
46. Balestrino R, Martinez-Martin P. Neuropsychiatric symptoms, behavioural disorders, and quality of life in Parkinson's disease. *Journal of the Neurological Sciences* 2017;373:173–8.
47. Ffytche DH, Creese B, Politis M, et al. The psychosis spectrum in Parkinson disease. *Nature Reviews. Neurology* 2017;13(2):81–95.
48. Nakum S, Cavanna AE. The prevalence and clinical characteristics of hypersexuality in patients with Parkinson's disease following dopaminergic therapy: a systematic literature review. *Parkinsonism & Related Disorders* 2016;25:10–6.
49. Balarajah S, Cavanna AE. The pathophysiology of impulse control disorders in Parkinson disease. *Behavioural Neurology* 2013;26 (4):237–44.
50. Martino D, Madhusudan N, Zis P, et al. An introduction to the clinical phenomenology of Tourette syndrome. *International Review of Neurobiology* 2013;112:1–33.
51. Stern JS. Tourette's syndrome and its borderland. *Practical Neurology* 2018;18 (4):262–70.
52. Eddy CM, Cavanna AE. Premonitory urges in adults with complicated and uncomplicated Tourette syndrome.

Behavior Modification 2014;38 (2):264–75.

53. Cavanna AE. Gilles de la Tourette syndrome as a paradigmatic neuropsychiatric disorder. *CNS Spectrums* 2018;23(3):213–8.
54. Evans J, Seri S, Cavanna AE. The effects of Gilles de la Tourette syndrome and other chronic tic disorders on quality of life across the lifespan: a systematic review. *European Child & Adolescent Psychiatry* 2016;25(9): 939–48.
55. Cavanna AE. *Pharmacological Treatment of Tics*. Cambridge: Cambridge University Press; 2020.
56. Cavanna AE, Eddy CM, Mitchell R, et al. An approach to deep brain stimulation for severe treatment-refractory Tourette syndrome: the UK perspective. *British Journal of Neurosurgery* 2011;25(1):38–44.
57. Pringsheim T, Wiltshire K, Day L, et al. The incidence and prevalence of Huntington's disease: a systematic review and meta-analysis. *Movement Disorders* 2012;27(9):1083–91.
58. Teixeira AL, de Souza LC, Rocha NP. Revisiting the neuropsychiatry of Huntington's disease. *Dementia & Neuropsychologia* 2016;10(4):261–6.
59. Albanese A, Bhatia K, Bressman SB, et al. Phenomenology and classification of dystonia: a consensus update. *Movement Disorders* 2013;28(7):863–73.
60. Zurowski M, McDonald WM, Fox S, et al. Psychiatric comorbidities in dystonia: emerging concepts. *Movement Disorders* 2013;28(7):914–20.
61. Cleymaet S, Nagayoshi K, Gettings E, et al. A review and update on the diagnosis and treatment of neuropsychiatric Wilson disease. *Expert Review of Neurotherapeutics* 2019;19 (11):1117–26.
62. Punukollu M, Mushet N, Linney M, et al. Neuropsychiatric manifestations of Sydenham's chorea: a systematic review. *Developmental Medicine and Child Neurology* 2016;58(1):16–28.
63. Medeiros GC, Smith FA, Trivedi MH, et al. Depressive disorders in HIV/AIDS: a clinically focused narrative review. *Harvard Reviews of Psychiatry* 2020;28(3):146–58.
64. Rubin LH, Maki PM. HIV, depression, and cognitive impairment in the era of effective antiretroviral therapy. *Current HIV/AIDS Reports* 2019;16(1):82–95.
65. Saylor D, Dickens AM, Sacktor N, et al. HIV-associated neurocognitive disorder – pathogenesis and prospects for treatment. *Nature Reviews. Neurology* 2016;12(4):234–48.
66. Nightingale S, Winston A. Measuring and managing cognitive impairment in HIV. *AIDS* 2017;31(Suppl 2): 165–72.
67. Gatchel J, Legesse B, Tayeb S, et al. Neurosyphilis in psychiatric practice: a case-based discussion of clinical evaluation and diagnosis. *General Hospital Psychiatry* 2015;37(5):459–63.
68. Friedrich F, Aigner M, Fearns N, et al. Psychosis in neurosyphilis: clinical aspects and implications. *Psychopathology* 2014;47(1):3–9.
69. Mai NT, Thwaites GE. Recent advances in the diagnosis and management of tuberculous meningitis. *Current Opinion in Infectious Diseases* 2017;30 (1):123–8.
70. Więdłocha M, Marcinowicz P, Stańczykiewicz B. Psychiatric aspects of herpes simplex encephalitis, tick-borne encephalitis and herpes zoster encephalitis among immunocompetent patients. *Advances in Clinical and Experimental Medicine* 2015;24 (2):361–71.
71. Munjal S, Ferrando SJ, Freyberg Z. Neuropsychiatric aspects of infectious diseases: an update. *Critical Care Clinics* 2017;33(3):681–712.
72. Koster MP, Garro A. Unraveling diagnostic uncertainty surrounding lyme disease in children with neuropsychiatric illness. *Child and Adolescent Psychiatry Clinics of North America* 2018;27(1):27–36.
73. Marrie RA, Reingold S, Cohen J, et al. The incidence and prevalence of psychiatric disorders in multiple sclerosis: a systematic review. *Multiple Sclerosis* 2015;21(3):305–17.
74. Vattakatuchery JJ, Rickards H, Cavanna AE. Pathogenic mechanisms of depression in multiple sclerosis. *Journal of Neuropsychiatry and Clinical Neurosciences* 2011;23(3):261–76.
75. Unterman A, Nolte JE, Boaz M, et al. Neuropsychiatric syndromes in systemic lupus erythematosus: a meta-analysis. *Seminars in Arthritis and Rheumatism* 2011;41(1):1–11.
76. Herken J, Pruss H. Red flags: clinical signs for identifying autoimmune encephalitis in psychiatric patients. *Frontiers in Psychiatry* 2017;8:25.
77. Al-Diwani A, Handel A, Townsend L, et al. The psychopathology of NMDAR-antibody encephalitis in adults: a systematic review and phenotypic analysis of individual patient data. *Lancet Psychiatry* 2019;6(3):235–46.
78. Young J, Murthy L, Westby M, et al. Diagnosis, prevention, and management of delirium: summary of NICE guidance. *BMJ* 2010;341:3704.
79. Maldonado JR. Neuropathogenesis of delirium: review of current etiologic theories and common pathways. *American Journal of Geriatric Psychiatry* 2013;21(12):1190–222.
80. Hshieh TT, Yue J, Oh E, et al. Effectiveness of multicomponent nonpharmacological delirium interventions: a meta-analysis. *JAMA Internal Medicine* 2015;175(4):512–20.
81. Meagher DJ, McLoughlin L, Leonard M, et al. What do we really know about the treatment of delirium with antipsychotics? Ten key issues for delirium pharmacotherapy. *American Journal of Geriatric Psychiatry* 2013;21 (12):1223–38.
82. Sachdev PS, Blacker D, Blazer DG, et al. Classifying neurocognitive disorders: the DSM-5 approach. *Nature Reviews. Neurology* 2014;10(11):634–42.
83. Lonie JA, Tierney KM, Ebmeier KP. Screening for mild cognitive impairment: a systematic review. *International Journal of Geriatric Psychiatry* 2009;24(9):902–15.
84. McKhann GM, Knopman DS, Chertkow H, et al. The diagnosis of dementia due to Alzheimer's disease: recommendations from the National Institute on Aging – Alzheimer's Association workgroups on diagnostic guidelines for Alzheimer's disease. *Alzheimers & Dementia* 2011;7 (3):263–9.
85. Dubois B, Feldman HH, Jacova C, et al. Advancing research diagnostic criteria for Alzheimer's disease: the IWG- 2 criteria. *Lancet. Neurology* 2014;13 (6):614–29.
86. Mayo MC, Bordelon Y. Dementia with Lewy bodies. *Seminars in Neurology* 2014;34(2):182–8.
87. Burrell JR, Hodges JR, Rowe JB. Cognition in corticobasal syndrome and progressive supranuclear palsy: a

review. *Movement Disorders* 2014;29 (5):684–93.

88. Mioshi E, Hsieh S, Savage S, et al. Clinical staging and disease progression in frontotemporal dementia. *Neurology* 2010;74(20):1591–7.
89. Burrell JR, Halliday GM, Kril JJ, et al. The frontotemporal dementia - motor neuron disease continuum. *Lancet* 2016;388(10047):919–31.
90. Zahr NM, Kaufman KL, Harper CG. Clinical and pathological features of alcohol related brain damage. *Nature Reviews. Neurology* 2011;7(5):284–94.
91. Isenberg-Grzeda E, Kutner HE, Nicholson SE. Wernicke-Korsakoff syndrome: under-recognised and under treated. *Psychosomatics* 2012;53 (6):507–16.
92. Jordaan GP, Emsley R. Alcohol-induced psychotic disorder: a review. *Metabolic Brain Disease* 2014;29(2):231–43.
93. Svanberg J, Evans JJ. Neuropsychological rehabilitation in alcohol-related brain damage: a systematic review. *Alcohol and Alcoholism* 2013;48(6):704–11.
94. Riper H, Andersson G, Hunter SB, et al. Treatment of comorbid alcohol use disorders and depression with cognitive-behavioural therapy and motivational interviewing: a meta-analysis. *Addiction* 2014;109 (3):394–406.
95. Hunt SA, Kay-Lambkin FJ, Baker AL, et al. Systematic review of neurocognition in people with co-occurring alcohol misuse and depression. *Journal of Affective Disorders* 2015;179:51–64.
96. Tang Y, Martin NL, Cotes RO. Cocaine-induced psychotic disorders: presentation, mechanism, and management. *Journal of Dual Diagnosis* 2014;10(2):98–105.
97. Fink M, Taylor MA. The catatonia syndrome. *Archives of General Psychiatry* 2009;66(11):1173–7.
98. Roncero C, Daigre C, Grau-López L, et al. Cocaine-induced psychosis and impulsivity in cocaine-dependent patients. *Journal of Addictive Diseases* 2013;32(3):263–73.
99. Gage SH, Hickman M, Zammit S. Association between cannabis and psychosis: epidemiologic evidence. *Biological Psychiatry* 2016;79(7): 549–56.
100. van Amsterdam J, Brunt T, van den Brink W. The adverse health effects of synthetic cannabinoids with emphasis on psychosis-like effects. *Journal of Psychopharmacology* 2015;29(3):254–63.
101. Gibbs M, Winsper C, Marwaha S, et al. Cannabis use and mania symptoms: a systematic review and meta- analysis. *Journal of Affective Disorders* 2015;171:39–47.
102. Badiani A, Belin D, Epstein D, et al. Opiate versus psychostimulant addiction: the differences do matter. *Nature Reviews. Neuroscience* 2011;12 (11):685–700.
103. Maremmani AGI, Rovai L, Rugani F, et al. Substance abuse and psychosis: the strange case of opioids. *European Reviews for Medical and Pharmacological Sciences* 2014;18 (3):287–302.
104. Eddy CM, Rickards HE, Cavanna AE. The cognitive impact of antiepileptic drugs. *Therapeutic Advances in Neurological Disorders* 2011;4 (6):385–407.
105. Piedad J, Rickards H, Besag FM, et al. Beneficial and adverse psychotropic effects of antiepileptic drugs in patients with epilepsy: a summary of prevalence, underlying mechanisms and data limitations. *CNS Drugs* 2012;26 (4):319–35.
106. Gunnell D, Knipe D, Chang SS, et al. Prevention of suicide with regulations aimed at restricting access to highly hazardous pesticides: a systematic review of the international evidence. *Lancet. Global Health* 2017;5(10): e1026–37.
107. Albano GD, Malta G, La Spina C, et al. Toxicological findings of self-poisoning suicidal deaths: a systematic review by countries. *Toxics* 2022;10(11):654.
108. Muelly ER, Moore GJ, Bunce SC, et al. Biochemical correlates of neuropsychiatric illness in maple syrup urine disease. *Journal of Clinical Investigation* 2013;123(4):1809–20.
109. Ritchie M, Yeap BB. Thyroid hormone: influences on mood and cognition in adults. *Maturitas* 2015;81(2):266–75.
110. Samuels MH. Psychiatric and cognitive manifestations of hypothyroidism. *Current Opinion in Endocrinology, Diabetes, and Obesity* 2014;21 (5):377–83.
111. Starkman MN. Neuropsychiatric findings in Cushing syndrome and exogenous glucocorticoid administration. *Endocrinology and Metabolism Clinics of North America* 2013;42(3):477–88.
112. Anderson NE, Chung K, Willoughby E, et al. Neurological manifestations of phaeochromocytomas and secretory paragangliomas: a reappraisal. *Journal of Neurology, Neurosurgery, and Psychiatry* 2013;84(4):452–7.
113. Anglin RE, Garside SL, Tarnopolsky MA, et al. The psychiatric manifestations of mitochondrial disorders: a case and review of the literature. *Journal of Clinical Psychiatry* 2012;73(4):506–12.
114. Urano F. Wolfram syndrome: diagnosis, management, and treatment. *Current Diabetes Reports* 2016;16(1):6.
115. Abdou E, Hazell AS. Thiamine deficiency: an update of pathophysiologic mechanisms and future therapeutic considerations. *Neurochemical Research* 2015;40 (2):353–61.
116. Cavanna AE, Williams AC. Neuropsychiatric symptoms in an early description of pellagra. *Journal of Neuropsychiatry and Clinical Neurosciences* 2010;22(4):451.e39.
117. Ghavanini AA, Kimpinski K. Revisiting the evidence for neuropathy caused by pyridoxine deficiency and excess. *Journal of Clinical Neuromuscular Disease* 2014;16(1):25–31.
118. Ramaekers V, Sequeira JM, Quadros EV. Clinical recognition and aspects of the cerebral folate deficiency syndromes. *Clinical Chemistry and Laboratory Medicine* 2013;51 (3):497–511.
119. Bremner JD, Shearer KD, McCaffery PJ. Retinoic acid and affective disorders: the evidence for an association. *Journal of Clinical Psychiatry* 2012;73(1):37–50.
120. Wright AD, Stevens E, Ali M, et al. The neuropsychiatry of scurvy. *Psychosomatics* 2014;55(2):179–85.
121. Noble M, Healey CS, McDougal LD-Chukwumah, et al. Old disease, new look? A first report of parkinsonism due to scurvy, and of refeeding-induced worsening of scurvy. *Psychosomatics* 2013;54(3):277–83.
122. Zimmermann MB. The effects of iodine deficiency in pregnancy and infancy. *Paediatric and Perinatal Epidemiology* 2012;26(Suppl 1):108–17.

Further Reading

Agrawal N, Faruqui R, Bodani M (eds). *Oxford Textbook of Neuropsychiatry*. Oxford: Oxford University Press; 2020.

Arciniegas DB, Yudofsky SC, Hales RE (eds). *The American Psychiatric Association Publishing Textbook of Neuropsychiatry and Clinical Neurosciences*. 6th ed. Washington, DC: American Psychiatric Association Publishing; 2018.

Cavanna AE. *Motion and Emotion: The Neuropsychiatry of Movement Disorders and Epilepsy*. New York: Springer; 2018.

David A, Fleminger S, Kopelman M, et al. *Lishman's Organic Psychiatry: A Textbook of Neuropsychiatry*. 4th ed. Hoboken, NJ: Wiley; 2009.

Trimble MR, George M. *Biological Psychiatry*. 3rd ed. Hoboken, NJ: Wiley; 2010.

Chapter 9

Autism

Ian A. Davidson, Mary Doherty and Clair Haydon

Neurodevelopmental conditions are distinct from mental illness. Traditionally framed in terms of deficit and impairment, a recent shift towards a neurodiversity-affirmative perspective is challenging the approach to assessment, diagnosis and management. Neurodiversity is a term publicised by Australian sociologist Judy Singer in 1998. It was inspired by the concept of biodiversity and relates to diversity in neurocognitive functioning. As we recognise that biodiversity is essential for a healthy ecosystem and a healthy planet, similarly there is increasing recognition that neurodiversity is beneficial for humanity.

The neurodiversity paradigm suggests that individual variations in neurocognitive functioning are part of the natural range of human diversity and that neurodevelopmental conditions are neurological differences rather than inherently pathological. Reframing the traditional deficit focus and tragedy narrative around neurodevelopmental conditions – and in autism in particular – towards a neurodiversity-affirmative approach may have particular benefits in terms of mental health.

One of the challenges in talking about neurodevelopmental conditions is the sheer range and variety of things that fall under that broad heading. This helps explain the wide variety of prevalence ranges cited, as it depends on what is included. Technically, it is any condition arising from differences in neurodevelopment, so it can include a wide range of speech and communication, motor and sensory differences – for example, visual things such as astigmatism clearly fall within the term as do multiple hearing, motor and coordination conditions from rare to relatively common such as dyslexia or congenital epilepsy. This is why it is often considered as too broad and too diverse to be clinically useful, but still it persists. DSM-5 and ICD-11 both seek to restrict the conditions defined within it, but both have a catch-all for 'other neurodevelopmental disorders'. ICD-11 and DSM-5 largely exclude sensory conditions (such as those linked with sight or hearing) and epilepsy from their neurodevelopmental categories but do include certain types of motor and communication disorders. The three most common in both classifications are intellectual/learning disability, ADHD and autism.

These are the ones most likely to be encountered by general psychiatrists. Although two or more neurodevelopmental conditions can occur in one person, they are very different, and so it is important that these are understood as separate conditions. If they do co-occur, then the interactions will be individual as for any other co-occurring conditions. For these reasons, there are separate chapters in this book on ADHD and Autism. (See also *Seminars in the Psychiatry of Intellectual Disability.*)

There is increasing awareness of neurodiversity in medicine more generally. This includes growing awareness of the needs of neurodivergent health care practitioners. Peer support and advocacy groups such as Autistic Doctors International (ADI) and The Association for Neurodivergent Doctors (AND) are growing rapidly, and they report a high proportion of psychiatrists among their members.

Introduction

We use the term 'autism' as an all-encompassing term as in the Autism Act 2009, and 'autistic people' is a term preferred by the autistic community in the United Kingdom.[1]

Autism is a neurodevelopmental condition, present from birth and lifelong. It is characterised by differences in reciprocal social interaction and communication, intense focal interests, repetitive movements and sensory sensitivities. There are no traits or sensitivities that are unique to autistic people, but the combination of features and the degree to which they occur is what characterises the condition. There is ongoing debate about whether autism is a disorder, a condition or a naturally occurring difference. Diagnostic manuals (ICD and DSM) use impairment-based language and class autism as a disorder.

Autism is not a mental illness or learning disability. Rather, it is a difference where traits and sensitivities can have positive and negative impacts on a person's life, and these impacts can change at different times or in different circumstances. Historically, clinical perspectives have focused on presenting difficulties and miss the positives. Autistic people experience the world differently and thus may identify solutions to problems that are not obvious to others and may show significant creativity, and their sensory sensitivities may enable them to notice changes in the environment that others might not. Autistic people are often methodical, consistent, loyal and reliable, and they can be excellent at researching topics of interest. They often have a strong sense of justice, including behaving honestly and expecting honesty from others, and they will advocate for those suffering injustice. They can be determined, tenacious and resilient. These traits are attributes that are beneficial in a variety of situations. Being different and having marked autistic traits and sensitivities can also lead to problems, disadvantages and needs, including all types of mental disorder. We recommend using the strengths, needs and aspirations approach to autism as to health assessments in general.

The ability to recognise autism is important because, in all branches of psychiatry, many patients, family members and colleagues of all disciplines will be autistic. The key clinical question for any type of clinical assessment is 'why this particular person is this particular way at this particular time'. Autism will be part of defining that individual (particular person), will modify how they present with physical and mental disorders (particular way) and may impact how they experience life circumstances (particular time). It is vital to recognise and understand autism in order to make reasonable adjustments to your assessment and treatment plan when treating co-occurring disorder in an autistic person.

Autistic people are more likely to experience adverse life events that directly contribute to greater risks of ill health, and they also currently face additional barriers to accessing health care compared to non-autistic people. This contributes to higher rates of co-occurring disorders and disabilities and reduction of life expectancy. Much of this is avoidable or at least can be mitigated by autism-informed services. The Parliamentary Post 2020 gives a good summary with key references on sociodemographic issues around autism.[2] In this chapter, we focus on the practical implications of recent advances in autism knowledge applicable to general psychiatrists.

Development of Autism as a Term of Classification

The concept of autism has evolved significantly. Early descriptions are usually attributed to Kanner and Asperger in the 1940s, although the syndrome was accurately described by Russian psychiatrist Sukhareva over 20 years earlier.[3] The contribution of Austrian psychiatrist George Frankl has been largely over-looked, but the fact that he worked with both Asperger in Vienna and Kanner in Baltimore casts doubt on the common assumption that the descriptions by Kanner and Asperger were unrelated and co-incidental. The fascinating history of autism is detailed in *NeuroTribes* (see further reading) and subsequent papers.[4-6]

Written by award-winning science journalist Steve Silberman, *NeuroTribes* is highly recommended reading for any clinician with an interest in autism. It is difficult to understand the contemporary issues and controversies that divide the autism community without an understanding of the history of the condition and the dehumanisation of autistic people in the past. Through painstaking research, Silberman chronicles the human stories behind the development of the concept of autism, from its earliest descriptions, through the eugenics programmes of Nazi Germany to the rise of behaviourism and the emergence of the autistic community.

The classic descriptions by Kanner and Asperger focused almost exclusively on boys, whereas Sukereva described a series of apparently autistic girls. Kanner described what is commonly referred to as 'classic autism', which he considered a rare condition. Initially thought to be a form of childhood schizophrenia, it was later recognised as a developmental condition and added as a new diagnostic category to DSM-III in 1980.

Asperger described a much wider range of presentations, including those without speech delay, and 'Asperger Syndrome' was added to ICD-10 in 1992 and DSM-IV in 1994, following introduction of his work to the English-speaking world by Lorna Wing in the 1980s. Differentiation between subgroups listed in DSM-IV were found to be inconsistent, and all prior subgroups were subsumed into the single category of 'autism spectrum disorder' in DSM-5 (2013). Although controversial at the time, this has been echoed in the WHO ICD-11. Research into the sub-division of the autistic spectrum or stratification biomarkers has not yielded robust groupings. Commonly used 'functioning labels' are unhelpful, so three levels of support needs were introduced in DSM-5. While, on a superficial level, the challenges associated with autism may appear to be bimodal, the reality is much more complex and fluctuant. Functioning labels have the effect of obscuring the support needs of those deemed 'high functioning' and underestimating the capabilities of others. Characterising individual strengths and specifying support needs is both more useful and more respectful.

Asperger was the first to consider the condition a manifestation of 'an extreme variant of male intelligence', a theory subsequently developed by psychologist Simon Baron Cohen. The characterisation of autism as the 'extreme male brain' has now largely been abandoned, but it excluded autistic women from diagnostic and support services for decades.

Even more problematic is the suggestion that autistic people lack empathy. This is probably the most damaging misconception of all, as the capacity for empathy is critical for human beings. The reality is that autistic people do have empathy, although how they respond to or display empathy is likely to be unconventional.

Theory of mind is the ability to infer mental states in other people, and the lack of theory of mind is another misconception about autistic people. This has arisen from the use of mentalising tests in young children, such as the 'Sally-Anne' test. Autistic children commonly 'fail' this test and are therefore deemed to lack theory of mind. The reality is that this ability may develop later for autistic than non-autistic children, and perspective taking is a skill that can be learned, even though it may remain a cognitive skill rather than intuitive for some.

Weak central coherence is the tendency to concentrate on constituent parts rather the whole. As this autistic tendency is a minority skill, it is traditionally framed as a deficit, whereas adopting a strengths-based approach highlights that strong pattern recognition and attention to detail is a vital skill in many contexts.

Theories of autism developed by autistic scholars and embraced by the autistic community such as the double empathy problem[7] and monotropism[8] have in recent years gained more prominence but are not well-known in general psychiatric practice.

The double empathy problem highlights the difficulty that non-autistic people have in understanding and empathising with autistic people, highlighting that apparent challenges are mutual, in contrast to the traditional view of the communication or empathy deficit being situated in the autistic person. Monotropism refers to a cognitive pattern common to autistic people, where attention tends towards a singular focus, which leads to challenges switching attention but allows autistic people to delve deeply into areas of special interest.

Research is interrogating the double empathy concept and determining that autistic peer-to-peer communication may be more effective than previously thought.[9] Non-autistic people tend to form negative impressions of autistic people, leading to social exclusion[10] and contributing to poor mental health outcomes. Therefore, efforts to improve autism understanding will reduce stigma and improve outcomes for autistic people. The growing adult autistic community, which is active both online and offline, is connecting autistic people from all walks of life, including autistic professionals and those who are non-speaking and have significant support needs. The contributions of autistic researchers are transforming the field of autism research.[11]

The concept of neurodiversity has transformed thinking around autism since the term was coined by Judy Singer in 1998. Recognising natural variability in neurocognitive functioning challenges the traditional deficit-based pathology paradigm and allows a focus on autistic strengths as well as challenges. Since co-occurring mental illness is a common issue for autistic people, primary prevention may be improved by avoiding the development of negative and deficit-focused self-perception. Encouraging autism acceptance and understanding among health and education professionals will promote the development of the supports required for families to thrive. This is relevant no matter what the level of communication difficulty or support need. Outcomes may be improved by approaches that work with the autistic person's natural strengths and communication style, rather than attempting to extinguish natural autistic behaviours and communication styles in an attempt to make an autistic person fit in or appear indistinguishable from peers.

Diagnostic Classification Systems (ICD, DSM, SNOMED)

Currently, in the UK, the default mode for diagnostic coding built into electronic patient records and reporting systems is ICD-10. Autism falls within the F84.x category. This chapter is not the place to discuss the merits of classification systems but, in relation to autism, both DSM-5 and ICD-11 have essentially removed the sub-categories as they were not robust or clinically useful, and both are now more explicit about the need to consider and list any co-occurring disorders (physical and mental disorders or learning disability). They have also both removed the specification that symptoms must be evident by age three from the criteria. DSM-5 follows DSM tradition in being more explicit about combinations of criteria needed to make a diagnosis, whilst ICD-11 follows ICD tradition of being more about a broad syndromal approach. Both are impairment-based but DSM more so than ICD, and DSM has categories of severity again based on more explicit criteria. It is not clear that the DSM severity criteria are useful in clinical practice as, in practice, people's needs will fluctuate over time and even within those broad categories. In the NHS, it is unclear if ICD-11 will directly replace ICD-10 in coding or whether it will be incorporated into SNOMED coding. As noted, there is considerable debate as to whether autism brings with it impairments or if those impairments are all due to co-occurring disorders or living in societies not set up for autistic people. We think it is a mixture of all of that. There is no one who is truly neurotypical just like no one is truly average in all domains, so everyone has strengths and weaknesses, and under differing circumstances, these can create benefits or impairments to a greater or lesser degree.

Aetiology

Autism is present from birth, so the aetiology of autism occurs prior to birth. Whilst there is a caveat that the majority of autistic people have not yet been identified, there is little dispute that it has high heritability (over 80 per cent) and that rates in close family members are higher than for general population. Despite that, it is (in common with most disorders) classed as multifactorial. Apart from a few specific and uncommon single genetic conditions that seem to have much higher rates of autistic traits, extensive genetic studies indicate that gene influence is polygenetic. There are weak correlations with issues in pregnancy and difficult births and with higher paternal age. In practical terms at the clinical level, all of this means that if there is an autistic person, there is a higher likelihood of other autistic people being in the family. It currently adds no clinical value, and obviously, if people have got specific genetic conditions that show higher rates of autistic traits, then management will be for that genetic condition. Otherwise, there are no management implications from current aetiological information. As noted, we do not know whether or not this will change as more autistic people are identified.

Prevalence

No single autistic trait or sensitivity is unique to autistic people as they are all common human traits. It is the frequency and magnitude of these traits that leads to an autism diagnosis. Autism is therefore a variant on a gradient rather than a distinct category, like height or blood pressure.

Until the late 1990s, the stereotype of autism being almost exclusively in boys with learning disability prevailed. Therefore, autism was not considered for others, leading to inaccurate prevalence rates.

Across the world, increasing research and, in particular, policy changes have led to more people being assessed for autism. One example is the Autism Act 2009, which committed the government to developing and publishing an autism strategy for England. Amongst other things, this committed public bodies to ensure a range of things including reasonable adjustments for autistic people but also to ensure that there was an autism diagnostic pathway in all areas of England. This, in turn, has led to a major surge in numbers of autistic people being diagnosed. The current version of the strategy is www.gov.uk/government/publications/national-strategy-for-autistic-children-young-people-and-adults-2021-to-2026.

Whilst other UK jurisdictions have differing rules and policies, similar changes have occurred across the whole UK. This is not limited to the UK, as similar things have happened across the world even though, again, policies and rules will vary. This has led to the realisation that, before 2010, most autistic people identified were from a subset who presented usually with other significant co-occurring conditions in childhood (intellectual/learning disability and ADHD being the most common), which in turn meant a number of theories about the nature and impact of autism were skewed by the skewed sample. Recent research (drawing on samples collected after 2010) is significantly changing the understanding of autism.

Currently in the UK, a prevalence rate of 1.1% is accepted as a minimum. Most autistic adults are still undiagnosed, but numbers have risen significantly recently. Reported prevalence rates in school-age children are higher (1.6% and above), although not all have had a formal assessment. If these school-based estimates are confirmed in diagnostic assessments, overall prevalence rates will increase. Evidence strongly suggests that the number of autistic people is not rising but that increasing numbers are now being identified. Increasing population density and cultural change will contribute to autistic people becoming more visible as they typically find enforced socialisation and rapid culturally enforced changes more stressful than the general population. Historically, it is likely that groups such as those diagnosed with simple schizophrenia or schizoid personality included people who were autistic. Currently, this occurs with personality disorder diagnoses, especially emotionally unstable personality disorder. Many people identified as 'treatment resistant' may be unrecognised as autistic, with lack of reasonable adjustments contributing to presentation and clinical course.

The percentage of autistic people with a learning disability has steadily fallen as diagnostic assessments became more widely available. Current estimates are that around 20% have learning disability, with some studies in Scotland and England indicating 15–18%. The percentage of males has fallen from over 90% to below 75% (and dropping) over 20 years.

The Recognition of Autistic People in Practice

As autism is a spectrum condition, every autistic person will present differently, and most won't have a diagnosis. It is important to recognise autistic traits, to consider autism in your clinical formulation where necessary and to adapt interactions and interventions. Table 9.1 illustrates some indicators of autism. As mental health symptoms may affect communication and social interaction, ascertaining what aspects of the presentation has changed and what traits may be lifelong – therefore, indicative of autism – is helpful.

Autism Diagnostic Assessments

Diagnostic services vary significantly across the UK, including having different access times, inclusion and exclusion criteria, tools used to assess and team professional make-up (e.g. psychiatrists, psychologists, occupational therapists, speech and language therapists, nurses). The National Institute of Health and Social Care Excellence (NICE) guidance CG142 indicates that a comprehensive autism diagnostic assessment should be team-based (i.e. have multi-professional input), assessors should be trained and competent and, wherever possible, should involve a family member, partner or other supporter to help to ascertain the person's developmental history and current and past behaviours.

The assessment should endeavour to identify core autistic traits and ascertain whether these are lifelong or can be explained by other life experiences or co-occurring conditions. It is important that the assessment report provides a formulation that clearly identifies the positive and negative impacts of the person's autistic traits on their life and functioning, the potential impacts of autistic traits in the future, any co-occurring conditions, sensory sensitivities and the person's strengths, needs and aspirations. In identifying the person's specific autistic traits and the impacts of these, this enables the identification of reasonable adjustments or strategies for overcoming or minimising the negative impacts of traits in order to support the person's optimum functioning and well being. Recording these explicitly in the report means they will be shared with the GP and the person being assessed, who may use them to access reasonable adjustments in other settings such as education or employment.

As adult autism diagnostic services in the UK can be limited in what can be offered after a diagnostic assessment, the assessment process should build in opportunities for the person being assessed (and their supporter where appropriate) to check that the assessment report is accurate and that a reasonable summary of the information provided and to correct or clarify information within the report before it is finalised. Best practice would also be to offer at least one post-diagnostic assessment review, to discuss the report, what the

Table 9.1 Autistic traits

Communication and social interaction differences	• Unconventional ways of integrating verbal and non-verbal communication (often appears 'odd' to a non-autistic person) • The use of social scripts in conversations that may appear more superficial and not used conventionally or well timed • Not demonstrating conventional patterns of listening • A longer time to process information • Repeated questions • Answers to questions may be unconventional – either too brief or too lengthy and detailed • Difficulty identifying or describing their own specific emotions, feelings or physical sensations • Literal interpretation of language • Missing common social cues or not recognising the conventional etiquette in a situation • Not picking up on subtle non-verbal cues from others • Lack of conventional eye contact, facial expression, intonation or gesture • Precise use of language • Dislike of small talk and less likely to initiate or reciprocate in a two-way conversation so you can end up feeling that you are interrogating them • Less likely to bring in social interest questions or comments • More likely to have a limited or no support network
Preferences for predictability, routine, repetition	• More likely to experience higher anxiety with regards to uncertainty, change, going into new situations and meeting new people • Needing extra details and time to plan and prepare • More rule-based so they typically expect things to happen as per the plan or the instructions set out • More likely to focus on intense or narrow interests • Repetitive behaviours including repetitive body movements, different body posture. These can be due to stimming (self-stimulating behaviours that help reduce stress and can look like elaborate fidgeting)
Sensory differences	• Hypersensitivity in any sensory modality can increase stress/distress whether caused from lighting, noise, touch, temperature, inactivity, smell and taste • May experience difficulties recognising hunger, thirst or the need to go to the toilet until it is urgent • More likely to experience pain differently (e.g. an oversensitivity or undersensitivity to pain)
Executive functioning issues	• Whilst most autistic people have generally good cognitive functioning, they may find it more difficult to initiate, sequence or plan tasks especially when stressed or faced with too many choices • They can get overstressed leading to difficulties with working memory, attention or organising tasks and may need a few minutes to compose themselves and reset

opinion means for them and what may be helpful for them in managing their future.

There are no agreed gold standard formal autism diagnostic assessments; the evidence and the information required to make a diagnostic decision can be obtained through interview and observation. However, many clinicians benefit from a tool or framework to complete the autism diagnosis process, and the following are frequently used to inform adult autism diagnostic assessments:

- **Royal College of Psychiatrists Diagnostic Interview Guide for the Assessment of Adults with Autism Spectrum Disorder** is a guide with prompts and questions for each diagnostic domain. The guide is designed to help clinicians to gather the relevant information, organise it and then come to a clinical judgement. No specific training is required to use this tool (autismwales.org/wp-content/uploads/2020/09/RC-Psych_Diagnostic-Interview-Guide-for-the-Assessment-of-Adults-with-ASD.pdf).
- **The Autism Diagnostic Observation Schedule (ADOS)** is a standardised assessment to specifically observe social interaction, communication, play and imaginative use of materials. The observational schedule consists of four 30-minute modules, each designed to be administered to different individuals according to their level of expressive language, and requires the person to complete set tasks with standardised instructions and prompts that are then scored. This assessment is usually completed in conjunction with a developmental history and informant information. Assessors require training to administer and score the assessment reliably, and the scores are only to be used to inform clinical judgement on whether someone may be autistic, as the evidence shows that it may be difficult to differentiate social and communication differences that may be attributable to autistic traits or co-occurring mental illness such as psychosis. The ADOS is most commonly used with children and young people or people with intellectual disabilities.
- **The Autism Diagnostic Interview-Revised (ADI-R)** is a standardised tool often used in conjunction with the ADOS to structure an interview with an informant (ideally a parent). Assessors are trained to use the tool, which is scored, and it asks questions relating to specific autistic traits at key developmental stages.
- **The Diagnostic Interview for Social and Communication Disorders (DISCO)** is a semi-structured interview designed to find out about the person's development, behaviour and skills from throughout their life. It is used with the person and should be used in conjunction with informant information, observations and other relevant information. Training is required to use the tool.

- **The Autism Quotient-10 items (AQ10)** is not generally used as part of a diagnostic assessment but is often used as a screening tool as to whether someone may have autistic traits to warrant a further specialist diagnostic assessment. The tool contains 10 statements, and the person is asked to consider whether they definitely agree, slightly agree, slightly disagree or definitely disagree. These items are then scored, and if the person scores 6 out of 10 or above, a more specialist assessment is indicated. As it is a self-assessment, no training is required. Some services include the AQ10 score of 6 or above as part of their eligibility criteria, although the evidence is unclear as to whether this is a reliable measure for predicting formal diagnosis, and where this criteria is strict, autistic people may be excluded from the diagnostic process.

Co-occurring Conditions

When assessing whether a person is presenting with autism or a co-occurring disorder, remember it can be both. Autistic people have high rates of co-occurring mental and physical health conditions.[12] These include other neurodevelopmental conditions such as attention-deficit/hyperactivity disorder (ADHD), intellectual disabilities or dyspraxia, and mental health conditions such as anxiety, depression, obsessive-compulsive disorder (OCD) and personality disorders. Co-occurring mental health conditions negatively impact a person's adaptive functioning, quality of life and employment. Higher risks of victimisation, maltreatment and more adverse life events occur.[13]

Increased physical health conditions include hypertension, diabetes, stroke, cardiovascular issues, gastrointestinal issues, epilepsy and Ehlers Danlos Syndrome or hyper-mobility. Such conditions can negatively impact a person's functioning and mental health.

Life expectancy is reduced. Autistic adults without co-occurring intellectual disability have a 16-year mortality gap compared to the non-autistic population, which rises to 30 years for autistic adults with intellectual disabilities. Autistic people are nine times more likely to die by suicide.[14]

Some co-occurring conditions are lifelong such as ADHD or epilepsy, whilst others are intermittent. Anxiety disorder, depression, hallucinations, delusions or suicidal ideation are not part of autism but are due to co-occurring conditions. Social networks are typically smaller, so when in difficulty, autistic people may lack access to informal support and advice, especially if a key trusted person is unavailable due to illness, death or relocation.

One key factor in determining whether a person is autistic or whether their presentation is better explained by another diagnosis is at what age patterns emerged. Autism is lifelong, so the traits and sensitivities emerge at relevant developmental stages. Late onset of such changes – particularly after significant illness – makes autism less likely, as does absence of distinct traits in any of the diagnostic domains of social communication, social interaction and intense focal interests. Sensory sensitivities, whether hypo- or hypersensitivities, tend to develop early.

Some autistic people develop coping strategies that make traits and sensitivities less obvious in non-diagnostic settings. Such 'masking' can be conscious or unconscious. This coping strategy can become overwhelmed due to acute stressors, leading to clinical presentation. A good developmental history shows the traits/sensitivities are long standing. The key point is to identify if a person meets the diagnostic criteria for another condition and to treat that condition, applying reasonable adjustments if the person is also autistic.

Common Co-occurring Mental Disorders and Differential Diagnosis

Whether a person is autistic or not, it is crucial to ask how they are feeling rather than determine this from non-verbal expression alone. Autistic people are much less likely to show conventional changes in non-verbal communication even when very distressed. All psychiatrists know that smiling or laughing is not evidence that someone is mentally well. Neither is it evidence that someone is not acutely suicidal; this applies to autistic people even more than to non-autistic people.

- **Anxiety Disorders:** It is not an inherent part of autism to experience more clinically significant anxiety than non-autistic people. Anxiety is a key part of normal defence mechanisms, but when it becomes excessive or seriously impairs functioning, it becomes a disorder, whether autistic or not. Excessive anxiety leads to lower quality of life, more learned helplessness and greater vulnerability to other health problems, and therefore, it needs appropriate care and treatment. There is a difference between being in your bedroom playing on computers because it is fun and a preferred lifestyle and being in your bedroom because anxiety makes it extremely difficult to leave. Do not assume that restricted lifestyles are a choice; they may be due to anxiety or other mental disorders. Ask why the restrictions are there.
- **Depression:** While common for autistic people, depression is neither inevitable nor an intrinsic feature of autism. There is emerging evidence that autistic people are more vulnerable to burnout, including the mood disorders linked to that.
- **Emotionally Unstable Personality Disorder:** The key aspects are difficulties in the domains of social communication and social interaction. EUPD is an acquired condition, usually secondary to major trauma such as abuse. People with EUPD will typically have had conventional social interaction and social communication until after the impact of trauma, when they develop coping strategies that over time become maladaptive. They don't typically have the focal and repetitive interests nor the

same range and depth of sensory sensitivities as autistic people. The social communication and social interaction difficulties are essentially learned behaviours, therefore amenable to interventions to develop alternatives, whereas autistic traits aren't learned behaviours, and forcing an autistic person to suppress them does harm not good. Autistic people can develop EUPD for all the same reasons as non-autistic people, but it is commonly a misdiagnosis.

- **Psychoses:** Psychosis is not a euphemism for schizophrenia. It is a key part of schizophrenia but can occur in multiple conditions (e.g. depression, epilepsy, delirium, sleep deprivation, sensory over-stimulation). Psychotic symptoms may occur in autistic people for a wide variety of reasons, and correct diagnosis is needed to deliver the correct interventions. Be careful about how symptoms are elicited – for example, 'do you hear voices' will almost certainly lead to an affirmative answer from an autistic person. If they have increased auditory acuity, they will say 'yes' to hearing voices other people don't hear. Use unambiguous language as they will answer a question precisely and usually no more than that. If psychosis is a long-term severe mental illness symptom, then standard treatment is appropriate with reasonable adjustments. Be alert for medication side effects.
- **Obsessive-Compulsive Disorder (OCD):** The key differential between a focal intense autistic trait and OCD is whether the interest/act is one that is interesting/ enjoyable to the person or one that must be done to prevent bad things from happening. Kicking a ball against a wall for hours on end because it is enjoyable and relaxing is an intense focal interest. Feeling a need to kick the ball against the wall to prevent harm to loved ones is a compulsion. Autistic people can develop OCD and, if left inadequately treated, OCD is not just a crippling illness, it can be fatal.
- **Catatonia:** Catatonia is a broad diagnostic category brought about by many underlying conditions. It is essentially a state of extreme hyperarousal. Look for the cause and treat accordingly. It is not a normal part of autism. At the very least, it indicates an extreme anxiety disorder with overwhelmed coping strategies, but it can also indicate other causes of catatonia.
- **Suicidal Feelings and Acts of Self Harm:** If you ask directly about suicidal thoughts, an autistic person will nearly always answer directly and precisely. If they say yes, then they mean it, and rates of suicide are higher than non-autistic population. Always ask when and under what circumstances because hospital admission for suicidal ideation is not beneficial when they are referring to future circumstances. If they are self-harming as a repetitive behaviour or stress-relieving mechanism, they generally can logically and precisely differentiate from suicidal intent. Self-harming without suicidal intent is a coping strategy; therefore, current stressors should be explored along with less harmful ways of addressing needs. Suicidal ideation in an autistic person is an emergency when they say it is likely in current or imminent circumstances.
- **Eating Disorders/Disorders of Eating:** Among those presenting to specialist eating disorder services, 20–30% may be autistic, a prevalence well above the population rate.[15] A complicating factor is that severe malnutrition can lead to non-conventional thinking and communication processes that impacts social communication and social interaction. However, increasing consensus is that this does not appear to account for the apparent excess presentation of autistic people. Everyone has strong preferences for certain foods/ drinks/tastes and strong dislikes for others. In autistic people, these preferences/dislikes can be much more intense and much more narrowly defined with greater reluctance to try new things. If this does not compromise a healthy dietary intake, it is not a disorder. Autistic people can develop classical eating disorders such as anorexia nervosa or bulimia nervosa; diagnostic criteria and aetiology are the same as for non-autistic people. However, autistic people are more likely to present with avoidant restrictive food intake disorder (ARFID). This can be life threatening but requires a different approach, as the core driver is not body image but rigidity about food types/ sensations. It varies from intense/rigid food preferences to an unhealthy restricted diet either in terms of quantity or lack of vital nutrients. People with ARFID may be as emaciated as those with severe anorexia nervosa but typically do not have altered body image. There are multiple factors, including sensory sensitivities, that can give rise to ARFID. The key is a good history, then identifying what will assist the person in gaining and maintaining a healthy diet.
- **Post-Traumatic Stress Disorder (PTSD):** Diagnostic criteria are the same whether autistic or not. As autistic people live in a world not well adapted for them and are more vulnerable to abuse and stigma, it is not surprising that they experience high rates of PTSD. In addition to this, many autistic people tend to be highly reflective. Over-reflection on traumatic experiences increases the risk of developing PTSD.
- **Dementia:** There is currently no robust evidence on whether autistic people have different rates of dementia than non-autistic people. As autistic people typically have smaller social networks and greater difficulty accessing help, they are more vulnerable to presenting with dementia at an advanced stage. In general, autistic people have difficulty adjusting to change, especially change outside their control. This includes difficulty coping with new people coming into their home and any changes of personnel or scheduling. They are more vulnerable to developing increased arousal and stress reactions, leading to presentations that others may see as challenging. Most

older autistic people have not been diagnosed, but identification as autistic with reasonable adjustments for their traits and sensitivities can avoid difficulties for themselves and carers.

- **Pathological Demand Avoidance:** This is neither a specific diagnosis nor is it diagnostic of autism. Pathological demand avoidance is common in people with chronic low self-esteem. It can occur early in life in some autistic people, which indicates low self-esteem from a very young age. People showing pathological demand avoidance patterns do not respond well to praise or reward-based interventions as fear of failure is a bigger driver than hope of success. They will avoid trying anything in case they fail and need help to avoid catastrophising normal experiences of failure, alongside support to learn the 'good enough' concept.

Treatment

Autism is not a condition needing or benefitting from treatment. It is a lifelong difference in thinking and interacting. Autistic people will benefit from help to learn skills and develop coping strategies that work for them, just like non-autistic people. The aim is to help the individual become a successful autistic person, not to try to appear as a non-autistic person. Developing a positive autistic identity is likely to help protect against mental illness.

The use of medication in autism is driven by treating co-occurring problems, not autism itself. It is very important to note that a major issue in the poor outcomes experienced by many autistic people is failure to treat those co-occurring disorders (whether mental or physical). No intervention works well for all human beings, and all can cause harms as well as benefits, but there is no evidence to justify withholding best practice treatments and interventions for co-occurring disorders from autistic people. Failure to treat typically leads to more complications and harms.

There has been justifiable concern that sometimes medications, especially antipsychotic medications, are used without there being an appropriate co-occurring disorder requiring treatment – hence, STOMP (stop the overprescribing of psychotropic medication) – but that should never be a reason for not using psychotropic medication appropriately when indicated for any co-occurring condition, whether these be common mental disorders or severe mental illness.

If a person is in distress and exhibiting distress behaviours, then treat the co-occurring disorder if it is present. The management of distress and behaviours linked to distress (whether the person is directing them at themselves or externally) are essentially as for anyone else. Non-pharmacological de-escalation is the best and safest way forward. For autistic people, this includes reasonable adjustments including giving them space and time to calm down. If medications must be used for rapid tranquillisation as the person is in such a highly aroused state that non-pharmacological interventions are not working and the risks are very high and imminent, then the usual trust/hospital policy should be followed (again making as many reasonable adjustments as the situation permits).

When treating co-occurring disorders, there is no evidence that any standard intervention (pharmacological, psychological, social or a combination) that works for non-autistic people does not provide similar benefits or produces more adverse events for autistic people. Therefore, co-occurring disorders should receive standard treatments. The worst approach is to fail to adequately manage treatable conditions just because the person is autistic. If first-line treatments do not work, then try alternatives as you would for non-autistic people. As with everyone, interventions should be person-centred, taking account of individual needs and preferences. For autistic people, the reasonable adjustments set out in this chapter and references will increase the likelihood of successful interventions.

Increasingly, 'autism hubs' and autism regional teams are being established, which can give advice about diagnosis or the best approach for a particular person. A wide range of other services and peer support can be accessed through the autism hubs where appropriate. The type of service varies within and between countries, and development is inconsistent but ongoing, so enquire what is available locally. In addition to generic advice such as CR228 from the Royal College of Psychiatrists, a range of other training and support is being developed in specialist services such as inclusion health, addiction services or eating disorders.

Challenges to Accessing Health Care

Early identification and intervention for mental health symptoms may prevent a crisis or acute phase of mental illness. However, autistic people face significant barriers to accessing health care. Reasons for autistic people not seeking help include not being understood, inappropriate exclusion from services and limited accessibility of mental health services.

Autistic people can find it difficult to identify symptoms of mental ill health, often due to issues with emotional recognition (e.g. alexithymia – difficulty in describing their emotional state in words)) or interoception, but it can also be due to low self-esteem, as they may feel unworthy of support. Stigma associated with autism and mental health can prevent help-seeking, as can previous negative experiences of accessing mental health services. Autistic people might not know when or how to seek help if this has never been explicitly explained. They often have limited support networks to recognise if they need to access mental health services or assist them to navigate referral pathways. Limited autism knowledge and experience of mental health professionals in dealing with autistic people can lead to misunderstandings and miscommunication. Commonly, autistic people don't feel listened to or taken seriously when communicating their mental distress. Autistic people have described difficulties navigating complex health systems, being bounced from one service to the next or having their primary mental health need overshadowed by autism and then being excluded from mental health care and treatment. In some cases, autistic people with above-average intelligence have been referred to learning disability services due to misconceptions about autism. General accessibility of GP surgeries and mental health services is an issue, especially for those who have difficulty using the phone, have executive functioning issues or sensory sensitivities.

Whilst there has been increased focus and provision of autism training for mental health professionals and general psychiatrists, there remains a lack of understanding of autism and confidence amongst health professionals in knowing how to effectively support an autistic person in their mental health recovery. Training and education for health care staff is the greatest need, in addition to awareness of the sensory environment in health care settings, autistic communication styles and the heterogeneity of people on the autism spectrum. Resources to improve health and health care self-efficacy are required, including information on how to navigate the health care system.

Statutory Responsibilities

In England, the Autism Act gives autism a unique standing over and above the general protections in the Equality Act. In other jurisdictions, the legal and policy frameworks will vary. In general, an autistic person is entitled to reasonable adjustments to mitigate disability or inequality of access to services and treatments.

In England, the reform of the Mental Health Act of 1983 seems likely to confirm that autism is legally neither a mental disorder nor a learning disability, so people should not be admitted to hospital because they are autistic but because they have a co-occurring disorder for which hospital treatment at that point is essential. Critically, they should not be denied admission because they are autistic if a non-autistic person with the same co-occurring disorder would be admitted.

Improving Access to Mental Health Services

Navigating complex care systems and knowing when or how to seek help when feeling unwell or distressed can be very stressful for autistic people, who may not have any social support or may find it difficult to use the phone, go to new or unfamiliar places, meet new people or clearly articulate their needs. It is important to consider how accessible your mental health services are. The NHS accessible information standard is not autism-specific but sets out the expected accessibility standards for NHS England.

- Use the mental health provider's website for health education on specific conditions including when and how to access support
- Allow people to communicate with services and make and attend appointments by different means (e.g. video, email, telephone, text and face to face)
- Provide online information about clinical environments, the booking process and other relevant information that may facilitate attendance, including public transport or parking
- Explicitly state whether a support person is welcome to attend an appointment
- Provide a quiet space to wait
- Offer flexibility with appointment times including asking for preferences and allowing longer appointment times

Reasonable Adjustments

Adjustments that improve accessibility, engagement and outcomes of mental health assessments and intervention must be reasonable to the person (person-centred) and reasonable to the service, such as not significantly impacting the ability to provide services to others.

If someone has an autism diagnosis, they may already have a health passport or alert on their electronic health record that lists their sensory or communication preferences. If autism is suspected but undiagnosed, or no information to inform reasonable adjustments is available, it is necessary to ask key questions about communication and social interaction; preferences for predictability, repetition or routine; sensory sensitivities; and how to respond effectively if they are in distress. Table 9.2 offers examples of reasonable adjustments that may be helpful for autistic people accessing mental health services.

Clinical Formulation and Using a Strengths-Based Approach

Access the autism diagnostic report, if available (especially if recent), to identify the person's traits and their impact on functioning and wellbeing. Ensure these are incorporated into the formulation or care plan alongside the person's strengths and how to build upon these to achieve their aspirations. Record preferences along with any trauma-related information or known triggers. It may be helpful to get information from someone who knows them as they may present differently in distress, in a new setting and with a new person.

Autistic people often have low self-esteem and may 'camouflage' or mask aspects of themselves from others, investing considerable effort daily in monitoring and modifying their behaviour to appear less autistic and conform to non-autistic social conventions.[16] For many autistic people, camouflaging is experienced as an obligation, rather than a choice. It takes significant energy, feels exhausting and can lead to depression and higher rates of suicidality. Camouflaging can also lead to misinterpretation as people can appear more capable or well; therefore, support may not be offered, and it is harder to ascertain if the treatment or intervention is successful. Camouflaging is hard to sustain and can lead to accusations of being 'manipulative' or inauthentic, leaving autistic people feeling misunderstood and that their needs haven't been taken seriously. It is imperative when care planning that specific

Table 9.2 Reasonable adjustments

Reasonable adjustments for communication	Ask which environment will be most comfortable to communicate in (e.g. a quiet space or 1:1 meeting as opposed to a group setting) Provide information in a variety of forms (e.g. written or visual information in addition to verbal communication where required) Encourage use of alternative and augmentative communication devices Check what you have communicated has been understood and check you have interpreted them correctly Ask specific questions and be explicit in your instructions/expectations Use semi-closed questions and options in lists rather than open questions Indicate directly when a question has been adequately answered Allow extra time to process information and make decisions, including extending appointment times Check that any humour, euphemism or metaphor has been interpreted correctly and be aware of the potential literal interpretation of language Avoid making assumptions based on non-verbal communication (e.g. intonation, facial expression, gesture) Understand that an autistic person may struggle to identify or express their emotions and ask for help Offer strategies for allowing an autistic person to communicate when they are distressed (e.g. wristbands or writing notes) and ask how best to respond Space out interactions as autistic people often feel overwhelmed and exhausted following a conversation due to the conscious effort it takes to correctly interpret others and be understood
Reasonable adjustments for sensory sensitivities	Ask if there are any sensory sensitivity or preferences to: Light – if they prefer the light on/off, blinds open/closed Touch – if they like to shake hands, like any touch (important to know how to respond with touch if they are distressed, especially in inpatient settings) Noise – prepare them for any fire alarm tests or other alarms that may go off, check background noises are not too distracting (radiator, open window) and make any changes where possible Smell – if any smells make them feel ill or cause distress (e.g. air freshener, cut flowers, food cooking) and make adjustments where possible Taste – if they have any strong aversions to food or taking medications and consider alternatives if needed Temperature – do they often feel warmer or colder than others, ask about preferred temperature, if they need a window open, if they would prefer to keep their coat on To put someone at ease, it may help to state that eye contact is not required Provide a selection of fidget tools that may assist concentration and relieve anxiety Consider interoception and whether the person receives signals from internal organs to know when to eat, drink, use the toilet or when they are experiencing an emotion such as anger
Reasonable adjustments for minimising uncertainty	Autistic people like details, especially details such as who they will see, how long for, where the meeting will take place, will this be a one-off or one of a number of appointments, what will happen if the session is late, and what will happen after the appointment Ensure roles, rules and expectations are clear and consistent Make sure you and your service keep your promises – don't promise what you can't deliver Ensure the person's treatment plan is explicit and consistent so it could be delivered in the same way by bank, agency or locum staff Ensure appointments are on time and, if an appointment is likely to be delayed, offer an option to leave completely and return at a later agreed time Wherever possible, allow the person to see the same clinician consistently and for appointments to be in the same location At the end of an appointment or interaction, be clear as to what has been decided or agreed and what will happen next Provide advanced warning of changes or new activities and allow time to plan and prepare

autistic traits are identified and a neurodiversity-affirmative approach adopted.

Criminal Justice System

It must be noted that who and why people come to the attention of the criminal justice system is very complex, and research is very difficult. Having said that, there are concerns about the interactions between autistic people and the criminal justice system. Many more autistic people will be victims than offenders, and they can find it extremely difficult to get effective help from the criminal justice system when needed. Reasons for this are similar barriers to those experienced by them in trying to access health services plus concerns that they may not make robust witnesses (whilst true for some, it is not true for all as with non-autistic people).

In relation to law breaking, autistic people are typically more likely to stick to the rules than non-autistic people, and this includes the laws. On the other hand, autistic people are people, and a proportion of people will break the law for a wide variety of reasons. It is therefore to be expected that a proportion of autistic people will break the law. What is less clear is whether this is a greater or lesser proportion than for non-autistic people, but the current belief is that it is a smaller proportion. As noted in this chapter, autism gives no protection against any other mental or physical disorder, so some autistic people will have co-occurring disorders such as ADHD, alcohol/substance misuse, psychopathy or other mental disorders that themselves are thought to have higher correlations with law breaking.

With all the caveats about limited identification of autistic people and hence skewed samples, it does appear that crimes based on special interests are rare even though they often attract high media interest.

Autistic people are more likely to confess than non-autistic people (as they are more likely to tell the truth) when they have done something and are confronted with it. They are also more likely to make false confessions if induced to do so (e.g. 'just say yes and you can leave') as panic leads to flight mode, and they may agree to anything to get away from the questioning. Hence, there is a need for appropriate safeguarding during questioning.

Autistic people can struggle with any interview situation especially where these are intense and lots of questions are asked or there is little time to process and reply to one question before the next one is asked. Reasonable adjustments apply just as much to criminal investigation interviews as to anything else.

If autistic people commit offences carrying an imprisonment tariff and get sent to prison, this is likely to be an even more challenging pace for them to be than it is for non-autistic people. If this is the verdict and sentence decided by the court, then again reasonable adjustments are needed in custodial settings but can be harder to do. If this is not done, then the risk of the person developing/exacerbating a co-occurring mental illness is much increased as is the risk of 'meltdowns', or overwhelming feelings of stress and fear leading to attempts at flight or fight to escape. Giving people quiet, safe places to calm down on their own usually quickly defuses meltdowns but can be very difficult to do in custodial settings.

See wrap.warwick.ac.uk/156472/7/WRAP-Working-community-learning-disabilities-autistic-risk-criminal-justice-system-2021.pdf for more information. Although this covers learning disability and autism – the bits on learning disability only apply to about 20 per cent of autistic people – it does give information more generally applicable to all autistic people.

Conclusion

The lifetime experiences of autistic adults through into older life are still largely unknown. It is important to treat co-occurring conditions in autistic people with the evidence-based treatments used for non-autistic people until and unless clear evidence emerges showing a different approach is preferable.

Further evolution of the concept of autism is likely and should build on prior collaborative work by autistic scholars and psychiatric experts in reaching consensus,[17] based on the lived experience of autistic people and familiarity with the autistic world.

References

1. Kenny L, Hattersley C, Molins B, et al. Which terms should be used to describe autism? Perspectives from the UK autism community. *Autism* 2016;20 (4):442–62. doi.org/10.1177/1362361315588200.
2. UK Parliament POST. *Postnote 612. Autism.* London: The Parliamentary Office of Science and Technology, 2020. post.parliament.uk/research-briefings/post-pn-0612/.
3. Manouilenko I, Bejerot S. Sukhareva – prior to Asperger and Kanner. *Nordic Journal of Psychiatry* 2015;69(6):479–82. doi.org/10.3109/08039488.2015.1005022.
4. Czech H. Hans Asperger, National Socialism, and 'race hygiene' in Nazi-era Vienna. *Molecular Autism* 2018;9:1–43. doi.org/10.1186/s13229-018-0208-6.
5. Muratori F, Calderoni S, Bizzari V. George Frankl: an undervalued voice in the history of autism. *European Child & Adolescent Psychiatry* 2021;30:1273–80. doi.org/10.1007/s00787-020-01622-4.
6. Baron-Cohen S, Klin A, Silberman S, et al. Did Hans Asperger actively assist the Nazi euthanasia program? *Molecular Autism* 2018;9:28. doi.org/10.1186/s13229-018-0209-5.
7. Milton DEM. On the ontological status of autism: the 'double empathy problem'. *Disability & Society* 2012;27 (6):883–7. doi.org/10.1080/09687599.2012.710008.
8. Murray D, Lesser M, Lawson W. Attention, monotropism and the diagnostic criteria for autism. *Autism* 2005;9(2):139–56. DOI:10.1177/1362361305051398
9. Crompton CJ, Ropar D, Evans-Williams CV, et al. Autistic peer-to-peer information transfer is highly effective. *Autism* 2020;24(7):1704–2. doi.org/10.1177/1362361320919286.
10. Sasson N, Faso D, Nugent J, et al. Neurotypical peers are less willing to interact with those with autism based on thin slice judgments. *Scientific Reports* 2017;7(1):1–10. doi.org/10.1038/srep40700.
11. Dwyer P, Acevedo SM, Brown HM, et al. An expert roundtable discussion on experiences of autistic autism researchers. *Autism in Adulthood* 2021;3(3):209–20. doi.org/10.1089/aut.2021.29019.rtb.
12. Croen LA, Zerbo O, Qian Y, et al. The health status of adults on the autism spectrum. *Autism* 2015;19 (7):814–23.
13. Griffiths S, Allison C, Kenny R, et al. The vulnerability experiences quotient (VEQ): a study of vulnerability, mental health and life satisfaction in autistic adults. *Autism Research* 2019;12:1516–28. doi.org/10.1002/aur.2162.
14. Hirvikoski T, Mittendorfer-Rutz E, Boman M, et al. Premature mortality in autism spectrum disorder. *British Journal of Psychiatry* 2016;208(3): 232–8.
15. Westwood H, Mandy W, Tchanturia K. Clinical evaluation of autistic symptoms in women with anorexia nervosa. *Molecular Autism* 2017;8(12). doi.org/10.1186/s13229-017-0128-x.
16. Cook J, Hull L, Crane L, et al. Camouflaging in autism: a systematic review. *Clinical Psychology Review* 2021;89. doi.org/10.1016/j.cpr.2021.102080.
17. Kapp SK, Ne'eman A. Lobbying autism's diagnostic revision in the DSM-5. In: Kapp SK (ed.) *Autistic Community and the Neurodiversity Movement: Stories from the Frontline.* Singapore: Springer; 2020: 167–94. doi.org/10.1007/978-981-13-8437-0

Further Reading

Doherty M, Haydon C, Davidson IA. Recognising autism in healthcare. *British Journal of Hospital Medicine*. 2021;82 (12):1–7.

Doherty M, Haydon C, Davidson IA. Autism: making reasonable adjustments in healthcare. *British Journal of Hospital Medicine*. 2021;82(12):1–11.

Fletcher-Watson S, Happé F. *Autism: A New Introduction to Psychological Theory and Current Debate*. 2nd ed. Abingdon: Routledge; 2019.

Kapp SK (ed.) *Autistic Community and the Neurodiversity Movement: Stories from the Frontline*. Singapore: Springer; 2020. Available open access from link .springer.com/book/10.1007%2F978-981-13-8437-0.

Royal College of Psychiatrists. *The Psychiatric Management of Autism in Adults* CR228; 2020. www .rcpsych.ac.uk/docs/default-source/improving-care/better-mh-policy/college-reports/college-report-cr228.pdf?sfvrsn=c64e10e3_2.

Silberman S. *NeuroTribes: The Legacy of Autism and the Future of Neurodiversity*. New York: Avery; 2015.

Chapter 10

Attention-Deficit/Hyperactivity Disorder

Marios Adamou

Introduction

Attention-deficit/hyperactivity disorder (ADHD) is a neurodevelopmental disorder characterised by inattention, hyperactivity-impulsivity or both. The literature for diagnosing and treating ADHD has grown vastly since Adam Weikard first described it in 1775.[1] In 1937, the efficacy of using amphetamine to reduce symptoms was serendipitously discovered, and by the 1940s, the brain was implicated as the source of ADHD-like symptoms. This was described as minimal brain damage resulting from an encephalitis epidemic. In 1980, the third edition of the *Diagnostic and Statistical Manual of Mental Disorders* (DSM) created the first reliable operational diagnostic criteria for the disorder. This was a result of studies that led the scientific community to view ADHD as a seriously impairing, often persistent neurobiological disorder of high prevalence that is caused by a complex interplay between genetic and environmental risk factors. These risk factors affect the brain networks' structural and functional capacity and lead to ADHD symptoms, neurocognitive deficits and a wide range of functional impairments.

Epidemiology of ADHD in Adulthood

ADHD is a common disorder. In 2007, a meta-analysis of more than 100 studies estimated the worldwide prevalence of ADHD in children and adolescents to be 5.3 per cent (95% Cl: 5.01–5.56).[2] This variability among studies was attributed to the choice of diagnostic criteria (not all studies used the same), the source of information used and the inclusion of a requirement for functional impairment and symptoms for diagnosis. After adjusting for these factors, a subsequent meta-analysis concluded that the prevalence of ADHD does not significantly differ between countries in Europe, Asia, Africa, the Americas and Australia.[3]

The diagnosis of ADHD is not 'for life'. Most children with ADHD will not continue to meet the full criteria for ADHD as adults. However, the likelihood of either functional impairment[4] or sub-threshold (three or fewer) impairing symptoms persisting into adulthood is high,[5] and meta-analyses[6] showed that the pooled prevalence of ADHD to be 2.5 per cent (95% Cl: 2.1–3.1) in adults. Overall, longitudinal studies supported the notion that approximately two-thirds of youths with ADHD retain impairing symptoms of the disorder into adulthood.[4]

In 2018, the National Institute for Health and Care Excellence (NICE) stated a prevalence of 3–4% of adults.[7] The number of diagnosed cases is substantially below these population estimates.

In the United Kingdom (UK), the results show fluctuations across time, with an increase recorded from 1998 to 2007 (6.9 and 12.2 diagnosed cases per 100,000 persons, respectively), followed by a decrease to 8.8 diagnosed cases per 100,000 persons in 2010. The incidence rate in adults was substantially lower when compared to children and adolescents, with the last available estimate of 0.9 diagnosed cases per 100,000 persons in 2010.[8]

Sociodemographic Factors

Sex, ethnicity and socioeconomic status are also important when considering the prevalence of ADHD. Regarding sex, for children and adolescents, ADHD predominantly affects males and exhibits a male-to-female sex ratio of 4:1 in clinical studies and 2.4:1 in population studies.[2] For adults, this sex discrepancy almost disappears,[9] possibly due to referral biases among treatment-seeking patients or sex-specific effects of the course of ADHD.

A large Swedish population-based cohort study of 811,803 individuals found that low family income predicted an increased likelihood of ADHD.[10] This could, however, be due to ADHD running in families who have educational and occupational underachievement rather than proving a direct link of socioeconomic status being causal. The over-representation of the socioeconomic disadvantage among ADHD families could be due to underemployment.[11]

In terms of ethnicity – although studies have not shown a difference in true prevalence – referral barriers and patterns reflecting different access to services may have disproportionately attributed an effect to particular ethnic groups.[12]

Gene and Environment Interactions

The evidence base suggests that ADHD runs in families. Both parents and siblings of people with ADHD show a 5-fold and 10-fold increased risk of developing the disorder compared with the general population.[13] In addition, twin studies place ADHD heritability between 70–80% in children and adults.[14] There is little or no evidence to suggest that the shared environment substantially influences this.[15]

According to the diagnostic criteria, ADHD is a categorical diagnosis. This disorder is influenced by stable genetic factors and those that emerge at different developmental stages from childhood to adulthood.[16] Thus, genes contribute to the onset, persistence and remission of ADHD, presumably through stable neurobiological deficits and maturational or compensatory processes that influence development.

It is not easy to clearly identify environmental causes of ADHD. Such associations can arise from other sources, such as the child's or parental behaviours that shape the environment. Children with ADHD might evoke styles of parenting that could be described as 'hostile', and that style may contribute to generating an ADHD presentation. In addition, if a child experiences severe early maternal deprivation, the risk of developing ADHD symptoms increases. The relationship between the length of deprivation and the risk of developing ADHD-like symptoms was dose-dependent.[17] Prenatal and perinatal factors include low birth weight, premature birth and maternal smoking and alcohol use. Exposure to environmental toxins such as polychlorinated biphenyls, organophosphate pesticides, zinc and lead are other associated environmental factors.[18]

Brain Mechanims in Adult ADHD

Cognitive deficits characterise ADHD in multiple, relatively independent domains. The deficits in executive functioning are well identified in visuospatial and verbal working memory, inhibitory control, vigilance and planning.[19] Studies of reward dysregulation show that patients with ADHD make suboptimal decisions,[20] prefer immediate rather than delayed rewards[21] and over-estimate the magnitude of proximal relative to distal rewards.[22] Other domains impaired in ADHD include temporal information processing and timing;[23] speech and language;[24] arousal and activation;[25] memory span, processing speed and response time variability;[26] and motor control.[27] For clinical practice, it is important to note that very few patients show deficits in all domains. Many will show deficits in one or two domains; some have no deficits at all.[28]

In terms of brain functioning, several brain regions and neural pathways have been implicated in ADHD. Functional MRI studies in patients with ADHD that used inhibitory control, working memory and attentional tasks have shown underactivation of frontostriatal, frontoparietal and ventral attention networks.[29] The purpose of the frontoparietal network is to mediate goal-directed executive processes, whereas the ventral attention network facilitates the reorientation of attention towards salient and behaviourally relevant external stimuli. Patients with ADHD show a lower ventral striatum activation in anticipation of reward than in controls.[30] ADHD is also associated with hyperactivation in somatomotor and visual systems,[29] which possibly compensates for impaired functioning of the prefrontal and anterior cingulate cortices.[31]

Regarding brain morphology, studies found structural brain alterations associated with ADHD. For example, ADHD is associated with a 3–5% smaller total brain size than controls;[32] this can be attributed to a reduction of grey matter.[33] Consistent with genetic data that support a model of ADHD as the extreme of a population trait, total brain volume correlates negatively with ADHD symptoms in the general population.[34] Patients with ADHD have smaller volumes across several brain regions, most consistently in the right globus pallidus, right putamen, caudate nucleus and cerebellum.[35] In addition, white matter is also affected, as widespread alterations in white matter integrity have been found, especially in the right anterior corona radiata, right forceps minor, bilateral internal capsule and left cerebellum.[36] Both structural and functional imaging findings are very variable across studies, suggesting that the neural underpinnings of ADHD are heterogeneous, which is consistent with cognition studies.

Clinical Diagnosis of ADHD

National and consensus guidelines for the treatment of ADHD in adults are similar across the world,[37] including guidance from the National Institute for Health and Care Excellence (NICE) in England and Wales.[7] These indicate that ADHD causes significant impairment across the lifespan, and efforts need to be made to recognise and treat ADHD in adults to reduce its impact on function and mental health in daily life.

The DSM criteria for ADHD include five components.[38] The A-criterion contains two symptom lists (inattention and hyperactivity/impulsivity), and an adult symptom count must exceed five symptoms on either list during the past six months. The A-criterion ensures that symptoms are stable and sufficiently elevated. The B-criterion requires symptom onset before age 12, establishing lifespan chronicity. The C-criterion requires that symptoms be present in multiple settings, ensuring contextual stability. The D-criterion requires that symptoms create significant impairment, providing clinical significance. Finally, the E-criterion requires that symptoms not be explained by another disorder, preserving the specificity of the diagnosis.

The currently relevant NICE guideline (NG87) was published in March 2018,[7] amending where appropriate the guidance CG72 published in September 2008.[39] The guidelines suggest that a specialist psychiatrist, paediatrician or other appropriately qualified health care professionals should make a diagnosis, based on a full clinical and psychosocial assessment of the person (which should include a discussion about behaviour and symptoms in the different life domains), along with developmental and psychiatric history, observer reports and assessment of the person's mental state.[28] The guidelines do not specify what a specialist is, but it would suggest that for such competency to be met, a specialist should have had supervised training in adult ADHD.

For a diagnosis of ADHD, symptoms of hyperactivity/impulsivity or inattention should meet the diagnostic criteria, cause at least moderate impairment, be pervasive and occur in two or more settings of everyday life (e.g. social, familial, educational or occupational settings). ADHD should be considered in all age groups, with symptom criteria adjusted for age-appropriate changes in behaviour.

As discussed earlier, there are no biomarkers or cognitive or neuroimaging tests with sufficient specificity and sensitivity to diagnose ADHD. For this reason, the cornerstone of an ADHD diagnostic assessment remains a detailed exploration of the clinical and behavioural presentation using a diagnostic interview supported by supplementary information.[40] This approach to the diagnosis of ADHD is endorsed by international guidelines, which all recommend the use of a diagnostic clinical interview.[41] The interview assessment should carefully evaluate the presence or absence of each of the 18 DSM or International Statistical Classification of Diseases and Related Health Problems (ICD)-11 symptoms, both currently and in childhood, as well as the additional criteria required for the diagnosis, such as the requirement for functional impairment. This interview mustn't be used as a simple tick-box exercise with binary 'yes' or 'no' answers regarding the presence or absence of a symptom. It should be a detailed interview probing DSM or ICD criteria for diagnosis. Careful probing is required to ensure that the individual expands in sufficient detail about specific examples for each diagnostic symptom criteria investigated, based on their experience in daily life and accompanied impairment directly attributable to these experiences.

In addition to the diagnostic interview, a critical additional component is to screen for other mental health and neurodevelopmental disorders and to evaluate whether another condition does not better explain the presenting symptoms. If another condition can explain these symptoms, an approach similar to what was suggested by Foulds should be taken, which is hierarchical.[42] This means that the other conditions will precede the diagnosis of adult ADHD. Indeed, psychiatric comorbidity is a clinically important dimension of ADHD heterogeneity. At one extreme, a small proportion of clinic-referred individuals are free of comorbidity; at the other end, some patients have a complex pattern of multiple problems, including substance use disorders,[43] anxiety disorders,[44] mood disorders,[44] communication disorders, sleep disorders,[45] intellectual disabilities,[44] specific learning disabilities,[44] disruptive behaviour,[44] tic disorders[44] and autism spectrum disorder.[46] Consideration of the patient's comorbidity profile is important as it will influence the matter of diagnosis as well as the treatment planning.

Treatment of ADHD

Not all people who meet the criteria for ADHD will choose to have or benefit from treatment. The symptom severity should be assessed, as the presence of comorbidities and the likelihood of reduction of impairment before treatment commences. The medications to treat ADHD should be prescribed seven days a week and throughout the year because the disorder affects aspects of life outside the workday, such as driving, socialising, academic studies and general functioning in the family environment.

The prescribing of medication starts by considering whether the patient will benefit from a stimulant or non-stimulant medication. Although both stimulant and non-stimulant medication effectively reduce ADHD symptoms,[47] on average, stimulants (amphetamine and methylphenidate) are more efficacious than non-stimulants (atomoxetine, guanfacine and clonidine).[48] Clinical guidelines, therefore, recommend stimulants as the first-line psychopharmacological treatment for patients of all ages with ADHD.

Pharmacological treatments are typically taken for many years, except for those patients who do not have a persistent course of ADHD. Taking treatment is important as this has been generally associated with improved outcomes. A systematic review of five randomised controlled trials (RCTs) and 10 open-label extension studies of adults with ADHD[49] support the view that stimulant therapy for ADHD has long-term beneficial effects and is well tolerated. Treating ADHD in children and adults is expected to bring improved long-term outcomes, although generally not to normal levels.[50] Although medication reduces ADHD symptoms and impairments in the short term, there is limited and inconsistent evidence for long-term medication effects on improved social functioning, academic achievement, employment status and psychiatric comorbidity.[51]

Medication

Stimulants

When choosing a stimulant, the first decision is whether to use a methylphenidate or an amphetamine product, both of which modulate the action of dopamine. Methylphenidate and amphetamine block the dopamine transporter, and amphetamine also promotes dopamine release and reverse transport. Although the efficacy of both classes of stimulants is similar, some patients preferentially respond to and tolerate one or the other.[48] However, it cannot reliably be predicted which patient will respond better to which stimulant. Both families of stimulants have short-acting (2–4 hours), intermediate-acting (6–8 hours) and long-acting (10–12 hours) formulations that enable tailoring the duration of coverage for each patient based on their needs. The best approach is to start on a low dose of stimulant and titrate at weekly intervals depending on response and adverse effects, according to the needs of the patient.[52] For all stimulant formulations, the duration of effect varies from patient to patient. Thus, titration of stimulants addresses the onset and duration of effect, overall efficacy and adverse events. For example, long-acting stimulants take 1–2 hours to begin working; thus, patients are told when to take the medication to secure benefits at the beginning of the workday. For some patients, the effects of long-acting stimulants can wear off by mid-to-late afternoon. Therefore, they might need additional pharmacological coverage or adjustment to the dose or formulation to help control symptoms later in the day.

The most reported side effects of stimulants are initial insomnia, decreased appetite, dysphoria and irritability. Sleep disturbances are very common in patients with ADHD, independent of stimulant use,[45] although not so much in adults. As appetite suppression usually occurs in the middle of the day, its effects can be mitigated by taking the medication after breakfast. If a person has dysphoria and irritability, managing these depends on whether they occur during the peak or trough of the bioavailability of the medication, as indicated by its pharmacokinetic curve.[53] If these symptoms occur during the peaks of drug bioavailability, switching to another stimulant is an option, as it may have a lower peak. If they occur during the troughs, they might be attributable to withdrawal or rebound effects, which can be mitigated by adding a small dose of a short-acting stimulant one hour before the symptoms occur or again by changing the stimulant formulation.

It is rare to have serious adverse effects with stimulants, although they do occur. These are reported as acute anxiety states, depression, mania and psychosis, in which treatment should be discontinued.[54] Evidence for the association of other serious adverse events with stimulant use for ADHD is less robust. Some studies raised concerns that stimulants cause sudden cardiac death, and one Danish study (n = 714,258) found that stimulant use was associated with an increased risk of any adverse cardiovascular event (with an adjusted hazard ratio of 1.83).

Non-stimulants

Regulatory agencies have approved two classes of non-stimulants for the treatment of ADHD. These include the selective noradrenaline re-uptake inhibitor atomoxetine[55] and long-acting formulations of two a2-adrenergic agonist drugs – clonidine[56] and guanfacine.[57] These drugs effectively manage ADHD, but the sedative effects of a2-adrenergic agonists limit their use in some patients.

Like stimulants, these medications require slow titration to avoid adverse effects by starting with a low dose and adjusting it based on outcomes. Atomoxetine can be prescribed once or twice daily.

Non-pharmacological Interventions

The treatment for ADHD is not limited to pharmacological options. Some patients do not respond well to medication and might experience, for example, poor symptom control, unmanageable adverse events or both. In addition, medication alone might not produce optimal results across all domains of ADHD-related impairment. Finally, there may be contraindications to medication either due to clinician concerns or policies limiting their access specific to their health care systems.

Behavioural interventions are the best established, most positively recommended and most commonly used form of psychological intervention.[58] The principles of positive and negative reinforcement and social learning provide the foundation for various techniques, often modified better to meet the needs of patients with adult ADHD.

More focused approaches improve specific areas of daily functioning, such as social or organisational skills.[59] Cognitive behavioural therapy and life-management skills coaching are recommended. These skills include self-instructional self-control training, compensatory strategies, problem-solving, diaries or time schedules.[60]

Effects of ADHD

ADHD impairs psychosocial functioning in a range of social, academic and occupational contexts, also affecting perceptions of wellbeing. Adverse outcomes include suicide attempts,[61,62] reduced occupational functioning, unemployment, and educational and vocational underachievement. Traffic accidents and violations are more frequent in drivers with ADHD[63] compared to those without the disorder. Family relationships involving individuals with ADHD might be characterised by discord and negative interactions compared with families not affected by ADHD.[64] Finally, patients with ADHD or a history of childhood ADHD have higher mortality rates than those without ADHD, as consistently documented in longitudinal studies[65] and a registry study.[66]

These functional impairments reduce the psychological and social wellbeing and health-related quality of life (HRQOL) of patients with ADHD.[67] Similarly, adults with ADHD have a low HRQOL in adulthood[68,69] as well as their retrospective reports from childhood.[70]

Treatments for ADHD reduce functional impairments and improve HRQOL. This evidence is, so far, almost entirely limited to pharmacological therapies. Epidemiological and clinical studies have found beneficial effects of medication on functioning and HRQOL for stimulants and atomoxetine.[71] These effects mirror, to some extent, medication effects on symptoms of ADHD, although with smaller effect sizes. Moreover, findings from national registry studies indicate that using medication – particularly stimulants – reduces the risk of accidents and trauma-related emergency department admissions and might have protective effects on substance abuse, suicidal and delinquent behaviour.[72] Given that there is little data available on longer-term treatment effects,[73] the extent to which changes in HRQOL are mediated by symptom changes, changes in functional impairment or other factors remain unclear.[49]

Summary

Traits and symptoms of ADHD, which can potentially lead to a diagnosis, are highly prevalent in the general population. In any typical town in the UK, there may be thousands of people who would potentially match the symptom descriptions set out in the diagnostic criteria. Such a screening approach could potentially pathologise normal human experience, or mislabel symptoms of a comorbid mental disorder that should take precedence in treatment.

There has been a sudden increase in the number of people seeking an assessment for adult ADHD – at least in the West – and a shift in their expectations about the outcome of their assessment. Demands of modern life may lead people to seek cognitive enhancement to allow them to perform. Some recent routes to seeking an assessment and treatment for ADHD may be linked to that; the ethics around neuroaugmentation are still being debated.[74]

In the minds of clinicians, ADHD should remain a clinical disorder that can only be reliably diagnosed if the specified number of pervasive symptoms is present, and another condition cannot better explain the impairment directly attributed to these. The primal purpose of this medical diagnosis is to provide access to evidence-based treatments aiming to reduce symptoms and not to validate a person's understanding of themselves through self-diagnosis. The consequences of a diagnostic label are not always positive.[75]

The lack of definition of what constitutes an ADHD specialist, the absence of consensus-based quality standards for a good diagnostic assessment and report, the heterogeneity of the adult ADHD presentation, and the potential for misattribution of reported benefits from treatment with stimulants from cognitive enhancement to symptom reduction all complicate the modern clinical practice in ADHD.

These service provision and clinical practice challenges will be the focus in the future.

References

1. Barkley RA, Peters H. The earliest reference to ADHD in the medical literature? Melchior Adam Weikard's description in 1775 of 'attention deficit' (Mangel der Aufmerksamkeit, Attentio Volubilis). *Journal of Attention Disorders* 2012;16(8):623–30.
2. Polanczyk G, de Lima MS, Horta B, et al. The worldwide prevalence of ADHD: a systematic review and metaregression analysis. *American Journal of Psychiatry* 2007;164(6):942–8.
3. Polanczyk GV, Willcutt EG, Salum G, et al. ADHD prevalence estimates across three decades: an updated systematic review and meta-regression analysis. *International Journal of Epidemiology* 2014;43(2):434–42.
4. Faraone, SV, Biederman J, Mick E. The age-dependent decline of attention deficit hyperactivity disorder: a meta-analysis of follow-up studies. *Psychological Medicine* 2006;36(2):159.
5. Biederman, J, Mick E, Faraone SV. Age-dependent decline of symptoms of attention deficit hyperactivity disorder: impact of remission definition and symptom type. *American Journal of Psychiatry* 2000;157(5):816–8.
6. Simon V, Czobor P, Bálint S, et al. Prevalence and correlates of adult attention-deficit hyperactivity disorder: meta-analysis. *The British Journal of Psychiatry* 2009;194(3):204–11.
7. National Institute for Health and Care Excellence. *Attention Deficit Hyperactivity Disorder: Diagnosis and Management*; National Institute for Health and Care Excellence; 2018. www.nice.org.uk/guidance/ng87.
8. Holden SE, Jenkins-Jones S, Poole CD, et al. The prevalence and incidence, resource use and financial costs of treating people with attention deficit/hyperactivity disorder (ADHD) in the United Kingdom (1998 to 2010). *Child and Adolescent Psychiatry and Mental Health* 2013;7(1):1–13.
9. Matte B, Anselmi L, Salum GA et al. ADHD in DSM-5: a field trial in a large, representative sample of 18- to 19-year-old adults. *Psychological Medicine* 2015;45(2):361–73.
10. Kieling C, Genro JP, Hutz MH, et al. The -1021 C/T DBH polymorphism is associated with neuropsychological performance among children and adolescents with ADHD. *American Journal of Medical Genetics Part B Neuropsychiatric Genetics* 2008;147B (4):485–90.
11. Biederman J, Petty CR, Fried R, et al. Educational and occupational underattainment in adults with attention-deficit/hyperactivity disorder: a controlled study. *Journal of Clinical Psychiatry* 2008;69(8):1217–22.
12. Lingineni RK, Biswas S, Ahmad N, et al. Factors associated with attention deficit/hyperactivity disorder among US children: results from a national survey. *BMC Pediatrics* 2012;12(1):1–10.
13. Biederman J, Faraone SV, Keenan K, et al. Further evidence for family-genetic risk factors in attention deficit hyperactivity disorder: atterns of comorbidity in probands and relatives in psychiatrically and pediatrically referred samples. *Archives of General Psychiatry* 1992;49(9):728–38.
14. Larsson H, Chang Z, D'Onofrio BM, et al. The heritability of clinically diagnosed attention deficit hyperactivity disorder across the lifespan. *Psychological Medicine* 2014;44 (10):2223–9.
15. Burt SA. Rethinking environmental contributions to child and adolescent psychopathology: a meta-analysis of shared environmental influences. *Psychological Bulletin* 2009;135(4):608.
16. Chang Z, Lichtenstein P, Asherson PJ, et al. Developmental twin study of attention problems: high heritabilities throughout development. *JAMA Psychiatry* 2013;70(3):311–8.
17. Stevens SE, Sonuga-Barke EJS, Kreppner JM, et al. Inattention/overactivity following early severe institutional deprivation: presentation and associations in early adolescence. *Journal of Abnormal Child Psychology* 2008;36(3):385–98.
18. Banerjee TD, Middleton F, Faraone SV. Environmental risk factors for attention-deficit hyperactivity disorder. *Acta Paediatrica* 2007;96(9):1269–74.
19. Willcutt EG, Doyle AE, Nigg JT, et al. Validity of the executive function theory of attention-deficit/hyperactivity disorder: a meta-analytic review. *Biological Psychiatry* 2005;57 (11):1336–46.
20. Sonuga-Barke EJ, Fairchild G. Neuroeconomics of attention-deficit/hyperactivity disorder: differential influences of medial, dorsal, and ventral prefrontal brain networks on suboptimal decision making? *Biological Psychiatry* 2012;72(2):126–33.
21. Luman M, Tripp G, Scheres A. Identifying the neurobiology of altered reinforcement sensitivity in ADHD: a review and research agenda.

Neuroscience & Biobehavioral Reviews 2010;34(5):744–54.

22. Scheres A, Lee A, Sumiya M. Temporal reward discounting and ADHD: task and symptom specific effects. *Journal of Neural Transmission (Vienna)* 2008;115 (2):221–6.
23. Toplak ME, Tannock R. Time perception: modality and duration effects in attention-deficit/hyperactivity disorder (ADHD). *Journal of Abnormal Child Psychology* 2005;33(5):639–54.
24. Tomblin JB, Mueller KL. How can the comorbidity with ADHD aid understanding of language and speech disorders? *Topics in Language Disorders* 2012;32(3):198.
25. Fair DA, Bathula D, Nikolas MA, et al. Distinct neuropsychological subgroups in typically developing youth inform heterogeneity in children with ADHD. *Proceedings of the National Academy of Sciences of the United States of America* 2012;109(17):6769–74.
26. Kuntsi J, Klein C. Intraindividual variability in ADHD and its implications for research of causal links. *Current Topics in Behavioral Neuroscience* 2012;9:67–91.
27. Fliers EA, Franke B, Lambregts-Rommelse NNJ, et al. Undertreatment of motor problems in children with ADHD. *Child and Adolescent Mental Health* 2009;15(2):85–90.
28. Coghill DR, Seth S, Matthews K. A comprehensive assessment of memory, delay aversion, timing, inhibition, decision making and variability in attention deficit hyperactivity disorder: advancing beyond the three-pathway models. *Psychological Medicine* 2014;44 (9):1989–2001.
29. Cortese S, Kelly C, Chabernaud C, et al. Toward systems neuroscience of ADHD: a meta-analysis of 55 fMRI studies. *American Journal of Psychiatry* 2012;169(10):1038–55.
30. Plichta MM, Scheres A. Ventral-striatal responsiveness during reward anticipation in ADHD and its relation to trait impulsivity in the healthy population: a meta-analytic review of the fMRI literature. *Neuroscience & Biobehavioral Reviews* 2014;38:125–34.
31. Fassbender C, Schweitzer JB. Is there evidence for neural compensation in attention deficit hyperactivity disorder? A review of the functional neuroimaging literature. *Clinical Psychology Review* 2006;26(4):445–65.
32. Durston S, Pol HEH, Schnack HG, et al. Magnetic resonance imaging of boys with attention-deficit/hyperactivity disorder and their unaffected siblings. *Journal of the American Academy of Child & Adolescent Psychiatry* 2004;43 (3):332–40.
33. Greven CU, Bralten J, Mennes M, et al. Developmentally stable whole-brain volume reductions and developmentally sensitive caudate and putamen volume alterations in those with attention-deficit/hyperactivity disorder and their unaffected siblings. *JAMA Psychiatry* 2015;72(5):490–9.
34. Hoogman M, Rijpkema M, Janss L, et al. Current self-reported symptoms of attention deficit/hyperactivity disorder are associated with total brain volume in healthy adults. *PLoS One* 2012;7(2): e31273.
35. Frodl T, Skokauskas N. Meta-analysis of structural MRI studies in children and adults with attention deficit hyperactivity disorder indicates treatment effects. *Acta Psychiatrica Scandinavica* 2012;125(2):114–26.
36. van Ewijk H, Heslenfeld DJ, Zwiers MP, et al. Diffusion tensor imaging in attention deficit/hyperactivity disorder: a systematic review and meta-analysis. *Neuroscience & Biobehavioral Reviews* 2012;36(4):1093–106.
37. Kooij SJ, Bejerot S, Blackwell A, et al. European consensus statement on diagnosis and treatment of adult ADHD: the European Network Adult ADHD. *BMC Psychiatry* 2010;10 (1):1–24.
38. American Psychiatric Association. Attention deficit/hyperactivity disorder. In: *Diagnostic and Statistical Manual of Mental Disorders: DSM-5™*, 5th ed. Arlington, VA: American Psychiatric Publishing, Inc.; 2013: 59–61.
39. National Institute for Health and Care Excellence. *Attention Deficit Hyperactivity Disorder: Diagnosis and Management of ADHD in Children, Young People and Adults, in NICE Clinical Guidance 72*. London: NICE; 2008.
40. Agrawal N, Faruqui R, Bodani M, *Oxford Textbook of Neuropsychiatry*. Oxford: Oxford University Press; 2020.
41. Schneider BC, Schöttle D, Hottenrott B, et al. Assessment of Adult ADHD in Clinical Practice: Four Letters – 40 Opinions. *Journal of Attention Disorders* 2023;27(9):1051–61.
42. Foulds GA, Bedford A. Hierarchy of classes of personal illness. *Psychological Medicine* 1975;5(2):181–192.
43. Bernardi S, Faraone SV, Cortese S, et al. The lifetime impact of attention deficit hyperactivity disorder: results from the National Epidemiologic Survey on Alcohol and Related Conditions (NESARC). *Psychological Medicine* 2012;42(4):875–87.
44. Biederman J, Newcorn J, Sprich S. Comorbidity of attention deficit hyperactivity disorder with conduct, depressive, anxiety, and other disorders. *American Journal of Psychiatry* 1991;148(5):564–77.
45. Cortese S, Faraone SV, Konofal E, et al. Sleep in children with attention-deficit/hyperactivity disorder: meta-analysis of subjective and objective studies. *Journal of the American Academy of Child and Adolescent Psychiatry* 2009;48 (9):894–908.
46. Antshel KM, Zhang-James Y, Faraone SV. The comorbidity of ADHD and autism spectrum disorder. *Expert Review of Neurotherapeutics* 2013;13 (10):1117–28.
47. Faraone SV, Glatt SJ. A comparison of the efficacy of medications for adult attention-deficit/hyperactivity disorder using meta-analysis of effect sizes. *The Journal of Clinical Psychiatry* 2009;71 (6):754–63.
48. Faraone SV, Biederman J, Spencer TJ, et al. Comparing the efficacy of medications for ADHD using meta-analysis. *Medscape General Medicine* 2006;8(4):4.
49. Fredriksen M, Halmøy A, Faraone SV, et al. Long-term efficacy and safety of treatment with stimulants and atomoxetine in adult ADHD: a review of controlled and naturalistic studies. *European Neuropsychopharmacology* 2013;23(6):508–27.
50. Shaw M, Hodgkins P, Caci H, et al. A systematic review and analysis of long-term outcomes in attention deficit hyperactivity disorder: effects of treatment and non-treatment. *BMC Medicine* 2012;10:99.
51. Van de Loo-Neus GH, Rommelse N, Buitelaar JK. To stop or not to stop? How long should medication treatment of attention-deficit hyperactivity

disorder be extended? *European Neuropsychopharmacology* 2011;21 (8):584–99.

52. Rostain A, Jensen PS, Connor DF, et al. Toward quality care in ADHD: defining the goals of treatment. *Journal of Attention Disorders* 2015;19(2):99–117.
53. Maldonado R. Comparison of the pharmacokinetics and clinical efficacy of new extended-release formulations of methylphenidate. *Expert Opinions on Drug Metabolism & Toxicology* 2013;9 (8):1001–14.
54. Wilens TE. ADHD: prevalence, diagnosis, and issues of comorbidity. *CNS Spectrums* 2007;12(S6):1–5.
55. Tanaka Y, Rohde LA, Jin L, et al. A meta-analysis of the consistency of atomoxetine treatment effects in pediatric patients with attention-deficit/ hyperactivity disorder from 15 clinical trials across four geographic regions. *Journal of Child and Adolescent Psychopharmacology* 2013;23(4):262–70.
56. Jain R, Segal S, Kollins SH, et al. Clonidine extended-release tablets for pediatric patients with attention-deficit/ hyperactivity disorder. *Journal of the American Academy of Child and Adolescent Psychiatry* 2011;50(2):171–9.
57. Biederman J, Melmed RD, Patel A, et al. Long-term, open-label extension study of guanfacine extended release in children and adolescents with ADHD. *CNS Spectrums* 2008;13(12):1047–55.
58. Pfiffner LJ, Haack LM. Behavior management for school-aged children with ADHD. *Child and Adolescent Psychiatric Clinics of North America* 2014;23(4):731–46.
59. Adamou M, Graham K, MacKeith J, et al. Advancing services for adult ADHD: the development of the ADHD Star as a framework for multidisciplinary interventions. *BMC Health Services Research* 2016;16(1):632.
60. Adamou M, Asherson P, Arif M, et al. Recommendations for occupational therapy interventions for adults with ADHD: a consensus statement from the UK adult ADHD network. *BMC Psychiatry* 2021;21(1):1–9.
61. Biederman J, Faraone SV. The effects of attention-deficit/hyperactivity disorder on employment and household income. *Medscape General Medicine* 2006;8 (3):12.
62. James A, Lai FH, Dahl C. Attention deficit hyperactivity disorder and suicide: a review of possible associations. *Acta Psychiatrica Scandinavica* 2004;110(6):408–15.
63. Chang Z, Lichtenstein P, D'Onofrio BM, et al. Serious transport accidents in adults with attention-deficit/ hyperactivity disorder and the effect of medication: a population-based study. *JAMA Psychiatry* 2014;71(3):319–25.
64. Biederman J, Monuteaux MC, Mick E, et al. Young adult outcome of attention deficit hyperactivity disorder: a controlled 10-year follow-up study. *Psychological Medicine* 2006;36 (2):167–79.
65. Klein RG, Mannuzza S, Olazagasti MAR, et al. Clinical and functional outcome of childhood attention-deficit/ hyperactivity disorder 33 years later. *Archives of General Psychiatry* 2012;69 (12):1295–303.
66. Dalsgaard S, Østergaard SD, Leckman JF, et al. Mortality in children, adolescents, and adults with attention deficit hyperactivity disorder: a nationwide cohort study. *Lancet* 2015;385(9983):2190–6.
67. Danckaerts M, Sonuga-Barke EJS, Banaschewski T, et al. The quality of life of children with attention deficit/ hyperactivity disorder: a systematic review. *European Child & Adolescent Psychiatry* 2010;19(2):83–105.
68. Agarwal R, Goldenberg M, Perry R, et al. The quality of life of adults with attention deficit hyperactivity disorder: a systematic review. *Innovations in Clinical Neuroscience* 2012;9(5–6):10–21.
69. Brod M, Pohlman B, Lasser R, et al. Comparison of the burden of illness for adults with ADHD across seven countries: a qualitative study. *Health and Quality of Life Outcomes* 2012;10:47.
70. Caci H, Asherson P, Donfrancesco R, et al. Daily life impairments associated with childhood/adolescent attention-deficit/hyperactivity disorder as recalled by adults: results from the European Lifetime Impairment Survey. *CNS Spectrums* 2015;20(2):112–21.
71. Coghill D. The impact of medications on quality of life in attention-deficit hyperactivity disorder: a systematic review. *CNS Drugs* 2010;24(10):843–66.
72. Ljung T, Chen Q, Lichtenstein P, et al. Common etiological factors of attention-deficit/hyperactivity disorder and suicidal behavior: a population-based study in Sweden. *JAMA Psychiatry* 2014;71(8):958–64.
73. Perwien AR, Kratochvil CJ, Faries DE, et al. Atomoxetine treatment in children and adolescents with attention-deficit hyperactivity disorder: what are the long-term health-related quality-of-life outcomes? *Journal of Child & Adolescent Psychopharmacology* 2006;16 (6):713–24.
74. Sahakian BJ, Morein-Zamir S. Neuroethical issues in cognitive enhancement. *Journal of Psychopharmacology* 2011;25 (2):197–204.
75. Sims R, Michaleff ZA, Glasziou P, et al. Consequences of a diagnostic label: a systematic scoping review and thematic framework. *Frontiers in Public Health* 2021;9:725877.

Chapter 11

Sleep Disorders and Psychiatry

Hugh Selsick

Introduction

Sleep is one of the great mysteries of human experience. It is a behaviour that is highly preserved throughout the animal kingdom, and it constitutes a third of our existence. It begins before birth and is with us throughout life. For a new-born baby, it is their predominant behaviour,[1] and sleep continues to occupy a large proportion of our lives as we age. It has long been suspected that it is essential for good mental and physical health, and in the last century, there has been growing scientific evidence to confirm this suspicion. Yet, we know very little about the functions of sleep and are only just beginning to understand the mechanisms that control it. In the past, it was commonly assumed that sleep had 'a function' but, the more we have come to understand, the clearer it has become that sleep performs multiple functions. Precisely what those functions are is still uncertain, and they may change across the lifespan or possibly even vary across different species. We know that sleep is essential for life, and total sleep deprivation for long enough is fatal,[2] and the fact that we spend a third of our lives in this vulnerable state underlines how important sleep must be.

Although our understanding of the mechanisms and functions of it is limited, any patient who has experienced a sleep disorder – or anyone who has been deprived of sleep – will be acutely aware of the distress and dysfunction that this causes. Given that we spend so much time sleeping, there is ample time for things to go wrong and, as sleep involves multiple physiological and psychological processes, it can go wrong in a wide variety of ways. This makes sleep medicine a truly multidisciplinary field of medicine, involving psychiatrists, psychologists, neurologists, respiratory physicians, dentists, medical technologists, anaesthetists and otorhinolaryngologists to name but a few. However, there is no doubt that, with the bidirectional relationship between sleep disorders and psychiatric disorders, sleep medicine is of great importance to mental health professionals and our patients.

Sleep Architecture

The development of the polysomnogram – comprising electroencephalogram (EEG), electrooculogram and electromyogram – allowed scientists to examine the structure of sleep in a way that was not possible before. It soon became clear that sleep is not a single state but rather a collection of different states with distinct EEG, physiological and psychological phenomena. These states are largely defined by their EEG characteristics and are broadly divided into two groups: rapid eye movement (REM) sleep and non-rapid eye movement (NREM) sleep. NREM is further divided into NREM1 (N1), NREM2 (N2) and NREM3 (N3). N3 is also referred to as delta sleep or slow wave sleep due to the slow delta waves on the EEG. Older texts divided NREM into stages 1, 2, 3 and 4. However, as stages 3 and 4 were both characterised by slow waves and the distinction between them was arbitrary, they have now been combined under the banner of N3.[3]

Wakefulness

In order to appreciate the changes across the different sleep stages, it is helpful to use the waking state as a baseline. In wakefulness, the EEG shows high frequency, low amplitude 14–30Hz waves with alpha waves (8–13z) when the eyes are closed. When we are alert, our eyes move rapidly, and muscle activity measured with an EMG is high. Attention is turned outwards, and the person is very responsive to external stimuli.[3]

NREM1 (N1)

This is a light stage of sleep characterised by reduced consciousness but still-significant awareness of external stimuli, with slow rolling eye movements, slowing of the EEG[3] and drifting, tangential thoughts. The EMG still shows significant activity. N1 does not appear to have any specific functions of its own and is generally thought to be a transitional stage between wake and sleep. The arousal threshold from this stage is low, and excessive NREM1 is a sign of disrupted or poor-quality sleep.[4]

NREM2 (N2)

This is the predominant form of sleep in adult humans as we spend approximately 50 per cent of the night in this stage.[1] It is characterised by the further slowing of the EEG but with distinctive waveforms: sleep spindles, which are 11–16Hz bursts of activity, and K-complexes, which are single high amplitude waves. N2 is a light stage of sleep with a low arousal threshold. Subjects woken from N2 will often report thinking rather than dreaming, though some dreams may occur in N2.[5]

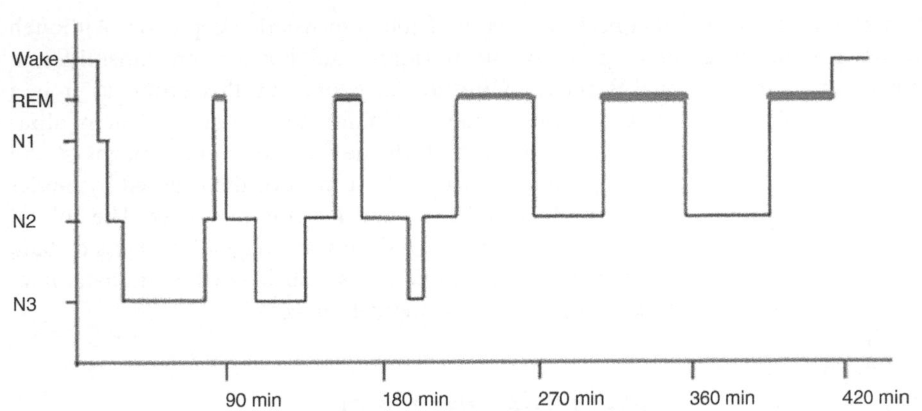

Figure 11.1 Hypnogram showing typical pattern of sleep stages.

NREM3 (N3)

N3 is the deepest stage of sleep with a high arousal threshold, and someone woken from N3 will generally take longer to become fully oriented than when woken from other sleep stages. This high arousal threshold is responsible for the parasomnias that arise from N3, as we'll see later on. The EEG shows high amplitude, slow waves. The muscle tone is lower than in N1 and N2, but there is still some muscle activity.[3] N3 is usually not associated with significant dreaming, though some simple, mental activity does occur.[5]

Rapid Eye Movement Sleep (REM/R)

REM sleep is perhaps the strangest and least understood sleep stage. The EEG looks very similar to that of the waking brain with high frequency, low amplitude waves. REM sleep is, contrary to popular belief, not a particularly deep stage of sleep, with the arousal threshold being somewhat variable.[5] There are characteristic rapid movements of the eyes, which give this stage its name, and there is an almost complete absence of muscle tone in all the muscles with the exception of the tiny muscles in the middle ear, the muscles of the eyes, the diaphragm and the sphincter muscles of the gastrointestinal and urinary systems. As a result, the EMG will be totally flat with only very occasional phasic twitches. This near-total paralysis is necessary as REM is when we do most (though not all) of our vivid, narrative dreaming. During dreaming, the motor cortex is active as the brain attempts to act out the dream, and the paralysis prevents this from occurring. Thermoregulation is suspended, whilst heart rate and blood become more variable. A penile erection occurs in men as well as clitoral and vaginal engorgement in women; this is a purely physiological phenomenon and is unrelated to dream content.[3]

The Sleep Cycle and the Progression of Sleep Across the Night

In adults, sleep is composed of periods of around 90 minutes where we cycle through the various sleep stages. On falling asleep, we first pass through N1 and then rapidly enter N2. We then enter the first period of N3, which is generally the longest N3 episode of the night. On emerging from N3, we re-enter N2 and then have the first episode of REM sleep, though this is generally very brief. With each successive cycle, the duration of N3 reduces and the duration of N2 and REM increase, and in the later cycles, there is often no N3 at all. As a result, N3 dominates the first part of the night while N2 and REM dominate the latter part. It should be noted that this is an idealised description, and individual nights rarely follow this pattern exactly. It is also common for there to be a few awakenings during the night, and as long as these awakenings are brief, this is entirely normal.[3]

Figure 11.1 shows a hypnogram that maps these sleep stages across the night and shows this typical pattern.

Sleep Architecture and Psychiatric Conditions

It has long been known that sleep architecture is altered in a significant proportion of patients with major depressive disorder (MDD). These changes include a reduced N3 sleep with the N3 more evenly distributed through the night rather than loaded towards the beginning of the night. Most striking, however, is the alteration to REM sleep. There is reduced latency to the first episode of REM sleep, with this episode of REM being longer than normal. There is an increased percentage of REM, though not an increased absolute amount of REM sleep. There are also more rapid eye movements within the REM periods than in controls.[6] These changes are not consistent enough to have diagnostic value, and reduced REM latency with increased rapid eye movements within REM are also seen in the manic phase of bipolar disorder. Consistent changes in sleep architecture are generally not a feature of anxiety disorders, psychotic disorders or obsessive-compulsive disorder (OCD). On the other hand, almost all psychiatric disorders have a negative impact on sleep continuity.[7]

The sleep architecture changes seen in MDD have led to some promising therapeutic applications. For example, partial sleep deprivation where patients are woken part way through the night, thus reducing their total REM sleep time, has long been known to lift mood in depressed patients.[8] On the other hand, partial N3 deprivation has also been shown to improve mood in depression,[9] demonstrating how much more we likely still have to learn about the complex relationship between sleep and mental health!

Impact of Psychiatric Medications on Sleep and Sleep Architecture

A wide range of neurotransmitters are involved in sleep-wake regulation, and therefore, any medications that act on these neurotransmitters in the central nervous system have the potential to affect sleep directly, for better or worse. It is worthwhile having an understanding of the most important neurotransmitters involved in regulating sleep so one is aware of the impact that psychiatric medications, which by their nature impact on central neurotransmitters, might have. In addition, the therapeutic effects and side effects of many medications can increase the risk of sleep disorders, thus indirectly impairing sleep.

The Neurotransmitters of Sleep and Wakefulness

Table 11.1[10,11] describes the most important neurotransmitters promoting wakefulness. Noradrenaline, serotonin and histamine activity levels are high during wakefulness, reduced in NREM sleep and absent in REM sleep. Acetylcholine activity is high in the waking brain, reduced in NREM but is also high in REM sleep. Thus, these four neurotransmitters are important for promoting wakefulness, but acetylcholine is also important for REM sleep, while noradrenaline, serotonin and histamine should be inactive in order for REM to occur. Consequently, medications that act on these neurotransmitters will act on sleep as a whole, but they will also affect the architecture of sleep. As an example, selective serotonin reuptake inhibitors (SSRIs) and serotonin and noradrenaline reuptake inhibitors increase serotonin and noradrenaline levels and promote wakefulness (insomnia is a common side effect) and suppress REM sleep. GABA can promote wakefulness in the pontine reticular formation but can promote sleep in other areas of the brain. Adenosine promotes sleep and may be the chemical expression of the homeostatic sleep drive. Although it is an endocrine hormone and not a neurotransmitter, it makes sense to include melatonin in this group as it is a sleep-promoting chemical in humans and one we can manipulate with medications. Caffeine is an adenosine antagonist and therefore inhibits sleep, whilst most of the licensed hypnotics are promotors of GABA and melatonin activity. The role of endogenous dopamine in sleep-wake regulation is less certain, but increasing dopamine levels – such as with amphetamine-based drugs – increases wakefulness.[10]

Table 11.1 Wakefulness promoting neurotransmitters

Neurotransmitter	Wakefulness	NREM Sleep	REM Sleep
Noradrenaline	++	+	-
Serotonin	++	+	-
Histamine	++	+	-
Acetylcholine	++	+	++
Orexin/hypocretin	++	-	-
Dopamine	++	+	++
Glutamate	++	+	++

Factors Affecting Sleep

The Two-Process Model of Sleep

Traditionally, the control of sleep has been attributed to the interaction between two physiological drives: the homeostatic sleep drive, also called Process S, and the circadian alerting drive, or Process C. The homeostatic sleep drive accumulates progressively during wakefulness and diminishes as we sleep. It is therefore very dependent on duration of wakefulness and the quality and duration of the preceding sleep episodes. Counteracting this is the circadian alerting drive, which is dependent on the innate circadian rhythm and is not particularly affected by sleep. The interaction between the two is shown in Figure 11.2.

In the morning, when we wake, the circadian alerting drive is low, but as the homeostatic sleep drive is even lower, we are awake. As the day progresses, the homeostatic sleep drive accumulates, but we do not fall asleep as the circadian alerting drive is also rising and remains higher than the sleep drive. The circadian alerting drive dips slightly in the early afternoon, and this is why we often feel sleepy at this time. In some cases, it may dip below the homeostatic drive leading to an unintended nap or a siesta. The circadian drive resumes its rise and stays ahead of the homeostatic sleep drive, peaking around 2100 hours. After this time, the circadian alerting drive starts to drop while the homeostatic sleep drive continues to rise. When the homeostatic drive becomes greater than the circadian drive, we fall asleep. During sleep, the homeostatic sleep drive diminishes, but we don't wake up as the circadian alerting drive is also dropping and stays below the sleep drive. The circadian alerting drive is at its lowest in the early morning and then starts to rise again. Once the circadian alerting drive becomes greater than the homeostatic sleep drive, we wake up and the cycle begins again.[12]

It is important to note that the times of the circadian peak and nadir vary from person to person depending on their chronotype. Some people are morning chronotypes, generally falling asleep early, waking early and being most alert in the mornings. Evening chronotypes prefer later bedtimes, later rising times and are more alert and productive in the evenings. Some people fall between these two extremes, and each person's degree of morning or evening preference is largely fixed through their lifespan.[13]

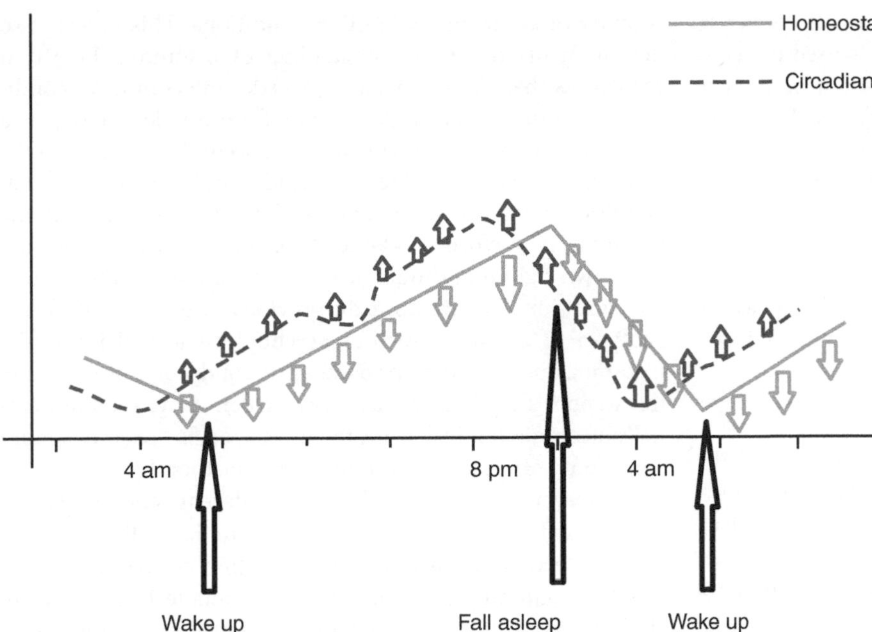

Figure 11.2 Two-process model of sleep.

Understanding the roles of the homeostatic and circadian drives is essential for evaluating and treating sleep problems. For example, anything that reduces the homeostatic sleep drive, such as napping in the day, will likely lead to poorer sleep at night. Attempting sleep at a time when the circadian drive is not conducive to sleep, as is the case for night-shift workers, is unlikely to be as successful as sleeping at night.

Other Factors Affecting Sleep

Although these two drivers underly the biology of sleep, they are clearly not the only factors.

Physical: Sleep can also be influenced by physical factors such as pain, urinary frequency, obstructive sleep apnoea (OSA) or restless legs.

Psychological: There is clearly an important role for psychological factors, which may be short or long term. Some short-term factors disrupting sleep include anxiety, excitement or any other cause of increased arousal. Conversely, low psychological arousal will be conducive to sleep. Long-term psychological influences that adversely affect sleep include psychiatric disorders or ingrained anxieties about sleep, while the absence of these factors and confidence in one's ability to sleep have the opposite effect.

Environmental: The environment can influence sleep in a variety of ways. Noise is a common disrupter of sleep, and excessive light can be a problem for some people. The temperature of the environment is an often-overlooked factor, with sleep being impaired by both excessively low and high ambient temperatures.[14]

Substances: Medications, alcohol, caffeine and recreational drugs all have the potential to impact on sleep. When determining the impact of a particular substance on sleep, one should consider the nature of the substance (e.g. is it stimulating or sedating), the initial dose of the substance, its pharmacokinetics and the timing of administration.

Sleep Investigations

The gold standard sleep investigation is the polysomnogram (PSG). The variables studied in a PSG will depend on the setting and what the investigators are looking for, but in a clinical setting, it typically involves the following:

- Electroencephalogram – to monitor brain activity, to quantify and stage sleep and detect awakenings
- Electrooculogram – to measure eye movements in order to stage sleep and monitor rapid eye movements in REM
- Submental electromyogram – to measure muscle tone, which aids in staging sleep
- Tibialis EMG – to detect limb movements
- Nasal airflow, chest movement sensors and abdominal movement sensors – to monitor breathing and detect apnoeas
- Pulse oximetry – to monitor oxygen saturations
- ECG – to screen for arrhythmias and determine heart rate
- Microphone – to detect snoring or vocalisations
- Video – to monitor behaviours in sleep and wakefulness and observe body position

The polysomnogram can be used overnight during habitual sleep time or for daytime studies to measure sleepiness or ability to avoid sleep.

In cases where one is screening specifically for obstructive sleep apnoea, home pulse oximetry or a limited study using only the respiratory channels may be used. Increasingly, technology is allowing for many more studies to be done outside of the sleep clinic – for example, at home or in a psychiatric ward.

Actigraphy uses an accelerometer worn on the wrist to monitor movement, and the movement data is used to determine when the subject is asleep or awake. It can be used to obtain longitudinal information about a person's sleep-wake patterns outside of the sleep clinic. As such, it may give a more realistic view of a person's sleep pattern than a polysomnogram performed in an inpatient setting over a single night.[15]

Commercially available technology such as smart watches has not yet been validated to the level where we can rely on it to diagnose sleep disorders, but this is likely to change as the technology matures and is subjected to more formal testing.[16]

Classification of Sleep Disorders

Although the International Classification of Diseases and the *Diagnostic and Statistical Manual of Mental Disorders* do list sleep disorders, the most comprehensive classification of sleep disorders is the *International Classification of Sleep Disorders, 3rd edition* (ICSD-3), which divides sleep disorders into six broad categories:

- Insomnia
- Sleep-related breathing disorders
- Central disorders of hypersomnolence
- Circadian rhythm sleep-wake disorders
- Parasomnias
- Sleep-related movement disorders[17]

There are 64 distinct sleep disorders and six sleep-related disorders listed in the ICSD-3, and it is beyond the scope of this chapter to examine all of them. However, we will look at the most important sleep disorders from each category, particularly those that have relevance to psychiatry.

Insomnia

Definition

Insomnia is a difficulty getting to sleep, staying asleep, waking up too early or a combination of these symptoms. The sleep is insufficient despite the patient having adequate opportunity, which distinguishes it from insufficient sleep syndrome (commonly referred to as sleep deprivation). It must also lead to daytime consequences such as tiredness, irritability, cognitive problems, academic or professional dysfunction or mood disturbance. These consequences distinguish insomnia from short sleep, which is a normal variant and describes those people who simply need less sleep than the average. Occasional insomnia symptoms are common, and so the symptoms should be present for at least three nights of the week to meet criteria for insomnia and should be present for at least six months to qualify as chronic insomnia.[17]

The way that we define insomnia has shifted significantly in recent years. One important change that has occurred recently is the shift from defining insomnia as either primary insomnia or insomnia secondary to other conditions to describing it as primary or comorbid with other conditions. This reflects two developments in our understanding of insomnia. Firstly, it recognises that insomnia often precedes the comorbid condition and – in the case of depression, for example – may play a role in the aetiology of that condition. Secondly, even when the insomnia is caused by the comorbid condition, treating that condition does not necessarily lead to the remission of the insomnia. Therefore, it is better to see insomnia as a condition in its own right that should be treated regardless of the comorbid condition. Furthermore, the previous emphasis on different subtypes of insomnia such as psychophysiological insomnia, insomnia due to medical or psychiatric conditions, or insomnia due to poor sleep hygiene has largely fallen away, as an individual's insomnia rarely falls neatly into a specific box and is more commonly caused by a combination of factors.[17]

However, more recently, two different phenotypes of insomnia have been proposed: insomnia with objective normal sleep duration and insomnia with objective short sleep duration. Although most insomnia patients feel that they are short sleepers, objective measures of sleep have shown that many insomnia patients have sleep durations that fall in the normal range. However, those who do have objectively short sleep appear to have a more severe phenotype with greater physiological arousal and stress response; poorer medical outcomes such as hypertension, diabetes and increased mortality; and are less likely to respond to treatment. It has therefore been proposed that this phenotype is more biological in origin as opposed to the normal sleep duration phenotype, which may be more psychological and behavioural in origin.[18]

Although I will demonstrate the role that insomnia plays in mental illness, it is important to point out that insomnia is a significant psychiatric condition in its own right. It has a similar impact on quality of life to chronic medical and psychiatric conditions such as congestive heart failure and major depressive disorder.[19] It will come as no surprise that insomnia is more common in the psychiatric population, but even in the general population, it is not uncommon. Prevalence rates in studies vary according to study methodology and the diagnostic criteria used, but in the general population, the prevalence of insomnia or insomnia symptoms with daytime consequences falls in the range of 4–15%.[20]

Insomnia and Psychiatric Conditions

There is a particularly close relationship between insomnia and major depressive disorder (MDD). In children, adolescents and adults with major depressive disorder, insomnia is reported in around two-thirds of patients.[21,22] Insomnia is one of the symptoms of depression, and depression increases the risk of developing insomnia, but it should not be assumed that the depression necessarily causes the insomnia. Indeed, when one looks at the timeline of depression and insomnia, depression precedes the insomnia in 23–29% of cases, and they occur simultaneously in 8–29% of cases. However, insomnia precedes the depression in 41–69% of cases, and insomnia is now recognised as a significant risk factor for depression, doubling the risk relative to good sleepers.[20] Furthermore, insomnia predicts increased incidence of depression decades later, making it unlikely that it is simply a prodromal symptom of depression.[23]

Nor is it certain that treating depression will resolve the insomnia. Insomnia is the most common residual symptom when depression resolves, and this residual insomnia is a risk factor for a relapse of the depressive disorder. It has long been known that insomnia is a marker for suicide risk, but more recently, the evidence has indicated that it is risk factor in its own right.

Assessment

The diagnosis of insomnia is made clinically and is often a diagnosis of exclusion. Patients generally present with a clear complaint of difficulty falling asleep or staying asleep, and this rapidly narrows down the differential diagnosis. However, you shouldn't assume that a patient who presents this way necessarily has insomnia. Firstly, you should ascertain whether the lack of sleep leads to daytime consequences – if not, then they may simply be someone who needs less sleep than the average but is anxious about this due to the widely held belief that we are supposed to sleep for eight hours. On the other hand, a number of other sleep disorders can mimic insomnia, such as restless legs, obstructive sleep apnoea and circadian rhythm disorders.[17] Therefore, it is essential to take a comprehensive sleep history to exclude other explanations for the poor sleep before you can be confident that the diagnosis is one of insomnia.

A sleep diary is immensely helpful in assessing insomnia as it allows you to see how variable the patients' sleep is, pick out patterns and plan behavioural interventions. Many patients now use smartphone apps and wrist accelerometers to monitor their sleep, but most of these have not been validated, and the quality of the data is affected by many other factors such as the specific phone they use or the presence of a bed partner.[16] It is also important to recognise that insomnia is a subjective disorder and objective measures of sleep in insomnia patients are inconsistent, and there are no pathognomonic findings on objective studies. Therefore, the patient's subjective experience of their sleep should determine the diagnosis and inform the treatment rather than any data from external devices. For the same reason, polysomnography is rarely indicated unless you suspect a comorbid sleep disorder.[24]

Treatment

Medication

The use of hypnotics to treat insomnia is a subject that is mired in controversy. There is a great deal of concern over the safety and efficacy of sleeping pills. Some of these concerns are justified, but the evidence from the scientific literature paints a more nuanced picture. The biggest concern is over the addictive potential of these medications, and there certainly are people who become addicted to or misuse them. However, the vast majority of patients who use these medications do not develop a dependence on them or misuse them.[25] Similarly, there is mounting evidence that these medications can remain effective in the long term in many patients, even with nightly use.[26,27]

When insomnia is likely to be time limited, then a short course of hypnotics can be effective and lead to rapid control of the symptoms,[28] but the situation is more complicated in chronic insomnia. Hypnotics treat insomnia but do not cure it, and once the hypnotic is stopped, the insomnia symptoms are likely to recur.[29] This recurrence of the symptoms often leads the patient to request more medication, and this is often mistaken for addiction rather than as the need for a chronic medication to treat a chronic condition. However, it does mean that if you are going to treat chronic insomnia with medication, you may need to prescribe the medication for many years.

The choice of which hypnotic to use is a complicated topic – beyond the scope of this chapter – but understanding some general principles can be helpful. In the majority of medications, the degree of sedation correlates closely with the plasma level of the drug. Therefore, the pharmacokinetics of the drugs acts as a guide to how quickly they act, how long they maintain their action and how likely residual sedation is the next day. Short-acting drugs are effective for sleep-onset insomnia but may not adequately treat middle of the night or early morning waking. Longer-acting drugs are more likely to maintain sleep through the night but raise the risk of daytime drowsiness.[30]

Insomnia comorbid with other psychiatric conditions can be successfully managed with the right choice of hypnotic. Benzodiazepines and z drugs are effective at treating insomnia in major depressive disorder and do not interfere with the action of antidepressants.[31] Indeed, eszopiclone and benzodiazepines may enhance the response to the antidepressant treatment.[32,33]

Non-Medical Treatments for Insomnia

Various non-medical interventions for insomnia have been proposed and trialled. However, the only intervention that has a strong evidence base is cognitive behaviour therapy for insomnia (CBT-I). CBT-I is composed of psychoeducation and behavioural and cognitive techniques. Although there is some overlap with cognitive behavioural techniques for other psychiatric conditions, there are a number of components that are specific to insomnia treatment. For example, some of the behavioural techniques are designed to optimise the physiological sleep drives by harnessing the circadian rhythm and the homeostatic sleep drive. Unlike medication, CBT-I leads to durable changes in sleep with improvements continuing well beyond the end of therapy.[34] However, there is a reduced response to CBT-I in patients with objectively short sleep, and this group can be challenging to treat.[35] The evidence for CBT-I is particularly strong in that CBT-I has been validated in multiple age groups and in the context of numerous comorbid medical conditions – such as chronic pain or cancer[36] – as well as in psychiatric conditions.[37]

The application of CBT-I in insomnia comorbid with other psychiatric conditions has benefits beyond improving the patient's sleep. CBT-I has been shown to reduce relapse rates in bipolar patients[38], to reduce post-traumatic stress disorder (PTSD) symptoms and increase remission rates in PTSD,[39] and reduce persecutory delusions in patients with psychosis.[40] However, the most consistent finding has been the positive impact of CBT-I on major depressive disorder. Not only does CBT-I lead to improvements in sleep and mood symptoms, but the improvement in mood symptoms may be as great as with CBT for depression.[41,42] This suggests that when patients have comorbid insomnia and depression, and therapy resources are limited, CBT-I should be prioritised over CBT for depression.

Movement Disorders

Sleep-related movement disorders include a diverse range of conditions such as restless legs syndrome, periodic limb movement disorder, sleep-related bruxism and sleep-related rhythmic movement disorder. Sleep-related bruxism – despite being common – has been the subject of very little research, and there are no well-validated treatment options so it will not be discussed further here. This section will focus on rhythmic movement disorder, restless legs syndrome and periodic limb movement disorder.

Sleep-Related Rhythmic Movement Disorder

Sleep-related rhythmic movement disorder is more common in babies and young children and can manifest as head banging, body rocking, leg banging or body rolling. These movements occur in drowsiness or sleep and are only considered problematic if they lead to sleep disruption, daytime symptoms or injury. In the majority of cases, they will resolve spontaneously as the child grows, and continuation of symptoms past adolescence is rare.[17] It is thought to be a self-soothing behaviour in some cases and so the treatment involves taking measures to prevent injury and providing alternative self-soothing strategies. In older children or adults, the use of short-term, gentle sleep restriction to accelerate sleep onset or a short course of hypnotics may be used. These strategies allow the patient to learn that they don't need the rhythmic movement to initiate sleep.[43]

Restless Legs Syndrome and Periodic Limb Movement Disorder

Although restless legs syndrome (RLS) and periodic limb movement disorder (PLMD) are separate conditions, they have a lot in common in terms of aetiology, investigation and treatment, and they often occur together.[44] They will, therefore, be examined together in this section.

Definitions

A diagnosis of RLS is made when the following criteria are met:

1. There is an urge to move the legs, or any other body part, usually due to an uncomfortable sensation that is:
   a. Worse at night or occurs exclusively at night
   b. Worse at rest
   c. Temporarily relieved by movement such as stretching or walking[17]

The discomfort and urge to move make it difficult to initiate sleep and can make it difficult to return to sleep when waking in the night. As a result, patients with RLS often present with a complaint of insomnia.[17]

A diagnosis of PLMD is made when highly stereotyped, repetitive limb movements occur in sleep. These movements are often associated with an arousal, leading to sleep disturbance and fatigue. The movements are usually observed in the lower limb with extension of the big toe and flexion of the ankle, knee and hip. Unlike restless legs – where the movement is volitional and is done in order to relieve the discomfort – periodic limb movements are not volitional, and the patient is often not aware that they are occurring. Therefore, unlike RLS – which can be diagnosed on history – PLMD requires polysomnography to make the diagnosis.[17]

RLS and PLMD have a number of potential causes including genetic predisposition, low iron, vitamin deficiencies, renal failure, pregnancy and neurological disorders. They can also be caused by multiple psychiatric medications such as selective serotonin re-uptake inhibitors, tricyclic antidepressants, lithium, antipsychotics and sedating antihistamines.[17,44] The fact that many medications that are used to treat insomnia, albeit often off label, can cause or exacerbate RLS and PLMD serves to emphasise the importance of excluding these conditions in patients who present with insomnia before initiating treatment. At the level of the central nervous system, there appears to be dysregulation of dopamine though the details of this are not well understood, but it may explain why bupropion – which is a dopaminergic antidepressant – does not exacerbate RLS.[45]

Although these conditions are more common with advancing age, it is not uncommon for them to begin in childhood, though it is often more difficult for children – particularly those with developmental delay – to describe their symptoms. As a result, RLS in children is often misdiagnosed as 'growing pains',[17] and the discomfort may lead to bed refusal and be misdiagnosed as a behavioural issue or as attention-deficit/hyperactivity disorder.[46]

RLS, PLMD and Psychiatric Conditions

It is now well established that RLS is associated with a significantly greater prevalence of mood and anxiety disorders, particularly major depressive disorder, generalised anxiety disorder, panic disorder and post-traumatic stress disorder.

The severity of the RLS is correlated with the severity of mood and anxiety symptoms, and there is some evidence to suggest that treating the RLS improves the mood symptoms.[17,46] Furthermore, 35 per cent of patients with RLS and depression report suicidal ideation as a result of the RLS.[47] Clearly, the situation is further complicated by the propensity for many psychiatric medications to worsen RLS and PLMD symptoms, as described earlier.

Another area of interest is the relationship between RLS/PLMD and ADHD. As mentioned earlier, RLS may be misdiagnosed as ADHD, and RLS is common in both paediatric and adult ADHD.[48] Whether the RLS plays a role in the aetiology of the ADHD or vice versa has yet to be established, though it is known that sleep disruption leads to attention deficit symptoms. However, both conditions may be related to dopamine dysregulation and so may have a common underlying cause.[46]

Assessment

As RLS occurs when awake and the patient is acutely aware of them, the diagnosis of RLS is a clinical one and seldom requires a sleep study.[17] It is surprisingly rare for patients to volunteer RLS symptoms, and they generally present with a complaint of 'insomnia', but a single question has been shown to have 100% sensitivity and 96.8% specificity for RLS in a neurology outpatient population: 'When you try to relax in the evening or sleep at night, do you ever have unpleasant, restless feelings in your legs that can be relieved by walking or movement?'[49]

However, in children, the diagnosis can be more challenging, particularly in children with neurodevelopmental conditions who may not be able to express their discomfort verbally. As there is often a genetic component, one should suspect RLS if a child with sleep difficulties has relatives with RLS. In children who are unable to describe their subjective sensations, a polysomnogram may be helpful, as a finding of PLMD would increase the likelihood that they also have RLS.[46]

Periodic limb movements are extremely difficult to detect on history unless they are sufficiently severe that they start before sleep onset. Therefore, a polysomnogram with EMG monitoring of the tibialis muscles and, ideally, video is required to make the diagnosis. PLMD should be suspected in patients who present with sleepiness or poor-quality sleep where no other clear cause has been established or the risk factors described previously are present.

Blood tests are often useful in RLS and PLMD to screen for low iron, low folate or vitamin B12, renal dysfunction, raised HbA1c (to screen for silent diabetic neuropathy)[50] and vitamin D deficiency.[51]

Treatment

The first step is always to correct any causative or exacerbating factors where possible, such as changing medications that may be contributing to the symptoms or supplementing iron and vitamins if they are low.

Because of the role of dopamine in generating RLS/PLMD, dopamine agonists such as pramipexole, ropinirole and rotigotine have long been the first line of treatment. However, these medications can have significant side effects such as nausea, compulsive behaviours and psychosis.[44,52,53] They also carry a risk of augmentation, which is a paradoxical worsening of RLS symptoms to a level one would not expect from the natural history of the condition.[54]

Augmentation is not a problem with α2δ-ligand medications gabapentin and pregabalin, which have a similar – or possibly better – efficacy than the dopaminergic drugs. As a result, the International Restless Legs Syndrome Study Group have recommended that, in most circumstances, the α2δ-ligand medications should be used as the first-line intervention.[54] Where α2δ-ligand and dopaminergic drugs have not been effective, opiates such as oxycodone, tramadol or methadone may be used. Clonazepam has also been widely used in the past, but evidence for its efficacy is equivocal.[53]

In children, there is a greater emphasis on optimising sleep hygiene, behavioural interventions and iron supplementation, with medication being reserved for children where these have not worked or are not possible. The use of medications in this population lacks a solid evidence base, but dopamine agonists, gabapentin and clonidine have all been used in clinical practice.[46,55]

Circadian Rhythm Disorders

Circadian rhythm disorders occur when there is a misalignment between the person's internal body clock and the external time or the social and occupational demands on that person. Advanced sleep-wake phase disorder (ASWPD) and delayed sleep-wake phase disorder (DSWPD) are conditions where the body clock is ahead or behind external time respectively, and this misalignment is stable over time. Non-24-hour sleep-wake disorder occurs when the body clock runs at slightly longer or, less commonly, slightly shorter than 24 hours. As a result, the internal clock and its related phenomena – such as sleep – rotate around the clock, and so there are periods when the person is in phase with the outside world and periods when they are out of phase. This is more common in certain types of blindness, as light is the most important factor in synchronising the body clock with the outside world. Irregular sleep-wake rhythm disorder, which is not uncommon in dementia, is a lack of any clear circadian rhythm with sleep, and wakefulness is equally spread across day and night.[17]

On the other hand, there are circadian rhythm disorders where there is nothing inherently wrong with the internal body clock, but it is the external time or demands that create the problem. Jet lag disorder occurs when the body clock is moved to a different external time by travel across times zones and is generally worse after eastward travel. Shift work disorder occurs when one works at times when one would normally be asleep and tries to sleep at times when one would

Table 11.2 Circadian rhythm sleep-wake disorders

Disorder	Description	Comments
Delayed sleep-wake phase disorder	Body clock is delayed relative to the outside world. Unable to initiate sleep until well past conventional bedtime and will sleep into late morning or afternoon if allowed to	More common in adolescents. Most alert at night and a struggle to function in mornings if woken before their natural waking time
Advanced sleep-wake phase disorder	Body clock is advanced relative to the outside world. Struggles to stay awake until conventional bedtime and wakes very early in morning	Leads to less educational or occupational dysfunction as they are rarely late for work or school and function well during normal work hours
Irregular sleep-wake rhythm disorder	Irregular sleep-wake episodes throughout the 24 hours. Has broken sleep at night and multiple naps in the day. There is no clear circadian rhythm	More common in neurodegenerative disorders (e.g. dementia) and in developmental disorders
Non-24-hour sleep-wake rhythm disorder	Circadian rhythm is slightly longer (or more rarely shorter) than 24 hours. Sleep period gets progressively later or progressively earlier and rotates around the clock	More common in blind patients who are unable to synchronise the body clock through light
Shift work disorder	Working shifts that overlap with normal sleep time leads to excessive sleepiness when awake and insomnia when trying to sleep between shifts. Total sleep time is reduced	Most commonly reported in workers who work night, early morning or rotating shifts
Jet lag disorder	Insomnia or excessive sleepiness with reduced total sleep time after travel across time zones	It is easier to adjust to westward travel than eastward travel as body clock has a natural tendency to delay
Circadian sleep-wake phase disorder not otherwise specified	Sleep-wake disruption due to circadian misalignment or alteration of the circadian rhythm that does not meet criteria for any of the above disorders	Can occur in neurodegenerative disorders

normally be awake, leading to sleepiness at work and insomnia when trying to sleep between shifts.[17]

The circadian rhythm disorders are summarised in Table 11.2.[56]

The most commonly encountered circadian rhythm disorder in clinical practice is delayed sleep-wake phase disorder, and we will examine this condition in more detail.

Delayed Sleep-Wake Phase Disorder (DSWPD)

Definition

DSWPD is a stable delay in the circadian rhythm that manifests as a delay in the night-time sleep period relative to the desired sleep time. The patient has difficulty initiating sleep at the preferred time, often falling asleep two or more hours later than the desired time. As a result, if they have to rise early in the morning to attend education or work, they will have insufficient opportunity to sleep and will experience sleep deprivation and daytime dysfunction. On the other hand, if they do not have to wake at a set time in the morning and can fall asleep late and wake up late, then they will generally sleep well and feel well in the day. Typically, people with DSWPD feel most sleepy and groggy in the morning and at their most alert late at night when others are getting ready for bed.[17]

DSWPD is most common in adolescents and young adults and will often resolve with increasing age, though it can be a lifelong condition. There is a strong genetic component, though it is likely that multiple genes are involved. As a result, patients with DSWPD tend to cluster in families, and they have a strong evening preference throughout their lives, even before developing DSWP or after the condition resolves. It is thought that some of the genes that predispose to DSWPD also predispose to depression, and there is a strong association between the two conditions.[12,57]

DSWPD and Psychiatric Conditions

There is a close relationship between circadian rhythm disorders and psychiatric conditions, and this is particularly the case for DSWPD. DSWPD has a strong association with depression, and this may reflect a common genetic predisposition. However, it has been hypothesised that depression may arise as a result of the DSWPD, due to repeated exposure to the circadian nadir. As described earlier, the circadian alerting drive is at its lowest in the early hours of the morning. The circadian alerting drive also correlates with the circadian variation in mood, and thus the lowest mood will tend to be in the early hours of the morning.[58] However, most people sleep through this period and are not exposed to that mood minimum. However, in DSWPD, the nadir occurs later in the morning when people are awake at school or work, and they are therefore repeatedly exposed to that mood minimum. Consequently, it is possible that this may mediate the relationship between DSWPD and depression. Treating the DSWPD leads to improvements in mood, supporting the idea that DSWPD may have a causative role in the depression.[59]

There is also evidence for an association between DSWPD and a number of other psychiatric conditions. For example, the delayed sleep seen in some schizophrenic patients, often attributed to a lack of structure in their day, may in fact be due to a delayed phase. DSWPD in schizophrenia leads to greater negative symptoms and poorer functional outcomes.[60] There is also an association between DSWPD and ADHD in children and adults, and treatment of the DSWPD may lead to improvements in the ADHD symptoms.[59]

Assessment

As the primary difficulty is one of falling asleep, it will often present as a sleep-onset insomnia. However, it is important to differentiate DSWPD from insomnia as the treatment of the two disorders is different. The diagnosis is largely made on history, but a sleep diary of seven days or longer and, if possible, actigraphy (a wrist-worn accelerometer) for a similar period are required to confirm the diagnosis. These records should cover work/education days as well as days off. It can also be helpful to have the patient fill out the Horne-Ostberg Morningness-Eveningness Questionnaire, which is freely available and provides a measure of the patients chronotype.

A history of strong evening preference, onset of symptoms in adolescence, and normal sleep when allowed to fall asleep late and wake up late are clues that one is dealing with DSWPD rather than insomnia. In sleep initiation insomnia, the age of onset is often later, and other forms of sleep disruption – such as difficulty getting back to sleep if woken in the night – are more common.

Treatment

The treatment of DSWPD does not involve hypnotic medication – although a hypnotic may induce sleep, it does not shift the circadian rhythm and so cannot reverse all of the daytime dysfunction caused by the circadian misalignment.[61] In order to advance the circadian rhythm of someone with DSWPD, melatonin is given in the evening, earlier than the time of the predicted endogenous melatonin secretion, which tends to occur around two hours prior to habitual sleep onset. The dose of melatonin needs to be high enough to have an effect but not so high that it acts as a hypnotic or that there is still residual melatonin in the bloodstream in the morning, which would serve to delay the circadian rhythm. As such, there is no universally agreed best dose for melatonin in DSWPD,[62] and so there is an element of trial and error in finding the right dose for each patient. Bright light – ideally daylight, though a seasonal affective disorder lamp can be used – is employed in the morning immediately after waking.[63]

Parasomnias

Parasomnias are unwanted experiences or behaviours that occur during sleep or on the boundaries of sleep and wakefulness. They are broadly divided into those that occur in NREM sleep, those that occur in REM sleep and those that are not related to a specific stage of sleep.[17] Some of the common parasomnias are listed in Table 11.3.[17]

Table 11.3 Common parasomnias

NREM parasomnias	REM parasomnias	Other parasomnias
Sleep terrors	Nightmares	Exploding head syndrome
Sleepwalking/eating	REM sleep behaviour disorder	Sleep-related hallucinations
Confusional arousals/ sexsomnia	Recurrent isolated sleep paralysis	Sleep enuresis

NREM Parasomnias

These are disorders that usually result from an incomplete arousal from N3 sleep.[64] As such, the brain is in a part wake–part sleep state, with the front of the brain showing characteristic N3 delta waves on EEG while the posterior part of the brain shows activity more characteristic of wakefulness.[65] This leads to the enactment of automatic behaviours, which can be remarkably complex. The episodes are not generally associated with dreaming, though some dreamlike mentation can occur. The person will usually not recall, or will at most have fragmentary recall for, the episodes the next morning. As these episodes arise from N3 sleep, they tend to cluster in the first third to the first half of the night. There is often a family history of parasomnias, particularly when they continue into adulthood. However, they are much more common in children and will generally resolve with time, so treatment is often not needed.

Sleep Terrors

The person will partially rouse from sleep with behavioural and physiological signs of extreme fear, such as screaming or crying or with tachycardia, tachypnoea, sweating and dilated pupils. The person is often inconsolable and unresponsive to external stimuli, but they may appear to be responding to hallucinations.[17,65]

Sleepwalking

The person gets out of bed and engages in complex behaviours that are often inappropriate, such as urinating in a drawer, walking outside in their pyjamas (or naked) or entering a stranger's house. It may include driving or, rarely, violent behaviours.[64] Because the arousal threshold in N3 is so high, they may sustain significant injuries without waking up. There are multiple recorded cases of patients dying or killing someone during a sleepwalking episode, though this is not the norm, and most patients do not cause or come to any harm. They will usually go back to bed or the couch, return to full sleep and have no recall of the events the next day.[17]

Sleep-Related Eating

The person will consume food in their sleep, often eating things they would not eat when awake, including hazardous substances.[17]

Confusional Arousals

The person wakes from N3 and remains in the bed without displaying any fear. However, their behaviour is confused, and this reflects underlying mental confusion. A variant of confusional arousals is sleep-related abnormal sexual behaviours or sexsomnia. The person engages in sexual behaviour, either with themselves or with the person next to them. The episodes that involve another person almost always involve someone right next to the sexsomnia patient. It is extremely rare for sexsomnia patients to leave their bed, sleepwalk to another's bed and then engage in sexual behaviour.[17]

NREM Parasomnias and Psychiatric Conditions

Patients or their families are often concerned that these parasomnias are a sign of mental illness. This is usually not the case, particularly in children where no association with psychopathology has been found. However, there is an association between NREM parasomnias and anxiety, obsessive-compulsive disorder and depression, though no causal relationship has been found.[17,64] It has long been thought that stress may precipitate episodes, and anecdotally, patients often report more frequent episodes when under stress. It is also thought that sleep deprivation and alcohol consumption increase episodes as can sleeping in an unfamiliar environment.[65]

Assessment

The diagnosis is often very clear from the history, and in children, further investigation is rarely needed. The history should look for precipitating factors such as poor sleep hygiene, sleep deprivation or stress. It is important to note that it is not uncommon for patients to exhibit more than one NREM parasomnia, and the nature of the parasomnias may change over time.

Care should be taken to exclude nocturnal panic attacks, which are reported in over a third of patients with panic disorder.[66] One also needs to exclude nocturnal epilepsy, which manifests as highly stereotyped movements that tend to occur three or more times a night, every night, and are often followed by an awakening. In contrast, NREM parasomnias occur one to three times a night, tend not to occur every night and are followed by a return to deep sleep. A polysomnogram may be helpful if the diagnosis is in doubt and should be performed in adults, particularly if there is a new onset of parasomnias. This is because parasomnias may be precipitated by other sleep disorders such as obstructive sleep apnoea.[65]

Treatment

In children, treatment is usually not required as they are likely to grow out of the parasomnias. Reassurance for the family and the child and ensuring their safety – for example, by locking the front and back door to prevent them leaving the house when sleepwalking – is often all that is required. As the parasomnias tend to occur early in the evening when the parents are still awake, it is unusual for children to leave the home unnoticed. Where treatment is warranted, anticipatory awakening – where the child is stirred from their sleep by the caregiver 15–30 minutes before they typically have the parasomnias – can be effective.[67] There is also evidence for the use of 5-HTP in the treatment of paediatric sleep terrors.[68]

In adults, the first intervention is often to treat any comorbid sleep disorders. Clonazepam up to 3 mg is widely used, and there is data from a case series to support this. There is also some evidence for paroxetine, imipramine and hypnotherapy.[28]

REM Parasomnias

Nightmare Disorder

Definition

Nightmare disorder is characterised by extremely distressing dreams that usually involve an element of threat or loss. These dreams disrupt sleep, and the patient becomes rapidly oriented on waking. There is clear recall for the dreams, and these dreams – or the resultant sleep disruption – lead to daytime dysfunction such as tiredness, cognitive problems, low mood, anxiety and fear of sleep.[17] As nightmares occur primarily in REM sleep, they are more frequent in the second half of the night, though they can occur during earlier REM sleep periods. However, it is important to note that nightmares can sometimes arise out of NREM sleep, particularly in PTSD.[69]

Occasional nightmares are normal and may confer an evolutionary advantage by allowing the brain to experience, and prepare for, frightening situations without being exposed to real physical hazards. They are more common in children and may be part of normal development as long as they do not become regular or lead to bed refusal or daytime dysfunction. However, persistent nightmares in children are often caused by psychological stressors and are the strongest predictor of persistent nightmares in adults.[17] Although the International Classification of Sleep Disorders does not specifically differentiate between PTSD-related nightmares and idiopathic nightmares, this distinction is frequently made in the research, and it is unclear how much of the research into PTSD-related nightmares can be extrapolated to idiopathic nightmares and vice versa.

Nightmare Disorder and Psychiatric Conditions

Eighty per cent of PTSD patients report nightmares, and the presence of nightmares following a traumatic event predicts the onset of PTSD. Furthermore, nightmares can persist once the other symptoms of PTSD have resolved and may continue throughout the patient's life. However, they are also associated with other psychiatric conditions such as schizophrenia, anxiety disorders and substance abuse. Nightmares can be caused by a number of medications used in psychiatry, including antidepressants and β-blockers, as well as by the withdrawal of these medications.[70]

However, the most important factor is the impact of nightmares on suicidality. Of all the sleep disorders, nightmares have the strongest association with suicide and suicidal ideation. Indeed, nightmares are associated with a five-fold increase in high suicidality. This relationship remains even when the comorbid psychiatric condition and the severity of that condition are accounted for, and this finding has been confirmed in multiple studies.[71,72] Although psychiatrists routinely ask about nightmares when screening for PTSD, this data suggests that asking about nightmares should be a part of the risk assessment in all psychiatric conditions.

Assessment

The diagnosis of nightmares is made on history, but a polysomnogram is useful to screen for other sleep disorders that may cause or exacerbate nightmares. For example, OSA can cause nightmares, and treating the OSA may improve or resolve the nightmares.[73] A number of medical and psychiatric drugs cause nightmares, and so, particular attention should be paid to the patient's medications and the temporal relationship between starting the medication and the onset of the nightmares. Obviously, it is important to screen for other signs and symptoms of PTSD. However, it is also important to differentiate between nightmares and negative dreams. Many normal dreams have a negative emotional tone, such as anxiety or embarrassment, but do not have the emotional intensity of nightmares and do not require treatment.

Treatment

It is sensible to treat any comorbid sleep disorders such as OSA, particularly as these treatments can often be rapidly initiated. It goes without saying that – where nightmares are a symptom of PTSD – the PTSD needs to be addressed, and this may improve the nightmares as well, though this is not universally the case. For example, venlafaxine – which is used to treat the daytime symptoms of PTSD – is not indicated for the treatment of PTSD-related nightmares.[69] It is therefore often necessary to specifically tackle nightmares in PTSD as well as in non-PTSD-related nightmares.

There are a number of evidence-based psychological treatments for nightmares, but the treatment with the strongest evidence base is imagery rehearsal therapy (IRT). In IRT, the patient recalls a nightmare and changes it in some way in order to make it more positive and less frightening. They then rehearse that new version of the dream repeatedly in the day. IRT has demonstrated efficacy in idiopathic and PTSD-related nightmares with reductions in nightmare frequency, which are maintained beyond the end of the therapy. Other options, albeit with a lower level of evidence, include progressive muscle relaxation, lucid dreaming training and a number of graded exposure treatments.[69]

Studies of medical treatments for nightmares have largely focused on PTSD-related nightmares, where there is strong evidence for the role of increased noradrenaline activity. Thus, medications that lower noradrenergic tone can be effective treatments. Prazosin, an α1 blocking antihypertensive, has been found to be successful in the treatment of PTSD-related nightmares in military and civilian populations. There is also some evidence for the efficacy of trazodone, atypical antipsychotics, topiramate, gabapentin and tricyclic antidepressants.[69] Although the evidence for these medications is of lower quality than for prazosin, the fact that some of them can be used to treat comorbid conditions such as pain, depression or psychosis – which may accompany the nightmares – make them worth considering.

REM Sleep Behaviour Disorder

REM sleep behaviour disorder (RBD) is caused by the absence of the normal muscle atonia that should be present in REM sleep. As a result, the patient acts out their dreams, and this manifests as repeated vocalisations and complex motor behaviours. Unlike in NREM parasomnias where the sleeper clearly interacts with their environment, in RBD, the person is interacting with their internal dream imagery. They may be observed to be running, fighting, laughing, shouting, talking or playing football, but as their eyes are closed if they grab an object or hit their bed partner, it is purely by chance. The observed actions will often correlate with the recalled dream content. It is very rare for patients to leave the bed and walk during an episode, though they may throw themselves out of bed, leading to injury. Indeed, injury to the self or the bed partner is often what triggers a referral to a sleep clinic.[17]

RBD is more commonly reported in men than in women,[17] though it is not certain if this reflects a true gender difference in prevalence or whether women – who tend to have less violent dreams and therefore less dramatic RBD – are less likely to come to medical attention.[74] It is predominantly a condition of middle and older age, though it can occur in younger adults or children who have narcolepsy, are on antidepressant medications or have a brainstem lesion.[17]

There is a remarkably strong association between RBD and neurodegenerative conditions, particularly α-synucleinopathies and multisystem atrophy. As many as 81% of idiopathic RBD patients will go on to develop Parkinson's disease/dementia.[75] Similarly, 40–60% of patients with established Parkinson's disease have RBD, and 72% of dementia with Lewy bodies patients have RBD.[74]

RBD and Psychiatric Conditions

Clearly, there will be an association between RBD and the psychiatric conditions associated with α-synucleinopathies, such as dementia with Lewy bodies and Parkinson's dementia. RBD patients may have a higher rate of mood disorders and active or past substance misuse.[66] The picture is complicated by the propensity for a number of psychoactive drugs to cause RBD. In particular, many antidepressants can cause RBD – regardless of the class of antidepressant – either whilst the drug is being taken or due to the REM rebound that occurs when the medication is stopped. It is not uncommon for RBD to be misdiagnosed as a psychiatric disorder or a sign of violent personality.[66]

Assessment

A single question has been shown to have 94% sensitivity and 87% specificity for RBD: 'Have you ever been told, or suspected yourself, that you seem to "act out your dreams" while asleep (for example, punching, flailing your arms in the air, making running movements, etc)?'[76] Although the diagnosis is often clear from the history, a polysomnogram to demonstrate a loss of REM atonia and associated behaviours in REM sleep are required to confirm the diagnosis.[17]

Treatment

Safety measures should be instituted immediately until the condition is well controlled. These include removing the bedside table and other objects around the bed that could lead to injury. The bed partner should sleep in a separate bed, if possible, though it is helpful if they can stay in the same room so they can monitor how the patient is responding to treatment.

Melatonin up to 12 mg nightly is effective at reinstating REM atonia and treating RBD with relatively few side effects. As such, it is now widely used as the first-line drug treatment. Clonazepam, despite not re-establishing atonia, is also effective but should be used with caution due to the potential for daytime sedation and falls.[77]

Recurrent Isolated Sleep Paralysis

Recurrent isolated sleep paralysis (RISP) occurs when the REM atonia starts before sleep onset or persists after waking from REM sleep. As such, the person experiences the paralysis on falling asleep or waking up with an inability to move or talk. It is often accompanied by frightening hallucinations, which may be visual, auditory, tactile or involve a sense of a malign presence in the room.[17] There may be a sense of not being able to breathe or someone pushing on their chest. This may be interpreted in a variety of ways depending on the person's cultural background, such as a ghost visitation, alien abduction, out-of-body experience or a stroke.[78]

Recurrent Isolated Sleep Paralysis and Psychiatric Conditions

An association between RISP and bipolar disorder has been identified,[17] and it is also thought to be more common in depression, PTSD and other anxiety disorders, but not in psychosis.[78] However, sleep deprivation, stress and irregular sleep-wake schedules are thought to be risk factors, and so, any psychiatric condition that affects sleep or stress levels has the potential to cause RISP.[17]

Assessment

The diagnosis is made on history, and a sleep diary can be particularly helpful. The diary can assist in identifying precipitants and should record not only sleep times and frequency of sleep paralysis, but also stress levels, caffeine and alcohol intake and the position the person is in when having the sleep paralysis. A polysomnogram is warranted to look for any causes of sleep disruption as anything that increases awakenings in the night increases the opportunity for sleep paralysis to occur. If the patient also experiences sleepiness or cataplexy, then a full screen for narcolepsy is required.

Treatment

There are few evidence-based treatments for RISP, and often, sleep hygiene advice, reassurance and patient education about the condition are all that is required. As it is more common in the supine position,[17] putting a tennis ball in the back of one's pyjamas to prevent the patient from lying on their back can be helpful. It would make sense that REM-suppressing antidepressants such as SSRIs and tricyclics would be useful, and they are not uncommonly used for this purpose in clinical practice, though there has been very little research to underpin this.[79]

Sleep-Related Breathing Disorders

This category covers obstructive sleep apnoea (OSA), hypoventilation, hypoxaemia and central sleep apnoea syndromes.[17] Hypoventilation, hypoxeamia and central sleep apnoea tend to be treated within respiratory medicine, while obstructive sleep apnoea is treated in sleep clinics. OSA is the most common of these disorders and the most relevant to psychiatry.

Obstructive Sleep Apnoea

OSA is the repeated complete or partial collapse of the upper airway during sleep. Complete collapses are termed apnoeas, and partial collapses are termed hypopnoeas. These collapses lead to repeated arousals in order to reopen the airway and can also lead to significant repeated oxygen desaturations. The patient may be aware of waking up choking or gasping for air, but often, the pauses in breathing are reported by their bed partner. As a result of the sleep disruption and oxygen desaturations, the patient will often usually complain of poor-quality sleep with daytime sleepiness, fatigue, low mood or insomnia symptoms. It is also a risk factor for multiple cardiovascular and metabolic conditions such as hypertension, coronary artery disease, cardiac arrhythmias, stroke and type 2 diabetes.[17]

In children, the most frequent cause of OSA is physical obstruction of the airway, such as having enlarged tonsils. In adults, this is less common, and obesity is the biggest modifiable risk factor. It is more common with increasing age, and having a first-degree relative with OSA doubles the risk of developing the condition.[17]

Obstructive Sleep Apnoea and Psychiatric Conditions

Psychiatric conditions may indirectly increase the risk of developing OSA, as obesity is more common in numerous psychiatric conditions, and weight gain is a side effect of numerous psychiatric medications.[80] OSA is more common in patients with psychiatric conditions, and it is therefore important for psychiatrists to be vigilant for the development of signs and symptoms of OSA.[81]

Conversely, there is also evidence of a role for OSA in the aetiology of psychiatric conditions. In the short term, OSA has a consistent negative impact on cognition. However, more worrying is that, in young children, untreated OSA can lead to longer-term cognitive deficits.[82] At the other end of the age range, OSA appears to be a risk factor for dementia, and effective treatment of the OSA can reduce this risk.[83] This may be a result of long-term sleep disruption or repeated oxygen desaturation events that lead to multiple cerebral infarcts.[84]

There is a complex relationship between OSA and depression. This is a difficult area to research as there is significant overlap between the symptoms of these conditions, and it is therefore difficult to determine whether a particular symptom is caused by depression, OSA or both. However, the rate of major depressive disorder is higher in OSA patients than in the general population, and treatment of OSA can lead to improvements in depressive symptoms. The relationship between OSA and bipolar affective disorder is less clear, but untreated OSA may lead to a poorer response to treatment in these patients.[81]

Anxiety disorders and PTSD come with an increased risk of OSA,[81] and the potential for OSA to exacerbate nightmares[73] increases the importance of screening for OSA in PTSD patients. Anxiety disorders can also have a negative effect on compliance with OSA treatment, and panic disorder – in particular – can make it difficult for patients to tolerate continuous positive airway pressure.[81]

OSA is also more common in schizophrenia than compared to the general population and to other psychiatric disorders. This may be due to lifestyle factors, such as increased rates of smoking or the weight gain from atypical antipsychotics. The burden of the cognitive, cardiovascular and metabolic effects of OSA may be greater in this population, who have negative symptoms and are already at higher of cardiovascular and metabolic disease.[81]

Assessment

A history of snoring, observed apnoeas, subjective experiences of waking up choking and poor-quality sleep should raise the possibility of obstructive sleep apnoea. The Epworth Sleepiness Scale, which measures subjective propensity to fall asleep in the day, is widely used as a screening tool and to monitor response to treatment with scores of 11 out of 24 and above indicative of excessive daytime sleepiness. However, it is important to note that not all OSA patients are sleepy in the day, and they can present with insomnia symptoms, fatigue, low mood and cognitive dysfunction rather than sleepiness.[17]

A sleep study is required to confirm the diagnosis. While it is sometimes useful to perform a full polysomnogram, it is much more common to do a respiratory sleep study, which involves monitoring air flow, pulse oximetry and chest and abdominal movements. Oximetry on its own can be done at home and is a useful screening tool with reasonably good specificity though less impressive sensitivity; a negative oximetry in the presence of a history suggestive of OSA should be followed by a more detailed study.[15] Newer technologies that can detect peripheral arterial tone as well as body position, snoring and other parameters are increasing the options available for home OSA testing and monitoring.[85]

The severity of the sleep apnoea is classified according to the apnoea/hypopnoea index (AHI), which is the average number of apnoeas and hypopnoeas per hour of sleep. An AHI below 5/hr is normal; an AHI of 5–14/hr represents mild OSA, 15–29/hr is moderate, and 30/hr or above is severe.[81]

Treatment

Weight loss is potentially curative, but this is often difficult to achieve. For milder cases of OSA, one can use a mandibular advancement splint, which is a jaw-guard-like device worn during sleep that pushes the mandible forward to open the upper airway. For moderate to severe OSA, the treatment is positive airway pressure – either a fixed pressure or one that adjusts to the patient's requirements automatically. These treatments do not cure the condition and so need to be used in the long term.[81]

Central Disorders of Hypersomnolence

This category of sleep disorders defines disorders where sleepiness is not caused by another sleep disorder such as OSA or PLMD. It covers a wide range of aetiologies including neurological, psychiatric and behavioural causes.

Insufficient Sleep Syndrome

Insufficient sleep syndrome or, more colloquially, sleep deprivation is characterised by excessive sleepiness due to curtailment of the habitual sleep period. The symptoms resolve once the sleep time is increased to meet that person's current sleep requirements. It is important to remember, however, that it can take multiple nights of recovery sleep to pay off the sleep debt that results from sleep deprivation. Therefore, one or two good nights' sleep may not be sufficient to improve daytime symptoms.[17]

Hypersomnia due to a Medical Disorder

Excessive daytime sleepiness can be a consequence of a number of medical disorders, including acquired brain injury, Parkinson's disease, tumours, infections or metabolic diseases. Ongoing sleepiness in obstructive sleep apnoea is also included in this category, and it is possible that this may reflect longer-term sequelae of hypoxic brain injury caused by the OSA prior to treatment.[17]

Hypersomnia due to a Medication or Substance

Hypersomnia may be caused by some drugs of abuse as well as sedating medications such as benzodiazepines, certain antidepressants and antipsychotics and opiates. It can also be caused by the withdrawal of alerting substances such as caffeine or amphetamines.[17]

Hypersomnia Associated with a Psychiatric Disorder

Hypersomnia associated with psychiatric conditions accounts for 5–7% of hypersomnia cases. It may be related to any psychiatric disorder but is particularly common in seasonal affective disorder, where it is present in over 50% of cases. In depression, the hypersomnolence may continue once the depression remits and is a risk factor for a depressive relapse.[17]

Narcolepsy

Narcolepsy is divided into narcolepsy type 1 (NT1) and narcolepsy type 2 (NT2). It can best be understood as a condition where REM sleep and its associated phenomena occur at the wrong times and contexts. Common to NT1 and NT2 is the symptom of excessive daytime sleepiness. Narcolepsy patients often feel refreshed on waking in the morning and on waking from daytime naps but then become progressively more sleepy until they nap again. Night-time sleep is often fragmented, and frequent hallucinations and sleep paralysis may occur at sleep onset and waking. When falling asleep at night or during the day, the patient will often rapidly enter REM sleep rather than following the normal pattern of passing through NREM stages N1, N2, N3 and N2 again before the first REM period. The hallucinations may be the superimposition of REM dreaming mentation on waking perception, and the paralysis is the normal REM atonia occurring prior to sleep onset or persisting after waking.

Narcolepsy type 1 is further characterised by either cataplexy (see later) or a low level of orexin/hypocretin in the cerebrospinal fluid. It is well established that NT1 is caused by the loss of orexin/hypocretin-producing neurons in the brain, usually secondary to an autoimmune reaction. It is found almost exclusively in people with the HLA DQB1*0602 subtype, and the absence of this HLA subtype casts doubt on a diagnosis of NT1.[17]

Cataplexy is the loss of muscle tone during wakefulness, usually in response to an emotion; laughter is the most common precipitant. The loss of tone is usually bilateral and lasts a few seconds to a couple of minutes. It may be subtle, with eyelid drooping, jaw slackness or head nodding, or as dramatic as a complete collapse to the floor.[17] It is a common misperception that narcoleptic patients are falling asleep in these episodes, but this is not the case. Again, it appears that cataplexy is the REM atonia occurring during wakefulness.[64]

Narcolepsy type 2 is diagnosed when the symptoms of narcolepsy are present with the exception of cataplexy and when the cerebral spinal fluid (CSF) orexin/hypocretin is normal or has not been measured. The underlying cause of NT2 is less well understood,[17] and there is some debate as to whether it would be better classified as a separate disorder altogether.

Idiopathic Hypersomnia

Idiopathic hypersomnia (IH) is a condition characterised by excessive daytime sleepiness despite often sleeping more than 11 hours at night, but without any cataplexy. IH differs from narcolepsy in a number of ways. In narcolepsy, nocturnal sleep is often disrupted, while IH patients tend to have very consolidated sleep. Narcolepsy patients often feel refreshed on waking in the morning or after naps, but IH patients commonly experience significant sleep inertia on waking. Sleep inertia is difficulty waking up, repeatedly falling back into sleep when woken, and feeling groggy and disoriented for an extended period after waking. The extended sleep time seen in IH patients is rarely seen in narcolepsy. The cause of IH is unknown.[17]

Central Disorders of Hypersomnolence and Psychiatric Conditions

Excessive daytime sleepiness is associated with a nearly three-fold risk of having depression and may be a risk factor for depression.[86] Hypersomnolence is associated with poorer outcomes, more lifetime suicide attempts and a poorer response to antidepressants. It is also significantly more common in bipolar depression than in major depressive disorder.[87] Narcoleptic patients appear to have a higher rate of major depressive disorder,[86] though this finding is not reproduced in all studies.[88] However, a third of narcoleptic patients meet diagnostic criteria for anxiety disorders, particularly social phobia. This may be due to the anxiety caused by the narcoleptic symptoms, such as uncontrolled sleepiness and the risk of having cataplectic attacks in public, but it has also been hypothesised that it is related to the loss of orexin/hypocretin that is involved in stress regulation.[88] The role of orexin/hypocretin in appetite regulation may also explain why most (though not all) studies have found a higher rate of binge eating disorders in narcolepsy.[86]

Assessment

Although a diagnosis of NT1 is often clear on history, objective studies are important in hypersomnolence cases. One needs to exclude other sleep disorders that may cause hypersomnolence, such OSA. If no other sleep disorder is found, this makes a central disorder of hypersomnolence more likely, and the studies are then useful in differentiating between the different central hypersomnolence syndromes.

The investigations in suspected central hypersomnolence include actigraphy followed by a nocturnal polysomnogram and daytime multiple sleep latency test (MSLT). The actigraphy uses an accelerometer on the wrist to measure sleep time in the home environment and should be performed for at least a week prior to the polysomnogram. This gives a picture of the patient's sleep quantity and quality in their home environment and ensures that they are not depriving themselves of sleep prior to the MSLT, which could lead to a false positive. They then come into the clinic for an overnight PSG to screen for other sleep disorders and, again, to ensure they get sufficient sleep prior to the MSLT. The next day, they remain in the clinic with the PSG array attached, and every two hours, they are given a 20-minute trial where they go to bed in a dark room and try to nap. The PSG is then scored to determine if and when the patient fell asleep and whether they experienced any REM sleep during the brief naps. The MSLT will generate a mean sleep onset latency across four or five naps, and any sleep observed will be scored to screen for the presence of REM sleep. A mean sleep onset latency of less than eight minutes is indicative of excessive daytime sleepiness. This short sleep onset latency in the presence of two or more REM episodes is indicative of narcolepsy, while a short sleep onset latency with one or no REM episodes suggests a diagnosis of IH.[89]

Treatment

The treatment for insufficient sleep syndrome simply involves increasing sleep opportunity. Where the hypersomnolence is related to medical or psychiatric disorders, then treating that disorder is clearly important, but this does not guarantee that the hypersomnolence will resolve.[17]

The treatment of hypersomnolence in narcolepsy and idiopathic hypersomnia relies on stimulant medications. Modafinil is widely used as a first-line drug, with methylphenidate and dexamphetamine also being used, usually as second- or third-line drugs.[86] More recently, pitolisant (an H3 autoreceptor inverse agonist)[90] and solriamfetol (a noradrenaline-dopamine re-uptake inhibitor)[91] have become available.

To manage the cataplexy, sleep paralysis and hallucinations in narcolepsy, the first-line treatment is REM-sleep-suppressing antidepressants (i.e. SSRIs, SNRIs and tricyclic antidepressants). If these are not effective, then sodium oxybate – taken at bedtime and in the middle of the night – can be used.[86]

References

1. Bliwise DL, Scullin MK. Normal aging. In: Kryger MH, Roth T, Dement WC (eds.) *Principles and Practice of Sleep Medicine.* 6th ed. Philadelphia: Elsevier; 2017: 25–38.
2. Everson CA, Bergmann BM, Rechtschaffen A. Sleep deprivation in the rat: III. total sleep deprivation. *Sleep* 1989;12(1):13–21. pubmed.ncbi.nlm.nih.gov/2928622/ (accessed 7 November 2021).
3. Arrigoni E, Fuller PM. An overview of sleep: physiology and neuroanatomy. In: Barkoukis TJ, Matheson JK, Ferber R, et al. (eds.) *Therapy in Sleep Medicine.* Philadelphia: Elsevier Inc.; 2012: 43–61.
4. Lee-Chiong T. *Sleep Medicine: Essentials and Review.* Oxford: Oxford University Press; 2008.
5. van de Castle RL. *Our Dreaming Mind.* New York: Ballantine Books; 1995.
6. Gehrman PR, Thase ME, Riemann D, et al. Depressive disorders. In: Winkelman J, Plante DT (eds.) *Foundations of Psychiatric Sleep Medicine.* Cambridge: Cambridge University Press; 2010: 247–65. www.cambridge.org/core/product/identifier/9780511777493%23c51511-15-2/type/book_part (accessed 14 November 2021).
7. Plante DT, Winkelman JW. Polysomnographic features of medical and psychiatric disorders and their treatments. *Sleep Medicine Clinics* 2009;4(3):407–19.
8. Schilgen B, Tölle R. Partial sleep deprivation as therapy for depression. *Archives of General Psychiatry* 1980;37 (3):267–71.
9. Landsness EC, Goldstein MR, Peterson MJ, et al. Antidepressant effects of selective slow wave sleep deprivation in major depression: a high-density EEG investigation. *Journal of Psychiatric Research* 2011;45 (8):1019–26.
10. Watson CJ, Baghdoyan HA, Lydic R. Neuropharmacology of sleep and wakefulness: 2012 update. *Sleep Medicine Clinics.* 2012;7(3):469–86. www.ncbi.nlm.nih.gov/pmc/articles/PMC3496285/ (accessed 8 September 2023).
11. McGinty D, Szymusiak R. Chapter 7 – Neural control of sleep in mammals. In: Krieger M, Roth T, Dement WC (eds.) *Principles and Practice of Sleep Medicine.* 6th ed. Philadelphia: Elsevier; 2017: 62–77.
12. Borbély AA, Daan S, Wirz-Justice A, et al. The two-process model of sleep regulation: a reappraisal. *Journal of Sleep Research* 2016;25(2):131–43.
13. Pack AI, Keenan BT, Byrne EM, et al. Chapter 31 – Genetics and Genomic Basis of Sleep Disorders in Humans. In: Krieger M, Roth T, Dement WC (eds.) *Principles and Practice of Sleep Medicine.* 6th ed. Philadelphia: Elsevier; 2017: 322–39.
14. Krauchi K, Deboer T. Thermoregulation in sleep and hibernation. In: Krieger M, Roth T, Dement WC (eds.) *Principles and Practice of Sleep Medicine.* 6th ed. Philadelphia: Elsevier; 2017: 220–8.
15. Kosky C. Sleep investigations. In: Selsick H (ed.) *Sleep Disorders in Psychiatric Patients.* Berlin, Heidelberg: Springer Berlin Heidelberg; 2018: 63–83. link.springer.com/10.1007/978-3-642-54836-9_4 (accessed 14 March 2019).
16. Kubala AG, Barone Gibbs B, Buysse DJ, et al. Field-based measurement of sleep: agreement between six commercial activity monitors and a validated accelerometer. *Behavioral Sleep Medicine* 2019;18(5):637–52. www.tandfonline.com/doi/abs/10.1080/15402002.2019.1651316 (accessed 15 November 2021).
17. American Academy of Sleep Medicine. *International Classification of Sleep Disorders – Third Edition (ICSD-3).* Darien, IL: AASM Resource Library; 2014.
18. Vgontzas AN, Fernandez-Mendoza J, Liao D, et al. Insomnia with objective short sleep duration: the most biologically severe phenotype of the disorder. *Sleep Medicine Reviews* 2013;17(4):241–54.
19. Katz D, McHorney C. The relationship between insomnia and health-related quality of life in patients with chronic illness. *The Journal of Family Practice.* 2002;51(3):229–35.

20. Lichstein KL, Taylor DJ, McCrae CS, et al. Insomnia: epidemiology and risk factors. In: Krieger M, Roth T, Dement WC (eds.) *Principles and Practice of Sleep Medicine*. 6th ed. Philadelphia: Elsevier; 2017: 761–8.
21. Fleming JAE. Insomnia: epidemiology, subtypes, and relationship to psychiatric disorders. In: Selsick H (ed.) *Sleep Disorders in Psychiatric Patients*. Berlin, Heidelberg: Springer Berlin Heidelberg; 2018: 99–107. link.springer.com/10.1007/978-3-642-54836-9_6 (accessed 14 March 2019).
22. Franzen PL, Buysse DJ. Sleep disturbances and depression: risk relationships for subsequent depression and therapeutic implications. *Dialogues in Clinical Neuroscience* 2008;10(4):473–81.
23. Chang PP, Ford DE, Mead LA, et al. Insomnia in young men and subsequent depression: the Johns Hopkins Precursors Study. *American Journal of Epidemiology* 1997;146(2):105–14. academic.oup.com/aje/article-lookup/doi/10.1093/oxfordjournals.aje.a009241 (accessed 27 December 2017).
24. Ong JC, Arnedt JT, Gehrman PR. Insomnia diagnosis, assessment, and evaluation. In: Krieger M, Roth T, Dement WC (eds.) *Principles and Practice of Sleep Medicine*. 6th ed. Philadelphia: Elsevier; 2017: 785–93.
25. Schonmann Y, Goren O, Bareket R, et al. Chronic hypnotic use at 10 years – does the brand matter? *European Journal of Clinical Pharmacology* 2018;74(12):1623–31. link.springer.com/article/10.1007/s00228-018-2531-4 (accessed 11 May 2021).
26. Roth T, Walsh JK, Krystal A, et al. An evaluation of the efficacy and safety of eszopiclone over 12 months in patients with chronic primary insomnia. *Sleep Medicine* 2005;6(6):487–95.
27. Roehrs TA, Randall S, Harris E, et al. Twelve months of nightly zolpidem does not lead to dose escalation: a prospective placebo-controlled study. *Sleep* 2011;34(2):207–12.
28. Wilson S, Anderson K, Baldwin D, et al. British Association for Psychopharmacology consensus statement on evidence-based treatment of insomnia, parasomnias and circadian rhythm disorders: an update. *Journal of Psychopharmacology* 2019;33(8):923–47.
29. Riemann D, Perlis ML. The treatments of chronic insomnia: a review of benzodiazepine receptor agonists and psychological and behavioral therapies. *Sleep Medicine Reviews* 2009;13(3):205–14.
30. Roehrs T, Roth T. Insomnia pharmacotherapy. *Neurotherapeutics* 2012;9(4):728. link.springer.com/article/10.1007/s13311-012-0148-3 (accessed 8 September 2023).
31. Howland RH. Sleep interventions for the treatment of depression. *Journal of Psychosocial Nursing and Mental Health Services* 2011;49:17–20.
32. Krystal A, Fava M, Rubens R, et al. Evaluation of eszopiclone discontinuation after cotherapy with fluoxetine for insomnia with coexisting depression. *Journal of Clinical Sleep Medicine* 2007;3(1):48–55.
33. Jindal RD. Insomnia in patients with depression: some pathophysiological and treatment considerations. *CNS Drugs* 2009;23(4):309–29. link.springer.com/article/10.2165/00023210-200923040-00004.
34. Trauer JM, Qian MY, Doyle JS, et al. Cognitive behavioral therapy for chronic insomnia: a systematic review and meta-analysis. *Annals of Internal Medicine* 2015;163(3):191–204.
35. Bathgate CJ, Edinger JD, Krystal AD. Insomnia patients with objective short sleep duration have a blunted response to cognitive behavioral therapy for insomnia. *Sleep* 2017;40(1).
36. Rybarczyk B, Lund HG. Comorbid insomnia. *Clinics in Sleep Medicine* 2018;4(4):571–82. dx.doi.org/10.1016/j.jsmc.2009.07.010.
37. Edinger JD, Olsen MK, Stechuchak KM, et al. Cognitive behavioral therapy for patients with primary insomnia or insomnia associated predominantly with mixed psychiatric disorders: a randomized clinical trial. *Sleep* 2009;32(4):499–510.
38. Harvey AG, Soehner AM, Kaplan KA, et al. Treating insomnia improves mood state, sleep, and functioning in bipolar disorder: a pilot randomized controlled trial. *Journal of Consulting and Clinical Psychology* 2015;83(3):564–77. doi.apa.org/getdoi.cfm?doi=10.1037/a0038655 (accessed 14 January 2018).
39. Ulmer CS, Edinger JD, Calhoun PS. A multi-component cognitive-behavioral intervention for sleep disturbance in Veterans with PTSD: A pilot study. *Journal of Clinical Sleep Medicine* 2011;7(1):57–68.
40. Myers E, Startup H, Freeman D. Cognitive behavioural treatment of insomnia in individuals with persistent persecutory delusions: a pilot trial. *Journal of Behavior Therapy and Experimental Psychiatry* 2011;42(3):330–6.
41. Cunningham JEA, Shapiro CM. Cognitive behavioural therapy for insomnia (CBT-I) to treat depression: a systematic review. *Journal of Psychosomatic Research* 2018;106:1–12.
42. Blom K, Jernelöv S, Rück C, et al. Three-year follow-up comparing cognitive behavioral therapy for depression to cognitive behavioral therapy for insomnia, for patients with both diagnoses. *Sleep* 2017;40(8).
43. Cogen JD, Loghmanee DA. Sleep related movement disorders. In: Sheldon SH, Ferber R, Kryger MH, et al. (eds.) *Principles and Practice of Pediatric Sleep Medicine*. 2nd ed. London: Elsevier Saunders; 2014: 333–6.
44. Allen RP. Restless legs syndrome/Willis Ekbom disease: evaluation and treatment. *International Review of Psychiatry* 2014;26(2):248–62.
45. Hornyak M, Scholz H, Kohnen R, et al. What treatment works best for restless legs syndrome? Meta-analyses of dopaminergic and non-dopaminergic medications. *Sleep Medicine Reviews* 2014;18(2):153–64. dx.doi.org/10.1016/j.smrv.2013.03.004.
46. Durmer JS. Restless legs syndrome, periodic leg movements and periodic limb movement disorder. In: Sheldon SH, Ferber R, Kryger MH, et al. (eds.) *Principles and Practice of Pediatric Sleep Medicine*, 2nd ed. London: Elsevier Saunders; 2014: 337–50.
47. Becker PM. The biopsychosocial effects of restless legs syndrome (RLS). *Neuropsychiatric Disease and Treatment* 2006;2(4):505–12.
48. Castaño-De La Mota C, Moreno-Acero N, Losada-Del Pozo R, et al. Restless legs syndrome in patients diagnosed with attention deficit hyperactivity disorder. *Revista de Neurologia* 2017;64(7):299–304. europepmc.org/article/med/28345734 (accessed 24 May 2021).
49. Ferri R, Lanuzza B, Cosentino FII, et al. A single question for the rapid screening of restless legs syndrome in

the neurological clinical practice. *European Journal of Neurology* 2007;14 (9):1016–21.

50. Klingelhoefer L, Bhattacharya K, Reichmann H. Restless legs syndrome. *Clinical Medicine Journal* 2016;16 (4):379–82.
51. Balaban H, Yildiz OK, Çil G, et al. Serum 25-hydroxyvitamin D levels in restless legs syndrome patients. *Sleep Medicine* 2012;13(7):953–7.
52. Hornyak M, Scholz H, Kohnen R, et al. What treatment works best for restless legs syndrome? Meta-analyses of dopaminergic and non-dopaminergic medications. *Sleep Medicine Reviews* 2014;18(2):153–64.
53. Deak MC, Winkelman JW. The pharmacologic management of restless legs syndrome and periodic leg movement disorder. *Sleep Medicine Clinics* 2010;5(4):675–87. linkinghub .elsevier.com/retrieve/pii/ S1556407X10000913 (accessed 29 March 2013).
54. Garcia-borreguero D, Silber MH, Winkelman JW, et al. Guidelines for the first-line treatment of restless legs syndrome/Willis-Ekbom disease, prevention and treatment of dopaminergic augmentation: a combined task force of the IRLSSG, EURLSSG, and the RLS-foundation. *Sleep Medicine* 2016;21:1–11. dx.doi .org/10.1016/j.sleep.2016.01.017.
55. Amos LB, Grekowicz ML, Kuhn EM, et al. Treatment of pediatric restless legs syndrome. *Clinical Pediatrics* 2014;53 (4):331–6. journals.sagepub.com/doi/ abs/10.1177/0009922813507997 (accessed 24 May 2021).
56. Selsick H, O'Regan D. Sleep disorders in psychiatry. *BJPsych Advances* 2018;24 (4):273–83. www.cambridge.org/core/ product/identifier/S2056467818000087/ type/journal_article (accessed 3 December 2018).
57. Kripke DF, Rex KM, Ancoli-Israel S, et al. Delayed sleep phase cases and controls. *Journal of Circadian Rhythms* 2008;6:1–14.
58. Wirz-Justice A. Diurnal variation of depressive symptoms. *Dialogues in Clinical Neuroscience* 2008;10 (3):337–43. www.tandfonline.com/doi/ full/10.31887/DCNS.2008.10.3/ awjustice.
59. Borodkin K, Dagan Y. Circadian rhythm disorders. In: Winkelman J, Plante D (eds.) *Foundations of Psychiatric Sleep Medicine.* Cambridge: Cambridge University Press; 2010: 186–202.
60. Poon YPYP, Kan CK, Yeung WF, et al. Delayed sleep-wake phase disorder and delayed sleep-wake phase in schizophrenia: clinical and functional correlates. *Schizophrenia Research* 2018;202(2018):412–3. doi.org/10.1016/ j.schres.2018.06.057.
61. Morgenthaler TI, Lee-Chiong T, Alessi C, et al. Practice parameters for the clinical evaluation and treatment of circadian rhythm sleep disorders: an American Academy of Sleep Medicine report. *Sleep* 2007;30(11):1445–59.
62. van Geijlswijk IM, Korzilius HPLM, Smits MG. The use of exogenous melatonin in delayed sleep phase disorder: a meta-analysis. *Sleep* 2010;33 (12):1605–14.
63. Dodson ER, Zee PC. Therapeutics for circadian rhythm sleep disorders. *Sleep Medicine Clinics* 2010;5(4):701–15. www.ncbi.nlm.nih.gov/pmc/articles/ PMC3020104/ (accessed 8 September 2023).
64. Leschziner G. Nocturnal Brain: Tales of Nightmares and Neuroscience. London: Simon & Schuster UK; 2019.
65. Eriksson S, Walker M. Non-REM parasomnias and REM sleep behaviour disorder. In: Selsick H (ed.) *Sleep Disorders in Psychiatric Patients.* Berlin, Heidelberg: Springer Berlin Heidelberg; 2018: 263–76. link.springer.com/10 .1007/978-3-642-54836-9_14 (accessed 14 March 2019).
66. Hurwitz TD, Schenck CH. Parasomnias. In: Winkelman J, Plante D (eds.) *Foundations of Psychiatric Sleep Medicine.* Cambridge: Cambridge University Press; 2010: 160–85.
67. Johnson CM, Lerner M. Amelioration of infant sleep disturbances: II. effects of scheduled awakenings by compliant parents. *Infant Mental Health Journal* 1985;6(1):21–30. onlinelibrary.wiley .com/doi/abs/10.1002/1097-0355% 28198521%296%3A1%3C21%3A% 3AAID-IMHJ2280060105%3E3.0.CO% 3B2-Q (accessed 26 May 2021).
68. Bruni O, Ferri R, Miano S, et al. L -5-Hydroxytryptophan treatment of sleep terrors in children. *European Journal of Pediatrics* 2004;163(7):402–7. link .springer.com/article/10.1007/s00431-004-1444-7 (accessed 26 May 2021).
69. Aurora RN, Zak RS, Auerbach SH, et al. Best practice guide for the treatment of nightmare disorder in adults. *Journal of Clinical Sleep Medicine* 2010;6 (4):389–401.
70. Arnulf I. Nightmares and dream disturbances. In: Kryger MH, Roth T, Dement WC (eds.) *Principles and Practice of Sleep Medicine*, 6th ed. Philadelphia: Elsevier; 2017: 1002–10.
71. Bernert RA, Nadorff MR. Sleep disturbances and suicide risk. *Sleep Medicine Clinics* 2015;10(1):35–9. dx .doi.org/10.1016/j.jsmc.2014.11.004.
72. Sjöström N, Waern M, Hetta J. Nightmares and sleep disturbances in relation to suicidality in suicide attempters. *Sleep* 2007;30(1):91–5.
73. Bahammam AS, Almeneessier AS. Dreams and nightmares in patients with obstructive sleep apnea: a review. *Frontiers in Neurology* 2019;10:1127.
74. Iranzo A, Santamaria J, Tolosa E. The clinical and pathophysiological relevance of REM sleep behavior disorder in neurodegenerative diseases. *Sleep Medicine Reviews* 2009;13 (6):385–401. dx.doi.org/10.1016/j.smrv .2008.11.003.
75. Schenck CH, Boeve BF, Mahowald MW. Delayed emergence of a parkinsonian disorder or dementia in 81% of older men initially diagnosed with idiopathic rapid eye movement sleep behavior disorder: a 16-year update on a previously reported series. *Sleep Medicine* 2013;14(8):744–8. www .sciencedirect.com/science/article/pii/ S1389945712003814 (accessed 20 August 2021).
76. Postuma RB, Arnulf I, Hogl B, et al. A single-question screen for rapid eye movement sleep behavior disorder: a multicenter validation study. *Movement Disorders* 2012;27(7):913–6.
77. Aurora RN, Zak RS, Maganti RK, et al. Best practice guide for the treatment of REM sleep behavior disorder (RBD). *Journal of Clinical Sleep Medicine* 2010;6(1):85–95.
78. Sharpless BA, Doghramji K. Sleep Paralysis: Historical, Psychological, and Medical Perspectives. Oxford: Oxford University Press; 2015.
79. Sharpless BA. A clinician's guide to recurrent isolated sleep paralysis. *Neuropsychiatric Disease and Treatment* 2016;12:1761–7. www.dovepress.com/a-clinicianrsquos-guide-to-recurrent-

isolated-sleep-paralysis-peer-reviewed-article-NDT (accessed 20 August 2021).

80. Lopresti AL, Drummond PD. Obesity and psychiatric disorders: Commonalities in dysregulated biological pathways and their implications for treatment. *Progress in Neuro-Psychopharmacology and Biological Psychiatry* 2013 Aug 1;45:92–9.

81. Jokic R. Obstructive sleep apnoea. In: Selsick H (ed.) *Sleep Disorders in Psychiatric Patients*. Berlin, Heidelberg: Springer Berlin Heidelberg; 2018: 213–38. link.springer.com/10.1007/978-3-642-54836-9_12

82. Krysta K, Bratek A, Zawada K, et al. Cognitive deficits in adults with obstructive sleep apnea compared to children and adolescents. *Journal of Neural Transmission* 2017;124(Suppl 1):187–201.

83. Dunietz GL, Chervin RD, Burke JF, et al. Obstructive sleep apnea treatment and dementia risk in older adults. *Sleep* 2021;44(9).

84. Morrell M. Changes in brain morphology associated with obstructive sleep apnea. *Sleep Medicine* 2003;4(5):451–4. linkinghub.elsevier.com/retrieve/pii/S138994570300159X (accessed 4 June 2014).

85. Pang KP, Gourin CG, Terris DJ. A comparison of polysomnography and the WatchPAT in the diagnosis of obstructive sleep apnea. *Otolaryngology – Head and Neck Surgery* 2007;137(4):665–8. journals.sagepub.com/doi/abs/10.1016/j.otohns.2007.03.015 (accessed 18 November 2021).

86. Shahid A, Shen J, Shapiro CM. Central hypersomnias. In: Selsick H (ed.) *Sleep Disorders in Psychiatric Patients*. Berlin, Heidelberg: Springer Berlin Heidelberg; 2018: 239–62. link.springer.com/10.1007/978-3-642-54836-9_13 (accessed 4 March 2019).

87. Murru A, Guiso G, Barbuti M, et al. The implications of hypersomnia in the context of major depression: results from a large, international, observational study. *European Neuropsychopharmacology* 2019;29(4):471–81.

88. Fortuyn HAD, Lappenschaar MA, Furer JW, et al. Anxiety and mood disorders in narcolepsy: a case-control study. *General Hospital Psychiatry* 2010;32(1):49–56.

89. Cao MT, Guilleminault C. Narcolepsy: diagnosis and management. In: Krieger M, Roth T, Dement WC (eds.) *Principles and Practice of Sleep Medicine*. 6th ed. Philadelphia: Elsevier; 2017: 873–82.

90. Dauvilliers Y, Bassetti C, Lammers GJ, et al. Pitolisant versus placebo or modafinil in patients with narcolepsy: a double-blind, randomised trial. *The Lancet Neurology* 2013;12(11):1068–75.

91. Subedi R, Singh R, Thakur RK, et al. Efficacy and safety of solriamfetol for excessive daytime sleepiness in narcolepsy and obstructive sleep apnea: a systematic review and meta-analysis of clinical trials. *Sleep Medicine* 2020;75:510–21.

Chapter 12

Eating Disorders*

Agnes Ayton

Introduction

Eating disorders are complex and serious illnesses that can result in physical and psychiatric comorbidities, medical emergencies and progressive health consequences. Although general psychiatrists may be called upon to assist in emergencies or differential diagnoses, training in this area has been limited. The author attempts to fill the gap by providing a summary of the most recent advances in the field of eating disorders in this chapter to help orient trainees and general psychiatrists. This chapter provides an overview of the most recent changes to the DSM-5 and ICD-11 diagnostic categories for eating disorders, as well as their epidemiology, aetiology and treatment, including the management of complications and life-threatening medical emergencies.

The chapter summarises recent advances in the genetic and neurobiological understanding of eating disorders, as well as emerging new research. These scientific advances have the potential to contribute to the development of new, more-effective eating disorder treatments in the future.

Feeding and eating disorders are characterised by a persistent disturbance of eating or eating-related behaviours that lead to decreased food consumption or absorption and significantly compromised physical health and psychosocial functioning. The *Diagnostic and Statistical Manual of Mental Disorders,* 5th edition (DSM-5)[1] introduced major changes in how eating disorders are classified. For the first time, childhood feeding and adult eating disorders are combined into a single category in DSM-5, and the International Classification of Diseases, 11th Revision (ICD-11)[2] follows the same structure. In addition to anorexia nervosa (AN) and bulimia nervosa (BN), binge eating disorder (BED) and avoidant restrictive food intake disorder (ARFID) were introduced. The AN criteria changed dramatically, whereas the BN criteria changed only slightly. The new category 'other specific feeding and eating disorders (OSFED)' now includes subtypes of AN, BN and BED, while the remaining group 'eating disorders not otherwise specified' has been renamed 'unspecified feeding or eating disorders (UFED)'. For a comparison, see Table 12.1.

Myths and Truths about Eating Disorders

Eating disorders are often stigmatised, both within health care and in society at large. In 2015, the Academy for Eating Disorders (AED) and several international advocacy groups released a document titled 'Nine Truths About Eating Disorders' to dispel common myths about eating disorders. The science underlying the nine truths is summarised in Table 12.2.

Epidemiology of Eating Disorders

Eating disorders are a global health concern. In Western societies, a significant proportion of young people and adults report having an eating disorder. A recent systematic review reported lifetime DSM-5 AN in 0.8–6.3% of women and 0.1–0.3% of men, BN by 0.8–2.6% of women and 0.1–0.2% of men, BED by 0.6–6.1% of women and 0.3–0.7% of men, other specified feeding or eating disorders by 0.6–11.5% of women and 0.2–0.3% of men, and unspecified by 0.2–4.7% of women and 0–1.6% of men. Gender and sexual minorities were especially vulnerable. Recent studies from Eastern Europe, Asia and Latin America revealed comparable high prevalence rates, and the incidence of eating disorders has continued to rise during the Covid-19 pandemic.[4]

Time Trends and Population Demographics

In the UK, there has not been a comprehensive population-based epidemiological study of eating disorders. The closest information we have is from the 2007 Adult Psychiatric Morbidity Survey and the 2019 Health Survey in England by NHS Digital.[5] Both of these studies used the SCOFF screening questionnaire,[6] which does not distinguish between the different types of eating disorders. SCOFF>2 indicates eating disorders (Box 12.1).[6]

In the 2019 Health Survey, 16% of adults aged 16 and over (19% of women and 13% of men) screened positive for a possible eating disorder in England. This included 4% (5% of women and 3% of men) who reported that their feelings about food interfered with their ability to work, meet personal responsibilities or enjoy a social life.[5] This represents a nearly three-fold increase since the 2007 APMS,[7] with the greatest

* Acknowledgements to James Downs, expert by experience; George Coates and Clair Gilbert, higher trainees, for their comments; and Janet Treasure for material adapted and utilised from her chapter in the 2nd edition of Seminars in General Adult Psychiatry.

Table 12.1 Similarities and differences between current and recent diagnostic systems for eating disorders

	ICD-10	DSM-5	ICD-11
Anorexia nervosa	F50.0 Anorexia nervosa F50.1 Atypical anorexia nervosa	Anorexia nervosa BMI<18.5 or 5th centile for children Subtypes: Restrictive Binge–purging Severity: Mild: BMI:17–18.5 Moderate: 16–16.9 Severe: BMI:15–15.9 Extreme: BMI<15 Full or partial remission	6B80 Anorexia nervosa 6B80.0 Anorexia nervosa with significantly low body weight (BMI between 14–18.5, or for children between 3rd and 5th centile) 6B80.1 Anorexia nervosa with dangerously low body weight (BMI<14, or <3rd centile) 6B80.2 Anorexia nervosa in recovery with normal body weight (one year) 6B80.Y Other specified anorexia nervosa 6B80.Z Anorexia nervosa, unspecified 6B80.x0 Restricting pattern 6B80.x1 Binge-purge pattern
Bulimia nervosa (BN)	F50.2 Bulimia nervosa F50.3 Atypical bulimia nervosa	Bulimia nervosa 307.51 Severity (frequency of compensatory behaviours): Mild: 1–3/week. Moderate: 4–7/week Severe: 8–13/ week. Extreme: >14/week. Full or partial remission	6B81 Bulimia nervosa
Binge eating disorder (BED)	F50.4 Overeating associated with other psychological disturbances	Binge eating disorder 307.51 Severity (frequency of binges): Mild: 1–3/week. Moderate: 4–7/week Severe: 8–13/ week. Extreme: >14/week. Full or Partial remission	6B82 Binge eating disorder
Rumination disorder	F50.5 Vomiting associated with other psychological disturbances	Rumination Disorder 307.53	6B85 Rumination-regurgitation disorder
PICA	F98.3 Pica of infancy and childhood	Pica	6B84 Pica
ARFID	F98.2 Feeding disorder of infancy and childhood Including: Rumination disorder of problems of new-born (P92.-)	Avoidant/restrictive food intake disorder Diagnostic criteria 307.59	6B83 Avoidant-restrictive food intake disorder
OSFED	F50.8 Other eating disorders Including: Pica in adults Psychogenic loss of appetite F50.9 Eating disorder, unspecified	Atypical anorexia nervosa: All of the criteria for anorexia nervosa are met except that, despite significant weight loss, the individual's weight is within or above the normal range. 2. Bulimia nervosa (of low frequency and/or limited duration) 3. Binge eating disorder (of low frequency and/or limited duration) 4. Purging disorder 5. Night eating syndrome	6B8Y Other specified feeding or eating disorders
UFED		Unspecified feeding or eating disorder	6B8Z Feeding or eating disorders, unspecified

increase occurring among young and middle-aged men. In parallel, the hospital admissions for severe eating disorders have quadrupled since 2007 (Figure 12.1).[8]

These findings may be surprising but are consistent with international epidemiological data.[9,10]

The 2019 Health Survey found that those with severe obesity and the lowest social income have the highest rates of eating disorders. This is consistent with international trends.[11] Furthermore, certain groups – such as people with diabetes, people in aesthetic sports (i.e. those that are focused

Table 12.2 The explanations behind the nine truths about eating disorders[3]

AED truths	Evidence & clinical implications
Truth 1: Many people with eating disorders look healthy yet may be extremely ill.	Eating disorders pose physical, psychological and social risks. Eating disorders cause medical consequences in the cardiovascular, gastrointestinal, musculoskeletal, dermatologic, endocrine, haematological and neurological systems. Many major somatic effects of eating disorders are invisible (including life-threatening electrolytes or glucose abnormalities, cardiovascular or neurological complications). Clinicians should screen for eating disorders.
Truth 2: Families are not to blame and can be the patients' and providers' best allies in treatment.	The assumption that parental characteristics or family dynamics are necessary and sufficient for the development of eating disorders (i.e. 'families are to blame') is an outdated psychological model that disregards contemporary aetiological evidence. In contrast, current guidelines recommend family-based treatment (FBT), in which parents reclaim control over their child's eating, as first-line treatment for adolescents with anorexia nervosa (AN). Family involvement can be also very helpful in supporting adults.
Truth 3: An eating disorder diagnosis is a health crisis that disrupts personal and family functioning.	An eating disorder is a severe health crisis that impacts every aspect of a person's life. Eating disorders are linked to developmental delays, psychological distress, isolation, stigma and difficulties with family and other interpersonal relationships. They also affect all aspects of social and economic wellbeing and can prevent healthy childhood and adolescent development. Clinicians should approach patients and families with compassion.
Truth 4: Eating disorders are not choices, but serious biologically influenced illnesses.	Neurobiological studies reveal altered reward pathways and gut-brain interaction, resulting in impaired appetite, high level of anxiety and self-control regulation. In addition, metabolic vulnerabilities have recently been identified in genetic studies. Chronic malnutrition is progressively harmful for all systems in the body.
Truth 5: Eating disorders affect people of all genders, ages, races, ethnicities, body shapes and weights, sexual orientations and socioeconomic statuses.	Although eating disorders are more common in females, they can affect both men and women, people of all ages and people of all races and ethnicities. LGBT people are especially vulnerable to eating disorders. It is important to recognise that men and minority groups are less likely to seek treatment, less likely to be diagnosed with an eating disorder despite presenting with identical symptoms as women, and less likely to access treatment despite having comparable clinical severity. Eating disorders are most common among people with severe obesity and low social classes.
Truth 6: Eating disorders carry an increased risk for both suicide and medical complications.	Eating disorders have an increased risk of premature mortality due to complications of malnutrition and suicide. Research indicates that the co-occurrence of eating disorders and suicide attempts may be attributable in part to common genetic variables. Clinicians should explore suicide risk in eating disorders and vice versa.
Truth 7: Genes and environment play important roles in the development of eating disorders.	Genes play a role in the familial occurrence of eating disorders. When compared to the general population, having a family history of anorexia nervosa raises the likelihood of developing anorexia four-fold. Twin studies have shown a significant genetic contribution in AN, BN, BED and ARFID.
Truth 8: Genes alone do not predict who will develop eating disorders.	Eating disorders are multifactorial in origin. Cultural and environmental factors can cause eating disorders in genetically predisposed people. The combination of environmental and protective factors affects a person's individual risk. According to twin studies, the risk of eating disorders is approximately 50% genetic, 40% non-shared and 10% shared environmental. Evidence-based treatment focusses on ongoing maintaining factors specific to the individual.
Truth 9: Full recovery from an eating disorder is possible. Early detection and intervention are important.	A substantial proportion of individuals with eating disorders achieve recovery, some without seeking treatment. Five-year clinical recovery rates have been estimated at 67% for AN and 55% for BN. By 10 years after onset, 70% of individuals recover. Treatment for an eating disorder typically includes psychological intervention and may include medication. For AN, weight restoration is the essential first step in treatment, which needs to be integrated with evidence-based psychological treatment.

on weight or appearance, such as ice skating, horse riding and marathon running), or those in performing arts – have a higher risk of eating disorders.[12] Sexual minority adults have higher rates of AN, BN and binge eating disorder than cisgender heterosexual adults. In a recent US study, the lifetime prevalence of eating disorders was 10.5% for transgender men and 8.1% for transgender women, including AN (4.2 and 4.1%) and BN (3.2 and 2.9%), respectively.[13] Body dissatisfaction may be a major stressor for transgender people. Treatment for gender dysphoria is helpful to improve body satisfaction.[14]

What societal factors changed in the last decades to cause the rise of eating disorders? The recent rise is clearly due to environmental changes. Eating disorders are linked to abuse and trauma, but they don't explain the rising trends.

Historically, it has been hypothesised that eating disorders are more prevalent in cultures that value thinness.[15] This was a very influential theory, but it has been called into question with the observation of increasing worldwide trends in eating disorders in parallel with industrialisation and the obesity epidemic.[16] One of the most significant changes over the past few decades has been the change in the food environment with the rise of industrial food processing, which has led to the replacement of traditional eating patterns.[17] Ultra-processed foods have an impact on gut microbiota, which result in appetite dysregulation and contribute to overeating and obesity.[18,19] In parallel, the diet and fitness industry has amplified the calorie in and calorie out hypothesis, which is also reinforced by digital technologies and social media, creating a perfect storm. Many people with eating disorders use smartphones and wearable devices to control their calories and exercise, which may reinforce the psychopathology.[20]

Box 12.1 SCOFF screening questionnaire

During the last year...

- have you lost more than one stone in a three-month period?
- have you made yourself be sick because you felt uncomfortably full?
- did you worry you had lost control over how much you eat?
- did you believe yourself to be fat when others said you were too thin?
- would you say food dominated your life?

The pandemic has had a further significant impact on the prevalence and severity of eating disorders across the age range.[4] The next Adult Psychiatric Morbidity Survey, due to be published in 2024, will give a more detailed picture of the changing trends in the UK.

Eating Disorders in Males

Recent research suggests that the prevalence of eating disorders among men is increasing. For example, the 2019 Health Survey found that the rate of self-reported eating disorders in young and middle-aged men has almost quadrupled since 2007. The cause is unknown, but a drive for muscularity has been identified as a specific concern in males.[21] Studies show that men with eating disorders often face unique challenges in seeking help, including stigma, a lack of awareness and understanding, and a lack of culturally sensitive treatment options.[22]

Anorexia nervosa is the least common but most dangerous form of eating disorder in men. A recent case-controlled study found that males with AN or BN had a lower rate of long-term survival than females.[23] This could be because men have lower fat reserves than women due to their different body composition. The mortality rate for inpatients with eating disorders, especially AN, is the highest.[24] However, the impact of BN, BED and OSFED can be severe. Certain groups, such as elite athletes or performance artists, are at higher risk of eating disorders. It is important for clinicians and services to recognise the signs and symptoms of eating disorders in men and to provide support and resources for those who need help without discrimination.

The Impact of Eating Disorders on the Individual and Wider Society

Eating is essential for life, so it should not be surprising that eating disorders and disordered eating have significant impact on an individual's nutritional status, physical and mental

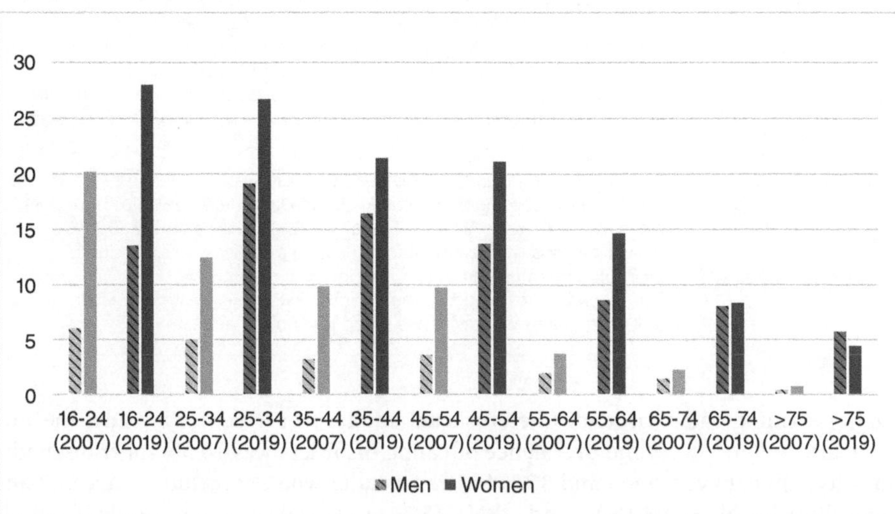

Figure 12.1 Changes of proportion of population screening positive for an eating disorder between 2007–2019 in adults over age 16 years.

health, social functioning, and – in the case of children – growth and development. A review of recent studies on the global burden of eating disorders in terms of mortality, disability, quality of life, economic cost and family burden in comparison to those without eating disorders estimated that over 3,300,000,000 healthy life years are lost annually due to eating disorders.[25]

In contrast to other mental diseases, years lived with disability have increased in AN and BN. Despite improvements in treatment, the premature death rates of AN and BN remain high. People with AN continue to have a mortality risk that is more than five times higher than that of age-matched general population. The mortality risks for BN and BED are lower but still approximately double those of healthy controls. In individuals with an eating disorder, the quality of life is diminished, annual health care costs are 48 per cent higher than in the general population, the presence of mental health comorbidity is associated with 48 per cent lower annual earnings, the number of offspring is decreased, and the risk for adverse pregnancy and neonatal outcomes is increased.[25]

The financial cost of eating disorders to the individual and the wider society is high. In fiscal year 2018–2019, the estimated one-year societal costs of eating disorders in the US – including health system expenses, individual and family productivity costs, lost wellbeing and other economic costs – was $64.7 billion.

A recent UK study estimated that the annual cost of eating disorders to the UK economy was approximately £9 billion in 2019–2020.[159] These findings highlight the importance of primary prevention and screening to identify emerging or early eating disorders in primary care, schools and workplaces as well as providing access to early evidence-based treatment to reduce complications and societal costs.

The Biology of Eating Behaviours

Despite a recent acceleration of research, the complex neurobiology of eating behaviours is still not fully understood.[26] The biological mechanisms can be explored in animal models. The most well-known example is the activity-based anorexia model in mice, which begins with daily unlimited chow for two hours or less and is followed by a running wheel, resulting in compulsive-like running, appetite suppression, voluntary food restriction, decreased anxiety-like behaviour, severe weight loss and death without intervention. This results in hypothermia, oestrus loss, increased hypothalamic-pituitary-adrenal axis activity, anhedonia, ulcers, and humoral, CNS, cardiovascular and gastrointestinal (GI) dysfunction – a plausible model for the behavioural and physiological components of AN.

Binge-like eating in animals can be triggered by stress, home-cage chow restriction and intermittent palatable food access (cafeteria diet). Intermittent reinforcement models induce the most robust binge-like eating without obesity because rodents restrict chow intake in anticipation of palatable food, which is similar to clinical presentations in humans. The cafeteria diet has a profound impact on the gut microbiome, which leads to features of metabolic syndrome and increased eating behaviours through the microbiota-gut-brain axis.[27,28] Furthermore, the combination of fats and sugars – which do not occur in natural foods – can override normal satiety mechanisms and may be relevant to binge eating.[29]

Recently, Small's group has proposed a two-stage model that combines biological and psychosocial factors that influence eating behaviours.[30] The first system uses metabolic signals from the gut that reach the brain and directly reflects the nutritional value of foods. This nutrient-sensing system appears to be important in regulating striatal dopamine, determining food value and driving food choice without conscious involvement. Perceptions such as flavour and beliefs about the caloric content, cost and healthfulness of foods are additional determinants of food choices in the second, conscious system. The latter is dependent on circuits in the prefrontal and insular cortex. This model is highly relevant to our understanding of the pathomechanisms underlying eating disorders, where unconscious metabolic and conscious psychological factors frequently conflict.

The General Principles of Assessment and Treatment: NICE and SIGN Guidelines

The NICE[31] and the more recent SIGN guidelines[32] are clear that services and commissioners should ensure that all people with eating disorders, as well as their parents or carers, have equal access to eating disorder treatments (including self-referral) regardless of age, gender or gender identity, sexual orientation, socioeconomic status, religion, belief, culture, family origin or ethnicity, where they live and who they live with, or any physical or other mental health problems or disabilities. These principles remain aspirational, and many services struggle to meet them.[33] The implementation of these national guidelines will require local needs assessment and targeted funding. The American Psychiatric Association have recently updated their eating disorder guidelines.[34]

Assessment

Eating disorders affect the person's physical and mental health, and therefore, both psychiatric and physical assessments are essential.

Compassionate and sensitive communication skills are critical when working with people with eating disorders. Patients often find it difficult or distressing to discuss their problems with health care professionals and are vulnerable to stigma and shame. When assessing a person suspected of having an eating disorder, it's crucial to address any misconceptions. Clinicians should provide information about the disorder's nature, risks and effects, as well as potential therapies and their benefits and limitations.

When discussing a person's weight and appearance, clinicians should keep in mind that both the patient and carers

Box 12.2 Example questions to elicit eating disorder psychopathology and behaviours as part of a mental state examination

- Has your weight changed recently? (Amount and rate of weight loss)
- What factors have contributed to this? (Illness, medication, lifestyle changes, weight loss on purpose)
- Do you worry about your weight and shape?
- What have you tried to control your weight and shape? (Dietary restrictions, exercise, laxatives, purging and so on)
- Do you try to control your weight? How? (Fasting, cleansing, laxatives and other substances, exercise – type, volume, frequency)
- What do you eat on a typical day? (It is important to elucidate the details, such as asking about dietary rules, avoiding certain foods, daily calorie limits, diet products, bingeing episodes and volume)
- Do you have a target weight that you'd like to achieve? Why? What is stopping you from achieving that? What are the risks and benefits? (If the patient is underweight, ask how they would feel if their weight was restored to a normal body mass index (BMI) of 20–25)
- What do you think of your shape? Is there any part of your body that you are unhappy with?
- How has your life and relationships been affected by your eating problem?
- What would you like to change with treatment?

may feel guilty and responsible for the eating disorder. It is essential to show empathy, compassion and respect and to deliver information in a style that is appropriate for them, particularly for younger patients or people with neurodiversity.

As a general rule, it is best to start the interview with open questions and move to the specific details (Box 12.2). All psychiatric patients should be screened for eating disorders, as they are common and often unrecognised in people who are not underweight.

Collaboration with carers is essential at any age. Families and carers may experience high levels of anxiety and distress when their loved one is ill with an eating disorder. If a family member or carer cannot attend an assessment or review, it can be helpful to send them written information or direct them to high-quality websites like RCPsych, BEAT (www.beateatingdisorders.org.uk/) and FEAST (www.feast-ed.org/) as well as to self-help books.[35] The amount of work with the family is dependent on the individual's developmental stage; more intensive involvement is necessary for children and young people. In all cases, including the patient's family in the initial assessment is necessary because they will have important collateral information about the patient's premorbid functioning, strengths and difficulties. General information about the illness, as well as specific advice, should be provided to the family. These are included in evidence-based psychological treatment models. When there is a moderate to high medical risk, it is best to explain it to the family and make sure they know how to deal with it and what to do in an emergency.

Risks should be assessed based on nutritional intake, speed of weight loss, compensatory behaviours, comorbidities. physical examination and investigations.

Outcome Measurement

A structured interview, the Eating Disorder Examination, is regarded as the gold standard method to measure symptoms for research.[36] EDE-Q is the most commonly used self-rating scale, which can also be used for monitoring treatment outcomes, both for therapy progress and for research. The Clinical Impairment Assessment (CIA)[37] is a helpful measure of social impairment due to eating disorders. In addition, monitoring anxiety and depression is usually done by GAD-7 and PHQ (which are shared with IAPT services). The SCOFF questionnaire (Box 12.1) is a brief screening questionnaire that has been used in several UK epidemiological studies, such as the 2019 Health Survey.

Weight and height monitoring: Monitoring the patient's weight is essential when managing severe eating disorders, particularly AN. Collaborative weighing is an integral part of CBT-E at each session, and it needs to be done sensitively. Psychoeducation is an important aspect of this: the clinician needs to explain the range of healthy weight for the individual and also explore unhelpful beliefs about weight changes that may maintain the illness (e.g. 'a BMI of 20 is high', 'if I eat freshly cooked meals, my weight will shoot up', 'laxatives help me lose weight'). As most patients are extremely concerned about minute changes in weight, it is helpful to reduce the sensitivity of scales to 0.5 kg, as any more detail is clinically insignificant. Focusing on the detail can be counterproductive. When measuring a patient's height, it is essential to ensure that they are standing straight. In cases of spinal deformities or immobility, the length of the ulna can provide an estimate of the patient's premorbid height that can be used for BMI calculations. The frequency of monitoring depends on the level of risk and type of treatment.

Treatment

Evidence-based psychological treatments focus on individual or family maintaining factors.[32,38,39] Out of these, family therapy has been shown to be most effective for adolescents[40] and cognitive behavioural therapy for adults.[39] Both of them are recommended across the diagnostic spectrum in line with Fairburn's transdiagnostic model,[41,42] which suggests that all eating disorders share the basic psychopathology of overevaluation of weight and shape and the individual's control[42] and that addressing these issues is essential in treatment. Alternative psychological treatment options are also available for adults with AN.[43–45] These include the Maudsley Model of Anorexia Treatment for Adults (MANTRA), Specialist

Box 12.3 The summary of psychological treatments approved by NICE and SIGN

- **Anorexia nervosa**:
  - FT-AN (1 year), <18-year-olds CBT-E as an alternative (SIGN)
  - CBT-E (40 wks)
  - MANTRA (30 wks)
  - SSCM (20-40 wks)
  - Focal psychodynamic therapy (40 wks)
- **Bulimia nervosa:**
  - FT-BN or CBT-E for adolescents (SIGN)
  - Guided self-help (16 wks)
  - CBT-ED (20 wks)
  - FT-BN (6 months) <18-year-olds
- **Binge eating disorder:**
  - FT or CBT-E for adolescents (SIGN)
  - Guided self-help (16 wks)
  - Group CBT-ED

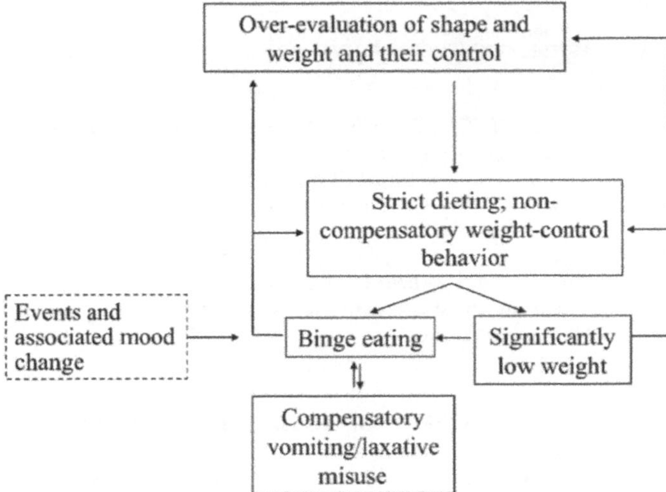

Figure 12.2 The transdiagnostic CBT-E formulation overview. Reproduced with permission from *Cognitive Behaviour Therapy and Eating Disorders* by Christopher G. Fairburn. Copyright 2008 by The Guilford Press.

Supportive Clinical Management (SSCM) and Focal Psychodynamic Therapy (FPT) for adults with AN. These will be discussed under the anorexia section. There is limited evidence for psychopharmacological treatment.[46]

People with eating disorders should receive evidence-based psychological treatment as soon as possible to reduce the risk of deterioration and complications. The content, structure and length of psychological treatments should be based on relevant manuals. Clinicians should have enough clinical supervision, and they should use standard outcome measures to track treatment response and progress. To ensure their competence, therapists should monitor treatment adherence (using, for example, session recordings and external auditing and scrutiny). The NICE and SIGN guidelines (see Box 12.3) recommend outpatient psychological treatment as first-line treatment, and clinicians are advised to consult other NICE guidelines for the management of comorbidities.

Transitions are known to increase patient risk; therefore, coordination of care is essential when a patient needs to transfer geographically or between services.[47]

Enhanced Cognitive Behavioural Therapy (CBT-E)

Cognitive behaviour therapy for eating disorders is the first-line recommended treatment across the diagnostic spectrum for adults, according to NICE and SIGN,[31,32] so we summarise the main principles here. Additional treatment options will be explored further within each diagnostic category. It was first developed by Professor Fairburn as an individual therapy for BN and tested in a number of randomised controlled trials.[48] It focusses on the personal maintaining factors of abnormal eating behaviours, as well as attitudes towards shape and weight.

CBT-E was revised in the early 2000s to make it appropriate for all types of eating disorders.[42] The resulting 'transdiagnostic' treatment is known as enhanced CBT. CBT-E is a flexible, personalised psychological model. It is based on the individual's formulation of their maintaining factors (www.CBTE.co/for-professionals/cbt-e-resources-and-handouts/) and can be modified as they progress. The CBT-E formulation diagram shows the main factors that keep the eating disorder going, and it can be adapted to fit the person's characteristics at the beginning of treatment (Figure 12.2).

CBT-E has been found to be effective for all types of eating disorders in adults,[49,50] has also been further developed for treating adolescents[51], and can offer a potential alternative to family-based therapy.[52]

CBT-E has been adapted for inpatient and day-care settings.[53]

CBT-E has four major goals:

- To engage patients in the treatment and involve them actively in the process of change
- To remove the eating disorder psychopathology and behaviours, such as dietary restraint and restriction (and low weight, if present), extreme weight-control behaviours and preoccupation with shape, weight and eating
- To correct the mechanisms maintaining the eating disorder psychopathology
- To ensure lasting change

Approximately 70 per cent of patients who are not significantly underweight (BN or BED) make a full recovery, and others respond partially.[50] Well-trained and supervised therapists produce better results. Longer duration of illness is predictive of a poorer prognosis across all diagnostic groups. This calls for further therapeutic research.

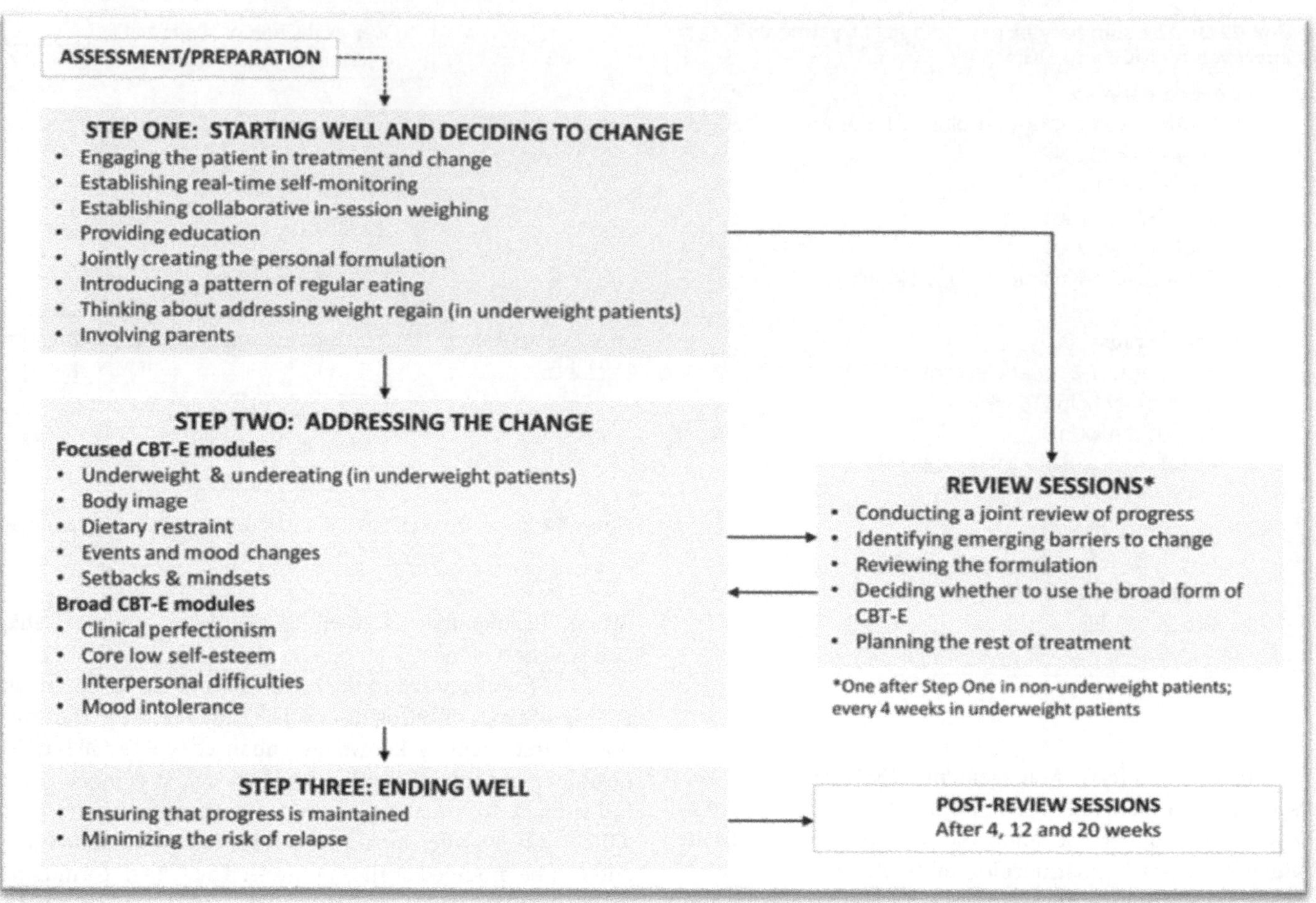

Figure 12.3 CBT-E process map. © Dalle Grave R, Eckhardt S, Calugi S, et al. A conceptual comparison of family-based treatment and enhanced cognitive behavior therapy in the treatment of adolescents with eating disorders. *Journal of Eating Disorders* 2019;7:42. doi.org/10.1186/s40337-019-0275-x. CC BY 4.0.

There is a treatment manual, self-help book and online training and handouts for clinicians available (www.credo-oxford.com/#topic6).

CBT-E has four stages (see the CBT-E map in Figure 12.3).

In Stage 1, the focus is on understanding and changing the person's eating pattern.

In Stage 2, progress is reviewed. Stage 3 involves weekly sessions that focus on the maintaining problems. Stage 4 focusses on the future after the therapy ends. For patients who are not significantly underweight, CBT-E is time-limited. It typically consists of an initial assessment consultation followed by twenty 50-minute therapy sessions spread out over 20 weeks, or 40 weeks for people who are underweight.

Comorbidities

All eating disorders have a high rate of comorbidities and complications. Common psychiatric comorbidities include affective and anxiety disorders, neurodevelopmental disorders, and suicidality across the diagnostic spectrum. Chronic malnutrition in AN leads to progressive multiorgan damage, which is reversible with weight restoration. Gastrointestinal and endocrine complications are common and will be discussed in more detail later. CBT-E has been adapted for managing comorbidities, and a manual is available for clinicians.[54]

Medical Emergencies in Eating Disorders

Severe eating disorders can present in life-threatening emergencies and, sadly, can result in avoidable deaths.[55] This is partially due to insufficient training during undergraduate and postgraduate medical education.[56] To fill this gap, the Royal College of Psychiatrists developed guidance on Medical Emergencies in Eating Disorders (MEED), which has also been endorsed by the Academy of Medical Royal Colleges.[57]

While AN is the most dangerous, all eating disorders can present in an emergency, either due to malnutrition or compensatory behaviours such as purging or medication or substance misuse. Furthermore, even if the patient is of normal weight, underlying physical illness – particularly type 1 diabetes – can have severe complications. Similarly, clinicians need to be aware of the increased risk of suicide in all eating disorders and the risks relating to purging. MEED Appendix 3 contains a summary of risk indicators and management decisions, which can be used as a quick reference for clinicians in emergency situations (Box 12.4).

Box 12.4 MEED Guidance. Appendix 3: Eating disorder risk checklist for emergencies[57]

Assessing

Does the patient have an eating disorder?

Yes   Anorexia nervosa – Bulimia nervosa – Other

Not sure: Request psychiatric review

Is the patient medically compromised?

- ☐ BMI <13 (adults); mMBI <70% (under 18)?
- ☐ Recent loss of >1kg for two consecutive weeks?
- ☐ Acute food or fluid refusal/intake <400 kcal per day?
- ☐ Pulse <40?
- ☐ BP low, BP postural drop >20 mm, dizziness?
- ☐ Core temperature <35.5°C?
- ☐ Na <130 mmol/L?
- ☐ K <3.0 mmol/L?
- ☐ Raised transaminase?
- ☐ Glucose <3 mmol/L?
- ☐ Raised urea or creatinine?
- ☐ Abnormal ECG?
- ☐ Suicidal thoughts, behaviours?

Is the patient consenting to treatment?

Yes

No: Mental health assessment requested

Refeeding

High risk for refeeding syndrome?

- ☐ Low initial electrolytes
- ☐ BMI <13 or mBMI <70%
- ☐ Little or no intake for >4 days
- ☐ Low WBC
- ☐ Serious medical comorbidities (e.g. sepsis)

High risk? Management:

- <20 kcal per kg per day
- Monitor electrolytes twice daily
- Build up calories swiftly
- Avoid underfeeding

Lower risk? Management:

- Start at 1,400–2,000 kcal per day (50 kcal/kg/day) and build by 200 kcal/day to 2,400 kcal/day or more
- Aim for weight increase of 0.5–1 kg/week
- Avoid underfeeding

Monitoring

- ☐ Electrolytes (especially P, K, glucose)
- ☐ ECG
- ☐ Vital signs
- ☐ BMI

Managing

Are medical and psychiatric staff collaborating in care?

Yes

No: Psych. consultation awaited

Are nurses trained in managing medical and psychiatric problems?

Yes

No and appropriately skilled staff requested/training in place

Are there behaviours increasing risk?

- ☐ Falsifying weight
- ☐ Disposing of feed
- ☐ Exercising
- ☐ Self harm, suicidality
- ☐ Family reaction to stress/anxiety
- ☐ Safeguarding concerns

Mobilise psychiatric team to advise on management

Note:

M%BMI = mean percentage of BMIPlease do not use BMI as a single indicator of risk

Patients who are at a high risk of complications require medical monitoring. This must be incorporated into active treatment for their eating disorder; otherwise, it is insufficient.

Anorexia Nervosa

Historical Background

Since ancient times, all religions have practised fasting. There are several historical accounts of people (mostly young women) starving themselves for prolonged periods. The causes and meaning attributed to such behaviour varied depending on the cultural context. The religious interpretation was that extreme piety led to this asceticism. Bell (1985),[58] in his book *Holy Anorexia*, described the practices of Italian holy women from the thirteenth century and noted the similarities with AN. However, if we look at the modern diagnostic criteria, one of the main features of typical anorexia was missing in these historical cases. The reason for the extreme dieting was religious rather than preoccupation with weight and shape. The starving saints might have had abnormally low body weight, hormonal abnormalities, abnormal eating behaviours, fear of fatness and even body-image distortion (as a sign of greed or gluttony). Nevertheless, as far as we can tell, the person's self-evaluation was not unduly determined by their weight and shape in historical cases. It is essential to recognise that the manifestation of most psychiatric disorders is heavily influenced by concurrent cultural belief systems. In other conditions, such as psychosis, the content of delusions varies depending on the dominant beliefs of the society in which the individual lives. These early descriptions of anorexia-like symptoms strongly suggest a biological basis for AN, which has recently been confirmed by genetic studies.

Richard Morton (1694)[59] is usually credited with the first medical descriptions of patients with AN. In his book on wasting illnesses, *Phthisiologia, Or, a Treatise of Consumptions*, he described two patients whose illness appeared to be due to voluntary food restriction. One was an 18-year-old girl who:

> *fell into a total suppression of her monthly courses from a multitude of cares and passions. ... From which time her appetite began to abate ... she was wont by her studying and continuing pouring upon Books to expose herself both day and night ... she was like a skeleton only clad with skin.*

This patient sadly died from the condition, but the second patient, a 16-year-old schoolboy who 'fell gradually into a total want of appetite, occasioned by studying too hard and the Passions of the Mind', was cured by advice, which was to 'abandon his studies, to go into the country Air, and to use Riding and a milk diet'. Morton observed a dramatic difference between the degree of emaciation and the level of mental and physical activity.

Unequivocal descriptions of AN appeared in the nineteenth century. Marcé (1860),[60] a young French psychiatrist, wrote of:

> *young girls who at the period of puberty become subject to inappetance carried to the utmost limits ... these patients arrive at the delirious conviction that they cannot or ought not to eat ... All attempts made to constrain them to adopt a sufficient regimen are opposed with infinite strategies and unconquerable resistance.*

Sir William Gull,[61] an English physician, and Charles Lasegue,[62] a French psychiatrist, brought the illness to the attention of the medical community between 1868 and 1888 with articles and case presentations. Lasegue's (1873) account is particularly vivid and well observed:

> *gradually she reduces her food further and further, and furnishes pretexts for so doing ... the abstinence tends to increase the aptitude for movement.*

He describes the lack of insight into the dangerousness of the weight loss and the patient gives a typical patient riposte when confronted: 'I do not suffer and therefore must be well.'

Attempts to classify the illness reflect some of the uncertainties that remain today:

> *the want of appetite is, I believe, due to a morbid mental state (Gull,1873)*[63]
>
> *the cases were not strictly insane; there was however something wrong in the nervous equilibrium, and usually something queer in the family history. (Ryle, 1936)*[64]

The name given to the disorder has changed over time as hypotheses about both the aetiology and the psychopathology have shifted. Gull (1868) argued that the deficit was central rather than peripheral and that 'AN' was the best term. In contrast, Simmonds in Germany proposed that a physical cause, 'pituitary insufficiency', was the explanation of the severe weight loss in some of these patients. In 1937, Sheehan described a similar picture in a woman, which was the result of damage to the pituitary gland during childbirth. Consequently, many patients who would be diagnosed as having AN today were diagnosed as suffering from Simmonds' or Sheehan's disease in the first part of the twentieth century in Europe, and the popularity of these diagnostic terms survived into the 1970s. Several case reports in the medical literature describe patients initially diagnosed with AN who were later diagnosed with various brain tumours, including pituitary gland tumours, so this remains an important differential diagnostic issue.

Another important historical record is the Minnesota study. Keys et al. (1950)[65] examined the effects that voluntary semi-starvation has on physiology and psychology during the Second World War. Although the project did not set out to examine AN, it remains the only systematic study of the consequences of chronic dietary restriction and controlled weight restoration on human physical and mental health, which are highly relevant to understanding the illness. The study has remained unique not only because current ethical regulations would prohibit its replication, but also because no one has since conducted a systematic study of the effects of self-induced starvation in healthy men. There is much less research on the consequences of AN in males, but the Minnesota study fills this gap. Anorexia nervosa and starvation have shared consequences. It is important to discuss the Minnesota study in order to understand which features are secondary to weight loss and hence will benefit from nutritional rehabilitation (Box 12.5).

In contrast to externally imposed starvation, which results in mental and physical lethargy, AN is characterised by increased activity despite weight loss. There is excessive exercise to 'burn off' calories. Others are driven by an obsession with cleanliness or orderliness.

In the 1960s, the morbid fear of fatness was described as a core feature of the disorder, which was regarded as a 'culture-bound syndrome' affecting mainly young women of higher social classes in Western countries.[66,67]

Clinical Presentations and Diagnosis

The hallmark of AN is deliberate insufficient dietary intake resulting in significant weight loss. The diagnostic criteria have changed significantly since 2013. Both the DSM-5 and ICD-11 retained the 'restriction of energy intake leading to significantly low weight in the context of age, sex, and developmental stage, driven by an intense fear of weight gain or becoming fat', 'the individual's self-evaluation is unduly influenced by weight and shape', 'there is a disturbance in how the body is perceived' and 'there is a persistent lack of recognition of the seriousness of the low body weight' as the main diagnostic features. The previous diagnostic requirement for amenorrhoea has been removed, as this is the consequence of malnutrition rather than being specific to AN.

The DSM-5 distinguishes between a restrictive and a binge eating and purging subtype of AN, depending on the presence or absence of compensatory mechanisms.

The BMI diagnostic threshold for adults is now 18.5 in accordance with WHO malnutrition categories (replacing 17.5); for children, it is below the 5th percentile.

Box 12.5 The Minnesota semi-starvation experiment

In the experiment, 32 healthy male conscientious objectors were given a diet of 1600 kcal/day and vigorous activity for six months (after a three-month initial control period) and were then followed up on for 12 weeks of rehabilitation. The participants lost 24 per cent of their pre-experiment weight (the average BMI before the experiment was 22). Both physical and psychological changes were observed.

Prior to this study, the physical effects of famines had been well documented, but the evaluation of psychological and behavioural changes associated with starvation and weight restoration was novel and ground-breaking.

The unexpected finding of the study was that many of the behavioural and psychological features of eating disorders emerged in healthy volunteers purely because of starvation. The men began to experiment with food – increasing the use of spices and salt – and to linger for two hours over a meal. Food became the main topic of their conversations and dreams, and their interest in food-related items increased. The men became emotionally unstable, irritable and aggressive. It was 'too much trouble' and 'too tiring' to participate in social activities. Sexual interest also dwindled, one man ruefully observing: 'I have no more sexual feeling than a sick oyster.' Furthermore, these symptoms persisted well beyond weight restoration.

These findings strongly suggest that starvation contributes to the symptoms of anorexia nervosa and perpetuates the vicious cycle. Many of the study's findings have been confirmed by later research on anorexia, so we now know that the findings also apply to women and young people.

The DSM-5 includes the following severity categories, based on the degree of malnutrition:

Mild: BMI>17
Moderate: BMI 16–16.9
Severe: BMI 15–15.9
Extreme: BMI<15

It also defines full and partial remission, if the person previously met the full diagnostic criteria.

The ICD-11 definitions are aligned with the DSM-5. The only difference is the definition of dangerous category (BMI<14; Table 12.1).

Atypical AN is interpreted differently: in the DSM-5, atypical AN is diagnosed in a person who meets all criteria except, despite severe weight loss, they are still within normal weight or overweight.

Course of Illness and Prognosis

The onset of AN is typically within a few years of puberty, at a median age of 18.[68] Recent genetic research supports a common variant genetic basis for age of onset and implicates biological pathways controlling menarche and reproduction. This is consistent with the highest sexual dimorphism among psychiatric disorders (10:1 female to male ratio).

Stress-related factors, such as bullying, sexual abuse, physical illness or dieting, are common precipitating factors.

The course of the illness varies. As a general principle, early intervention can reduce complications and improve outcomes.[69] A recent study found that approximately 70 per cent of individuals with AN experience remission within 10 years of onset, whereas 20–30% develop a chronic course.[70] For those patients who require hospitalisation, remission rates are generally lower and relapse rates and mortality are higher.[24,71] This is related to the severity of the illness and additional comorbidities and complications. The standardised mortality ratio is about 5, but this is higher in certain populations, such as physical or psychiatric comorbidities and level of severity.[25,71] The leading causes of death are malnutrition-related medical complications and suicide.[72] However, many of these deaths are avoidable with timely treatment.

In about half of AN cases, there is a migration towards BN and other sub-threshold eating disorders before recovery.[41]

Factors that are associated with poor outcome are:

- Malnutrition-related factors: extreme malnutrition, chronic malnutrition, failure to attain normal weight
- High volume of compensatory behaviours (vomiting, over-exercise)
- Additional comorbidities
- Poor premorbid psychological adjustment
- Social isolation

Differential Diagnosis and Comorbidity

If the presenting symptoms are atypical (e.g. onset after age 40 years, males or absence of the characteristic preoccupation with weight and shape), other causes of low body weight or significant weight loss should be excluded in the differential diagnosis.

Weight loss may be caused by gastrointestinal disease, hyperthyroidism, occult malignancies, pituitary tumours and AIDS. In addition, acute weight loss caused by a medical condition may be followed by the onset or recurrence of AN, which may be overshadowed by the medical condition. Anorexia nervosa can rarely develop post-bariatric surgery or with some medications. These may include aripiprazole, topiramate or SLGT inhibitors.

Ehlers-Danlos syndrome (EDS) and hyper mobility: the link between hyper mobility and eating disorders is often missed.[73,74] Patients with hyper mobility and EDS have significantly more gastrointestinal symptoms and food allergies or intolerances than controls, as well as a higher prevalence of eating disorders and a lower BMI. GI symptoms in EDS raise the risk of ED. Although the aetiological mechanisms underlying the comorbidity of EDS and GI disorders are unknown, it is possible that connective tissue abnormalities cause

Box 12.6 Common comorbidities and their impact on mortality risk

	Physical comorbidities	SMR	Psychiatric comorbidities	SMR
Anorexia nervosa & atypical presentations	• Malnutrition: acute & chronic	5–6	• Depression	12
	• Amenorrhoa		• Bipolar	
	• Fertility problems		• Anxiety	
	• Reduced bone density		• OCD	
	• Cardiovascular		• Personality disorder	
	• Electrolyte abnormalities		• ASD	
	• Endocrine		• Alcohol and substance misuse	11–35
	• Delayed development		• Suicide attempt/suicide	18
	• Gastrointestinal			
	• Type 1 diabetes	14.5		

alterations in GI tract motility, biomechanics and gut-brain interaction. Autonomic dysfunction is common in EDS patients and has been linked to GI issues. Patients seen in psychiatric or psychological clinical settings who are suspected or diagnosed with ED and present with joint hyper mobility (JH) and musculoskeletal pain should be evaluated for an underlying connective tissue disorder.

Psychiatric disorders should be assessed both as differential diagnoses and as comorbidities (see Box 12.6). Most individuals with AN have additional psychiatric morbidity. Depression is the most common. People suffering from major depressive disorder may lose weight, but this is due to a loss of appetite rather than a strong desire to lose weight or a strong fear of gaining weight. Treatment of co-occurring depression is difficult because antidepressants have not been found to be effective in underweight patients. Weight restoration is the first line of treatment. CBT-E can include behavioural activation or addressing low self-esteem, which can be helpful.

Similarly, patients with schizophrenia may have unusual eating habits and lose weight, but they rarely have the fear of weight gain and distorted body image that are symptoms of AN. A few patients with schizophrenia develop full-blown AN after taking aripiprazole. There is a genetic overlap with schizophrenia, which may explain near-delusional beliefs in some patients.

A recent study in a tertiary centre found that 11.3% of patients with AN had bipolar disorder(BD).[75] These patients had more severe clinical profiles in terms of anxiety, depression and dietary symptoms, as well as other lifetime comorbidities. These findings highlight the importance of early detection of BD and mood disorders in people with severe AN. It is often misdiagnosed as emotional unstable personality disorder (EUPD) if there is a history of suicide attempt or self harm. The correct diagnosis is essential for providing the best possible care.

Obsessive-compulsive disorder (OCD), social anxiety disorder (social phobia) and body dysmorphic disorder commonly co-occur with AN, and they may need additional treatment in their own right. If the patient is severely malnourished, weight restoration should be the first step, and the relevant NICE guidelines should be followed. The recent genome-wide association study (GWAS) discoveries that show a genetic overlap with OCD have important therapeutic implications: more attention needs to be given to intrusive thoughts and compulsions (e.g. exercise compulsion) in treatment.

There is a growing interest in the possibility that AN and autism spectrum disorders are phenotypically and etiologically linked.[76] It remains unclear whether the elevation of autistic traits precede AN in early childhood. In a large population-based cohort study of 5,987 individuals (52.4% female), parents reported autistic traits at ages 9 and 18. There was a marked increase in restricted/repetitive behaviours and interests in individuals with acute AN. A less-pronounced elevation was observed for social communication problems, but there was no clear evidence of increased autistic traits in children who later developed AN.[77] These findings are consistent with the lack of association in GWAS. Future research should use specific measurements to determine whether autistic traits are best understood as a consequence of the acute AN phase or whether these symptoms represent autism as a clinically verifiable neurodevelopmental disorder.[77]

Nevertheless, adopting the treatment and the hospital environment to meet the needs of people with neurodevelopmental disorders can be helpful.[76]

Personality Disorders

When AN is dominant, it is best to avoid diagnosing personality disorder for a number of reasons. Firstly, it is difficult to accurately assess the personality of patients with AN because many features may be the result of malnutrition or eating-disorder psychopathology. These include heightened sensitivity to rejection, emotional dysregulation and even self harm. Furthermore, making a diagnosis of personality disorder in such patients is particularly difficult because, due to the adolescent onset, most do not have a period of adult life free of the disorder's impact. CBT-E can be tailored to patients with complex difficulties by using the modules from the broad version, such as the mood intolerance, clinical perfectionism and core low self-esteem, or marked interpersonal difficulties modules depending on the individual's formulation.

Substance Misuse

Individuals who use appetite suppressants (e.g. cocaine, stimulants) and fear gaining weight should be thoroughly evaluated for the possibility of comorbid AN, as substance abuse may be a component of the desire to lose weight.

Epidemiology

Anorexia nervosa was extremely rare in the past. The first epidemiological studies were conducted in the 1960s in the USA. By the 1970s, there had been a 400 per cent increase in incidence, but the incidence rate was still around 5 out of 100,000 people.[78] Thirty years later, a UK study showed a further increase in incidence rates of AN to approximately 20 out of 100,000 people.[79] Recent epidemiological studies estimate 0.4–1% prevalence rates in Western countries.[80,81] Incidence of AN is lower in the Far East than in Western countries, but trends are increasing.[16,82-84] The changing diagnostic criteria present an additional challenge when comparing historical trends.

Demographics

The female to male ratio is 10:1, which is the highest sex difference for any mental disorder. It was a historically held view that AN is more common within the upper social classes. However, this may reflect a referral bias as population-based studies do not confirm the association but instead suggest a relationship with educational achievement.

Aetiology

The aetiology of AN is not fully understood; however, it is likely to be multifactorial (see Box 12.7). Historical explanations included various theories on family functioning.[85] Rigidity (resistance to change), enmeshment, conflict avoidance and overprotection were described as features of the family of a child with AN.[86] However, these hypotheses have not stood the test of time. Recent studies have found that these features may be a non-specific response to a severe illness.

Crisp (1980)[87] suggested a conflict relating to sexual maturation and identity, and in clinical practice, we see a high rate of history of sexual abuse and an overrepresentation of the LGBT community. However, these associations are neither sufficient nor specific to eating disorders.

Genetic Factors

Female relatives of those with AN are 11 times more likely to develop AN compared to female relatives of those without AN (four-fold increase in total for both sexes). Specific eating disorder manifestations are not inherited, which is consistent with the observed diagnostic fluctuation. First-degree relatives of people with AN and BN have an increased risk of full and partial AN syndrome, as well as DSM-IV eating disorder not otherwise specified (EDNOS).

Twin study heritability estimates range from 0.28 to 0.74 for AN. This wide range is due to different disease definitions, with narrower definitions yielding higher heritability estimates. Diagnostic transitions between AN and BN are explained in part by shared genetic factors, with genetic correlations ranging from 0.46 to 0.79 based on twin studies.[26] According to bivariate twin studies of AN with major depression and OCD, genetic correlations of 0.34 and 0.52, respectively, reflect shared genetic factors.[88]

The psychiatric genomic consortium identified one genome-wide significant locus on chromosome 12 that had previously been implicated in type 1 diabetes and rheumatoid arthritis, both of which are autoimmune diseases.[89] This is a significant finding because autoimmune diseases are more common in AN, and type 1 diabetes is associated with an increased risk of eating disorders, so it opens up new research. They also found significant genetic correlations between AN and other psychiatric disorders such as schizophrenia, personality traits such as neuroticism, and educational attainment. Tissue-enrichment analysis of AN-associated genes revealed a significant association with the central nervous system.[90]

GWAS revealed significant genetic correlations with metabolic, lipid and anthropometric traits, indicating that metabolic mechanisms may be responsible for physiological resistance to healthy body weight (Figure 12.4).[88] Particularly intriguing were the positive genetic correlations with high-density lipoprotein cholesterol and the negative genetic correlations with body mass index (BMI), obesity, fasting insulin and glucose. Overall, these findings have led to the proposal of reclassifying AN as a metabo-psychiatric disorder. They also

Box 12.7 Summary of common aetiological factors

	Biological	Psychological	Social
Predisposing	Genetic factors	Perfectionism, low self-esteem	Cultural factors, family factors
Precipitating	Stresses: dieting, illnesses, infections, emotional stress	Bullying, exams	Lifecycle transition, peer group, media, family models
Maintaining factors	Dysregulation of neuroendocrine system and gut-brain interaction Disruption of microbiome?	Cognitive impairment, low mood, denial	Family factors, isolation, peer group

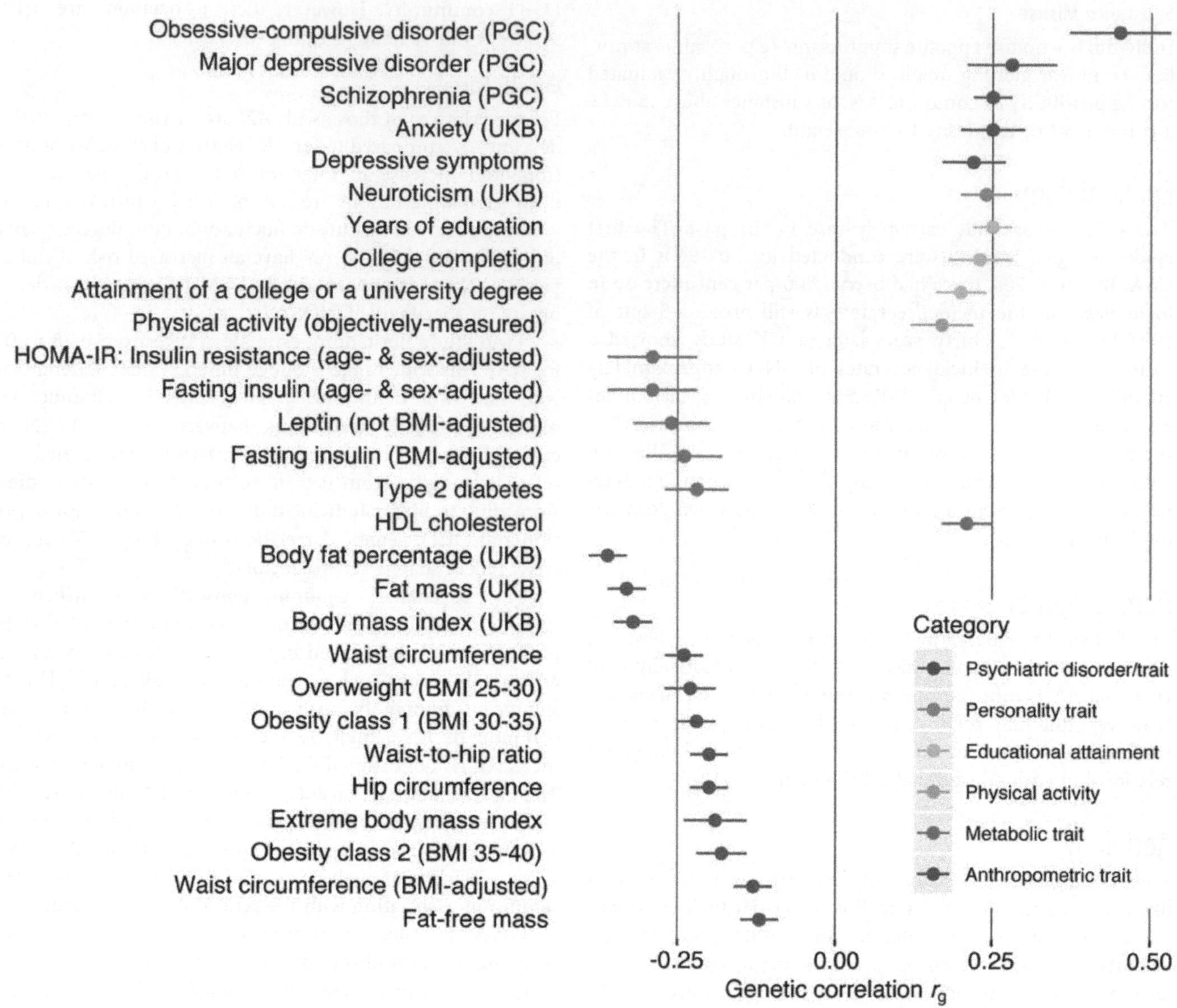

Figure 12.4 Bonferroni significant genetic correlations (SNP-rgs) and standard errors (error bars) between anorexia nervosa and other phenotypes as estimated by LD score regression.[89]. Only traits with significant P-values following Bonferroni correction are shown. Correlations with 447 phenotypes were tested (Bonferroni-corrected significance threshold $P>1.11\times10^{-4}$). PGC – psychiatric genomic consortium. UKB – UK BioBank. HOMA-IR – homeostatic model assessment-insulin resistance.

have therapeutic implications: psychoeducation can include the fact that AN patients are less likely to become overweight or obese than the general population. This metabolic signature may also explain why atypical antipsychotics, such as olanzapine, with known metabolic side effects rarely cause weight gain in AN.

Genes associated with autoimmunity have been replicated in recent studies.[91] This is consistent with a large population-based cohort study; autoimmune and auto-inflammatory diseases increased AN risk by 36 per cent.[91,92] Coeliac disease is much more common in AN patients. Men have a higher rate of autoimmune and auto-inflammatory diseases. Because ED symptoms are similar to those of chronic inflammatory GI and endocrine diseases such as inflammatory bowel disease and type 1 and type 2 diabetes, clinicians should consider these in their differential diagnoses and treatment.

Reconceptualising Anorexia Nervosa

Historically, AN was viewed as a primarily psychological problem with physical consequences. It is becoming evident that both psychological and metabolic factors are required for the development of AN. A new emphasis on integrating metabolic factors may improve treatment efficacy, and future interdisciplinary research in the fields of obesity and metabolism may lead to the development of novel treatments. The concurrent study of genetics, the external environment (including the impact of food choices on the gut microbiome) and their interactions has already begun and will likely accelerate in the coming years.[93]

Psychosocial Factors

Perfectionism and obsessive-compulsive behaviours are common antecedents of AN. In a clinical sample of patients with AN and atypical AN, obsessiveness was positively correlated with a drive for thinness, a key aspect of AN symptomatology.[94] Evidence from a three-year prospective study of 615 pairs of twins in the United States suggests that elevated risk for AN is associated with higher levels of depression and anxiety combined with a strong desire to be thin, rather than either risk factor alone.

Puberty is a critical period for the development of ED in both males and females. Increased production of sex hormones, particularly oestrogen, during puberty has been linked to the onset of EDs. Early puberty is strongly associated with an increased risk of ED development in both young males and females, according to research. Early-onset AN was significantly genetically correlated with younger age at menarche, while typical-onset AN was significantly negatively genetically correlated with anthropometric traits. Genetic risk scores for age of onset and early-onset AN derived from independent GWASs significantly predicted age of onset. Mendelian randomisation analysis revealed a link between younger age at menarche and early-onset AN.[68]

It has been argued that if an adolescent experiences changes in their body shape associated with menarche at a younger age than their peers, this may lead to increased body dissatisfaction, which may contribute to the early onset of eating disorders; however, recent genetic studies implicate biological pathways regulating menarche and reproduction.

Medical Consequences

All organ systems are affected by chronic malnutrition. There are some parallels with diabetes: if blood sugar levels are chronically abnormal, it has long-term damage on all organs and the person's mental health. Malnutrition triggers protein and fat catabolism, which reduces cellular volume and function, causing heart, brain, liver, intestinal, kidney and muscle atrophy.[95] These medical complications worsen with the severity of the patient's nutritional intake and severity of malnutrition.

It is helpful to inform the patient and their carers that the majority of medical complications are fully reversible if the patient is supported in regaining and maintaining a healthy weight, but chronic malnutrition is progressively harmful. Young people tend to underestimate the severity of the long-term consequences of malnutrition, so it can be helpful to highlight visible or immediate complications – such as dry skin, hair loss, feeling cold, loss of periods and sexual interests, or low mood – that are meaningful in the present.

Dermatological

Severe malnutrition results in hair loss, dry hair and fragile nails, which most patients notice and worry about, which can help them engage in treatment. The skin also becomes dry, fragile and bleeds easily. Lanugo hair is common and is thought to be an adaptation to prevent heat loss. Slow wound healing may result in decubitus ulcers over bony prominences, and the loss of subcutaneous fat exacerbates bruising. For this reason, bed rest is best avoided. Patients are frequently cold sensitive and develop acrocyanosis due to poor circulation.

Cardiovascular

Bradycardia and hypotension are indicators of the severity of malnutrition. Tachycardia at rest is a red flag sign because it may indicate secondary infection. Refeeding and weight restoration normalises blood pressure and heart rate in a few weeks.

On echocardiography, 22–71% of patients have silent pericardial effusion.[95] This could be caused by a low BMI, rapid weight loss, low T3 and IGF-1 levels. Several studies have found lower left ventricular mass as well as reduced cardiac output, diastolic and systolic dimensions.

Arrhythmias other than bradycardia may complicate AN. QT prolongation and dispersion may indicate an increased risk of sudden cardiac death, and medications known to increase QT interval should be closely monitored. QT prolongation may be caused by hypokalaemia and vagal activity. Takotsubo cardiomyopathy, a rare reversible acute heart failure caused by stress-induced catecholamine elevations, can be caused by severe malnutrition.

Respiratory System

Rarely, emphysema or pulmonary insufficiency can be found in AN. Pneumothorax and pneumomediastinum are uncommon but potentially fatal complications. Acute gastric rupture in patients who self-induce vomiting can result in spontaneous tension pneumoperitoneum and pneumothorax.

Gastrointestinal

Food restriction can cause slow gastric emptying or gastroparesis if the weight falls below 15–20% of the ideal. Severe bloating, upper quadrant pain and early satiety are the most common symptoms. Acute gastric dilation is an extreme and uncommon complication of delayed gastric emptying. If left untreated, extreme stomach dilatation can lead to gastric necrosis, perforation and death. If the patient has severe left upper quadrant pain or significant vomiting, an abdominal X-ray is recommended. Bloating caused by slow gastrointestinal transit may be exacerbated by high-fibre diets. A nuclear medicine gastric emptying study may be required in rare cases of prolonged symptomatology.

Constipation is a common complication of dietary restrictions. Patients should be reassured that this can be resolved by restoring their weight. Diarrhoea is a red flag; in addition to laxative abuse, underlying disorders like IBD and IBS malabsorption syndromes must be investigated.

Almost half of all patients have abnormal AST and ALT levels due to starvation, which can cause AST and ALT levels to rise by two to three times the normal level. If a high carbohydrate content is used, steatosis (mild transaminase elevation) can occur early in refeeding. Severe AN raises transaminase (4–30 times normal) before refeeding, indicating multiorgan failure; this resolves with nutrition but usually takes several weeks. A liver ultrasound can help distinguish between starvation-induced and refeeding-induced enzyme elevations. On ultrasound, refeeding hepatitis may show a fatty liver. Elevations caused by starvation are more likely in patients weighing less than 12 kg/m^2. The pathomechanism remains unknown. The first step should be safe refeeding; if the problem persists, consult a gastroenterologist.

The superior mesenteric artery (SMA) syndrome is a severe complication caused by the loss of fat around the SMA, compressing the duodenum posteriorly between the aorta and spine and the SMA anteriorly. It causes upper quadrant abdominal pain, early satiety, nausea and post-meal vomiting, and an abdominal CT or upper GI series can be used to diagnose it.

Protein-energy malnutrition can rarely be associated with dysphagia, which can lead to aspiration. Aspiration pneumonia can result from poor swallowing and food bolus transfer. The diagnosis can be confirmed with bedside speech therapy or video fluoroscopic swallowing. Dysphagia and aspiration may necessitate changes in food consistency or the use of a feeding tube until weight gain improves swallowing.

Refeeding can occasionally result in acute pancreatitis. Pancreatitis manifests as posterior epigastric pain, nausea, vomiting and elevated pancreatic enzymes (amylase and lipase) during early refeeding.

Microbiome

The involvement of the gut microbiota in AN and eating behaviours in general is a topic of active research.[96,97] Changes in the composition of the gut microbiota have been demonstrated to influence brain function, including the regulation of hunger and satiety signals, and may contribute to the emergence of disordered eating patterns. Additionally, the gut microbiota can influence the body's metabolism and energy homeostasis, which may alter body weight and eating behaviours. More research is needed to elucidate the gut microbiome's function in eating behaviours as well as the role of genetic and environmental factors, including food choices. Patients with AN have significant changes in their gut microbiome that persist even after weight restoration. In some studies, polyunsaturated fatty acids (PUFA) administration have been found to be beneficial in the treatment of AN, affecting the microbiome, body weight and executive functions. A large study is currently underway to investigate the effects of PUFA nutritional supplementation on the gut microbiome and body mass index (BMI) in AN patients.[98]

Endocrine Abnormalities

Malnutrition causes widespread endocrine consequences. It increases cortisol secretion and decreases metabolic clearance, potentially extending cortisol's half-life. Elevated cortisol levels in AN may contribute to bone loss, high levels of anxiety and poor emotional regulation. IGF-1 levels are lower, indicating growth hormone resistance.

Diabetes insipidus and AN can lead to a variety of complications. Electrolyte imbalance, dehydration and hyponatraemia can occur. Hyponatraemia, also known as 'water intoxication', can develop as both a symptom and a complication of AN.

Both euthyroid sick syndrome and AN are characterised by low levels of T4 and T3. Nutritional rehabilitation normalises thyroid function, rendering thyroid hormone replacement therapy unnecessary and dangerous. Due to the association between autoimmune thyroiditis and eating disorders, patients should be screened for these conditions.

Glucose metabolism abnormalities and hypoglycaemia are caused by hepatic glycogen depletion and the disruption of gluconeogenesis. Severe hypoglycaemia and death can occur as a result of liver failure and substrate depletion. Hypoglycaemia in AN lowers insulin levels, and refeeding can occasionally result in reactive hypoglycaemia as part of refeeding syndrome.

The combination of type 1 diabetes and AN is extremely dangerous, complicating treatment and increasing mortality. Poor control of glucose can lead to irreversible microvascular complications, such as diabetic retinopathy and nephropathy. This concern is relevant over prolonged uncontrolled illness. During initial refeeding, a glucose level below 14 mmol/L for a few weeks is unlikely to be harmful. Short-term 'permissive hyperglycemia' can improve therapeutic engagement during refeeding, but long-term treatment should focus on optimal glucose control in collaboration with the diabetic team.

Male and female sex hormones, such as GnRH, LH, FSH, oestrogen and testosterone, are suppressed by malnutrition. Sexual interest, libido, fertility, potency, bone density and mood are all affected by these abnormalities. Women with AN develop a temporary hypothalamic-pituitary disorder resulting in amenorrhoea. Despite this, unexpected ovulation can occur, and therefore, contraception is advised to prevent unwanted pregnancies. Women of childbearing age need to be informed that pregnancy and new-born complications include miscarriages, premature birth and small-for-gestational-age infants if the mother's nutritional state is suboptimal.

Metabolic Rate and Hypothermia

The Minnesota study described the reduction of basal metabolic rate by as much as 30 per cent and hypothermia in malnutrition, which both conserve energy. This could explain why some patients with chronic AN can maintain their weight with very little dietary intake. Refeeding improves both basic metabolic rate and temperature, but it also means that dietary intake must be adjusted for ongoing weight gain. Warming patients may be beneficial because it reduces high stress hormone levels.[99]

Haematological Consequences

Malnutrition causes bone marrow suppression and, in extreme cases, leads to hypoplastic anaemia, gelatinous atrophy and pancytopenia. Anaemia and leukopenia affect one-third of patients, and thrombocytopenia affects 10 per cent of patients. Petechiae, purpura and a mildly elevated serum INR can be caused by liver damage and impaired coagulation factor synthesis.

There is no increase in susceptibility to infectious diseases despite the pancytopenia. However, individuals with AN may not exhibit fever or elevated white blood cell counts; therefore, vigilance and a lower infection threshold are recommended.

Immune-mediated conditions, such as asthma, allergies and acne, improve with weight loss and worsen with weight restoration. This needs to be explained to the patient, and appropriate treatment should be offered during treatment.

Bone Health

Bone density is reduced by chronic malnutrition. This is a slow, approximately one-year-long, process that can become progressive if the patient remains chronically malnourished. Pathological fractures are more likely and can be severely debilitating (e.g. spinal compression fractures), but they usually take many years to develop. It is important to note that these changes are partially reversible with full weight restoration and weight-bearing exercise (patients need to avoid high-impact exercise due to the risk of fractures). Long-term outcomes studies are needed, but calcium or vitamin D supplements seem ineffective. Because bone accrual continues until the mid-20s, adolescents with AN may never reach peak bone mass. Men with AN are at increased risk of osteoporosis due to a decrease in testosterone caused by malnutrition.[95]

Neurologic

The severity of malnutrition correlates with brain atrophy. On an MRI, the enlarged ventricles and decreased cortical substance of severe AN may resemble Alzheimer's disease. This may explain cognitive problems, social withdrawal and low mood in severe AN. Although complete recovery is possible, gaining weight does not immediately normalise MRI brain scans, particularly grey matter.

Peripheral neuropathy is common in malnutrition and can be especially dangerous in cases of vitamin B and folate deficiencies, such as pellagra, beriberi or B12.

Males with Anorexia Nervosa

Anorexia nervosa is less prevalent in men than in women. Men with AN may experience stigma and gender-based stereotypes that discourage them from seeking treatment. Recent studies indicate differences between men and women with AN presentation and worse prognosis for men.[23] Because they have less body fat and more lean muscle than women, men develop ketosis and protein breakdown faster after losing weight. They often present after severe weight loss, with more severe clinical and laboratory findings. Loss of sexual function and drive is a common complication due to reduced testosterone in malnutrition.

According to research, gay men may be more likely than heterosexuals to develop AN, particularly as a secondary diagnosis.[100] This risk may be increased by stigma, discrimination, minority stress and body dissatisfaction. Accessing and receiving appropriate eating disorder treatment may be particularly difficult for gay men due to provider insensitivity and ignorance as well as barriers to affirming and inclusive treatment environments. These barriers can delay treatment, thereby worsening the condition and outcomes.

Further research is necessary to better understand, diagnose and treat AN in men and to raise awareness of the condition. Clinicians must provide care that is culturally sensitive and inclusive.

Assessment

The initial assessment should include a thorough psychiatric assessment and physical examination, and if the clinical picture changes, these need to be revisited.

The psychiatric history should focus on family history, early development, premorbid functioning, dietary intake before and since the onset of the illness and any potential contributory factors. Medical and drug and alcohol histories aid in the identification of any potentially complicating factors. The details of dietary and fluid intake and compensatory mechanisms are essential both for the assessment of risk and treatment.

Mental State

During the first meeting, the clinician must keep in mind that the person in front of them is usually ashamed, terrified of being judged and frightened of change or the possibility of being forced to receive treatment. For successful engagement, assessment and treatment, a sensitive and compassionate approach is essential. Opening a discussion about the specific nature and details of their eating difficulties, as well as their impact on the person's life and ability to function, is important for both engagement and risk assessment, which will serve as the foundation for treatment.

In addition to the standard mental state examination, it is important to ask about dietary restrictions, compensatory behaviours, preoccupation with weight and shape, fear of weight gain and self-evaluation.

The physical examination is summarised in Box 12.8.

Investigations

Initial investigations should focus on tests that screen for differential diagnoses and risks. These include full blood count (FBC), urea and electrolytes (U&E), liver function tests (LFT), thyroid function tests (TFT), Ca, Mg, phosphate, C-reactive protein (CRP), B12, folate, weight and height and

Box 12.8 Physical examination outline

Height, Weight = BMI
Weight centile for children

Appearance
Pallor, Jaundice
Peripheral cyanosis
Oedema

Skin
Tattoos / Bruises / Scars / Turgor / Dryness of skin
Russell sign
Lanugo

Observations
BP sitting and standing
Pulse rate / Rhythm / Volume
O_2 saturation
Temperature
Respiratory rate

Orobuccal
Parotid

Thyroid

Cardiovascular
ECG

Respiratory

Abdomen

Neurological (General)
Muscle mass & atrophy
Squat test / Sitting up test
Sensation
Tone & clonus
Power
Coordination
Reflexes

Cranial Nerves

electrocardiogram (ECG). The frequency of blood tests should be determined by the level of malnutrition and associated risks, including compensatory behaviours. When the risk of refeeding syndrome is high at the start of weight restoration (usually two to three weeks), twice-weekly monitoring of U&E and Ca/Mg phosphate may be required. Because most community services cannot provide this level of monitoring on a regular basis, hospitalisation may be necessary if the risk is significant. Refeeding complications are more likely if the patient is severely malnourished (BMI <14), experiencing rapid weight loss, abusing laxatives or alcohol, or has physical comorbidities.

Treatment

Since ancient times, refeeding has been used to treat AN. The classical treatment, advocated by Gull, was to remove the patient from her home environment and place her in a nursing home, where 'moral management' would be applied. Until the 1980s, patients were treated using operational conditioning principles, which included forced bed rest and having to 'earn privileges' by weight gain. These practices are counterproductive and have no place in modern clinical practice.

The psychological treatment of AN has been transformed over the past 30 years. The main treatment models that are approved by international guidelines include family-based treatment for children and young people, CBT-E, MANTRA, SSCM and FPT for adults. A recent systematic review and network meta-analysis found specific psychological treatments for adult outpatients with AN improve clinical course and quality of life, but there is no reliable evidence to prove their superiority or inferiority.[101] CBT-E had half of the all-cause drop-out rate compared with psychodynamic-oriented psychotherapies. Integrated CBT-E for severe AN has been shown to achieve much improved outcomes,[102] but comparative studies with high-quality outpatient treatment are lacking. New research is urgently needed to develop and improve treatment for AN.

Family-Based Treatment

For children and adolescents with AN, FT-AN usually consists of 18–20 sessions spread out over a year. The progress is evaluated four weeks after treatment begins and then every three months to determine how frequently sessions should be held and how long treatment should last. The importance of the family's role in the young person's recovery is emphasised in this treatment model. The introduction includes education about the consequences of malnutrition. In the first phase, it is critical to encourage the parents or carers to play a central role in assisting the child or young person with eating while emphasising that this is a temporary task. In the second phase, the goal is to establish a strong therapeutic alliance with the young person, as well as with their parents or carers and other family members. In the final phase, the focus is on establishing a level of independence appropriate for the young person's developmental level as well as working on relapse prevention and post-treatment plans. Separate appointments from family members or carers for children and adolescents with AN can be beneficial, especially if there are concerns about high-expressed emotions. It is important to determine whether family members or carers need help on their own.

CBT-E

CBT-E for outpatient treatment of AN requires approximately 40 sessions. CBT-E can also be integrated into day and hospital treatments, which will be discussed later.

MANTRA

For adults with AN, MANTRA[43] typically consists of 20 sessions, with weekly sessions for the first 10 weeks and a flexible schedule after that, with up to 10 extra sessions for people with complex problems. The modules of MANTRA are delivered flexibly and when the person is ready; they cover nutrition, symptom management and behaviour change. The goal is to encourage the person to develop a 'non-anorexic identity'. It entails family members or carers assisting the individual in understanding their condition and the problems it causes – as well as the connection to the larger social context – and changing their behaviour.

SSCM

SSCM for adults suffering from AN should typically consist of 20 or more weekly sessions, depending on the severity of the disorder. Developing a positive relationship between the individual and the therapist is key. The goal is to assist the patient in regaining weight by providing psychoeducation and nutritional education and advice – as well as physical health monitoring – establishing a weight range goal, and developing healthy eating habits. Progress is reviewed collaboratively on a regular basis, and the patient is encouraged to play an active role in determining what else should be included in their therapy.

Focal Psychodynamic Therapy (FPT)

FPT was recently developed in Germany as a manualised psychodynamic treatment for AN.[45] The 'Anorexia Nervosa Treatment of Out Patients' (ANTOP) study compared FPT to either CBT-E or treatment as usual (structured care from a family doctor) over a 10-month period (averaging 40 sessions each). All outpatient treatment groups improved weight and eating disorder psychopathology, but there were no significant differences. CBT-E had the highest rate of treatment completion. At the five-year follow-up, 41% patients recovered fully, 41% had partial recoveries and 18% remained chronically ill. BMI at the five-year follow-up was predicted by baseline BMI, illness duration and baseline depression. These predictors of the long-term course of AN indicate that we must treat patients at an earlier stage of the disease, with a clear emphasis on weight gain and consideration of other comorbidities.[103]

The long-term results of the ANTOP trial indicate that, despite receiving specialised outpatient treatment, a significant proportion of patients with AN have a poor overall outcome. This is consistent with clinical experience and calls for further research improving treatment.

Treatment of Complex Comorbidities

Clinicians should provide a comprehensive treatment approach for patients with AN given the prevalence of physical and psychiatric comorbidities. Recently, Dalle Grave published a guide for clinicians on the treatment of common comorbidities.[54]

Inpatient Treatment and Integrated Care

In both the UK and internationally, there is a growing demand for inpatient treatment of severe eating disorders.[8,104,105] However, hospitalisation for severe eating disorders is still controversial owing to poor long-term outcomes. Inpatient treatment should be available for those who do not respond to outpatient treatment, but the threshold for admission – as well as the length and model of treatment – varies greatly depending on local historical arrangements.[106]

Historically, hospital treatment programmes were based on operant conditioning techniques, in which the patient was placed on complete bed rest and given small privileges like going to the bathroom alone as a reward for eating or weight gain. These approaches create conflict and are counter-productive. Bed rest is still widely used in acute hospitals even though there is an increasing recognition of harm. Because of the risk of physical and psychological harm, bed rest should be used only on rare occasions and for as short a time as possible.[107] A team psychological approach is essential for positive patient experience and successful treatment.

Treatment Models

Current inpatient treatment programmes in the UK generally adhere to the NHSE Standard Contract for Specialised Eating Disorder Services and the NICE guidelines. The contract requires both the NHS and independent providers commissioned by NHSE to meet the contract's standards.

The NHSE contract is based on consensus and specifies three types of admissions:

1. Unplanned or urgent admissions with 'modest weight restoration'
2. Short-term admission for 'medical stabilisation' or symptom relief
3. Admissions for symptom recovery include weight restoration to 'a normal weight or weight at which the patient can reliably continue independent weight restoration or weight maintenance with less intensive input', as well as improved eating habits and psychological understanding

In routine practice, these admission types are rarely distinct. The recommended combination of multi-disciplinary interventions was developed independently for outpatients and have never been tested in combination in inpatient settings, and the potential risk is in giving contradictory messages to the patient. This may explain why disengagement and self-discharge are so common – up to 60 per cent in some studies. Furthermore, unplanned admissions are common, and most patients are discharged before achieving a healthy weight. A 2013 multicentre cohort study of short-term outcomes of hospital treatment including 137 adults with AN reported a mean admission BMI of 14 and discharge BMI of 17.3. Only 22 per cent of patients were discharged at BMI >19 despite the lengthy admissions (average length of stay for inpatient treatment was 184 days and 126 days for day treatment).[108] A study in Scotland reported similar results.[109]

Integrated or Multistep CBT-E

Dalle Grave's team in Garda, Italy, developed a whole system inpatient programme based on CBT-E to improve patient experience and outcomes. This programme's clear theoretical foundation distinguishes it from eclectic models and focusses on the individual formulation of the patient, encouraging autonomy and recovery. This has many advantages. Even when patients are severely ill, patient autonomy and therapeutic optimism helps engage them. It is a whole system approach: all team members are CBT-E-trained, and interventions follow the same principles. The team helps the patient overcome her eating disorder rather than forcing her to do so. Treatment intensity is determined by patient need (outpatient, intensive day treatment or hospital treatment). Treatment is time-limited and consists of 13 weeks admission followed by 7 weeks of day treatment and ongoing outpatient aftercare. Psychological treatment begins before admission and continues for 40 sessions to ensure continuity and stepped care (Figure 12.5).

Dalle Grave's manual[53] and papers on the method and outcomes show superior outcomes and completion rates compared to traditional eclectic models.[110] The model has been implemented in Oxford and demonstrated much improved outcomes compared with other alternatives, including treatment as usual (TAU) and crisis admission.[102] The differences between TAU and I-CBT-E include (Box 12.9):

- Integrated CBT-E across the care pathway without any interruption
- Time-limited and planned admission
- Full weight restoration, 1.5 kg/week
- Recovery focus
- Seven weeks intensive support for weight maintenance
- Ongoing outpatient CBT-E without interruption

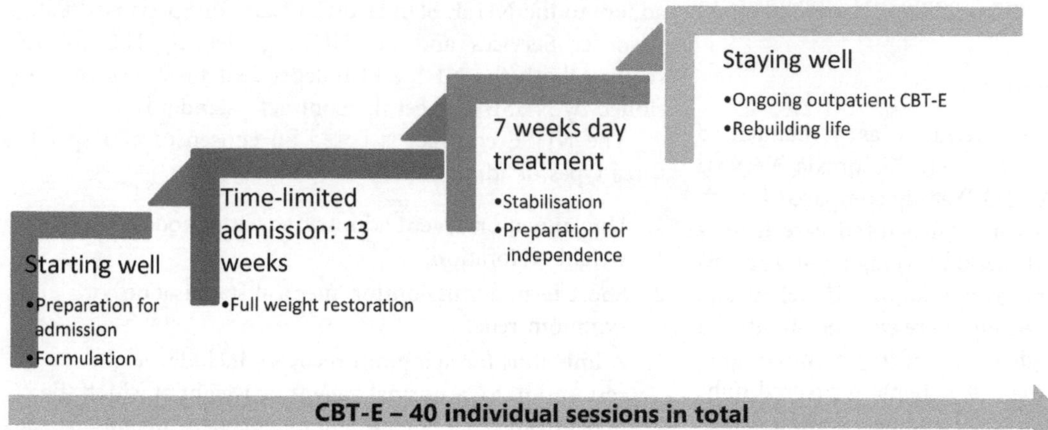

Figure 12.5 Stepped care.

Box 12.9 Comparison between inpatient treatment models and outcomes[102]

		I-CBT-E	Crisis management	TAU
Preparation for admission	Admission planning	yes	yes	variable
	CBT-E formulation	yes	yes	rarely
	Jointly agreed goals	yes	yes	variable
	Agreed timescale	13 weeks	6–8 weeks	undetermined
Inpatient treatment	Psychological treatment	CBT-E groups, formulation and individual therapy	CBT-E groups, formulation	Eclectic groups and individual psychology
	Speed of weight gain	1–1.5 kg/week	1–1.5 kg/week	0.5–1kg/week
	Agreed weight restoration	Min BMI: 20	6–9 kg weight gain (Min BMI 16)	variable
Day treatment	Day treatment	7 weeks	NA	variable
Aftercare	Outpatient psychological treatment	20 weeks (40 sessions in total)	variable	variable
Outcomes[102]	Length of stay (days)	125	50	132
	Admission BMI	14.6	14.2	14.6
	Discharge BMI	19.7	16.0	17.0
	Remission after 1 year	**70%**	**<5%**	**<5%**
	Readmission rate	**14%**	**44%**	**44%**

Admission Preparation

Even for physically compromised patients, inpatient CBT-E requires admission preparation. Patients with AN are often fearful and ambivalent about treatment and recovery. Diet, weight and shape control are central to psychopathology, so premature discharge is a risk unless the patient is fully committed to treatment. If possible, patients should start psychological treatment before admission or have a care coordinator coordinate inpatient and outpatient treatment. The patient and carers should be able to visit the unit and the team to learn about the treatment. This helps manage anxiety and engagement. Admission preparation may require more than one visit, but it is time well spent.

Refeeding

Extremely malnourished patients require safe refeeding. Underfeeding is as dangerous as refeeding syndrome,[57] which tends to occur when the patient has significant comorbidities. This is highlighted in the MEED guidelines[57] (see Box 12.4). Usually, patients tolerate well an introductory 30–40 kcal/kg/day diet and gradually increasing it, depending on weight gain. According to NICE guidelines, the expected rate of weight gain in a hospital setting is approximately 0.5–1 kg per week. Slower weight restoration would lengthen the hospital stay and is associated with poor outcomes. Faster weight restoration (approximately 1.5 kg/week) is completely safe biologically and has been recommended by Dalle Grave.[53]

The frequency of blood test monitoring is best determined based on the patient's risk. It is critical to understand that patients who are severely malnourished frequently have normal blood test results in restrictive AN. The body will try to maintain a normal blood calcium level, for example, even if it means depleting calcium from the bones and other tissues. The most common abnormality in blood tests found in patients who purge is a low potassium level and low magnesium.

Hypophosphatemia and thiamine deficiency are the most common refeeding complications. Pabrinex can be helpful to prevent Korsakow syndrome. Refeeding oedema can develop, and it can be especially severe if the patient uses large amounts of laxatives.

The dietician and the patient usually discuss the diet, with medical input if there are any specific concerns. Patients with severe anorexia usually require intensive nursing support at mealtimes.

Patients with AN who have insulin-dependent diabetes require joint working between the diabetic and inpatient teams.

Artificial Nutrition

Nasogastric (NG) feeding has been controversial, with some people regarding it as 'horrific' and 'inhumane'. If the patient is unable to complete the required dietary intake and NG feeding is necessary, it is essential to engage and reduce anxiety. After adequate explanation and anxiety management, most patients accept NG feeding as a necessary medical intervention, just as they would accept a drip or blood test. If the team works well with the patient, it is extremely rare that NG feeding is administered against the patient's will. The aim is to manage fears and make reasonable adjustments for autistic patients. NG feeding is always a short-term intervention, and it is critical to encourage the patient to resume normal eating as soon as possible. According to the NICE guidelines, NG feeding against the patient's will should only be administered by a highly skilled team and within the legal framework.

In exceptional cases, a percutaneous endoscopic gastrostomy (PEG) tube may be required as a temporary solution. The PEG may allow the person to be discharged from the hospital as long as she or he willingly accepts the feed through the PEG. In the author's experience, outcomes are poor, so all efforts should be made to help the patient resume eating food normally. Similarly, long-term use of nutritional supplements can reinforce the psychopathology and is counter-productive.

Mealtime Support

Dietary restriction is a major maintaining factor in eating disorders. Therefore, introducing regular meals is an essential component of treatment, both physically and for addressing psychopathology. Regular eating is one of the most important CBT-E interventions, and inpatient units can assist patients in regaining normal eating patterns. Most specialist units in the United Kingdom provide intensive nursing support and supervision during mealtimes. Anxiety management is a critical component of this and requires a collaborative team effort.[111] Smaller, but more frequent, meals are easier to digest for severely malnourished people at the beginning of weight restoration, and eating every few hours helps maintain energy levels; hence, most units have three main meals and three snacks. Later on, however, having three larger main meals and one snack is fine, and it is easier to maintain after discharge.[53] Dalle Grave recommends live self-monitoring and using distraction strategies to manage intrusive thoughts during mealtimes. These can be incorporated into NHS settings too, instead of under nursing supervision.

In preparation for discharge, it is essential to include a variety of foods that reflect family traditions and lifestyles and to practise eating outside of the hospital.

Compulsory Treatment

Most countries have legal frameworks in place that allow for the compulsory treatment of people suffering from mental illnesses. The Care Quality Commission (CQC) issued a 'Guidance Note on the Treatment of Anorexia Nervosa under the Mental Health Act 1983 in England and Wales' to assist clinicians with treatment decisions when the patient refuses treatment. They state in general, 'compulsory measures are unnecessary in the treatment of AN because they may be counter-productive to patient autonomy in the long term', but they acknowledge that in 'rare cases', when the patient's 'physical health or survival is seriously jeopardised by food or fluid refusal, compulsory treatment may be required'. In this document, the patient's physical risk is prioritised. Anorexia nervosa has a high suicide rate, so risks to oneself or others (e.g. while driving) also need to be taken into account. Treatment needs to be as collaborative as possible, even for the detained patient.[112,113] NICE recommends 'feeding against the patient's will only in the context of the Mental Health Act (MHA) or the Children's Act'. The NICE guidelines advise against using parental consent 'indefinitely' to override a young person's treatment refusal. If both the AN patient and those with parental responsibility refuse treatment, NICE recommends seeking legal advice to pursue Children's Act action.

Compulsory treatment is rarely studied. Long-term outcomes studies do not support the presumption that compulsive treatment is inherently harmful, but additional research is required for this population of patients at extremely high risk.[114]

Transition and Prevention of Relapse

The risk of relapse after discharge is highest in the first year, particularly within the first 60–90 days.[115] Integrated treatment produces better results. A recent longitudinal cohort study in the UK showed that integrated CBT-E performed significantly better in real-world settings than traditional inpatient treatment models. Seventy per cent of patients with severe and extreme AN who received integrated CBT-E throughout the care pathway had good outcomes at least one year later, compared to less than 5 per cent who received treatment as usual or through crisis pathways. The integrated CBT-E, discharge BMI and legal status were the most important predictors of good outcomes, but not age, comorbidity or admission BMI.[102] These findings suggest that weight restoration to a healthy weight range is necessary but not sufficient for good outcomes. Integrated CBT-E and ongoing psychological treatment are needed for long-term changes. Alternative transition models are being investigated.[116,117]

Medication

Medication is not recommended as a sole treatment for AN due to insufficient effectiveness, but they may be used for significant comorbidities.[31] Before making any treatment decisions, the potential side effects and benefits must be carefully balanced. Anxiolytics are frequently used in hospitals as a temporary measure to alleviate the anxiety associated with initial weight restoration. They have never been tested for AN in formal clinical trials, but there is no evidence of harm in the literature, so they can be helpful in managing severe anxiety and distress in the short term if used cautiously.

There is some evidence that olanzapine can be beneficial as part of a comprehensive treatment plan for severe cases of AN. Olanzapine (or other atypical antipsychotics) may be used if patients are extremely distressed and agitated or if anorexic beliefs are almost delusional in intensity and resistant to rational discussion. It can help reduce intense anxiety and mood swings, as well as delusional levels of preoccupation.[118] In underweight patients, the most common side effects of olanzapine are drowsiness and low blood pressure. In the author's experience, depot olanzapine is well tolerated and provides better stability than the oral preparation, but this needs further study. Olanzapine is known to cause metabolic side effects in other patient populations, such as those with psychosis or bipolar disorder, but this rarely happens in AN. This should reassure patients, who often fear weight gain. Thus, olanzapine may be used to supplement weight restoration if the patient is highly distressed, beginning with low doses of 2.5–5 mg/d in adults and 1.25 mg/d in adolescents and increasing to a maximum of 20 mg/d if necessary. Side effects and treatment responses need to be carefully monitored. The optimal length of AN treatment is unknown, but it is likely to be several months. Risperidone can be a helpful alternative if there is underlying autism and high level of anxiety and severe obsessional symptoms. Aripiprazole can cause weight loss, so it is best avoided in this patient population.

Comorbidity is common in AN, such as underlying depression or obsessive-compulsive disorder. These issues may require medication treatment, especially if psychological treatment is ineffective. Despite the high prevalence of comorbid depression, the jury is still out on whether antidepressants are beneficial for malnourished people. Furthermore, these medications may increase the risk of self harm, particularly in adolescents and young adults, so they need to be carefully monitored. The risk of harm, for example, from the consequences of QT prolongation needs to be weighed against the negligible evidence of benefit from antidepressants, antipsychotics and antihistamines in patients with low weight.

Interestingly, OCD responds to the usual pharmacological approaches in AN, although often requiring augmentation of selective serotonin re-uptake inhibitors (SSRIs).

Comorbid bipolar illness needs to be diagnosed and treated with mood stabilisers. Lithium can be very helpful if the patient complies appropriately with monitoring.

Physical Consequences and Comorbidities

As patients are significantly malnourished, it is helpful to use a good multivitamin and mineral supplement, such as Forceval or Centrum Gold, to prevent gross vitamin deficiencies. Vegan patients will require B12 supplementation. In addition, thiamine and zinc supplementation can be helpful in the first few months of refeeding. Essential fatty acid supplementation is an area of further study.[98]

Full weight restoration with a nutritionally balanced diet is the most effective osteoporosis prevention. Vitamin D supplementation may be necessary if levels are low.

Weight-bearing exercise after weight restoration may be helpful.

Abdominal discomfort is common during weight loss. Reflux, constipation and abdominal bloating are examples. It is important to keep gastroenterological medication to a minimum; most problems resolve with time. Fox's Glacier Mints, which contain peppermint oil, have successfully relieved abdominal discomfort on our unit. Macrogols should be the first-line treatment for constipation.

Controversies

The notion of 'terminal anorexia'[119,120] and withdrawing treatment for patients with severe eating disorders raises significant ethical concerns and is deeply controversial.[121,122] It suggests that some lives may not be deemed valuable or deserving of medical care, which goes against the principle of equal treatment for all patients. Withdrawing treatment is also against the principles of evidence-based medicine. The limited effectiveness of treatment for severe eating disorder should not be a reason to give up on patients but rather a call to increase resources and funding for research to improve treatment options. Improving treatment for these disorders requires more resources, capacity and training, not limiting access to care. Clinicians must work to provide the care and support needed by patients with long-standing eating disorders to overcome their illnesses. Equal treatment and appropriate care should be given to all patients, regardless of the severity of their illness.

New Treatments

New psychological approaches include:

Radical Openness Behavioural Therapy (RO-BPT): RO-BPT is a type of behavioural therapy that focusses on promoting openness and flexibility in thinking and behaviour.

Acceptance and Commitment Therapy (ACT): ACT is a form of cognitive behavioural therapy that emphasises acceptance and mindfulness as a way of reducing psychological suffering.

Compassion-Focused Therapy (CFT): CFT is a form of therapy that focusses on increasing self-compassion and compassion for others.

There is some evidence suggesting that RO-BPT, ACT and CFT may be helpful in the treatment of anorexia nervosa, but the evidence base is still limited, and more research is needed to fully understand their potential as treatments for AN.

In terms of biological approaches, leptin, oxytocin and deep brain stimulation (DBS) are three areas that have garnered some interest in recent years. These are still in their early stages, and more research is needed to fully understand their potential role in the disorder and their effectiveness as treatment options.

Avoidant Restrictive Food Intake Disorder

Avoidant restrictive food intake disorder (ARFID) (ICD-11) is a new category, first introduced in DSM-5 in 2013. It is characterised by food intake of insufficient quality or variety to meet needs, resulting in significant weight loss, nutritional deficiencies or otherwise negatively affect physical health with significant functional impairment. Weight loss or gain is not motivated by preoccupation with body weight or shape, nor is it the result of a lack of food or the manifestation of another medical condition.

This category replaces and expands the DSM-IV diagnostic of feeding disorder of infancy or early childhood. Prior to that, the presentation was classified as atypical AN in adults, selective eating in children by the ICD-10, or EDNOS (eating disorder not otherwise specified). The key diagnostic characteristic is avoidance or restriction of food intake, as shown by clinically significant failure to meet nutritional needs or inadequate oral energy intake. At least one of the following must be present:

- Severe weight loss
- Considerable nutritional deficiency (or related health consequence)
- Dependency on enteral feeding or oral nutritional supplements
- Significant impairment of psychosocial functioning

The evaluation of whether a weight loss is significant is based on clinical judgement; children and adolescents who are still growing may not maintain weight or height gains throughout their developmental trajectory rather than losing weight.

Prevalence

As ARFID is a relatively new diagnostic category, its prevalence is not well established. Nevertheless, some studies estimate that ARFID affects between 2 and 5 per cent of the general population and that it may be more prevalent in certain populations, such as children and adolescents than in adults.[123] Avoidant/restrictive food intake associated with autism spectrum disorder is more prevalent in males than in females and with those with a history of gastrointestinal diseases.

Differential Diagnosis

Differential diagnoses include organic causes, such as malignancies and chronic inflammation or infections, such as inflammatory bowel disease (IBD), HIV or Covid. Other mental disorders, such as specific phobias, depression or schizophrenia, need to be excluded.

Because patients present with malnutrition, the evaluation follows a pattern very similar to that of AN. Due to selective eating, vitamin deficiencies such as scurvy and pellagra are more common, and appropriate supplementation is necessary.

Aetiology

A recent twin study estimated 79 per cent heritability and 21 per cent non-shared environmental factor.[124] Further genetic studies are under way.

Treatment

NICE has not yet recommended a treatment due to insufficient research. CBT can be adapted for ARFID, and therapeutic research is ongoing. Current practices include a multidisciplinary approach, including dieticians, psychologists and medical practitioners.

Bulimia Nervosa

History

The word 'bulimia' is derived from the Greek 'bous', meaning 'ox', and 'limos', meaning 'hunger'. A state of pathological voracity has been recognised for centuries. However, in many accounts, the bulimia was considered to be a symptom of a physical disorder. In August 1979, Professor Gerald Russell[125] published 'Bulimia Nervosa: An Ominous Variant of Anorexia'. He recounted 30 cases from the previous eight years. Christopher Fairburn[126] was a junior doctor in Edinburgh at the time, and he writes later:

> *Two of Gerald Russell's suggestions were off:*
>
> *He implied bulimia nervosa was rare. I was unknown, but I had seen almost as many cases as he had. I also noticed that many of these patients had hidden their problem for years. I thought bulimia nervosa was common but hidden.*
>
> *He called the disorder 'intractable' . . . I never found it intractable. Half my patients responded completely, and many others improved significantly.*

Building on these early observations, Fairburn spent the rest of his career developing psychological treatments for eating disorders. The diagnosis was added to DSM in 1980.

Clinical Presentation and Diagnosis

The main distinction from the AN binge–purging subtype is that people suffering from BN are of normal or above-average weight. According to the DSM-5, BN is characterised by the following key features:

- Recurrent episodes of binge eating
- Recurrent inappropriate compensatory behaviours to prevent weight gain
- Self-evaluation that is unduly influenced by body shape and weight

Binge eating and inappropriate compensatory behaviours must occur at least once per week on average for three months to qualify for the diagnosis. An 'episode of binge eating' is defined as consuming a greater quantity of food in a discrete period of time than the average person would consume in a similar period of time under similar conditions. The clinician's assessment of whether the intake is excessive may be influenced by the context of eating (such as feasts at festivals versus eating alone in secret). Bingeing has not been clearly defined, but there is a move to use operational criteria such as objective overeating (1,000 kcal or much more) accompanied by a sense of loss of control, followed by feelings of shame and disgust. Fairburn also distinguishes objective and subjective binges (in the latter, a person may feel guilty about eating something outside of their dietary rules). The content of binges varies from an array of 'forbidden' hyperpalatable foods[127] to foodstuffs that would normally be regarded with disgust (leftovers or food from the dustbin). The most common triggers for binges are violations of self-imposed dietary restrictions or feelings of depression, anxiety, loneliness or boredom. Binges tend to occur at night, suggesting that there may be a disturbance of diurnal rhythm in BN. The preoccupation with weight and shape concerns is the driving force behind disordered eating, which can interfere with concentration and socialisation. Common compensatory behaviours include self-induced vomiting, laxative abuse, prolonged fasting and excessive exercise. The extent of these can be extreme and can put the patient at significant distress and risk.

Severity is defined according to the frequency of binge–purging cycles.

Epidemiology

The lifetime prevalence of BN is estimated to be 1–3%.[71,81] Population studies show that up to 3% of females and more than 1% of males suffer from this disorder during their lifetime. While epidemiological studies in the past mainly focused on young females from Western countries, AN and BN are reported worldwide among males and females from all ages. The rate of BN has been increasing globally and is similar in industrialised nations such as the USA, Canada, Europe, Australia, Japan, New Zealand and South Africa. In specialist services in the UK, white female patients are predominant, but other ethnic groups have comparable rates. Males and ethnic minorities are underrepresented in treatment-seeking populations due to stigma and barriers to accessing services. This is an important challenge for service organisations.

Aetiology

The aetiology of BN is still poorly understood but involves a complex interaction of biological, psychological and environmental factors. The following are among the most well-known risk factors for the development of BN:

Genetic and Neurobiological Factors

Twin studies have reported BN heritability estimates ranging from 28 per cent to 83 per cent.[26,128] Several studies are currently underway to recruit people suffering from BN and BED for genome-wide studies as part of a global effort led by the Psychiatric Genomics Consortium.[128] Molecular genetics research in the genome-wide era is improving our understanding of the biology behind eating disorders' heritability and may help find new treatments.

BN pathophysiology has been studied using a variety of biological systems, including serotonergic genes, dopaminergic genes, opioid genes, appetite regulation genes and endocannabinoid genes. The serotonergic system is of interest because BN patients have abnormalities in peripheral serotonin uptake, and medications acting on 5-HT pathways have shown efficacy in BN patients.[26] The dopaminergic system is also implicated in BN,[129] with neuroimaging studies showing abnormalities. Opioid peptides influence feeding behaviour, and their genes are likely to influence BN. In comparison to AN, studies on appetite regulation genes in BN have been limited, and conflicting results have been obtained regarding the association with plasma leptin levels. Hormone secretion, such as PYY and GLP-1, has been found to be reduced in BN patients. This may indicate abnormalities in satiety regulation. The endocannabinoid system may also play a role in BN control through central and peripheral mechanisms.

Psychological Factors

Individuals with BN are more likely to have low self-esteem and a need for control, as well as neurodiversity. In addition, traumatic experiences and stressful life events can increase the likelihood of developing BN. A large case-controlled study found that those with eating disorders were more likely than controls to have experienced stressful life events. Specifically, rape, other forms of sexual assault, and emotional abuse were significantly more prevalent among those with a history of binge eating/purging ED subtypes than among controls. In addition, a history of life-threatening illness and the death of a close relative, partner or friend were associated with certain subtypes of ED. Multiple events increased the risk. Clinical experience supports this, but the pathomechanism needs clarification.[130]

Social Factors

Social factors can contribute to the development of body dissatisfaction and the motivation to lose weight. Dieting is a long-recognised risk factor for bulimic pathology.[131] In a large longitudinal cohort study, higher weight suppression at baseline predicted higher bulimic symptoms at the 20-year follow-up, controlling for demographic variables, baseline bulimic symptoms, body mass index and drive for thinness. An increased desire for thinness mediated this effect at 10-year follow-up. This finding suggests that weight suppression has a long-term effect on bulimic symptoms, and preoccupation with thinness may maintain this association. On the positive side, two-thirds of patients recovered.[132]

In conclusion, the aetiology of BN is likely complex and multifactorial, and different people may have different risk factors. These may include premorbid dieting and related risk factors and general psychiatric disorder risk factors. Effective interventions must investigate individual maintaining factors.

Comorbidities

Physical

People with type 1 and type 2 diabetes are prone to BN and BED.[133] The co-occurrence of diabetes and eating disorders suggests the potential shared pathomechanisms. Insulin may be a common denominator: its involvement in diabetes is well-known, and it has a significant impact on satiety and eating behaviour.[134] A recent study found that 98 per cent of individuals with type 1 diabetes engage in disinhibited eating during perceived episodes of hypoglycaemia, which is related to a mismatch of the dose of insulin and dietary carbohydrate intake, and up to 50 per cent develop disturbed eating behaviours after the diagnosis of diabetes and commencement of insulin treatment.[135]

A number of models have been proposed for the maintenance of eating disorders in type 1 diabetes, which consider the biological and metabolic effects of insulin and disruption of hunger and satiety regulation in addition to traditional psychological factors.[136,137]

Diabulimia as a term is controversial,[138] and the current preferred name in the UK is T1DE (type 1 disordered eating).

Research has shown that people with diabetes and eating disorders do not respond to standard eating disorder treatment and have high drop-out rates from psychological therapies and high risk of irreversible complications.[136,139]

Psychiatric

Affective disorders are common in eating disorders, and BN is no exception.[140] They include atypical depression or bipolar illness. Overeating is typical in significant depression, as is the focus on body shape and weight of BN. If the criteria of both disorders are met, both diagnoses should be provided. It is important to be aware that the risk of suicide is elevated in BN.[81,141]

Substance Misuse

Twin studies reveal shared genetic variance between liabilities to eating disorders and substance use, with the strongest associations between symptoms of bulimia nervosa and problem alcohol use.[142] Comorbid alcohol and substance misuse is not uncommon and greatly increases the risk of physical complications and suicide, and it is essential that patients receive integrated care across various agencies.

Personality Disorder

Emotionally unstable (borderline) personality disorder has been a topic of much debate.[143] Binge eating is included in the impulsive behaviour criterion that is part of the borderline personality disorder definition. Clinical experience suggests that successful treatment of the eating disorder often improves emotional dysregulation,[54] but further research is needed.

The link between ADHD and BN has been recently recognised.[144] ADHD is often missed in patients with eating disorders. Patients with comorbid ADHD and BN are more impulsive and inattentive, have more severe disordered eating patterns, and

Box 12.10 Common comorbidities and risk of mortality in BN

	Physical comorbidities	SMR	Psychiatric comorbidities	SMR
Bulimia nervosa	• Overweight and obese • Fertility problems • Cardiovascular • Electrolyte abnormalities • Endocrine • Gastrointestinal • Reduced bone density • Type 1 and type 2 diabetes	**2–3**	• Depression • Bipolar • Anxiety • PTSD • Personality disorder • ADHD • Alcohol and substance misuse • Suicide attempt	**3.4** **4** **3–7**

have more general psychopathological symptoms than those without ADHD. Psychostimulants have been found to reduce BN symptoms in patients with comorbid ADHD. A summary of common comorbidities in BN is found in Box 12.10.

Assessment

Clinicians need to be aware that patients often feel intense shame and embarrassment about their bingeing and purging, so a compassionate and sensitive approach is essential. In depth exploration of the eating pathology and the methods of weight control should be included as a part of the psychiatric assessment. The presence of any other psychiatric comorbidity should be established, as this may influence treatment. Social difficulties and current life stresses should be also sought, as they may play a role in maintaining the illness.

It is important to ascertain during history taking whether there are any significant underlying medical conditions or medical consequences. The enquiry should cover teeth, salivary glands, gastrointestinal function (bleeding, regurgitation) and kidney and endocrine function. A physical examination and a screen for electrolyte abnormalities are also required.

Physical Complications and Risk Indicators

Even if the patient is at a healthy weight, BN can result in serious, life-threatening complications. These include electrolyte imbalances and dehydration, which can lead to arrhythmias, kidney and heart damage, weakness and fatigue, cognitive disturbances or seizures. Gastrointestinal problems, such as acid reflux, abdominal pain, inflammation of the oesophagus, gastric dilation and bowel complications due to laxative abuse, can be dangerous. Tooth decay and gum disease from exposure to stomach acid during purging are common and need treatment. Hormonal imbalances, such as irregular menstruation, can also occur in BN.

Differential Diagnosis

Binge eating/purging subtype of AN: Patients whose binge eating behaviour happens solely during periods of AN should be diagnosed with AN, binge eating purging type, and should not be diagnosed with BN as well. For individuals with AN who binge and purge but no longer satisfy the entire criteria for AN, binge eating/purging type (e.g. when weight is normal), a diagnosis of BN should be made only after all criteria for BN have been met for at least three months.

Binge eating syndrome: If the person binge eats without inappropriate compensatory behaviours on a regular basis, binge eating disorder diagnosis should be considered.

Purging disorder (OSFED): Recurrent purging behaviour to influence weight or shape (e.g. self-induced vomiting; misuse of laxatives, diuretics or other medications) in the absence of binge eating.

Uncommon medical conditions: Abnormal eating behaviours in certain neurological or other medical diseases, such as Kleine–Levin syndrome or gastroparesis, but the typical psychological aspects of BN – such as over-concern with body form and weight – are not present.

Treatment

The NICE[31] guidelines advocate a step care model, based on severity.

The first step is BN-nervosa-focused guided self-help, which use cognitive behavioural self-help materials[35] and are supplemented by brief supportive sessions (e.g. four to nine sessions lasting 20 minutes each over 16 weeks). If this is unacceptable, contraindicated or ineffective, CBT-E should be considered (see earlier). Both use the CBT model of the individual formulation of BN as shown in Figure 12.2. CBT delivered in a self-help or guided self-help format seems to be almost as efficacious as a full course of CBT (usually 20 sessions).[145] Recently, the shorter form of CBT-ED has been found sufficient for some patients, and research on online delivery shows encouraging results.[146,147]

Medication is less effective than psychological treatments, and the combination of medication and psychological treatment seems to be more effective than either treatment on its own but has higher drop-out rates. Most studies have focused on SSRIs, such as fluoxetine (60 mg/d). Higher doses than are typically used in depression produce a positive effect on the number of binge-purge episodes. Treatment for two years is recommended by some authors,[148] although RCT evidence is lacking. Other substances currently being studied in RCT include the opioid antagonist naloxone, which is administered intranasally, and lisdexamfetamine.

Outcome

Course Development

Bulimia nervosa typically starts in adolescence or early adulthood. It is unusual for symptoms to appear before puberty or after the age of 40. Binge eating usually starts during or after a period of dieting to reduce weight. Multiple stressful life events might potentially precipitate the onset of BN.

Common associated psychological features include depression, guilt, irritability and poor concentration. A subgroup of BN share the same compulsive behaviours as seen in AN. Social impairment can be significant. A disruption in the social network is common, as people with BN become unpredictable; for example, they let people down and arrive late because of their tendency to spend long periods of time checking their body. The profound change in mood can result in neglect and disinterest in friendships or avoidance because of the fear of eating with others, while in work situations, mood changes can result in impaired concentration, missing school and increased sick leave. People with BN are more likely to get involved in romantic relationships than those with AN, but these relationships may be impaired by the disorder. Because the illness has a later onset, often when people have left home, there is less family involvement. Otherwise, problems may arise over the use of the bathroom or eccentric behaviours around food, including stealing from others.

Long-term follow-up studies are scarce. Steinhausen found that, based on 27 studies with three outcome criteria (recovery, improvement and chronicity), nearly 45% of patients recovered from BN, 27% improved significantly and 23% had a chronic, prolonged course.[149] Early treatment of BN improved outcomes. The severity of psychiatric comorbidities predicts a poorer long-term prognosis of BN.[150]

Individuals with BN have a significantly increased risk of mortality (all-cause and suicide). The following are risk factors for BN mortality:

Electrolyte imbalances: severe purging behaviours can result in life-threatening electrolyte imbalances, dehydration and cardiac complications such as arrhythmias or heart failure.

Digestive system: Purging can cause damage to the digestive system, including the oesophageal tears and stomach, which can result in serious health problems.

Suicide: People suffering from BN are more likely to die by suicide or engage in self-harming behaviours. The risk is increased with a previous history of self harm and comorbid psychiatric disorders, including substance misuse.

Binge Eating Disorder

Clinical Presentation and Diagnosis

Binge eating disorder is similar to BN, with the exception of compensatory behaviours. BED includes recurrent episodes of binge eating without compensatory behaviours. An episode of binge eating is characterised by the following:

- Eating, in a discrete period of time (e.g. within any two-hour period), an amount of food that is definitely larger than what most people would eat in a similar period of time under similar circumstances. The binge eating episodes are associated with three (or more) of the following:
    - Eating much more rapidly than normal
    - Eating until feeling uncomfortably full
    - Eating large amounts of food when not feeling physically hungry
    - Eating alone because of feeling embarrassed by the amount eaten
    - Feeling disgusted with oneself, depressed or very guilty afterward
- A sense of lack of control over eating during the episode (e.g. a feeling that one cannot stop eating or control what or how much one is eating)
- Marked distress
- The binge eating occurs, on average, at least once a week for three months
- The binge eating is not associated with the recurrent use of inappropriate compensatory behaviour as in BN and does not occur exclusively during the course of BN or AN

People with BED are often obese and have obesity-related complications. Depression is common.

Epidemiology

Although population-based epidemiological studies are limited, BED is increasing. A recent Australian population-based study focusing on trends between 1995 and 2015 found that the prevalence of both obesity (19 to 33%) and binge eating (3 to 11%) increased significantly. The highest increases were observed in the prevalence of obesity with comorbid binge eating (7.3-fold) and obesity with comorbid very strict dieting/fasting (11.5-fold) (Figure 12.6).[11]

Furthermore, the association between diabetes and eating disorders, particularly BN and BED, is increasingly recognised.[92,151] A recent systematic review and meta-analysis found that the risk of type 2 diabetes is approximately three times higher among people with BN and BED, whilst the risk of developing type 2 diabetes is reduced in AN.[152]

The pandemic had a further impact. In a sample of 35,000 UK residents, those with psychiatric disorders, ethnic minority status, unemployment or pandemic anxiety were more likely to binge eat, have suicidal or self harm thoughts, or self harm for the first time.[153] This shows that a high level of stress triggers BED in vulnerable people. For a summary of comorbidities with BED, see Box 12.11.

Aetiology

Many of the risk factors for BN are shared by people with BED. Genetics and metabolic factors are under investigation.

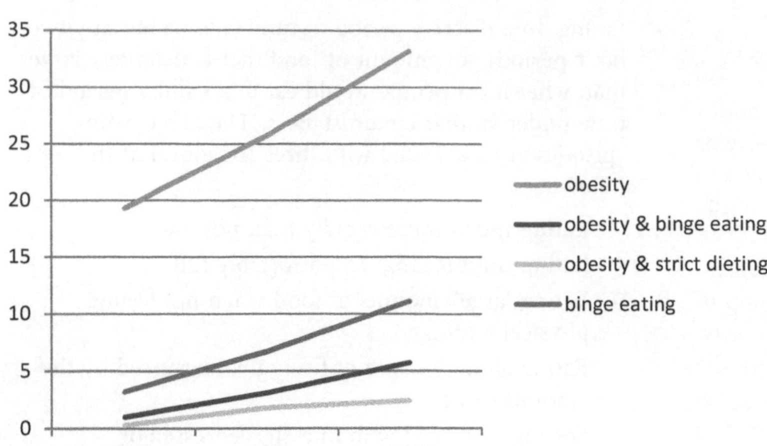

Figure 12.6 Prevalence of obesity and comorbid eating disorder behaviours in South Australia from 1995 to 2015.[11,29]

Box 12.11 Comorbidities and BED

	Physical comorbidities	SMR	Psychiatric comorbidities	SMR
Binge eating disorder	• Obesity • Respiratory disorders • Musculoskeletal • Gastrointestinal disorder • Type 2 diabetes, endocrine • Metabolic disorder • Fatty liver • Cardiovascular	**1.5–2**	• Depression • Bipolar • Anxiety • PTSD • Alcohol and substance misuse • Suicide attempt	

A recent UK BioBank study found that people with binge-type eating disorders had higher polygenic scores than controls for other psychiatric disorders, including depression, schizophrenia and attention-deficit/hyperactivity disorder, and higher polygenic scores for body mass index, which is consistent with clinical observations.[154] A systematic review found that bulimia nervosa and binge eating disorders are associated with decreased insulin sensitivity.[155]

Treatment

Most of the treatments applied in BN, such as self-help approaches using CBT manuals have been applied to people with BED. NICE (2017) also suggests the possibility of group or individual CBT-ED. Efficacy in terms of reduction in binge eating is good, although there is usually little success in terms of weight loss for those who are obese. Further work is needed to address both the metabolic and psychological factors in treatment.

Medication

Lisdexamfetamine is approved for the treatment of BED in several countries, including the United States. It is also approved for the treatment of ADHD. There are good indications of efficacy for SSRIs (citalopram, fluvoxamine, fluoxetine and especially sertraline), with special emphasis on the positive effect on impulse control and the treatment of comorbid anxiety and depression. The dose is high, as is common in the treatment of obsessive-compulsive disorder. Among the SSRIs, sertraline has the best evidence for treating BED (off label). Topiramate, an anticonvulsant, has also been found to be effective in the treatment of BED in terms of weight loss and reduction of BED symptoms; however, it has significant side effects and is not always tolerated.[148]

Outcome

Binge eating disorder is often hidden and long-standing. In clinical samples, it is not uncommon to have a delay of treatment seeking by decades. Work is under way to develop online self -help programmes to reduce this treatment gap.[156]

Medical complications are related to obesity, which can increase the risk of various health problems, including cardiovascular complications, type 2 diabetes, high blood pressure, high cholesterol and sleep apnoea. Joint pain and mobility problems can develop due to obesity complications. Patients with lifetime AN have higher complexity as well as physical and psychiatric comorbidities, including gastrointestinal disorders and comorbid anxiety, depression and ADHD.[157] Risk of suicidal ideation and suicide attempts is significantly increased.[158]

References

1. American Psychiatric Association. *Diagnostic and Statistical Manual of Mental Disorders: DSM-5.* Washington, DC: American Psychiatric Association; 2013.
2. World Health Organization. *ICD-11: International Classification of Diseases (11th revision).* Geneva: World Health Organization; 2019.
3. Schaumberg K, Welch E, Breithaupt L, et al. The science behind the Academy for Eating Disorders' Nine Truths About Eating Disorders. *European Eating Disorders Review* 2017;25 (6):432–50.
4. Silen Y, Keski-Rahkonen A. Worldwide prevalence of DSM-5 eating disorders among young people. *Current Opinion in Psychiatry* 2022;35(6):362–71.
5. NHS Digital. *Health Survey for England, 2019.* digital.nhs.uk/data-and-information/publications/statistical/health-survey-for-england/2019/health-survey-for-england-2019-data-tables (accessed 15 December 2022).
6. Kutz AM, Marsh AG, Gunderson CG, et al. Eating disorder screening: a systematic review and meta-analysis of diagnostic test characteristics of the SCOFF. *Journal of General Internal Medicine* 2020;35(3):885–93.
7. McManus SM, Meltzer H, Brugha T, et al. *Adult Psychiatric Morbidity in England, 2007: Results of a Household Survey.* London; 2009.
8. Ayton A, Viljoen D, Ryan S, et al. Risk, demand, capacity and outcomes in adult specialist eating disorder services in South-East of England before and since COVID-19. *BJPsych Bulletin* 2022;46 (2):89–95.
9. Galmiche M, Dechelotte P, Lambert G, et al. Prevalence of eating disorders over the 2000–2018 period: a systematic literature review. *American Journal of Clinical Nutrition* 2019;109(5):1402–13.
10. Nolan E, Bunting L, McCartan C, et al. Prevalence of probable eating disorders and associated risk factors: an analysis of the Northern Ireland Youth Wellbeing Survey using the SCOFF. *British Journal of Clinical Psychology* 2022;62(1):180–95.
11. da Luz FQ, Sainsbury A, Mannan H, et al. Prevalence of obesity and comorbid eating disorder behaviors in South Australia from 1995 to 2015. *International Journal of Obesity (London)* 2017;41(7):1148–53.
12. Flatt RE, Thornton LM, Fitzsimmons-Craft EE, et al. Comparing eating disorder characteristics and treatment in self-identified competitive athletes and non-athletes from the National Eating Disorders Association online screening tool. *International Journal of Eating Disorders* 2021;54(3):365–75.
13. Nagata JM, Ganson KT, Austin SB. Emerging trends in eating disorders among sexual and gender minorities. *Current Opinion in Psychiatry* 2020;33 (6):562–67.
14. Ferrucci KA, Lapane KL, Jesdale BM. Prevalence of diagnosed eating disorders in US transgender adults and youth in insurance claims. *International Journal of Eating Disorders* 2022;55 (6):801–9.
15. Swartz L. Anorexia nervosa as a culture-bound syndrome. *Social Science & Medicine* 1985;20(7):725–30.
16. Pike KM, Dunne PE. The rise of eating disorders in Asia: a review. *Journal of Eating Disorders* 2015;3:33.
17. Monteiro CA, Moubarac JC, Cannon G, et al. Ultra-processed products are becoming dominant in the global food system. *Obesity Reviews* 2013;14(Suppl 2):21–8.
18. Tobias DK, Hall KD. Eliminate or reformulate ultra-processed foods? Biological mechanisms matter. *Cell Metabolism* 2021;33(12):2314–5.
19. Hall KD, Ayuketah A, Brychta R, et al. Ultra-processed diets cause excess calorie intake and weight gain: an inpatient randomized controlled trial of ad libitum food intake. *Cell Metabolism* 2020;32(4):690.
20. Eikey EV, Reddy MC, Booth KM, et al. Desire to be underweight: exploratory study on a weight loss app community and user perceptions of the impact on disordered eating behaviors. *JMIR mHealth uHealth* 2017;5(10):e150.
21. Ghaderi A, Bulik C, Myralf M, et al. Anonymous online survey on disordered eating, drive for muscularity, sexual orientation, and satisfaction with life in young Swedish males. *Archives of Sexual Behavior* 2022;51(7):3457–65.
22. Downs J, Mycock G. Eating disorders in men: limited models of diagnosis and treatment are failing patients. *BMJ* 2022;376:o537.
23. Fichter MM, Naab S, Voderholzer U, et al. Mortality in males as compared to females treated for an eating disorder: a large prospective controlled study. *Eating and Weight Disorders* 2021;26 (5):1627–37.
24. Hoang U, Goldacre M, James A. Mortality following hospital discharge with a diagnosis of eating disorder: national record linkage study, England, 2001-2009. *International Journal of Eating Disorders* 2014;47(5):507–15.
25. van Hoeken D, Hoek HW. Review of the burden of eating disorders: mortality, disability, costs, quality of life, and family burden. *Current Opinion in Psychiatry* 2020;33(6):521–7.
26. Bulik CM, Coleman JRI, Hardaway JA, et al. Genetics and neurobiology of eating disorders. *Nature Neuroscience* 2022;25(5):543–54.
27. Mack I, Penders J, Cook J, et al. Is the impact of starvation on the gut microbiota specific or unspecific to anorexia nervosa? A narrative review based on a systematic literature search. *Current Neuropharmacology* 2018;16 (8):1131–49.
28. Mack I, Cuntz U, Gramer C, et al. Weight gain in anorexia nervosa does not ameliorate the faecal microbiota, branched chain fatty acid profiles, and gastrointestinal complaints. *Scientific Reports* 2016;6:26752.
29. Ayton A, Ibrahim A. The Western diet: a blind spot of eating disorder research? – a narrative review and recommendations for treatment and research. *Nutrition Reviews* 2020;78 (7):579–96.
30. Small DM, DiFeliceantonio AG. Processed foods and food reward. *Science* 2019;363(6425):346–47.
31. National Institute for Health and Care Excellence. *Eating Disorders: Recognition and Treatment. NICE Guideline (NG69).* London: NICE; 2017.
32. Scottish Intercollegiate Guidelines Network. *SIGN 164: Eating Disorders.* Edinburgh: Heathcare Improvement, Scotland; 2022.
33. Viljoen DK, King E, Harris S, et al. The alarms should no longer be ignored: A survey of the demand, capacity and provision of adult community eating disorder services in England and Scotland. *PsyArXiv* 2022. psyarxiv.com/6eszj/.

34. American Psychiatric Association. *The American Psychiatric Association Practice Guideline for the Treatment of Patients with Eating Disorders*. Washington, DC: American Psychiatric Association; 2023.

35. Fairburn CG. *Overcoming Binge Eating*. 2nd ed. New York, London: The Guilford Press; 2013.

36. Cooper Z, Fairburn C. The eating disorder examination: a semi-structured interview for the assessment of the specific psychopathology of eating disorders. *International Journal of Eating Disorders* 1987;6(1):1–8.

37. Bohn K, Doll HA, Cooper Z, et al. The measurement of impairment due to eating disorder psychopathology. *Behavior Research and Therapy* 2008;46 (10):1105–10.

38. Hilbert A, Hoek HW, Schmidt R. Evidence-based clinical guidelines for eating disorders: international comparison. *Current Opinion in Psychiatry* 2017;30(6):423–37.

39. National Institute for Health and Care Excellence. *NICE Guidance 69. Eating Disorders: Recognition and Treatment*. London: NIHCE. www.nice.org.uk/guidance/ng69 (accessed 14 September 2023).

40. Lock J. Family therapy for eating disorders in youth: current confusions, advances, and new directions. *Current Opinion in Psychiatry* 2018;31(6): 431–5.

41. Milos G, Spindler A, Schnyder U, et al. Instability of eating disorder diagnoses: prospective study. *British Journal of Psychiatry* 2005;187:573–8.

42. Fairburn CG, Cooper Z, Shafran R. Cognitive behaviour therapy for eating disorders: a 'transdiagnostic' theory and treatment. *Behavior Research and Therapy* 2003;41(5):509–28.

43. Schmidt U, Ryan EG, Bartholdy S, et al. Two-year follow-up of the MOSAIC trial: a multicenter randomized controlled trial comparing two psychological treatments in adult outpatients with broadly defined anorexia nervosa. *International Journal of Eating Disorders* 2016;49(8):793–800.

44. McIntosh VV, Jordan J, Luty SE, et al. Specialist supportive clinical management for anorexia nervosa. *International Journal of Eating Disorders* 2006;39(8):625–32.

45. Zipfel S, Wild B, Gross G, et al. Focal psychodynamic therapy, cognitive behaviour therapy, and optimised treatment as usual in outpatients with anorexia nervosa (ANTOP study): randomised controlled trial. *Lancet* 2014;383(9912):127–37.

46. Monteleone AM, Pellegrino F, Croatto G, et al. Treatment of eating disorders: a systematic meta-review of meta-analyses and network meta-analyses. *Neuroscience & Biobehavioral Reviews* 2022;142:104857.

47. National Institute of Care and Excellence. *Transition between Inpatient Mental Health Settings and Community or Care Home Settings (NG 53)*. London: NICE; 2016.

48. Fairburn CG, Jones R, Peveler RC, et al. Three psychological treatments for bulimia nervosa. A comparative trial. *Archives of General Psychiatry* 1991;48 (5):463–9.

49. Fairburn CG, Bailey-Straebler S, Basden S, et al. A transdiagnostic comparison of enhanced cognitive behaviour therapy (CBT-E) and interpersonal psychotherapy in the treatment of eating disorders. *Behavior Research and Therapy* 2015;70:64–71.

50. Fairburn CG, Cooper Z, Doll HA, et al. Transdiagnostic cognitive-behavioral therapy for patients with eating disorders: a two-site trial with 60-week follow-up. *American Journal of Psychiatry* 2009;166(3):311–9.

51. Dalle Grave R, Calugi S, Doll HA, et al. Enhanced cognitive behaviour therapy for adolescents with anorexia nervosa: an alternative to family therapy? *Behavior Research and Therapy* 2013;51 (1):R9–R12.

52. Le Grange D, Eckhardt S, Dalle Grave R, et al. Enhanced cognitive-behavior therapy and family-based treatment for adolescents with an eating disorder: a non-randomized effectiveness trial. *Psychological Medicine* 2020:1–11.

53. Dalle Grave R. *Multistep Cognitive Behavioral Therapy for Eating Disorders*. Plymouth, UK: Jason Aronson; 2013.

54. Dalle Grave R, Sartirana M, Calugi S. *Complex Cases and Comorbidity in Eating Disorders*. New York: Springer; 2021.

55. Parliamentary and Health Service Ombudsman. *Ignoring the Alarms: How NHS Eating Disorder Services Are Failing Patients*. London: Parliamentary and Health Service Ombudsman, 2017.

56. Ayton A, Ibrahim A. Does UK medical education provide doctors with sufficient skills and knowledge to manage patients with eating disorders safely? *Postgraduate Medical Journal* 2018;94(1113):374–80.

57. Nicholls D, Robinson P, Ayton A, et al. *Medical Emergencies in Eating Disorders (MEED): Guidance on Recognition and Management. CR233*. London: Royal College of Psychiatrists; 2022.

58. Bell RM. *Holy Anorexia*. Chicago, IL: The University of Chicago Press; 1985.

59. Morton R. *Phthisiologia: Or, a Treatise of Consumptions*. London: Smith and Walford; 1694. *English translation of*;1689.

60. Marcé L-V. On a form of hypochondriacal delirium occurring consecutive to dyspepsia, and characterized by refusal of food. *Journal of Psychological Medicine and Mental Pathology* 1860;13:264–66.

61. Gull WW. Address in medicine. *British Medical Journal* 1868;2(397):131.

62. Lasegue EC. On hysterical anorexia. *Dialogues in Philosophy, Mental & Neuro Sciences* 2016;9(1).

63. Gull W. Anorexia hysterica (apepsia hysterical). *British Medical Journal* 1873;2:1873.

64. Ryle JA. Anorexia nervosa. *Lancet* 1936;2:893.

65. Keys A, Brožek J, Henschel A, et al. *The Biology of Human Starvation* (2 vols). Minneapolis: University of Minnesota Press; 1950.

66. Russell GF. The changing nature of anorexia nervosa: an introduction to the conference. *Journal of Psychiatric Research* 1985;19(2–3):101–9.

67. Prince R. The concept of culture-bound syndromes: anorexia nervosa and brain-fag. *Social Science & Medicine* 1985;21 (2):197–203.

68. Watson HJ, Thornton LM, Yilmaz Z, et al. Common genetic variation and age of onset of anorexia nervosa. *Biological Psychiatry Global Open Science* 2022;2 (4):368–78.

69. Austin A, Flynn M, Shearer J, et al. The first episode rapid early intervention for eating disorders – upscaled study: clinical outcomes. *Early Intervention in Psychiatry* 2021;16(1):97–105.

70. Dobrescu SR, Dinkler L, Gillberg C, et al. Anorexia nervosa: 30-year outcome. *British Journal of Psychiatry* 2020;216(2):97–104.

71. van Eeden AE, van Hoeken D, Hoek HW. Incidence, prevalence and mortality of anorexia nervosa and bulimia nervosa. *Current Opinion in Psychiatry* 2021;34(6):515–24.

72. Keshaviah A, Edkins K, Hastings ER, et al. Re-examining premature mortality in anorexia nervosa: a meta-analysis redux. *Comprehensive Psychiatry* 2014;55(8):1773–84.

73. Ishiguro H, Yagasaki H, Horiuchi Y. Ehlers-Danlos syndrome in the field of psychiatry: a review. *Frontiers in Psychiatry* 2021;12:803898.

74. Sharp HEC, Critchley HD, Eccles JA. Connecting brain and body: transdiagnostic relevance of connective tissue variants to neuropsychiatric symptom expression. *World Journal of Psychiatry* 2021;11(10):805–20.

75. McAulay C, Hay P, Mond J, et al. Eating disorders, bipolar disorders and other mood disorders: complex and under-researched relationships. *Journal of Eating Disorders* 2019;7:32.

76. Li Z, Halls D, Byford S, et al. Autistic characteristics in eating disorders: treatment adaptations and impact on clinical outcomes. *European Eating Disorders Review* 2022;30(5): 671–90.

77. Dinkler L, Taylor MJ, Rastam M, et al. Anorexia nervosa and autism: a prospective twin cohort study. *Journal of Child Psychology and Psychiatry* 2021;62(3):316–26.

78. Jones DJ, Fox MM, Babigian HM, et al. Epidemiology of anorexia nervosa in Monroe County, New York: 1960–1976. *Psychosomatic Medicine* 1980;42 (6):551–8.

79. Micali N, Hagberg KW, Petersen I, et al. The incidence of eating disorders in the UK in 2000-2009: findings from the General Practice Research Database. *BMJ Open* 2013;3: e002646. doi:10 .1136/ bmjopen-2013-002646.

80. Udo T, Grilo CM. Prevalence and correlates of DSM-5-defined eating disorders in a nationally representative sample of U.S. adults. *Biological Psychiatry* 2018;84(5):345–54.

81. Keski-Rahkonen A, Mustelin L. Epidemiology of eating disorders in Europe: prevalence, incidence, comorbidity, course, consequences, and risk factors. *Current Opinion in Psychiatry* 2016;29(6):340–5.

82. Nakamura K, Yamamoto M, Yamazaki O, et al. Prevalence of anorexia nervosa and bulimia nervosa in a geographically defined area in Japan. *International Journal of Eating Disorders* 2000;28 (2):173–80.

83. Tong J, Miao S, Wang J, et al. A two-stage epidemiologic study on prevalence of eating disorders in female university students in Wuhan, China. *Social Psychiatry and Psychiatric Epidemiology* 2014;49(3):499–505.

84. Tsai MC, Gan ST, Lee CT, et al. National population-based data on the incidence, prevalence, and psychiatric comorbidity of eating disorders in Taiwanese adolescents and young adults. *International Journal of Eating Disorders* 2018;51 (11):1277–84.

85. Selvini-Palazzoli M, Viaro M. The anorectic process in the family: a six-stage model as a guide for individual therapy. *Family Process* 1988;27 (2):129–48.

86. Minuchin SR, Baker BI. *Psychosomatic Families: Anorexia Nervosa in Context.* Harvard, MA: Harvard University Press; 1978.

87. Crisp A, Hsu L, Harding B, et al. Clinical features of anorexia nervosa: a study of a consecutive series of 102 female patients. *Journal of Psychosomatic Research* 1980;24(3–4):179–91.

88. Watson HJ, Yilmaz Z, Thornton LM, et al. Genome-wide association study identifies eight risk loci and implicates metabo-psychiatric origins for anorexia nervosa. *Nature Genetics* 2019;51 (8):1207–14.

89. Duncan L, Yilmaz Z, Gaspar H, et al. Significant locus and metabolic genetic correlations revealed in genome-wide association study of anorexia nervosa. *American Journal of Psychiatry* 2017;174(9):850–8.

90. Berthold N, Pytte J, Bulik CM, et al. Bridging the gap: short structural variants in the genetics of anorexia nervosa. *International Journal of Eating Disorders* 2022;55(6):747–53.

91. Johnson JS, Cote AC, Dobbyn A, et al. Mapping anorexia nervosa genes to clinical phenotypes. *Psychological Medicine* 2023;53(6):2619–33.

92. Hedman A, Breithaupt L, Hubel C, et al. Bidirectional relationship between eating disorders and autoimmune diseases. *Journal of Child Psychology and Psychiatry* 2019;60 (7):803–12.

93. Bulik CM, Flatt R, Abbaspour A, et al. Reconceptualizing anorexia nervosa. *Psychiatry and Clinical Neurosciences* 2019;73(9):518–25.

94. Penas-Lledo E, Bulik CM, Lichtenstein P, et al. Risk for self-reported anorexia or bulimia nervosa based on drive for thinness and negative affect clusters/ dimensions during adolescence: a three-year prospective study of the TChAD cohort. *International Journal of Eating Disorders* 2015;48(6):692–9.

95. Cass K, McGuire C, Bjork I, et al. Medical complications of anorexia nervosa. *Psychosomatics* 2020;61 (6):625–31.

96. Bulik CM, Carroll IM, Mehler P. Reframing anorexia nervosa as a metabo-psychiatric disorder. *Trends in Endocrinology & Metabolism* 2021;32 (10):752–61.

97. Igudesman D, Sweeney M, Carroll IM, et al. Gut-brain interactions: implications for a role of the gut microbiota in the treatment and prognosis of anorexia nervosa and comparison to type I diabetes. *Gastroenterology Clinics of North America* 2019;48(3):343–56.

98. Keller L, Dempfle A, Dahmen B, et al. The effects of polyunsaturated fatty acid (PUFA) administration on the microbiome-gut-brain axis in adolescents with anorexia nervosa (the MiGBAN study): study protocol for a longitudinal, double-blind, randomized, placebo-controlled trial. *Trials* 2022;23 (1):545.

99. Carrera O, Gutierrez E. Hyperactivity in anorexia nervosa: to warm or not to warm. That is the question (a translational research one). *Journal of Eating Disorders* 2018;6:4.

100. Feldman MB, Meyer IH. Comorbidity and age of onset of eating disorders in gay men, lesbians, and bisexuals. *Psychiatry Research* 2010;180(2–3):126–31.

101. Solmi M, Wade TD, Byrne S, et al. Comparative efficacy and acceptability of psychological interventions for the

treatment of adult outpatients with anorexia nervosa: a systematic review and network meta-analysis. *Lancet Psychiatry* 2021;8(3):215–24.

102. Ibrahim A, Ryan S, Viljoen D, et al. Integrated enhanced cognitive behavioural (I-CBTE) therapy significantly improves effectiveness of inpatient treatment of anorexia nervosa in real life settings. *Journal of Eating Disorders* 2022;10(1):98.

103. Herzog W, Wild B, Giel KE, et al. Focal psychodynamic therapy, cognitive behaviour therapy, and optimised treatment as usual in female outpatients with anorexia nervosa (ANTOP study): 5-year follow-up of a randomised controlled trial in Germany. *Lancet Psychiatry* 2022;9(4):280–90.

104. Matthews A, Kramer RA, Peterson CM, et al. Higher admission and rapid readmission rates among medically hospitalized youth with anorexia nervosa/atypical anorexia nervosa during COVID-19. *Eating Behaviors* 2021;43:101573.

105. NHS Digital. *Finished Admission Episodes (FAEs) with a Primary or Secondary Diagnosis of Eating Disorder.* digital.nhs.uk/data-and-information/find-data-and-publications/supplementary-information/2018-supplementary-information-files/finished-admission-episodes-faes-with-a-primary-or-secondary-diagnosis-of-eating-disorder.

106. Kaye WH, Bulik CM. Treatment of patients with anorexia nervosa in the US – A crisis in care. *JAMA Psychiatry* 2021;78(6):591–2.

107. Ibrahim A, Cutinha D, Ayton A. What is the evidence for using bed rest as part of hospital treatment of severe anorexia nervosa? *Evidence-Based Mental Health* 2019;22(2):77–82.

108. Goddard E, Hibbs R, Raenker S, et al. A multi-centre cohort study of short term outcomes of hospital treatment for anorexia nervosa in the UK. *BMC Psychiatry* 2013;13:287.

109. Morris J, Simpson AV, Voy SJ. Length of stay of inpatients with eating disorders. *Clinical Psychology & Psychotherapy* 2015;22(1): 45–53.

110. Dalle Grave R, Conti M, Calugi S. Effectiveness of intensive cognitive behavioral therapy in adolescents and adults with anorexia nervosa. *International Journal of Eating Disorders* 2020;53(9):1428–38.

111. Gardner L, Trueman H. Improving mealtimes for patients and staff within an eating disorder unit: understanding of the problem and first intervention during the pandemic – an initial report. *BMJ Open Quality* 2021;10(2).

112. Tan JOA, Stewart A, Fitzpatrick R, et al. Attitudes of patients with anorexia nervosa to compulsory treatment and coercion. *International Journal of Law and Psychiatry* 2010;33(1):13–9.

113. Ayton A, Keen C, Lask B. Pros and cons of using the Mental Health Act for severe eating disorders in adolescents. *European Eating Disorders Review* 2009;17(1):14–23.

114. Ward A, Ramsay R, Russell G, et al. Follow-up mortality study of compulsorily treated patients with anorexia nervosa. *International Journal of Eating Disorders* 2015;48(7):860–5.

115. Walsh BT, Xu T, Wang Y, et al. Time course of relapse following acute treatment for anorexia nervosa. *American Journal of Psychiatry* 2021;178(9):848–53.

116. Treasure J, Oyeleye O, Bonin EM, et al. Optimising care pathways for adult anorexia nervosa. What is the evidence to guide the provision of high-quality, cost-effective services? *European Eating Disorders Review* 2021;29(3):306–15.

117. Adamson J, Cardi V, Kan C, et al. Evaluation of a novel transition support intervention in an adult eating disorders service: ECHOMANTRA. *International Review of Psychiatry* 2019;31(4):382–90.

118. Han R, Bian Q, Chen H. Effectiveness of olanzapine in the treatment of anorexia nervosa: a systematic review and meta-analysis. *Brain and Behavior* 2022;12(2): e2498.

119. Mack RA, Stanton CE. Responding to 'Terminal anorexia nervosa: three cases and proposed clinical characteristics'. *Journal of Eating Disorders* 2022;10(1):87.

120. Gaudiani JL, Bogetz A, Yager J. Terminal anorexia nervosa: three cases and proposed clinical characteristics. *Journal of Eating Disorders* 2022;10(1):23.

121. Riddle M, O'Melia AM, Bauschka M. First, do no harm: the proposed definition of 'terminal anorexia' is fraught with danger for vulnerable individuals. *Journal of Eating Disorders* 2022;10(1):81.

122. Downs J, Ayton A, Collins L, et al. Untreatable or unable to treat? Creating more effective and accessible treatment for long-standing and severe eating disorders. *Lancet Psychiatry* 2023;10 (2):146–54.

123. Lindvall Dahlgren C, Wisting L, Ro O. Feeding and eating disorders in the DSM-5 era: a systematic review of prevalence rates in non-clinical male and female samples. *Journal of Eating Disorders* 2017;5:56.

124. Dinkler L, Wronski ML, Lichtenstein P, et al. Etiology of the broad avoidant restrictive food intake disorder phenotype in Swedish twins aged 6 to 12 years. *JAMA Psychiatry* 2023;80 (3):260–9.

125. Russell G. Bulimia nervosa: an ominous variant of anorexia nervosa. *Psychological Medicine* 1979;9(3):429–48.

126. Fairburn CG, Cooper Z, Doll HA, et al. The natural course of bulimia nervosa and binge eating disorder in young women. *Archives of General Psychiatry* 2000;57(7):659–65.

127. Ayton A, Ibrahim A, Dugan J, et al. Ultra-processed foods and binge eating: a retrospective observational study. *Nutrition* 2021;84:111023.

128. Bulik CM, Thornton LM, Parker R, et al. The Eating Disorders Genetics Initiative (EDGI): study protocol. *BMC Psychiatry* 2021;21(1):234.

129. Donato K, Ceccarini MR, Dhuli K, et al. Gene variants in eating disorders. Focus on anorexia nervosa, bulimia nervosa, and binge-eating disorder. *Journal of Preventive Medicine and Hygiene* 2022;63(2 Suppl 3):E297–E305.

130. Lie SO, Bulik CM, Andreassen OA, et al. Stressful life events among individuals with a history of eating disorders: a case-control comparison. *BMC Psychiatry* 2021;21(1):501.

131. Fairburn CG, Welch SL, Doll HA, et al. Risk factors for bulimia nervosa. A community-based case-control study. *Archives of General Psychiatry* 1997;54 (6):509–17.

132. Eddy KT, Tabri N, Thomas JJ, et al. Recovery from anorexia nervosa and bulimia nervosa at 22-year follow-up. *Journal of Clinical Psychiatry* 2017;78 (2):184–9.

133. Winston AP. Eating disorders and diabetes. *Current Diabetes Reports* 2020;20(8):32.

134. Fanelli G, Franke B, De Witte W, et al. Insulinopathies of the brain? Genetic overlap between somatic insulin-related and neuropsychiatric disorders. *Translational Psychiatry* 2022;12(1):59.

135. Wisting L, Reas DL, Bang L, et al. Eating patterns in adolescents with type 1 diabetes: associations with metabolic control, insulin omission, and eating disorder pathology. *Appetite* 2017;114:226–31.

136. Treasure J, Kan C, Stephenson L, et al. Developing a theoretical maintenance model for disordered eating in Type 1 diabetes. *Diabetic Medicine* 2015;32 (12):1541–5.

137. Peterson CM, Fischer S, Young-Hyman D. Topical review: a comprehensive risk model for disordered eating in youth with type 1 diabetes. *Journal of Pediatric Psychology* 2015;40(4):385–90.

138. Wisting L, Snoek F. Terminology matters: 'diabulimia' is insufficient to describe eating disorders in individuals with Type 1 diabetes. *Diabetic Medicine* 2020;37(6):1075–6.

139. Goddard G, Oxlad M. Caring for individuals with type 1 diabetes mellitus who restrict and omit insulin for weight control: evidence-based guidance for healthcare professionals. *Diabetes Research and Clinical Practice* 2022;185:109783.

140. Appolinario JC, Sichieri R, Lopes CS, et al. Correlates and impact of DSM-5 binge eating disorder, bulimia nervosa and recurrent binge eating: a representative population survey in a middle-income country. *Social Psychiatry and Psychiatric Epidemiology* 2022;57(7):1491–503.

141. Cucchi A, Ryan D, Konstantakopoulos G, et al. Lifetime prevalence of non-suicidal self-injury in patients with eating disorders: a systematic review and meta-analysis. *Psychological Medicine* 2016;46(7):1345–58.

142. Munn-Chernoff MA, Johnson EC, Chou YL, et al. Shared genetic risk between eating disorder- and substance-use-related phenotypes: evidence from genome-wide association studies. *Addiction Biology* 2021;26(1): e12880.

143. Miller AE, Trolio V, Halicki-Asakawa A, et al. Eating disorders and the nine symptoms of borderline personality disorder: a systematic review and series of meta-analyses. *International Journal of Eating Disorders* 2022;55 (8):993–1011.

144. Yilmaz Z, Quattlebaum MJ, Pawar PS, et al. Associations between attention deficit hyperactivity disorder symptom dimensions and disordered eating symptoms in adolescence: a population-based twin study. *Behavior Genetics* 2023;53(2):143–53.

145. Jenkins PE, Luck A, Violato M, et al. Clinical and cost-effectiveness of two ways of delivering guided self-help for people with an eating disorder: a multi-arm randomized controlled trial. *International Journal of Eating Disorders* 2021;54(7): 1224–37.

146. Wade TD, Ghan C, Waller G. A randomized controlled trial of two 10-session cognitive behaviour therapies for eating disorders: An exploratory investigation of which approach works best for whom. *Behavior Research and Therapy* 2021;146:103962.

147. Toro CT, Jackson T, Payne AS, et al. A feasibility study of the delivery of online brief cognitive-behavioral therapy (CBT-T) for eating disorder pathology in the workplace. *International Journal of Eating Disorders* 2022;55(5):723–30.

148. Himmerich H, Kan C, Au K, et al. Pharmacological treatment of eating disorders, comorbid mental health problems, malnutrition and physical health consequences. *Pharmacology & Therapeutics* 2021;217:107667.

149. Steinhausen HC, Weber S. The outcome of bulimia nervosa: findings from one-quarter century of research. *American Journal of Psychiatry* 2009;166 (12):1331–41.

150. Franko DL, Tabri N, Keshaviah A, et al. Predictors of long-term recovery in anorexia nervosa and bulimia nervosa: data from a 22-year longitudinal study. *Journal of Psychiatric Research* 2018;96:183–8.

151. Garcia-Mayor RV, Garcia-Soidan FJ. Eating disoders in type 2 diabetic people: brief review. *Diabetes & Metabolic Syndrome* 2017;11(3):221–4.

152. Nieto-Martinez R, Gonzalez-Rivas JP, Medina-Inojosa JR, et al. Are eating disorders risk factors for type 2 diabetes? A systematic review and meta-analysis. *Current Diabetes Reports* 2017;17(12):138.

153. Davies HL, Hubel C, Herle M, et al. Risk and protective factors for new-onset binge eating, low weight, and self-harm symptoms in >35,000 individuals in the UK during the COVID-19 pandemic. *International Journal of Eating Disorders* 2023;56(1):91–107.

154. Hubel C, Abdulkadir M, Herle M, et al. One size does not fit all. Genomics differentiates among anorexia nervosa, bulimia nervosa, and binge-eating disorder. *International Journal of Eating Disorders* 2021;54(5):785–93.

155. Ilyas A, Hubel C, Stahl D, et al. The metabolic underpinning of eating disorders: a systematic review and meta-analysis of insulin sensitivity. *Molecular and Cellular Endocrinology* 2019;497:110307.

156. Milton AC, Hambleton A, Dowling M, et al. Technology-enabled reform in a nontraditional mental health service for eating disorders: participatory design study. *Journal of Medical Internet Research* 2021;23(2):e19532.

157. Pawar PS, Thornton LM, Flatt RE, et al. Binge-eating disorder with and without lifetime anorexia nervosa: a comparison of sociodemographic and clinical features. *International Journal of Eating Disorders* 2023;56(2):428–38.

158. Bulik CM, Bertoia ML, Lu M, et al. Suicidality risk among adults with binge-eating disorder. *Suicide and Life-Threatening Behavior* 2021;51 (5):897–906.

159. Virgo H, Hutchison E, Mitchell E, et al. *The Cost of Eating Disorders in the UK 2019 and 2020.* Hearts and Minds and Genes Coalition for Eating Disorders. 2021. www.yumpu.com/en/document/read/65877873/the-cost-of-eating-disorders-in-the-uk-2019-and-2020-with-annex.

Chapter 13

Perinatal Psychiatry*

Joanna Cranshaw, Gertrude Seneviratne and George Stein

Among the very earliest descriptions of serious mental illness occurring after childbirth is Hippocrates' account of puerperal insanity. Hippocrates, who lived in the fifth century BC in ancient Greece, cited the case of 'the wife of Epicrates, in the town of Cyzicus, who gave birth to twins, then developed severe insomnia, became restless on the 6th day, delirious on the 11th day, speechless on the 16th day and died on the 17th day'. Hippocrates offered two explanations: first, that the lochia had been suppressed and redirected to the brain, which had caused mania; second, that the mania was the result of an influx of blood into the breast. He also described five fatal cases of infective delirium, but the distinction between infective and non-infective delirium was to come much later.[1]

Many more clinical descriptive accounts followed over the next 2,000 years. Occasional case histories were found in textbooks of general medicine and obstetrics,[1] but the modern era probably starts with Esquirol's[2] account in the early nineteenth century, based on his work at the Salpêtriére during the Napoleonic era. He described 92 cases, of which 37 started within two weeks of childbirth. Of the 92 cases, 49 were of mania, 35 melancholy and monomania, whereas 'dementia' (probably schizophrenia) occurred in only 8 – a pattern not dissimilar to the diagnostic profile of present-day admissions. In 1829, Gooch[3] – a lecturer in midwifery at St Bartholomew's Hospital in London – made the important distinction between fatal and non-fatal delirium, the fatal type being due to sepsis and the non-fatal variety being caused by insanity.

Esquirol had a brilliant pupil, Marcé,[4] who in 1858 wrote the first substantive textbook on the subject, *Traité de la folie des femmes encientes, des nouvelles accoucheés et des nourrices.* ('Treatise on the insanity of pregnant women, the recently delivered and the breast feeding women'). He described 310 cases, of which 79 were his own; 9% started in pregnancy, 58% had an early puerperal onset and 33% had a later onset and were termed 'lactational psychosis'. He considered ways in which these illnesses both resembled and differed from non-puerperal mental disorder, which was to be a recurring conundrum of the twentieth-century literature.

Patients with a puerperal psychosis were admitted to the new asylums of the nineteenth century, often for one or two years, until their illnesses remitted spontaneously. This comprised around 7% of all admissions.[1] They suffered from a high mortality, of around 10%, usually the result of debility, infection or suicide. However, coinciding with the introduction of electroconvulsive therapy (ECT) in the 1940s, there was a dramatic fall in the mortality of the illness. Today, the prognosis is much better, with recovery taking up to 6 to 12 months and most severe symptoms improving within 2 to 12 weeks,[5] although there are still occasional suicides (the biggest single cause of maternal mortality in the first postpartum year).

An important innovation in the management of puerperal mental disorder was made by Thomas Main (1958),[6] a psychoanalyst, when he arranged for the first joint admission of a mother and baby to the Cassel Hospital in London and so ushered in the modern era of joint admissions for mothers with their babies.

The more recent developments in perinatal psychiatry have focused on pre-conceptual involvement, the early detection of illness and consideration of psychological interventions during this vulnerable period. Postpartum disorders are today the province of the perinatal psychiatric team, but prior to the establishment of this sub-speciality, such cases comprised a significant portion of the case load of any catchment area team. The conditions covered in this chapter will include:

1. The postpartum psychoses, which follow around 1–2 out of 1,000 deliveries[7]
2. The postnatal depressions and other related affective disorders, which occur in around 12 per cent of women[8]
3. The 'maternity blues', which occurs in around 40 per cent of women[9] so are considered a normal reaction and not a clinical disorder
4. Miscellaneous other syndromes, such as postpartum post-traumatic stress disorder and effects of stillbirth
5. Child abuse, due to it being a complex factor frequently requiring consideration in perinatal psychiatry

Puerperal Psychoses

The onset of puerperal psychoses may be abrupt and frightening, both for the patient and for those around them. Sometimes, but not always, the first two to three days are relatively symptom free, and then the illness either gradually

* Acknowledgements to Dr Madeleine Bonney-Helliwell for her helpful comments.

appears or can – more often – just abruptly come on. It thus declares itself between days three and seven, with the peak time of onset being around days five and six. In the days when parturient women remained in hospital for seven to ten days, the onset was in hospital, whereas in the modern era, when hospital stays after childbirth are very brief, the onset now is most often at home – and relatives are usually very alarmed by the rapid deterioration they see. Most cases will have started in the first two weeks, although a small number may start at any time in the first six months, occasionally coinciding with the first premenstrual phase or with the onset of weaning. The initial presentation is usually one of delirium with an undifferentiated, rapidly changing psychotic state. Karnosh and Hope[10] provide an early description of puerperal delirium in 1937:

> panic, sudden aversion and mistrust of relatives, misidentification, hallucinosis, sing song chat, and disintegration of poor affect, together with a rapid pulse and fever ranging from 99°–102°F. This delirium usually abates but mania, depression, schizophrenia, occasionally normality and rarely even death may ensue.

The main symptoms of a puerperal psychosis at its onset included restless activity, disinhibition, fleeting anger and negativistic behaviour, and a profound insomnia, anxiety and a state of fear. The most prevalent symptoms of postpartum psychosis were irritability (73%), abnormal thought content (72%) and anxiety (71%). Suicidal pre-occupations were present in 19% and infanticidal ideation in 8% of patients.[11] Delusions and hallucinations often had a negative content. Because many women are experiencing the maternity blues at this time, the initial diagnosis is sometimes confused with severe blues, but the appearance of bizarre psychotic material will generally alarm relatives or midwives and result in an emergency psychiatric referral.

The presence of an elevated temperature ('milk fever') may occasionally feature at the onset of a psychosis and may also be a source of diagnostic confusion. In higher-income countries, puerperal infections are rare, but blood cultures and other tests for infection are still required. However, in the lower-income countries, postpartum infections are far more common. Although puerperal sepsis and mania may both present with delirium and fever, in sepsis, the fever is usually higher – in the range of 39.5°C or above – and there may be rigours, tachycardia, breathlessness, as well as abdominal pain and obstetric causes of acute infection. Exclusion of sepsis is by blood tests, blood culture for bacteria, white blood cell count and other markers of infection. The initial undifferentiated picture of delirium in postpartum psychosis usually passes fairly rapidly into a more classical psychotic picture.

Affective Disorders

Puerperal Mania

Puerperal mania is among the most florid conditions encountered in psychiatric practice, and the motor symptoms of mania, hyperactivity and distractibility are marked. The onset may be abrupt, but more often, there is increasing irritability or elation, with severe blues around the fourth or fifth day postpartum. Sleep is invariably severely disturbed, with patients waking in the early hours and then displaying typical manic symptoms. Some women may present with grandiosity with associated uncharacteristic behaviours such as sexual disinhibition, but many may describe a sense of feeling persecuted and questioned about their current feelings and intentions. These behaviours are usually quite out of character, and therefore, this can be a distressing experience for the affected woman and their loved ones.

A recent study[11] comparing puerperal mania with non-puerperal mania found postpartum episodes had a significantly higher incidence of perplexity and excessive self-reproach. Classic manic symptoms, specifically pressured speech and increased sociability, were significantly less frequent in postpartum manic episodes. Overall, there were significantly fewer manic symptoms and significantly more depressive symptoms in the postpartum episodes than in the non-postpartum episodes.

Postpartum Psychotic Depression

Severe depression usually presents sub-acutely, in the first 10 days. It is often confused with severe blues, but the mood fails to lighten, and depressive delusions appear, such as delusions concerning the baby (e.g. that the baby would be better off dead), nihilistic delusions, infanticidal urges or declarations that the baby should be removed from them. These may be accompanied by severe psychomotor retardation, depressive stupor or suicidal thoughts or acts. Thoughts of worthlessness and hopelessness may also coincide with such a presentation. Although the diagnosis is usually obvious, the condition is extremely dangerous – much more so than the rather more florid manic conditions. Such women may also present with poor motivation and self-neglect, and as a result of this, the relationship between them and their baby may be affected.

Hospitalisation for such depression may occur as an emergency at the request of relatives, carers or professionals who are fearful for the life and safety of both mother and baby. These severe depressions follow around 1 per 1,000 births. A diagnosis of psychotic depression lies behind the majority of the perinatal tragedies of maternal suicide and infanticide. Women with severe personality disorder, multiple social problems and difficulties in functioning may also require admission to mother and baby units. These women may also present with life-threatening situations, although their depressions are generally less severe, and the relative absence of the biological symptoms of depression makes the diagnosis of a non-psychotic disorder more likely.

Puerperal Schizophrenia and Schizoaffective Disorder

Puerperal schizophrenia is rare, and rates of 4–16% in series of women with puerperal psychoses are given in most UK studies.[12] Higher rates are reported from some non-Western countries, such as 22–34% in India,[13] even when Western diagnostic criteria are used. Most cases of puerperal schizophrenia are the result of pregnancies occurring in women with previous schizophrenia, although in some instances, the schizophrenia may start after childbirth. Although rare, the long-term outlook is much worse than for puerperal affective disorder, and the ability to care for the new-born infant is often severely impaired.

As with the other puerperal psychoses, schizophrenia may have a delirious onset, and this may progress through both manic and melancholic phases before the full picture of 'dementia' emerges;[14] the disorder is then often indistinguishable from non-puerperal schizophrenia. Delusions and hallucinations often focus around the baby. Thus, one woman with previous paranoid delusions believed her baby to be a cat. Another, with catatonic features and marked echolalia, began to scream loudly every time her baby cried.

Most authorities do not believe that puerperal schizophrenia comprises a separate schizophrenic subgroup, but at least in the early phases, there often is an affective colouring to the clinical picture. Although pure pictures of mania, depression or schizophrenia may occur in the postnatal period, many cases present with a mixed picture of both schizophreniform and affective features. Sometimes, it is possible to discern a classic schizo-manic or schizo-depressive picture, in which case a diagnosis of schizoaffective disorder should be made.

Case Example

Jane became confused immediately after delivery. She gradually became more depressed and was admitted five days after delivery. She expressed a delusional belief that her husband was an imposter. She also feared that her baby would be sexually abused and asked her doctor to teach her baby not to talk to strangers. She was unable to cope with the day-to-day management of her baby because she said opposing forces were inserting clicks into her mind. After a four-month admission with little improvement, the addition of lithium to her antipsychotic drugs led to a rapid resolution of her illness, and her diagnosis was changed from schizophrenia to schizoaffective disorder.

Mixed manic and depressive pictures or mixed affective states are also quite common, with some women showing rapid switches in and out of mania and depression in a single day, while a more common pattern is for some women to present initially with mania and then, after a few weeks, switch into a state of depression.

In most of the published series, these mixed pictures are usually classed as 'psychotic disorder not otherwise specified'. An Edinburgh[12] study found 10% fitted this picture, a Dutch study[13] gave a figure of 30% and an Indian series[15] gave a figure of 47% for such mixed pictures. The presence of a large number of patients with these mixed pictures was one of the arguments used to support the notion that puerperal psychosis was a unique and distinct category of psychosis and should be listed separately in official schemes, although such a view has little support today. Thus DSM-5[16] does not have a separate specifier for schizophrenia starting after childbirth whereas it does for depression.

Brief Psychosis

A small number of patients are admitted during the puerperium in a psychotic state that resolves rapidly after a few days, and these patients are said to have a brief psychosis. DSM-5 has a category of brief psychosis 'with peri-partum onset', and episodes should last more than a day but less than a month. In ICD-11,[17] this comes under the heading of 'acute and transient psychosis', but there is no specific postpartum category. The main features include an abrupt onset, psychotic symptoms such as delusions and hallucinations and sometimes grossly disorganised thinking or catatonia. By definition, brief psychosis requires full remission between episodes and usually has minimal implications for later childcare.

Nosology

The nosological status of postpartum psychosis was once a contentious issue, mainly because there is no universally accepted definition of 'postpartum psychosis'. Although postpartum psychosis has a superficial appearance of being a unitary category with its own specialist perinatal services and their teams, for the greater part, these illnesses are episodes of other more common psychoses, particularly bipolar disorder but are triggered by the events occurring after childbirth. Arguments in favour of having a separate category are that this would facilitate research into postpartum illness and appropriate service provision, specifically perinatal services, as well as training for obstetric and mental health staff. Absence of a category would mean data on such cases would be lost amid the vast numbers of people with other psychotic episodes admitted to hospital. The argument against a separate category is that such illnesses show only minor differences from other psychotic episodes, and current opinion today is that these illnesses do not merit a separate category. The present position as described in both DSM-5 and ICD-11 is that childbirth acts as a trigger and that when the illness fulfils diagnostic criteria of another illness such as schizophrenia or mania, it should be diagnosed as such. In other cases and for major depression, the DSM-5 adds that the perinatal onset specifier is added in 'with peripartum onset' for cases with a pregnancy onset and for those commencing up to four weeks after delivery.

ICD-11 has three categories starting within six weeks of delivery: 'mental or behavioural disorders associated with pregnancy, childbirth or the puerperium with psychotic features', (6E21), the second being 'mental or behavioural disorders associated with pregnancy, childbirth or the puerperium without psychotic features', (6E20), with the subtype forming the third category of 'postnatal depression not otherwise specified (NOS)', also coded as 6E20.

Epidemiology

Puerperal psychosis is not a common disorder, and Marcé's[4] original estimate of 2.2 per 1,000 deliveries has stood the test of time. There is some variation in the reported rates – for example, in the Edinburgh series, Kendell[12] reported a rate of 1 per 1,000 births, while Jansson[18] in Sweden found an admission rate of 4.8 per 1,000 deliveries admitted to a university hospital. Presumably, the increased availability of hospital beds and lower threshold of severity required for admission may explain some of this variation. Although in the literature there are many reports of uncontrolled case series, there are very few proper epidemiological studies (i.e. which examine cases only from a defined catchment area).

Paffenbarger[19] examined all the case notes of women aged between 15 and 47 who were admitted to either public or private hospitals in Hamilton County, Ohio, during the years 1940–1958 and identified 314 cases. Of interest was a relatively low rate of admission during pregnancy, at 7–9 per month, which was lower than the rate for non-pregnant women, but this rose dramatically in the first month after delivery to 164 cases, giving an 18-fold increased risk for the first month, and there was a total of 242 admissions during the first six months. In the Edinburgh study,[12] information was matched from the Edinburgh psychiatric case register with data from the Scottish maternity discharge computer for all women who had delivered in Edinburgh during 1970–1978. As in Paffenbarger's study, this also showed the relative risk of admission during pregnancy was decreased (RR = 0.65). However, the risk of psychiatric admission for a psychotic or mood disorder was 22 times greater in the first month following delivery compared to before pregnancy. This risk was further increased among women who were primiparous (i.e. had given birth to their first baby), with psychiatric admissions being 35 times more likely. Risk factors of this magnitude are unusual in medicine and almost unheard of in psychiatry and are presumably due to some unknown, possibly biological factor associated with childbirth.

Link with Bipolar Disorder

Several studies[11] have shown that more than 40 per cent of women affected by postpartum psychosis have no previous history of severe psychiatric illness. The remainder present with a recurrence of a pre-existing condition, predominantly of a psychotic or mood disorder. Evidence robustly indicates a strong and specific relationship with bipolar disorder, suggesting that in most cases, postpartum psychosis may be a manifestation of bipolar disorder in women vulnerable to the puerperal trigger. Among women with schizophrenia or any other mood or psychiatric disorder, the risk of admission for psychotic (RR = 4.6) or severe mood episodes (RR = 3.0) was elevated within the first three months following childbirth compared to a sample of non-mothers matched for psychiatric diagnosis. However, this elevation was relatively small compared to that found amongst women with bipolar disorder. Thus, the risk of psychiatric admission for a recurrence of bipolar disorder in the postpartum period is especially high, being 37 times more likely than in women who had never given birth.[5] In a more recent study,[20] psychiatric admissions within the first six weeks of childbirth are most commonly for a severe recurrence of bipolar disorder (14.4%), while other psychiatric disorders accounted for a considerably lower proportion of all admissions (ranging from 1.4% to 7.2%). A recent meta-analysis estimated that as many as one in five women (20%) with bipolar disorder are affected postnatally by a psychotic or manic episode, a rate considerable higher than that observed in the general population (1–2 in every 1,000 deliveries) and for other psychiatric disorders.[20]

Aetiology

As with other psychoses, the aetiology of postpartum psychosis remains unknown but is likely to be explained as a complex interaction of biological, psychological and social factors. In recent years, there has been some progress in understanding the role of particular genes. There is an obvious interest in whether obstetric factors are associated. Of all obstetric factors investigated, only primiparity has been reliably associated with the onset of postpartum psychosis. However, nineteenth-century physicians such as Marcé,[4] writing when multiparous birth was much more common, suggested a multigravid predominance. At a clinical level, it is striking how very few women – even those with extremely difficult and complex labours – develop psychiatric sequelae and how often the deliveries of patients with severe psychoses have been completely normal.

In most European studies, the sex of the child was unrelated. However, in one South African study,[21] there was an association with having a male child, whereas in a study from India, having a female infant was associated[15] as appears to be the case with postnatal depression as well.

Genetics

'It is a fact', wrote Savage[14] in 1875, 'that the neuroses of pregnancy and childbirth are often associated with a hereditary tendency', and this is confirmed by the family studies of the last century. Thus, Thuwe[22] – pooling the data of 10 series published between 1911 and 1973 – found that, in 40% of 614 cases, there was a family history of mental illnesses. The disorders found in the relatives were not confined to the psychoses, but rather there was a mixture of depression, bipolar disorder, psychopathy, alcoholism and suicide. Thuwe also found that around 10% of the children of patients with puerperal psychosis developed acute psychotic illnesses later in life, and this was a six-fold increase over the rate in the control groups.

In the UK, a large family study[21] reported that for female probands with a puerperal affective disorder, the risk for any affective disorder amongst siblings was 10%, and for parents, it was 14.7%, figures which are similar to those reported for probands with non-puerperal affective disorder.

Evidence shows that as many as 40–50% of women with a history of postpartum psychosis screen positive for a family history of mood disorders among first- and second-degree relatives, a much higher rate than that observed in the general population. A specific vulnerability to the childbirth trigger of severe mood episodes may also be familial,[23] with findings further suggesting postpartum psychosis may be a marker for a genetically heterogenous subtype of bipolar disorder. Thus, a comparison between the postpartum course of bipolar women with a family history of a puerperal psychosis with that of women without such a history found that a puerperal episode occurred in 20 out of 27 women (74%) who had a family history of puerperal psychosis, but it occurred in only 38 out of 125 women (30%) where such a family history was absent.[23] When only first episodes were considered, the odds ratio rose to 6, indicating that childbirth acts as an extremely potent trigger for psychosis in a subgroup of patients with a bipolar affective disorder who may possibly carry an inherited liability to postpartum psychosis. Modern DNA genome analysis has also begun to yield several candidate genes that have been targeted for further investigation, including variations in the 5-HTT serotonin transporter gene, the expression of which is known to be influenced by hormones.

Social Factors

Although social factors are important in the aetiology of the less-severe pregnancy and postpartum depressions, there is also evidence that they play a role in the more severe psychotic illnesses. Savage[14] remarked on how few cases 'could be traced back to fright, grief or losses', and more systematic studies of life events in the UK initially failed to establish any links between recent life events and severe postpartum depression,[24] but this has since been refuted.[25,26] Nor have any particular personality typologies been associated with these illnesses.

Treatment

'Tonics and a change of scenery are useful' wrote Savage[14] in 1875, and the same principles apply today, although the tonics of today are the modern psychotropics and 'the change of scenery' is nowadays the local mother and baby unit. In severe cases, hospital admission is always advisable and will sometimes require the immediate implementation of a section of the Mental Health Act. If possible and where facilities are available, the baby should be admitted with the mother unless there is sufficient evidence from family members and from objective assessment that the baby remaining with the mother is itself a risk to the mother or baby.

Soon after admission, blood tests that screen for organic illness such as infective states and thyroid abnormalities (both hypo and hyperthyroid states can occur) is advisable, whilst alcohol and drug screens should be able to detect drug toxicity or withdrawal states. Rarely, urea cycle abnormalities occur and can be detected by raised plasma ammonia levels. The use of common psychotropics and their side effects is similar to their use in non-puerperal episodes, and drug treatments for depression are outlined in Chapter 3.3, for mania in Chapter 4.1 and for psychosis in Chapter 5.3. A recent review[27] by a Dutch team has proposed that lithium monotherapy sometimes works, but more commonly, lithium is used as an adjunctive therapy in cases that have not responded to an initial antipsychotic or antidepressant. Antidepressants can trigger subjects into manic states, but when lithium is co-prescribed, there may be greater mood stability. Similarly, mood instability can occur with antipsychotic monotherapy but does not occur with lithium monotherapy.[27] If lithium is used, women should be advised to stop breast feeding because of the risks of neonatal lithium toxicity. When ECT first came in the 1940s, it had a dramatic and beneficial effect on postpartum psychosis, and a fall in the mortality of the condition occurred. However, today it is rarely used because medication is generally able to clear the vast majority of cases with little need to revert back to ECT. A recent small study of five resistant cases of both puerperal mania and depression showed a good response to ECT,[28] so this remains a reserve treatment for resistant cases.

Prognosis and Recurrence

Following treatment, recovery from an initial episode of postpartum psychosis is usually excellent for most women, but this has not always been the case. Thus the natural history of the untreated condition as described by nineteenth-century authors is of a rather lengthy illness, although it usually eventually did remit. Savage,[14] writing in 1875, found that among 84 women with puerperal psychosis, only a third were better after six months. Among the 54 women with melancholia, 50% were better by six months and 85% by one year – but 8% had died. The introduction of ECT and modern psychopharmacology led to dramatic improvements. Thus, a Swedish study in 1964 showed that these figures had much improved and found that 75% of patients with puerperal psychosis had admissions of less than six weeks, 15% were ill for 6–12 weeks and only 3% for more than six months, and there were no deaths.[18]

For those who go on to have further children, more than 50% are at risk of the recurrence of a perinatal mood episode. Amongst women with bipolar disorder type 1 who had given birth at least once and who also had a perinatal history of mania or psychosis, 43% relapsed after a subsequent pregnancy.[29] This is compared to approximately 10% of women with bipolar I disorder and 2% of those with bipolar II disorder without such previous perinatal history. In a family study,[30] women with a bipolar disorder who had both previous puerperal and non-puerperal episodes were at greater risk (50%) of a subsequent puerperal breakdown than those with only a previous puerperal episode, for whom the rate was 36%.

It is noteworthy that there are a few women who developed a depression after every single pregnancy. These women gain relief from their depression only during pregnancy, and this may explain why they find themselves in a repeated cycle of pregnancy → postnatal depression → pregnancy. Identifying these women early on may be helpful as the pattern can be reversed by counselling and long-term antidepressant treatment.

There are two recent and large studies on recurrence. The first, on 887 women with bipolar disorder and schizoaffective disorder in the UK,[5] gave an overall rate for a first lifetime episode of 28% for this large bipolar sample. For those who had a postpartum episode following their first pregnancy, the rate was 55% following their second pregnancy; for women with bipolar disorder even without a previous postpartum episode, rates were still high at 34% in their second pregnancies with similar rates for bipolar I and bipolar II. A recent meta-analysis[20] involving more than 4,023 subjects with a previous postpartum admission found an overall postpartum relapse risk of 35%, or around 1 in 3. Possibly this is the best figure to offer patients as it is based on a very large sample size.

Puerperal schizophrenia is a far less common condition, and there are therefore very few reports on its recurrence rate. Protheroe[21] gave a figure of 47%, while Yarden[31] gave a figure of 45%. His team also investigated whether pregnancy had any longer-term deleterious effect on the course of schizophrenia and, in a controlled study, showed there was no difference in subsequent admission rates among women with schizophrenia who became pregnant and a matched control group with schizophrenia who had never been pregnant.

There also appears to be a longer-term risk of further puerperal and non-puerperal episodes. Thus, a Dutch study[32] followed 119 women who had an admission for a postpartum disorder and found that 66 (55%) had a later non-puerperal episode over the next 20 years. A 23-year UK follow-up study[33] found that 75% had a further episode, most of which were non-puerperal, and around one-third of this sample experienced at least three further episodes, indicating that the puerperal episode frequently represented the opening phase of a recurrent affective disorder.

Prophylaxis

After an episode of puerperal psychosis or severe depression, many women will wish to have more children and will seek advice on the risks of recurrence (detailed earlier) and the possibility of prevention. The scientific literature on this important practical matter is relatively sparse, but a recent Cochrane review[34] concluded that postnatal psychosis occurred in one to two of every 1,000 new mothers with an abrupt onset within a month of childbirth. Affected mothers develop frank psychosis, cognitive impairment and disorganised behaviours. Factors that increase risk include primiparous mothers who are single, women who are older, those with a past psychiatric history and family history of affective psychosis, prenatal depression and autoimmune thyroid dysfunction. The risk of a future postnatal recurrence is 25 to 57 per cent. Preventive interventions for postnatal psychosis aim at identifying women with risk factors, early recognition of imminent psychosis through screening, and preventive drug therapy. Mood stabilisers, antipsychotic drugs and hormone therapy may be beneficial in the prevention of postnatal psychotic episodes in women at risk.

Non-psychotic postnatal depression also showed a recurrence rate of 50 per cent following second pregnancies where mothers had depression following their first pregnancy. Although the clinical pictures of both episodes were not identical, they showed similar polarity, shared many features and also tended to have a similar time of onset.

Hamilton[35] gave a mixture of oestrogen and testosterone in oil to 40 women and noted that none had a recurrence. Given that oestrogen may sometimes cause malignant changes in uterine cells and deep vein thrombosis, it is best avoided and so is not used today. Wisner et al.[36] conducted a randomised, double-blind, placebo-controlled trial of 50 mg nortriptyline started immediately after birth and then continued for 20 weeks. Relapse rates of 25 per cent were found in both the placebo and the nortriptyline-treated women, so the drug appeared to offer no protection. However, a later placebo-controlled study of sertraline[37] found a significant prophylactic effect. Of the 14 subjects who took sertraline, only 1 (7%) experienced a relapse, but of the eight subjects who took the placebo, 4 (50%) relapsed, an effect which was statistically significant. This is the only controlled trial in the literature to date to document a positive prophylactic effect for an antidepressant administered after delivery.

As most puerperal illnesses are thought to be affective, Stewart[38] administered lithium to 25 women with previous manic or schizo-manic illnesses, and only two women (8%) relapsed, which was lower than the expected rate of around 35%. In some cases, the bipolar disorder is so severe that lithium must be taken in pregnancy and, although episodes are not completely abolished, around 23% on lithium relapsed compared to 66% who were not on prophylactic lithium.

The same group reported on the use of lithium starting after delivery. Thus, 70 pregnant women at high risk for postpartum psychosis because of previous episodes were referred to the psychiatric outpatient clinic. Women who were initially medication free were advised to start lithium prophylaxis immediately postpartum, and their outcome was compared to similar women who declined to take lithium prophylaxis. Four of the nine (44%) who declined prophylaxis relapsed compared to *none* of the 20 (0%) of women who took lithium immediately after delivery relapsed.[39] On this basis, the authors recommend initiating prophylactic lithium treatment immediately after delivery in women with a history of psychosis limited to the postpartum period, and by commencing postpartum, they are able to avoid *in utero* foetal exposure to medication.[39]

A Strategy for Relapse Prevention

When women seek prophylactic advice, a careful history of the previous episode or episodes should be obtained, because puerperal relapses are usually remarkably similar to the original index illness. If this is completed before the woman has become pregnant, it is more commonly called 'pre-conceptual counselling', and this is offered by perinatal mental health services. Critical information includes:

- The time of onset – so that a prophylactic regimen can be instituted for this
- The diagnostic category, as indicated in the case notes – so that drugs known to ameliorate this particular disorder can be selected
- Whether any particular treatments appeared to work well in the previous episode
- The severity, duration, dangerousness and the amount of harm incurred by the previous illness to establish how necessary prophylaxis will be
- The feeding choices the woman may have for her baby once it is born

Armed with this information, it is usually possible to give an estimate of the likely risks of a recurrence as described earlier. It is also relatively easy to select which medications may be beneficial and decide when they should be started and how long they should be taken. In cases where the first experience of perinatal illness was significant for the woman, the need for a prophylactic regimen may be of considerable importance to them. In other cases, the illness may have been relatively brief – perhaps lasting for only a few days or weeks – or may have improved following a short course of medication and supportive psychological interventions. For women who have had these milder episodes, prophylaxis may be perceived to be more optional, with women using their previous experiences of illness and recovery as potential pointers that a recurrence may not occur.

Whether this assessment is completed pre-conceptually or antenatally, the risks of a recurrence and possible treatment regimens should be outlined to the patient. Ideally, a care plan and recommendations should be agreed before the woman becomes pregnant (if pre-conceptually) but certainly by the end of the pregnancy. Wherever possible, the patient's partner should also be involved. Because most of the more serious illnesses are bipolar in origin (both mania and depression), lithium and antipsychotic mood stabilisers may have a role to play in the prophylaxis.

The following regimens are offered, and they should all start on the first night after delivery.

For Previous Mania, or Schizomania

A small dose of an atypical antipsychotic (e.g. 5 mg olanzapine) can be prescribed at night after the first day, but oversedation can occur. A small Indian study[40] of olanzapine prophylaxis found that two (18.2%) of the women in the olanzapine group experienced a postpartum mood episode, whereas eight (57.1%) of the women who did not take olanzapine did fall ill. Lithium is also usually helpful, and a small Dutch trial[39] supports its use, but breast feeding is contraindicated because lithium is expressed in breast milk and can result in neonatal lithium toxicity and thyroid dysfunction of the neonate. If lithium is used, a lithium level should be taken after a few days and the dosage then adjusted to be in the lower therapeutic range. Also, if lithium is taken throughout pregnancy, then high-resolution ultrasound and echocardiography should be performed at 6 and 18 weeks of gestation. In the third trimester, total body water increases; an increasing dose of lithium may be required to maintain the lithium level. However, requirements return abruptly to pre-pregnancy levels immediately after delivery. Lithium plasma levels should be monitored every month during pregnancy and immediately after birth. Neonatal goitre, hypotonia, lethargy and cardiac arrhythmia can occur in the infant.

Whatever regimen is implemented, the patient should be monitored very closely in the first 10 days after delivery because this is the peak time when a relapse may occur. Some patients taking these drug regimens will develop mild, attenuated illnesses with broken sleep, and this could be managed using techniques described in Chapter 11, along with considering an increase in dosage of the antipsychotic or adding in a hypnotic. These minor mood swings and insomnia indicate that a recurrence has probably occurred, but it is being suppressed or masked by the medication, and so the early detection and swift treatment of these premonitory symptoms will be essential to prevent more serious developments.

For Previous Depression

If the previous illness responded well and without significant side effects to a particular SNRI, SSRI or tricyclic and the patient has confidence in that particular drug, then the same drug should be used to prevent the next episode, and this could be started antenatally or postnatally. If an SSRI is used, the drug is started in full dosage (e.g. 50 mg sertraline or 20 mg fluoxetine) from the first day, and the dose may need to be increased dependent on the symptoms the woman presents with. If tricyclics are used, then dosage titration upwards will help avoid side effects. Breast feeding is safe with both tricyclics and SSRIs, but it is worth considering the relative infant dose (RID) of the antidepressant into breast milk when facilitating the woman's informed choice as described later in this chapter. Paediatric advice may be necessary if the baby is born pre-term as this may reflect on the infant's ability to metabolise medication passed through breastmilk. Fortnightly monitoring is usually sufficient, but this should continue for at least three months because many illnesses have a later onset. Breast feeding is safe with sertraline as foetal blood levels are usually low.

Completed Suicide

Suicide is presently rare in pregnancy in the UK, but this has not always been the case. In the years 1900–1947, 12.6% of all women of childbearing age who died by suicide were pregnant; this figure then fell to 1.3% for the years 1943–1980.[41] For many centuries and right up to the middle of the twentieth century, there was much shame associated with being an unmarried mother, and such women were commonly rejected by their families and their communities; these societal attitudes would have contributed to the raised suicide rates of pregnant women during this era.

Presumably, the advent of contraception – and a change in attitude of society towards single motherhood and unwanted pregnancy – explain much of this fall. The UK suicide statistics for 1973–1984 also suggest a very low standardised mortality ratio (SMR) for suicide of 0.17 for pregnancy, in comparison with an age- and sex-matched general population group. However, concerningly, there were certain vulnerable high-risk groups – pregnant teenagers, single mothers, those with stillbirths and mothers with a mental illness – among whom the methods of suicide used were commonly violent.[42]

In a seminal and methodologically sound study of the Danish national psychiatric case register[43] for the two decades of 1973–1993, it was found that the SMR for suicide for women who had a hospital admission for a postpartum psychiatric disorder was raised 70-fold. When only the first two postpartum years were considered, the SMR for this group was raised 19-fold, but this high risk persisted over a 15-year period, at 17-fold.[43] Thus, although postpartum illness is rare, it carries a substantial risk of both early and late suicide, and these risks will be present with each recurrence (whether puerperal or non-puerperal). The increased risks of late suicide for women hospitalised for a postpartum depression indicates that these illnesses comprise a more severe and dangerous form of depression both during the postpartum period as well as in later life – even long after the childbearing years – so they should be viewed with seriousness and treated vigorously.

In 2015, new World Health Organization[44] guidelines included postpartum suicide as a direct cause of maternal mortality, thus expanding these cases and leading to an increase in published maternal mortality rates. As noted earlier, the suicide mortality rate in postpartum women is lower than that in women of the same age who have not been pregnant.[45] Information on perinatal suicide is now available from many countries, and in the later section, rates of suicide per 100,000 live births are given in parenthesis from two recent reviews.[45,46] In the USA, there is variation between states: the rate for the state of Washington (1.4) was very low, but it was higher for Colorado (4.6). By comparison, for Finland, it was 5.9, and in Taiwan, it was 6.9. The Taiwanese study[45] showed a 20-fold increased risk for both suicide attempts and completed suicide compared to non-pregnant women. Studies related to the entire perinatal period (i.e. pregnancy and the year following childbirth) yielded figures for Canada (2.6), the UK (2.0) and Sweden (3.7). The US National Violent Death Reporting System reported a rate of 2.0.[47] Whilst these figures are relatively low, every one of these suicides is an unspeakable tragedy for the families concerned.

Factors associated with a completed maternal suicide include lower education level, low infant birth weight and a diagnosis of anxiety or mood disorder. The methods of suicide used during the perinatal period are distinct in their violent nature – such as by hanging or by jumping from height – as compared to female suicides at other periods of life, implying high intent as these methods are more likely to result in death. The more violent methods employed may also reflect the psychotic intensity underlying some of the delusions and the hallucinatory experiences that underlie such suicides. In some countries, including the UK, suicide is the main causes of maternal mortality in the year following childbirth. However, it is noteworthy that, in both the UK and Australia, the reduction in maternal mortality rates in recent years have not been paralleled by a similar decrease in the rate of maternal deaths by suicide.

Attempted Suicides in the Postpartum Period

The rate of attempted suicide in the UK may be reduced after childbirth, having a relative risk of around 0.43 for the first postpartum year in comparison with age-matched non-perinatal women.[42] A recent Israeli study[46] confirmed this reduction in the rates for suicide attempts; thus the rate for non-postpartum women was three- to five-times higher than that for postpartum women. In the state of Washington, USA, over a 15-year period, the rate for suicide attempts averaged at around 43.9 for every 100,000 live births, whilst in Israel, the rate reached a peak of 42 per 100,000 live births in 2011. In Taiwan, the rates were much lower at around 9.9, but this may have been a methodological artefact because only cases presenting to hospital were counted. Social factors associated with suicide attempts postpartum tended to be country specific – for example, in Israel, emigres from the former Soviet Union and Israeli Arab women were at greater risk of suicide attempts. In the UK, those with personality disorder and social crises were at an increased risk. Other factors associated with attempted suicide include never having married, being widowed or divorced, having a caesarean delivery or a previous history of suicide attempts.

Although pregnancy is associated with a lower rate of suicide than the postpartum period (SMR = 0.05), suicides still occur in pregnancy and appear to be more prevalent in societies with higher levels of violence such as the USA, where intimate partner conflict and violence may play an important role. A study based on 2,083 female suicide victims found that mental health, substance use and intimate partner conflict[47] were associated with pregnancy-associated suicide. A second study based in Georgia reported[48] on 94 counts of pregnancy-associated suicide and 139 counts of pregnancy-associated homicide, yielding pregnancy-associated suicide and homicide rates of 2.0 and 2.9 deaths per 100,000 live births, respectively. Victims of pregnancy-associated suicide were significantly more likely to be older, white or Native American when compared with all live births in the National Violent Death Reporting System. Pregnancy-associated homicide victims were significantly more likely to be African American and at the extremes of the age. A key finding in this study was that *intimate partner conflict* was associated with 54.3% of pregnancy-associated suicides and 45.3% of pregnancy-associated homicides. Intimate partner violence is also widely prevalent in the UK, with 6.9% of women experiencing domestic abuse in the year ending March 2022, according to the Office for National Statistics.[49] Domestic abuse should be routinely enquired about in maternity care and, if present, should be further investigated and addressed, never ignored, as partner violence can result in tragic outcomes.

Although completed suicide is uncommon in pregnancy, suicidal thoughts are very frequent. In some American-based studies, up to 33% of subjects report such thoughts. Rates were high in urban communities at 23–33%, with a lower prevalence for those residing in suburban communities (3–4%). There was a small tendency for younger women below 20 years of age to be more affected.[50] Associated social factors included having a current or past history of psychiatric disorders; being young, unmarried or unemployed; having an unplanned pregnancy that was eventually terminated with an induced abortion; being addicted to illicit drugs or alcohol; having a lack of effective psychosocial support; or having suffered from episodes of sexual or physical violence. The most common primary diagnoses were unipolar depressive disorders (68.5%), and almost two-thirds also had comorbid anxiety disorders. A striking 22.6% had bipolar disorders.[51]

At a national level, some countries such as Israel[46] have instituted mandatory national screening programmes using the Edinburgh Postnatal Depression Scale (EPDS) both in pregnancy and in the postpartum period to identify those with depression. At an individual level, clinicians are able to identify those with depression and psychosis who are at greatest risk and therefore should endeavour to protect these women from their own suicidality and bring their depressions to a close as quickly as possible.

Postnatal Depression (PND)

There has been increasing recognition and interest in the milder, non-psychotic depressions found in routine community surveys and in psychiatric outpatient clinics. Community surveys in the UK and many other countries reveal that around 10–17% of women are depressed postnatally, and around 1.6% will be referred to psychiatric outpatient clinics; the account later focuses more on the clinic cases that lie at the more severe end of the spectrum because this is the group with which the psychiatric team will be more likely to work.

Presentation and Symptoms

The illness presents as an ordinary depression (see Chapter 3.1) and syndromally does not differ markedly from depression occurring at other times. Outpatients will usually lack the severe and life-threatening delusions of the rare cases of psychotic depression that may have resulted in a hospital admission. The illness may start during pregnancy, straight after delivery or first appear on the fourth or fifth day as the maternity 'blues' that have apparently failed to resolve, or it may insidiously creep on in the first few weeks after delivery. A few cases have an onset with the first premenstrual phase or with weaning.

Low mood, depressive thoughts and feelings of inadequacy are common. Tearfulness is also very common, and the frequency of this usually reduces as the illness resolves with this reduction serving as a simple clinical marker of any progress in treatment or otherwise. Anhedonia is an almost universal complaint in PND and usually presents as a failure to gain any pleasure from caring for the new-born infant. A postnatal mother in the absence of the onset of mental illness may have increased emotional lability during her first few weeks, but unless she is also suffering from a depression, she will still usually derive much pleasure from caring for her baby. As well as emotional lability, some women with PND have increased irritability, aggression and hostility, which may be towards the partner but occasionally at older children or the new-born baby.

Feelings of exhaustion, poor concentration, psychomotor retardation and confusion are also common; these result in difficulties in task completion, including the practical aspects of mothering like feeding or changing the baby. Some mothers will vacillate in a state of indecisiveness. Others are perplexed and complain of feeling confused about the different advice they receive from different health professionals or their own families. Completion of activities of daily living may seem impossible, especially in cases where there is severe hypersomnia leading to neglect of routine activities and childcare duties.

Depressive sleep disorder – with difficulty getting off to sleep – early morning wakening and occasional nightmares should be distinguished from the broken sleep resulting from the demands of the infant. Diurnal mood variation is common; depression may be worse in the morning, but some patients report being worse in the afternoon or evening. Weight loss may be an unreliable sign because this is fluctuant throughout the perinatal period and changeable postnatally. Some women may be actively trying to restore their pre-pregnancy weight after their baby is born, and a small number of women may also have comorbid eating disorders. A few women may comfort eat and so gain weight.

Suicide is rare in non-psychotic PND, but suicidal thoughts are common and frighten the patient, their family and other carers, which may act as a trigger for referral. Infanticidal thoughts are even less common, such as imagining placing a cushion briefly over the baby's face or considering drowning the baby in the bath, but they usually accompany suicidal thoughts. Some women who have not otherwise abused their babies may describe brief attacks where infanticidal urges have been half-heartedly acted on but not been carried through. They may only report such episodes years later, usually with much remorse. Infanticide today is extremely rare, and a declaration of such thoughts should alert the clinician more to a risk of suicide.

A decrease in libido is common after childbirth, but during postnatal depression, this is almost universal. The return of sexual feelings is usually delayed until well after the resolution of any underlying depression and may be further delayed by the use of antidepressant drugs such as SSRIs.

Complex Cases

Most published studies are based on community samples, and they paint a picture of a mild, self-limiting disorder that responds readily to a few sessions of counselling or a short course of an antidepressant. While such a benign picture may apply to women detected in a community screening programme, many of those attending the psychiatric clinic present with a more complex and challenging picture. Whilst it is not possible to cover all possible types of presentations case, some of the more problematic types of case are outlined here.

Some women are troubled with severe morbid thoughts, distressing nightmares or strange obsessions or near delusional thoughts, even though they are not psychotic. Small doses of an atypical antipsychotic such as olanzapine (2.5–5 mg) at night or quetiapine (25–50 mg) may be helpful in these cases. A small minority of new mothers have severe depression, which may be complicated by suicidal or infanticidal thoughts; however, for a variety of social reasons (e.g. other small children at home or a lack of hospital beds), they cannot be admitted to hospital or hospital admission has itself proved to be unhelpful. In these cases, the input from the perinatal community team should be high, with frequent visits as is practised by crisis teams. The support of other family members or friends who can stay with the patient and help with childcare should be enlisted. Drug therapy should be more vigorous, perhaps using higher doses of antidepressants, with an earlier consideration of lithium augmentation. If a day hospital or other day facilities are available, they may be useful to provide more intensive support and respite. In some cases, there appear to be risks to the baby or more commonly older children in the family, and in these cases, social services should be involved.

Patients with borderline personality disorder, or those with pre-existing borderline traits that are exacerbated by a postnatal depression, may present with severe distress and face particular challenges in treatment. These women may not respond as well to antidepressants, experience mood lability and impulsivity and may self harm. They may have difficulties in their relationships, which could include their family and partners but also therapists and professionals. Some of these women may experience repeated emotional and social crises, which the team should anticipate through provision of support in their care plan. Women with personality difficulties may have experienced domestic abuse and trauma in their past, including sexual trauma, and these specific vulnerabilities should also be considered when making trauma-informed care plans.

Treating women in the perinatal period with comorbid substance misuse issues also presents specific challenges; these are expanded upon in detail later in this chapter. As well as the impact of substances on foetal development and the potential to induce withdrawal states in the new-born, substance misuse issues affect the physical and mental wellbeing of both the mother and the child, impacting on the mother's ability to provide safe care of the infant and can have a detrimental effect on her mental state (see also Chapter 14).

In contrast to these severe illnesses, some women have prolonged milder puerperal illnesses that can nevertheless be unresponsive to both pharmacological and psychotherapeutic approaches; these disorders sometimes persist for three or four years. Occasionally, there is an associated medical disorder such as a hypothyroidism or hypopituitarism, and in these cases, supportive interviews accompanied by trials of different antidepressants in conjunction with treatment of the organic disorder may prove helpful until such time as the illness resolves spontaneously – which it usually does.

Reactions to the baby are not always joyful. Some women became very anxious or self-critical of their skills to care for their baby. This may even present as a near-phobia of looking after their baby; however, they seem to function quite well otherwise. In these cases, infant care may be delegated to other relatives or child-minders. These women sometimes benefit from interventions focused on improving the bond with their babies and peer support, but these women often relate better to their offspring when they are young children and already talking. An early return to work is also sometimes helpful in such cases.

Having a medically ill or very premature baby may naturally provoke anxiety; however, women in these situations have not been found to have a raised rate of depression. However, if they do develop depression, the content of the depression may revolve around their infant's health, and there may be wide variations in mood that follow all the ups and downs of the child's medical progress. Associated trauma from the delivery or any obstetric complications may also contribute to the woman's difficulties. Antidepressants can help dampen the severity of these mood swings, and these women usually welcome any psychological support as well.

In contrast, women with babies born with a significant disability may have overpowering feelings of hurt and anger ('Why me?', 'Why my baby?'), but despite their distress, they rarely seek psychiatric help. Again, psychological support may be of benefit for these women.

During a postnatal illness, once menstruation has resumed, a premenstrual exacerbation of almost any premenstrual symptom is common, particularly towards the end of the first postpartum year. As the postnatal depression recedes, the premenstrual tension becomes more distressing because the abrupt deterioration in mood occurring premenstrually is less well tolerated than the more continuous depression of the earlier PND.

Epidemiology and Aetiology

Most epidemiological research into postnatal depression is based on the use of the EPDS. Cox[52] devised this scale by adapting questions from the Hospital Anxiety and Depression Scale[53] but excluded physical symptoms because after childbirth, these symptoms are common and are of physical rather than psychological origin. The scale has 10 questions, each with four levels of severity, and the score ranges from 0 to 30, with a score of 12 or above usually indicating a depressive disorder. Lower prevalence figures are obtained when a stricter interview-based definition of PND is applied and where only cases fulfilling criteria for major depressive disorder are counted. Thus, when the three-month time window is considered and both major and minor depressions are included, the period prevalence is 19.2% and the point prevalence is 12.9%.[54] When major depression alone is considered, the three-month postpartum period prevalence is 7.1% (4.7% point prevalence), and the 12-month period prevalence is 21.9% (3.9% point prevalence).[54] Depending on the cut-off score used for various depression severity ratings, recent data suggest that 7–14% of women in the general population will screen positive for depression at four to six weeks postpartum. Interestingly, while 40% of postpartum women with depression report the episode onset during the postpartum period, as many as 33.4% report antenatal onset and 26.5% report onset before pregnancy.[54]

The Edinburgh scale is far easier to apply than interviews for major depression and so has been widely applied in many countries and among many different ethnic groups. These studies have shown that postnatal depression is a universal phenomenon. A large meta-analysis of 291 studies[55] from 56 countries found a global pooled prevalence rate of PND was 17.7%, ranging from a low of 3% in Singapore to a high of 38% in Chile. Higher PND rates were found in countries with significantly higher rates of income inequality (R2 = 41%), maternal mortality (R2 = 19%), infant mortality (R2 = 16%) or women of childbearing age working more than 40 hours/week (R2 = 31%). Together, these mainly socioeconomic factors explained 73% of the international variation in the prevalence of PND. However, this does not mean the wealthy are spared from getting PND.

The DSM-5 uses the phrase 'with perinatal onset up to 4 weeks postpartum' because many cases actually start in pregnancy. This is borne out by a recent large Czech study[56] where the prevalence of depressive symptoms *before* delivery was 12.8%, at six weeks post-delivery was 11.8% and six months after delivery was 10.1%. Significant risk factors for PND in this study were a family history of depression in *both* parents of the expectant mother, an unintentional pregnancy, feelings of unhappiness about being pregnant, primary education only, mothers opting not to breast feed and mothers living without partners. Family savings were identified as a protective factor. None of the obstetric variables were significantly associated with an increased risk for postnatal depression in these relatively small studies.

This is in line with clinical experience where the vast majority of those with PND report a normal experience of labour, whilst most of those with prolonged difficult or complicated labours do not develop PND, although a small number do get post-traumatic stress disorder. A much larger population (N = 392,458) based cohort study using Danish national registers[57] compared those with and those without PND. The only significant obstetric associations were for hyperemesis, gestational hypertension, pre-eclampsia and caesarean section.

Hormone levels or the sharpness of postpartum falls show no differences between those with and without PND. All that is known is that there are some women who are especially sensitive to hormone withdrawal effects, and they may develop depression when high levels of sex hormones are abruptly withdrawn. Evidence to support this is provided by a seminal study, in which the supraphysiologic levels of oestrogen and progesterone typically observed in pregnancy were simulated in a sample of women with and without a history of postpartum depression. Following blind withdrawal of these steroids, 62 per cent women with a history of postpartum depression developed symptoms of mood disorder, compared to none in the control group.[58]

Hereditary factors may be important. A recent large twin study based on the Swedish National Twin register[59] applying the lifetime version of the Edinburgh Postnatal Depression Scale in 3,427 Swedish female twins found the heritability of perinatal depression was estimated at 54 per cent with the remaining variance attributable to non-shared environment. A second study in the same paper, based on a Swedish population-based cohort of 580,006 sisters also in this register, separated those with clinical diagnoses of depression into two groups: (i) those with perinatal depression and (ii) those without perinatal depression. In this sibling study, the heritability of perinatal depression was estimated at 44% and the heritability of non-perinatal depression at 32%. The authors concluded that 12% of the genetic contribution to PND was unique to PND and not shared with those who did not have perinatal depression.

Psychological models such as the stress diathesis model and the cognitive behavioural model of PND emphasise the role of psychological stressors such as 'father abandonment', 'financial strain' and 'underlying cognitive vulnerabilities' – such as a negative attributional style – and the ameliorating role of psychosocial resources such as social support and self-esteem. These theories posit that pregnancy, childbirth and new parenthood are stressors for many mothers. A comprehensive recent review of all the biological and psychosocial factors that may contribute to PND[60] found that social factors in PND related to those occurring in depression generally but also specifically highlighted issues related to infants and partners.

Consequences of PND

In an elegant meta-study of 122 eligible controlled studies where the controls were mothers without PND from all over the world, Slomian[61] reviewed all the physical and mental consequences of PND to the mothers, to their partners and their infants up to three years of age, and the account here is drawn from this masterly review.

For physical health, they found that apart from a slightly greater degree of weight retention after delivery, there were otherwise no adverse physical health consequences to mothers with PND. Also, many of the psychological associations were part and parcel of the depression itself. Thus, mothers with PND had higher rates of suicidal ideation, which correlated with higher depression scores, higher rates of thoughts of self harm and higher rates of imagining infanticidal acts. They also had lower self-esteem, increased anger scores and more negative life events.

On the social front, PND mothers had more financial problems, more illness amongst close relatives, greater levels of homelessness and more relationship difficulties, but the review made no distinction as to whether these factors were causes or consequences of the PND. Rates of returning to work were unaffected.

Mothers with depression also reported more partner relationship difficulties, a non-significant rise in break-ups and a decreased rate of return to previous sexual activity. With regard to addictive behaviour, there were increased rates of returning to smoking after pregnancy and the use of illicit drugs but not of drinking alcohol. Breast feeding was also adversely affected as 16 out of 22 studies reported an early discontinuation of breast feeding and more breast feeding problems amongst mothers with PND, but four studies did not find any adverse effect.[61]

Maternal PND and Its Effects on Infants

This was the area of greatest interest. Infant physical health was adversely affected in 9 out of 10 cohort studies, with significantly more diarrheal episodes per year. Increased rates of febrile episodes were found in studies from Ghana and Cote d'Ivoire; there was also a three-fold raised infant mortality for PND mothers, but this has not been found in European studies.

Two out of three infant sleep studies showed an increased incidence of infant night-time wakenings, and a third study found less adherence to the recommended 'back-to-sleep position' amongst mothers with PND.

Cognitive development has been the focus of many studies, and of 11 studies, seven showed a negative association between cognitive development and maternal PND, but three did not. At 36 months post-delivery, 6 out of 13 studies on language development found a direct association with poorer language skills, but some studies ascribed this to the quality of overall maternal caregiving, an effect which was strongest for lower socioeconomic groups. One American study examined high infant vocalisations, a presumed indicator of infant distress, and found that maternal PND predicted less silence and more high positive infant vocalisations, which were maintained for longer periods of time than amongst non-depressed mothers. One study showed that mothers with PND tended to sing faster to their infants than mothers without PND, presumably due to raised levels of maternal anxiety. However, it should be noted that three studies showed no effect on language development.

With regard to emotional development, four out of five studies found fear and anxiety scores in infants of mothers with PND to be higher. Interestingly, one study found no association with infant separation anxiety and PND, which is not the case for older children. Ten out of 12 studies showed negative behavioural traits and an increased rate of behaviour problems years later, as well as less mature regulatory behaviours amongst toddlers aged two years. Dysregulated behaviour in infants was more prevalent in one study but only when the PND was associated with maternal personality disorder. In many studies, it was noted that PND had greater effects when the whole home environment was adversely affected with less maternal warmth.

A total of 11 studies showed a negative effect on mother-to-infant bonding. All mothers showed improvement in bonding scores by six months, and in some studies, an effect on bonding was no longer detected at 14 months. Women with PND showed less closeness, warmth and sensitivity; lower levels of mutual attunement; and more difficulties in the relationship with their child in the first postpartum year compared to non-depressed women.

Children of mothers with depression were also found to be less likely to have completed immunisation programmes at the expected times. They were also more likely to have visited A&E departments and more often consulted their GPs or paediatricians for non-routine care. Maternal care was also affected with a tendency towards low nurturance and high discipline regimes. Mothers with PND more often had a negative perception of their infant (e.g. 'he has a difficult temperament') and more frequently complained of their infant having crying or sleep problems. One American study found mothers with depression were 4.2 times more likely to spank their child whilst a Japanese study revealed higher rates of worrying about parenting, including worries about being an abusive parent.

Given that the majority of the studies in this review depended on self-report, it is not surprising that there was little data on child maltreatment, and accurate data in this sensitive area can only depend on interview-based studies. However, there is no evidence that mothers with PND are more likely to harm their infants; when it occurs, it seems likely to be due to other known risk factors. Chronic depression where it was studied showed a greater impact on infants than transient episodes of depression, and severe depression had greater effects than mild depression. Social support seemed to have protective effects, but mothers with PND presented with lower levels of perceived social support than mothers without depression. The overall impression is that PND has a negative impact on mothers and their new-born infants, but specific effects will vary according to country and culture.

Treatment of Postnatal Depression

The initial diagnostic consultation is often the most important and offers many useful opportunities for therapy and support. Patients usually present with a diffuse set of complaints – including depressive symptoms, disappointment in motherhood, sleep disorder or shame associated with their morbid thoughts – which seem to be out of character for the person concerned. The act of sharing such thoughts with a professional may provide an immediate cathartic relief. For other symptoms – such as panic attacks, obsessions or an episode of depersonalisation, all of which may be a novel and frightening experience for the new mother – a 'medical explanation' in itself may be reassuring.

During the initial interview, the patient's present family set-up and family background should be explored to give some idea of what sources of support are available to them. Towards the end of the initial consultation, if there is evidence of a clear-cut depressive episode, it should be discussed with the patient as being likely that of 'postnatal depression'. This simple act of naming the condition appears to have a beneficial effect for many women, as it provides an explanation for their feelings of confusion and any sense of failure they may have. This initial discussion and formulation of their situation may help with the validation of the mother with PND's current experiences.

Perinatal services are encouraged to offer all partners a signposting service.[62] Partners will often be seen and offered recommendations such as support groups. Partners are also usually reassured that the cause is a treatable medical disorder with a mainly benign outcome. It is usually helpful to also see the partner who may themselves have become depressed, as they too may present with symptoms that might benefit from appropriate signposting of services. Because relationships often go through difficult patches during this period but may improve later, joint sessions with both partners may sometimes be helpful. There is also a nationally led drive to employ male and female peer supporters within perinatal teams.

Psychotherapy

An Israeli study[63] found that the preferred mode of treatment of PND clients was psychotherapy delivered by a skilled psychologist or physician. Next in popularity came group approaches; thirdly, medication; and the least popular modes were internet and Skype-based treatments. There are now many reports showing that psychotherapy in the form of cognitive behavioural therapy (CBT) or interpersonal psychotherapy is effective in postnatal depression. One trial of interpersonal therapy found around a third (37%) of those who received therapy recovered compared with only 13% of the waiting-list controls.[64] In this trial, although the effects of psychotherapy were positive, the majority of women (63%) with major depression did not improve, and for these women, pharmacological therapies are indicated.

A UK-based study[65] has shown that many different types of psychotherapy – such as counselling, CBT and psychodynamic therapy – are all equally effective for postnatal depression. As in other conditions, what probably matters more than the theoretical basis of a particular psychotherapeutic technique is the empathic quality of the therapeutic relationship. In conducting psychotherapy with postnatal women, due allowance should be made for real practical difficulties such as illnesses in babies and the needs of other children in the family. During the early stages of psychotherapy – and particularly with the more severe illnesses – most women prefer to talk mainly about their symptoms, and sympathetic listening, permission to talk expansively on symptomatic distress and a cognitive approach are beneficial. Feelings of rejection or hostility directed at the partner or other children are commonplace, and some new mothers also complain of an inability to experience warmth towards the baby. As the depression lightens, the more traditional psychotherapeutic themes of relationships with parents and other family members begin to emerge. Motivation to remain in psychotherapy varies. It may last only for the duration of the depression, but once the depression lifts, women may cease contact. Long-term, dependent relationships with therapists are now relatively unusual in the NHS, especially with Improving Access to Psychological Therapy services where therapy resources are restricted to numbers of sessions indicated for specific conditions. This is not always the case, however, in other NHS and private psychological services.

Group therapy, where all the participants are experiencing postnatal depression, can provide a highly supportive environment that many women find helpful. These groups are usually led by a psychologist or mental health worker. Women improve their strategies for coping with depressive symptoms by learning from the way other group members have dealt with their symptoms. Group interventions can give mothers a feeling that they are not alone but rather part of a group coping with difficulties of PND. The social aspect of the group is itself of great importance, with many women building supportive relationships with other group members. However, as many women prefer individual therapy, this should always be on offer as well.

Drug Therapy for Postnatal Depression

Some women, particularly those with brief or mild episodes of postnatal depression, will neither wish for nor require pharmacotherapy. O'Hara[64] found that 40 per cent of women with postnatal depression in the community would reject drug treatment. However, as noted in his trial of psychotherapy, around 63 per cent of subjects failed to respond to psychotherapy and will require another approach such as medication. Those referred to specialist services appear to have more severe illnesses and are usually more willing to take medication; they may even have started it before they are seen. The NICE guidelines[66] suggest that when an antidepressant is considered, the main side effects and risks need to be discussed, as well as the risks associated with starting and stopping these drugs abruptly. The NICE text mentions three groups of antidepressants – TCAs, SSRIs and SNRIs – but in practice, the vast majority of prescriptions are for the SSRIs, especially for sertraline. Antidepressant therapy at this time is similar to antidepressant therapy at other times and is described in Chapter 3.3, but a few points deserve mention.

Both SSRIs and tricyclics are effective in postnatal depression and safe in mothers who are breast feeding (see later). The more benign side-effect profile of the SSRIs has led to them becoming the drugs of first choice in the treatment of PND in most instances. Tricyclics and mirtazapine may be useful in cases where sleep disturbance is prominent because of their sedative effects, and they also have an advantage in that dosage can be gradually titrated upwards, starting from very low doses, where side effects are minimal. Many patients will respond to relatively low doses (e.g. for amitriptyline in the 30–75 mg range). However, certain tricyclic side effects are particularly problematic in the perinatal period, such as daytime drowsiness and dizziness, which can interfere with caring for the baby. Toxicity in overdose is another major concern with the use of tricyclics, and this is another reason that SSRIs are often preferred.

Failure to respond to the initial prescription is quite common, and this should be picked up and acted early on because shortening the overall duration of the depression is a treatment priority. Increasing the dose or switching to a drug of a different group may be helpful. Lithium augmentation (with either a tricyclic or an SSRI antidepressant) is often a useful strategy in resistant cases, possibly because the more severe puerperal cases may have an underlying bipolar diathesis. If lithium is used, breast feeding should cease, but most of those with a severe resistant depression will have already given up breast feeding by this stage.

Once the condition has resolved, drug therapy should continue for a further 6–12 months because case register studies have shown that morbidity remains high in the second postpartum year. Drug tapering should be gradual and supervised closely, as relapses are common and not always easy to treat. Relapses after further pregnancies are common, with an approximate risk of 50 per cent. Antidepressants can be used prophylactically and started immediately after delivery to minimise the risk of recurrence – as described earlier for puerperal psychosis – although there is only RCT support for sertraline.

Hormonal approaches to treating PND have an obvious attraction because they fit well with the known massive hormonal falls after childbirth. In the 1960s, London-based GP Katherine Dalton advocated the widespread use of progesterone for the treatment of both PND and premenstrual tension, but double-blind trials were not supportive.[67] Allopregnanolone is a progesterone metabolite found in small quantities in the central nervous system (CNS) and is a neuroactive steroid, or a neurosteroid, and it can be synthesised from steroid hormone precursors, such as progesterone, or synthesised *de novo* from cholesterol. Neurosteroids are positive allosteric modulators at $GABA_A$ receptors, a property which is thought to mediate the therapeutic effects of these compounds. Intravenously administering a single dose of a synthetic derivative of allopregnanolone, called brexanolone, showed a significant antidepressive effect in a placebo-controlled trial,[68] and this effect lasted a month. Intravenous antidepressant treatment is never likely to catch on, but oral preparations have been developed, so it remains to be seen whether the new generation of allopregnanolone-based treatments will prove to be useful.

Breast Feeding and Psychotropic Drugs

The benefits for the child from breast feeding are well-known. However, many women who are prescribed psychotropic medications may be concerned about the safety of breast feeding whilst taking these medications. In addition, the severity of mental illness may also impact on a woman's ability to breast feed, and women with severe illness may need additional help and support if they wish to breast feed. Preconception counselling is an ideal opportunity for women to discuss their medication and feeding preferences so that appropriate plans can be made to suit the woman's needs, weighing up the risks and benefits.

All psychotropic drugs are small molecules and are highly fat soluble; they enter the breast milk to a variable degree and also cross the infant's blood–brain barrier. Most of the commonly used psychotropic drugs appear to be 'relatively safe', but no drug is completely safe; although, by the same token, none is absolutely contraindicated. This means that the psychiatrist will need to be knowledgeable of the existing evidence regarding the various psychotropic drugs. This is described in full in the Maudsley guidelines[69] on prescribing. The psychiatrist will need to be able to advise mothers who wish to breast feed whilst taking a psychotropic on its safety. A summary is presented in Table 13.1.

A critical measurement in evaluating a drug's merit or otherwise in breast feeding is the maternal plasma to foetal plasma ratio for each drug, and this is known as the relative infant dose (RID), which should be less than 10 per cent. Breast feeding while taking a psychotropic drug should be avoided where the infant has a hepatic, renal or neurological disorder; is premature; or has some other contraindication. Maternal drug dosages should be kept to a minimum, as there is uncertainty regarding how new-born infants can handle the higher plasma levels of psychotropic drugs. It should be noted that there will always be a small proportion of mothers (and presumably infants as well) who may be slow metabolisers,

Table 13.1 Database on breast feeding and psychotropic drugs[69,70]

Drug	Summary of reported findings
Tricyclics	Generally well tolerated by mothers and infants
Amitriptyline	Milk to serum ratio 0.7–1.6, mean around 1. Infant plasma levels low or undetected. Relative infant dosage = 2.8%. Sedation and poor suckling reported with amitriptyline The use of 10 mg tablets allows for dosage titration to ensure minimum effective dosage. Widely used in the pre-SSRI era
SSRIs	
Fluoxetine	Hendrick et al.[71] found infant fluoxetine levels low or undetectable, but norfluoxetine was detected (n = 20). Relative infant dose = 1.6–14.6%. Maternal dosage was critical: at 20 mg/day, mean fluoxetine and norfluoxetine level was 8.9 ng/ml; at 30 mg, the mean level was 62.5 ng/ml. Colic, excessive crying, diarrhoea, somnolence and hypotonia have been observed in the infants. Single case of seizures reported. A serotonin-like syndrome reported in one infant whose mother was on fluoxetine 60 mgs
Sertraline	Small amounts only in breast milk. Relative infant dose low at 0.5–3%. Undetected in infant plasma, but desmethyl sertraline present at 24%. Significantly higher levels in women on 100 mg daily or above. Serotonergic overstimulation reported in one pre-term infant. Probably today the antidepressant of first choice in breast feeding women who need an antidepressant
Paroxetine	Levels of paroxetine and its metabolite were undetectable in infant blood.[72] No adverse reports. Not used today because of difficulties in withdrawal
Citalopram	Relative infant dosage = 3–10% Infant blood levels higher than sertraline but lower than for fluoxetine. In infants, sleep disturbance and colic resolved when maternal dose reduced
Escitalopram	Relative infant dose = 3–8%. One case of necrotising enterocolitis from *in utero* exposure. Seizures reported in one case
Mirtazepine	Relative infant dose = 0.5-4.4%. Infant levels were low at 0.2 ng/ml. Elevated incidence of poor neonatal adaption syndrome amongst infants who were breastfed
SNRIs	Venlafaxine: relative infant dosage = 6–9%. At birth, jitteriness, rapid breathing and poor suckling alleviated by breast feeding after one week. Little used today
Antipsychotics	
Chlorpromazine	Maternal plasma to breast milk ratio 0.5. One report of lethargy. Commonly used before SGAs
Haloperidol	Present in breast milk. Relative infant dose = 0.2–12%. One report of hypersomnia, poor feeding and slowed movements. One report of delayed development in a woman breast feeding on chlorpromazine and haloperidol, but infants exposed to haloperidol alone did not show this
Quatiapine	Relative infant dose = 0.09–0.1%. Infant blood levels undetected. No adverse effects reported
Clozapine (avoid)	Estimated relative infant dosage = 1.4%. Infants had sedation, agranulocytosis, decreased suckling, irritability and cardiovascular instability. Avoid because of high risk of serious side effects
Risperidone	Relative infant dosage = 2.8–9.1%. Infant blood risperidone undetectable. Infants: one case of hypersomnia
Amisulpiride	Relative infant dosage = 4–7% No infant side effects reported
Sedative antipsychotics	
Thioxanthenes	May improve breast feeding (possibly by increasing prolactin). No adverse reports. Sulpiride has limited data
Olanzapine	Limited data. One report of jaundice and drowsiness
Aripiprazole	No information, but because of this and theoretical risks, manufacturers advise to avoid. Extrapyramidal effects noted in the neonates
Mood stabilisers	
Lithium	Maternal plasma to milk ratio 0.3–0.7. Infant lithium levels highly variable. Lithium toxicity in infants is a known hazard, presenting as cyanosis, lethargy, hypothermia and hypotonia. Close infant lithium monitoring may not be sufficient to prevent toxicity as any inter-current illness (e.g. infant diarrhoea) can rapidly cause electrolyte imbalance and toxicity. Because there is a definite risk of neonatal lithium toxicity, lithium should not be given to breast feeding women. Hence 'Avoid'
Valproate	Breast milk levels 1–10% of maternal plasma levels. Infant blood levels low at 4–12% of maternal blood levels. One report of thrombocytopenia and anaemia, which reversed on stopping the valproate. However, valproate no longer advisable in women during their reproductive years and is prohibited in some jurisdictions
Carbamazepine	Breast milk levels 7–95% of maternal blood levels. Infant levels 6–65% of maternal levels. Adverse reports: two cases of hepatic dysfunction, one report of drowsiness and irritability. Seizures reported in one case of an infant whose mother was on fluoxetine, carbamazepine and buspirone, indicating the increased risks to infants of mothers on polypharmacy
Lamotrigine	Limited data but appears to be safe and so, if an antiepileptic or mood stabiliser is needed, lamotrigine is the drug of choice recommended by NICE but monitor blood lamotrigine levels
Benzodiazepine sedatives	Relative infant doses: diazepam 0.88%–7%, clonazepam 2.8%, lorazepam 2.6%–2.9%, oxazepam 0.28%–1%. Maternal milk to plasma ratios 16–30%. NICE recommends a short-acting benzodazepine such as lorazepam if a sedative is required. Infants present with sedation/drowsiness or floppy infant syndrome

and because metaboliser status will be unknown to the prescriber, the level of psychotropic drugs in the maternal breast milk may be highly variable and hence in the infant as well.

The main risk to the infant is of drug toxicity, and although full-blown toxicity syndromes are rare, women on psychotropics often report their babies are lethargic, sleepy or irritable. The psychiatrist should make specific enquiry about these symptoms and the infant's general welfare at each visit. If the infant's symptoms appear to be clinically significant, maternal drug dosage should be reduced or alternatives to breast feeding should be considered.

Psychiatric Disorder in Pregnancy

The NICE guidelines[66] on treating a mental health problem in pregnancy specify:

1. It should be delivered by competent practitioners who should receive regular high-quality supervision
2. Clients should be seen within two weeks of referral

Epidemiological data suggest that the prevalence of minor and major depression is 18% during pregnancy and 19% during the first three postpartum months, with higher rates among low-income women (27% and 23%, respectively). The prevalence of any anxiety disorder during pregnancy and the postpartum period is 13%. These rates are similar to those found in the non-perinatal population. Women with psychiatric conditions (all conditions) are also significantly more likely to experience pre-term birth (i.e. birth prior to 37 weeks gestation), lower than average birth weight infants (i.e. <2,500 g), an increased rate of caesarean delivery and an increased likelihood that their infant will be admitted to the neonatal care unit. Risks for antenatal depression are increased by lifestyle, poor nutrition and socioeconomic factors, particularly poverty. Of concern and amenable to intervention is antenatal depression associated with poor maternal self care, contributing to the increased risk for pre-term birth, low birth weight and intra-uterine growth restriction. Also, studies have shown that antidepressant medication use during pregnancy results in a small but significantly increased risk for low birth weight and pre-term birth.

Approximately 3.5 per cent of all pregnant women in the Western world use psychotropic drugs during pregnancy. All psychotropics cross the placenta, and new-born infants are therefore exposed to a drug withdrawal syndrome, the severity of which may be dependent on the particular drug and its dosage. Because fears of causing birth defects are very high during pregnancy, it is not surprising that around 39 per cent of women reported being non-compliant with their medication, and this varies according to the type of medical treatment. Compliance was highest for anti-HIV medication as women saw this as being helpful and preventing their baby from getting HIV. Discontinuing antidepressant medication treatment is of itself associated with worse clinical outcomes. Discontinuation rather than treatment resistance is the main cause of treatment failure for pregnancy depressions and, in America, this has been associated with lower socioeconomic status and being single, black and Hispanic.[70]

There is good RCT evidence for the efficacy of CBT and IPT in pregnancy and post-partumdepression,[73] and so where this is readily available, this may be a good first option. However, if this fails to provide relief or is only available after a long wait, there is also good data supporting the use of SSRIs to treat the depression. Treatment discontinuation is common for both antidepressants and psychotherapy but is less when both treatments are combined. In the UK, although CBT may not be available for all, whenever women are being treated with an antidepressant, if possible they should also be offered support from a member of the perinatal team, as it appears that the combined pharmacological and psychotherapeutic approach has lower discontinuation rates and hence ultimately better outcomes.

Schizophrenia in pregnancy. A large study[74] based on the Finnish national register compared singleton pregnancies amongst women with schizophrenia against controls. The main findings pointed to higher rates of gestational diabetes, possibly a consequence of antipsychotic usage. These effects had not previously been observed to any great extent for first-generation antipsychotics (FGAs), and some authorities have even recommended either using FGAs for new cases of schizophrenia or switching women to FGAs in pregnancy, but this has not caught on. Guidelines[69] suggest sticking to the same antipsychotic if this is working well. Risks were also increased for more rapid foetal growth, premature contractions, hypertension and pregnancy-related hospitalisations. The study also found that suspected damage to the foetus from comorbid alcohol/drugs was significantly more common among women with schizophrenia than controls. The possible teratogenicity of antipsychotics is discussed later in this chapter.

Women commonly request a discontinuation of their antipsychotics in pregnancy, but it is known that the abrupt discontinuation of antipsychotics in pregnancy often leads to relapses in both bipolar disorder and schizophrenia. Therefore, if discontinuation is to occur, it should be both supervised and tapered. Depots are not generally recommended except in cases where women were non-concordant with oral medication and have had a good response to depot medication.[69] The decision whether to discontinue or not, must be individualised, and the latest NICE guidelines – apart from recommending discussion with the patient – do not offer any specific guidance. However, if drugs are stopped, continued observation and contact with the perinatal team is essential as symptoms can return at any time, and a psychotic relapse in late pregnancy or the early postpartum period may be hazardous.

It may be appropriate to strongly advise a continuation of medication throughout pregnancy where previous episodes have been disruptive, distressing or dangerous but, as with all such situations, a balanced approach providing information for and against continuation to enable the patient to come to a decision is much more likely to lead to a positive outcome.

Postpartum Obsessive-Compulsive Disorder

Obsessional symptoms are common and worrying and occasionally merit a separate diagnosis of an episode of obsessive-compulsive disorder. More frequently, the obsessional symptoms are part and parcel of the depression and tend both to appear and to resolve together with the depression. Obsessional phenomena among postnatal women may seem both unusual and frightening and may include intrusive, repetitive thoughts and images of harming or even killing the baby, which can be graphic and disturbing. Themes of sexual abuse are also quite common. Although it is extremely rare for a patient to act on an obsessive thought, they are not always harmless. For example, one woman had an obsession about wasting water and, as a consequence, refused to cool the baby's feed down with running cold water and instead gave the baby over-heated feeds.

A Turkish study[75] gave the incidence of OCD at six weeks postpartum at 4%. The most common obsessions in women with postpartum OCD were contamination (75%), aggression (33.3%) and symmetry/exactness (33.3%), and the most common compulsions were cleaning/washing (66.7%) and checking (58.3%). In comparison with non-puerperal OCD, those with postpartum OCD had significantly more frequent aggressive obsessions but less-severe obsessive-compulsive symptoms. PND was commonly associated with the OCD, and both the OCD and the PND responded well to SSRIs in most cases. Personality predictors of a postpartum onset for OCD in this study were avoidant and obsessive-compulsive personality disorder traits.

Anxiety Disorders

A wide spectrum of anxiety disorders may also present postnatally, but usually they appear together with the depression and remit as the depression resolves. Generalised anxiety disorder is the most common and presents with a picture of mixed anxiety and depression, with the content of the anxiety usually relating to issues of infant care and infant health. The high rate of anxiety disorders and mixed anxious-depressive pictures led Pitt[76] in 1968 to apply the term 'atypical depression' to postnatal depression, but today, these illnesses are not regarded as atypical or significantly different from major depressive disorder as occurring at other times, which is also often accompanied by anxiety. Tokophobia is an anxiety disorder presenting as an extreme fear of childbirth. It can be highly distressing and disabling for women, and in extremis, may even result in women seeking to terminate their pregnancy due to fear of the birth process itself. If tokophobia is detected, this should lead on to a referral to a health care professional with expertise in providing perinatal mental health support.

During pregnancy, up to 5 per cent of women may experience panic disorder and as many as 10 per cent have generalised anxiety disorder (GAD). Panic disorder and panic attacks may be particularly frightening, and some women may also have separation anxiety with their partner and loved ones when faced with being alone, as this can often trigger a panic attack. In most cases, the panic occurs in women with a previous history of panic attacks, but new onset cases are also reported in the first three months after delivery. In a meta-analysis[77] of studies on panic disorder in 215 pregnancies, 89 (41%) were associated with improvement of panic disorder in pregnancy, while 38% exhibited new onset or exacerbation of panic disorder in the postpartum period, and so it is unclear if the perinatal period has any influence on the course of panic disorder.

Agoraphobia may sometimes start for the first time after childbirth, but this generally resolves as the depression improves, although a more severe chronic agoraphobia can occasionally start in the perinatal period.

Acute depersonalisation which commonly starts with the depression usually resolves as the depression remits, but in a few cases, it may fail to remit and can sometimes turn into a chronic depersonalisation syndrome without depression, which may take some years to resolve but this too usually also eventually remits.

Eating Disorders

There is no uniform behaviour that occurs when a woman with an eating disorder discovers she is pregnant.[78] For some women, concern for their unborn child motivates a complete cessation of eating disorder behaviours, but this is not always the case. Women may reduce certain behaviours – for example, moving from binge-purging to binge eating alone. For many women, there is no change in symptoms, and in some cases, their symptoms may worsen during pregnancy. Eating disorder behaviours in pregnancy are linked to poor maternal and neonatal outcomes, and therefore, specialist intervention should be offered where possible (see Chapter 12). For mothers, complications may include miscarriages, significant morbidity, increased mortality, pre-eclampsia, depressive symptoms during pregnancy and postnatal depression. For infants, there may be low birth weight as well as impaired attachment and maternal bonding.[61]

The NICE guidelines for Mental Health in Pregnancy for those with Eating Disorders[79] recommend:

1. Assess the need for foetal growth scans
2. Discuss the importance of healthy eating during pregnancy and the postnatal period
3. Advise the mother about feeding the baby
4. Consider more intensive prenatal care for pregnant women with current or remitted anorexia nervosa to ensure adequate prenatal nutrition and foetal development

Postpartum Post-traumatic Stress Disorder (PP-PTSD)

Although relatively uncommon, classical post-traumatic stress disorder has been increasingly recognised as a complication of difficult or traumatic deliveries, and the account here draws on a recent review.[80] The prevalence of a postpartum diagnosis of PTSD varies widely between studies depending on differing methodologies and exactly how long after childbirth the study took place. This is because most of the symptoms fade rapidly in the first three months after childbirth. Published rates are in the range of 0–6.9% (2% on average), but significant levels of symptoms of the sub-threshold PTSD could be present in a much greater number. Overall, the prevalence rates of PP-PTSD, in its acute form (between one and three months postpartum) were 5–8% in community samples. Cluster modelling revealed four distinct symptom groups in line with PTSD occurring at other times:

1. Reliving, or re-experiencing, symptoms, namely nightmares and flashbacks
2. Avoidance coupled with unwanted memories (other re-experiencing symptoms)
3. Negative cognitions and mood disturbances
4. Hyperarousal reactivity

In some women with a previous history of trauma, the PTSD symptoms occurring after childbirth are a continuation of their previous symptoms. For the majority, however, this will be a new onset after a difficult delivery. The subjective experience of the traumatic event is a more important factor in predicting PTSD than its objective stressor severity, so a negative subjective experience of a traumatic childbirth is commonly associated with PP-PTSD.

PP-PTSD has a significant influence on the mother and baby's daily and long-term functioning. It has a high comorbidity rate with other mental disorders, especially postnatal depression, and it may fade as the depression itself recedes. The condition remains poorly recognised and is usually untreated in routine clinical services. Consequences of PP-PTSD include a refusal to breast feed the new-born, attachment problems, partner and intimacy avoidance, low self-esteem and low self-adequacy. These women may associate their delivery with pain, fear or depression, or sometimes display traumatic amnesia.

Risk factors for postpartum PTSD after delivery are mostly the same as for PTSD after any other trauma, but with some specificity related to the event of childbirth. Possible pre-traumatic factors risk include personality traits, tokophobia, history of previous psychological problems or the number of previous deliveries. Risk factors related to delivery include the mode and duration of delivery, obstetric factors and complicated deliveries, pain and epidural analgesia, intensive fear for own or baby's life, sleep disturbances or peri-partial dissociation. Treatment is as for PTSD in other circumstances (see Chapter 6.2).

Is prevention possible? A recent review[81] showed that a few interventions work. Measures considered were debriefing, structured psychological interventions, expressive writing, encouraging skin-to-skin contact with healthy new-borns immediately postpartum and holding or seeing the new-born after birth. Two RCTs showed that debriefing had no preventive effect. However, one study of a psychological intervention including elements of exposure and psycho-education seemed to lead to fewer post-traumatic stress disorder symptoms in women who had delivered via emergency caesarean section.[81]

Postnatal Neonatal Adaption Syndromes

Approximately 3.5 per cent of all pregnant women in the Western world use psychotropic drugs during pregnancy. All psychotropics cross the placenta, and therefore, many infants are exposed to psychotropic drugs, so a withdrawal syndrome termed poor neonatal adaptation (PNA) may sometimes occur. Midwifery staff should be on the lookout for this amongst infants delivered from a mother who has had psychotropics in the third trimester of pregnancy. The symptoms are largely similar after exposure to antidepressants, antipsychotics and benzodiazepines and consist of mostly mild neurologic, autonomic, respiratory and gastrointestinal abnormalities. Most symptoms develop within 48 hours after birth and last for two to six days. Breast feeding is presumably at least partially protective for development of PNA. Drug dosage does not seem to be related to the risk of PNA, and this applies to all types of psychotropic drugs. When PNA symptoms are present and observable, admission to the special care baby unit (SCBU) and care of the paediatrician is advisable, and observation of the infant takes place until the symptoms are fully resolved. In most cases, symptoms are non-specific, which requires that other neonatal diagnoses – such as infection or neurologic problems – have to be excluded. Most cases of PNA are mild, of short duration and self-limiting without need for treatment. Supportive measures such as frequent small feedings, swaddling and increase of skin-to-skin contact with the mother is usually sufficient.

Maternity Blues

Transient mild depression and crying spells after childbirth are frequent and have been called the baby blues, third-day blues, the maternity blues and the transitory syndrome – the latter term capturing the evanescent nature of the mood swing. The syndrome is reviewed in detail by Stein.[82] Crying spells are the hallmark of the maternity blues and are reported in 50–70% of new mothers. Women will often cry after delivery, which may be accompanied by feelings of happiness or tears of joy, but around 10% of women describe feeling acutely depressed, strange or depersonalised immediately after delivery. Women may experience more severe and prolonged crying spells in the subsequent days after the birth, which sometimes occurs with an altered mood, although the mood is not necessarily depressed. Anxiety, elation, irritability or a state of emotional lability may also be present.

More severe depressive feelings, sometimes with a violent or bizarre content and reminiscent of the thought pattern observed in depressive illness, occur in around 10% of women and are more common among those with previous depression. The severity of the blues can be measured with the Stein Maternity Blues scale.[83] This more intense depression usually lasts only for a few hours and rarely for the whole day, but it may recur in bouts on two or three successive days. Irritability or angry feelings directed at the partner or hospital staff are common, while transient negative feelings towards the baby and an early lack of maternal affection can be elicited in up to 40% of women. These usually resolve without any adverse consequences. Although forgetfulness, confusion and poor concentration are common complaints, psychometric testing has failed to detect any objective measure of cognitive impairment. Elation is present in over 80% of women on day one, but this falls to 40% by day four, although a few women are elated every day. This elation falls far short of hypomania. Emotional lability, particularly on the blues day, is also common.

Insomnia, dreaming and nightmares are common, while transient hallucinations on wakening (hypnopompic hallucinations) occur in around 10% of women. Rapid eye movement and stage IV sleep are decreased in pregnancy, but they may show a rebound increase on nights two and three postpartum, approximately coinciding with the blues.[84] A mild headache – generally bilateral and frontal – occurs in around a third of women, usually between days three and six, and this appears to be more common among those women with a personal or family history of migraines.[85] For most women, the maternity blues is a brief acute episode lasting no more than a few hours and for one or two days only, but a few women may have a rather more continuous pattern of disturbance. Just occasionally, a very severe, brief, almost psychotic episode occurs for two to three days as a part of the maternity blues, and this was the original 'milk fever'.

The only established clinical associations with the maternity blues are anxiety and depression during late pregnancy, previous premenstrual tension and a subsequent postnatal depression. Parity, social factors and obstetric complications do not appear to be related. The condition only needs to be distinguished from the prodrome of a psychotic illness and the onset of an episode of postnatal major depression. There is no need to treat 'the blues' as it is so transient, although reassurance may be comforting, and the use of supportive measures such as simple analgesia for headaches may be useful. There is an abrupt loss of body weight at around the onset of the maternity blues.[82]

Stillbirth

Ten countries account for 66 per cent of the world's stillbirths with most (98%) occurring in low-income and middle-income countries. The stillbirth rate in sub-Saharan Africa is approximately 10 times that of developed countries (29 vs 0.3 per 1,000 births), and most of it is due to remediable factors.[86] For a high-income country, the UK has one of the highest rates. In 2017, the stillbirth rate in England and Wales was 4.2 per 1,000 total births. Stillbirth has been termed an 'invisible death' due to being neglected as a public health issue of importance to society and health policy makers. The UK government's ambition is to halve the stillbirth rate in England by 2025, which would require the rate to fall to 2.6 per 1,000 total births.[87] Poverty and socioeconomic factors are potentially remedial factors; for England for 2017, the stillbirth rate in the most-deprived areas was 5.5 per 1,000 total births, compared with 3.0 per 1,000 total births in the least-deprived areas.

Grief following perinatal loss is a normal phenomenon, and for the most part, women should be allowed to grieve without psychiatric intervention. The pattern is usually one of initial shock followed by numbness, disbelief and denial. Guilt may be prominent as women desperately search for an explanation. Some women may subject themselves to overly harsh self-criticism (e.g. for minor peccadillos during pregnancy, such as drinking small amounts of alcohol, eating the wrong foods or failing to follow certain medical advice) when there may be no indication that these considerations are causal. It is important to distinguish normal grief from complicated grief and depression because there is significant overlap between the symptoms of psychiatric disorder and grief. Women who experience a perinatal loss have four-fold higher odds than women with a live birth of screening positive for depression. The highest risk is for women with a loss occurring after 20 weeks of gestation, and the most commonly reported psychiatric disorder is adjustment disorder.

Clarke and Williams[88] found that, although rates of depression among women who had had a stillbirth were increased at three months postpartum, by six months, the rate was no higher than among non-pregnant women.. Thus, while women with recurrent miscarriages, foetal death after 20 weeks of gestation and a previous history of depression are at increased risk of depression/adjustment disorder in the year following perinatal loss, this risk gradually declines later on.

Perinatal loss is also associated with an increased risk of anxiety disorders. At nine months after perinatal death (stillbirth and infant death), women with a perinatal death had more than twice the odds for generalised anxiety disorder and social phobia even after adjusting for demographic factors, current depression and previous history of psychiatric disorders. PTSD rates are increased after all types of perinatal loss. Longer gestational ages are associated with greater severity of PTSD. Nine months after a stillbirth or neonatal death, women have a seven-fold higher rate for screening positive for PTSD when compared with women with live births,[89] but there is no increase in rates of maternal suicide.

At one time, bereaved mothers of stillborn babies were largely ignored, and the stillbirth was treated as a non-event, but this has changed in recent years. In a large Swedish study of stillbirth,[90] of the 314 women who gave birth to a stillborn child, nearly every mother had seen her child, and 80% had caressed her baby. More than 90% of the mothers stated that the medical staff showed respect, and about 80% of the mothers stated that staff exhibited tenderness towards their dead children and that mothers were valued and had properly taken photographs. Feelings of sadness and having been deeply hurt or angered by the medical staff's behaviour were reported by 37% of the women, but 70% of women reported that the hospital had good routines to support mothers of stillborn children. An area of controversy has been whether to hold their baby after death, with some women reporting that too much pressure was put on them to do so whilst others said that they were not sufficiently encouraged to hold their baby. Ratings of satisfaction with the decision to hold the infant were uniformly high, and all studies that measured this outcome found higher rates of satisfaction among women who held their stillborn baby (85–99%) compared with those who did not. In addition, this study[88] noted that while holding their stillborn infant, women retrospectively reported feeling warmth (94%) and pride (81%), although this was mixed with feelings of insecurity (48%), discomfort (39%) and fear (35%).

Studies of counselling with a professional after a stillbirth have suggested that couple counselling may be helpful. It can give partners an opportunity to express their grief, which may otherwise lead to depression, relationship issues or dysfunctional behaviours (e.g. excessive drinking). However, most women prefer instead to seek support from fellow sufferers through organisations such as the Stillbirth and Neonatal Death Society (SANDS). There is national development of maternal loss services[91] as part of a drive to increase support for these women. Many regions in 2023 were planning and recruiting for their services – using the 'Thrive' service in Kent as a model of good practice – such that more women could be offered psychologically based services coming from existing perinatal teams.

Stillbirth is a traumatic experience, with reports of adverse psychosocial effects such as anxiety, depression, shame, suicidal thoughts, post-traumatic stress disorder (PTSD) and guilt. The overwhelming impact on parents can be long-lasting and ripples outwards to siblings, grandparents, extended family and friends. In the long term, it affects couples' relationships, older children, subsequent children, social life, career and work colleagues.

Infanticide and Neonaticide

Filicide refers to the homicide of children aged under 16, neonaticide to the killing of infants very soon after delivery (usually on the first day) and infanticide to the killing of infants under one year of age. Of these types of homicide, infanticide is the most strongly associated with psychiatric disorder, especially postpartum psychosis and depression. In England and Wales, the Infanticide Act 1938[92] provides for a verdict of infanticide if:

> the mother causes death of her child under the age of 12 months by wilful act or omission, but at the time of the act or omission the balance of her mind was disturbed by reason of her not having fully recovered from the effect of her having given birth to the child or by reasons of the effect of lactation consequent on the birth of the child.

It is usually dealt with leniently by the courts, with the offence being classed as manslaughter rather than murder and then dispensed with either by a probation or hospital order. The Infanticide Act does not apply in Scotland nor is there any similar legislation in the USA. In these countries, when mental illness is thought to have contributed, a plea of diminished responsibility is submitted, and a verdict of manslaughter rather than murder is given.

Human infanticide has been described ever since history has been recorded and was common in England in the Middle Ages. Hopwood[93] examined 166 women admitted to Broadmoor following an infanticide verdict between 1900 and 1927, and they comprised 42% of all female admissions; indeed, this was the most common reason for a female admission to Broadmoor at that time. Around 70% of the cases occurred during lactation rather than in the very early puerperium, and these women had what Hopwood termed an 'exhaustional psychosis'. The clinical picture at the time of the homicide comprised of symptoms of restlessness, insomnia, delusions, hallucinations, confusion, depression, disorientation and occasionally stupor – a picture consistent with an untreated puerperal psychosis today. In addition to 'exhaustion psychoses', 13% had manic depression, 10% 'dementia' (i.e. schizophrenia) and 5% epilepsy – these women killed their child during an epileptic automatism (e.g. in a confused state; one mother placed her child in the fire and the kettle in the cradle). Most cases (60%) of 'exhaustion psychoses' resolved spontaneously fairly quickly, but 30% of these women also attempted suicide and 6% died.

Hopwood's study teaches us that an untreated or undertreated puerperal psychosis is a very dangerous condition, and these risks extend through the whole of the first postpartum year. However, human infanticide in the UK is rare today. Combining two series of six years each,[94,95] there were a total of 385 infant homicides over 11 years, giving an average UK annual rate for infanticide of 35. Receiving an infanticide verdict in court is much less frequent, and this occurred in around eight cases per year, and a further 15% received a verdict of some other type of manslaughter.[95] The frequency of the infanticide verdict appears to be unchanged because, in the decade of 1976–1985, the rate was also around seven cases per year.

Infants under one year of age appear to be at greatest risk of being victims, with the risk being four times that of the general population, and within the first year, it is the first six months that appear to be the most dangerous.[96] Those between one and five years of age have the same risk, whilst children between 5 and 15 years have a lower risk.

Mothers are most commonly responsible for early homicides and fathers and step-fathers for the later cases. Although UK studies do not show any links with socioeconomic factors, a study from South Korea[97] found links with the unemployment rate to infanticide rates showing a lag of two quarters from the unemployment rate, and levels of wealth inequality also correlated. Perinatal psychiatric services should aim to eliminate or at least minimise those infanticides associated with acute psychoses and postnatal depression.

Neonaticide

Neonaticide is rather more of a social and historical phenomenon than the result of psychiatric disorder. In ancient Sparta, weak or sickly new-born infants were left to die at the foot of Mount Taygetus. In eighteenth-century Japan, peasants would kill some new-born infants by suffocating them with wet paper, a procedure known as *makibi* ('thinning out'), and this was used as a means of population control. In nineteenth-century Europe, young single mothers would often conceal illegitimate pregnancies and then either smother or drown their new-born infant.

Preferences for male offspring over females still persist in some Asian societies. The picture is particularly stark in India, where a recent study entitled 'Missing Girls in India: Infanticide, Foeticide and Made to Order Pregnancies?'[98] reported a sex ratio of 933 girls to 1,000 boys for the year 2001 and, on this basis, postulated there were 44 million women missing from Indian society. This deficit was caused by a combination of neglect of infant females and women resulting in early death, selective female foeticide, female infanticide and antenatal sex determination, which became widespread with the introduction of ultrasound scans in 1980. However, the relative contribution of each of these factors to the societal gender imbalance is not known.

Neonaticide is rare in the UK today but does still occur. Between 1995 and 1999, there were 27 infant homicides on the first postpartum day, which comprised around 16 per cent of the total number of infant homicides. Neonaticides may be influenced by feelings of intense shame and severe practical difficulties of raising a child. In earlier times when neonaticide was more common, societal rejection of illegitimate birth was the most common cause. In Western Europe, the main maternal psychological features of neonaticide were a denied or concealed pregnancy followed by concealment of the deceased baby, a non-hospital delivery, a relative absence of pain during labour and a previous history of physical or sexual abuse. For individual cases, it is usually too late to prevent a neonaticide since the potential individuals are unknown to the services at the critical time, but efforts to ameliorate the problem have been made on a broader societal level.

In some countries, a warmed baby hatch is placed in designated locations – such as the walls of a hospital or in a local fire station – where women can drop off an unwanted baby in anonymity, and this was implemented by law in the USA in 1999. In Austria, which for a period had a relatively high neonaticide rate, a law was passed in 2001 that permitted anonymous birth so that a woman could have a hospital delivery without declaring their name or showing any form of identity, and this law was given widespread publicity on TV and the newspapers at the time. Prior to this law, the police reported for the decade prior to the anonymity law, there was an average annual neonaticide rate of 7.2/100,000 births, but in the decade following the passing of this law, this rate fell to 3.1/100,000.[99] The UK has neither a system of safe baby hatches nor any anonymity law, and newspapers continue to publish reports of new-born infants being found in telephone kiosks or other unsuitable places.

Teratogenicity of Psychotropic Drugs

In 1957, a drug called thalidomide was introduced as a non-addictive, non-barbiturate sedative – by the German pharmaceutical company, Chemie-Grunenthal – as an over-the-counter sleeping remedy. This was soon found to be an effective anti-emetic in pregnancy and was heavily marketed as being safe. It was not until 1961 that thalidomide was reported by Lenz in Germany and McBride in Australia to be the cause of probably the largest man-made medical disaster in history.[100] Large numbers of women gave birth to infants with severe birth defects, mainly phocomelia, in their offspring. This was a severe developmental abnormality of the limbs, and many thousands of infants were affected. The drug was then withdrawn in 1962 but remains in use today for inflammatory disease associated with leprosy, as a chemotherapeutic agent in the treatment of multiple myeloma, and sometimes for Crohn's disease, HIV and other conditions.

The thalidomide scandal as it is now known has left a deep and indelible mark on the minds of all pregnant women from that time forward, as well as on the medical profession and the pharmaceutical industry. For pregnant women, this has meant a huge reluctance to take any medication at all in pregnancy, although polypharmacy remains an issue.[101] For the medical profession, it has meant any doctor who prescribes for a pregnant woman must be knowledgeable about all the possible teratogenic risks of any drug suggested (for further information, see the UK Teratology Information Service).[102] For the pharmaceutical industry, it has led to a regulatory requirement for extensive drug testing in pregnancy in several different mammalian species to obtain a licence, as well as a high degree of frankness about any and all side effects of any new drug. We review the data on the more common psychotropics as well as the effects of substances of abuse taken in pregnancy.

Antipsychotics

The most recent meta-analysis of antipsychotic use in in pregnancy[103] was based on 6,289 antipsychotic-exposed pregnancies (all antipsychotics) and was compared to 1,618039 unexposed pregnancies and gave an overall increased relative risk (RR = 2.12) for major malformations with no significant difference between typicals and atypicals. The most commonly affected organ was the heart with an RR = 2.09. The study found a small but significant rate of pre-term delivery (RR = 1.86) and a slightly lower birth weight (−57.9 g) but no increased risk for stillbirth.

First-generation antipsychotics (FGAs). Most data originate from studies that included primarily women with hyperemesis gravidarum (a condition itself associated with an increased risk of congenital malformations) who were treated with low doses of phenothiazines. The modest increase in risk identified in some of these studies, along with no clear clustering of congenital abnormalities, suggest that the condition being treated may be responsible rather than the drug treatment itself. Risks from FGAs are generally thought to be low.[69] Neonatal dyskinesia and neonatal jaundice was been reported amongst new-born infants with phenothiazines.[69]

Second-generation antipsychotics (SGAs). The extent of placental passage is highest for olanzapine, followed by risperidone and then quetiapine. Olanzapine has been associated with both increased and lowered birth weight and an increased risk of neonatal intensive care admission. It is also associated with an increased risk of gestational diabetes secondary to weight gain. Use in early pregnancy has been associated with a small increased rate of cono-truncal heart defects including Fallot's tetralogy. Although olanzapine seems to be relatively safe with respect to congenital malformations, it has been associated with a range of problems including hip dysplasia, meningocele, ankyloblepharon (this is partial or complete adhesion of the ciliary edges of superior and inferior eyelids) and neural tube defects. Significantly, there is no clustering of any particular malformation. Limited data suggest that neither risperidone, quetiapine or clozapine are major teratogens in humans, but clozapine is associated with gestational diabetes and neonatal seizures, but NICE accepts its use in pregnancy. The general consensus appears to be that antipsychotics are safe in pregnancy.[69]

Antidepressants. Foetal exposure to tricyclics (via the umbilicus and amniotic fluid) is high when they are used in pregnancy. Prior to the advent of the SSRIs, TCAs were widely used throughout pregnancy with no apparent detriment to the foetus, but there is a small increased risk of pre-term delivery. Use of TCAs in the third trimester is associated with neonatal withdrawal effects: agitation, irritability, seizures, respiratory distress and endocrine and metabolic disturbances. However, tricyclic usage has now faded.

The SSRIs are the most commonly used psychotropics in pregnancy: 63–85% of pregnant women who take a drug in pregnancy will take an SSRI. They may be associated with a small elevation in miscarriage rates. They have usually been held to be safe, but some abnormalities and cardiac malformations have been noted for a number of years. A recent meta analysis combining data for all SSRIs covering more than 9 million pregnancies[104] gave a relative risk (RR) of 1.1 for major abnormalities where a relative risk of 1.0 means no increased risk. However, for cardiac abnormalities, the RR was 1.24, and for individual SSRIs, the figures were:

For citalopram: RR for all abnormalities 1.20; for congenital heart disease 1.24

For fluoxetine: RR for all abnormalities 1.17; for congenital heart disease 1.28

For sertraline: RR for all abnormalities 1.1; for congenital heart disease 1.42

It appears that most of the cardiac abnormalities were for septal defects, and the RRs for individual SSRIs for septal defects were citalopram (1.81), fluoxetine (1.65) and sertraline (2.69). Confidence limits were wide, and so it was not possible to determine if any one drug was better or worse than another. Other abnormalities noted were cystic kidney disease (2.96), abdominal wall defects (1.81) and neural tube defects (1.49), and although other defects occurred in this study, their RRs were only a little above 1, making it impossible to determine if they were truly caused by the SSRI or not.

These figures may be helpful in the common clinical situation where a depressed pregnant woman is reluctant to take an SSRI antidepressant. Women can be reassured that for most major malformations, the risk is no greater than taking no antidepressant, but there may be a small increased risk for congenital heart disease. The base rate for congenital heart disease (CHD) in the population is around 8 cases per 1,000 births, which gives the risk of CHD happening *without* any drug as 0.8%, and sertraline will increase this to around 11 per 1,000 births (1.1%), making the absolute increase in risk of around 0.3%.

This is still a very low risk, and in the discussion with the patient, the physician should compare this low risk to all the adverse sequelae that may follow on from an untreated or undertreated depression in pregnancy, which can result in adverse maternal and child outcomes for the pregnancy. For mothers, this would include raised rates of spontaneous abortion, decreased rates of breast feeding initiation and increased rates of postpartum depression; increased uterine artery resistance; for their labour, more premature labours, more operative deliveries and labour being experienced as more painful, which means they require more epidural analgesia; and for infants, lower APGAR scores, increased need for special neonatal care, neonatal growth restriction, babies with smaller head circumference and increased rates of cognitive, emotional and behavioural problems in children. Hopefully, this list will serve as a counter argument for the depressed mother's reluctance to taking an antidepressant.

SSRIs have also been associated with decreased gestational age (mean 1 week), spontaneous abortion and decreased birth weight (mean 175 g). Three groups of symptoms are seen in neonates exposed to antidepressants in late pregnancy: those associated with serotonergic toxicity, those associated with antidepressant discontinuation symptoms and those related to early birth. Third-trimester exposure to any SSRI has been associated with a low risk of persistent pulmonary hypertension in the new-born.[69] Sertraline has been associated with reduced early APGAR scores at birth. SNRIs and tricyclics may be associated with an increased risk of pre-eclampsia and postpartum haemorrhage. Data on duloxetine, venlafaxine and trazodone are insufficient to confirm safety, but there are no reports of major adverse effects either.

Lithium has been associated with cardiac abnormalities, particularly Ebstein's anomaly affecting the Tricuspid valve, though more recent studies have not shown an increased risk.[105] Further recent studies and reviews of data has suggested that maternal mental illness itself may present as a risk of heart defects rather than lithium use.[106] Rarely, other malformations of the external ear, diaphragmatic hernia and increased rates of miscarriage are reported whilst transient arrythmias have sometimes been found in the new-born. Neurodevelopmental studies on exposed infants are inconclusive.

Antiepileptics. Most data relating to carbamazepine and valproate come from studies in epilepsy, a condition itself associated with increased neonatal malformation. Both carbamazepine and valproate have a clear causal link with an increased risk of a variety of foetal abnormalities, particularly spina bifida. *In utero* exposure to valproic acid is associated with an increased risk of major congenital malformations, dysmorphic features, behavioural issues in childhood, autism and developmental delays, including lowering of IQ. Effectively, valproate is contraindicated in women of child-bearing age because of the risks of severe malformations. Both drugs should be avoided, if possible, and an antipsychotic prescribed instead. Lamotrigine does not appear to be associated with any major malformations or neonatal syndromes, and if a mood stabiliser is required, it may be the drug of choice.[69]

Benzodiazepine use in pregnancy is uncommon now, with no more than 0.8% of women taking them.[107] At one time, there was thought to be an increased risk of oral clefts in new-borns, but subsequent studies failed to confirm this. The most recent study[107] found an association with the Dandy–Walker malformation (RR = 3.1). This is an abnormality of the CNS resulting in hydrocephalus, with giant cell lesions in the maxilla and mandible resulting in facial abnormalities. Aprazolam[107] has been linked to anophthalmia and micro-ophlamia (OR = 4.0).

Maternal use of benzodiazepines during pregnancy was associated with a significantly increased risk of pre-term delivery (RR = 6.79) and with increased risks of low birthweight, low APGAR score, neonatal intensive care unit (NICU) admissions and respiratory distress syndrome. Third-trimester use is commonly associated with neonatal difficulties (floppy baby syndrome). Promethazine has been used in hyperemesis gravidarum and appears not to be teratogenic, although data are limited. NICE recommends the use of low-dose chlorpromazine or amitriptyline instead.

ADHD medications (usually stimulants) taken in early pregnancy[108] are associated with infants having increased rates of gastroschisis (OR = 2.9), omphalocoele (OR = 4.0) and transverse limb deficiency (OR = 3.3).

Substances of Abuse Taken in Pregnancy

Internationally, large numbers of pregnant women smoke,[109] with rates between 12 per cent and 22 per cent in high-income countries and rates probably being even higher in developing economies. Smoking in pregnancy is associated with increased risks of miscarriage, stillbirth, prematurity, low birth weight, raised perinatal morbidity and mortality, neonatal and sudden infant death, infant respiratory problems, cleft palate and poorer infant cognition. There are adverse infant behavioural outcomes, especially in terms of externalising behaviours, oppositional behaviours extending through childhood and ADHD-like symptoms.

Older children (6–16 years) who had been exposed *in utero* display similar behavioural issues, including aggression, oppositional defiance and delinquency, and it appears that no level of tobacco consumption is safe. Passive smoking, or as it is now called secondary smoking, seems to be associated in new-borns with a 1.5 fold increased risk of cleft palate.[109] Pregnancy is probably the one event that most often motivates female smokers to try quitting. In the UK, over 50 per cent of pregnant smokers will try to stop and seek help from NHS smoking cessation clinics, and the government intends to try and reduce the rates of smoking in pregnancy from the present rates of 12% to 6% by 2024.

Ordinary tea and coffee drinking appears to be quite safe, but excessive caffeine in pregnancy appears to be associated with obesity amongst the offspring. Around 7 per cent of a large cohort of women reported an intake greater than 200 mgs/daily, and 3 per cent had an intake greater than 300 mgs daily.[110] Infants of these mothers had increased weight velocity gain and a greater risk of obesity at three years and five years, but this did not persist at eight years except for with mothers who had consumed 300 mgs or more daily.

Alcohol. Taken to excess in pregnancy, alcohol can result in foetal alcohol syndrome (FAS). These infants have a characteristic facial abnormality showing microcephaly (small head), micro-ophthalmia (small eyes), short palpebral fissures, a thin upper lip and flattening of the maxillary area. Sometimes, there is a cleft palate and poor sucking. A whole constellation of other developmental abnormalities may also be associated including congenital heart defects, liver and kidney problems, deafness and a variety of bone abnormalities. However, the most important abnormalities relate to the brain and result in intellectual impairment and developmental delays. In FAS, the estimated average IQ is 65.7. Prospective studies establishing the level of *in utero* exposure have found that increasing amounts of maternal alcohol consumption led to progressively lower intellectual functioning in childhood. Estimates of the prevalence of the full FAS picture vary, but one recent review gave a figure of 9 out of 1,000 live births in the USA. In some countries, the prevalence of FAS may be considerably higher – for example, in South Africa where rates of alcoholism in women are very high. The consumption of only moderate levels of as little as one to two drinks per day of alcohol during pregnancy has been found to be associated with later childhood attention deficit disorders and behavioural problems.[16,111] The prevalence of foetal alcohol spectrum disorders – that is the milder degrees of cognitive deficit and behavioural problems – has been estimated to be somewhere between 2–4% in European populations.[111]

It is thought that up to 90% of children with prenatal alcohol exposure develop some neurological deficits, and the DSM-5 now discusses a syndrome entitled 'neurobehavioural disorder associated with prenatal alcohol disorder' amongst its conditions[16] for further study for possible inclusion in its main glossary. Foetal alcohol syndrome is now the most common preventable cause of intellectual disability. Women identified as using alcohol by antenatal services should be advised about the harmful consequences of the alcohol and, if agreeable, referred on to local alcohol treatment programmes.

Cocaine. The consumption of cocaine amongst young people is high, and a study in the USA amongst women of reproductive age (18–44) found 3.4 per cent of pregnant women used cocaine in the last month. Data on cocaine consumption in pregnancy in the UK is not known, but it is likely to be similar. Pregnancy may increase the cardio-toxicity of cocaine.[112] Cocaine rapidly crosses the maternal and foetal blood–brain barrier and the placenta by simple diffusion, causing generalised vasoconstriction by directly affecting foetal and maternal blood vessels. Cocaine toxicity in mothers may cause severe hypertension, hyperreflexia, proteinuria, oedema and seizures, which can be easily confused with pre-eclampsia. Beta-adrenergic antagonists, including labetalol and propranolol, should be avoided as they may create unopposed alpha-adrenergic stimulation and are associated with coronary vasoconstriction. Maternal complications of cocaine use in pregnancy include cardiovascular complications such as hypertension, myocardial infarction and ischaemia; renal failure; hepatic rupture; cerebral ischaemia/infarction; and maternal death. Obstetric complications include abruptio placentae and various antenatal and postnatal complications including prematurity, and in the foetus, intra-uterine growth retardation, cerebral haemorrhage and sudden infant death. Cocaine use puts women at increased risk for adverse perinatal outcomes: pre-term delivery, low birth weight (<2,500 gms), small for gestational age infants, earlier gestational age at delivery and reduced birth weight. There is disagreement on whether cocaine use increases the risk of structural malformations, although some studies show an increase in urinary tract anomalies, and other studies show an increase in vascular disruption-type abnormalities, including limb reduction and intestinal atresia. However, systematic studies have proved to be elusive because the majority of pregnant cocaine users do not declare their use. In contrast to alcohol, there is no specific syndrome in new-borns attributable to cocaine usage. Some studies have found that children who have had prenatal exposure to cocaine have dysregulated behaviour, impaired growth, inhibitory control, attentional deficit and abstract reasoning impairment. However, a systematic review did not establish that these changes were exclusively due to cocaine as opposed to other confounding factors, such as other maternal comorbidities including low socioeconomic status.

Khat. This is another stimulant widely used in East Africa and Yemen. In affected regions, khat chewing is found in around 15 per cent of pregnant women. Khat chewing appears to be associated with an increased risk of premature rupture of membranes (OR = 1.5) and hence premature labour.[113] In a study of women who chewed khat while breast feeding, 75% women who chewed khat four or more times a week also had a history of a child dying compared to only 7% of women who chewed khat once a week. It is unknown whether this is a direct toxic effect of cathinone (the active ingredient of khat), which is an amphetamine and may be concentrated in breast milk, or whether this is due to secondary effects such as over-sedation in the mother impacting on care giving. There are insufficient medical records and literature in this area at present to establish whether or not khat has teratogenic effects.

Heroin.[114] Heroin does not appear to have a specific teratogenic effect. However, non-obstetric adverse effects are legion and include physical symptoms (malnutrition, poor dental hygiene, infections), psychological symptoms (feelings of blame and guilt, self harm, depression) and social difficulties (relationship difficulties, domestic violence, involvement in crime). Specific obstetric complications include antepartum haemorrhage, low birth weight and higher neonatal mortality, as well as non-specific complications including premature rupture of membranes, premature birth and intra-uterine growth retardation. Infants born to mothers who have taken opiates in pregnancy are highly liable to have a neonatal abstinence syndrome (NAS). Typical characteristics of opioid NAS are irritability, high pitched cry, vomiting, diarrhoea, hypertonicity, tremor, tachypnoea and, in severe case, seizures. Most cases of opioid NAS only require supportive treatment measures in the special care baby unit, but severe cases will need pharmacological treatment in a tapering opiate regime to counter opiate withdrawal with other opiates. There are no long-term effects apart from a predisposition to opiate addiction in later life.

Mother and Baby Units and Perinatal Community Services

Perinatal psychiatry is one of the more recent sub-specialities of adult general psychiatry and is better developed in the UK than in most other countries. Much progress has been made since Thomas Main (1958), a psychoanalyst, arranged for the first joint admission of a mother and baby to the Cassel Hospital in London. There is a specialist perinatal community team in almost all districts of the UK, and there are 19 mother and baby units (MBUs), each with between 4–12 beds, giving a total of 150 beds in the UK.[115] Joint mother and baby admission is now common practice in the UK, Australia and New Zealand but is rather uncommon elsewhere. Australia has two types of units: MBUs similar to the UK dealing with severe mental illness as well as 'residential early parenting services', which often have long waiting lists. A study based in the state of Victoria found 0.9% of all mothers were admitted to MBUs and around 5% to a parenting unit, a rather high proportion of all births, indicating that Australians take the problems of early parenting very seriously.

The USA has no designated mother and baby units or facilities for joint admission. This may be because acute admissions in America are paid for through private insurance and Medicare, Medicaid and private means, with admissions of more than seven days rarely being funded. As the average UK joint MBU admission is for 56 days, it can be seen that conjoint admissions are never likely to take off in the USA, but the USA has many community-based services mainly for postnatal depression. The system for treating puerperal psychosis in most countries remains a separation of mother from their baby, with the psychotic mother being admitted and treated in the general psychiatric ward whilst the infant is cared for either by the partner, other relatives or social services for the duration of the mother's hospitalisation.

The Royal College of Psychiatrists in the UK outlined in their recommendations for perinatal services in 2021[62] that all perinatal mental health services have a dual function to both assess and treat maternal mental illness, as well as assess and actively support the mother-infant relationship. They recommend that 'all women requiring mental health admission in the last trimester of pregnancy or after delivery should be admitted to a specialist mother and baby unit, unless there are compelling reasons not to do so'.

The indications for admission are shown in Box 13.1.

Surveys of admission diagnoses show that unipolar depression (often psychotic depression) is the most frequent diagnosis, followed by bipolar disorder (usually mania/hypomania) and fewer cases of schizophrenia and a miscellany of other diagnoses. Medical treatments are similar to managing non-puerperal cases as described in Chapters 3.3, 4.2 and 5.3 earlier in this book.

However, the management of the mother and baby dyad is unique in this setting. In the vast majority of cases, women are able to be successfully treated on the unit along with their baby and continue to provide parental care on the unit. In some cases of particularly severe illness (for example, an acute manic episode), high levels of staff supervision may be required initially (for example, 1:1 or 2:1 staff supervision at all times) to ensure the safety of the woman and her baby, whilst enabling essential bonding to take place. This level of observation can be reduced over time once staff have observed that it is safe to do so. In cases where the risks are deemed too high to be manageable on a mother and baby unit, it may be that the mother and baby need to be separated temporarily whilst the mother is treated on a general acute psychiatric unit. In the UK, it is recommended that all attempts are made to avoid this so that ideally the mother and baby can remain together. If separation is required, this should be for the minimum amount of time before a mother can be moved to a suitable mother and baby unit and reunited with her infant.

Box 13.1 Admission to a mother and baby unit should be considered if the mother shows any of the following[116]

- Rapidly changing mental state
- Suicidal ideation (particularly of a violent nature)
- Pervasive guilt and hopelessness
- Significant estrangement from the infant
- New or persistent beliefs of the inadequacy as a mother
- Any evidence of psychosis

Whilst on the unit, staff can observe and support with all aspects of care of the infant as needed. Mother and baby unit staff include psychiatrists, specialist mental health nurses, psychologists, occupational therapists, social workers and nursery nurses who are experts in infant care.

Major psychiatric disorder can have significant effects on parenting abilities. Mothers with severe depression, with psychomotor retardation or difficulties in concentration and feelings of exhaustion may have insufficient energy to complete the daily practical tasks required for infant care. Women who may have hostile, violent or suicidal thoughts may require particular support, as well as an increased level of observation if they are felt to pose a potential risk to themselves or their infant. The safety of both the mother and the infant are paramount on the unit, and as described earlier, intensive levels of observation can enable a mother who may be having these thoughts to continue to provide loving care for their infant, with the close support of staff in a safe environment. Delusional beliefs can result in harm to the baby, and so this should be explored with sensitivity by staff and the appropriate level of support and supervision offered.

Women experiencing an acute manic phase may also pose a risk of inadvertent harm to their infant due to distractibility, irritability and other symptoms such as grandiosity. Distraction can make caring for an infant very difficult or impossible. However, as concentration improves, the woman may be able to care more consistently for her baby. Unusual behaviours could also lead to inadvertent harm to the infant – for example, making unsafe feeding choices for the baby's age. Irritability may be directed towards their partner or staff but occasionally might be directed towards the baby. Women experiencing acute mania may require intensive monitoring during their admission in order to support them to provide safe baby care, whilst treating their affective symptoms.

Schizophrenia or other forms of psychosis thought disorder may interfere with the woman's ability to carry out practical tasks, while negative symptoms such as apathy and emotional blunting can impact on their ability to provide emotionally sensitive infant care. Distraction can result in potentially dangerous mistakes, especially, for example, when feeding or bathing the infant – providing feeds of the wrong temperature or becoming distracted during bathing and allowing the baby to slip under the water. The presence of negative symptoms, which may be long-lasting, is a poor prognostic sign.

Delusions may preoccupy a woman's mind to such an extent that the infant is excluded or neglected. Delusions and hallucinations that focus around the baby may be particularly dangerous, as women may act on the basis of their delusions.

Postpartum psychosis usually responds well to medication, often within a matter of days, although in some cases, improvements are less rapid.

The nurses on mother and baby units serve many crucial functions. Perhaps most importantly, when the mother is obviously struggling or the situation is dangerous, they may need to intervene and speedily remove the infant from the mother. They also need to observe and support the mother for her primary psychiatric disorder, as well as provide instruction and review of the woman's ability to safely care for her baby. The ward may also have access to perinatal nursery nurses who are invaluable in providing this type of support. Primigravid women may have the dual impact of experiencing a psychosis alongside facing the challenges of being a new mother with little parenting experience. Learning new skills is often difficult during a psychotic episode, with sedative psychotropic medication being an additional impeding factor. It is sometimes better to wait until more florid psychotic symptoms have subsided before focusing on basic parenting skills. However, often supervised contact between mother and baby will be encouraged and facilitated after appropriate risk assessments have been completed. This can begin to improve the mother and baby relationship even when the woman is very unwell. Nursery nurses are commonly employed solely to look after the babies when mothers are unable to do so or to provide an essential element of respite (for example, providing night care so that a sleep-deprived mother can have therapeutic rest). The experienced nursery nurses can also support anxious or underconfident new mothers with parenting skills. Many nurses may also have their own experiences of childcare which can be very valuable. Multi-agency working is an essential part of the MBU, and this includes liaison with child and family social services. Some mother and baby units – in addition to offering treatment for mental health problems – can also provide formal parenting assessments for the local authority to help inform decisions around social care proceedings.

During admission, assessment and treatment should be focused on the following domains:

- *Parenting skills and mother-infant relationship:* Enhancing the mother-infant relationship and supporting the mother to optimise her parenting skills are a key part of treatment. As described earlier, staff including nursery nurses can provide intensive support and feedback on parenting skills. Some units have access to developmental psychologists, who can provide expert feedback on mother-infant interactions and help women to further develop the bond with her baby.
- *Treatment of mental health symptoms:* A holistic treatment plan should be created collaboratively with the woman, and any family and carers she would like involved, to treat any mental health symptoms (e.g. psychotic symptoms or mood symptoms) considering biological, psychological and social aspects of treatment, involving all members of the MDT.
- *Risk assessment:* Safety of both mother and baby is paramount, and staff are responsible for ongoing dynamic risk assessment. This would include ensuring that appropriate levels of supervision are in place and that safeguarding procedures are followed for any concerns regarding neglect or abuse. Units should ensure good communication with any other agencies involved – for example, child and family social services, obstetricians, GP, health visitors, midwives and adult and perinatal community mental health services.
- *Physical health:* The physical health of both mother and baby should be optimised during admission. Units should work closely with local obstetric, maternity and paediatric teams to ensure that women and babies receive the right physical health care – for example, antenatal and postnatal checks as well as referring women if there are concerns about physical health requiring investigation/treatment in the general hospital. Appropriate monitoring of psychotropic medication should be conducted as per guidelines. Suspected organic causes of puerperal mental disorders must be ruled out.

Community Services

An effective perinatal mental health service should consist of both inpatient mother and baby units and community perinatal mental health teams. The NHS 5-year forward view published in 2016[117] highlighted that, despite great need, only 15 per cent of localities in England had an effective community perinatal service in place, and more than 40 per cent had no community perinatal service at all. As a result of this, major investment (an additional £1 billion in funding for mental health services) has led to the development of new perinatal community services across England, such that, by 2019, every area of England had access to a community perinatal team. In other parts of the UK and elsewhere in the world, this is yet to be achieved.

The Royal College of Psychiatrists recommend that all community services should endeavour to provide care to all pregnant and postpartum women who are either experiencing significant mental illness or are at high risk of developing a severe postnatal illness.[117] This treatment should involve (but is not limited to) pre-conceptual counselling, assessment of the mother-infant relationship, providing crisis support, prioritising the management of women on leave from or recently discharged from MBUs, and providing partner and carer support. Women should be offered a range of evidence-based treatment including medication, psychological therapies (which could include individual and group therapies) and psychosocial interventions. Specialist support may be offered for specific groups – for example, teenage mothers. Referrals to perinatal community teams come from a wide variety of sources mostly from antenatal clinics, other psychiatric specialty teams and social services.

Collaborative working with other services is a key part of the role of a community perinatal team. Take, for example, a woman who is pregnant, has depression and is opiate dependent. The drug team might make the initial referral to perinatal services but would continue to provide treatment throughout the pregnancy. The perinatal team might offer psychological therapy – for example, CBT. The obstetric team and midwives would be involved due to the higher risk of complications associated with opiate use. Once the baby is born, the paediatric team may need to provide detoxification and special care, if needed. Throughout the pregnancy and once the baby is born, social services would be involved to ensure that the mother is able to provide safe care for the infant. If there are concerns about the mother's ability to care for her child safely, this could also involve social services and the courts.

The perinatal team will usually need to maintain contact with all these agencies as well as the client mother until the infant is around a year old when most perinatal services cease involvement (although extension to 24 months has been proposed[62]), and if further psychiatric care is required, the case is handed back to the local CMHT (or in a case such as this, the drug and alcohol team). It can be seen that such a complicated trajectory could lead to miscommunications between the various services, making high-quality teamwork an essential requirement for safe perinatal psychiatry.

Midwives now screen new bookings for psychiatric disorder in the antenatal clinic, and they are then assessed in a joint obstetric/psychiatric liaison clinic. One study[118] showed that this was a good way of identifying women at high risk or ultra-high risk of a puerperal relapse, especially where there was a previous or family history of psychosis as well as also identifying those women with more severe depression in pregnancy requiring further intervention from the perinatal team.

Most units arrange for pre-birth planning meetings at around 32 weeks of pregnancy to which the relevant professionals, the patient and key relatives are invited. This meeting should cover (amongst other things) medication plans during pregnancy and after delivery, any potential risks, and plans for infant placement and additional support once the baby is born. For women at high risk of relapse following birth, the possibility of admission to a mother and baby unit should be discussed. For women with social services involvement, a discussion should be had about whether the mother is able to provide infant care independently when the baby is born or whether, for example, the mother should be admitted to a residential mother and baby unit for a planned parenting assessment, or if any additional support needs to be in place at home. In some cases, the courts may have decided that a baby will be removed from the mother straight after birth.

In addition to providing medical treatment, perinatal psychiatrists are also increasingly becoming involved in parenting assessments of mothers with mental illness for the courts where psychiatric issues are important, a task they share with child psychiatrists and occasional forensic psychiatrists or others, and this is described in the next section.

Child Abuse and Neglect

Colossians 3:21 Fathers do not exasperate your children so they will not lose heart.

Even though child cruelty was common in the ancient world, this quote from the New Testament – probably written by Paul – shows an early insight into the adverse effects of parental emotional abuse on children. Parents in ancient Greece or Rome had absolute rights over their child's life with children having no rights of their own. The problem of child abuse did not raise much concern until the mid-twentieth century, although the first legislation on child labour was in 1880. This can readily be understood in the light of the very high infant and child mortality rates existent right up until the end of the nineteenth century. Large numbers of children died of mainly infectious diseases and so being beaten by a parent was not seen as matter of great significance. However, by the 1930s, with the advent of universal clean drinking water, the high child mortality rates due to infections fell dramatically, and it is soon after this when modern awareness of child abuse begins.

Paediatricians were first alerted to parental child abuse in 1946 through a report by Caffey,[119] a paediatric radiologist, who saw puzzling radiographs of six infants who presented with the unusual combination of multiple fractures of their long bones and subdural haematomas. The fractures were all at different stages of healing, which suggested the infant had received multiple episodes of trauma over a prolonged period, and this was combined with bilateral subdural haematomas, which were presumed to be due to a shaking injury. In all cases, the parents denied any history of injury. Kempe[120] drew further attention to the problem in a famous paper entitled 'The Battered Child Syndrome', which suggested the phenomenon was quite widespread.

Child abuse has been documented in all societies where it has been looked for, and the overall lifetime prevalence is high. In the UK, data from the National Crime survey[121] for the year ending in March 2019 gave the following figures: around 1 in 5 adults between ages 18–74 (around 8.5 million or 20.7% of the population) had experienced some form of child abuse, and around half (52%) of those who experienced it below the age of 16 then went on to experience domestic abuse later in life compared to 13% lacking such an earlier experience. In terms of type of abuse, the most frequent was witnessing domestic violence (9.8%), followed by emotional abuse (9.3%), physical abuse (7.6%) and sexual abuse (7.5%). In March 2019, there were 49,570 children in England (41 per 10,000) who were being looked after by their local authority because of abuse and neglect. The overall worldwide estimated prevalence rates[122] for self-reported maltreatment studies (mainly assessing maltreatment ever experienced during childhood) were 127/1,000 for sexual abuse (76/1,000 among boys and 180/1,000 among girls), 226/1,000 for physical abuse, 363/1,000 for emotional abuse, 163/1,000 for physical neglect and 184/1,000 for emotional neglect.

Procedures for Dealing with Child Abuse and Neglect in the UK

In the UK, the Department for Education is responsible for policy on child protection. Section 11 of the Children Act (2004) placed a statutory duty on certain agencies to safeguard and promote the welfare of children: these being the local authorities, NHS services, police and probation. People working in these agencies have a *mandatory* duty to always report suspected cases of abuse and neglect, and failure to do so may result in disciplinary action but not criminal charges. In addition, since 2016, health and social care professionals and teachers in England are obliged to report 'known cases' of female genital mutilation (FGM) in under 18s to the police.

Other people (non-professionals) should phone the police if they think a child is in imminent danger, but if there is no immediate risk, they should either follow the safeguarding procedures of their organisation or phone the local child protection services. A social worker is then delegated to do a preliminary investigation within 24 hours to determine whether:

- The child requires immediate protection, and urgent action is required
- The child is in need and should be assessed under Section 17 of the Children Act 1989[123]
- There is reasonable cause to suspect that the child is suffering or likely to suffer significant harm, and whether enquires must be made and the child assessed under Section 47 of the Children Act 1989
- If any services are required by the child and family and what type of services are needed

A Section 47 enquiry refers to Section 47 of the Children Act 1989 and involves social workers gathering evidence and speaking with the child, family and other relevant professionals to determine if any interventions may be beneficial to the child's welfare. All assessments should be completed within 45 working days. Psychiatric opinions are sometimes sought as part of the Section 47 enquiry.

If significant harm to the child is thought to be present, a child protection conference with the relevant professionals is convened. This can also be for an unborn child. At the case conference, relevant professionals can share information, identify risks and outline what needs to be done to protect the child. In England, this must happen within 15 working days of the strategy discussion. Professionals draft a child protection plan that they will develop and implement, and the core group for this may also include family members.

In some cases, professionals may conclude the parents are not able to provide safe and appropriate care and so decide to take the child into care, usually under Section 20 of the Children Act (1989), which is voluntary. At the initial hearing, the court may decide to award an Interim Care Order (ICO) to the social services, which is initially for eight weeks but is renewable, so the social workers have the legal power to decide on the child's placement. Rehabilitation then aims to return the child to the birth family, but if this fails, the court can make a full care order, which gives the social services the options of a long-term fostering arrangement or adoption. The legal criteria for a full care order is discussed next.

Legal Criteria for a Care Order

The court will only make a full care order if they are convinced:

- The child is suffering, or is likely to suffer, significant harm
- Making an order would be better for the child than making no order and that the level of harm is due to either:
  - The care the child is receiving or likely to receive if the care order is not made
  - The child is beyond parental control

Child Maltreatment

The main categories of child maltreatment are physical abuse, neglect, sexual abuse, psychological abuse and emotional harm. Each category will be considered in the following sections.

Physical Abuse

Common presentations of physical abuse are bruises, especially if multiple and not accounted for properly, as well as fractures and multiple fractures, especially when occurring in infants. Children aged below one year of age are defenceless and non-ambulatory, making it difficult for them to fall over and give themselves factures. Because they are also unable to communicate, diagnosis for this age group is difficult. Therefore, fractures below this age are highly likely due to non-accidental injury (NAI). In one recent study,[124] 32% of fractures in children aged below one year were due to NAI whereas only 5% of fractures in children aged one to two years were reported as NAI. Sixteen of 19 (84%) patients reported for abuse had multiple fractures; 15 of these patients were aged under one year. Fractures due to NAI become more suspicious if they occur in different parts of the body or there is other evidence of physical abuse such as burns. Injuries around the mouth are common – with split lips, lacerations of mucus membranes, torn frenulum or injuries to the palate – presumably related to attempts to stop the infant screaming. Blows on the head may rupture the eardrum and cause deafness or damage the external ear. A series of non-accidental injuries tends to cause multiple complex fractures at different stages of healing, whereas genuine accidents are more likely to cause single, linear fractures. Blows to the abdomen may cause visceral injuries such as ruptured spleen, kidney, stomach or bowel and may have a high mortality. Sub-periosteal haematomas may result from pulling limbs, while shaking can cause both retinal haemorrhages and bilateral subdural haematomas. Bite marks are always suspicious but may be misleading because they are sometimes inflicted by an older sibling. Burns, scalds and chemical burns may all occur, while simple trauma may cause widespread bruising and petechial haemorrhages. The diagnosis of physical abuse and making the distinction between NAI from more genuine accidents, which are commonplace in the lives of most children, is the responsibility of the paediatrician and sometimes the radiologist.

No specific psychopathology apart from a few cases of antisocial personality disorder has been linked to physical abuse, and the majority of the perpetrators almost always deny any involvement. Most do not have a previous psychiatric history or evidence of current psychiatric disorder, and so psychiatrists play little role in this category.

Child Neglect

Child neglect is an act of omission and is rather more common among the infants of mothers with psychiatric disorder. Federal law in the USA defines abuse and neglect as 'Any recent act or failure to act on the part of a parent or caretaker which results in death, serious injury, emotional harm, sexual abuse, exploitation or an act or failure to act which presents an imminent risk of serious harm'. In the UK, 'harm' is defined in the Children Act 1989 as 'ill-treatment or the impairment of health or development'. Subsequently, another clause was added in to clarify the definition of harm which includes 'impairment suffered from seeing or hearing the ill-treatment of another'. This addition was made because of a growing realisation that even just witnessing parental domestic violence could be very harmful to children.

Neglect may involve a failure to protect the child from exposure to any kind of danger or a failure to carry out important aspects of the child's care. Each of the main categories of neglect is considered here.

- **Physical neglect.** This includes failure to provide adequate food to prevent malnourishment. Many forms of severe mental illness (for example, depression and schizophrenia), as well as substance misuse disorders, can result in self-neglect and may also result in a parent being unable to meet their child's physical needs.
- **Appropriate shelter.** To give protection from common hazards or provide adequate housing. Housing may be lacking in basic amenities or be unhygienic.
- **Poor hygiene.** There may be evidence of severe nappy rashes, after babies have been left in wet nappies for too long or even being left alone unsupervised. Infections and other illnesses may be more frequent because the house may be unclean and minimum standards of hygiene are not maintained, while the accompanying emotional neglect may cause developmental delays. Sometimes, clothing is not appropriate; either too little so infants are cold, sometimes too much so infants become over-heated.
- **Failure to gain weight** that is not due to some medical disorder. 'Non-organic failure to thrive' is one of the most common presentations of physical neglect, and in around a third of such cases, no medical condition is found. These infants seem mute and lifeless at home, but they thrive, gain weight and become happy and playful in hospital. Such cases are less dramatic than those of physical abuse, but neglect can also result in considerable long-term damage. Neglect is usually detected initially by health visitors, social workers or general practitioners, but the psychiatrist will become involved if mental illness is suspected as a cause.
- **Adequate supervision.** This is essential, but UK law does not stipulate any particular age that a child can be left alone. However, the National Society for the Prevention of Cruelty to Children (NSPCC) provides a guideline which states:
  1. Children under 12 are rarely mature enough to be left alone for a long period of time
  2. Children under 16 should not be left alone overnight
  3. Babies, toddlers and very young children should never be left alone

  Whilst the physical presence of a parent in the household is important, the parent must also be in a mentally fit enough state to pay attention to their adventurous toddler. Being distracted by hallucinations, for example, or sedated by psychotropic medication or illicit drugs may impact on a woman's ability to care for her infant, which could put the child at risk of accidental injury.
- **Medical neglect.** This refers to either a failure or delay to consult a medical professional during a child's illness or accident as well as a failure to institute a prescribed treatment. Also, there is commonly a failure to ensure infants are up-to-date with their vaccination programme or attend for vaccinations. Social workers always investigate this because it is usually clearly documented, so easy to prove for legal purposes, and is often an indicator of many other types of neglect as well.
- **Dental neglect.** This is also common, presenting as dental abscesses and premature loss of teeth, and is caused by a failure to take the child to the dentist and a failure to control excess sugar in the diet.

Neglect is a multifaceted complex phenomenon and is often chronic. This is because maternal factors predisposing to neglect often fail to improve. Designating whether it has occurred is usually the responsibility of the social services, who may then proceed to further investigation and legal action, which may include psychiatric assessments and sometimes to child removal. Likely indicators of physical neglect is listed in Box 13.2.

Child neglect is a social problem, and there is no single or specific psychiatric cause of child neglect, rather a wide variety of maternal psychiatric disorders may contribute, but sometimes no disorder at all is present or responsible.

Psychological maltreatment. This includes emotional neglect, psychological neglect and psychological abuse.

Emotional neglect refers to a lack of warmth or affection, and such parents may be emotionally unavailable to their children.

Box 13.2 Likely indicators of physical neglect[125]

1. Lack of adequate medical or dental care
2. Chronic sleepiness or hunger
3. Poor personal hygiene, dirty clothing, inappropriate clothing for weather conditions
4. Evidence of lack of supervision or poor supervision
5. Home conditions that are a health hazard
6. Home lacks basic utilities, water, electricity or poor plumbing
7. The presence of fire hazards (e.g. due to maternal hoarding behaviours)
8. Poor or inadequate sleeping arrangements
9. Refrigerator has either little or no food, or it is spoiled

Mental health neglect occurs when the parent(s) are failing to comply with a recommended treatment programme or delay in seeking it. It presents as emotional and behavioural difficulties in the child, usually in middle childhood.

Psychological abuse is a more serious and malignant problem, and the American Professional Society on the Abuse of Children[126] defined this as meaning 'a repeated pattern of caregiver behaviour or incidents that convey to children that they are worthless, flawed, unwanted, unloved, endangered and only of value when meeting another person's needs'. It comprised six main categories of parental behaviours.

Spurning includes rejecting behaviours such as belittling, shaming, publicly humiliating or repeatedly singling out one child in a sibship for punishment.

Terrorising is a label given to parents who threaten a child or those he loves or their possessions with violence or abandonment.

Isolating refers to placing a child in a confined space and depriving them opportunities to socialise with others.

Exploiting and corrupting behaviours include training a child to commit crimes such as stealing or forcing them to engage in sex work.

Making negative attributions to the child, when these abusive parents more often see negative intentions in their children's behaviour than do normal parents – for example, 'He is such a sneaky child' is repeated so often that the child eventually comes to believe it of themselves and so undermines their confidence. Such parents more often have unrealistic expectations of what is developmentally appropriate. They tend to find even normal infant or child behaviour more stressful. They may also have *age-inappropriate expectations,* such as accusing a three-year-old who picks something up that is not theirs of stealing.

The vast majority of normal, loving parents will have indulged in some of these strategies on occasions, but it is the repetition with a high frequency over a prolonged period that will inflict a damaging effect. Distinguishing what is normal parenting or normal child behaviour from behaviours arising out of a child psychiatric disorder or from the effects of parental psychological abuse is far from straightforward and is rightly the province of the child psychologist or child psychiatrist.

Educational neglect. This is usually defined as a failure to meet legal requirement of school attendance. Schools must register all attendance and so this is readily quantifiable and expressed as a percentage of all possible attendances. Because it is generally associated with other types of neglect, this figure is sometimes used as measure of the overall functionality of the household, with changes in attendance reflecting progress or otherwise in reducing neglect. There are many complex social reasons why a child may not attend school. These may include disorganisation or disruption at home, parental financial or mental health difficulties or a lack of understanding of the importance of education.

Background Causal Factors

Child abuse and neglect is a social phenomenon and not a medical disorder. It has a multiplicity of causes that all probably interact with each other. These include distal societal causes, child factors, individual and family causes, which include parental mental illness. The most important distal cause is poverty. Rates are much higher in households with low family income than amongst affluent families, and this effect can also be seen geographically. Thus, children from poor neighbourhoods in the USA were found to be six times more likely to suffer abuse or neglect than those from affluent neighbourhoods.[127] Poverty is usually associated with high unemployment rates, which may independently cause frustration, increased rates of depression and substance abuse. Rates are much higher for single mothers, and this may be linked to the poverty of single parenthood. It is noteworthy that the majority of psychiatric assessments in care proceedings are for single parents. Similarly, some children from large families may be at increased risk, and this may also be linked to the poverty of very large families.

Certain risk factors are related to the child. Thus, being female, younger, having a physical disability, learning difficulties, a difficult temperament and a childhood psychiatric disorder are all associated with a raised rate of physical abuse, but it should be noted that the vast majority of children even within these categories are brought up by loving parents and are not subject to abuse.

Child abuse appears to be able to transmit across generations. A striking clinical finding is the high number of abusing parents who were themselves abused as children. Oliver[128] demonstrated that cycles of familial violence and abuse of children could be established; that is, the abused children became abusive parents, and this pattern might extend over several generations. Personality disorder, mental illness, suicide attempts, drug and alcohol dependence in both mothers and fathers, epilepsy, learning disability and criminality were all conspicuous features in these families. However, there is no clear understanding of the mechanism or what exactly is transmitted from one generation to another.

Each parent may make a different contribution. In the USA, 40% of children were maltreated only by their mother, 18% were maltreated only by their father and 17% were maltreated by both parents.[122] Physical discipline (corporal punishment) has increasingly been recognised as a form of child abuse and is now legally banned in many European countries, but in many parts of the world, it is still widely believed to be an essential part of normal parenting. Thus, only 4% of parents in Albania believed it to be essential compared to 93% in Syria.[122] Children with conduct problems, attentional difficulties and non-compliance – the so-called externalising behaviours – are at greater risk of being at the receiving end of corporal punishment, which itself can further exacerbate such behaviours. Social factors such as low family income also contribute whilst low parental educational levels are associated with a seven-fold increase in rates of corporal punishment.

How large is the contribution of each factor? A quantitative meta-analysis of over 1.5 million children[122] in the USA yielded the following data: parental experience of maltreatment in his or her own childhood ($d = 0.47$, d being a measure of effect size), low socioeconomic status of the family ($d = 0.34$), dependent and aggressive parental personality ($d = 0.45$), intimate partner violence ($d = 0.41$) and higher baseline autonomic nervous system activity ($d = 0.24$).

Does intervention work? The umbrella review of interventions to prevent or reduce child maltreatment showed only modest effectiveness ($d = 0.23$) for interventions targeting child abuse potential or families with self-reported maltreatment and ($d = 0.27$) for officially reported child maltreatment cases.[122]

In the UK, the parents of a large cohort of children were screened with a 12-item checklist of factors thought to predispose to child abuse.[129] Five years later, 0.7% of the children had become the focus of a social service enquiry into suspected or actual maltreatment or neglect. The most important risk factor was a history of family violence (12.4%), followed by the parent being abused or neglected as a child (7.6%); indifferent, intolerant or overanxious parents (7%); a history of mental illness, drug or alcohol addiction (5.2%); single or separated parent (5.0%); socioeconomic problems such as unemployment (3.9%); step-parent or cohabitee present (3.2%); and mother below 21years (2.8%). The following infant-related factors all had a significant but low contribution of below 3%: prematurity, low birth weight, separation for more than 24 hours after birth, a mentally or physically handicapped child and less than 18 months between births of children.

Socioeconomic factors and child-related factors are said to be static causes and cannot be changed. They are of academic interest but are not of immediate concern to child protection teams because they cannot be changed. However, parental causes are sometimes amenable to improvement, and these include psychiatric disorder, where sometimes successful treatment can lead on to safer and better parenting.

Consequences of Child Abuse and Neglect

Many thousands of studies have been published on the adverse effect of all types of child abuse, and the literature is not easy to interpret, but some guidance is offered in a comprehensive review of longitudinal cohort studies.[130] Diverse populations and methodologies have prevented meta-analyses, but there is a general consensus that child maltreatment is variably associated with almost all classified psychiatric disorders. A major confounding factor is that many of the social factors associated with child abuse – such as poverty, poor housing or poor parental education – are also factors associated with adult mental illness, and it is almost impossible to factor out these variables from the majority of studies.

Child abuse has differing effects according to the age and maturity of the individual. For infants and toddlers, the main effects appear to be difficulties in self-regulation, emotional regulation and poor attachment. The main features of poor attachment are shown in Box 13.3.

Children of primary school age sometimes manifest disorder at school. There is poor motivation to learn, poor concentration, poor academic achievement, low self-concept and poor attendance. Boys may display externalising behaviours such as angry outbursts, aggression or bullying, whilst girls may present as anxious with social withdrawal and somatic symptoms such as headaches and stomach pains.

Adolescents who have experienced abuse may have depression, anxiety or social withdrawal. In addition, adolescents who live in violent situations tend to run away to what they perceive to be safer environments. They engage in risky behaviour such as smoking, drinking alcohol, early sexual activity, using drugs, prostitution, homelessness, gang involvement, and in America, even carrying guns. General hospital admission rates for substance abuse and self harm are three times

Box 13.3 Features of attachment disorder

- An aversion to touch and physical affection: The child might flinch, laugh or even say 'ouch' when touched; rather than producing positive feelings, touch and affection are perceived as threats.
- Control issues: The child might go to great lengths to prevent feeling helpless and remain in control; such children are often disobedient, defiant and argumentative.
- Anger problems: Anger might be expressed directly, in tantrums or acting out, or through manipulative, passive-aggressive behaviour; the child might hide his or her anger in socially acceptable actions, like giving a high-five that hurts or hugging someone too hard.
- Difficulty showing genuine care and affection: The child might act inappropriately affectionate with strangers while displaying little or no affection towards his or her parents.
- An underdeveloped conscience: The child might act like he or she does not have a conscience and might fail to show guilt, regret or remorse after behaving badly.

more likely; psychiatric admission rates for any disorder are twice as likely compared to non-abused children.

Poverty is an important determinant on all forms of child abuse and many childhood psychiatric disorders. However, does poverty relief change the situation? A partial answer to this issue comes from an eight-year naturalistic follow-up of a group of 9- to 13-year-old Native American children raised initially in poverty but with a dramatic change for the better in their material circumstances.[131] The key event was the establishment of a casino in the American Native Reserve, which brought great wealth to the whole community and all families within it. There was a reduction in the rates of conduct disorders among the children, but there was no subsequent reduction in anxiety or depression. It seems that the effects of early adversity may not be so easily reversed by the removal of poverty alone.

It is now thought that child abuse, neglect and child sexual abuse act as non-specific causes resulting in a general increase in all types of mental disorder, mainly for the onset of the disorder rather than its persistence and with a modest effect size. Adverse childhood events (ACEs) figure prominently in the literatures on aetiology of most adult mental disorders. Evidence is better for some disorders than for others. Depression is correlated with all types of abuse, but particularly with childhood sexual abuse (CSA); the prevalence of depression increases with the severity, intrusiveness and frequency of the sexual abuse in a dose-response fashion.

PTSD, substance abuse, general anxiety disorder and panic disorder all show a similar dose-response pattern to CSA. Social anxiety disorder is also associated with CSA, but it is the chronicity that is associated with CSA. Personality disorder – particularly borderline personality disorder in women – and eating disorders are both strongly associated with CSA, also in a dose-response pattern.

Role of the Adult Psychiatrist and Writing Reports

The decision on whether to remove a child in care proceedings is made by the court and not by the doctor, but psychiatrists become involved where parental mental disorder is present, or suspected to be present. A generation ago, the social worker would write to the local clinician caring for the mother and seek their opinion on their patient's capacity to parent a child. However, this practice led to clinicians being placed in an impossible position of either telling the truth and risk offending their patient, who might terminate their medical contact, or to plead on the mother's behalf and so potentially place the child at risk. Today, the vast majority of these assessments are done by an independent psychiatrist, and this is often a perinatal psychiatrist, but sometimes a child or a forensic psychiatrist, none of whom will have any vested interest in maintaining a relationship with the mother.

The request to see a mother usually arrives with a few kilograms of paper termed 'the bundle' and a letter of instruction, both of which are now highly formalised. The assessing psychiatrist will need to understand why the case has come about, and the necessary reading for this is 'the social workers report', where the onus is on the social services to provide evidence that the threshold for *significant harm* has been reached and so justify the proceedings.

The interview should be prefaced by the independent psychiatrist introducing themselves and explaining to the mother that the normal doctor–patient confidentiality code is waived in court work, and whatever is said may enter the report and seen by all the participants used in the court case. However, if there is anything the client does not wish to disclose, they should just state so – for example, 'I don't want to talk about my previous relationship' – and then only a statement of this kind will be included in the report.

The interview often lasts between one to two hours and should be as thorough as possible but conducted in a warm empathic fashion, regardless of the circumstances of the case. There should be no criticism or admonishment of the parent, even in cases of apparent cruelty. It should cover the same ground as a routine clinical interview (see Chapter 2), but certain areas are of special interest: in particular, all the factors known to be associated with child abuse as covered earlier such as the mother's own family of origin, any abuse in their own childhood, relationships with partners, their substance abuse history and any previous psychiatric history.

It is also necessary, preferably towards the end of the interview, to cover the problematic behaviours and events as described in the social workers report that led up to child removal but to do this in a non-critical and non-confrontational way – for example, 'It says here in the social workers report that the fridge was always empty... I don't wish to criticise you, but I would just like to hear what you make of this remark'. Almost always there will be a strong rebuttal that this was untrue, but the assessor should remain impartial throughout. It is important to record what the social worker found as well as how the mother deals with criticisms, whether she has any insight or remorse or has any ability to change.

The report should conclude with a diagnosis, but the main interest for the judge and the court is whether the psychiatric disorder carries any risks for the child and whether any treatment will be able to alleviate or improve the situation.

For Mothers with Schizophrenia

For women with schizophrenia, the decision of whether or not to take antipsychotic medication may be highly relevant. In many cases, antipsychotic medication may be recommended long term by medical professionals, but this may not align with the patient's wishes. Considering the benefits and drawbacks of oral versus depot medication may be helpful, as many women find depot medications more convenient than having to remember to take oral medications. Ultimately, it may be that psychotic symptoms are unable to be controlled adequately without the use of regular antipsychotic medication and, therefore, not taking medication could increase the chance of a woman being unable to care adequately for her child. One study[132] found that only one of 17 mothers who had an admission for PSE-defined schizophrenia during the puerperium was able to retain her children. By contrast, another UK study[133] examined a group of mothers who had a psychosis (mostly schizophrenia but also some with affective disorders) found that 90 per cent kept their children, although they often lived under impoverished and unsatisfactory conditions; long-term fostering arrangements or child removal were required only for the other 10 per cent. This was associated with the mothers being of younger age, being involuntarily admitted, having a criminal record and – in the particular district studied (Southwark, in London) – being of Black African origin.[133]

In bipolar disorder, the issues revolve around the severity of the mania. Severe untreated mania as in bipolar disorder type 1 is unlikely to be compatible with independent safe parenting whilst the woman is in the acute manic phase. However, mothers with milder hypomania, which is neither too severe nor too frequent and is occurring in an otherwise stable family setting with a supportive partner, can sometimes successfully parent their children. Unfortunately, the effects of the disorder may mean that relationships are lost or damaged, which means that the woman may not have the support she needs to effectively parent. Most women with a puerperal psychosis who are admitted to a mother and baby unit have bipolar disorder, and the majority of these mothers seem to retain the care of their babies. Mothers and babies are protected during the acute psychotic phase, but once this has passed, it is unusual for child maltreatment to occur.

Mothers with transient or brief psychoses will require a full appraisal, but as the condition usually has a benign long-term outcome, in the presence of a supportive partner, parenting is often successful.

Personality disorders. Every individual case should be assessed within its own specific context. For the greater part, the classical personality subtypes as described in DSM-5 and ICD-11 are not encountered but present with mixtures of psychopathology and are best diagnosed as 'personality disorder NOS (not otherwise specified)'.

A frequent presentation is with a picture of emotionally unstable personality disorder but variably having other features such as antisocial, paranoid, aggressive or rejection sensitivity traits. There may be a family history of major mental disorder, and the childhood history is often one of severe abuse, followed by a very disturbed adolescence of being taken into care themselves and failures in the fields of school, work and relationships. There may also be comorbid depression and drug and alcohol misuse. Relationships are often of a poor quality and characterised by domestic abuse. However, a traditional borderline picture is uncommon as core borderline features such as 'abandonment fears', 'dysphoria' and 'recurrent self-damaging behaviours' are rarely encountered. Sometimes, it is the mother's recurring aggressive outbursts that have led to the destruction of childcare, and in these instances, the aggression will sometimes respond well to SSRI therapy. It is worth picking out such cases as some, though not all, will benefit from an SSRI or psychological therapy.

Women with classical paranoid personality disorder may present certain challenges to work with. The nature of the condition means that they may have fallen out with other professionals and may be engaged in litigation against the social services or the education authorities. Paranoid ideation is pervasive but usually non-delusional and not responsive to medication. Their life story is usually of a normal non-abusive upbringing and successful early life, a marriage, but then a gradual deterioration with increasing isolation and a presentation in their mid-30s with suspiciousness, conspiracy theories and morbid jealousy. An example might be where jealous rages destroy marriages, the partner is charged with domestic violence and served with non-molestation orders and, at least initially, social workers and lawyers take the mother's side. However, once the child becomes enmeshed in the mother's paranoid thinking and begins to share her strange ideas with others at school, the diagnosis becomes much clearer. Some mothers with paranoid personality disorders sometimes remove their children from school because of their paranoid beliefs (e.g. that the teachers or other pupils were sexually abusing their own child). There is no treatment for paranoid personality disorder, and the psychiatrist will serve the court well by making the diagnosis (which the client will always object to) and indicate that the natural history is one of slow deterioration, with no known effective treatment, and in so doing will support the social services and the court in the removal of the child. This is often to the previously ex-partner. Sometimes the mother is granted contacts after the child's removal, but these contacts must be closely supervised as there may be continued attempts to undermine the placement with the ex-partner. Some of these mothers may also have been vindictive towards their child, and so sometimes, their children will refuse to see their paranoid mother even in a supervised contact setting.

Avoidant personality disorder. This is not uncommon but a clue as to whether this is present is repeated non-attendance at important appointments and failure to engage with social services. These women are frightened of contact, relationships may be brief or with a married man who is unavailable for cohabitation, and they often have no social contacts. The avoidant behaviour can result in medical neglect (e.g. failure to take the child to the doctor or dentist or their immunisation programme). It should always be actively diagnosed if present because it is now considered one of the 'schizophrenia spectrum personality disorders' and may be difficult to treat or to change.

Antisocial personality disorder. In child protection cases, this is much more common amongst men than women, and it can present with serious physical abuse (e.g. fractures in the infant) and an associated personal and family criminal history. If there is a history of callous crimes, parenting is contraindicated, but milder cases – perhaps with a previous history of minor criminality – are more difficult to decide on. Some women who themselves are adequate mothers either cannot break with an abusing psychopathic partner or repeatedly select violent partners and so place their children in harm's way. Sometimes, dynamic psychotherapy that explores the mother's own childhood can help to reduce this specific vulnerability, although such psychotherapy is not always available, nor does it always work.

Alcoholism and substance abuse. This presents a major challenge. Some women are able to give up their drink in the face of a threat of losing their children, but others are so truly addicted, so they fail to do so. Both alcohol and drugs are obviously harmful to the foetus, the infant and the growing child. Substance abuse assessments require a detailed history of the various substances abused including possible aetiology, severity and previous treatment efforts, and there should also be a search for any other potentially treatable comorbid psychiatric disorders. The courts are interested in the client's risk to their children, treatability and their future outlook. Alcohol and substance misuse disorders in mothers pose significant risks to their infants and toddlers, both from the physical effects of the substance (e.g. drowsiness or intoxication, meaning they are unable to safely supervise their child) or from the emotional lability caused by the substance resulting in outbursts. The goal should be abstinence from all substances in order for mothers to stand the best chance of retaining custody of their children and, most importantly, ensuring their safety. The courts will want to know from the assessing psychiatrist the likelihood of the mother achieving and maintaining sobriety, and sometimes the assessor is asked almost impossible questions such as 'What is the likelihood of the mother being sober until the child reaches their minority?' To answer such a question too optimistically has the risk of exposing the child to the harmful effects of a substance misuse disorder in their mother, but to be overly pessimistic runs the risk of undermining the mother and her current attempts at abstinence. Psychiatrists are not parenting experts, and so perhaps, it is best to respond by deferring and saying this is a question best redirected at a parenting expert as this is not an area of the psychiatrists' expertise.

The psychiatric assessment of mothers in care proceedings is probably amongst the most important type of psychiatric assessment undertaken by our profession because so much is at stake and so it must be done with care. At all times, it is important to bear in mind that the child's needs come first. Because the decision as to whether to remove a child or not has lifelong consequences, getting the report right is a matter of great importance. The decision is made by the judge and not the psychiatrist, but the judge will be guided by the medical evidence. Being overkind to a neglectful parent and so leaving the child in an unsafe environment may have grave risks, sometimes even to the child's life. However, also to wrongly remove a child from a loving and reasonably competent parent will leave both mother and child bereft for life – yet both such outcomes still occur today. By contrast, in personal injury litigation, the end result is usually the award of a certain amount of money, a little more if the medical report is good and a little less if it is not so good. In such childcare assessments, the child's needs come first, but since this is often the only time a mother will encounter a psychiatrist, it is important also to be on the lookout for any treatable psychiatric condition.

References

1. Brockington I. *Motherhood and Mental Health.* Oxford: Oxford University Press; 1996.
2. Esquirol J. Observations sur l'aliénation mentale à la suite de couches. *Journal Général de Médicine, de Chirurgie et de Pharmacie Françaises et Étrangères* 1818;2(1):148–64.
3. Gooch R. *Puerperal Psychosis.* Oxford: Oxford University Press; 1829.
4. Marcé L. Traité de la folie des femmes enceintes, des nouvelles accouchées et des nourrices: et considérations médico-légales qui se rattachent à ce sujet. Baillière; 1858 (accessed 5 October 2017).
5. Di Florio A, Gordon-Smith K, Forty L, et al. Stratification of the risk of bipolar disorder recurrences in pregnancy and postpartum. *The British Journal of Psychiatry* 2018;213(3):542–7.
6. Main T. Mothers with children in a psychiatric hospital. *The Lancet* 1958;272(7051):845–7.
7. VanderKruik R, Barreix M, Chou D, et al. The global prevalence of postpartum psychosis: a systematic review. *BMC Psychiatry* 2017;17(1):272.
8. Woody CA, Ferrari AJ, Siskind DJ, et al. A systematic review and meta-regression of the prevalence and incidence of perinatal depression. *Journal of Affective Disorders* 2017;219:86–92.
9. Rezaie-Keikhaie K, Arbabshastan ME, Rafiemanesh H, et al. Systematic review and meta-analysis of the prevalence of the maternity blues in the postpartum period. *Journal of Obstetric, Gynecologic & Neonatal Nursing* 2020;49(2):127–36.
10. Karnosh LJ, Hope JM. Puerperal psychoses and their sequellae. *American Journal of Psychiatry* 1937;94(3):537–50.
11. Gordon-Smith K, Perry A, Di Florio A, et al. Symptom profile of postpartum and non-postpartum manic episodes in bipolar I disorder: a within-subjects study. *Psychiatry Research* 2020;284:112748.
12. Kendell R, Chalmers J, Platz C. Epidemiology of puerperal psychoses. *The British Journal of Psychiatry* 1987;150(5):662–73.
13. Klompenhouwer J, Van Hulst A. Classification of postpartum psychosis: a study of 250 mother and baby admissions in the Netherlands. *Acta Psychiatrica Scandinavica* 1991;84 (3):255–61.
14. Savage GH. Observations on the insanity of pregnancy and childbirth. *Guy's Hospital Reports* 1875;20:83–117.
15. Agrawal P, Bhatia M, Malik S. Postpartum psychosis: a study of indoor cases in a general hospital psychiatric

clinic. *Acta Psychiatrica Scandinavica* 1990;81(6):5715.

16. American Psychiatric Association. *Diagnostic and Statistical Manual of Mental Disorders: DSM-5*. Washington, DC: American Psychiatric Association; 2013.
17. World Health Organization. *ICD-11: International Classification of Diseases (11th revision)*. Geneva: World Health Organization; 2019.
18. Jansson B. Psychic insufficiencies associated with childbearing. *Acta Psychiatrica Scandinavica. Supplementum* 1964;172:1+.
19. Paffenbarger Jr RS. Epidemiological aspects of parapartum mental illness. *British Journal of Preventive & Social Medicine* 1964;18(4):189.
20. Wesseloo R, Kamperman AM, Munk-Olsen T, et al. Risk of postpartum relapse in bipolar disorder and postpartum psychosis: a systematic review and meta-analysis. *American Journal of Psychiatry* 2016;173 (2):117–27.
21. Protheroe C. Puerperal psychoses: A long term study 1927–1961. *The British Journal of Psychiatry* 1969;115 (518):9–30.
22. Thuwe I. Genetic factors in puerperal psychosis. *The British Journal of Psychiatry* 1974;125(587):378–85.
23. Jones I, Craddock N. Familiality of the puerperal trigger in bipolar disorder: results of a family study. *American Journal of Psychiatry* 2001;158(6): 913–7.
24. Dowlatshahi D, Paykel E. Life events and social stress in puerperal psychoses: absence of effect. *Psychological Medicine* 1990;20(3):655–62.
25. Meltzer-Brody S, Larsen JT, Petersen L, et al. Adverse life events increase risk for postpartum psychiatric episodes: a population-based epidemiologic study. *Depression and Anxiety* 2018;35 (2):160–7.
26. Nager A, Johansson LM, Sundquist K. Neighborhood socioeconomic environment and risk of postpartum psychosis. *Archives of Women's Mental Health* 2006;9(2):81–6.
27. Bergink V, Rasgon N, Wisner KL. Postpartum psychosis: madness, mania, and melancholia in motherhood. *American Journal of Psychiatry* 2016;173(12):1179–88.
28. Forray A, Ostroff RB. The use of electroconvulsive therapy in postpartum affective disorders. *The Journal of ECT* 2007;23(3):188–93.
29. Perry A, Gordon-Smith K, Jones L, et al. Phenomenology, epidemiology and aetiology of postpartum psychosis: a review. *Brain Sciences* 2021;11(1):47.
30. Dean C, Williams R, Brockington I. Is puerperal psychosis the same as bipolar manic-depressive disorder? A family study. *Psychological Medicine* 1989;19 (3):637–47.
31. Yarden PE, Max DM, Eisenbach Z. The effect of childbirth on the prognosis of married schizophrenic women. *The British Journal of Psychiatry* 1966;112 (486):491–9.
32. Schöpf J, Rust B. Follow-up and family study of postpartum psychoses Part I: overview. *European Archives of Psychiatry and Clinical Neuroscience* 1994;244:101–11.
33. Robling S, Paykel E, Dunn V, et al. Long-term outcome of severe puerperal psychiatric illness: a 23 year follow-up study. *Psychological Medicine* 2000;30 (6):1263–71.
34. Essali A, Alabed S, Guul A, et al. Preventive interventions for postnatal psychosis. *Cochrane Database of Systematic Reviews* 2013(6). Art. No.: CD009991. DOI: 10.1002/14651858. CD009991.pub2. Accessed 18 December 2023.
35. Hamilton J. *Postpartum Psychiatric Problems. St.* Louis, MO: Mosby; 1962.
36. Wisner KL, Perel JM, Peindl KS, et al. Prevention of recurrent postpartum depression: a randomized clinical trial. *Journal of Clinical Psychiatry* 2001;62 (2):82–6.
37. Wisner KL, Perel JM, Peindl KS, et al. Prevention of postpartum depression: a pilot randomized clinical trial. *American Journal of Psychiatry* 2004;161(7):1290–2.
38. Stewart D, Klompenhouwer J, Kendell R, et al. Prophylactic lithium in puerperal psychosis: the experience of three centres. *The British Journal of Psychiatry* 1991;158(3):393–7.
39. Munk-Olsen T, Liu X, Viktorin A, et al. Maternal and infant outcomes associated with lithium use in pregnancy: an international collaborative meta-analysis of six cohort studies. *The Lancet Psychiatry* 2018;5 (8):644–52.
40. Sharma V, Smith A, Mazmanian D. Olanzapine in the prevention of postpartum psychosis and mood episodes in bipolar disorder. *Bipolar Disorders* 2006;8(4):400–4.
41. Kleiner GJ, Greston WM. Overview of demographic and statistical factors. In: Kleiner GJ, Greston WM (eds.) *Suicide in Pregnancy*. Chichester: John Wright; 1984: 23–40.
42. Appleby L. Suicide during pregnancy and in the first postnatal year. *British Medical Journal* 1991;302 (6769):137–40.
43. Appleby L, Mortensen PB, Faragher EB. Suicide and other causes of mortality after post-partum psychiatric admission. *The British Journal of Psychiatry* 1998;173(3):209–11.
44. World Health Organization. *Maternal Mental Health*. Geneva: World Health Organization; 2015.
45. Weng S-C, Chang J-C, Yeh M-K, et al. Factors influencing attempted and completed suicide in postnatal women: a population-based study in Taiwan. *Scientific Reports* 2016;6(1):25770.
46. Glasser S, Levinson D, Gordon E-S, et al. The tip of the iceberg: postpartum suicidality in Israel. *Israel Journal of Health Policy Research* 2018;7(1):1–12.
47. Gold KJ, Singh V, Marcus SM, et al. Mental health, substance use and intimate partner problems among pregnant and postpartum suicide victims in the National Violent Death Reporting System. *General Hospital Psychiatry* 2012;34(2):139–45.
48. Palladino CL, Singh V, Campbell J, et al. Homicide and suicide during the perinatal period: findings from the National Violent Death Reporting System. *Obstetrics and Gynecology* 2011;118(5):1056.
49. Office for National Statistics. *Statistical Bulletin, Domestic Abuse in England and Wales Overview: November 2022*. www.ons.gov.uk/peoplepopulationandcommunity/crimeandjustice/bulletins/domesticabuseinenglandandwalesoverview/november2022 (accessed 23 March 2023).
50. Gelaye B, Kajeepeta S, Williams MA. Suicidal ideation in pregnancy: an epidemiologic review. *Archives of*

Women's Mental Health 2016;19:741–51.

51. Nock MK, Borges G, Bromet EJ, et al. Cross-national prevalence and risk factors for suicidal ideation, plans and attempts. *The British Journal of Psychiatry* 2008;192(2):98–105.

52. Cox JL, Holden JM, Sagovsky R. Detection of postnatal depression: development of the 10-item Edinburgh Postnatal Depression Scale. *The British Journal of Psychiatry* 1987;150(6):782–6.

53. Zigmond AS, Snaith RP. The hospital anxiety and depression scale. *Acta Psychiatrica Scandinavica* 1983;67 (6):361–70.

54. Kim DR, Epperson CN, Weiss AR, et al. Pharmacotherapy of postpartum depression: an update. *Expert Opinion on Pharmacotherapy* 2014;15(9):1223–34.

55. Hahn-Holbrook J, Cornwell-Hinrichs T, Anaya I. Economic and health predictors of national postpartum depression prevalence: a systematic review, meta-analysis, and meta-regression of 291 studies from 56 countries. *Frontiers in Psychiatry* 2018;8:248.

56. Fiala A, Švancara J, Klánová J, et al. Sociodemographic and delivery risk factors for developing postpartum depression in a sample of 3233 mothers from the Czech ELSPAC study. *BMC Psychiatry* 2017;17:1–10.

57. Meltzer-Brody S, Maegbaek M, Medland S, et al. Obstetrical, pregnancy and socio-economic predictors for new-onset severe postpartum psychiatric disorders in primiparous women. *Psychological Medicine* 2017;47 (8):1427–41.

58. Bloch M, Schmidt PJ, Danaceau M, et al. Effects of gonadal steroids in women with a history of postpartum depression. *American Journal of Psychiatry* 2000;157(6):924–30.

59. Viktorin A, Meltzer-Brody S, Kuja-Halkola R, et al. Heritability of perinatal depression and genetic overlap with nonperinatal depression. *American Journal of Psychiatry* 2016;173 (2):158–65.

60. Yim IS, Tanner Stapleton LR, Guardino CM, et al. Biological and psychosocial predictors of postpartum depression: systematic review and call for integration. *Annual Review of Clinical Psychology* 2015;11:99–137.

61. Slomian J, Honvo G, Emonts P, et al. Consequences of maternal postpartum depression: a systematic review of maternal and infant outcomes. *Women's Health* 2019;15:1745506519844044.

62. Royal College of Psychiatrists. *Perinatal Mental Health Services: Recommendations for the Provision of Services for Childbearing Women. CR232.*–www.rcpsych.ac.uk/docs/default-source/improving-care/better-mh-policy/college-reports/college-report-cr232—perinatal-mental-heath-services.pdf?Status=Master&sfvrsn=82b10d7e_4 (accessed 8 March 2023).

63. Simhi M, Sarid O, Cwikel J. Preferences for mental health treatment for post-partum depression among new mothers. *Israel Journal of Health Policy Research* 2019;8:1–8.

64. O'Hara MW, Stuart S, Gorman LL, et al. Efficacy of interpersonal psychotherapy for postpartum depression. *Archives of General Psychiatry* 2000;57 (11):1039–45.

65. Cooper PJ, Murray L, Wilson A, et al. Controlled trial of the short-and long-term effect of psychological treatment of post-partum depression: I. Impact on maternal mood. *The British Journal of Psychiatry* 2003;182(5):412–9.

66. National Institute for Health and Clinical Excellence. *Antenatal and Postnatal Mental Health: Clinical Management and Service Guidance.* London: NICE; 2006.

67. Wyatt K, Dimmock P, Jones P, et al. Efficacy of progesterone and progestogens in management of premenstrual syndrome: systematic review. *BMJ* 2001;323(7316):776.

68. Kanes S, Colquhoun H, Gunduz-Bruce H, et al. Brexanolone (SAGE-547 injection) in post-partum depression: a randomised controlled trial. *The Lancet* 2017;390(10093):480–9.

69. Taylor DM, Barnes TR, Young AH. Pregnancy and breastfeeding. In: Taylor DM, Barnes TR, Young AH (eds.) *The Maudsley Prescribing Guidelines in Psychiatry.* Oxford: John Wiley & Sons; 2021: 679–702.

70. Kornfield SL, Kang-Yi CD, Mandell DS, et al. Predictors and patterns of psychiatric treatment dropout during pregnancy among low-income women. *Maternal and Child Health Journal* 2018;22:226–36.

71. Hendrick V, Stowe ZN, Altshuler LL, et al. Fluoxetine and norfluoxetine concentrations in nursing infants and breast milk. *Biological Psychiatry* 2001;50(10):775–82.

72. Hendrick V, Fukuchi A, Altshuler L, et al. Use of sertraline, paroxetine and fluvoxamine by nursing women. *The British Journal of Psychiatry* 2001;179 (2):163–6.

73. Nillni YI, Mehralizade A, Mayer L, et al. Treatment of depression, anxiety, and trauma-related disorders during the perinatal period: a systematic review. *Clinical Psychology Review* 2018;66:136–48.

74. Simoila L, Isometsä E, Gissler M, et al. Schizophrenia and pregnancy: a national register-based follow-up study among Finnish women born between 1965 and 1980. *Archives of Women's Mental Health* 2020;23:91100.

75. Uguz F, Akman C, Kaya N, et al. Postpartum-onset obsessive-compulsive disorder: incidence, clinical features, and related factors. *Journal of Clinical Psychiatry* 2007;68(1):132.

76. Pitt B. "Atypical" depression following childbirth. *The British Journal of Psychiatry* 1968;114(516):1325–35.

77. Hertzberg T, Wahlbeck K. The impact of pregnancy and puerperium on panic disorder: a review. *Journal of Psychosomatic Obstetrics & Gynecology* 1999;20(2):59–64.

78. Fogarty S, Elmir R, Hay P, et al. The experience of women with an eating disorder in the perinatal period: a meta-ethnographic study. *BMC Pregnancy and Childbirth* 2018;18:1–18.

79. National Institute for Health and Clinical Excellence. Eating disorders: recognition and treatment (NICE guideline No. 69). In: *Conception and Pregnancy for Women with Eating Disorders.* Section 1.9; 2017: 27.

80. Dekel S, Stuebe C, Dishy G. Childbirth induced posttraumatic stress syndrome: a systematic review of prevalence and risk factors. *Frontiers in Psychology* 2017;8:560.

81. de Graaff LF, Honig A, van Pampus MG, et al. Preventing post-traumatic stress disorder following childbirth and traumatic birth experiences: a systematic review. *Acta Obstetricia et Gynecologica Scandinavica* 2018;97 (6):648–56.

82. Stein G. S. The maternity blues. In: Brockington IF, Kumar R (eds.) *Motherhood and Mental Illness.* Cambridge, MA: Academic Press; 1982: 119–39.

83. Stein GS. The pattern of mental change and body weight change in the first post-partum week. *Journal of Psychosomatic Research* 1980;24(3–4):165–71.

84. Karacan I, Williams RL, Hursch C, et al. Some implications of the sleep patterns of pregnancy for postpartum emotional disturbances. *The British Journal of Psychiatry* 1969;115(525):929–35.

85. Stein GS. Headaches in the first post partum week and their relationship to migraine. *Headache: The Journal of Head and Face Pain* 1981;21(5):201–5.

86. Bhat A, Byatt N. Infertility and perinatal loss: when the bough breaks. *Current Psychiatry Reports* 2016;18:1–11.

87. Kingdon C, Roberts D, Turner MA, et al. Inequalities and stillbirth in the UK: a meta-narrative review. *BMJ Open* 2019;9(9):e029672.

88. Clarke M, Williams A. Depression in women after perinatal death. *The Lancet* 1979;313(8122):916–7.

89. Turton P, Hughes P, Evans C, et al. Incidence, correlates and predictors of post-traumatic stress disorder in the pregnancy after stillbirth. *The British Journal of Psychiatry* 2001;178 (6):556–60.

90. Rådestad I, Säflund K, Wredling R, et al. Holding a stillborn baby: mothers' feelings of tenderness and grief. *British Journal of Midwifery* 2009;17(3):178–80.

91. NHS England. *New Maternal Mental Health Services Supporting Hundreds of Expectant, New, or Bereaved Mothers to Get Mental Health Support.* www.england.nhs.uk/mental-health/case-studies/perinatal-mental-health-case-studies/new-maternal-mental-health-services-supporting-hundreds-of-expectant-new-or-bereaved-mothers-to-get-mental-health-support/#thrive (accessed 8 March 2023).

92. HM Government. *Infanticide Act: UK Public General Acts.* London: HMG; 1938.

93. Hopwood JS. Child murder and insanity. *Journal of Mental Science* 1927;73(300):95–108.

94. Marks M, Kumar R. Infanticide in England and Wales. *Medicine, Science and the Law* 1993;33(4):329–39.

95. Brookman F, Maguire M. *Reducing Homicide: A Review of the Possibilities: Home Office Research, Development and Statistics Directorate*; 2003.

96. Marks M. Characteristics and causes of infanticide in Britain. *International Review of Psychiatry* 1996;8(1):99–106.

97. Baek S-U, Lim S-S, Kim J, et al. How does economic inequality affect infanticide rates? An analysis of 15 years of death records and representative economic data. *International Journal of Environmental Research and Public Health* 2019;16(19):3679.

98. Sahni M, Verma N, Narula D, et al. Missing girls in India: infanticide, feticide and made-to-order pregnancies? Insights from hospital-based sex-ratio-at-birth over the last century. *PLoS ONE* 2008;3(5):e2224.

99. Klier CM, Grylli C, Amon S, et al. Is the introduction of anonymous delivery associated with a reduction of high neonaticide rates in Austria? A retrospective study. *BJOG: An International Journal of Obstetrics & Gynaecology* 2013;120(4):428–34.

100. McBride WG. Thalidomide and congenital abnormalities. *Lancet* 1961;2 (1358):90927–8.

101. Anand A, Phillips K, Subramanian A, et al. Prevalence of polypharmacy in pregnancy: a systematic review. *BMJ Open* 2023;13(3):e067585.

102. UK Teratology Information Service. *Best Use of Medicines in Pregnancy.* www.medicinesinpregnancy.org/ (accessed 5 April 2023).

103. Coughlin CG, Blackwell KA, Bartley C, et al. Obstetric and neonatal outcomes after antipsychotic medication exposure in pregnancy. *Obstetrics and Gynecology* 2015;125(5):1224.

104. Gao S-Y, Wu Q-J, Sun C, et al. Selective serotonin reuptake inhibitor use during early pregnancy and congenital malformations: a systematic review and meta-analysis of cohort studies of more than 9 million births. *BMC Medicine* 2018;16(1):1–14.

105. McAllister-Williams RH, Baldwin DS, Cantwell R, et al. British Association for Psychopharmacology consensus guidance on the use of psychotropic medication preconception, in pregnancy and postpartum 2017. *Journal of Psychopharmacology* 2017;31 (5):519–52.

106. Boyle B, Garne E, Loane M, et al. The changing epidemiology of Ebstein's anomaly and its relationship with maternal mental health conditions: a European registry-based study. *Cardiology in the Young* 2017;27 (4):677–85.

107. Tinker SC, Reefhuis J, Bitsko RH, et al. Use of benzodiazepine medications during pregnancy and potential risk for birth defects, National Birth Defects Prevention Study, 1997–2011. *Birth Defects Research* 2019;111(10):613–20.

108. Metz TD, Gordon AJ. Stimulant use in pregnancy – An under-recognized epidemic among pregnant women. *Clinical Obstetrics and Gynecology* 2019;62(1):168.

109. Sabbagh HJ, Hassan MHA, Innes NP, et al. Passive smoking in the etiology of non-syndromic orofacial clefts: a systematic review and meta-analysis. *PLoS ONE* 2015;10(3):e0116963.

110. Papadopoulou E, Botton J, Brantsæter A-L, et al. Maternal caffeine intake during pregnancy and childhood growth and overweight: results from a large Norwegian prospective observational cohort study. *BMJ Open* 2018;8(3):e018895.

111. Sayal K. Alcohol consumption in pregnancy as a risk factor for later mental health problems. *BMJ Mental Health* 2007;10(4):98–100.

112. Meyer KD, Zhang L. Short-and long-term adverse effects of cocaine abuse during pregnancy on the heart development. *Therapeutic Advances in Cardiovascular Disease* 2009;3(1):7–16.

113. Yadeta TA, Egata G, Seyoum B, et al. Khat chewing in pregnant women associated with prelabor rupture of membranes, evidence from eastern Ethiopia. *Pan African Medical Journal* 2020;36:1.

114. Namboodiri V, George S, Boulay S, et al. Pregnant heroin addict: what about the baby? *Case Reports* 2010;2010: bcr0920092246.

115. NHS England. *Better Births Four Years On: A Review of Progress.* www.england.nhs.uk/wp-content/uploads/2020/03/better-births-four-years-on-progress-report.pdf (accessed 8 March 2023).

116. Humphreys J, Obeney-Williams J, Cheung RW, et al. Perinatal psychiatry: a new specialty or everyone's business? *BJPsych Advances* 2016;22(6):363–72.

117. NHS England. *The Five Year Forward View for Mental Health. A Report from the Independent Mental Health Taskforce to the NHS in England.* London: NHS England; 2016.

118. Magon R, White R. Specialist community perinatal screening clinic: service evaluation. *The Psychiatrist* 2010;34(11):492–5.

119. Caffey J. Multiple fractures in the long bones of infants suffering from chronic subdural hematoma. *American Journal of Roentogenology* 1946;56:163–74.

120. Kempe CH, Silverman FN, Steele BF, et al. The battered-child syndrome. *JAMA* 1962;181(1):17–24.

121. Office for National Statistics. *Crime in England and Wales.* www.ons.gov.uk/peoplepopulationandcommunity/crimeandjustice/bulletins/crimeinenglandandwales/yearendingseptember2021 (accessed 8 March 2023).

122. van IJzendoorn MH, Bakermans-Kranenburg MJ, Coughlan B, et al. Annual research review: umbrella synthesis of meta-analyses on child maltreatment antecedents and interventions: differential susceptibility perspective on risk and resilience. *Journal of Child Psychology and Psychiatry* 2020;61(3):272–90.

123. HM Government. *The Children Act: UK Public General Acts.* London: HMG; 1989.

124. Leaman LA, Hennrikus WL, Bresnahan JJ. Identifying non-accidental fractures in children aged< 2 years. *Journal of Children's Orthopaedics* 2016;10(4):335–41.

125. McCoy ML, Keen SM. *Child Abuse and Neglect.* London: Psychology Press; 2013.

126. American Professional Society on the Abuse of Children. *Psychosocial Evaluation of Suspected Psychological Maltreatment in Children and Adolescents. Practice Guidelines.* Chicago, IL: American Professional Society on the Abuse of Children; 1995.

127. Lansford JE, Godwin J, Tirado LMU, et al. Individual, family, and culture level contributions to child physical abuse and neglect: a longitudinal study in nine countries. *Development and Psychopathology* 2015;27(4pt2):1417–28.

128. Oliver J. Successive generations of child maltreatment: social and medical disorders in the parents. *The British Journal of Psychiatry* 1985;147(5):484–90.

129. Browne K. Child protection. In: Rutter MJ, Taylor EA (eds.) *Child and Adolescent Psychiatry.* Oxford: Blackwell Publishing; 2002;1158–74.

130. Fryers T, Brugha T. Childhood determinants of adult psychiatric disorder. *Clinical Practice and Epidemiology in Mental Health* 2013;9:1–50.

131. Costello EJ, Compton SN, Keeler G, et al. Relationships between poverty and psychopathology: A natural experiment. *JAMA* 2003;290(15):2023–9.

132. Da Silva L, Johnstone EC. A follow-up study of severe puerperal psychiatric illness. *The British Journal of Psychiatry* 1981;139(4):346–54.

133. Howard LM, Kumar R, Thornicroft G. Psychosocial characteristics and needs of mothers with psychotic disorders. *The British Journal of Psychiatry* 2001;178(5):427–32.

Chapter 14

Substance Use Disorders

Ed Day and Zainab Bashir

Introduction

Human beings have prepared and used psychoactive substances for thousands of years. Alcohol was produced by the earliest civilisations and has played some part in most cultures throughout history. Other psychoactive substances have been extracted from local vegetation for specific reasons. For example, hill farmers working at high altitudes in Peru began to chew coca leaves for their stimulant effects, the Ancient Greeks used opium poppy extracts in medical poultices, and the hallucinogenic effects of mescaline from the peyote cactus became part of the religious ceremonies of indigenous people in Mexico. Technological advances have meant that some substances have become more readily accessible, and so their associated harms have become more apparent. Humankind's relationship with these substances has always generated strong emotions, both for and against, and there has been a concerted drive by the wealthiest countries to prohibit the use of many psychoactive substances ('illicit drugs') whilst promoting others (alcohol). Although the use of particular substances tends to wax and wane, it is important to see this in the wider historical context, as use of psychoactive drugs has increased every decade since the Second World War. More importantly, people's first introduction to drugs occurs at a younger age, and this is important because earlier use is associated with an increased risk of developing significant problems.

Of importance to the psychiatrist, a proportion of individuals develop an 'addiction' to these psychoactive substances whereby their ability to control the frequency and extent of their consumption becomes eroded. Psychoactive substance use occurs across a wide spectrum, from occasional social use through to use that starts to cause biological, psychological and social problems and to dependence. Dependence can be thought of as the iceberg visible above the water, with a much larger potential issue lurking below the waterline. Alcohol consumption is directly or indirectly associated with many health conditions, and 5.3 per cent of all global deaths in 2016 were estimated to be attributable to alcohol,[1] a greater cause of mortality than that caused by diseases such as diabetes, tuberculosis and HIV/AIDS. Illicit drug use has much in common with the use of legal substances such as tobacco and alcohol, but the illegality of this drug use adds new problems such as the risk of legal sanctions. Although the neurobiological and psychological understanding of addiction has increased dramatically in the past 30 years,[2,3] substance use disorders remain a heavily stigmatised problem.

All health care professionals should be able to take a basic history and signpost the individual with a substance use disorder towards help and support. The medical perspective on this issue is just one of many, and effective responses to people who struggle with the use of psychoactive substances incorporate a wide range of interpersonal, familial, community and societal strategies. This chapter will focus on the broad principles of assessment and diagnosis and will outline the current structure of specialist treatment services and the interventions that they deliver.

Defining Substance Use Disorders

Use of psychoactive substances occurs across a spectrum. The World Health Organization has defined three categories of substance use:[4]

- *Hazardous use*: A pattern of substance use that increases the risk of harmful consequences for the user. In contrast to harmful use, hazardous use refers to patterns of use that are of public health significance despite the absence of any current disorder in the individual.
- *Harmful use*: A pattern of psychoactive substance use that is causing damage to health. The damage may be physical or mental, and there will commonly be adverse social consequences. This is an ICD-10 and ICD-11 diagnostic term.
- *Dependence*: A cluster of behavioural, cognitive and physiological phenomena that may develop after repeated substance use. Dependence exists at different levels of severity, and the concept is useful for determining treatment strategies and prognosis. The full ICD-10 criteria are listed in Table 14.1, alongside the simplified version in ICD-11.

The latest version of the *Diagnostic and Statistical Manual* (DSM-5) has removed the category of dependence for a variety of technical reasons.[5] *Substance use disorder* (SUD) in DSM-5 combines the DSM-IV categories of substance abuse and substance dependence into a single disorder measured on a continuum from mild to severe – a problematic pattern of alcohol

Table 14.1 ICD-10 and ICD-11 diagnostic criteria for alcohol dependence, with recommended prompt questions to illicit these symptoms

ICD-10	ICD-11	Questions to elicit these diagnostic criteria
(a) A strong desire or sense of compulsion to drink alcohol (an essential characteristic)	Impaired control over alcohol, including craving	*Have you wanted a drink so badly you could not think of anything else?*
(b) Difficulties in controlling drinking behaviour in terms of onset, termination or levels of consumption		*Have you wanted/tried to cut down or stop drinking but couldn't?* *Have you had times when you ended up drinking more, or for longer, than you intended?*
(c) A physiological withdrawal state when drinking ceases or is reduced, evidenced by the characteristic alcohol withdrawal syndrome; or use of a closely related substance with the intention of relieving or avoiding withdrawal symptoms (e.g. benzodiazepines)	Physiological features caused by pharmacological tolerance and withdrawal	*Have you found that, when the effects of alcohol are wearing off, you experience withdrawal symptoms such as shakiness, nausea or sweating?*
(d) Evidence of tolerance, such that increased quantities of alcohol are required in order to achieve the effects originally produced by lesser amounts		*Do you have to drink much more than you used to in order to get the effect you want? Have you found that your usual alcohol consumption had much less effect than before?*
(e) Progressive neglect of alternative pleasures or interests because of alcohol consumption, increased amount of time necessary to obtain or drink alcohol or to recover from its effects	Alcohol becomes increasingly prioritised in life, often despite problems	*Have you given up or cut back on activities that were important, interesting or pleasurable to you in order to drink?*
(f) Persisting with drinking alcohol despite clear evidence of overtly harmful consequences, such as liver damage, depressive mood or impaired cognitive functioning.		*Have you found that drinking, or being ill from drinking, has often interfered with taking care of your home, family or other responsibilities?* *Have you continued to drink even though it was causing trouble with your family or friends?* *Have you continued to drink even though it was making you feel depressed or anxious or adding to another health problem?*

use leading to clinically significant impairment or distress, as manifested by at least two of the following within a 12-month period:

Physiological correlates of alcohol use: (1) tolerance, (2) withdrawal symptoms, (3) craving

Loss of control over alcohol use: (4) drinking longer/larger amounts than intended, (5) unsuccessful attempts to cut down/control use

Alcohol taking over meaningful activities: (6) increasing time spent in activities related to alcohol, (7) other activities given up because of alcohol

Problems resulting from alcohol use: (8) failure to fulfil role obligations, (9) social or interpersonal problems, (10) physical or psychological problems, (11) use in situations that are physically hazardous

Mild SUD is diagnosed if two or three are present, moderate SUD if four or five are present and severe SUD if six or more are present. The ICD-10 concept of dependence is closest to severe SUD, as moderate SUD can be diagnosed when only problems resulting from use of the substance are present.

Definitions in Practice: The Example of Alcohol

The spectrum of use and harms may be used to understand the extent of issues with alcohol or other drugs within the general population, as well as creating target populations for interventions. With this in mind, the UK Department of Health has defined four categories of alcohol use based on weekly alcohol consumption or the Alcohol Use Disorder Identification Test (AUDIT) score. These are shown in Table 14.2, alongside the equivalent WHO category and two methods of defining the group: units of alcohol per week (see Box 14.1) and score on the AUDIT (see later in chapter).[6] The current Chief Medical Officer for England's guidance around alcohol is summarised in Box 14.2.

Table 14.2 Level of consumption of alcohol and associated risk defined by the UK Department of Health[63]

	Description	AUDIT score
Low risk	No amount of alcohol consumption can be called 'safe', but risks of harm are low if below 14 units/week	≤7
Increasing-risk consumption (hazardous use)	A pattern of alcohol consumption in excess of the recommended levels (14 units/week) but without experiencing harm	8–15
Higher-risk consumption (harmful use)	A pattern of consumption in excess of the recommended levels (14 units/week) and experiencing health-related harms	16–19
Dependence	Drinking alcohol above recommended levels whilst experiencing harm and symptoms of dependence	≥20

As the level of daily and weekly alcohol consumption goes up, so the risk of physical, psychological and social problems increases. Therefore strategies that reduce average consumption

Box 14.1 Calculating units of alcohol

A drink's alcohol content is usually expressed by the standard measure 'Percentage Alcohol by Volume' or %ABV. This is a measure of the amount of pure ethanol as a percentage of the total volume of liquid in a drink. In the UK, it is found on the labels of cans and bottles by law. This means that 5 per cent of the volume of a can of cider labelled as '5% ABV' is pure alcohol.

The number of units in any drink can be calculated by multiplying the total volume (in ml) by its ABV and dividing the result by 1,000.

For example, the number of units in a pint (568 ml) of strong cider (ABV 7.5%):

(568 x 7.5)/1,000 = 4.3 units

Keeping track of units is important, as the increasing strength of many alcoholic drinks and larger glass sizes served in many bars mean that people are often drinking more alcohol than they realise. Units calculators are available:

https://alcoholchange.org.uk/alcohol-facts/interactive-tools/unit-calculator

Box 14.2 The Chief Medical Officer's advice in England

Since 2015, the advice[64] from the UK Department of Health is that in order to minimise the risk of health harms associated with drinking:

- Both men and women should drink no more than 14 units of alcohol per week, no more than 3 units in any given day, and have at least 2 alcohol-free days a week
- Pregnant women or women trying to conceive should not drink alcohol at all. If they do choose to drink, they should not drink more than 1–2 units of alcohol once or twice a week and should not get drunk
- Children should not drink alcohol at all, but if they do, they should be at least 15 years old, never drink more than once a week, be supervised by a parent or carer, and never exceed the recommended adult daily limits

across the whole population by a small amount produce considerable health benefits. Increasing the cost of alcohol relative to earnings has been consistently associated with reduction in alcohol-related harm, and a minimum cost for a unit of alcohol has been implemented in both Scotland and Wales.[7]

Levels of Alcohol and Drug Consumption in the UK

The Health Survey for England 2018 reported that alcoholic drinks were consumed by 82% of the population in the past year. Although most (61% men, 72% women) either consumed no alcohol or drank within the recommended levels described earlier, it is estimated that a quarter of the adult population of England drank in a way that is potentially or actually harmful to their health. The 2014 Health Survey for England reported that 16% of the population were non-drinkers, 59% drank at lower-risk levels (≤14 standard units per week), 21% at increasing-risk levels (>14 units to <35 units per week for women and <50 units per week for men) and 3% at higher-risk levels (≥35 for women and ≥50 to <75 units per week for men).[8] Increasing-risk and higher-risk drinkers are responsible for more than 75% of the total self-reported alcohol consumption. Best estimates suggest that, in England, there are just over 600,000 dependent drinkers,[9] and less than 20% of these are receiving treatment.

In terms of numbers, it is therefore clear that most alcohol-related problems occur in hazardous and harmful drinkers rather than people with alcohol dependence. From a public health perspective, secondary prevention aims to detect health problems at an early stage and intervene to produce positive changes in behaviour. This has been called the 'prevention paradox' – the greatest impact at a population level is likely to come from reducing (not necessarily stopping) consumption in hazardous and harmful drinkers rather than focusing on the heaviest, dependent drinkers. Most hazardous and harmful drinkers are unaware of their alcohol-related risk or harm, and so a screening mechanism is required to detect them. There is a strong evidence base for the effectiveness of screening and brief interventions for people who are drinking at risky levels but who are not actively seeking treatment for alcohol problems.[27]

In 2019, approximately 3.2 million people (9.4%) adults in the UK aged 16 to 59 reported taking an illicit drug in the last year.[10] Cannabis was the most commonly used illicit drug, with powder cocaine being second. Around 1 in 25 (3.7%) adults aged 16 to 59 had taken a Class A drug (mainly heroin and crack cocaine) in the past year, equating to around 1.3 million people. Although less than 1% of people reported opiate use, heroin users make up the largest proportion of the specialist treatment population.

Assessment of Substance Use Disorders

The process of assessment follows a similar pattern to that of any psychiatric history, and it is essential to identify needs and start the process of developing the goals of treatment with the patient. Assessment of risk and the development of a plan to mitigate this risk is also important. The following broad areas should be covered:[11]

Presenting Problem: Substance Use

The three key elements of assessment of alcohol or drug consumption are *quantity*, *frequency* and *route*.

Alcohol: Frequency of drinking is a more accurate measure than quantity. A simple but reasonably accurate approach is to ask the individual how many times they drank alcohol in a given time period. The 'past month' strikes a balance between a period that is long enough to be representative but short enough to be remembered. Accurate data about quantity are harder to collect and may be best captured prospectively using a 'drink diary' (see Box 14.1 regarding how to calculate alcohol units). Biological markers such as blood or breath alcohol concentration, mean corpuscular volume (MCV), serum gamma-glutamyltransferase (GGT), aspartate aminotransferase (AST), alanine aminotransferase (ALT) or carbohydrate deficient transferrin (CDT) are objective but are not very specific or sensitive to alcohol use.

Drugs: As with alcohol, frequency of use is much easier to capture than quantity. With the emergence of 'novel psychoactive substances' (at one point known as 'legal highs'), it can even be challenging to accurately name an illicit substance. In this case, it is easier to determine the effect of the drug using the seven broad categories in Mark Adley's 'Drugs Wheel' (www.thedrugswheel.com) as a guide:

- Stimulants: amphetamine, cocaine, mephedrone, khat
- Opioids: heroin, methadone, buprenorphine, codeine
- Depressants: benzodiazepines, gabapentin, pregabalin
- Cannabinoids: cannabis, 'Spice', 'Mamba'
- Psychedelics: LSD, mescaline, psilocybin
- Empathogens: MDMA (ecstasy), MDA, PMA
- Dissociatives: ketamine, PCP, nitrous oxide

It is useful to have an awareness of the names that people use for each substance (street names, which tend to vary regionally), and some suggestions are given in Table 14.3.

The variable and unknown purity of illicit drugs means that capturing a quantity is not often helpful, and asking about how much the individual spends each day is often the best guide. There are multiple potential routes of use, and drugs may be swallowed, snorted, smoked, inhaled, injected (subcutaneously, intramuscularly or intravenously) or inserted rectally. Each route has its own advantages and disadvantages, with intravenous injection bringing the best value for money but also the highest risk of accidental overdose or the spread of blood-borne pathogens.

There is often concern about how truthful a history of substance use is. In reality, this may vary as a function of how well the patient is known to the assessor and what the implications of the assessment are. Patients may exaggerate use to obtain a prescription but minimise it if there are implications such as child protection issues. It is essential to follow up history taking (including an assessment of the degree of problem use and dependence) and physical examination with objective drug testing. Oral mucosal fluid (saliva) and urine are the two most available body fluids to test, and both instant (near patient) and laboratory-based methods are available. For a full review of testing methods, see Wolff et al.[12]

History of Presenting Problem

A screening list for the main substances should be administered (i.e. have you ever used?), followed by establishing the age of first use, presence of dependence (see Table 14.1) and any periods of abstinence (and the circumstances). It is important to consider the patient's efforts at controlling or stopping their problematic use and not to forget mutual aid groups such as those of the twelve step fellowships (e.g. Alcoholics Anonymous, Narcotics Anonymous). Past episodes of treatment should also be noted, including any medications prescribed and the outcome.

Past Psychiatric History

The relationship between alcohol or drug use and symptoms of mental health disorders is often complex, and a comprehensive psychiatric screen is useful. Substance use can be the cause, consequence or mimicker of symptoms such as low mood or anxiety, and it is often hard to disentangle the various elements of a person's presentation. One UK study found that 44% of patients attending a Community Mental Health Team reported past-year problem drug use or harmful alcohol use, and 75% of drug service and 85% of alcohol service patients had a past-year psychiatric disorder.[13] Co-existing mental illness and substance use should be considered the norm rather than the exception, though it is often unrecognised and associated with poorer outcomes, and provision of care is often criticised as inadequate.[14] Heavy drinking or drug use can contribute to non-compliance with, or interaction and reduced efficacy of, medical and other treatments. Personality disorder, self harm, history of abuse or trauma, depression, anxiety and severe and enduring mental illness should all be considered, along with any past episodes of treatment.

Family and Personal History

Substance use disorders are best understood by looking at the interaction between biological, psychological and social factors. This complex and dynamic interplay partly explains why not everyone who drinks or experiments with drugs will develop problems. The personal history should include consideration of problems in personal relationships (including domestic violence and abuse), family, housing and living arrangements, education, employment, benefits and financial problems. Safeguarding considerations mean it is important to enquire about childcare issues, including parenting, pregnancy and child protection. Stone and colleagues have summarised the evidence base for both risk and protective factors for substance use disorders in childhood and young adulthood,[15] and it is helpful to structure the personal history around them:

Risk Factors

In general, the younger the individual is when they first use psychoactive substances, the more likely they are to develop a long-term problem. Emotional distress, aggression, or

Table 14.3 Information about five common substances of abuse in the UK

Drug type	Cocaine	Heroin	Benzodiazepines	Cannabis	Synthetic cannabinoid receptor agonists
Forms	Crack (freebase form of cocaine that can be smoked)	AKA Diamorphine hydrochloride Other opiates: Codeine (metabolised to morphine)	Alprazolam (Xanax) Diazepam (Valium) Flunitrazepam (Rohypnol: *'date rape drug'*) Nitrazepam (Mogadon) Temazepam	Skunk: high THC content cannabis	Known as synthetic cannabinoids, but in reality, not really cannabis-like. May have an 'official' name based on an international naming standard, but it is usually referred to by the names below
Street names	Cocaine: *Coke, Charlie, Snow, White, Nose candy* Crack: *Base, Freebase, Rocks, Stones, Bones, White*	*Brown, Gear, Smack, Skag, Dope, Junk, Shit, H, Horse*	AKA 'Downers' Alprazolam: *Xs* Diazepam: *Vallies, Blues* Flunitrazepam: *Rohies, Rufies* Nitrazepam: *Moggies* Temazepam: *Temazies, Jellies*	*Marijuana, Hash, Pot, Weed, Blow, Black, Draw, Dope, Herb, Grass, Bud, Bhang*	*Spice, Black Mamba, Man Down, Pandora's Box, Exodus Damnation, Cherry Bomb and many others*
Mode of use	Cocaine: snorting, injecting, rubbing on gums Crack: smoking (through pipe or spliff), injecting (along with heroin, known as 'snowball')	Smoking on foil ('chasing the dragon' or 'booting') Injecting Rectally	Orally Rectally Injecting (potentially very harmful)	Smoke: a) Spliff or joint: cannabis cigarette usually mixed with tobacco b) Bongs: pipe is heated, and the cannabis is inhaled as smoke through water c) Others such as 'hot knives, lungs', vape Edibles: eating or drinking, such as cakes ('hash brownies'), lollipops, yoghurt, tea	Smoke: dried plant material is sprayed with a synthetic cannabinoid, a chemical that mimics the action of THC or CBD at brain cannabinoid receptors. This is then smoked in a spliff, but also pipes and bongs. Vaping is also growing in popularity
Effects	Powerful stimulant. Heightened energy, happy, excited, alert, powerful, in control, euphoria, sexually aroused, confident Physical: vasoconstriction, increased heart rate and blood pressure, pupillary dilatation	Powerful pain killer. Euphoria, profound wellbeing, content, relaxed, absence of worry, sleepiness	CNS depressant: sedating, anxiolytic effects, 'chill out', aids sleep after stimulant use, amnesiac. Slurred speech, clumsiness and confusion. Can cause paradoxical overexcitement and violence	Variable (depending on dose/type). Relaxation, euphoria, excitability, light-headedness, hilarity, anxiety, confusion, paranoia, lethargy, increased appetite	Strength of street synthetic cannabinoids varies enormously. Euphoric, stoned, detached feeling. Altered perception and a feeling of relaxation and calm
Duration of action	Cocaine: effects start after 5–30 mins, last for 20–30 mins Crack: effects immediate, lasts 10–15 mins	Smoking: effects start after a few minutes, lasts for an hour	Variable depending on type. Longer acting ones (e.g. Diazepam) has a half-life of 20–50 hours	*Smoking*: effects take a few minutes and tend to wear off within an hour *Edibles*: gut absorption is slower, and effects can take up to 1 hour but can last several hours	Usually up to an hour May be longer, with unpleasant 'comedown' period
Withdrawal features	Anxiety, paranoia and low mood	'Cold turkey': sweating, tearing and runny nose, anxiety, restlessness, irritability, joint/bone ache, muscle spasms, tremor, goose flesh, GI upset	Abrupt withdrawals: insomnia, anxiety, restlessness, agitation, tremors and convulsions. Potentially death (rare)	Irritability, nausea, shaking, diarrhoea, insomnia, poor appetite	Sweating, shakes, nausea and vomiting, abdominal pain
Problems associated with use	Nasal septal perforation, gum disease and cavities, COPD, arrhythmias, myocardial infarction, stroke, ulcers, gangrene, depression, psychosis, HIV and other BBV infections	Physical withdrawal syndrome. Overdose potentially leading to death Physical: damage to blood vessels, femoral aneurysms, DVT, infective endocarditis, BBV infections, abscesses, cellulitis. Social problems: self-neglect, crime, violence	Effects depend on age and other drugs taken: drowsiness, light-headedness, dizziness confusion, unsteadiness, slurred speech, muscle weakness, memory problems Increased risk of fatal overdose with other sedative drugs Paradoxical effects (more common in children/older adults): anxiety, agitation, aggressive behaviour, delusions, depersonalisation/derealisation, disinhibition, personality change	Psychosis, depression, short-term memory loss, lung damage	Psychiatric: anxiety, severe panic, low mood, disorientation, fear, aggression, hallucinations, depersonalisation, derealisation and delusional states Physical: tachyarrhythmia or bradycardia, respiratory distress, raised body temperature. Paralysis, limb rigidity uncontrollable movements, sensory loss in limbs, reduced sensitivity to pain Seizures, loss of consciousness and amnesia post incident

'difficult' temperament in childhood and adolescence are associated with substance use, as are rebellious activities. A positive attitude towards alcohol or drugs combined with limited perception of risk often predates problematic use.

It is important to enquire about peers, friends or family members who used alcohol or drugs around the patient in childhood or adolescence. Family history of substance use that was both persistent and generalised, or substance use disorders in close family members, should be noted, as substance use disorders consistently show a heritability of approximately 50 per cent. Certain types of parenting style/ability are also an important risk factor – for example, an inability to set clear expectations for behaviour; failure to supervise and monitor children; or excessively severe, harsh or inconsistent punishment. Parents with positive attitudes to drugs or approval of drug use increase the risk of use, as does family discord – conflict between parents or between parents and children (including abuse or neglect).

Academic failure beginning in primary school and a general lack of commitment to, or enthusiasm for, school is a common precursor to heavy or regular substance use. The ready availability of alcohol and drugs in the local community is a risk factor, alongside social norms that promote the acceptability of substance use in young people. Finally, community disorganisation evidenced by high population density, lack of natural surveillance of public places, physical deterioration and high rates of adult crime have a strong association with problematic substance use, as does low parental socioeconomic status (as determined by education, income and occupation).

Protective Factors

The risk factors are counter-balanced by protective factors that should also be considered. Social, emotional, behavioural and moral competence in childhood and early adolescence is important, including interpersonal skills that allow a young person to integrate feelings, thinking and actions to achieve social and interpersonal goals. Self-efficacy and resilience (i.e. the capacity to adapt to change or stressful events in flexible and healthy ways) are protective factors, as is attachment and commitment to, and positive communication with, family and the wider community. Marriage or a committed relationship and living with a partner who does not use alcohol or drugs problematically can be helpful, as can involvement in spiritual or religious practices. Parents (and teachers or other community members) who provide recognition for effort and achievements can motivate individuals to engage in positive behaviours. Family, school and community norms that communicate clear and consistent expectations about not misusing drugs are also protective, as are developmentally appropriate opportunities to be involved with others.

Forensic History

Criminal involvement, offending and other legal issues must be explored, including arrests, fines, outstanding charges and warrants, probation, imprisonment and violent offences. Prosecution for driving under the influence of drink or drugs is often a first sign of dependence, and shoplifting and other acquisitive crimes are associated with the need to feed an expensive addiction. For example, it is estimated that a typical dependent heroin user spends 2–3 times the average mortgage payment on drugs each month.

Past Medical History

The risk of alcohol-related harm increases with the amount of regular alcohol consumption. Short-term health risks include accidents and injuries, and alcohol is a causal factor in more than 60 medical conditions.[16] Heavy drinkers have more than twice the mortality rate of the general population. No organ system in the body remains unaffected by the direct toxic effects of chronic alcohol consumption, and many of these effects are compounded by dietary insufficiency associated with the 'empty calories' of alcohol (for a detailed review, see Day et al.[17]). Intoxication with alcohol increases the risk of soft-tissue injuries, fractures, head injuries and other trauma. Physical health issues associated with more sustained alcohol consumption include hypertension, stroke, obesity, alcoholic liver disease (including fatty liver, hepatitis and cirrhosis), cancer, aspiration pneumonia, pancreatitis, cognitive deficits, alcohol-related brain damage, epileptic seizures, peripheral neuropathy, foetal alcohol syndrome and sexual dysfunction.

The route of drug use has an impact on the harms caused. Smoking cannabis is associated with changes in lung function, but unlike tobacco, it appears to increase the risk of severe bronchitis at quite low exposure but not lead to chronic obstructive pulmonary disease.[18] Inhaling cocaine predisposes users to infection of the upper respiratory tract, including sinusitis and septal abscesses. Acute respiratory symptoms develop within minutes to hours of smoking crack cocaine, including a cough accompanied by the production of black sputum, chest pain (sometimes with shortness of breath), haemoptysis and an exacerbation of asthma.[19] The risk of pulmonary tuberculosis (including drug-resistant cases) appears to be increased among drug users as a result of crowded living conditions, delays in diagnosis, poor adherence to treatment and the prevalence of HIV infection or AIDS.

Injecting is most common when supplies of a drug are limited, and this may also be associated with riskier injecting practices such as increased frequency of injecting, sharing equipment or groin injecting. The greatest public health concern comes from the transmission of blood-borne bacterial and viral infections via shared equipment. In the UK, over half of the people who inject drugs (PWID) report recent symptoms of a bacterial infection, and approximately one in every 100 PWID is infected with HIV, one in every 200 PWID with hepatitis B (HBV), and around one in every 4 PWID with hepatitis C (HCV).[20] Most acute infections remain undiagnosed, and the consequences include AIDS (HIV) or cirrhosis and hepatocellular carcinoma (HBV and HCV).

Infective endocarditis is another serious complication of injecting. Right-sided endocarditis is more frequent (over 50 per cent of cases involve the tricuspid valve) and may cause pulmonary pathology, including abscesses. Repeated injection of drugs and adulterants using unsterile, contaminated equipment produces hyperpigmented 'tracks' along the path of veins; the inflammation of the veins (thrombophlebitis), local infections, abscesses, ulcers and septicaemia are all common. Opioid overdose can result from simultaneous use of more than one drug or fluctuations in the purity of an illicit drug. It often follows a period of abstinence, when tolerance to the drug's respiratory depressant effects falls.

Combining psychoactive substances is the norm and may create further complications. Up to two-thirds of people who take cocaine combine it with alcohol, as the combination prolongs cocaine's euphoric effect and decreases its unpleasant consequences such as agitation and dysphoria. Combining cocaine and heroin in the same syringe creates a 'speedball'. Cocaine's stimulant effects wear off quicker than the sedating effects of the heroin, increasing the risk of delayed respiratory depression. Illicit drugs are often mixed with both inert and active substances to increase the apparent quantity of the street drug or to enhance its effect. Such adulterants are likely to increase the risk of adverse effects.

Presenting symptoms of any physical health concern should be gathered, alongside past medical history including operations, injuries and periods in hospital. Women should be asked about relevant contraception history, cervical screening and menstrual and pregnancy history. Everyone should be asked about sexual health and sexually transmitted infections (including any partners with HIV or hepatitis C). Problems with oral health are especially common in users of heroin and crack cocaine.

Medication

Current prescribed and non-prescribed medication must be recorded, including over-the-counter medicines.

Monitoring the Outcome of Treatment

Another way of structuring the personal history is to consider potential areas of improvement as treatment progresses. Four areas are often identified as key outcomes: substance use, health, criminal activity and social functioning. The first three have already been covered, and key social factors are housing, employment and relationships. Alcohol and drugs are often implicated in relationship breakdown, domestic violence and poor parenting, including child neglect and abuse. Both alcohol and drugs contribute to absenteeism from work, financial problems, accidents in the workplace and decline in work performance, as well as being linked to unsafe sex, unplanned pregnancy and homelessness. The long-term stressful impact of substance use disorder on family members also produces significant harms.[21] The annual cost of illicit drug misuse in the UK is estimated to be nearly £11 billion per year,[22] and alcohol-related harm is estimated to cost England approximately £21.5 billion per year.[23] These costs include lost productivity, crime, policing and the NHS.

Recovery from addiction is often about an accumulation of social capital. Therefore, it is important to explore the patient's personal, family, social and other strengths. An assessment of the social network can be particularly helpful in developing the goals of treatment,[24] as can establishing the details of past successes and difficulties in achieving stability or in making improvements. The final component of the assessment is to understand the patient's motivation for change and their preferred treatment options.

Box 14.3 Key elements of the physical examination and investigations[11]

- Measurement of weight and blood pressure – baseline measurements can be useful in monitoring progress
- Detailed examination of gastrointestinal system, with particular focus on signs of chronic liver disease
- Neurological examination (indications = loss of sensation, organic causes of confusion, forgetfulness, convulsions, blackouts)
- Assessment of injection sites in all limbs and inguinal areas, particularly if the patient reports current injecting or has injected in the past
- Electrocardiogram (ECG)
- Chest X-ray
- Pulmonary function tests such as peak flow and FEV/FVC
- Pregnancy test
- Blood tests to assess liver function, thyroid function, renal function, haematological indices, B12 and folate
- Blood test for HIV, hepatitis C (including PCR testing for the presence of HCV RNA) and hepatitis B infection
- Urine testing for markers of conditions such as diabetes and infection
- Urine (or oral mucosal fluid) test for drugs of abuse

Physical Examination

Physical examination should include a general assessment of respiratory, cardiovascular and other body systems, paying attention to any symptoms offered and complaints described (which can lead to a more detailed examination of that system or signposting the patient to their GP for this). Box 14.3 summarises the key areas to focus on.

Treatment of Alcohol or Drug Dependence

Use of alcohol or drugs is common but not always problematic. If the harmful consequences of use begin to outweigh the benefits, attempts may be made to cut down or stop use. If these attempts are unsuccessful, the individual may seek help from a professional health care agency. The helping response required to overcome mild to moderate alcohol or drug problems may be brief and designed to mobilise the individual's motivation to change. However, severe substance use disorders

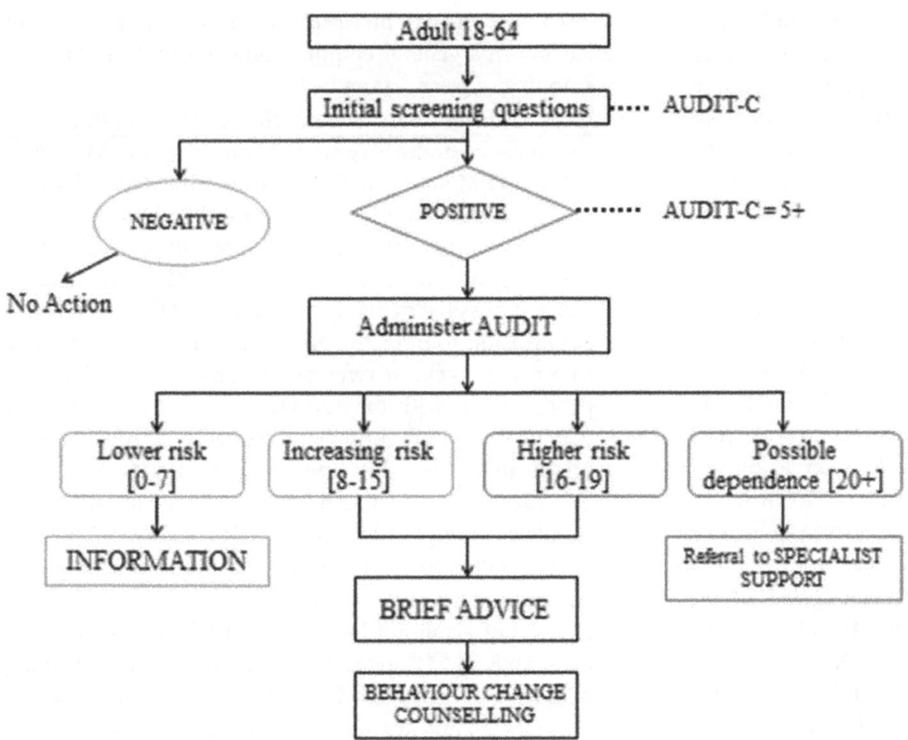

Figure 14.1 A flowchart to guide the process of a brief intervention for alcohol using AUDIT.

often require interventions that are complex, multifaceted and sustained over many years. Dependence can be very hard to overcome once established, and two-thirds completing a successful episode of treatment will have lapsed or relapsed within 12 months. Such is the stigma and shame surrounding the issue, people are often reluctant to return to the original treatment provider, allowing significant problems to develop. The framework for providing health care should therefore adopt a chronic care rather than an acute care model.[25]

Treatment is often presented in a polarised manner, with 'harm reduction' strategies as one option and abstinence as the other. In reality, the ideal treatment system includes both elements in equal measure. In considering the correct treatment strategy and intensity, it is important to consider risks, capacity to consent to treatment, the experience and outcome of previous episodes of treatment, motivation for change and other existing problems, including harm to others. Six broad treatment approaches will be considered: harm reduction, brief interventions, medically assisted withdrawal (sometimes known as detoxification), opioid assisted treatment (OAT, sometimes known as maintenance treatment or opioid substitution treatment, OST), psychosocial interventions designed to bring about behaviour change, and relapse prevention medication. Figure 14.1 shows how these may be sequenced within the wider biopsychosocial treatment model described later.

Harm Reduction

Although dependence is a chronic condition, many (and probably a majority) of people become abstinent in the long term. However, the process may take years, and mortality rates in people dependent on alcohol, heroin or cocaine are considerably higher than those who are not. Therefore, a simple all-or-none approach to treatment that views abstinence as the only marker of success is unhelpful. The harm reduction approach refers to policies, programmes and practices that aim to reduce the harms associated with the use of psychoactive substances in people unable or unwilling to stop. The focus is on prevention of harm rather than the prevention of substance use itself, but this approach is compatible with reducing the overall level of use.

Alcohol: Individuals who are experiencing shaking, sweating, nausea or headache after several hours without a drink should be advised not to stop drinking suddenly due to the potentially serious consequences (seizures or delirium). The goal should be to cut down and gain some control by using alcohol as a 'medicine'. Information about the daily pattern of consumption from a drink diary is used to space out the drinks, focusing on the middle of the day whilst keeping consumption at the beginning and the end stable. Once daily intake has been stabilised for seven days, it is possible to start to cut down slowly (e.g. by 10 per cent every four days).

Tips to help patients reduce their alcohol intake include:

- Switching to a lower strength (%ABV) drink
- Using a measuring cup to ration drinks more accurately
- Adding water or a mixer to drinks
- Alternating soft drinks with alcohol
- Dietary measures (e.g. limiting sugar intake, eating brown rice/wholemeal bread to reduce the impact of thiamine deficiency)
- Keeping well hydrated

It is always good to enlist positive support from family and friends in this exercise. Experiencing a seizure, becoming confused or starting to experience hallucinations, double vision or unsteadiness should prompt seeking emergency help.

Opiates and other drugs: The risk of spreading blood-borne viruses (BBV) such as hepatitis B and C and HIV through the sharing of drug-injecting paraphernalia is a major public health risk. Needle and syringe programmes (NSPs) provide needles, syringes and other injecting paraphernalia, as well as a safe place to return used equipment. NSPs deliver opportunistic education to help people to understand the potential harms of injecting and to inject more safely (e.g. avoiding groin injecting, using better sterile technique). UK drug treatment services have provided a very successful HBV vaccination programme, leading to very low levels of the disease. However, HCV remains a major concern. New treatments provide a realistic expectation of cure from HCV, but the challenge remains getting those at risk to access them.

Accidental overdose is the commonest cause of death in heroin users, and 40 to 70 per cent of injecting users have experienced at least one overdose.[26] The majority of heroin overdoses are witnessed by other drug users, and so education about how to avoid and manage an overdose is supplemented by the provision of the full opioid antagonist naloxone. This must be administered parenterally and so requires some initial training (at the time of writing, intranasal versions are starting to be used but are expensive). In the absence of opioids, it has no pharmacologic action and so has little potential for misuse. In 2005, naloxone was added to the list of prescription-only medicines that anyone (not just health care professionals) can administer by injection for the purpose of saving a life, similar to epinephrine in an 'Epipen'. Legislation in October 2015 meant that it could be supplied to individuals by drug services without prescription. Users are advised to administer naloxone intramuscularly, and it is available in the UK in prefilled syringes (0.4 mg per 1 ml) with an attachable needle.

Brief Interventions for Alcohol Use

All health care professionals should be comfortable and confident in raising the topic of alcohol consumption in a consultation, and NICE recommends that alcohol screening should form part of routine practice across the NHS.[27] Providing even a few minutes of advice in a structured manner has a number needed to treat (NNT) of 8 where the goal is drinking at lower-risk levels.[27] All clinicians should be aware of the facts about alcohol consumption and health-related harms (see Box 14.2). It is important to avoid stigmatising terms like 'alcoholic', emphasising instead the increased risk with higher levels of consumption and suggesting cutting down to a lower-risk level rather than necessarily stopping. Brief interventions have three stages:[28]

Stage 1 – Raise the issue: Discussing alcohol consumption can produce indifference, uncertainty about 'healthy' levels of drinking, and sometimes defensiveness and irritability. It may be easiest to embed questions about alcohol in a general enquiry about lifestyle factors (e.g. smoking, diet and exercise)

Stage 2 – Administer and score the AUDIT questionnaire: The most cost-effective way of screening for AUD is by using a valid and reliable questionnaire. The **'Alcohol Use Disorders Identification Test'** (AUDIT, Table 14.4) consists of 10 questions about drinking frequency and intensity, alcohol-related problems and signs of possible dependence.[6] The AUDIT score guides the decision to offer the patient a 'brief intervention' or to make a specialist referral (see Figure 14.1). The process starts with the administration of the first three AUDIT questions (known as AUDIT-C). A score of 5 indicates a high likelihood of drinking at an 'increasing-risk' level, and the full AUDIT questionnaire should be completed. A full AUDIT score of 7 or less should be fed back in a positive manner, pointing out that people who exceed these levels increase their chances of alcohol-related health problems. A score between 8 and 19 suggests that the individual's drinking pattern is in the increasing-risk or higher-risk band (see Table 14.2), and the clinician should move to stage 3.

Stage 3 - Deliver structured brief advice: An open-ended 'transitional' statement such as 'how important is it for you to change your drinking?' can be useful, accompanied by a 'readiness ruler' between 1 and 10. A structured episode of brief advice may only last 5–10 minutes and is best guided by a structured tool (such as available at https://www.gov.uk/government/publications/health-matters-preventing-ill-health-from-alcohol-and-tobacco/health-matters-preventing-ill-health-from-alcohol-and-tobacco-use). This makes use of the FRAMES structure for brief interventions (feedback, responsibility, advice, menu, empathy, self-efficacy)[29] by providing *feedback* on the patient's level of drinking when compared to others, a *menu* of options to support the attainment of their preferred drinking goal, and *advice* on units and the common effects of alcohol. The clinician must ensure that the individual takes *responsibility* for making the change (re-stating the need to reduce risk and encouraging an immediate start), whilst also showing *empathy* (e.g. 'It can be very difficult to make these changes if everyone around you is drinking heavily'). At the same time, it is important to boost confidence and *self-efficacy* ('You mentioned you were going to drink a non-alcoholic drink first when you get home in the evening. That sounds like an excellent start.'). Ideally, the individual should be offered a follow-up appointment to assess their progress in reducing their alcohol consumption. A referral is made to specialist alcohol treatment services if the patient asks for this help, is already showing signs of significant alcohol-related harm, or has an AUDIT score of 20 or more.

Table 14.4 The Alcohol Use Disorders Identification Test (AUDIT)[6]

ALCOHOL USE DISORDERS IDENTIFICATION TEST (AUDIT)			
1. How often do you have a drink containing alcohol? (0) Never (1) Monthly or less (2) 2 to 4 times a month (3) 2 to 3 times a week (4) 4 or more times a week	☐	6. How often during the last year have you needed a first drink in the morning to get yourself going after a heavy drinking session? (0) Never (1) Less than monthly (2) Monthly (3) Weekly (4) Daily or almost daily	☐
2. How many units of alcohol do you have on a typical day when you are drinking? (0) 1 or 2 (1) 3 or 4 (2) 5 or 6 (3) 7, 8 or 9 (4) 10 or more	☐	7. How often during the last year have you had a feeling of guilt or remorse after drinking? (0) Never (1) Less than monthly (2) Monthly (3) Weekly (4) Daily or almost daily	☐
3. How often do you have 6 or more units if female, or 8 or more units if male, on a single occasion in the last year? (0) Never (1) Less than monthly (2) Monthly (3) Weekly (4) Daily or almost daily	☐	8. How often during the last year have you been unable to remember what happened the night before because you had been drinking? (0) Never (1) Less than monthly (2) Monthly (3) Weekly (4) Daily or almost daily	☐
4. How often during the last year have you found that you were not able to stop drinking once you had started? (0) Never (1) Less than monthly (2) Monthly (3) Weekly (4) Daily or almost daily	☐	9. Have you or someone else been injured as a result of your drinking? (0) No (2) Yes, but not in the last year (4) Yes, during the last year	☐
5. How often during the last year have you failed to do what was normally expected from you because of drinking? (0) Never (1) Less than monthly (2) Monthly (3) Weekly (4) Daily or almost daily	☐	10. Has a relative or friend, doctor or another health worker been concerned about your drinking or suggested that you cut down? (0) No (2) Yes, but not in the last year (4) Yes, during the last year	☐
TOTAL SCORE	☐		

Medically Assisted Withdrawal (MAW)

Failed episodes of withdrawal reduce self-efficacy, and preparation work is crucial. It is important to assess readiness for abstinence, learning points from previous attempts to stop, and coping strategies other than pharmacotherapy for dealing with withdrawal symptoms. Throughout the preparation phase, patients should stabilise or slowly reduce their substance use with the assistance of a drink/drug diary. In the community setting, a friend/family member should be identified to support and monitor the withdrawal period. The best marker of long-term success is the development of clear plans and social supports to sustain abstinence following withdrawal, including a programme of activities or work to prevent boredom and ideas on how to replace the role of alcohol or drugs.

The default position for a planned episode of MAW is the community, but this depends upon an assessment of the risks involved. This means an understanding of the withdrawal syndrome of the substance(s) in question (see Table 14.3), potential interactions with medications, and the physical and mental health of the patient. It is important to consider a history of seizures or delirium, high dosages (particularly with short-acting depressant drugs such as lorazepam) or polypharmacy, and pre-existing conditions (e.g. hypertension, ischaemic heart disease, significant liver or renal impairment, diabetes, mental illness including organic brain damage, or pregnancy). Risks relating to the available levels of support and supervision will also influence the treatment plan, such as the lack of a non-using support person or a person willing to supervise medicine, childcare difficulties or the distance to the treatment centre.

Alcohol: Minor degrees of alcohol withdrawal are common and can be managed with information, reassurance, adequate fluid intake and diet. About six to eight hours after an abrupt

Table 14.5 Medications used to reduce the symptoms and signs of opiate withdrawal

Autonomic symptoms (sweating, tachycardia, myoclonus)	• Lofexidine 0.2 to 0.6 mg oral every 6 hours; hold dose if blood pressure <90/60 mmHg (0.4 mg four times daily is usual in the outpatient setting) *Recommend test dose (0.4 mg oral) with blood pressure check 1 hour post dose, obtain daily blood pressure checks, increasing dose requires additional blood pressure checks. Re-evaluate in 3 to 7 days, taper to stop, average duration is 15 days*
Anxiety, dysphoria, lacrimation, rhinorrhea	• Promazine 25 mg up to 6-hourly (and 50 mg nocte) • Diphenhydramine 25 mg every 6 hours as needed • Small doses of benzodiazepines may be useful (e.g. diazepam 2–5mg up to 8-hourly), but there is high addiction potential *Anxiety levels are an important feature of the opioid withdrawal syndrome. Providing good information prior to withdrawal can reduce this, alongside reassurance and other non-pharmacotherapeutic techniques*
Myalgia	• NSAIDs (e.g. ibuprofen 400 three times daily) • Paracetamol 1 g every 6 hours as needed • Topical medications like menthol/methylsalicylate cream
Sleep disturbance	• Zopiclone 7.5 mg orally at bedtime • Nitrazepam 10 mg orally at bedtime *Difficulty sleeping is common with opioid dependence, and medication will only provide limited help. Sedating antidepressants such as mirtazapine or trazadone may be useful, but they are not without side effects and not licenced as hypnotics*
Nausea	• Prochlorperazine 5 to 10 mg every 4 hours as needed • Promethazine 25 mg orally or rectally every 6 hours as needed • Ondansetron 4 mg every 6 hours as needed
Abdominal cramps	• Dicyclomine 20 mg every 6 to 8 hours as needed
Diarrhoea	• Loperamide 4 mg orally initially, then 2 mg with each loose stool, not to exceed 16 mg daily

reduction in alcohol intake, most people with severe alcohol dependence experience hyperactivity, anxiety, tremor, sweating, nausea and retching, increased heart rate, high blood pressure and mildly raised temperature. These symptoms usually peak over 10–30 hours and subside by 48–72 hours. More seriously, seizures may occur in the first 12–48 hours (and rarely after this), and characteristically frightening auditory and visual hallucinations can occur in the first 48 hours. Delirium tremens occurs in up to 5 per cent of people, and it usually starts 48–72 hours after cutting down/stopping drinking. Major symptoms include coarse tremor, agitation, fever, rapid heart rate, profound confusion, delusions and hallucinations. Moderate to severe alcohol withdrawal symptoms require medication to reduce symptom severity and reduce the risk of seizures and delirium tremens. Long-acting benzodiazepines (chlordiazepoxide or diazepam) are the drug of choice. Rating scales such as the Clinical Institute Withdrawal Assessment for Alcohol (CIWA-Ar) are used to measure the severity of the withdrawal symptoms and more accurately adjust the dose. The use of such a 'symptom-triggered' regimen is only recommended if trained staff are available (e.g. in an inpatient setting).[30,31]

Opiates: Opiate withdrawal symptoms present less threat to life than severe alcohol withdrawal, but those that have experienced them will go to great lengths to avoid them. The MAW process is most likely to be successful if the individual is well engaged in treatment or mutual aid interventions and actively addressing issues relating to drug use, including stabilising the amount used, resolving life problems, cutting links with other drug users and developing strategies for relapse prevention. Opiate withdrawal can actually increase the risk of mortality from overdose as opiate tolerance disappears rapidly after abstinence is achieved.[32] Careful monitoring of withdrawal symptoms is necessary using standardised scales – for example, the Short Opiate Withdrawal Scale (SOWS) or Clinical Opiate Withdrawal Scale (COWS). Monitoring throughout MAW may reveal either physical or mental illness previously masked by substance use and which may require referral to an appropriate specialist.

There are two broad MAW strategies that might be adopted:

1. *Abrupt opiate discontinuation and symptomatic relief*: stop the use of illicit opiates abruptly and manage the resulting withdrawal symptoms. Making the patient aware of the inevitability of some physical or psychological discomfort prior to commencing MAW reduces distress and discomfort,[33] and medications useful for reducing opiate withdrawal symptoms are listed in Table 14.5.
2. *Stabilisation followed by taper from buprenorphine or methadone*: This approach is recommended as the first-line MAW treatment in NICE Clinical Guidance.[34] *Buprenorphine* has the benefit that it is straightforward to convert to stabilisation or maintenance prescribing if the MAW is unsuccessful. It binds to the opioid receptor long after elimination from the blood which means mild protracted residual withdrawal symptoms similar to (but of less severity than) methadone. Patients already stabilised on buprenorphine should receive a gradual dose reduction – for example, reduce by up to 2 mg each time

until 4 mg is reached, 0.4 mg each time until 0.4 mg is reached, then halve the dose and stop. The actual rate should depend on the psychological preparedness of the individual. Adjunctive medications are not typically needed, although a hypnotic maybe useful for the 10-day period around termination of the dose. Patients not already stabilised on buprenorphine (i.e. using heroin) may benefit from a brief period of stabilisation followed by a reduction over a 10- to 14-day period. Stabilisation may occur over one to two days at between 8 and 16 mg/day, followed by a steady reduction to zero over the next 10 days. At the time of writing, long-acting depot buprenorphine is being introduced to the UK and may offer a further way of slowly withdrawing from opiates.

After stabilisation with *methadone*, the dose can be reduced at a rate that will result in cessation in around 12 weeks (usually a reduction of 5 mg every 7 to 14 days). The limited evidence base suggests that a rate directed by the patient is most likely to be successful,[35] and a period of reduction followed by stabilisation is most often successful. A significant number of patients supplement their methadone prescriptions with other opiates when the dose falls below 20 mg daily, and so this regimen is best suited to more stable patients with well-established positive alternatives to drug use and plenty of social support.

Opioid Agonist Treatment (OAT)

The manifestations of heroin dependence are both medical and social (e.g. unsafe injecting, criminal activity and family and relationship dysfunction). Treatment with a long-acting opioid agonist (sometimes called opioid substitution treatment or 'maintenance' therapy) aims to manage these problems, allowing the patient to tackle other issues without having to deal with the daily cycle of intoxication and withdrawal. The aim of a prescription is to bring about stability in four domains: substance use, physical and psychological health, social functioning, and offending.

Methadone is a synthetic μ-opioid receptor agonist with similar activity to morphine. Its pharmacological profile makes it ideal for OAT: the oral route avoids the risks associated with injecting, its long half-life allows it to be taken as a single daily dose, and accumulation in the body means that steady-state plasma levels are easily achieved after repeated administration. No serious long-term effects have been associated with continued treatment over 30 years. At steady state, the elimination half-life is roughly 24–36 hours, but there is considerable individual variation (10 to 80 hours). In contrast, the half-life of morphine is about 3 hours, so heroin users need to use the drug at least two to three times per day. In stabilised patients, methadone does not have the pronounced euphoric or sedative effects seen with shorter-acting opioids such as heroin. The 1 mg/1 ml solution used in routine practice has low potential for use by injection. Potential side effects are nausea and vomiting, constipation, drowsiness, respiratory depression and hypotension. Alongside other drugs used in psychiatry, methadone has a dose-related effect in prolonging the QTc interval.[36] Patients with known heart or liver disease, electrolyte abnormalities, a known history of ECG abnormalities (particularly prolonged QTc interval) or taking medication known to inhibit the CYP3A4 system in the liver should therefore be monitored carefully.

Buprenorphine is both a partial μ-opioid receptor agonist and ƙ-opioid receptor antagonist, and its low intrinsic agonist activity gives a milder, less euphoric and less sedating effect than full opioid agonists. Taken sublingually, it has an onset of effect within one hour and peak effect within four hours. Buprenorphine's high affinity for μ-opioid receptors means that doses of 12 mg or more reduce the impact of additional 'on top' heroin use by preventing receptor occupation. Doses many times greater than normal therapeutic doses rarely result in clinically significant respiratory depression. However, the safety of buprenorphine is not clear when it is mixed with high doses of other sedative drugs such as alcohol or benzodiazepines. The sublingual tablets can be crushed to snort or inject, with significantly more potent effects.

Buprenorphine's high affinity for the opioid receptor means that it competitively removes full agonists occupying brain receptors, and the resulting partial agonist effect is experienced as opiate withdrawal. Patients should be therefore cautioned about the possibility of 'precipitated' opiate withdrawal symptoms if buprenorphine is commenced within 12 hours of heroin or 72 hours of methadone use. It also follows that buprenorphine should be used with caution in people with recurrent acute or chronic pain conditions requiring opioid analgesia with a full opioid agonist. Buprenorphine is available with the opioid antagonist naloxone in a combined sublingual tablet (buprenorphine-naloxone in a 4:1 ratio). When taken sublingually as intended, the naloxone has low bioavailability and does not diminish the therapeutic effect of the buprenorphine. However, if injected, the naloxone has high bioavailability and is liable to precipitate withdrawal in an opioid-dependent patient, therefore discouraging further misuse. A monthly depot version of the drug has recently become available in the UK.

The minimum criteria for commencing OAT are ICD-11 opioid dependence AND at least three months regular opioid use OR high-risk behaviour OR failed attempts at abstinence. An OAT prescription should never be started in a new patient that does not have an oral fluid/urine test positive for opioids (although be aware of the limitations and potential false positives associated with each type of testing[12]). The assessment process should establish the initial aims of OAT, and two broad strategies might be considered:

1. *Short- or medium-term stabilisation*: OAT can be a means of achieving stability and lifestyle changes that will lead to abstinence. The aim is to replace the illicit drugs with opioid medication, thus completely relieving or preventing any withdrawal symptoms. The ultimate aim is to achieve abstinence from all opioid drugs by moving towards a

withdrawal phase once stability has been reached. If MAW is unsuccessful, it may be necessary to switch to strategy 2.

2. *Longer-term maintenance treatment*: This requires doses greater than those required for stabilisation in order to extinguish opioid craving and block the reinforcing effects of illicit opioids. Outcomes are improved by understanding that the goal of maintenance is acceptable in its own right, rather than treating it as a stepping stone to abstinence.

An extensive body of evidence shows that long-term higher-dose (>60 mg/day) methadone prescribing programmes produce better outcomes than short-term, low-dose programmes.[37] However, there are successes from short-term, low-dose programmes, and a 'one-size-fits-all' approach does not always apply. UK prescribing guidance recommends maintaining individuals on a daily dose of methadone between 60 mg and 120 mg.[11] Higher doses can reduce heroin consumption, but caution needs to be observed if there is associated alcohol or other benzodiazepine dependence. Receiving a prescription for OAT at an early stage in the treatment process may be a key factor in engaging the person in treatment, but it is important to remember that other approaches may also be useful. In particular, starting a substitute prescription is likely to remove some of the drivers that led the individual to seek help in the first place, and so it is important to work closely with the patient to continue the momentum towards recovery in the first three months of treatment. The service should present a positive, optimistic attitude at the point of initial assessment, emphasising the patient's strengths and existing 'recovery capital' and possible exits out of treatment.[38] An early meeting with someone with lived experience of recovery can inspire hope, and all potential pharmacological, psychological and social options should be presented prior to the first meeting with a prescriber.

Psychosocial Interventions

Interventions based on psychological or social processes of change are a mainstay of treatment for alcohol or drug use disorders. Evidence-based treatments include:

Motivational interviewing (MI): This uses a guiding style to engage with patients, elicit and reinforce their strengths and goals, and evoke their own motivational statements for change in their patterns of substance use. It has been shown to promote behaviour change in many health care settings and lead to better outcomes for patients.[39] MI has been incorporated into a manual-based intervention for alcohol use disorders, which has been shown to be effective in large research trials in the USA and the UK.

Cognitive behavioural therapy (CBT): Cognitive techniques (e.g. identifying and challenging negative thinking) and behavioural 'experiments' are used to help achieve specific goals (e.g. cutting down or stopping use). 'Relapse Prevention' is one example of an individual- or group-based CBT programme that may include identifying high-risk situations and triggers for craving, developing strategies to avoid such situations, enhancing skills to manage cravings and painful emotions without using alcohol, learning to cope with lapses, and increasing pleasurable sober activities and relationships.[40]

Contingency management: Operant conditioning theory suggests that some consequences strengthen behaviour, whilst others weaken it. The Community Reinforcement Approach is based on the principle that individuals have their own positive reinforcers in their environment, which maintain both their using and non-using behaviours. By altering these reinforcement contingencies (and involving the patient's social network in this process), the individual can make changes in their lifestyle that will support abstinence from alcohol.[41]

Family and social interventions: These can be grouped into three areas: (1) working with family members to encourage people with SUD into treatment – for example, the Community Reinforcement and Family Training (CRAFT),[42] (2) involving the social network or family members in the treatment of people with SUD,[43] and (3) treatment of family members in their own right – for example, the 5-Step Method.[44] It is often said that the opposite of addiction is 'connection', so paying close attention to the social environment can be a crucial part of effective treatment.

Mutual aid/self-help approaches: Alcoholics Anonymous (AA) and Narcotics Anonymous (NA) are self-help fellowships that provide support, friendship and a structured programme of recovery. The 12 Steps lay out a process that individuals are recommended to follow, based on the belief that substance dependence is a disease and can be treated by lifelong abstinence. Although the main text of AA asserts that recovery is achieved through 'spiritual awakening', findings from studies on mechanisms of behaviour change suggest this may be true for only a minority of individuals with high SUD severity.[45] In fact, AA's beneficial effects appear to be achieved mainly by social, cognitive and affective mechanisms similar to those mobilised in formal treatment, but it is able to do this over an extended period for free and in the community in which the individual lives. Manual-driven Twelve Step Facilitation approaches guide professionals through the process of effectively linking their patients to mutual aid meetings, with the aim of maintaining abstinence whilst in treatment and sustaining gains made after treatment concludes. Other mutual-help groups such as SMART Recovery are also increasingly available in the UK. All psychiatrists should attend at least one 12-Step meeting as a learning experience.

Although research suggests that such treatments lead to improved outcomes when compared to no treatment at all, the evidence favouring one type of psychosocial intervention over another is less clear.[46] Other factors such as therapist characteristics and service variables are also important.[47] There is wide variation in the uptake and implementation of psychosocial approaches in the UK, and most practices involve an eclectic approach that combines strategies from various psychological approaches that typically last 12 weeks. Psychological treatments can also be used to help people experiencing harmful substance use or dependence to address co-existing problems such as anxiety and depression.

Relapse Prevention Medication

Alcohol: *Acamprosate* and the opioid antagonist *naltrexone* are both effective in increasing the time to first drink and to relapse in people with alcohol dependence who have achieved abstinence.[48] Both should be started as soon as possible after withdrawal and always in combination with a parallel psychosocial intervention. They may be prescribed for six months or more depending on perceived benefit. *Disulfiram* is a deterrent that works by interfering with the metabolism of alcohol, leading to an unpleasant set of symptoms including hypertension and a throbbing headache if alcohol is drunk after taking it. It should be used with caution in pregnancy, severe mental illness, stroke, heart disease or hypertension. *Nalmefene* is licenced for reducing alcohol consumption in adults with alcohol dependence who continue to drink more than 7.5 units/day (men) and 5 units/day (women) but without physical withdrawal symptoms or the requirement for immediate medically assisted withdrawal.

Opiates: The opioid antagonist *naltrexone* is also used to help prevent relapse to opiate use following MAW. It provides 72 hours of blockade of opioid receptors with little intrinsic action of its own. If the patient takes the naltrexone tablets as prescribed, any use of heroin or other opioid drugs will have no effect. It therefore provides protection against a sudden urge to use opioids, although it will not stop cravings to use heroin or maintain motivation to remain abstinent. However, the loss of tolerance produced by naltrexone means that an individual's usual dose of injectable heroin may now prove fatal. Furthermore, there is a risk of overdose if a patient who has taken naltrexone in the previous few days tries to take larger doses of heroin in order to overcome the blockade and achieve a pleasurable effect. Although only a minority of opioid-dependent people seek naltrexone treatment, a significant proportion of those who comply with the treatment for three months or more remain abstinent from heroin. Depot and implantable forms of naltrexone are available, but they are not yet licenced in the UK.

Integrating the Components of Treatment

Various attempts have been made to summarise and coordinate these components into a treatment system for alcohol[49,50] or drug use disorders.[51] Large-scale national evaluations and clinical trials show that longer periods of treatment are associated with better outcomes. Furthermore, outcome research suggests that reliable behavioural change only appears after about three months of treatment. Despite extensive efforts to understand which characteristics of patients entering the 'black box' of treatment predict the best results, no clear pattern has been established. However, when the treatment process is broken down into stages (similar to the well-known 'Stages of Change'[52]), some useful predictors of retention in treatment and subsequent outcomes emerge. For example, patients with higher levels of motivation and readiness for treatment at the start of the episode tend to have better results. There are three stages of treatment:

1. *Early Engagement*: patients entering treatment must participate (i.e. attend treatment sessions) and begin forming positive therapeutic relationships. These indicators of early engagement are especially important in the first two months after treatment admission and are associated with patient motivation and treatment readiness.
2. *Early Recovery*: indicators of early recovery such as behaviour change (i.e. substance use) and psychosocial change (i.e. addressing problems in housing, relationships) by month three are directly related to the level of early engagement shown by patients.
3. *Retention/Transition*: positive early recovery indicators predict better retention in treatment.

Different outcome measures are important at each stage of the journey, and psychosocial and other interventions should be tailored to the relevant stage. These approaches have been summarised and packaged in a node-link map form[53] and are available from www.gov.uk/government/publications/routes-to-recovery-from-substance-addiction. The process of treatment may be seen as a journey from interventions delivered by experts-by-training to peer- and community-led strategies. Whereas the initial goal may be reduction of risks, as engagement builds, there is a shift to behaviour change and a reconfiguration of the patient's physical and social environment towards one that supports abstinence, citizenship and self-efficacy (Figure 14.2).

Recovery and Recovery Orientated Integrated Systems of Care (ROISC)

Alcohol or drug dependence is a chronic condition that usually involves cycles of abstinence and relapse over many years. With a lesser degree of severity, remission may end a chapter in the person's life that never recurs. In more severe cases, remission requires a move from being immersed in the 'culture of addiction' to the 'culture of recovery'.[54] This change in outlook and identity fundamentally alters how an individual thinks about themselves, and such people describe themselves as being 'in recovery'.[55] Recovery is underpinned

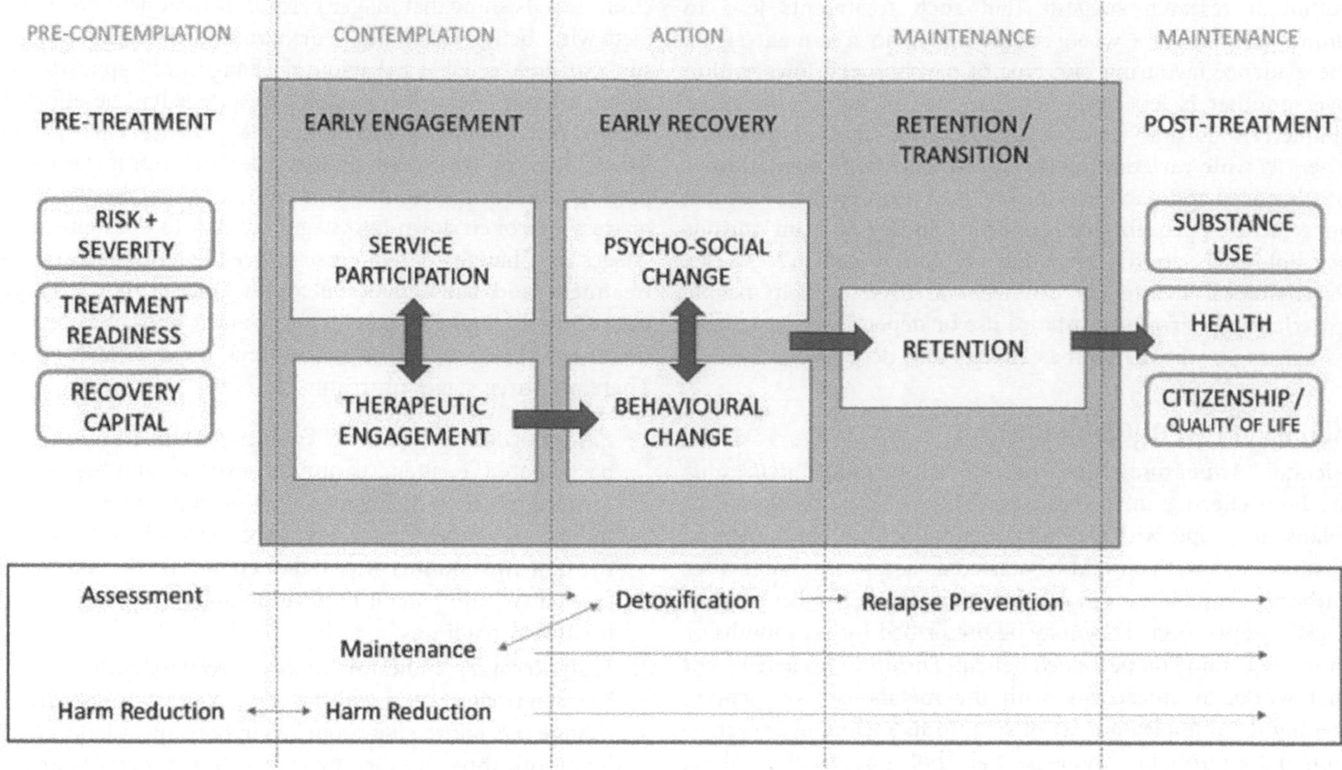

Figure 14.2 The 'black box' of treatment showing the stages that must be negotiated, with the relevant potential treatment strategies shown at the bottom.

by a new sense of 'hope' that things will be better in the future and requires the building of personal and social assets by the individual and those around them. It might utilise a variety of different forms of formal and informal support or may occur without any external help: one size does not fit all. Recovery is a process and not a single event, takes time to achieve and effort to maintain, and must be voluntarily sustained in order to be lasting. It has three important elements:[56]

1. A comfortable and sustained freedom from compulsion to use substances. For many people, this will require abstinence from the problem substance or all substances, but for others, it may mean abstinence supported by prescribed medication or consistently moderate use of some substances (e.g. the occasional alcoholic drink).
2. Optimised health and wellbeing, encompassing both good physical and mental health as far as they may be attained for a person.
3. A satisfying and meaningful life, as defined by the person themselves, involving participation in the rights, roles and responsibilities of society. For many people, this is likely to include being able to participate fully in family life and be able to undertake work in a paid or voluntary capacity.

Recovery looks different for different people, and appropriate interventions and resources should be matched to the relevant point in an individual's journey. Spirituality, peer support and family support and involvement are all important components.[57] A chronic disease often requires both intensive and extensive treatment to bring about remission, and the ideal system of care blends both professional treatment services and peer-led recovery support services in a seamless Recovery Oriented Integrated System of Care (ROISC).[38,58] Professional treatment services and peer-led recovery support services (RSS) are organised into a framework that incorporates the whole health and social care system. The ROISC should be easy to navigate, transparent and responsive to the cultural diversity of the community in which it is grounded.

The ROISC framework avoids the polarised debate that often develops between harm reduction and abstinence-based approaches, as well as between 'experts by training' and 'experts by experience'. As Figure 14.3 shows, the system has both elements, with a gradual transition towards self care and peer support as recovery develops. The emphasis is placed on each group of services delivering their component of the system to the highest level, with assertive linkage between professional and recovery support services and resources within the surrounding community. Professional treatment of SUD is often conceptualised as an acute intervention, and if success rates are considered in terms of episodes of abstinence, treatment is successful 20–60% of the time.[59] However, when combined with long-term recovery support, outcomes improve dramatically.[60]

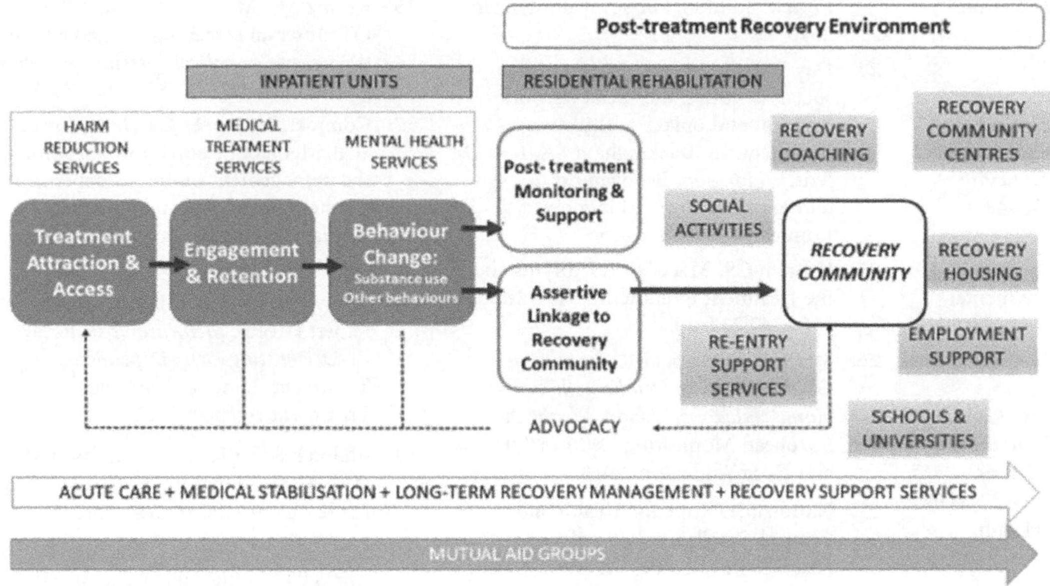

Figure 14.3 A schematic diagram showing a Recovery Orientated Integrated System of Care (ROISC). Services led by 'experts by training' are shown on the left, and those led by 'experts by experience' are on the right.

Conclusions

Problems relating to alcohol or drugs occur across a spectrum of levels of consumption and may be physical, psychological or social in nature. At one extreme, there is a small but significant proportion of people who develop dependence and may require both intensive and extensive support. However, on a population level, huge reductions in the harm caused by psychoactive substances could be made if everyone was encouraged to use a bit less. All health and social care professionals should be able to screen for potential alcohol use disorders, deliver brief advice and refer on to specialist services where appropriate. They should also have an awareness of the common illicit drugs and the potential problems they are associated with. The evidence base for treatment of substance use disorders has developed over the past 30 years, and clinicians should be positive and optimistic that meaningful change in behaviour can be achieved. Prompt referral to the right level of support and treatment may prevent future problems. Recovery support services play a crucial part in sustaining any gains made in treatment, and many people recover without using professionally directed treatment at all. It is estimated that approximately 10 per cent of the population of the USA is in remission from a substance use disorder of any severity.[61,62]

References

1. World Health Organization. *Global Status Report on Alcohol and Health 2018*. Geneva: WHO Press; 2018.
2. Volkow ND, Koob GF, McLellan AT. Neurobiologic advances from the brain disease model of addiction. *New England Journal of Medicine* 2016;374 (4):363–71.
3. West R, Brown J. *Theory of Addiction*. 2nd ed. Chichester: Wiley Blackwell; 2013.
4. World Health Organization. *Lexicon of Alcohol and Drug Terms*. Geneva: World Health Organization; 1994. www.who.int/publications/i/item/9241544686.
5. Hasin DS, O'Brien CP, Auriacombe M, et al. DSM-5 criteria for substance use disorders: recommendations and rationale. *American Journal of Psychiatry* 2013;170:834–51.
6. Babor TF, Higgins-Biddle JC, Saunders JB, et al. *AUDIT: The Alcohol Use Disorder Identification Test. Guidelines for Use in Primary Health Care*. Geneva: World Health Organization; 2001.
7. Rice P, Drummond C. The price of a drink: the potential of alcohol minimum unit pricing as a public health measure in the UK. *The British Journal of Psychiatry* 2012;201 (3):169–71.
8. Sheron N, Gilmore I. Effect of policy, economics, and the changing alcohol marketplace on alcohol related deaths in England and Wales. *BMJ* 2016;353: i1860.
9. Pryce R, Buykx P, Gray L, et al. *Estimates of Alcohol Dependence in England based on APMS 2014, including Estimates of Children Living in a Household with an Adult with Alcohol Dependence: Prevalence, Trends, and Amenability to Treatment*. London: Public Health England; 2017.
10. NHS Digital. *Statistics on Drugs Misuse, England, 2019: Health and Social Care Information Centre*. digital.nhs.uk/data-and-information/publications/statistical/statistics-on-drug-misuse/2019/part-3-drug-use-among-adults.
11. Clinical Guidelines on Drug Misuse and Dependence Update 2017 Independent Expert Working Group. *Drug Misuse*

and Dependence: UK Guidelines on Clinical Management. London: Department of Health; 2017.

12. Wolff K, Welch S, Strang J. Laboratory investigations for assessment and management of drug problems. In: Day E (ed.) *Clinical Topics in Addiction*. London: RCPsych; 2007: 130–48.
13. Weaver T, Madden P, Charles V, et al. Comorbidity of substance misuse and mental illness in community mental health and substance misuse services. *British Journal of Psychiatry* 2003;183:304–13.
14. Public Health England. *Better Care for People with Co-occurring Mental Health and Alcohol/Drug Use Conditions. A Guide for Commissioners and Service Providers*. London: Public Health England; 2017.
15. Stone AL, Becker LG, Huber AM, et al. Review of risk and protective factors of substance use and problem use in emerging adulthood. *Addictive Behaviors* 2012;37(7):747–75.
16. Anderson P, Baumberg B. *Alcohol in Europe: A Public Health Perspective*. London: Institute of Alcohol Studies; 2006.
17. Day E, Khurmi S. Alcohol. In: Gray D, Cormac I (eds.) *Essentials of Physical Health in Psychiatry*. London: RCPsych Publications; 2012: 301–15.
18. Gracie K, Hancox RJ. Cannabis use disorder and the lungs. *Addiction*. 2020;116(1):182–90.
19. Haim DY, Lippmann ML, Goldberg SK, et al. The pulmonary complications of crack cocaine. *A Comprehensive Review. Chest* 1995;107:233–40.
20. Public Health England. *Shooting Up: Infections Among People Who Inject Drugs in the UK, 2018: An Update, December 2019*. London: Public Health England; 2019.
21. Copello A, Templeton L, Powell J. The impact of addiction on the family: estimates of prevalence and costs. *Drugs: Education, Prevention and Policy* 2010;17(Suppl 1):63–74.
22. Burkinshaw P, Knight J, Anders P, et al. *An Evidence Review of the Outcomes That Can Be Expected of Drug Misuse Treatment in England*. London: Public Health England; 2017.
23. Public Health England. *The Public Health Burden of Alcohol and the Effectiveness and Cost-Effectiveness of Alcohol Control Policies: An Evidence Review*. London: Public Health England; 2016.
24. Day E. Building bridges to positive social identities: the social network diagram and opiate substitution treatment. In: Buckingham SA, Best D (eds.) *Addiction, Behavioural Change and Social Identity*. Abingdon: Routledge; 2017: 172–95.
25. O'Brien CP, McLellan AT. Myths about the treatment of addiction. *The Lancet* 1996;347:237–40.
26. Strang J, McDonald R. *Preventing Opioid Overdose Deaths with Take-Home Naloxone*. Lisbon, Portugal: European Monitoring Centre for Drugs and Drug Addiction; 2016.
27. National Institute for Health and Clinical Excellence. *Alcohol-use Disorders: Preventing the Development of Hazardous and Harmful Drinking*. London: NICE; 2010.
28. Day E, Copello A, Hull M. Assessment and management of alcohol use disorders. *BMJ: British Medical Journal* 2015;350.
29. Miller WR, Sanchez VC. Motivating young adults for treatment and lifestyle change. In: Howard G (ed.) *Issues in Alcohol Use and Misuse by Young Adults*. Notre Dame, IN: University of Notre Dame Press; 1993: 55–82.
30. National Institute for Health and Clinical Excellence. *Alcohol-Use Disorders: Diagnosis and Clinical Management of Alcohol-Related Physical Complications (CG100)*. London: NICE; 2010.
31. Day E, Daly C. Clinical management of the alcohol withdrawal syndrome. *Addiction* 2021;117(3):804–14.
32. Strang J, McCambridge J, Best D, et al. Loss of tolerance and overdose mortality after inpatient opiate detoxification: follow up study. *BMJ* 2003;326(7396):959–60.
33. Green L, Gossop M. Effects of information on the opiate withdrawal syndrome. *British Journal of Addiction* 1988;83:305–9.
34. National Treatment Agency for Substance Misuse. *Drug Misuse: Opioid Detoxification. Report No.: Clinical Guideline 52*. London: NICE; 2007.
35. Nosyk B, Sun H, Evans E, et al. Defining dosing pattern characteristics of successful tapers following methadone maintenance treatment: results from a population-based retrospective cohort study. *Addiction* 2012;107(9):1621–9.
36. Krantz MJ, Martin J, Stimmel B, et al. QTc interval screening in methadone treatment. *Annals of Internal Medicine* 2009;150(6):387–95.
37. Connock M, Juarez-Garcia A, Jowett S, et al. Methadone and buprenorphine for the management of opioid dependence: a systematic review and economic evaluation. *Health Technology Assessment* 2006;11(9):1–171.
38. Recovery Orientated Drug Treatment Expert Group. *Medications in Recovery: Re-Orientating Drug Dependence Treatment*. London: National Treatment Agency; 2012.
39. Rollnick S, Butler CC, Kinnersley P, et al. Motivational interviewing. *British Medical Journal* 2010;340:1242–5.
40. Mitcheson L, Maslin J, Meynen T, et al. *Applied Cognitive and Behavioural Approaches to the Treatment of Addiction: A Practical Treatment Guide*. Chichester: Wiley-Blackwell; 2010.
41. Meyers RJ, Miller WR. *A Community Reinforcement Approach to Addiction Treatment*. New York: Cambridge University Press; 2001.
42. Meyers RJ, Miller WR, Hill DE, et al. Community reinforcement and family training (CRAFT): engaging unmotivated drug users in treatment. *Journal of Substance Abuse* 1999;10:291–308.
43. Copello A, Orford J, Hodgson R, et al. *Social Behaviour and Network Therapy for Alcohol Problems*. London: Routledge; 2009.
44. Copello A, Templeton L, Orford J, et al. The 5-Step Method: principles and practice. *Drugs: Education, Prevention, and Policy* 2010;17(s1):86–99.
45. Kelly JF. Is Alcoholics Anonymous religious, spiritual, neither? Findings from 25 years of mechanisms of behavior change research. *Addiction* 2017;112(6):929–36.
46. Day E, Mitcheson L. Psychosocial interventions in OST services: does the evidence provide a case for optimism or nihilism? *Addiction* 2017;113 (8):1329–36.
47. Miller WR, Moyers TB. The forest and the trees: relational and specific factors in addiction treatment. *Addiction* 2014;110(3):401–13.
48. National Institute for Health and Clinical Excellence. *Alcohol-use Disorders: Diagnosis, Assessment and*

Management of Harmful Drinking and Alcohol Dependence. London: NICE; 2011.

49. Department of Health, *National Treatment Agency for Substance Misuse. Models of Care for Alcohol Misusers (MoCAM)*. London: National Treatment Agency for Substance Misuse; 2006.
50. Rush B. A systems approach to estimating the required capacity of alcohol treatment services. *British Journal of Addiction* 1990;85:49–59.
51. Simpson DD. A conceptual framework for drug treatment process and outcomes. *Journal of Substance Abuse Treatment* 2004;27:99–121.
52. Prochaska JO, DiClemente CC. Transtheoretical therapy: toward a more integrative model of change. *Psychotherapy Theory Research and Practice* 1982;19 (3):276–88.
53. Day E. *Routes to Recovery via the Community*. London: Public Health England; 2013.
54. White WL. *Pathways from the Culture of Addiction to the Culture of Recovery*. 2nd ed. Center City, MN: Hazelden; 1996.
55. US Department of Health and Human Services (HHS) Office of the Surgeon General. *Facing Addiction in America: The Surgeon General's Report on Alcohol, Drugs, and Health*. Washington, DC: Health and Human Services; 2016.
56. UK Drug Policy Commission Recovery Consensus Group. *A Vision of Recovery*. London: UK Drug Policy Commission; 2008.
57. Davidson L, White W. The concept of recovery as an organizing principle for integrating mental health and addiction services. *Journal of Behavioral Health Services & Research* 2007;34(2):109–20.
58. Ashford RD, Brown AM, Ryding R, et al. Building recovery ready communities: the recovery ready ecosystem model and community framework. *Addiction Research & Theory* 2020;28(1):1–11.
59. National Institute on Drug Abuse. *Principles of Drug Addiction Treatment: A Research-Based Guide*. Bethesda: National Institute on Drug Abuse; 2018. Contract No.: 05/06/2020.
60. Simoneau H, Kamgang E, Tremblay J, et al. Efficacy of extensive intervention models for substance use disorders: a systematic review. *Drug and Alcohol Review* 2018;37(S1):S246–S62.
61. Kelly JF, Bergman B, Hoeppner BB, et al. Prevalence and pathways of recovery from drug and alcohol problems in the United States population: implications for practice, research, and policy. *Drug and Alcohol Dependence* 2017;181:162–9.
62. White WL. *Recovery/Remission from Substance Use Disorders: An Analysis of Reported Outcomes in 415 Scientific Reports, 1868–2011*. Chicago/Philadelphia: Philadelphia Department of Behavioral Health and Intellectual Disability Services & Great Lakes Addiction Technology Transfer Center; 2012.
63. Office for Health Improvement & Disparities. *Guidance Alcohol: Applying All Our Health*; 2022. www.gov.uk/government/publications/alcohol-applying-all-our-health/alcohol-applying-all-our-health (accessed 14 September 2023).
64. NHS. *Alcohol Advice*. www.nhs.uk/live-well/alcohol-advice/ (accessed 14 September 2023).

Chapter 15

Suicide and Self Harm

George Stein

More than three-quarters of a million people die through suicide worldwide each year, and the problem of suicide is central to psychiatry. The topic is also very old, and there are descriptions in the Egyptian literature that predate the Old Testament (OT) by many centuries. However, the OT is unique in presenting a collection of several case histories of suicide, suicidal thoughts and self harm, all within the confines of a single volume and so perhaps provides the 'first chapter' on the topic of suicidology.[1] The OT views the topic with equanimity; there is no law banning it nor is there any blame or moral condemnation for the act. It was duly recorded by the scribes of the day when it occurred in a person of some importance, such as a king. In this brief introduction, an account is given of how our attitudes to suicide have changed over the last three millennia.

Life in the ancient world was much more of a chance affair than today, and so attitudes to death were far more fatalistic. Today, most people can expect to reach old age, and the average life expectancy in the UK is around 85 for a man and 88 for a woman. Life expectancy in the ancient world is unknown because there were no records, but parish records, which start in the Middle Ages, suggest a life expectancy of around 28 to 30 years; this is unlikely to have been any better in biblical times. A premature death lurked round the corner for all as a result of wars, famine, epidemics or some untreatable medical condition, or death in childhood. In such a world, a self killing might be a painless way out, and so neither the Bible nor the much larger Greek literature on suicide gives any suggestion of blame or moral condemnation.

Barraclough,[2] a psychiatrist who did some of the first rigorous research into suicide, lists 11 biblical suicides and 15 descriptions of suicide in the Bible. Around four of these are the deaths of defeated kings: Saul, Abimelech, Samson and Zimri. There are also the suicides of shame and betrayal: Ahithopel, Macron and, in the New Testament, Judas Iscariot. There are two suicide-martyrdom deaths. Of these, the death of King Saul is the best known, and the Bible has three separate accounts of his death following his defeat at the hands of the Philistines at Mt Gilboa.

Then Saul said to his armour bearer:

> draw your sword and thrust me through with it, so that these uncircumcised may not come and thrust me through and make sport of me. But his armour bearer was unwilling, for he was terrified, *so Saul took his own sword and fell upon it.*[5] When his armour bearer saw that Saul was dead, he also fell upon his sword and died with him. (1 Sam. 31:4–6)

Saul is frightened of his uncertain future at the hands of the Philistines, who were the victors, and he believed that death was a better option. Similar thinking can occur in a modern suicide where, following a serious loss such as a broken relationship or the loss of a job, death seems preferable to the uncertain future, although few today can boast of such a grand loss as a defeat by the Philistines. Some 500 years later, the book of Chronicles (*circa* 400BCE) gives a similar account of the death of Saul but gives a different theological reason for it:

> So Saul died for his unfaithfulness. He was unfaithful to the Lord in that he did not keep the command of the Lord, moreover he had consulted with a medium seeking guidance from the Lord. Therefore the Lord put him to death and turned the kingdom over to David, son of Jesse. (1 Chr. 10:13)

In this account, it is God who has caused the suicide. The chronicler thus transforms Saul's defeat by the Philistines and his suicide into an act of divine judgement. Saul's unfaithfulness, of course, anticipates the unfaithfulness that will be practised by many later kings and many other individuals as well, and this is the origin of the idea that suicide is an act of God.

The suicide of Samson and his death also has modern parallels. Once Samson had been captured, the Philistines blinded him. The story is told in the book of Judges.

> 27Now the house was full of men and women; all the lords of the Philistines were there, and on the roof there were about three thousand men and women, who looked on while Samson performed. v28Then Samson called to the LORD and said, 'Lord GOD, remember me and strengthen me only this once, O God, so that with this one act of revenge I may pay back the Philistines for my two eyes.' v30Then Samson said, 'Let me die with the Philistines.' He strained with all his might; and the house fell on the lords and all the people who were in it. So those he killed at his death were more than those he had killed during his life. (Judges 16:27–30)

Today many people who have attempted suicide often give a story of revenge against a rejecting partner, an overly harsh employer or some other oppressor as the cause of their suicidal act. The motivation behind the modern suicide bomber who carries out his deadly deed in a large hotel or in the public market has the clear intention of causing the maximum number of deaths, sometimes in the name of religion or some political cause, and in many ways, this resembles the suicide of Samson, and such revenge suicides have been termed *Samsonic.*

Some of the Biblical suicides are planned events, such as that of Ahithopel.[1] He was David's chief advisor, but during the revolt of Absalom (David's son), he switched sides and joined Absalom. However, his advice was not followed, and Absalom was defeated.

> When Ahithopel saw that his counsel was not followed, he saddled his donkey and went off home to his own city. He set his house in order and hanged himself: he died and was buried in the tomb of his father. (2 Sam. 17:23)

When viewed from a modern psychiatric perspective, the most authentic feature of the Ahithopel saga lies in the very minor detail that '*he set his house in order*'. Sometimes, those who plan their suicide will have a short delay between their decision and the execution of the act itself, usually used to arrange their affairs – for example, by writing a suicide note to explain their actions or to arrange their financial matters. During this delay, they may become calm, and later whilst in a settled state, they take their own lives, and this is what Ahithopel seems to have done.

In ancient Greece, suicide was viewed as a mainly stoic phenomenon. The most famous of the Greek suicides was that of Socrates who drank hemlock, and Plato records his discussions with Socrates on the topic of suicide in his tract *Phaedo.* Socrates expresses his value for life, which he argues should not be taken away lightly.

> The Gods are our guardians and we humans are the possessions of the Gods. If one of your possessions should go on to kill itself when you had not intended that you wished it to die, would you not be angry with it and punish it?[3]

However, Socrates then went on to argue that there were certain circumstances when the taking of one's life become permissible, as in his own case, because he was already under a sentence of death. 'It is not unreasonable to say that a person must not kill themselves until the Gods send some necessity (*anangke*) upon him – such as has now come upon me.' Socrates then came to view his forthcoming suicide positively and indeed urged every person 'with an interest in Philosophy to come after me as quickly as they can'. Many famous Greeks ended their lives through suicide, and this was not impulsive but was planned and done in a state of calm. Within this hall of fame were Pythagoras aged 82, Anaxagoras at 72, Epicurus at 70, Diogenes at 80 and most ostentatiously, Empedocoles, who at 71 flung himself into the volcano Mt Etna. Elderly males are known to have a high suicide rate, but there is no modern equivalent list of such intellectual heavyweights to have perished at their own hands.

Such positive attitudes to suicide seemed to be more common in the ancient world than today and probably led to some people seeking martyrdom, initially amongst the Jews as a way of preserving their identity and faith whilst living in the Persian diaspora and later amongst the early Christians also as an act of devotion to demonstrate their faith.

Two sects in the early Church, the Montanists of the second century and then the later Donatists, an extreme North African Christian sect of the fourth and fifth centuries CE, displayed florid suicidal behaviours. This turned the opinion of the Catholic church under Augustine against the moral acceptability of suicide. Almost as a reaction, Pope Augustine decreed suicide was to be separated from martyrdom and identified more with murder, and this is set out in the Augustinian text *Against Gaudentium* (a Donatist Bishop) as well as in his book *The City of God.*[4]

Augustine based his case against suicide on similar arguments that Socrates had expounded in *Phaedo*, namely that to sever the bonds between body and soul prematurely usurped a privilege belonging only to God. To do so would be an act of murder and so also violated the sixth commandment of the Decalogue (thou shalt not kill). From that time on, Christianity has regarded suicide as a form of murder – an immoral act alongside other major sins such as apostasy and adultery.

A series of church synods over the next few centuries gradually hardened the Church's attitude to suicide. Thus, in the council of Arles (452 CE), suicide was denounced as the work of the devil. The synod of Braga (536 CE) decreed that full burial rites should be denied to those who died through suicide. Attempted suicide was to be punished at the synod of Toledo (693 CE) by exclusion from church practice. In 1284 CE, the synod of Nimes denied the rite of burial in consecrated ground to those who died through suicide. This led to suicide victims being buried just outside the walls of the churchyard.

Colt (1987)[5] has described some of the rituals performed on those who died through suicide practised in more primitive societies, and these include decapitation, burying the corpse outside the city limits, and publicly burning the corpse of the suicide victim. These primitive rituals were gradually incorporated by the organised church, ultimately leading to laws penalising survivors. Suicide was a crime against God; someone had to be punished for it, and since the deceased was gone, the punishment was meted out to the surviving family, who were to be disinherited and sometimes even fined as well. Eventually, it was decreed that the body of a suicide had to be buried outside the town, preferably at a crossroads, sometimes with a stake driven though their heart and a stone placed over the face. The logic of a burial at the crossroads was that the traffic going over two roads was heavier than that passing over only one, and this would make it much more difficult for the ghost of the suicide to escape and return to haunt the survivors. Driving a stake through the victim's heart gave added protection by preventing the ghost of the suicide victim from escaping.

This led to relatives doing their best to conceal the body and the subject's mode of death. By the later Middle Ages, the expropriation of the properties gradually ceased. There were no punishments for the relatives, but this was replaced by stigma, which was wrapped up in the prevailing fears of the day: superstitions and prejudices connected to insanity. During the seventeenth century, there was a realisation that many people who died through suicide were insane and so the courts had to make a decision as to whether the person was insane and therefore innocent of the crime (*non compos mentis)* or guilty of a crime against themselves (*felo de se*). Suicide became a crime against the state as well as a crime against God.

By the nineteenth century, some countries began to publish suicide statistics, and Morselli had demonstrated that Catholic countries had lower suicide rates than Protestant ones, a finding that was confirmed by the French sociologist Durkheim (1897) in his great book '*Le Suicide*'.[6] Durkheim began to apply statistical methods to the epidemiology of suicide and is now considered the father of modern sociology as well as suicidology. The observation that many people who died through suicide were mentally ill at the time led to an expectation that good treatment of mental illness would reduce its rate. This ownership of the suicide domain was thrust upon psychiatry in the first part of the twentieth century, but many prominent anti-psychiatrists such as Szasz[7] rejected the notion that suicide 'belongs to Psychiatry' and viewed this as no more than a medicalisation of life's problems and that the medical profession bears no responsibility for suicide. At the same time, in the early decades of the twenty-first century, the issues of euthanasia and medically assisted suicide have drawn the medical profession to the centre of a sometimes-heated debate. In countries that have legalised euthanasia – such as Canada, Belgium and the Netherlands – euthanasia now accounts for up to 5 per cent of all deaths. The issue of so-called psychiatric euthanasia, in which a physician kills a person with a severe and enduring psychiatric illness (without a terminal medical condition) at their request is now a subject of deep ethical reflection. Up until the 1950s, most suicide research focused on case histories from psychoanalytic practice, but this was then almost completely eclipsed by the modern statistical approach. Today, almost all research is based on an evidential base. Sociodemographic items such as age, social class, marital or employment status or national gross domestic product (GDP) are fixed and may be correlated with suicide rates. Underlying the modern statistical approach is the notion that external causation is responsible for suicide, but what actually drives a person to take the final step is internal pain. Psychodynamics can offer some insight into this pain. Menninger remarks that both murder and suicide are unnatural killings, but it is murder that has attracted a huge curiosity as evidenced by articles in newspapers, TV programmes and the like, whereas, until recently, very little was written in the public domain about suicide, but this has been changing (see discussion medica guidelines later).

The Suicide Verdict

The World Health Organization's definition of suicide is 'the act of deliberately killing oneself'.[8] However Farmer[9] has stated that the first problem encountered in the study of suicide is its definition in linguistic terms. The word 'suicide' appeared in the English language only in 1635.[10] The nineteenth-century French sociologist Durkheim[6] proposed the following definition of suicide:

> The term suicide is applied to all cases of death resulting directly or indirectly from a positive or negative act of the victim himself, which he knows will produce this result.

Of course, any definition has to address the issue of intent, and this can be problematic to assess retrospectively. Rabbi Akiva, a famous Jewish sage of the first century CE, provides a clear exposition of intent and exactly what comprises an act of suicide:

> What is accounted for a suicide: it is literally one who destroys himself? It is not one who climbs to the top of a tree or the top of the roof and falls to his death. Rather it is one who says 'Behold I am going to climb to the top of the tree or the top of the roof and then I will throw myself down to my death.' And thereupon others see him climb to the top of the tree or the top of the roof and see him fall to his death, such a one is presumed to be a suicide.[11]

Suicide statistics from official figures are derived from what is essentially a legal process. This differs from the way in which a clinical diagnosis is reached. In England and Wales, a coroner brings in a verdict of suicide only when there is explicit evidence of suicidal intent. In the case of self-inflicted death where there is insufficient evidence of an intention to die, the coroner will give either an open verdict or, increasingly, a narrative verdict or one of accidental death or death by misadventure (legally, the last two terms are synonymous). There is no doubt that the majority of cases returned as open verdicts are in fact suicides.[12] A recent innovation in cases of doubtful intent has been the use of narrative verdicts. These were introduced in 2004 in England, Wales and Northern Ireland, and this enabled coroners to give a verdict at an inquest that records only the factual circumstances of the death, instead of one of the standard short verdicts such as 'accidental death' or 'unlawful killing'. Information reviewed in 2012 suggested that the use of narrative verdicts remains relatively low, but individual coroners vary in their use of them. Another recent change is that the level of evidence needed by coroners to conclude whether a death was caused by suicide was changed from the criminal standard of 'beyond all reasonable doubt' to the civil standard of 'on the balance of probabilities' on 26 July 2018. This legal change has not resulted in any significant change in the reported suicide rate in England and Wales, but both changes may be important in rates reported at local levels.

Methods of Suicide

The choice of method of suicide depends on availability, ease of use, social acceptability, cost, symbolism, scope for second

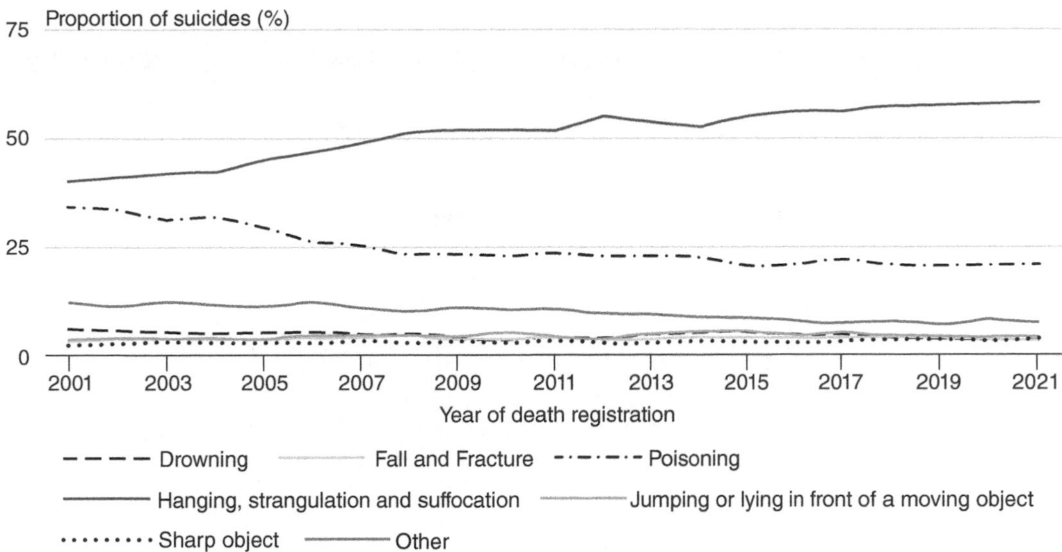

Figure 15.1 Proportion of suicides by method, England and Wales, registered between 2001 and 2021. Office for National Statistics (ONS), released 6 September 2022, ONS website, statistical bulletin, Suicides in England and Wales: 2021 registrations. Open Government Licence v3.0

thoughts and chances for intervention. In England and Wales, self-poisoning is the most common method of suicide for women but is the second most common method for men, after hanging,[13] and is increasing in proportion (see Figure 15.1).[14]

This was a cause for concern, particularly as reducing the availability of hanging is not really feasible, except possibly in a restricted environment such as a hospital ward.

Action taken through a national initiative based on the Confidential Inquiry into Suicide and Homicide sought to remove ligature points in psychiatric ward settings and appears to have had a significant impact on rates of suicide in inpatient settings in the years following. Hanging is the most common method used in Asia, as well as among Asian migrants in the USA.

In low- and middle-income countries, pesticide ingestion is the most common method of committing suicide, and it is thought that one-third of all suicides worldwide are through this method, resulting in between 230,000 to 400,000 deaths per year in 2009. Pesticides usually result in lung damage, which can be fatal.

In the USA, firearms are the chosen method in 60 per cent of suicides.[16] Jumping from tall buildings applies in some Asian-Pacific countries such as Hong Kong, Taiwan and Singapore, where much of the population lives in high rise apartments. Prevention of suicide by restricting access to the means to die through suicide is discussed towards the end of the chapter.

International Suicide Rates

Suicide is a global problem, and insights sometimes gained from changing rates in one country may be applicable in other nations but sometimes they are not. In 2019, an estimated 703,000 people died by suicide and the global age standard rate was 9 per 100,000.[15] The range was between 2 and 80 per 100,000. More than 1.3 per cent of all deaths in 2019 were the result of suicide, which was more than is attributable to malaria, breast cancer, HIV/AIDs, war or homicide. Rates derived from WHO data in a selection of countries is shown in Table 15.1.

The Office of National Statistics[14] reported that, in 2018 in the UK, there were 11.2 deaths from suicide per 100,000 population. Rates in men were 17.2 per 100,000 and in women were 5.4 per 100,000. The male rate exhibited a significant increase from that observed in 2017, while the female rate has been stable for around 10 years. The highest completed suicide rate is seen in both men and women aged 45–49 years (27.1 per 100,000 in men and 9.2 per 100,000 in women). Since the 1980s, there has been a gradual decline in the overall suicide rate. However, the suicide rate in women aged under 25 years has significantly increased since 2012 to its highest ever recorded level of 3.3 per 100,000. Suicide rates in men aged 80–84 years were also significantly higher in 2018 than in 2017 (17.2 per 100,000 vs 9.1 per 100,000). It has been observed around the world that suicide rates tend to increase in the oldest age groups for both men and women, with factors such as psychiatric illness, deterioration of physical health and functioning, and social factors believed to be contributory.

In the 20 years between 2000 and 2019, the global age standard suicide rate decreased by 36%. In the Eastern Mediterranean region, the decrease was 47%; in Europe, 49%; and Australasia, 49%. Only in the Americas did the rate rise by 17%.[15]

Suicide rates vary widely between nations, but this probably relates to factors including culture, substance use, unemployment, urbanicity, migration as well as geography (e.g. effects on social isolation). For individual countries, rates

Table 15.1 International suicide rates for 2019[15] (WHO data)

Suicide rates per 100,000	Both sexes	Female	Male	Data quality
Algeria	2.5	1.8	3.1	4
Ghana	6.6	1.2	11.8	4
Nigeria	3.5	1.9	5.0	4
Egypt	3.0	2.0	4.0	3
Iran	5.2	2.7	7.7	2
Iraq	3.6	1.9	5.2	3
South Africa	23.5	9.8	37.6	
Argentina	8.4	3.3	13.7	2
Brazil	6.9	3.0	10.9	1
Canada	11.8	6.1	17.6	1
Mexico	5.3	2.2	8.5	1
USA	16.1	7.5	25.0	1
Pakistan	8.9	4.3	13.3	4
Europe				
Austria	14.6	6.7	22.8	1
Belarus	21.2	7.7	36.7	1
Bulgaria	9.7	4.4	15.3	2
Czech Republic	12.2	4.8	19.8	1
Denmark	10.7	6.5	14.9	1
Estonia	14.9	6.9	24.3	1
Finland	15.3	7.6	23.6	1
Hungary	16.6	8.3	25.9	1
Latvia	20.1	7.0	35.5	1
Lithuania	26.1	9.6	45.4	1
Russia	25.1	9.1	43.6	2
Ukraine	21.6	6.5	39.2	2
Norway	11.8	8.3	15.8	1
Sweden	14.7	9.5	19.9	1
United Kingdom	7.9	4.0	11.8	1
Spain	7.7	4.1	11.4	1
Netherlands	11.8	8.3	15.5	1
Italy	6.7	3.5	10.1	1
France	13.8	7.6	20.4	1
Germany	12.3	6.2	18.6	1
Asia				
India	12.7	11.1	14.1	4
Indonesia	2.4	1.1	3.7	4
China	8.1	6.2	9.8	4
Japan	15.3	9.2	21.8	1
Sri Lanka	14.0	6.2	22.3	2
South Korea	28.6	16.9	40.2	1
Australia	12.5	6.4	18.6 1	
New Zealand	11.0	5.8	16.5	1

Data quality: Quality 1 = Multiple years of death registration available, and time series can be used for policy evaluation; Quality 2 and 3 = Multiple years of data available. Low quality completeness and issues with cause of death; level 2 denotes moderate quality issues and level 3 denotes severe quality problems; Quality 4 = Death registration data unavailable or unusable due to quality issues.

Table 15.2 Comparison between suicide rates in four European countries (Greece, Ireland, Italy, Portugal) and four Middle Eastern Arab countries[18]

Country	Suicide rate/million	Undetermined deaths	Accidental deaths
Four European countries	66	56	57
Egypt	1	119	33
Jordan	3	60	14
Saudi Arabia	2	174	7
Iraq	1	331	18

tend to be stable over time, and the rank order of countries changes little over time as well. This relative stability of rates was also shown for individual regions as was demonstrated by Durkheim in his studies of the Catholic and Protestant provinces of Germany. Studies of immigrants who have died through suicide in the USA have shown that rates tend to be higher amongst immigrants than in the native born and tend to follow their country of origin, rather than that of their new domicile.[16] Each country will have their own narrative about their suicide rates, whether they are rising or falling, and possible reasons for their distribution, and these are given in a recent large volume,[17] which for reasons of space cannot be given here. However, two situations will be discussed further: the low rates of Middle Eastern Arab countries and the special case of Hungary, at one time the suicide capital of the world.

In Islam, suicide is considered to be a sin. It is *haram* or forbidden. A suicide will bring much shame to the family and so not surprisingly suicide rates appear to be very low in Islamic countries. However, this varies between different Muslim countries, and this effect is not shown in Muslim countries of the former Soviet Union such as Azerbaijan, Kazakhstan, Turkmenistan and Uzbekhistan; the very low reported rates are found only in Middle Eastern Arab nations. A recent study compared the rates for verdicts for suicide, undetermined death and accidental deaths (deaths due to falls, drowning and poisoning) in Muslim countries with the mean rate in four European countries (Ireland, Italy, Greece and Portugal), all of whom also have a strong religious culture (see Table 15.2).

It can be seen that verdicts other than suicide, such as undetermined or accidental deaths, are much preferred instead of suicide in these Middle Eastern countries. Possibly because of the shame associated with a suicide, families bring pressure on to coroners to avoid a suicide verdict whenever possible.

Hungary

Hungary is an interesting case. For many decades, Hungary had the highest suicide rates in the world – in 1987, the rate was 66.1 per 100,000 while at the same time in England and Wales, the rate was 12.1 per 100,000.[19] The problem was mainly male and rural suicide rather than urban, but the explanation was obscure. Earlier hypotheses proposed a lack of treatment of depression especially in men, and this was an early example of 'the unrecognised/untreated male depression' narrative. A Hungarian sociologist, Moksony[20] studied 600 rural villages in Hungary. He visited many of them and found those villages that were economically backward with little development often had a suicide subculture and had much higher rates of suicide than those villages that had high levels of socioeconomic development. People who had lost their position were especially vulnerable; Protestants had higher rates than Catholics. The Hungarian suicide rate peaked in the late 1980s just before the collapse of communism and then began to fall throughout the 1990s, had a brief rise following the 2008 financial crises, and thereafter continued its downward trend. A more recent study[21] addressing the question of why rates have fallen in the 1990s to the present time has to some extent validated the earlier socioeconomic explanation offered by Moksony. Thus, the fall in suicide numbers appeared to correlate with a change in population demographics as the number of people with higher education in the population greatly increased. This resulted in a one-third decrement in the male suicide rate between 1990 and 2011, but amongst women, the decrease in suicide attributable to rising educational levels was only about a tenth. The authors concluded that there was an inverse relationship between suicide rates and educational level and that the data supported the suggestion that educational policy was an indirect health policy.

Epidemiology and Associated Factors

Societal Factors

The first attempt to produce a sociological theory of suicide was made by Durkheim, who examined the suicide rates in various European countries in the mid-nineteenth century.[6] Finding a remarkable stability in ranked order of national suicide rates over successive five-year periods, he suggested that suicide results primarily from social factors. Durkheim argued that the society in which people live exerts control over them in two ways: individuals are integrated into the values and norms of their social group, and in turn, society regulates their goals and aspirations.

Durkheim proposed four types of suicide: egoistic, altruistic, anomic and fatalistic. Egoistic suicide results from poor integration into society as a result of the way an individual behaves for example, by virtue of their mental illness. In altruistic suicide, there is an over-integration into society. An example is the act of *hara-kiri*, in which the customs of feudal Japanese society obliged an individual to die through suicide in certain circumstances. Anomic suicide occurs if the bonds between people have been loosened, as in an inner-city area, and norms regulating behaviour no longer apply. In fatalistic suicide, there is an excessive regulation by society, so that individual feel they have no personal freedom and therefore no hope. An example would be the suicide of a slave.

Mental Illness

Although psychiatric illness is an important aetiological factor, causal mechanisms leading to suicide are usually multifactorial. Depression is undoubtedly important, but at the same time, we know that the vast majority of people who have suffered a depressive episode will not kill themselves. Durkheim described his view that the various '... states that make up mental illness cannot account for the collective tendency to suicide in general'(p.46).[6] Whilst the individual characteristics of a person will influence their response to events, there are wider sociological factors in play as well. Adverse aspects of a person's life and the meaning they ascribe to their situation should always be assessed because they often play a central role in the development of suicidal despair, whatever the precise categorisation of psychiatric illness. The importance of social factors can be illustrated by the fact that the incidence of suicide in pregnancy and the puerperium appears to have fallen dramatically in the previous hundred years, so that now the incidence is lower than the rate expected in the general population, even though the puerperium is a time of major biological and psychological stress (see also Chapter 13). Such a reduction in morbidity may be due to changes in social attitudes to pregnancy, the availability of contraception and abortion (thereby reducing the likelihood that the pregnancy will be unwanted) and the lessening of stigma attached to an unwanted pregnancy. Socioeconomic factors, such as financial crises, can also lead to fluctuations in suicide rates.

Sex and Suicide

In most countries, there is a male predominance in suicide rates. An exception to this has been until recently China, where there was a female predominance, although now men predominate. The reason for the female predominance in China for many decades was high rates of young women in rural China ingesting highly lethal pesticides, but this problem has come under some control in recent years, and so there are fewer female suicide fatalities, and the more common picture of a small male excess of suicides has now appeared. Surveys of suicidal thoughts and attempted suicide usually show a female predominance in contrast to fatal suicides, which are more frequent in men.

In certain cultures, voluntary death occurs, such as *sati* in India where the Hindu widow was expected to climb on to the funeral pyre of her deceased husband. Cultural factors and gender role expectations, 'the good wife', seem to play the significant role as opposed to formal mental illness.[22] Although the practice was outlawed during colonial rule in 1829, it continued in some places, with the most recent legislation banning the practice passed in the Indian Parliament in the Sati Prevention Act (1987). The picture is also confused by suspicious deaths of women due to domestic fires from open cooking stoves. This phenomenon has been reported in India, Iran, Sri Lanka, South Africa and Zimbabwe.

In almost all countries, suicide rates are higher amongst men than women. Most male suicides occur during depressive episodes, yet depression is diagnosed twice as often in women. The reasons for this paradox are unclear, but it has been suggested that men are more alexythymic – that is, unable to express or report their emotions, especially their depression, as well as women. The male response to stress is commonly different to women, and male depressions are more strongly linked to aggression violence and suicidality. As an example of this, the suicide rate in the first year following a divorce is seven times higher in Danish men than Danish women following an identical stressor.

Marital Status

It is well-known that marriage and family tend to be protective against suicide and are associated with lower suicide rates, especially amongst men. US data shows rates of suicide from highest to lowest are widowed, divorced, single or never married and married with children. A majority of studies, though not all, also show this pattern.

What is there about being married and having a family that seems to protect against suicide? Probably many factors contribute. Certainly there is less social isolation for those who are married. Those with a family can enjoy intimacy and may be better motivated to live, work and earn money. Possibly those who are able to sustain a marriage are both physically and mentally more robust than those who fail to engage with others. What is known is that disruptions in marital and family life – such as divorce, widowhood, estrangement, break-ups and abandonment – are times of increased stress and raised rates of suicide attempts and completed suicide. However, in spite of increased rates of marital breakdown in the UK, suicide rates have been decreasing.

The Young

Suicide can and does occur in children, but US data shows that it is rare between the ages of 5–14, and the rate is around 3 per 100,000. Below age five, even though a child may die at his own hand, they are probably unable to formulate a suicidal intent, or a concept of death as being a final event. However, adolescents are able to form an intent and make large numbers of attempts, and there are fatalities as well. The suicide rate in England and Wales for 15-to-19-year-olds showed a gradual decline from 6.21 per 100,000 in 1998 to 4.62 in 2016 but then increased again so that, by 2021, the rate was 6.2 per 100,000. There are particular concerns for the rise in rates in young women under 24. In the earlier US study, a previous attempt, stressful life events, severe depression, alcohol abuse and parental alcohol abuse and antisocial behaviours (boys more than girls) are associated, and 40 per cent had a family history of suicide in a first- or second-degree relative. Psychological autopsy studies suggest that interpersonal conflict, shame and a sense of humiliation all play a role. Seeking an understanding of this recent rise in the UK will require a number of perspectives, with probably no single simple 'cause'.

Suicide in the Elderly

In most countries, suicide rates increase with age and are particularly high among the elderly, especially those aged 70 and over. Late life suicide is characterised by less warning, higher lethality and a greater prevalence of depression and physical illness.[23] In younger people, suicide is more often impulsive and communicative, but in the elderly, it is often long planned and frequently involves highly lethal methods. In the elderly, the ratio between attempts and successful suicide is four to one, whereas amongst the young, it is 100–200 to one.[24] Suicide attempts in the elderly are therefore particularly predictive of risk of completion.

Many causes can explain the increased elderly suicide risk. These include factors associated with the social and interpersonal relationships of their earlier life, such as sexual abuse, social exclusion and lack of social support, economic insecurity, access to lethal means, stressful life events and traumatic life experiences. Individual risk factors, including major depression and other mental disorders, physical illnesses, bereavements and loss of independence, are all also important. Functional impairments, personality traits such as neuroticism, hopelessness, difficulties in decision-making and cognitive inhibition, cognitive rigidity and obsessional traits have all been linked.

At the national level, a number of health-related indicators, markers of socioeconomic status and health care are correlated with suicide rates for the elderly. The risks in major depression are increased in the presence of alcohol dependence, Cluster B personality disorder and high levels of impulsivity and aggression. In jurisdictions that allow euthanasia or assisted dying, over time, the proportion of deaths declared due to this tend to rise – for example, as seen in the Netherlands, where voluntary euthanasia or assisted dying accounted for 4.4% of all deaths in 2017.[25]

In China, there is a large rural excess of suicides (rural vs urban, OR = 3.35) possibly due to there being large numbers of 'left behind elderly' because younger people have migrated to work in the cities, leaving their elderly parents on their own,[26] and the main method used is insecticide poisoning, a very lethal method. In other densely populated areas in Asia, the most common method is jumping off a high building, a method with obvious high lethality.

Protective factors for the elderly include good physical and mental health, as well as good social relationships, which seem to promote greater longevity. The good news is that rates for the elderly are probably in decline in most parts of the world. The WHO (2017) burden of disease study[27] found a 29 per cent decline in elderly suicide rates globally between 1970 and 2017. These changes correlated with improvements in the sociodemographic index, a composite measure of sociodemographic developmental status. However, there was considerable variation between countries with the largest decreases for elderly suicides being found in Chile and most of Western Europe, but there were rises in Armenia and South Korea and a few other countries. Reasons for these welcome decreases are not really understood, but possible explanations include the more widespread use of SSRIs, which are better tolerated than the previous generation of antidepressants (the tricyclics) and improvements in the socioeconomic position of many pensioners.

Many elderly people who are isolated and live on their own give no notice of their distress, and the first information of their suicidality comes with the discovery of their body in their flat; in such cases, intervention is not possible. However, others may make an unsuccessful attempt or present with suicidal thoughts in the context of a depression, which must be taken seriously, and any depression needs to be treated vigorously and brought to an end quickly with antidepressants, hospitalisation and, if necessary, ECT.

Mental Illness

When a suicide occurs, it sometimes appears to be a mystery to those around as to why the individual chose to end their life at that particular time. For many centuries, it has been known that insanity lay behind some episodes, and personal unhappiness lay behind many others. The coroner will conduct an inquest with the main aim of establishing whether or not suicidal intent was present or not to confirm that a verdict of suicide can be given. However, the inquest may reveal many other reasons as being possibly causal since suicide is a multicausal event. Top of this list is mental disorder, but a broad definition of mental disorder encompasses a wide range of conditions, including the tautologous ('he died through suicide because he must have been mentally disordered', for example) – a point made by Durkheim: 'There are suicides, and a great number of them, which are not the product of folly [insanity]' *('qui ne sont pas vésaniques')* (p.45).

Over several decades in the UK, the National Confidential Inquiry has examined suicide and homicide in people in contact with services, building a large database that now stands at over 144,000 deaths by suicide in the general population, including over 36,000 patients, and publishing biennial reports, most recently in 2021.[28] These reports highlight key trends and themes – for example, the risks associated with certain groups, such as those living alone or the raised risks in those recently discharged from hospital.

The psychological autopsy approach can study individual cases in a more detailed way. Here, as much information about the deceased's last few months and their mental state is obtained by interviewing relatives and friends, as well as examining their medical and police records. Any diagnoses of mental disorder are made according to standardised recognised criteria. However, although this detailed and time-consuming approach has faded from the research literature and the most recent meta-analyses of psychological autopsies

Table 15.3 Diagnostic distribution of suicides in psychological autopsy studies, compared to control groups,[29] N = 3,275 suicides

Diagnostic Category	Odds Ratio
Psychoses	6.6
Depressive disorders	6.2
Bipolar disorders	3.2
Personality disorders	4.5
Substance abuse problems	3.5
Anxiety disorders	2.4
Adjustment disorders	1.3
Any mental disorder	10.5

date from the early 2000s, the more comprehensive but focused methodology of the Confidential Inquiry based on psychiatric completion of reports has replaced it. Arsenault-Lapierre in 2004[29] found that around 79 per cent of all suicides had a psychiatric diagnosis at the time of their death, indicating that mental illness makes an important (and potentially reversible) contribution to suicide. Psychoses appear to be the most lethal disorders, followed closely by affective disorders, especially depression, as shown in Table 15.3. Numerically, because depression is by far the most common affective disorder, the majority of suicides will be related to depression.

Previous meta-analyses produced approximately similar figures. The picture for the UK is also broadly similar. Thus, Hunt (2006)[30] reported on a four-year sample of UK suicides (N = 4,859) where there had been a recent (less than one year contact) with mental health services, and the most common mental disorder had been depressive disorders(34%). Next came schizophrenia (20%), personality disorder (9%), alcohol dependence (9%), bipolar disorder (8%) and anxiety disorders (4%). Dementia (0.5%) had a protective effect, and earlier studies had shown that learning difficulties also had lower rates.

The logic of the exploration of the link between mental disorder and suicide is that improvements in the treatments of mental disorder has the potential to reduce suicide due to mental disorder. One futuristic study[31] suggested that if treatment effectiveness for major mental disorders reached 50 per cent effectiveness, this could potentially result in a projected 20 per cent reduction in overall suicide rates. This study was published around 20 years ago, and since then, there has been a reduction in suicide rates, at least in Europe – but no study has so far been able to link this with improved services or the more widespread use of antidepressants or any other factor.

Suicide in Particular Mental Disorders

Depression

Earlier series and meta-analyses found that 19 per cent of deaths amongst people with depression were accounted for by suicide. However, these figures were based on depression found amongst hospital inpatients where the depression was usually very severe. More recent figures point to lower rates: 8% for those admitted for suicidality, 4% for those admitted for any affective disorder (but not suicidality) and 2% for mixed inpatient and outpatient depressed populations. Rates for suicide for depression encountered in general practice are much lower than for hospital-based cases.[32]

A genetic element may be operating since offspring of probands with suicidal attempts had much higher rates of suicide attempts (RR = 6.5) when compared to offspring of probands lacking such a history. The symptomatic profile of those people with depression who die through suicide more often have features of DSM-5 melancholia; more guilt, which is often inappropriate; insomnia; appetite and body weight disturbance; poor concentration; and impulsive and aggressive behaviours. Comorbid alcohol and drug abuse and anxiety disorders may also be present. Two other emotions, hopelessness and shame, have now been recognised as important drivers of suicidality, and they are discussed later. However, whenever we are considering the clinical judgements that arise, it is as well to see clinical judgement as the complex exercise of multiple iterations of Bayes' Theorem (i.e. complex probability assessments with imprecise data) and to retain some humility and caution about the judgements that we make.

Hopelessness

On the basis of his own observations in long-term psychotherapy with suicidal patients, Aaron Beck[33] wrote, 'Suicidal preoccupations seem to be related to the patient's conceptualisation of their situation as untenable or hopeless. The suicidal patient could see no solution to the problem and they could only see suicide as the solution for their "desperate" or "hopeless situation"'. His team devised a specific 'hopelessness scale' and investigated the relationship between hopelessness, depression and suicidality in a large sample of people who had made a serious attempt on their lives but recovered. They found that the bulk of the variance between suicidality and depression was accounted by hopelessness as measured on their scale. If hopelessness emerges as a significant theme in a diagnostic assessment, then Beck recommends exploring the cognitive distortions that lie behind this, in addition to the depression or the suicidality.

Shame

Lansky (1991)[34] writes:

> Shame is the most significant affect in suicidal patients, while depression, guilt and anger are secondary to the shame in driving the suicide. Shame is the feeling associated with the failure to live up to ideals and to achieve important aspirations and goals. Shame is a response to feedback from others indicating incompetence or inefficiency and maybe indistinguishable from hopelessness.

Sometimes it is also associated with exhibitionism and falling short in the context of an ambitious driving quality, as in the case of some brilliant students who feel they have not lived up to their expectations. Excessive primitive shame triggered by the experience of incompetence or inadequacy or lack of control can provoke cognitive impairment and bodily reactions and even a sense of self-disintegration. Shame maybe related to the loss of, or impossibility of meaningful bonding.

The role of shame in heightening the risk of suicide in those charged with sexual offences against children has been highlighted.[35] This group may at times not elicit much sympathy from services, even if they do approach requesting help, and an awareness of this risk needs to be kept in mind when such input is requested.

Suicide in Schizophrenia

Around 5 per cent of people with schizophrenia die through suicide. Suicide mortality is typically lower for females than for males possibly because suicide attempts are less common, and women use less lethal means. A meta-analysis[36] of 35 studies with 16,747 individuals with schizophrenia found the pooled lifetime prevalence of suicide attempts was 26.8%, while the one-year prevalence was 3.0%. High-income countries in North America, Europe and Central Asia had significantly higher suicide attempts. In a UK follow-up investigation, most suicides occurred within the first two years of the onset of the psychotic disorder.

Demographic and clinical factors associated with the risk of suicide attempts in schizophrenia included an earlier age of onset, comorbid depressive symptoms, comorbid substance use, a family history of suicide, multiple hospitalisations and more severe psychotic symptoms, all of which increased the risk of suicide attempts. Adverse childhood experiences (ACEs) are common in the general population (around 30 per cent), but suicide attempts are more frequent amongst people with schizophrenia who also had ACEs.

Assessment of suicidal ideation amongst people with schizophrenia should cover recent life events, losses and social isolation. In the mental state, the intensity of the suicidal ideation must be gauged. Agitation is common and may be the precipitating emotion. People with schizophrenia sometimes die through suicide in response to auditory hallucinations, which give them instructions to kill themselves – often by violent or bizarre means – and if these are severe, loud or intrusive, this will serve as an indication for treatment, some times for admission, and if necessary, under section.

There are now indications that treatment, especially clozapine, may sometimes help to reduce suicidality. An 11-year follow-up study in Finland[37] found a lower overall mortality for treatment with any antipsychotic versus no drug (hazard ratios HR = 0.8) and, for clozapine, mortality was reduced even further (HR = 0.74). Specifically for attempted or completed suicide, there was a reduction for clozapine HR = 0.64 in a Finnish cohort and HR = 0.66 in the Swedish cohort. No other antipsychotic was associated with a reduced risk of attempted or completed suicide. In the same study, benzodiazepines and Z-drugs (zopiclone/zolpidem) were associated with an increased risk of attempted or completed suicide: benzodiazepines (HR = 1.30) and Z-drugs (HR = 1.33).

A case could be argued that the more widespread use of clozapine might reduce the overall suicide rate in schizophrenia, and perhaps a single or multiple suicide attempts (the best predictor of a subsequent suicide) should be considered as a possible indication for clozapine, but this has not been formally adopted so far.

Suicide in Bipolar Subjects

Suicide is an established risk for bipolar disorder. In the analysis of Harris and Barraclough,[38] the suicide mortality for bipolar disorder was 15 times that of the general population, and a Swedish study similarly found a standardised mortality ratio (SMR) of 15 for males and 22 for females. Rates were high, especially in the first year after diagnosis.[39]

A comprehensive recent meta-analysis[40] of 141 studies of bipolar disorder and suicide or suicide attempts and completed suicide found the following associations. *Sex*: Bipolar women are three times more likely than men to attempt suicide. However, for completed suicide, the picture is less clear. Studies based on the follow-up of army veterans in both the USA and Sweden also found higher rates for female than male veterans, but no clear picture emerges for general populations studies. *Age*: A large American study based on over 30,000 bipolar suicides did not find any significant pattern of age distribution, but suicide attempts were more frequent amongst younger BP subjects. *Ethnicity:* There were no discernible trends for ethnicity. *Single and divorced people* had higher rates as did single parents of either sex.

An earlier age of onset and *greater duration of illness* were both associated with increased numbers of attempts. *Depressive polarity* at onset and also where depressive polarity was most frequent were also associated with raised rates of attempts. *Mixed episodes* are associated with a higher lifetime risk of attempts, and in one study, this was 60 per cent compared to only 17 per cent for those with pure mania. However, because the vast majority of bipolar episodes are depressive, most of the suicide attempts and deaths occurred during phases of major depression. No particular trend was observed for the presence of psychosis, nor have significant differences been found between BP-I and BP-II disorders.

Comorbidity

Comorbid anxiety disorders, especially panic, are associated with raised rates of suicide attempts, but the picture is less clear for other anxiety disorders. *Borderline personality disorder*, amongst BP subjects, is also associated with raised rates of attempts as is a lifetime history of *anorexia nervosa* (OR = 3.7) or a *family history of suicide* (OR = 2.8). A suicide death is a much less frequent occurrence than an attempt, but this is also associated with a positive family history of suicide. *A family history of bipolar disorder and bipolar spectrum disorder* is also strongly associated with a death from suicide (OR = 4.9), but numbers were small in these samples. A large Finnish cohort of bipolar subjects found a *previous suicide attempt* increased the risk (OR = 3.93). *A history of child abuse*, both physical and sexual, also raised the risk. The review also included a single study of 67 suicide deaths in children and, compared to matched controls, found raised rates for *mixed states* (OR = 9.0) and for *comorbid substance abuse* (OR = 17.0), but numbers in these categories were small.

The good news is that lithium seems to help prevent suicide, although this is not undisputed.[41] A meta-analysis of 31 studies[42] involving a total of 85,229 person-years of risk-exposure to either lithium or other drugs found the overall risk of suicides and attempts was five times less among lithium-treated subjects than among those not treated with lithium (RR = 4.91). Risks of completed and attempted suicide were consistently lower, by approximately 80 per cent, during treatment of bipolar and other major affective disorder patients with lithium for an average of 18 months. These benefits were sustained in randomised as well as open clinical trials. At points in recent decades, lithium had fallen out of favour – mainly because of its risk of long-term renal damage – and valproate became more prominent in prophylaxis. As the teratogenic effects of valproate became more widely recognised and more recent prophylactic trials are also showing superiority for lithium, lithium is returning to favour. Recent large-scale population-based studies appear to have further conformed this association for other mood stabilisers but with the strongest effect for lithium.[43] There is, however, widespread variation in rates of prescribing lithium across the UK, and there are differences between counties. This reflects individual variation in clinical practice as well as the fluctuating currents of opinion on the optimal longer-term treatment for major mood disorders. There is always a balance between potential increases in rates of longer-term physical conditions, such as impaired renal and thyroid function, with the psychiatric benefits of any treatment. A case can be made that longer-term treatment with lithium now has a strong evidence base to support its use despite the need for ongoing review of its costs and benefits in the individual case.

Its efficacy against suicide, which appears to be quite large, should also be taken into account in the long-term management of bipolar disorder. The NICE bipolar guideline[44] recommends offering lithium as the first-line, long-term treatment for all bipolar subjects (subject to discussion of risks and benefits and suitability).

Personality Disorder and Suicide

Borderline personality disorder is strongly associated with suicide attempts, but it is also associated with suicide deaths. It is a mistake to think that a suicide threat or attempt by someone with BPD is without any danger because there are an appreciable number of fatalities.

Borderline personality disorder is often comorbid with depression, and in BPD subjects, this is often a chronic depression with guilt, hopelessness and worthlessness. Stone[45] followed up his series of 200 DSM-III BPD subjects for 10–23 years and found an overall suicide rate of 9%. A particularly high rate was found for those who were comorbid for schizoaffective disorder (23%) and for more severe BPD. Thus, of the 15 subjects who satisfied all eight DSM - III criteria, six subjects (36%) died through suicide. A UK-based study[46] examined the files of patients in the National Confidential Inquiry of Suicides in Hospital for the year of 2013 and found that, out of 1,601 people who died through suicide, 154 had a diagnosis of personality disorder, most often borderline PD, and they comprised around 10 per cent of the hospital-based suicides in that year.

The mean age of all patients at the time of death was 42 years; 95% had a history of self harm, which might be expected since this is one of the diagnostic criteria of BPD, 66% had a history of alcohol abuse and 52% had a history of substance abuse. A stressful life event was the most common precipitant, and most had been in contact with the psychiatric services in the year prior to the suicide, either as a brief admission or through the crisis team or some other part of the service. Only a few patients had received the psychologically more-intensive treatments such as dialectical behaviour therapy and mindfulness based therapy prior to their death, and the authors speculated whether more widespread availability of such therapy might have had an impact on suicide in BPD subjects.

A psychological autopsy study[47] of recruits to the Israeli Defence force who had died through suicide found strong narcissistic and perfectionistic traits in around 25% of those who killed themselves, while 40% showed schizoid or avoidant traits, and their parents often described them as 'isolative individuals'. Some people diagnosed with 'borderline' personality also present with intense anger, and it is this group that many professionals and services struggle to engage successfully with therapeutic approaches. There are particular difficulties with regard to patients with personality disorders complicated by depressive symptoms, adverse life events and past histories of trauma and resulting challenging behaviours. It may be tempting to withdraw from such a clinical dilemma on the assumption that such patients are 'not ill' and 'should take full responsibility' for what they do. The person 'having capacity' is sometimes cited as a justification to withdraw services or to avoid efforts to engage with a distressed individual.[48] The use of this rationalisation appears to be growing, perhaps symptomatic of the very real, distressing clinical dilemmas that are faced by clinicians every day. However, such a clinical problem commonly precedes suicide, and professionals must reflect on this, and any risk should be assessed, acknowledged and managed appropriately. Morgan coined the term 'malignant alienation' to describe the negative dynamic that he saw developing in some cases between the individual who died through suicide and the teams and individuals involved in their care. Psychoanalysts, viewing the same phenomena, write about the patients' 'provocative' behaviours resulting in 'hate in the counter-transference'. Understanding the reasons for the anger and distress through a collaborative assessment can enable a plan to be drawn up collaboratively to address the needs and wishes expressed (see Chapter 7.2).

Alcohol Dependence, Harmful Drinking and Suicide

Alcohol dependence and alcohol-related difficulties are strongly associated with suicide (see Chapter 14). An early meta-analysis[38] of 32 studies found the suicide risk for alcohol dependency was almost six times greater than that expected. This meta-analysis also found that the suicide risk for females (x20) was very much greater than for males (x4); suicide risk among alcohol-dependent individuals has been estimated to be 7 per cent.[49] Of 40,000 Norwegian conscripts who were followed prospectively for over 40 years, the probability of death by suicide was 4.76 per cent (RR = 6.9) among those classified as alcohol abusers compared to veterans who were not. There was also an association between suicide attempts, unemployment, separation or divorce and fewer years of education in this cohort.

Norström[50] reported that the effect of per capita consumption of alcohol on suicide was stronger in Sweden than in France. The Northern Europe pattern of misuse is mainly spirit drinking with a discontinuous pattern including binge drinking that may result in drunkenness. The Southern Europe pattern is mainly wine drinking usually with food and is daily and continuous with infrequent episodes of drunkenness. An analysis[51] of vodka sales in Russia between 1980 and 2005 found coincident trends between the level of vodka sales and suicide rates: an effect that was greater for men than for women. The analysis suggests that a one-litre increase in vodka sales per capita would result in a 5% increase in violent mortality rate, an 11.3% increase in accidents and injuries mortality rate, a 9.2% increase in suicide rate, a 12.5% increase in homicide rate and a 21.9% increase in fatal alcohol poisoning rates. Only vodka drinking resulted in an increased rate of alcohol-related psychoses. These findings indicate that a restriction of vodka availability can be considered as an effective measure for suicide prevention in countries with high spirit consumption and high suicide rates. Studies of samples of completed suicides indicate that people with alcohol dependencies account for 20–40% of all suicides. Follow-up studies suggest that people with alcohol dependence may be between 60 and 120 times more likely to complete suicide than those free from psychiatric illness. Among people with alcohol dependencies, the lifetime risk of suicide is about 10–15%, and the majority of suicide attempts occurred in the context of impulsiveness and current alcohol misuse. Depression and alcohol dependence were comorbid in 85% of 100 cases of completed suicide.

Sociological explanations for the strong association between alcohol dependence and suicide include the hypothesis that acute alcohol use leads to increased social deterioration and anomie, unemployment, debts and social isolation. Biological explanations emphasise impaired physical and mental functioning, as well as interactions with other psychotropic drugs. Disinhibition, in which alcohol acts to remove psychological barriers to self harm, may also be a relevant factor.

Patients who have alcohol dependence should be assessed for suicidal ideation whenever they exhibit a significant level of depressive symptoms, whenever they have a relapse of their alcohol or drug use, or whenever they have experienced a recent interpersonal loss or a loss of housing or employment.

Double Suicide and Suicide Pacts

When his armour bearer saw that Saul was dead, he also fell upon his sword and died with him...
(1 Sam. 31:5)

There is no further comment in the Bible on the death of Saul's armour bearer. Van Hooff[3] discusses such double suicides in the ancient world and classifies them as *devotees* and *Fides*. (Fides means 'reliability', a sense of trust between two parties). The *devotees* were virtual slaves, women or other low-ranking friends towards their masters.[3] In Japanese culture, this type of suicide is called *Junshi*. Amongst the Celts, soldiers would pledge their life and soul to their leader to such a degree that they would share death with them.

Today, suicide pacts are uncommon but still occur, and Fishbain[52] found the most common combination had one terminally ill partner with the other being well but dependent on them and sometimes being coerced into it. In their study of 5,895 suicides in Dade County, Florida, his group found 20 such pairs (40 suicides), giving an overall prevalence of 0.6 per cent for suicide pacts amongst all suicides.

Suicide and Violence

There are strong known associations between violence and suicide. A study of 50 habitually aggressive men in a forensic facility found 15 (30%) had made previous suicide attempts.[53] A survey of a school population in South Carolina showed that those with severe suicidal behaviours also had high rates of assaultive behaviours towards fellow pupils and teachers.[54] Amongst hospitalised adolescent psychotic patients, 67% were violent, 43% were suicidal and 27% were both violent and suicidal. A study of a large number of patients in Missouri mental hospitals found that suicidal thoughts were the highest single predictor of homicidal ideas, and the reverse was true as well.[55] This association between suicidal and homicidal thoughts is important as a small number of murders are committed by depressed men who then go on to die through suicide. In the majority of murder-suicides, men kill women. These commonly occur as the extreme manifestation of a relationship consisting of high levels of pre-existing domestic violence and coercion. On occasions, other family members such as children are also victims of homicide in these circumstances, with often-shocking accounts leading to national news coverage. Domestic violence as a risk factor for suicide in women is increasingly recognised. In the particular case of murder-suicide, a pre-existing history of acts of domestic violence in the perpetrator is usually present, often over an extended period of time. Other factors such as alcohol misuse, personality disorder and sometimes depression may also be present. Occasionally, a perpetrator may be suffering from a psychotic mental illness, though this is exceptional. Most of these final and terrible acts are perpetrated by coercive and controlling men consumed with rage and jealousy at the potential loss of the object of their control. In the routine assessments of suicidal patients, it is always necessary to enquire whether they are also harbouring any thoughts of 'wanting to take someone with them' and take appropriate warning actions if homicidal thoughts are also present

Suicide in Prisons

All deaths in prison custody are subject to a police investigation and a coroner's inquest. Statistical updates for England and Wales are provided via Gov.uk, and prior to the pandemic, a three-monthly update on safety in custody was released.

Between 2012 and 2020, the rate of self-inflicted deaths in white prisoners increased from 0.8 to 1 per 1,000, with some year-to-year fluctuation, and a high of 1.7 per 1,000 in 2016.[56] The rates in other ethnic groups ranged between 1 and 5 per year, so are harder to interpret statistically due to the small numbers. In 2020, there were 57 self-inflicted deaths in white prisoners. Comparison of prison suicide rates with those in the general population is problematical because it is necessary to match population subgroups precisely to achieve any meaningful findings.[57] Furthermore, accurate evaluation of the denominator is difficult, given the mobile and rapidly changing nature of much of the prison population. The most common method of prison suicide is hanging using bedclothes and window bars, and it usually occurs at night.

More recent information is available from a large meta-analysis of 77 studies from 28 countries comprising 35,351 suicides deaths.[58] The five strongest factors associated with prison suicide were suicidal ideation during current period in prison (OR = 15.2), previous suicide attempt (OR = 8.2), a history of self harm (OR = 7.1), single-cell occupancy (OR = 6.8) and current psychiatric diagnosis (OR = 6.1). Several criminological variables were also associated with suicide risk, including remand status (OR = 3.6) and offence type, particularly homicide (OR = 3.1). A diagnosis of depression carried an increased risk (OR = 4.9) as well as alcohol misuse (OR = 2.9). Based on only two studies, the item 'having no social visits' had a small but significant increased risk (OR = 1.9). An absence of visits might reflect a poor supportive social network. There were only two studies of female prison suicide, and these showed an association between remand status, violent offending and states of drug withdrawal, but numbers were small.

A decreased risk for suicide was found for those serving for drug offences (OR = 0.4) and for already having been sentenced (OR = 0.3) when compared to being on remand. Presumably, once a person's case has been settled, an 'already sentenced prisoner' has less anxiety than a remand prisoner, who waits in limbo before judgement.

The Home Office clearly would seek to minimise suicide in custodial settings, but the reports of the Chief Inspector of Prisons explain why conditions, (e.g. lack of space, exercise and occupation) make this particularly difficult. The prison population is overwhelmingly male and marginalised. Prisoners often have a complex mixture of social disadvantage, interpersonal problems and mental disorder, including substance misuse, as well as many other difficulties associated with raised risk of suicide. Various approaches have been developed, including screening on reception into custody and various other initiatives. These have included in some places placing prison health services within the remit of local Trusts, the development of 'buddy' systems (involving developing skills within the prisoner population) and wider staff training. Nonetheless, this remains a significant problem again without easy solutions.

Poverty, Occupation and Unemployment

Relative poverty is associated with an increased risk of suicide. In the UK between 1991 and 1993, the standardised mortality ratio (SMR) for suicide was four times higher in men aged 20–64 from social class V than in men of a similar age from social class I.[59] The reasons for this are complex, but they include the direct effects of mental illness on material deprivation, acute financial losses, bankruptcy, house repossession, higher levels of unemployment and job insecurity and downward social migration by people who develop mental illness. There may also be lower levels of social support amongst the poor. Such factors may lead directly or indirectly to mental health problems such as depression, anxiety and binge drinking, any of which might also predispose to suicidal behaviours.

Measures likely to help include targeted interventions for unemployed people, membership of social organisations and responsible media reporting. Good primary care and mental health services are needed to cope with increased demand in times of economic recession, but some administrations – such as the UK, in the aftermath of the Banking crisis – reduced health care spending as an austerity measure following the 2008–2009 banking crisis.

Effects of Occupation

Earlier studies – based on proportional mortality rates – showed that for men, certain occupational groups stood out as being particularly vulnerable to suicide; these included farmers, dentists, veterinary surgeons, sales representatives

Table 15.4 Standard mortality ratios (SMRs) for specific occupations. Base rate = 100

Occupation	SMR
Low-skilled construction occupations	369
Call centre occupations	290
Roofers	266
Musicians	252
Actors/entertainers	241
Plasterers	234
Farmworkers	221
Bakers	205
Gardeners and landscape gardeners	201
Care workers and home carers	192
Waitresses	156
Primary and nursery education teaching	142
Nurses	123

After Windsor-Shellard and Gunnell[60]

and medical practitioners; for women, they include medical practitioners, housekeepers, vets, waitresses and nurses.[13] The explanations given at the time was that those in the medical and allied professions have both knowledge of and access to drugs. Similarly, farmers have relatively easy access to firearms and pesticides.

More recent studies based on standard mortality rates (SMR) for suicide published by the Office for National Statistics has reversed this order, and now it appears that those in the building construction and related industries have the highest SMRs for suicide, but even rates for nurses are elevated. Table 15.4 shows the SMRs for some common occupations.

Low-skilled construction workers had the highest SMRs and accounted for 17 per cent of all male suicides. Skilled tradesman had an SMR of 135, but because there were a large number of people working as skilled tradesmen, they accounted for 29 per cent of all male suicides in the UK. The explanation is unclear, but job insecurity and alcoholism are also high in these trades. Amongst women, the highest rates were found amongst carers and care workers, possibly because many more poor people are engaged in these occupations, and it may be a very draining work type of work.

The earlier studies of the 1980s and 1990s, which found doctors and dentists had high rates of suicide, were based on a different statistic – the proportional mortality data (PMR). The PMR establishes whether the proportion of total deaths due to a specific cause (e.g. suicide) is higher or lower than deaths due to that cause in the general population. The main limitation of the PMR is that higher-income, highly educated populations tend to be healthier, with lower rates of cardiovascular and cancer deaths, and so the denominator is greatly lowered – hence, suicide as a proportion of all deaths among these higher-income occupations will seemingly be high, leading to a spuriously high estimate of the risk.

This is why occupations that had previously been of concern in PMR-based studies – such as farmers, doctors and dentists – have not been identified in SMR population-based studies to have elevated rates. Thus, for farmers, the SMR was 101, and for male doctors, the SMR was 84. Although for female medical workers the rate was raised at 124, this was mainly because of high rates amongst female nurses. It is now thought that methodological problems in terms of numerator/denominator errors account for these differences.

There is now some recognition of the risks for mental health issues in the building trades. Thus, in Australia, a training programme called 'MATES in Construction' has been developed to improve knowledge of mental health issues and help-seeking behaviours. Their literature points out that a construction worker is six times more likely to die by suicide than through an industrial accident. Training for managers can have a positive impact on employee sickness levels.

Economic Crises

It is well-known that unemployment is a risk factor for suicide. From time to time, there are major economic crises that sweep through nations or even the whole world, resulting in increases in unemployment. Paradoxically, the Great Depression of the 1930s in America resulted in an increase in lifespan, but there was also an increased suicide rate of 2 per cent.[61] The fall of communism in Russia in the early 1990s was followed by a decade of economic chaos and unemployment, resulting in an increase in suicides particularly in working age men, possibly also related to increased spirit consumption in this period. The 1997 Asian economic crisis is thought to have resulted in over 10,000 excess suicide deaths. The 2008 banking crisis, which led to collapsing stock markets all over the world, resulted in an excess of 34 million unemployed people in 2009 compared to 2007, and its effects on suicide rates has been the focus of numerous studies.[62] Using data supplied from the WHO database, mainly from Europe and North America, there were an estimated 4,884 excess suicides, with rates increasing by 4.2% in Europe and 6.4% in America. Amongst women, there was no rise in Europe and only a small rise (2%) in America. Men in the 45–64 age group were most affected, and the rise showed some correlation with rising unemployment rates.

In recent years, 'the Euro crisis' impacted most sharply on Greece, which went into a deep recession and was required to bring in severe austerity measures. Greece had joined the Euro in 2002, and the country greatly overspent on the back of Euro loans. This was associated with a temporary decrease in suicide rates (−27%), but the Greek economy was insufficiently robust to sustain its loan repayments, and as a result, severe austerity measures were introduced in June 2011. These plunged the country into a deep recession with high rates of unemployment. Over a 30-year period, the highest months of suicide in Greece occurred in 2012, and there was significant, abrupt and sustained increases in total suicides (+35.7%) and male suicides (+18.5%).[63] Suicides by women in Greece also underwent an abrupt and sustained increase in May 2011 following austerity-related events (+35.8%). These observations show that national suicide rates are closely linked to economic prosperity, and that austerity measures can result in increases in suicide at a population level.

Religion and Religiosity

A strong affiliation to religion is generally also held to have a protective effect against suicide. The initial observation was made in 1881 by Morselli,[64] who found that the Catholic states in Germany had consistently lower suicide rates (6 per 100,000) than Protestant states (19 per 100,000), and this was later confirmed by Durkheim.[6] The explanation offered at that time was that the Catholic religion had many more beliefs, rituals and practices than Protestantism and hence demanded a much greater degree of religious participation, and it was the strength of affiliation that gave protection from suicide.

A review of the 162 studies on the topic completed between 1882 and 2008 found that 82 per cent reported a protective effect for religion on suicide but 18 per cent did not.[65] Religion also offers some protection from depression, which is the most common mental disorder linked to suicide. However, the protective effect against suicide is very complex. It seems to operate both at the national and individual levels. Thus, nations dominated by religions that strongly condemn suicide, such as Catholicism and Islam, appeared to have lower rates of both completed and attempted suicide. At an individual level, the picture is also complicated, and the protective effect does not appear to derive from the religion itself but from the individual's degree of religiosity – that is, the degree of religious commitment, strength of belief and frequency of church attendance. It is also thought that regular meetings with co-religionists provide helpful social interactions and 'a moral community', where there is very little in the way of deviant behaviour of any sort, combined with a much lower level of suicide acceptability than is found in the wider community. For those who have religious beliefs, discussions with priests or a spiritual approach to their problems is sometimes helpful.[66] However, it is probable that under-reporting of suicide, because of the stigma involved, contributed significantly to the rates reported.

Other Possible Causes: War, Pandemics and Gambling

Durkheim observed the differences in suicide rate between times of war and times of peace. These upheavals produce often profound ways in which social groups and nations view themselves, and these clearly will impact on the behaviour of individuals within these societies at these times of change.

The Covid-19 pandemic, which developed from the end of 2019, produced huge disruption and responses, including economic disruption caused by 'lockdowns'. Initial data do not indicate an increase in suicide rates during the pandemic in the UK, but we are still at a very early stage of understanding its ramifications.

The rise of the legalised gambling industry in recent years has also been suggested as contributing to suicide risk in the population of people who gamble. Organisations such as the Samaritans and charities such as Gambling with Lives have highlighted this, citing supportive data from the ONS Psychiatric Morbidity Study, with over 400 suicides a year classified as possible gambling-related suicides.[67] See specific coverage of these issues in Chapter 7.3.

Assessment of Suicidality

Interviewing

A full psychiatric history and mental state examination is necessary for every patient, and the account here is taken from the previous edition of this textbook.[68] The suicidal state of mind frequently includes despair, a sense of humiliation and ambivalence concerning whether to live or die. The latter has been referred to as the 'Janus-faced' quality of suicidality. It explains how suicidal individuals may appear to appeal for help at the same time as feeling true despair and being at high risk. An attitude of hopelessness generated by a sense of defeat, entrapment and inability to escape is another important feature leading to both a disinclination to seek help and loss of hope.[69] Forming an understanding, empathic relationship with the individual and promoting mutual trust are essential to generating hope. Listening and allowing discussion of important issues are crucial features in establishing such rapport, though too-liberal reassurance may merely confirm a person's fears that others do not understand what it means to have lost hope. Suicidal individuals often declare their intention to die to a number of people before killing themselves, and it is a fallacy to assume that those who talk about such ideas are less likely to die through suicide. Attempting to guess whether someone is 'genuine' or challenging them is an ill-advised venture. Rather, it is better to accept the word of the person at face value, explore with them any ambivalence they are expressing, and find ways, if possible, to develop a collaborative approach to managing the distress they are expressing.

Although suicide risk questionnaires may be a useful prompt to ensure all relevant areas are covered, they cannot and should not replace a full psychiatric assessment, which is much more than a simple gathering of information from a checklist. In day-to-day clinical care, careful assessment of an individual's mental state, recent behaviour and relationship with others against the background of a thorough clinical history affords the most reliable means of evaluating the immediate degree of risk, and a checklist or a risk score should not be used to determine access to care or otherwise. Standardised questionnaires may then add useful back-up data. An interesting study showed that the worst-ever degree of suicidal ideation as assessed by questionnaire may be as useful as the current level in predicting risk.[70] This emphasised the importance of the previous history in clinical assessment.

It is advisable to lead into the topic of suicidal ideation gradually. In this way, the interviewer signals sensitivity to the individual's distress. The approach should take the form of a series of open questions, although it may be necessary to ask some leading questions to ensure that all the items are covered (see Box 15.1). Current suicidal thoughts or activities are the most important risk factor for suicide in psychiatric patients. A case-control study of psychiatric inpatient suicides[71] concluded that attempts to define a clinical stereotype of suicide are unrealistic. Predicting a suicide on the basis of current knowledge of predictors is just not possible today.

Whilst it is sometimes possible to identify a person as in a higher-risk group demographically, this in fact says little about the specific individual risk or its immediacy, and even less about the risk over longer periods of time. Working out the 'when' and the 'where' of the act is just not possible, making elimination of suicide an aspiration that is ultimately unlikely to be achieved without over-embracing custodial and coercive approaches that would ultimately be impossible within a democratic country with respect for the rights of individuals. Even if such an approach were attempted, it is likely it would fail; the demographics and statistics are such that the majority of suicides occur in groups that would be classed as 'lower risk'. Although being discharged from a psychiatric inpatient unit raises the risk of suicide, most people who die through suicide have not been recently discharged from a psychiatric hospital. Similarly, most people who die through suicide are not currently involved with mental health services. Sensitive, compassionate, face-to-face evaluation of each patient, based on attempting to establish a therapeutic alliance, is the only way of potentially modifying an individual risk that is impossible to quantify precisely.

Box 15.1 Potential prompt questions in exploring suicidal ideation and motivation

- Do you hope that things will turn out well?
- Do you get pleasure out of life?
- Are you able to face each day?
- Do you ever despair about things?
- Do you feel life is a burden?
- Are you feeling entrapped, defeated, hopeless?
- Do you wish you were dead?
- Why do you feel this way (e.g. to be with a person who has died, bleak life, morbid guilt)?
- Do you have thoughts of ending your life? (If so, are they intermittent or more persistent?)
- Have you ever acted on these ideas?
- How strongly are you able to resist these ideas? Is there anything that makes them worse or alleviates them?
- Assess how likely the person is to kill himself/herself (intent, detailed plans made, method considered and available)
- Assess the ability of the patient to give assurance about safety – for example, until next appointment if the patient is to remain in the community
- Assess the willingness of the patient to seek help in crisis
- Review sources of help and how to activate them
- Look at options other than suicide
- Assess risk to others (e.g. are others included in the patient's sense of hopelessness? Is there a possibility of an associated homicide? Is there aggressive behaviour related to personality difficulties or psychotic mental illness?)

Difficulties in Assessment

Difficulties in assessment are described in Box 15.2. The degree of risk is sometimes underestimated despite the communication of suicidal ideas and intent.[72] The Confidential Inquiry reported that in 80 per cent of inpatient suicides, the patients were regarded as being of no or low risk.[73] It is now accepted that attempting to stratify risk in this way is not helpful although resource allocation – for example, who to admit, voluntarily or compulsorily, and what level of support and supervision is required at home or in hospital – requires such assessments and judgements to be made and communicated.

Suicidal patients may exhibit behaviour that is perceived sometimes as provocative or uncooperative by staff. The emotional reactions of staff – in psychodynamic terms, the 'counter-transference' – influenced by their own experience and emotional life, may manifest as a loss of sympathy or outright hostility and criticism. This in turn can lead to interactions in which the patient experiences this criticism and lack of validation in ways that increase their sense of rejection and, in turn,

Box 15.2 Difficulties in suicide risk assessment

- The inherent uncertainty in assessing risk of suicide in any individual
- Variability in degree of distress and intent (ambivalence towards suicide, removal from stress factors)
- Misleading improvement due to final decision to kill self or removal from stressful situation
- Deliberate denial of suicidal ideas
- Difficulties in engaging in a therapeutic assessment
- Anger and resentment, sometimes displaced on to staff
- Staff assumptions that talk of suicide is no more than a manipulative threat
- Staff fears that direct discussion of suicide might precipitate it
- Surveillance difficulties
- Physical hazards in hospital ward surroundings
- Malignant alienation
- Setting over-ambitious goals, which foster sense of failure

increase their suicidality. Suicidal patients may exhibit provocative or uncooperative behaviour, which needs to be explored and understood. As a result, others – including health care professionals – may lose sympathy and become critical of a person at real risk of suicide, who then in turn perceives staff as unhelpful and rejecting. Similarly, recurrent relapse can lead to staff frustration and breakdown of the therapeutic relationship. This process has been termed 'malignant alienation' and deserves identification and consideration before treatment runs into difficulties.

A further problem worthy of special mention is short-lasting and misleading improvement, which has been previously reported occurred in 45 per cent of inpatient suicides.[72] This may be related to temporary disengagement from stressful situational factors, and care should be taken to address such problems adequately before arranging leave or discharge, which might otherwise trigger relapse. Lack of overt distress may also follow a final decision to die through suicide, with a resulting freedom from states of agonising indecision.

Overall Assessment of Risk

It has already been noted that the known correlates of suicide are imperfect indicators of risk at an individual level, particularly in the short term (a list of factors can be found in Box 15.3). They should inform rather than replace the face-to-face clinical assessment, which must encompass the widest possible perspective. Risk assessment instruments have not been demonstrated to be helpful, and the focus should be on individualised dynamic formulation.[73] The use of categories such as low, medium and high has also been criticised as being poorly predictive and static.[74]

Critical information required in the risk assessment is given below:

- Previous history (e.g. of self harm and level of suicidal ideation)
- Personality characteristics (especially traits of aggression and impulsivity)
- Evaluation of current mental state, with particular attention to detailed and systematic assessment of suicidal ideation and intent

Such an approach helps to distinguish the degree to which an openness to help is present and can be met for an unequivocal wish to die, which may require immediate intervention. In most cases, a degree of both apply. Environmental hazards should also be monitored constantly. The overall approach should take into account the balance between risk and protective factors.

Psychiatric Inpatients

Background Data

Selected data concerning the large series of inpatient suicides from England and Wales, as reported by the Confidential Inquiry[76,77] are set out in Box 15.4.

Box 15.3 Risk factors for suicide[75]

Demographic factors
- Male
- Increasing age
- Low socioeconomic status
- Unmarried, separated, widowed
- Living alone
- Unemployed

Background history
- Self harm (especially with high suicide intent)
- Childhood adversity (e.g. sexual abuse)
- Family history of suicide
- Family history of mental illness

Clinical history
- Mental illness diagnosis (e.g. depression, bipolar disorder, schizophrenia)
- Personality disorder diagnosis (e.g. borderline)
- Physical illness, especially chronic conditions or those associated with pain and functional impairment (e.g. multiple sclerosis, malignancy, pain syndrome)
- Recent contact with psychiatric services
- Recent discharge from psychiatric inpatient facility

Psychological and social factors
- Hopelessness
- Impulsiveness
- Low self-esteem
- Life event
- Relationship instability
- Lack of social support

Current context
- Suicidal ideation
- Suicide plans
- Availability of means
- Lethality of means

There Should Be Thorough Admission Procedures

The National Confidential Inquiry into Suicide and Homicide by People with Mental Illness is a large government-led inquiry, which publishes reports every one to two years. The raw data used are submissions made after every suicide or homicide that has occurred in England and Wales who had been an inpatient or recently discharge from mental health services. The report of 2001 stated that, for admitted patients, 24 per cent of suicides occurred during the first week after admission. Inadequate admission procedures present serious hazards; policies need to be clear and fully understood by all staff.[76] The Confidential Inquiry also advised that staff should attend skills training programmes at least every three years. Such clinical skills involve accurate evaluation of the mental state and of current as well as previous risk factors for suicide

Box 15.4 Data from the confidential enquiry into inpatient suicide deaths

- Sixty-four per cent of patients dying by suicide are male
- Patients dying by suicide as inpatients tended to be more morbid than those dying by suicide overall (79% had affective disorders or schizophrenia, with higher rates of previous self harm and violence as well as multiple previous admissions)
- By far, the most frequent method was hanging (42%). Other common methods were jumping from a height or in front of a moving vehicle (27%), drowning (8%) and overdose (11%)
- For hanging, the most common ligature used was a belt, and the most common suspension point was a curtain rail
- Of those suicides that occurred on the ward, 74% were by hanging
- Overall, 31% of patient suicides occurred on the ward, 53% at a distance from the ward and 14% otherwise in or around the hospital
- Around a third were on agreed leave, and a quarter had left the ward without staff agreement
- Of all patients dying by suicide, 28% were detained under the Mental Health Act
- Of all patients dying by suicide, 23% were under non-routine observation
- Particularly vulnerable times were the first week after admission (24% of deaths) and when discharge was planned (41% of deaths)
- Though most patients (76%) had been in contact with a staff member in the 24 hours before death, in only 15% were suicidal ideas detected
- Problems identified by staff included the need for close supervision, patient non-compliance, insufficient staff numbers and the need for better staff training and communication

Source: Data drawn from 754 patients in England and Wales, in the National Confidential Inquiry[76,77]

Hospital Admission

Bed pressures are a reality for most mental health services, and so pre-emptive and respite admission are generally unavailable. However, admission should always be obtained when the risks appear to be high or the patient is acutely psychotic, if necessary, under the Mental Health Act. The main purpose of the admission is to prevent access to the means of committing suicide, and legal detention is required to prevent the subject from leaving the ward because access to lethal means is much easier outside the hospital. Bed shortages have been accompanied by a huge rise in 'out-of-area' admissions, and this has been highlighted as a potential risk factor for post-discharge suicide.

Supportive Observation

A clear care policy for suicidal patients is imperative, inherent in which should be the principle that increased risk must be matched by more-intensive care in terms of relationship with staff, provision of appropriate physical security (including control of exits and removal or at least control of hazards in the ward and wider hospital environment) and provision of adequate numbers of staff. The aim should be to establish a supportive alliance with the patient *against* suicidal ideas and behaviour. The terminology should be explicit and unambiguous; words such as 'close' or 'special' convey little to newcomers or to those who work in other hospital units and are a recipe for confusion. At the same time, this requires more than a custodial approach – being constantly observed is intrusive, often distressing and can be counter-productive. The process should therefore be one of intense support for the patient rather than unwelcome intrusive surveillance. Levels vary, with intensive face-to-face supervision at all times for patients at the highest risk (when there is also a risk of violence, more than one staff member may need to be present). Engaging the patient in collaboratively developing their plan rather than simply imposing it can foster the essential therapeutic alliance between staff and patient. Once the risk is perceived to be less, observations can be decreased to 15 minutes, then 30 minutes, hourly, and to a point where the nurse is only required to visualise the patient at certain intervals, and considerations of leave may be made. Such judgements require collaborative assessment between medical and ward staff, with the person themselves and, where appropriate, their carer.

Occasionally, the risk is high, yet the patient appears and says that they feel better. The Confidential Inquiry[76] found that around a quarter of inpatient suicides occurred during non-routine observation (48% of these had left the ward, 11% with staff agreement) and suggests that intermittent observation is of unproven value. However, it is important to stress that regular, face-to-face contact with a patient at risk needs to be a supportive alliance of therapeutic value rather than impersonal policing; the value of such support must surely be hard to gainsay when treating patients who are struggling against being overwhelmed by suicidal ideas.

Working with the Suicidal Patient

It is necessary to move as quickly as possible towards establishing a close, supportive relationship, one that may even need to be assertive and controlling, especially at times of crisis. Identifying the painful reality of depressive symptoms is a useful early step. Similarly, it can be very helpful to indicate an understanding of feelings of ambivalence and even anger towards others. Isolating the suicidal drive by seeing it as part of an illness, agreeing on ways of minimising it (having identified what may worsen or relieve it), and explaining how depressive symptoms usually resolve with time and the manner in which they can distort ways of thinking all help to regenerate hope.

When relatives become included in morbid depressive thinking concerning the need to die, or in any other form of psychotic ideation, risks to their safety should also be carefully evaluated, as suicides are occasionally accompanied by homicides (see earlier). Failure to respond to therapy should lead to a review of medication, as well as a fresh look at how to deal with adverse events and situations that appear intractable. The therapist should be consistent in what is said and done and needs to see the patient regularly and predictably. Even the most despairing patients can derive considerable comfort from another person's willingness to listen and sit with them. This sharing of a space can provide the thread of a connection that enables the person to alter their perspective.

Use of Medication

If medication is judged to be necessary, it is important to target it carefully. Collaboration with medication may be seen as crucial to progress, but a negotiated approach – where possible – is most likely to reduce confrontation and lead to progress.

Individuals who proceed to die through suicide often receive inappropriate medication in a low and ineffective dose during the last few weeks of their lives.[78] The state of depression also may not be recognised.[79] Liquid medication will prevent patients from hoarding tablets. Medication-induced akathisia can be mistaken for a state of agitation related to the mental illness, and all clinicians should be vigilant for this..

On discharge, follow-up is expected within 48 hours of discharge. Supplies of medication should be limited if there is any concern at potential risk of overdose.

Factors liable to complicate risk management have been set out in Box 15.3. If alienation of staff occurs, it is wise to discuss this openly so that attitudes of frustration and hostility directed towards the patient can be dealt with objectively. Negotiating limits to the behaviour that is acceptable is sometimes necessary, particularly for psychiatric inpatients with personality disorders and adolescents, but arbitrary imposition can exacerbate confrontation.

These are, however, challenging areas of practice. Given the uncertainty that exists in assessing risk of suicide, limit setting in the face of disturbed behaviours can be one of the most taxing tasks in clinical psychiatry. The patient's management will require frequent discussions within the whole clinical team, attempting to maintain team consistency whilst making ongoing efforts to maintain and extend a collaborative, respectful approach with the patient.

Control of hazards in the hospital environment is a most important issue. Recognition that a high proportion of inpatient suicides were due to hanging through the National Confidential Inquiry led to identifying approaches to reduce this through identifying ligatures and potential ligature points and removing them. Future designs of inpatient units should incorporate designs that 'design-out' as far as possible these hazards, paying attention to shower rails, bed and window frames, door handles, piping and access to potential ligatures. Among the elderly, plastic bags are a particular hazard. Many so-called hangings by inpatients are more in the nature of strangulation and do not involve bodily suspension from a height. This means that it is necessary to be vigilant about a wide variety of items found on a typical ward (e.g. shoelaces or anything that can be tied) when an individual's suicide risk is high. These findings have implications for observation techniques: so-called hanging can occur in a supine position (25 per cent of suicides of detained patients occurred despite observations every 15 minutes).

A suicide prevention strategy should seek to identify and address wider environmental hazards. Acute wards should ideally be on the ground or first floor, staircases should be safe, windows should open only to a limited degree, and access to motorways or bridges in the immediate vicinity should be limited as far as possible – for example, by the use of barriers. If a suicide occurs, the investigation should seek to comprehend the whole system within which the death has occurred, take into account the perspective of the bereaved relatives and look for areas of potential improvement for the service as a whole. The aim should be towards the design of a service that is founded on safe, compassionate foundations that acknowledges the degree of uncertainty in clinical practice. It should avoid, if possible, an approach intended to apportion blame, though sometimes an adversarial approach develops in the context of litigation or a coroner's inquest.

In those cases where an inpatient or outpatient suicide has occurred, documentation of medical decisions and nurses' observations, levels set and concordance with Trust policies will be examined, and explanations of these decisions may be sought by relatives and coroners.

Treating the Unwilling Patient

When the immediate risk escalates such that it cannot be controlled adequately because the patient is unable to comply with treatment, it may become necessary to act against his or her will – for example, by preventing self-discharge and administering medication or other forms of treatment. The prevention of self harm is given as one of the three reasons for which patients may be detained under the Mental Health Act 1983 (the legislation was specifically devised to cope with this situation), but this is not always successful. A review[80] by the Mental Health Act Commission of 168 suicidal deaths of detained patients found that 41% occurred in a public place while the patient was on approved leave, and 28% of the patients had gone absent without leave. These findings again draw attention to the need to review observation and leave strategies.

Discharge and Leave

The Confidential Inquiry[76] found that 41% of inpatient suicides occurred when discharge was being planned and another 32% within two weeks of discharge, most commonly in the first week. Decisions concerning leave and discharge clearly need to be made very carefully. For patients who have been detained under the Mental Health Act, great care should be taken to ensure that leave agreements are consistent with the Act's requirements in each instance. In particular, it must be remembered that section 17 of the Act directs that the relevant consultant (i.e. the responsible clinician) must give specific permission for any leave arrangements. The Confidential Inquiry advised that individual care plans should specify action to be taken if a patient is non-compliant or fails to attend. It found that 40% of post-discharge suicides occurred before the first follow-up appointment.[76]

The Inquiry recommended an appointment within seven days of discharge from hospital for every patient with severe mental illness or a history of self harm in the previous three months, and this has since developed into the policy of 'two-day follow-up' of everybody discharged from psychiatric inpatient care. This illustrates two important points: firstly, the identification of patterns from a case series and, secondly, the imprecision of trying to identify a subgroup of people at 'high risk'. Recognising the high-risk status and trying to look for broad approaches to manage this is crucial. Enlisting the help of relatives and friends is often beneficial if it can be done.

Early Twentieth Century Psychoanalytic Perspectives on Suicide

Cognitive behavioural theories and interventions have been discussed previously in this chapter, but there have been psychodynamic perspectives that have informed the understanding of suicidal behaviour. Freud never had a unitary theory of suicide, but where suicide or suicidal thoughts appeared in his cases, he wrote about the analysis of these individuals. In 1920, in his paper 'Beyond the Pleasure Principle',[81] he proposed the presence of two opposing instincts: the more familiar life instinct *(Eros)* and opposing this was a death instinct *(Thanatos)*, which were in constant tension with each other. He regarded guilt as important, especially in regard to hostile impulses towards the parents; some patients would reproach themselves for the death of their parents. Freud himself was deeply affected by the death of his own father, and in his self-analysis, he found emotions of hostility, guilt feelings, as well as admiration for his father. These feelings were temporarily transferred onto his friend and mentor, Fleiss. During the grieving period following his father's death, he found he had become increasingly irritable with Fleiss and speculated that this was a transference phenomenon.

Freud only expressed suicidal thoughts once in his life, and this was in his letters to his fiancée, Martha, in the thought that he might possibly lose her. He eventually married her, but he drew parallels between being in love and suicide as, in both instances, the ego (the person, their reality) becomes overwhelmed by the object, though in different ways. In the case of the Rat Man, a person with serious OCD, the analysis revealed that the suicidal impulses were punishments for rage and jealousy directed towards his rivals. Freud wrote, 'We find that the impulses of suicide in a neurotic turn out to be self-punishment for wishes for someone else's death.' In his classic 1915 paper, 'Mourning and Melancholia',[82] Freud explains how depression and aggression, directed at the self, occur when psychic energy is withdrawn from a lost object. It is relocated in the ego (introjection), and this recreates the loved person in the ego and then becomes a permanent feature of the self. At a later date, there is identification of the ego with the lost object, and the ego turns in on itself and with murderous impulses attacks the object. This oft quoted idea may or may not be true, but Littman, reviewing this theory,[83] considered that more recent concepts of regression, disorganisation and ego splitting would allow one part of the ego to initiate an attack on another part.

Menninger[84] considered that suicide was a very complicated act driven by more powerful forces than external reality, and it was far more than the random act of an insane person. Rather, suicidal individuals construct a predicament in their life pattern from which they cannot perceive of an escape except through suicide. He also wrote there were three elements to the suicidal impulse: (i) the element of dying, (ii) the element of killing and (iii) the element of being killed. These forces play out in both the conscious and unconscious, but they are not of equal strength. Thus, for example, we know from those who survive, the wish to kill and its associated anger is much stronger than the wish to be dead because many survivors of serious suicide attempts are grateful to have survived and not be dead. The wish to kill is in part related to the innate aggressive drives and is directed at a hated person, and as Freud had previously pointed out, many suicides are disguised murders. Menninger suggested that the wish to be killed was an act of extreme submission, possibly similar to what might occur in the sexual act, but it can also stimulate unconscious guilt for which a deserved punishment should be applied, and this would be a self-inflicted death penalty.

In another paper, Freud speculated on the symbolic meaning of different methods of suicide as possibly being sexual wish fulfilments. Thus, to poison oneself might symbolise to become pregnant, to drown was to bear a child, and to throw oneself off a high building was to be delivered of a child. Whilst Menninger[84] wrote that suicide by gunshot was a masculine way of dying, representing the sexual act; poisoning and drowning were female methods reflecting a passive role that females have in the sexual act; he also described self mutilation as a partial suicide

Rescue Fantasies

Almost all psychiatrists will have encountered patients who have attempted suicide but survived thanks to someone else intervening 'as if by chance'. A closer look at such attempts reveals that the suicidal person has often left a note or other clues about their intention and their location to the rescuer, who then has an active role to save the patient. Suicide is a social phenomenon and quite often a dyadic act with the involvement of another person, and in the attempt, the suicidal person plays a game of Russian roulette with the person selected as their rescuer, 'Will I or won't I be rescued and saved?'

The other person may be a spouse or may be the therapist who ultimately symbolises the parents. Sometimes the fantasy of being rescued is conscious, but more often, it is unconscious and not apparent. The prototype for this type of relationship probably exists in the earlier mother/infant dyadic relationship.

Menninger suggests that the relative selected as 'rescuer' sometimes fails to recognise their part and may have guilt about their role. If this concept of being rescued in suicide is valid, the original trauma is of the abandoned infantile ego, and the underlying fantasy is an attempt to restore the original relationship between the primary object and the person, and the ego of the suicidal person

A variety of other fantasies may also lie behind a suicide, including reunion fantasies especially after a bereavement. Vengeful and murderous fantasies can occur amongst those who feel wronged. Guilt and self-punishment were found to be prominent in the treatment of suicidal PTSD subjects following the Vietnam War. Similarly, self-punishment features prominently amongst university students who are convinced they have failed to attain the high academic standards expected of them. Fantasies of control and omnipotence may underlie conditional threats of suicide – for example, 'I cannot live unless I get into this particular university' or 'I must die, if my affection is not reciprocated by my ex-partner'. Both conscious and unconscious motivation is most likely to be manifest in the weeks before, or in a failed suicide attempt in its immediate aftermath. Understanding and conveying the meaning of the attempt to the suicidal individual may bring relief and so help to diminish their suicidal drive.

Psychotherapy with the Suicidal Subject

Shneidman,[85] an American suicidologist and also a psychoanalyst, wrote extensively on the topic in the 1960s. He said, 'Suicide is an event and not a disease, and succour can be obtained by many different kinds of people apart from physicians.' He suggests there are two key words that need to be considered by anyone trying to understand and treat suicide. These are *perturbation* and *lethality*. Perturbation refers to agitation, anxiety, depression, and how upset the person is, whether due to a social situation or a psychiatric illness; lethality refers to the dangerous thoughts or acts of the suicidal person. Any suicidal act has the potential for lethality, but sometimes an act has obvious high lethality. The way to decrease lethality is to decrease the perturbation. He later wrote[85] about the ultimate cause of suicide as '*psyche-ache*', an unbearable degree of psychological pain that led people down the path to suicide.

Psychotherapy with a suicidal person has a very different aim from that of more general psychotherapy where the aim is to increase comfort. With the suicidal subject, the aim is no more than the preservation of life. He found that there were four components that the therapist needs to deal with in the therapy: (i) heightened inimicality, by which he means hostility; (ii) elevated perturbation; (iii) constriction of intellectual focus and (iv) the idea of death as a solution.

The suicidal patient is constricted in thought and can only think of death, and so the therapist must seek to widen the range of possible thoughts and fantasies to move the patient out of his dyadic concept (life or death) to at least three options or, if possible, more. He should also attempt to decrease the level of perturbation. How does one do this with a highly suicidal person?

Shneidman thought this can be done by doing anything and everything to cater for the infantile idiosyncrasies, dependency needs, hopelessness and helplessness the individual is experiencing. The therapist may need to go along with the patient that life is often a choice between only lousy alternatives, but wisdom is to choose the least lousy alternative that is attainable.

He also writes about the intensity of consultations with suicidal people – of the transferences and countertransferences – and the exhaustive and depletive effects of working with highly suicidal people, that such cases should be shared, and therapists should only see a few such cases at a time. He also says that confidentiality is not sacrosanct in such cases, especially when homicidal thoughts are expressed, and the therapist is under a duty to report these.

Hendin[86] writes: 'It is important not to confuse management with therapy.' By management, he means active attempts to prevent access to meet the methods, hospitalisation and compulsory admission because, at the end of the day, nothing will stop a determined suicidal individual, whereas helping the individual with his problems can help reduce his perturbation and lethality. Hendin also examined cases in therapy where the therapy had failed and the person had gone on to die through suicide, and he identified three possible areas where things had gone wrong. Firstly, there was a failure to tolerate infantile regression; second, the therapist himself may have become despondent about the progress of the therapy and the client has picked this up; thirdly, an outside event of great significance to the patient had occurred that the therapist had failed to recognise. This need not be a momentous event, but something like the patient's spouse not replying to a letter might have great significance to the client but would not have registered with the therapist.

Some Common Errors in Working with Suicidal Patients

The vast majority of suicidal patients are treated as outpatients. To start with, the fragmented (or 'functional') nature of many modern services can present challenges that services need to acknowledge and seek to address. Common errors in talking to suicidal subjects include:[87]

i. Being overly reassuring: A tendency to reassure may be helpful in many situations, but for suicidal individuals, it tends to negate their powerful feelings of despair. It is better to ensure these feelings are fully vented.
ii. Inadequate assessment of suicidality: This is common, but if someone talks about going to a railway bridge or a coastal cliff, it is important to explore this further and act on such information.
iii. Failure to recognise or discuss the precipitating event: Subjects are usually distressed by some recent rejection or slight, and this should be explored in detail.
iv. Advice giving: The patient's immediate problem cannot be solved by the therapist (e.g. 'I think you must leave your wife'), but through collaborative working and problem solving, the client will be helped to reach their own solution.
v. Being too passive: Repeatedly saying 'Aha' or 'Yes, I can see that' without interacting. Engagement is essential if anxiety levels are to be reduced.
vi. Being overly defensive: Some patients issue repeated provocative challenges to the therapist's authenticity, competence or sincerity. A reply is demanded immediately, and the therapist must avoid entering into a tit-for-tat dispute but reply in a non-challenging, non-defensive fashion (e.g. 'Well, I have not been suicidal myself, but I think I can still help you by exploring the problem with you.')

(Maris et al. chapter 21, pp. 521–2)[87]

Working with Suicidal Outpatients

Risk assessment and management is an ongoing process with patients and responsive to the individual's changing circumstances and mood. Central to management is collaborative evidence-based[88] safety planning, which will be done in conjunction with the therapeutic team, but the psychiatrist usually has a major role in drawing up, reviewing and implementing it. It enables a collaborative approach with the person themselves, their family and carers and the mental health team. Components that seem most acceptable to patients in a plan include individual warning signs, coping strategies (things that I can do that help), social settings that reduce stress, people whom the patient can ask for help during a crisis, professionals or agencies to contact during a crisis, things that make the patient's environment safer.

Where suicidality is a component of complex emotional needs (personality disorder), patients frequently present as distressed and angry, anticipating – from previous experience – negative responses from those they meet. With these challenging individuals, it is important to convey that you do not believe that the person is exaggerating – more often minimising – their distressing experiences. This will include what happened to them in the past. They are not speaking falsely but instead telling you the truth as they see it. As Marsha Linehan – the developer of dialectical behaviour therapy – has stressed, it is the validation of the individual that is critically important in itself, and this validation helps to develop the working relationship (see more detail in Chapter 7.2).

Suggestion and Imitation

Suicide can sometimes be contagious and occur in clusters, and this is sometimes known as 'the Werther effect'. This is the name given to media influence on social suicidal behaviour. The Werther effect is based on an apparent epidemic of suicides, by shooting, which occurred soon after the publication of Goethe's book[89] *The Sorrows of Young Werther*, in which the hero dies by shooting himself when his love for a woman is not reciprocated. This led to an epidemic of suicide across Europe, and this alarmed authorities to such an extent that the book was banned from Italy, Leipzig and Copenhagen.

Phillips reviewed[90] the problem in 1974 and found that, in the first two months after the suicide of a famous person, there was often a small rise in the number of suicides; however, this did not prove that the publicity had caused the suicide. To do this, he selected a series of well-known suicides in America, and similarly in Britain, and he examined the suicide rates in the aftermath of the event. American suicides, which had only been publicised in the American newspapers, caused an elevation of the suicide rate in America, but not in Britain. Similarly, the suicides of famous British people caused a small elevation in the total number of suicides in Britain, but not in America. The only satisfactory way to explain this was that it was the intervention of the newspapers that had caused the rise in suicide rates in each country.

A recent meta-analysis[91] analysed 31 studies and found the effect size of imitation was an elevation of 13% (range 8–18%) in suicide rates occurring in the first two months after the suicide of a well-known person. The study also found that when the method of suicide used by the celebrity was published, this was associated with a 30% increase in suicides by the same method. However, a Werther effect was only found in 36% of famous suicides reported in the press.

It is now generally accepted that the reporting of suicide can occasionally trigger a suicide by imitation, and the underlying mechanism appears to depend on identification with the deceased person, especially if they were of high social standing; the increased media reporting of the suicide act, resulting in a normalisation of suicide as an acceptable way to deal with life's difficulties; and information on the suicide methods, which might influence the choice of suicide by a vulnerable person.

The authors recommend responsible reporting of suicides, and there are now guidelines for the media reporting of suicide that form a part of most national suicide prevention strategies. Typically, the guidelines include specific suggestions about ways to minimise harm – for example, by avoiding glorification of the suicide, avoiding mention of specific methods employed and avoiding repeated reporting of the same suicide. Also, they recommend that the report should always include information about the role of treatment in mental illness, where and how to ask for help for depression, including giving practical help in the form of telephone crisis numbers and helping agencies, as well as imparting a message of hope that treatment is possible and that suicide is usually preventable.

The written press and TV broadcasters are nowadays more or less compliant with these regulations, but the newer social media such as Facebook, Twitter and the like – which are unregulated – permit the publicising of uncensored material. They have 'suicide' and 'self mutilation sites', which are unregulated and sometimes glorify suicide and provide detailed instructions on how to die through suicide, and these sites are potentially dangerous. Younger patients should always be asked whether they have visited any such sites. Even though the tech companies try and remove these sites, they reappear very speedily, and there is much debate at a political level as to how to enforce better regulation of the internet with regard to such harmful sites. The UK parliament is currently debating a law that will not only ensure that tech platforms close these sites down, but that failure to do so will result in hefty fines.

Non-fatal Self Harm (SH)

History and Definition of SH

In the UK, before the Suicide Act 1961, any suicide attempt was punishable under the law. Up until that time, the number of reported episodes was small, but now it is so large that it represents a major challenge in health care, particularly for those working in A&E departments and in general hospital settings.

There is continuing debate about the relative merits of the terms 'self harm', 'parasuicide' and 'attempted suicide', which are often used synonymously. The WHO has defined parasuicide usefully as the following:

> An act with non-fatal outcome, in which an individual deliberately initiates a non-habitual behaviour that, without intervention from others, will cause self-harm, or on purpose ingests a substance in excess of the prescribed or generally recognized therapeutic dosage, and which is aimed at realising changes which the subject desired via the actual or expected physical consequences.

For many years, suicide and 'attempted' suicide were regarded as varieties of the same behaviour, and Stengel et al. (1958)[92] showed that – although they were different – they did overlap. The difficulty in using the term 'attempted suicide' is that it implies an intention to die that may not be present; some authors have suggested that people who deliberately harm themselves and display significant suicidal intent should be described separately as 'suicide attempters'.

DSM-5 has advanced the debate a little further and has two new categories, *suicidal behaviour disorder* and *non suicidal self injury*, which are not included in the main text but in its 'appendix of conditions for further study'.

Suicidal Behaviour Disorder

This is defined as 'within the last 24 months, the individual has made a suicide attempt and the act does not meet criteria for non-suicidal self injury. It does not occur in states of confusion.'

Essentially, this is the same as a suicide attempt, and there should be evidence of a wish to die. In ICD-11, this is classified according to the method used – whether by a violent means or not, or a method with high lethality – and the degree of planning. It is considered to be *current* if it is not more than 12 months since the last attempt and in *early remission* if it is 12–24 months since the last attempt. Some 25–30% of subjects will go on to further attempts, and the main risk is for a later completed suicide. Suicide attempts usually occur in the context of a mental disorder (anxiety, depression, schizophrenia, PTSD, anorexia nervosa, BPD and substance abuse – especially alcohol) and are unusual in people without any mental disorder except in cases of terminal illness.

Non-suicidal Self Injury (NSSI)

This is defined in DSM-5 as 'Intentional self-inflicted damage to the skin which is likely to induce bleeding, bruising, pain (e.g. by cutting, bruising, stabbing, hitting, or excessive rubbing) with the expectation that injury will lead only to minor or moderate physical harm' – there is no suicidal intent. The main motivation for this is to obtain relief from a state of tension, a negative feeling or a negative cognitive state – or to resolve an interpersonal issue – and to induce a positive feeling. The bulk of the available literature on self harm concerns both these subtypes together and does not separate them out.

Epidemiology of Self Harm

After the deciminalisation of suicide in 1961, the UK witnessed a sharp increase in the incidence of SH. The rise continued during the 1970s, but rates increased during the latter part of the 1980s, only to show another rise in the 1990s.[93] The 2014 Adult Psychiatric Morbidity Survey[94] reported that, in England, the proportion of people aged 16–74 years who reported having ever self-harmed increased from 2.4% in 2000 to 3.8% in 2007 and to 6.4% in 2014. This increase was observed in both men and women and across age groups. Around one in every four 16-to-24-year-old women (25.7%) reported having self-harmed at some point, more than twice the rate for men in this age group (9.7%). The rate in women aged 25–34 years was 13.2%. In 2014, 5.4% of 16-to-74-year-olds reported suicidal thoughts in the past year, compared with 3.8% reporting this in 2000. Around one in every 20 men and one in every 12 women have *attempted* suicide at some point, with highest rates in women aged 16–24 years and men aged 25–34 years.

Many other European countries as well as the USA and Australia have also shown similar trends. SH research also needs to distinguish rates for persons from rates of number of episodes.

Overall, the prevalence in European countries is between 3–5%, but an international survey[95] found some variation in prevalence between nations: Puerto Rico was highest at 5.9%, France 5%, New Zealand 4.4%, Estonia 3.6%, West Germany 3.4%, Korea 3.2%, Brazil 3.1%, China 2.4% and 0.8% in Taiwan. Vietnam was lowest at 0.4%. Actual prevalence in the UK today is difficult to ascertain because many cases do not present to A&E, others are treated in general practice and many do not seek treatment at all and are therefore not counted. One figure[96] that may be helpful is that for every completed suicide, there are 48 cases of SH.

Self harm has a significant financial impact on the health care system. In the UK, for 2013, each episode on average cost £809 per self-harm presentation, with an approximate extrapolation to England of an impact on the NHS budget of approximately £162 million each year.[97] In one study in England,[82] SH was the third most frequent reason for acute general hospital admissions; 10% of admissions for SH resulted in psychiatric inpatient care, and 10% of patients were readmitted over the following 12 months with a repeated episode of SH. A systematic review[98] of the literature on hospital-treated SH indicated a 16% rate for non-fatal repetition and a 2% suicide rate after one year.

Age and Gender

In contrast to the pattern of a male predominance for completed suicide rates, the rates of SH among females are higher than those among males for all age groups (female to male = 1.5–2 to 1). The peak for females occurs in the 15–24 year age group, and for males is in the 25–34 year age group.[99] The average ratio of SH to a completed suicide in females is 21:1, but this decreases steeply with age, starting at 61:1 in the 15–24 year age group to 5:1 in those aged over 55. The ratio of SH to suicide in the USA is lower than in the UK, and it has been suggested that this is because of the more frequent use of firearms in attempting suicide.

Social Factors

Rates of SH are higher among people in social class V,[100] and factors associated with social instability and poverty are prominent. Well-established associations with SH are female sex, youth, single, being separated or divorced, lower educational level and unemployed people. Psychiatric disorder is also associated, particularly depression, but also substance abuse, borderline and antisocial personality disorders, severe anxiety – especially panic disorder – and physical illness. Certain psychological traits are also commonly reported, particularly impulsivity, aggression, impaired decision-making and poor problem solving.[101]

Methods of SH

Mostly non-violent methods are used in SH, as violent methods often lead to death at the first attempt. The vast majority of SH episodes in the UK involve self-poisoning by drug overdose. In one Oxford-based study,[99] around 88% of all the episodes of SH involved self-poisoning, 8% involved self injury and 4% involved both; paracetamol overdoses were more common in first-time attempters and young people, whereas overdoses of antidepressants and tranquillisers were more common in repeaters and older people. These differences may reflect the differential availability of the various medications. The WHO/EURO study reported similar findings: 64% of males and 80% of females used self-poisoning, whereas self injury was the method chosen by 17% of males cases and 9% of female cases.[101] In some poorer countries, self-poisoning by weed killers and insecticides (organophosphates) is common, but following recent bans (e.g. in Sri Lanka) on the sales of these compounds, death rates have been falling.

Self Injury

As indicated earlier, self injury is the second most common method of SH. Hawton (1989)[101] classified self cutting as superficial, deep or self mutilation. In the study of Favazza and Conterio,[102] the most common method of self injury was cutting (72%), burning (35%), hitting or punching parts of body (22%), interfering with wound healing (22%), scratching (22%), hair pulling (10%) and breaking bones (8%). In the same study, the most common site for the cutting was the wrist and arms (74%), the legs (44%), the abdomen (25%), head (23%), chest (18%) and the genitalia, including the vagina (8%). The onset is usually in the late teens, and the behaviour persists for 5 to 10 years. More than half of their sample had wounded themselves on more than 50 occasions. Sometimes, there is a history of childhood physical and sexual abuse, but in many instances, the early background is unremarkable.

Superficial self cutting tends to be associated with less suicidal intent, and to qualify for the DSM-5 category of '*non suicidal self injury*', there should be no suicidal intent. Carving on the skin and picking at a wound are the most commonly reported types of self mutilation. These occurred in about a third of a sample of US adolescents presenting with SH, often to dermatology clinics. Some subjects positively enjoy their self mutilation; Kafka[103] described a young female cutter who reported 'the exquisite border experience of coming alive at the moment of cutting' and later explained how the 'flow of blood has been like a voluptuous bath with pleasant warmth spreading all over her body' and then added 'why everyone did not indulge in blood baths routinely especially as they were so readily available by simply unzipping one's skin'.

Those with self mutilation were more likely to be diagnosed with oppositional defiant disorder, major depression or dysthymia. They also had higher scores on measures of hopelessness, loneliness, anger, risk taking, reckless behaviour and alcohol use.[104] Self mutilators appear to have more persistent suicidal ideation and to perceive their behaviour as less lethal than it actually is.[105]

Deep cutting sometimes involves major blood vessels, nerves and tendons, and it is sometimes (although not necessarily) associated with serious suicidal intent; it is, though, usually associated with severe psychiatric disorder. Psychotic self mutilation is rare and may affect the eyes, tongue or genitalia.

Oedipism (as distinct from the Oedipus complex) is defined as 'self-inflicted injury to the eye', though some authors restrict it to cases of self enucleation alone.[106] According to legend, Oedipus killed his father, King Laius of Thebes, and married his mother, Jocasta, unaware of the identity of either. Pestilence descended on Thebes, and Oedipus consulted an oracle, who told him that his incest and the murder of his father were the cause of pestilence. In a state of horror, Oedipus tore out his eyes and became a blind, wandering beggar.

Self-inflicted damage to the eyes is rare but occasionally presents to ophthalmology clinics. A recent study[106] described five cases where patients tried to get at the source of intrusive auditory hallucinations, which they believed were coming from inside their heads, either by repeatedly hitting the sides of their face or by poking their fingers into the sides of their eyes to enucleate them. Self-inflicted traumatic cataracts, detached retinas and lens dislocations have also been reported.

Major self mutilation includes removing eyes or a testicle, severing the penis or amputating a portion of a limb. An Australian survey[107] found that 143 of 189 cases (76%) had a psychiatric illness, and of these 119 (83%) were diagnosed with a schizophrenia spectrum disorder and 90% were men. Of those who amputated their genitalia who were not psychotic, the largest group had gender identity disorder, and a second group of Asian men believed that penile amputation would result in their death and so were probably suicidal and depressed. Around 80% of the schizophrenic subjects described a delusional belief. The most common delusions involved a false belief that the amputated organ was evil (43%), that the organ had special – usually threatening – supernatural powers such as the ability to spread evil (28%) or that it needed to be sacrificed to save the patient or others (20%). Around half of the self mutilation took place in their first episode of psychosis when it is known that the risks of schizophrenic homicide are thought to be particularly high (x 20), and the authors likened these episodes to schizophrenic homicide.

Attempting suicide by burning is rare in Europe. Self-immolation rarely occurs in developed countries, but it is more prevalent in developing countries such as Iran, Sri Lanka and India. More than 90 per cent of burn cases that result in death occur in developing countries. One study[107] reported that SH by burning constituted 1 per cent of all admissions to a burns unit, and that among these cases, there was high incidence of prior psychiatric illness.

The relationship between the severity of suicidal intent and the lethality of the method used is not clear, but if either is present, then the later risk of a suicide is high, and this should be taken into account in the treatment plan.

Biological Factors in Suicide and Self Harm

The biological aetiological factors in SH and completed suicide are similar, and the small literature on the topic is considered here. It has long been known that suicide may be familial but unclear whether this was through a genetic or environmental mechanism. Roy[108] combined several twin studies giving 399 twin pairs; 17 (13.2%) of the 129 MZ twins were concordant for suicide compared to only 2 (0.7%) out of the 270 DZ pairs, suggesting a strong effect for genetics.

A large Australian population twin study (N = 6,000) assessing both severe suicidal thoughts and attempts found that after controlling for psychiatric disorder, childhood trauma and religious affiliation, a history of suicide attempts or persistent thoughts in the respondent's co-twin remained a powerful predictor in MZ pairs (OR = 3.9) but was not consistently predictive in DZ pairs. Overall, these investigators estimated that genetic factors accounted for approximately 45 per cent of the variance in suicidal thoughts and behaviours.[109]

There is always a difficulty in ascertaining whether a familial effect can be inherited or is learnt, but adoption studies – mostly based on data from the Danish adoption registers – can help tease out what is nature and what is nurture. The register had 57 adoptees[110] who had died through suicide, and they were matched with 57 control adoptees. A total of 269 relatives of each group were identified, and 12 (4.5%) of the 269 biological relatives of the suicide adoptees had died through suicide compared to only 2 (0.7%) of the 269 relatives of the control group ($p < 0.01$). This suggest that the familial effect for suicide is largely genetic.

Low cholesterol levels have been repeatedly reported amongst patients admitted with an episode of SH. Amongst major depressive disorder (MDD) subjects, suicide attempters compared to non-attempters had lower cholesterol. A recent meta-analysis confirmed these observations, that there was an association with total cholesterol and low-density lipoprotein cholesterol (LDL-C), but there were no differences for high density lipoprotein cholesterol (HDL-C), cholesterol or for triglycerides.

The main neurochemical hypothesis to explain this revolve around serotonin in that there is an association between low cholesterol concentrations, poor serotonin uptake and a decrease in the viscosity of brain-cell membranes.[111] Abnormalities in the serotonergic system correlate with high levels of impulsivity and have been implicated in suicidal behaviour. Research today is now focused on genes possibly related to suicide and those related to serotonin, but results are too inconclusive to add anything useful at present.

Treatment of Self Harm

There is no specific treatment for SH since it may have multiple and diverse causes, and many different treatments may be needed. Because some subjects with SH present with challenging and even abusive behaviours, as a group they have developed a poor reputation particularly amongst A&E staff,

Box 15.5 The NICE quality standard for self harm (2013)[112]

- People are treated with compassion, respect and dignity.
- They receive an initial assessment of physical health, mental state, social circumstances and risk of suicide.
- They receive a comprehensive psychosocial assessment.
- They receive the monitoring they need to keep them safe.
- They are cared for in a safe physical environment.
- Collaborative risk management plan is in place.
- They have access to psychological interventions.
- There is a transition plan when moving between services.

occasionally resulting in hostile staff responses. This issue was addressed in the first clause in the last set of NICE guidelines, given above in Box 15.5.

Most of the psychological treatment programmes that have been tried are CBT-based; problem solving has been found to be poorly developed amongst those prone to suicide attempts but can be improved with basic CBT. A majority of those who attempt suicide are depressed, and so CBT for depression (see Chapter 3.4) is sometimes also used as is dialectical behaviour therapy for BPD. Manual-assisted CBT is a relatively cheap option, but few patients stuck to the manual, so this method was not effective in preventing relapse. Suicide cards give patients an emergency telephone number they can contact if they are distressed and feel they are going to make an attempt. A controlled trial of interpersonal therapy,[113] where nurses visited patients in their own homes for four weeks, starting one week after their suicide attempt, is one of the few trials to demonstrate a significant effect for psychotherapy. A Cochrane review in 2016 of the treatment of self harm concluded that CBT-based psychological therapy can result in fewer individuals repeating SH,[114] but evidence is limited and more rigorous studies are needed.

Suicidal Thoughts

Suicidal thoughts are very common, and an epidemiological study[115] gave data on the annual incidence of particular suicidal thoughts as follows: Felt life not worth living (7.8%), wished you were dead (5.0%), thoughts of taking one's life (2.3%) and – this is the most commonly quoted figure – seriously considered taking one's life (1.5%) and made a suicide attempt (0.4%). Other negative thoughts such as 'no one loves me', 'I have no future', 'my life has no meaning', 'I would be better off dead', 'no one understands my depression', 'there will never be an end to my misery' and similar thoughts are also commonly reported.

Fewer than 1 in 200 (or 500 per 100,000) of those suffering from suicidal thoughts go on to complete suicide, but this is still 45 times more than the 14 per 100,000 base rate for suicide in the general population. Amongst those with depression, around 40% may also have suicidal thoughts but, for those in the depressed phase of a bipolar disorder, this figure rises to 72%, indicating that bipolar depressed subjects are at a much greater risk. Surveys of suicidal thoughts separate out simple suicidal thoughts from those where there are thoughts associated with suicide planning, which is taken as a more dangerous sign. A routine psychiatric assessment of a suicidal patient will always entail enquiring whether subjects are actively planning such an outcome and how far they have progressed in this endeavour.

What is less well-known is the extent and degree of intrusiveness of such thoughts. One study[116] found that many suicidal patients experienced a repetition of their suicidal thoughts several hundred times a day, and the total amount of time these suicidal thoughts intruded into their mind sometimes amounted to 10 or 15 hours a day. In times of crisis, such suicidal thoughts would keep them awake and account for their distressing insomnia, and some even reported the impossibility of stopping their suicidal thoughts, and this proved to be the tipping point for their suicide attempt. Suicidal auditory hallucinations, which give the subject an instruction to die through suicide, may also have an intrusive, repetitive quality, and sometimes patients give in to the instructions of their suicidal hallucinations. Certain features in suicidal thoughts point to a higher risk, and these include hopelessness, high levels of anxiety, insomnia and depression, very intense emotions and rarely psychotic features, such as hearing voices or having depressive delusions. Thoughts associated with suicide planning are especially dangerous.

Accounts from survivors of attempts that would be expected to be lethal (e.g. a follow-up of a cohort of people who jumped from the Golden Gate bridge in San Francisco, which has over a 97 per cent fatality rate) suggest that, even in the seconds after the expected lethal attempt, regret is common.[117] Follow-up of survivors of such attempts also suggest that the great majority do not end their lives through suicide.

Suicide Prevention

The act of a suicide results in a death and is final and irreversible. This means that preventative strategies must operate early, reduce risk factors and pre-empt the final deed. Many people who die from suicide do not seek any prior treatment nor have they made a previous attempt and are therefore unknown to services. Hence, they can only be reached through population-based strategies that reduce the causes and means for suicide. Prevention at a national level has therefore focused on education, reducing access to methods of suicide and – at an individual level – on treating people with mental illness and the consequent risk of suicide and, if necessary, hospitalisation.

Preventing Access to the Means for Suicide

Perhaps the most successful preventative strategy in the modern era has been the switch from coal gas to natural gas in the 1960s, which had little or no carbon monoxide. This single move practically abolished carbon monoxide poisoning, and suicide rates due to gas inhalation reduced from 50% in 1960 to 0.2% in 1976 and were not replaced by other methods in the UK.[118] Another helpful innovation came with the introduction of catalytic converters in exhausts to get rid of noxious gases. Thus, the Clean Air Act 1970 led to the first catalytic converters being introduced in 1975 in the USA, resulting in a suicide reduction from 10 to 5 per million person-years between 1968 and 1988. In the UK in 1993, new legislation required all petrol vehicles to be fitted with catalytic converters, reducing carbon monoxide emissions, so suicides due to motor vehicle exhaust inhalations subsequently declined.

Reduction of the Availability of Medication

In most countries, overdoses of medication, usually psychotropics, remain the most common method of suicide. In the 1970s, an Australian research team noted that suicide rates correlated highly with the number of barbiturate prescriptions, and legislation was brought in to tighten up barbiturate prescribing, restrict repeat prescriptions and individually wrap tablets, so it was no longer possible to take a handful of tablets. This led to a reduction in rates of barbiturate poisoning.[119]

Paracetamol overdose can result in fatal liver failure, and rates of this complication were reduced by restricting the sales of large quantities of paracetamol over the counter. Today, Panadol sales are restricted to no more than eight grams per sale in France and 12 grams in the UK, and this had a marked effect in reducing paracetamol overdoses and admissions for paracetamol-induced liver failure.[120]

Most overdoses today are with anxiolytic-hypnotic prescriptions, and a campaign[121] was instituted in Sweden to limit their use but fell short of banning them completely. Even so, the campaign resulted in a 25% reduction in suicide rates and attempts, 12% reduction in repeat prescriptions and 40% reduction in anxiety hypnotic drug abuse.[121] Restricting prescriptions clearly works, but apart from reducing paracetamol availability, this method has not been more widely applied.

Gunshot is a common method of suicide amongst men, particularly in the USA. Gun control has been highly controversial and limited in America, but in Canada, which for a period had a similar access to guns as America, a law was passed in 1977 to regulate gun ownership with fairly strict licensing criteria. Initially, there was no obvious effect, but a 20-year follow-up[122] showed a fall in all suicides, but most especially gunshot suicides, which was not replaced by suicide by other means. The fall applied mainly to younger suicides, where the suicide was more often impulsive, but rates for elderly suicides were unaffected. In Tasmania in 1966, there was a gunshot massacre of 36 people, resulting in the Australian government bringing in strict gun control measures, and this resulted in a reduction of all gunshot deaths including suicide.[123] Legal gun control measures seem to work, but there is a difficulty is getting such measures through legislatures, particularly in America, because of opposition from campaigning by gun control lobbies such as the National Rifle Association.

Pesticide Control

In low- and middle-income countries, pesticide ingestion is the most common method of committing suicide, and it is thought that one-third of all suicides worldwide are through this method.[124] Some pesticides have low lethality, such as chlorpyrifos which has a lethality of 8%, while others such as paraquat and aluminium hydroxide have very high lethalities of around 70%. Pesticides usually result in lung damage, which can be fatal.

There are around 2 million hospital admissions per year for pesticide poisoning, mainly in low- and middle-income countries, and these often result in lengthy stays in intensive care beds, indicating that the problem is a major consumer of scarce health service resources. Treating pesticide poisoning is medically difficult because there are so many different pesticides, each requiring their own antidote or mode of treatment. Also, in rural India and rural China where most of these episodes occur, there is a lack of expertise to treat pesticide poisoning, so many suicide attempts become suicide deaths even though this was never intended.[125]

In 1996, paraquat was introduced into Samoa, and this led to a rise in suicide rates in Samoa. However, in 2003, its use was abolished in Sri Lanka,[124] and this led to a fall in suicide rates. Both these examples show that death by paraquat overdosing was closely linked to its availability. Many ideas have been proposed as ways to reduce pesticide deaths, and these include banning the use of the most lethal pesticides, increasing taxes according to the pesticide lethality, requiring farmers to keep them in safe boxes or in a community safe and so making them difficult to obtain, and increasing knowledge of the dangers of pesticides, but implementation of these measures has only had partial success.

Suicide in Rural China

Suicides in China account for 26% of all global suicides, and pesticide ingestion is the most common method used in China. Pesticide poisoning rates are strongly correlated with the amount of pesticide sold and associated management policies. However, a report in 2014[125] has shown some decrease in recent years from 62% to 49%, but it is still the leading cause of suicide. Self-poisoning with pesticides, especially among women, may be used to gain attention, express distress or seek revenge, but not necessarily to end life. Traditionally, suicide is an influential method for people – particularly women and those with low status – to prove their innocence or protest against unfair treatment, and commonly, pesticides found in their homes or farms are used. Most of these rural suicides are unplanned (57%) and impulsive, and pesticide ingestion was the most common method employed in unplanned suicides. Young women in China who attempt suicide have a similar profile as the 'attempted suicide population' found in Western nations such as the UK. Thus, in one study of 147 women suicide attempters in rural China[125] aged under 35, the method used was pesticide ingestion in 88% of the cases, family conflict was present in 60%, and there were no signs of mental disturbance in 62% of the subjects. They also cite similar reasons for their suicide attempt, except in rural China – rather than swallowing too many Valium tablets, which has a very low lethality – they ingest a very toxic pesticide with a high fatality rate, with women being more often affected than men and the fatal outcome usually being unintended.

This may explain why the sex ratio for suicide in China showed a female predominance for several decades, although in the last decade, the pattern has reverted to the more usual pattern of men more commonly committing suicide than women, as found in the rest of the world.

Suicides by Jumping

In Hong Kong, Taiwan and Singapore, there are many high buildings, and suicide in these countries is commonly by jumping. In Taipei, Taiwan, 35% of the population live on the sixth floor or above, and 20% of all suicides are by jumping. In Hong Kong, the figure for 2014 was 50%, and in Singapore, the figure was even higher at 75%.[126] In the UK, death from jumping from a height only occurs in 4% of suicides.[127] It has been shown that the placing of high barriers, of at least 1.5 metres, combined with reducing media coverage of such events has reduced the rates.

Charcoal Burning

In Hong Kong in 1998, a woman was reported as having killed herself by burning charcoal in her room and dying from carbon monoxide poisoning. The phenomenon was widely reported in the local media and on the internet, and the method became increasingly popular in Hong Kong, Taiwan and southern coastal China.[128]

In a confined place such as a closed room of a small flat, charcoal burning will result in high levels of carbon monoxide. Charcoal burning was perceived as being an easily accessible, effective and painless means of killing oneself, and this led to epidemics in Japan and Korea amongst young people. Charcoal is used for recreation, barbeques and religious ancestry worship and so is freely available in shops in the Far East. It had a low mortality rate of 3 per cent, but amongst the survivors, globus pallidus necrosis (a known complication of non-fatal carbon monoxide poisoning) occurred in almost 60 per cent of subjects.[128] An attempt was made to reduce access by removing it from the shelves of supermarkets and shops and placing it in a store at the back of the shop, and this is thought to have led to some reduction in rates.

Alcohol

Alcohol can be used as an agent both to die through suicide but also as an adjunct to other methods and is commonly found in the blood of suicide victims. In Sweden, alcohol was present in 45% of victims, Finland 40%, Sri Lanka 31%, America 29% and in Holland 20%.[129] Suicide rates tend to follow levels of alcohol consumption, which can be regulated – where the will exists – by increasing taxation. When this is done, a fall in suicide rates does seem to occur.

During the collapse of the Soviet Union, Mikhail Gorbachev, as a part of his perestroika reforms, sought to reduce alcohol consumption. He imposed a large increase in the price of spirits, and this resulted in a 32% decrease in suicide rates for men and 19% for women. Unfortunately, the Russian public did not take kindly to this price rise and still wanted their vodka, so the policy was scrapped, and thereafter suicide rates began to rise again.[130]

These examples show that reducing the availability of the means to a suicide can lead to a reduction in rates – but instituting such measures is not straightforward. Thus, the chances of Americans giving up their guns or Russians their vodka any time soon is not great. In the UK, however, managing the cost and availability is feasible and being advocated to the government.

Crisis Hotlines

From his small church, St. Stevens, in the city of London, the Reverend Chad Varah, who founded the Samaritans wrote, 'When I made it known to the press that from 2nd November 1953, people contemplating suicide were invited to telephone me ... I did not think of myself as founding an organisation, let alone a world movement.' In his own words, the service was just 'a man willing to listen with a base and an emergency telephone'.[131] Today, the Samaritans is an organisation with more than 20,000 volunteers in the UK, and it is now estimated that over a hundred thousand volunteers staff suicide hotlines.

Assessing whether they are effective or not has been difficult to prove because a prevented suicide yields no data for analysis. A study[132] of silently monitoring calls reported that empathy, respect and good contact, and a collaborative approach, could be observed, and most calls ended on a positive note. However, during the calls, there were infrequent attempts to assess suicide risk. Another study showed that caller distress decreased in 43% of the calls. In a veteran's administration study, 84% had a satisfactory outcome in that either a reduction of the distress concerning the specific issue occurred within the call or that there was a referral to a mental health facility.[133] However, 16% of calls ended in an unresolved state. A Dutch study[134] found little change in suicidality during the interview: in around 3%, it got better; in 30%, it stayed the same; and in 3%, it got worse. There was no difference between volunteer and paid call responders provided they had each done more than 140 hours of telephone responding work. A Hong Kong-based study of those who had died through suicide found that 14% had previously contacted the hotline, indicating that the contact had not prevented a suicide, although it is possible it might have delayed it, but it did confirm that the callers to such services comprise a very high risk group.[135]

Educational Approaches

A variety of educational programmes targeted at schools mainly in America have been devised. Some are targeted at teachers, counsellors and those in direct contact with adolescent pupils with the aim of enhancing their abilities in recognising at pupils at risk. Some skills-based programmes are used to train pupils to handle their emotions of depression, anger or loneliness. In other cases, questionnaires are given to pupils to screen out those who are currently depressed or suicidal, who are then referred on for treatment. These programmes are not used in the UK, but almost all secondary schools now have school counsellors to deal with suicidal and other emotional problems amongst teenagers. Educational programmes targeted at GPs to ensure better detection and treatment of depression have also been tried. One of the best known was the Gotland Program. Rutz[136] offered a structured education programme to help GPs in the recognition and treatment of depressive disorders on the island of Gotland in Sweden. The authors found that this led to a significant reduction in the number of suicides on this Swedish island. Three years after the programme had ended, the authors returned to Gotland,[137] only to find that the suicide rate had risen back to its old pre-training course level. This suggests that if an education programme has some success, it needs to be maintained over the longer term to preserve any gains made.

Because suicide is a very evocative topic, politicians and other 'influencers' have become involved, and there have been national campaigns to encourage suicide awareness and its prevention such as Defeat Depression 1992–1996 in the UK, Beyond Blue in Australia 2001 and the National Strategy for Suicide Prevention in the USA, as well as several others,[138] including the more recent 'Zero Suicide' approach. Whilst these campaigns give those participating a feeling that 'something is being done', accruing evidence for their effectiveness or otherwise is not straightforward and perhaps is not a question amenable to simple scientific enquiry. The issue loops back to the sociological factors and wider societal influences that Durkheim described as influencing suicide rates.

Grassroots campaigns to try to promote suicide prevention and help disenfranchised groups access support, such as those organised through networks associated with professional sport for both players and their communities – for example, the charity 'State of Mind' in Rugby League – might be postulated to have some beneficial impact, though demonstrating this beyond individual cases is difficult. In Durkheimian terms, it could be seen as an effort to build greater social cohesion and address 'anomie' or alienation at a local social level.[139] There is a risk also that use of phrases such as 'Zero Suicide' may be counter-productive; whilst setting a clear goal for prevention, it can be argued that it may make it harder to get people to work with suicidal individuals.

Suicide Survivors

A person's death is not only an ending but also a beginning – for the survivors, whose lives are changed forever –
Edwin Shneidman[139]

Who then are the survivors? It is usual to consider both parents, siblings and close friends as survivors, and Shneidman estimated there were on average around six survivors for every single suicide. However, once more distant relatives, such as grandparents, and school teachers and classmates were counted, the numbers become much larger as many people will be affected.

Professionals who have known the patient can also be seen as survivors in this sense, and the impact of suicide and other serious events on professionals is a significant but often unspoken issue.

A suicide stirs up strange feelings amongst those around the event. Although much of the overt stigma has now gone, relatives have often internalised this stigma, and it forms a part of their grief. Incidents such as the suicide of a patient under the care of mental health services are likely to lead to further investigation as a 'serious incident'. Such deaths are a small minority of deaths of all patients, but they are deaths that invoke powerful emotions and the human need to attempt to understand. How organisations approach their duties to investigate contribute to the culture of their organisation significantly. All such deaths will also be subject to a coroner's inquest. Organisations have to try to promote a culture of safe care and so examining the individual case is crucial to identify any processes or systems that could have contributed, as well as whether there were any major individual errors in the clinical care. This requires some objective review of what happened. At the same time, such reviews need to hold in mind that they commence the review from a point of knowledge of what has happened that was not available to the professionals prior to the suicide. Danish philosopher Kierkegaard (1813–1855) conveyed this observation as: 'Life can only be understood backwards; but it must be lived forwards'.

Organisations also have to be aware of the need to provide a framework of support to staff who are involved in delivering care and making decisions moving forward in time, without the knowledge of what will happen in the future. The balance that organisations achieve with these approaches may influence factors crucial to good patient care, such as staff recruitment and retention.[140]

American studies[141] have shown that around a half of all practising psychiatrists in the USA have experienced the loss of a patient under their care to suicide, and around half of these psychiatrists experienced symptoms on the PTSD checklist, with younger trainee psychiatrists being more affected than 'older seasoned professionals'. Some psychiatrists also sought counselling at the time as well. A Gibbons et al. study[140] in four Trusts in England suggested that around 80 per cent of their sample of psychiatrists had had the experience of a patient suicide, with many reporting adverse impacts on their wellbeing and future practice.

More recently, there has been a number of studies that have examined how a suicide bereavement differs from a bereavement following a death due to natural causes. Feelings of sadness, loneliness and loss may follow in any bereavement. In a suicide bereavement, however, these are often magnified by feelings of guilt, confusion, shame and anger. Rates of complicated grief may be elevated following a suicide bereavement where healing is either slow or does not occur. Most suicide survivors are plagued by the need to understand the suicide, that perhaps they should have done something to prevent the suicide, or by the shame that it happened in their family. Those with complicated grief after suicide had the highest rates of lifetime depression, pre-loss passive suicidal ideation, self-blaming thoughts, and impaired work and social adjustment.[142] Social stigma may sometimes be associated with a suicide bereavement, and this may complicate the grieving process amongst the suicide survivors. Does this matter, and does suicide survivor status confer greater risks of mental ill health and suicide itself?

There is limited data, but a recent large South Korean study[143] performing psychological autopsies on adolescent suicide survivors found that up to 95 per cent of subjects showed psychiatric difficulties meeting clinical criteria. Some of those with psychiatric morbidity were referred to mental health services, and they had a significantly better outcome than those who were not referred. The latter group subsequently had a 2.08 times higher risk of death by suicide.

Although there is no specific treatment for 'suicide survivors', many subjects found attending ordinary bereavement groups was both upsetting and unhelpful, preferring to attend specific suicide survivor groups. These originally started in the USA in the 1970s, the first probably being 'The Ray of Hope', founded by Elizabeth Ross in Iowa City.[144] Since then, more than 300 such groups have been established in the USA. In the UK, there is an organisation called 'Survivors of Bereavement by Suicide' (SOBS) , founded in 1991[145] by Alice Middleton following the death of her brother. Finding little support was locally available at the time, she placed an advert in her local paper seeking to make contact with others who had been similarly bereaved by suicide, and the first support group started from her living room in Hull. This has grown to become a national charity providing dedicated support to adults who have been bereaved by suicide, and their literature states they have helped over 7,000 subjects to come to terms with their loss and to connect with others.

Conclusion

Suicide is a tragedy for the individual concerned as well as for their families, who may suffer greatly, sometimes for the rest of their lives. Tackling suicide will require much more than psychiatry can offer, and it will involve many additional agencies of society as described in the Suicide Prevention Strategy for England published in 2023.[146] Psychiatry, though, has a special responsibility for suicide attempts and completed suicide for those with mental illness. All psychiatrists should acquire the skills needed to assess suicidal risk and be able to talk to suicidal patients, helping to reduce their suicidality and distress. Modern suicidology research has generated vast quantities of numerical data, and root causes are well understood. However, usable prediction remains beyond our reach, and key questions as to why and when certain individuals will take their lives without specific identified reason or in the face of common life events that the vast majority of people negotiate without resorting to suicide remain unanswered. In the UK and Western Europe, rates are currently slowly falling, but it is unknown how much this is due to the efforts of psychiatrists and suicide prevention programmes or to sociodemographic and economic changes such as greater prosperity or more equality in society.

Proving that a suicide prevention programme works is almost impossible, but it is likely that some programmes – especially those that reduce the availability of lethal agents in the environment – are reducing the total numbers of people who die through suicide. Suicide prevention is a worthwhile venture, but its status at the moment is best described as no more than 'a work in progress'.

References

1. Stein GS. Suicide, suicidal thoughts and self-mutilation in the Bible. In: *The Hidden Psychiatry of the Old Testament.* Falls Village, CT: Hamilton Books; 2018: 231–89.
2. Barraclough BM. The Bible suicides. *Acta Psychiatrica Scandinavica* 1992; 86(1):64–9.
3. Van Hooff AJL. *From Autothanasla to Suicide. Self Killing in Classical Antiquity.* Abingdon: Routledge; 1990.
4. Augustine A. *The City of God Against the Pagans. 426 AD* (trans. RW Dyson). Cambridge: Cambridge University Press; 1998.
5. Colt GH. The history of the suicide survivor: the mark of Cain. In: Dunne EJ, Mackintosh JL, Dunne-Maxim K (eds.) *Suicide and Its Aftermath: Understanding and Counselling the Survivors.* London: Norton; 1987: 3–18.
6. Durkheim E. *Le Suicide* (trans. JA Spaulding and G Simpson as *Suicide: A Study in Sociology* 1952). Abingdon: Routledge & Kegan Paul; 1897.
7. Szasz T. *Suicide: What is the clinician's responsibility.* Unpublished paper presented at the Harvard Medical School. In: Maris R, Berman AL, Silverman MM (eds.) *Comprehensive Textbook of Suicidology.* New York: Guilford Press; 1985: 495.
8. World Health Organization. *Preventing Suicide: A Global Imperative.* Geneva: World Health Organization; 2014.

9. Farmer RDT. Assessing the epidemiology of suicide and parasuicide. *British Journal of Psychiatry* 1988;153(1):16–20.
10. Alvarez A. *The Savage God. A Study of Suicide.* London: Norton; 1990.
11. Babylonian Talmud. *Semahot.* Cited in: Siegel S. *Religion: a Jewish view.* In: Hankoff LD, Einsidler B (eds.) *Suicide: Theory and Clinical Practice.* London: PSG Publishing; 1979: 83–90.
12. Linsley KR, Schapira K, Kelly TP. Open verdict v. suicide – importance to research. *British Journal of Psychiatry* 2001;178(5):465–8.
13. Kelly S, Bunting, J. Trends in suicide in England and Wales, 1982–1996. *Population Trends* 1998;92:29–41.
14. Office of National Statistics. *Suicides in England and Wales: 2021 Registrations.* www.ons.gov.uk/peoplepopulationandcommunity/birthsdeathsandmarriages/deaths/bulletins/suicidesintheunitedkingdom/2021registrations.
15. World Health Organization. *Suicide Worldwide in 2019: Global Health Estimates.* Geneva: World Health Organization; 2021.
16. Kushner HI. *American Suicide. A Psychocultural Exploration.* New Brunswick: Rutgers University Press; 1991.
17. Wasserman D, Wasserman C. *The Oxford Textbook of Suicide Prevention A Global Perspective.* Oxford: Oxford University Press; 2009.
18. Pritchard C, Iqbal W, Dray R Undetermined and accidental mortality rates as possible sources of underreported suicides: population-based study comparing Islamic countries and traditionally religious Western countries *British Journal of Psychiatry Open* 2020;6(4):e56.
19. Diekstra RFW. An international perspective on the epidemiology and prevention of suicide. In: Blumenthal SJ and Kupfer D (eds.) *Suicide Over the Life Cycle.* Washington, DC: American Psychiatric Press, 1990: 536–7.
20. Moksony F. Age patterns of suicide in Hungary. *Suicide Research* 1995;1 (4):217–22.
21. Balint L, Fuzer K, Gonda X, et al. Estimation of the relationship between the persistent decrease of the suicide rate in Hungary between 1990 and 2011. *PLoS ONE* 2020;15(10):e0241314.
22. Bhugra D. Sati: A type of nonpsychiatric suicide. *Crisis* 2005;26(2):73–7.
23. Salih E, Rahim S, El-Nimr G, et al. Elderly suicide: an analysis of coroners inquests into 200 cases of elderly suicide in Cheshire 1989–2001. *Medicine, Science, and the Law* 2005;45(1):71–80.
24. Leo D, Padovani W, Lonnqvist J et al. Attempted and completed suicide in older subjects: results from the WHO/EURO multi-centre study of suicidal behaviour *International Journal of Geriatric Psychiatry* 2001;16(3): 300–10.
25. Groenewoud AS, Atsma F, Arvin M, et al. Euthanasia in the Netherlands: a claims data cross-sectional study of geographical variation. *BMJ Supportive & Palliative Care* 2021.
26. Li M, Katikireddi SV. Urban-rural inequalities in suicide among elderly people in China: a systematic review and meta-analysis *International Journal of Equity Health* 2019;18:2.
27. World Health Organization. *Burden of Disease Study.* Geneva: World Health Organization; 2017.
28. The National Confidential Inquiry into Suicide and Safety in Mental Health. *Annual Report: England, Northern Ireland, Scotland and Wales.* Manchester: University of Manchester; 2021. documents.manchester.ac.uk/display.aspx?DocID=55332 (accessed 18 February 2023).
29. Arsenault-Lapierre G, Kim C, Tureki G. Psychiatric diagnoses in 3,275 suicides, a meta-analysis. *BMC Psychiatry* 2004;4:37.
30. Hunt IM, Kapur N, Robinson J et al. Suicide within 12 months of mental health contact in different age and diagnostic groups. National Clinical Survey. *British Journal of Psychiatry* 2006; 188:135–42.
31. Bertolote JM, Fleischman A, Leo D et al. Suicide and mental disorder: do we know enough *British Journal of Psychiatry* 2003;182(5):382–3.
32. Lonnqvist J. Major psychiatric disorders in suicide and suicide attempters. In: Wasserman D, Wasserman C (eds.) *Oxford Textbook of Suicidology and Suicide Prevention: A Global Perspective.* Oxford: Oxford University Press, 2009: 275–286.
33. Beck AT, Steer RA, Brown G. Dysfunctional attitudes and suicidal behavior in psychiatric outpatients. *Suicide and Life-Threatening Behaviour* 1993;23(1):11–20.
34. Lansky M. Shame and the problem of suicide: a family systems perspective. *British Journal of Psychotherapy* 1991;7 (3):230–42.
35. Key R, Underwood A, Farnham F, et al. Suicidal behavior in individuals accused or convicted of child sex abuse or indecent image offenses: Systematic review of prevalence and risk factors. *Suicide and Life-Threatening Behavior* 2021;51(4):715–28.
36. Lu L, Dong M, Zhang L, et al. Prevalence of suicide attempts in individuals with schizophrenia: a meta-analysis of observational studies. *Epidemiology Psychiatry and Science* 2020;29:e39.
37. Taipale H, Lähteenvuo M, Tanskanen A, et al. Comparative effectiveness of antipsychotics for risk of attempted or completed suicide among persons with schizophrenia. *Schizophrenia Bulletin.* 2021;47(1):23–30.
38. Harris EC, Barraclough B. Suicide as an outcome for mental disorders. A meta-analysis. *British Journal of Psychiatry* 1997;170;205–28.
39. Osby U, Brandt L, Correia N, et al. Excess mortality in bipolar and unipolar disorder in Sweden. *Archives of General Psychiatry* 2001;58(9):844–50.
40. Schaffer A, Isometsä ET, Azorin J, et al. A review of factors associated with greater likelihood of suicide attempts and suicide deaths in bipolar disorder: Part II of a report of the International Society for Bipolar Disorders Task Force on Suicide in Bipolar Disorder. *Australian and New Zealand Journal of Psychiatry* 2015;49 (11):1006–20.
41. Wortzel HS, Simonetti JA, Oslin D, et al. Lithium use for suicide prevention, revisited. *Journal of Psychiatric Practice* 2023;29(1):51–7.
42. Baldessarini RJ, Tondo L, Davis P, et al. Decreased risk of suicides and attempts during long-term lithium treatment: a meta-analytic review. *Bipolar Disorder* 2006;8(5 Pt 2):625–39.
43. Chen, P-H, Tsai, S-Y, Chen, P-Y, et al. Mood stabilizers and risk of all-cause, natural, and suicide mortality in bipolar disorder: a nationwide cohort study. *Acta Psychiatrica Scandinavica* 2023;147(3):234–47. DOI: 10.1111/acps.13519.

44. National Collaborating Centre for Mental Health. *Bipolar Disorder: The NICE Guideline on the Assessment and Management of Bipolar Disorder in Adults, Children and Young People in Primary and Secondary Care (CG185).* 2020. www.nice.org.uk/guidance/cg185.
45. Stone MH. *The Fate of Borderline Patients.* New York: Guilford Press; 1990.
46. Flynn S, Graney J, Nyathi T, et al. Clinical characteristics and care pathways of patients with personality disorder who died by suicide British *Journal of Psychiatry Open* 2020;6(2): e29.
47. Apter A. Bleich A, King R, et al. Death without warning? A clinical study of 43 Israeli male suicides *Archives of General Psychiatry* 1993;50(2):138–42.
48. Beale C. Magical thinking and moral injury: exclusion culture in psychiatry. *BJPsych Bulletin* 2022;46(1):16–9.
49. Borges G, Bagge C, Cherpitel CJ, et al. A meta-analysis of acute alcohol use and the risk of suicide attempt *Psychological Medicine* 2017;47(5):949–57.
50. Norström T, Rossow I. Alcohol consumption as a risk factor for suicidal behaviour: a systematic review of associations at the individual and at the population level. *Archives of Suicide Research* 2016;20(4):489–506.
51. Razvodovsky YE. The structure of alcohol sale and violent mortality: time series analysis. *Psychiatry* 2009;1:6–12.
52. Fishbain DA, Achille L, Barsky S, et al. A controlled study of suicide pacts. *Journal of Clinical Psychiatry* 1984:45 (4):154–7.
53. Hillbrand M. Self-directed and other-directed aggressive behaviour in a forensic service. *Suicide and Life-Threatening Behaviour* 1992;22 (3):333–40.
54. Garrison CZ, Mckeown RE, Valois RF, et al. Aggression, substance abuse and suicidal behaviours in high school students. *American Journal of Public Health* 1993;83(2):179–84.
55. Altmann H, Slett W, Eaton ME, et al. Demographic and mental status profles: Patients with homicidal, assaultive suicidal, persecutory and homosexual ideation. The Missouri Automated Standard System of Psychiatry. *Psychiatric Quarterly* 1971;45(1):57–64.
56. Ministry of Justice. *Self-inflicted Deaths in Prison Custody.* www.ethnicity-facts-figures.service.gov.uk/crime-justice-and-the-law/prison-and-custody-incidents/self-inflicted-deaths-in-prison-custody/latest (accessed 5 February 2023).
57. Gore S. Suicide in prisons. Reflection of the community served or exacerbated risk? *British Journal of Psychiatry* 1999;175:50–5.
58. Zhong S, Senior M, Yu R, et al. Risk factors for suicide in prisons: a systematic review and meta-analysis. *Lancet Public Health* 2021;6(3): e164–e174.
59. Gunnell D, Peters T, Kammerling M, et al. The relation between parasuicide, suicide, psychiatric admissions, and socio- economic deprivation. *British Medical Journal* 1995;311 (6999):226–30.
60. Windsor Shellard B, Gunnell D. Occupational specific suicide risk in England: 2011–2015. *British Journal of Psychiatry* 2019;215:594–9.
61. Granados J, Roux A. Life and death during the Great Depression. *Proceedings of the National Academy of Sciences USA* 2009;106(41):17290–5.
62. Chang S, Shuckler D, Gunnell D. Impact of 2008 global economic crisis on suicide: time trend in 54 countries. *British Medical Journal* 2013;347:f5239.
63. Branas C, Kastanaki AE, Michalodimitrakis M, et al. The impact of economic austerity and prosperity events on suicide in Greece: a 30-year interrupted time-series analysis *British Medical Journal Open* 2015;5(1):e005619.
64. Morselli H. *An Essay on Comparative Mortality Statistics.* London: Kegan Paul; 1881.
65. Stack S, Kposowa AJ. Religion and suicide: integrating four theories cross-nationally. In: O'Connor RC, Platt S, Gordon J (eds.) *International Handbook on Suicide Prevention Research Policy and Practice.* Chichester: Wiley Blackwell; 2011: 241–57.
66. Cook CH, Powell A, Sims A. *Spirituality and Psychiatry.* London: Royal College of Psychiatrists; 2009.
67. Samaritans. *Policy Brief: Gambling and Suicide.* media.samaritans.org/documents/Samaritans_gambling_policy_position_April_2021.pdf (accessed 18 February 2023).
68. Vassilas CA, Morgan G, Owens J, et al. Suicide and non-fatal self-harm. In: Stein G, Wilkinson G (eds.) *Seminars in Adult General Psychiatry,* 2nd ed. London: Gaskell; 2007: 142–66.
69. Williams JMG, Pollock LR. Psychological aspects of the suicidal process. In: van Heeringen K. (ed.) *Understanding Suicidal Behaviour: The Suicidal Process Approach to Research, Treatment and Prevention.* Hoboken, NJ: Wiley; 2001: 76–93.
70. Beck AT, Brown GK, Steer RA. Suicide ideation at its worst point: a predictor of eventual suicide in psychiatric outpatients. *Suicide and Life-Threatening Behaviour* 1999;29(1):1–9.
71. Morgan HG, Stanton R. Suicide among psychiatric in-patients in a changing clinical scene: suicide ideation as a paramount index of short term risk. *British Journal of Psychiatry* 1997;171:561–3.
72. Morgan, HG, Priest, P. Suicide and other unexpected deaths among psychiatric in-patients. *British Journal of Psychiatry* 1991;158(3):368–74.
73. Chan MK, Bhatti H, Meader N, et al. Predicting suicide following self-harm: systematic review of risk factors and risk scales. *British Journal of Psychiatry* 2016;209(4):277–83.
74. Large MM, Ryan CJ, Carter G, et al. Can we usefully stratify patients according to suicide risk? *BMJ* 2017;359:j4627.
75. Department of Health. *National Mental Health Risk Management Programme. Best Practice in Managing Risk.* London: Department of Health; 2009.
76. Department of Health. *Safety First: Five Year Report of the National Confidential Inquiry into Suicide and Homicide by People with Mental Illness.* London: Department of Health; 2001.
77. Meehan J, Kapur N, Hunt IM, et al. Suicide in mental health in-patients and within 3 months of discharge. National clinical survey. *British Journal of Psychiatry* 2006;188:129–34.
78. Isometsä ET, Aro HM, Henriksson MM, et al. Suicide in major depression in different treatment settings. *Journal of Clinical Psychiatry* 1994;55 (12):523–7.
79. Rihmer Z, Barsi J, Katona CLE. Suicide rates in Hungary correlate negatively with reported rates of depression. *Journal of Affective Disorders* 1990;20 (2):87–91.

80. Mental Health Act Commission. *Deaths of Detained Patients in England and Wales.* London: Mental Health Act Commission; 2001.

81. Freud S. *Beyond the Pleasure Principle (The Standard Edition 1920)* (trans. J Strachey). New York: Liveright Publishing Corporation; 1961.

82. Freud S. Mourning and melancholia. In: Strachey J (ed.) *The Standard Edition of the Complete Works of Sigmund Freud 1917, Vol (10)* (trans. J Strachey). London: Hogarth Press; 1962: 243–58.

83. Littman RE. Sigmund Freud on suicide. In: Shneidman E (ed.) *Essays on Self Destruction.* London: Science House; 1967: 324–44.

84. Menninger K. *Man Against Himself.* San Diego, CA: Harcourt Brace World; 1938.

85. Shneidman ES. *Suicide as Psyche Ache. A Clinical Approach to Self-Destructive Behaviour.* Lanham, MD: Jason Aronson; 1993.

86. Hendin H. *Suicide in America.* London: Norton; 1982.

87. Maris RW, Berman AL, Silverman MM. Treatment and prevention of suicide. In: Maris RW, Berman AL, Silverman MM (eds.) *Comprehensive Textbook of Suicidology.* New York: Guilford Press; 2000: 522.

88. Stanley B, Brown GK, Brenner LA, et al. Comparison of the safety planning intervention with follow-up vs usual care of suicidal patients treated in the emergency department. *JAMA Psychiatry* 2018;75(9):894–900.

89. von Goethe JW. *Die Lieden Jungen Werther's (The Sorrows of Young Werther).* Leipzig: Weygand'sche; 1787.

90. Phillips DP. The influence of suggestion on suicide: substantive and theoretical implications of the Werther effect *American Sociological Review* 1974;39 (3):340–54.

91. Niederkrotenthaler T, Braun M, Pirkis J, et al. Association between suicide reporting in the media and suicide: systematic review and meta-analysis. *British Medical Journal Open* 2020;368:575.

92. Stengel E, Cook NG, Kreeger I. *Attempted Suicide: Its Social Significance and Effects.* Maudsley Monograph No. 4. London: Chapman & Hall; 1958.

93. Hawton K, Fagg J, Simkin S, et al. Trends in self-harm in Oxford, 1985–1995. *British Journal of Psychiatry* 1997;171(6):556–60.

94. Office for National Statistics. *Adult Psychiatric Morbidity Survey: Survey of Mental Health and Wellbeing, England.* digital. nhs.uk/data-and-information/publications/statistical/adultpsychiatric-morbidity-survey/adult-psychiatric-morbiditysurvey-survey-of-mental-health-and-wellbeing-england-2014 (accessed 14 May 2022) (Archived at www.webcitation.org/78W1SNSJl).

95. Platt S, Bille-Brahe U, Kerkhof A, et al. Parasuicide in Europe: the WHO/EURO Multicentre Study on Parasuicide. I. Introduction and preliminary analysis for 1989. *Acta Psychiatrica Scandinavica* 1992;85 (2):97–104.

96. Tschristas A, Geulayov G, Casey D, et al. Incidence and general hospital costs of self-harm across England based on the multi-centre study of self-harm. *Epidemiology and Psychiatric Sciences* 2020;29(e108):1–23.

97. Owens D. Self harm patients not admitted to hospital. *Journal of the Royal College of Physicians of London* 1990;24(4):281–3.

98. Hawton K, Arensman E, Townsend E, et al. Deliberate self harm: systematic review of efficacy of psychological and pharmacological treatments in preventing repetition. *BMJ* 1998;317 (7156):441–7.

99. Townsend E, Hawton K, Harriss L, et al. Substances used in deliberate self-poisoning 1985–1997: trends and associations with age, gender, repetition and suicide intent. *Social Psychiatry and Psychiatric Epidemiology* 2001;36 (5):228–34.

100. Schmidtke A, Bille-Brahe U, De Leo D et al. Attempted suicide in Europe: rates, trends and sociodemographic characteristics of suicide attempters during the period 1989–1992. Results of the WHO/EURO Multicentre Study on Parasuicide. *Acta Psychiatrica Scandinavica* 1996;93(5):327–38.

101. Hawton K, Kirk J. Problem solving. In: Hawton K, Salvkovskis PM, Kirk J, et al. (eds.) *Cognitive Behaviour Therapy for Psychiatric Problems: A Practical Guide.* Oxford: Oxford University Press, 1989: 406–27.

102. Favazza A, Conterio K. Female habitual self-mutilation. *Acta Psychiatrica Scandanavica* 1989;79(3):283–89.

103. Kafka JS. The body as a transitional object: a psycho-analytic study of a self-mutilating patient. *British Journal of Medical Psychology* 1969;42(3): 207–12.

104. Stanley B, Gameroff MJ, Michalsen V, et al. Are suicide attempters who self-mutilate a unique population? *American Journal of Psychiatry* 2001;158 (3):427–32.

105. Brown R, Al-Bachari M, Kambhampati K. Self-inflicted eye injuries *British Journal of Ophthalmology* 1991;75 (8):496–8.

106. Large M, Babidge N, Andrews D, et al. Major self-mutilation in the first episode of psychosis. *Schizophrenia Bulletin* 2009;35(5):1012–21.

107. Krummen DM, James K, Klein RL. Suicide by burning: a retrospective review of the Akron Regional Burn Center. *Burns* 1998;24(2):147–9.

108. Roy A. Genetics, biology and suicide in the family. In: Maris RW, Berman AL, Maltsberger JT, et al. (eds.) *Assessment and Prediction of Suicide.* New York: Guilford Press; 1992: 574–88.

109. Statham, DJ, Heath AC, Madden PA, et al. Suicidal behaviour: an epidemiological and genetic study. *Psychological Medicine* 1998;28(4); 839–55.

110. Kety S. Genetic factors in suicide: family, twin and adoption studies. In: Blumenthal SJ, Kupfer D (eds.) *Suicide over the Life Cycle.* Washington, DC: American Psychiatric Press; 1990: 127–43.

111. Li H, Zhang X, Sun Q, et al. Association between serum lipid concentrations and attempted suicide in patients with major depressive disorder: a meta-analysis. *PLoS ONE* 2020;15(12):e0243847.

112. National Institute for Clinical Excellence. *Self-harm Quality Standard, 2013.* www.nice.org.uk/guidance/qs34.

113. Guthrie E, Kapur N, Mackway-Jones K, et al. Randomised controlled trial of brief psychological intervention after self-harm. *British Medical Journal* 2001;323;135–8.

114. Hawton K, Witt KG, Taylor Salisbury TL et al. (2016). Psychosocial interventions for self-harm in adults. *Cochrane Database of Systematic Reviews* 2016(5), [CD012189]. DOI: 10.1002/14651858.CD012189.

115. Paykel ES, Myers JK, Lindenthal JJ, et al. Suicidal feelings in the general

population. *British Journal of Psychiatry* 1974;124(582):460–9.

116. Kerkoff A, Spijker B. Worrying and rumination as proximal risk factors for suicidal behaviour. In: O'Connor RC, Platt S, Gordon J (eds.) *International Handbook on Suicide Prevention Research Policy and Practice*. Oxford: Wiley Blackwell; 2011: 199–210.
117. Newman E. *A Lesson from 29 Golden Gate Suicide Attempts*. ennyman.medium .com/a-lesson-from-29-golden-gate-suicide-attempts-a42f4ef3f970 (accessed 18 February 2023).
118. Clark DC, Lester D. *Suicide: Closing the Exits*. Berlin: Springer-Verlag; 2013.
119. Oliver R, Hetzel B. Rise and fall in suicide rates in Australia. *The Medical Journal of Australia* 1972;2(17):919–23.
120. Morgan G, Majeed A. Restricting paracetamol in the United Kingdom to reduce poisoning. *Journal of Public Health* 2005;27(1):12–8.
121. Leenaars A, Lester D, Baquedano C, et al. Restrictions of access to drugs and medication in suicide prevention. In: Wasserman D, Wasserman C (eds.) *Oxford Textbook of Suicidology and Suicide Prevention: A Global Perspective*. Oxford: Oxford University Press; 2009: 573–6.
122. Leenaars AA, Lester D. The impact of gun control on suicide and homicide across the life span. *Canadian Journal of Behavioural Science/Revue canadienne des sciences du comportement* 1997;29 (1):1.
123. Chapman S, Alpers P, Aklo K, et al. Australia's 1966 gun law reforms: faster falls in firearm deaths, firearms suicides and a decade with mass shootings. *Injury Prevention* 2006;12(5):365–72.
124. Phillips MR, Gunnell D. Restrictions of access to pesticides in suicide prevention. In: Wasserman D, Wasserman C (eds.) *Oxford Textbook of Suicidology and Suicide Prevention: A Global Perspective*. Oxford: Oxford University Press; 2009: 583–7.
125. Pearson V, Phillips MR, He F, et al. Attempted suicide amongst young women in the People's Republic of China: possibilities for prevention. *Suicide and Life-Threatening Behaviour* 2002;32(4),359–69.
126. Chen Y, Yip P. Prevention of suicide by jumping experiences from Taipei City (Taiwan), Hong Kong and Singapore. In: Wasserman D, Wasserman C (eds.) *Oxford Textbook of Suicidology and Suicide Prevention: A Global Perspective*. Oxford: Oxford University Press; 2009: 569–71.
127. Joyce J, Fleminger S. Suicide attempts by jumping. *Psychiatric Bulletin* 1998;22 (7):424–7.
128. Chan K, Yip P, Lee D. Charcoal burning suicide in post-transition Hong Kong. *British Journal of Psychiatry* 2005;186 (1):67–73.
129. Ku H, Huang H, Hsu W, et al. Incidence rate and predictors of globus pallidus necrosis after charcoal burning suicide. *International Journal of Environmental Research and Public Health*, 2019;16 (22):4426.
130. Wasserman D, Hadlaczky G. Restriction of alcohol consumption in suicide prevention. In: Wasserman D, Wasserman C (eds.) *Oxford Textbook of Suicidology and Suicide Prevention: A Global Perspective*. Oxford: Oxford University Press; 2009: 599–602.
131. Varah, C. *Before I Die Again: The Autobiography of the Founder of Samaritans*. London: Constable; 1992.
132. Mishara B, Chagnon F, Daigle M, et al. Comparing models of helper behaviour in actual practice in telephone crisis intervention: a silent monitoring study of calls to the US 1-800 SUICIDE network. *Suicide and Life-Threatening Behaviour* 2007;37(3):291–7.
133. Britton PC, Kopacz MS, Stephens B, et al. Veterans crisis line callers with and without prior VHA service use. *Archives of Suicide Research* 2016;20(3):314–22.
134. Mokkenstorm JK, Eikelenboom M, Huisman A, et al. Evaluation of the 113 Online suicide prevention crisis chat service: outcomes, helper behaviours and comparison to telephone hotlines. *Suicide and Life-Threatening Behaviour* 2017;47 (3):282–96.
135. Chan CH, Wong HK, Yip PS. Exploring the use of telephone helpline pertaining to older adult suicide prevention: a Hong Kong experience. *Journal of Affective Disorders* 2018;236:75–9.
136. Rutz W, von Knorring L, Walinder L. Long term effects of an educational programme for general practitioners given by the Swedish Committee for the Prevention and Treatment of Depression. *Acta Psychiatrica Scandinavica* 1992;85(1):83–8.
137. Rutz W, Walinder J, Knorring L, et al. Prevention of depression and suicide by education and medication: impact on male suicidality, an update from the Gotland study. *International Journal of Psychiatry in Clinical Practice* 1997;1 (1):39–46.
138. Dietrich S, Pfeiffer-Gerschel T, et al. Education and awareness programmes for adults. In: Wasserman D, Wasserman C (eds.) *Oxford Textbook of Suicidology and Suicide Prevention: A Global Perspective*. Oxford: Oxford University Press; 2009: 495–500.
139. Shneidman E. Cited in McIntosh JL. Survivors of suicide: a comprehensive bibliography update, 1986–1995. *Omega-Journal of Death and Dying* 1996;33(2):147–75.
140. Gibbons R, Brand F, Carbonnier A, et al. Effects of patient suicide on psychiatrists: survey of experiences and support required. *BJPsych Bulletin* 2019;43(5):236–41.
141. Ruskin R, Sakinofsky I, Bagby RM, et al. Impact of patient suicide on psychiatrists and psychiatric trainees. *Academic Psychiatry* 2004;28(2):104–10.
142. Young T, Iglewicz A, Gioroso D, et al. Suicide bereavement and complicated grief. *Dialogues in Clinical Neuroscience* 2012;14(2):177–86.
143. Kim J, Hong SH, Hong HJ. The impact of referral to mental health services on suicide death risk in adolescent suicide survivors. *Journal of the Korean Academy of Child and Adolescent Psychiatry* 2020;31(4):177–84.
144. Jobes DA, Luoma LA, Hustead T, et al. In the wake of suicide and postvention. In: Maris RW, Berman AL, Silverman MM (eds.) *Comprehensive Textbook of Suicidology*. New York: Guilford Press; 2000: 542.
145. Survivors of Bereavement by Suicide. uksobs.org/ (accessed 1 February 2023).
146. Department of Health and Social Care. *Suicide Prevention Strategy for England: 2023 to 2028*. London: Department of Health and Social Care; 2023. www .gov.uk/government/publications/ suicide-prevention-strategy-for-england-2023-to-2028 (accessed 17 September 2023).

Chapter 16

Physical Health Care

Paul Rowlands and John Wass

Summary

Psychiatrists, before they become psychiatrists, are doctors with medical training. Before they commence their formal training in psychiatry, they have acquired theoretical and practical experience of physical medicine and bring their knowledge and skills in these matters to their practice of psychiatry. This chapter will begin by making some general comments about the taking of a medical history and then set these into the context of patients with serious or severe mental illness. We then describe a multilevel approach to attempting to make a difference in the mortality outcomes that have been clearly documented in this patient group for nearly two hundred years. We conclude with fourteen broad, practical areas for achievable interventions to make a difference, retaining an approach founded on collaborative optimism.

> The first and always most important method of examination is that of *conversation* with the patient.
>
> —Karl Jaspers, *General Psychopathology*[1]

Introduction

Taking a history is an essential part of the assessment process. In mental health conditions, gaining an understanding of an individual's physical health is integral to a full assessment. No assessment can be regarded as complete unless this has been considered. At the end of the assessment – in the majority of patients – one will have a fairly clear idea as to a diagnostic formulation, including the physical health issues. It is essential that the process is thorough and based around organising principles but also relaxed and conversational in manner. Patients vary in their abilities to recount their story, and clinicians also vary in how well they grasp the patient's account. Honesty, humour and humility need to be exhibited, and at all stages, jargon – which the patient will not or may not understand – should be avoided. Skill and competence in doing this is achieved only with practice blended with a theoretical framework: 'organising principles'.

Preparation and Meeting the Patient

Prior to meeting the patient, the practitioner should carefully read the referral notes and all the available information. The clinician should be clear what the background to the problem is, ensuring that the patient realises that the practitioner has properly prepared.

A polite, respectful and friendly introduction is important: 'Hello, my name is. . .' (a form of words championed by a geriatrician and patient, the late Kate Granger) is as good a form to use as any. The patient should be made comfortable and put at ease because they will commonly be anxious about the consultation.

Doctors should be observant: What is the demeanour of the patient? Is he or she anxious? What is the appearance of the patient, including facial expressions, which can give so much information away without a word being spoken? How are they clothed? Are they clean and reasonably presented or dirty and dishevelled? Observing their hands, are there marks or scars visible that may be of significance? Are their nails clean or not?

Taking the History

A medical history is a fundamental component of any psychiatric history and assessment. Without this, any holistic psychiatric assessment will be incomplete.

Where this sits within any assessment though will vary depending on what the patient brings to the consultation at any given point, but the clinician must keep in mind the importance of this domain. Seeking an integrated, holistic assessment is the goal.

When conducting any assessment, it begins with setting the scene. This is just like a theatre: we need the scenery. After checking the name and age and properly introducing oneself, the clinician might attempt to put the patient at their ease with some neutral, friendly discussion. The next matter is then to ascertain why the patient thinks they are there and what medical or other issues you can solve together. All histories need to include the social context: family relationships, occupation, income and wider social networks, but the timing for the gathering of this information needs to be judged in each individual case.

Initially, after setting the scene, the patient needs to be allowed to speak uninterrupted and tell his or her story. This is done first because this is the most important aspect of the patient, and they will have come prepared to tell you. Some clinical method books talk about everything else before the history, but we are very clear this is the first thing to do. During this process, notes are made, and the clinician should aim to impose himself or herself as little as possible on the patient. Taking of notes is a way of conveying that matters are being taken seriously, and without note taking, it can be difficult to recollect the details of complex histories. A history is guided by the individual and is not a checklist or a form, though forms can be useful as an aide-memoire.

After this initial phase concludes, the clinician should fill the gaps and go through the story that the patient has told, ascertaining more relevant details. Clarifying the nature and extent of reported symptoms is likely to be necessary: If there is pain, when is it, how bad is it on a scale of 0–10 and where does it go? Headaches? When did they start, where are they in the head, what makes them worse, what alleviates them and are they associated with vomiting or other symptoms? Similarly, all other reported symptoms affecting other systems will require clarification and some degree of quantification.

Having filled the gaps of the history, a systematic enquiry is important, covering the major systems including appetite, weight, micturition, bowel function and exercise tolerance. How well does the patient sleep? Enquiry is made regarding any sexual dysfunction, and for women, a menstrual history should be taken. A detailed drug history is important and smoking and alcohol history likewise.

The past medical illnesses are important including operations, hospitalisations and accidents as well as details of past mental illness and contacts with mental health services.

The next part of the history is the family history. Weight, blood pressure, autoimmune thyroid disease and early cardiac problems are important aspects of this. The social history is likewise important: What is the family set-up? Who is around day-to-day? How do they spend their days? Are there stresses in the family?

At the end of the history taking of the general medical aspects, it is important to summarise the main points and get a list of the important aspects of the medical situation moving forward. This means listing the patient's most important symptoms first together along with all the other issues that need to be sorted out, in terms of investigation and treatment.

Taking a history is intellectually satisfying and obviously essential for the diagnosis. It should be comprehensive and thorough. Without it, we cannot move forward to help the patient or their family.

The Medical History and Severe Mental Illness

Physical and mental illness is inter-related and always occurs in a social context. It has been known for many years that there is an excessive death rate in patients with serious mental illness. Indeed, this was well-known in the nineteenth century. Bucknill and Tuke[2] (pp.139–143) discussed mortality using data from the 1872 Lunacy Report (which contained returns from asylums) and demonstrated the differences with the general population mortality, coming to estimates of premature mortality remarkably similar to those that persist today, as has been demonstrated by Brown's[3] systematic analysis of 25 years of Case Register data. Solutions moreover remain elusive, and the whole situation remains a substantial cause for concern. Social influences are of fundamental importance, but therapeutic pessimism or nihilism needs to be avoided.[4]

Apart from suicide in patients with severe mental illness – rates of which are increased – the largest numbers of deaths in patients with severe mental illness are caused by diseases that occur in the general population. However, they affect patients at an earlier age, leading to significant disability. In part, this may be due to marginalisation, stigmatisation and low quality of care. Access to care may be less easily available, services may be less well resourced and the behaviour and attitudes of staff may be negative. There is socioeconomic imbalance, and in people with serious mental illness (SMI), there is a higher prevalence of smoking and obesity and lower levels of physical exercise.

There are thus many reasons for increased rates of the main causes of preventable deaths: cardiac disease, type II diabetes, obesity, vitamin D deficiency, respiratory disease, cancer and liver disease. All these common diseases are more prevalent and occur commonly, and the underlying reasons for this are complex with no single solution likely to address them. There is also geographical variation, with likelihood of dying before age 75 varying across Upper Tier Local Authority Areas (UTLAs) between 2.5 and 7.2 times that of the general population. The extent of this disparity varies by age: it is most marked for those between age 30 and 49: between these ages those with SMI are seven times as likely to die as their peers in the general population. Data on this is regularly summarised and updated on the Government GOV.UK website.

In looking to prevent and manage these problems, there needs to be a holistic approach, with information available at the point of care that is person-centred. Open and willing attitudes are important in all the health care professionals involved. Knowledge is key, and it is important that this is kept up to date. Training is important, and this domain of holistic care needs continuous attention and a spirit of continuous quality improvement that avoids too much introspective self-criticism of individuals and the services attempting to make a difference. Equally, a nihilistic externalising of the issue onto 'society' is likely to create a sense of hopelessness in clinicians, which is ultimately unhelpful. Clinicians deal with individuals, and the individual's individual outcome cannot be assumed from the overall group outcome.

However, the reasons why disability occurs earlier in the group of patients with severe mental illness are many. There may include lifestyle issues – which are discussed later – social aspects and inequality. The care of patients in institutions looking after patients with severe mental illness need to attend not only to mental but physical aspects of care. There may often be delays in the diagnosis of serious conditions, worsening the likelihood of a good outcome. Once diagnosed, the patient may not access optimal care for many reasons.

Understanding the Main Issues: Individuals, Networks, Systems and Approaches

What Are the Main Conditions That People Working in Mental Health Services Need to Understand?

'Common things occur commonly' is a truism in medicine and psychiatry. Looking out the window, do I see magpies or

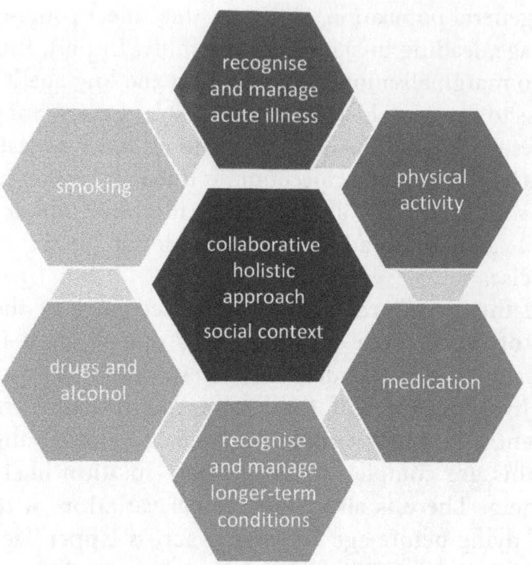

Figure 16.1 Holistic approach to assessment.

eagles? Whilst there is satisfaction in understanding a speciality at a deep level such that rare conditions are recognised when they present, the foundational need is for a good understanding of the common conditions commonly seen. In mental health, where patients are often disengaged from proper primary care services, it is important that all staff at the point of care appreciate this. As doctors, all psychiatrists should have received a good grounding in understanding physical health and disease. Other disciplines within the mental health team may have received more limited training in physical health, and the psychiatrist within any team should recognise that they are likely to have an important role in educating the wider team about the importance of good integrated health care for individuals. Particular approaches to increasing awareness and utilising workplace-based opportunities for teaching have been described (e.g. 'Bite Size Teaching' HEE 2019[5]). However, psychiatrists need to steer a careful course here: their role is not to substitute for general physicians or GPs but rather to be aware of the issues and act as advocates for their patients, looking to facilitate access to the right practitioner and the level of care that patients require.

There are three broad areas that need to be addressed (see Figure 16.1).

Recognition of Presentations of Acute Physical Illness and Their Immediate Management

All mental health teams need to be able to recognise acute physical illness in their patients or the deterioration of long-term physical health conditions. The particular setting of mental health care may impact on this, however, with a lack of knowledge or impaired situational awareness leading to conditions being missed. This 'diagnostic overshadowing' can occur anywhere – settings that are used to seeing certain conditions, such as acute mental health units, can be so used to seeing the 'mental health' presentation that they are not attuned to seeing the less common 'physical health' condition.

Team-based approaches to training can be of use, particularly where the background depth to training is not deeply embedded in an understanding of physical health. An example of this is the use of simulation training to increase staff awareness, knowledge and skills.[6]

Recognition of Longer-Term Conditions

a. Those comorbid and 'unrelated' to the psychiatric condition
b. The influence of psychiatric treatments (e.g. antipsychotics, lithium)
c. The influence of modifiable behaviours (e.g. diet, smoking, alcohol use, use of drugs, exercise and other behaviours)
d. The influence of the wider environment and other factors
e. The engagement of the individual in the management of their conditions
f. Advocacy to attempt to ensure that patients access equivalent services to the general population

Management of Longer-Term Conditions

The management of comorbid physical conditions, which are extremely common in patients with mental health problems, requires development of a standard approach to care that takes note of physical health and promotes prevention, good management, improvement and wider social interventions. As a way of evaluating a risk profile for an individual patient, calculators such as QRISK3[7] can be used, which uses a large real-world sample from UK General Practices to show the average risk for a patient with the same entered characteristics – such as of heart attack or stroke – over the following 10 years. This is expressed as a percentage (or probability) of the unwanted event over the following 10 years: 'the 10 years risk'. The Primary Care Quality and Outcomes Framework (QoF) 2021–2022[8] covers the common conditions that underlie most morbidity and mortality – many patients will be covered under more than one category, and again, this emphasises the importance of a holistic, integrated approach. The rewarded measures do alter between iterations, but the 2021–2022 QoF saw the reintroduction of three indicators focused on patients with a serious mental illness to promote improved uptake in all six elements of the SMI physical health check.

Whilst there are commonalities to the general approach, with many shared underlying aspects, an understanding of the main specific conditions using a systems-based approach is a helpful mental template to hold (see Box 16.1). There are many excellent medical textbooks available that will cover particular conditions in depth, and an up-to-date version of one of these should be available in the hospital library or the local post graduate centre.

Box 16.1 Specific areas to be addressed – common things that occur commonly – 14 potential areas for intervention

1. Smoking cessation (SMOK002, SMOK005)
2. Increased physical activity
3. Reduced use of alcohol (MH007)
4. Control of blood pressure (HYP001, BP002)
5. Prevention and control of diabetes (QoF MH012, QoF diabetes indicators)
6. Control of blood lipids (QoF MH011)
7. Reduction in obesity and improved diet (QoF MH006)
8. Identification and treatment of atrial fibrillation (AF001)
9. Management of chronic kidney disease (CKD indicators, lithium)
10. Management of chronic obstructive pulmonary disease (COPD) (QoF COPD items)
11. Management of the consequences of prescribed medication (corticosteroids, antipsychotics, lithium) (QoF lithium items, diabetes items, obesity items)
12. Cancer screening (an emphasis in QoF of earlier diagnosis)
13. Reduced use of drugs of misuse
14. Ensure uptake of flu and Covid vaccination

Developing an Integrated Approach

Can anything be done to reduce the mortality gap between the SMI population and the general population? The major risk factors for premature mortality in people with mental illness are, unsurprisingly, the same as the general population. The following are domains for intervention that can impact across a range of conditions: The list is not exhaustive but gives some practical pointers. Most morbidity and mortality are multifactorial, and therefore, attempting to assess holistically and integrate interventions in a patient-centred manner is key. The Quality and Outcomes Framework 2021–2022[8] for primary care provides domains to consider as part of the annual review in primary care for people with serious mental illness, and the psychiatric services need to work on developing integration with what primary care is providing by complementing and developing approaches to increase access to services and increase access to broad-based interventions. Secondary care should seek better integration and not necessarily simply seek to replicate and duplicate what primary care is set-up and paid to do. Nonetheless, simply assuming it is 'the responsibility of primary care' is a recipe for disaster and not the right approach. There is much work needed to make the aspiration of integrated approaches between primary and secondary care a reality. As well as having systems and processes in place that support this, clinicians need to work on approaches that break down barriers that may be present – not an easy task, and one that cannot be accomplished by diktat, although the explicit statement of policy around this is welcome. The cultivation of local constructive partnerships and relationships must form a substantial part of this, and recent NICE guidance on rehabilitation for adults with complex psychosis[9] and other related documents emphasise the need for services and commissioners to think systematically about these issues.

Mirroring the QoF domains, mental health assessment and intervention should consider the following. Bear in mind the question is how to ensure access to assessment and intervention based around the needs of the individual patient. The aim of the comprehensive annual physical health check in primary care is 'to identify and address risk factors for cardiovascular disease (CVD)'. Whilst this sounds simple, it is complex in practice and – because of the way that QoF is structured (for example, allowing exclusions or coding for 'remission') – it is easy for patients to slip out of this framework of review and intervention.

The Lester Tool[10] mantra, 'Don't just screen, intervene', is a rallying cry for services as is the caution within QoF for coding 'remission' from serious mental illness. Recognising the reality that serious mental illness can be a long-term condition should not mean that this inevitably leads to a pessimistic approach to its management.

Smoking Cessation

Smoking represents the largest single modifiable risk factor for many physical health conditions. Rates have fallen greatly in the general population – in 1974, over 50% of men smoked and over 40% of women, but by 2019, this had fallen to 15.9% of men and 12.5% of women. The rates, however, have not fallen in the same way for groups such as people with serious mental illness, with the prevalence of smoking remaining around 40%, according to PHE and GP data. This disparity is likely to widen already existing health inequalities. Smoking is common in patients with severe mental illness. It is estimated that those with severe mental illness lose 14.9 years of life[11] and that smoking may account for up to two-thirds of the difference in life expectancy between smokers with severe psychological illness and never-smokers.

System-wide interventions such as adoption of 'smoke-free' wards need to be complemented by adoption of other approaches, recognising the barriers that many people will face in accessing appropriate individual interventions.

Gilbody and colleagues[12] explored whether a bespoke intervention for heavy smokers with SMI would improve cessation compared to usual care and found significant differences at six months (14% vs 6%) but non-significant differences at 12 months, suggesting a need for attention to be paid to sustaining quitting. The fall in general population rates, however, do suggest that huge inroads can be made into rates of smoking. In clinical settings, brief and ultra-brief interventions around this (Do you smoke? Have you thought of quitting?) and a willingness to have a non-judgemental discussion on the part of the clinician can open

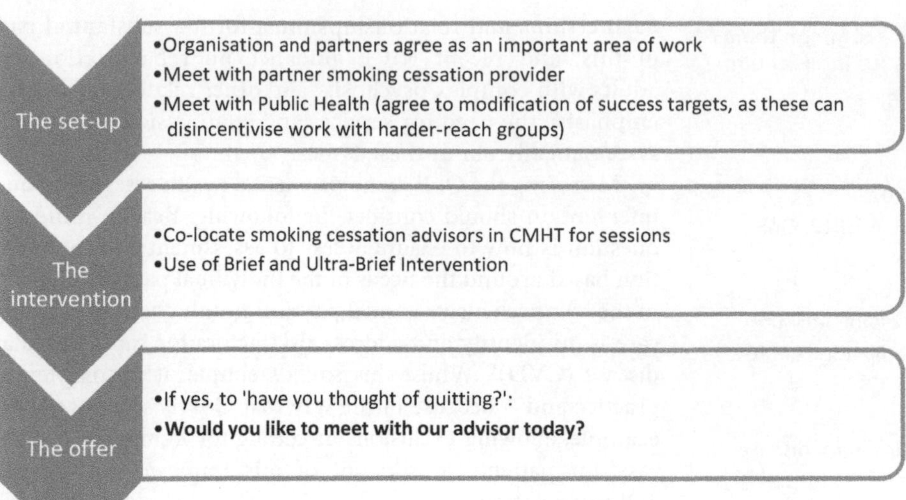

Figure 16.2 Smoking cessation.

up possible routes. Working to ensure there is awareness of local resources and adopting a motivational interviewing approach can be easily adopted within busy clinical settings. Working with partner services such as smoking cessation services to make it easier for people to access the service can help with making incremental improvements; pre-pandemic, co-locating a smoking cessation service within a clinic setting offered easy access to a bespoke approach, building on 'treatment as usual' to try to look at improving accessibility (see Figure 16.2).

Other interventions in recent years at a strategic level – in addition to moving to smoke-free inpatient units – include an on-going tax policy on tobacco, increasing costs to its consumers, although this policy may potentially then lead to increased organised crime activity in the illegal import of tobacco products.

Physical Activity

In adults, there is strong evidence to demonstrate the protective effect of physical activity on a range of many chronic conditions, including coronary heart disease, obesity and type II diabetes, mental health problems and social isolation. Even small increases in activity can have health benefits. A mix of aerobic and strengthening activities is recommended, and balance and flexibility exercises become especially important as people grow older (see guidelines in Table 16.1).

There are many examples across the country of the charitable arm of professional football clubs (often called a 'community trust' or similar). Examples include Everton in the Community (evertoninthecommunity.org/) or Chesterfield FC Community Trust (spireitestrust.org.uk), using the corporate brand of the professional club to promote community engagement and choices around physical activity and health. An understanding of behavioural economics (e.g. 'Nudge' theory[13]) is helpful in understanding this concept of 'choice architecture' that may influence the way individuals make these decisions in their lives.

Table 16.1 UK Chief Medical Officers issued guidelines for all adults on physical exercise in 2019[14]

Physical activity guidelines for adults aged 19 to 64
Adults should do some type of physical activity every day. Any type of activity is good for you. The more you do, the better.
Adults should:
• Aim to be physically active every day. Any activity is better than none, and more is better still
• Do strengthening activities that work all the major muscles (legs, hips, back, abdomen, chest, shoulders and arms) on at least 2 days a week
• Do at least 150 minutes of moderate-intensity activity a week or 75 minutes of vigorous-intensity activity a week
• Reduce time spent sitting or lying down, and break up long periods of not moving with some activity

Reduce Use of Alcohol

As with smoking, brief and ultra-brief intervention is possible to begin the process of change for people in whom this is an issue needing to be addressed. The WHO estimate that harmful use of alcohol is implicated in 5.3% of all deaths, and there are an estimated number of dependent drinkers in excess of 500,000 in the UK. The numbers of drinkers exceeding recommended safe levels runs into the millions – around a quarter of all adults regularly exceed the recommended safe levels. Excess alcohol use is associated with many conditions, including mouth, throat, stomach, liver and breast cancers, high blood pressure, cirrhosis of the liver and depression.

Again, exploring this area with patients need not take long, and the evidence base (mainly from primary care) supports its effectiveness. Making non-judgemental exploration of this a natural part of the therapeutic conversation can empower patients to acknowledge and begin addressing any issues that may be present.

Control Blood Pressure

Hypertension (140/90 mmHg or higher for those under 80) rarely causes noticeable symptoms, but around a third of adults have high blood pressure defined at his level. It is a risk factor for ischaemic heart disease, cerebrovascular disease and vascular dementia; chronic kidney disease; and the full range of other vascular conditions. It is associated with other modifiable risk factors commonly present in psychiatric populations including obesity, smoking, lack of physical exercise, excessive alcohol consumption, excessive caffeine consumption as well as age, ethnicity and wider socioeconomic deprivation. At a population level, controlling and reducing the level of dietary salt has a marked impact on population rates of hypertension.

Again, exploring this with the individual patient is not difficult but equally is often not addressed. In psychiatric settings, all inpatients should have this checked on admission. In certain clinic-based settings – such as clozapine clinics – it will form part of the standard operating procedure, but in general outpatient clinics, it may not. However, in the outpatient setting, simple approaches can ensure that this is being managed appropriately. All adults between the age of 40 and 74 are entitled to the NHS Health Check, every five years, which is aimed at those who are not receiving regular follow-up already for pre-existing conditions such as heart disease, hypertension, chronic kidney disease or diabetes. Many patients in general psychiatric settings will have comorbid physical health problems in the groups that are entitled to regular follow-up. Being on the Severe Mental Illness Register also entitles the patient to this. However, many patients may not be accessing this care at the right level – the requirement on GPs is to *invite* the patient to the review, and there is no requirement for proactive, assertive follow-up if a patient does not attend, beyond sending out a further invitation. Needless to say, this means the most marginalised and disengaged are less likely to receive review and care at the right level. The Lester Tool[10], a variation of the NHS Health Check and covering the same domains, provides a handy visual diagram of what needs to be assessed and done. The mantra, 'Don't just screen, intervene', is a powerful call to action.

In the mental health service setting, a simple question 'Have you had a physical review recently with your GP or nurse?' begins the discussion. If the patient has recently had this done, the clinician can review the results, if available, and continue to explore the issue, looking at the wider picture.

If the answer is no, then discussion can follow as to how the patient views this, and a plan can be agreed. It may be that a one-off check can be conducted, if appropriate, there and then, but it may be more important to look at the issue more widely and consider how the patient can be engaged at the appropriate level and in the right setting for these issues to be systematically addressed. Doing a one-off check of a patient's blood pressure outside of a systemic approach is unlikely to be of much use, but for disengaged groups, setting up bespoke services tailored to their particular needs – preferably using co-production approaches – can improve access to care.

Prevent and Control Diabetes

Type II Diabetes Mellitus (T2DM) is associated with premature mortality and poor physical health. In most countries, it is a leading cause of mortality, affecting around 1 in 15 of the UK population. In studies of people with serious mental illness, the prevalence of diabetes may be between 2 and 5 times higher than this – the national diabetes audit suggested it was twice as common in people with SMI than in the general population. The reasons as ever are complex and multifactorial but include obesity, poor diet, hyperlipidaemia, smoking, hypertension and lower levels of physical activity. Adverse effects of antipsychotic drugs also contribute, whether directly via metabolic disruption or indirectly via weight gain. Some studies have suggested an increase of prevalence in first-episode patients, potentially suggesting some factor intrinsic to schizophrenia itself.

Once T2DM is present and identified, patients may not be engaged with the same level of intervention and monitoring as their peers in the general population. In the general population, many people with T2DM are not identified as such, and the same applies in psychiatric populations. Again, the same general principles apply: make it easy, keep it simple and look at the wider system and the social context.

The individual clinician needs to see each contact as a point at which they can 'add value' to the individual patient's management. They need to be aware and to watch for the expected as well as the unexpected. For T2DM, this means:

1. Could this person have this common condition? Are they at increased risk?
2. Have they had any recent blood tests? Can I access these online easily whilst with the patient? If not, why not and what will I do to ensure that I can?
3. What are the results of these tests? What do they mean?
4. Are there processes and systems in place to address this in this patient group?
5. If this person has the condition (e.g. T2DM), are they accessing the correct care, including group-based approaches, screening and the most appropriate medical management?
6. Is the care around this being implemented holistically, in a patient centred way, breaking down barriers to accessing what is needed?
7. Is the approach looking to wider networks to improve social connection and addressing physical health more widely? The condition cannot be seen in isolation.

Control Blood Lipids

Raised LDL cholesterol and raised triglycerides are associated with a raised risk of ischaemic heart disease and associated mortality. Whilst a small number of cases are associated with familial hyperlipidaemias from a young age, LDL cholesterol rises with age in men especially after the mid-forties and in women especially after menopause. Risk may be higher if there is a close family history of heart disease or raised cholesterol at a young age. Certain antipsychotics – notably clozapine and olanzapine, but also others – are associated with dyslipidaemias.

In those without a familial hyperlipidaemia, there will be no symptoms or signs beyond the lipid profile blood test. Overlapping risk factors with other conditions mean that the same multifactorial approach is required with simple approaches integrated into the holistic assessment.

The starting point is knowing the numbers: Do you and the patient know what their total cholesterol/HDL ratio is?

Do you and they know what this means and what it therefore implies needs to be done? Does it require intervention with a statin? What lifestyle and dietary changes might help– a diet higher in vegetables and oily fish, for example – but what if your patient does not eat fish?

Whilst the Primrose study examining statin prescribing in people with SMI[15] did not show a benefit for treatment over control on the primary endpoint measure (lower cholesterol), it did show improvement in both groups, suggesting that statin treatment is broadly acceptable to patients with SMI. Those in the intervention group also occupied fewer inpatient beds over the 24 months of the study, an intriguing finding.

Actions that follow from exploring this area with patients must be part of a wider plan integrating the approach to both physical and mental health, including increasing the patient's knowledge and sense of agency over the management of their health.

Reduce Obesity and Improve Diet

Nearly two-thirds of adults in England are overweight or obese, some of the worst figures in Europe. Patients who have severe mental illness and such illnesses as schizophrenia are more likely to be overweight or obese and to lead sedentary lifestyles. There is also a higher prevalence of type II diabetes and cardiovascular disease, and these issues undoubtedly contribute to reduced life expectancy. Jaspers in *General Psychopathology*[1] described 'fluctuations in body-weight' that can 'reach an extraordinary degree' in patients with schizophrenia before the antipsychotic era (p.247), and Kraepelin's textbook makes explicit reference to these issues with weight in his patients (pp.87–88 in *Dementia Praecox and Paraphrenia*). There may be a shared vulnerability genetically to obesity and serious mental ill health, though unquestionably, there is also a significant contribution to this from prescribed antipsychotic medication. Treatment of patients with severe obesity can be even more difficult in the context of severe mental illness than with ordinary patients with obesity, and there are no good studies looking at this aspect of care. Despite this, outward-looking inpatient and community teams need to allocate resource and time to understand their own local landscape of opportunities.

The NHS Long Term Plan[16] notes that obesity is linked with type II diabetes; high blood pressure; high cholesterol; increased rates of respiratory, musculoskeletal and liver disease; and certain types of cancer.

The NHS Long Term Plan commits to a targeted offer of support and access to weight management services in primary care for people with a diagnosis of hypertension or type II diabetes with a BMI >30, amongst other actions to reduce obesity. NICE has produced multiple guidelines on clinical and public health approaches to this issue, which has been further highlighted as a major risk factor for serious morbidity and raised mortality in the Covid pandemic. Locally, services need to ensure that people with SMI receive fair access to these specialist services and are not excluded.

The prescribing of glucogan-like peptide-1 receptor agonists (GLP-1 agonists) has received substantial publicity recently with increased availability through commercial services as well as through the NHS. Although the real-world benefits have been debated,[17] the use of these agents has increased greatly, not only in the population of people with established type II diabetes. The role of these agents in managing, for example, antipsychotic-induced weight gain will require further careful evaluation in the coming years.

Being overweight at any point increases risk of death. Obesity is one of a number of inter-related risk factors that coalesce and together drive differences in mortality between different groups. Specific underlying factors may be present, specific interventions may be available, and this approach can bear fruit, but integrating interventions and empowering the individual is again key. Understanding something of behavioural economic theories (e.g. 'Nudge' theory) can provide insights. There are a number of other things that can help to bring the issue into focus. Broadly similar intervention approaches apply to many of these areas but specifically for obesity (see Figure 16.3).

1. Measuring and recording weight and BMI should be a standard part of any assessment. Are there scales in every clinical room? How do you integrate this effortlessly into the approach to the assessment and follow-up appointment?
2. How do you explain potential effects on appetite of medication that you are prescribing?
3. How do you monitor this – for example, do you a have a standard organisational approach to implementing the Lester Tool for new antipsychotic prescriptions?
4. What links do you have to mainstream healthy lifestyle interventions for your patients?
5. How does your team approach this and build its links?
6. Are there other specific interventions that might help? What specialist advice would be required for prescription of anti-obesity medication as part of a wider strategy?

Such prescribing would not ordinarily fall under the remit of a general psychiatrist, but medications such as orlistat,

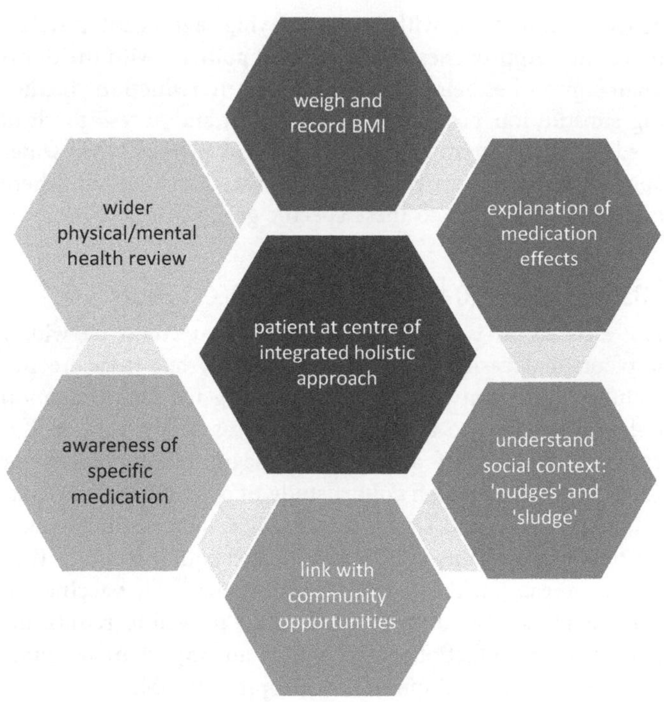

Figure 16.3 Holistic/multilevel approach to care: example of obesity.

metformin, glucagon-like peptide (GLP-1) agonists (e.g. liraglutide) and topiramate are sometimes prescribed for patients elsewhere, who are also attending psychiatric clinics. Occasionally, patients request that the psychiatrist prescribe the anti-obesity medication, and sometimes, patients obtain them directly from online pharmacies. The psychiatrist should be familiar with these and the developments in weight management services and the management of diabetes but should, without question, remain within their own areas of competence and knowledge in prescribing matters. This is a rapidly changing area of medical practice.

Identify and Treat Atrial Fibrillation and Identify At-Risk Cardiac Rhythms

Screening of patients with ECG prior to prescribing antipsychotic or other psychotropic medication has never been standard practice, but concerns about the potential risks of QT interval prolongation and the ease of obtaining rapid reporting of ECGs means this is an area that could potentially improve rapidly. Atrial fibrillation (AF) is common, with prevalence increasing with age, and is seen in men more commonly than women. In people aged over 65, prevalence is 7.2%. In people with identified AF, a stroke risk calculator is used (by primary care) to determine the need for stroke prophylaxis, but clearly, many people in the population may have unidentified AF, which raises the risk of stroke. AF may be paroxysmal and may be asymptomatic or symptomatic. If present, it can be identified at the radial pulse, but if paroxysmal, AF may be missed.

It is increasingly easy for individuals and professionals to access ECGs and the reporting of ECGs – from the use of apps and smartphones through to rapid virtual reporting of the standard 12-lead ECGs. Psychiatrists and mental health professionals need to enable their patients to access investigations as easily as anyone else can, bearing in mind that patients may have barriers to accessing such things that are not there for other members of the general population. Psychiatrists will undoubtedly have a role in breaking down any commissioning barriers that might hinder this.

Ensure Proper Management of Chronic Kidney Disease

it is common to see impairment of renal function occurring in patients treated with lithium. Overall, the evidence suggests that patients on lithium have improved outcomes in terms of their physical health compared to the general population, but the regular monitoring of renal function means that this impairment is commonly identified at an early stage.

The QoF Framework[8] suggests that an estimate of the overall population prevalence of CKD (diagnosed and undiagnosed) is 4.3 per cent of the population over 18, with the prevalence rising with age and female sex. Because of lithium's known effectiveness in prophylaxis of major mood episodes and suicide prevention, decisions around its continued use in people showing CKD are not straightforward. Shared, informed decision-making is key.

Ensure Proper Management of COPD

With smoking rates higher than the general population, COPD rates are higher in the SMI than in the general population. The optimal treatment of COPD can be viewed at many levels, and the London Respiratory Network developed an effective visualisation of this, emphasising the importance of the simple, low-cost approaches such as flu vaccination, smoking cessation and pulmonary rehabilitation as the foundation on which other specific medical interventions, such as tiotropium, long-acting β agonists (LABA), and 'triple therapy' are based.

Monitor and Manage the Consequences of Prescribed Medication (Corticosteroids, Antipsychotics, Lithium)

All medicine prescribing requires a balance to be struck between adverse effects and harms and potential benefits. The risks should be carefully explained alongside the possible benefits, and the patient should be central to the decision-making. Involving the patient as an active participant in monitoring of the impact of the medication is important. Recording results and encouraging patients to access their medical records and become knowledgeable about their condition will develop a collaborative shared approach between patient and clinician. Understanding the Quality and

Outcomes Framework Mental Health measures and developing collaborative approaches across service boundaries to maximise uptake is part of the wider approach to addressing physical health issues.

Ensure Proper Access to Cancer Screening

In the course of the Covid pandemic beginning in 2019, there was huge disruption to normal NHS services, including treatment for cancers. The 2021–2022 QoF guidance states that 'all tumour types have seen a drop in the number of first treatments; however, those where there has been the most significant decrease include the other most common cancers – breast, colorectal and prostate – as well as skin, bladder, head and neck, kidney and uterine'. Increasing early-stage diagnosis of cancer to improve outcomes of treatment had been a priority before the pandemic, and regaining ground lost will be a priority moving forward. QoF reiterates the ambition of the NHS Long Term Plan, setting out an ambition that, by 2028, the proportion of cancers diagnosed at stages 1 and 2 will rise from around half now to three-quarters of cancer patients. NHS England estimates that achieving this will mean that – from 2028 – 55,000 more people each year will survive their cancer for at least five years after diagnosis. For most cancers, survival is much greater at both one and five years if detected at stage 1 – highlighting the need for early diagnosis. People with serious mental illness have multiple barriers to overcome, and practices have been encouraged to include a focus on inequalities in screening in their assessment, particularly for those at risk and with low uptake, which might include people with serious mental illness. Again, awareness and the willingness to try to do 'something' is key. A systems-based understanding and efforts to co-ordinate and integrate are necessary to effect change – merely pointing out the inequality achieves little beyond raising awareness. A study from South-West London[18] found that outcomes were worse in people with mental health history compared to the whole cohort, although in this study, the stage of cancer at presentation was not different.

Address Issues Associated with Use of Drugs of Misuse

Drug misuse compounds physical health issues. As a subset of people with mental health problems, people with comorbid substance misuse have extremely poor outcomes and often multiple morbidities combined with their mental health difficulties. Direct 'drug-related deaths' have risen year on year but remain across the population at around 50 per million per year. This, however, conceals a far larger number of people with substance misuse problems dying prematurely from wider physical health problems. Even taking into account confounding factors such as deprivation, long-term drug use is associated with several decades of life lost compared to the general population, with accompanying significant physical morbidity. Approaches aim at various points – with the dominant approaches being variations on 'harm reduction', including substitution programmes, education and access to clean needles, and attempts to engage people in the wider approaches to improving their health discussed elsewhere but possibly tailored to these specific groups.

Ensure Access to Flu and Covid Vaccination

Flu vaccination is a simple approach that could be widely implemented easily for people with SMI, but they are not included at present within the groups targeted for vaccination unless they fall into another category (as many may do, for example, because of a comorbid diagnosis of diabetes or COPD). A large Danish cohort study of over 800,000 patients, 11,343 of whom had SMI, showed a 52% increase in all-cause mortality for patients with SMI admitted with infections, with a 71% increase for those with schizophrenia.[19] Flu vaccination and Covid vaccination programmes are proven to reduce the risk of severe infection and are thus an important potential area for service development for people with SMI.

Summary

Exploring both the physical and psychological health of individual patients and setting this in the context of their social environment and influences has been at the heart of medical practice for millennia, evidenced throughout the surviving works of Hippocrates, Galen and Avicenna. A psychiatry that recognises this need for the 'whole picture' must work at multiple levels to make this integration a reality. To make inroads into the morbidity and mortality associated with physical illness in patients with mental health problems requires rounded clinicians who are comfortable in considering these aspects and who are willing to work collaboratively across service boundaries. This is not simple, but continuing to work on continuous improvement around this essential aspect of management with an optimistic spirit is crucial as is continuing to work on the common problems that cause the great majority of morbidity and mortality in the general population. Viewing this as a 'work in progress', with associated staff training, educational and quality improvement initiatives as needed, can develop the 'can-do' culture that is a prerequisite for progress to be made in this crucial area of practice.

However, the individual point of contact with a patient is still the crucial building block of wider outcomes. This point of contact can be supported or hindered, and the work at this 'point of care' can be done well or badly. Approaching the system of care in an optimistic spirit whilst recognising the complexity and difficulty of these issues offers a constructive way of approaching this immensely important domain of practice.

Appendix 16.1: Some Examples of Common Conditions that Practitioners Should Be Aware of

Cardiac: ischaemic heart disease, hypertension, atrial fibrillation, cardiac failure

Respiratory: COPD, asthma, lung cancer

Metabolic/Endocrine: diabetes, dyslipidaemias, obesity, thyroid disorders

Blood: anaemias, leukaemias

GI: liver disease, cirrhosis, inflammatory bowel disease, bowel cancer

Renal: chronic kidney disease, lithium nephropathy

Joint: arthritis, chronic pain

Neurological: multiple sclerosis (MS), brain tumours, motor neurone disease (MND), encephalopathy, dementias, delirium, epilepsy

Skin: psoriasis, drug-induced conditions including Stevens-Johnson, stigmata of systemic disease

Nutritional disorders: anaemias, avitaminoses, malnutrition

Auto immune conditions: systemic lupus erythematosus (SLE), Guillain-Barre syndrome, vasculitis

Manifestations of metastatic cancer: bone, liver, lung, peritoneum, adrenal, skin, muscle

References

1. Jaspers K. *General Psychopathology* (trans. J Hoenig and MW Hamilton 1963). Manchester: Manchester University Press; 1959:826.
2. Bucknill JC, Tuke DH. *A Manual of Psychological Medicine, Containing the Lunacy Laws: the Nosology, Aetiology, Statistics, Description, Diagnosis, Pathology, and Treatment of Insanity, With an Appendix of Cases*. New York: Lindsay and Blakiston; 1879.
3. Brown S, Kim M, Mitchell C, et al. Twenty-five year mortality of a community cohort with schizophrenia. *British Journal of Psychiatry* 2010;196:116–21.
4. Firth J, Siddiqi N, Koyanagi A, et al. The Lancet Psychiatry Commission: a blueprint for protecting physical health in people with mental illness. *Lancet Psychiatry* 2019;6(8): 675–712.
5. Health Education England. *Bitesized Teaching*. www.hee.nhs.uk/our-work/mental-health/bitesized-teaching.
6. Health Education England. *The RAMPPS Course Handbook*. www.yorksandhumberdeanery.nhs.uk/sites/default/files/the_rampps_course_handbook.pdf (accessed 20 March 2023).
7. ClinRisk. *QRISK3*. qrisk.org/.
8. NHS England. *Quality and Outcomes Framework, 2021–2022*. digital.nhs.uk/data-and-information/publications/statistical/quality-and-outcomes-framework-achievement-prevalence-and-exceptions-data/2021-22.
9. National Institute of Health and Social Care. *Rehabilitation for Adults With Complex Psychosis; NICE Guideline [NG181]*. www.nice.org.uk/guidance/ng181.
10. Shiers DE, Rafi I, Cooper SJ, et al. *2014 Update (with Acknowledgement to the Late Helen Lester for Her Contribution to the Original 2012 Version) Positive Cardiometabolic Health Resource: An Intervention Framework for Patients with Psychosis and Schizophrenia*. London: Royal College of Psychiatrists; 2014.
11. Tam J, Warner KE, Meza R. Smoking and the reduced life expectancy of individuals with serious mental illness. *American Journal of Preventative Medicine* 2016;51(6):958–66.
12. Gilbody S, Peckham E, Bailey D, et al. Smoking cessation for people with severe mental illness (SCIMITAR+): a pragmatic randomised controlled trial. *Lancet Psychiatry* 2019;6 (5):379–90.
13. Arno A, Thomas S. The efficacy of nudge theory strategies in influencing adult dietary behaviour: a systematic review and meta-analysis. *BMC Public Health* 2016;16:676.
14. UK Chief Medical Officers. *Physical Activity Guidelines*. assets.publishing.service.gov.uk/government/uploads/system/uploads/attachment_data/file/832868/uk-chief-medical-officers-physical-activity-guidelines.pdf.
15. Osborn DP, Hardoon S, Omar RZ, et al. Cardiovascular risk prediction models for people with severe mental illness: results from the prediction and management of cardiovascular risk in people with severe mental illnesses (PRIMROSE) research program. *JAMA Psychiatry* 2015;72(2): 143–51.
16. NHS England. *The NHS Long Term Plan*. London: NHS England; 2019. www.longtermplan.nhs.uk/.
17. Weiss T, Yang L, Carr RD, et al. Real-world weight change, adherence, and discontinuation among patients with type 2 diabetes initiating glucagon-like peptide-1 receptor agonists in the UK.

BMJ Open Diabetes Research and Care 2022;10(1):e002517.

18. Chang C-K, Hayes RD, Broadbent MT, et al. A cohort study on mental disorders, stage of cancer at diagnosis and subsequent survival. *BMJ Open* 2014;4(1):e004295.
19. Ribe AR, Vestergaard M, Katon W, et al. Thirty-day mortality after infection among persons with severe mental illness: a population-based cohort study in Denmark. *American Journal of Psychiatry* 2015;172 (8):776–83.

Chapter

17

Culture, Mental Health and Mental Illnesses

Dinesh Bhugra, Max Pemberton, Sam Gnanapragasam and Daniel Poulter

Introduction

Human beings are born, live and die in a culture or a combination of cultures. We are not born with a culture but into one. Cultures mould our beings, thinking and functioning. Over our lifetime, we accumulate cultural capital. Cultures influence our world view and cognitive and social development. The way children are brought up depends very much on cultures, and their development is strongly influenced by parenting, family structures and social interactions. Cultures are an integral part of our beings and affect our identities, our attitudes, as well as the way we behave with others. In addition, cultures dictate certain ingrained characteristics and our emotional expressions. The way cultures mould our physical and emotional responses is significant. Cultures also influence our diet, physical activity and other factors, which may contribute to the wellbeing of individuals as well as communities.

The role of cultures in psychiatric conditions and their presentation, explanatory models and help-seeking is crucial. Cultural factors can influence the way an individual identifies and labels psychiatric symptoms but also where, when and from whom help is sought. There is every likelihood that individuals may well accept help from social and informal sources depending upon a number of factors including access and availability but, perhaps more importantly, depending on explanatory models.

As cultures influence human behaviour and define normality, it is crucial that mental health professionals are aware of cultural variations in epidemiology, presentation and therapeutic engagement. Cultures mould every sphere of an individual's life. In this chapter, we propose to highlight some of the key factors that influence the contents of psychiatric disorders and how these can be identified and utilised in clinical encounters. Every individual has a culture within which they have micro-identities reliant upon, and interfacing with, various components of wider cultures and society. In this chapter, we will provide an overview of the role that cultures play in the genesis, perpetuation, precipitation and prevention of psychiatric disorders and offer some practical suggestions for managing individuals from cultures other than that of the clinician.

Definitions

Culture is defined as a complex whole including knowledge, beliefs, arts, laws, morals and customs, which may include the capabilities and mindsets acquired from being a member of any society.[1] Culture is shared attributes, meanings, beliefs, norms and values.[2,3] Culture has been seen as a web that is created by human beings.[4] Kleinman notes that culture is a result of lived daily experiences, activities, communications, rhythms, rituals and patterning of social relationships.[5] Individuals and cultures are interconnected, and both are dynamic in each other's development. Cultures also set rules that the individuals must follow, and these rules can thus by attribution define what is deviant or abnormal, which is perhaps much more relevant in the practice of clinical psychiatry.[6] It is obvious that individuals carry with them a number of micro-cultures that inform their micro-identities. For example, cultures of a place of training or workplace can influence cognitive development, which will affect attitudes. These micro-cultures may create conflict within the individual or with others or may lead to an accumulation in a more supportive manner.

Kirmayer notes that culture has various distinctive applications. From the original use of the term to describe cultivation, it also reflects certain standards of conduct and refinement.[7] It can also describe a way of life and institutions. As individuals, cultures give us a sense of belonging and a sense of purpose.

Historically, there was a time when the upper social strata were seen as being 'cultured'. The high culture of art and letters affected the definitions of culture. The collective identity as embedded in culture was based upon tradition, language and common ancestry, and it carries with it a way of life, values, customs, beliefs, knowledge and humanly structured and socially transmitted aspects of the environment.[8] Institutions within cultures carry their own cultures. It can be argued that cultures carry their own personalities, as do nations, and these characteristics have been moulded by historical traditions in the same way a child's development affects their cognitive and social responses in their adulthood and beyond.

Boas saw cultures as a manifestation of the social habits of a community.[9] Culture has been seen as an intervening variable between the human organism and the environment.[10] Kirmayer points out that definitions of cultural psychiatry are thus influenced by historical traditions.[7] Cultures carry with them a common heritage and shared meanings,[3] but it is both interpretive and experiential. It derives from daily lived experiences and activities, as well as the communication (languages) between the individual and the society.[5]

Culture is defined as learned behaviours and their consequences, but the components (of these behaviours) are shared with a group of people and transmitted.[11] Hofstede sees culture as a collective programming of the mind distinguishing one category (or group) of people from another.[12] This definition therefore takes into account various professional groups and their cultures. There is no doubt that cultures carry within them different perspectives and dimensions, which is what makes them unique. However, it is important to recognise that not all individuals from the same culture will carry with them all cultural characteristics.

DSM-5 defines culture as systems of knowledge, concepts, rules and practices which are learnt and transmitted across generations.[13] Cultures include language, (organised) religion, spirituality, family structures, lifestyle stages, ceremonial rituals and customs as well as moral and legal systems. Cultures are dynamic and change individuals but also change themselves in response to individuals. Thus, cultures can have an extraordinary amount of influence on an individual's functioning. However, more importantly, cultures define what is normal and what is abnormal or deviant, of particular importance in psychiatry and identifying and diagnosing psychiatric disorders. Cultures do set standards of actions and behaviours but also help interpret other people's actions as normal, abnormal or deviant. It is well recognised that cultures can precipitate, perpetuate and influence presentation of illnesses.

Cultural psychiatry is a branch of psychiatry that deals with the impact of cultural factors on the genesis, presentation, perpetuation and outcome of various psychiatric disorders. Cultures are key influencers in the social and cognitive development of individuals. They affect child rearing, religious practices, values and taboos and help develop an individual's world view. These factors can influence rates of various psychiatric disorders, how they present and where people seek help from when they are distressed and stressed. Cultures mould our explanatory models of distress, and it is the explanatory models of individuals, their families and informal carers that dictate where they seek help from. There is no doubt that the culture of the individual may clash with the culture of the institutions where people train, work and play.

These cultural dimensions can be important in human development. Hofstede described various dimensions, and these are worth recognising even though often there is a danger in stereotyping individuals and the cultures they come from, thereby creating both stigma and discrimination.[14,15] In an interesting overview, UNESCO includes spiritual features along with emotional features of the society as part of the culture. This definition also refers to material features and lifestyle, among others.[16] As Eshun and Gurung note, cultures include ethnicity, race, religion, age, sex, family values, similar physical characteristics (e.g. hair, skin colour), similar psychological characteristics (e.g. hostility) and common superficial characteristics.[17] Thus, there may be community or kinship characteristics and individual cultural values and traits. Both objective and subjective aspects of culture are relevant to this.

Culture can be defined as a highly specific pool of information categories, rules for categorisations of inter-subjective meanings, collective representations, and ways of knowing, understanding and interpreting stimuli as a result of a common history, thus appearing to be broader in its vision and history (see Table 17.1).[18] Culture has its capital, which is described later. Basic characteristics of culture are set out in Figure 17.1.

Cultural psychiatry remains primarily concerned with the cultural aspects of human behaviour, mental health,

Table 17.1 History and evolution of cultural psychiatry

Primitive psychiatry
Pre-scientific psychiatry
Ethnopsychiatry
Folk-psychiatry
Anthropological psychiatry
Cultural psychiatry
Transcultural/Cross-cultural psychiatry
Comparative psychiatry

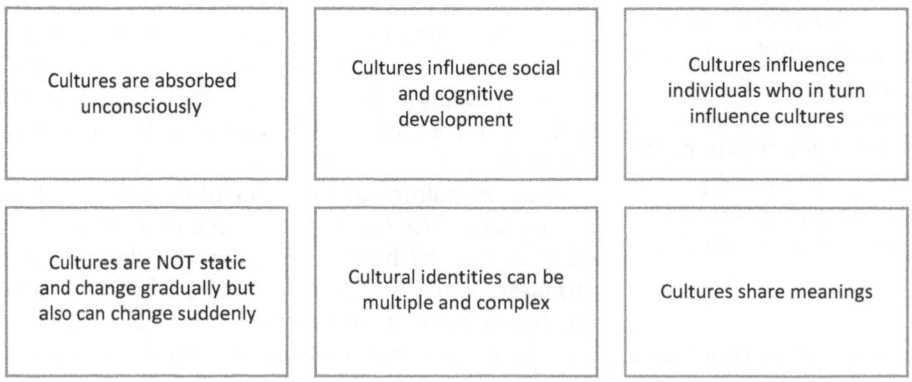

Figure 17.1 Basic characteristics of culture.

psychopathology and treatment. Its knowledge is crucial for a number of reasons. An understanding of culture works at different levels. These are (i) clinical level: culturally relevant care, (ii) theoretical: cross-culturally valid theories, and perhaps more importantly, (iii) research that focuses on cultural factors that are likely to affect human behaviour, psychopathology and healing, including therapeutic alliance. These levels have very often been ignored in the past. This has led to various racial, cultural and minority groups being excluded from research studies. Then, the tragedy is that findings from one group are blindly applied to other groups without taking cultural variations into account.

While interest in cross-cultural studies had started at the beginning of the twentieth century among migrant groups to America, on the other side of the world, colonisation in the eighteenth and nineteenth centuries led to natives being seen as primitive and exotic, creating a model where – in many colonised countries – the traditional systems of medicine were ignored or actively discouraged.

Clinical applications of cultural factors started in real earnest in the twentieth century. For example, early studies of Odegaard that compared rates of schizophrenia in Norwegians who had migrated to the USA and those who had stayed in Norway found differential rates of schizophrenia.[19] This study did start a trend. It was observed that rates of schizophrenia varied between London and New York. This led to the US-UK project, which looked at differential rates of schizophrenia and manic-depressive psychosis between London and New York (see also Chapter 5.2). The International Pilot Study of Schizophrenia (IPSS) and Determinants of Outcome in Severe Mental Disorders (DOSMED) took it one step further.[20,21] The recent spate of surveys around the world have raised some interesting questions. Although these studies have been criticised on a number of aspects, they did indicate similarities and differences in rates. In order to focus on similarities, differences are often forgotten even within the same country.

Individual identity can carry with it multiple micro-identities, and some of these are very strongly influenced by cultural factors. These cultural identities work by creating the world view held by the individual. This internal world view will also contribute to alienation and distress. Similarly, professionals carry their own cultural identities depending upon the institution they have been trained in, as well as the organisation or the institution they work in – each is likely to have its own culture. The major cultural impact of training and workplace is important in helping mould an individual's identity and, regrettably, often gets ignored in therapeutic interactions with patients and their families. Thus, a psychiatrist trained in China, India or Nepal may have a completely different world view in comparison with those trained in Australia, the USA or Brazil. In addition, the cultures of universities in the same country are likely to impact upon the inner world of the clinician but also how they select their speciality. Training across universities is broadly similar, but subtle nuances will make a difference in how training needs are absorbed by the individuals. It will also affect the way they practise, deal with the patients and understand them following various schools of thought if they are working in different cultures. Hence, cultural identity not only has various aspects and components, it is also important at multiple levels.

Classification and Dimensions of Culture

Cultures differ from one another on a number of parameters and perspectives. Various dimensions place different and varying emphasis on aspects of individual and social development and functioning. However, it is worth noting that, even within the same cultures, a vast degree of heterogeneity may occur alongside differing child development and peer pressures and other social and psychological determinants. It is helpful to explore some of these dimensions in this section. Comparing cultures can be problematic. Hofstede uses the term 'mental programmes' associated with values and culture.[14,15] Building on the General Hierarchy of Systems,[22,23] Hofstede noted that of the nine levels, humans are at level 7, human organisations are at level 8 and transcendental systems are at level 9. Each higher level adds a degree and a level of complexity to the previous one. He observes that the levels of uniqueness can be seen at individual, collective and universal levels. Hofstede describes five value dimensions attributed to culture.[14,15] These are identity (collectivism or individualism), hierarchy (large or small power distance), gender (femininity or masculinity), truth (strong or weak uncertainty avoidance) and virtue (long-term or short-term orientation). Although it is possible that there can be some overlap between these types and dimensions, Hofstede argues that – if present – such an overlap is minimum. Hofstede emphasises that the dimensions of collectivism and individualism as well as masculinity and femininity are independent of each other.[24] He observes that masculine/feminine is rooted in the power balance between the father and mother at home. These dimensions deserve further exploration to understand links with the epidemiology of physical and psychiatric disorders and characteristics of families, institutions and behaviours.

Collectivist/Individualistic Cultures

The identity dimension of culture is divided into collectivist (sociocentric)/individualistic (egocentric) (see Table 17.2). Individualistic cultures are verbal, self-centred and defensive, and they experience stress in a physical way. Egocentric cultures may use others by virtue of their usefulness, and friendships can be based on usefulness or links that are related to schools they went to, universities attended or clubs they belong to. The focus is on the self, me, I-ness, with loyalty to the immediate nuclear family, although occasionally parents may be included in this. Extreme collectivist cultures are kinship- or tribe-based. These are particularly close emotionally, with a clear emphasis on maintaining harmonious relationships. These cultures carry with them a degree of

Table 17.2 Features of collectivist (sociocentric) and individualistic (egocentric) cultures[14,15,24]

Collectivist (sociocentric)	Individualistic (egocentric)
We-ness. We consciousness, collective identity, emotional interdependence, group solidarity, sharing duties and obligations, need for stable and predetermined friendships, group decisions	I-ness. I consciousness, autonomy, emotional independence, individual initiative, right to privacy, pleasure seeking, financial security, need for specific friendships
Common good/social harmony	Related to high levels of gross national product
Individuals bound by relationships	Good at entering and leaving new social groups
Others put first before themselves	Having substantial levels of migration, most social and geographical mobility
Concession/compromise	Great skills in forming new in-groups and superficially appear more sociable
Justice and institutions are seen as an extension of the family	Yield less to group norms
Paternalism and legal moralism	High levels of crime, suicide, divorce, child abuse, emotional stress and physical and mental illness

dynamics in which the focus is on the collective good. By and large, these cultures keep the out-groups at a distance and, thus, may be averse to learning new things.

Masculine/Feminine Cultures

There are clear challenges in such a classification as it can often lead to stereotypes and expectations that people and cultures will fit into these narrow dimensions and categories.

Using work goals as a dimension, Hofstede and colleagues define the Mas/Fem or Masculine/Feminine dimension of cultures using a number of parameters (see Table 17.3).[24] He argues that feminine societies carry dominant values that aim at caring for others. People and warm relationships between individuals are seen as important. Both men and women are allowed to be tender and have sympathy for the weak, which is positively encouraged. In general, sex and violence in the media are taboo and frowned upon. Both boys and girls are allowed to cry. Mothers and fathers deal with both facts and feelings. The educational system focuses on learning and not necessarily on achievement and ambition. Characteristics of schools appear to focus on being average, and failure is seen only as a minor setback. Teachers are supposed to be friendly, and boys and girls are encouraged to take the same subjects. People work in order to live, and in the workplace, there is a clear emphasis on equality and quality of work life. Any conflicts, be they personal or workplace-related, are supposed to be resolved by negotiation and compromise. In politics, society looks after the weak, paying particular attention to the preservation of the environment and high levels of foreign aid. Embedded equality means there are often more women in elected posts in these societies. On the other hand, masculine societies see money and material possessions as important, with men being ambitious, tough and assertive. Women in masculine societies are encouraged to be tender and take care of relationships. Fathers tend to deal with facts whereas mothers deal with feelings. Boys are not supposed to cry, and girls are not encouraged to fight. Failing in school is seen as a disaster. Ambition is encouraged, and

Table 17.3 Differences between masculine and feminine societies[14,15,24]

Masculine	Feminine
Equality	Equity
Focus on winning	Society focus on performance
High spend on armies	Low expenditure on army
Assertiveness	Negotiation permissive
Focus on economic growth	Preservation of environment
Unequal share of work at work and home	Men and women do equal share of work and home
Live to work	Work to live

pressure to achieve can be high. Masculine cultures show the dominant values of material success, possibly related to the perception of men as being assertive. Once again, it must be reiterated that not all individuals belonging to one culture will behave in exactly the same way.

It can be argued that there is a degree of stereotyping of masculine societies and an idealisation of feminine societies. Hofstede does present findings from 40 countries confirming these observations.[14,15]

Scandinavian counties such as Norway, Finland, Denmark and Sweden are seen as feminine cultures, whereas Latin American counties are seen as 'mas' or masculine cultures. It must be recognised that cultures everywhere are beginning to change as are stereotypes, and these observations by Hofstede are over 40 years old, but there are clear lessons here that clinicians must be aware of.

Low/High Uncertainty Cultures

The dimension related to truth has uncertainty avoidance as a characteristic of cultures. Hofstede notes that uncertainty is an important aspect of life everywhere.[14,15] Many cultures try to avoid these by developing and setting up a number of strategies. There are also key differences between traditional and modern societies in the avoidance of uncertainties. These can be measured using an index, which includes employment stability and

Table 17.4 Differences between low and high uncertainty countries[14,15]

Low uncertainty	High uncertainty
Low anxiety – ready to live day by the day	Higher levels of anxiety
Low job stress	High job stress
Loyalty to employer	Stay with employer
Hope for success and strong achievement motivation	Fear of failure
More risk taking	Less risk taking
Broad guidelines are enough	Need clear instructions
Higher tolerance for ambiguity	Low tolerance for ambiguity
Optimism	Pessimism

stress level – measured by rates of psychosis, suicide, caffeine consumption, alcohol intake, accidents, coronary heart disease, divorce, murder and other crimes in the society as a whole. These differences are illustrated in Table 17.4.

Hofstede notes that young democratic nations such as Austria, Finland, France, Germany and Japan show high rates of uncertainty avoidance, whereas old democracies like Australia, Belgium, Canada, Denmark, Britain and the USA are more likely to show low levels of uncertainty avoidance.[14,15]

The dimension related to hierarchy as described by Hofstede has to do with the distance to the centre of power. This is reflected in the inequality in society. Such inequalities can occur in a variety of areas. These include wealth, power, social status and prestige, laws and physical and mental characteristics. Hofstede sees privileges allocated to or taken by certain individuals as private laws. Low power distance countries focus on high levels of independence rather than conformity. In the counties that illustrate low power distance, the focus often is on the reduction of inequality, interdependence and equal rights, with stress on reward and latent harmony. Hofstede offers a historical perspective on the development of power distance norm.[14,15,25]

Culture, therefore, has to be seen as a multi-faceted entity that penetrates every human being, with some features susceptible to change and others not.

Other Cultural Types

Pelto divided societies into two types: tight or loose cultures.[26] This is seen as the degree to which social entities themselves are tight or loose. In tight societies, rules are strongly enforced, and there is little tolerance to deviant behaviours. In loose societies, there are far fewer rules, and there appears to be a greater tolerance for deviance.[27] Thus, tight societies appear to have more authoritarian rulers who impose tight rules that are strictly enforced, and the independence of the traditional – as well as social – media is limited, with high levels of restriction. Consequently, these societies have fewer civil liberties and high levels of severe punishment measures, including the death penalty. Gelfand and colleagues point out that, in tight societies, a very restricted range of behaviours is permitted.[28] Their citizens are encouraged and expected to be more dutiful with higher levels of impulse control and self-monitoring. Interestingly, they are expected to have a higher need for structures. It may be difficult to tease out whether the need for structures and strictures is enforced by the rulers or demanded by the populations or perhaps both. These authors argue that these societies face more disasters and more territorial threats. Again, it is difficult to know whether this tight nature emerges from facing disasters or the two are independent of each other. In addition, these societies appear to have a higher population density and high levels of communicable diseases and air pollution. Thus, it may be that these are more traditional societies, which may have been ruled by monarchs in the past and by dictators now, which may have contributed to the tightness of norms. Interestingly, these societies also show higher levels of child mortality (but perhaps also high rates of population growth). The correlation between these factors and types of society deserves further exploration in order to understand cultural relativism and, consequently, cultural differences. It is likely that the tragedy of global mental health is the imposition of Western models, which often do not transfer well from high-income countries to low- and middle-income countries.

Loose societies are likely to tolerate a wider variety of behaviours. It is worth emphasising that although superficially it sounds attractive that loose cultures are more likely to have egocentric members, that would be a gross generalisation and also feeds an erroneous assumption that egocentric members do not require social connection or social support. They may have laws imposed to correct this looseness as has been shown in modern societies. It is also worth exploring as to why tight societies have higher levels of pollution, infant mortality and infectious diseases, which is in contrast with the observation by Gelfand and colleagues.[28] These high rates of infection may be due to the increased population density, poor public health conditions related to population density and poor access to clean water. A possible conjecture is that tight societies may have faced higher territorial threats in the past, and this may well encourage a need for developing and building strong social norms. It is also likely that, as collectivist and traditional societies are more kinship- and tribe-based, they are likely to create networks that can create increased population density and the tight nature of society. As Harrington and Gelfand note, loose societies can afford deviant behaviour perhaps because they have fewer ecological threats.[27] Thus, any model that combines various dimensions can give very complex perspectives that need to be teased out in the context of an individual sense of belonging and identities. For example, tight cultures are likely to be traditional and sociocentric, and the laws may not be entirely explicit. In their study of 33 nations, Gelfand and colleagues had used a number of methods to ascertain characteristics of culture.[28] They observed that the structures of tightness–looseness were clearly related to everyday recurring situations but also with the historical contexts for that particular country. These cultural differences, along with specific characteristics, require further careful and detailed exploration, particularly in understanding the characteristics and dimensions of various cultures such as overlap of collectivist and tight cultures or individualistic and loose cultures. Furthermore, the role of feminine and masculine cultures and these dimensions needs careful study to ascertain how these affect the formation of the worldviews of individuals and the individual's cognitive and social development. These are likely to play a major role in settling down after migration and undergoing processes of acculturation. Gelfand and colleagues compared rates of Covid-19 across countries and found that loose cultures had nearly five times the rates of infections compared with tight cultures.[29] This may reflect the perceived and the real role of the governments, which can 'dictate' behaviours. In some ways, this study goes contrary to earlier observation about high rates of infection in tight cultures but offers an interesting perspective on the way the governments and leaders convey their messaging and ensure population compliance at times of perceived national emergency.

Linear, Multi-active or Reactive Cultures

Another classification of cultures has been put forward by Lewis, who divides cultures into linear active, multi-active or reactive cultures.[30] A linear active culture encourages its people to focus on doing only one thing at a time and do so with total concentration – thus in a linear way. These actions have to be done within a scheduled period with patience and quiet, with fixed hours, timetabled activities and by sticking to plans. Individuals are encouraged to be job oriented, unemotional, procedural. Countries like Germany, Austria and the Scandinavian countries are given as prime examples of this type of culture. On the other hand, multi-active cultures have almost the opposite characteristics: generally extroverted individuals with an inquisitive nature, gregarious and talkative who work any hours and have unpredictable habits. They may be multi-tasking, doing several things at the same time, and they may not be able to concentrate and may be more emotional. Various countries that have been described as multi-active cultures include the Czech Republic, Latin American countries and India.

Reactive cultures combine characteristics of both groups in response to the environment. They are quiet, caring, respectful and people oriented and consequently very good listeners. They may use subtle body language. The model is often shown as a triangle or a tripod with countries ranged along lines between two vertices. Lewis notes that linear active countries are colder countries and multi-active countries are often hotter, but north European countries are also likely to include a reactive dimension.[30] Again, a note of caution is needed to confirm that not all individuals will fit into a single model, and care must be taken into avoiding stereotyping countries as well as individuals.

Another note of caution is put forward by Hofstede and colleagues, who remind us of potential problems in aspects of culture such as the complex and dynamic nature of culture.[31] They also point out that culture may not be seen as a universally accepted notion and 'once you begin considering culture, there is the problem of knowing when to stop' (p.40). They argue that people in the culture may not be able to describe the culture accurately, perhaps because values are implicit and defy conscious reflection. Culture is not personality, and various dimensions of one person may be in conflict with another individual thereby creating tensions. Those from individualistic cultures may attribute culture-based behaviour to personal character.

Cultural Variations

Often it is easy to argue that cultures are homogenous. They are to a degree, but there are additional differences that need to be considered. Harrington and Gelfand point out that even within what is perceived as a homogenous culture (e.g. American), variations in tightness and looseness occur, and this is likely to be related to huge variations in ecological and historical conditions and personality characteristics.[27] Using previously validated methods for assessing these, they studied severity of punishment, permissiveness, moral order and members of foreign-born populations in individual states. They were able to show that tight states had not only greater ecological vulnerabilities, but they also had fewer natural resources. These states also positively related to all indicators of disease prevalence as well as low urban dwellings, and they showed an increased level of military presence (perhaps due to the perception of threat). Of particular interest from a cultural perspective is the variation of personality across these states. Harrington and Gelfand have postulated that living in loose or tight states is likely to affect the development of certain psychological traits, which will mould personality. It is also likely to mould world view and cognitive development. In their study, tight states showed higher levels of conscientiousness and lower openness, which was related to greater cautiousness, as well as low levels of cultural openness, which may reflect a level of introversion. Although it is clear that certain ecological features play a role in the moulding of cultural values, inevitably they will also affect social and cognitive development and eventually personality traits.

There is a clear danger that the classification of cultures may well lead to stereotypes of national characters and hence create negative attitudes towards them. With a much-increased level of exposure and resulting assimilation of other cultures through exposure to television, the internet and social media, the cultural differences at one level are beginning to shift, and there is a degree of similarity beginning to emerge. On the other hand, there is a tendency in many cultural settings to revert to perhaps more rigid cultural norms.

These changes can be seen in third-generation migrant individuals (although technically they are not migrants) in many cultures. Furthermore, it is clear that as cultures mould certain psychological traits, historical factors along with child rearing can influence cognitive development, and in return, these characteristics will go on to re-frame cultures. The maintenance of cultural differences is, therefore, of great interest both in the historical longitudinal sense, but also in the horizontal sharing of cultural values. The ecological and historical bases can play a role in human cultural development.

In order to highlight some of the life stages, we will now illustrate cultural variations in brief. There are, of course, some major generalisations in this.

Birth

The birth of a child is celebrated in different ways with specific cultural rituals. For the new mother, often there will be dietary recommendations and dietary restrictions. These will often allow the mother to recover. In some cultures, new mothers will be confined to her bed or room for nine days, whereas in other cultures, it will be 'doing the month'. The purpose is to create a recuperative and supportive atmosphere. In some cultures, the naming of the child will not occur until the 9th, 13th or 15th day. Other rituals may well include shaving the head or dressing the boys in girls' clothes. These rituals are meant to deflect superstitions and evil eye.

In some cultures, male children are to be preferred over female children, which in itself, can be attributed to cultural values. For new mothers, different systems may emerge whether they are in a collectivist or individualist society. Family and household structures will provide a level of support that may be relatively more medicalised in Western European countries. Joint families or nuclear families will vary in their responses to childbirth, as will urban/rural locations. One-parent families have their own specific issues. Bearing children and fertility can be extremely important in some cultures. Hsu described the axis of loyalty and affection bonds in families and noted that there are clear variations across cultures.[32] The axis may be built on husband–wife (Europe), father–son (Asian cultures), mother–son (India, Jewish, Italian, Muslim groups), brother–brother (sub-Saharan Africa) and brother–sister (Micronesia) dyads. Thus, nature and a degree of conflict and competition can vary across cultures. There is every likelihood that, depending upon different types of emphasis on dyads, different family systems can emerge. Cross-cultural studies of child development can highlight varying cultural emphasis. Attachment patterns vary across cultures along with attachment objects, which will influence brain development.

Ageing

Ageing occurs across all cultures, but the role of the older individuals and their responsibilities, along with respect accorded to these characteristics, can vary across cultures. Ageing can be physical, psychological or social.[33] Each of these has varying levels of importance across cultures. Attitudes towards ageing can be positive (filial piety) or negative (ageism). Attitudes to age and ageing vary – for example, in the USA, the emphasis is on youth, beauty and achievement, whereas in countries like India, respect for the older individual is important. Coping with ageing landmarks, such as menopause, can be difficult in some cultures. Adulthood and expectations of how adults behave rely on the type of culture and cultural expectations they are brought up in. The gender roles and gender role expectations for young people, for adults and older adults are dictated by cultures.

In an interesting survey, Bengtson and colleagues found that the concept of ageing varied across different ethnic groups in southern California.[34] Mexican Americans in this study saw themselves as old at age 57 whereas, for African Americans, this age was 63 and, for Caucasian Americans, it was 70. This may reflect their experiences of hardship that they may have gone through.[35] Similarly, it can be postulated that middle-age crisis and adjustment will vary across cultures. Bodily changes and social changes such as employment, growing family and changes in relationships can all contribute to this mid-life crisis. Socioeconomic and educational factors will play a role in this adjustment. Coming up to retirement and the 'artificial' age of giving up work can have differential impact on people's functioning and mental health.

Marriages

Marriages in many cultures, especially traditional and kinship-based societies, are conducted between families rather than individuals. In many traditional cultures, arranged marriage is still the norm whereas, in others, it is individual choice and increasingly, in others, a mix of the two approaches is prevalent. There are clear variations between egocentric and sociocentric cultures.

Death

Cultures contribute to views about death and dying. The notions about the dead, death and dying are contributors to rituals that influence attitudes about death. In parts of Africa, the dead join the ancestors, thereby becoming venerable, and the whole village is expected to participate in the funeral.[36] In some cultures, the dead have to be buried before the next sunset whereas, in others, it may be necessary to take time before burial takes place. Religion and culture will play a major role in choosing the method of disposal of the body. Various rituals have to accompany this act, and there may be a clear timeline for various rites and rituals to take place.

Attitudes to death and whether it is celebrated or mourned have changed over the years. Grief as a result of loss, which is an emotional event, can be significant. However, rituals are devised to help individuals cope with the loss. Expression of grief also varies across cultures. In some cultures, total silence is to be observed whereas, in others, wakes will be held with loud music and chatter. The psychiatric diagnosis of abnormal grief reaction, therefore, must be seen in a cultural context. For example, among Hindus, after death, various rites have to be carried out on specified days, and for 11 months after the death, no joyous activities such as marriage are to be conducted. However, with culture in transition, this is beginning to change, which illustrates both a shift in the expression of grief and social expectations. Clinicians, therefore, must take into account the cultural notions of grief before reaching a diagnosis of abnormal grief reaction.

Cultural Capital

There is a clear distinction between social capital and cultural capital. Social capital is seen as bonds between individuals, and these relationships are based on a number of factors, including friendships and work relationships with colleagues and peers as well as personal relationships in the family, kinships and larger community. Social capital can assist and help an individual to form bridges or connections between acquaintances and distant friends, which more often than not provide support along with a sense of belonging and purpose, which will influence the degree of self-esteem. Social media has changed the way people form and see friendships, communicate and support each other; thus the concept of social capital needs to be revisited and perhaps redefined. As social capital can include linkages with peers, colleagues and employers, the type of culture as described by Hofstede may influence social capital.

Developed in the 1970s, the concept of cultural capital was described by Bourdieu, and it emerged from the field of education, but it can equally well fit into the field of health, especially mental health.[37] The core components of cultural capital fall into three categories: the first one of which constitutes objective components such as books, arts, folk tales and music with which an individual is familiar and may have grown up with. They may subsequently learn and acquire some of these tastes. The acquisitions of these components may well have changed, especially if the individual and their family have moved across cultures – or in a closely connected world, through social media, television and web. People in different cultures are likely to acquire tastes which were probably not traditionally part of their cultural upbringing. The second set of components is to do with embodied aspects, which include diet, language and dress. These are perhaps most likely to change as a result of migration, coming in contact with other cultures directly or indirectly and consequent acculturation. The third component of cultural capital is seen as the institutional ones, which include degree, training, other qualifications and skills. From an acculturation perspective, these (degrees, qualifications, and training) can help open certain doors, especially in relation to educational attainment, employment and other opportunities.

From a cultural perspective, an understanding and knowledge of these components of cultural capital is important because the culture of the institutions can play an instrumental role in helping develop micro-identities. Other components of cultural capital appear to include emotional, subcultural and national aspects. These national or cultural characteristics can sometimes lead to national and cultural stereotypes and consequent negative attitudinal shifts creating stigma, discrimination and xenophobic racism. It is conceivable that as Bourdieu and colleagues had predicted, cultural capital can give status and power to the individual.[38] Our contention is that cultural capital too is transmitted across generations. The child gathers values, beliefs, skills and knowledge through the process of child rearing. Cultural capital is an important part of the individual's identity. However, it needs to be remembered that institutions and organisations transmit their core values through knowledge, training and skills, which award qualifications. These can contribute to both individual and collective identity and cultural capital, so this may be seen as a two-way process.

Cultural capital can be understood at different levels, and a knowledge of each level is critical for the process of acculturation by migrants. These three levels are at individual, group or kinship and institutions.[39,40] The concept can be criticised on a number of grounds, especially if it is seen only at a superficial level.

Thus, it is self-evident that every individual carries with them what can be called core cultural capital. Wherever they are, they will carry this core with them, if not all total aspects of cultural capital. These values thus contribute to developing personal, community and institutional dimensions attributable to a particular culture. Individual members will carry their cultural capital, which gives them a sense of belonging and purpose but also self-esteem. It is important for the clinicians to be cognisant of the cultural capital of the individual they are seeing.

Race and Racism

WHO described racism as the belief that there is an inherent connection between perceived, hereditary and cultural traits and that some groups see themselves as superior to others.[41] On the other hand, prejudice is negative attitudinal, behavioural and emotional beliefs set against an individual or group based purely on selected social or cultural characteristics. Ethnocentrism is the overvaluing of one's own culture in comparison with other cultures, thereby leading to biased judgements.

It is worth recalling that racism has preceded the concept of race. The discrimination and prejudice are often to do with perceived or real power and 'the otherism', which may be misogyny, homophobia or Islamophobia. Bethencourt takes a similar view and notes that racism existed at the time of the Crusades and continues to the present.[42] Raising the question that the same person can be considered black in the USA, coloured in the Caribbean or South Africa and white in Brazil, Bethencourt defines racism as prejudice concerning ethnic descent coupled with discriminatory action. The concept of racism is of Western interest, although a degree of 'otherness' exists in all countries. The question of racism based on skin colour thus remains problematic, but the reality is that it exists and creates a kind of hierarchy that brings with it certain privileges. Even though prejudice concerning ethnic descent coupled with discrimination existed in various parts of the world and various periods of history, it is conceivable that the so-called scientific framework provided by the theory of race made it not only more obvious but perhaps acceptable. Throughout history, notions of blood and descent have existed in identification as terms such as 'blue blood' have indicated, but Bettencourt notes that the modern ethnic and racial divide was largely inspired by (and influenced by) traditional religious antagonism. Prejudices even in ancient Greece are said to be more cultural. Consistent and systematic discrimination forms a crucial aspect of racism.

Sowell notes that the term 'race' was once widely used to distinguish the Irish from the English or the Germans from the Slavs, as well as groups more sharply different based on skin colour, hair texture and so forth.[43] Sowell notes that this application has become obvious since the Second World War, and the distinction is based on external appearances. Race is a powerful social concept. The notion of classification is not new either. People have been classifying each other on various bases for millennia. Even technological advances can lead to those who are familiar with the web and those who are unfamiliar or left behind. That can lead to class distinction – again, a form of arbitrary classification.

The concept of race emerged as a means of classifying 'the other' based on superficial – often, observable – physical characteristics. Its spread and acknowledgement were partly placed on the colonialists, who saw the native as exotic and 'the other' and created categories. Race is thus often constructed as a physical characteristic, as they are easy to observe, and erroneously attributed solely to biological factors such as skin colour or body shape. This concept of race carries with it a set of different meanings. As Thompson and Carter have illustrated, it can have stereotypes of racial ideology and systems of racial meanings.[44,45] Through the processes and experiences of socialisation, individuals tend to be imbued with messages that determine the appropriateness as well as inappropriateness of their roles as social beings.[46] These roles, whether they are perceived or real, in turn can influence identity and how the individuals see themselves but also how they perceive others seeing them. Racial identity emerges from the contextualised experiences of race as a pattern of attitudes, beliefs and behaviours.[44]

Race is not a biological or scientific fact but a social construct.[47] Spickard blames the European scientists who chose to identify people by virtue of geography as well as physical characteristics.[48] These were subsequently modified according to tribes or clans, languages spoken or other characteristics.[49] This classification reflects the basic human interest and tendency to divide things into groups. In many cultures (e.g. in India, Jamaica), individuals with lighter skin are looked upon favourably and tend to hold higher positions in the social hierarchy. Hays notes that colonialists saw light-skinned Christians to be superior to the dark-skinned natives.[50] This, in itself, may have contributed to the two key factors of religion and skin colour to artificially give them power. As Hays notes, until relatively recently, in the USA, 'white blood' was seen as separate and perhaps superior and special so was not to be tainted by 'black blood'; thereby, in many states, inter-racial marriages were banned and illegal. Racial distinctions are not genetically discrete.[51] Many physical characteristics are common enough across cultures and communities. Linking race with IQ is not only erroneous, but racist in itself. Thus, the creation and recognition of race on a genetic basis is problematic as it creates erroneous perceptions of similarities as well as differences. It is often the case that migrants who look different are likely to be treated differently, but even the slightest differences in accent, language or way of dressing can create otherness by the new community, which can lead to rejection or being ignored or even the community becoming hostile to the newcomers. The clear and obvious distinction thus is physical by virtue of skin colour or physical appearance, which is visible.

Helms defines racial identity as a sense of group or collective identity based on a perception that the individuals share a common heritage with that social group.[52] Race has been defined as a social construction by white Europeans and Americans to establish social demarcation, elevate the white race and justify the oppression and exploitation of certain ethnic groups who are seen as and presumed to be inferior on a number of measures including intelligence, physicality, morality and culture.[44] This unscientific but persistent nature of the concept appears to have given legitimacy to the creation of further divisions and subdivisions within humanity. According to Thompson and Carter, not surprisingly, the concept of race is often confused with culture and ethnicity, thereby recognising that there may be a degree of overlap and confusion about these inter-related observations.

The concept of race carries with it a significant community and personal impact, even though there is no clear biological or scientific basis, but this is a purely social construction and perhaps that is why the notion carries such strong feelings and emotions. This social value is loaded with meaning and can lead to discrimination and exclusion at a number of levels. These negative attitudes not surprisingly affect the mental health and wellbeing of individuals as well as their social and personal functioning.[13]

Race is not a particularly useful or helpful concept, but its social persistence and existence continues to create 'the other' and also the 'in' and 'out' groups. In addition, race is often seen as leading to certain privileges for the in-group and disadvantages for the out-group. Racism can be seen as an ideology and belief to do with the self- identified superior race not only holding on to certain privileges such as wealth, education and power, but also building on these for their own gains. One type of racism is institutional racism, which as a concept, has had its ups and downs in the UK. It is defined as an enforcement of racism maintained by legal, cultural, religious, educational, economic and political institutions in maintaining the differential in access and advancement on the basis of race. Many other types of racism have been described. In the clinical settings, perhaps the most hideous racism is missionary racism, where the clinician sees people from other cultures being unable to make decisions for themselves, and actions are taken on behalf of the perceived inferior individual, conveying a message that the clinician knows what is good for them. 'Colour blindness' is another form of racism where all minority individuals are seen as similar as are their needs. This could be construed as universalist phenomenon, which sees all cultures as similar with no individual or cultural variation. In our view, cultures are relativist as there are clear differences across cultures but equally importantly within the so-called same cultures as shown earlier in Harrington and Gelfand's work. For example, even within a metropolitan place such as London or New York, there are clear differences across boroughs, and each borough has its own subtle cultural nuances, be they dialects or behaviours. Individuals belonging to the same culture may not be entirely alike and carry certain subtle and not-so-subtle differences in cultural values and expressions.

Nearly 30 years ago, Cohen observed that language plays a role in conveying racism and anti-racism ideas.[53] Racism can be seen as institutionalised false consciousness, as irrational prejudice, as white power, as class rule or as rational self-interest. All of these observations can play a major role in institutions providing education and health care. Rattansi, in the same volume, defines institutional racism as signifying 'all the myriad, taken for granted ways in which routine institutional procedures, whatever their original purposes, end up discriminating against (ethnic) minorities'.[54] This is of particular importance in clinical psychiatry, where 'clinicians can deprive people with mental illness their liberty and force them to have treatment against their will'. Race has been conceptualised as an unstable and decentred complex of social meanings constantly being transformed by political struggle.[45]

Although race may be seen as a major expression of culture, it forms only a small component. It is the culture that is the most important facet in an individual's life, which makes them who they are by moulding their child rearing and social and cognitive development. However, it is important to recognise that not every individual will imbibe or absorb the cultural values the same way, and their individual characteristics may well differ from others in the same culture. As mentioned earlier, often race and culture are confused, and unconscious bias towards race gets transferred to a particular culture, which is then seen as particularly inferior. Race is obviously seen as a physical characteristic and therefore seen as easy to identify. However, cultural aspects of race can be influenced by the external features of religion and taboos, but also by factors such as diet. Economic, political, social and educational or occupational aspects and perspectives are crucial in our understanding of culture.

In psychiatry too, perhaps for historical reasons, often race has been defined on the basis of pure physical characteristics, whereas anthropologists have used the term 'geographical race' to indicate a group with distinctive genetic make-up.[55] Races remain socially and culturally constructed categories, and there is little doubt that, even within the same race, there are major genetic differences.[56] The validity of race as a biological term has been discredited, but it persists in many countries.[57] Thus, the racial discrepancy is attributable to colonial, historical, social, economic and political circumstances.

Racism is about the feelings of prejudicial discrimination against a minority group by a majority group on the basis of physical appearances. The practice of clinical psychiatry is often strongly influenced by social mores and societal expectations. For example, until recently, homosexuality was seen as a mental illness (it still is in many countries), and in the nineteenth century USA, drapetomania (desire to run away as a slave) was seen as a psychiatric illness. Pinderhughes also defines racism as a relatively constant pattern of prejudice and discrimination.[58] Such prejudice and discrimination occur between one party who is idealised and favoured, perhaps by being in a majority position, whereas the other is generally a minority that is devalued and exploited. In spite of educational equivalence, social class may also play an important role in the development of racism and discrimination. Thomas and Comer define racism as a belief that race or identifiable physical characteristics are key determinants of basic human behaviour.[59] There is every likelihood that racism will affect accomplishment and achievements. This inherent superiority of certain races to others is part of a racist belief system.[60] Allport argues that the human potential for prejudgement (the latter becoming prejudices if they are not reversible in the face of new knowledge) is based on misconception. Prejudice and racism are targeted at individuals as well as groups, especially if they are out-groups, leading to anti-Semitism, homophobia and Islamophobia. Kerner sees the attitudes of the white majority towards blacks, American Indians and others as perceived white privilege and superiority and black inferiority.[61] The white population's attitudes to other whites based on the 'within in-groups' attitudes may reflect discrimination of one kind or another.

Racism needs to be differentiated from ethnocentrism in that ethnocentrism accepts people from other communities whereas racism focuses on one or more communities as inferior. Racist views are not seen as pathological by those who hold them. Although recently this has been challenged, there is considerable evidence that institutional racism exists and focuses on institutional privileges that restrict the choices of a minority or out-group in comparison with in-group or the majority. Institutional racism appears to support individual racism. It needs to be emphasised that racist institutions are not necessarily headed by racist individuals,[62] but the structures are such that these make it difficult to get rid of institutional racism. Frederickson points out that institutional racism appeared to break down between 1945 and 1994 (largely in response to Nazism) and goes on to highlight that, in medieval times, religion was the key instrument for institutional racism.[63] The perceived superiority of Christianity and the need to convert natives created a superior class and a system that may have embedded institutional racism.

Impact of Institutional Racism on Services

If any of the services, especially health care related, are institutionally racist, they are far less likely to be used by minority groups. This may lead to delays in help-seeking, and the longer the delay, the worse the long-term outcome. Furthermore, even if they access services – due to institutionalised racism – individuals may not collaborate with any therapeutic interventions, reject these interventions or drop out of treatment. Delays in help-seeking cause poor outcomes. If services are not perceived to be racist, individuals can seek help readily. Racism in mental health care can lead to misunderstandings and increase the likelihood of compulsory detentions. In a randomised controlled trial from South London, Bhugra and colleagues reported that black patients who worked with a black charity after discharge when compared to treatment as usual showed higher levels of engagement and satisfaction.[64] This was attributed to the organisation being culturally sensitive, offering appropriate interventions and materials for such things as make-up or a suitable diet.

Causes of Institutional Racism

Causes of institutional racism are complex and varying according to a number of factors. In general, institutions are organisations that are formed of individuals and traditions and not buildings alone. Institutions can be extremely powerful. Institutions reflect the interlocking of people and of social practice.[65] A commonality of cultural systems is essential, and there are different levels of institutions as observed.[66] Thus, their inherent culture expects its members to behave in a certain way. In the end, racism is about overt and covert power. It is a multidimensional complex concept.[67]

Impact of Institutional Racism on Individuals

In addition to institutional racism, in their daily lives, individuals from minority groups will experience life events, some of which may be classed as racial life events, which may cause ongoing minority stress. This may precipitate psychiatric disorders and contribute to poor functioning.[68] Many social determinants are attributable to institutional discrimination. These include poverty, unemployment and poor housing. Repeatedly, studies have shown that all things being equal, those with foreign-sounding names are less likely to be shortlisted for job interviews and less likely to be appointed. This may well lead to low self-esteem and differential attainments and pay gaps. It has been suggested that institutional racism can lead to schizophrenia.[69,70]

It has been observed that not only actual discrimination, but also its perception that can contribute to mental ill health.[71] Feeling trapped or a loss of locus of control may act as mediating factors.

Personal prejudice can be expressed in many ways, both directly and indirectly. Systemic discriminations can lead to non-engagement and physical assault, whereas personal discrimination can add to a sense of alienation on the part of the minority individual. Another insidious manifestation of prejudice is described as adjectival racism,[72] which is attaching a racial or ethnic identifying adjective to a person or group confirming a stereotype. In providing and accepting health care, this may lead to exclusion and non-availability of various treatments and therapies and increased loss of status.

Clinicians may carry their own prejudices and unconscious bias, and at an individual level, the clinician may also stereotype other cultures and unwittingly reject the minority individual. They may feel threatened or under attack or may be seen as threatening by the migrant, who may have different expectations of the clinical encounter, thus creating a double-bind. Racism itself, be it individual or institutional, will act as a chronic difficulty and a stressor. Racism thus creates differential social status with differential health consequences, differential exposure and impact on a minority individual's social and personal functioning and mental wellbeing.

The role that politics (and politicians) play in shaping racial and ethnic attitudes and policies is an important one. Political ideologies influence social acceptance or social rejection of ideas and policies. Political power can contribute to institutional racism, which then excludes those vulnerable individuals who need maximum support. Political manoeuvrings can lead to or deepen bipolarisation and divides. These may offer short-term gains to individuals but may well be corrosive to the society as a whole. The role that doctors and mental health professionals can play under these circumstances can be crucial. Both as specialists and as members of the society, they are well placed to challenge this division and, more importantly, propose solutions that can be long-term and long-lasting. In democracies everywhere, often the politicians are looking at the next election and at the short-term gains, so they may end up playing the race/culture/ethnicity card. The social impact of xenophobic nationalism can be devastating on the mental health and wellbeing of minority communities.

Ethnicity

Ethnicity has also been defined as the group's concept of 'peoplehood', including the 'common ancestry through which individuals have evolved shared values and customs'.[73] Ethnicity may have some shared biological or genetic heritage, but its most important aspects are socially constructed.[50] Ethnic groups are often labelled very broadly and widely. Phinney urges that ethnicity is not to be conceptualised as a discrete categorial variable.[74]

In the UK, ethnicity is self-ascribed. Ethnic groups have been defined as a self-perceived group of people who have common folk and religious beliefs, language, common ancestry and historical continuity.[75] Ethnicity thus is a culturally constructed group identity that defines peoples and communities[13] that may be rooted in geographical settings and origins, common history and other characteristics such as religion or language. This may have clearly identified geographical origins of individuals but will also include other characteristics. Furthermore, it is worth noting that the concept of geographical heritage varies. For example, in the USA, Asian often refers to Far East Asian origins including Chinese, Cambodians or Vietnamese whereas, in Britain, Asian generally refers to those from South Asia.

Acculturation

Acculturation has been defined by Sam and Berry at both group and individual levels.[76] Redfield and colleagues had previously defined the process of acculturation as a mixture of cultural and psychological changes that can occur when two cultures come into contact with each other.[77] Although individual beings are carriers of such communication, it is worth recalling that, in current times, globalisation and social media provide a strong degree of inter-connectedness – both directly and indirectly – which can effectively melt cultural boundaries. From collective acculturation to individualised acculturation, certain aspects of one's culture can easily give way to another even though they may or may not be totally replaced. Thus, some parts of cultural capital may be exchanged more readily than others. For example, language, diet and dress may change more rapidly than others. Skills and knowledge may also develop and be exchanged more readily, but beliefs and certain tastes such as arts, books and music may not. Various outcomes of acculturation have been described as assimilation, biculturalism, deculturation (marginalisation) or integration.[78]

Individual identity and its role in acculturation are of particular interest in psychiatry. It can be seen to have multiple components. For example, micro- identities relate to gender, religion and sexual orientation. Phinney and Baldelomar see identity at an individual level with language and one's heritage or ethno-cultural background.[74,79] The second level is identification with the majority or the dominant group. For each of these, one or more components of cultural capital may be needed to explain, exploit and exchange.

Acculturation as the process of cultural and psychological change can occur through a number of processes. The reach of American television, for example, has not only led to people following American fashions but also speaking with an American accent. Graves introduced the concept of psychological acculturation, in which the individual is influenced both by external factors (related generally to the dominant culture) but also to changes within personal culture (revealing in general to be non-dominant).[80] Sam and Berry suggest that cultural and psychological changes may need to be kept separate because cultural change may occur at the community level and psychological change at an individual level, and this is articulated in a framework.[76] This process of acculturation influences the identity of an individual.

Types of Acculturation

Berry describes four acculturation strategies and consequences. These are integration, assimilation, separation and marginalisation.[78] Each of these outcomes is influenced by the degree, distance and nature of the contact between the two cultures influencing the individual. An interesting concept put forward by Camilleri and Malewska-Payne draws a distinction between what an individual wants to be in an ideal sense (value identity) and what the individual really is (their real identity).[81] These can be similar or very different. This discrepancy can lead to negative thoughts and low self-esteem. This concept has been described by Bhugra and colleagues when comparing achievement and expectation in different domains such as social standing, employment and education.[82] Such a comparison can give a level of discrepancy between an individual's aspirations and achievement, which if widely different, can lead to depression or other psychiatric disorders. It is likely that not all but some migrants may face a degree of acculturative stress if the actual process of acculturation itself is difficult.[83] Berry sees this process as having three sub- processes: culture shielding, culture learning and culture conflict. The first two involve the selective, accidental or deliberate loss of certain behaviours (as embedded in cultural capital). Culture conflict occurs when two cultures have varying values that do not fit in with each other, and this process itself can lead to acculturative stress.

i. Adaptation can be both psychological and sociocultural; hence, this has to be seen at an individual level and the community level. Acculturation can also include processes of cultural identification leading on to cultural, structural, behavioural, civic and moral adjustments. Very often, language may need to be learnt, including nuances, dialects and subtleties. Dress may need to be adapted depending upon factors such as weather and environment. Similarly, diet may need to change in order to adapt to availability of certain types of food but also trying to fit in with the majority culture. For migrants, this process of acculturation is often lifelong. In addition, the family members may acculturate at different speeds and use different processes, thereby creating internal cultural conflict and tensions within the family. Children of migrants may go through a different, faster process of adjustment through schools and education.
ii. Biculturalism: Some groups settle down fairly rapidly in the new culture and are equally comfortable in both the culture of origin and their new culture. They may be able to speak both languages fluently, and attitudes are modified accordingly.
iii. Deculturation: Due to invasion, wars or conflict, one culture may be overwhelmed, and the new culture

imposed. This may lead to loss of language, tradition and arts, as well as artefacts.

iv. Assimilation: This may be seen as giving up some cultural aspects and being absorbed into the new culture.

Cultural Consonance

Cultural consonance has been defined as the degree to which individuals in their own beliefs and behaviours approximate the shared expectations encoded in cultural models.[84] Measured as cultural domains and lifestyle along with social support, Dressler and his research group have illustrated that these shared models affect health and wellbeing in a number of ways.[85–90] What is interesting is to note that these models appear to be consistent over a decade, at least as found by their research. Recent developments go on to look at national identities, family life, occupational and educational aspirations and food. Dressler and colleagues have reported gene-environment interaction in depressive conditions and have illustrated that childhood adversity-gene interaction may be mediated by cultural consonance in family life.[91] This may be attributed to the learning of cultural models and cultural consonance in the family. The concept is an attractive one and is needed to study the impact of culture on health and health behaviours.

Cultural contraction is the process by which the individual may voluntarily or otherwise give up parts of their culture. Cultural expansion, on the other hand, is when aspects of new culture are adapted and absorbed, especially if some common features already exist.

Disease and Illness

Eisenberg made a distinction between disease and illness.[92] Disease can be considered as 'dis-ease' and is focused on pathology. This is what clinicians are trained to identify, diagnose, manage and treat. Illness, on the other hand, is the social impact of disease – the social functioning of the individual as a result of disease, which is what patients, their carers and families are interested in. The disease can cause the patient to lose their job, housing or relationships, thus converting it into an illness, which is what patients appear to be interested in managing. Patients can live with their symptoms provided they have a degree of independence, financial activity, housing and relationships. The shaping of the response to disease into illness is very strongly influenced by culture. Identifying the distress and consequent 'symptoms' does not automatically turn individuals into patients. The illness behaviour is moulded by culture and the cultural expectations of an individual's role by the society. These will, undoubtedly, vary between egocentric and sociocentric cultures and societies as noted earlier. Tseng and Streltzer also propose that disease is a reflection of biological or physiological changes in the individual.[93] Of course, these changes are likely to affect functioning, whereas illness is about the perceptions of patients and their experiences and understanding of their 'dis-ease'. Contrary to illness, the term 'sickness' is often used by society to describe and regulate illness behaviours, such as the duration of statutory sick leave and sick pay with or without medical intervention.

Individuals often have some idea about what has gone wrong in their body or mind and why something has gone wrong. This explanation is likely to be very strongly influenced by culture. Inevitably, factors such as educational, economic and social status will modify the developing and sharing of these explanations. In traditional societies, people with mental illnesses may blame the evil eye by jealous neighbours or not carrying out rituals for the ancestors, thus offering supernatural explanations. Tseng described these explanations in the following categories: supernatural, physical, psychological, social natural or a mixture of two or more.[94] He further posited that these explanations may reflect the type of society a person lives in, and these explanations may further change as societies and cultures evolve and become more modern.

Idioms of Distress

Idioms of distress are what individuals use to express distress. These may be perceptions as well as metaphors. These use physical, psychological, spiritual and supernatural words as potential explanations. For example, among Punjabi women, the idiom of distress can be 'my heart is sinking', which can be seen as similar feelings to 'butterflies in my stomach'. If the latter, for example, is translated into another language, this may have very different meaning. Similarly, explanatory models (see Table 17.5) may include the supernatural, natural, medical, social, psychological or a mix of explanations. These may vary according to type of society. For example, more traditional cultures may have more supernatural or natural explanations. As cultures change, these may change. Table 17.5 illustrates factors that clinicians must be aware of when attempting to explore cultures.

Explanatory Models

Kleinman described the concept of explanatory models.[95] Weiss noted that an understanding of explanatory models on the part of the clinicians is absolutely vital in improving therapeutic alliance and engagement (see Table 17.6).[96]

It is worth remembering that both idioms of distress and explanatory models can change as a result of acculturation. Both of these will not necessarily fit neatly into any diagnostic category.

Table 17.5 Basic assessment of culture

1. Be aware of cultural background and beliefs
2. Be cognisant of strengths and weaknesses of own and other cultures
3. Be sensitive to different styles of communication
4. Be sensitive to metaphors being used in expressing idioms of distress
5. Be aware of the purpose of assessment

Table 17.6 Illustration of what is needed while exploring an explanatory model

What do you call your problem? Why has it occurred now?
What do you think has caused it?
What do you think are its consequences for you?
How does it affect others around you?
How serious do you think it is?
How worried are you? How worried are others around you?
What is needed for you to get better?
What happens if it does not?

Table 17.7 Relationship between patients, clinicians and teams

Patient	Doctor	Team member(s)
Race	Race	Race
Culture	Culture	Culture
Gender	Gender	Gender
Orientation	Orientation	Orientation
Religious beliefs	Religious beliefs	Religious beliefs
Explanatory models: **Illness**	Explanatory models: **Disease**	Explanatory models: **Disease**
Treatment **Accepted**	Treatment **Offered**	Treatment **Offered**
Alliance	Alliance	Alliance
Adherence	Adherence	Adherence

The interaction between physical and psychological experiences is important. In many cultural models of illness, Cartesian mind-body dualism does not exist; hence, the individual may express psychological distress in physical terms.

Cultures of the patient and the clinician may well differ on subtle parameters, even if they both come from the same country. The variations can be nuanced. However, an additional point worth noting is that, in a clinical context, psychiatrists have additional power on behalf of the state to detain and treat patients against their will. Prejudice and unconscious biases on behalf of the clinician and the patient can create tensions and distrust, which may well lead to a reluctance to work together. Another complicating factor can be the culture of the institution where the clinicians work. In that case, the patient's or their families' past experiences can create problems in engagement. This variation may further contribute to tensions within the team. The hierarchy, be it explicit or implicit in the team, may add to disenchantment in the patient and team and can create difficulties in engagement. Various team members may ally with or go against those from their own cultures. Gender, race, religion and sexual orientation may inform hierarchies within the team. Each discipline and team member will have their own culture, which will need to be negotiated. Matters related to confidentiality and privacy may take on different meanings in different cultures. For a summary on the relationship between patients, clinicians and teams, see Table 17.7.

It is worth reminding ourselves of what Sam and Moreira pointed out nearly a decade ago;[97] they emphasised that culture and mental illnesses are more or less embedded in each other. In order to understand any type of mental illness and its impact on the individual, family and kinship, as well as society at large, it is important to explore cultural aspects. Culture can precipitate certain psychiatric disorders (P), affect the way they present (A), influences the reactions (R) individuals with symptoms have, the responses (R) of their carers and family members, and their engagement (E) with services and treatment (T) outcome (PARRET). The outcome of therapeutic intervention depends upon whether the cultures prefer pharmacotherapies, psychotherapies or a mixture of the two. Castillo highlighted the ways in which culture influences mental health through not only personal experiences of illness and its expression, but also how these symptoms are expressed and treated.[98]

There are challenges in our understanding and exploration of cultures in that clinicians and researchers take what anthropologists see as either culturally universalist positions (where <u>all</u> cultures experience and express psychiatric disorders in the same way) or culturally relativist positions (where cultures vary, and their responses vary). Rather tragically, there appears to be a tilt in the recent global mental health movement towards a more universalist position, assuming that mental illnesses not only occur across cultures – which is true – but with their argument that the contents and characteristics are the same, which is patently not true. Eshun and Gurung make a distinction between absolutist and universalist positions, seeing the former as a more extreme position, which is something clinicians and researchers need to be aware of.[17]

It is worth remembering that cultures shape our perceptions of reality and influence societal forms of conflict, behaviour and psychological disorders.[99] In order to understand the role of culture, clinicians need to be culturally competent and familiar with investigating stress, its impact on individuals and illness behaviours and particular variations across cultures. Coping strategies will vary across cultures at different levels: personal, family, kinship or societal. At each of these levels, the coping and resilience will be influenced by a number of additional factors such as education, previous experiences, social and economic status. When examining psychopathology, it is helpful to look at coping strategies too. Descriptive and phenomenological aspects of the distress should be explored along with dynamic factors and support systems, which can then guide the clinician into finding a suitable therapeutic intervention. Cultural competence is about making sure that the culture of the individual remains centre stage in any assessment and treatment. Often, there is an assumption that minority individuals and migrants are the only ones that have a 'culture', as opposed to broader society including the clinician themselves, which is obviously untrue. The relationship between various disciplines and cultural psychiatry is illustrated in Figure 17.2.

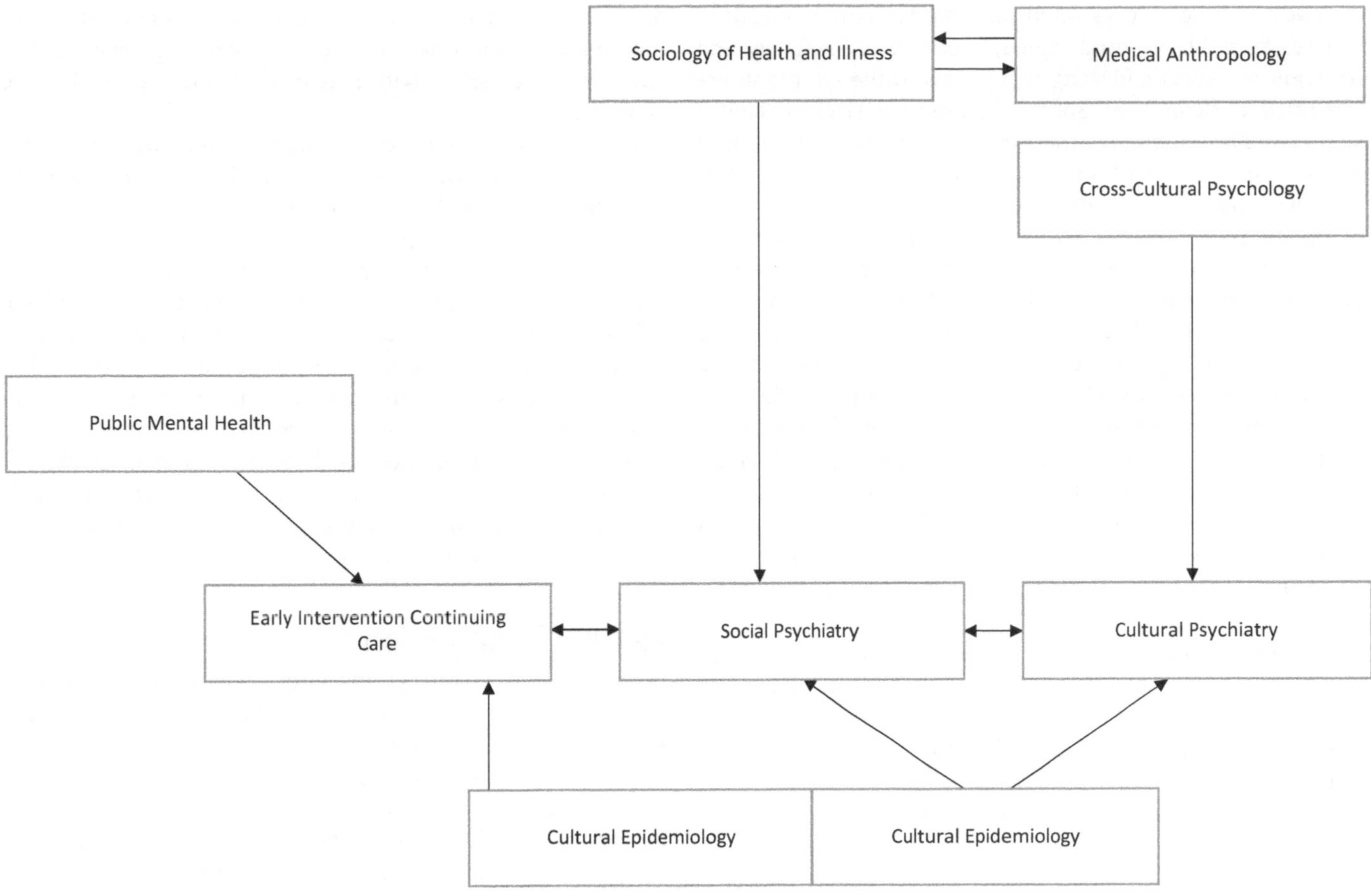

Figure 17.2 Domains of academia and practice that relate to culture, psychiatry and mental health.

In contrast with culture, society can be seen as a social institution with a particular visible organisation structure composed of a collective group of members.[57] Cultures form part of the society and, within them, carry subcultures with its own set of rules and expectations of its members. Furthermore, people may undergo changes in the periphery of their culture or at the core in response to a number of factors, both external and internal. Health care professionals need to be crucially sensitive to cultural nuances and the roles that culture plays in the lives of the individuals they are dealing with.

Cultures can influence mental illnesses in the following ways:[94]

i. Pathogenic: Cultures can cause illness (e.g. culture bound syndromes)
ii. Pathoreactive: Modifies beliefs (e.g. conversion disorders)
iii. Pathoselective: Selective pathology (e.g. symptom content varying)
iv. Pathoplastic: Modification of symptoms (e.g. somatisation)
v. Pathoelaborating: Elaborates symptoms (e.g. alcohol abuse, suicide)
vi. Pathofacilitating: facilitates symptoms (e.g. conversion disorders)

Thus cultures can precipitate, present and perpetuate psychiatric symptoms.

Basic Principles of Mental State Exam

Psychiatry as a specialty relies on mental state assessments and confirmatory corroborative history from informants. For assessing the mental state of individuals from different cultures (especially if they differ from that of the clinician), certain factors must be taken into account. Ideally, clinical assessment should take more than one session with the collection of clear third-party information. If the language of the clinician and the patient differ and interpreters are used, certain steps must be taken (see later for further details). The clinical assessment will carry with it different challenges depending upon the purpose of assessment and where it takes place. For example, assessing a patient at home for detention may carry different imperatives with it in comparison with a patient being assessed in a police station or the court. In psychiatric assessments, both verbal and non-verbal patterns of communication are important and will be influenced by cultures. For examples, in some cultures, physical distance between doctor and patient can be seen as intimate even if they are just in the same room whereas, in some cultures, physical closeness will be seen as important. Verbal communications will be affected by cultural capital, knowledge of language and its nuances, dialect and slang as well as how the symptoms are identified and conveyed. Subtle differences may create confusion, so clinicians must be sensitive to these. Prolonged periods of assessment may be required, and hence, it is important not to rush these assessments.

As mentioned earlier, where the patient is assessed will be important so care must be taken to ensure privacy. The purpose of the assessment should be clear. Non-verbal communication is important but is likely to vary across cultures. Eye contact, facial expressions, gestures, language, dialect and emotional expressions all play a role in communicating distress. Mistry and colleagues, in a small survey of psychiatrists from different counties, found varying responses to the question of assessing women who were wearing niqab, thus covering their faces during consultation.[100] Some psychiatrists were very comfortable in carrying out mental state assessments under these circumstances, whereas others were reluctant to do so.

Verbal communication will convey distress but may need clarification if accents, colloquialisms, style and dialect are difficult to follow.

Tseng points out that normality and abnormality are an essential distinction by clinicians. Assessment of functioning, thought and mood are important, and crucially, all are culturally influenced.[101]

Working with Interpreters

It is important to know how to work with interpreters (see Table 17.8). Sometimes, the interpretation can be conducted using the telephone or video links rather than in person. Some interpreters may wish to protect their cultures by holding back information from the patient, whereas others may exaggerate.

Using Assessment Tools

Using assessment tools across cultures, especially if they have been developed in one culture, must be done with care. Firstly, these should have cultural validity and sensitivity. They need to have conceptual equivalence in the new language in order to avoid category fallacy. Lin and Kleinman proposes that tools developed in one culture can create categories that may not exist in other cultures, thereby imposing categories which can be seen as false.[102] In spite of following standard recommendations, often questionnaires can create difficulties and deliver false positive or false negative results. The tools must also have criterion and conceptual validity. Thus, clinicians may need to familiarise themselves with specific assessment tools that are culture specific.

The instruments developed from within the culture are called emic (deriving from the linguistics term 'phonemic'), and these are most likely to identify pathology. Etic instruments are those developed from outside the culture – again, the term originating from 'phonetic' (meaning 'sounds like'). It is important to recognise that all assessment tools must have cultural validity for the culture in which they are going to be used. Conceptual equivalence is important to ensure that cross-cultural comparisons can be made. In the past, culture brokers, culture mediators and cultural ambassadors have been used for helping individual patients traverse the clinical care and pathways, but there is no reason why such individuals cannot advise researchers and clinicians to help develop cultural validity in assessment tools.

Cultural Formulation

In DSM-5,[13] the concept of cultural formulation has been described at some length. Lewis-Fernández and colleagues see it as a set of guidelines for clinicians.[103] The purpose of cultural formulation is to assist and enable the clinician to systematically evaluate the impact an individual's culture has on their mood, thoughts and behaviours. It assesses the cultural context of their illness experience and enables clinicians to develop and deliver culturally sensitive and appropriate strategies.

DSM-5 describes a review of the patient's cultural background, the cultural context of how symptoms are being experienced by them, how their distress is expressed and how these differences affect the clinical and therapeutic relationship. Exploring symptoms, any precipitating factors, levels of behavioural and social dysfunction, previous experiences and patterns of help-seeking are all culturally influenced and form part of the cultural formulation (see Table 17.9).[104]

Cultural identity will need to be explored carefully, as some individuals may be reluctant to share this as it may be seen as inferior or stigmatising. In order to explore cultural identity, various aspects such as cultural capital, migration, reasons for migration, path taken, age at migration, whether migration happened alone or in a group, language spoken and other such

Table 17.8 Working with interpreters

Where possible, use the same interpreter and always try to work with interpreters who are trained
Always talk to the patient not to the interpreter
Use simple language and clarify as much as needed
Try not to use family members or children for interpretation unless it is an absolute emergency

Table 17.9 Cultural formulation of distress and health seeking[104]

How is the distress experienced?
How is it identified as a problem?
How is this problem defined culturally?
What are the cultural perceptions?
What are the cultural factors that are providing support?
How is help sought?
Similar questions may need to be asked of family members or informants.

factors may be assessed by the clinician. Aspirations, achievements and discrepancies must be explored.

Cultural competence includes an awareness of the cultures of the key players in the therapeutic interaction, between that of the physician/psychiatrist and the patient. The environment of the interaction of the institution as well as the clinical disciplines will have their own cultures. The emphasis on clinical diagnosis and treatment algorithms may create problems in therapeutic engagement. The medical culture in some settings will insist on fixed appointments, whereas patients and their families may prefer drop-in. In clinical psychiatry, the culture of the team inspired and installed by its leadership will also play a major role in engaging with the patient and their families. Shifting the emphasis to patient engagement and team decisions may be seen as difficult in some cultures. A psychiatrist's biases will influence their openness to patient experiences.

Cultural sensitivity means a recognition of being aware of the strengths and weaknesses of the patient's culture and potentially divergent views. Thus, it is necessary to be aware that patients may experience and express distress in different ways than described in textbooks as it depends upon cultural experiences. The patient and their carers and families carry attitudes, beliefs and ways of addressing problems, and their value systems will influence therapeutic interaction and engagement.

Cultural empathy is defined as an ability to understand the patient's cultural perspectives and engaging in the patient's emotional experience, which can be extremely helpful in therapeutic engagement. This engagement is based on cultural empathy.[58]

Cultural Knowledge

In developing cultural sensitivity and empathy, cultural knowledge is crucial. Clinicians may not know the details and subtle nuances of all the cultures they come across, but it is critical that they are aware of access to resources. Culture brokers, cultural mediators or advocates can help advise the team about norms and mores of the community, but they can also inform the community about the role of the team and institution. Careful judgement will be required to ascertain the accuracy of information being conveyed.

Culturally appropriate interactions will influence cultural transference and counter transference. It is worth noting that a patient may belong to a majority community and a therapist to a minority one, which will bring different sets of issues of engagement. The power differential between the patient and the therapist will vary across cultures, as interpersonal relationships are defined and regulated by cultural norms. Attitudes towards authority vary across cultures as do expectations from a medical encounter. Ethnic matching of the patient and clinician is superficially very attractive but, apart from initial engagement, it is unlikely that long-term outcomes will differ, especially if the clinicians are culturally competent. Even if the patient and the clinician are from the same culture, the patient may choose to hide or give misleading information in order to prevent bringing the culture and community to disrepute and shame. Language and meanings in cultural content are important.

Professional–Patient Interaction

The individual identifies their distressing experiences into symptoms and seeks help for them. The social angle of such distress provides potential failure into meeting social obligations but also dissatisfaction with interpersonal relationships. In some cultures, individuals will not present these dissatisfactions to doctors because it might be seen as bringing shame to the family. It is well recognised that patients will present to doctors what they see the purpose of the doctor or actual point of consultation is. These views are likely to be very strongly influenced by cultural values and expectations. What also matters to the patient is their own view of getting better or recovery. In some cases, this may cause a discrepancy between what they see as having recovered or what the doctor sees as recovery. There are differential perceptions of recovery and illnesses between Black Americans and White Americans.[105] Social and cultural determinants of health will play a role in not only the presentation to medical professional services, but also to therapeutic engagement and outcome. It must be restated that doctors and other clinicians need to go beyond symptoms and look at social processes, which may or may not be directly related to the symptoms. It has been shown that doctors may be approached for both health and non-health problems, but doctors also may be approached as the village elder - wise and judicious.[106]

In order to make an appropriate diagnosis, the clinician must bear in mind whether the cluster of symptoms the individual is presenting with is culturally influenced and, if so, how. The role cultures play in verbal and non-verbal communication in expressing distress may be taken into account. In addition, whether the symptoms are seen as abnormal by the family and those around them should also be noted. It is also important to recognise whether the patient's presentation can be understood in the context of their culture along with the social, economic and political pressures on them. When people seek help and advice from faith healers or practitioners of traditional medicine, it is important to recognise that such interventions often see individuals 'as a whole person' and may, therefore, be preferred by their families and carers. When modern medicine is exported to traditional societies, it fails to provide the necessary ritual and philosophic basis considered necessary for such societies.[107] Of course, a lot has changed in the past 45 years, but one thing remains the same. When we look at all those who come to the health services, it is very rare that health services go to where our patients are. The therapeutic encounter is strongly influenced by both patient and the clinician's respective explanatory models and mutual expectations of

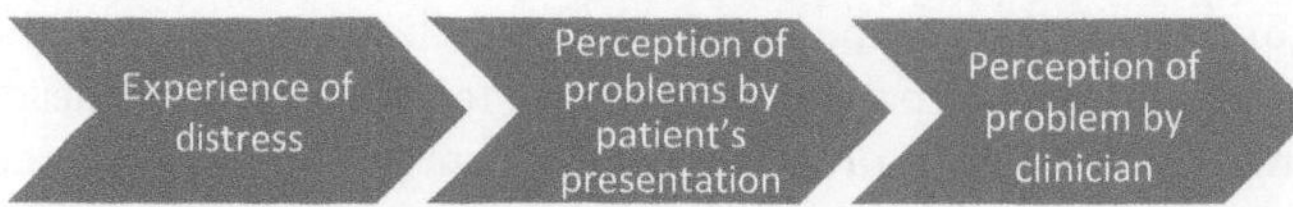

Figure 17.3 Cultural assessment.

each other (see Figure 17.3). Furthermore, the culture of the institutions and micro-identities will play a role in engagement and potential outcome.

Outpatient Psychiatry

A vast majority of psychiatric consultations take place in outpatient settings. In addition to the cultural aspects of patients, clinicians and the institution itself, there are challenges related to the purpose and the process of the assessment itself. If it is for a simple assessment, the patient's and family's feelings and expectations will need to be addressed and managed appropriately. If the patient has been brought there from elsewhere, such as courts or prison, then the interaction will vary. In the UK, with many services offering early intervention, the clinical assessment may take place at home. On the other hand, for such an assessment, some individuals from other cultures may be too welcoming while others may resent the intrusion into their personal space. It is important that patients are approached with empathy, which includes not only understanding but also the regular framing of the symptoms and problems with the patient and their carers. There is sometimes a danger and tendency to blame everything on culture. Understanding explanatory models and confirming that the clinician is cognisant is important. It is worth remembering that patients from the same culture may still not have similar experiences.

Inpatient Psychiatry

Inpatient psychiatry will need a clear understanding of the culture of the ward. There is no doubt that, in the UK, ethnic minorities are over-represented in acute admission wards, as well as medium and high secure units. They are also more likely to be admitted under a compulsory detention order and treated by force. Any plans to offer culturally sensitive inpatient units must include training for staff to provide things like culturally appropriate diet or make-up. If it is not possible to do so, then working with local third sector organisations can help build community engagements and also support for patients after they are discharged. Needs assessments of patients must include cultural needs. Staff recruitment, retention and training must reflect local populations.

Liaison Psychiatry

Cultural factors are particularly important for patients being seen in consultation liaison services. As mentioned earlier, they may be presenting psychological distress with physical symptoms. This may lead to unnecessary and expensive investigations and interventions, creating further distress for the patient. It is also important that the members of the multidisciplinary team are trained in cultural competence. Patients from many countries and settings may present with somatisation or conversion disorders. These will require careful assessment and management. Comorbidity between depression and medical conditions such as hypertension and diabetes is well recognised, and both conditions will need proper investigation and treatment, particularly if the patients are to be taken seriously. The culture of the physician and their team is likely to affect engagement with the patient and their carers. Chronic medical illnesses will bring their own challenges, and the consultation liaison psychiatrist will need to remain up to date with developments.

In comorbid conditions, like any other condition, families can play a major role and thus will require education as well as support. Psychiatrists need to be aware of culturally specific evidence of therapeutic interventions and ensure that there are individually tailored.

Table 17.10 Culturally competent history taking in addictions-related care

Do you feel you have a problem?
Do family members criticise your drinking or drug use/behaviour?
Did the family use alcohol or substances?
When did you start using. . .?
Did you experience any problems? If so, what were these?
What do you think has caused these?
How do you think you should manage these?
Are there people who will support you?

Addiction Psychiatry

Culture can play a significant role in the recognition and management of substance abuse. In many cultures, alcohol is prohibited, but illegal distillation can lead to its use and consequent problems. In countries where cannabis has been legalised, it is likely that the use will be higher with resulting complications. Socialisation varies across cultures, and knowledge about various psychoactive substances or alcohol will depend upon cultures. Pathogenic patterns will vary across cultures and within cultures. Addiction to the internet and social media are being described and recognised regularly. Any intervention will have to be culturally appropriate. Religion and spiritually can play an important role in contributing to the management of certain patients. Some key questions are illustrated in Table 17.10. These will also include exploring and understanding explanatory models that the patient and their carers carry. In addition, clear third-party information (collateral) can help establish diagnosis. A distinction would need to be made between normative and deviant use of alcohol and drugs.

Another challenge in assessing drug use is to ascertain whether there are ceremonial uses or secular ones. Group versus individual decisions can push an individual towards using drugs. In some cultures, children or adolescents will be introduced to alcohol as part of growing up, and these cultures tend to have lower rates of binge diving and alcoholism. Timely and careful exploration of cultures is essential in assessing alcohol and substance abuse.

Child and Adolescent Psychiatry

Nearly three-quarters of psychiatric disorders in adulthood start below the age of 24; hence, it is helpful to be aware of adolescence patterns across cultures. Cultures influence child development very strongly. Child development is not only physical but psychological, emotional and cognitive too. All these components will be influenced by culturally influenced dietary factors but external and environmental factors too. Genetic and hereditary factors will influence physical growth. Other cultural factors can lead to the development of identity and the world view. Different gender roles and gender role expectations will be significant in the development of identity in many cultures. Rituals undertaken at puberty will be of importance in some cultures and will thus carry important meanings. As mentioned earlier, in feminine cultures, both parents play an equal role in childcare. However, child neglect and abuse can be seen across culture – its prevalence may vary. In some cultures, children are worshipped, but neglect and abuse still occur. Neglect can be both physical and emotional. Rates of various psychiatric disorders such as eating disorders vary. These conditions are rare in traditional societies, but these are beginning to change as cultures are changing. Transfer of care from child and adolescent services to adult services will need to be done very carefully.

Cultural sensitivity is a must when addressing child-rearing patterns and the upbringing of a child. In addition, many cultures are hierarchical as far as children and their roles are concerned. Similarly, schooling and the role and responsibility of teachers will be important factors in working with schools and parents. Furthermore, the expectations from a child regarding their future careers and marks of success will vary across cultures. Often, migrant parents will want their children to achieve more, and this may put an inordinate amount of pressure on them. Teachers may be given extraordinary powers and responsibilities, and children will be expected to follow these teachers. Working with the family is important and can be tricky. Parents may feel extraordinary pressure if the child has a mental illness, and emotions of guilt and shame will be important to manage. Subtle pressures and the roles of fathers and mothers may need to be navigated very carefully. Access and availability of services should be prioritised. In these settings, mediators can be extremely helpful in educating both the community and the team.

Intellectual Disability

Adults with intellectual disability are likely to have been diagnosed in childhood, but cultural meanings and causes and perceptions of intellectual disability will be important and need to be explored carefully. In addition, sensitivity is required to explore consanguineous marriages. Daily living skills, educational needs and clinical needs will have to be explored very carefully. Similarly, interventions will need to be carefully designed. Information about conditions may need to be presented in specific languages.

Culture, Ageing and Old Age Psychiatry

Cultures have varying attitudes towards normal ageing and older individuals. In many cultures, families are expected to look after the older adults as they are seen as important sources of wisdom. Ageing can be seen as chronological age. In some low-income countries, people can retire at 55 or 58, and their role in the family may well change. For migrants, it is possible that some older adults may be secondary migrants and may find it difficult to acculturate and settle, particularly as they may have difficulties in forming friendships and may also face problems related to things such as diet and language. This may contribute to social isolation and loneliness. In addition, there may be tensions and cultural conflict in the family where the younger generation may already be better settled in the new culture.

In clinical assessment, it is important to put the individual in their cultural context and not see their behaviour as automatically abnormal. Family can and should be encouraged to be part of therapeutic engagement. Intergenerational and cultural issues must be ascertained. Cognitive assessments must be conducted in a careful and culturally sensitive manner. Norms may need to be adjusted. Similarly, handover from adult services to old age services may create difficulties.

Forensic Psychiatry

For forensic psychiatrists, it is crucial to be aware of subtle cultural variations that can define normality or deviance. Between medium and high secure units for admission, a careful assessment of behaviour and abnormality needs to be carried out. Stigma associated with involuntary hospitalisation and compulsory treatment can be really problematic and needs careful decision-making. An awareness of the legal system is a must. Cultural evaluation and sensitive interpretation after recognising abnormal behaviour is also a must. Cultural and ethical expectations must be explored, and the clinician must seek information if they are not familiar with cultural nuances.

Folk Explanations

No matter which culture people belong to, folk explanations of distress and stress may exist and vary. For a considerable period in the history of humankind, mental illnesses were seen as the purview of religious institutions. Folk explanations are offered by religious and community leaders and need to be taken into account. These explanations are not simple but can be both descriptive and logical in their own way.[108] These explanations are both cultural and personal and can include supernatural explanations – for example, object intrusion, soul loss, spirit intrusion and spirit possession, breach of taboos and sorcery, among others. Distress can be attributed to the lack of worship of ancestors, possession by ghosts or jinns or casting an evil eye – all those supernatural and natural explanations.[57,94] Other folk explanations include natural explanations such as the disharmony of natural elements, incompatibility with natural principles, philosophical explanations and noxious factors in the environment.

Folk explanations are likely to change as cultures change in response to a number of factors. The role culture plays in cognitive and social development through child rearing and schooling cannot be underestimated. The customs of a particular culture beliefs – whether they are religious or cultural – will influence behaviour and functioning within that culture and society. Individual psychology will also be influenced by cultural values, norms and expectations. However, that does not mean that all members of one culture will behave exactly in the same way. Taboos, customs, rituals and etiquette will all influence various rites of passage and personal development.

Collective Mental Disorders

Collective mental disorders can be defined as those in which more than one or a group of individuals share psychopathology. These occur in a contagious way in a short period of time in a particular social setting in an epidemic fashion.[57] This epidemic may start from one individual and involve dozens or hundreds of vulnerable individuals. This transmission or communication is closely related to social atmosphere. Often these may lead to mass hysteria, panic attacks, group or mass suicide, folié à famille or Koro. Koro is an interesting syndrome where men are frightened that their penis is shrinking, and they may tie weights to stop that from happening. Often seen in South-East Asia, it can be related to social tensions. Similarly, mass hysteria has been shown to affect large groups of people around the globe as have collective delusions. Mass panic reactions are not unknown. In the olden days in Northern India, women may commit jauhar (to avoid falling into enemy hands) by jumping into wells or fire. Various other group suicides have been described from around the world. In a 100-year period (1872–1972) Sirois identified 78 episodes of epidemic hysteria overall, more often in Malaysia. The underlying explanations may include group identity, individual psychological vulnerability, social isolation and crowd response.[109] More recently, some have suggested that the distressing symptoms experienced by American diplomats based in Havana (hearing a noise prior to cognitive challenges including memory problems), initially thought to be due to an 'acoustic weapon', may be the result of mass psychogenic illness.[110] It will be interesting to see how the social media and resulting inter-connectedness can affect the development and presentation of these collective mental disorders, especially as cultures change due to globalisation.

Traditional Folk Medicines

In many cultures – due to a number of factors like increased availability and easy access, affordability and the use of a whole person approach – often individuals will seek help from traditional medicine practitioners. Very often, the models in these do not follow mind-body dualism, and they also take into account factors such as environment, diet and seasons; they are therefore closer to folk explanations and thus more acceptable. Ayurvedic medicine classifies ill health as physical, mental and accidental.[111] The Chinese system sees causes of ill health to be external, internal or others. The concept of yin and yang focusses on the balance between positive and negative forces that are complementary to each other, and these are fairly understandable. Their theory of five elements proposes that everything in the universe is one of five categorical elements: wood, water, fire, earth and metal.[57] These are interlinked, thereby requiring not only an interconnecting approach but also a holistic one.

Islamic-Greek medicine follows humoural theory. In these types, it is observed that ill health occurs as a result of the imbalance between humours, and external and internal factors play a role. These are illustrative examples of theories from traditional medicine. Clinicians, therefore, need to be aware of potential interactions leading to potential side effects, and these combined with dietary taboos can create additional difficulties in therapeutic engagement. Medical systems outside formally recognised systems are seen as traditional, though there is official recognition of the Chinese system in China and Ayurveda in India. It is entirely possible that migrants from these cultures will have these models in their mind when seeking help.

Culture Bound Syndromes

Various terms such as 'culture bound syndromes'[112] or 'culture specific disorders'[113] have been used in the past and, to a certain extent, continue to be used to describe psychiatric syndromes that are defined as being confined in certain cultures and localities. Seen as an expression of aberrant behaviour, these conditions express patterns of distress often seen as exotic and unusual, especially by the outsiders. These may not fit into traditional psychiatric diagnosis categories. The original concept put forward by Yap suggested using psychological processes, which could be seen as reactive and severe.[112] Vulnerable individuals expressed abnormal reactions in response to unmanageable stress and distress. Yap argued that these were neither exotic nor rare, and individual cultures formed these variations that did not fit in the Western classificatory systems. In the early years after recognition of culture bound syndromes, the numbers were over 100, but in the most recent edition of DSM-5, the number has gone down to nine. These are now called cultural syndromes. Also recognised as cultural idioms of distress and cultural explanations or perceived causes, these syndromes and their presentation may have changed as a result of globalisation and perhaps cultural transitions.

Cultural syndromes should be seen as such if these are well defined discrete syndromes.[114] Gaw notes that distress is labelled as such in the cultural context and points out that obesity, type A behaviour patterns, petism, shoplifting and anorexia nervosa should be seen as culture bound syndromes of the West.[115–117] Some of these disorders are now being seen in clinical settings in many low- and middle-income countries.

The symptoms and aberrant behaviour seen in *amok* in the Malayan peninsula can express itself in indiscriminate shootings in the USA and yet not be recognised as such. Similarly, semen loss anxiety (*dhat*), although commonly reported from the Indian subcontinent, existed in Britain and the USA in the eighteenth and nineteenth centuries, and various treatments were offered and advertised.[118,119]

Assessment of culture bound syndromes should include:

- Thorough repeated mental state assessments with corroborative information
- Check if these are culturally expected and accepted idioms of distress
- Meaning of symptoms to the individual, their family and others may not necessarily meet diagnostic criteria

We have chosen to use 'culture bound syndromes' as this term is commonly understood, but perhaps a better or more specific term should be 'culturally influenced syndromes'. Tseng and McDermott recommend using culture-related specific psychiatric syndromes.[120] DSM-5[13] recommends that concepts of syndromes, idioms and explanations are more relevant to clinical practice than the old concepts of culture bound syndromes. In these syndromes included in DSM-5, anxiety lies at the core of the symptoms and presentation. It is worth bearing in mind that even the symptoms of anxiety and its presentations will vary across cultures, and normal responses to stress should not be medicalised or pathologised. Further descriptions and details of various syndromes are beyond the scope of this chapter; see associated references.[118,121]

Sexual Variations

Although it is well recognised that LGBTQA+ individuals exist across all cultures, attitudes to sexual minorities and sexual variations vary tremendously. In nearly one-third of countries around the world, same-sex behaviour is illegal and, in a portion, punishable by the death penalty. Bullough divided cultures into sex positive and sex negative cultures.[122] Sex positive cultures are those where the purpose of sexual activity is for fun whereas sex negative cultures are those where the main purpose of sex is procreation only. Religious attitudes will influence these attitudes and expectations. Curative therapies are recommended in many settings. Often, sexual orientation and sexual behaviour get confused. Depending upon the availability of same-sex partners in boarding schools and prisons, heterosexual men may participate in same-sex behaviour. Attitudes to gender also vary across cultures as do attitudes to disability and chronic physical or psychiatric conditions.

Attitudes to individuals with mental illness will vary across cultures, leading to stigma and subsequent discrimination, which may get embedded in law. Cultural attitudes are likely to influence legal systems. It is because the definition of deviancy and deviant behaviour will be due to these attitudes and practices, as well as social expectations. Socioeconomic and educational status may provide a degree of support and protection in many cultures.

Cultural Competence

Cultural competence is defined as an ability to be cognisant of and understand and use cultural factors of the patients, their families and carers to engage them in any therapeutic intervention. It can be argued that cultural competence is, at heart, good clinical practice, which should be used by clinicians to understand social, cultural, religious factors and attitudes and behaviours. This also means that clinicians are comfortable with understanding explanatory models that the patient has about their illness as well as the carers and family's expectations.

The clinicians need to be culturally competent, but as they function and practice within the institutions, these must be culturally competent too. Part of being culturally competent is being aware of one's own culture – its strengths and weaknesses – as well as that of the patients being seen. Cultural competence is to ensure that the clinician is aware of the patient's culture and is skilled at not disrespecting cultural values and nuances even if they appear to be odd. Such an awareness is the key to better patient engagement as well as working with the patient's family and other informal carers. Being aware of these cultural factors can be particularly helpful as they will play an important role in defining normalcy and deviance, which are particularly important factors in clinical psychiatry.

Two previous models have been described and are worth noting. These are LEARN (listen, explain, acknowledge, recommend treatment and negotiate)[123] and CRASH (consider culture, respect, assess differences, sensitivity and humility).[124] In any therapeutic encounter, it is worth remembering that cultural influences may not be entirely apparent or clear at the initial encounter. Individual components and micro-identities will play a major role in therapeutic engagement as will cultural knowledge and attitudes towards others. Cultural competence can help therapeutic engagement and subsequent alliance.

In DSM-5,[13] cultural formulation is defined as bringing together aspects of history, psychopathology and investigations within the context of culture as well as interventions. According to Gaw, this includes the cultural identity of the individual, cultural explanations of the individual's illness, psychosocial and cultural environments, and culturally embedded elements in the therapeutic encounter.[114] The aim of cultural formulation is for the clinician to use cultural analysis as an ongoing process in the therapeutic encounter. The cultural background of the individual, their cultural context of expression of symptoms, the influence of the cultural differences (if any) on the therapeutic encounter, all of these form part of cultural formulation. Using the associate interview technique, where the individual in distress is free to speak with limited subtle directions by the interviewee and collaborative third-party interviews, can allow for cultural influences of distress to be ascertained.[95]

Cultural formulation will consist of the cultural definition of the distress or problem, cultural perceptions of cause context and support, and cultural factors defining self-coping and help-seeking. Cultural identity will include gender, race, ethnicity, heritage, culture of origin, languages spoken and places where the identities are used (e.g. home, work, leisure), sexual orientation, religion, education, employment (places and type of work), migration, acculturation, as well as degree of comfort in new culture and in our culture.

DSM-5 recommends that cultural concepts should be carefully applied to reaching the diagnosis.[13]

There are several culture-related principles that need to be considered in the context of therapeutic interactions in mental health:

- Cultural competence is good clinical practice, where the clinician sees each patient in the context of the patient's culture as well as their own cultural values and prejudices. Often, it is erroneously assumed that only minority patients have cultures
- Cultural sensitivity
- Cultural knowledge
- Cultural empathy
- Culturally appropriate interactions
- Cultural awareness (own)
- Cultural formulation: cultural identity of the individual and their beliefs and values
- Symptoms in cultural context
- Relationship with the environment
- Reinforcing factors
- Distress due to the problems and its explanations
- Shared understanding of the problems
- Shared plan for addressing the problems
- The nature of the interaction

Psychopharmacology and Culture

Medication is often a key part of the therapeutic encounter, and it can be prescribed and, in many countries and cultures, easily available over the counter without prescription. The explanatory models of the patients and their carers will seek medication either by itself or as part of the overall intervention. The role of the medication, its impact and side effects will all be affected by the patient's explanatory models and biological differences. The use of medication and especially its acceptance will depend upon a number of cultural factors. In cultures where the concept of hot and cold substances exists, the patients will inevitably ask of the prescriber whether the medication is hot or cold and whether it is to be taken with hot or cold liquids and what dietary things are to be avoided. For factors to explore prior to prescribing medications, see Table 17.11.

Table 17.11 Factors to explore prior to prescribing medication

Check weight, BMI, ethnicity-diet-taboo and religious taboo
Check medication history, especially complementary alcohol, nicotine, caffeine and other substance intake

Many drug trials are conducted in different cultures, and recommended doses may not be applicable to other cultures. Cultures also have varying attitudes to the colour and size of pills. Some cultures prefer big tablets, whereas others prefer a small size as these are considered to have more concentrated compound and hence be more potent.[118] In some cultures, liquid medication is preferred whereas, in others, injections are seen as more potent. In many cultures, patients will continue to take complementary and alternative medicines at the same time, and these may thus increase the likelihood of drug interaction and likely to stop prescribed medication. Nicotine, alcohol, food additives and pollution are some of the other factors that may affect the pharmacodynamics and pharmacokinetics of drugs.

The pharmacodynamics of a drug (i.e. its effect on an organism) affect the neurotransmitters and the neurophysiological and psychosocial effects of drugs, which are strongly influenced by enzymes.

Pharmacokinetics is the effect of the absorption and metabolism of a drug on a biological organism. Thus, some individuals may be fast metabolisers and others slow ones, and the same dose of medication may produce different responses and varying side effects. The variation in enzymes has been reported across ethnic groups. Thus, dietary patterns will affect the metabolism of drugs and consequently their effect.

Doses of antipsychotics, antidepressants and mood stabilisers should be carefully titrated according to ethnicity. Substances and spices like black pepper, nutmeg, mace, cinnamon, turmeric, white pepper and sage have been shown to cause inhibition of various enzymes, affecting metabolism and leading to increased side effects.[125] While implementing therapeutic medication, clinicians must work with the patients, their carers and families and provide as detailed information in as simple language as possible (see Table 17.12). Written information in relevant languages can be very helpful. Regular monitoring and follow-up and the impact of cultural and physical factors on the success of medication and side effects of the medication should be considered on a regular basis (see Table 17.13).

Table 17.12 Factors to consider when prescribing

Start with lowest dose
Monitor side effects
Adjust doses carefully
Give verbal and written information to patient/carers/family

Table 17.13 Factors to consider after prescribing

Regular monitoring levels
Regular monitoring of side effects
Teach staff and family to identify side effects and compliance
Check serum levels
Check changes in diet/habits

Psychological Therapies and Culture

Psychotherapy is a mode of intervention applying various principles of human relationships, which are used to bring about a permanent or sustained change in an individual's cognitions, their inner world and functioning. The therapist attempts to understand and explore the patient's inner world and works with the patient to explore cognitions and conscious and unconscious minds, depending upon the type of therapy. The principle is to bring about the change in functioning – an outcome generally agreed in the early stages of intervention. Psychotherapy can be supportive, re-educative and constructive.[126] A majority of psychotherapies tend to be ego-based, which may be problematic for their use across cultures, especially in collectivist or sociocentric cultures. Folk therapies use restructuring of meaning by the patient in order to control their emotional distress and alleviate symptom.[127] Frank described expectant faith effect, which is the perceived effectiveness of the healer's approach by that of the patient.[128] Such an expectation can lead to the formation of a charismatic relationship between the patient and the healer. It may be that such an impact results from transference. Again, it can be argued that such approaches are more effective in traditional or sociocentric approaches. Such expectant faith effect uses healing symbols, and the healer in general is more in tune with the patient.

Medication may be seen as a symbol in Western or allopathic therapeutic encounters. Universal elements of psychotherapy include the joint clarification of problems with exploration of cultural factors and an agreement to work on the intervention together.[120] Cultural transference and cultural counter transference play an important role. Understanding and exploring unconscious bias on the part of both the patient and the therapist is a must. Therapeutic outcomes will reduce symptom severity and improve social functioning. The outcome of therapy needs to be agreed upon and checked on follow-up.

The question and importance of race in psychotherapy may be raised by the patient. The therapist must be sensitive to it and respond accordingly. The impact of race must be explored and differentiated from mental state assessment.

Specific Therapies: Behaviour therapy may work better in certain instances with individuals from certain ethnic minority groups. Cognitive behaviour therapy can work if the therapist is aware of differences in the cultural cognitive development. Similarly, supportive therapies may depend upon diagnosis and ethnicity. Involving family members and carers may require additional careful exploration of knowledge, attitudes and behaviour.

Couple, marital and family therapies with patients from minority ethnic groups have different sets of challenges. In mixed ethnicity relationships, there may be challenges related to minority/majority cultures and degrees of acculturation. Previous and past experiences and states of marriage – whether arranged or not – will be important to explore. Universal elements of therapy will include identifying the problem and exploring precipitating and perpetuating causes as well as explanatory models. It is helpful to clarify the expectations of therapy and the understanding of the processes.

Clinicians and therapists must be aware of their own prejudices, strengths and weaknesses, as well as individual and cultural transference and counter transference and the likelihood of idealising one or other cultures. The therapist must not be colour blind in assuming that all minority patients are the same as the majority. They must not place blame on race and be aware of cultural paradigms as well as nuances.

Family status and roles and responsibilities of individual members must be explored. Gender roles and gender role expectations within the family must be enquired into carefully. Family members can provide information about the patient and culture but also work as co-therapists and support. For minority individuals and families, acculturation levels must be ascertained.

Culture and Social Determinants

As mentioned earlier, all cultures involve shared meaning, attitudes towards certain things which then go on to influence behaviours, and ways of identifying abnormality and deviance. The attitudes in a culture may focus on the advancement of the group or that of the individual at a cost to the larger society. Cultural attitudes also vary towards education and occupations. Migrants, be they political or economic (asylum seekers and refugees), carry their cultures and cultural capital with them. Voluntary migration is the common type, but involuntary migration is increasing in response to changing geopolitical and social determinants. This is likely to be exacerbated with climate-related changes around the world. Non-European migrants have played significant roles in many cultures and transformed their economies. Sowell defines cultural receptivity of people to new technologies and new ideas.[43] He argues that the diffusion of technology is not simply a process of making information available but more than simply transferring technology to other hands. People have to be willing to learn and accept new technologies and utilise them.

Culture itself is a major factor in the acceptance and receptivity of individuals and their behaviours, especially those of migrants. The recent rise in xenophobic racism and nationalism in many countries blames migrants as the 'other', particularly abusing them by saying that they take jobs away from the local people and forgetting that there are no fixed numbers of jobs. These jobs expand and retract depending upon the state of economy. In many economic systems, migrants tend to pay in more with taxes than they take. The social consequences of facing another culture need further detailed teasing out. Families of migrants, possibly in the first or second generation, are likely to be perhaps more clannish and seen as such and also likely to be seen as cliquish and sticking together. The younger generations may choose to develop relationships with the larger society. Cultural differences between groups are also reflected in their roles in different jobs and professions. These variations then go on to lead to pay gaps and attainment gaps, with race often the most common factor used to make these distinctions. It is also likely that different migrant cultural groups could possibly differ in their skill-sets and behaviours. In racially and culturally heterogenous societies, employment prospects for migrant groups and individuals vary, not only with their own skills and work patterns, but also with their acceptability to co-workers, customers and employers.[43] Often, migrants may start in menial jobs, and they or their children then work their way up, although that is not always universal. Discrimination may play another role in obstructing promotion and achievement. Cheap homebased labour has given way to a lot of what is seen as 'dross' work. The homebased labour has been exported to low-income countries as a result of globalisation. Poor employment is likely to lead to poor housing, overcrowding and lack of green spaces, creating poor social determinants and subsequently poor mental health.

Conclusion

The role culture plays in the development, presentation and outcome of various psychiatric disorders is often ignored in clinical practice as well as during medical training. Clinicians need to be cognisant of the impact culture can have on therapeutic engagement and therapeutic alliance. Therefore, the services and the clinicians need to be flexible, sensitive and appropriate (in cultural context) in engaging with patients and their carers as well as offering appropriate therapeutic interventions. Explanatory models and perspectives from the patient, their family or carers may well vary from that of the clinician, but that does not make it less valid. Hence, the clinicians need to be open-minded and culturally sensitive. Such a variation in the explanatory models also does not diminish the patient's need for care or support for autonomy in decision-making. Cultural competence means that the patient is at the core of the therapeutic interaction, and their experiences must be seen in the context of their culture and the health care professional's own culture and unconscious biases but also prejudices. Due acknowledgement of beliefs and social processes can facilitate engagement and improve outcomes. With recognition of community mental health interventions and consequent services, it is essential that curricula and training include cultural psychiatry and that its components and cultural competence are seen as an integral part. Mental health services need to be culturally appropriate and sensitive and accessible to ensure that the mental health needs of all individuals are met in a non-discriminatory and equitable manner.

References

1. Tylor EB. *Primitive Culture: Researches into the Development of Mythology, Philosophy, Religion, Art and Custom.* London: J. Murray; 1871.
2. US Department of Health and Human Services. *Mental Health: Culture, Race, and Ethnicity.* Rockville, MD: US Department of Health and Human Services. Substance Abuse and Mental Health Services Administration, Center for Mental Health Services, National Institutes of Health, National Institute of Mental Health; 2001.
3. US Department of Health and Human Services. *Mental Health: A Report of the Surgeon General.* Washington, DC: Department of Health and Human Services, US Public Health Service; 1999.
4. Geertz C. *The Interpretation of Cultures.* New York: Basic Books; 1973.
5. Kleinman A. How is culture important for DSM-IV? In: Mezzich JE, Kleinman A, Fabrega Jr H, et al. (eds.) *Culture and Psychiatric Diagnosis: A DSM-IV Perspective.* Washington, DC: American Psychiatric Press; 1996: 15–25.
6. Haviland WA. *Cultural Anthropology.* Chicago: Holt, Rinehart and Winston; 1990.
7. Kirmayer LJ. Cultural psychiatry in historical perspective. In: Bhugra D, Bhui K (eds.) *Textbook of Cultural Psychiatry.* 2nd ed. Cambridge: Cambridge University Press; 2018: 1–17.
8. Kuper A. *Culture: The Anthropologists' Account.* Harvard, MA: Harvard University Press; 2000.
9. Boas F. *Race, Language, and Culture.* Chicago: University of Chicago Press; 1982.
10. Kroeber AL, Kluckhohn C. *Culture: A Critical Review of Concepts and Definitions. Papers. Peabody Museum of Archaeology & Ethnology.* Harvard, MA: Harvard University; 1952.
11. Linton R. *The Cultural Background of Personality.* New York: Appleton-Century-Crofts; 1945.
12. Hofstede G. National cultures and corporate cultures. In: Samovar LA, Porter RE (eds.) *Communication Between Cultures.* Belmont, CA: Wadsworth 1984;51: 51.

13. APA. *Diagnostic and Statistical Manual of Mental Disorders: DSM-5™*, 5th ed. Arlington, VA: American Psychiatric Publishing, Inc.; 2013.
14. Hofstede G. *Culture's Consequences: Comparing Values, Behaviors, Institutions and Organizations Across Nations*. London: Sage Publications; 2001.
15. Hofstede G. *Culture's Consequences: International Differences in Work-Related Values*. London: Sage Publications; 1980.
16. Matsuura K. Universal declaration on cultural diversity. *Diogenes* 2005;52 (1):141–5.
17. Eshun S, Gurung A. Introduction to culture and psychopathology. In: Gurung RA, Eshun S (eds.) *Culture and Mental Health: Sociocultural Influences, Theory, and Practice*. New Jersey: Wiley and Sons 2009: 1–17.
18. Landrine H, Klonoff EA. The schedule of racist events: a measure of racial discrimination and a study of its negative physical and mental health consequences. *Journal of Black Psychology* 1996;22(2):144–68.
19. Odegaard O. Emigration and insanity: a study of mental disease in Norwegian born population in Minnesota. *Acta Psychiatrica et Neurologica Scandinavica* 1932;4(Suppl):1–206.
20. World Health Organization. *Schizophrenia: An International Follow-up Study*. Chichester: Wiley; 1979.
21. Jablensky A, Sartorius N, Ernberg G, et al. Schizophrenia: manifestations, incidence and course in different cultures. A World Health Organization Ten-Country Study. *Psychological Medicine Monograph Supplement* 1992;20:1–97.
22. von Bertalanffy L. *General Systems Theory: Foundations, Developments, Applications*, revised ed. New York, NY: George Braziller, Inc; 1968.
23. Boulding KE. General systems theory – the skeleton of science. *Management Science* 1956;2(3):197–208.
24. Hofstede GH, Hofstede G, Arrindell WA, et al. *Masculinity and Femininity: The Taboo Dimension of National Cultures*. London: Sage; 1998.
25. Hofstede G. *Geert Hofstede: culture's consequences* (abridged edition) 1984, Beverly Hills, London and New Delhi: Sage. 325 pages. *Organization Studies* 1984;5(4):96.
26. Pelto PJ. The differences between 'tight' and 'loose' societies. *Trans-action* 1968;5(5):37–40.
27. Harrington JR, Gelfand MJ. Tightness–looseness across the 50 united states. *Proceedings of the National Academy of Sciences* 2014;111(22):7990–95.
28. Gelfand MJ, Raver JL, Nishii L, et al. Differences between tight and loose cultures: a 33-nation study. *Science* 2011;332(6033):1100–4.
29. Gelfand MJ, Jackson JC, Pan X, et al. The relationship between cultural tightness–looseness and COVID-19 cases and deaths: a global analysis. *The Lancet Planetary Health* 2021;5(3): e135–e44.
30. Lewis R. *When Cultures Collide: Leading Across Cultures*: London: John Murray Press; 2018.
31. Hofstede G, Pedersen P, Hofstede G. *Exploring Culture: Exercises, Stories and Synthetic Cultures*. Yarmouth, ME: Intercultural Press; 2002.
32. Hsu FL. Kinship and ways of life: an exploration. In: Hsu FL (ed.) *Psychological Anthropology*. Cambridge: Schenkman; 1972: 509–72.
33. Birren JE, Renner VJ. Research on the psychology of aging: principles and experimentation. In: Birren JE, Schaie KW (eds.) *Handbook of the Psychology of Aging* 1977: 1.
34. Bengtson VL, Kasschau PL, Ragan PK. The impact of social structure on aging individuals. In: Birren JE, Schaie KW (eds.) *Handbook of the Psychology of Aging* 1977: 327–53.
35. Jackson JJ. Aged Negroes: their cultural departures from statistical stereotypes and rural-urban differences. *The Gerontologist* 1970;10(2):140–5.
36. Opoku KA. African perspectives on death and dying. In: Berger A, Badham P, Kutscher H, et al. (eds.) *Perspectives on Death and Dying*. Philadelphia: The Charles Press Publishers; 1989: 14–23.
37. Bourdieu P. The forms of capital. In: Richardson JG (ed.) *Handbook of Theory and Research for the Sociology of Education*. Westport, CT: Greenwood; 1986: 241–58.
38. Bourdieu P, Nice R. The production of belief: contribution to an economy of symbolic goods. *Media, Culture & Society* 1980;2(3):261–93.
39. Bhugra D, Watson C, Ventriglio A. Migration, cultural capital and acculturation. *International Review of Psychiatry* 2021;33(1–2):126–31.
40. Bhugra D. *Culture and Self-harm: Attempted Suicide in South Asians in London*. London: Psychology Press; 2004.
41. World Health Organization. *Lexicon of Cross-cultural Terms in Mental Health*. Geneva: World Health Organization, 1997.
42. Bethencourt F. *Racisms: From the Crusades to the Twentieth Century*. Princeton: Princeton University Press; 2014.
43. Sowell T. Race and culture: a world view. *National Interest* 1994;38:97–100.
44. Thompson CE, Carter RT. *Racial Identity Theory: Applications to Individual, Group, and Organizational Interventions*. Mahwah, NJ: Lawrence Erlbaum Associates Publishers; 1997.
45. Omi M, Winant H. *Racial Formation in the United States. From the Sixties to the Nineties*. New York: Routledge, 1986.
46. Carter RT. *The Influence of Race and Racial Identity in Psychotherapy: Toward a Racially Inclusive Model*. Oxford: John Wiley & Sons; 1995.
47. Sternberg RJ, Grigorenko EL, Kidd KK. *Intelligence, Race, and Genetics*. Washington, DC: American Psychological Association; 2005.
48. Spickard PR. The illogic of American racial categories. In: Root MPP (ed.) *Racially Mixed People in America*. Newbury Park, CA: Sage; 1992: 12–23.
49. Thomas A, Sillen S. *Racism and Psychiatry*. Toronto: Ontario Citadel Press; 1972.
50. Hays PA. *Addressing Cultural Complexities in Practice*. Washington, DC: American Psychological Association; 2008.
51. Smedley A, Smedley BD. Race as biology is fiction, racism as a social problem is real: anthropological and historical perspectives on the social construction of race. *American Psychologist* 2005;60(1):16.
52. Helms JE. *Black and White Racial Identity: Theory, Research, and Practice*. Westport, CT: Greenwood Press; 1990.
53. Cohen P. Its racism what dunnit: hidden narratives in theories of racism. In: Donald J, Rattansi A (eds.) *Race,*

Culture and Difference. London: Sage; 1992: 62–100.

54. Rattansi A. Changing the subject? Racism, culture and education. *Race, Culture and Difference* 1992;1:11–48.
55. Hoebel EA. Religion and myth: symbolic ideology. In: Hoebel EA (ed.) *Anthropology: The Study of Man*, 4th ed. New York: McGraw-Hill; 1972: 571.
56. American Anthropological Association. AAA statement on race. *American Anthropologist* 1998;100(3):712–13.
57. Tseng W-S. *Clinician's Guide to Cultural Psychiatry*. Cambridge, MA: Academic Press; 2003.
58. Pinderhughes EB. Teaching empathy: ethnicity, race and power at the cross-cultural treatment interface. *American Journal of Social Psychiatry* 1984;4 (1):5–12.
59. Thomas CS, Comer JP. Racism and mental health services. In: Willie C, Kramer B, Brown B (eds.) *Racism and Mental Health*. Pittsburgh, PA: University of Pittsburgh; 1973: 165–84.
60. Allport GW, Clark K, Pettigrew T. *The Nature of Prejudice*. Reading, MA: Addison-Wesley; 1954.
61. Kerner C. *The Kerner Report: National Advisory Commission on Civil Disorders Report*. Princeton: Princeton University Press; 1969.
62. Pettigrew TF. Racism and the mental health of white Americans: a social psychological view. In: Willie C, Kramer B, Brown B (eds.) *Racism and Mental Health*. Pittsburgh, PA: University of Pittsburgh; 1973: 269–98.
63. Frederickson G. M. *2002–Racism: A Short History*. Princeton, NJ: Princeton University Press, 1998.
64. Bhugra D, Ayonrinde O, Butler G, et al. A randomised controlled trial of assertive outreach vs. treatment as usual for black people with severe mental illness. *Epidemiology and Psychiatric Sciences* 2011;20(1):83–9.
65. Harré R. *Social Being: A Theory for Social Psychology*. Lanham, MD: Rowman and Littlefield; 1980.
66. Guala F. *Understanding Institutions*. Princeton, NJ: Princeton University Press; 2016.
67. Bhui K, Bhugra D. Racism in psychiatry: paradigm lost – paradigm regained. *International Review of Psychiatry* 1999;11(2–3):236–43.
68. Bhugra D, Ayonrinde O. Racism, racial life events and mental ill health. *Advances in Psychiatric Treatment* 2001;7(5):343–49.
69. Littlewood R, Lipsedge M. Psychiatric illness among British Afro-Caribbeans. *BMJ: British Medical Journal* 1988;297 (6641):135.
70. Perera R, Owens D, Johnstone E. Disabilities and circumstances of schizophrenic patients – a follow-up study. Ethnic aspects. A Comparison of three matched groups. *The British Journal of Psychiatry. Supplement* 1991 (13):40–2, 44.
71. Jackson JS, Brown TN, Williams DR, et al. Racism and the physical and mental health status of African Americans: a thirteen year national panel study. *Ethnicity & Disease* 1996;6 (1–2):132–47.
72. Cochrane R. Race, prejudice and ethnic identity. In: Bhugra D, Cochrane R (eds.) *Psychiatry in Multicultural Britain*. London: Gaskell; 2001: 75–90.
73. McGoldrick M, Giordano J, Garcia-Preto N. *Ethnicity and Family Therapy*. New York: Guilford Press; 2005.
74. Phinney JS. When we talk about American ethnic groups, what do we mean? *American Psychologist* 1996;51 (9):918.
75. De Vos G. Ethnic pluralism: conflict and accommodation. In: DeVos G, Romanucci-Ross L (eds.) *Ethnic Identity: Cultural Continuities and Change*. Palo Alto, CA: Mayfield Publishing Company; 1975: 5–41.
76. Sam DL, Berry JW. *The Cambridge Handbook of Acculturation Psychology*. Cambridge: Cambridge University Press; 2006.
77. Redfield R, Linton R, Herskovits MJ. Memorandum for the study of acculturation. *American Anthropologist* 1936;38(1):149–52.
78. Berry JW. Acculturation as varieties of adaptation. In: Padilla AM (ed.) *Acculturation: Theory, Models and Some New Findings*. Boulder, CO: Westview Press; 1980: 25.
79. Phinney JS, Baldelomar OA. Identity development in multiple cultural contexts. In: Jensen LA (ed.) *Bridging Cultural and Developmental Approaches to Psychology: New Syntheses in Theory, Research, and Policy*. Oxford: Oxford University Press; 2011: 161–86.
80. Graves TD. Psychological acculturation in a tri-ethnic community. *Southwestern Journal of Anthropology* 1967;23 (4):337–50.
81. Camilleri C, Malewska-Peyre H. Socialization and identity strategies. *Handbook of Cross-cultural Psychology* 1997;2:41–67.
82. Bhugra RM, Julian Leff, Dinesh. Schizophrenia and African-Caribbeans: a conceptual model of aetiology. *International Review of Psychiatry* 1999;11(2–3):145–52.
83. Berry JW. Acculturation and adaptation in a new society. *International Migration* 1992;30(s1):69–85.
84. Dressler WW. *Culture and the Individual: Theory and Method of Cultural Consonance*. Abingdon: Routledge; 2017.
85. Dressler WW. Culture and the risk of disease. *British Medical Bulletin* 2004;69 (1):21–31.
86. Dressler WW, Balieiro MC, Dos Santos JE. Finding culture change in the second factor: stability and change in cultural consensus and residual agreement. *Field Methods* 2015;27(1):22–38.
87. Dressler WW, Balieiro MC, Dos Santos JE. The cultural construction of social support in Brazil: associations with health outcomes. *Culture, Medicine and Psychiatry* 1997;21(3):303–35.
88. Dressler WW, Balieiro MC, Santos JEd. Culture and psychological distress. *Paidéia (Ribeirão Preto)* 2002;12:5–18.
89. Dressler WW, Balieiro MC, Santos JED. Culture, socioeconomic status, and physical and mental health in Brazil. *Medical Anthropology Quarterly* 1998;12(4):424–46.
90. Dressler WW, Oths KS. Cultural determinants of health behavior. *Handbook of Health Behavior Research I: Personal and Social Determinants* 1997;1:359–78.
91. Dressler WW, Balieiro MC, de Araújo LF, et al. Culture as a mediator of gene-environment interaction: cultural consonance, childhood adversity, a 2A serotonin receptor polymorphism, and depression in urban Brazil. *Social Science & Medicine* 2016;161:109–17.
92. Eisenberg L. Disease and illness distinctions between professional and popular ideas of sickness. *Culture, Medicine and Psychiatry* 1977;1(1):9–23.

93. Tseng W-S, Streltzer J. *Culture and Psychotherapy: A Guide to Clinical Practice*. Washington, DC: American Psychiatric Pub; 2008.
94. Tseng W-S. *Handbook of Cultural Psychiatry*. Cambridge, MA: Academic Press; 2001.
95. Kleinman A. *Patients and Healers in the Context of Culture*. Berkeley, CA: University of California Press; 1980.
96. Weiss M, Somma D. Explanatory models in psychiatry. In: Bhugra D, Bhui K (eds.) *Textbook of Cultural Psychiatry*. Cambridge: Cambridge University Press; 2007: 127–40.
97. Sam DL, Moreira V. Revisiting the mutual embeddedness of culture and mental illness. *Online Readings in Psychology and Culture* 2012;10 (2):2307-0919.1078.
98. Castillo RJ. *Culture & Mental Illness: A Client-centered Approach*. Pacific Grove, CA: Thomson Brooks/Cole Publishing Co; 1997.
99. Kiev A. *Transcultural Psychiatry*. New York: Free Press; 1972.
100. Mistry H, Bhugra D, Chaleby K, et al. Veiled communication: is uncovering necessary for psychiatric assessment? *Transcultural Psychiatry* 2009;46 (4):642–50.
101. Tseng W-S, Streltzer J. *Culture and Psychopathology: A Guide to Clinical Assessment*. New York: Brunner/Mazel; 1997.
102. Lin K-M, Kleinman AM. Psychopathology and clinical course of schizophrenia: a cross-cultural perspective. *Schizophrenia Bulletin* 1988;14(4):55–67.
103. Lewis-Fernández R, Aggarwal NK, Bäärnhielm S, et al. Culture and psychiatric evaluation: operationalizing cultural formulation for DSM-5. *Psychiatry: Interpersonal and Biological Processes* 2014;77(2):130–54.
104. Caraballo A, Lee J, Lim R. Applying the DSM-5 outline for cultural formulation and the cultural formulation interview. In: Lim RF (ed.) *Clinical Manual of Cultural Psychiatry*. 2nd ed. Washington, DC: American Psychiatric Publishing; 2015: 43–76.
105. Andersen RM, Mullner RM, Cornelius LJ. Black-white differences in health status: methods or substance? *Milbank Quarterly* 1987;65(Suppl 1):72–99.
106. MacCarthy B, Craissati J. Ethnic differences in response to adversity. A community sample of Bangladeshis and their indigenous neighbours. *Social Psychiatry and Psychiatric Epidemiology* 1989;24(4):196–201.
107. Chen PC. Medical systems in Malaysia: cultural bases and differential use. *Social Science & Medicine* 1975;9(3):171–80.
108. Good BJ, Good M-JD. Toward a meaning-centered analysis of popular illness categories: 'fright illness' and 'heart distress' in Iran. In: Marsella AJ, White G (eds.) *Cultural Conceptions of Mental Health and Therapy*. New York: Springer; 1982: 141–66.
109. Kerckhoff AC, Back KW. Sociometric patterns in hysterical contagion. *Sociometry* 1965;28(1):2–15.
110. Baloh RW, Bartholomew RE. *Havana Syndrome: Mass Psychogenic Illness and the Real Story Behind the Embassy Mystery and Hysteria*. New York: Springer Nature; 2020.
111. Bhugra D. Psychiatry in ancient Indian texts: a review. *History of Psychiatry* 1992;3(10):167–86.
112. Yap PM. Classification of the culture-bound reactive syndromes. *Australian and New Zealand Journal of Psychiatry* 1967;1(4):172–9.
113. Jilek WG, Jilek-Aall L. Culture-specific mental disorders. In: Henn F, Sartorius N, Helmchen H, et al. (eds.) *Contemporary Psychiatry*. New York: Springer; 2001: 965–93.
114. Gaw A. *Concise Guide to Cross-cultural Psychiatry*. Washington, DC: American Psychiatric Press; 2001.
115. Littlewood R, Lipsedge M. Culture-bound syndromes. In: Granville-Grossman K (ed.) *Recent Advances in Clinical Psychiatry*. Edinburgh: Churchill Livingstone; 1985: 105–42.
116. Ritenbaugh C. Obesity as a culture-bound syndrome. *Culture, Medicine and Psychiatry* 1982;6(4):347–61.
117. Winzeler RL. *Latah in South-East Asia: The History and Ethnography of a Culture-Bound Syndrome*. Cambridge: Cambridge University Press; 1995.
118. Ventriglio A, Ayonrinde O, Bhugra D. Relevance of culture-bound syndromes in the 21st century. *Psychiatry and Clinical Neurosciences* 2016;70(1):3–6.
119. Sumathipala A, Siribaddana SH, Bhugra D. Culture-bound syndromes: the story of dhat syndrome. *The British Journal of Psychiatry* 2004;184(3):200–9.
120. Tseng W-S, McDermott JF. *Culture, Mind, and Therapy: An Introduction to Cultural Psychiatry*. New York: Brunner/Mazel; 1981.
121. Bhugra D, Bhui K. *Textbook of Cultural Psychiatry*. Cambridge: Cambridge University Press; 2018.
122. Bullough VL. *Sexual Variance in Society and History*. New Jersey: John Wiley & Sons; 1976.
123. Berlin EA, Fowkes Jr WC. A teaching framework for cross-cultural health care – application in family practice. *Western Journal of Medicine* 1983;139 (6):934.
124. Rust G, Kondwani K, Martinez R, et al. A crash-course in cultural competence. *Ethnicity & Disease* 2006;16(2 Suppl 3): S3–29.
125. Henderson D, Vincenzi B. Ethnopsychopharmacology. In: Lim RF (ed.) *Clinical Manual of Cultural Psychiatry*, 2nd ed. Arlington: American Psychiatric Publishing; 2015: 495–530.
126. Wolberg LR. *The Technique of Psychotherapy*. New York: Grune & Stratton; 1954.
127. Castillo RJ. Lessons from folk healing practices. In: Tseng WS, Streltzer J (eds.) *Culture and Psychotherapy: A Guide to Clinical Practice* Washington, DC: American Psychiatric Pub; 2001: 81–101.
128. Frank JD. The faith that heals. *The Johns Hopkins Medical Journal* 1975;137 (3):127–31.

Chapter

18 Psychiatry in Primary Care

Linda Gask and Safi Afghan

The Scope of Psychiatry in Primary Care

Unlike the corresponding chapter in the previous edition of this book, this version is titled psychiatry in 'primary care' not 'general practice'. However, we've retained 'psychiatry' rather than change to the broader term 'mental health'. That's because we will address not only how general practitioners (GPs) and other professionals in primary care manage those who form the majority, by far, of people with mental health problems in the community, but also the role that psychiatrists can play in working in collaboration with primary care.

Primary care is the local, universally available, essential, and – according to the World Health Organization (WHO) – '*first point of contact with the health system, based on practical, scientifically sound and socially acceptable methods and technology at a cost the community and country can afford*'.[1] In many – but not all – high-income countries, this is provided by a GP (or family doctor or primary care physician) working with a team, which in the United Kingdom, usually consists of practice nurses, health visitors, midwives, community nurses, new physician associates and other attached staff – often related to mental health (e.g. psychologists, counsellors) – alongside a team of administrative staff, not least the practice manager. Extensive international research has shown that when systems are organised around primary care, outcomes are better, with improved equity and lower costs.[2] However, the very person-centred model of care that a GP traditionally provides in the UK – with continuity of care, close relationships with family and depth of knowledge of a community – has been considerably challenged by developments in the last couple of decades.[3]

Primary care has assumed a considerable international importance for both the recognition and the treatment of mental health problems worldwide.[4] ***Primary care mental health*** has been a developing area of interest both within general practice and psychiatry since the middle of the last century, when Michael Shepherd at the Institute of Psychiatry General Practice Research Unit declared that '*The cardinal requirement for improvement of mental health services . . . is not a large expansion of and proliferation of psychiatric agencies, but rather a strengthening of the family doctor in his/her therapeutic role*'.[5] The interface between psychiatry and primary care became not only a focus for epidemiological research, but also a setting for innovative ways of providing mental health services in the community – developments that continue to this day (see later).

Epidemiology of Mental Illness in Primary Care

The Pathways to Care model, first described by Goldberg and Huxley in 1980,[6] provides a useful framework for understanding how the prevalence of mental illness in the community (particularly for common mental disorders such as anxiety and depression) is distributed, as well as how this changes according to the way that health care systems are organised (see Figure 18.1).

Level 1 refers to all psychiatric disorders in the population – data for this level are collected through large surveys of the population such as the UK Psychiatric Morbidity Surveys. Level 2 refers to all psychiatric disorders in the primary care setting, even if the GP has not diagnosed a disorder, and data here comes from surveys of those attending. To pass through filter 1, a person has to make the decision to consult the doctor. Filter 2 is governed by the GP's recognition and diagnosis, so level 3 is a 'conspicuous' or diagnosed psychiatric disorder. Filter 3 is governed by the GP's decision to refer to secondary care, and level 4 is the prevalence of morbidity in that setting (both inpatient and outpatient).

In health care systems where people can consult specialists directly – and the GP does not act as a gatekeeper – this will have an impact on data collected from 'secondary' care settings (which are, in effect, then primary). People with a psychotic disorder may also not enter services via their GP but rather through Emergency Departments or via the police. However, early intervention may still be flagged up through a GP visit or a family expressing concerns. The model is also complicated by the role increasingly played by the voluntary sector in providing mental health care in the community over recent years and self-referral to psychological therapy services with the aim of both reducing stigma and increasing access to care. The concept of 'candidacy'[7] clarifies how many underserved communities, such as people from ethnic minorities and older people, don't seek mental health care from their GP. They may be better served by the voluntary sector[8] with which joint working is essential. The 'decision to consult' (filter 1) may also be determined not only by the severity of symptoms but also by perceived stigma of mental illness and whether a person might consider themselves a 'candidate' for receiving care.

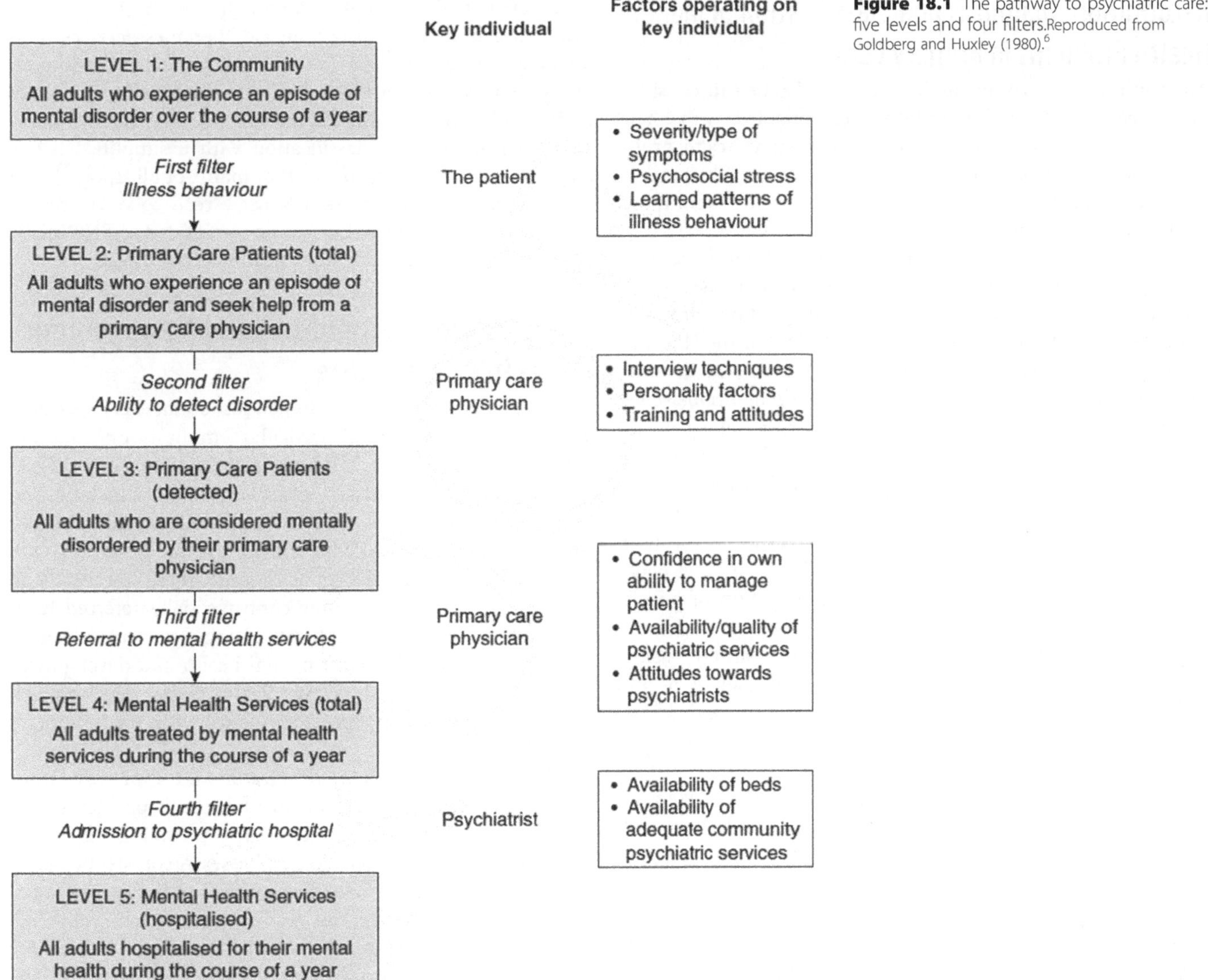

Figure 18.1 The pathway to psychiatric care: five levels and four filters. Reproduced from Goldberg and Huxley (1980).[6]

National prevalence figures make it possible to assess roughly how many people with mental illness might be identified on the average list size (2,000) of a GP in the UK.[9] In such a population, one would expect, at any one time, a GP to have about 76 people with depression, 14 people with a psychotic illness and around 26 people with dementia. There will also be approximately 132 people with generalised anxiety disorder (GAD), 88 patients screening positive for post traumatic stress disorder (PTSD), 128 patients who report self harming and a further 170 or so with milder degrees of depression and anxiety, not meeting the more specific diagnostic criteria. On an individual level, people with a diagnosis of schizophrenia and dementia may experience the greatest degree of disability. At the level of the community and in primary care, however, common mental health problems such as anxiety, depression (which commonly occur together) and substance misuse pose the greater challenge to public health.[10,11] These differing perspectives – from the outpatient clinic and the GP practice – can sometimes lead to conflict over the distribution of resources between psychiatrists, who work with people most disabled by mental illness, and GPs, burdened by the high demand for care from people with common mental health problems. Both are important, and the complexity of helping those with what sometimes are dismissed as having 'common mental health problems' (or even being called the 'worried well') is often underestimated by those who have not worked in primary care. Social (deprivation, unemployment, stigma), biological (chronic physical illness and disability) and psychological (health beliefs, sequelae of early abuse, interpersonal stresses and family dynamics) factors may play a part in preventing a person with an apparently 'common' problem such as depression from accessing care or making an uncomplicated recovery.[12]

Recognition, Diagnosis and Classification of Mental Health Problems in Primary Care

Although much early research in this field failed to consider the impact of GPs' longer-term relationships with their patients on their rate of recognition of mental health problems, we do know that there is variation in this rate.[13] A doctor's consultation style plays a key part in determining both whether a person will disclose how they are feeling during a consultation[14] and whether the doctor is able to identify emotional distress[15] – as determined by agreement between the patient's score on a self-rated questionnaire such as the General Health Questionnaire (GHQ)[16] or the Hospital Anxiety and Depression Scale (HADS).[17] Those who demonstrate empathy can pick up on the patient's emotional cues (both verbal and non-verbal) and move from asking open-ended questions early in the interview to closed questions later on are much better at detecting emotional distress. Most research has been carried out on recognition of depression. However, the GP – as noted earlier – may be crucially involved in the early recognition of psychosis,[18] and primary care plays a key role in early identification and investigation of people with possible dementia (see later).[19]

Evidence does not generally support simply using screening questionnaires to detect common mental health problems such as depression in the primary care setting[20] as it does not lead, in usual practice, to significant changes in management and, therefore, improved outcomes.

Patients in primary care settings are much less likely to present with clearly identifiable diagnostic syndromes and commonly come with a wide variety of symptoms – often a mixture of physical, social and emotional problems. These may not only be 'undifferentiated' – as originally described by Michael Balint[21] – but, at first presentation, unrehearsed by prior discussion with those versed in the language of diagnosis. Those attending with emotional symptoms in primary care are generally less distressed, less likely to have an identifiable mental disorder and less impaired than are cohorts of psychiatric patients within secondary care.[22] However, although symptoms may often be transient, some become recurrent or chronic. There is a link between persistent depressive symptoms and social disadvantage, abuse and higher levels of overall morbidity and disability,[23] with considerable morbidity occurring in people with long-term physical illness such as diabetes, heart disease and chronic obstructive pulmonary disease.[24]

Diagnosis is a contested field in primary care, which is not surprising given that diagnostic systems are generally developed in specialist settings and may not fit well with morbidity in primary care settings. The very nature of that diagnosis and its differentiation from distress can be a source of considerable disagreement between practitioners,[25] and some have even advocated a move away from diagnosis altogether – a non-categorical approach based on achieving a shared understanding of their problems, symptoms and social situation with the patient.[26] Although the PHQ-9 scale for depression is used by psychological therapies services, it is no longer expected that GPs will ask patients to complete rating scales as part of the Quality and Outcomes Framework.[27] Meanwhile, the ICD-11 will have its own international primary care classification with a simplified list of diagnoses in comparison to the main publication.[28] For decades, primary care in the UK used 'read codes' to record symptoms and diagnoses but has now migrated to SNOMED-CT to be compatible with other health care settings.

Some Specific Recognition and Management Issues in Primary Care

'Primary care' psychiatry touches on just about every speciality in psychiatry, but with a particular emphasis on common mental health problems. It is beyond the scope of this chapter to provide a comprehensive overview, which can be found elsewhere,[29] but we have selected aspects of particular problems relevant to the work of a *general psychiatrist* liaising with primary care. The frequency and, sometimes, complexity in primary care of what are now controversially referred to as 'medically unexplained symptoms', eating disorders, substance misuse, child and adolescent mental health and development problems and learning difficulties illustrate the need for much broader liaison across specialities and with the voluntary sector (see later).

The National Institute for Health and Care Excellence (NICE) guidance for common mental health problems provides advice on a range of key issues, including improving access to services, identification and assessment, stepped care, treatment and referral and developing local care pathways. However, it then refers the reader on to each individual guideline for each diagnosis, which is less then helpful for primary care where disorders may be less differentiated. The most common presentation in primary care is 'mixed anxiety and depression'[30] and, as with other NICE guidance, individual guidelines provide only limited advice for what a GP should be able to offer when working in this common scenario of 'multimorbidity'.

Depression

Depression and chronic physical conditions such as diabetes and cardiovascular disease are often inter-linked in this setting with a clear dose-response relationship between the number of long-term physical conditions (which may be mediated by self-perceived health-related quality of life) and depressive symptoms.[24] This comorbid depression may go unrecognised in primary care settings[31] or be difficult to treat.

Grief is very common, but when it becomes *complicated* (a particular problem during the Covid pandemic), it may be indistinguishable from major depression and may benefit from treatment as depression alongside psychological interventions for grief.

Antidepressant medication remains controversial. Even though the prevalence of depression has been consistent in the last few decades, the rates of prescribing antidepressants has risen markedly in primary care. According to Dowrick,[32] in England, antidepressant prescribing increased by over 10 per cent each year between 1998 and 2010, mainly due to an increase in long-term prescriptions. There is no doubt that a significant number of people remain on them for longer periods than perhaps necessary,[33] and there is new guidance available on withdrawal,[34] which is usually carried out in primary care.

Collaborative care (see later) is the most effective way of treating depression and common mental health problems in primary care – particularly for older people[35] – and has been widely adopted across the world, but not in the UK, where there has instead been major investment in stand-alone or attached psychological therapy services (in England by Improving Access to Psychological Therapy – IAPT).[36]

It has been estimated that 10 per cent of people prescribed antidepressants in primary care for anxiety or depression turn out to have unrecognised bipolar disorder.[37] It is, therefore, essential for GPs assessing patients for depression to ask about possible symptoms of bipolar disorder such as previous periods of elevated mood, overactivity or disinhibited behaviour lasting for four days or more.

Brief psychological therapy – cognitive behavioural therapy (CBT) informed guided self-help, behavioural activation and problem-solving therapies – may be provided by GPs themselves but more commonly by attached psychological therapists (in-person or online). According to current NICE guidance, these therapies should be the first-line treatment in mild depression, an option in moderate and provided with medication in severe depression. Referral for more formal CBT or psychodynamic therapy should also be available, but the latter, in particular, is now often harder to access without payment.

Social prescribing is a practical, preventive and holistic alternative in primary care to medical interventions with a range of mental health problems (including those who are lonely or isolated), chronic and long-term conditions and social difficulties (homelessness, debt, unemployment). These services are local and often provided by voluntary or community sector organisations. Link workers can provide a key 'bridge' between the GP and community, where previously GPs were limited by the number of relationships they could build with the different community groups.[38]

Suicide Prevention in Primary Care

In the UK, it is known that nearly three-quarters of people who complete suicide were expected to be supported by primary care (GP) and were not open to secondary care mental health services. GPs have a vital role in managing the self harm and suicide risk among the patients registered with them. It is essential that they acquire appropriate expertise, skills and confidence to be able to carry out targeted assessments, safety planning and signposting for people at risk of suicide. GPs are also expected to be aware of their local crises care pathway for referring people needing urgent psychiatric assessment.

From a case control study comparing people who died of suicide to living patients in primary care during the 10-year period for the years 2002–2011, the National Confidential Inquiry into Suicide and Homicide by People with Mental Illness (NCISH) concluded:[39]

- In primary care patients who die by suicide, mental illness (depression) is frequently unrecognised.
- Suicide risk is associated with frequent attendance of GP consultations, increasing attendance and non-attendance. The non-attenders were primarily young males. Suicide risk increased with increasing number of GP consultations, particularly in the two to three months prior to suicide. In those who attended more than 24 times, risk was increased 12-fold.
- Markers of risk in those attending includes frequent consultation, multiple psychotropic drugs (four or more at a time) and specific drug combinations such as benzodiazepines with antidepressants. These markers could be the basis of a 'flag' alert in primary care records, leading to further assessment.
- The current Health Check in primary care should be amended to include mental health as a step to identifying risk in non-attenders.
- Suicide prevention in primary care non-attenders will have to rely on other agencies, including the voluntary sector and internet-based supports, who may be better able to maintain contact with young people at risk.

Personality Disorders

About 4 per cent of the general population meet the diagnostic criteria for personality disorder,[40] but the prevalence is much higher in primary care attenders.[41] Common mental health problems such as depression, anxiety and substance misuse are more common in people with personality disorder, are more difficult to treat and have worst outcomes.

GPs find patients with a diagnosis of personality disorder quite challenging, difficult to manage, unpredictable and place excessive demands on their time. In a recent qualitative study, they reported experiencing difficulties in engaging those with personality disorders or monitoring their mental health. GPs specifically highlighted having limited knowledge about the type of treatment or management approach they could utilise.[42] The GPs' views on the effectiveness of IAPT for helping them with their patients with this diagnosis was not very positive or convincing. Moreover, IAPT rejected many referrals due to high risk. However, some were not accepted by the mental health services due to symptoms not reaching the threshold or, in some cases, were discharged due to poor engagement with services. The majority of people with the diagnosis fell into the gap between primary care and secondary mental health services. Some GPs managed to access independent sector or commissioned therapists to manage them in primary care. Some GPs recognised the need for dedicated time and continuity of care. They also needed an opportunity to open up and ventilate their distress.

Although GPs have limited skills and time to effectively manage people with a diagnosis of personality disorder, they can provide initial support and management, with consideration given to the following principles:

- Explore treatment options in an atmosphere of hope and optimism
- Build a trusting relationship with an open and non-judgemental manner
- Have services be accessible, consistent and reliable as most of the patients have had past experiences of trauma and abuse
- Work in partnerships to help develop autonomy, encouraging those in treatment to find solutions to their problems.

Severe and Enduring Mental Illness

Most GPs in the UK see only one or two people with first-episode psychosis each year. Despite this low number, the role of primary care is important for a number of reasons. GPs are frequently consulted at some point during the patient's first episode of psychosis and are the most common final referral agent to mental health services in the patient pathway.[43]

The primary care management of severe mental illness is usually in partnership with specialist care, with emphasis on physical health or sequelae of the psychiatric illness.[32] GPs need to look at the consequences of reduced volition and negative symptoms, which affect lifestyle – such as smoking, obesity and substance misuse – and lead to increased risk of heart and respiratory diseases. They also need to be aware of the side effects of treatment with new-generation antipsychotics such as clozapine and olanzapine in their patients, which can lead to an increased risk of weight gain and reduced insulin sensitivity, leading to diabetes and the possible emergence of tardive dyskinesia in the longer term. The combination of these problems results in a 20-year mortality gap in the life expectancy compared to the general population.

NICE guidance states that GPs and other primary care professionals should monitor the physical health of people with severe mental illness at least once a year.

GPs have often known the person as a child before the illness developed, and many people who will not attend psychiatric clinics are still happy to go to their own doctor's surgery for care.[44] There are, however, several obstacles in the management of schizophrenia in primary care:

- *Education and learning*: GPs often need up-to-date information and practical advice on the management of schizophrenia. Similarly, practice nurses – the majority of whom are registered general nurses – have little or no mental health training. Mental health courses for practice nurses are almost exclusively directed towards counselling for anxiety and depression.
- *Reactive nature of primary care*: General practice is essentially reactive, as GPs wait for people to come and see them. This approach will work for people with psychotic disorders in remission or are stable on treatment and have the insight to present themselves for a review. However, a proportion of people with schizophrenia and psychotic conditions do not see their GP from one year to the next and need to be sought out for a review. GPs and practice nurses need to be aware of people who do not ask for their antipsychotic medication (repeat prescriptions) or review in order to alert the community mental health teams (CMHT) to find out whether those individuals are unwell or running into problems.
- *Limited time for assessments*: Due to a limited consultation time in primary care (10 minutes), GPs and practice nurses need a strategy to identify important problems or changes in people with schizophrenia quickly and efficiently. Traditionally, GPs have been taught that the most efficient consulting style is to start with an open question and encourage the person to set the agenda. However, many people who have a diagnosis of schizophrenia with prominent negative symptoms are not likely to bring their problems to their GP's attention.

In this regard, it may be worthwhile to have a template for a 10-minute consultation that could include the following areas (see Box 18.1)

Box 18.1 Template for a ten-minute consultation in primary care for a person with severe and enduring mental illness

- Treatment adherence
- Symptoms of relapse (delusions, hallucinations, thought disorder)
- Physical health (smoking, screening for metabolic syndrome)
- Substance/alcohol misuse
- Social factors (housing, finances, employment)
- Red flag symptoms:
  a. Self neglect
  b. Social withdrawal
  c. Human rights abuse, exploitation
  d. Risk to self (usually secondary to psychotic symptoms, depression) presenting with self harm and suicidal ideation or intent
  e. Risk to others (usually delusional driven) and presenting as aggressive or violent

Burns and Kendrick[45] also identified the following key indicators as important for shared-care discussions (see later):

- Persistent symptoms
- Sudden or gradual changes in behaviour
- 'Any problem that the GP cannot deal with'

Shiers et al.[46] have produced an easy-to-read leaflet for GPs and primary care staff entitled 'Ten Top Tips to Protect the Physical Health of People Experiencing Psychosis', which provides practical guidance and advice including useful references for GPs to screen and manage the physical health of the patients with severe mental illness.

A new training resource developed by the NHS for practice nurses can be found at: www.southeastclinicalnetworks.nhs.uk/phsmi/

Dementia

One in every 14 of the population aged 65 years and over have dementia,[47] and GPs consistently report limited skills and confidence in the diagnosis and management of dementia.

In an online survey of GPs in which 1,011 responded,[48] GPs felt that they had not had sufficient basic and post-qualifying training in dementia and acknowledged that their overall knowledge about dementia was low. The GPs who had qualified before 1990 appeared more confident in diagnosing dementia, giving advice about it and managing dementia-related symptoms. However, the same group were not convinced that early diagnosis was beneficial and more likely to feel that the patients with dementia can be a drain on resources with poor prognosis. On the contrary, younger GPs (born after 1990) were more positive about the patient's outcomes and were optimistic that much could be done to improve their quality of life.

Similarly, Iliffe and Wilcock[49] studied the impact of educational interventions and policy changes aimed at promoting timely or early diagnosis of dementia syndrome. They analysed data from 476 group practices (covering a sample of 1,3338,659 patients aged 60 years or over) covering a period of 14 years (1997–2011). The study results were discouraging as they showed that educational interventions did not appear to change the recorded incidence of dementia syndrome. There appeared to be no impact of incentives or memory clinic activity. The memory clinics were seeing more patients, but fewer were being diagnosed with dementia. There were however some improvements in the documentation of consultations with people with dementia.

Nevertheless, GPs are increasingly aware of their potential role in the assessment and management of patients with dementia and the benefits of collaborative care programmes. The evolving and pragmatic view is that the diagnosis of dementia is a shared responsibility between the GP and specialist. However, it would be beneficial if the GPs explore the patient's ideas and concerns about their symptoms prior to referral and carry out informed discussion about the probable diagnosis.

Once the diagnosis has been established, the GP should provide support to the patient and their families to come to terms with living with dementia, and the systematic follow-up of both the person and their carers should be integrated into primary care.[32] Primary care teams can enhance the quality of care for people diagnosed as having dementia by carrying out an annual dementia review, underpinned by the Quality Outcomes Framework in the UK.[50] Reviews can also include assessment for depression and the need for medication for cognitive and psychotic symptoms.

A user-friendly educational resource for GPs entitled 'Dementia Diagnosis and Management: A Brief Pragmatic Resource for General Practitioners' is available from the NHSE[51] and provides guidance on diagnosis of dementia, an overview of subtypes and reasons for referral to the specialist mental health team. It also includes flexible choices for the GPs to consider undertaking for cognitive assessment, from the shortest (one minute) to 15-minute planned reviews with several clinical scenarios relevant to primary care.

Working at the Interface between Primary and Secondary Mental Health Services

Effective working at the interface not only ensures that those people who require specialist care are able to access it but also supports the GP in managing the majority of people with mental health problems.

'Traditional' Ways of Working: The Community Mental Health Team

After the closure of the asylums, new ways of working in the community led to the development of multi-disciplinary community mental health teams. GPs detect when people have mental health problems, managing them within primary care as far as possible, then referring on to the CMHT when indicated.

However, this is not only heavily dependent on the GP's interest in and knowledge of mental health, but the capacity of the service to manage the demand. The patient must agree to attend a clinic that may be experienced as a very stigmatising experience. If the service has limited access to those with 'serious mental illness' (SMI, generally interpreted as psychosis), then many – particularly those with severe depression – which the GP feels unable to treat but don't meet criteria for referral, as well as those with a personality disorder diagnosis whom the specialist service deems unable to help, will fall through the gaps in the system. This inevitably leads to dissatisfaction with services and conflict at the interface.[52,53] Various approaches have been used to try and improve how the interface works.

Managing Demand

Demand for a service can be managed by limiting access to the service or increasing the flow through the service by increasing the availability of therapists. CMHTs have operated 'gate-keeping' and 'triage' models to more tightly (and bureaucratically) manage the interface.[54] These have included single consultations only or initial telephone assessment of referrals through to 'single point of access' models. This latter system has been widely implemented despite only limited evaluation. In a study in London, GPs compared it to 'referral into a void'[55] because neither they nor the patient had any idea who the patient would be seen by, if at all, and existing relationships with professionals – especially between psychiatrists and GPs – were severed.

In primary care in the United Kingdom, counsellors were introduced to increase the availability of therapists,[56] but these have largely been superseded in England (though not the other nations of the UK) by Improving Access to Psychological Therapy (IAPT) services,[57] with the aim of providing not only increased access but managing demand for care for people with anxiety and depression. However, waiting times have continued to be a problem, and they have been criticised for a lack of integration with other services. Scotland has introduced Clinical Associates in Applied Psychology (CAAPs) to work closely with primary care.

Restructuring the Care Pathway

This involves implementing guidelines and 'stepped' models of care,[58] as in NICE (National Institute for Health and Care Excellence) and SIGN (Scottish Intercollegiate Guidelines Network), into service redesign. Implementation of guidelines has not, on its own, been shown to improve patient outcomes in primary care.[59] However, enhanced collaboration (see later) – particularly between primary and secondary care professionals and managers in face-to-face meetings to develop care pathways – paired with treatment guidelines or protocols has been shown to be superior to either intervention alone in major depression.[60] In Wales, the Mental Health Measure incorporates new primary care-based mental health teams into a stepped care model.

Improving Communication

The most important method of improving communication is for both primary and specialist mental health professionals to have opportunities to meet each other regularly to solve practical problems, have joint educational sessions and simply to get to know, and trust, each other. In the UK, this seems to happen much less frequently than it did in the past. One of us demonstrated many years ago that whether or not GPs knew the psychiatrist to whom the patient was referred had a significant impact on their degree of satisfaction with the outcome of referral.[61]

Patient-held records were suggested as a way of improving access to information but not demonstrated to be effective.[62] In some systems, specialist services can access primary care records electronically when a patient is referred, and both GPs and psychiatrists get easy electronic access to the results of tests and investigations. In some parts of the world – especially in rural and remote areas of Australia and North America (but also in the Scottish islands) – telemedicine is also becoming much more widely used to enhance communication across the interface, both for doctor–patient and doctor–doctor interactions. It provides many opportunities for closer collaboration in psychiatry[63] and is likely to be even more widely used post-Covid-19.

Integrated and 'Shared' Care

The term 'shared care' can have many different meanings – from collaboration between professionals working in different organisations who agree to a protocol for the shared management of people between primary and specialist care, to complex integrated models such as 'collaborative care'. Shared care may be formalised with each professional having particular responsibilities agreed by all involved. This should ideally include clarity over who oversees the patient's ongoing physical health care, health promotion activities and routine blood tests, such as for lithium levels. What 'shared care' is NOT is simply instructing the GP to carry out a list of tests and investigations. Arrangements may be at the service rather than practitioner level. For example, a psychiatrist based in a specialist service will retain responsibility for psychotropic medication, monitoring and management of adherence, response and side effects, with the GP prescribing, undertaking mental health monitoring and assessments as agreed as well as attending to routine health care. Problems occur where the patient fails to attend appointments with specialist care or disengages altogether or where the patient fails to attend primary care. Physical health care may then be over-looked unless the patient is proactively re-engaged with the GP.

In the UK, 30 per cent of people on registers for severe and enduring mental illness in primary care are not under the care of specialist services,[64] and there is confusion or disagreement about who is responsible for certain aspects of care unless these arrangements are formalised.

Link-Working

Link-working may involve limited clinical intervention but not expert clinical advice or structured liaison. A member of the CMHT links with a particular GP practice. The most comprehensive randomised controlled trial (RCT) of link-working[65] went beyond this remit and used meetings between general practice and community mental health workers, a link worker, the creation of registers of patients with severe mental illness and recall systems facilitated by payments to GPs. Patients in the practices receiving the intervention had fewer psychiatric relapses and improved review and recall, and intervention providers reported improved satisfaction.

Co-Location

The 'shifted outpatient clinic'[66] was once a common way of moving mental health care into the community and has been utilised not only by consultants but also by other members of the mental health team, including nurses and psychological therapists. This leads to more effective working at the interface, but only if professionals from each team are able to meet face-to-face, which doesn't always occur if space is only occupied by mental health professionals during the period of the day when GPs are no longer in clinic. A meta-analysis of 42 studies[67] found that a positive outcome occurred when on-site mental health workers provided psychological and psychosocial interventions in primary care practices. On-site mental health workers were associated with significant reductions in primary care provider consultations, psychotropic prescribing, prescribing costs and rates of mental health referral. Co-location 'normalises' accessing mental health care and can reduce the burden of travel to additional services.

Consultation–Liaison

In the consultation–liaison model, a mental health specialist provides expert advice that is different from the usual referral relationship. The original model as described by Creed and Marks[68] consisted of:

- Regular face-to-face contact between psychiatrist and a primary health care team (PHCT)
- Referral only after a discussion at a face-to-face meeting
- Some cases are managed by the PHCT only
- When referral does take place, there is feedback to, and management by, the PHCT

A specialist may carry out an assessment and limited treatment with some educational input, but clinical responsibility for the patient remains with the GP. Consultation–liaison services have been offered in combination with brief therapeutic contact, and in rural areas, consultation–liaison has been provided successfully via teleconferencing. Consultation– liaison differs from the other models in that it challenges the way that professionals relate to each other across organisational boundaries. There is also no evidence that it has an impact on outcomes although it may be an important way of improving professional relationships across the interface.[69] Tom Burns in London set up group liaison meetings between the CMHT and GPs in order to discuss problems primarily relating to patients with longer-term mental health problems that they had in common.[70] These meetings are still taking place.

Safi Afghan writes:

> *In my experience as a consultant adult psychiatrist serving a catchment area based on 6 GP practices (traditional sector model) in the West Midlands of England, I have been involved in organising face to face meetings (and more recently following Covid-19, online meetings) with my sector GPs at regular intervals. A typical meeting involves the consultant psychiatrist and team members with the general practice (group of GPs alongside the practice manager). These meetings have been professionally rewarding in improving closer communication and foster a professional relationship with the practice, especially the lead GP.*
>
> *A typical meeting lasts for approximately one hour to 90 minutes and may cover a range of areas especially discussion of mutual patients (patients from the practice currently open to secondary mental health care including open to CPA /CMHTs).*
>
> *The consultant psychiatrist and his team undertake preparation for the meeting in the form of updating the shared caseload (names, diagnosis, treatments, date last seen, date of upcoming review etc) and sharing the updated list with the GP practice manager before the scheduled meeting. The preparation also involves identifying patients from the caseload who have remained stable and can now be stepped down to primary care, as well as identifying patients who are unstable or currently presenting with crises, risks or challenging behaviours.*

Box 18.2 Typical format of meeting between a consultant psychiatrist & GP (and primary care)

Agenda

- Informal and open-ended discussion on the access, response, communication, quality of care and any operational changes to the access and design of service
- Discussion on the identified (flagged-up) patients who have remained stable from a mental health perspective and achieved a good degree of recovery. To arrive at a consensus for stepping them down to primary care
- Discussion relating to unstable, complex and high-risk patients, including their engagement with the primary or secondary care
- Accessing information from the GP/practice manager if the individual patients are picking up their repeat prescriptions (indirect indicator of medication adherence)
- Consultation/liaison: Discussion and advice on new (and potential) referrals and using the opportunity to reduce unwanted referrals to secondary case. Providing advice where indicated on the pharmacological, psychological or social interventions (including social prescribing)
- Seeking written feedback from the GP on the quality of care provided by the psychiatrist and mental health team including accessibility, responsiveness, communication (including written communication such as clinic letters and discharge summaries)

The usual areas covered in these meetings, resources and advantages have been summarised in Box 18.2.

Benefits of meetings include:

- Meetings provide an opportunity for fostering and building positive relationships with GPs and primary care
- Meetings help with prompt decision-making (e.g. stepping down of stable/recovered patients back to primary care)
- GPs and psychiatrists have better awareness of patients' physical and psychosocial difficulties
- Improving quality of care for patients

Collaborative Care

Collaborative care is based on the principles of chronic disease management[71] and involves the addition of new staff ('case managers') who work directly with patients and liaise with primary care professionals and specialists in order to improve the quality of care for people with common mental health problems (see Box 18.3).

Case managers provide support, medication management and brief psychotherapies directly to patients, while liaising with the primary care and receiving support from a specialist. Collaborative care also differs that people are systematically followed up, and failure to attend is not assumed to be a reason for discharge – quite the opposite – and attempts are made to re-engage. Considerable efforts are made to work closely with primary care, including regular access to and entry in GP records, and supervision (clinical and case management) is methodically organised and delivered by more experienced (and specifically trained) mental health professionals.

This approach was developed and extensively researched in Seattle. There is now considerable evidence for its effectiveness for anxiety and depression,[72] especially for older people and also for those with comorbid physical health problems, and it has been rolled out in North America. It has now also been successfully tested out in two large UK randomised controlled trials – the CADET[73] and COINCIDE[74] studies. In these studies, psychological wellbeing practitioners (PWP) were successfully trained and supervised to deliver collaborative care and situated within primary care. The quality, delivery and organisation of supervision is essential to this process, and the routine collection of outcome data in collaborative care fits with the demands of IAPT. However, the supervision and management team are ideally multi-professional, with medical input too, enabling management of more complex problems.

Collaborative care has also been utilised for people with severe mental health problems in the USA (particularly for bipolar disorder),[75] focusing on improving their physical health care with a primary care service embedded within mental health services (the Integrated Behavioural Health Home model[76]). In the UK, the focus has been on step-down/seamless step-back-up services for people with severe mental illness who are moving back to primary care.

Box 18.3 Key element of collaborative care

- **Multi-professional and systematic approach to patient care** provided by a case manager who is working with the GP while under regular supervision from specialist mental health clinician(s)
- **A structured management plan** of medication support and the provision of brief psychological therapy
- **Scheduled patient follow-ups** with attempts to contact if they do not attend
- **Enhanced inter-professional communication** including patient-specific written feedback to GPs via electronic records and personal contact

A naturalistic study in East London[77] of 'enhanced primary care' (EPC) has demonstrated its utility. The service model was aimed to enable the recovery of patients and to safely discharge them to primary care settings with a view of addressing their mental health needs. The model was an alignment and partnership of a specialist mental health service with clinical commissioning groups/primary care teams, and their working groups included GPs, consultant psychiatrists, community psychiatric nurses, psychologists and social work leads. The key elements of the EPC pathway were:

- Regular GP reviews, recovery care plan development, practice nurses administering depot injections, physical health assessments and signposting to healthy lifestyle groups
- Consultant psychiatrist providing enhanced support to primary care and attending regular practice-based mental health multi-disciplinary meetings
- Training and education to GPs on managing SMI in primary care, as well as for practice nurses on treatment with antipsychotic medication including administration of depot medication

After three years, it was indicated that 31% (N = 717) of patients (N = 2,310) with SMI (who had previously been under secondary care service for an average of 10 years) were transferred to primary care. However, 10% of cases from the EPC had to be transferred back to secondary care. The patient and staff satisfaction with the EPC model was high.

In the UK, the Partners2 study has adapted the principles of collaborative care for people with serious mental illness discharged to primary care or with low needs in secondary care. The intervention incorporates a recovery framework and employs coaching as the psychosocial intervention delivered by the case manager or 'care partner'. These workers were as far as possible embedded in primary care and worked not only on patient goals, but in liaison with primary care, voluntary and other community agencies and secondary care. Patients might be stepped up back to crisis services or the CMHT, or discharged to primary care, but remain in limited contact with the care partner.

The study, conducted across four sites in England, did not significantly improve quality of life for the patients over the limited timescale of just under a year, but crucially, shifting the focus of care to primary care did not result in any adverse events.[78]

A comprehensive review of the literature on ways of improving work at the interface carried out in Australia by Fuller and colleagues[79] strongly supports the use of a *range* of linkage combinations in primary mental health care. The strongest body of evidence seems to be for those interventions that use a combination of the approaches described earlier but *always including collaborative care.*

Current Policy Developments in the NHS in England

The community mental health framework for adults and older adults is derived from the NHS long term plan and is an ambitious plan to infuse much-needed resources to bolster mental health service provision nationally. We are focusing on the developments in England at this point because the proposed changes are radical and recognise the need to strengthen the resources for the community mental health teams alongside enhancing the capacity of primary care and proposes a new 'place-based' community mental health model.

One of its key objectives will be to develop new and integrated models of primary and community mental health care that will support adults and older adults with severe mental illnesses. The framework has broadened the scope of mental health service provision in such that it is not limited to the people with long-term severe mental illness but also focuses and recognises the needs of people who are deemed too severe for the IAPT services but not severe enough to meet secondary care thresholds including, for example, eating disorders and complex mental health difficulties associated with the diagnosis of personality disorder.

The plan envisages a different way of working for community-based psychiatrists, with much more focus on working not only with primary care but also voluntary sector organisations.

It states that '*the new community-based offer which will include access to psychological therapies, improved physical health care, employment support, personalised and trauma informed care, medicines management and support for self-harm, and co-existing substance use and proactive work to address racial disparities. Local areas will be supported to redesign and reorganise core community mental health teams to move towards a new place-based multidisciplinary services across health and social care aligned with primary care networks*'.[80]

GP practices across England have come together in around 1,300 geographical primary care networks (PCNs), each covering a population of approximately 30,000–50,000 patients. NHS England's expectation are that the PCNs will be one of the main channels for delivering many of the commitments in the long-term plan in providing a wider range of services to the patients.

Although the community mental health framework produced by NHS England[81] illustrates a broad direction of travel for community mental health services in England, it still needs much more specific detail and direction to build the capacity within primary care and demonstrate improved connection and joined-up working across primary care and mental health services. Much of that detail might be informed by the research, new models and ways of working across the interface that we have described earlier.

Education and Training

Training GPs and Practice Nurses about Mental Health

The Royal College of General Practitioners (RCGP) curriculum statement describes the comprehensive range of knowledge and skills that GPs in training are expected to acquire.[82] However, less than a half of GPs in practice have received specific training in a mental health post.[83] GP attachments in psychiatry have not always been viewed positively, with trainees reporting too much emphasis on inpatient care of people with psychotic illness (and their physical health care too) instead of getting experience in more appropriate community settings.[84]

Training for GP registrars in psychiatry should focus on the common problems they are going to see in primary care[85] – anxiety, depression, people with medically unexplained symptoms, alcohol and drug problems and common mental health problems of childhood and old age, in addition to cultural factors that determine access to, presentation and treatment of mental health problems. They need to know about the symptoms of early psychosis, mental health law and the physical health of people with severe mental illness as well as how the interface between primary and specialist care works, but they will be bored and disinterested in the finer points of psychopathology discussed during postgraduate training in psychiatry. Training in the interview skills required to recognise and manage people with common mental health problems can be delivered using role play and videofeedback,[86] while Balint groups are still popular with some GPs (sometimes facilitated by a psychotherapist) – originating through Balint's work in general practice. Any postgraduate training event is always best planned, organised and delivered in collaboration with experienced GPs who will understand the needs of the audience and how best to encourage attendance – and engage them.

Practice nurse experience and involvement in mental health remains variable with a limited evidence base,[87] despite their potentially important role in improving the physical health care of people with severe mental illness.[88] Tom Burns and colleagues carried out a trial of teaching practice nurses who delivered depot injections to carry out brief structured assessments and to bring any problems to their GP's attention.[89] However, outcomes did not improve as problems uncovered by the nurses were not always dealt with by the GP. More recently, the PRIMROSE study demonstrated that primary care nurses and health care assistants can deliver cardiovascular disease risk-reducing interventions to people with SMI. They reported that the intervention was well attended, and this resulted in fewer inpatient admissions; however, there was no impact on the primary outcome of total cholesterol level.[90]

Training Psychiatrists about Primary Care

In our experience, health professionals who work with primary care must take the view that they are there to work with, and learn from, primary care – not to direct, teach or dictate to primary care. They must be familiar with the evidence base for what does and does not work in terms of treatment of common mental health problems and interventions at the interface as well as willing to learn a range of brief psychological therapies applicable in primary care to be able to assist in the supervision of other workers. Flexibility and approachability are essential attributes. The timetable of primary care differs from specialist care, and scheduling a rigid time to discuss medication issues with a consultant once a week between 11.30 and 12 noon will not be met favourably.

In current training, most psychiatrists now will have had experience of general practice during foundation training. However, more opportunities are needed for psychiatric trainees to spend time in primary-care-based teams to develop the knowledge, attitudes and skills to fill the role of a 'primary care psychiatrist'. Many years ago, an experiment at St George's hospital in London – which gave psychiatric trainees a six-month period in general practice[91] – did not, as hoped, help to develop their consultation skills, but it did provide them with an appreciation of the work involved in becoming an expert generalist and helped to develop their broader clinical skills.

Conclusion

The psychiatry of primary care, and the work that GPs do, has expanded as a field of interest for psychiatrists, beyond its early roots in epidemiological research and studies into the detection of mental disorders by general practitioners. An understanding of the key role of the primary care team in managing often-complex mental health problems in the wider community as well as how to work effectively at the interface in partnership and joint work with GPs is essential, not only for general adult psychiatrists but other specialists too, as policy makers – both local to the UK and internationally – continue to recognise its importance.

References

1. Starfield B, Shi L, Macinko J. Contribution of primary care to health systems and health. *The Milbank Quarterly* 2005;83(3):457–502.
2. World Health Organization. *Declaration of Alma-Ata*. Geneva: World Health Organization; 1978.
3. Gerada C, Riley B. The 2022 GP: our profession, our patients, our future. *British Journal of General Practice* 2012;62(604):566–7.
4. World Health Organization, World Organization of Family Doctors (Wonca). *Integrating Mental Health into Primary Care: A Global Perspective*. Geneva: World Health Organization; 2008.
5. Shepherd M. *Psychiatric Illness in General Practice*. Oxford: Oxford University Press; 1981.
6. Goldberg D, Huxley P. *Mental Illness in the Community: The Pathway to Psychiatric Care*. London/New York: Tavistock; 1980.
7. Dixon-Woods M, Cavers D, Agarwal S, et al. Conducting a critical interpretive synthesis of the literature on access to healthcare by vulnerable groups. *BMC Medical Research Methodology* 2006;6 (1):1–3.
8. Gask L, Bower P, Lamb J, et al. Improving access to psychosocial interventions for common mental health problems in the United Kingdom: narrative review and development of a conceptual model for complex interventions. *BMC Health Services Research* 2012;12(1):1–3.
9. Thomas L, Lewis G. The epidemiology of mental illness. In: Gask L, Kendrick T, Peveler R, et al. (eds.) *Primary Care Mental Health*. Cambridge: Cambridge University Press; 2018: 12–23.
10. Andrews G, Henderson S (eds.) *Unmet Need in Psychiatry: Problems, Resources, Responses*. Cambridge: Cambridge University Press; 2000.
11. Das-Munshi J, Goldberg D, Bebbington PE, et al. Public health significance of mixed anxiety and depression: beyond current classification. *British Journal of Psychiatry* 2008;192(3):171–7.
12. Ronalds C, Creed F, Stone K, et al. Outcome of anxiety and depressive disorders in primary care. *British Journal of Psychiatry* 1997;171:427–33
13. Üstün TB, Sartorius N (eds.) *Mental Illness in General Health Care: An International Study*. Oxford: John Wiley & Sons; 1995.
14. Davenport S, Goldberg D, Millar T. How psychiatric disorders are missed during medical consultations. *The Lancet* 1987;330(8556):439–41.
15. Goldberg DP, Jenkins L, Millar T, et al. The ability of trainee general practitioners to identify psychological distress among their patients. *Psychological Medicine* 1993;23 (1):185–93.
16. Goldberg D, Williams P. *General Health Questionnaire Manual*. Windsor: National Foundation for Educational Research; 1982.
17. Snaith RP, Zigmond AS. *Hospital Anxiety and Depression Scale (HADS). Handbook of Psychiatric Measures*. Washington, DC: American Psychiatric Association; 2000.
18. Skeate A, Jackson C, Wood MB, et al. Duration of untreated psychosis and pathways to care in first-episode psychosis: investigation of help-seeking behaviour in primary care. *British Journal of Psychiatry* 2002;181(S43):s73–7.
19. Iliffe S, Wilcock J. The UK experience of promoting dementia recognition and management in primary care. *Zeitschrift für Gerontologie und Geriatrie* 2017;50 (2):63–7.
20. Thombs BD, Coyne JC, Cuijpers P, et al. Rethinking recommendations for screening for depression in primary care. *Canadian Medical Association Journal* 2012;184(4):413–18.
21. Balint M. *The Doctor, His Patient and the Illness*. London: Pitman; 1964.
22. Mattisson C, Bogren M, Horstmann V, et al. The long-term course of depressive disorders in the Lundby Study. *Psychological Medicine* 2007;37 (6):883–91.
23. Gunn J, Elliott P, Densley K, et al. A trajectory-based approach to understand the factors associated with persistent depressive symptoms in primary care. *Journal of Affective Disorders* 2013;148(2–3):338–46.
24. Gunn JM, Ayton DR, Densley K, et al. The association between chronic illness, multimorbidity and depressive symptoms in an Australian primary care cohort. *Social Psychiatry and Psychiatric Epidemiology* 2012;47(2):175–84.
25. Geraghty AW, Santer M, Beavis C, et al. 'I mean what is depression?'A qualitative exploration of UK general practitioners'

perceptions of distinctions between emotional distress and depressive disorder. *BMJ Open* 2019;9(12).

26. Byng R, Groos N, Dowrick C. From mental disorder to shared understanding: a non-categorical approach to support individuals with distress in primary care. *British Journal of General Practice* 2019;69(680):110–1.
27. NHS Quality and Outcomes Framework. *2019/20 General Medical Services (GMS) Contract Quality and Outcomes Framework (QOF).* www.england.nhs.uk/wp-content/uploads/2019/05/gms-contract-qof-guidance-april-2019.pdf.
28. Goldberg DP, Prisciandaro JJ, Williams P. The primary health care version of ICD-11: the detection of common mental disorders in general medical settings. *General Hospital Psychiatry* 2012;34(6):665–70.
29. Gask L, Kendrick T, Peveler R, et al. (eds.) *Primary Care Mental Health.* Cambridge: Cambridge University Press; 2018.
30. Shevlin M, Hyland P, Nolan E, et al. ICD-11 'mixed depressive and anxiety disorder' is clinical rather than sub-clinical and more common than anxiety and depression in the general population. *British Journal of Clinical Psychology.* 2021;61(1):18–36.
31. Coventry PA, Hays R, Dickens C, et al. Talking about depression: a qualitative study of barriers to managing depression in people with long term conditions in primary care. *BMC Family Practice* 2011;12(1):10.
32. Dowrick C. Update on advances in psychiatric treatment in primary care. *BJPsych Advances* 2016;22(2):99–107.
33. Lewis G, Marston L, Duffy L, et al. Maintenance or discontinuation of antidepressants in primary care. *New England Journal of Medicine* 2021;385(14):1257–67.
34. RCPsych. *Stopping Antidepressants.* www.rcpsych.ac.uk/mental-health/treatments-and-wellbeing/stopping-antidepressants.
35. Unützer J, Katon W, Callahan CM, et al. Collaborative care management of late-life depression in the primary care setting: a randomized controlled trial. *JAMA* 2002;288(22):2836–45.
36. Clark DM. Implementing NICE guidelines for the psychological treatment of depression and anxiety disorders: the IAPT experience. *International Review of Psychiatry* 2011;23(4):318–27.
37. Hughes T, Cardno A, West R, et al. Unrecognised bipolar disorder among UK primary care patients prescribed antidepressants: an observational study. *British Journal of General Practice* 2016;66(643):e71–7.
38. Aughterson H, Baxter L, Fancourt D. Social prescribing for individuals with mental health problems: a qualitative study of barriers and enablers experienced by general practitioners. *BMC Family Practice* 2020;21(1):1–7.
39. National Confidential Inquiry into Suicide and Homicide by People with Mental Illness (NCISH). *Suicide in Primary Care in England: 2002–2011.* Manchester: University of Manchester; 2014.
40. Coid J, Yang MI, Tyrer P, et al. Prevalence and correlates of personality disorder in Great Britain. *British Journal of Psychiatry* 2006;188(5):423–31.
41. Moran P, Jenkins R, Tylee A, et al. The prevalence of personality disorder among UK primary care attenders. *Acta Psychiatrica Scandinavica* 2000;102(1):52–7.
42. French L, Moran P, Wiles N, et al. GPs' views and experiences of managing patients with personality disorder: a qualitative interview study. *BMJ Open* 2019;9(2):e026616.
43. Skeate A, Jackson C, Wood MB, et al. Duration of untreated psychosis and pathways to care in first-episode psychosis: investigation of help-seeking behaviour in primary care. *British Journal of Psychiatry* 2002;181(S43):s73–7.
44. Kendrick T. Management of people with schizophrenia in primary care. *Advances in Psychiatric Treatment* 1998;4(1):46–72
45. Burns T, Kendrick T. The primary care of patients with schizophrenia: a search for good practice. *British Journal of General Practice* 1997;47(421):515–20.
46. Shiers D, Pandey S, Campion J. *Ten Top Tips to Protect the Physical Health of Patients Experiencing Psychosis.* London: Royal College of General Practitioners; 2017.
47. Prince M, Knapp M, Guerchet M, et al. *Dementia UK: Update.* London: Alzheimer's Society; 2014.
48. Ahmad S, Orrell M, Iliffe S, et al. GPs' attitudes, awareness, and practice regarding early diagnosis of dementia. *British Journal of General Practice* 2010;60(578):e360–5.
49. Iliffe S, Wilcock J. The UK experience of promoting dementia recognition and management in primary care. *Zeitschrift für Gerontologie und Geriatrie* 2017;50(2):63–7.
50. Connolly A, Iliffe S, Gaehl E, et al. Quality of care provided to people with dementia: utilisation and quality of the annual dementia review in general practice. *British Journal of General Practice* 2012;62(595):e91–8.
51. NHS England. *Dementia Diagnosis and Management. A Brief Pragmatic Resource for General Practitioners.* www.england.nhs.uk/wp-content/uploads/2015/01/dementia-diag-mng-ab-pt.pdf (accessed 16 September 2023).
52. Chew-Graham C, Slade M, Montana C, et al. A qualitative study of referral to community mental health teams in the UK: exploring the rhetoric and the reality. *BMC Health Services Research* 2007;7(1):117.
53. Chew-Graham C, Slade M, Montana C, et al. Loss of doctor-to-doctor communication: lessons from the reconfiguration of mental health services in England. *Journal of Health Services Research & Policy* 2008;13(1):6–12.
54. Gask L, Khanna T. Ways of working at the interface between primary and specialist mental healthcare. *British Journal of Psychiatry* 2011;198(1):3–5.
55. Raine R, Carter S, Sensky T, et al. 'Referral into a void': opinions of general practitioners and others on single point of access to mental health care. *Journal of the Royal Society of Medicine* 2005;98(4):153–7.
56. Rowland N. Counselling for mental health and psychosocial problems in primary care. *Cochrane Database of Systematic Reviews* 2011(9). Art. No.: CD001025. DOI: 10.1002/14651858.CD001025.pub3.
57. NHS England. *IAPT at 10: Achievements and Challenges.* www.england.nhs.uk/mental-health/adults/iapt/.
58. Richards DA, Hill JJ, Gilbody S, et al. Collaborative care and stepped care. In: Gask L, Kendrick T, Peveler R, et al. (eds.) *Primary Care Mental Health.* Cambridge: Cambridge University; 2018: 401.
59. Croudace T, Evans J, Harrison G, et al. Impact of the ICD-10 Primary Health Care (PHC) diagnostic and management guidelines for mental disorders on detection and outcome in primary care: cluster randomised

controlled trial. *British Journal of Psychiatry* 2003;182(1):20–30.

60. Craven MA, Bland R. Better practices in collaborative mental health care: an analysis of the evidence base. *Canadian Journal of Psychiatry* 2006;51(6):1S.
61. Gask L. What happens when psychiatric out-patients are seen once only? *British Journal of Psychiatry* 1986;148(6):663–6.
62. Lester H, Allan T, Wilson S, et al. A cluster randomised controlled trial of patient-held medical records for people with schizophrenia receiving shared care. *British Journal of General Practice* 2003;53(488):197–203.
63. Fortney JC, Pyne JM, Turner EE, etal. Telepsychiatry integration of mental health services into rural primary care settings. *International Review of Psychiatry* 2015;27(6):525–39.
64. Reilly S, Planner C, Hann M, et al. The role of primary care in service provision for people with severe mental illness in the United Kingdom. *PLoS ONE* 2012;7 (5):e36468.
65. Byng R, Jones R, Leese M, et al. Exploratory cluster randomised controlled trial of shared care development for long-term mental illness. *British Journal of General Practice* 2004;54(501):259–66.
66. Gask L, Sibbald B, Creed F. Evaluating models of working at the interface between mental health services and primary care. *British Journal of Psychiatry* 1997;170(1):6–11.
67. Harkness EF, Bower PJ. On-site mental health workers delivering psychological therapy and psychosocial interventions to patients in primary care: effects on the professional practice of primary care providers. *Cochrane Database of Systematic Reviews* 2009(1). Art. No.: CD000532. DOI: 10.1002/14651858. CD000532.pub2.
68. Creed FR, Marks B. Liaison psychiatry in general practice: a comparison of the liaison-attachment scheme and shifted outpatient clinic models. *Journal of the Royal College of General Practitioners* 1989;39(329):514–7
69. Bower P, Gask L. The changing nature of consultation-liaison in primary care: bridging the gap between research and practice. *General Hospital Psychiatry* 2002;24(2):63–70.
70. Midgley S, Burns T, Garland C. What do general practitioners and community mental health teams talk about? Descriptive analysis of liaison meetings in general practice. *British Journal of General Practice* 1996;46(403):69–71.
71. Wagner EH, Austin BT, Von Korff M. Organizing care for patients with chronic illness. *The Milbank Quarterly* 1996;74(4):511–44
72. Archer J, Bower P, Gilbody S, et al. Collaborative care for depression and anxiety problems. *Cochrane Database of Systematic Reviews* 2012(10).
73. Richards DA, Hill JJ, Gask L, et al. Clinical effectiveness of collaborative care for depression in UK primary care (CADET): cluster randomised controlled trial. *BMJ* 2013;347:f4913.
74. Coventry P, Lovell K, Dickens C, et al. Integrated primary care for patients with mental and physical multimorbidity: cluster randomised controlled trial of collaborative care for patients with depression comorbid with diabetes or cardiovascular disease. *BMJ* 2015;350:h638.
75. Woltmann E, Grogan-Kaylor A, Perron B, et al. Comparative effectiveness of collaborative chronic care models for mental health conditions across primary, specialty, and behavioral health care settings: systematic review and meta-analysis. *American Journal of Psychiatry* 2012;169(8):790–804
76. Druss BG, von Esenwein SA, Glick GE, et al. Randomized trial of an integrated behavioral health home: the health outcomes management and evaluation (HOME) study. *American Journal of Psychiatry* 2017;174(3):246–55.
77. Röhricht F, Waddon GK, Binfield P, et al. Implementation of a novel primary care pathway for patients with severe and enduring mental illness. *BJPsych Bulletin* 2017;41(6):314–9.
78. Byng R, Creanor S, Jones B, et al. The effectiveness of a primary care-based collaborative care model to improve quality of life in people with severe mental illness: PARTNERS2 cluster randomised controlled trial. *British Journal of Psychiatry* 2023;222(6): 246–256.
79. Fuller JD, Perkins D, Parker S, et al. Effectiveness of service linkages in primary mental health care: a narrative review part 1. *BMC Health Services Research* 2011;11:72.
80. NHS England, NHS Improvement and National Collaborating Central for Mental Health.*The Community Mental Health Framework for Adults and Older Adults*. 2019. www.england.nhs.uk/wp-content/uploads/2019/09/community-mental-health-framework-for-adults-and-older-adults.pdf.
81. NHS England, NHS Improvement, National Collaborating Centre for Mental Health. *The Community Mental Health Framework for Adults and Older Adults*. London: NHSX; 2019.
82. Royal College of General Practitioners. *Curriculum Topic Guides*. www.rcgp.org .uk/mrcgp-exams/gp-curriculum/ clinical-topic-guides.
83. England E, Nash V, Hawthorne K. GP training in mental health needs urgent reform. *BMJ* 2017;356:j1311.
84. Williams K. Self-assessment of clinical competence by general practitioner trainees before and after a six-month psychiatric placement. *British Journal of General Practice* 1998;48(432):1387–90.
85. Ratcliffe J, Gask L, Creed F, et al. Psychiatric training for family doctors: what do GP registrars want and can a brief course provide this? *Medical Education* 1999;33(6):434–8.
86. Gask L, Goldberg D, Lewis B. Teaching and learning about mental health In: Gask L, Kendrick T, Peveler R, et al. (eds.) *Primary Care Mental Health*. Cambridge: Cambridge University Press; 2018: 423–38.
87. Halcomb EJ, McInnes S, Patterson C, et al. Nurse-delivered interventions for mental health in primary care: a systematic review of randomized controlled trials. *Family Practice* 2019;36(1):64–71.
88. Hardy S. Improving physical health in people with severe mental illness. *Practice Nursing* 2020;31(11):456–60.
89. Burns T, Millar E, Garland C, et al. Randomized controlled trial of teaching practice nurses to carry out structured assessments of patients receiving depot antipsychotic injections. *British Journal of General Practice* 1998;48 (437):1845–8.
90. Osborn D, Burton A, Hunter R, et al. Clinical and cost-effectiveness of an intervention for reducing cholesterol and cardiovascular risk for people with severe mental illness in English primary care: a cluster randomised controlled trial. *The Lancet Psychiatry* 2018;5 (2):145–54.
91. Burns T, MacDonald L, Sibbald B, et al. Educational assessment of general practice experience for psychiatric trainees. *Medical Education* 1995;29 (2):159–64.

Chapter

19 Psychiatry in the General Hospital

Parashar Ramanuj and Alice Ashby

Consultation-liaison (CL) psychiatry is one of the newer sub-specialties of adult psychiatry and is concerned with the practice of psychiatry in non-psychiatric settings. Typically, this means in general hospital wards and outpatient clinics, although in some countries, it also includes liaison with primary care. This chapter provides an outline of the development and the practice of CL psychiatry, as well as possible future directions, along with some illustrative examples of the practice of psychiatry in non-psychiatric settings.

History

Exactly when the sub-specialty started is difficult to define, but the need for psychiatric expertise to assess patients who could not easily fit into a straightforward single medical diagnosis was already recognised towards the end of the nineteenth century, when J J Putnam, a Harvard neurologist working at the Massachusetts General Hospital, was assigned the task of 'evaluating medical patients whose complaints defied diagnoses'. Initially grounded in psychoanalytic and psychodynamic theories, the field of psychosomatic medicine was developed in the USA. From the 1930s onwards, general hospital psychiatry became established in the USA, and Edward Billings at the Colorado General Hospital first coined the term 'liaison psychiatry'. As liaison psychiatry services gradually developed during the twentieth century, it became clear that psychiatrists working in a general hospital had an important educational role to play, teaching a holistic approach to medical students and other health care workers, training primary health care workers to identify and manage psychiatric disorders as well as establishing close links between medicine and psychiatry, and the consultative aspects of general hospital psychiatry was developed. The first edition of the *Massachusetts General Hospital Handbook of General Hospital Psychiatry* was a landmark text that established the practice of psychiatry in the general hospital. This was because it was written not only for psychiatrists but also for physicians, surgeons and professionals in other disciplines who worked in the general hospital.

In the UK, dedicated liaison psychiatry services remained virtually unknown until the 1970s, although psychiatric outpatient clinics and wards had been established in a few general hospitals – mainly within neurology departments – during the first half of the twentieth century. The Suicide Act of 1961 decreed that suicide was no longer a crime, and this was soon followed by a recommendation by the Ministry of Health (following the Hill report) that all cases of attempted suicide brought to a hospital should have a psychiatric assessment before discharge. This resulted in a rapid increase in the amount of contact between psychiatrists and general hospital departments.

In 1983, the UK Liaison Psychiatry Special Interest Group was established at the Royal College of Psychiatrists in response to the growing interest in and need for psychiatric services in general hospitals. In addition to the management of suicide attempts, psychiatrists contributed to important developments in the fields of nephrology, transplantation, cardiology, HIV and pain management, which are beyond the scope of this brief review to cover. However, particularly significant developments occurred in the treatment of delirium, neurology, perinatal mental health and cancer care. At the same time, liaison psychiatry in Britain was building on its historical roots with neurology, and the new discipline of neuropsychiatry was forged in the 1970s with the publication of the seminal work of Alwyn Lishman, *Organic Psychiatry*.[1] Similarly, general adult and liaison psychiatrists had always treated women in the perinatal period, but driven by new epidemiological and clinical research on the under-provision of care culminating in a series of national reviews, the Perinatal Section of the Royal College of Psychiatrists became a fully-formed faculty in 2014, thus giving rise to the sub-specialty of perinatal psychiatry.[2] A similar evolution is currently occurring in cancer care. The psychological effect of cancer surgery was first pointed out in 1952, and there is now a whole sub-specialty of psycho-oncology emerging, with consideration given to the psychological impact of the different cancer treatments, identification of clinical depression in cancer patients, and improved communication between staff and patients.

As the field has evolved, two central responsibilities of the psychiatrist in the general hospital setting have developed: consultation and liaison.[3] Consultation refers to a response to a request from a patient's primary physician to evaluate and make recommendations about psychiatric issues affecting the patient's management. Psychiatric liaison has increasingly come to mean joining a care team in an ongoing fashion, both within and without the hospital. The benefits that psychiatric services can offer general hospital settings have been increasingly recognised. The importance of the joint working between physicians/surgeons and psychiatrists has been highlighted in national reports by NHS England 2016[4] and by the Royal College of Emergency Medicine,[5] by the Care Quality Commission and by the National Enquiry into Patient Outcome and Death.[6] These reports highlight the need for doctors and nurses in general hospitals to possess adequate skills in psychological care, as well as the need for all general hospitals to have a specialised liaison psychiatry service. The manner in which CL psychiatrists, physicians and surgeons work jointly in inpatient, outpatient and emergency settings varies from a free-standing psychiatric service for the general hospital (consultation model) to a fully integrated medical–psychiatric service.[7] Although much has changed between the chapter in the 2nd edition of this book in 2007 by Akagi and House,[8] most of the basic knowledge of CL psychiatry as practised today was formulated in the latter part of the twentieth century, and so we have also drawn on this previous chapter.

An economic evaluation of the Rapid Assessment Interface and Discharge (RAID) liaison psychiatry team set up at City Hospital in Birmingham by Tadros and colleagues was a turning point in recognising the cost effectiveness of CL psychiatry.[9] The evaluation concluded that the service, which has cost £0.8 million per year, saved the hospital £3.55 million in reduced bed use (particularly around the team assisting with earlier discharge of older people), approximately equating to £4 saved for every £1 spent. In England, these developments were taken forward in the NHS 5 Year Forward View,[4] and the more recent Long Term Plan[10] has supported significant investment and expansion in CL psychiatry, particularly in the acute and emergency medicine field. A similar revolution is now required in the non-emergent branches of medicine, such as orthopaedics, rheumatology and other elective services.

Relation between Physical Disease and Mental Disorder

The Biomedical versus the Biopsychosocial Model of Illness

The biomedical model of disease, the dominant model in which medicine came to be practised during the twentieth century, assumes that disease can be understood in terms of deviation of a biological variable from the norm. Such a model has the advantage of simplicity and of facilitating scientific investigation into disease. However, the assumption that the nature and extent of biological disease alone will determine illness as well as the subjective experience of the disease ignores the way that social, psychological and behavioural factors influence susceptibility to disease, differences in help-seeking behaviour and the manner in which symptoms are reported, as well as the response to treatment. A patient's experience of a disease will rarely correlate directly with underlying pathophysiological processes.

Engel[11] proposed an alternative biopsychosocial model, which takes into account how biological, psychological and social factors contribute to illness. Here, we examine each of these aspects in patients with co-occurring physical and mental disorders.

Biological Factors Contributing to Psychological Change in Physical Disease

Mental function can be disturbed by physical disease either as a direct result of structural brain damage or as a consequence of brain dysfunction from systemic causes (Box 19.1). The structural brain damage could be focal (cerebral tumour, stroke) or diffuse (degenerative disorders, infections, multiple sclerosis); these disorders are more extensively described in Chapter 8. The systemic causes can include infection, endocrine disorders and metabolic disorders, which can lead to psychiatric symptoms (see also Chapter 16). Mood disorders may also be a paraneoplastic manifestation of cancer. Delirium is a common but often under-diagnosed mental complication of a wide variety of physical diseases.

An organic cause should be suspected in people presenting with a new mental disorder who are already known to have a premorbid co-existing physical disorder. In these instances, comparing the timing of the onset of the mental symptoms with the nature of the physical disease, its onset and treatment may provide valuable clues. If the underlying physical condition can be treated or ameliorated, then the mental disorder may also show some improvement. However, it is not always clear whether the presenting mental symptoms are the result of the underlying physical disease or are a consequence of treatment, such as steroid treatment in systemic lupus erythematosus where there is cerebral involvement. Correlating measures of physical disease activity (where these are available) with the course of the mental disorder may help to clarify whether the disease process or the treatment is the likely cause.

Box 19.1 Physical diseases causing mental disorder

Structural brain disease

- Focal – cerebral tumour, abscess, stroke, subdural haemorrhage
- Diffuse – degenerative disorders, infections, multiple sclerosis, hydrocephalus

Systemic disturbances

- Infection
- Endocrine disorders
- Metabolic disorders
- Paraneoplastic manifestation of cancer

Mental Disorder as a Direct Side Effect of Medical Treatment

Many drugs are associated with mood disorder or cognitive impairment. Some examples are listed in Box 19.2.

The assessment of a mental disorder in a medically ill person should include a comprehensive recent drug history, and drug-induced disorders should be considered in the differential diagnosis. As with physical disease, the temporal relation between the drug therapy and the onset of mental symptoms should be noted. Non-pharmacological treatments that may affect mood or cognitive function include cranial irradiation and renal dialysis.

Physical Disorder as a Consequence of Psychiatric Disorder

Psychiatric disorders have been shown to predispose individuals to some physical disorders. For example, the increased risk of cardiovascular and cerebrovascular disease in people with mental disorder has been known for many decades.[12–14] Some of the increased risk of physical disorders may be associated with treatments for psychiatric disorders. Michelson[15] described the increased risk of reduced bone mineral density in women with a current or past history of major depression, although SSRIs have been subsequently found to also significantly reduce bone mineral density independent of the incidence of depression itself.[16] Similarly, the increased risk of diabetes with second-generation antipsychotics has now been conclusively proven, although people with schizophrenia already have an increased prevalence of impaired glucose homeostasis at the onset of the disorder, before antipsychotics are prescribed.[17] Therefore, the psychiatric and physical disorders may share common risk factors, including genetic risk and early developmental risk factors such as premature birth and early childhood adversity. There appears to be a particularly strong link between psychiatric disorders and physical disorders associated with impaired inflammatory responses – for example, people with depression are more likely to develop psoriatic arthropathy and rheumatoid arthritis (and vice versa) even when controlling for other factors.[18,19] Importantly, the treatment of depression reduces this risk,[20] leading to the inflammatory hypothesis of depression[21] and schizophrenia.[22] In both conditions, the hypothesis postulates that inflammation is often neurotoxic. In acute states, as in acute encephalitis, this can be life-threatening, whereas in chronic inflammation, this can lead to long-term impairments – sometimes termed 'smouldering inflammation'.[23] Elevated levels of pro-inflammatory chemicals such as cytokines have been found in the blood and cerebrospinal fluid with depression and schizophrenia.[24,25]

Box 19.2 Drugs associated with mental disorders

Drugs associated with depression

- Beta-blockers
- Calcium channel blockers
- H_2 receptor antagonists
- Proton pump inhibitors
- Anti-Parkinsonian drugs
- Corticosteroids
- Cancer chemotherapeutic drugs
- Interferon
- Roaccutane

Drugs associated with psychosis or delirium

- Anti-Parkinsonian drugs
- Digoxin
- Beta-blockers
- Anticholinergic drugs
- Anticonvulsants
- Corticosteroids
- Thyroxine
- Opiates
- Hypnotics

Psychological Factors in Physical Disease

Lloyd[26] categorised the factors influencing the psychological response to physical disease in three ways: those related to the patient, those related to the nature of the illness and those related to the social environment. Patient factors include premorbid attitudes or personality, age and life experiences before and at the onset of the illness. In terms of illness factors, the chronicity of physical illness may be a major influence on the persistence of the psychiatric disturbance. However, the psychological meaning the condition has for the patient appears to matter more than its objective severity. This is true of both psychiatric and physical disorders, but it is particularly important in the former given the epistemic factors and stigma associated with psychiatric disorders as well as the central importance that meaning-making has on wellbeing and health. Epistemic factors refers to the credibility that others, usually people in positions of power (like health care professionals), give to those who offer a different explanation for their experience.[27] Social factors may include those people the patient considers significant, the life stage the person is at, and the presence or absence of litigation, as well as background cultural factors (further discussed in Chapter 17).

There are three main theoretical approaches to understanding a person's psychological reaction to a physical disease: the first has its focus on the cognitive approach, the second on psychodynamic mechanisms and the third weighs the influence of social and behavioural factors.

The Cognitive Approach

Understanding the cognitive approach is important, particularly if cognitive-behavioural methods are to be used in treatment. The key factors influencing patients' reactions to illness are their thoughts, attitudes and beliefs about the illness,[28] that is, the way people come to make sense and give meaning to their experiences. This concept is of central importance in CL psychiatry. Sociologists have also tried to analyse the reasons that lie behind the differences in people's responses to their symptoms and also used the concept of patient attribution to explain important phenomena such as 'illness behaviour'.[29]

A valid explanation of the diversity of the psychological reactions to illness will need to encompass a broad range of cognitions and patient beliefs and then to link them to coping behaviours and functional outcome, as well as to the patient's emotional response to the illness.[30] The self-regulatory model of illness as described by Leventhal[31,32] is useful in this respect. It views illness as 'a problem' and the patient's behaviour or reaction to it as an attempt to 'solve the problem'. In response to a health threat, this model postulates that individuals will pass through three stages. First, they generate a representation in their mind (the patient's own interpretation of the physical problem), and this representation will be linked to their emotional response. Second, these representations will then determine the patient's coping strategy. Third, the patient will appraise the outcome of their strategy. This process goes on in parallel at both a cognitive and an emotional level, and these may also interact. Thus, the initial representation or emotional reaction is crucial in determining the type of coping strategy, but the way the patient appraises the outcome may also feedback onto the illness representation and so modify it (Figure 19.1).

The model hypothesises that there are three processes influencing the way individuals form illness representations, react emotionally and choose the coping strategy they employ as well as how they interpret (appraise) the outcome. First, there are memories of previous illness episodes, which may provoke emotional reactions or physical symptoms (schematic memory). Second, there are memories about other illness episodes, which will determine how the individual will label emotions and illness (conceptual memory). Third, there is the information the individual receives about the illness, which may come from health professionals or other sources – such as family, the media and so on.

Illness representation has at least five attributes:[32]

1. Identity (the disease label and its symptom indicator)
2. Timeline (acute, cyclic or chronic)
3. Consequences (physical, social and economic)
4. Antecedent causes (injury, infection, genetic weaknesses)
5. Potential for cure and control

This model provides a useful framework for understanding the patient's cognitive, behavioural and emotional responses to disease and hence is a good guide to planning psychological interventions. Patients should be questioned in the five areas suggested in the model to gain a picture of their internal model of the illness. These illness models shape people's health-protective behaviour, how they recover and their perceptions of disability. In a study of patients with a first episode of myocardial infarction, the patient's initial perceptions of the illness were important determinants of attendance at cardiac rehabilitation, return to work, functional disability and sexual dysfunction.[33] Among patients with rheumatoid arthritis, chronic obstructive pulmonary disease or psoriasis, these illness perceptions, coping variables and the expected medical variables were all significantly related to functional outcome.[34] This is true not just for chronic illnesses, but also in the acute phase after traumatic life-changing injury, in which appraisals as described here mediate the response to the consequences of the injury, adaptation to disability and long-term distress.[35] For women who have had a mastectomy, those with an avoidant style of coping tended to have more long-lasting depression as well as a greater loss of libido.[36] A patient's belief system will also influence concordance with treatment: medication beliefs are more powerful predictors of reported concordance than clinical sociodemographic factors.[37]

The Psychodynamic Approach

The psychodynamic concept of defence mechanisms provides another way of making sense of the ways in which patients react to their illness. Psychiatric referrals may be made for patients who seem – to the clinical team – to be reacting to their illness in an unusual or inappropriate way. A defence mechanism (or a combination of defence mechanisms) may

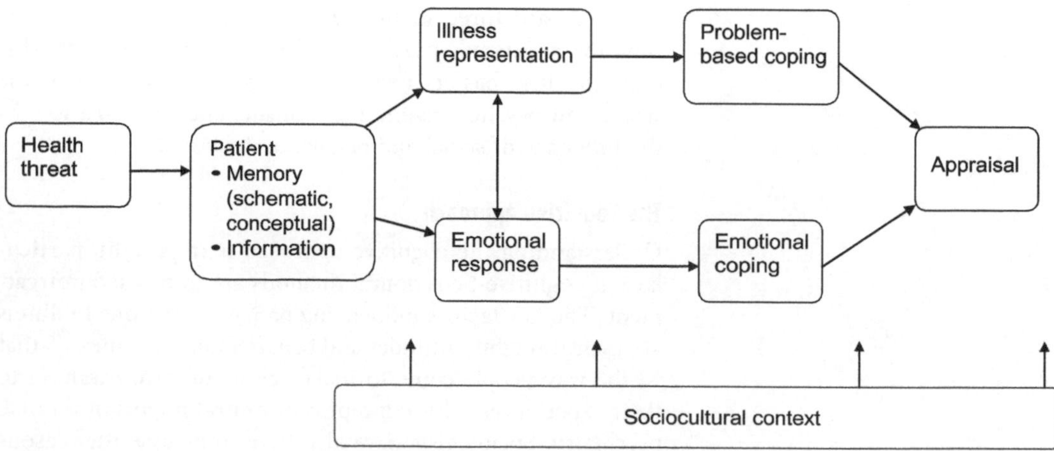

Figure 19.1 Cognitive model of reaction to illness. (adapted from Leventhal et al.[32])

be used to manage the difficult emotions provoked by a physical illness.

- Denial refers to a common defence mechanism in which patients may not take in a serious diagnosis, or not deal with it appropriately, and this may lead to a referral from the medical team. Denial can also serve as a short-term adaptive mechanism, enabling the patient to continue to function. Where it leads to delay in seeking medical help – or interferes with treatment adherence or establishing therapeutic relationships – it becomes maladaptive.
- Regression refers to the patient adopting a pattern of behaviour appropriate to an earlier stage of development. Some patients exhibit a child-like dependency on staff, which may be adaptive if it permits them to accept the care and help they need, but it can equally interfere with processes that require more active patient involvement, such as rehabilitation.
- Displacement refers to the transfer of powerful emotions from situations or objects with which they are normally associated to other objects that will give rise to less distress. In tandem with projective mechanisms, this may result in the distress being directed at clinical staff rather than at the illness itself. This may take the form of patients becoming angry or hostile with the staff caring for them for no apparent or logical reason. Staff understandably feel bewildered by such strange and hostile responses and may seek guidance.

Social Factors

Social Factors Influencing Morbidity

In a biopsychosocial model of understanding illness, factors beyond the individual – principally family, community and societal influences – also need to be taken into account. At its broadest, the relation between health and social circumstances is well established. The Whitehall study of British civil servants highlighted the relation of both morbidity and mortality to socioeconomic status.[38] This association between socioeconomic status and mortality is observed where the former has been measured in a variety of different ways, such as occupation, income, material assets, education or composite indices of deprivation.[39] The relationship is also observed for a range of health outcomes and holds for both sexes. The reasons underlying this association are complex and multifactorial. Social factors correlate with health-risk behaviours such as smoking. There may be differences in investment in health care. Social circumstances determine the availability of social support. Adverse social conditions are likely to increase exposure to psychosocial stressors. Feldman[40] found that mood disorders in medically ill inpatients were associated with several different social problems: financial troubles, dissatisfaction with social life, housing problems, dissatisfaction with being out of work and dissatisfaction with living alone. Of particular interest to a CL psychiatrist is the relationship between social factors and help-seeking behaviour as well as the relationship between psychosocial stressors and psychiatric and physical morbidity.

Social Factors Influencing Help-Seeking Behaviour

Mechanic was among the first to recognise that illness and illness experience are shaped by sociocultural and social-psychological factors. He proposed the term 'illness behaviour', which he defined as 'the ways in which given symptoms may be differently perceived, evaluated and acted (or not acted) upon by different kinds of persons'. He studied how attentive the subjects were to pain and symptoms, which processes affected the way pain and symptoms were defined, what meaning was given to the symptom, how it was labelled socially, the extent to which help was sought, how it changed the patient's lifestyle and what demands were made on others.[29]

Key social factors that may influence a patient's reaction to a medical condition are emotional responses of significant people around the patient (usually the family), the timing of the illness in relation to stages of life, the quality of the doctor–patient relationship, and the possibility of litigation.[26] Sociocultural factors may also influence illness representation, and this in turn will affect the way the illness presents, the health-seeking behaviours and the treatment.[32] In particular, strife, emotional turmoil and family disorganisation increase the risk of treatment non-concordance, while a good doctor–patient relationship can improve concordance.[41]

The emotional response of the key people in the patient's life would have been shaped by their own personal experiences or illness beliefs or shaped as a consequence of the patient's current illness and the effect the present episode is having on the mental health of the family and carers. The way in which the illness behaviours are conceptualised in wider society may also have some bearing on how the patient is perceived by the community.[29] Society sanctions or expects certain behaviours in an ill person. Parsons[42] termed this the 'sick role' and suggested that it has four components:

1. Exemption from normal social responsibilities
2. The right to care and help from others
3. An expectation that the sick person will want to recover
4. An obligation to seek and cooperate with appropriate treatment

Conflict in patient–staff or patient–family relationships may arise when patients are not perceived to be acting in accordance with their expected role. On the one hand, there may be denial of the medical condition and associated non-concordance. On the other hand, conflict can arise when clinical staff or the family perceive that the patient is exaggerating the sick role by becoming overly dependent and demanding. A perceived lack of will to recover is another issue that can strain patient–staff relationships. An example of role conflict can be seen in patients in end-stage renal failure who are undergoing chronic haemodialysis. The patient is wholly dependent on the dialysis for survival and must comply with fluid and dietary restriction, yet the patient is theoretically restored to normality between treatments. This creates uncertainty over whether the patient is sick or healthy and results in a mismatch in the expectation of roles between patients and carers. Role confusion of this type can lead to conflicts over issues of compliance and autonomy in patients undergoing haemodialysis.[43]

Relation between Psychosocial Stressors and Morbidity

An association between a traumatic or stressful life event and onset of serious illness, both physical and psychiatric (such as heart attacks, strokes, AIDS, cancers and depression) is a common enough observation to link the two. The pathways linking exposure to the stressful life event with onset of disease have been extensively studied and include alterations in health behaviours (e.g. health care utilisation), emotional regulation (e.g. fear, anxiety responses) and neurochemical systems (e.g. cortisol), as well as the direct effect of the autonomic nervous system on physiology. The risk of disease incidence appears to be correlated to multiple adverse events (i.e. a cumulative effect), the magnitude of trauma associated with the event (major or catastrophic being more traumatic than lifetime-associated events) and duration (chronic stressful events being worse than acute).[44] However, establishing a causal link is difficult.[45] There is little agreement on what is a significant life event, and there are various other uncertainties: How does one capture chronic stressors as well as discrete events? How can these events be identified and recorded? Are there different degrees of seriousness? What appears to be important is the appraisal the individual makes of the event on their wellbeing and future outcomes, rather than the event itself.

It is important to remember, however, that most people exposed to stressful events do not become ill. In an experiment by Cohen,[46] stressful events were recorded for a sample of 276 healthy participants using the Life Events and Difficulties Schedule. These people were then inoculated with a common cold rhinovirus. As expected, those reporting an enduring stressful life event were more likely to develop a common cold than those who did not report a stressful life event. However, of the 75 participants who reported a stressful life event, 38 (51%) did not develop a common cold. This phenomenon is true even when the event is particularly traumatic. So, stressful life events may not actually trigger the pathogenesis of disease in healthy people but may be one final common pathway, exacerbating already established risk. The relationship is further complicated because stressful life events can have enduring effects. For example, adverse childhood experiences (ACEs) such as childhood maltreatment or exposure to domestic violence can influence subsequent development of disease. A recent large, well-conducted systematic review and meta-analysis published in *The Lancet* found a dose-dependent relationship between ACEs and increased adult risk of harmful substance use and mental disorders (OR >5), cancer, cardiovascular disease, respiratory disease (OR 2–3) and diabetes (OR 2).[47] To complicate things further, life stressors have different impacts and effects depending on gender and life course. For example, losing a spouse is more strongly associated with negative outcomes when it occurs earlier than in later life.[48] These impacts are thought to be more driven by socialised roles and expectations than biological vulnerability; for example, men are more likely to report achievement-related negative experiences as stressful (such as loss of a job), and women are more likely to report interpersonal stressful experiences – for example, on caregiving[49] – which appears to be mediated by socialised gender roles.[50]

The Epidemiology of Physical and Psychiatric Comorbidity

The burden of physical and psychiatric comorbidity to the health service and society as a whole is very large. The prevalence of psychiatric disorders in different medical populations may vary, but epidemiological studies are not well suited to the description of the complex and multifactorial problems encountered in CL psychiatry. Difficulties arise in the realms of case definition, agreed diagnostic criteria, assessment measures, population bias and heterogeneity, as well as the absence of appropriate controls, because suitable control groups are difficult to identify.[51] Additionally, the psychological response to a physical illness is rarely static; different problems emerge at different phases of the illness. Delirium and anxiety may be seen early in response to an acute illness, whereas depression may appear only at a later stage. Mood may improve with recovery from acute illness, but there may be persistent psychological problems in chronic illness.

Case Definition

The continuous distribution of emotional distress means that there will always be a grey area between the normal response to an illness and a pathological reaction (disorder). A psychiatric diagnosis itself will cover different degrees of severity, and epidemiological studies vary in the case definitions and severity thresholds used. In addition, conditions that fail to reach a diagnostic threshold for psychiatric disorder may still be clinically significant in a medical setting. These subclinical conditions may impair quality of life, lead to inappropriate or excessive consultation, result in poor concordance with treatment or an unnecessarily poor physical outcome, and have a destructive effect on family or other relationships.[52] Thus, it may not always be helpful to categorise the psychological problems of medical patients solely in terms of a clinical psychiatric diagnosis, and the role of the psychiatrist in a general hospital setting should not be limited merely to managing risk or assessing and treating psychiatric disorder, but also in helping the multi-disciplinary team alleviate psychological distress where it is impacting upon a patient's recovery.

In practice, it is the psychiatric formulation (which should incorporate all the key psychological, physical, behavioural and social dimensions) that forms the cornerstone of the psychiatric assessment, rather than the formal diagnosis. This formulation should describe the way all the key causal factors interact, as well as provide some sort of an estimate of their relative weighting and so provide an accurate description of psychiatric and physical comorbidity, especially if it is to form the basis of the treatment plan.

Rates in Different Populations

Psychological distress is particularly common in people in general hospitals, affecting 38 per cent of people one month after an emergency admission.[54] Mood disorders such as depression, severe psychiatric conditions such as schizophrenia, and alcohol and substance abuse appear to cluster with a range of physical health conditions, particularly cardiovascular disease, chronic respiratory conditions, cancer, diabetes and musculoskeletal conditions, as well as with chronic infections such as HIV.[42,55] A population-based study of the frequency of psychiatric care before and then again after acute medical admissions found that the numbers receiving psychiatric care increased in the year following admission for a wide range of medical conditions (acute chest pain, cancer, diabetes mellitus and myocardial infarction).[56] These studies suggest that psychiatric disorder is both an early and a late consequence of a medical episode.

In England, the Adult Psychiatric Morbidity Survey 2014 reported that 39 per cent of adults aged 16–74 years were accessing mental health treatment, either through their GP or from more specialist services.[57] Of these, the vast majority (over half) were receiving support for mood and anxiety disorders in the community. About two-thirds of people with a common mental health disorder like depression or an anxiety disorder have at least one other physical health condition, and prevalence rises with age and socioeconomic deprivation, so that 86 per cent of adults aged 45–64 years with a mental health condition living in the most socially deprived areas of England have at least one physical health condition.[58] Thus, it is far more common for a person with a mental health condition to have a concurrent physical health condition than not. The most common of these are chronic painful musculoskeletal conditions (like arthritis), hypertension and asthma.[59]

In those with more serious or complex mental health needs, admission to a psychiatric unit is associated with an elevated risk of mortality for more than five years after discharge. Death from medical causes (particularly vascular events) far exceed death from suicide or other unnatural causes,[60] suggesting that deterioration in mental health is associated with deterioration in physical health. Supporting this hypothesis is a large Australian population-based linkage study that has demonstrated increased rates of hospitalisation for potentially preventable physical health conditions (such as the complications of diabetes, or illnesses that could be prevented through screening or vaccination efforts) in those requiring specialist mental health input in the community.[61] CL Psychiatrists therefore have an important role in supporting the mental health needs of those admitted for physical health conditions and, equally, the physical health needs of those with serious mental health conditions.

Individual Psychiatric Conditions in the Medical Setting

Depressive Disorder

The combination of depression and physical illness is the most common comorbid problem facing the CL psychiatrist.[62] A review of the literature[63] provided a range of estimates for the prevalence of depressive disorder in general hospital inpatients of between 4% and 32%, with a median prevalence of 12%. This is twice that in the general population, for which international studies suggest an average 12-month prevalence of about 5%.[64] Prevalence varies based on condition and setting. Wang et al.[65] found a pooled prevalence of depressive disorder or depressive symptoms of 27% in general hospital outpatients, which was over three times the prevalence in healthy controls. Prevalence varied between 17% and 53% based on specialty, with ENT (53%), dermatology (39%) and neurology (35%) outpatients having the highest prevalence of either depression or depressive symptoms. Importantly, prevalence also varied depending on method of assessment: the Beck Depression Inventory provided higher estimates than the Hospital Anxiety and Depression Scale, and both provided higher estimates than the clinical interview, according to a study conducted in people with cancer.[66]

There may be phenotypical differences in the presentation of depression in general hospital settings compared to in the community or in mental health settings. In 1990, Hawton[67] compared the prevalence of symptoms that met the criteria of the Present State Examination (PSE) in medical patients with and without affective disorder to identify which were the most useful for distinguishing those with an affective disorder in the medical population. Depressed mood, diurnal variation and hopelessness provided a reasonable discrimination for depression; nervous tension, free-floating anxiety and panic attacks, as well as simple phobias, provided an almost-perfect discrimination for anxiety disorder.[67] A later study[68] found anhedonia, low positive affect and psychomotor agitation to be more common in medical inpatients with depression, whereas negative cognitions were more common in depressed psychiatric inpatients. A more recent study from China has reported that weight change, hypersomnia and a tendency of denying emotional or cognitive symptoms are more common in patients with major depressive disorders in general hospitals compared to psychiatric hospitals; although, the results should be interpreted within the context of how depression manifests across different cultures.[69]

Some of the difficulty in diagnosing depression in medically unwell patients may lie in the commonality of somatic symptoms between depression and certain physical conditions. Thus, three of the nine listed key symptoms (weight changes, insomnia and fatigue) for the diagnosis of ICD-11 major depression are somatic symptoms, and they all commonly occur in people who are medically ill. Boland[70] points out that there is consequently a risk of over-diagnosing major depression in these populations. This is of most concern when the presumption of depression delays other medical, neurological or psychological evaluations. Nonetheless, somatic symptoms may still be a helpful pointer to depressive disorder in physically ill patients because these symptoms may arise from both physical and psychological reasons. Forty per cent of those judged not to have a depressive disorder had other psychiatric conditions, particularly dementia, delirium and anxiety disorders.

Other sources of confusion may be an associated grief or other adjustment reaction or the behavioural manifestation of a serious medical condition, both of which may be incorrectly attributed to affective disorder. For example, in a sample of 368 individuals with type 1 diabetes, significant depressive symptomatology as described on the Patient Health Questionnaire was found in more than half of cases, attributed to the emotional distress associated with managing a demanding chronic disease and other life stressors and not necessarily to underlying psychopathology.[71] It should be noted that irrespective of aetiology, psychological distress remains within the preserve of the hospital psychiatrist to help alleviate, and therefore, need is not determined by diagnosis.

Adjustment Disorders

Adjustment disorder is one of the most commonly made psychiatric diagnoses in general hospital settings, particularly after traumatic injuries.[72,73] It is at least as prevalent as depressive disorders. A multi-site, international study found that adjustment disorder could definitely be diagnosed in 12 per cent of consultations, with a further 11 per cent identified as possible cases.[74]

Adjustment disorder was previously considered a subsyndromal condition with multiple, vague symptoms that were difficult to distinguish from a normal reaction to a stressful situation. However, adjustment disorder can have serious implications and is highly associated with suicidality.[75] To counteract these problems, the ICD-11 clearly defines adjustment disorder as a maladaptive reaction, which usually emerges within one month of a significant life stressor and presents with two major aspects:

- Preoccupation with the stressor or its consequences: recurring distressing thoughts, constant worry or rumination
- Failure to adapt: generalised stress response (for example, sleep disturbances or concentration problems) resulting in significant problems in important areas of functioning

The symptoms should not be better explained by another psychiatric disorder and usually resolve within six months, unless the duration of the stressor is longer.

Many stressors, such as the diagnosis of a serious illness or the consequences of traumatic injury in the consultation-liaison setting, persist for many years. In these situations, the Adjustment Disorder – New Module can be used as a screening instrument.[76-78]

Phobic Anxiety Disorder

Specific phobias may develop in the course of a medical illness or their treatment and may persist beyond the illness. Some phobias may be serious enough to interfere with medical investigations or treatment, such as needle phobia or claustrophobia in patients undergoing magnetic resonance imaging or computerised tomography. Conditioned phobic responses may sometimes develop during courses of chemotherapy or radiotherapy and so compromise these treatments.

Organic Mental Disorder

Just under a fifth of people referred to psychiatrists in general hospital settings are because of organic mental disorders, making these among the most common causes for psychiatric referral.[79] Older studies have suggested that the prevalence of organic disorders, as defined by the Mini-Mental State Examination,[80] in general medical wards across all ages is between a quarter and a third of all inpatients.[81] This has been corroborated by more recent epidemiological studies investigating causes of mental incapacity on general medical wards.[82] This is far in excess of rates found in the general population, where cognitive dysfunction is rare below 65 years of age. Structured psychiatric interviews identify cognitive dysfunction in 13–69% of medical admissions of all ages, with acute confusional state (delirium) being the most common, followed by dementia or a combination of both.[83] Acute confusional states occur in up to 80 per cent of critically ill patients requiring intensive care.[84] Across all general hospital settings, acute confusional state is associated with increased mortality and morbidity, increased length of stay in hospital, and discharge to non-residential settings. Administration of potent sedative medication, especially benzodiazepines, is most consistently associated with an increased risk of delirium, whereas early identification and mobilisation/activity reduces burden.

Eating Disorders

Significant eating disorder may result in physical problems from malnutrition or metabolic disturbance from vomiting or purgative and diuretic abuse, requiring medical admission. These complications are described in more detail in Chapter 12. Excessive eating due to psychological problems may result in obesity and other health problems. An abnormal eating pattern may also complicate the management of diabetes mellitus, especially among those who are insulin dependent. Significantly increased rates of eating disorders (15%) and intentional insulin under-treatment (12%) have been reported in young females with diabetes.[51] However, when appropriate non-diabetic control populations were included in an interview-based study of young females with diabetes, the latter did not have a higher prevalence of clinical eating disorders.[85] Nevertheless, the comorbidity of an eating disorder with insulin-dependent diabetes mellitus poses a major therapeutic challenge, as there will be difficulties in obtaining good glycaemic control and dangers of either diabetic ketoacidosis or hypoglycaemia. The same study confirmed that disordered eating was common, and the under-use of insulin with an intention to control weight was widespread, even among those without an obvious eating disorder.

Post-traumatic Stress Disorder

The hospital admission itself may have been caused by an incident that was both physically and psychologically traumatic – for example, a serious accident, an assault or a natural disaster – or the trauma may have occurred during the course of hospital treatment, such as a traumatic obstetric delivery or the memory of a frightening episode of delirium.

One prospective follow-up study of a consecutive series of inpatients on a burns unit[86] found a prevalence of 35.3% for post-traumatic stress disorder at 2 months, with higher rates at 6 and 12 months. The development of the disorder did not correlate with the severity of the burns but with less perceived emotional support and with greater emotional distress immediately after admission. This suggests that the individual's psychological state immediately following the event may be more predictive of the outcome than the degree of trauma.

Alcohol-Related Disorders

Alongside mood and adjustment disorders and organic mental disorders, alcohol use disorders are among the most common reasons for referral to psychiatrists in general hospital settings. The World Health Organization defines several disorders of alcohol use:

- Hazardous drinking is not a diagnostic term but a pattern of alcohol consumptions that increases someone's risk of harm. Currently, the National Institute for Health and Care Excellence (NICE) suggests that drinking more than 14 units of alcohol a week – by either men or women – increases risk of harm.
- Harmful drinking is a pattern of alcohol consumptions that is causing mental or physical damage. Some also include harmful social consequences as evidence of harm. NICE recommends considering alcohol-related harms when a man drinks more than 50 units a week and a woman more than 35.
- Alcohol dependence is a syndrome of behavioural, cognitive and physiological features that include a strong desire to consume alcohol and difficulties in controlling its use.
- Intoxication and withdrawal are other alcohol-related disordered states.

Box 19.3 The CAGE questionnaire

- Have you ever felt you should **C**ut down on your drinking?
- Have people **A**nnoyed you by criticising your drinking?
- Have you ever felt bad or **G**uilty about your drinking?
- Have you ever had a drink first thing in the morning or to get rid of a hangover (**E**ye-opener)?

Scoring: one point for yes to each question.

The original paper[121] suggested that one positive response should lead to further enquiry. Generally, a score of two or more is considered to be clinically significant and found to have good sensitivity and specificity for alcohol misuse or dependence.[122]

The Alcohol Use Disorders Identification Test (AUDIT) was developed by the WHO to screen for these condition (see also the CAGE questionnaire in Box 19.3).[87] Approximately one in five patients in UK hospitals is using alcohol harmfully, and one in ten is alcohol-dependent according to a systematic review conducted in 2019.[88] These figures are eight and ten times greater respectively than the rates in the general population of the UK, according to the most recent Adult Psychiatric Morbidity Survey.[89] Alcohol misuse and dependence may lead to a variety of health problems, including heart, liver, pancreatic, cerebral and vascular diseases, accidents and suicide. Also, the complications of alcoholism may cause management difficulties in the general hospital, especially behavioural problems as a result of intoxication and alcohol withdrawal. The latter sometimes goes unrecognised and untreated because staff are unaware of the extent of the patient's dependence or the degree of cognitive impairment, and these patients may present with an apparently unexplained confusional state of acute onset.

The Impact of Physical and Psychiatric Comorbidity

Psychological and physical comorbidity may increase the burden on the individual, the family and the health care system, as well as influence the outcome of the physical condition itself (see Box 19.4).

Survival and Disease Outcome

There has been increasing interest in whether psychological factors influence the outcome of a variety of physical diseases, such as cancer and myocardial infarction (MI). Psychological factors studied have ranged from diagnosable psychiatric disorder to psychological responses to the disease, such as coping strategies or adjustment to illness. A prospective cohort study of women with early-stage breast cancer indicated that a high score on the Hospital Anxiety and Depression (HAD) scale and the helplessness/hopelessness score on the Mental Adjustment to Cancer (MAC) scale had quite a large

Box 19.4 Impact of physical and psychological comorbidity

Patient

- Survival and disease outcome
- Functional disability
- Quality of life
- Suicide

Family

- Relationships
- Mental health
- Financial/occupational status

Health care use

- Medication non-adherence
- Length of hospital stay
- Frequency of consultations

detrimental effect on five-year survival rates.[90] Helplessness/hopelessness as defined by the MAC scale affected event-free survival at five years with a hazard ratio of 1.55, and HADS-defined depression (score equal to or over 11) influenced five-year survival with a hazard ratio of 3.59.

With regard to survival after MI, studies have also suggested that sub-threshold psychiatric disturbance (as seen by raised Beck Depression Inventory scores in the absence of definitive diagnosis) may also have a significant influence on the outcome of MI. The risk associated with depression was greatest in patients with frequent premature ventricular contractions, which suggests that an arrhythmic mechanism may be the link between psychological factors and sudden cardiac death. A more recent study of patients who developed depression after MI found that high levels of social support, through an alleviation of depressive symptoms, may protect patients from the negative cardiovascular consequences of a depressive episode.[91] The TRIUMPH study is a recent observational multicentre American cohort study that enrolled 4,062 patients aged ≥18 years with acute myocardial infarction (AMI) from 24 US hospitals. Overall, 759 (18.7%) patients met PHQ-9 criteria for depression, and 231 (30.4%) were treated. Compared with 3,303 patients without depression, the 231 patients with treated depression had one-year mortality rates that were not significantly different (6.1% vs 6.7%). By contrast, the 528 patients with untreated depression had higher one-year mortality when compared with patients without depression (10.8% vs 6.1%, adjusted hazard ratio R=1.91). The authors concluded that, although depression in patients with AMI is associated with increased long-term mortality, this association may be confined to patients with untreated depression. The study highlights the importance of detecting and treating depression following MI, but further work is needed to establish the efficacy of such an intervention.[92] Delirium is now a well-recognised risk after open heart surgery. Recent data suggest an age-dependent incidence of post-cardiac surgery delirium: 21.4% of patients aged ≥65 suffered from post-operative delirium (POD), and POD was observed in 33.5% of patients aged >80. Patients with delirium are more likely to have a prolonged hospitalisation, a pre-existing dementia and to die during hospitalisation.[93]

Functional Disability and Quality of Life

Psychiatric comorbidity can influence perceived health status as well as functional ability, and it may also impair social and occupational function. A prospective follow-up study of patients with MI in Oxfordshire found that initial emotional distress (as defined by a HAD score of over 19) predicted poor symptomatic, psychological and social outcome at 3 and 12 months after MI,[94] as assessed by the 36-item Medical Outcomes Study short form (SF-36) and HAD scales.

Functional ability and quality of life are particularly relevant in patients with chronic medical conditions. A large cross-sectional study of patients enrolled in a study funded by the US Veterans Administration looked at the relation between depressive symptoms and scores on the Health Related Quality of Life (HRQoL) scale.[95] Among 1,252 patients who completed relevant questionnaires, 59 per cent had significant depressive symptoms as determined by Hopkins' Symptoms Checklist 20 (SCL-20) using a cut-off of 1.75. Those with depressive symptoms had worse scores on both general health measures (SF-36) and disease-specific measures (Seattle Obstructive Lung Disease Questionnaire – SOLDQ), which were both statistically and clinically significant. Linear regression analysis indicated that 11–18% of the variance in physical functioning could be attributed to depressive symptoms alone. The contribution of depression to the variance in HRQoL score was greater than those due to age, educational level, marital status, smoking history or the number of comorbid medical conditions. The results were compatible with previous observations that the correlation between objective measures of pulmonary function, such as spirometry and quality of life as measured by the HRQoL, was weak and that depression or anxiety (or both) accounted for a significant amount of the variance of the HRQoL scores.

Psychological factors, cognitive responses and coping style may have an important influence on outcome. Scharloo[34] looked at the influence of coping strategies and illness perceptions on the levels of daily functioning in patients with rheumatoid arthritis, chronic obstructive pulmonary disease or psoriasis in a cross-sectional study of 244 patients. Coping strategies were assessed using the Utrecht Coping List, and illness perceptions were assessed by an interview and the Illness Perception Questionnaire. They found that a strong illness identity, passive coping, a belief in a long illness duration, a belief in strong consequences and an unfavourable score on medical variables were associated with worse outcomes in the areas of physical and social function. In contrast, coping behaviours involving seeking social support as well as beliefs in the controllability/curability of the disease were significantly associated with better functioning. In a prospective study of the initial perception of MI, belief that the illness could be controlled or cured was a factor influencing attendance at a cardiac rehabilitation course, whereas the perception that the illness would last a long time and have serious consequences was associated with a delay in return to work.[33] These findings emphasise that the way patients think and feel about their physical disorder may have a profound influence on outcome and, therefore, needs to be taken into account in the treatment plan.

Suicide

Physical health conditions have long been associated with increased risk of suicide.[96–98] A case-control study of 2,674 people who had died by suicide across eight mental health networks in the USA, compared with controls who had died by other means, found that nearly all physical health conditions significantly increased risk of suicide, even when controlling for the co-occurrence of mental health and substance use disorders.[99] The risk was highest for people with traumatic brain injury, sleep disorders and HIV/AIDS. Similarly, almost all physical health conditions are associated with an increased risk of first suicidal ideation with cardiovascular, cerebrovascular, non-cancer painful conditions and respiratory conditions being associated with suicidal acts, as well as epilepsy, cancer and heart attack/stroke being associated with planned attempts.[100] The association appears to be dose-dependent: having more than one physical health condition increases risk further (although the additional risk conferred by each individual condition decreases).

Given these statistics, it should come as no surprise then that those discharged from general hospitals are three times more likely to die by suicide within a year of discharge than those discharged from psychiatric hospitals.[101] Almost a quarter of these deaths occur within three months of discharge; therefore, the psychiatrist in the general hospital has an important role in educating general health care professionals, helping to identify those with suicidal risk factors and providing appropriate evaluation and follow-up.

Treatment Non-concordance

CL psychiatric referrals are sometimes made when there is non-concordance to treatment that could have serious consequences. The problem is widespread. In one study based at a university hospital, more than a third of the patients in a medical clinic took less than the prescribed amount of one or more medications.[102]

Stoudemire and Thompson[41] have reviewed the literature on the multiplicity of factors influencing concordance. They found no consistent correlation between the severity of the illness and sociodemographic factors with concordance. Lack of basic knowledge about their medication, more complex regimens and unpleasant side effects all increased the risk of non-concordance. Certain side effects – in particular, excessive sedation, gastrointestinal distress, anticholinergic symptoms, sexual dysfunction and changes of physical appearance – were found to be much more likely to lead to a complete discontinuation of medication.

Patients' beliefs about their illness, the attitudes of other family members and the quality of the doctor–patient relationship may also influence treatment adherence. Concordance is higher if patients felt susceptible to the illness or its complications, if they believed the illness might have severe consequences for their life, if they also believed that the prescribed medication would probably be effective, and if they saw no major obstacle in engaging with the treatment. However, simple attempts at patient education about their illness as a sole measure were not effective. Concordance was better when the doctor and patient agreed on the treatment approach, the doctor–patient relationship was good, and there was good communication between the two. Strife, emotional turmoil and family disorganisation increased the risk of non-concordance, whereas a close and stable family or other social support facilitated it. Psychiatric disorders (major depression, bipolar disorder, schizophrenia, dementia/delirium and alcoholism), personality disorders and the maladaptive defence mechanism of denial were the main psychiatric factors associated with poor adherence, through a variety of different mechanisms.

Health Care Use

The addition of psychiatric comorbidity to a physical illness increases health service utilisation; this has been confirmed in several health care systems. However, the pattern of use varies. A review by the Health Foundation of England's 2013/14 hospital admissions data found that people with mental ill health had three times more Accident & Emergency (A&E) attendances and five times more emergency inpatient admissions than people without mental disorders.[103] Only a fifth of the emergency attendances were to support their mental health.

Correspondingly, people with mental disorders had less planned inpatient care, and for common inpatient procedures, they were more likely to be admitted as emergencies rather than planned admissions. These findings suggest that opportunities for planned care are being missed for people with mental disorders. The disparity appears to be highest among the younger age groups; a population-wide linkage study in New South Wales found that rates of potentially preventable hospitalisations (such as for vaccine preventable illnesses) in people aged 20–29 with mental disorders were equivalent to rates in over-60-year olds without mental disorders.[61]

When admitted, people with mental disorders are more likely to have a prolonged length of stay, increasing their risk of hospital-acquired infections and increasing health care costs. A retrospective study of 16,898 admissions of patients with a primary diagnosis of lung or colorectal cancer, chronic obstructive pulmonary disease, type 2 diabetes, ischaemic heart disease and stroke between 2010 and 2015 found a mean length of stay that was 8 to 109 per cent longer than for those without mental disorder for the same physical health condition.[104]

Psychiatric Assessment in the General Hospital Setting

Assessment by Non-psychiatrists

Most depression in the community, especially of mild to moderate severity, is now routinely diagnosed and treated by general practitioners. For episodes occurring in the medical setting, it is the physicians, surgeons, nursing and other clinical staff who are in the best position to recognise the signs of possible comorbidity and respond to the patient's psychological needs. However, research suggests that over half of all medical patients who have a diagnosable psychiatric disorder will have the latter undetected by the medical or nursing staff caring for them.[40,105–107] There are several reasons for this: patients may not give any clues suggestive of a psychological disorder, attention may focus exclusively on the somatic disorder during a medical interview, lack of privacy may inhibit patients from admitting to psychological difficulties, there is commonly also a lack of awareness that a psychiatric disorder may exacerbate a patient's physical symptoms, and finally, some clinicians lack the confidence to assess a patient's mental state.[108]

Maguire[109] identified a number of 'distancing tactics' when observing doctors and nurses who were talking to real or simulated patients suffering from a terminal illness. Medical staff may not enquire directly about emotional difficulties, on the assumption that patients would disclose them if they were present. They may try to alleviate distress by explaining that it is understandable or likely to be experienced by anybody in the same predicament. False reassurances may be made by making more positive statements than are warranted by the circumstances. On those occasions when a patient mentions both physical and psychological difficulties, the doctor may follow up only on the physical symptoms or deflect difficult questions by advising the patient to seek advice from someone else. Doctors and nurses tend to spend less time with patients who are dying and may even avoid them altogether. Clinical staff are usually unaware that they have adopted such strategies, yet they will tend to discourage patients from disclosing their inner anxieties and so create a barrier to effective psychological care.

Screening and Standardised Tests

Screening tests have been suggested as one way to help clinicians identify those with a psychiatric disorder. Instruments used to screen for common mental disorders include the Patient Health Questionnaire 9,[110] the Hospital Anxiety and Depression Scale (HADS),[111] the Beck Depression Inventory (BDI),[112] the Geriatric Depression Scale[113] and the Symptoms Check List 8[114] (see also the Abbreviated Mental Test Score in Box 19.5).

Box 19.5 The Abbreviated Mental Test Score[123]

- Age
- Time [correct to nearest hour]
- Three-item address (e.g. 42 West Street) [registration and recall at end of test]
- Month
- Year
- Name of place [If not in hospital, ask type of place or area of town]
- Date of birth
- Start of First World War
- Name of present monarch
- Count from 20 to 1 (backwards)

Score: abnormal when six or less.

Screening patients prior to their consultation allows for more efficient assessment, improved recognition of patient concerns and more actions being taken to address those concerns.[115] There are, however, a number of difficulties in using these screening instruments. First, some patients may have difficulty in completing a questionnaire. Second, the sensitivity and specificity will depend on the cut-off scores used, and the prevalence of the condition in the population will determine the positive predictive value of the test.[116] The positive predictive value (the proportion of those tested positive who have the condition) of screening instruments in different medical conditions can vary very widely; Meakin[117] gave the range as 19–92%, with a median figure of around 60%. This means that between a third to a half of the patients scoring above the cut-off may not actually have the psychiatric condition identified by the screening instrument. Positive results should prompt the clinician not only to make further enquiries about other symptoms of mood disorder and attempt to make a psychiatric diagnosis, but also to assess whether any of the items contributing to the raised score could be explained by the medical condition itself and whether the distress was only of a transient nature. It should also be borne in mind that because the specificity of a screening test rarely reaches 100 per cent, some patients with a definite psychiatric disorder will score below the cut-off and therefore be missed.

Despite a huge amount of effort in devising these screening instruments and considerable research enthusiasm aimed at detecting psychiatric disorders, it appears that the routine administration of anxiety and depression questionnaires in non-psychiatric settings does not translate into an increased rate of intervention or improved outcomes. Most screening questionnaires are designed for one specific problem, and so multiple questionnaires would be necessary to screen general hospital patients for all mental disorders. The need for a multiplicity of questionnaires (in different formats and requiring the handling of many sheets of paper) would make it difficult, if not impossible, to implement paper-based routine screening in a busy general medical setting. Incorporating these questionnaires on to data platforms with touch screens may be a better option and has begun to be implemented in clinical settings.[118]

Two-stage screening procedures (see later in this chapter) might be of use for patients at higher risk of mental disorder in the general hospital setting. Thus, patients with frequent admissions, longer length of stay, poor disease control, intolerance to drugs and poor pain control probably should be screened because, in these groups, it may be important not to miss cases of psychiatric disorder. Another approach is to use screening tools in conjunction with clinical interview to improve identification of mental disorder; when combined with care coordination, screening has promise in improving outcomes for people with co-occurring mental and physical health conditions, although the approach is resource intensive.[119,120]

Referrals to CL Psychiatry

Referrals to CL psychiatry generally come from clinicians in other medical specialties, usually from a member of the medical or nursing staff, or occasionally from other disciplines, such as physiotherapy or occupational therapy. Because the patient is already under clinical care for a physical problem, which some patients will strongly believe to be entirely physically caused, there will sometimes be a reluctance to accept a psychiatric referral. Some patients may interpret these referrals as 'They don't believe me' or 'They think this is all in my mind' or 'They think I am being a nuisance' or 'I am being palmed off' and so forth. This makes it even more important for the general hospital clinician making the referral to allow adequate time, which may mean fitting in the assessment between investigations or treatment sessions. A few patients cannot tolerate a full interview, and in these cases, more than one visit may be required.

Box 19.6 outlines the elements of the assessment. It is often helpful to open the CL psychiatry interview by enquiring how the patient felt about the referral, as this will elicit any fears or misunderstandings surrounding a psychiatric referral. It is important to address these issues from the outset and engage the patient in the interview and generally clear the air. Starting with the medical problem will often entail initially taking an extended physical history, and this may be especially helpful when engaging patients with suspected somatoform disorders, who will appreciate the time spent eliciting and understanding their physical symptoms. This may also facilitate moving on to other aspects of the history. In cases where it seems that the physical illness has led to the psychiatric disorder, the time course of the mental symptoms should be clearly noted in relation to other events, such as the development of the physical problems, their investigation and treatment. If medication is suspected as a cause of the mental symptoms, it is important to record the present medication(s), as well as when they were this started or stopped.

Box 19.6 Consultation-liaison psychiatry assessment

1. Understand the purpose of the referral from the referrer
2. Engage the patient, and allow time to discuss the purpose and nature of the assessment
3. Assess the patient:
   - History of the physical problems
   - Nature, time course, treatments, impact of the physical condition
   - Psychiatric history, including relationship between life events, physical problems and psychological symptoms
   - Assessment of coping styles, risk factors
   - Patient's understanding of physical/psychological difficulties
4. Interview significant others
5. Review medical notes/medication chart
6. Formulate a management plan
7. Feedback to patient and referrer

Looking at the current drug chart can also help tell whether the patient is following the prescribed drug regimen.

CL Psychiatry Assessment

Psychiatric assessments of hospital inpatients are often conducted on general wards, which are usually very busy places. It is better practice to find a private room where the assessment can take place without risk of interruption or being overheard. The patient's medical needs will also have to be taken into account, and time to explain the reasons for the referral and why a psychological approach may help the patient. If the referral is for bodily distress disorder (formerly somatoform disorder), for example, it is important to emphasise to the patient that the referral does not negate the reality of the symptoms in question, but its purpose is more to widen the scope for understanding how the symptom(s) came about and to find better ways of managing them. The liaison psychiatrist must also be quite clear about the reasons for the referral (Box 19.7), and this may necessitate a discussion with the referrer before the assessment. Seeking the views of the nursing staff who care for the patient and access to the medical notes will also provide important additional information.

The main part of the assessment should then continue, covering the usual items in a standard psychiatric interview. A common mnemonic to assess pain is SOCRATES (site, onset, character, radiation, associated features, timing, exacerbating/relieving factors, severity). This mnemonic can be modified to allow for a brief but satisfactory assessment of psychological factors:

- Symptoms (of a mental disorder)
- Onset

Box 19.7 Reasons for referral to consultation-liaison psychiatry

- Suspected mental illness and/or advice on treatment
- Assessment of risk, especially in relation to a patient who has suicidal or paranoid ideas or who is aggressive towards others
- Disturbed or disruptive behaviour from suspected mental disorder
- Refusal of treatment or erratic adherence to treatment
- Help with assessment of capacity to consent to or refuse treatment
- Non-organic symptoms
- Request for transfer to a psychiatric unit

- Course: fluctuating, constant, worsening
- Response (of the individual): impact on social/occupational functioning, activities of daily living
- Associated features: sleep disturbance, fatigue, drug misuse (of prescribed and non-prescribed substances)
- Timing: independent or aligned to physical health condition for which the patient is in the general hospital
- Exacerbating/relieving factors: medicine, rest, activity
- Suicidality: thoughts vs acts, active or passive wish to die/escape

The family and previous psychiatric history are important, as a biological predisposition to recurrent psychiatric disorder would increase the risk of a relapse during periods of physical disease. There is a strong association between a history of psychiatric illness and affective disorder in general medical in- patients.[40] The personal and social history as well as premorbid personality also contribute to the assessment of personality, and it is useful to know the coping style the patient has shown during previous stressful points in life.

The assessing psychiatrist is often concerned with elucidating a diagnosis, but presenting problems may not always fit into a neat psychiatric category, and significant psychological morbidity may still be present in the absence of a conventionally diagnosable mental disorder. It is important to explore patients' beliefs concerning their symptoms, diagnosis and treatment; their reaction to the illness; their understanding of the prognosis; and how they feel they have been dealt with by the medical profession. A similar range of issues should be covered with the patient's family or carers. In cases where cognitive impairment is suspected, a history from an informant is essential. It may also be helpful to obtain further information from the general practitioner, especially where there is complicated or extensive medical or psychiatric history.

Diagnosis

As previously discussed, it is often neither possible nor useful to categorise the patient's problem under a single diagnosis, and it may be preferable to use a multidimensional system. A formulation that covers the biological, individual psychological and social factors that have contributed to the presenting problem helps to make sense of the patient's current problems and should be recorded in the medical notes (Figure 19.2). If this can then be shared with the patient and the referrer, it will help to establish a good therapeutic relationship.

In formulating a management plan, the patient's medical needs and the reason for the referral need to be taken into account. The plan may include suggestions for psychological input and psychotropic medication or whether there is any need for further follow-up by the psychiatrist. There should also be guidance to the ward staff on how to manage difficult behaviours or how to meet the patient's emotional needs. There may also be recommendations for family support or social input, which may involve professionals or other voluntary agencies outside the medical and liaison psychiatry team.

It is essential to let the referrer know precisely what information has been given to the patient. The written plan should also clarify who is expected to take responsibility for each item in it. For outpatient assessments, the summary letter should include the formulation, the management plan and an outline of the patient's perspective, and this should be forwarded to the relevant clinical team(s) as well as the patient's general practitioner.

Management of Liaison Psychiatry Patients

Correct diagnosis and correct weighting of the various aetiological factors are essential in preparing a useful formulation in CL psychiatry, and this is a major part of the skill of the CL psychiatrist. The other important skill is the ability to carry the hospital clinical staff along with the treatment plan. This will entail spending time with the medical and nursing team and discussing the psychiatric and psychosocial aspects of the case with them and, in some cases, involving the family as well. Teaching, training and upskilling hospital clinical staff is an important responsibility of the liaison psychiatrist, and sometimes, managing the anxiety of the referrer is as important as managing the symptoms in the referred.

Psychotropic Medication

Psychotropic medication will be considered where there is immediate significant risk to the patient or others; this may be suicidal risk or result from behavioural disturbance or severity of the mental illness. In a physically ill patient, it is particularly important to pay attention to the potential for medication to exacerbate particular physical symptoms, to drug interactions and the potential for drug toxicity. Therefore, it is important to take a full medical and drug history, paying particular attention to any history of cardiovascular disease, hepatic and renal dysfunction, epilepsy or cognitive dysfunction. Any proposed drug should be cross-checked for its use in the presence of organ dysfunction as well as the patient's existing medication with, for example, the current *British National Formulary* or the *Psychotropic Drug Directory* (Box 19.8).[124] The starting dose of

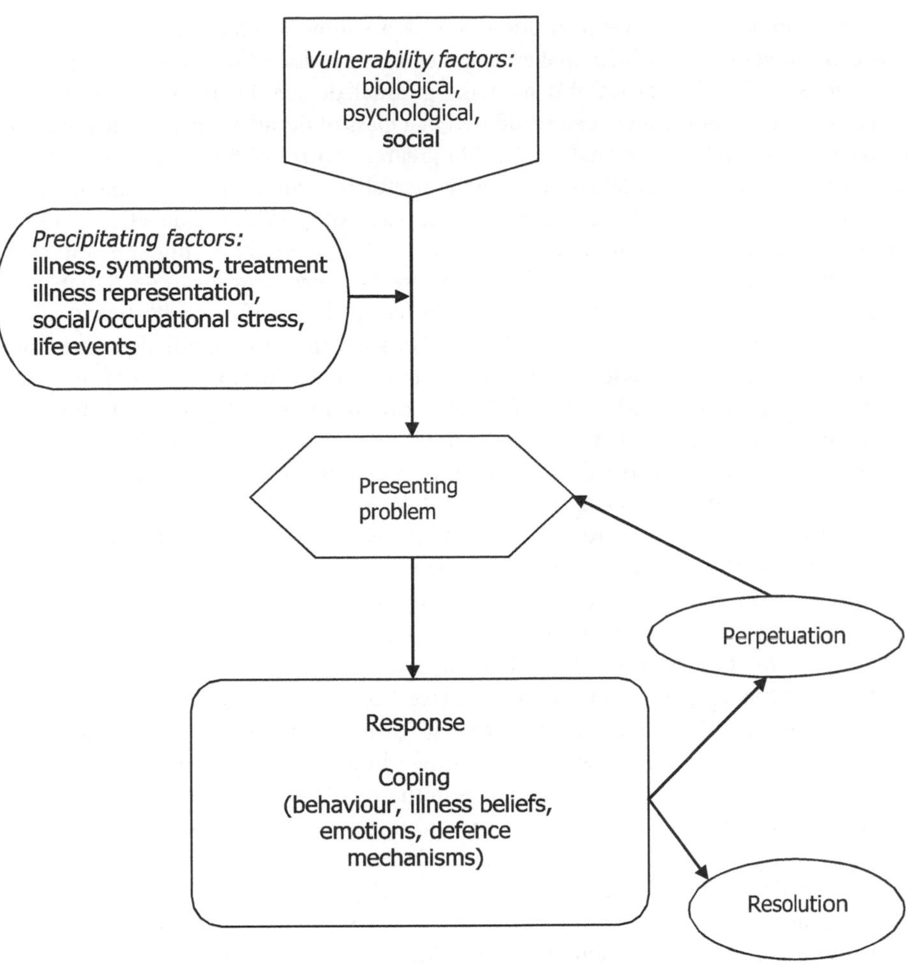

Figure 19.2 Diagnostic formulation in consultation-liaison psychiatry.

Box 19.8 Use of psychotropic medication in the medical setting

Consider Existing Physical Disease

Will the psychotropic medication exacerbate existing problems, such as:

- Cardiac dysfunction
- Hypertension/postural hypotension
- Glycaemic control in diabetes mellitus
- Weight gain/loss
- Gastrointestinal bleeds
- Neurological disorders, including epilepsy

Are there conditions that require dose adjustment?

- Reduced absorption (intestinal disease or surgery, malabsorption)
- Altered distribution (hypoproteinaemia)
- Reduced metabolism/excretion (hepatic/renal dysfunction)

Guidance on Prescribing in Specific Physical Illnesses

- *British National Formulary* (especially appendices on liver disease, renal impairment, pregnancy and breast feeding)
- *Bazire Psychotropic Drug Directory*

Consider Drug Interactions

- *British National Formulary*'s appendix on interactions

psychotropic drugs may need to be reduced in medically ill patients as they are especially likely to be sensitive to the side effects of psychotropic drugs.

Antidepressants

In a patient with mild depression of recent onset, the first course of action will be watchful waiting with a review after a couple of weeks, rather than proceeding directly to psychotropic medication. It is helpful to address any other psychosocial factors identified at the first assessment, such as ensuring a good understanding of the medical condition; assisting adjustment to the illness or coming to terms with the consequences of treatment, such as loss or disfigurement; encouraging helpful coping behaviour and so on, while also monitoring the mood.

Antidepressants need to be considered for patients who present with major depression where a psychotherapeutic approach may be inappropriate or insufficient. When used appropriately, they increase the chance of reduction in depressive symptomatology, with possible associated improvements in the physical condition. The principles of the use of antidepressants for the medical population is not as different from that for other psychiatric patients (see Chapter 3.3), especially for those patients in whom the underlying medical condition is well controlled. However, it is important to pay attention to medical cautions and contraindications and the frequent need for dose adjustment, in response to either side effects or impaired drug metabolism in medical patients.

Generally, SSRIs are used as first-line antidepressants, as the older tricyclic antidepressants are less well tolerated because of their higher incidence of side effects, especially anticholinergic ones. SSRIs should be avoided if possible, or used with caution, in patients aged over 80 years, those with prior upper gastrointestinal bleeding, and in those taking aspirin or another non-steroidal anti-inflammatory drug.[125] SSRIs vary in their effect on the hepatic cytochrome P450 system and may affect metabolism of other drugs prescribed at the same time.[126] Citalopram and sertraline have the least problems in this respect. It is also important to be aware of the possibility of serotonin syndrome with other serotonergic medications (e.g. pethidine/pentazocine perioperatively, 5-HT agonists - triptans - for migraine).

It is important to ensure close follow-up over the first few weeks after patients have started on antidepressants to monitor any side effects and address any other concerns the patient may have, in order to facilitate adherence. Some patients are anxious about starting and staying on antidepressant medication, as they may believe their problems are 'physical' and either do not understand or have difficulty accepting their need for psychotropic medication. If the patient started on the medication as an inpatient, it is important to clarify the follow-up arrangements, whether the general practitioner will be expected to monitor the antidepressant treatment or whether the patient will be followed up in the CL psychiatry outpatient clinic. There may also be a need for other clinicians (both hospital and primary care) to be made aware of any medical consequences of introducing the antidepressant medication. For instance, patients on high-dose venlafaxine may need their blood pressure to be monitored, while those with an increased risk of gastrointestinal bleeding prescribed SSRIs may need to be prescribed a proton pump inhibitor. These issues should be communicated clearly to both the treating clinician and the patient's general practitioner.

Intolerance of side effects is common in medical patients. For patients who are already experiencing physical discomfort from their medical condition or treatment, additional problems due to the introduction of antidepressants may be especially distressing. Some patients become hypervigilant of physiological changes, and they may mistakenly report these as side effects. It is all too easy then to become caught in multiple changes of antidepressants in response. If it is anticipated that side effects may become a problem, it may be best to start patients on low doses and gradually increase the dosage. Several antidepressants are now available in a liquid form, which makes it easier to introduce them at sub-therapeutic doses and to make gradual dose adjustments. The fact that these can be diluted in a glass of liquid appears to help patients feel that they are in greater control of how the antidepressant is taken, and this is useful for those who are anxious about taking medication because of previous side effects. Liquid formulations are also useful when the antidepressant needs to be withdrawn. There is a growing awareness that some patients may suffer prolonged or difficult withdrawal symptoms, even when SSRIs are withdrawn gradually. The Royal College of Psychiatrists and the National Institute of Health and Care Excellence now promotes a tapered withdrawal in which dose reductions are made proportionally to the prescribed dose. Liquid preparations may be very useful in allowing for a tapered dose reduction.

Treatment resistance is also commonly observed, and as with any patients, the first steps to take are to check the dose, concordance with prescriptions and the duration of treatment. It is prudent to list all the other medications the patient is currently taking, in case they are taking a drug known to worsen depression (see Box 19.2) or reduce the effectiveness of antidepressants. In these instances, it may be helpful to liaise with the treating clinician to see whether there is any scope for a change in the medication prescribed for the physical condition. It is also important to explore whether there are any unaddressed psychosocial factors that may be perpetuating the disorder, as antidepressants are rarely sufficient on their own to treat depression in medical patients. Rarely, augmentation with lithium or other mood stabilisers may be needed. Lithium is contraindicated in patients with impaired renal function, and if it is used among those with hypothyroidism, closer monitoring of thyroid function is indicated.

Antipsychotics

Antipsychotics may be required in the medical setting for the treatment of mania and other psychotic states and in controlling acute behavioural disturbance. For patients who are behaviourally disturbed, the initial priority is to try to defuse the situation by creating a safe and calm environment, ensuring safety for both the patient and others. As soon as this is achieved, it is essential to look for medical causes for the disturbed behaviour - such as a reaction to medication or the presence of infection - and deal with them. However, medication may be required to contain acute and serious disturbance, and the most commonly used medications in these situations are antipsychotics such as olanzapine or aripiprazole or short-acting benzodiazepines (e.g. lorazepam). In cases of delirium tremens, benzodiazepines such as chlordiazepoxide are indicated. Where antipsychotics are required in addition to benzodiazepines, haloperidol is recommended in the short term - especially if an intramuscular injection is required - as it is less likely to cause hypotension or respiratory depression; however, it requires cardiac monitoring because of its highly cardiotoxic nature so it may not always be practicable. Antipsychotics and short-acting benzodiazepines should not be used in the treatment of delirium, except to manage acute behavioural disturbance that presents a risk to the patient or others. In people with delirium, there is unclear evidence of benefit from antipsychotics and benzodiazepines; they do not reduce the duration of delirium, and there is strong evidence of harm, including increased mortality.[127] They should be avoided as much as possible in people with dementia, where they have been shown to increase risk of falls, stroke and all-cause mortality.[128]

Longer-acting depot preparations, such as acuphase, should not be used in the acute management of behavioural disturbance on a medical ward. The clinical state of disturbed and physically ill patients may fluctuate rapidly and require regular adjustment of psychotropic dose, which is not possible with these preparations.

Anxiolytics

As indicated earlier, short-acting benzodiazepines may be used in controlling acute behavioural disturbance on the ward if non-pharmacological strategies have failed. They may also be helpful when severe or phobic anxiety (e.g. needle phobia) has resulted in refusal of key investigations or treatments, and non-pharmacological anxiety management methods are not possible. When benzodiazepines are given parenterally, vital signs should be monitored closely, and flumazenil – a competitive benzodiazepine antagonist – should be available on the ward in case significant respiratory depression should occur. Whenever benzodiazepines are recommended by the CL psychiatry team, it is essential that the recommendation should include their indications as well as guidance on the frequency and total duration of their use. This is because prescriptions are sometimes started on the medical ward and then repeated without clear instructions, leading to long-term use and dependence. Care should be taken in the use of benzodiazepines in the presence of significant respiratory illness, owing to the risk of compromising respiratory function even further.

Patients often request night sedation in hospital. It is important to find out whether any worries or physical discomfort is interfering with sleep; sometimes the short-term use of hypnotic medication may be necessary.

Electroconvulsive Therapy

Electroconvulsive therapy (ECT) may sometimes be required in depressed medical patients for the same indications as for psychiatric patients with depression, which include immediate high risk of suicide, severe psychomotor retardation, risk of dehydration due to limited oral intake or any other condition where a rapid relief of severe symptoms is required (for example, intractable catatonic stupor). Special attention should be paid to any relative contraindications such as raised intracranial pressure, recent myocardial infarction or cerebrovascular accident, acute respiratory infection, retinal detachment and phaeochromocytoma. The risks and benefits of the general anaesthetic and ECT should be weighed carefully in discussion with the patient and family, the medical team and anaesthetist and clearly documented in the notes. The topic is discussed in Chapter 3.3.

Alcohol Detoxification

Alcohol detoxification may be required on the medical ward when a patient with alcohol dependence is admitted. However, in a minority of patients, the alcoholism is unknown, and – when these patients are admitted as an emergency or on the day of their elective surgery – they may abruptly show behavioural disorders apparently occurring without any obvious precipitant, consistent with delirium tremens (DTs). This is a dangerous condition, and a comprehensive account of detoxification regimens and the DTs is given in Chapter 14. Screening, brief intervention and referral to treatment (SBIRT) approaches in emergency departments have been shown to reduce alcohol use in low to moderate users, reduce injuries in all users and reduce repeat emergency visits.[129] Because of the high frequency of alcohol problems, it is important for the medical and psychiatric liaison teams to agree on the protocol for the management of alcohol withdrawal; this protocol should clearly delineate the responsibilities of each team. Many hospitals now have dedicated substance misuse liaison services that support patients, families and staff when alcohol (or other drug misuse) occurs together with altered health status.

Psychological Treatments

A high proportion of emotional distress identified in an acute medical setting is of a mild and transient nature.[40] For these patients, formal referral to psychiatrists or psychologists is inappropriate, and first-line psychological support is best provided by the doctors and nurses who are presently caring for them. However, general hospital staff often have difficulty in identifying psychological problems and, more importantly, in handling them. Therefore, the liaison psychiatry team will play an important role in training and supporting the clinical staff, helping them manage minor affective disorders more effectively and with greater confidence.

The basic psychological skills that general hospital clinicians should possess in order to facilitate the psychological care of their patients comprise the following abilities:

- To communicate clearly with patients, discuss their concerns, elicit any misapprehensions and correct them
- To break bad news
- To facilitate the grieving process by patients and their relatives
- To discuss psychological symptoms and distress without embarrassment

- To discuss the need for specialist psychiatric help without seeming dismissive
- To use antidepressants rationally

General hospital staff who are interested or have greater responsibility in managing the emotional wellbeing of people with physical conditions may want to champion such approaches by becoming proficient in communication techniques such as motivational interviewing or brief (so-called 15-minute) cognitive behavioural therapy (CBT).

Psychological intervention may be aimed at improving mood, addressing the psychosocial stressors that are maintaining the mental disorder, addressing cognitive or motivational factors that are interfering with medical treatment, or dealing with any interpersonal difficulties that have arisen as a consequence of the illness.

There are undoubtedly constraints to the delivery of psychotherapy in a general hospital setting or where patients are significantly ill, are cognitively impaired or have difficulty attending sessions regularly – for physical reasons – and so treatment should be tailored to the needs of the individual patients and delivered more flexibly. However, it is possible to deliver psychological treatments on busy medical wards even with the difficulties inherent in doing so. For example, Prof Deborah Cabaniss at Columbia University in New York has modified psychodynamic psychotherapy to be deliverable in brief sessions on busy medical wards by training psychiatrists on these fundamental principles: careful assessment of ego function, formulation to guide the psychiatrist (and the team) and support to bolster functioning in the patient.[130] The focus on ego functioning is a core principle of supportive psychotherapy also, which can easily be delivered on general medical wards and has been shown to improve outcomes in patients with coronary artery disease, certain gastrointestinal conditions, HIV infection and certain cancers.[131] The goals of supportive psychotherapy on helping patients understand emotional experiences, improve affect-regulation and reality testing, make use of their most effective coping strategies and engage in collaborative problem solving should be inherent to all psychiatrists. Some more specialised therapies are shown later – access to them may involve referral to community services. Across England, all GPs have access to Increasing Access to Psychological Therapies (IAPT) services, to which patients can self-refer. The CL psychiatrist should be able to prescribe psychological treatment as competently as pharmacological therapies and should be able to discuss with the patient the most appropriate therapy for them. These include:

- Problem-solving therapy[132]
- Cognitive behavioural therapy
- Motivational interviewing[133]
- Interpersonal psychotherapy[134,135]
- Psychodynamic interpersonal therapy[136]
- Couples therapy
- Family therapy
- Group therapy

Does Psychological Intervention Influence the Course of Emotional or Physical Outcome?

Evidence suggests that psychological treatments can be effective for a range of outcomes in the management of physical health conditions, including asthma, diabetes and pain disorders,[137] but psychological treatments are not a panacea and so should be combined with other physical and psychiatric treatments. Psychological treatments can be used to:[138]

- Treat the emotional consequences of physical illness
- Co-occurrence of mental disorder with physical illness
- Symptoms of the physical illness itself (e.g. fatigue in cancer, breathlessness in asthma)
- Improve concordance with treatment or self-management of the physical condition

The ultimate aim is to improve quality of life.

Cognitive behavioural therapy (CBT) has the strongest evidence base. A meta-analysis of 30 studies demonstrated that CBT has a small to moderate effect in improving anxiety, fatigue and depression that co-occurs with chronic physical illnesses.[139] The greatest effect was on fatigue and the smallest on anxiety. Longer duration of treatment appeared to be associated with stronger effect sizes. This meta-analysis did not find an impact on pain from CBT, but a more rigorously conducted Cochrane review of 75 studies found good quality evidence that CBT has a very small to small effect on reducing pain, disability and distress associated with fibromyalgia, chronic low back pain, rheumatoid arthritis and mixed chronic pain.[140] Behavioural therapy as well as acceptance and commitment therapy (ACT) may also have beneficial effects on pain, but the quality of the evidence was too poor to be certain. So, it appears that CBT targeted at the most disabling symptoms in selected conditions has the greatest chance of success. Similarly, a CBT-based intervention targeted at fatigue following remission from cancer greatly improved fatigue and functional impairment in an RCT of 112 cancer survivors.[141]

A randomised controlled trial of 238 patients with COPD and moderate anxiety/depression showed that CBT given weekly for eight weeks improved quality of life and reduced anxiety and depression symptoms.[142] However, CBT was no more effective than COPD education, and there was no impact on COPD outcomes or health service use. Psychological therapies have a small effect in improving depression symptoms associated with inflammatory bowel disease, and CBT also improves quality of life according to a meta-analysis of 14 RCTs including 1,196 patients. However, effects were short-lived and disappeared after the end of therapy.

What is evident then is that psychological therapies have small and, in most cases, short-term benefits in physical illnesses. However, these effects can act in a cumulative manner when combined with more standard approaches to management of physical health conditions. CL psychiatrists are sometimes asked to help patients and physicians in the management of their chronic illness in a more collaborative manner. Such an approach – developed on the basis of social learning and self-regulation theories and, to some extent, using methods developed to manage long-term mental illness – aims to define the patient's problems collaboratively, to set goals and targets, and to plan action. This collaborative care approach has good evidence for improving both mental and physical health outcomes in people with co-occurring mental and physical conditions like diabetes or cardiac disease.[119] It has been used in the NHS to improve depressive symptoms, anxiety, quality of life and role functioning in people with poor prognosis cancer[143] and is now endorsed by NICE in the management of depression and anxiety co-occurring with physical health conditions, but it is still poorly provided.[144]

Consent, Capacity and the Mental Health Act in the General Hospital

The following refers to the law in England and Wales. The procedures and considerations around capacity, consent and the Mental Health Act are slightly different in Scotland and Northern Ireland.

Box 19.9 Consent and capacity

Valid Consent Is That Which Is:

- Based on adequate knowledge of –
  - The nature of the treatment
  - The risks associated with the treatment
  - The consequences of not having the treatment
- Voluntary – the patient was not under undue influence of others
- Given by a patient who has the capacity (see below) to decide.

Assessment of Capacity (Mental Capacity Act, 2005)

If there is an impairment in the functioning of mind or brain, a person is deemed to have capacity, if they can:

- Understand the nature, purpose and reason for the treatment
- Understand the benefits, risks and alternatives and the consequences of not receiving the treatment
- Retain the information for long enough to use it and weigh it in the balance in order to arrive at a decision
- Communicate the decision

Assessment of Capacity to Consent to Medical Treatment

Any procedure carried out in the medical setting from examination to investigation to treatment requires consent by the patient. Consent is:

> the voluntary and continuing permission of the patient to receive a particular treatment, based on an adequate knowledge of the purpose, nature, likely effects and risks of that treatment including the likelihood of its success and any alternatives to it. (Mental Health Act 1983; see also the *Mental Health Act 1983 Code of Practice*, Department of Health & Welsh Office, 1999)

The law around capacity is laid out in the Mental Capacity Act (MCA) 2005. The presumption is that adult patients have the capacity to decide whether to consent to or refuse the proposed medical intervention, even where a refusal may result in harm to themselves or even in their own death. A patient with capacity to decide is also free to withdraw consent at any stage. The withdrawal of consent is legally-binding in a capacitous person (provided they cannot be detained under the Mental Health Act), whereas a request for treatment does not have to be complied with but should be considered by a clinician (for example, the request for antibiotics to treat a viral illness).

A child under 16 may give valid consent to medical treatment if he or she is assessed to be 'Fraser competent'; that is, he or she has the capacity to make the decision to have the proposed treatment and is of sufficient understanding and intelligence to be capable of making up his or her own mind. Children of 16 or over may give consent to treatment, and it is not necessary to obtain parental consent. However, if a patient under 18 lacks capacity, those with parental responsibility may give consent on that patient's behalf. No adult can give or withdraw consent for another adult unless they have Lasting Power of Attorney or there is an Advanced Directive giving them the power to consent.

It is the responsibility of each clinician to ensure that valid consent is obtained for any treatment proposed (this may be written or otherwise, non-verbal or verbal, see Box 19.9). Informed consent requires a clinician to give information about the treatment, to be satisfied that the patient has the capacity to make the decision, and to allow the patient to make a voluntary choice without undue influence from others. It is essential for the practice of medicine that all clinicians are able to adequately assess a patient's capacity to consent to treatment. Under the MCA, the person proposing the treatment, procedure or intervention is responsible for assessing the capacity.

A patient lacks capacity only if some impairment or disturbance of mental functioning renders the person unable to decide whether to consent to or refuse treatment.

The patient has the capacity to decide on the treatment if he or she:

- Understands the nature, purpose and reason for the treatment
- Understands its benefits, risks and alternatives and the consequences of not receiving the treatment
- Is able to retain the information for long enough to use it and weigh it in the balance in order to arrive at a decision
- Can communicate their decision to the clinician (this does not have to be verbally; it can also, for example, be the withdrawal of an arm when attempting to take blood)

When there has been any doubt as to the capacity of the patient to consent to treatment, the patient should be questioned on each of the above items. It is important to record the verbatim responses of such an assessment in the medical notes, as the question of capacity can later become a legal issue or even a matter for the courts.

The presence or absence of capacity is not an all-or-none matter; it is a time-specific and decision-specific measure. Patients may temporarily become incapable of giving consent due to lost or impaired consciousness, fear, fatigue, shock, pain, drugs or alcohol. Some may have longer-term impairment from learning disability or dementia. In either case, a patient may have the capacity to consent to some treatments and not others, and it is important that the presence or absence of capacity is considered on each relevant issue.

Although all clinicians are expected to be able to assess a patient's capacity to make treatment decisions, a psychiatrist may be asked to assist in such an assessment. In these cases, the psychiatrist must make sure not to unduly influence the patient or pronounce on the nature of capacity outside her/his competence. However, a psychiatrist can clarify whether the patient has been given adequate information about the proposed treatment. In particular, the psychiatrist may be best placed to assess whether a mental disorder is present and, if so, to make a judgement as to whether it has any bearing on the patient's ability to comprehend the information given, believe it, retain it and weigh up the options needed to come to a decision.

Where patients are refusing treatment, especially where this may have serious consequences for their health, it is vital that their capacity to make treatment decisions is assessed carefully and that senior clinicians should be involved in this type of assessment. Discussion of the reasons for refusal may sometimes reveal some small practical or interpersonal issue that has made the selected treatment unacceptable to the patient. In these instances, it may be possible to make alternative arrangements or select a different but equally effective treatment that the patient can accept. Even when the patient is assessed as being capable of refusing a treatment, it is important that there is ongoing discussion and negotiation about management where possible – involving family (if the patient allows this) – while respecting the patient's autonomous decision, as he or she may change the decision with time.

Overdose

Psychiatrists covering the emergency department or medical wards are sometimes consulted about patients who have taken an overdose and are refusing treatment. This is a complex legal issue over which there has been considerable debate.[145–147] The initial action in this situation should be to assess the patient's capacity to make treatment decisions, and there should also be an attempt to lower levels of emotional arousal to permit further discussion with the aim of persuading the patient to accept treatment. If the patient lacks capacity to consent to treatment, the decision to treat should be taken in the patient's best interest (see later). Capacity in these patients may be impaired for a variety of reasons, such as alcohol intoxication, direct effect of drugs taken in overdose affecting the levels of consciousness, or a very high degree of distress that impairs concentration and the ability to weigh up options.

If the patient has been detained under the Mental Health Act for a mental disorder and the overdose is considered to be due to the underlying mental disorder, then the medical treatment for the overdose can be given as an ancillary treatment under section 63. Under the Act, this treatment should be under the direction of the responsible medical officer. However, where the patient is not detained under the Act and has been assessed to have capacity to make treatment decisions, the patient's wish cannot be overridden. As with any other significant treatment refusal, senior clinicians should be involved in the assessment of the patient. Even in such circumstances, the patient may accept admission for further observation or may permit clinicians to contact the family, which will facilitate the monitoring of the patient's physical condition and leave open the possibility of a change of mind in due course. In this, as in all medical situations, the clinician's overriding duty is to make decisions that promote the safety and wellbeing of the patient while upholding any decisions made by a patient who has capacity.

Patients Who Lack Capacity

The treatment of patients lacking capacity is covered under the MCA 2005. In patients lacking capacity, no other person can give or withhold consent on their behalf, but the treating clinician will have the responsibility to make medical decisions that are in the best interest of the patient. For a treatment to be allowed, the doctrine of necessity should be applied. This states that a treatment given to a patient who lacks capacity should be necessary to save life or alleviate or prevent deterioration in the patient's physical or mental health, that the benefit of the treatment should outweigh the burden, and that the decision would be supported by a responsible body of medical opinion in the field. The MCA also makes it clear that any decision made in a person lacking capacity should be the least restrictive option.

In making the decision of 'best interest', there is a strong presumption of preservation of life, although the best interest may be framed in terms of medical, emotional or other welfare issues. It is also good practice in these fraught situations to consult close relatives to clarify the patient's best interest, although any such enquiry should be mindful of the duty of confidentiality owed to the patient.[148] Where there is a need to restrain a patient who lacks capacity in the general medical setting, this may be permitted under common law, provided the action taken is necessary, reasonable and in the patient's best interest.

If the patient had a valid advance directive while he or she had capacity to make it, this should be respected, provided the decision is applicable to the procedure in question and there is no reason to believe that the patient had changed his or her mind.

Questions about capacity also arise in situations where a patient is refusing to go to the hospital for a physical disorder. If the patient lacks capacity to make a decision about going into hospital and it is in the person's best interest to receive the treatment for that medical condition in hospital, the common law doctrine of necessity allows conveyance to hospital.

The Mental Capacity Act 2005 provides a legal framework for England and Wales, which enshrines these common principles, sets out a test for assessing capacity and provides a checklist for decisions in the best interest for those who lack capacity. It makes provisions for those having lasting powers as the final arbiter for capacity matters. The Act also makes provision for an 'independent mental capacity advocate' (IMCA) to support those who lack capacity, allows for advance decisions to refuse treatment to be utilised, introduces a new criminal offence of ill treatment or neglect of a person who lacks capacity and sets parameters for research involving such persons. The Mental Capacity Act Code of Practice provides practical guidance in the application of the Act.

In October 2004, the European Court of Human Rights ruled in the Bournewood case that detention in hospital of a patient lacking capacity, under the common law doctrine of necessity, 'where the patient is under continuous supervision and control', infringed Article 5 of the European Convention of Human Rights. This has come to be known as the 'Bournewood gap', and the UK government closed this gap by amending the Mental Capacity Act 2005 by putting in place Deprivation of Liberty Safeguards (DoLS). By 2018, DoLS had become overly complicated and bureaucratic and so were replaced by Liberty Protection Safeguards. These safeguards refer to the issue of detention alone and not to medical treatment of incapacitated patients. Non-therapeutic or controversial treatments (e.g. non-therapeutic utilisation, organ donation, withdrawal of nutrition in patients in a persistent vegetative state, bone marrow donation) in patients lacking capacity should be referred to the Court of Protection.

Mental Health Act 1983 in the General Hospital

The Mental Health Act 1983 in England and Wales allows compulsory detention and treatment of mental disorder where it is in the interest of the patient's health, safety or the safety of other persons and where voluntary admission is not possible. The Act also allows treatment of physical disorder where it has given rise to mental disorder and it is necessary to treat the physical disorder in order to treat the mental disorder (e.g. treatment of thyroid disease that has given rise to severe depression or psychotic illness, refeeding of patients with severe anorexia nervosa). However, where there is a temporary mental disorder – such as delirium arising from an underlying physical disorder – which results in the patient temporarily losing capacity to consent to treatment, it is more appropriate to consider treatment under the Mental Capacity Act 2005.

The procedure for application for detention of a patient under the Mental Health Act is the same in the general hospital setting as it is in the mental health setting. If an inpatient needs to be held on the ward in an emergency under the Act, the medical holding power of section 5(2) may be considered. The consultant with medical responsibility may exercise the power (usually through a deputy) to detain the patient for up to 72 hours while awaiting a full assessment under the Act. The Act allows the consultant to nominate a deputy to carry out the detention, but this person must be a fully registered medical practitioner (thus a Foundation Year 1 doctor cannot take on this role). Any medical team using the section 5(2) holding power should be advised to contact the psychiatric services as soon as possible. Patients detained under the temporary holding power cannot be moved to another hospital under this power.

As section 5(2) is applicable only to inpatients, patients in the accident and emergency department usually cannot be held under it, as they will not have been formally admitted (although patients in Acute Assessment Units and Clinical Decision Units can). Patients who lack capacity to consent to remain will need to be held under the Mental Capacity Act 2005 once it has been established it is in their best interest to remain in the emergency department to receive treatment (see earlier). The nurses' holding power (section 5(4)) can be used only by appropriately registered nurses, with training in mental health or learning disabilities, on informal inpatients already being treated for mental illness and would not normally be applicable in a general hospital setting. The liaison consultant psychiatrist will be perceived by the rest of the hospital staff as the most knowledgeable concerning these medico-legal conundrums, and his or her opinion will often be sought. Thus, whenever a patient is being treated without consent, it is important for the liaison psychiatrist to know exactly under which Act, doctrine or law such treatments are taking place.

The Provision of Consultation-Liaison Psychiatry Services

The need for mental health input to general hospital services has been recognised for many years, formalised in joint reports from the Royal Colleges of Physicians (2003)[149] and Surgeons (1997)[150] and the Royal College of Psychiatrists. This described a need for the clinical staff in general hospitals to possess basic psychological skills as well as the need for wards to have facilities in which staff can see patients privately and safely. These reports advocated that CL psychiatry services should become an integral part of acute medical services, and there should also be special services for alcohol counselling and for patients who have harmed themselves. In practice, however, the development of services often floundered on commissioning issues: Who was responsible for their funding? Which organisations would benefit from the funding of these teams? All might agree on their value, but out of whose budget should the funding come? Demonstration of potential cost savings to general medical services from enhanced liaison services through models such as Rapid Assessment Interface and Discharge (RAID) began to stimulate interest in commissioners and providers.

However, despite demonstration that such services could save costs and improve care, implementation required strategic planning, collaboration and joint working that was not always easy to develop quickly. The Strategic Clinical Network for Mental Health, Dementia and Neurological Conditions South West commissioned a report in 2014, which set out four effective models for liaison psychiatry in use in the UK, and this scheme was adapted into NICE Guidance by NHS England. The Five Year Forward View for Mental Health objective added further strategic impetus to this by stating that by 2020/21, all acute hospitals would have all-age mental health liaison teams in place, and at least 50 per cent of these will meet the 'Core 24' service standard as a minimum. Movement towards this aspiration was of course interrupted by the pandemic, but this remains an important statement of policy intent. NICE set out its implementation guidance for 'Achieving Better Access to 24/7 Urgent and Emergency Mental Health Care' in 2016, codifying this work that had been developing over many years and describing suggested team composition.

Models of Service

The Standard Requirements for a CL Service

The CL psychiatry service should be led by a consultant who specialises in liaison psychiatry. This person should have responsibilities for direct clinical work (consultation and liaison), clinical supervision of psychiatric trainees and those from other disciplines, and the administrative and organisational work.

All of these models recognised the need for a multidisciplinary service, incorporating a team of doctors, nurses and other allied health professionals, as well as sufficient administrative support:

- Core Liaison Psychiatry Services, working hours, or extended hours only
- Core24 Liaison Psychiatry Services, 24 hours, seven days a week
- Enhanced24 Liaison Psychiatry Services, 24 hours, seven days a week, with extensions to fill local gaps in service and some outpatient services
- Comprehensive Liaison Psychiatry Services, 24 hours, seven days a week, enhanced with inpatient and outpatient services to specialties at major centres

NHS England recommended in 2016 that 'Given that services need to provide 24/7 care, only the core 24, enhanced 24 and comprehensive models should be considered by commissioners where Eds in general hospitals operate on a 24/7 basis. All liaison mental health services within hospitals providing regional and supra-regional services should aim to implement the comprehensive service model' (see Table 19.1).

Table 19.1 Staffing approaches with different service models[151]

Staff	Core 24	Enhanced 24	Comprehensive (illustrative for a 2,000-bed hospital)
Consultants	2	4	5
Other medical	2	2	2
Nurses	6 band 7	3 band 7	2 band 8b
	7 band 6	7 band 6	17 band 6
			10 band 5
Other therapists	4	2	16
Team manager	1	1	
Clinical lead	0.4	0.4	1
Admin and business support	3	3	13

The Consultation Model

In this model, the general hospital clinician refers the patient to a mental health professional, who provides a psychosocial or psychiatric assessment and gives advice to the patient and the clinical team regarding management. A service of this type relies on clinical staff for the detection of potential mental disorders. The effectiveness of the consultation model is also influenced by the quality of the communication between the referrer and mental health professionals.

There are four models of consultation:[152]

1. *A patient-oriented consultation*, in which the patient is the direct focus. The consultation should incorporate a diagnostic interview and evaluation of the patient's personality, reaction to illness and other psychological aspects.
2. *A crisis-oriented therapeutic consultation*, in which there is a rapid assessment of the presenting problem and coping style as well as active therapeutic intervention, as might occur following an episode of parasuicide. The therapist may give guidance on techniques such as active problem solving or other cognitive methods to help the patient through the crisis.
3. *A referrer-oriented consultation*, which focuses on the referrer's problem with a given patient – for example, where the clinicians may be left feeling very anxious or angry in cases of treatment refusal.
4. *A situation-oriented consultation*, which looks at the interaction between the patient (and sometimes the family) and the clinical team, as may occur in cases where conflicts or disagreements arise over the treatment plan.

The Liaison Model

In this model, the psychiatrist meets with the general clinicians in ward rounds or joint clinics. This gives an opportunity to discuss individual patients as well as more general topics, such as the psychosocial contribution and the psychological care of patients, and this provides a forum for educating and training the clinical team. The pure liaison model is very demanding in terms of the consultant psychiatrist's time, and most services work with a mixture of the two models. Thus, individual consultations will follow on referral from a clinician, but there may also be specific links with medical clinical teams to facilitate liaison work.

Service Needs

A liaison psychiatric service will be needed for the emergency department, as well as the inpatient and outpatient departments. referrals are predominantly for physical and psychological comorbidity; for persistent, medically unexplained physical symptoms; and for problems arising in patient management as a result of psychosocial factors, as well as for self harm. annual referral rates in these settings have been estimated from both published and unpublished reports for a district general hospital of 600 beds serving a population of 250,000: self harm, 500 per annum; accident and emergency, 150 per annum; ward referrals, 150 per annum; and outpatient contacts, new 50–100, follow-up 500 per annum. However, these figures may vary depending on the type and size of the hospital and the availability and popularity of the liaison service.[153]

A more recent study[154] from a CL service in a large Italian general hospital in Perugia of a 1,000 consecutive CL referrals gave the following figures. First examinations: the largest number of referrals (29.5%) were requested by the accident and emergency unit (A&E) and the other (70.5%) came from other hospital units. Medical units provided 53.1% of requests for psychiatric consultation, surgical units provided 8.8% and specialist units provided 38.1%. The most common reasons for requesting consultation were anxiety (18.9%), symptoms of depression (18.2%), confusion (13.4%), unexplained somatic symptoms (11.2%), suicide attempt/risk (11.2%), psychomotor agitation (10.9%) and history of psychiatric illness (14.4%). The CL interview was the main intervention in most cases (83%), and 60% were prescribed a psychotropic drug, mainly an antidepressant or a benzodiazepine. The main liaison intervention was raising awareness among medical and nursing staff in the unit where they were being treated. The fact that the main intervention was the actual CL interview means that the person and the knowledge of the CL psychiatrist are crucial to the operation of the CL service. Although these figures are from an Italian hospital, it is likely that CL services in the UK are similar.

The type of CL service that can be offered will depend on a number of factors:

- *The consultation time available.* This will depend on the composition of the team providing the service (as will the range of disciplines and skills available within it). This can range from a single general adult psychiatrist, whose primary responsibility is a community sector but who provides a few liaison sessions, through to a full consultant-led multi-disciplinary team.
- *Any other established services provided to the hospital.* There may be pre-existing services provided by the psychiatric or psychology departments, covering areas such as psychiatry for the elderly, substance misuse, eating disorders, sexual dysfunction, HIV-related disorders and neuropsychiatry/rehabilitation. The CL service may work independently of the other services without overlap or work in conjunction with them.
- *Expectations of other professionals.* Clinical staff in the general hospital and psychiatrists working in the community will have different expectations about exactly what the CL services should be providing. General hospital staff want easy and rapid access, an expectation of a single referral point with a quick response, and an efficient self harm assessment service. General psychiatrists working in the community live in the hope that the CL service will deal with all the general hospital referrals, so that the sector teams can be free to concentrate their resources on their patients in the community sector. Good liaison with both groups is important, and the support of general hospital clinicians and psychiatric colleagues will be essential when seeking resources for a new or expanded CL service. The views and needs of the service users and carers should also be taken into account in service planning.

Some CL services have dedicated inpatient wards in a medical setting, where patients with complex physical and psychiatric needs may be assessed and managed. This may be the best setting for managing those with severe chronic disorders, who are often reluctant to engage in psychiatric services, who are too disabled for outpatient care and who need all the skills of a multi-disciplinary team for the assessment and management of their condition.

Links with Other Services

Consultation-liaison psychiatry services will need to have links with other services within the mental health field, such as psychodynamic therapy, cognitive behavioural therapy, the drug and alcohol services, eating disorder services and perinatal psychiatry. In some cases, psychological care can more appropriately be provided by those working in the hospital, such as the clinical team, the palliative care team or specialist nurse counsellors. Links with the voluntary sector may also facilitate referrals to services in this sector, such as self-help groups and patient organisations (Figure 19.3).

Specialty-Based Services

As mentioned under the liaison model, CL psychiatric teams may develop specific services for a particular medical specialty, such as oncology, diabetes, neurology, renal dialysis, transplantation, intensive care, a pain clinic or a fatigue clinic. The liaison aspect of this link may take the form of:

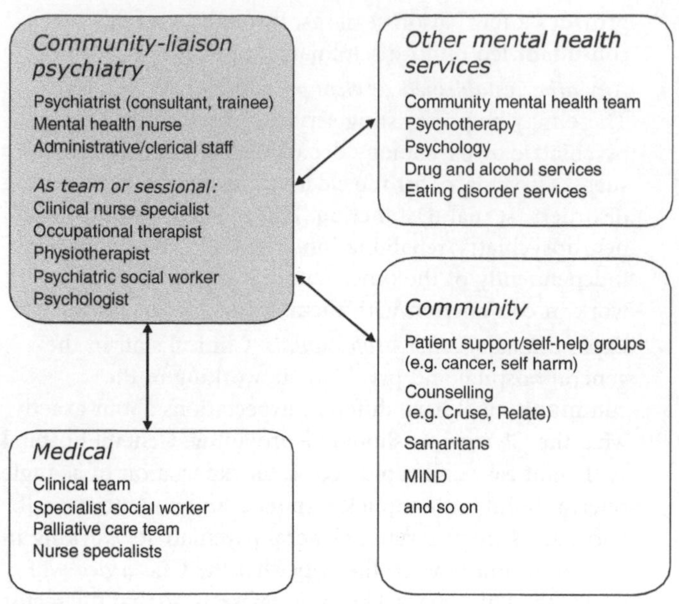

Figure 19.3 Links between a consultation–liaison psychiatry service and other services.

- A joint service, joint clinic or joint ward round
- A case review meeting or case conference with the multi-disciplinary staff on the ward/clinical area
- Psychological supervision or training for medical and paramedical staff in the specialist unit

It is beyond the scope of this brief overview to give an account of services in the many different specialist settings, but these are described in detail in the book by Peveler.[155]

Conclusions

In recent years, there have been important changes in general medicine relevant to CL psychiatry. There is now a much wider recognition of the high prevalence of psychiatric and physical comorbidity and how this influences consultation frequency, service utilisation, treatment adherence, the physical prognosis and probably the overall cost as well. There has also been recognition of the high prevalence of non-organic complaints among general medical patients and an awareness of the high costs of investigating these patients, which has led on to a search for better ways to manage this group of patients.[156] This means that a liaison psychiatrist should be an integral part of any medical service, from the viewpoint of both quality of care and cost. Making a clear case for the need and providing a realistic service model that meets these needs will prove to be important in sustaining and developing CL services.

References

1. Lishman WA. *Organic Psychiatry. The Psychological Consequences of Cerebral Disorder*. 2nd ed. Oxford: Blackwell Scientific Publications; 1987: 127.
2. Humphreys J, Obeney-Williams J, Cheung RW, et al. Perinatal psychiatry: a new specialty or everyone's business? *BJPsych Advances* 2016;22(6):363–72.
3. Muskin PR, Skomorowsky A, Shah RN. Co-managed care for medical inpatients, C-L vs C/L psychiatry. *Psychosomatics* 2016;57(3):258–63.
4. NHS England. *Mental Health Task Force. Five Year Forward View*. London: NHS England.; 2016.
5. Royal College of Psychiatrists, Royal College of Nursing, Royal College of Emergency Medicine, Royal College of Physicians. *Side by Side: A UK-wide Consensus Statement on Working Together to Help Patients with Mental Health Needs in Acute Hospitals.* 2020. www.rcpsych.ac.uk/docs/default-source/members/faculties/liaison-psychiatry/liaison-sidebyside.pdf (accessed 16 September 2023).
6. National Enquiry into Patient Outcome and Death. *Treat as One: Bridging the Gap Between Mental and Physical Healthcare in General Hospitals.* London: National Enquiry into Patient Outcome and Death; 2017.
7. Sharpe M, Protheroe D, House A. Joint working with physicians and surgeons. In: Peveler R, Feldman E, Friedman T (eds.) *Liaison Psychiatry: Planning Services for Specialist Settings.* Berlin/Heidelberg: Springer Science & Business; 2000: 195–206.
8. Akagi H, House A. Psychiatry in the general hospital. In: Stein G, Wilkinson G (eds.) *Seminars in Adult General Psychiatry.* London: Gaskell; 2007: 408–31.
9. Parsonage M, Fossey M. *Economic Evaluation of a Liaison Psychiatry Service.* London: Centre for Mental Health; 2011.
10. NHS England. *The NHS Long Term Plan.* London: NHS England; 2019.
11. Engel GL. The need for a new medical model: a challenge for biomedicine. *Science* 1977;196(4286):129–36.
12. Wulsin LR, Vaillant GE, Wells VE. A systematic review of the mortality of depression. *Psychosomatic Medicine* 1999;61(1):6–17.
13. Ford DE, Mead LA, Chang PP, et al. Depression is a risk factor for coronary artery disease in men: the precursors study. *Archives of Internal Medicine* 1998;158(13):1422–6.
14. Pratt LA, Ford DE, Crum RM, et al. Depression, psychotropic medication, and risk of myocardial infarction. Prospective data from the Baltimore ECA follow-up. *Circulation* 1996;94 (12):3123–9.
15. Michelson D, Stratakis C, Hill L, et al. Bone mineral density in women with depression. *New England Journal of Medicine* 1996;335(16):1176–81.
16. Zhou C, Fang L, Chen Y, et al. Effect of selective serotonin reuptake inhibitors on bone mineral density: a systematic review and meta-analysis. *Osteoporos International* 2018;29(6):1243–51.
17. Pillinger T, Beck K, Gobjila C, et al. impaired glucose homeostasis in first-episode schizophrenia: a systematic review and meta-analysis. *JAMA Psychiatry* 2017;74(3):261–9.
18. Lewinson RT, Vallerand IA, Lowerison MW, et al. Depression is associated with an increased risk of psoriatic arthritis among patients with psoriasis: a population-based study. *Journal of*

Investigative Dermatology 2017;137 (4):828–35.

19. Vallerand IA, Patten SB, Barnabe C. Depression and the risk of rheumatoid arthritis. *Current Opinion in Rheumatology* 2019;31(3):279–84.
20. Tohid H, Aleem D, Jackson C. Major depression and psoriasis: a psychodermatological phenomenon. *Skin Pharmacology and Physiology* 2016;29(4):220–30.
21. Halaris A. Inflammation and depression but where does the inflammation come from? *Current Opinion in Psychiatry* 2019;32(5):422–8.
22. Müller N, Weidinger E, Leitner B, Schwarz MJ. The role of inflammation in schizophrenia. *Frontiers in Neuroscience* 2015;9:372.
23. Kutzelnigg A, Lucchinetti CF, Stadelmann C, et al. Cortical demyelination and diffuse white matter injury in multiple sclerosis. *Brain* 2005;128(Pt 11):2705–12.
24. Dowlati Y, Herrmann N, Swardfager W, et al. A meta-analysis of cytokines in major depression. *Biological Psychiatry* 2010;67(5):446–57.
25. Anderson G, Berk M, Dodd S, et al. Immuno-inflammatory, oxidative and nitrosative stress, and neuroprogressive pathways in the etiology, course and treatment of schizophrenia. *Progress in Neuro-psychopharmacology and Biological Psychiatry* 2013;42:1–4.
26. Lloyd GG. Psychological reactions to physical illness. *British Journal of Hospital Medicine* 1977;18 (4):352,355–8.
27. Crichton P, Carel H, Kidd IJ. Epistemic injustice in psychiatry. *BJPsych Bulletin* 2017;41(2):65–70.
28. Sensky T. Patients' reactions to illness. *BMJ* 1990;300(6725):622–3.
29. Mechanic D. *Medical Sociology*. New York: Free Press; 1978.
30. Horne R, Weinman J. Illness cognitions: implications for the treatment of renal disease. In: McGee HM, Bradley C (eds.) *Quality of Life Following Renal Failure: Psychological Challenges Accompanying High Technology Medicine*. London: Psychology Press; 1994: 113–32.
31. Leventhal H, Nerenz DR, Steele DJ. Illness representations and coping with health threats. In: Baum A (ed.) *Handbook of Psychology and Health Social Psychological Aspects of Heath*. Hillsdale, NJ: Lawrence Erlbaum Associates; 1984: 219–52.
32. Leventhal H, Diefenbach M, Leventhal EA. Illness cognition: using common sense to understand treatment adherence and affect cognition interactions. *Cognitive Therapy and Research* 1992;16(2):143–63.
33. Petrie KJ, Weinman J, Sharpe N, et al. Role of patients' view of their illness in predicting return to work and functioning after myocardial infarction: longitudinal study. *BMJ* 1996;312 (7040):1191–4.
34. Scharloo M, Kaptein AA, Weinman J, et al. Illness perceptions, coping and functioning in patients with rheumatoid arthritis, chronic obstructive pulmonary disease and psoriasis. *Journal of Psychosomatic Research* 1998;44 (5):573–85.
35. Scholten EWM, Simon JDHP, van Diemen T, et al. Appraisals and coping mediate the relationship between resilience and distress among significant others of persons with spinal cord injury or acquired brain injury: a cross-sectional study. *BMC Psychology* 2020;8 (1):51.
36. Maguire P, Parkes CM. Surgery and loss of body parts. *BMJ* 1998;316 (7137):1086–8.
37. Horne R, Weinman J. Patients' beliefs about prescribed medicines and their role in adherence to treatment in chronic physical illness. *Journal of Psychosomatic Research* 1999;47 (6):555–67.
38. Marmot MG, Smith GD, Stansfeld S, et al. Health inequalities among British civil servants: the Whitehall II study. *Lancet* 1991;337(8754):1387–93.
39. Carroll D, Sheffield D. Social psychophysiology, social circumstances, and health. *Annals of Behavioral Medicine* 1998;20(4):333–7.
40. Feldman E, Mayou R, Hawton K, et al. Psychiatric disorder in medical in-patients. *Quarterly Journal of Medicine* 1987;63(241):405–12.
41. Stoudemire A, Thompson TL. Medication noncompliance: systematic approaches to evaluation and intervention. *General Hospital Psychiatry* 1983;5(4):233–9.
42. Parsons T. *The Social System*. London: Routledge and Kegan Paul; 1951.
43. Pritchard M. Psychological pressure in a renal unit. *British Journal of Hospital Medicine* 1982;27(5):512–6.
44. Brown GW, Harris TO. *Life Events and Illness*. New York: Guilford; 1989.
45. Cohen S, Murphy MLM, Prather AA. Ten surprising facts about stressful life events and disease risk. *Annual Review of Psychology* 2019;70:577–97.
46. Cohen S, Frank E, Doyle WJ, et al. Types of stressors that increase susceptibility to the common cold in healthy adults. *Health Psychology* 1998;17(3):214–23.
47. Hughes K, Bellis MA, Hardcastle KA, et al. The effect of multiple adverse childhood experiences on health: a systematic review and meta-analysis. *Lancet Public Health* 2017;2(8):e356–e66.
48. Shor E, Roelfs DJ, Curreli M, et al. Widowhood and mortality: a meta-analysis and meta-regression. *Demography* 2012;49(2):575–606.
49. Helgeson VS. Gender, stress, and coping. In: Folkman S (ed.) *The Oxford Handbook of Stress, Health, and Coping*. Oxford: Oxford University Press; 2011: 63–85.
50. Dedovic K, Wadiwalla M, Engert V, et al. The role of sex and gender socialization in stress reactivity. *Developmental Psychology* 2009;45 (1):45–55.
51. Rodin G, Daneman D. Eating disorders in patients with diabetes. *American Journal of Psychiatry* 1991;148(7):957.
52. Mayou R. Introduction: the relationship between physical and psychiatric pathology. In: Mallinson C (ed.) *Psychiatric Aspects of Physical Disease*. London: Royal College of Physicians; 1995: 3–7.
53. Patel V, Chatterji S. Integrating mental health in care for noncommunicable diseases: an imperative for person-centered care. *Health Affairs* 2015;34 (9):1498–505.
54. Faessler L, Kutz A, Haubitz S, et al. Psychological distress in medical patients 30 days following an emergency department admission: results from a prospective, observational study. *BMC Emergency Medicine* 2016;16(1):33.
55. Murray CJ, Vos T, Lozano R, et al. Disability-adjusted life years (DALYs) for 291 diseases and injuries in 21 regions, 1990-2010: a systematic

analysis for the Global Burden of Disease Study 2010. *Lancet* 2012;380 (9859):2197–223.

56. Mayou R, Seagroatt V, Goldacre M. Use of psychiatric services by patients in a general hospital. *BMJ* 1991;303 (6809):1029–32.

57. McManus S, Bebbington PE, Jenkins R, et al. *Mental Health and Wellbeing in England: The Adult Psychiatric Morbidity Survey 2014*. NHS Digital; 2016.

58. Hodgson K, Stafford M, Fisher R. *Inequalities in Health Care for People with Depression and/or Anxiety*. London: Health Foundation; 2020.

59. Smith DJ, Court H, McLean G, et al. Depression and multimorbidity: a cross-sectional study of 1,751,841 patients in primary care. *Journal of Clinical Psychiatry* 2014;75(11):1202–8; quiz 8.

60. Swaraj S, Wang M, Chung D, et al. Meta-analysis of natural, unnatural and cause-specific mortality rates following discharge from in-patient psychiatric facilities. *Acta Psychiatrica Scandnavica* 2019;140(3):244–64.

61. Sara G, Chen W, Large M, et al. Potentially preventable hospitalisations for physical health conditions in community mental health service users: a population-wide linkage study. *Epidemiology and Psychiatric Sciences* 2021;30:e22.

62. Scott G, Beauchamp-Lebrón AM, Rosa-Jiménez AA, et al. Commonly diagnosed mental disorders in a general hospital system. *International Journal of Mental Health Systems* 2021;15(1):61.

63. Walker J, Burke K, Wanat M, et al. The prevalence of depression in general hospital inpatients: a systematic review and meta-analysis of interview-based studies. *Psychological Medicine* 2018;48 (14):2285–98.

64. Kessler RC, Bromet EJ. The epidemiology of depression across cultures. *Annual Review of Public Health* 2013;34:119–38.

65. Wang J, Wu X, Lai W, et al. Prevalence of depression and depressive symptoms among outpatients: a systematic review and meta-analysis. *BMJ Open* 2017;7(8): e017173.

66. Mitchell AJ, Chan M, Bhatti H, et al. Prevalence of depression, anxiety, and adjustment disorder in oncological, haematological, and palliative-care settings: a meta-analysis of 94 interview-based studies. *Lancet Oncology* 2011;12 (2):160–74.

67. Hawton K, Mayou R, Feldman E. Significance of psychiatric symptoms in general medical patients with mood disorders. *General Hospital Psychiatry* 1990;12(5):296–302.

68. Clark DA, Cook A, Snow D. Depressive symptom differences in hospitalized, medically ill, depressed psychiatric inpatients and nonmedical controls. *Journal of Abnormal Psychology* 1998;107(1):38–48.

69. Cui L, Wang C, Wu Z, et al. Symptomatology differences of major depression in psychiatric versus general hospitals: a machine learning approach. *Journal of Affective Disorders* 2020;260:349–60.

70. Boland RJ, Diaz S, Lamdan RM, et al. Overdiagnosis of depression in the general hospital. *General Hospital Psychiatry* 1996;18(1):28–35.

71. Fisher L, Hessler DM, Polonsky WH, et al. Prevalence of depression in Type 1 diabetes and the problem of over-diagnosis. *Diabetic Medicineh* 2016;33 (11):1590–7.

72. Reed GM, Mendonça Correia J, Esparza P, et al. The WPA-WHO global survey of psychiatrists' attitudes towards mental disorders classification. *World Psychiatry* 2011;10(2):118–31.

73. O'Dronnell ML, Alkemade N, Creamer M, et al. A longitudinal study of adjustment disorder after trauma exposure. *American Journal of Psychiatry* 2016;173(12):1231–8.

74. Strain JJ, Smith GC, Hammer JS, et al. Adjustment disorder: a multisite study of its utilization and interventions in the consultation-liaison psychiatry setting. *General Hospital Psychiatry* 1998;20 (3):139–49.

75. Casey P, Jabbar F, O'Leary E, et al. Suicidal behaviours in adjustment disorder and depressive episode. *Journal of Affective Disorders* 2015;174:441–6.

76. Einsle F, Köllner V, Dannemann S, et al. Development and validation of a self-report for the assessment of adjustment disorders. *Psychology, Health & Medicine* 2010;15(5):584–95.

77. Maercker A, Bachem RC, Lorenz L, et al. Adjustment disorders are uniquely suited for eHealth interventions: concept and case study. *JMIR Mental Health* 2015;2(2):e15.

78. Liang L, Ben-Ezra M, Chan EWW, et al. Psychometric evaluation of the Adjustment Disorder New Module-20 (ADNM-20): a multi-study analysis. *Journal of Anxiety Disorders* 2021;81:102406.

79. Huyse FJ, Herzog T, Lobo A, et al. Consultation-liaison psychiatric service delivery: results from a European study. *General Hospital Psychiatry* 2001;23 (3):124–32.

80. Folstein MF, Folstein SE, McHugh PR. 'Mini-mental state'. A practical method for grading the cognitive state of patients for the clinician. *Journal of Psychiatric Research* 1975;12(3):189–98.

81. Mayou R, Hawton K. Psychiatric disorder in the general hospital. *British Journal of Psychiatry* 1986;149:172–90.

82. Raymont V, Bingley W, Buchanan A, et al. Prevalence of mental incapacity in medical inpatients and associated risk factors: cross-sectional study. *Lancet* 2004;364(9443):1421–7.

83. Mukadam N, Sampson EL. A systematic review of the prevalence, associations and outcomes of dementia in older general hospital inpatients. *International Psychogeriatrics* 2011;23 (3):344–55.

84. Vasilevskis EE, Han JH, Hughes CG, et al. Epidemiology and risk factors for delirium across hospital settings. *Best Practice & Research Clinical Anaesthesiology* 2012;26(3):277–87.

85. Fairburn CG, Peveler RC, Davies B, et al. Eating disorders in young adults with insulin dependent diabetes mellitus: a controlled study. *BMJ* 1991;303(6793):17–20.

86. Perry S, Difede J, Musngi G, et al. Predictors of posttraumatic stress disorder after burn injury. *American Journal of Psychiatry* 1992;149(7):931–5.

87. Saunders JB, Aasland OG, Babor TF, et al. Development of the Alcohol Use Disorders Identification Test (AUDIT): WHO collaborative project on early detection of persons with harmful alcohol consumption – II. *Addiction* 1993;88(6):791–804.

88. Roberts E, Morse R, Epstein S, et al. The prevalence of wholly attributable alcohol conditions in the United Kingdom hospital system: a systematic review, meta-analysis and meta-

regression. *Addiction* 2019;114 (10):1726–37.

89. NHS Digital. *Adult Psychiatric Morbidity Survey: Survey of Mental Health and Wellbeing, England*, 2014. digital.nhs.uk/data-and-information/publications/statistical/adult-psychiatric-morbidity-survey/adult-psychiatric-morbidity-survey-survey-of-mental-health-and-wellbeing-england-2014 (accessed 14 May 2022) (Archived at www.webcitation.org/78W1SNSJl).

90. Watson M, Haviland JS, Greer S, et al. Influence of psychological response on survival in breast cancer: a population-based cohort study. *Lancet* 1999;354 (9187):1331–6.

91. Frasure-Smith N, Lespérance F, Gravel G, et al. Social support, depression, and mortality during the first year after myocardial infarction. *Circulation* 2000;101(16):1919–24.

92. Smolderen KG, Buchanan DM, Gosch K, et al. Depression treatment and 1-year mortality after acute myocardial infarction: insights from the TRIUMPH registry (translational research investigating underlying disparities in acute myocardial infarction patients' health status). *Circulation* 2017;135 (18):1681–9.

93. Sadlonova M, Vogelgsang J, Lange C, et al. Identification of risk factors for delirium, cognitive decline, and dementia after cardiac surgery (FINDERI-find delirium risk factors): a study protocol of a prospective observational study. *BMC Cardiovascular Disorders* 2022;22 (1):299.

94. Mayou RA, Gill D, Thompson DR, et al. Depression and anxiety as predictors of outcome after myocardial infarction. *Psychosomatic Medicine* 2000;62 (2):212–9.

95. Felker B, Katon W, Hedrick SC, et al. The association between depressive symptoms and health status in patients with chronic pulmonary disease. *General Hospital Psychiatry* 2001;23 (2):56–61.

96. Stenager EN, Stenager E. Suicide and patients with neurologic diseases. Methodologic problems. *Archives of Neurology* 1992;49(12):1296–303.

97. Feinstein A. Multiple sclerosis, depression, and suicide. *BMJ* 1997;315 (7110):691–2.

98. Breitbart W, Krivo S. Suicide. In: Holland C (ed.) *Psycho-Oncology*. Oxford: Oxford University Press; 1998: 541–7.

99. Ahmedani BK, Peterson EL, Hu Y, et al. Major physical health conditions and risk of suicide. *American Journal of Preventive Medicine* 2017;53(3):308–15.

100. Scott KM, Hwang I, Chiu WT, et al. Chronic physical conditions and their association with first onset of suicidal behavior in the world mental health surveys. *Psychosomatic Medicine* 2010;72(7):712–9.

101. Dougall N, Lambert P, Maxwell M, et al. Deaths by suicide and their relationship with general and psychiatric hospital discharge: 30-year record linkage study. *British Journal of Psychiatry* 2014;204:267–73.

102. Brody DS. Physician recognition of behavioral, psychological, and social aspects of medical care. *Archives of Internal Medicine* 1980;140(10):1286–9.

103. Dorning H, Davies A, Blunt I. *Focus On: People with Mental Ill Health and Hospital Use. Exploring Disparities in Hospital Use for Physical Healthcare. Quality Watch.* London: The Health Foundation and Nuffield Trust; 2015.

104. Siddiqui N, Dwyer M, Stankovich J, et al. Hospital length of stay variation and comorbidity of mental illness: a retrospective study of five common chronic medical conditions. *BMC Health Services Research* 2018;18(1):498.

105. Moffic HS, Paykel ES. Depression in medical in-patients. *British Journal of Psychiatry* 1975;126:346–53.

106. Bridges KW, Goldberg DP. Somatic presentation of DSM-III psychiatric disorders in primary care. *Journal of Psychosomatic Research* 1985;29:563–9.

107. Seltzer A. Prevalence, detection and referral of psychiatric morbidity in general medical patients. *Journal of the Royal Society of Medicine* 1989;82 (7):410–2.

108. Goldberg D. Identifying psychiatric illness among general medical patients. *British Medical Journal (Clinical Research Ed)* 1985;291(6489):161–2.

109. Maguire P. Barriers to psychological care of the dying. *British Medical Journal (Clinical Research Ed)* 1985;291 (6510):1711–3.

110. Kroenke K, Spitzer RL, Williams JB. The PHQ-9: validity of a brief depression severity measure. *Journal of General Internal Medicine* 2001;16 (9):606–13.

111. Zigmond AS, Snaith RP. The hospital anxiety and depression scale. *Acta Psychiatrica Scandinavica* 1983;67 (6):361–70.

112. Beck A, Steer R, Brown G. *BDI-II, Beck Depression Inventory: Manual.* San Antonio, TX: Psychological Corp; 1996.

113. Yesavage JA, Sheikh JI. 9/Geriatric depression scale (GDS) recent evidence and development of a shorter version. *Clinical Gerontologist* 1986;5(1–2):165–73.

114. Fink P, Ørbøl E, Hansen MS, et al. Detecting mental disorders in general hospitals by the SCL-8 scale. *Journal of Psychosomatic Research* 2004;56 (3):371–5.

115. Velikova G, Booth L, Smith AB, et al. Measuring quality of life in routine oncology practice improves communication and patient well-being: a randomized controlled trial. *Journal of Clinical Oncology* 2004;22(4):714–24.

116. House A. Mood disorders in the physically ill – problems of definition and measurement. *Journal of Psychosomatic Research* 1988;32(4-5):345–53.

117. Meakin CJ. Screening for depression in the medically ill. The future of paper and pencil tests. *British Journal of Psychiatry* 1992;160:212–6.

118. Rayner L, Matcham F, Hutton J, et al. Embedding integrated mental health assessment and management in general hospital settings: feasibility, acceptability and the prevalence of common mental disorder. *General Hospital Psychiatry* 2014;36(3):318-24.

119. Katon WJ, Lin EH, von Korff M, et al. Collaborative care for patients with depression and chronic illnesses. *The New England Journal of Medicine* 2010;363(27):2611–20.

120. Thompson H, Faig W, Gupta N, et al. Collaborative care for depression of adults and adolescents: measuring the effectiveness of screening and treatment uptake. *Psychiatric Services* 2019;70 (7):604–7.

121. Ewing JA. Detecting alcoholism: the CAGE questionnaire. *JAMA*;252 (14):1905–7.

122. Hearne R, Connolly A, Sheehan J. Alcohol abuse: prevalence and detection in a general hospital. *Journal of the Royal Society of Medicine* 2002;95 (2):84–7.

123. Hodkinson HM. Evaluation of a mental test score for assessment of mental impairment in the elderly. *Age Ageing* 1972;1(4):233–8.

124. Bazire S. *Psychotropic Drug Directory 2014: The Professionals' Pocket Handbook and Aide Memoire.* Cheltenham: Lloyd-Reinhold Communications; 2014.

125. Bulletin DaT. Do SSRIs cause gastrointestinal bleeding? *Drug and Therapeutics Bulletin* 2004;42(3):17–88.

126. Anderson IM, Edwards JG. Guidelines for choice of selective serotonin reuptake inhibitor in depressive illness. *Advances in Psychiatric Treatment* 2001;7(3):170–80.

127. Inouye SK, Marcantonio ER, Metzger ED. Doing damage in delirium: the hazards of antipsychotic treatment in elderly persons. *Lancet Psychiatry* 2014;1(4):312–15.

128. Maust DT, Kim HM, Seyfried LS, et al. Antipsychotics, other psychotropics, and the risk of death in patients with dementia: number needed to harm. *JAMA Psychiatry* 2015;72 (5):438–45.

129. Barata IA, Shandro JR, Montgomery M, et al. Effectiveness of SBIRT for alcohol use disorders in the emergency department: a systematic review. *Western Journal of Emergency Medicine* 2017;18(6):1143–52.

130. Cabaniss DL, Cherry S, Douglas CJ, et al. *Psychodynamic Psychotherapy: A Clinical Manual.* 2nd ed. Chichester, West Sussex: John Wiley; 2017.

131. Van Den Beldt HM, Ruble AE, Welton RS, et al. Contemporary supportive therapy: a review of history, theory, and evidence. *Psychodynamic Psychiatry* 2021;49(4):562–90.

132. Wood BC, Mynors-Wallis LM. Problem-solving therapy in palliative care. *Palliative Medicine* 1997;11 (1):49–54.

133. Miller WR, Rollnick S. *Motivational Interviewing: Helping People Change.* New York: Guilford Press; 2012.

134. Klerman GL, Weissman MM. *Interpersonal Psychotherapy of Depression: A Brief, Focused, Specific Strategy.* Lanham, MD: Jason Aronson, Incorporated; 1994.

135. Markowitz JC, Klerman GL, Perry SW. Interpersonal psychotherapy of depressed HIV-positive outpatients. *Hospital & Community Psychiatry* 1992;43(9):885–90.

136. Barkham M, Guthrie E, Hardy GE, et al. *Psychodynamic-Interpersonal Therapy: A Conversational Model.* London: SAGE Publications Ltd; 2017. sk.sagepub.com/books/psychodynamic-interpersonal-therapy-a-conversational-model.

137. Sperry L. *Psychological Treatment of Chronic Illness: The Biopsychosocial Therapy Approach.* Washington, DC: American Psychological Association; 2006.

138. Graham CD, Gouick J, Krahé C, et al. A systematic review of the use of Acceptance and Commitment Therapy (ACT) in chronic disease and long-term conditions. *Clinical Psychology Review* 2016;46:46–58.

139. Bernard P, Romain A-J, Caudroit J, et al. Cognitive behavior therapy combined with exercise for adults with chronic diseases: systematic review and meta-analysis. *Health Psychology* 2018;37(5):433.

140. Williams ACC, Fisher E, Hearn L, et al. Psychological therapies for the management of chronic pain (excluding headache) in adults. *Cochrane Database of Systematic Reviews* 2020;8:CD007407.

141. Gielissen MF, Verhagen S, Witjes F, et al. Effects of cognitive behavior therapy in severely fatigued disease-free cancer patients compared with patients waiting for cognitive behavior therapy: a randomized controlled trial. *Journal of Clinical Oncology* 2006;24(30):4882–7.

142. Kunik ME, Veazey C, Cully JA, et al. COPD education and cognitive behavioral therapy group treatment for clinically significant symptoms of depression and anxiety in COPD patients: a randomized controlled trial. *Psychological Medicine* 2008;38(3):385–96.

143. Walker J, Hansen CH, Martin P, et al. Integrated collaborative care for major depression comorbid with a poor prognosis cancer (SMaRT Oncology-3): a multicentre randomised controlled trial in patients with lung cancer. *Lancet Oncology* 2014;15(10):1168–76.

144. Ramanuj PP, Pincus HA. Collaborative care: enough of the why; what about the how? *British Journal of Psychiatry* 2019:1–4.

145. Hassan TB, MacNamara AF, Davy A, et al. Lesson of the week: managing patients with deliberate self harm who refuse treatment in the accident and emergency department. *BMJ* 1999;319 (7202):107–9.

146. Hewson B. The law on managing patients who deliberately harm themselves and refuse treatment. *BMJ* 1999;319(7214):905–7.

147. Hull A, Haut F. Managing patients with deliberate self harm who refuse treatment in accident and emergency departments. (Letter – author reply 917). *BMJ* 1999(319):916.

148. British Medical Association & Law Society. *Assessment of Mental Capacity,* 2nd ed. London: BMJ Books; 2004.

149. Royal College of Physicians & Royal College of Psychiatrists. *The Psychological Care of Medical Patients (Council Report CR108).* London: Royal College of Psychiatrists; 2003.

150. Royal College of Surgeons of England & Royal College of Psychiatrists. *Report of the Working Party on the Psychological Care of Surgical Patients (Council Report CR55).* London: Royal College of Surgeons of England & Royal College of Psychiatrists; 1997.

151. National Institute of Health and Social Care. *Achieving Better Access to 24/7 Urgent and Emergency Mental Health Care – Part 2: Implementing the Evidence-based Treatment Pathway for Urgent and Emergency Liaison Mental Health Services for Adults and Older Adults – Guidance.* London: National Institute of Health and Social Care; 2016.

152. Lipowski ZJ. Consultation-liaison psychiatry: the first half century. *General Hospital Psychiatry* 1986;8(5):305–15.

153. House A, Hodgson G. Estimating needs and meeting demands. In: Benjamin S, House A, Jenkins P (eds.) *Liaison Psychiatry: Defining Needs and Planning Services.* Berlin/Heidelberg: Springer Science & Business; 1994: 3–15.

154. De Giorgio G, Quartesan R, Sciarma T, et al. Consultation-liaison psychiatry—from theory to clinical practice: an observational study in a general hospital. *BMC Research Notes* 2015;8(1):1–6.

155. Peveler R, Feldman E, Friedman T. *Liaison Psychiatry: Planning Services for Specialist Settings.* Berlin/Heidelberg: Springer Science & Business; 2000.

156. Creed F, Morgan R, Fiddler M, et al. Depression and anxiety impair health-related quality of life and are associated with increased costs in general medical inpatients. *Psychosomatics* 2002;43 (4):302–9.

Chapter

20 Adult Mental Health Services*

David Kingdon and Paul Rowlands

Mental health services are intended to provide the means to deliver interventions and care to people experiencing mental health problems. This can only be achieved if the staff and resources to provide interventions and care are available. These form 'the tools of the trade' for psychiatrists working in leadership roles in mental health teams, and their influence on the shape and prioritisation of provision is fundamental to maximising the effectiveness of services. Unfortunately, the current design and resourcing of services can seriously interfere with this happening. Services have evolved over centuries, and many practices are determined by convention and limited by resources, particularly the availability of staff in sufficient numbers and with appropriate skills. This chapter focuses on general adult services in the UK, with specialist perinatal, general hospital, substance misuse, eating disorders, personality disorder and services in general practice described elsewhere in the book. The complexity of these services and their interfaces will be discussed in this chapter.

Assessing the Evidence Base for Mental Health Services

The evidence base for mental health services comprises randomised controlled trials, cohort and observational studies, which can be qualitative or quantitative. Where a specific defined intervention is being considered, it can be possible to use randomised control trials (RCT), but such service-based RCTs are relatively unusual. Individual RCT studies have investigated size of caseloads,[1] employment services,[2] assertive outreach[3] and early intervention.[4] Positive results have been obtained, but limitations on the length of the investigation period (especially important due to the long-term and relapsing nature of many conditions), variability of the interventions offered, control of extraneous factors and the difficulty in performing and funding multiple studies to develop interventions (as might happen with specific therapies, e.g. drug or psychological) mean that RCTs are difficult to conduct and, sometimes, to interpret and generalise. They cannot therefore be considered the 'gold standard' for evaluating all mental health service interventions. Innovation in services and durability has probably been more important in shaping them, relying on the clinical experience of multiple individuals' outcomes accounting for variation with multiple conditions and severities. Political, philosophical and social attitudes and pressures – and changes in these – have shaped service development hugely. As an example, the nineteenth-century legislative reform driven by evangelical political figures such as Lord Shaftesbury as well as twentieth-century policies on deinstitutionalisation[5] have been seminal. However, the risk of developing services in this way is that practices become established as a result of political direction, convention and convenience, and they can be removed for financial reasons; research methods involving meaningful patient and carer input and effective advocacy are essential to minimise this. Research funding agencies (e.g. the Research Councils, NHS Research and Development and other funding agencies) need to prioritise further development of such methodologies and investment to evaluate services.

Evolution of Services

There was very little organised care for people with mental illness before the eighteenth century with the exception of the Bethlem hospital in London, which was founded in 1247. General population mortality was high, and prior to the nineteenth century, around half of the people born died before puberty. England had a small, largely rural population of around five and a half million people in the early eighteenth century. The numbers of people confined for mental illness remained small throughout the eighteenth century, but small, private 'madhouses' developed. Concern at the nature of these and the inhumanity of many of the practices led to legislative reform, and by the middle of the nineteenth century, the 1845 Lunacy Act and the County Asylums Act mandated the establishment of public asylums by every county and borough to provide asylum treatment for its 'pauper lunatics'. This Act also set up the lunacy commission to oversee asylums nationally. These initially were successful with a majority of patients discharged within a year but then, as they expanded – against the huge population growth and shifts of the nineteenth century – they became more crowded, conditions deteriorated and discharge rates declined. Over time, 'incurable' patients accumulated, giving the asylum its characteristic feel and reputation in the public consciousness. Treatments involved bloodletting and purges aimed at altering the hypothesised

* Acknowledgements to Letsie Tilley for advice on the funding section.

organic basis of mental illness, and vivid descriptions of these methods and associated cruelty remain etched in public awareness. Roy Porter[6] described how:

> Those horror stories of lunatics chained in underground dungeons in France, whipped in Germany and jeered by ogling sightseers in London's Bedlam – all are true. But 'moral' (meaning psychological and social) management was also used, notably at the Retreat in York, based on the belief that many forms of madness arose from life experiences and could be cured by psychosocial means. It emphasised kindness, minimisation of coercion and encouragement of productive activity. In some asylums, for paying patients, conditions were positively comfortable.

The foundation of the asylums in the nineteenth century was associated with legislation requiring the head of the asylum to be a qualified medical practitioner. In 1841, Dr Samuel Hitch, resident superintendent of the Gloucestershire General Lunatic asylum, organised a meeting for asylum doctors that led on to the formation of the 'Association of Medical Officers of Asylums and Hospitals for the Insane'. This was the world's first national psychiatric association. This became the Medico-Psychological Association (1865–1926) when it acquired a Royal Charter and became the Royal Medico-Psychological Association (RMPA, 1926–1971). However, the emergence of the Royal College of Psychiatrists was not without serious birth pangs at the time. A group of then-junior doctors at the time known as the Petitioners objected to the hold the Royal College of Physicians had over the RMPA, as well as the inability of the RMPA to facilitate training. This dispute was eventually resolved with the formation of the Royal College of Psychiatrists in 1972, with the prominent academic Sir Martin Roth becoming its first president.

In 1853, the Association of Medical Officers of Asylums and Hospitals for the Insane started to publish *The Asylum Journal*, which then cost a grand total of 6 pence. In its first editorial, its editor Sir John Bucknill argued strongly that the care of the insane should remain in the province of medicine.[7]

> The physician is now the responsible Guardian of the Lunatic, and ever must remain so unless by some calamitous reverse the progress of the world in civilisation should be turned back to the direction of practical barbarism... Since the public in all civilised countries have recognised the fact that Insanity lies strictly within the domain of medical science new responsibilities and new duties have devolved to those who have devoted themselves to its investigation and treatment..." (*The Asylum Journal* 1853;1:1)

This is the origin of psychiatry as a medical speciality in the UK. In France, these doctors were known as the alienists. The alienists of France and asylum doctors of the UK can be described as the first 'true' psychiatrists as they were the first doctors to work full time with the mentally ill.

After a few years in 1858, the *Asylum Journal* became the *Journal of Mental Science*, a name which remained for more than 100 years, until in 1962 the name changed to become the *British Journal of Psychiatry*.

Informal admission to an asylum became possible only with the Mental Treatment Act of 1930, which also encouraged local authorities to develop outpatient clinics and aftercare services, which again Shaftesbury had championed towards the end of his life in the late nineteenth century. Hospital numbers peaked in Britain and in the USA in the mid-1950s, although substantially later in many other countries – for example, Japan, where numbers remain very high. The reduction in numbers that then occurred in the USA and UK reflected major changes in society post-war, including the introduction of the NHS and establishment of a Royal Commission: 'The Percy Commission' from 1954–1956. The introduction of therapeutic community principles (e.g. at Dingleton Hospital in the Borders), antipsychotic medication, the opening of hospital doors (e.g. Mapperley in Nottingham) and subsequently the major revisions to the Mental Health Act 1959 consolidated this. The Minister of Health at the time, Derek Walker-Smith, stated that 'One of the main principles we are seeking to pursue is the reorientation of the mental health services away from institutional care towards care in the community'.[8] His successor Enoch Powell's 'Water Tower' speech in 1961[9] at the National Association for Mental Health (forerunners of MIND) set a target of reducing psychiatric bed numbers from around 150,000 to 75,000 over 15 years, called for the old asylums to be torn down and demanded a 'transformation' in how people thought about care for the mentally ill.

By 1975, the focus had moved away from the asylum to the development of psychiatric units in local general hospitals with a range of community services as described in *Better Services For The Mentally Ill.*[10] The thrust of policy was then to move towards community-based services with a gradual replacement of the institutions. Basaglia, a psychiatrist in Trieste, Northern Italy, led the most radical changes in inpatient care with the Italian parliament in 1978 focusing on human rights for patients, limiting provisions for involuntary detention and closing the local mental hospitals.[11]

The numbers in hospitals in Britain peaked in the mid-1950s (estimated at 155,000 in England). It has dropped substantially since, with rehabilitation and long-term care for general adult (as opposed to forensic) patients in the UK now provided in community settings, albeit some remaining on premises previously used by the mental hospital. The rapid decline in bed numbers initially focused on long-stay beds. The past decade has included acute beds, but this has been unevenly and inadequately replaced by alternative services. This led to a lack of systematic care and support in the community, increasing family/carer burden and major concerns about the number of people with mental illness who were homeless or residing in prison. The relationship between prisoner numbers and mental hospital patient numbers is a complex issue, but across decades and across countries, an inverse correlation has been observed.[12] As psychiatric bed numbers fall, numbers of people with mental illness in prison rise.

The hospital closure programme was assessed by research studies during the period when the numbers in institutions were reducing. The Team for the Assessment of Psychiatric Services (TAPS) compared populations in two hospitals (Claybury and Friern in North London), which progressed at different rates of resettlement, and they published a large series of papers describing process and outcomes.[13] The studies suggested that those who move into reasonably good-quality residential care generally showed similar clinical and symptomatic outcomes compared with matched cohorts who remained in hospital, but had better social outcomes, had enhanced social networks, showed decreased behavioural problems and improved medication compliance, and were much happier with their living situations.[14] There was no evidence of increased death rates, suicide, crime or vagrancy. The cost of care in the community was generally slightly less than of continuing care in hospital, but it showed significant increases with increasing levels of disability.[15]

The argument has been made that rather than deinstitutionalisation occurring, we have now seen trans-institutionalisation.[16] In other words, the asylum has effectively been replaced by a range of forensic and residential accommodation and homeless hostels/prison. The latter was recognised in the early 1990s, and homeless mental illness and prison in-reach teams were developed to mitigate this occurrence. Statutory mental health accommodation, at levels much lower than at the peak of asylum bed numbers, can be argued from TAPS evidence to be more suited to needs and desires (see Box 20.1). There seems little evidence however that reductions in overall prevalence of this population have been occurring, and we now have a dispersed population living in a range of settings, some impoverished and inappropriate, in ways that can have historical resonance with the pre-asylum era.

Box 20.1 Asylums[17]

Advantages of the asylums:

- spacious – internal (unless overcrowded) and especially, external
- range of facilities within the hospital grounds
- peace and tranquillity
- easy to admit and discharge

Disadvantages:

- stigmatisation by the local community
- often remote from home due to central or peripheral location in cities or counties
- for patients, not an alternative to home compared to community residence
- difficult for visitors to access
- community teams available based locally and able to visit at home and more accessible in an emergency
- lack of access to a primary care team

As the case was accepted that mental health services can be effective using evidence-based psychopharmacological and psychosocial treatments and provide support local to the persons home, services have increasingly been deemed responsible for the absence or unavailability of effective interventions or treatment when things have gone wrong. This has particularly related to circumstances where homicides were committed by people with mental illnesses but has increasingly come to include people in contact with services who have died from suicide. A further widening of this perceived responsibility has included focus on the raised overall mortality of people with mental health problems.

An instance of homicide of a mental health social worker associated with a patient under mental health care led to the *Report of the Committee of Inquiry into the Care and Aftercare of Miss Sharon Campbell* (1988). This stipulated that a clinical system for providing safe and effective care outside hospital be defined and implemented. This became known as the *Care Programme Approach* (1990, see later). Subsequently, the Mental Health (Patients in the Community) Act 1995 introduced supervised discharge, which was compulsory aftercare but not compulsory treatment. In due course, compulsory treatment orders were introduced in the Mental Health Act (2008) and have been used a great deal, far more than originally estimated, but they have not been demonstrated to be effective in their goal of improving outcomes or reducing overall relapse rates.[18] In 2020–2021, there were 6,070 new community treatment orders (CTOs); the rate in 'Black or Black British' people was 78.9 per 1,000,000, 10 times the rate for the 'White' group – 7.8 per 1,000,000.[19]

Health of the Nation in 1991 prioritised mental health as one of five key areas, with objectives set to reduce suicide rates by 10 per cent over 10 years (which was achieved) and improve the health and social functioning of mentally ill people (see outcome measurement later). Population surveys were also instituted – the Office for National Statistics (ONS) National Psychiatric Morbidity Survey (NPMS) and a measure of Attitudes to Mental Illness. These have been repeated and was used to assess and monitor prevalence and the effectiveness of mental health promotion initiatives (see later[20]). The NHS Plan in 2000[21] provided new funding for 'evidence-based' teams (Assertive Outreach, Early Intervention in Psychosis, Crisis and Home Treatment and Primary Care Liaison Teams). This did not directly provide additional resources for core community mental health teams, but responsibility for patients who were presenting with signs of early psychosis, were difficult to engage or were presenting in crisis moved to the new specialist 'functional' teams. A variety of frameworks and guides followed, including policy implementation guides to the specialist teams and CMHTs[22] as well as statements of intent around issues such as management of personality disorder.[23] They remain broadly relevant in terms of definitions and descriptions of current service components. The National Institute for Health and

Social Care (NICE) and Health Improvement Scotland (SIGN) Clinical Guidelines and Evidence Reviews initially started with schizophrenia in 2002 and have now been issued and updated for all the common and severe mental disorders. They have been influential, although specific funding has not directly accompanied recommendations and so implementation have generally been inadequately resourced.

The Community Mental Health Framework,[24] launched immediately prior to the pandemic, represented an attempt to reground services and again re-engineer the structure of service delivery, emphasising the importance of community connectedness. It is too early to say how this will unfold against a background of mental health and primary care services still struggling with the consequences of prolonged austerity and the impacts of the pandemic. Its call for 'transformation' echoes the calls of policy reformers dating back more than half a century.

Care Programme Approach

As concerns about public safety progressed (see earlier), the *Care Programme Approach* (CPA) was established in 1991[25] in England, with similar provisions elsewhere in the UK, to ensure that a safety net of care was provided for people with severe mental illness, and recent developments have recognised that it has broadened its principles to all served by mental health services.[26] The 1990 circular establishing CPA set out requirements for health and social care assessment, including risk assessment, and for involving patients, carers, the multi-disciplinary team and other agencies in response to the Spokes Inquiry into the death of Isobel Schwarz, a social worker. She had sadly died at the hands of a person with severe mental illness whose care had not been provided in an organised and effective multi-disciplinary way.

Patients accepted by mental health services were required to have a key worker, care plan and a review date, in consultation with the patient, carers and other involved professionals. It initially described two levels, basic and enhanced; in practice, this generally meant that patients on basic CPA were those seen by a single practitioner, often a doctor in outpatients, and for enhanced, a doctor, a non-medical care coordinator and sometimes other agencies. Targets were set by government (Monitor and now NHS Improvement) that all CPA patients had a care plan completed every year and, under the National Commissioning for Quality and Innovation (CQUINs) payments framework (replaced by the Quality and Outcomes Framework), received a minimum of an annual physical health check. The number of people on CPA has sometimes been used as a proxy for the severity of individuals on caseloads and for use in service redesign. Numbers reported as 'on CPA' have varied hugely between organisations and often appear to have been driven by other bureaucratic demands.

Services have now progressed such that the broad principles of CPA are fully accepted by professionals and regulatory bodies, as reiterated in the NHS Position Statement on CPA in 2021.[26] However, there is no evidence that CPA criteria have been applied consistently across services or that this has improved over the years. Recent figures from the Mental Health Intelligence Network 'Fingertips' tool[27] range from 1.7 to 23.5 per cent of patients allocated to CPA, which is not proportional to morbidity. Similarly, there is no sign that the quality as opposed to quantity of care plans or health checks and interventions is adequate. The CPA definition is broad and subjective, and applying a 'tick box' approach to care plans and physical health checks is at best only a first step to improving their application. Dichotomising patients into CPA or not is overly simplistic, and allocation of resources has not explicitly followed, although managers probably give consideration to providing increased resource and time for increased need (whether on CPA or not). It has also contributed, despite the emphasis on its being primarily a clinical process, to an administrative rather a person-focus:

> care plans were described as administratively burdensome and were rarely consulted. Carers reported varying levels of involvement. Risk assessments were central to clinical concerns but were rarely discussed with patients. Patients valued therapeutic relationships with care coordinators and others, and saw these as central to recovery.[28]

When it was introduced, CPA was also intended to lead to a prioritisation of service delivery to people according to their needs. The allocation to enhanced CPA can be argued to have initially achieved this, and refocusing on CPA provided further reinforcement. Such prioritisation remains necessary, but allocation to CPA is a blunt instrument to do this. In practice, applying targets to CPA has also been a disincentive to allocating patients to it. This has now been accepted by NHS England in its CPA position statement,[26] CMHT transformation proposals and its proposed move to a pathways-based funding system.

So, the principles of CPA have been accepted as the essential foundation to improving quality of community services, and broad consensus about their application has developed. However, CPA may not have led to the movement from these principles to practice in the systematic application of the evidence-based clinical guidelines and quality standards that have been developed since CPA originated. The National Institute for Health and Clinical Excellence (NICE) has described these for the range of clinical conditions, and they have been operationalised into care pathways describing 'what should happen and when'. This requires allocation of individuals to care pathways going beyond a dichotomous 'severe' and 'less severe' definition. Quality standards and outcome measures (see later) relevant to the pathways can now be implemented and monitored. Briefly clinical measures (see later) such as the HoNOS and Patient Rated Measures such as DIALOG[29] and ReQoL[30] support this and are relatively simple and quick to use and can be used in service benchmarking.[31]

So it is argued that CPA has been invaluable in setting principles and practice to follow as services in the community

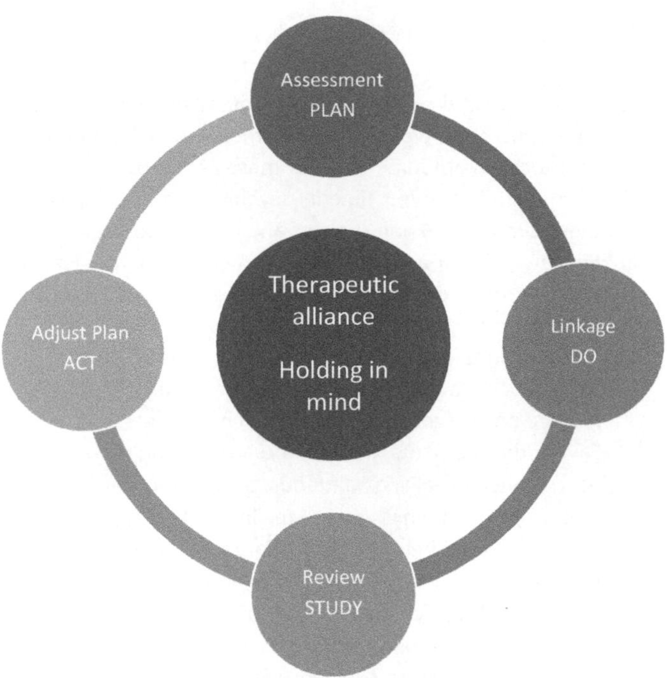

Figure 20.1 Quality Improvement PDSA cycle.

have developed, but mental health services now need to move beyond it.[32] CPA has done an invaluable job, but as time has passed, more individualised and sophisticated pathway-based systems should now be adopted. The fundamental principles though are sound. People should have an assessment, an agreed plan and agreed follow-up of that plan over time by an agreed individual within an agreed timeframe within a trusting therapeutic alliance. If it is not to be reviewed, that too should be agreed, and changes in the plan should also be negotiated and agreed. This can be conveniently summarised as a Quality Improvement PDSA cycle (Figure 20.1).

Who Needs Mental Health Services?

Mental health problems, illnesses or disorders are extremely common but usually self-limiting or managed within social networks. Help may be sought from local community organisations, faith organisations, voluntary and support groups and also national groups (e.g. Samaritans, Alzheimer's society, MIND and RETHINK Mental Illness) and also groups dealing with specific issues (e.g. domestic violence, cancer or gender identity). Such sources are non-stigmatising and connect people with flexible support that may sustain over time. Where these are not contacted or insufficient, local councils and general practitioners (see Chapter 18) provide a next level of support for an estimated 90 per cent or more of mental health presentations. Mental health services therefore provide care and treatment to only a small proportion of those with mental health issues.

These will be people with more severe or persistent mental health issues, but social circumstances and physical illness and access to specialised services may also be a major contributor to the need for mental health service involvement. Severe mental illness is generally preferred to 'serious', which can be misconstrued in terms of importance rather than referring to severity. This term is often used to describe psychosis and bipolar disorder; however, other conditions can also present severe problems. About one in 200 people have psychosis or bipolar disorder[33] – some need high levels of support and skilled interventions, but many with the right support will recover and manage their lives well. As described elsewhere, depression or anxiety disorders (including post-traumatic stress disorder and obsessive-compulsive disorder) can also be very distressing and debilitating, as can eating disorders and severe emotional needs/difficulties, alternatively described as personality disorder – borderline occurring in about 1 in 100.[33] Only 6 per cent of those accessing serious mental illness (SMI) services in 2018/2019 received inpatient care.[34] One in four adults experiences at least one diagnosable mental health problem each year, and mental illness costs the UK economy £105bn annually. In 2018/2019, more than 3.2 million people in England accessed the Improving Access to Psychological Therapies (IAPT) programme and serious mental illness (SMI) services.

Many people have a number of different conditions at the same time (comorbidities): physical illness, substance misuse,[35,36] psychoses and emotional difficulties. Social issues include estimated unemployment rates amongst individuals with severe mental illness are up to 95 per cent.[2] Nearly half (24,429) of all patients with disabilities accessing Supporting People housing-related support in 2008/2009 had a mental health disability. Of these, 50 per cent were subject to the Care Programme Approach (CPA). People with mental health conditions are more likely to live in rented accommodation than to be owner occupiers. People with mental health conditions are twice as likely as those without mental health conditions to be unhappy with their housing and four times as likely to say that it makes their health worse. Mental ill health is frequently cited as a reason for tenancy breakdown. Housing problems are frequently cited as a reason for a person being admitted or readmitted to inpatient care: finding appropriate accommodation is a major reason for delays in discharge.[37] People with severe problems die on average 20 years earlier than the general population[38] (see Chapter 16). Effects of mental health issues on the parenting of children are highly significant; interventions may be effective, though limited evidence exists[39] – care needs to be 'vertically integrated' (working with parents and children individually and collectively). Working towards stability and eventual recovery from mental health problems usually requires all these issues to be taken into account, which is where mental health services can contribute.

Prevention and De-stigmatisation

Prevention rather than cure remains a key aim of health care, and this should particularly be the case with mental health issues,[40] where social factors (e.g. poverty, inequality, physical illness, trauma and relationships) have been demonstrated to have such major impacts. Changes in society or health care that improve or lead to deterioration will impact on individuals and subsequently services and have costs for society itself.[41] Prevention may seem unrealistic for severe mental disorders such as schizophrenia or bipolar disorder and alleviation more reasonable. However, the argument is made that severe and apparently intractable illnesses, such as smallpox, have been eradicated, and the social antecedents of severe mental illnesses, especially childhood trauma and drug misuse, may similarly be amenable in time with changes in society. Depression and anxiety are natural responses to loss and threat, so prevention of their occurrence may be less practical, but improvements in adjustment and coping along with reduction in severity, recurrence and persistence are reasonable.

Public mental health is a major area of development (e.g. see Bhugra et al.)[42] Mental disorder prevention can be:

- Primary: interventions that prevent mental disorders from arising
- Secondary: early intervention for mental disorders and the associated impacts to minimise their effects
- Tertiary: intervention for people with established mental disorders to prevent relapse and the associated impacts to minimise disability

Mental wellbeing promotion can be:

- Primary: promotion of protective factors for mental wellbeing
- Secondary: early promotion in people with recent deterioration in mental wellbeing
- Tertiary: promotion in people with long-standing poor mental wellbeing

Campion and colleagues provide multiple examples of how prevention, promotion and resilience can be developed and reasons why this has not occurred in the past.[43] Implementing such initiatives has been assessed to be highly cost-effective.[43,44]

The evidence that specific approaches to individual wellbeing prevent mental health problems is however harder to demonstrate, but the Office for Science in 2008 produced a report proposing 'Five Ways to Wellbeing',[45] which has been widely advocated and can be readily communicated to people at risk or experiencing mental health problems (see Box 20.2). These changes involve individual choice, group and family support, as well as local and national political initiatives. The psychiatrist's role may be through individual support and influence at a local level or collectively through local and national organisation (e.g. Royal College of Psychiatrists and BMA).

Stigma and discrimination is widespread[46] (e.g. in employment). This can be particularly pronounced for ethnic minority and LGBTQ+ communities – where prevalence of mental illness is often higher in combination with distrust of mental health services; help may also not be received in a timely way.[47] Evidence is most promising for intensive public awareness campaigns, but these require organisation and resourcing at a regional or national level.[48] 'Time to Change' was a major country-wide anti-stigma campaign using individual stories that was evidence-based.[49] It aimed to change behaviour as well as attitudes and may have had economic benefits.[50] Significant increases in positive attitudes related to prejudice and exclusion occurred after the Time to Change campaign.[20]

Box 20.2 Five ways to wellbeing

1. Connect: With the people around you. With family, friends, colleagues and neighbours. At home, work, school or in your local community. Think of these as the cornerstones of your life and invest time in developing them. Building these connections will support and enrich you every day.
2. Be active: Go for a walk or run. Step outside. Cycle. Play a game. Garden. Dance. Exercising makes you feel good. Most importantly, discover a physical activity you enjoy and that suits your level of mobility and fitness.
3. Take notice: Be curious. Catch sight of the beautiful. Remark on the unusual. Notice the changing seasons. Savour the moment, whether you are walking to work, eating lunch or talking to friends. Be aware of the world around you and what you are feeling. Reflecting on your experiences will help you appreciate what matters to you.
4. Keep learning: Try something new. Rediscover an old interest. Sign up for that course. Take on a different responsibility at work. Fix a bike. Learn to play an instrument or how to cook your favourite food. Set a challenge you enjoy achieving. Learning new things will make you more confident as well as being fun.
5. Give: Do something nice for a friend, or a stranger. Thank someone. Smile. Volunteer your time. Join a community group. Look out, as well as in. Seeing yourself, and your happiness, as linked to the wider community can be incredibly rewarding and creates connections with the people around you.

Office of Science, 2008[45]

Mental Health Commissioning

Each commissioning area of the country has a duty to fund mental health care provision for its population, but this has become increasingly complicated as functionalisation of services and reduction in acute inpatient beds has been accompanied by a rise in Out-of-Area placements, increased provision of secure locked rehabilitation from private providers and a proliferation of service providers for the

'Increasing Access to Psychological Therapies' (IAPT – 'Talking Treatment') services. Demarcation disputes between teams and services over who is 'responsible' for leading the care of an individual have arisen. As competitive tendering has allowed provider units to win contracts in areas of the country that have sometimes been distant from their main base, this has produced further confusion. The process has not been demonstrated to improve quality of services nor reduced costs but has led to services being increasingly difficult for patients and families and professionals to understand and access. Concepts such as continuity of care over time have in some areas been given less priority than immediate access to assessment and short-term intervention. This loss of a sense of continuity and the experience of having to constantly retell one's story is a frequent theme from service users. There is now however a move back towards greater integration and less competition, but this has yet to produce major improvements.

Integrated Care Systems (ICS)[51] to combine primary, secondary, mental health and social care commissioning were introduced in 2022 – 42 in total in England – each covering just over a million population. The system elsewhere in the UK over the past few years has differed, but Scotland, Northern Ireland and Wales have generally been able to retain the more integrated approaches now advocated for England. Most commissioning areas have at least one provider unit (NHS Trusts) for general adult psychiatry. There may be separate units for more specialist services (e.g. eating disorders, substance misuse and autism).

Improving Access to Psychological Treatment (IAPT – Talking Treatments) may also be provided separately, often in conjunction with one or more third sector organisation (i.e. a voluntary or private provider). The pattern of provision nationally is similar, described later, due to requirements set by the government, Care Quality Commission (CQC) and National Institute for Health and Social Excellence, but resources in terms of staffing levels and physical provision may vary. The quality of services is regulated through CQC, which visit health and social services and rank them in terms of whether they provide people with safe, effective, compassionate, high-quality care; they will make recommendations and take action where necessary. It is also influenced by Health and Wellbeing boards of local councils and coroners who can make Reports to Prevent Future Deaths. Each ICS/STP area will have available assessments of the needs of the local community (on council websites) and the demand for mental health services in the Joint Strategic Needs Assessment (JSNA), which have been drawn up for each area.[52]

Government mental health and capacity legislation is not discussed in this book due to the specialist detail, changing nature of legislation and differing laws in each of the nations in the UK. Training and refresher courses are provided and regulated and are a requirement for psychiatrists approved to use their provisions. Likewise, specific commitments to improve services by government evolve and change, but there has been a sustained focus for people with SMI on addressing effects of diversity (see Chapter 17), improving physical health care (Chapter 16) and crisis response and community services.

Funding

In the UK, as elsewhere, much informal care is provided by family, friends, neighbours and the community, including non-statutory 'voluntary' agencies (e.g. MIND and RETHINK Mental Illness). However, the vast majority of statutory care is provided through national funding for health care and local government for social care. Private funding for adult mental health care is only a small percentage of overall spend, but funding to private hospitals is substantial, estimated at £2 billion in 2022[53] (this will include services for organic disorders). A recent systematic review of the cost of mental disorders internationally[54] found developmental disorders (this includes autism), schizophrenia and intellectual disabilities to be the highest individual cost but noted that other disorders were prevalent and so contributed substantially to total costs.

Health care therefore comes through the National Health Service and is funded through national taxation, with the planned spending for health and social care in England in 2021–2022 totalling £190.3 billion, of which over 70 per cent is allocated to the NHS. In turn, the central NHS structures allocate this budget largely through NHS England and NHS Improvement down to the local commissioners (previously Clinical Commissioning Groups, now Integrated Care Systems) with responsibility to distribute these funds to the front-line services. This commissioning process can be complex and, whilst some funding was initially allocated for nationally prioritised plans (such as the NHS Plan teams from 2000 onwards, creating the specialist early intervention, crisis and AO teams, and later perinatal teams), much of it is not spending as part of these plans.

In 2016, the government committed to increasing investment in mental health services by at least £1bn (in real terms) by 2021 to deliver the Five Year Forward View for Mental Health.[55] In the 2019 NHS Long Term Plan,[56] there was a further commitment given that funding for mental health services should grow faster than the overall NHS budget. A new ringfenced local investment fund known as the Mental Health Investment Standard was created, which was planned to rise to at least £2.3 billion a year by 2023/2024.[57]

Mental health spending is competing also against other budget lines for health spending and currently comprises only around 11 per cent of all health spending,[58] despite accounting for nearly a quarter of all morbidity. The proportion given by the NHS Mental Health Dashboard is higher (14.8 per cent in 2021/2022) but includes funding for dementia and LD.

Whilst, in general, configuration of mental health services is not a source of political disagreement, quantity and direction of funding is politically determined and will be directed and announced in a way to maximise demonstrable benefit to the party funding it. This can be frustrating to clinicians but which should also be a motivator to demonstrate effectiveness of new and expanded services through research and then clinical outcome measurement (e.g. as has been the case with Improving Access to Psychological Treatment services).

NHS England is responsible for determining how much money is allocated to each local commissioner each year. This allocation process is designed to reflect local health care needs and intended to help reduce inequalities. This is done by using a 'weighted capitation formula' that allocates resources based on the size of the local population, an assessment of their health needs and level of deprivation. The formula is also adjusted for unavoidable higher costs of delivering health care due to higher staff and building costs, known as the market forces factor. There are separate weighted populations for need for general and acute services, mental health services, community services, maternity services and prescribing, which are combined into a single need-weighted population.

Mental health services provided by the NHS have been funded through local commissioners (formerly Clinical Commissioning Groups and latterly Integrated Care Systems),[59] who are required to assess the needs of the population and to commission services that will provide the best health outcomes for that population. Most (but not all) of the mental health services have been funded on some form of 'block contract' basis. Over the next few years, the intention is to move over to an 'aligned payment and incentive approach', which is a type of blended payment with a fixed element based on funding an agreed level of activity and a variable element to increase or reduce payment based on the actual elective activity levels and to reflect performance against quality measures. In practice, substantial discretion is possible – for example, in terms of funding for mental and physical health – although direction from government occurs. Reference costs (which are the unit costs of providing defined services) are submitted by Trusts and then aggregated to produce a national average unit cost, which can be used as a broad comparator. These are used to guide allocations through a mental health allocations formula, but major differences exist because of inequitable, quite often historical, funding distributions and the vagaries of individual commissioners. There are also – frequently short-term – funding initiatives targeting particular developments (e.g. perinatal or IAPT services).

Nowadays, funding for mental health services has been predominantly by block contracts modified by some funding provided only when certain quality standards are met (e.g. Commissioning for Quality Improvement – CQUIN) or when specific services are provided, but 'payment by results' has never been implemented in mental health. This has meant that cuts in mental health care have probably been easier to implement than in physical health care, where payment for number of patients treated (though not for results) has been common. It has also helped to conceal inefficiency and uneven distribution of workloads between teams and individuals. Payment for pathways groups in the NHS is now being proposed[60] with some similarities to Health Resource Groups used elsewhere in health care, although HRGs currently do not generally include outcome measurement. This application to mental health services may better protect and form a basis for outcome measurement (see the NHS England website, likely to be updated over time, for initial proposals[61] and information on finance and payment – considerations for mental health, community and non-acute services[62]). Mandatory collection of patient-level information and costing systems (PLICS) data from 2022 in mental health services as well as acute and community should also make resource allocation more transparent and equitable. Unit costs are applied to individual-level resource use data to calculate total costs per participant. The unit costs for most health and social care services are obtained from the most recent versions of NHS Reference costs,[63] Unit Costs of Health and Social Care[64] and the Prescription Cost Analysis.[65] Linking this to pathway groups could then provide much more meaningful data for use in achieving parity and understanding as well as comparing resource usage and managing services.

Waiting lists and access standards have also disproportionately driven funding in the past away from mental health services; the introduction of such standards can be seen as a mixed blessing as they impose pressures on services that may not be financially fully compensated, are impeded by lack of appropriately trained staff or distort clinical priorities. Nevertheless, over time, they can counter-balance funding moving elsewhere. Standards introduced in 2022 similar to those in IAPT were:

- People in the community receive help within four weeks for non-urgent treatment
- Patients of all ages with an urgent mental health need would be seen by community crisis teams within 24 hours
- Those who present to A&E with mental health needs have a face-to-face assessment by specialist mental health liaison teams within one hour of being referred by an emergency department

Over much of the period since the austerity crisis of 2008/2009, the NHS has also had a system of 'efficiency savings', which has imposed the re-investment of Trust income by arbitrarily cutting a percentage paid to the provider (NHS Trust) with the intention of improving cost effectiveness of services. The finance released came from reducing costs of, or simply closing, 'inefficient or unnecessary' services, which was then to be reinvested by commissioners to develop new services to meet new developments or needs, though not necessarily in mental health from which it was taken. In practice, this has occurred over a period when demand has outstripped provision, funding has not accounted for health service inflation, and this has led to, for example, the virtual disappearance of day hospitals and day care, and increase in caseloads/discharge of patients and an arbitrary and large reduction in bed numbers without sufficient development of supporting community services. The expensive placement of patients in the private sector away from their homes has been a result of this (recently estimated at £2 billion per year) and exacerbated the reduction in trained mental health staff available to provide local NHS services. This lack of trained staff has had a major influence on quality, in terms of personal contact and continuity of care, as well as quantity of services, and it has held back developments and availability of evidence-based care dependent on trained people being available, especially psychotherapies and social approaches. Funding of mental health services has been prioritised nationally under the NHS Long Term Plan[56] according to NHS England, but this has rarely been perceived as occurring by local services providers.

There is also substantial funding that comes through local authorities for social care, some funded from local council tax based on property values and a large but substantially shrinking proportion from central government. The difference between health and social care may be discernible at the extremes (e.g. hospital care compared to domestic support) but in practice is a continuum with interdependence. Lack of social support and loneliness undoubtedly affects mental health.[66] Deprivation indexes, such as Jarman-8 and York indices for psychiatric funding[67] and Mental Health Investment Standard, have been proposed to provide parity of esteem and therefore funding for mental health services.[68] Substance misuse services, transferred from NHS to local authority funding, have major health components (see Chapter 14).

Staffing

The NHS as a whole employs around 1.4 million staff and the social care sector around 1.6 million. In the NHS workforce, around half of the staff hold a professional qualification. Of the professionally qualified staff, in mental health, nurses continue to be the largest professional group, especially in inpatient units, but unqualified health care support workers provide a large contribution to patient care both on wards and in the community. Occupational therapists and psychologists and, less frequently, physiotherapists and dietitians work in wards and community teams. Pharmacists are employed for inpatients and increasingly also provide input to community teams. Clinical psychology has grown and become focused on training, supervising and providing therapy. Psychological measurement – for example, neuropsychological evaluation and administration of personality disorder inventories – is now provided much less than previously. Increasingly, peer support workers (i.e. people with personal experience of mental health services or mental distress) are being employed to enhance explicitly the way services understand and address the needs of the people they see.[69]

There have been shortages in all these professions despite the popularity of psychology and medicine in universities. Workforce surveys do show some surprising facts. For example, around 20,000 'psychological professionals' (psychologists of various kinds) are employed within the NHS in England. The Royal College of Psychiatrists conduct regular workforce surveys and, in 2021, reported a headcount of 7,056 consultants, of whom 3,584 were full time (around 50 per cent). These numbers compare with 2,920 reported FTE consultant psychiatrists in 2003, a dramatic increase on paper in available numbers. Yet, despite this, the same issues with demand are still present and continue to provide challenges to developing a workforce able to meet the requirements of delivering sustainable service provision.

Despite the objective increase in posts, government funds regulate the number of psychiatry training places and clinical psychology places, which have always been lower than NHS-assessed need; numbers in medicine have also been lower than need but are also distorted towards physical health care, where even greater expansion has occurred at the expense of mental health disciplines. Other factors including changes in attitudes and legislation on hours of work and patient expectation, as well as some electronic record systems being unfit for purpose and hindering the efficient delivery of care,[56] have also contributed to perceptions of demand exceeding resource. The College has been having some success by addressing this through a psychiatric workforce plan and strategy (as, encouragingly, is also happening in the USA), which has led to 100 per cent of core posts being filled in 2022 and 75 per cent of higher trainee places. However, whilst consultant posts have increased by 6.4 per cent from 2012 to 2022 (4,472 posts – 2,634 in general adult psychiatry), vacancies have increased as well (10.4% in GAP), and there has been an increase in locums filling posts. The high number of psychology graduates interested in psychological therapies has led to the employment of many as psychology assistants, and there have also been attempts to recruit and train them to work in ward and community teams.[70] Other new professional roles are developing, including that of the advanced clinical practitioner, providing routes to senior clinical responsibility – and higher pay bands – for professions other than psychiatry and psychology.

Since the days of the asylum medical superintendent, the psychiatrist's role has changed substantially. Community care, the expansion of the numbers of people in contact with mental health services, profound changes in attitude and wider society has led to large community caseloads and rival ideological approaches to the various issues. In the early 2000s, '*New Ways of Working*'[71] described the issues and potential solutions to the major challenges and opportunities that multi-disciplinary working, clinical leadership and shortage of trained staff had created. It reviewed ways of working in multi-disciplinary teams (MDTs) to improve effective working through care coordination and skill mix, such as the use of pharmacists and nurse practitioners, with the psychiatrist taking more of a role as 'consultant' to the team. This was intended to ensure that urgent and complex situations could be reviewed by the psychiatrist promptly – for example, in outpatient clinics or community, in supervision or team meetings – and that more routine care could be transferred to care coordinators who might also be able to provide continuity and more frequent and regular input. Primary care liaison was also expected to receive greater emphasis (see Chapter 18). In practice, there has been change in the ways of working, but workload pressures have impacted on the ability of primary care to provide mental health care, community mental health teams (CMHTs) to support patients, psychologists to provide therapy and psychiatrists to see patients and consult. Factors such as staff turnover and burnout (see later) have also impacted. Pressures to reduce caseload (e.g. in outpatient clinics) have led to the discharge of patients when 'stable' despite the value that longer-term – albeit brief and infrequent – contact and monitoring can provide. Re-presentation has then occurred in 'crisis' with consequent distress and increasing disability after failure to detect and intervene when deterioration has occurred. This feeds a cycle of high-cost inpatient spending with the marginal savings made through the discharge of stable patients with severe problems being drowned out by the costs of managing relapse, notwithstanding the human costs also associated.

The NHS Benchmarking surveys make this starkly clear (Table 20.1).

It is now easy to understand how for many years cutting beds became the preferred option for dealing with financial pressures on the NHS, and this may be why the UK has ended up with so few beds compared to its European neighbours and a reason why politicians extol the virtues of care in the community. It is, of course, harder to measure costs saved as opposed to costs incurred – just as in a football match, measuring goals scored is easier than measuring goals prevented. Nonetheless, this is a crucial area for services to be considering as the consequences of not doing so will be a continued reliance on crisis management and a sense for staff of working within a system about to collapse that, whilst a perennial theme in the psychiatric service literature for decades, has become particularly pertinent.

More recent innovations in relation to staffing include training in psychosocial approaches, with increasing numbers of staff developing competencies (e.g. Competency Frameworks for psychological treatments[72]). The non-statutory (mainly private and voluntary) sector has a myriad of functions from befriending, day-to-day care, crisis housing, counselling and specific social and financial functions (e.g. Citizen's Advice Bureaus). In many areas, social prescribing[73] or community navigators are being developed to assist people to find services relevant to their social needs, which have a profound effect on the problems they encounter with housing, benefits and emotional needs, and so help prevent the mental health problems that they might otherwise develop. The Centre For Workforce Intelligence Report (2014)[74] described a number of potential future scenarios and potential roles of psychiatrists within these scenarios. Two of the scenarios described 'peer led' scenarios, one with low psychiatrist numbers focusing on statutory work, the other with psychiatry having a much wider remit. Prediction is difficult, especially about the future, as Niels Bohr, the great physicist, said.

Table 20.1 Cost per year of care (NHS Benchmarking 2021)

	Cost per year (£)	Relative cost per year of care
Adult Acute IP	142,557	41
PICU	286,022	82
Eating Disorders IP Unit	178,843	52
Mother And Baby IP Unit	257,497	74
Low Secure	164,322	48
Medium Secure	206,674	60
Generic CMHT	3,459	1

Greater involvement of doctors, including psychiatrists, in management roles has developed over the past few decades, accelerated by the Griffiths Report in 1983. Roles of medical and clinical directors have been established in Trusts, but there have also been specific responsibilities for a wide range of clinical issues, such as the Mental Health Act, information officers, ECT administration and directors of research and development, as well as clinical tutor, responsibilities for continuing personal development for existing staff as well as programmes for new psychiatric trainees, although much of this is achieved in the regional deaneries nowadays. Medical involvement is generally highly valued and very important in achieving responsive and effective systems but is not without its cost in time and frustration levels.

Burnout

Burnout is a self-reported job-related syndrome increasingly recognised as a critical factor affecting physicians and their patients,[75] affecting between 4 and 7 per cent of the working population. GPs have the highest rates of burnout in the medical profession – for example, amongst Danish general practitioners, a 25 per cent prevalence was found. Key features include emotional exhaustion, feelings of depersonalisation, feelings of low personal accomplishment, increased mental distance from one's job, or feelings of negativism or cynicism related to one's job as well as reduced professional efficacy. Depression is commonly associated, and some have argued that burnout should be considered a form of depression. However, there may be advantages to considering burnout as a distinct entity because this *avoids pathologising* the workers' emotional reactions to their jobs

Consequences of burnout include impaired life satisfaction, raised rates of cardiovascular diseases, increased rates of suicidal ideation, depressive symptoms, occupational disability, job dissatisfaction and low commitment to their organisation and lower work performance. There is considerable overlap with depression, particularly with high exhaustion burnout. Chronic stress is defined as persistent demands that threaten to exceed the individual's resources. This is considered the proximal cause of burnout symptoms; more specifically, chronic work-related stress is a cause of burnout symptoms.

Causation models focus on excessive job demands. According to the job demands-resources model, burnout develops when job demands (e.g. workload, time pressure, conflict) are high, while resources (e.g. autonomy, social support, positive relationship with supervisor) are poor or limited. Resources are therefore not able to buffer the negative impact of high demands on stress reactions. Job demands and resources have also been linked to specific burnout symptoms; thus, emotional exhaustion is caused by high workload and emotional demands, whereas cynicism, reduced professional efficacy and disengagement have been associated with a lack of resources. Burnout can be measured and sometimes diagnosed using a version of the Maslach Burnout Inventory (MBI),[76] but the scale does not distinguish between job-related and non-job-related stress.

The main studies of burnout amongst psychiatrists are from the American Veteran Administration Hospitals[3]. These found four work-environment characteristics consistently associated with significantly lower burnout rates: (1) 'My workload is reasonable [*reasonable workload*];' (2) 'I have the appropriate supplies, materials, and equipment to perform my job well [*I have resources for the job*];' (3) 'It is worthwhile in my workgroup to speak up because something will be done to address our concerns [*supervisor addresses concerns*]' and (4) 'I am given a real opportunity to improve my skills [*skill building*]'. Psychiatric nurses are by far the largest group of psychiatric professionals in the NHS, and research findings show psychiatric nurse burnout is associated with unsupportive management, a lack of a formal orientation programme or continuing education for staff, looking after high risk and acutely ill patients, too much paperwork and inadequate numbers of staff.

In considering management within the psychiatric services, it is important to recognise when burnout is occurring because of its adverse consequences to both the individual and the service.[77] Usually, it is self-diagnosed, and complaints to a medical or clinical director that 'the doctor is cracking up under the strain of the workload' must be taken seriously and not dismissed with a reply such as 'I think you should increase your antidepressants' but instead 'let's explore your workload and working conditions'. It is better to understand the psychiatric professional as a worker with burnout instead of as a patient with depression so as not to medicalise the problem.

Making adjustments to workload – for example, by adding extra sessions of another doctor to the team [*workload alleviation*] or making specific changes requested by the doctor to the way the team operates may also alleviate the problem [*improved resources*]. Some of the daily work could be done by clerical or clinical support staff [*task-shifting*]. Having an unreasonable workload represented the strongest and most consistent predictor of burnout.

General Adult Psychiatry Services

Services should form a continuum of care across acute, rehabilitation and a range of community services, with the latter providing by far the greater share of care but the former – acute and rehabilitation – being more intensive and with a greater concentration of resources. The emphasis over the years has been to provide increased services in the community near to patients' localities or homes, but this has often been driven or complicated by cost considerations rather than solely improving the quality and acceptability of services.

Acute Inpatient Care

The evidence base for inpatient care is remarkably limited, although the need for it as part of a comprehensive service is rarely questioned. Inpatient care is universal and usually the most expensive component of mental health systems (60% of inpatients typically are experiencing psychotic episodes). There were 23,447 consultant-led mental health beds in 2010–2011 and 17,610 in 2020–2021, a reduction of 5,837 (25%), and UK bed numbers are very low internationally.[78] For more hospital statistics, see Table 20.2.

Lengths of stay vary, with an average of 30 days (England) compared to 7–14 days in the USA (which has very different systems and funding mechanisms). There is also a cohort of patients who will spend substantially longer in inpatient units. Acute inpatient length of stay was 60 days or above in about 15 per cent of cases in 2018/2019, some of which will be related to severity but most to inefficiency in flow between different areas of care due to lack of necessary support and housing. A clear indication for admission would be where risk of serious harm to oneself or others is so likely that leaving a person on their own would be considered a danger to their own or another's life or that serious harm might result. In 2019–2020, out of a total of 171,575 admissions, there were 50,893 new detentions under the Mental Health Act of which 32,320 took place at the point of admission to hospital with a further 14,576 that occurred following admission (there are data quality issues)[80] – this is worth noting as this is only 30 per cent of all admissions, much less than most psychiatrists would estimate it to be. Detention usually indicates a risk of significant harm to self or others, with the legally defined criteria being risk of harm to the self or others. However, where this indication has been questioned and resources made available – from families or agencies – which is sufficient to provide protection, it has been possible for a person to receive monitoring and support in their own home by family or services or a combination to prevent harm occurring in some of the most complex situations. The degree of monitoring will vary with the severity and nature of the risk and, for example, the size, ingenuity and strength of the individual if coercion is considered necessary. For example, very wealthy families have been known to engage sufficient trained personnel to manage individuals around the clock for sometimes lengthy periods within their homes.

Table 20.2 Hospital statistics 2019–2020[79]

Primary diagnosis: summary code and description		Finished consultant episodes	Admissions	Male	Female	Gender unknown	Emergency	Waiting list	Planned	Other admission method	Mean time waited	Median time waited	Mean length of stay	Median length of stay	Mean age
F00–F09	Organic, including symptomatic, mental disorders	78,231	36,554	34,125	44,092	14	32,398	2,712	712	732	16	6	19	9	81
F10–F19	Mental and behavioural disorders due to psychoactive subst.	79,141	50,531	55,219	23,893	29	48,160	593	1,376	402	55	25	6	1	46
F20–F29	Schizophrenia, schizotypal and delusional disorders	33,067	20,706	20,193	12,850	24	16,227	750	2,365	1,364	38	9	75	26	44
F30–F39	Mood [affective] disorders	28,953	21,041	12,779	16,167	7	17,349	788	1,851	1,053	60	44	33	12	49
F40–F48	Neurotic, stress-related and somatoform disorders	27,722	22,352	10,682	17,023	17	18,948	1,576	1,401	427	46	27	9	1	46
F50–F59	Behavioural syndromes associated with physiological disturbances and physical factors	6,677	4,516	1,014	5,656	7	2,969	690	686	171	64	35	27	7	28
F60–F69	Disorders of adult personality and behaviour	13,624	11,063	4,251	9,084	289	7,561	1,682	1,212	608	122	87	26	7	33
F70–F79	Mental retardation	589	430	362	227	0	211	83	92	44	37	31	241	39	34
F80–F89	Disorders of psychological development	2,960	2,671	1,825	1,133	2	810	1,149	651	61	55	32	47	3	15
F90-F98	Behavioural and emotional disorders with onset usually occurring in childhood and adolescence	1,515	1,323	860	654	1	889	167	210	57	40	23	17	2	19
F99–F99	Unspecified mental disorder	648	570	304	341	3	520	10	17	23	36	36	16	1	40

So, the question arises: Shouldn't it be possible to provide such support and therefore avoid any need for compulsory or indeed any inpatient care? There are a few considerations that need to be taken into account, which include the individual's wishes and rights, and hospitalisation may provide the least intrusive and most therapeutic approach. The legal framework that governs such situations is, of course, of relevance in such situations involving confinement and removal of liberties whether at home or hospital. There is also evidence that day hospitals can be used with suicidal patients,[81] where support in the home can be provided (see Chapter 15, which discussed risk management).

Inevitably, however, it is the human resources and expertise availability to provide individualised service that currently precludes this. Such resources are not available in the public sector, so inpatient care remains for acute episodes, especially where high risk to others or self is involved. For psychosis, this can be where psychotic symptoms are distressing or endangering self or others, often in the context of non-acceptance of medication but can also occur due to breakdown in social circumstances and unavailability of alternatives. Stays have become shorter – often a few days in the US or three to four weeks in Europe – but in the latter, accommodation issues and provision of community support can seriously prolong stays. Ready availability of community resources, especially housing and support, could improve use of beds, but pressuring services and patients into discharge when services are not available or over-stretched is counter-productive. Out-of-Area placements have developed for acute care, including psychiatric intensive care and some specific groups – those with eating disorders or personality disorder – and have also increased in the number for routine admissions, an indication of under-provision of NHS psychiatric beds. These lead to multiple problems for individuals and their carers due to geographical distance dislocating connections from home, friends, education, employment, primary care and community teams. This aggravates the problems involved and interrupts therapeutic relationships, which often need to be medium- to long-term. Distress and disability are increased with prolongation of lengths of stay – often therapy is either interrupted or not commenced until return to the home area. However, structural changes in UK health services, including movement of funding and attraction of staffing from private to NHS services, will be needed to enable change. Concerns over other detrimental aspects of this overuse of Out-of-Area beds led to a wish to end the practice, which is yet to materialise. Targets are recognised as frequently having unintended consequences. There is concern that preventing the use of private beds will simply block off a safety valve that covers the lack of beds required for necessary admissions to hospital – with negative effects on patients and staff as detailed previously.

So, inpatient care remains an integral and indispensable part of all mental health systems, but its role has been changing rapidly. Admission has been described as uniquely able to provide constant observation, enforce treatment where necessary and tolerate behaviour that would be unmanageable or unacceptable in the community with the potential for providing high levels of interpersonal contact and therapeutic engagement.[82,83] Admission criteria vary considerably, particularly where effective teams are operating (e.g. CMHTs, Assertive Outreach or especially home treatment, see later) and where effective bed management strategies and resources are in place. Unnecessary hospitalisation is damaging to the individual's coping abilities and often their self-esteem but may be appropriate, though currently rarely available, for treatment and respite as well as having a protective function. Respite, asylum, was well recognised as a function of hospitals but, in most circumstances and increasingly due to the hospital ward environment, is no longer conducive to this. Nevertheless, there are circumstances where wards may still have this function (e.g. where accommodation has abruptly broken down), carers are unavailable (e.g. though illness amongst themselves) and no immediate solution (e.g. a crisis house or supported accommodation) is available that night or for a few days. It is noteworthy that a crisis house is only available in half of all catchment areas.[84] For further discussion of reasons that determine hospital admission, see Box 20.3.

Teams working with inpatients for their mental health care include nurses, student nurses, psychiatrists and their trainees – who commonly become 'the ward doctor' at least for the duration of their stay – and unqualified support workers. Most wards should have occupational therapy and pharmacy input, and some units have access to psychological services and physiotherapists. A range of inpatient settings exist: most commonly acute admission, psychiatric intensive care and rehabilitation units but also low, medium and high secure forensic wards. There are also a small number of specialist units for such needs as eating and perinatal disorders. There will be some differences in the type of crises presenting in these different settings, with risk issues being more prominent and complex with the higher secure environments. However, the underlying issues giving rise to crises are likely to be similar in each of these environments. In rehabilitation settings, similarities to acute inpatient settings will be greater where a higher level of nursing staff are available, especially if they are sited on hospital premises. As the levels of support reduce, so the similarities lessen, and crisis presentations in rehabilitation units are managed essentially as crises in the community.

Most patients use acute inpatient services because they are in a crisis and cannot be adequately supported at home. The very process of going into hospital can be traumatic, particularly if the admission is not voluntary. Inpatients are out of their own environment, although they may still maintain contact with it through leave arrangements. This work involves the most vulnerable and distressed patients, but sadly, the status of inpatient units in mental health services has become relatively low with retention of nursing staff on the wards a particular difficulty in many areas. The growth of specialist teams has attracted many of the most experienced

Box 20.3 Reasons that determine admission

- Significant risk of serious harm to self or others: expressed suicidal intent, expressed homicidal intent or serious threat of physical harm to others; suicidal planning or serious harm to others with uncertainty about intent; suicidal thinking where there is concern that this might abruptly change to intent (e.g. where there is foreknowledge of catastrophic news affecting the person or past history of this occurring), command hallucinations with demonstrated 'control over-ride' (i.e. the person believes they have to act in accordance with the commands of the voice(s) and does something to make this apparent), severe physical neglect (e.g. caused by anorexia nervosa, mania or presents late with depression or psychosis) or as an alternative to living at home or where homeless.
- Home treatment is not possible without a home. However, admission to hospital cannot be the best option in these circumstances although its convenience is such that it is frequently used. Better alternatives may be to use the local homelessness provision and work with the local housing department. Discussions about temporary options (e.g. friends and family) may be possible – sometimes with the practitioner assisting with direct contacts to set this up and provision of an appropriate support package for the patient and any carer.
- Few services have respite options available (e.g. supported flats or crisis accommodation). It may be more sensible, economic and less damaging to fund guest house accommodation, 'foster' homes, crisis houses or crisis beds in hostel accommodation.
- Intensive or specialised care required: for example, commencement on the antipsychotic clozapine may be safer to do in hospital because of potential adverse reactions, but partial hospitalisation or community options, especially with home treatment support, may be better; ECT – where there is concern about physical status, although day patient options can be explored.
- Patient preference for hospital admission: Previous positive experience or a feeling of need for the perceived safety of admission, 'unable to cope' with demands of home life or escape from home circumstances where they may feel at risk or under pressure from family (including domestic violence), carers are no longer able to cope, alternatives not available or acceptable to patient or carer (although this may not seem sufficient reason, at times not agreeing can lead to a greater crisis, increased risk or the carer not being prepared to continue that role).
- Combined risk, preference and other considerations – for example, comorbid physical illness, presence or absence of assertive outreach or home treatment service (see later) – may make admission inevitable and appropriate.

nursing staff away from the wards. Wards in many areas depend on temporary staff from recruitment agencies that may not know the patients and are unable to offer continuity of care at a time when it is most needed.

Patients report serious concerns about inpatient units[85] regarding the poor physical and psychological environment for care, including lack of basic necessities and arrangements for safety, privacy, dignity and comfort. Often, there is insufficient information on their condition and treatment and on how the ward and service operates; lack of involvement and engagement in the planning and reviewing of their own care and in how the ward is run; inadequate staff contact, particularly one-to-one contact with staff; insufficient attention to the importance of such key factors as ethnicity and gender and protection from harassment/abuse; lack of 'something to do', especially activity that is useful and meaningful to recovery; and lack of psychological treatment.

There have been attempts to respond to these concerns: the environment provided by some units has improved and can now be very good – clean, tidy and homely – but in many, it is still poor, and this is certainly a factor in aggravating and even precipitating crises. Distress will be increased in poor surroundings; behaviour can worsen, and nursing care can be that much more difficult. Not surprisingly, patients will also be reluctant to be admitted to these units, leading to unnecessary use of compulsory measures at times. Once someone is admitted to inpatient care, it is easy for community staff to fall into the trap of believing that crisis management or prevention is over. However, the circumstances of acute wards and the nature of the problems that people are admitted with mean that crises will often continue. Many patients do not want to be there – either because there is nowhere more suitable for them to go because of accommodation shortages or because they are detained under mental health legislation. Resurgence of psychotic symptoms or suicidality, panic or behavioural disorder occurs on a day-to-day basis, and management of these crises is necessary.

The bulk of input, at least initially, on wards is focused on refining diagnoses and the future management plan as well as supporting patients to manage crises, adjust to treatments and prepare for living elsewhere. Many units have adapted ways of working to emphasise the importance of planning the purpose of the admission from day one or even before with active daily review (e.g. purposeful inpatient admission – PIPA)[86] and taking a 'whole system' approach, with inpatient care just one component of a wider system:

- Advice on medication on admission
- Social issues (e.g. housing to manage exit strategy, named community worker)
- Risk management
- Family issues – key member of family to liaise
- Community support for discharge and attention to the feasibility of plans
- Responsible community consultant and coordinator to communicate with

Initial Ward Management

For some patients, there is also a need to protect them from the risk to self or others. A new admission is likely to be a person in crisis, and that person is likely to have had at least one assessment if not several in the 24 hours or so before admission. The initial work on the ward involves engagement with them and the introduction to the new environment for the patient, including collecting vital information together and establishing the level of support and observation that will be needed as well as attempting to allay current symptomatic distress. A psychiatric and nursing assessment will occur from which nursing care plans will be established and then built up with the patient over time and after discussion in nurse meetings and multi-disciplinary ward reviews. There can be advantages to being in a new place and away from the previous sources of distress. Some patients talk of the help they get from having the 'time out' that came from being in hospital, to be able to adjust while being away from the pressures of everyday life.

The decision about the level of observation of the patient required will be a joint one between nursing staff and admitting doctor supervised by senior staff. This should not be affected by staff levels available, but where staffing is too low to provide the levels determined, it is important to involve more senior doctors and nurse managers to safely resolve the situation. Their reassessment of risk may lead to a decision that high levels of observation are not required or that other staff can be drafted in from elsewhere or that the patient needs to be nursed in a safer environment (e.g. a psychiatric intensive care or low secure unit). Good documentation of risk together with the proposed levels of nursing observations is essential, as tragedies can occur, resulting in later litigation with allegations of inadequate nursing supervision. Levels are described in each Trust's guidelines, for example, as:

- General: location of patient known to staff at all times, contact with staff at each shift
- Intermittent: location checked every 15–30 minutes, exact time specified
- Within eyesight: day or night
- Within arms length: more than one member of staff may be needed

Many of the principles and practice described elsewhere for management of, for example, self harm, depression and psychotic symptoms are applicable in inpatient units, although the circumstances and lack of staff can mean that taking time out to work through a crisis with someone can be difficult but necessary. It may be that partial and sequential working through occurs as and when the psychiatrist and other staff members can assist – having a good memory and structured and evolving crisis management plans can make such a difficult situation possible.

Difficulties in Ward Management

There are a number of key problems for managing crises in an inpatient setting, which are about the setting itself. People associate hospitals with medical symptoms and approaches; the focus on managing the crisis in such a setting can be biological and focused on medication. This can be reinforced by psychiatric and nursing attitudes, but the mere fact of being in hospital may invite the patient to see their distress in medical terms. They may ignore the relevance of the precipitating factors that led up to the episode unless they are specifically invited to. The social and psychological circumstances involved in hospitalisation will inevitably need to be addressed if discharge is to occur and readmission avoided. The person in hospital may behave in an institutional way – this can be like a person in hospital is 'meant' to behave, such as a patient or a recipient of care. This can lead to a passivity, which can frustrate the staff. There are also other institutional behaviours that can impede recovery, such as patients feeling rebellious against a, seemingly or actual, authoritarian regime and becoming verbally aggressive or persistently rule breaking. This is more likely to be the case if staff take a parental/patronising approach to patients who are inpatients. Some principles (such as used in transactional analysis) can be helpful in keeping 'adult to adult' interactions going rather than the 'parent–child' roles that develop so easily. The patient is often disempowered by the hospital setting, and collaboration in care planning can be problematic – this can be due to the dominance of the 'ward round' in the planning of care. These have often been relatively large meetings involving doctors, nurses, students, an OT and a pharmacist and, somewhere within, the voice of the patient. Options include nurses or doctors countering this problem by helping patients articulate, perhaps write down their views beforehand, and by the use of advocates in ward reviews. Patient time in a smaller gathering (e.g. with the psychiatrist and key nurse alone) to discuss important issues may be more profitable than the 'grand round'. Involvement of community agencies in discharge planning, the requirements of training and multi-disciplinary review can lead to large meetings, but the needs and wishes of the individual patient should always have priority.

Discharging Patients and CTOs

Decisions about discharge, especially when the patient expresses the wish to go – 'I want to leave now' – may depend on determination of risk issues but also availability of housing, care and support. They may be amenable to stay if that is judged clinically appropriate or consideration may be made in relation to continuing or initiating use of the Mental Health Act.

Community Treatment Orders

Sometimes patients leave hospital and rapidly become non-adherent to their medication and aftercare, relapse and are then readmitted to hospital. As discussed earlier, community treatment orders (CTOs) were brought in as amendments to the Mental Health Act (2007) with the aim of providing some sort of compulsory supervision in the community. A CTO can only be applied if a patient is detained under Section 3 or Section 37 or a notional Section 37. This effectively suspends the pre-existing Section. There are two 'statutory' conditions – the patient must make themselves available for a meeting with their Responsible Clinician (RC) for the purposes of considering a renewal and make themselves available for review by a Second Opinion Appointed Doctor (SOAD). Other non-statutory conditions can be added, but medication cannot be administered against a patient's consent in the community. A patient who defaults on his CTO can be recalled by the RC back to hospital for an initial period of 72 hours during which assessment can be made regarding options, including reversion to Section 3, revocation of the CTO or continuation of the CTO – though the case law around what constitutes grounds for recall continues to evolve – and then placed on a Section 3 and be readmitted. The hope was that the number of readmissions due to non-compliance would reduce, but as described previously, a large study showed that this was not the case.[18] However, CTOs continue to be widely used with an increase in the number of new CTOs per year of nearly 50 per cent since their introduction (4,107 in 2008 to 6,070 in 2021).

Such consideration has to be long- and short-term. For example, continuing an admission when substances have been misused contrary to contract/agreement or behaviour has been verbally or physically aggressive or simply obstructive (e.g. in relation to finding alternative housing) may seem safer in the short-term for the individual. However, by protecting the person from the consequences of their behaviour, this can lead to it continuing and making the inevitable rejection by services, and society more generally, more devastating and dangerous at that time. The potential damage to others within the ward, both patients and staff, also has to be weighed up. Continuing support is usually appropriate to offer where inpatient admission has been deemed appropriate initially. Sometimes, where admission has occurred unplanned or out-of-hours and no continuing mental health support will help, continuing admission may not be appropriate. Discharging when someone wants to stay can be difficult and risky; it will then involve both inpatient and community team identifying and negotiating with them and formal and informal carers regarding what support they need.

Section 117 Aftercare

For those admitted on Section 3 (or where a Section 2 has progressed to a Section 3) or those admitted under S(37), the Mental Health Act itself provides an entitlement to aftercare. This section is deliberately imprecise to enable an individual tailoring of the aftercare plan, but it is explicit in stating this as an entitlement. S117 places an enforceable duty on both health (ICS, previously Clinical Commissioning Group (CCG)) and social (local authority/council (LA)) services to provide aftercare services. This has been further emphasised by the inclusion of this group of patients within the group of people entitled to Personal Health Budgets.

What happens post-admission when responsibility for the patient gets passed back to community services depends on a range of factors. This may be for short-term follow-up, day care, outpatient care or for more long-term support or therapy. The patient may be referred to a specialist team directly if they are assessed as having a very specific problem (e.g. an eating disorder) or a need for rehabilitation services. They may have been involved with those teams prior to admission and be well supported there. Hospital discharge does not necessarily mean crisis resolution has occurred and indeed many patients are returning to the same social stresses they had prior to admission. Suicide rates increase in the week after discharge (peaking at three days) and remain elevated over the next year, and therefore adequate follow-up is vital in crisis prevention.

Aggressive Behaviours

Training in management of aggressive behaviour is a part of mandatory training for health care staff and focusses on listening, negotiation, discussion and de-escalation. Where control and restraint are necessary, specific competency with appropriate training is a necessary precursor to involvement in situations where it may be used. Organisations are obliged to monitor this carefully, reporting and recording incidents and reviewing safe practice. Policy is needed regarding liaison with police and other agencies and clear guidelines around supporting staff. There needs to be an agreed organisational policy and approach for pursuing criminal prosecution, as rarely occurs, in appropriate cases. Hospital is the one setting where response to aggressive behaviour can include seclusion; restraint is also more likely to occur, but these responses need to be in accordance with an agreed policy, proportional to the risks involved, necessary (the principle of necessity under English common law applies) and documented appropriately.

Prevention of the escalation of distress and disturbance to circumstances in which restraint is required and seclusion needs to be used is the ultimate goal and having sufficient trained staff to enable this to happen. Attention also needs to be paid to the interpersonal consequences of patient behaviour on the ward. A code of conduct should be in place to identify clearly unacceptable behaviour such as racial or sexual harassment or theft. This should also cover ward rules – negotiated with patients – regarding housekeeping issues such as management of noise (TVs, radios, etc) and how disputes – often crises – over such matters are to be resolved, taking into account often-complex capacity issues. Unfortunately many patients and staff members experience wards as unsafe and overly restrictive – a continuing focus of CQC attention.

Psychiatric Intensive Care Units

Psychiatric intensive care units manage those who are acutely unwell, so many patients will be experiencing mania or psychosis, especially where complicated by drug misuse or aggression. Although acutely ill, patients are frequently open to engage in therapeutic negotiating approaches and formal interventions (e.g. CBT and trauma work) which can instil hope, defuse agitation, reduce distress and improve collaboration. Medication certainly has a role, but the process of enforcing it can increase alienation and confusion; shared decision-making on type and dose can assist even where compulsion is eventually necessary. Details of how rapid tranquillisation and the various drugs are used is given in Chapter 5.3. People with borderline personality disorder/complex emotional needs are generally considered not to be helped by admission to PICUs as self harm often seems to exacerbate with the confinement involved, but short stays do occur with the intention of de-escalation or preventing increasing harm – often from transfers that occur out-of-hours. There is a danger that short stays then become longer and problems more intractable – with transfer Out-of-Area to private hospitals sometimes occurring. Early discussions, psychological treatment and safety planning between patient and their psychiatric, nursing and psychology teams can avert this or at least reduce the chance of exacerbation. Standards and skills for working in PICUs have been set out by the National Association of PICUs and Royal College of Psychiatrists Quality network for PICUs.

Habitation, Rehabilitation and Recovery

In the early phases of the closure of the mental hospitals, extensive systems of rehabilitation and resettlement were developed to overcome the detrimental effects of institutionalisation as well as of the conditions themselves. As the mental hospitals began to be replaced by community accommodation in the 1960s and 1970s, most services developed resettlement teams to assist support patients over this transitional period, and eventually many of these converted to become rehabilitation teams. These teams have offered a service to patients with mental health problems who need long-term support to be able to manage in the community, including those patients with symptoms of psychosis that are recurrent and interfere significantly with their lives – and also for those with severe depression, OCD, bipolar and personality disorders. These teams have, in many areas, been going through further transition, and some have converted to assertive outreach teams or merged with CMHTs. Some areas, often those without historically having a nearby county asylum, have never had rehabilitation services as such. In the era of the asylum and particularly in the latter half of the twentieth century, social psychiatry developed; training in daily living and social skills was provided to enable individuals to return to community living. Employment was provided in sheltered workshops with payments made for goods produced. As the focus changed from support in leaving hospital to community living, rehabilitation services have become community based, with a range of facilities from 24-hour nursed accommodation to support in individual flats or houses by community teams – in some areas specified as rehabilitation teams but with varying overlap with assertive outreach teams (AOT), crisis resolution and home treatment (CRHT) and CMHTs. NICE issued guidance on the development of services for people with complex psychosis in 2020[87] – an important statement of principles at a time when much uncertainty was present regarding the implementation of the new Community Mental Health Framework and discussed in more detail later.

Mental health rehabilitation services specialise in working with people whose long-term and complex needs cannot be met by general adult mental health services. Over 80 per cent supported by rehabilitation services have a diagnosis of schizophrenia, but only 1 per cent of people with this diagnosis – supported by secondary mental health services – require inpatient rehabilitation at any given time.[88,89] Most of this group experience severe 'negative' symptoms that impair their motivation, organisational skills and ability to manage everyday activities (self care, shopping, budgeting, cooking) and place them at risk of serious self-neglect.[88,89] Most have symptoms that have not responded to first-line medications and require treatment with complex medication regimes.[88] Around 20 per cent have comorbidities such as other mental disorders, physical health problems and substance misuse problems that complicate their recovery further.[89] Most require an extended admission to inpatient rehabilitation services and ongoing support from specialist community rehabilitation services at least initially, and there are some for whom this lasts many years,[90] although this may be influenced by the availability of community rehabilitation teams and expert interventions.

Despite their problems, with appropriate rehabilitation and support, there is good evidence that two-thirds of people with complex and long-term mental health needs who are supported by rehabilitation services can progress to successful community living within five years, and around 10 per cent will achieve independent living within this period.[91] Those who receive support from rehabilitation services are eight times more likely to achieve or sustain successful community living than people with similar problems who were receiving support from generic community mental health services.[92]

An aim of most rehabilitation teams is to avoid crises occurring for team patients by providing effective support and prompt access to it. However, where nevertheless crises arise, they provide crisis management, as described elsewhere – at times with the support of other teams and facilities (e.g. home treatment and inpatient settings). Maintaining patients in their own accommodation, at least in the crisis, is usually an aim, with review of their needs at a later stage. As in all mental health settings and, paradoxically, avoidance of the possibility that crisis can occur can mean that patients are sometimes held back from moving forward towards recovery and more independent living. Low expectations of abilities to cope have limited referrals for employment and self-supporting accommodation where patients themselves may prefer to take the risk of relapse to improve their quality of life.

Rehabilitation teams have tried to counter this by actively promoting recovery in their patient group rather than focusing solely on the long-term nature of their patients' problems. Many do this by working towards social inclusion – for example, by organising groups to access local community facilities from the cinema, gyms and walking groups to ordinary activities such as watching the local professional sports teams. Encouraging participation in programmes located at local sports venues or other mainstream community activities or actively exploring work opportunities, both paid and voluntary, and encouraging activities of the person's own choosing helps in the development of structure, meaning, social relationships and self-esteem. The creative use of support workers in rehabilitation teams can offer patients a choice between services set up for people with mental health problems or accessing community facilities – the latter is the aim, but the former may be necessary as a stepping stone or, if unable to take the next step, longer-term support. This approach can offer effective support to those people with long-term problems who may have family responsibilities or who wish to take up voluntary work, for example, as a first step back to paid employment. There may be more formal work going on in rehab teams, either cognitive therapy for psychosis or structured family work or work on patients' own plans for recovery and how they would define and achieve this. Personal recovery has emerged as an important concept that can be contrasted with clinical recovery, which tends to focus on symptoms, signs or behaviour.

> The principal factors influencing personal recovery are hope, control and opportunity ... recovery of a valued pattern of life and living, with or without ongoing symptoms and difficulties, linked to an active personal commitment to working on recovery[93]

The move away from the long-stay hospital system meant that there were a large number of patients who had led institutionalised lives, and rehabilitation teams catered well for this group. In more recent times, they – and assertive outreach teams – have had to adapt to offer services to younger people moving on from early intervention teams with persistent psychotic symptoms, including many who misuse substances or have had forensic involvement. This has presented challenges as services appropriate to younger people can be radically different to those enjoyed by more mature patients. It has also led to new forms of structured work, such as awareness of how drug use and personality issues affects symptoms in positive and negative ways. Newer medications with different side effects – which can be less debilitating and overtly stigmatising in terms of tremor, rigidity and involuntary movements – have offered greater life opportunities to patients who need medication long term, so again rehabilitation teams can be active in promoting this by giving access to skills that lead to employment or other fuller social inclusion such as confidence building and social skills training.

NICE guidelines for rehabilitation for people with complex psychosis[87] have recently been developed and require that rehabilitation services should be offered as soon as complex psychosis is identified. This includes schizophrenia, bipolar affective disorder, psychotic depression, delusional disorders and schizoaffective disorder with severe and treatment-resistant symptoms and cognitive and functional impairment. It will particularly include people with recurrent admissions or extended stays in acute wards or in 24-hours staffed accommodation where the placement is breaking down. Management includes assessment, prevention and treatment of physical health issues. Inpatient and community rehabilitation services should be staffed by multi-disciplinary teams and include access to specialists in substance misuse, physical exercise, employment, welfare rights, diet, podiatry, speech and language therapy and physiotherapists. Work with primary care and staff working in supported accommodation will be necessary. Unfortunately, despite the face validity of rehabilitation services, the NICE research review into these services found rehabilitation services to be seriously under-evaluated. Long-term rehabilitation from severe mental illness does not lend itself easily to the RCT paradigm, however, and RCTs are unlikely to be the best approach to evaluating their success or otherwise. Other measures including patient satisfaction, patterns of service utilisation over time (a proxy for costs as well as morbidity) and social outcomes such as employment, settled accommodation and carer stress may provide a better framework for evaluation. Local ICSs will need to consider these issues of evaluation, and psychiatrists working clinically should contribute to ensure appropriate approaches are taken.

Day Hospitals and Day Care

Community services and mental health units on general hospital sites were established in most areas as the gradual replacement of the large mental hospitals occurred and provided alternative support and treatment to reduce hospitalisation or, if it occurred, happened locally rather than in, often remote, rural settings. These were first described in Moscow in the 1930s and then the Marlborough Day Hospital in Paddington in London.

Day hospitals initially were often established on hospital sites, then in localities, and were popular with patients and clinicians with an evidence base that suggested that they were effective.[81,94] They provided support to carers who might be able to monitor and support patients over evenings and weekends but could not do so continuously during work hours or where their family commitments took priority. The advantage of maintaining community support sometimes included maintaining employment.

In the USA, day hospitals have been described as partial hospitalisation. The International Clubhouse Model has also proved a very popular approach with many patients and emphasises mutual cooperation and consensus between staff and members in the development of the programme and the importance of meaningful occupation both within and outside the clubhouse.[95] Specific employment projects have been demonstrated to be effective, especially using intensive placement and support models.[2,96]

Day hospitals and day care as previously constituted are available in few areas now, but the varied functions have shifted into a looser and less well-defined landscape that can appear confusing. The over-arching terms such as 'day services' is sometimes used to include this wide range of community-based groups and locations with a far looser definition than the old day hospitals and social care day services. Rather like inpatient units, as new teams have emerged and taken staff from existing day hospitals, they have often become depleted of staff and attention. The term, day hospital, tends to be used to mean a place where the focus is on people who have relatively acute symptoms and who attend for a relatively brief period of time. Generally, this means no more than three to six months although frequently exceptions are made. Sometimes, they are in the same building as inpatient wards or alongside a community mental health centre or separately located in a community setting. Group and individual activities are provided for the purposes of, for example, anxiety management, assertiveness, art or occupational therapy, recreation and social skills with the objective of providing an alternative to admission to hospital. It has been demonstrated that they can be effective in doing this and reduce pressure on inpatient services. They may also provide intensive input to manage, for instance, depressive symptoms. They may support the provision of outpatient ECT.

Day care, by contrast, tends to mean services provided in day centres or clubs, often run by social service departments or non-statutory organisations (such as MIND), which provide a range of social, creative, occupational and other therapeutic activities. Some will run groups on symptom management or relaxation and have services for particular groups of patients (e.g. women, men, black people or younger people). There may be assistance with vocational advice and associated skills. Patients attend for as long as their mental health problems warrant it, and many day centres can become a long-term lifeline for patients. They meet a need for company and meaningful occupation, and some are open at weekends or evenings when patients may need support.

Day care has been described as support during the day that has tended to be longer term and provided social interaction. In practice, therefore, local social service departments in councils and voluntary groups have provided it. The latter often receiving some funding from the councils. They have also offered occupation and employment initiatives and been popular with patients.

Day services therefore can provide support for people who have presented in crisis, and also, patients and staff may encounter and manage such crises in these settings. In fact, some patients attend day services several times a week, and it is therefore to the day services that a patient may turn if they are experiencing difficulties, and their advice to other teams about problems for the patient can be valuable. Patients may develop roles within them, such as providing peer support, running user-led groups or advocacy. The Community Mental Health Framework[24] promotes the development of variants of the day service approach. In many places, large third sector organisations such as Rethink and MIND have taken substantial roles in facilitating peer recovery and peer led groups and a large role in developing the wider approach to community engagement explicit in the model.

Day services can frequently manage crises themselves but may ask for help from the patient's care coordinator in other teams. The principles and practice described elsewhere apply here. Managing and having the confidence to manage crises effectively can mean that maintaining support for individuals after the crisis occurs is possible. Unfortunately, crises can lead to exclusion from facilities. Whilst disruption to activities and others' equilibrium needs to be considered, if day care and day hospitals are to be most valuable for those who can most benefit from them, coping effectively with crises and minimising turbulence are necessary skills for staff to develop with the appropriate support and training. Often, explanations to other group members in general or specific terms – where patients give permission – can allay their anxieties and enlist their support to help the patient avoid or cope better with future crises.

Unfortunately, in general adult psychiatry in the UK today, day hospitals and day care have virtually disappeared despite reasonable evidence about their effectiveness. This is almost certainly because they have proved very easy targets for managing budgets where systematic slicing through efficiency savings has occurred. Council funding has been reduced by the substantial and relentless cuts in central government support. In the NHS, efficiency savings – whereby a fixed sum is removed from budgets each year by managers – promoting efficiency – and reinvested in new evidence-based approaches. This is on the surface of it logical and may have been beneficial in some circumstances. Sadly, as an example, recovery has been cited as a reason to remove day care on the basis that the latter has not been sufficiently integrated with the community (i.e. providing sufficient 'throughput'/move on). Firstly, this misunderstands the nature of persistent mental health issues and stigmatisation that still exists in the community; secondly, personal choices should be inherent in defining recovery; thirdly, removal of support often eventually leads to crises, which in turn lead to much more damage to the individual and require expensive interventions by crisis services and inpatient care. The money released often hasn't been invested in alternative mental health provision that meet the functions lost and instead contributed to reductions in funding in mental health services. The process of moving funding from services is related to the lack of protest or power of the patients and carers – and professionals – who are losing services and the ignoring/minimising of the evidence base for sustaining them.

Crisis and Intensive Home Treatment Teams

Crisis has been recognised as a time when the effect of the distress involved can bring about significant and meaningful change, especially where enhanced by therapeutic intervention. The NHS (England) provides a dedicated phone line (111) or in emergency (999) and website for advice in crisis, which can provide valuable information on physical and mental health issues and which links to mental health helplines and services. Such services include crisis resolution and home treatment (CRHT) teams, which were established by many services from 2000 onwards when specified funding was made available under the NHS Plan to develop such services in every area of England.[84] These were expected to provide intensive treatment as an alternative to admission to hospital. The evidence for their effectiveness has come from a range of sources[83] Stein and Test[97] in Wisconsin developed a programme for intensive home treatment, which demonstrated effectiveness in comparison with the current services provided and had influence internationally. Adherence criteria to the model of care were described. Intensive home support, including assertive community treatment, is used to reduce hospitalisation although the evidence for this has been mixed. It is however very positively regarded by patients and caregivers.[3] Home treatment teams (also known as crisis resolution teams) have evolved from services developed in the 1980s and 1990s in the USA, Australia and the UK. However, as with all the new teams described in this chapter, the research base is for an approach that appears to combine assertive community treatment, home treatment and, to some degree, early intervention, although the latter does have its own literature to support it.

Home treatment teams would be expected to provide precisely what their name says, treatment in the patient's own home, which includes providing additional short-term support to patients in supported accommodation, group homes or hostels. However, in practice, telephone contacts and visits to team bases make up the majority of contacts. Services may provide more intensive support (e.g. daily contact) but, very rarely, anything resembling 'hospital at home', as an alternative to admission to hospital but also variable amounts of less intensive and less frequency contact. Home treatment is provided as a service for most types of CMHTs – those established to focus on early intervention, assertive outreach, rehabilitation or the local community – depending on the resources available to them. Services are more effective if they provide 24-hours 7-days-a-week cover, but emergency out-of-hours teams may be able to supplement daytime services. However, the latter are often established to respond to emergencies rather than to monitor, support and prevent development of crisis or manage higher levels of risk in the community. They can also help to support collaboration with treatment where disorganisation, ambivalence or forgetfulness is addressed by delivery of daily medication to them at home to reduce relapse and admissions from missing medication. They are also limited in their ability to provide access to services outside working hours, which has been expressed as a major concern by patients.

Dedicated home treatment teams were developed to provide sufficient staff to provide a rostered service around the clock and varied experience – nurses, social workers, doctors, occupational therapists and psychologists with support and administrative staff – to provide input in the home. They may be the 'gateway' (although can also be a barrier) to inpatient services, acting as an assessment filter to ensure that admissions occur only when other community alternatives have been explored and either found to be unsuitable, ineffective or having unacceptable risks. Crisis Resolution and Home Treatment (CRHT) teams have therefore been considered as best placed to decide which cases can be best treated in the community and so decide on inpatient admission and provide support for early discharge. However in 2018/2019, inpatient admissions were reported to be the sole responsibility of CRHT teams in only 58.2 per cent of Trusts, usually because CMHT medical staff have resisted this occurring. Such loss of admission oversight has been seen as an infringement to their autonomy and professionalism, but it has also been argued that their longer-term knowledge of the patient justifies them taking admission decisions influenced sometimes by the adequacy of the service offered, which may include concern about the absence of a CRHT medical assessment or of adequate home support.

Medical involvement in supervision and team discussions of all patients under their care is usual to ensure that appropriate treatment and care plans are in place and that risks are assessed (including whether consideration of use of the Mental Health Act is needed). Visits to the home can enhance engagement with the team and assessment of mental and physical state, negotiation about medication and involvement of family. Lone working policies exist for safeguarding of staff because of potential serious risks that might arise.

Home treatment was developed as an alternative to admission primarily because of pressure on hospital beds, their expense and the expressed preference by most users of service to receive care based in their own homes. However, there is a case for home treatment to be used for intensive therapy where admission is not considered an option; patients who can potentially benefit from intensive work with them in the home include those who have:

- Agoraphobia
- Psychosis, including delusions of reference and negative symptoms
- Severe depression and amotivation.

Daily visiting can enable these patients to make progress in a way not possible without such sustained input. Regular support at home may also allow respite for carers, who are then able to leave the home or allow themselves to leave the home. There should be a continuum established as resources allow between local mental health teams and home treatment input enabling this to happen. Generally, however, the decisions to be made are: If the service were unavailable, would this person need hospital admission? Can they be supported by the team safely and effectively without such admission (see reasons for admission under inpatient care earlier)?

Assessment continues after the initial phase where a decision is made about offering care and it is likely that further valuable information will emerge. Monitoring will be offered – but what does that mean? It can seem rather sinister 'checking up on me'. How is it done? It should be a combination of listening and observation. What's happened since we last met and particularly since you last met one of the team? Discussion needs to be about social issues and family events as well as symptom occurrence and medication issues. What impact have those events had or are going to have? Discuss any key problems and progress or otherwise with them. Symptoms are important to discuss. Are they worsening or improving? Have any new symptoms emerged? What about basic functions – sleep or appetite? How are they? How do you feel? How are you getting on with medication? What side effects are you getting? Continuing reassessment needs to be made of expressions of mental state – signs of anxiety, agitation, confusion, anger or depression. Observation of the environment can allow detection of incipient crises by looking for changes that may be relevant: neglect, sign of a lot of money being spent. Observations of the carer can be informative. How are they coping? Therapy may be relevant and possible, non-directive listening to engage with them, problem-solving – especially solution-focused (DIALOG+[98]) – couples or family work or cognitive behaviour therapy.

Work with other agencies around crisis can be productive and improve the delivery and coordination of services to individuals. 'Crisis Cafes/Havens' in some areas provide assessment and support usually by peer workers, often out-of-hours, who can link to statutory services.[84] Safety and Crisis plans (see chapter 15) compiled by the patient with support from care coordinators or key workers prior to crises developing can mean that those providing support are aware of how the individual is experiencing the crisis and what and who can help, as well as what makes things worse. Where the patient is prepared to share the plan or parts of it with other agencies, who can then develop their role in responding, this enhances coordination. Systems to coordinate agency responses have been developed with mental health, substance misuse, emergency – A&E, police and ambulance – and social services, and shared information protocols are established so that when individual services are involved, they can respond in a way most likely to involve and benefit the patient.[99] This can avoid approaches that are likely to be counter-productive[100] (e.g. involving the police in antisocial behaviour orders) by providing alternative routes for all involved agencies to manage distress.

Assertive Outreach

The research on assertive community treatment has been highly influential in the development of services. As a concept, it has found general acceptance, but there has been more controversy over whether it should be applied as part of a CMHT using the Care Programme Approach or as specific teams working to the original programme for assertive community treatment developed in Wisconsin, USA, in the early 1970s.[97] There has been debate about the applicability of the US model to the UK and other health systems, and the nature of the health systems have meant that differences exist although, given that the issues encountered with patients are much the same, similarities are more common. In England under the NHS Plan in 2000,[21] assertive outreach teams were funded and set up according to a policy implementation guide alongside CMHTs, whereas in the USA, they seem to have been effectively stand-alone with very limited services available to those with SMI in the community and so differences would be expected to be more marked. Teams consisted of psychiatrists, nurses, social workers and health care support workers, with psychologists employed in many and occupational therapists in some.

Assertive outreach is a description of a way of taking a less passive response to service delivery than has been traditional in most mental health services involving follow-up with patients in their own homes and neighbourhoods improving support and reducing the likelihood of loss of contact with services. Assertive outreach teams maintain a high staff member to patient caseload ratios (usually under 10:1), provide cover out-of-hours and tend to maintain team knowledge of patients so that reliance on one individual care coordinator does not compromise follow-up. Assertive outreach is therefore appropriate for patients who do not reliably attend outpatient or clinic appointments or avoid organised home visits and who frequently do not collaborate with services or treatments because they have practical difficulties – for example, have financial problems, have homelessness, are too disorganised, are too unwell, are unwilling, are substance misusing, are vulnerable to being 'led astray' or exploitation or have a combination of these problems.

Assertive outreach, as a principle, involves going to the patient rather than waiting for them to come to services and working to develop a relationship, which allows collaborative assessment and management. Often, the focus is on helping them manage the social problems described; this may involve doing practical tasks with them, even for them, or at least arranging for them to be done, acting and advocating as well as working with them to reduce or cope with symptoms through the use of medication and psychosocial approaches. Taking medication can be a problematic issue as patients often have very negative views about it. In some cases of medication non-compliance, it is helpful for the assertive outreach worker to administer the medication on their visit and observe the patient taking it and so deal with the patient's medication non-compliance without getting into any arguments. Instead, this can lead to an informative discussion about the fears, concerns and doubts about the need for medication that the patient has – which it may be possible to allay. Working with this, including considering shared decision-making about dose, administration and precise drug offered (see Chapter 5.3) can be key to effective intervention, recovery from this crisis and prevention of the next.

Crises with patients who are being supported by assertive outreach teams tend to be those related to significant social problems, substance misuse and behavioural presentations with psychosis or, often, a combination of these factors. Depression and anxiety can also be important and remediable issues but may be neglected because other issues seem more significant. Paranoia, voices and substance misuse, for example, may be responses to social causes of distress. Engagement issues are often underlying factors that need to be considered, developing collaboration over treatment issues, as previously discussed, and a focus on developing an effective trusting relationship that can be more than just a foundation to work from and can become therapeutic in its own right. Feeling that you are not totally alone in the world, as patient or carer, and that there are people on your side trying to help you resolve the problems you see around you can have a major therapeutic effect on what seems like a crisis.

The team approach that AOTs tend to take to their patient group makes it very much easier to prevent and manage crises as all team members are likely to have a prior knowledge of the patient and their particular social circumstances, and initial assessment and engagement has already happened. The practitioner hearing of the crisis knows the background, and it is only the more recent circumstances that need exploration. AOTs tend to deal with their own crises themselves unless they request an assessment for compulsory admission. If the home treatment team acts as a gateway to hospital beds, the AOTs may need to liaise with them over alternatives to admission. Psychological consultation, supervision and treatments should be available – for example, CBT for psychosis or depression and treatment for trauma or substance misuse (see relevant chapters elsewhere) – but has frequently not been the case.

As noted, in England, assertive outreach teams were also set up alongside community rehabilitation/resettlement teams focusing on those with more severe and, specifically, long-term conditions, particularly psychosis. Caseloads came from these, wards and CMHTs. Evidence exists for effectiveness in terms of patient preference and engagement with services but not for reduction in hospital admission or symptoms.[101] In many CMHTs, a pattern of working assertively using AO principles within the CPA framework was already in place, and the main distinguishing factor between the teams was caseload size, so it was perhaps unsurprising that the UK services did not show the dramatic impact of the original American AO studies. At the beginning of the 2010s when the requirement to have them was relaxed, many services disbanded them as a result of cost pressures/cuts rather than redistribution of resources, citing this research. This occurred especially in areas where the case for integration with generic CMHTs was stronger due to geographical and morbidity characteristics. However, some inner-city areas have retained them because of the expertise that had developed in working with engagement, maintaining contact with services and comorbid substance misuse.

Early Intervention

Early intervention and outreach have been an ostensible aim of local mental health teams since they were first established, but work with referred and current patients has inevitably taken precedence. However, early intervention can begin as soon as a crisis is identified and management commenced. The carer, patient or referrer may not be considering longer-term issues when they present, but it can nevertheless be a window of opportunity to make a major difference.

Early intervention is relevant for all mental disorders for which effective interventions exist and will be described in a broad context. Early treatment may be able to reduce distress, disability and even death (from suicide in particular), although varying evidence exists on its effectiveness in affecting this or improving outcome. Early intervention in depression and anxiety disorders (through Improving Access to Psychological Treatment – Talking Treatment – services, discussed later) and psychosis (EIP) is now established in the UK and some other high income countries. EIP has strong evidence[4] in reducing duration of untreated psychosis[102,103] and cost effectiveness.[104] There remain some issues about the long-term effects of EIP; the OPUS study in Scandinavia saw a reduction in benefits at five years after the initial two-year intervention had finished.[105] (OPUS offered modified assertive community treatment, family involvement and social skill training but not CBT for psychosis, which is a standard component in UK EIP.) The duration of untreated psychosis (DUP) can be reduced by measures that include early intervention teams and mental health promotion campaigns.[106] Increased length of DUP correlates positively with severity of illness, treatment response and health and social outcomes. Reduction can be expected to have long-term benefits in terms of cost and health gain, including recovery.[107]

EIP services have a number of key features beyond the early detection of psychosis, including a strong recovery-oriented psychosocial approach, a focus on the unique needs of younger adults, an emphasis on family support, and attention to the impact of interrupted development and the social consequences of serious mental illness. First contact within mental health services through adult generic community mental health team or child and adolescent services predicts longer overall DUP and delayed access to early intervention in psychosis teams. First contacts involving acute treatment facility or early intervention teams (EIT) predicted significantly shorter delays in accessing treatment, which could reduce DUP to from 90 to 60 days.[108] Maintenance of gains made with EIT may be lost with transfer to CMHTs or primary care[109–111] – continuing engagement, support and psychosocial intervention needs to be considered.

EIP has involved provision of assertive outreach to individuals and caregivers presenting to mental health services and increased intensity of case management. Use of medication, family work and social support is offered early by a multidisciplinary team of doctors, nurses, social workers, occupational therapists and psychologists with health care support workers and often employment workers. Psychological interventions are made available, although there has been variability in approaches offered. In the UK, CBT for psychosis provided by psychologists and nurse therapists has been the preferred individual modality. In the USA (e.g. in RAISE),[102] the NAVIGATE programme has been offered, which does include some elements of CBT provided by team members.[112] EIP teams were established and funded under NHS plan[21] in 2000 as the case was made for their effectiveness at that stage. As a group, the teams established outcome measures and collected data, but unfortunately, this was not taken up nationally and was never used in the way that later occurred with IAPT to shape and expand services (see later in this chapter). However, after initially working with the age range 14–35, they have expanded to accept those up to 65 in recent years. Links with children and adolescent services and skills within teams to work with adolescents have therefore been necessary. Guidance on ways of working were provided with the initial Policy Implementation Guidance and later developed with the EIP framework (2016),[113] which also introduced access and waiting time standards that more than 50 per cent of people experiencing first-episode psychosis will be treated with a NICE-approved care package within two weeks of referral and specified outcome measures including DIALOG[30] and recovery scales.

Early intervention (EI) involves providing services when they are first needed and likely to be effective. The primary reason for this is that the distress and disability that so many patients and carers experience should be alleviated or at least reduced as soon as possible. Secondarily, this may have an effect on the longer-term outcome of the problem. A major issue is how to identify patients early who are likely to benefit from EI. Primary care has been a particular focus for this with some success in the detection of mental health issues. However, even established services only estimate that they reach a minority of people who eventually go on to have psychotic illnesses. Orientating services towards EI requires similar changes to those involved in preventing and responding to crises. Detecting early signs of psychosis in those presenting for the first time is the focus, but it is also important to do so in those re-presenting, even when they have had other diagnoses. Many patients who are eventually given a diagnosis of psychosis initially present and may be managed with an alternative diagnosis of, for example, drug misuse, borderline personality disorder or depressive illness.

With psychosis, the trigger for intervention tends to be potential positive symptoms, especially where combined with vulnerability – for example, shy or very sensitive personality (schizoid or paranoid), family history, and increasing social withdrawal or generally deteriorating performance. the latter, emerging negative symptoms, may become the main focus of concern but are often identified late. the main indicators of the prodrome of psychosis, which will be the focus of the EI service, include a family history of psychosis, transient psychotic phenomena – brief limited intermittent psychotic symptoms (BLIPS) and attenuated symptoms. Symptoms can often present initially during episodes of substance misuse and then become persistent. With possible bipolar disorder, the emergence of disinhibition and impulsivity that is out of keeping with normal behaviour may be the signal for involvement. With other disorders, the point at which early intervention by mental health services is appropriate may be more difficult to determine (e.g. with depression) – this is probably after first-line measures in primary care have been offered (e.g. antidepressant therapy or counselling) or, with anxiety, after basic counselling, self-help and problem-solving to deal with issues. If psychotic symptoms or risk issues are present, patients should always be advised not to make any life changing decisions whilst acutely ill. Current meaningful activity (e.g. work, education or leisure) can be identified and maintained:

- For work or education, this may mean contact and negotiation with employers or education providers – adjustments or deferral may preserve posts
- For friendships, establishing who the current friends are and then working out how to maintain contact
- For self-respect/esteem and respect of others, needs identifying as an issue early and appropriate measures used to preserve this
- For physical health, maintaining or developing exercise and dietary patterns early to combat the risks of this deteriorating

Carers can provide invaluable information and need the opportunity to do so. Where a decision is made to intervene, providing them with information – taking into account confidentiality issues – is likely to be helpful to all concerned. Where intervention is not thought to be appropriate, careful explanation of why not is needed. However, it is important to describe where doubts exist: 'although that is the position at the moment, some of the things he/she said, e.g. [specify what was said] may be early signs of problems' or 'it is possible that he/she is not telling me about their concerns'.

An explanation for the behaviour, where it is not thought to be due to significant mental health problems, is useful: 'He/she may be stressed by exams, falling out with friends, etc', 'He/she may be behaving like this because you aren't getting on too well together at the moment – as often happens in adolescence', 'This may be his/her way of beginning to develop his/her own adult identity – sometimes they push those close to them away so that they can become more confident and independent'.

Most important is to either inform that 'I will come back or speak to you on the telephone on . . . [day] at . . .[time] to see how things are progressing' and 'If things deteriorate, please contact us at [tel. nos. for day & out-of-hours use]'. It may be helpful to specify possible signs of deterioration – for example, increasing depression, distractibility or fear – changes in behaviour such as in eating patterns or increasing isolation or hostility. Communication with the original referrer of decisions is important – and again to make contact if circumstances change or don't improve.

Community Mental Health Teams (CMHTs)

When CMHTs were initially established, their remit was very broad and could be very variable – essentially all patients with mental illness referred by a doctor to them from inpatient wards, primary care, general hospital clinics and emergency departments within a defined geographical area or from specified primary care teams. They took the place of the previous consultant-based outpatient services, where the consultant for an area ran the service with one or two CPNs. Gradually and variably self-referral systems developed, and sources such as social services and the criminal justice services extended this. However, also services to provide specialist eating disorder and perinatal care, earlier intervention for psychosis and common mental disorders and liaison/emergency/crisis services evolved. Services for people with substance misuse have changed with mixed results (see Chapter 14).

Generic CMHTs now often express concern that, over the years with the new developments of specialist teams and redefinition of the roles of older peoples and child and adolescent mental health services, they are now essentially working with people who just don't fit into other teams, rather than seeing the CMHT as having a very worthwhile role in its own right. This has affected recruitment to them and priority for funding. Caseloads now focus on people who may have been initially seen by IAPT or EIP services and been discharged or transferred and who have persistent or relapsing depression, bipolar disorder, psychosis, Complex PTSD and personality disorder. Increasingly, they are asked to see people with neurodevelopmental disorders, perhaps after brief assessments from specialist services or whilst people are waiting for specialist assessment. There may also be local agreements that they continue to provide care for older people whose needs are unlikely to be better met by transfer to old age services. The Community Mental Health Framework[24] has been introduced to address many of these issues. Overall the number of community contacts in 2019 was 31,095/100,000 population with 1,685/100,000 on caseloads.

Care and treatment offered varies considerably. Care plans will usually include pharmacological, social and psychological components; practical support, including facilitating access to housing and finance; family and caregiver advice; social contact; and prescription and support in taking medication. Meaningful activity, which includes work but can involve other activities such as hobbies, social activities with family and friends, exercise, sport and other leisure activities, as well as more structured activities including educational and vocational courses, may also be included. Some of these activities can be provided at day centres or support groups, but increasingly, mental health services make links with mainstream community resources to develop collaborative approaches to involve patients in accessing courses (e.g. colleges) and other community facilities (e.g. gyms).

A community mental health team (CMHT) will be staffed by a number of professionals from different disciplines who will bring their particular expertise to the team. In a typical team, there are likely to be mental health nurses, social workers, psychiatrists, occupational therapists, psychologists, administration staff and support workers. Within this group of staff, there may well be individuals who take a particular role – for example, in group work or in working with patients who are involved in the criminal justice system, as well as others who manage the interface with forensic services. Patients are often seen in their own homes, and practitioners work with patients to produce support packages that promote recovery and maximise quality of life. A community team manager or individuals within the team will also often hold a budget for the purchase of care for patients in that area (e.g. for domiciliary care packages, residential care or sometimes transport costs for patients to access services). As for health and social care everywhere, resources are limited, and priorities have to be set. However, it is worth noting that despite this, that teams score 87 per cent satisfaction on the 'Friends and Family' test (2019).

Most teams work with those people who have severe and enduring mental health problems. They are also likely to have referrals of those who are being discharged from inpatient care. Some teams are in a position to do more work that is preventative in nature, maybe by running clinics in primary care settings or by short-term work with people who are becoming unwell. Whatever the size and breadth of the individual team, it is certainly in this sort of team that the majority of patients will receive their mental health care. It is usually to these teams that a GP will initially refer a patient with problems, and it is often the decision of this team to refer the patient on to specialist teams that exist in the locality. Teams are likely to offer the following:

- Assessment of new referrals of people with potential mental health difficulties – urgent, immediate or routine
- Short and long-term psychosocial interventions by care coordinators for those with severe or enduring mental health problems
- Some group work, maybe around particular issues (e.g. abuse or hearing voices) or around skills (e.g. assertiveness or anxiety management)
- Gate keeping for services such as day services or care management
- Some therapies: psychological, guided self-help and maybe complementary therapies
- Psychiatric outpatient and domiciliary services and medication management
- Depot medication administration and Clozapine clinics
- Support of carers
- Support in accessing occupation and leisure activities
- The provision of a duty service

- Supervision of people on Community Treatment Orders[18]
- Physical wellbeing assessment and intervention collaborating with primary care

Crises in CMHTs tend to be managed by a duty service or worker unless the patient is already known and allocated to a worker within the team, who happens to be available. The duty service means a practitioner (or a number of practitioners) who have put time aside from their usual work to deal with any new referrals, general inquiries, requests for advice or indeed any crisis presentations that may come up. The staff that cover this service are likely to be qualified (and usually) non-medical staff. There is then usually a parallel system of medical duty cover, although increasingly these are being integrated in a multi-disciplinary way. As most crisis presentations come to the CMHT, it is at this point that the decision gets made about who is to respond to the situation and undertake the necessary assessment. We will discuss some guidelines for deciding who should provide the initial assessment later in this chapter, but the important role for the CMHT duty worker is the 'triage' role, the gathering of the initial information, often over the telephone, which will inform that end decision.

Psychiatric outpatients have formed the backbone of psychiatric services over many years but recently have come under scrutiny, partly as a result of the reconsideration of the psychiatrists role in *New Ways of Working*[71] but also as a result of pressures on CMHTs leading to increased emphasis on discharge of patients to allow space for new referrals. The role of the psychiatrist as consultant to the team has been promoted as a more efficient way to use the scarce skills that they have available. A balance certainly seems necessary, but most psychiatrists do seem to still see a role for outpatients as a time-efficient way to provide and manage care to complex patients, monitor mental and physical state and reduce likelihood of relapse but very much in coordination with the MDT. Face-to-face contact has a vital role alongside consultation and remote contact (e.g. phone and video especially during and since the Covid pandemic). Contact with primary care and community support services, whether by team or psychiatrist, cannot be over-looked, and referral letters copied or addressed to patients are generally very positively received.

Meaningful Activity

Meaningful activity includes work but can involve other activities such as hobbies, social activities with family and friends, exercise, sport and other leisure activities, as well as more structured activities including educational and vocational courses. Some of these activities can be provided at day centres, but increasingly, mental health services make links with mainstream community resources to develop collaborative approaches to support patients to access courses (e.g. colleges) and other community facilities (e.g. gyms).

There is strong evidence for the effectiveness of social interventions,[114] and social prescribing[73] is a mechanism – usually via primary care – for linking patients with non-medical sources of support within the community. These might include opportunities for arts and creativity, physical activity, learning new skills, volunteering, mutual aid, befriending and self-help, as well as support with, for example, employment, benefits, housing, debt, legal advice or parenting problems. Schemes may include 'exercise on prescription' or 'prescription for learning' or 'books on prescription',[115] although there is a range of different models and referral options.[116]

Employment Support

Despite the high rate of unemployment, it has been reported that most patients with severe mental illness want to work.[117,118] Individual Placement and Support (IPS) employment programmes place patients on competitive jobs without extended preparation. Rapid job search and attainment by matching patients to jobs based on their interests and skills take place prior to teaching them new skills to prepare for future jobs.[119] There is international evidence that people supported into regular employment via IPS had fewer, shorter stays in hospital with an associated reduction in cost than those who were not supported.[120] However, in recent studies, IPS wasn't able to have the positive effect on employment in the UK setting seen in the USA and other European countries, possibly because of factors related to the welfare benefit system,[121] and the job vacancy rate, at the time, can also be influential.

The IPS model uses assertive outreach, based on the assertive community treatment case-management model for severe mental illness,[97] and is the most widely studied approach to supported employment.[122] In IPS, employment specialists provide a full range of vocational services to each patient, including engagement in services, job interests identification and vocational assessment, job finding and job support.

The emphasis on providing community-based services in IPS may be especially critical for the retention of patients in vocational services, whose motivation to work may fluctuate over time[123] and for whom assertive outreach may provide a critical bridge to maintaining continuity of services. Although IPS helps people get jobs, IPS may not help them retain them.[122] Nearly half of supported employment participants do not obtain competitive work at any time during the periods studies have covered.[124]

Social firms provide employment and are a popular European model.[125,126] Clubhouse – US user-led projects – in two studies had good employment outcomes with better tenure and pay than the comparison IPS intervention.[120]

Accommodation

Housing support services[127–129] lower the frequency of unplanned admissions into psychiatric wards (and speed discharge) and lower the rates at which community mental health services are used, reduce the rates at which the people with severe problems became homeless (reducing the use of homelessness shelters) and the rates at which they were arrested, improve wellbeing among people with severe problems, and reduce other welfare and health system costs (US research).

Homelessness is a complex multi-faceted social problem with a lengthy history, and subsumed within this lies the history of the destitute mentally ill – the 'pauper lunatics'. In Tudor times, the first poor laws were passed in 1601, and they established a system of subsistence for the 'impotent poor' – infants, the elderly and the infirm who would literally be licensed to beg in certain towns, while consigning 'able-bodied' adults to local workhouses. Even in the early days, it was estimated that around 25 per cent of the workhouse population were pauper lunatics.[130] Conditions were appalling in the workhouses and resulted in numerous scandals, leading a parliamentary commission of 1807 to investigate the situation of the pauper lunatics. The commission found that 92 per cent were living in the poor houses, and only 4.8 per cent resided in the private madhouses. The vagrancy act of 1824 directed local parishes to care for vagrants and beggars in their districts.[130]

In the latter part of the nineteenth century, other non-statutory bodies such as the Salvation Army[130] developed their hostels for the homeless, the Rowton Houses and the Temperance and Friendly societies became involved with the care of the homeless as part of their crusades against alcoholism, and this led to a gradual replacing of many of the workhouses. Some workhouses, particularly those in working-class districts of cities survived and became reception centres for homeless men, and this pattern of care extended right into the mid-twentieth century, as described eloquently in George Orwell's 1931 essay 'The Spike'. London had one very large reception centre, the 900-bedded Camberwell reception centre, which covered the whole of London.

A study by Griffiths Edwards of the residents of this centre in 1968 found that 25 per cent had a previous mental hospital admission.[131] A study of acute admissions to a Birmingham city centre psychiatric ward[132] found that 25 per cent gave their address as 'No Fixed Abode' – a euphemism for homelessness, indicating that many homeless men had mental illness. Many of the residents at reception centres were found to be suffering from severe malnutrition, so this pattern of care was not really working.

A more formal government commitment to care for the homeless came with the post-war Attlee government,[130] which passed the National Assistance Act (1948) and set up the National Assistance Board. This abolished all the previous poor laws, closed all the remaining workhouses and provided a safety net for those who could not work – the disabled, the unmarried mothers, as well as for the homeless and other disadvantaged groups. This protection was the forerunner of our modern benefits system, including universal credit. The National Assistance Board was to administer this and, with regard to the homeless, their stated aim was 'to get the previously homeless and those leading an itinerant life to settle down into a fixed and stable domicile'.

The causes of homelessness today are legion but broadly speaking can be divided into two over-lapping groups: those with psychiatric disorders and those afflicted by economic or social catastrophes. This latter group includes redundancies, foreclosures, divorce, serious illnesses, loss of support networks, evictions, poverty or natural disasters such as floods, fires and hurricanes. Amongst young people, an increasing number of adolescents flee impulsively from abusive situation without any specific plans where to stay and so find themselves living on the streets. For most of these groups, a solution is usually readily at hand, and the homelessness is unlikely to become chronic. However, for these with psychiatric difficulties, the solution is more complicated as they will usually require treatment before they can be accepted for social housing, and they may not present or cooperate with treatments even if treatments are readily available, which often they are not.

The problem is worldwide, and Fazel[133] conducted a meta-analysis of 29 studies based in the USA, Europe and Australia, of which 28 reported on psychotic illness. They estimated that around 1 million people worldwide were homeless. In the UK, this was around 38,000, the majority of whom were accommodated in various hostels; in the USA, the figure was 780,000, but around 300,000 of these individuals were actually sleeping rough on any given night.

Alcohol dependence was the most common cause with a pooled prevalence rate of 37.9%, but the prevalence rate varied widely between studies from 8–54%. The meta-analysis noted a trend for rates of alcohol-related homelessness to increase in recent decades. Psychotic illness was present in around 12% (3–42%). This is substantially greater than community prevalence rates reported for psychosis, which are usually in the range of 1–2%. Personality disorders had a mean prevalence of 23% (2–71%) and drug dependence 24%(4.7–54%). There was only one study reporting on homeless women (N = 33), but the rates for drug addiction were high at 24%. For major depression, the pooled prevalence rate was 11.4% (0.0–41%), which – though greater than community prevalence rates for depression – was not as grossly elevated as the other disorders. All these disorders are amongst the most difficult to treat in psychiatry and, even when mentally ill homeless persons receive adequate mental health services, a range of unmet welfare and housing needs may remain, implying that normal community mental health service provision is usually insufficient.[133]

Homeless people have a reduced life expectancy. A Danish study[134] reported on a whole nation survey of the homeless in Denmark. They found that 62.4% of the men and 58% of women had a registered psychiatric disorder. The standardised mortality ratios for homeless men was 5.6 and for women was 6.7. The remaining life expectancy at age 15–24 was 21 years lower for men and 17 years lower for women when compared to a general population cohort. Those with drug abuse had the greatest reduction in mortality. Physical conditions, which are a particular risk for homeless people, appear to be TB, bacterial pneumonia, hepatitis B and HIV, all of which can nowadays be treated.

Mitigating against a solution to the problem is the severe loss of social housing started by Mrs Thatcher's right to buy policy, where tenants of council housing who had been paying rent for three years had the right to buy their house, and this resulted in a serious depletion of the social housing stock, since – despite promises of the local authorities – these houses were not replaced. At the same time, there was a closure of the older reception centres. Thus, in 1981, there were 9,751 bed spaces in the UK for traditional hostels for the homeless, but they had appalling physical conditions and were difficult to run because of staff shortages and a lack of financial support. By now, they were under local authority control, and they were gradually phased out without any adequate reprovision.

Different political philosophies governed the treatment of the poor, so with it came a variable generosity/meanness in the funding of initiatives for the homeless. The left, drawing on ideas from France, viewed the poor and destitute as a marginalised group in society who needed support to obtain greater inclusion in society.[130] By contrast, the US right wing were heavily influenced by the writings of Charles Murray, who wrote that society had a whole underclass of people (including the homeless) who had become over-dependent and addicted to welfare whereas, in reality, they were responsible for their own fate, and the solution was a withdrawal of welfare benefits to encourage greater self-reliance and to find their own solutions to their predicament. Such views dominated thinking for a period in many America municipalities and so, needless to say, the problem of homelessness is far worse in America than the UK or Europe – where it is probably better than in the UK because of better welfare provision in most European countries.

Economic forces, policy decisions particularly in housing, budget priorities, societal trends and attitudes about public assistance all contribute to the causes and cure of homelessness. In recent history, economic and financial circumstances related to the Great Recession of 2008–2010 – the worst global recession since the Great Depression – resulted in high rates of mortgage foreclosures, evictions and unemployment. As a result, may people were pushed out of their homes in America. In the UK, the government's austerity programme from 2010–2020, combined with the depletion of social housing, resulted in a much-increased homeless problem, which is still with us.

The Department of Health's Homeless Mental Illness initiative in the early 1990s established outreach teams of social workers, nurses and psychiatrists with relatively low caseloads who successfully reduced the amount of homelessness in their localities, but with ever present funding problems, such teams have sometimes been disbanded with the task being delegated to the local assertive outreach team – where they exist – or CMHTs. Inner-city districts such as the London borough of Westminster, Sheffield and Southampton, which have high rates of homelessness, have been able to hold on to such teams over the longer term. In addition, it is noteworthy that at the beginning of the Covid-19 pandemic lockdown, the government decreed that all those sleeping rough were to be provided with hotel accommodation, indicating that if there was a necessity to eliminate the problem, it could be done.

Personalised Care

Social inclusion: Six broad categories for 'action' include stigma, health/social care in reintegration, employment, local community participation, basics (housing, finance, transport) and implementation. There is evidence that community projects are effective at reducing stigma and promoting inclusion when community development practitioners, supported through various partnerships, bring people together to address both their individual concerns, as well as creating new community-led resources and connections between individuals, groups and organisations.[135]

Peer providers: Peer support is becoming more widespread, with patients working together to support themselves and each other in a variety of settings. Peer support has also been used to improve the effectiveness of self-management.[136] There are, however, a wide variety of definitions within peer support projects and not all have been found to be empowering or indeed genuinely peer led, some being run or led by professionals rather than patients.[137] One study has shown that peer support reduces inpatient bed use[138] and another that peer worker-facilitated psychiatric advance directives are specifically effective in decreasing compulsory hospital admissions and increasing some mental health outcomes (self-perceived symptoms, empowerment and recovery).[139]

For black and minority ethnic groups,[47] the main barriers can be grouped into sociocultural difficulties (health beliefs and mistrust of services), systemic problems (lack of culturally competent interventions), economic issues and individual barriers (shame, stigma)(see Chapter 17).[140] Stigma is thought to be created and maintained due to a complex interplay of social-structural, interpersonal and psychological factors.[141]

The most important choices that patients wish for have been described:[142,143]

- **A service-user centred user-professional relationship**
  - Dignity and respect in the partnership (i.e. clear communication)
  - Valuing the individual perspective (person-centred communication skills)
- **Immediacy of help**
  - More flexible ways to get access quickly
- **Range of choices available**
  - More options, including 'talking treatments' and community and social care help
  - Opportunities to regain employment
  - Focus on recovery

  - Cultural and spiritual needs[144] considered
  - Practices and mental health services acting as community resources (i.e. community services based within same premises)
- **Education on self-management**
  - Knowledge and support on ways to help self
  - Self-help groups

Care for most people experiencing psychosis occurs in community settings and will involve support by case managers, psychiatric nurses, social workers or occupational therapists, with psychiatrists and psychologists providing expert support, supervision and treatment. Peer workers have an important role in many services and can provide social support to counter loneliness,[66] including befriending[145,146] and guidance through the labyrinth of financial benefit and housing networks. Physical health care is also a key issue as life span is substantially reduced (standardised mortality ratios are two to three times higher) in people with severe mental health problems due particularly to life style issues such as poor diet, lack of exercise, smoking and substance misuse, and failure to detect and act upon early signs of illness (see Chapter 16).[38] When asked, patients/patients prioritise these social and physical care issues over treatment; quality of life and recovery are dependent on these needs being addressed. Treatments can certainly be important in dealing with distress and disability as well as overcoming obstacles but only where these primary needs are being met. Numerous studies have shown that users emphasise the importance of practical help, housing, money, physical health care, while professionals tend to rate interventions, treatment, support and symptom control as being most important. The approach that has emerged from this now goes beyond controlling illness to working alongside individuals to develop an active, meaningful life in the community in a way that leads towards their personally defined 'recovery' (see previously).[148] Various instruments for measuring need exist (e.g. DIALOG[29]), which has now been adapted and evaluated to include a solution-focused intervention.[98]

Statutory teams outside mental health services also play an important role. In crisis work, there will often be a need to co-work with colleagues from other teams – for example, the learning disability services or from the children and families teams. In assessments that are to consider compulsory measures, there is usually a rota of available qualified staff to undertake these on a geographical basis. In the UK, this is often organised by approved social workers employed by the local social services department or other approved practitioners who cover all patient services and ages.

Crisis management sometimes involves a number of specialist teams within the main service, and there may be problems mainly regarding the interface and demarcation ('who does what') between the different teams. When service planning is at its worst, patients can end up being passed from team to team in a crisis, perhaps being 'assessed' three or four times before a plan of support is drawn up. People do not come in one dimensional 'packages' – a patient may need an alternative to admission but also have an eating disorder and a substance misuse problem. If the patient was then pregnant as well, the whole system can snarl up! However, when service planning is at its best, having specialist teams can ensure that patients in specific circumstances receive a tailor-made service that really meets their needs.

Support for Carers

Support from families, friends and carers can have a strong influence on recovery, supporting a crisis and relapse prevention. Good social support has been found to reduce carers' perceived responsibilities,[148] but this is not easy to deliver, and many carers feel excluded and marginalised.[149–151] Carers views have rated 'get listened to and involved in all decisions as equal partners' as a high priority, and in a large survey of people with severe problems, carers and professionals found that each group had differing views about what information should be shared.[151] Confidentiality requirements do not prevent information being received by staff or general advice being given. The concept of a 'triangle of care'[152] involves listening to and providing advice for all carers, with more formal psycho-education for many and then family work offered to those who can and wish to participate. Carers are entitled to carer's allowances at different rates through the benefits system.

Improving Access to Psychological Therapies (Talking Treatments)

Services to Improve Access to Psychological Therapies (IAPT – Talking Treatments) were funded and introduced in 2008. These were to provide psychological treatments for people with mild to moderate depression or anxiety disorders. Previously, general practitioners themselves or counsellors that they employed provided some services, but these were not available in many areas or variable in quality. The impetus to develop these services came from the Layard Report, which was an economic assessment of the costs to the community of depression and anxiety. Professor Lord Layard (2007)[153] from the London School of Economics argued that a lot of money spent on benefits could be saved by ensuring that effective treatments were freely available on the NHS for these conditions to help people get back to work. Secondary care mental health services have been focusing services on those with more severe problems, so this group of patients with milder disorders either visited private therapists if they could afford it or, if not, received either inadequate and no services at all. There have been difficulties in determining responsibility for specific patients, and in many areas, IAPT and secondary care psychologists/CMHT managers have attempted to resolve differences and allocate responsibilities. Patients diagnosed with personality disorder, psychosis or recurrent depression or anxiety are not generally accepted by IAPT. However, bodily distress disorder (formerly 'medically unexplained symptoms' – see Chapter 6.6) are now a focus.

IAPT services offer a range of NICE-recommended therapies for depression and anxiety disorders since 2008 in line with a stepped-care model, when appropriately indicated.[154] Low-intensity interventions (guided self-help, computerised CBT and group-based physical activity programmes) have been identified as being effective for sub-threshold depressive symptoms and mild to moderate depression, as well as some anxiety disorders. For people with persistent sub-threshold depressive symptoms or mild to moderate depression who have not benefited from a low-intensity intervention, NICE recommendations include the following high-intensity psychological interventions: CBT, interpersonal psychotherapy (IPT), behavioural activation, couple therapy for depression, brief psychodynamic therapy and counselling for depression. IAPT services have dealt with over a million people per year with 8,000 practitioners. Assessment and outcome measurement includes use of the Patient Health Questionnaire–9 items (PHQ-9), Generalised Anxiety Disorder scale–7 items (GAD-7) and the Work and Social Adjustment Scale (WSAS). These are used to monitor individual therapy but also overall achievement of local services, and there are also targets for the numbers of patients seen assessed for each area using prevalence data. Of these, 50 per cent of patients recover, and 70 per cent were improved at completion.

The services were carefully regulated and generally accessed by self-referral. They provide cognitive behaviour therapy, counselling or couples therapy. There is an initial telephone triage process, which will usually provide initial problem-solving and only if that is unsuccessful are patients offered evidence-based therapies.

Interface and Continuity Issues

Changes in service delivery have led to increasing discontinuities in care in primary and secondary care, including mental health services, and this is frequently referred to by patients, and there is now research evidence that this does have negative impacts on outcome.[155] This was much less common with the previous model of a one sector psychiatrist and one team than with the newer models of service provision, which have been unable to retain continuity of care as a key therapeutic ideal: a similar process has happened across medicine as sub-specialties have developed. Crises often raise issues of responsibility for provision of assessment and continuing services, but this can also occur on referral or re-referral to services. Crises or serious, sometimes irremediable, delays leading to deterioration may be caused by such issues where services are unilaterally withdrawn or disputes between teams and service members arise. Conflict can arise as a result of age demarcation disputes between general adult and children's or older peoples teams and also with between CMHTs and functional teams (i.e. CRHT, AOT and EIPs) and with specialist perinatal teams, eating disorders services, drugs and alcohol teams and general hospital liaison teams. Overly rigid specialist team criteria can lead to the patient and carer 'falling through the cracks' and cause unnecessary distress and disability – and risk.

Much can be prevented by prioritising continuity, including caution in relation to discharge, and developing agreed service protocols and readily available reconciliation processes which clearly define:

- Where responsibility lies
- How transfers should occur
- Which teams also provide for shared services where this may be appropriate

The key determinant should be the needs of the individual patient and carers, but this inevitably will be balanced by considerations of how best to provide a service to the population as a whole. This has not been helped by the separation of area services between different organisations – one process that the integrated care systems are intended to remedy. As an example, a woman of 67 in part-time employment who has become depressed for the first time might be best served by adult rather than old age services. A young man of 20 who has never worked, living at home with parents, presenting after a family crisis might be assessed as likely to benefit from the family work, career advice and links with education services that a child and adolescent service can provide. However, although for the individual, a case might be made for these services, provision of services could become chaotic if such a course was followed. Extending the age range to 70 for adult services might make sense, although moving that of children's services to 20 probably wouldn't – unless, for example, a full adolescent service for under 25s is established. Consideration of such issues in protocols, building in defined flexibility, can assist in crisis situations. Arguments between service teams undoubtedly worsen crises and can lead, and indeed have led, to catastrophes. Old age services have greater experience in dealing with organic mental disorders, and their assistance in assessing and then taking on management of them is generally appropriate for the individual and for services. However, younger patients with dementia may be difficult to nurse in old age wards and accommodation, so assistance from adult services may be needed under shared care arrangements. Alternatively, older people who are in employment and physically fully active may benefit from community supports that adult services are aware of and have access to. Adolescents who have left school and are at least potentially seeking employment, especially where they have developed mental health problems that are likely to require support and management well into adult life (e.g. psychotic illnesses) may benefit from early transfer to adult services; issues sometimes arise about inpatient care where this is needed (see earlier). Collaboration between adult and adolescent services in early intervention can also share skills and access to facilities effectively, but differing criteria for teams can cause confusion and gaps in services.

If a patient is already working with a particular service, then if they experience a problem – whether of crisis proportions or not – they will normally contact the people who they know and who support them. Those practitioners are best placed to manage the situation. However, there are times when the interface between services causes difficulties, such as when a person is not allocated to a service. This becomes worse for a patient who may have been formerly working with a team and has had their 'case' closed. The patient contacts, for example, an early intervention or a perinatal team in need of help but gets sent back to their family doctor who is told to ring the CMHT.

Where services are stretched, there can be lengthy discussions about which service should take the patient, and it can lead to the patient being passed around, which increases both distress and risk. A patient can end up being assessed by several teams before being accepted by one, which is wasteful of resources and disrespectful to a patient having to tell their story repeatedly. This can also happen where a person is allocated to a team, and the allocated worker or duty worker wishes to enlist another team's support to manage a crisis. In reality, the teams that the practitioner will want are likely to be the home treatment service or the inpatient team, though it can be the case that requests for joint assessments with other teams can be made. The interface problems here come if the other teams do not accept the assessment of the allocated worker. Either the original practitioner is left having to put in a plan that is not the one indicated by their assessment, or the patient has to be assessed again by the other team, which makes the original worker's assessment a waste of time.

The issues are essentially about criteria for acceptance to a particular service and how advice can be readily accessed from other services. There are two principles to start from in examining how to improve interface disputes when supporting people in crisis.

- We should all be interested in helping the patient requesting assistance.
- We should wish to avoid the patient having multiple assessments, for the sake of their wellbeing and for the sake of limited mental health resources.

No system can ever be perfect, but the following guidelines could help the process:

- If each team has a clear statement about their criteria for acceptance that they then stick to (unless the person needs help but falls in the gap between the different services criteria)
- If a patient meets the criteria for a team, such as for home treatment, that team accepts a triage style assessment from the referring team to avoid duplication or else does a joint assessment where eligibility for the service is in question
- Duty workers in all teams are trained in triage assessment, knowing what information to get over the phone to pass on
- All teams having somebody available to offer advice on their particular specialist area to colleagues from other teams seeking help in a crisis
- Operational management need to examine patterns of activity and ensure a fair distribution of workload

Multi-agency Working

Psychiatrists work in complex systems across health and social care. This requires them to be able to work comfortably with a wide range of different professionals and agencies outside of traditional boundaries. Whilst psychiatrists deal with the immediacy of patient contact, they have to also work as part of a team. The team will also relate to a wider organisation, and the organisation is embedded within a wider network of agencies, organisations and institutions at local, regional and national levels. Psychiatrists will work and contribute across all of these different levels.

This complexity is illustrated well with some of the issues that can arise in relation to safeguarding of children and of adults (see also Chapter 13, which discusses child abuse and neglect). Legislative frameworks exist that have been developed to approach some of this complexity. However, frameworks to guide and shape how this develops are implemented at local levels and provide the means of supporting this difficult and challenging work within the Rule of Law.

Section 42 of the Care Act 2014 outlines duties in relation to the Safeguarding of Adults. This is the equivalent for those aged 18 and over of legislation applying to the safeguarding of children outlined in the Children Act (1989, 2004) and provides an example of legislation in this area that is applicable in day-to-day practice, often requiring multi-agency approaches. All local authority areas will have a Safeguarding Adults Board to draw all the strands together and ensure appropriate local implementation.

The intention of the Act is to ensure that if concerns are identified, they are addressed in a person-centred way, taking into account the views of the person. It runs alongside other statutory responsibilities that might relate to many other Acts of Parliament (see Box 20.4).

The six key principles in the Care Act 2014 are:

- Empowerment
- Prevention
- Proportionality

Box 20.4 Examples of statutes of relevance to adult care

- Care Act 2014
- Mental Capacity Act 2005
- Human Rights Act 1998
- Mental Health Act 1983
- Modern Slavery Act 1998
- Equality Act 2010
- Children and Families Act 2014
- NHS Act 1946
- National Insurance Act 1911, 1946

- Protection
- Partnership
- Accountability

At local levels, agencies are mandated to ensure proper processes are in place to address the potential areas using a collaborative multi-agency approach. Authorities will have local processes that might have different names (e.g. Vulnerable Adults Risk Meetings, VARMs) but all should be under the overview of the local Safeguarding Adults Board.

If a patient is deemed to lack capacity within the terms of the MCA (2015) or requires detention under the MHA (1983, 2007), then these pieces of legislation take priority. However, there are many situations where concerns can arise but where these pieces of legislation cannot be used. Capacity, for example, is decision- and time-specific, and people may have capacity in relation to some decisions but not for others. Their capacity may vary.

The Care Act allows for a proportionate response across agencies where the MHA and MCA do not necessarily apply but where there may identified needs for care and support in a setting of significant concerns at potential risk.

The areas of concern are grouped in the Care Act under the following headings:

Risk of:

- Neglect
- Physical abuse
- Financial abuse
- Psychological abuse
- Self-neglect
- Domestic abuse
- Sexual abuse
- Organisational abuse
- Discriminatory abuse
- Modern slavery

Example of a local VARM process:[156]

Local VARM processes are intended to create a process to manage risks which may arise within specific circumstances when working with adults deemed to have capacity to make decisions for themselves, but who are at risk of serious harm or death through:

- Self-neglect (Care Act 2014)
- Risk taking behaviour/chaotic lifestyles
- Refusal of services

The VARM is a multi-agency adult assessment risk management process to:

- Identify the relevant risks for the individual
- Discuss and agree agency responsibilities/actions
- Record, monitor and review progress with the agreed action plan
- Agree when the risks have been managed and evaluate the outcome

The aim of the VARM policy and practice guidance is to provide professionals with useful information and a framework to facilitate effective multi-agency working with adults who are at significant risk.

The local Safeguarding, VARM or similar process should therefore allow any professional in any agency to raise a concern and convene a multi-agency review to consider all the relevant issues and construct an appropriate plan centred around the individual. The multi-agency approach can ensure involvement of many agencies (e.g. housing, fire service, social care, mental health service, primary care, police, probation) that can then develop creative solutions to the immediate issues. The process should facilitate this flexible person-centred way of working in which agencies are not disconnectedly working in isolation from each other in ignorance of each other's perspective and should ensure that a process of review is in place.

Quality Improvement

Not all doctors will undertake research projects, but all will be involved – frequently – in quality improvement initiatives.[157] These may be part of statutory processes (e.g. Care Quality Commission inspections) or internal organisational processes. The Royal College Centre for Quality Improvement (CCQI) hosts quality networks, accreditation, national clinical audits (e.g. medication use), psychosis, anxiety and depression, and research and evaluation. Standards for a range of settings – inpatient, community or rehabilitation – provide detailed guidance on good practice for services who may then seek accreditation.

Individual projects can arise from concerns about delivery of services – for example, prescription of antipsychotics, completion and standard of physical health checks, implementation of specific NICE guidelines or patient issues about communication. There are general principles[158] (e.g. teamwork and feedback), some excellent examples and a range of tools available to assist (see East London Mental Health NHS Trusts' QI website or the Cambridge Centre for Engineering Better Health Care).[159]

Outcome Measurement

Use of routine outcome measurement in adult mental health services is virtually absent with the exception described of IAPT services. Many measures have been developed for specific syndromes but are only used in research. This means that assessing outcomes of services and individual treatments has not occurred routinely, which reduces the effectiveness and credibility of services and has failed to generate appropriate and certainly not equitable funding with physical health services.[160] It can be argued that the latter also have neglected outcome measurement, but the obvious effect of a surgical intervention or the more rapid and recognisable effect of medications used has proved convincing and has biased funding towards these services. The Improving Access to Psychological Services project (see service description earlier) has demonstrated that it is feasible to use clinical measures with other available information (e.g. relapse or disengagement from services) to reflect recovery or improvement using a balance of increased satisfaction levels, symptoms, functioning and other needs. They have, as a result of demonstrable improvements, been funded to extend services to provide evidence-based interventions to broader groups of patients – those with physical symptoms of uncertain cause.

Outcome measurement should be centred on the needs of patients and self-rating instruments; 'Patient Rated Outcome Measures' (PROMs) allow this and are also convenient to administer. However, there is also an essential role for clinician assessment – Clinician Rated Outcome Measures (CROMs). This may be more specific to the objectives of treatment and, for example, with psychosis or OCD, or where some outcomes may be important although the patient may not prioritise them. There are therefore broad measures such as the Health of the Nation Outcome Scales and Clinical Global Improvement (CGI) and specific symptomatic measures that can be used in clinical practice to complement the PROMs available (e.g. DIALOG[29] and ReQoL,[30] see Box 20.5).

Developments in funding services using pathways (see earlier) may promote the use of these measures, but this will only occur if systems are put in place so that the information generated is developed, used and disseminated meaningfully to those collecting the data.[161]

Box 20.5 Outcome measures

Health of the Nation Outcome Scale Clinician Rating (0–4)

- Overactive or aggressive behaviour
- Non-accidental self injury
- Problem drinking or drug-taking
- Cognitive problems
- Physical symptoms
- Problems associated with hallucinations or delusions
- Problems with depression
- Other symptoms – specify
- Problems with relationships
- Daily living
- Living conditions
- Occupation & activities

DIALOG

How satisfied are you with your . . .

- mental health?
- physical health?
- job situation?
- accommodation?
- leisure activities?
- friendships?
- partner/family?
- personal safety?
- medication?
- practical help you receive?
- consultations with mental health staff

Rated for each item: totally satisfied to totally dissatisfied, and if any additional help needed.

ReQol (Recovering Quality of Life)

1. I found it difficult to get started with everyday tasks
2. I felt able to trust others
3. I felt unable to cope
4. I could do the things
5. I wanted to do
6. I feel happy
7. I thought my life was not worth living
8. I enjoyed what I did
9. I felt hopeful about my future
10. I felt lonely
11. I felt confident myself

Rated: none of the time to most of the time (0–4).

Please describe your physical health: no problems to very severe problems.

Digital Technology, Data Management and Interventions

The past two decades have transformed the process of care through digital innovations,[162] and the recent pandemic has greatly expanded the use and acceptability of video and telephone interviewing.[163] The smartphone and computers now diarise, measure activity and provide access to a breadth of information, including journals, guidelines and resources. Electronic patient records replace, often illegible, writing with copious and detailed records that can overwhelm clinicians with multiple-alerts and time-consuming mandatory data field entry. However, they have undoubtedly improved accessibility from multiple sites and have a potential to radically improve outcome measurement and indeed outcomes – but clinician input (not just designated clinical information officers) is constantly needed to make them fit for purpose. Natural language processing may be a route forward in obtaining meaningful information from records for planning and research.

Data to guide service delivery is also becoming much more available to clinical managers and individual clinicians with most Trusts having Chief Clinical Information Officers (CCIO) to promote usage. This means data on individual activity – for example, caseloads, number of patients seen, frequency and time taken, discharge rates and medication usage, but less on consultation, supervision and training and performance, which is more difficult to measure. Interpretation of such data can be difficult: How do you define an optimal – and dynamic – balance, good practice, especially without meaningful outcome data? The complexity of caseloads and practice in a multi-disciplinary team also makes individual performance assessment difficult, if not impossible. Mental health services are complex, but using approaches from other disciplines can provide useful insights: the use of network analysis approaches and the mathematics of graph theory can be applied to the flow of patients through services and yield insights from routinely gathered activity data. Such approaches to data will be increasingly developed and, as it becomes more sophisticated, can usefully inform clinical practice and management. Much of this data will be available within Trusts using systems analysis and, increasingly, presenting comparisons for clinician use, and there are also systems readily available for comparison across Trusts (e.g. NHS Digital,[164] RCPsych[165] and DHSC Mental health data and analysis)[166] as a guide for health professionals, including reference to the Mental Health Intelligence Network 'Fingertips' tool.[167] Individual Trusts gather and receive NHS Benchmarking data annually, which allows for comparison with other Trusts, and further information is made available through national websites (e.g. NHS Digital for Out-of-Area placements).

Finally, computerised assessment tools and therapies have advanced – for example, for training and disseminating CBT approaches and use of apps for early intervention in psychosis and relapse prevention. Use of avatars has now been successfully adapted for work with hallucinations and virtual reality for phobias and paranoia. Do we need to be wary of 'systems that are able to converse and interact with human users using spoken, written, and visual languages' – chatbots – as rivals or welcome them as allies? Patients generally seem to have positive perceptions of them.[168] Digital technologies will undoubtedly become more important – with benefits to patients and psychiatrists – but with a new set of issues (e.g. effect on the therapeutic relationship) to consider.

References

1. Burns T, Creet F, Fahy T, et al. Intensive versus standard case management for severe psychotic illness: a randomised trial. UK 700 Group. *Lancet* 1999;353:2185–9.
2. Burns T, Catty J, Becker T, et al. The effectiveness of supported employment for people with severe mental illness: a randomised controlled trial. *Lancet* 2007;370(9593):1146–52.
3. Killaspy H, Bebbington P, Blizard R, et al. The REACT study: randomised evaluation of assertive community treatment in north London. *BMJ* 2006;332(7545):815–20.
4. Correll CU, Galling B, Pawar A, et al. Comparison of early intervention services vs treatment as usual for early-phase psychosis: a systematic review, meta-analysis, and meta-regression. *JAMA Psychiatry* 2018;75(6):555–65.
5. Bewley T. *Madness to Mental Illness: A History of the Royal College of Psychiatrists*. London: RCPsych Publications; 2008.
6. Porter R. *The Faber Book of Madness*. London: Faber & Faber; 1991.
7. Alfred HR, Ida M. *Three Hundred Years of Psychiatry, 1535–1860: A History Presented in Selected English Texts*. Oxford: Oxford University Press; 1963.
8. Jones K. *Asylums and After: A Revised History of the Mental Health Services: From the Early 18th Century to the 1990s*. London: Athlone; 1993.
9. Powell E. *Enoch Powell's Water Tower Speech 1961*. studymore.org.uk/xpowell.htm (accessed 20 July 2022.).
10. Department of Health and Social Security. *Better Services for the Mentally Ill*. London: HMSO; 1975.
11. Mezzina R. Community mental health care in Trieste and beyond: an 'open door-no restraint' system of care for recovery and citizenship. *Journal of Nervous and Mental Disease* 2014;202(6):440–5.
12. Wild G, Alder R, Weich S, et al. The Penrose hypothesis in the second half of the 20th century: investigating the relationship between psychiatric bed numbers and the prison population in England between 1960 and 2018–2019. *The British Journal of Psychiatry* 2022;220(5):295–301.
13. Trieman N, Leff J. Closing psychiatric hospitals – some lessons from the TAPS project. In: Jack R (ed.) *Residential versus Community Care: The Role of Institutions in Welfare Provision*. Basingstoke: Macmillan; 2016: 41C.
14. Beecham J, Johnson S. The European Socio-Demographic Schedule (ESDS): rationale, principles and development. *Acta Psychiatrica Scandinavica Supplement* 2000;405:33–46.
15. Leff J, Trieman N. Long-stay patients discharged from psychiatric hospitals. Social and clinical outcomes after five years in the community. The TAPS Project 46. *British Journal of Psychiatry* 2000;176:217–23.
16. Priebe S, Badesconyi A, Fioritti A, et al. Reinstitutionalisation in mental health care: comparison of data on service provision from six European countries. *BMJ* 2005;330(7483):123–6.
17. Goffman E. *Asylums: Essays on the Social Situation of Mental Patients and Other Inmates*. New York: Doubleday (Anchor); 1961.
18. Burns T, Rugkåsa J, Molodynski A, et al. Community treatment orders for patients with psychosis (OCTET): a randomised controlled trial. *Lancet* 2013;381(9878):1627–33.
19. NHS Digital. *Mental Health Act Statistics, Annual Figures, England, 2020–2021*. files.digital.nhs.uk/ED/8F6815/ment-heal-act-stat-eng-2020-21-summ-rep.pdf (accessed 20 February 2023).
20. Evans-Lacko S, Corker E, Williams P, et al. Effect of the Time to Change anti-stigma campaign on trends in mental-illness-related public stigma among the English population in 2003-13: an analysis of survey data. *Lancet Psychiatry* 2014;1(2):121–8.
21. NHS *The NHS Plan: A Plan for Investment, a Plan for Reform*. London: Department of Health; 2000.
22. Department of Health, Community Mental Health Teams. *Mental Health Policy Implementation Guide*. London: Department of Health; 2002.
23. National Institute for Mental Health in England. *Personality Disorder: No Longer a Diagnosis of Exclusion:*

Policy Implementation Guidance for the Development of Services for People with Personality Disorder. London: National Institute for Mental Health in England; 2003.

24. NHS England, NHS Improvement, National Collaborating Centre for Mental Health. *The Community Mental Health Framework for Adults and Older Adults*. London: NHSX; 2019.
25. Kingdon D. Care programme approach: recent government policy and legislation. *Psychiatric Bulletin* 1994;18 (2):68–70.
26. NHS England. *Care Programme Approach: Position Statement*. www.england.nhs.uk/publication/care-programme-approach-position-statement/ (accessed 19 May 2022).
27. Office for Health Improvement & Disparities. *Public Health Data 'Fingertips' Tool: Mental Health*. fingertips.phe.org.uk/profile-group/mental-health (accessed 19 July 2022).
28. Simpson A, Hannigan B, Coffey M, et al. Recovery-focused care planning and coordination in England and Wales: a cross-national mixed methods comparative case study. *BMC Psychiatry* 2016;16:147.
29. Priebe S, McCabe R, Bullenkamp J, et al. Structured patient-clinician communication and 1-year outcome in community mental healthcare: cluster randomised controlled trial. *British Journal of Psychiatry* 2007;191:420–6.
30. Keetharuth AD, Brazier J, Connell J, et al. Recovering Quality of Life (ReQoL): a new generic self-reported outcome measure for use with people experiencing mental health difficulties. *British Journal of Psychiatry* 2018;212 (1):42–9.
31. Mosler F, Priebe S, Bird V. Routine measurement of satisfaction with life and treatment aspects in mental health patients – the DIALOG scale in East London. *BMC Health Services Research* 2020;20(1):1020.
32. Kingdon D. Care programme approach - time to move beyond? *BJPsych Bulletin* 2019;43(3):101–3.
33. NHS Information Centre. *Adult Psychiatric Morbidity in England, 2007: Results of a Household Survey*. London: NHS Information Centre; 2009.
34. Davidson I. *Mental Health – Adult Crisis and Acute Care. NHS GIRFT Programme National Specialty Report*. gettingitrightfirsttime.co.uk/wp-content/uploads/2021/09/Mental-Health-Sept21i.pdf (accessed 22 February 2023).
35. Koskinen J, Lohonen J, Koponen H, et al. Rate of cannabis use disorders in clinical samples of patients with schizophrenia: a meta-analysis. *Schizophrenia Bulletin* 2010;36 (6):1115–30.
36. Koskinen J, Lohonen J, Koponen H, et al. Prevalence of alcohol use disorders in schizophrenia – a systematic review and meta-analysis. *Acta Psychiatrica Scandinavica* 2009;120 (2):85–96.
37. Tulloch AD, Fearon P, David AS. Timing, prevalence, determinants and outcomes of homelessness among patients admitted to acute psychiatric wards. *Social Psychiatry and Psychiatric Epidemiology* 2012;47(7):1181–91.
38. Brown S, Kim M, Mitchell C, et al. Twenty-five year mortality of a community cohort with schizophrenia. *British Journal of Psychiatry* 2010;196:116–21.
39. Fraser C, James EL, Anderson K, et al. Intervention programs for children of parents with a mental illness: a critical review. *The International Journal of Mental Health Promotion* 2006;8 (1):9–20.
40. Newton J. *Preventing Mental Ill-health: Informing Public Health Planning and Mental Health Practice*. Abingdon: Routledge; 2013.
41. Knapp M, McDaid D, Parsonage M, et al. *Mental Health Promotion and Mental Illness Prevention: The Economic Case*. London: Department of Health; 2011.
42. Bhugra D, Bhui K, Wong SYS, et al. *Oxford Textbook of Public Mental Health*. Oxford: Oxford University Press; 2018.
43. Campion J, Javed A, Lund C, et al. Public mental health: required actions to address implementation failure in the context of COVID-19. *Lancet Psychiatry* 2022;9(2):169–82.
44. McDaid D, Park A-L, Wahlbeck K. The economic case for the prevention of mental illness. *Annual Review of Public Health* 2019;40(1):373–89.
45. Foresight. *Foresight Mental Capital and Wellbeing Project: Final Project Report*. London: The Government Office for Science; 2008.
46. Thornicroft G. *Shunned: Discrimination against People with Mental Illness*: Oxford: Oxford University Press; 2006.
47. Institute of Medicine. *Unequal Treatment: What Healthcare Providers Need to Know About Racial and Ethnic Disparities in Healthcare*. Washington, DC: The National Academies Press; 2002.
48. Lloyd-Evans B, Crosby M, Stockton S, et al. Initiatives to shorten duration of untreated psychosis: systemic review. *British Journal of Psychiatry* 2011;198:256–63.
49. Henderson C, Thornicroft G. Stigma and discrimination in mental illness: Time to Change. *Lancet* 2009;373 (9679):1928–30.
50. Sharac J, McCrone P, Clement S, et al. The economic impact of mental health stigma and discrimination: a systematic review. *Epidemiologia e Psichiatria Sociale* 2010;19(3):223–32.
51. Kings Fund. *Integrated Care Systems Explained: Making Sense of Systems, Places and Neighbourhoods*. www.kingsfund.org.uk/publications/integrated-care-systems-explained (accessed 19 July 2022).
52. Department of Health. *Joint Strategic Needs Assessment and Joint Health and Wellbeing Strategies Explained. Commissioning for Populations.* assets.publishing.service.gov.uk/government/uploads/system/uploads/attachment_data/file/215261/dh_131733.pdf (accessed 22 February 2023).
53. Guardian. *NHS Paying £2bn a Year to Private Hospitals for Mental Health Patients*. www.theguardian.com/society/2022/apr/24/nhs-paying-2bn-pounds-a-year-to-private-hospitals-for-mental-health-patients (accessed 11 April 2023).
54. Christensen MK, Lim CCW, Saha S, et al. The cost of mental disorders: a systematic review. *Epidemiology and Psychiatric Sciences* 2020;29:e161.
55. NHS England. *The Five Year Forward View for Mental Health. A Report from the Independent Mental Health Taskforce to the NHS in England*. London: NHS England; 2016.
56. NHS England. *The NHS Long Term Plan*. London: NHS England; 2019.

57. NHS England. *NHS Mental Health Dashboard.* www.england.nhs.uk/mental-health/taskforce/imp/mh-dashboard/#:~:text=To%20support%20the%20ambitions%20within,a%20year%20by%202023%2F24.

58. Kings Fund. *Has the Government Put Mental Health on an Equal Footing with Physical Health?* www.kingsfund.org.uk/projects/verdict/has-government-put-mental-health-equal-footing-physical-health (accessed 20 February 2023).

59. Fund K. *Integrated Care Systems Explained: Making Sense of Systems, Places and Neighbourhoods.* www.kingsfund.org.uk/publications/integrated-care-systems-explained (accessed 19 July 2022.).

60. Kingdon D. Outcome-based providing and commissioning: pathways and standards. *BJPsych Bulletin* 2019;43(6):282–86.

61. NHS England, NHS Improvement. *Mental Health Currency Review: A Proposed New Approach to Counting Mental Health Activity.* www.england.nhs.uk/wp-content/uploads/2021/02/21-22_Mental_health_currency_review.pdf (accessed 23 February 2022).

62. NHS England, NHS Improvement. *2022/23 Finance and Payment – Considerations for Mental Health, Community and Non-acute Services.* www.england.nhs.uk/wp-content/uploads/2021/09/22-23-finance-and-payment-engagement_Non-acute-recording.pdf (accessed 23 February 2023).

63. NHS Digital. *Reference Costs.* digital.nhs.uk/data-and-information/data-collections-and-data-sets/data-collections/reference-costs (accessed 23 February 2023).

64. Personal Social Services Research Unit. *Unit Costs of Health and Social Care 2020.* www.pssru.ac.uk/project-pages/unit-costs/unit-costs-2020/ (accessed 22 February 2023).

65. NHS Business Services Authority. *Prescription Cost Analysis – England 2020/21.* www.nhsbsa.nhs.uk/statistical-collections/prescription-cost-analysis-england/prescription-cost-analysis-england-202021 (accessed 23 February 2023).

66. Wang J, Mann F, Lloyd-Evans B, et al. Associations between loneliness and perceived social support and outcomes of mental health problems: a systematic review. *BMC Psychiatry* 2018;18(1):156.

67. Glover GR. Money for mental health care in 2003/4. *Psychiatric Bulletin* 2003;27(4):126–9.

68. Fund. K. *Funding and Staffing of NHS Mental Health Providers: Still Waiting for Parity.* www.kingsfund.org.uk/publications/funding-staffing-mental-health-providers (accessed 19 July 2020).

69. White S, Foster R, Marks J, et al. The effectiveness of one-to-one peer support in mental health services: a systematic review and meta-analysis. *BMC Psychiatry* 2020;20(1):534.

70. Kingdon D. The mental health practitioner – bypassing the recruitment bottleneck. *Psychiatric Bulletin* 2002;26(9):328–31.

71. Department of Health. *New Ways of Working for Psychiatrists: Enhancing Effective, Person-centred Services Through New Ways of Working in Multidisciplinary and Multiagency Contexts.* London: Department of Health; 2005.

72. University College London. *Competence Frameworks.* www.ucl.ac.uk/pals/research/clinical-educational-and-health-psychology/research-groups/competence-frameworks (accessed 23 February 2023).

73. Friedli L. *Social Prescribing for Mental Health – a Guide to Commissioning and Delivery.* London: Care Services Improvement Partnership; 2008.

74. Kosicka A, Fitzner G. *In-depth Review of the Psychiatrist Workforce - Main Report.* London: Centre for Workforce Intelligence; 2014.

75. Rotenstein LS, Torre M, Ramos MA, et al. Prevalence of burnout among physicians: a systematic review. *JAMA* 2018;320(11):1131–50.

76. Maslach C, Jackson S, Leiter M, et al. *Maslach Burnout Inventory Manual.* Menlo Park, CA: Mind Garden, Inc; 2016.

77. Zivin K, Chang MUM, Van T, et al. Relationships between work-environment characteristics and behavioral health provider burnout in the Veterans Health Administration. *Health Services Research* 2022;57:83–94.

78. NHS Benchmarking Network. *International Mental Health Comparisons 2019.* s3.eu-west-2.amazonaws.com/nhsbn-static/Other/2019/International-MH-report-31-October-2019.pdf (accessed 23 February 2023).

79. NHS Digital. *Hospital Admitted Patient Care Activity.* digital.nhs.uk/data-and-information/publications/statistical/hospital-admitted-patient-care-activity (accessed 24 February 2023).

80. NHS Digital. *Mental Health Act Statistics, Annual Figures England, 2019–2020.* files.digital.nhs.uk/99/3916C8/ment-heal-act-stat-eng-2019-20-summ-rep%20v1.1.pdf (accessed 23 February 2023).

81. Priebe S, Jones G, McCabe R, et al. Effectiveness and costs of acute day hospital treatment compared with conventional in-patient care: randomised controlled trial. *British Journal of Psychiatry* 2006;188:243–9.

82. Bowers L, Chaplin R, Quirk A, et al. A conceptual model of the aims and functions of acute inpatient psychiatry. *Journal of Mental Health* 2009;18(4):316–25.

83. Johnson S, Dalton-Locke C, Baker J, et al. Acute psychiatric care: approaches to increasing the range of services and improving access and quality of care. *World Psychiatry* 2022;21(2):220–36.

84. Dalton-Locke C, Johnson S, Harju-Seppänen J, et al. Emerging models and trends in mental health crisis care in England: a national investigation of crisis care systems. *BMC Health Services Research* 2021;21(1):1174.

85. Baskind R, Kordowicz M, Chaplin R. How does an accreditation programme drive improvement on acute inpatient mental health wards? an exploration of members' views. *Journal of Mental Health* 2010;19(5):405–11.

86. Crisp N, Smith G, Nicholson K. *Old Problems. New Solutions: Improving Acute Psychiatric Care for Adults in England.* London: NHS Providers; 2016. nhsproviders.org/media/1750/otdb-independent-commission-on-acute-adult-inpatient-psychiatric-care-final-report.pdf (accessed 16 September 2023).

87. National Institute of Health and Social Care. *Rehabilitation for Adults with Complex Psychosis NICE Guideline [NG181].* www.nice.org.uk/guidance/ng181.

88. Holloway F. *The Forgotten Need for Rehabilitation in Contemporary Mental*

Health Services: A Position Statement from the Executive Committee of the Faculty of Rehabilitation and Social Psychiatry. London: Royal College of Psychiatrists; 2005.

89. Killaspy H, Rembarran D, Bledin K. Mental health needs of clients of rehabilitation services: a survey in one trust. *Journal of Mental Health* 2008;17:207–18.
90. Edwards TR, Meaden A, Commander M. A 10-year follow-up service evaluation of the treatment pathway outcomes for patients in nine in-patient psychiatric rehabilitation services. *BJPsych Bulletin* 2023;47(1):23–7.
91. Killaspy H, Zis P. Predictors of outcomes of mental health rehabilitation services: a 5-year retrospective cohort study in inner London, UK. *Social Psychiatry and Psychiatric Epidemiology* 2013;48 (6):1005–12.
92. Lavelle E, Ijaz A, Killaspy H. *Mental Health Rehabilitation and Recovery Services in Ireland: A Multicentre Study of Current Service Provision, Characteristics of Service Users and Outcomes for Those with and without Access to These Services*. Dublin: Final Report for the Mental Health Commission of Ireland; 2011.
93. Roberts G, Boardman J. Understanding 'recovery'. *Advances in Psychiatric Treatment* 2013;19(6):400–9.
94. Marshall M, Crowther R, Maraz-Serrano A, et al. Day hospital versus admission for acute psychiatric disorders. *Cochrane Database of Systematic Reviews* 2003;1.
95. McKay C, Nugent KL, Johnsen M, et al. A systematic review of evidence for the clubhouse model of psychosocial rehabilitation. *Administration and Policy in Mental Health and Mental Health Services* 2018;45(1):28–47.
96. Drake RE. Introduction to supported employment. *Epidemiology and Psychiatric Sciences* 2020;29:e185.
97. Stein LI, Santos AB. *Assertive Community Treatment of Persons with Severe Mental Illness*. New York: Norton; 1998.
98. Priebe S, Kelley L, Omer S, et al. The effectiveness of a patient-centred assessment with a solution-focused approach (DIALOG+) for patients with psychosis: a pragmatic cluster-randomised controlled trial in community care. *Psychotherapy and Psychosomatics* 2015;84(5): 304–13.
99. Department of Health and Social Care. *Consensus Statement for Information Sharing and Suicide Prevention*. www.gov.uk/government/publications/consensus-statement-for-information-sharing-and-suicide-prevention (accessed 24 February 2023).
100. Royal College of Psychiatrists. *RCPsych Calls for Urgent and Transparent Investigation into NHS Innovation Accelerator and AHSN Following HIN Suspension*. www.rcpsych.ac.uk/news-and-features/latest-news/detail/2021/06/14/rcpsych-calls-for-urgent-and-transparent-investigation-into-nhs-innovation-accelerator-and-ahsn-following-hin-suspension (accessed 24 February 2023).
101. Killaspy H, Kingett S, Bebbington P, et al. Randomised evaluation of assertive community treatment: 3-year outcomes. *British Journal of Psychiatry* 2009;195(1):81–2.
102. Kane JM, Robinson DG, Schooler NR, et al. Comprehensive versus usual community care for first-episode psychosis: 2-year outcomes from the NIMH RAISE early treatment program. *American Journal of Psychiatry* 2016;173(4):362–72.
103. Stafford MR, Jackson H, Mayo-Wilson E, et al. Early interventions to prevent psychosis: systematic review and meta-analysis. *BMJ* 2013;346:f185.
104. McCrone P, Craig TKJ, Power P, et al. Cost-effectiveness of an early intervention service for people with psychosis. *British Journal of Psychiatry* 2010;196:377–82.
105. Bertelsen M, Jeppesen P, Petersen L, et al. Five-year follow-up of a randomized multicenter trial of intensive early intervention vs standard treatment for patients with a first episode of psychotic illness: the OPUS trial. *Archives of General Psychiatry* 2008;65(7):762–71.
106. Lloyd-Evans B, Crosby M, Stockton S, et al. Initiatives to shorten duration of untreated psychosis: systematic review. *British Journal of Psychiatry* 2011;198 (4):256–63.
107. Hegelstad WT, Larsen TK, Auestad B, et al. Long-term follow-up of the TIPS early detection in psychosis study: effects on 10-year outcome. *American Journal of Psychiatry* 2012;169 (4):374–80.
108. Birchwood M, Connor C, Lester H, et al. Reducing duration of untreated psychosis: care pathways to early intervention in psychosis services. *The British Journal of Psychiatry* 2013;203 (1):58–64.
109. Norman RMG, Manchanda R, Malla AK, et al. Symptom and functional outcomes for a 5 year early intervention program for psychoses. *Schizophrenia Research* 2011;129(2–3):111–15.
110. Gafoor R, Nitsch D, McCrone P, et al. Effect of early intervention on 5 year outcome in non-affective psychosis. *British Journal of Psychiatry* 2010;196:372–6.
111. Bertelsen M, Jeppesen P, Petersen L, et al. Five-year follow-up of a randomized multicenter trial of intensive early intervention vs standard treatment for patients with a first episode of psychotic illness. *Archives of General Psychiatry* 2008;65 (7):762–71.
112. Mueser KT, Penn DL, Addington J, et al. The NAVIGATE Program for first-episode psychosis: rationale, overview, and description of psychosocial components. *Psychiatric Services* 2015;66(7):680–90.
113. National Institute of Health and Social Excellence. *Implementing the Early Intervention in Psychosis Access and Waiting Time Standard: Guidance*. www.nice.org.uk/guidance/qs80/resources/implementing-the-early-intervention-in-psychosis-access-and-waiting-time-standard-guidance-2487749725 (accessed 24 February 2023).
114. Killaspy H, Harvey C, Brasier C, et al. Community-based social interventions for people with severe mental illness: a systematic review and narrative synthesis of recent evidence. *World Psychiatry* 2022;21(1):96–123.
115. Reed BC. Review of 'Prescription for a Healthy Nation: A New Approach to Improving Our Lives by Fixing Our Everyday World'. *JAMA: Journal of the American Medical Association* 2005;293 (22):2797–2801.
116. North West Development Centre. *Social Prescribing for Mental Health – a Guide to Commissioning and Delivery*. London: Care Services Improvement Partnership; 2006.

117. Hatfield B, Huxley P, Mohamad H. Accommodation and employment: a survey into the circumstances and expressed needs of users of mental health services in a northern town. *British Journal of Social Work* 1992;22:61–73.

118. Shepherd G, Murray A, Muijen M. *Relative Values: The Differing Views of Users, Family Carers & Professionals on Services for People with Schizophrenia in the Community.* London: The Sainsbury Centre for Mental Health; 1994.

119. Mueser KT, Clark RE, Heines M, et al. The Hartford study of supported employment for persons with severe mental illness. *Journal of Consulting and Clinical Psychology* 2004;72 (3):479–90.

120. Crowther R, Marshall M, Bond G, et al. Vocational rehabilitation for people with severe mental illness 18. *Cochrane Database of Systematic Reviews* 2001(2): CD003080.

121. Lloyd-Evans B, Johnson S. An evaluation of the implementation of an IPS employment support service in a UK catchment area: the WISE study. *Psychiatrische Praxis* 2011;38.

122. Bond GR, Drake RE, Becker DR. An update on randomized controlled trials of evidence-based supported employment. *Psychiatric Rehabilitation Journal* 2008;31(4):280–90.

123. Mueser K, Salyers M, Mueser P. A prospective analysis of work in schizophrenia. *Schizophrenia Bulletin* 2001;27(2):281–96.

124. Twamley EW, Jeste DV, Lehman AF. Vocational rehabilitation in schizophrenia and other psychotic disorders: a literature review and meta-analysis of randomized controlled trials. *Journal of Nervous and Mental Disease* 1993;191(8):515–23.

125. Spear RB, E. *The Role of Social Enterprise in European Labour Markets. Working Papers Series, no. 03/10.* Liège: EMES European Research Network; 2003.

126. Savio M, Righetti A. Cooperatives as a social enterprise in Italy: a place for social integration and rehabilitation. *Acta Psychiatrica Scandinavica* 1993;88 (4):238–42.

127. Culhane DP, Metraux S, Hadley T. Public service reductions associated with placement of homeless persons with severe mental illness in supportive housing. *Housing Policy Debate* 2002;13 (1):107–63.

128. Tsemberis S. Housing first: ending homelessness and transforming lives. *Schizophrenia Research* 2010;117(2-3):163–4.

129. Metraux S, Marcus SC, Culhane DP. The New York-New York housing initiative and use of public shelters by persons with severe mental illness. *Psychiatric Services* 2003;54(1):67–71.

130. Timms P. Homelessness and mental health. In: Bhugra D (ed.) *Homelessness and Mental Health.* Cambridge: Cambridge University Press; 1996: 11–25.

131. Whiteley JS. Down and out in London; mental illness in the lower social groups. *Lancet* 1955;269(6890):609–10.

132. Berry C, Orwin A. 'No fixed abode': a survey of mental hospital admissions. *British Journal of Psychiatry* 1966;112 (491):1019–25.

133. Fazel S, Khosla V, Doll H, et al. The prevalence of mental disorders among the homeless in western countries: systematic review and meta-regression analysis. *PLoS Med* 2008;5(12):e225.

134. Nielsen SF, Hjorthøj CR, Erlangsen A, et al. Psychiatric disorders and mortality among people in homeless shelters in Denmark: a nationwide register-based cohort study. *Lancet* 2011;377 (9784):2205–14.

135. Seebohm P, Gilchrist A. *Connect and Include: An Exploratory Study of Community Development and Mental Health.* London: National Social Inclusion Programme; 2008.

136. Crepaz-Keay D, Cyhlarova E. A new self-management intervention for people with severe psychiatric diagnoses. *Journal of Mental Health Training, Education and Practice* 2012;7 (2):89–94.

137. Franke CCD, Paton BC, Gassner L-AJ. Implementing mental health peer support: a South Australian experience. *Australian Journal of Primary Health* 2010;16(2):179–86.

138. Lawn S, Smith A, Hunter K. Mental health peer support for hospital avoidance and early discharge: an Australian example of consumer driven and operated service. *Journal of Mental Health* 2008;17(5):498–508.

139. Tinland A, Loubière S, Mougeot F, et al. Effect of psychiatric advance directives facilitated by peer workers on compulsory admission among people with mental illness: a randomized clinical trial. *JAMA Psychiatry* 2022;79 (8):752–9.

140. Fitch C, Wilson M, Worrall A. *Improving In – Patient Mental Health Services for Black and Minority Ethnic Patients: Recommendations to inform accreditation standards.* London: Royal College of Psychiatrists; 2010.

141. Link B, Phelan JC. Conceptualizing stigma. *Annual Review of Sociology* 2001;27:363–85.

142. National Institute for Health and Care Excellence. *Service User Experience in Adult Mental Health: Improving the Experience of Care for People Using Adult NHS Mental Health Services.* London: National Institute for Health and Care Excellence; 2011.

143. Department of Health North East Regional Government Office, the North East Health Development Authority, the North East NHS Region, et al. *Mental Health Promotion in Primary Care.* London: Department of Health, 2005.

144. Gilbert P. *Spirituality and Mental Health Care.* Brighton, UK: Pavilion; 2011.

145. Siette J, Cassidy M, Priebe S. Effectiveness of befriending interventions: a systematic review and meta-analysis. *BMJ Open* 2017;7(4): e014304.

146. Priebe S, Chevalier A, Hamborg T, et al. Effectiveness of a volunteer befriending programme for patients with schizophrenia: randomised controlled trial. *British Journal of Psychiatry* 2020;217(3):477–83.

147. Davidson L, Rakfeldt J, Strauss J. *The Roots of the Recovery Movement in Psychiatry: Lessons Learned.* Oxford: John Wiley & Sons; 2011.

148. Awad AG, Varuganti LN. The burden of schizophrenia on caregivers: a review. *Pharmacoeconomics* 2008;26(2):149–62.

149. Seloiwe ES. Experiences and demands of families with mentally ill people at home in Botswana. *Journal of Nursing Scholarship* 2006;38(3):262–8.

150. Chien WT, Chan SW, Morrisey J. The percieved burden among Chinese family caregivers of people with schizophrenia. *Journal of Clinical Nursing* 2007;16(6):1151–61.

151. Morgan J, Lowe J, Lowe L, et al. Editorial: an international perspective

on what carers want – the professional's dilemma. *International Journal of Social Psychiatry* 2010;56(3):211–6.

152. Worthington A, Rooney P, Hannan R. *The Triangle of Care: Carers Included: A Guide to Best Practice in Mental Health Care in England.* Rugby: Carers Trust; 2013. www.england.nhs.uk/wp-content/uploads/2017/11/case-study-supporting-well-carers-included.pdf (accessed 16 September 2023).
153. Layard R, Clark DM, Knapp M, et al. *Cost-Benefit Analysis of Psychological Therapy*. London: Centre for Economic Performance; 2007.
154. NHS England. *The NHS Talking Therapies Manual.* www.england.nhs.uk/publication/the-improving-access-to-psychological-therapies-manual/ (accessed 24 February 2023).
155. Macdonald A, Adamis D, Craig T, et al. Continuity of care and clinical outcomes in the community for people with severe mental illness. *The British Journal of Psychiatry* 2019;214(5):273–8.
156. Derbyshire Safeguarding Adults Board. *Vulnerable Adult Risk Management (VARM).* www.derbyshiresab.org.uk/professionals/vulnerable-adult-risk-management.aspx (accessed 11 April 2023).
157. Boland B. Quality improvement in mental health services. *BJPsych Bulletin* 2020;44(1):30–5.
158. Shah A. How to move beyond quality improvement projects. *BMJ* 2020;370: m2319.
159. University of Cambridge. *Centre for Engineering Better Health Care.* cebc.eng.cam.ac.uk/ (accessed 21 February 2023).
160. Freedland KE, Zorumski CF. Success rates in psychiatry. *JAMA Psychiatry* 2023;80(5):407–8.
161. Ryland H, Carlile J, Kingdon D. A guide to outcome measurement in psychiatry. *BJPsych Advances* 2021;27(4):263–71.
162. Torous J, Bucci S, Bell IH, et al. The growing field of digital psychiatry: current evidence and the future of apps, social media, chatbots, and virtual reality. *World Psychiatry* 2021;20 (3):318–35.
163. Greenhalgh T, Wherton J. Telepsychiatry: learning from the pandemic. *British Journal of Psychiatry* 2022;220(5):257–61.
164. NHS Digital. *Mental Health Hub.* digital.nhs.uk/data-and-information/data-tools-and-services/data-services/mental-health-data-hub (accessed 24 February 2023).
165. Royal College of Psychiatrists. *Mental Health Watch.* mentalhealthwatch.rcpsych.ac.uk/ (accessed 24 February 2023).
166. Office for Health Improvement and Disparities. *Mental Health Data and Analysis: A Guide for Health Professionals.* www.gov.uk/guidance/mental-health-data-and-analysis-a-guide-for-health-professionals#severe-mental-illness (accessed 24 February 2023).
167. Office for Health Improvement and Disparities. *Fingertips: Public Health Data. Mental Health, Dementia and Neurology.* fingertips.phe.org.uk/profile-group/mental-health (accessed 24 February 2023).
168. Abd-Alrazaq AA, Alajlani M, Ali N, et al. Perceptions and opinions of patients about mental health chatbots: scoping review. *Journal of Medical Internet Research* 2021;23(1): e17828.

Index

Note that page numbers in **bold** represent tables, while those in *italics* represent figures.

abbreviated mental test score, 750
Abdurrachid, N., 399
ablative neurosurgery, 178
abnormal involuntary movement scale (AIMS), 264, 265
abnormal phenomena, 36
abreaction, 381
absolute poverty: definition, 94
Academy for Eating Disorders (AED), 565
Academy of Medical Royal Colleges, 58, 572
acamprosate, 649
acceptance and commitment therapy (ACT), 288, 397, 587, 756
accommodation, 57, 228, 282, 288, *431*, 769, 771, 779, 780, 783, 784, 786, 791–3, 795
acculturation, 704, 706, 710–11
  types, 710–11
acetylcholine, 244
acetylcholinesterase inhibitors, 502, 503
aciclovir, 492
acid-sensing ion channels (ASICs), 309
acquired brain injury (concept), 469
acromegaly, 517
actigraphy, 550, 560
  definition, 555
acuphase, 755
acupuncture, 397
acute alcoholic poisoning, 505
acute and transient psychotic disorder (ATPD), 200, 217
acute assessment units, 759
acute confusional state: same as 'delirium' (*qv*), 746
acute inpatient care
  admission (reasons), 780
  admission criteria, 779
  bed numbers, 777
  crisis management, 780
  environment, 780
  expertise (availability), 779
  general adult psychiatry services, 777–80
  input, 780
  legal framework, 777
  length of stay, 777, 779
  patient concerns, 780
  role (changing rapidly), 779
  statistics (2019-2020), **778**
  teams, 779
  traumatic process, 779
  whole system approach, 780
acute intermittent porphyria, 514
acute mania (case J.N.G. No 555), 49
acute myocardial infarction, 748
Adamou, M., 539–43
adaptive fear, 474
Addenbrooke's cognitive examination (ACE), 463, 501
addiction psychiatry, 716–17
Addis, M., 158
Addison, T., 517
Addison's disease, 172, 517
adenosine, 548
ADHD, *See* attention-deficit/hyperactivity disorder
adjusted hazard ratio (aHR), 251
adjustment disorder: new module, 746
adjustment disorders: general hospital setting, 746
Adley's drugs wheel, 639
adolescence, 446, 456
  onset of mental health problems, 105
adolescent psychiatry: culture, 717
adolescents, 454, 470
  bipolar disorder (drug treatment guidelines), 172
adoption studies, 678
adrenoleukodystrophy, 514
adult care: statutes of relevance, 796
adult mental health services, 767–99
  accommodation, 791–3
  assertive outreach, 787–8
  burnout, 776–7
  CMHTs, 790–1
  cost per year of care, **776**
  crisis and intensive home treatment teams, 785–7
  day hospitals and day care, 784–5
  digital technology, 798–9
  early intervention, 788–90
  evidence base, 767
  evolution of services, 767–70
  funding, 773–5
  IAPT, 794–5
  interface and continuity issues, 795–9
  meaningful activity, 791–3
  mental health commissioning, 772–3
  multi-agency working, 796–7
  need, 771
  outcome measurement, 797–8
  personalised care, 793–4
  prevention and de-stigmatisation, 771–2
  psychiatry services (general), 777–84
  quality improvement, 797
  staffing, 775–6
  support for carers, 794
Adult Psychiatric Morbidity Survey, 14, 91, 95, 168, 315, 448, 747
  (2007), 565
  (2014), 676, 745
adult psychiatry, 414
adult psychiatry services, *See* general adult psychiatry services
adult separation anxiety disorder (ASAD)
  diagnosis, 294
advanced (clinical) practitioner, 59
advanced directive, 757
advanced sleep-wake phase disorder, 553
adverse childhood experiences (ACEs), 44, 97, 98, 629, 663, 744
  personality disorder, 421
adverse life events, 44, 104
  psychosis risk factor, 228
adynamia, 31
ÆSOP-10 study, 230, 231, 232, 233, 234
aetiology, 18
  Alzheimer's disease, 502
  anorexia nervosa, 577
  ARFID, 588
  ASPD, 446–7
  autism, 529
  BDD, 391
  binge-eating disorder, 591–2
  bipolar disorder, 169–70
  bulimia nervosa, 588
  functional neurological disorder, 376–8
  gambling, 454
  hypochondriasis, 394
  OCD, 340–6
  paranoid personality disorder, 448–9
  personality disorder, 421–2
  postpartum psychosis, 601
affect disorders, 207–8
  anhedonia, 208
  blunted affect, 207
  depression, 207–8
  incongruous affect, 207
affective disorders, 599–600
  case example, 600
  postpartum psychotic depression, 599
  puerperal mania, 599
  puerperal schizophrenia, 599
  schizoaffective disorder, 599
Afghan, S., 726–36
Africa, 492, 494, 705
African Americans, 454
age: depression differences, 93–4
ageing, 717
agitated behaviour scale (ABS), 464
agitated depression
  clinical presentation (symptom profiles), 77
  'not clearly defined', 77
  'not recognised diagnosis', 77
agitation, 71–2
agnosia, 469
agomelatine, **109**, 114–15, 130, **132**
  pharmacokinetics, 115
  side effects, 115
agoraphobia, 295, **325**, 325, 326, 327, 329, 330, 614
  onset and course, 327
agranulocytosis, 270
agraphaesthesia, 466
Agras, S., 327
Ahithopel: suicide, 655
Akagi, H., 740
akathisia, 72, 672
  definition, 53, 265
  motor side effect (antipsychotics), 265
Akiskal, H. S., 162
Akiva, Rabbi, 656
Alameda, L., 228
Albania, 628
Alcaro, A., 423
alcohol
  assessment (three key elements), 638

alcohol (cont.)
consumption advice (Chief Medical Officer, England), 638
global mortality (2016), 636
harm reduction, 643–4
pregnancy, 620–1
prevention paradox, 638
relapse-prevention medication, 649
suicide prevention, 681
alcohol dependence, 747
diagnostic criteria (ICD-10, ICD-11), **637**
homelessness, 792
suicide risk, 665
alcohol detoxification: liaison psychiatry patients, 755
alcohol units: calculation, 638
alcohol use, 52, 631
integrated approach, *692–3*
medically assisted withdrawal, 645–6
whether any link with depression, 100–1
alcohol use disorder identification test (AUDIT), 637, **640**, 644, 747
alcohol withdrawal delirium, 508
alcohol withdrawal syndromes, 508–9
alcoholic hallucinosis, 508
Alcoholics Anonymous, 639, 648
alcohol-induced amnesia: definition, 506
alcohol-induced hypoglycaemia, 508
alcohol-related brain damage, 505–9
acute manifestations, 506–7
alcohol withdrawal syndromes, 508–9
chronic manifestations, 507–8
epidemiology and pathophysiology, 505–6
neuropsychiatric manifestations, **506**
presentation, 505
subacute manifestations, 507
alcohol-related disorders: general hospital setting, 747
alexia
definition, 468
two forms, 468
Allen, H. A., 214
Allitt, B., **399**
allopregnanolone, 611
Allport, G. W., 708
alopecia areata, 354
alpha mannosidosis, 514
alternative model for personality disorders (AMPD), **408**, 408
altitude-related hypoxia, 514
Altman self-rating mania scale, 168
aluminium hydroxide, 680
aluminium intoxication, 511
Alzheimer, A., 501, 504
Alzheimer's disease, 19, 210, 468, 473, 501–3
aetiology, 502
course, 502
diagnosis, 502
neuropathological features, 502
presentation, 502
replacement therapy, 502
subdivisions, 502
symptoms (behavioural and psychological), 502
Alzheimer's Society, 771
ambitendence, 209
American Medico-Psychological Association
later APA (*qv*), 46
American Neuropsychiatric Association, 461
American Professional Society on Abuse of Children, 627
American Psychiatric Association (APA), 45, **46**, 283, 408. *See also* DSM
eating disorders, 569
OCD, 349
American Veteran Administration Hospitals, 777
AMI, *See* acute myocardial infarction
amiloride, 175
amisulpride, 250, **612**
efficacy, 246, 247
amitriptyline, 111, 511, **612**, 620
amok, 719
amphetamines, 228, 541
Amsterdam, 229
anabolic androgenic steroid (AAS), 167
anaemia, 520
analysts, 43
analytic epidemiology: central concern, 7
anamnesis, 33
anankastia, 451
definition, 409, 419, 427
ancient Greece, 162, 707, 718
Anderson, I. M., 64–86
Andreasen, N. C., 207
Andrews, P. W., 152
anger, 68
anger management, 456
Angst, J., 80, 162
anhedonia, 67
definition, 208
disorders of affect, 208
animal phobia, **325**
ankyloblepharon: definition, 619
anomic aphasia, 468
anorexia nervosa, 339, 573–87, 663
assessment, 581
bone health, 581
Bonferroni-significant genetic correlations, *578*
clinical presentations and diagnosis, 574–5
comorbidities, 586
comorbidities (impact on mortality risk), **576**
controversies, 587
course and prognosis, 575
demographics, 577
differential diagnosis, 575–6
endocrine abnormalities, 580
epidemiology, 577
factors (aetiological), **577**
genetic factors, 577–8
haematological consequences, 581
historical background, 573–4
investigations, 581
males, 581
metabolic rate and hypothermia, 580
microbiome, 580
Minnesota semi-starvation experiment, 575
neurologic evidence, 581
physical consequences, 586
physical examination outline, 581
psychosocial factors, 579
reconceptualisation, 578
suicide rate 'high', 586
treatments (new), 587
anorexia nervosa (medical consequences), 579–80
cardiovascular, 579
dermatological, 579
gastrointestinal, 579–80
respiratory, 579
anorexia nervosa (treatment models), 583–7
admission preparation, 585
artificial nutrition, 585
comparison, **584**
compulsory treatment, 585
mealtime support, 585
medication, 586
refeeding, 585
stepped care, *584*
transition and prevention of relapse, 586
anorexia nervosa (treatment), 582–3
CBT-E, 582, 583, 585
comorbidities, 583
family-based, 582
FPT, 583
inpatient treatment and integrated care, 583
integrated CBT-E, 583, 584, 586
MANTRA, 582
SSCM, 583
anorexia nervosa treatment of outpatients (ANTOP), 583
anosodiaphoria, 466
anosognosia, 466
anoxic brain injury, 514
anterograde amnesia, 373, 466
anterograde memory, 463
anticholinergics, 112, 511
side effects, 267–8
anticipatory anxiety, 474
anticonvulsants, 171
antidepressants, 39, 108–17, 128, 479
adequate trial, 129
agomelatine, 115
augmentation treatment, 135, 136
augmentation treatment (with non-antidepressant medication), 135
bupropion, 114–15
cessation of treatment, 131–4
combination treatment, 135, 136
cross tapering, **109**, **132**
delay in onset, 129
dose adjustment, 129
level monitoring 'not commonly used', 129
liaison psychiatry patients, 753–4
liquid form, 754
'little efficacy' in treating bipolar disorder, 162
MAOIs, 113–14
miscellaneous, 114–17
NaSSAs, 112–13
reboxetine, 115–16
relapse prevention, 134
'remain controversial', 729
side effects, 557
SNRIs, 110–11
SSRIs, 108–10
switching (third way), 135, 136
teratogenicity, 619–20
terminological fluidity, 108
trazodone, 116
tricyclics, 111–12
vortioxetine, 116–17
antidopaminergic drugs, 484, 485
antiepileptic hypersensitivity syndrome, 176
antiepileptics, 119–20, 270, 477, 479, 480, 510
examples, 119
mechanism of action, 119
monitoring, 119
teratogenicity, 620
antihistamines, 111
acute psychosis treatment, 246
antiinflammatories, 123
antimuscarinic side effects (antipsychotics), 267
antipsychiatry, 38–9
antipsychotic polypharmacy, 248
antipsychotics, 34, 112, 117–18, 136, 171, 243, 435, 480, **612**
absorption and food effect, 272
acute psychosis treatment, 246–7
background, 117
catatonia treatment, 260
classification, 246
discussion with patients and carers, 246
dosage, 247, **248**
effectiveness in negative symptoms, **254**
efficacy, 246
evidence from pragmatic trials, 247
examples, 117
liaison psychiatry patients, 754–5
mechanism of action, 117
outcome, 232–3
pharmacokinetics, 117
rapid tranquilisation, 257–8
teratogenicity, 618–20
terminological inconsistency, 108
tolerability, 247
antipsychotics (adherence), 248–50
breakthrough symptoms and dopamine supersensitivity, 249
dose reduction and discontinuation, 249–50
long-acting injectables, 249
antipsychotics (side effects), 262–71
anticholinergic side effects, 267–8
cardiac side effects, 266–7
diabetes, 268
dyslipidaemia, 269
hyperprolactinaemia and sexual dysfunction, 263
impaired glucose tolerance, 268
motor side effects, 263–6
obesity, 268–9
other side effects, 269

sedation, 262–3
antisocial personality disorder, 444–7, 630
aetiology, 446–7
birth complications, 446
clinical features, 444–5
epidemiology, 446
treatment, 447
Anton syndrome, 467
anxiety, 68, 344, 345, 346
macro-circuitry and micro-circuitry, *297*
anxiety disorders, 293–310, 474, 614
anxiolytic drugs (potential developments), 309–10
autism, 532
benzodiazepine anxiolytics, 301–4
beta blockers, 305–9
buspirone and related azapirones, 305
causes, 296–300
diagnosis and differential diagnosis, 295–310
differential diagnoses, 294, **294**
epidemiology, 296
gabapentinoids, 304–5
perinatal loss, 616
pharmacological treatment (general considerations), 300–1
anxiety disorders (causes), 296–300
generalised anxiety disorder, 296–7
panic disorder, 297–8
separation anxiety disorder, 299–300
social anxiety disorder, 298–9
anxiety disorders (diagnosis and differential diagnosis), 295–310
specific phobias, 294
anxiety disorders (diagnosis)
adult separation anxiety disorder, 294
generalised anxiety disorder, 293
panic disorder, 293
social anxiety disorder, 294
anxiety disorders (epidemiology), 296
generalised anxiety disorder, 295
panic disorder, 295
separation anxiety disorder, 296
social anxiety disorder, 295–6
anxiety hierarchy, 347
anxiolytic drugs
ideal properties, **300**
liaison psychiatry patients, 755
potential developments, 309–10
anxiolytic-hypnotic prescriptions, 680
anxious depression: clinical presentation (symptom profiles), 76
anxious personality disorder, 326
AOTs, *See* assertive outreach teams
apathy, 71, 474
aphasia, 467–8
aphonia (functional mutism), 375
apnoea/hypopnoea index (AHI), 559
appearance, 71
bipolar disorder, 165
mental state examination, 53
appetite, 70
Appleby, L., 406, 411
applied relaxation (AR), 308
apraxia, 468–9
aprazolam, 620
arcuate fasciculus, 468
Aretaeus of Cappadocia, 162
ARFID, *See* avoidant restrictive food intake disorder
Argyll Robertson pupil, 490
Arias, F., 326
aripiprazole, 117, 118, 135, 136, 137, 171, 172, 244, 754
'best avoided' (specific instance), 586
co-prescription (augmentation), 248
long-term prophylaxis, 172
to be avoided by breast feeding women, **612**
Aristotle, 31
Armenia, 661
Arsenault-Lapierre, G., 662
arsenic poisoning, 511–12
art therapy, 438
ascertainment bias: form of observer bias, 24
Asher, R., 397
Ashkenazi Jews, 515
Asia, 492
Asian economic crisis (1997), 667
ASPD, *See* antisocial personality disorder
Asperger, H., 528
Asperger's syndrome, 528
assertive community treatment, 786
assertive outreach, 787–8, 791
definition, 787
principle, 787
assertive outreach teams, 784, 787, 788
patient crises, 788
assertiveness training, 155
assessment, 61
assessment interview, 42
Association for Neurodivergent Doctors (AND), 527
Association of Medical Officers of Asylums, 768
associations (measures of strength), 12–13
astereognosia, 466
ASWPD, *See* advanced sleep-wake phase disorder
Asylum Journal, 768
asylums, 34, 43, 767, 768, 769, 783
atenolol, 305
definition, 306
atomoxetine, 354, 541, 542
atrial fibrillation: identification and treatment, 695
at-risk mental state (ARMS), 244–5
attachment anxiety, 299
attachment avoidance
definition, 299
attachment disorder, 628
attention-deficit/hyperactivity disorder, 2, 167, 539–43, 589
brain mechanisms, 540
clinical diagnosis, 540–1
comorbidities, 541
effects, 542
epidemiology, 539
gene and environment interactions, 539
sociodemographic factors, 539
treatment, 541–2
attention-deficit hyperactivity disorder (treatment)
non-stimulants, 542
stimulants, 541–2
attenuated psychotic syndrome, 48
attitudes to mental illness, 769
attrition, 23, 92
atypical antipsychotics, 349, 480
atypical depression, 67, 137
clinical presentation (symptom profiles), 77
definition, 137
uncertainty about concept value and definition, 77
auditory disorders: sensory FND, 372
auditory hallucinations, 54, 71, 203
augmentation: definition, 135
Augustine, St., 655
Australia, 43, 95, 170, 183, 228, 232, 316, 320, 454, 605, 618, 621, 667, 676, 678, 680, 701, 703, 732, 734, 745
birth cohort study, 94
Austria, 618, 703, 704
autism, 2, 527–37
adverse life events, 528
aetiology, 529
age of onset, 532
anorexia nervosa link, 576
characteristics, 527
clinical formulation (strengths-based approach), 535–6
co-occuring conditions, 532
criminal justice system, 536–7
development as term of classification, 528–9
diagnostic assessments, 530–2
diagnostic classification systems, 529
differential diagnosis, 339
health care access (challenges), 534–5
key clinical question, 528
life expectancy, 532
mental health services (improving access), 535
prevalence, 529–30
reasonable adjustments, 535, **536**
statutory responsibilities, 535
traits, **531**
treatment, 534
autism (co-occuring mental disorders and differential diagnosis), 532–4
anxiety disorders, 532
catatonia, 533
dementia, 533
depression, 532
eating disorders, 533
EUPD, 532
OCD, 533
pathological demand avoidance, 534
psychoses, 533
PTSD, 533
suicide and acts of self harm, 533
Autism Act (2009), 527, 530, 535
autism diagnostic interview: revised (ADI-R), 531
autism diagnostic observation schedule (ADOS), 531
autism hubs, 534
autism quotient: 10 items (AQ10), 532
autism regional teams, 534
Autistic Doctors International (ADI), 527
autistic spectrum disorder, 168, 449
autoimmune encephalitis: organic psychotic disorders, 261
autoimmune encephalopathies, 497
autoimmune neurological disorders, 495–7
autoimmune encephalopathies, 497
multiple sclerosis, 495–6
systemic lupus erythematosus, 496–7
automatisms (epilepsy), 478
autotopoagnosia: definition, 466
avatars, 288, 799
average causal effect, 20
Avicenna, 696
avoidant behaviours, 392
avoidant personality disorder, 326, 450–1, 630
avoidant restrictive food intake disorder, 533, 587
aetiology, 588
differential diagnosis, 587
prevalence, 587
Avon longitudinal study of parents and children (ALPSAC), 18, 91, 94
AVPD, *See* avoidant personality disorder
Ayton, A., 565–92
Ayurvedic medicine, 718
azapirones, 305

BA, *See* behavioural activation
babies, 552
Babinski sign, 371
baby hatches, 618
backwards spelling test, 463
bacteria, 35
Baillarger, 162
Baldelomar, O. A., 710
Baldwin, D. S., 293–310
Bálint syndrome, 466, 467
Balint, M., 728, 735
Bandelow, B., 309, 342
Bangladesh, 511
banking crisis (2008), 666, 667, 793
Bantick, S. J., 396
Bárány Society criteria for PPPD, 374, **375**
barbiturate prescriptions, 680
Barcelona group psychoeducation programme, 191, **191**
Barraclough, B. M., 654, 663
barriers to housing and services (domain), 95
Bashir, Z., 636–51
Bass, C., 390, 398, 399
Batinic, B., 326
Bayes' theorem, 662
Bazett formula, 266

Bazire Psychotropic Drug Directory, 753
BDD, *See* body dysmorphic disorder
Beard, G., 34
Beards, S., 228
Bear-Fedio questionnaire, 480
Beck depression inventory (BDI), 464, 745, 750
Beck, A. T., 44, 68, 101, 104, 147–8, 152, 153, 329, 330, 662
  cognitive model of depression, 147
bed closure, 1
bed rest, 583
Bedi, G., 207, 215
beer potomania, 522
behaviour
  bipolar disorder, 165
  mental state examination, 53
behavioural activation, 153
behavioural couple therapy (BCT), 155
behavioural immune theory, 345
behavioural inhibition, 300
  definition, 296
behavioural techniques (CBT), 149
  activity scheduling, 149
  behavioural experiments, 149
  graded task assignment, 149
  mastery and pleasure ratings, 149
behavioural therapy, 756
Belgium, 656, 703
Bell, R. M.: *Holy Anorexia* (1985), 573
belongingness: definition, 438
Bengtson, V. L., 705
benign ethnic neutropaenia, 270
benign paroxysmal positional vertigo (BPPV), 374
Bentovim, A., 398
benzodiazepines, 39, 130, 301–4, 330, **612**, 755
  acute psychosis treatment, 246
  catatonia treatment, 259
  dependence (risk factors), 302
  dependence and withdrawal (management principles), **303**
  dosages, **304**
  effects (beneficial), 301
  efficacy, 302
  pharmacokinetic parameters, **301**
  potency, 302
  prescribing correlates, **301**
  rapid tranquilisation, 257
  side effects, 302
  tolerance, 302
  UK information, **640**
  withdrawal (clinical features), **303**
bereavement, 40, 48
bereavement-related depression, 81–3
Berger, H., *462*
beriberi, 519
Berrios, G. E., 199
Berry, J. W., 710
Bertillon classification of causes of death, 45
Bertillon, J., 45
Bertillon, L. A., 45
best interests, 758, 759
beta blockers, 121
  anxiety disorders, 305–9
  panic disorder, 307–9
  separation anxiety disorder, 309
  social anxiety disorder, 309
Bethencourt, F., 706
Better Services for Mentally Ill (1975), 768
beyond blue campaign (Australia, 2001), 682
Bhugra, D., 699–722
bias, 7, 10, 12, 21, 23–5
  classification, 23
  definition, 23
  information bias, 24–5
  selection bias, 23–4
Bible: suicides, 654–5
biculturalism, 710
big 5 personality traits, 418
bilateral medial temporal lobe lesions, 466
Billings, E., 739
binge-eating disorder, 590, 591–2
  aetiology, 591
  CBT-ED, 592
  clinical presentation and diagnosis, 591
  comorbidities, **591**
  epidemiology, 591
  medication, 592
  outcome, 592
  treatment, 592
Bini, L., 124, 125
binomial nomenclature, 31
Binswanger, O., 504
biological disadvantage, 36
biological mechanisms: psychosis (course and outcome), 234–6
biomedical model, 44, 740
Bion, 426, 432
biopsychosocial model, 44, 388, 447, 643, 740, 743
  now called 'holistic model', 45
bipolar disorder, 83, 85, 162–78, 601, 630, 679
  aetiology, 169–70
  clinical features, 165–7
  cognitive behavioural model (hypomania and depression relapse), *186*
  comorbidity, 162, 170
  comorbidity (physical illnesses), 170
  comorbidity (prevalence), 193
  depression in, 83
  diagnosis, 162–5
  diagnostic issues (DSM-5 versus ICD-11), 165
  differential diagnosis, 167–8
  ECT, 177
  genetic heritability, 102
  history, 162
  measurement of mania, 168
  medication-induced, 167
  mixed features (with depressive disorders), 83
  natural history, 168–9
  neurodiverse populations, 168
  other medical conditions, 167
  other physical treatments, 177–8
  outcome, 169
  suicide, 663
  transcranial magnetic stimulation, 177
  vagus nerve stimulation, 177–8
  young people, 168
bipolar disorder (aetiology), 169–70
  family history and genetics, 169
  neurodevelopmental and psychosocial factors, 169–70
bipolar disorder (clinical features), 165–7
  history, 165
  mental state examination (bipolar depression), 165
  mental state examination (mania and hypomania), 165–6
  self-reports, 166–7
bipolar disorder (drug treatment guidelines), 170–2
  bipolar depression, 171
  children and adolescents, 172
  manic episodes, 170–1
  mixed episodes, 171–2
  mood episodes (prophylaxis), 172
bipolar disorder (drug treatment)
  carbamazepine, 176–7
  guidelines, 170–2
  lithium, 172–6
  oxcarbazepine, 177
  valproate, 176
bipolar disorder (natural history), 168–9
  age of onset, 168
  episodes (duration), 168
  episodes (frequency), 168
  episodes (number), 168
  prevalence, 168
bipolar disorder treatment
  best practice, 183
  cognitive behavioural therapy, 192
  collaborative recovery focused approach, 183–4
  cultural and family approaches, 185
  developmental and life-course perspectives, 184–5
  early warning signs (EWS), 187–9
  family therapy and prevention programmes, 193
  holistic approach, 184
  ISRT, 192
  key learning points, 195
  mood-monitoring, 190
  neuropsychological function, 189
  physical health care, 193–5
  positive psychology (resilience, capability, recovery), 189
  psychoeducation, 191–2
  psychological approaches, 193
  psychological interventions, 190–1
  psychological, social, physical health approaches, 183–95
  psychosocial approaches (historical development), 183
  relapse (EWS), **188**
  remediation (cognitive or functional), 192
  self-esteem and explanatory style, 187
  stressors (other types), 186–7
  stressors (psychosocial), 185–6
bipolar I disorder (diagnosis), 163–5
  antidepressant drug treatment, 164
  hypomanic episode, 164
  major depressive episode, 164
  manic episode, 163–4
  mixed states, 164–5
  rapid cycling, 165
  sub-classes, 163
bipolar II disorder
  diagnosis, 165
  differentiation from borderline personality disorder, 167
bipolar spectrum disorder
  distinguishing characteristics, **163**
  types, **163**
Bipolar UK, 183, 188
Birken, M., 435
Birmingham, 792
Birmingham: City Hospital, 740
birth asphyxia: effect on schizophrenia, 15
birth cohort study (BCS70, UK), 91
birth cohorts, 90, 96
Bisson, J. I., 314–21
bitopertin, 244
black and minority ethnic groups, 389
blepharospasm, 487
Bleuler, E., 34, 35, 162, 198, 199, 200, 205, 214, 282, 449, 457
  Dementia Praecox or Group of Schizophrenias (1911), 34
Bleuler, M., 231
blinding, 24
Bloch, F., 461
blood, 174
blood and injury phobia, **325**
blood lipids: control, 693–4
blood oxygenation level-dependent contrast (BOLD), 462
blood phobia, 328
blood pressure: control (integrated approach), 693
blood-brain barrier, 306, 488, 611, 621
Boas, F., 699
bodily distress disorder, 387–92
  aetiology, 391
  course, 389–90
  diagnostic requirements, 389
  epidemiology, 390–1
  exclusions (ICD-11), 387
  ICD-11, 387
  management, 391–2
  prognosis, 391
  severity, 389
  specialist treatment, 392
  terminology 'major issue', 388
  types in hospital clinics, **390**
bodily distress syndrome (BDS), 388
  'broader than BDD', 391
body dysmorphic disorder, 335–6, 350–2
  cognitive behavioural model, *351*
  ERP, 351–2
  'poor insight', 350
  psychological treatment, 351–2
  psychopharmacology, 350–1
  Ryan case study, 351–2
  treatment, 350–2
  treatment outcome, 352
Bohr, N., 776

Boland, R. J., 746
Bolton, D., 42
bone marrow, 174
bones, 174
Bonferroni correction, 27
Bonhoeffer, K., 461
borderline controversy, 406–7
borderline personality disorder, 167, 404, 405, 406–7, 408, 409, 410, 418, 436, 437, 607, 663
  classification (if not 'personality disorder'), 407
  dangers, 407
  heterogeneity, **407**
  presentation, 406
  suicide, 664–5
  whether 'personality disorder', 406–7
borderzone aphasia, 468
Bose, K. C., 241
Boswell, J., 392
boundary disorders, 80, 83
  bipolar disorders, 83
  primary psychotic disorders, 83
Bourdieu, P., 706
Bournewood gap, 759
bovine spongiform encephalopathy, 494
Bowden, C. L., 162
Bowlby, E. J. M., 154
  attachment theory, 81
Bradford-Hill, A., 19
  criteria for causation, 19
brain, 89, 98, 99, 112, 125, 220, 221, 249, 297
  ASPD, 446
  Bayesian, 378
  Broca's area, 286
  dopamine signalling, 242
  MRI scans, 461
  OCD, 341, 342, 343, 344
  structural abnormalities, 199
brain abnormalities, 449
brain damage, 398
brain intoxicants, 511–14
brain lesions: location, 470
brain mechanisms: adult ADHD, 540
brain mythologies, 33
brain nuclei, *297*
brain structural abnormalities, 235
brain syndromes with regional connections, 464–7
  corpus callosum, 467
  frontal lobe, 464–5
  parietal lobe, 466–7
  temporal lobe, 465–6
brain tumours, 475–6
brain-derived neurotropic factor (BDNF), 376
Bratiotis, C., 353
Brazil, 228, 677, 701, 706
breast cancer, 263, 747
breast carcinoma, 475
breast feeding, 609, 611–13, 615, 619, 621
  database on psychotropic drugs, **612**
brexanolone, 611
brexpiprazole, 244
brick mother (Rey), 428, 433
Bridgman, P. W., 35
brief limited intermittent psychotic symptoms (BLIPS), 789
brief psychiatric rating scale (BPRS), 234, 253
brief psychosis (puerperal), 600
brief psychotic disorder, 200
  definition, 217
Briquet, P.: *Treatise on Hysteria* (1859), 387
Briquet's syndrome, 387, 450
Bristol stool chart, 270
British and Irish Group for Study of Personality Disorder (BIGSPD), 415, 435
British Association for Psychopharmacology (BAP), 135, 136, 170, 177, 254, 348
British Journal of Mental Science, 30
British Journal of Psychiatry, 30, 768
British National Formulary, 112, 114, 752, 753
British Neuropsychiatry Association, 461
British Psychological Society, 430
Broadmoor, 617
Broca, P., *464*, 465
Broca's aphasia, 467
Broca's area, 464, 468
Brodmann areas, 467
broken heart syndrome, 82
Brown, S., 689
Brown, T., 401
Brugada's syndrome, 172, 174
buccofacial apraxia, 469
Buckinghamshire, 215
Bucknill, J. C., 32, 34, 43, 48, 689, 768
Bucy, P., 466
bulimia nervosa, 84, 339, 588–91
  aetiology, 588
  assessment, 590
  CBT-E, 590
  clinical presentation and diagnosis, 588
  comorbidities (personality disorder), 589
  comorbidities (physical), 589
  comorbidities (psychiatric), 589
  comorbidities (risk of mortality), **590**
  comorbidities (substance use), 589
  course, 591
  differential diagnosis, 590
  epidemiology, 588
  history, 588
  mortality (risk factors), 591
  outcome, 591
  pathophysiology, 589
  physical complications, 590
  psychological factors, 589
  risk indicators, 590
  social factors, 589
  treatment, 590
bulimia: etymology, 588
Bullough, V. L., 719
bullying, 98, 104
  definition, 98
buprenorphine, 646, 647–8
bupropion, **109**, 114–15, 130, **132**, 134, 135, 137, **273**, 552
  background, 114
  contraindications, 115
  interactions, 115
  mechanism of action, 114
  pharmacokinetics, 114
  side effects, 114
  toxicity in overdose, 115
Burgess, J., 162–78
Burkauskas, J., 324–31, 334–59
burnout, 776–7
Burns, T., 731, 733, 735
Burton, R., 392
  Anatomy of Melancholy (1621), 64, 81, 367
Bush-Francis Catatonia Rating Scale, 259
buspirone, 120, 305
  contraindications, 120
  elimination half-life, 120
  mechanism of action, 120
  overdoses, 120
  side effects, 120
butane, 513
Butler, A. C., 152
Butler, M., 366–81

Cabaniss, D., 756
Cade, J. F., 170
CADET, 734
caffeine, 48, 272, 510, 548, 620
Caffey, J., 624
CAG repeats, 485
CAGE questionnaire, 52, 747
calcium channels, 112, 123
calcium deficiency, 521
California, 705
Cambridge behavioural inventory (CBI), 501
Camilleri, C., 710
camouflaging, 535
camphor, 124
Campion, J., 772
Canada, 183, 446, 605, 656, 680, 703
cancer, 193, 394, 739, 740, 747, 757
cancer-screening, 696
candidacy (concept), 726
cannabidiol (CBD), 229, 244
cannabis, 716
  neuropsychiatric manifestations, 510
  UK information, **640**
cannabis use, 21, *22*, 52, 220, 233, 235, 641
  causal association with psychosis (confounder), 21
  'cries out for preventive approach', 230
  prospectively linked with depression (some evidence), 100–1
  psychosis risk factor, 228–9
Cannon, M., 227
capacity, 757–9
capacity to consent
  assessment, 757–8
  Mental Capacity Act (2005), 757
  overdose, 758
  patients lacking, 758–9
  valid consent, 757
Capgras syndrome, 219, 469
carbamates, 513
carbamazepine, 171, 175, 272, 456, 471, **612**, 620
  combination with lithium (risk), 174
carbamazepine (treatment of bipolar disorder), 176–7
  doses, 176
  drug interactions, 177
  pharmacokinetics, 177
  side effects, 176
carbon dioxide, 298, 300
carbon disulphide, 512
carbon monoxide, 92, 514, 680, 681
carbon tetrachloride, 512
cardiac rhythms: at-risk (identification), 695
cardiac side effects (antipsychotics), 266–7
  general assessment, 266
  orthostatic hypotension, 267
  QT interval prolongation, 266–7
  tachycardia, 267
Cardiff, 320
cardiomyopathy, 271
cardiovascular disease, 112
Cardno, A. G., 224
Care Act (2014), 796, 797
  areas of concern, 797
  key principles, 796
care homes, 498
care in community, 776
care programme approach (CPA), 733, 769, 770–1, 788
  established in 1991, 770
Care Quality Commission (CQC), 60, 585, 740, 773, 797
carer support and intervention: psychosocial management of psychosis, 288–9
carer's allowances, 794
carers, 789, 794
cariprazine, 137, 171, 244
Carlsson, A., 241, 242
Carpenter, W. T., 213
Carroll, L.: Alice's Adventures in Wonderland, 512
Carson, A., 368, 460–522
Carter, R. T., 707
case register data, 689
case-control studies, 16, 22, 90
  most important issue, 16
  prevalence bias, 24
  selection bias, 23, 90
case-history approach, 32–3, 48, 49
Casetta, C., 224–36
Caspi, A., 104
Castillo, R. J., 712
catalytic converters, 680
cataplexy, 560, 561
catatonia, 2, 208–9, 212, 259–60, 533
  case example, 209
  clinical presentation (symptom profiles), 75–6
  course, 199
  current understanding, 201
  definition, 72, 199, 208, 259
catatonia treatment
  antipsychotics, 260
  benzodiazepines, 259
  complications (prevention), 260
  electroconvulsive therapy, 259
  lorazepam challenge test, 259
  management strategy, 259
  other treatments, 260
CATEGO, 35
Catholicism, 668
CATIE trial, 247, 255, 263
cauda equina, 376
causal effect, 22, 23
causal inference, 7, 19, 20, 23, 25

causal inference (cont.)
contemporary versus traditional techniques, 8
causal pathway, *22*, 22
causation, 13, 19–27
bias, 23–5
chance, 25–7
confounding, 21–2
cornerstone issue, 19
multifactorial, 90
negative findings (points to consider), 27
reverse causation, 25
cause
definition, 89
identification, 90
'necessary' versus 'sufficient', 89
Cavanna, A. E., 460–522
Cawley, R., 348
Cawley, R. H., 36
CBT, *See* cognitive behavioural therapy
celecoxib, 123
censoring, 23
census data, 12, 46
central nervous system, 447, 490
lithium side effects, 173
organic psychotic disorders, 261–2
central nervous system infections (other), 492–5
Creutzfeldt-Jakob disease, 494–5
cysticercosis, 492
long Covid, 495
Lyme disease, 493
malaria, 494
subacute sclerosing panencephalitis, 492
toxoplasmosis, 493
trypanosomiasis, 493
typhus, 493
Whipple's disease, 492
central pontine myelinolysis, 509
Centre for Workforce Intelligence (2014 report), 776
cerebral cortex, 199
cerebrotendinous xanthomatosis, 514
cerebrovascular disease, 473–5
Cerletti, U., 124, 125
Chagas' disease, 493
chance, 21, 25–7, 92
hypothesis testing, 26
type 1 and type 2 error, 25–6
chaos of detail, 50
charcoal-burning (suicide prevention), 681
Charcot, J-M., 367
Iconography, 367
Charpentier, P., 241
Chartonas, D., 406, 411
chatbots, 799
Chesney, E., 241–72
chest medicine, 36
Chesterfield FC Community Trust, 692
Cheyne, G.: *English Malady* (1733), 392
Chicago follow-up study, 231
chief clinical information officers (CCIO), 798
Chief Inspector of Prisons, 666
child abuse, 398, 664, 717
child abuse and neglect, 624–31
adult psychiatrist (role), 629, 631
causal factors, 627–8
consequences, 628–9
definition (federal law, USA), 626
mothers with schizophrenia, 629
report-writing, 629
child abuse and neglect (UK procedures), 625–7
child care order (legal criteria), 625
child maltreatment, 625–7
child care order (legal criteria, UK), 625
child maltreatment, 625–7
neglect, 626–7
physical abuse, 625–6
child maltreatment (psychological abuse), 627
age inappropriate expectations, 627
exploiting and corrupting behaviours, 627
isolating, 627
making negative attributions to child, 627
spurning, 627
terrorising, 627
child maltreatment (psychological maltreatment), 626–7
emotional neglect, 626
mental health neglect, 627
psychological abuse, 627
child neglect, 626–7
adequate supervision, 626
appropriate shelter, 626
dental neglect, 626
educational neglect, 627
failure to gain weight, 626
medical neglect, 626
physical neglect, 626
poor hygiene, 626
child protection conferences, 625
child psychiatry: culture, 717
childhood adversity
definition, 227
psychosis (risk and mediating factor), 233
psychosis risk factor, 228
childhood autoimmune neurological syndrome (CANS), 344
childhood neglect and adversity, 407
childhood sexual abuse (CSA), 629
childhood trauma, 186
children, 375, 378, 446, 447, 470, 552, 553
bipolar disorder, 193
bipolar disorder (drug treatment guidelines), 172
capacity to consent to medical treatment, 757
Children Act (1989), 625, 796
definition of 'harm', 626
Children Act (2004), 625, 796
Children Act (date unspecified), 586
children and young people's mental health surveys (England), 95
Chile, 608, 661
China, 305, 317, 455, 488, 513, 660, 677, 680, 681, 701, 718, 745
rural suicide, 680–1
suicide (elderly people), 661
Chinese classification of mental disorders (CCMD), 45
chlordiazepoxide, 754
chlorinated pesticide compounds, 513
chlorpromazine, 34, 111, 170, 234, 241, **612**, 620
Chodoff, P., 48
cholecystokinin (CCK), 298
cholera, 6
cholestanol, 514
cholesterol, 694
chorea: definition, 485
chromosomes, 102
chronic alcoholic hallucinosis, 507
chronic kidney disease (CKD), 173
proper management, 695
chronic obstructive pulmonary disease (COPD), 695, 756
chronic pain, 395–7. *See also* pain
ICD-11, 396–7
chronic primary pain, 397
definition (ICD-11), 396
chronic traumatic encephalopathy, 473
Cicero, 64
cimetidine, 112
circadian alerting drive (process C), 548, 549
circadian rhythm, 100, 115, 187
circadian rhythm disorders, 553–5
descriptions and comments, **554**
Cirnigliaro, G., 324–31, 334–59
citalopram, 108, 109, 110, 113, 116, 134, 348, 349, 511, **612**, 754
cardiac side effects, 134
risk of abnormalities, 619
CJD, *See* Creutzfeldt-Jakob disease
CL, *See* consultation-liaison psychiatry
Clare, A., 43
Psychiatry in Dissent (second edition, 2012), 39
Clark, D. M., 329, 330
Clarke, M., 616
classification, 31–4
aetiologically-based, 32
case-history approach, 32–3
culture (role), 39
history, 31–2
Kraepelin, 33–4
symptom-based, 32
Clean Air Act (USA, 1970), 680
cleanliness and clutter scale, 353
Cleare, A., 108–38
Cleckley, H.: *Mask of Sanity* (second edition, 1941), 444, 445
clinical assessment schemes: development, 48–9
Clinical Associates in Applied Psychology (CAAPs), 732
clinical commissioning groups, 773
clinical decision units, 759
clinical depression: term 'best avoided', 72
clinical epidemiology, 6–28. *See also* epidemiology
clinical global impression-schizophrenia scale (CGI-S), 234
clinical global improvement, 798
clinical high-risk (CHR) state, 245
clinical impairment assessment (CIA), 570
Clinical Institute withdrawal assessment for alcohol (CIWA-Ar), 646
clinical interview schedule-revised (CIS-R), 9
gold standard, **9**
clinical interview: risk of violence, 53
clinical observation, 37
clinical opiate withdrawal scale (COWS), 646
clinical skills, 2
clinician rated outcome measures (CROMs), 798
clock drawing test, 463
clomipramine, **109**, **132**, 138, 334, 342, 346, 348, 349, 350, 484
OCD, 341
side effects, 348
clonazepam, 558, **612**
Huntington's disease, 485
clonidine, 113, 541, 542
clozapine, 117, 137, 171, 234, 242–4, 249, 262, 342, 482, 511, 619, 693, 694, 730, 780
alternatives, 251
discovery (1959), 241
plasma levels, 250–1
resistance, 251
side effects, 269–71
to be avoided by breast feeding women, **612**
treatment-resistant schizophrenia, 250–1
withdrawal, 251
clozapine augmentation strategies, 251–2
adding antidepressant, 251
adding mood stabiliser, 252
adding second antipsychotic, 251
non-pharmacological options, 252
novel treatments, 252
novel treatments (most promising), **252**
cluster analysis, 214, 221
CMHF, *See* community mental health framework
CMHTs, *See* community mental health teams
coarse brain disease, 54
cocaine, 54, 228, 509, 641, 642
pregnancy, 621
UK information, **640**
Cochrane reviews, 122, 127
antidepressant use, 254
ASPD, 447
bipolar disorder (pharmacotherapy), 435
bipolar disorders (psychological interventions), 438
CBT, 756
personality disorder (psychological therapies), 436
postnatal psychoses, 603
psychological therapies, 330
schizophrenia and schizoaffective disorder, 253
self harm (2016), 679

treatments for depression in schizophrenia, 253
CODES trial, 380
cognition
approach to deficits, **255**
impairment in psychoses, 255
cognitive behavioural therapy, 44, 105, 147–52, 283, 729
ADHD, 542
antidepressant medication, 153
behavioural techniques, 149
bipolar disorder, 192
case illustration, 152
characteristics, 148
cognition (change strategies), 149–52
consideration of alternative views, 151
cultural issues, 721
definition, 147
dysfunctional thought record, **151**
efficacy, 152
facing up to worst fear, 152
FND, 380
gambling, 454–5
generalised anxiety disorder, 287, 307
hypochondriasis, 395
invented by Beck, 101
management of physical health conditions, 756
OCD, 346, 347
OCD (outcome), 347
pain, 397
panic disorder, 298, 308
perinatal depression, 613
personality disorder, 436
postnatal depression, 610
preventative strategies, 152
relapse prevention, 152
self harm, 679
social anxiety disorder, 309
substance use disorders, 648
thinking errors, 148
third-wave, 347
weekly activity schedule, **150**
without trauma focus, 319
cognitive behavioural therapy (techniques), 149
behavioural techniques, 149
cognitive techniques, 149
preventative strategies, 149
cognitive behavioural therapy for eating disorders (CBT-E), 570, 571–2, 582
process map, *572*
stages, 572
transdiagnostic overview, *571*
cognitive behavioural therapy for insomnia (CBT-I), 551
cognitive behavioural therapy for psychosis (CBTP), 283–4, 288, 788, 789. *See also* psychological treatment
assessment, 284
negative symptoms, 287
cognitive behavioural therapy with trauma focus (CBT-TF), 318
PTSD, 318
cognitive disturbances (COGDIS) criteria, *245*
cognitive function
impaired, 69
mental state examination, 54–5
cognitive impairment (schizophrenia), 209–10
attention, 210
executive function, 210
memory, 210
origin and time course, 210
cognitive restructuring: definition, 150
cognitive styles questionnaire, 101
cognitive techniques (CBT)
negative automatic thoughts (challenging), 149
negative automatic thoughts (identification), 149
cognitive theories: OCD, 345–6
cognitive therapy (CT), 147
cognitive-perceptive basic symptoms (COPER) criteria, 245
Cohen, P., 708
Cohen, S., 744
Cohen, S. B., 528
Cohen's kappa, 8
cohort studies, 15, 22, 90, 94, 609
cause-and-effect estimates (strengthening), 92–3
key strength, 15
limitations, 91–2
non-response bias, 23
same as 'longitudinal studies' (*qv*), 91
utility, 15
cohort: definition, 91
coin tosses, 25
COINCIDE, 734
collaborative care, 729, 732, 734
key elements, 734
collaborative care approach, 757
collective mental disorders, 718
College Handbook on ECT, 125
collider, 23
collider bias, 23
example, *23*
colour blindness, 708
Colt, G. H., 655
coma, 505
comate, 31
combination: definition, 135
Comer, J. P., 708
command hallucinations, 71
commissioning for quality improvement, 774
committee of famous professors principle, 31
common cold, 744
common factor theory, 417, 418
common law, 61, 758
doctrine of necessity, 759, 782
common mental disorders (CMD), 94
community based (probation) order, 61
community mental health framework, 425, 783, 785, 790
launched immediately prior to pandemic, 770
community mental health teams, 159, 426, 428, 624, 639, 731, 733, 735, 769, 776, 786, 788, 790–1
assertive outreach, 787, 788
budgets, 790
care and treatment offered, 790
caseloads, 790
crises, 791
local agreements, 790
patients, 790
remit, 790
role, 790
staffing, 790
support packages, 790
community perinatal mental health services, 623–4
role, 623
community perinatal mental health teams, 623
community perinatal teams
collaborative working, 623
maintaing contact with other agencies, 624
pre-birth planning meetings, 624
community reinforcement and family training (CRAFT), 648
community reinforcement approach, 648
community treatment orders, 781–2
comorbidity, 42–3
bipolar disorder, 170
definition, 83
comorbidity (physical and psychiatric), 744–5
case definition, 744–5
impact, 747–50
rates in different populations, 745
comorbidity in depressive disorders, 83–4
medical comorbidity, 84
psychiatric comorbidity, 84
compassion-focused therapy (CFT), 288, 587
complex emotional needs, 410, 420
complex psychosis, 783
complex PTSD (CPTSD), 314, 408, 420, 430
ICD-11 symptom criteria, 315
treatment, 320–1
complicated grief, 82
synonyms, 82
composite international diagnostic interview (CIDI), 390
comprehensive assessment of at-risk mental states (CAARMS), 245
compulsions: definition, 334
compulsory treatment orders (CTOs), 769
computed tomography, 461
main characteristics, **461**
computerised CBT (cCBT), 152
conceptual memory, 742
concurrent validity, 9
sensitivity and specificity, 9–10
conditional logistic regression, 13
conduction aphasia, 468
confidence intervals, 26
confidentiality, 758
'not sacrosanct', 674
confounders, 8
controlling for, *21*
definition, 21
confounding, 14, 16, 21–2, 23, 90
basic structure (causal diagram), *21*
threat to cohort studies, 92
confounding (five methods to overcome), 21–2
1. restriction, 21
2. matching, 21
3. stratification, 22
4. regression adjustment, 22
5. randomisation, 22
confounding-by-indication, 22
confusion assessment protocol (CAP), 464
confusional arousals, 555
congenital heart disease (CHD), 619
Consensus Statement on Personality Disorder, 416
consent, 757–9
patients who lack capacity, 758–9
CONSORT statement, 17
construct validity, 9
construction workers: suicide risk, 667
constructional apraxia, 469
consultation-liaison model, 733
consultation-liaison psychiatrists, 743, 756
commonest comorbid problem, 745
role, 744, 745, 746, 749
skills, 752
consultation-liaison psychiatry, 739, 744
assessment, 751–2
assessment checklist, 751
central concept, 741
conclusions, 762
diagnosis, 752
diagnostic formulation, *753*
history, 739–40
referrals, 751
referrals (reasons), 752
consultation-liaison psychiatry services (consultation model), 760
crisis-oriented therapeutic consultation, 760
patient-oriented consultation, 760
referrer-oriented consultation, 760
situation-oriented consultation, 760
consultation-liaison psychiatry services (determining factors), 761
consultation time available, 761
expectations of other professionals, 761
other established services provided to hospital, 761
consultation-liaison psychiatry services (provision), 759–62
consultation model, 760
liaison model, 760
links with other services, 761
models of service, 760–1
service needs, 761
speciality-based services, 761
staffing, **760**
standard requirements, 760
container-contained (Bion), 426–7
definition, 426
Conteiro, K., 677

contemporary causal inference, 20
content validity, 9
continuous performance test (CPT), 210
conversation, 688, 692
conversion disorder. *See also* functional neurological disorder
term with 'baggage', 368
Cookson, J., 162–78
Cooper, B., 6
Cooper, D., 39
copy number variations (CNVs), 226, 227, 235
core consciousness, 422, 424
Core Values for Psychiatrists (CR204), 3, 4
Cormack. A., 461
coroner's inquest, 682
corporal punishment, 628
corpus callosum, 467, 470, 507
correlation does not imply causation, 7
cortical signs: schizophrena, 211
corticosteroids, 194, 261
cot death, 159
Cotard delusions, 69
Côte d'Ivoire, 609
Cougnard, A., 229
counterfactual scenario, 20, 22
County Asylums Act, 767
Court of Protection, 759
Courvoisier, S., 241
Cousins, D., 162–78
Covid-19 pandemic, 43, 44, 59, 345, 378, 456, 495, 565, 568, 591, 668, 694, 696, 728, 732, 793
'loose' versus 'tight' cultures, 704
PTSD, 316
vaccination, 696
Cox, J. L., 608
CPA, *See* care programme approach
CQUIN, *See* commissioning for quality improvement
crack, **640**
crack cocaine, 641
craniopharyngiomas, 476
Cranshaw, J., 598–631
CRASH, 719
c-reactive protein (CRP), 98
Creed, F., 394
Creed, F. R., 733
Creutzfeldt, H. G., 494
Creutzfeldt-Jakob disease, 494–5
Crick, F., 460
criminal justice system, 536–7
Criminal Procedure (Insanity and Unfitness to Plead) Act (1991), 61
crisis and home treatment teams (CHTTs), 434
crisis hotlines (suicide prevention), 681–2
crisis resolution and home treatment (CRHT), 786
Crisp, A., 577
criterion-related validity, 9
Cronbach's α, 9
cross-cultural studies, 701
cross-sectional studies, 14–15, 90
advantages and drawbacks, 91
prevalence bias, 24
CT, *See* computed tomography
CTE, *See* chronic traumatic encephalopathy
CTOs, *See* community treatment orders
Cuijpers, P., 152, 155
Cullen, W., 64
Synopsis Nosologica Methodicae, 31
cultural assessment, *715*
cultural capital, 699, 706, 710, 714
cultural competence, 715, 716, 719–20, 722
definition, 719
history-taking (addictions-related care), **716**
cultural consonance, 711
definition, 711
cultural empathy, 715
cultural formulation, 714–15, 719
components, 720
distress and health-seeking, **714**
cultural knowledge, 715
cultural psychiatry, 2
evolution, **700**
prime concern, 700
role, 700
cultural sensitivity, 715, 717
culture, 389, 699–722
addiction psychiatry, 716–17
ageing and old-age psychiatry, 717
assessment tools, 714
basic assessment, **711**
characteristics, *700*
child and adolescent psychiatry, 717
classification and dimensions, 701–6
collective mental disorders, 718
conclusion, 722
criterion for assessing psychiatric classification systems, 41
definitions, 699–701
disease and illness, 711
domains of academia and practice relating to psychiatry and mental health, *712*
explanatory models, 711–13
explanatory models (what is needed), **712**
folk explanations, 717
forensic psychiatry, 717
idioms of distress, 711
inpatient psychiatry, 716
intellectual disability, 717
liaison psychiatry, 716
'linear active' versus 'reactive' (Lewis), 704
'loose' versus 'tight', 703–4
mental state examination (basic principles), 713–14
outpatient psychiatry, 716
professional-patient interaction, 715–16
psychological therapy, 721
psychopharmacology, 720
relationship between patients, clinicians, teams, **712**
role in diagnosis and classification systems, 39
sexual variations, 719
social determinants, 721–2
traditional folk medicines, 718
value dimensions (Hofstede), 701
working with interpreters, 714, **714**
culture (value dimensions)
collectivist versus individualist, 701, **702**
low versus high uncertainty, 702–3
masculine versus feminine, 702
culture bound syndromes, 718–19
cumulative incidence, 11–12
definition, 11
formula, 11
Currie, A., 162–78
Cushing, H., 516
Cushing's syndrome, 516
CutlaSS RCT, 263
cutting (self-injury method), 677
cyberchondria, 336, 355
cyclothymia: definition, 83
cyproheptadine, 110, 114
cystathione synthase defects, 515
cysticercosis, 492
cytochrome P450 (CYP) enzymes, 272, 348
induced by tobacco smoke, 272
inhibited by grapefruit juice, 272
interactions with antipsychotics, **272**
pharmacogenomics, 272
cytochrome P450 enzymes, 112
Czech Republic, 608, 704

D'Espine, M., 45
classification of diseases, 45
Dagonet. M., 444
Dale, O., 414–39
Dalle Grave, R., 583, 585
Dalton, K., 611
Damasio, A., 422, 464
Dandy-Walker malformation, 620
Danish College of General Practitioners, 391
dark traits, 445
Davidson, I., 527–37
Davies, C., 227
day care
definition, 785
providers, 785
virtual disappearance (UK), 785
day hospitals
use of term, 785
virtual disappearance (UK), 785
day hospitals and day care, 784–5
day services, 785
crisis management, 785
Day, E., 636–51
days/months backwards test, 463
DBS, *See* deep brain stimulation
DBT, *See* dialectical behavioural therapy
DCR-10, 46
dead salmon experiment, 24
Decision-Making and Consent (GMC guidance), 4
deculturation, 710
deep brain stimulation, 126–7, 482, 485, 587
mechanism of action, 126
OCD, 349
side effects, 126
deep dyslexia, 468
deep magnetic stimulation (DTMS), 350
default mode network (DMN), **298**, 298, 378
defeat depression campaign (UK, 1992-6), 682
Delay, J., 241
delayed sleep-wake phase disorder, 553, **554**, 554–5
assessment, 555
definition, 554
psychiatric conditions, 554
treatment, 555
delirium, 497–500, 740, 759
aetiology, 500
causes, **498**
clinical features, **498**
cognitive symptoms, 498
course, 499
definition, 497
detection rates, 499
direct side effect of medical treatment, 741
disturbances to attention, 498
emotional lability, 499
management, 500
outcome, 499
pharmacotherapy, 500
predisposing and precipitating factors, **499**
synonyms, 498
delirium rating scale (DRS), 464
delirium tremens, 508, 509, 646, 754, 755
delta sleep, 546
delusional disorder, 198, 200, 218–19
case example (Ernst Wagner), 219
definition, 218
delusional perception, 54
delusions, 69–70, 287, 491, 678
Jasperian definition, 283
mental state examination, 54
schizophrenia, 204–5
dementia, 473, 498, 500–5
aetiology, 500
autism, 533
causes, 500
diagnostic criteria, 501
differential diagnosis, 500
epidemiology, 500
intellectual impairment (patterns), 500
main syndromes, **500**
mild neurocognitive disorder, 501
neurodegenerative dementias, 501–4
neurodegenerative versus non-neurodegenerative, 500
other types, 504–5
overview, 500–1
Parkinson's disease, 483
primary care, 731
treatment, 501
dementia caused by infective agents, 505
dementia paranoides, 212
dementia praecox, 34, 198, 212
later 'schizophrenia', 33
dementia with Lewy bodies, 503, 557
differential diagnosis, 503
pharmacotherapy, 503
presentation, 503
Dempster, E. L., 226
denial (defence mechanism), 743
Deniker, P., 241

Denmark, 191, 228, 231, 339, 542, 605, 608, 660, 678, 696, 703, 792
denominator error, 12
dependent personality disorder, 451
depersonalisation, 38, 614
depersonalisation, derealisation (DPDR), 71
depressed mood, 66–7
depression, 1, 24, 454
affect disorders, 207–8
autism, 532
biopsychosocial causation (integrating stressors and vulnerability), 104
causes, 89–105
clinical presentation (symptom profiles), 75–8
controversies and implications, 65–6
dimension of psychopathology in schizophrenia, 213
direct side effect of medical treatment, 741
epilepsy (aetiology), 479
frequency of different symptoms, **66**
genetics, 102–4
increased prevalence since 1993 (UK), 91
inflammatory hypothesis, 741
longitudinal studies, 91
OCD, 338
other specified depressive disorders, 80
persistent depressive disorders, 79–80
physical health problems (bidirectional association), 99
post-stroke, 474
poverty factor, 94–5
primary care, 728–9
rating scales, **86**
selection bias (case-control studies), 90
self-help books, 158
sleep problems, 99–100
specific phobia comorbidity, 326
suicide, 662
treatment (systematic approach), 128–38
treatments (drugs), 108–24
treatments (physical), 124–8
vicious circles, 148
websites and apps, 158
depression (clinical presentation)
agitated depression, 77
anxious depression, 76
atypical depression, 77
catatonia, 75–6
melanchoic depression, 76–7
mixed depressive and anxiety disorder, 76
psychotic depression, 75–6
depression (history), 64–5
1. antiquity to Renaissance, 64
2. seventeenth to nineteenth centuries, 64–5
3. twentieth century to today, 65
depression (psychological management principles), 156–9
change techniques, 158–9
cognitive behavioural techniques, 158
education about depression and medication, 157–8
engaging patient and maintaining therapeutic relationship, 156–7
guidance and advice, 159
indications for therapies, **159**
interviewing family members, 158
psychological aspects of assessment process, 156
depression (psychological therapies), 147–55
behavioural activation, 153
cognitive behavioural therapy, 147–52
interpersonal therapy, 153–4
psychodynamic therapy, 154–5
third-wave CBT, 153
depression (related disorders), 80–3
grief and bereavement, 81–3
premenstrual dysphoric disorder, 80–1
depression (risk factors), 96–101
adverse childhood experiences, 97
alcohol and cannabis use (evidence discussed), 100–1
bullying, 98
family history of depression, 97
inflammation, 98
loneliness, 100
obesity, 99
origins in early life, 96
parental depression, 97
perinatal risk factors, 97
sedentary behaviour, 99
stress response, 97–8
stressful life events, 97
depression differences
ethnicity, 95–6
gender and age, 93–4
sexual orientation and gender identity, 96
socioeconomic background, 94–5
depression treatment (general principles), 128–34
dose adjustment, 129
making diagnosis, 128–9
relapse prevention, 134
response monitoring, 129–30
side-effect management, 130–1
stopping effective treatment (when and how), 131–4
switching treatment, 130–1
depression treatment (monitoring)
drug factors, 130
illness factors, 130
patient factors, 130
depression treatment (psychological and social), 147–59
conclusions, 155
group and systemic therapies, 155
psychological management (principles), 156–9
conclusions, 159
psychological therapies, 147–55
social interventions, 156
depression treatment (systematic approach), 128–38
atypical depression, 137–8
comorbid chronic pain, 138
general principles, 128–34
hepatic impairment, 138
renal impairment, 137–8
special cases, 137–8
unipolar depression (with psychotic symptoms), 136–7
unipolar depression (without psychotic symptoms), 134–6
depression vulnerability, 101–4
environmental stressors and response, *104*
psychological theories, 101–2
depression with onset in later life, 78–9
depressive disorders
assessment (relevant features), **85**
clinical features, 64–86
comorbidity, 83–4
epidemiology, 84–5
general hospital setting, 745–6
natural history, 85
primary versus secondary, 72
rating scales, 85–6
depressive disorders (affective symptoms), 66–8
anhedonia, 67
anxiety, 68
depressed mood, 66–7
hopelessness, 67
irritability and anger, 68
worthlessness, shame, guilt, 67–8
depressive disorders (behavioural features), 71–2
altered psychomotor function, 71–2
appearance, 71
catatonia, 72
dissociative and histrionic behaviour, 72
general functioning, 72
lack of motivation and apathy, 71
depressive disorders (cognitive symptoms), 68–70
delusions, 69–70
hypochondriasis (illness anxiety), 69
impaired cognitive function, 69
obsessive-compulsive phenomena, 69
repetitive, intrusive, distressing thoughts, 69
thoughts of death and suicide, 68
worry and rumination, 69
depressive disorders (perceptual symptoms), 71
depersonalisation, derealisation (DPDR), 71
hallucinations, 71
depressive disorders (physical symptoms), 70
appetite and weight, 70
fatigue and lack of energy, 70
sleep, 70
depressive disorders (somatic symptoms): loss of libido, 70
depressive disorders (symptoms and signs)
affective symptoms, 66–8
cognitive symptoms, 68–70
perceptual symptoms, 71
physical symptoms, 70
somatic symptoms, 70
depressive episodes, 72. *See also* major depressive episodes
definition, **73**
timing of onset, 78–9
with short-duration hypomania., 48
depressogenic schemas: definition, 148
deprivation of liberty safeguards (DoLS), 759
Descemet's membrane, 487
descriptive psychopathology, 49
desipramine, 111
desmethylimipramine, 111
desvenlafaxine, **109**, 110, **132**
detachment: definition, 419, 427
determinants of outcome in severe mental disorders (DOSMED), 701
developmental psychopathology
personality disorder, 422–5
prognosis and life course (personality disorder), 425
developmental psychopathology (clinicopathological description), 424–5
borderline and relational psychosis, 425
dissociative experiences, 424
emotional intensity and impulse disorders, 424
impairments of mentalisation, 424
negative affectivity, 425
problems of self-actualisation, 425
dhat (semen loss anxiety), 719
Di Forti, M., 220
diabetes, 194, 271, 589, 591
antipsychotics side effect, 268
prevention and control (integrated approach), 693
diabetes mellitus, 518, 519
di-acetyl morphine: same as 'heroin' (*qv*), 34
diagnosis, 30–62
advances (mid-C20), 34
bipolar I disorder, 163–5
bipolar II disorder, 165
depression treatment, 128–9
dimensions and disease definition, 36
factitious disorders, 399–400
FND, 369–70
operational criteria, 35
personality disorder, 429–30
primary care, 728
psychosis (risk and mediating factor), 233
purpose, 36–7
stigma, 40–1
diagnosis (criticisms and disadvantages), 37–9
dehumanisation, 38
mental illness 'myth', 38–9
reductionism, 37
unreliability, 38
validity lacking, 37–8
Diagnostic and Statistical Manual of Mental Disorders, See DSM
diagnostic category: describes condition (rather than labels person), 37
diagnostic interview for social and communication disorders (DISCO), 531

diagnostic nihilism, 41
diagnostic systems: mental disorders, 41
dialectical behavioural therapy, 381, 400, 422, 426, 429
  personality disorder, 436–7
  self harm, 679
DIALOG, 284, 770, 789, 794, 798
diazepam, 39, 171, 257
dichloro-diphenyl-trichloroethane (DDT), 513
dicyclomine, **646**
DIDMOAD: key to abbreviation, 518
Diem's, 211
diet: improvement (integrated approach), 694–5
diffusion tensor imaging (DTI), 461
digit span test, 463
digital technology, 798–9
Dilthey, W., 32, 49
dimensional assessments (listed), 201
Diogenes syndrome, 448
diphenhydramine, **646**
directed acyclic graphs (DAGs), 20
  acyclic element, 20
  definition, 20
  directed element, 20
  introduction, 20–1
  nodes and edges, 20
disability-adjusted life years (DALYs): definition, 85
disclosure, 428
discontinuation syndrome, 131
disease entity, 35, 37
disease odds ratio, 13
disease risk ratio, 13
diseases, 35
  definition (Scadding), 36
disgust sensitivity, 345
disinhibition, 491
  definition, 419, 427
disorder
  features (quantitative definition), 35
  morbid risk, 10
  post-test odds, 10
  post-test odds (formula), 9
  post-test probability, 10
  post-test probability (formula), 9
  pre-test odds, 10
  pre-test odds (formula), 9
  symptomological approach, 36
disorder frequency
  incidence, 11–12
  prevalence, 10–11
disorganisation
  dimension of psychopathology in schizophrenia, 213
  schizophrenic symptom, 212
displacement (defence mechanism), 743
dissociality, 445, 446
  definition, 419, 427
dissociation, 379
  ICD-11, 379
dissociative amnesia, 373
dissociative experiences, 424
dissociative neurological symptom disorder, *See* functional neurological disorder
dissociative seizures, 481
distress, 50
  key element to qualify as disorder, 48
disulfiram, 649
DIT, *See* dynamic interpersonal therapy
divorce, 169
dizygotic (DZ) twins, 102, 224
dizziness, 374
DNA methylation (DNAm), 226
doctors
  primary task, 30
  suicide risk exaggerated, 667
domestic violence, 607, 666
Dominguez, M-G., 216
donepezil, 472
dopamine, 194, 199, 234–5, 487, 541, 553
dopamine active transporter (DAT) scan, 264
dopamine antagonists, *See* antipsychotics
dopamine D2 receptor gene (DRD2), 224
dopamine receptors, 242
dopamine supersensitivity, 249
dopamine transporter SPECT imaging (DaTscan), 462
dopamine transporter single-photon emission computed tomography (DAT-SPECT), 371
dorsolateral syndrome, 465
double depression, 79
double empathy problem: definition, 529
double orientation, 205
Dowrick, C., 729
drama triangle, 427, 429
dressing apraxia, 469
Dressler, W. W., 711
Driver and Vehicle Licensing Agency, 173
drug interactions: treatment of psychoses, 271–2
drug treatments for depression (classification), 108–24
  'augmentory' medications, 117–22
  antidepressants, 108–17
  antiepileptics, 119–20
  antipsychotics (dopamine antagonists), 117–18
  buspirone, 120
  experimental medications, 122–4
  ketamine, 121–2
  lithium salts, 118–19
  pindolol, 120–1
drug use, 52, 509–10, 696
  cannabis, 510
  hallucinogens, 510
  opiates, 510
  stimulants, 509–10
drugs
  assessment (three key elements), 639
  association with mental disorders, 741
Drummond, L. M., 324–31, 334–59
DSM-I, 46
  published (1952), 47
DSM-II, 47
DSM-III, 35, 41, 47, 65, 356
  ADHD, 539
  ASPD, 447
  autism, 528
  BPD, 664
  bulimia nervosa, 588
  impulse control disorders, 453
  personality disorder, 408
  PTSD, 314
  published (1980), 200
  specifications, 47
  switch to symptom-based definitions, 47
DSM-IV, 8, 39, 46, 47, 48, 370
  anorexia nervosa, 577
  ASPD, 447
  Asperger's syndrome, 528
  eating disorders, 587
  gambling, 453
  hypochondriasis, 394
  impulse control disorders, 452, 453
  malingering, 400
  pain disorders, 396
  personality disorder, 404, **408**, 408, 409, 447, 448
  PTSD, 315
  published (1994), 48
  specific phobia, 324
  STPD, 449
DSM-5, 2, 31, 39, 40, 42, 43, 401, 444
  ADHD (five components), 540
  alcohol use in pregnancy, 621
  anorexia nervosa, 574–5
  ARFID, 587
  ASPD, 446, 447
  autism, 527, 529
  autism spectrum disorder, 528
  AVPD, 450
  BDD, 387
  bipolar disorder, 162
  brief psychosis (puerperal), 600
  bulimia nervosa, 588
  cultural formulation, 714, 719, 720
  culture, 700
  culture bound syndromes, 718, 719
  dependent personality disorder, 451
  depressive disorders (classification), 72, **73**
  depressive disorders (principal severity and course descriptors), 74
  diagnostic categories, 47
  eating disorders, 565
  excoriation disorder, 355
  factitious disorders, 397, 398, 399, 400
  functional neurological disorder, 368–9, 370
  gambling, 453, 454
  gaming disorder, 455
  history, 46–8
  hoarding disorder, 353
  hypochondriasis, 356
  impulse control disorders, 452
  intermittent explosive disorder, 456
  kleptomania, 457
  major depressive disorders (principal severity and course descriptors), 74
  melancholia, 662
  mild neurocognitive disorder, 501
  mood episode qualifiers and specifiers, 75
  narcissistic personality disorder, 450
  neurodevelopmental disorders, 527
  non-substance addictive disorders, 453
  non-suicidal self injury, 676, 677
  obsessive-compulsive personality disorder, 451, 452
  other personality disorders, 452
  pain disorders, 396
  paranoid personality disorder, 448
  personality change due to medical condition, 452
  personality disorder, 404, 406, 407, 416
  personality disorders (clusters A, B, C), 447–8
  PND, 608
  postpartum psychosis, 600
  PTSD, 314–15
  published (2013), 200
  puerperal schizophrenia, 600
  pyromiania, 457
  schizophrenia, 201
  schizophrenia spectrum and other psychotic disorders, 200–1
  somatic symptom and related disorders, 388
  specific phobia, 324, 325
  STPD, 449
  substance use disorder (SUD), 636
  suicidal behaviour disorder, 676
  ultimate origins (1840), 46
  used in USA, 62
DSWPD, *See* delayed sleep-wake phase disorder
dual action uptake inhibitors, *See* serotonin and noradrenaline re-uptake inhibitors
duloxetine, **109**, 110, 111, **132**, 135
  diverse effects, 110
  not to be prescribed to liver-disease and narrow-angle glaucoma patients, 111
dura mater, 469
duration of untreated psychosis (DUP), 216, 232, 236, 788
  psychosis (risk and mediating factor), 233
Durkheim, É., 7, 659, 660, 661, 668, 682
  suicide, 6–7
  Suicide (1897), 656
  suicide (four types), 659
dynamic interpersonal therapy (DIT), 154, 155
dyscalculia, 469
dysfunctional assumptions, 101–2
dysfunctional attitudes scale, 101
dysgraphia, 469
dyskinesia
  orofacial, 211
  tardive, 211
  trunk-and-limb, 211
dyslexia, 468
dyslipidaemia, 269
dysthymia, 79, 83, 84, 85
  'relatively little clinical recognition', 79
dysthymic disorder, 79
dystonia, 486–7

definition, 486
motor FND, 371
motor side effect (antipsychotics), 264–5
symptoms (behavioural), 487
treatment, 487

early intervention, 786, 788–90
longer-term outcome, 789
early intervention (psychosis), 788
early intervention in psychosis (EIP), 24
early intervention teams (EITs), 788
early maladaptive schemas, 437
ease of use: criterion for assessing psychiatric classification systems, 41
East Africa, 621
East Asia, 84
Eastern Europe, 488
eating disorder examination (EDE-Q), 570
eating disorders, 2, 533, 565–92
anorexia nervosa, 573–87
ARFID, 587–8
assessment, 569–70
binge-eating disorder, 591–2
biology, 569
bulimia nervosa, 588–91
CBT-E, 571–2
comorbidities, 572
diagnostic systems (DSM-5, ICD-10, ICD-11), **566**
epidemiology, 565
general hospital setting, 746–7
impact on individual and society, 568–9
males, 568
medical emergencies, 572–3
nine truths (explanations), **567**
outcome measurement, 570
perinatal psychiatry, 614
psychopathology (example questions), 570
time trends and population demographics, 565–8
treatment, 570–1
Ebstein's cardiac anomaly, 174
écho de la pensée, 202
echocardiography, 579, 604
echolalia: definition, 72
echopraxia, 208
definition, 72
ecological bias, 14
ecological fallacy, 14
ecological studies, 14
economic crises: suicide risk, 667–8
ECT, *See* electroconvulsive therapy
Edinburgh, 600, 601
Edinburgh postnatal depression scale (EPDS), 606, 608
EDNOS (eating disorder not otherwise specified), 587
educational history, 51
Edwards, M. J., 378
effect modification, 14
effect sizes, 18
power calculations, 27
ego-boundary disturbance, 53
Ehlers-Danlos syndrome, 327, 532
Einheit psychosen (unitary psychosis), 32
Eisenberg, L.: 'disease' versus 'illness', 711
elaborate belief systems, 338
electoral register data, 12
electrocardiogram (ECG), 170, 695
electroconvulsive therapy, 137, 252, 598, 602
bipolar disorder, 177
catatonia treatment, 259–60
liaison psychiatry patients, 755
electroconvulsive therapy for depression, 124–6
background, 124–5
contraindications, 126
mechanism of action, 125
side effects, 125
electroencephalography (EEG), 372, 446, 462, 504
OCD, 343
purpose, 549
electrolytes, 520–2, 591
electronic patient records (EPRs), 57, 58
electrooculogram: purpose, 549
elevated mood, 162
Ellis, A., 44
Emery, G., 330
emic and etic instruments, 714
Emminghaus, H., 44
emotional dysregulation, 407, 408, 427, 435
emotional regulation groups (ERG), 429
emotionally-unstable personality disorder, 339, 532, 576, 589, 630
empathy, 50, 528
employment, *see* employment stress; employment support; jobs
employment stress, 159
employment support, 791
Enara, A., 324–31, 334–59
encephalitis, 491–2
cause, 491
diagnosis (essential steps), 492
presentation, 491
treatment, 492
endocannabinoid system, 244
endocrine disorders, 516–18
endogenous psychosis (Group II mental disorders), 33
endophenotypes: definition, 225
Engel, G. L., 43, 740
England, 84, 91, 95, 96, 105, 228, 397, 530, 676, 683, 694, 729, 732, 768, 773
children looked after by local authorities, 624
law, 457
psychological problems (2014), 76
self harm (annual cost to NHS), 677
England and Wales, 194, 195, 420, 540, 585, 659, 666, 670, 757, 759
coroner's court (narrative verdict), 656
coroner's court (suicide verdict), 656
stillbirth rate, 616
young people (suicide rate), 660
English longitudinal study of ageing, 15
enhanced CBT, 571
enhanced primary care (EPC), 734
key elements, 734
enhancing neuroimaging genetics through meta-analysis (ENIGMA), 235, 342
environmental risk factors (psychosis), 227–30
advanced paternal age, 227
adverse life events, 228
cannabis and other substance use, 228–9
childhood adversity, 227–8
conclusion, 229–30
cumulative effect, 229
gene-environment interaction, 229
pregnancy and birth complications, 227
social adversities and trauma, 227–8
social geography, 228
ephedrine, 511
epidemics: etymology, 6
epidemiologic catchment area studies (USA), 338
epidemiology, 6–28, 89
ADHD, 539
alcohol-related brain damage, 505–6
anorexia nervosa, 577
anxiety disorders, 295–6
ASPD, 446
associations (measures of strength), 12–13
BDD, 390–1
binge-eating disorder, 591
branches, 7–8
bulimia nervosa, 588
causation, 19–27
critical appraisal, 27
definition, 6
depressive disorders, 84–5
eating disorders, 565
exposures, outcomes, confounders, 8
functional neurological disorder, 369
gambling, 454
hypochondriasis, 394
internal versus external validity, 27
measures of disorder frequency (prevalence and incidence), 10–12
measures of impact, 13–14
mental illness (primary care), 726–8
OCD, 340
paranoid personality disorder, 448–9
physical and psychiatric comorbidity, 744–5
puerperal psychoses, 601
self harm, 676–7
study designs, 14–19
suicide, 659–62
trichotillomania, 354
epidemiology measures (reliability), 8–9
inter-item reliability, 9
inter-rater reliability, 8
test-retest reliability, 8
epidemiology measures (validity), 9–10
concurrent validity (sensitivity and specificity), 9–10
formulae, 9
types, 9
epigenetics, 226, 421
definition, 226
epigenome-wide association studies (EWAS), 226
epilepsy, 112, 115, 194, 372, 373, 466, 476–81, 620
diagnosis, 476
ictal and peri-ictal phenomena, 477–8
interictal disorders, 478–81
management (main line), 476
organic psychotic disorders, 260
psychological and behavioural approaches, 477
psychosis (aetiologies), **261**
epilepsy (interictal disorders), 478–81
anxiety and affective disorders, 478–80
cognitive impairment, 480–1
forced normalisation, 480
Gastaut-Geschwind syndrome and aggressive behaviours, 480
psychogenic nonepileptic attacks, 481
schizophrenia-like psychosis, 480
types, **479**
epileptic auras, 476
epileptic psychoses, 478
epileptic seizures
definition, 476
elements, 476
prevalence, 476
epileptic seizures (types)
absence seizures, 476
focal seizures, 476
generalised seizures, 476
motor seizures, 476
non-motor seizures with focal onset, 476
epinephrine, 644
episodic memory: definition, 463
epistemic trust, 416, 424
Epworth sleepiness scale, 559
Equality Act (England), 535
Erklaren (explanation), 43, 44
eros (life instinct), 673
error-related negativity (ERN), 343
erythromycin, 194
escitalopram, 109, 129, 348, 349, 350, 612
titration (rapid), 134
Eshun, S., 712
esketamine, 121
Esquirol, J., 598
essential blepharospasm, 486
Estonia, 677
ethnicity, 295
definition, 709
depression differences, 95–6
ethnocentrism, 708
definition, 706
ethylene glycol, 512
EUFEST trial, 247
EUPD, *See* emotionally unstable personality disorder

European Court of Human Rights, 759
euthanasia, 656
euthymia, 157
Evans, S., 415
event-related potential (ERP), 343
Everton in Community, 692
evidence, 28
evidence-based psychological therapies
depression, 147–55
Excellence by Design (GMC framework), 3
excess rate, 12
excess risk, 12
exchangeability, 22
excoriation disorder, *See* skin-picking disorder
definition, 336
executive function testing, 463
executive network, **298**, 298
exogenous steroid administration, 517
experimental studies: causation, 19
experimental study designs, 7
explanatory style, 187
exposure and response prevention (ERP), 346
BDD, 351–2
OCD, 346–7
OCD (outcome), 347
exposure frequency, 19
exposure odds ratio, 13
exposure risk ratio, 13
exposure status, 15
exposures
range, 8
same as 'risk factors' (*qv*), 91
exposures and outcomes, 7, 12
association (causal diagram), *22*
causal association, 13
individual level, 14
expressed emotion (EE), 186, 289
extended consciousness, 422, 424
externalising behaviours, 628
extrapyramidal side effects (EPSEs), 254, 255, **255**, 258, 261, 263–4, 265
extrapyramidal syndromes, 503
eye movement desensitisation and reprocessing (EMDR), 284, 308, 318
PTSD, 318–19
Eysenck, H. J., 328

Fabry disease, 515
face validity, 9
Facebook, 676
facial expression, 71
factitious disorders, 390, 397–400
diagnosis, 399–400
diagnostic evidence (categories), 398
imposed on self, 397–8
malingering, 400
Muchausen by proxy (FII), 398–9
psychopathology, 400
factitious illness imposed (FII) on another, 398–9, 400
DSM-5, 399
falsification (types), 399
intention of perpetrator, 400
perpetrators (classification), 400
psychopathology, 400
factual scenario, 20
Fahr, K. T., 488
Fahr's disease, 488
Fairburn, C. G., 570, 571, 588
faith healer, 721
Fallon, B. A., 395
Fallot's tetralogy, 619
Falret, J-P., 32, 162, 393
false suffocation alarm (FSA), 298
familial basal ganglia calcification (Fahr's disease), 488
familial hyperlipidaemia, 694
family, 185
family history, 51, 664
bipolar disorder, 169
family poverty, 94
family studies: OCD, 341
family therapy, 155, 400, 721
bipolar disorder, 193
family-based treatment, 582
famous professor principle, 31
Farmer, A. E., 214
Farmer, R. D. T., 656
Farr, W., 45
classification of diseases, 45
Farran-Ridge, C., 211
Farrington, D. P., 447
fasting, 573
fatigue, 70
Favazza, A., 677
Fazel, S., 792
fear: 'crucial for survival', 324
fear-circuit, 298
Feighner, J. P., 35, 47, 65
Feldman, E., 743
female genital mutilation (FGM), 625
filicide: definition, 617
Fineberg, N. A., 324–31, 334–59
finger agnosia: definition, 469
Finland, 118, 232, 241, 250, 345, 605, 613, 663, 664, 681, 703
first episode of psychosis (FEP), 230–1, 232, 233, 234
first-generation antipsychotics (FGAs), 254, 255, 263, 264, 265, 267, 613, 619
first-rank symptoms, 54, 201
Fish, F., 49
Fishbain, D. A., 665
fitness to be detained, 61
fitness to be interviewed, 61
fitness to plead, 60, 61
Pritchard criteria (1836), 61
flex-ext sign, 371
flexibilitas cereus (waxy flexibility), 208
flight of ideas, 53
fludeoxyglucose, 462
fluent aphasia, 467
flumazenil, 171, 259, 755
fluorescent treponemal antibody absorption (FTA-Abs), 490
fluorinated hydrocarbons (freons), 513
fluoxetine, 17, 108, **109**, 112, 117, 122, **132**, 134, 171, 272, 348, 350, 456, 590, 604, **612**
combination with olanzapine, 136
hypochondriasis patients, 395
propensity to cause violent episode, 131
risk of abnormalities, 619
fluphenazine, 241
fluvoxamine, **109**, **132**, 134
side effects, 109
FND, *See* functional neurological disorder
FND Action, 380
FND Hope, 380
focal dystonias, 486, 487
focal psychodynamic therapy (FPT), 571, 583
foetal alcohol syndrome (FAS), 48, 620, 621
foetal valproate syndrome, 176
folk explanation, 717–18
Folstein, M. F., 463
Fonagy, P., 154
Food and Drug Administration (FDA, USA), 242, 265, 270
Fore tribe, 494
Foreman, E., 158
forensic psychiatry, 717
formal thought disorder, 53
formulation, 42, 56, 61, 156
definition, 430
five Ps, 42
personality disorder, 430
power threat meaning framework, 430
formulation (five Ps), 430
perpetuating factors, 430
precipitating factors, 430
predisposing factors, 430
presenting problem, 430
protective factors, 430
Foucault, M., 38, 39
Foulds, G. A., 541
FPT, *See* focal psychodynamic therapy
FRAMES structure (alcohol), 644
France, 45, 48, 228, 241, 453, 494, 665, 677, 680, 703, 768
Frances, A., 47
Frank, A., 493
Frank, J. D., 721
Frankl, G., 528
Fraser competence, 757
Frederickson, G. M., 708
free will, 38
Freedom of Information Act (2005), 58
Freeman, W., 464
Frégolie syndrome, 219
Freud, S., 32, 44, 47, 65, 154, 286, 328, 334, 344, 367–8, 422, 460
Beyond Pleasure Principle (1920), 673
'Mourning and Melancholia', 81, 427
Neuro-Psychoses of Defence (1894), 367
on suicide, 673
oral-dependent characters, 451
Studies in Hysteria (1895), 367
Freudian psychoanalysis, 43, 450
Fridericia formula, 266
Fromm, E., 353
frontal assessment battery (FAB), 463
frontal lobe, 464–5, 477
frontal lobotomies, 464
frontotemporal dementia
age of onset, 503
diagnosis, 503
familial cases, 504
neuropathology, 504
presentation, 503
semantic dementia phenotype, 504
temporal lobe variants, 504
frusemide, 175
functional amnesia, 373–4
functional cognitive disorder
symptoms (distinguished from dementia), **374**
functional cognitive disorders, 373
functional coma, 375
definition, 375
functional disability, 748–9
functional magnetic resonance imaging (fMRI), 24, 342, 462
functional mutism (aphonia), 375
functional neurological disorder, 366–81
associated symptoms, 370
comorbidities, 370
conclusions, 381
diagnosis, 366
history, 366–8
modern world, 368
prognosis, 376
subtypes, **368**
functional neurological disorder (aetiology and risk factors), 376–8
biological effects of maltreatment, 377
biological risk, 376
childhood maltreatment, 377
evolution from physical insults or injuries, 377
precipitating factors, 377–8
predisposing factors, 377
social contact (epidemic functional illness), 377–8
functional neurological disorder (clinical features), 368–70
classification (DSM-5-TR and ICD-11), 368–9
epidemiology, 369
functional neurological disorder (diagnosis), 369–70
investigations, 369–70
positive clinical signs, 370
taking history, 369
functional neurological disorder (mechanistic hypotheses), 378–9
Bayesian brain, 378–9
dissociation, 379
neuroimaging (structural and functional), 379
functional neurological disorder (other functional syndromes), 374–6
dizziness, 374
functional coma, 375
functional speech disorders, 374–5
functional urological syndromes, 375–6

persistent postural-perceptual dizziness (PPPD), 374
functional neurological disorder (subtypes), 370–6
functional amnesia, 373–4
functional cognitive disorder, 373
functional seizures, 372–3
motor FND, 370–2
sensory FND, 372
functional neurological disorder (treatments), 379–81
CBT, 380
general principles, 379–80
medication, 381
non-medical treatments, 381
physiotherapy, 380
psychodynamic therapy, 380–1
psychoeducation, 380
psychological therapy, 380–1
functional Parkinsonism, 371–2
functional remediation: bipolar disorder treatment, 192
functional seizures (FND), 372–3
functional stupor, *See* functional coma
functional urological syndromes, 375–6
funding, 1

gabapentin, 304–5
class C controlled substance (2019), 304
gabapentinoids, 304–5
non-prescribed use (principles of clinical management), **305**
property, 304
uses, 304
Gage, P., 464, 465
Gail, M. H., 13
Galen, 64, 366, 696
Galenic syndrome, 420
Gall, F., 460
Gamblers Anonymous, 455
gambling, 453–5
aetiology, 454
CBT, 454–5
comorbidity, 454
definition, 453
epidemiology, 454
treatment, 454–5
Gambling with Lives, 668
gameChange (automated VR cognitive therapy), 283
gaming disorder, 455–6
gamma hydroxybutyrate (GHB), 302
gamma-aminobutyric acid (GABA), 235, 301, 316, 327
Ganser syndrome, 501
GAP study, 231, 232, 233, 234
Gask, L., 726–36
Gastaut, H., 480
Gastaut-Geschwind syndrome, 479, 480
Gates, W. H., 44
Gaughran, F., 241–72
Gaupp, R., 219
Gaw, A., 719
Gedankenlautwerden, 54, 202
Gee, H., 427
Gelfand, M. J., 703–4, 708
gender, 701, 717
depression differences, 93–4, 96
gender roles, 721, 744
gene disorders, 89
gene-environment correlation, 103–4
definition, 103, 229
gene-environment interaction, 104
psychosis risk factor, 229
general adult psychiatry services, 777–84
acute inpatient care, 777–80
aggressive behaviour, 782
community treatment orders, 781–2
intensive care units, 782–3
patient discharge, 781
patient disempowerment, 781
rehabilitation, 783–4
section 117 aftercare, 782
ward management (difficulties), 781
ward management (initial), 781
general health questionnaire (GHQ), 9–10, 728
general hierarchy of systems, 701
general hospital setting, 745
liaison psychiatry patients (management), 752–7
Mental Health Act (1983), 757–9
psychiatry, 739–62
general hospital setting (psychiatric assessment), 750–2
assessment by non-psychiatrists, 750
CL psychiatry assessment, 751–2
diagnosis, 752
referrals to CL psychiatry, 751
screening and standardised tests, 750–1
general hospital setting (psychiatric conditions), 745–7
adjustment disorders, 746
alcohol-related disorders, 747
depressive disorder, 745–6
eating disorders, 746–7
organic mental disorder, 746
phobic anxiety disorder, 746
PTSD, 747
general medicine, 35
general paralysis of insane (GPI), 34, 36
general practitioners, 9, 10, 58, 726
average list size, 727
burnout, 776
consultation style, 728
NHSE dementia resource, 731
training about mental health, 735
General Register Office of England and Wales, 45
generalised anxiety disorder (beta blockers)
exercise, 307
medications after non-response, 307
pharmacological treatment (long-term), 306
pharmacological treatment (short-term), 306
psychological interventions, 307
generalised anxiety disorder (GAD), 330, 474, 614
beta blockers, 306–7
causes, 296–7
diagnosis, 293
epidemiology, 295
onset predicted by phobic disorders, 326
generalised anxiety disorder scale-7 items (GAD-7), 795
Generic Professional Capabilities (GMC framework), 3
genetics, 89, 410, 421
bipolar disorder, 169
OCD, 340–1
studying heritability (other methods), 341
genetics of depression, 102–4
candidate genes, 102
genes and environments (correlation and interaction), 103–4
GWAS, 102–3
major concern, 102
twin studies, 102
genius (artistic), 169
genome-wide association studies, 169, 341, 576, 577
genetics of depression, 102–3
psychosis risk factors, 225
sample sizes, 102
geriatric depression scale, 750
Germany, 34, 48, 84, 109, 199, 327, 574, 583, 618, 668, 677, 703, 704, 768
domination in psychiatric nosology (C19), 32
Gerstmann syndrome, 466, 469, 475
Gerstmann, J., 469
Gerstmann–Sträussler syndrome, 494
Geschwind, N., 460, 480
Ghana, 609
Gianino, A., 423
Gibbons, R., 683
Gilbert, P., 158
Gilbody, S., 691
Gillespie, R., 393
girls, 488
Glasgow antipsychotic side-effect scale for clozapine (GASS-C), 270
Glasgow coma scale, 470
global aphasia, 468
Global Burden of Disease, 89
globus hystericus, 393
globus pallidus necrosis, 681
glucagon-like peptide (GLP-1) agonists, 694, 695
glutamate, 342
Gnanapragasam, S., 699–722
Goddard, S. ('Adam Ant'), 166
Goldberg, D., 726
Goldberger, J., 7
Gooch, R., 598
Good Medical Practice, 3, 4
good psychiatric management, 425
Goodman, W. K., 342
Goodwin, F. K., 162
Goodwin, G. M., 328
Google Play, 158
Gorbachev, M., 681
Gotland Programme, 682
Gottesman, I. I., 224
GPs, *See* general practitioners
Granger, K., 688
grapefruit juice, 272
Graves, T. D., 710
Gray, J., 398
Great Depression (1930s), 667
Great Smoky Mountains longitudinal study, 92
Greece, 667
Green, B., 399
Greenberger, D., 158
Greenland, S., 20, 26
grief, 154, 705, 728
perinatal loss, 616
grief-related depression, 81–3
complicated grief, 82
normal grief, 81–2
Griesinger, W., 32, 199, *461*
grievance: role in avoiding grieving, 427
Griffiths Report (1983), 776
group A beta-haemolytic streptococci, 343
group psychotherapy: personality disorder, 437–8
group suicides, 718
group therapy, 155
guanfacine, 541, 542
guilt, 67–8
Guislain, J., 64
Gull, W. W., 574, 582
gun control, 680
Gurung, A., 712
gustatory hallucinations, 54
GWAS, *See* genome-wide association studies

Hachinski, V., 504
haemorrhagic stroke, 473
hair pulling disorder, *See* trichotillomania
Hallopeau, F., 354
hallucinations
definition, 71
definition (strictest), 204
mental state examination, 54
schizophrenia, 203–4
hallucinogens: neuropsychiatric manifestations, 510
haloperidol, 124, 171, 211, 233, 258, 349, 612, 754
Hamilton depression scale, 129, 464
Hamilton, J., 603
Hamilton, M. W., 49
Hamilton, S. F., 167
Han Chinese, 176
hand drop test, 375
hanging, 514, 657, 666, 671, 672
Hannon, E. L., 226
haptic hallucinations, 54
Harding, C. M., 216
Hare, R. D., 445, **445**
Harlow, J., 464
Harper, S., 435
Harrington, J. R., 703, 704, 708
Harris, E. C., 663
Harrow, M., 231
Hartman, T. C., 391
Hartnup disease, 519
Havana, 718
Hawton, K., 677, 745
head injuries, 452
ASPD (earlier onset), 446
Headspace, 158
health anxiety, 392
definition, 393

health anxiety (cont.)
  measurement, 394
health anxiety questionnaire, 394
Health Check, 729
Health Education England, 59, 415
Health Foundation of England, 749
Health of Nation (1991), 769
health of nation outcome scales, 798
health resource groups (HRGs), 774
Health Survey for England
  (2014), 638
  (2018), 638
  (2019), 565, 566, 568, 570
health: definition (WHO), 39
Healthcare Safety Investigation Branch, 56
healthcare use, 749–50
health-related quality of life (HRQoL), 542, 748
Hearing Voices groups, 289
heart disease: most possible causes 'neither necessary nor sufficient', 89
hebephrenia, 199, 212
Hecker, E., 199
Hegel, G. W. F., 49
Heidelberg School, 41, 43
Helbich, M., 14
Helms, J. E., 707
help-seeking behaviour: social factors, 743–4
hemidystonia, 487
Hempel, C. G., 35
Henderson Hospital, 414, 415
Henderson, D. K., 444
Hendin, H., 674
hepatic encephalopathy, 508
hepatic impairment, 138
hepatitis, 641, 642, 644
hepato-lenticular degeneration (Wilson's disease), 487
heritability, 341
Hernan, M., 8, 20, 21, *23*
heroin, 641, 644
  OAT, 647–8
  pregnancy, 621
  relapse-prevention medication, 649
  UK information, **640**
herpes simplex virus, 491
Heschl's gyrus, 465
hierarchy, 701
  diagnostic, 42–3
high culture, 699
high density lipoprotein cholesterol (HDL-C), 678
Hindus, 706
Hinshelwood, R. D., 417, 418
hippocampus, 466
Hippocrates, 6, 64, 162, 460, 478, 598, 696
Hirsch, S. R., 207
histrionic personality disorder, 450
Hitch, S., 768
HIV, *See* human immunodeficiency virus
HM Prison and Probation Service, 415
hoarding, 452
hoarding disorder, 352–4
  management, 353–4
  OCRD, 336
Hoenig, J., 49
Hofstede, G., 700, 701–3, 704, 706
holistic approach, 739
  fourteen potential areas for intervention, 691
  physical health conditions (assessment), *690*
  severe mental illness (comorbid physical conditions), 688–97
holistic approach (issues facing mental health teams), 690
  1. acute physical illness (recognition of presentations), 690
  2. longer-term conditions (recognition), 690
  3. longer-term conditions (management), 690
Hollander, A-C., 6
Holzman, P. S., 207, 211
home treatment, 786, 796
home treatment teams, 786
homelessness, 521, 780, 787
  history, 792
homeostatic sleep drive (process S), 548, 549
HOMES multi-disciplinary risk assessment, 353
homicide cases, 61
homlessness, 791–3
homocystinurias, 515
homosexuality, 38, 47, 337
Hong Kong, 340, 657, 681, 682
Hoover's sign, 370
Hope, J. M., 599
hopelessness, 67
  suicide, 662
hopelessness (challenged), 156–7
  cost-benefit analysis of suicide, 157
  review of depressive episodes and euthymia, 157
  time projection, 157
Hopwood, J. S., 617
hormone withdrawal effects, 608
Horne-Ostberg morningness-eveningness questionnaire, 555
Horwitz, A. V., 46
hospital anxiety and depression scale (HADS), 608, 728, 745, 747, 748, 750
hospital wandering, 398
hospitalisation: psychosis outcome indicator, 232
hot and cold (cultural concept), 720
Hounsfield, G., 461
House, A., 740
housing, 94, 771, 777, 779, 782, 791–3
Howe, A., 414–39
Hsu, F. L., 705
Hughlings-Jackson, J., 460
Hui, C. L. M., 249
human immunodeficiency virus, 261, 488–90, 641, 642, 644
  antiretroviral therapy, 490
  anxiety, 489
  cognitive impairment, 489
  dementia, 489, 490
  depression, 488
  later stages (psychiatric disorders, epilepticc seizures), 489
  mania, 489
  psychiatric disorders (bidrectional relationship), 489
  psychiatric symptoms, 488
  psychopharmacology, 489
  psychotic symptoms, 489
humoral theory, 64, 718
Hungary: suicide, 659
Hunt, I. M., 662
huntingtin protein (Htt), 485
Huntington, G., *485*
Huntington's disease, 265, 485–6
  cause, 485
  depression (clinical manifestations), 486
  juvenile form, 485
  organic psychotic disorders, 261
  presentation, 486
  psychosis, 486
  treatment, 485
Husserl, E., 49
Huxley, P., 726
hydrocephalus, 505
hygiene, 345
hyperadrenalism, 516
hyperemesis gravidarum, 519, 619, 620
hyperglycaemia, 518
Hypericum perforatum (St. John's wort), 122
hyperkalaemia, 521
hypermagnesaemia, 521
hypernatraemia, 521
hyperparathyroidism, 517
hyperprolactinaemia, 263
hypersalivation, 270
hypersomnia, 559, 606
hypersomnolence disorders, 559–61
  assessment, 560
  hypersomnia associated with psychiatric disorder, 560
  hypersomnia due to medical disorder, 559
  hypersomnia due to medication or substance, 559
  idiopathic hypersomnia, 560
  insufficient sleep syndrome, 559
  narcolepsy, 560
  psychiatric conditions, 560
  treatment, 561
hypertensive crisis, 114, 115
hyperthyroidism, 516
hypervitaminosis A, 520
hypnotics, 551, 555
  choice, 551
hypocalcaemia, 521
hypochondrial region, 392
hypochondriasis, 35, 355–9, 392–5
  aetiology, 394
  case history (Ash), 357–9
  classification, 356
  clinical features, 393–4
  definition, 69, 336
  definition (literal), 392
  differential diagnosis, 394
  epidemiology, 394
  ICD-11, 393
  location in major classification systems, **356**
  management, 394–5
  measurement, 394
  psychopharmacology, 356
  reassurance, 395
  recent (C19-) understanding, 393
  therapy chart, *358*
  treatment, 356–9
  treatment (psychological), 357–9
  Whiteley index, 394, 395
hypocretin, 560
hypoglycaemia, 518
hypokalaemia, 521
hypomagnesaemia, 521
hypomania, 630
  mental state examination, 165–6
hypomanic episodes (bipolar I disorder), 164
  1. elevated mood, 164
  2. associated symptoms, 164
  3. change in functioning, 164
  4. observable to others, 164
  5. impairment of functioning, 164
  6. not consequence of other medical condition, 164
hyponatraemia, 521, 522
hypoparathyroidism, 517
hypophosphataemia, 521
hypopituitarism, 517
hypopnoeas, 558
hypothalamic-pituitary-adrenal (HPA) axis, 99, 100, 123, 170, 185, 228, 235, 298, 377, 500
hypothesis testing, 26, 92
hypothyroidism, 516, 521, 754
hypoxic brain injury, 514
hysteria, 366, 367
hysterical seizures, 481

IAPT, *See* improving access to psychological therapies
ICD scheme, 45–6
ICD-6 (1948): first WHO version, 46
ICD-8 (1968), 35, 46
ICD-9 (1979), 46, 65
ICD-10, 8, 41, 46
  alcohol dependence (diagnostic criteria), **637**
  Asperger's syndrome, 528
  autism, 529
  AVPD, 450
  BDD, 387
  depressive disorders (classification), 72, **73**
  eating disorders, 566, 587
  impulse control disorders, 452, 453
  pain disorders, 396
  personality disorder, 404, 406, **408**, 409, 419, 448
  published (1992), 65
  somatoform disorders, 388
ICD-11, 2, 31, 42, 43, 46, 65, 401, 444
  acute and transient [puerperal] psychosis, 600
  ADHD, 541
  adjustment disorder, 746
  alcohol dependence (diagnostic criteria), **637**
  anankastia, 451
  anorexia nervosa, 574–5
  approved (2019), operational (2022), 200
  ARFID, 587
  ASPD, 446
  autism, 527, 529
  autism spectrum disorder, 528
  AVPD, 450
  BDD, 387

chapter six (mental, behavioural or neurodevelopmental disorders), 46
chronic primary pain, 396–7
depressive disorders (classification), 72, 73
depressive disorders (principal severity and course descriptors), 74
eating disorders, 565
factitious disorders, 397, 398, 400
functional neurological disorder, 368–9
gambling, 453
gaming disorder, 455
hypochondriasis, 356, 393
intermittent explosive disorder, 456
internet gaming disorder, 452
major depression, 746
major depressive disorders (principal severity and course descriptors), 74
mood episode qualifiers and specifiers, 75
neurodevelopmental disorders, 527
non-substance addictive disorders, 453
opioid dependence, 647
other personality disorders, 452
personality disorder, 426, 447, 448
personality disorder (implications of new classification), 404–11
personality disorder classification, 419–25
post-partum psychosis, 600
primary care classification, 728
PTSD, 314–16
pyromiania, 457
ratification (2019), 45
schizophrenia, 201–2
schizophrenia and other primary psychotic disorders, 200–1
specific phobia, 324–5
STPD, 449
suicide attempts, 676
used throughout world (except USA), 62
ICD-11 for Mortality and Morbidity Statistics (online, 2022), 46
ictal dissociative symptoms, 478
ictal emotions, 477
ictal flashbacks, 478
ictal psychiatric symptoms, 477
ictal violence, 478
ideational apraxia, 468
identity, 701
identity disturbance, 405
ideomotor apraxia, 469
idiopathic hypersomnia, 560
idiopathic psychosis, 260
Idiots Act (UK, 1886), 40
Ikkos, G., 396
Illiffe, S., 731
illness
biomedical versus biopsychosocial models, 740
cognitive model of reaction (Leventhal), *742*
illness anxiety, *See* hypochondriasis
illness attitude test, 394
illness behaviour, 742
definition (Mechanic), 743
illness perception questionnaire, 748
illness representations
attributes, 742
processes, 742
illusions: schizophrenia, 203–4
imagery rehearsal therapy (IRT), 557
imipramine, 111, 241
Impey, B., 293–310
Improving Access to Psychological Therapies, 39, 59, 155, 156, 159, 289, 392, 610, 729, 732, 735, 756, 771, 773, 788, 789, 794–5, 798. *See also* talking treatments
impulse control disorders, 335, 452–3
inception cohort, 16
incidence, 11–12
definition, 11
incidence density sampling, 13
incidence measures: calculation, *11*
incidence rate, 10, 11–12
definition, 11
formula, 11
incidence rate ratios, 13
independent mental capacity advocate (IMCA), 759
index of multiple deprivation (IMD), 95
India, 241, 340, 488, 513, 600, 601, 604, 660, 678, 680, 701, 704, 705, 707, 718, 719
infanticide, 618
individual placement and support (IPS), 791
individuals, 690
interviewed within own home, 15
individuation, 422
inequalities, 703
infant mortality, 608
infanticide, 617–18
definition, 617
Infanticide Act (England and Wales, 1938), 617
infants: effects of maternal PND, 609–10
infectious diseases, 488–95
CNS infections (other), 492–5
encephalitis, 491–2
human immunodeficiency virus, 488–90
meningitis, 491
syphilis, 490–1
inflammation, 98, 99, 100, 194
infliximab, 123
influenza vaccination, 696
information bias, 24–5
definition, 24
observer bias, 24–5
recall bias, 24
types, 24
informed consent, 428, 435, 757
Ingraham, L. J., 224
inhibitors, 511
injection phobia, 328
injury phobia, 328
inpatient costs, 282
insecticide poisoning (suicide method), 661
insight: mental state examination, 55
insomnia, 156, 550–2
assessment, 551
CBT-I, 551
comorbidity, 550, 551
definition, 550
link with major depressive disorder, 550–1
prevalence, 550
psychiatric condition in own right, 550
types, 70
insomnia (treatment), 551–2
medication, 551
non-medical, 551–2
instinctual affects, 423
Institute of Group Analysis, 437
Institute of Psychiatry, 726
institutional racism, 708–9
causes, 709
definition, 708
impact on individuals, 709
impact on services, 709
instrumental variable analysis, 92
insufficient sleep syndrome, 550, 559
insulinomas, 518
integrated behavioral health home, 734
integrated care systems (ICS), 773
integrated psychosis, 214
integrated psychotic disorder, 221
intellectual disability, 717
intensive care units (psychiatric), 782–3
interface and continuity issues, 795–9
interim care order (ICO), 625
interleukin 6 (IL-6), 98
intermittent explosive disorder, 456–7
management of aggression, 456–7
internal validity (of research studies), 27
International Classification of Diseases, See ICD
International Classification of Sleep Disorders, 550, 556
international clubhouse model, 784
International Congress of Alienists (Paris, 1867), 32
International League Against Epilepsy, 373
International Pilot Study of Schizophrenia (IPSS), 35, 203, 233, 701
International Restless Legs Syndrome Study Group, 553
International Society for Traumatic Stress Studies, 317, 319, 320
International Statistical Congress (Brussels, 1853), 45
internet, 716
internet gaming disorder, 48
internet-based CBT (iCBT), 152, 307, 308, 309
interpersonal and social rhythm therapy (ISRT), 192
interpersonal dysfunction, 405
interpersonal model, 45
interpersonal psychotherapy (IPT), 795
perinatal depression, 613
interpersonal therapy, 153–4, 158
clinical application, 153
efficacy, 154
managing depressive state, 154
targeting problem areas, 154
theoretical framework, 153
inter-rater reliability, 24, 38
tests (basis), 35
interviewing style, 57
intimate partner violence (IPV), 421, 606
intraclass correlation coefficient, 8
intra-rater reliability, 38
inventory of gambling situations, 455
iodine deficiency, 521
ioflupane, 462
Iowa City, 683
iproniazid, 34
first antidepressant (1952), 113
hepatotoxicity, 113
IPT, *See* interpersonal therapy
Iran, 660, 678
iron deficiency, 521
irregular sleep-wake rhythm disorder, 553
irritability, 68
ischaemic heart disease, 394
ischaemic stroke, 473
Islam, 659, 668, 718
isocarboxazid, 113
isolated phobias, 294
isomorphic process, 425
isoniazid, 113, 519
isopropanol vapour, 512
Israel, 605, 606, 610, 664
ISTSS, *See* International Society for Traumatic Stress Studies
Italy, 228, 241, 377, 583, 761, 768
iTunes, 158

Jablensky, A., 41
Jacobson, N. S., 153
Jakob, A. M., 494
Jamaica, 707
James. W., 462
Jamison, K. R., 162
Janet, P., 367, 379
Jansen, J., 353
Jansson, B., 601
Japan, 296, 305, 618, 659, 665, 681, 703, 768
Jaspers, K., 30, 34, 35, 37, 41, 43, 44, 56
classification of psychiatric disorders, *33*
General Psychopathology (1913, 1959), 32, 33, 41, 49, 50, 54, 688, 694
Jastrowitz, M., 465
jauhar, 718
Jeffery, A., 6–28
jet lag disorder, 553
job demands-resources model, 777
jobs, 25, 449, 453, 722, 776, 791. *See also* employment
joint strategic needs assessment (JSNA), 773
Jones, A., 396
Jongsma, H. E., 16
judgement thoughts, 437
jumping from tall buildings (suicide method), 657, 661, 681
Jung, C., 414, 422

Kafka, J. S., 677
Kahlbaum, K., 162, 199
Kandola, A., 18
Kanner, 528
Kant, I., 30, 49
Karnosh, L. J., 599
Karpman, S., 427
Kasanin, J., 198, 217, 218
Katz, J., 396
Kayser-Fleischer rings, 487
Kempe, C. H., 624
Kendell, R. E., 36, 38, 41, 601
Kendler, K. S., 31, 65
Kendrick, T., 730
Keown, P., 14
Kępińska, A. P., 224–36
Kernberg, O. F., 154
Kerner, C., 708
ketamine, 121–2, 136, 244, 381, 510
  contraindications, 122
  interactions, 122
  mechanism of action, 121
  pharmacokinetics, 121
  side effects, 121
  toxicity in overdose, 122
Kety, S. S., 224, 462
Keys, A., 574
khat: pregnancy, 621
kidney: lithium side effects, 173
Kierkegaard, S., 682
Kingdon, D., 1–2, 30–62, 282–90, 387–401, 767–99
Kingston-upon-Hull, 683
Kirby, G.: Guide for Clinical Examination of Psychiatric Cases (1921), 43, 49
Kircher, T., 207
Kirkbride, J. B., 6–28
Kirmayer, L. J., 394, 699
Klein, D. F., 298
Klein, M., 154
Kleine-Levin syndrome, 590
Kleinman, A., 699, 711
Kleinman, A. M., 714
Kleist, K., 41
kleptomania, 457
Klerman, G. L., 153
Klüver, H., 466
Klüver-Bucy syndrome, 466
Knights, A., 207
Knowledge and Understanding Framework (KUF), 415
knowledge base, 2
Korea, 677, 681
koro syndrome, 718
Korsakoff syndrome, 506, 507, 585
Korsakoff, S., *506*, 506
Kraepelin, E., 32, 35, 41, 42, 64, 77, 162, 168, 198, 199, 211, 212, 214, 224, 694
  clinical description, 49
  contribution to classification, 33–4
  dementia praecox (essential feature), 199
  Lehrbuch der Psychiatrie, 33
Krafft-Ebing, R. von, 64
Krahn, L. E., 398
Kräupl-Taylor, F., 36
Kretschmer, E., 448, 450
Kübler-Ross, E., 81
Kukopoulos, A., 162
kuru epidemic, 494
labelling, 38, 148, 150. *See also* stigma
Laborit, H-M., 241
lack of capacity (legal defence), 61
Lacroix, F. B. de, 31
lactic acidosis, 518
Laing, R. D., 39
Lally, J., 231
Lambeth early onset trial, 233
lamotrigine, 171, 172, 418, 435, 456, 511, **612**, 620
  antiepileptic agent, 270
  long-term prophylaxis, 172
Lancet, 744
Landolt phenomenon, 480
Lange, C., 64
language, 37, 40, 463, 708
Lansky, M., 662
large cell carcinoma, 475
Lasegue, C., 574
Lashley, K., 460
lasting power of attorney, 757
late luteal phase disorder, 81
Latin America, 492, 702, 704
laudanum, 34
law of retaliation (*lex talionis*), 416
Lawlor, D. A., 20
Layard, R., 794
LDL cholesterol, 693
lead poisoning, 512
leaden paralysis, 70
League of Nations, 46
LEARN, 719
learned helplessness theory, 101
learning about thinking emotions & relationships (LATER), 430
lecanemab, 19
leeches, 407
Leeds, 454
Lellouch, J., 327
Leonard, 162
Lépine, J-P., 327
lesions, 35
Lester tool, 691, 693, 694
letter-by-letter dyslexia, 468
Leucht, S., 232, 283
leucotomy, 34, 128, 464, 466
Leventhal, H., 742, *742*
levetiracetam, 511
  contraindicated in TBI cases, 471
levodopa-responsive dystonia (Segawa syndrome), 487
levothyroxine, 172
Lewis, A., 35, 49, 334
Lewis, G., 406, 411
Lewis, Gemma, 89–105
Lewis, Glyn, 89–105
Lewis, R., 704
Lewis-Fernández, R., 714
Lewy bodies: definition, 503
Lewy, F. H., 503
LGBT, 96, **567**, 577, 719
LGI1 antibodies, 497
Li, T. C. W., 435
liaison consultant psychiatrists: medico-legal conundrums, 759
liaison psychiatry, 392, 716
  term coined by Billings, 739
liaison psychiatry patients (management), 752–7
  alcohol detoxification, 755
  ECT, 755
  psychological intervention (influence on outcome), 756–7
  psychological treatments, 755–6
  psychotropic medication, 752–5
Liaison Psychiatry Special Interest Group (RCP, 1983-), 739
liberty protection safeguards, 759
Liddle, P. F., 198–221
  three syndrome model, 213
Lieb, R., 390
Liepmann, H., 468
life events and difficulties schedule, 744
life expectancy, 415
  homeless people, 792
  psychosis outcome, 231–2
life stages
  1. birth, 705
  2. ageing, 705
  3. marriages, 705
  4. death, 705
  LIST, 706
lifetime prevalence, 10
light therapy, 127
likelihood ratio (LR), 10
  formula, 9
limbic encephalitis associated with CASPR2 antibodies, 497
limbic system, 465, 466
Lin, K-M., 714
Lindqvist, M., 241
Linehan, M., 407, 436, 675
Linnaean system, 31
Linnaeus, C.
  Genera Morborum (1763), 31
  System Naturae (1735), 31
liothyronine, 120
Lipowski, Z. J., 393
liraglutide, 695
lisdexamfetamine, 592
Lishman, W. A.: *Organic Psychiatry* (1987), 739
Lissauer, H., 469
Lissek, S., 298
lithium, 34, 44, 118–19, 129, 135, 137, 170, 172, 456, 457, 600, 602, 603, 604, 611, **612**, 664, 695
  contraindicated (patients with impaired renal function), 754
  definition, 172
  gold standard for treating bipolar disorder, 162
  gold-standard agent (long-term prophylaxis), 172
  interactions, 119
  mechanism of action, 118
  renal impairment cases, 138
  side effects, 118
  toxicity in overdose, 119
lithium (side effects), 173–4
  blood and bone marrow, 174
  cardiovascular effects, 174
  central nervous system, 173
  gastrointestinal, 173
  kidney, 173
  mental and cognitive effects, 173
  metabolic effects and weight gain, 174
  neuromuscular transmission, 174
  parathyroid, bones, teeth, 174
  respiratory effects, 174
  sexual function, 174
  skin, 173
  thyroid, 173
lithium (toxicity), 175–6
  clinical features, 175
  diagnosis, 175
  factors, 175
  outcome, 175
  symptoms, **175**
  treatment, 175
lithium (treatment of bipolar disorder), 172–6
  contraindications, 172
  doses, 172
  pregnancy, 174–5
  side effects, 172–4
lithium carbonate, 172
  pharmacokinetics, 118
lithium citrate, 118, 172
lithium combinations, 171
Lithium Information Center (Wisconsin), 174
lithium salts, 118–19
  contraindications, 119
  mechanism of action, 118
  monitoring, 119
litigation risk, 781
Littman, R. E., 673
liver disease, 111
Liverpool HIV drugs interaction checker, 261
Lloyd, G. G., 741
local authorities, 793, 796
lofepramine, 111
lofexidine, **646**
London, 229, 230, 231, 454, 630, 681, 696, 701, 708, 732, 733, 734, 769, 792
  Institute of Psychiatry, 243
  Marlborough Day Hospital (Paddington), 784
London Respiratory Network, 695
London: Bethlem Hospital, 767, 768
London: Cassel Hospital, 414, 415, 598, 621
London: Maudsley Hospital, 16, 224
London: St Bartholomew's Hospital, 598
London: St George's Hospital, 736
London: Westminster, 793
loneliness, 100
  definition, 100
  risk factor for depression, 100
long Covid, 495
long-acting injection (LAI), 172
  antipsychotics, 234, 249
long-acting β agonists (LABA), 695
longitudinal studies, 25, 589, 628
  determinants of illness, 90–3
  dysfunctional assumptions (Beck) and learned helplessness (Seligman) theories, 101–2
  nature and value, 91
  sleep and depression, 100
long-term memory, 463
loperamide, **646**
lorazepam, 171, 256, 257, 258, **612**, 754
  catatonia (challenge test), 259
loss to follow-up, *23*, 23

low and middle-income countries (LMICs), 717, 719
  psychosis (course and outcome), 235–6
low density lipoprotein cholesterol (LDL-C), 678
loxapine, 256, 257
  salbutamol inhaler should be available, 259
Lubin, J. H., 13
Luborsky, L., 154
Lucini, G., 353
Lucock, M. P., 394
Lunacy Act (1845), 767
Lunacy Report (1872), 689
lurasidone, 118, 136, 171, 172
  absorption with food, 272
Luria test, 463
Luria, A., 461
Lyme disease, 493
lysergic acid diethylamide (LSD), 242, 243, 510

Machiavellianism: definition, 445
MacLean, P., 465–6
Macmillan, D., 448
macro-circuitry: definition, 296
macropsia: definition, 204
magnesium deficiency, 521
magnetic resonance imaging (MRI), 297, 461
  main characteristics, **461**
magnetic resonance spectroscopy (MRS), 342, 343, 462
magnetoencephalography (MEG), 462
Maguire, P., 750
Main, T. F., 424, 598, 621
  'Ailment' (1957), 415, 418
major depression, 35
  clinical presentation (symptom profiles), 75–7
major depressive disorder, 552
  link with insomnia, 550
  sleep, 547
major depressive episodes
  bipolar I disorder, 164
  defined by timing of onset, 78–9
  definition, **73**
major depressive episodes (defined by timing of onset)
  depression with onset in later life, 78–9
  peripartum depression, 78
  seasonal affective disorder, 78
major histocompatibility complex (MHC), 225
makibi (Japan, 'thinning out' of neonates), 618
malaria, 494
Malaysia, 718
Malewska-Payne, H., 710
malignant alienation (Morgan), 664, 670
malignant melanoma metastases, 475
malingering, 390, 398, 400
malnutrition, 580
management plan, 56, *57*
manganese intoxication, 512
mania, 112
  measurement, 168
  mental state examination, 165–6
manic depression: now known as 'bipolar disorder', 40
manic episodes (bipolar I disorder), 163–4
  1. elevated mood, 163
  2. associated symptoms, 163
  3. impairment of functioning, 163
  4. not consequence of substance abuse, 163
manic episodes: drug treatment guidelines, 170–1
manic-depressive insanity, 33, 198
MAOIs, *See* monoamine oxidase inhibitors
maple syrup urine disease, 515
Marcé, L., 574, 601
  Traité de la folie des femmes encientes (1858), 598
Marchiafava-Bignami disease, 507
Marie, P., 504
market forces factor, 774
Marks, B., 733
Marks, I. M., 328
  Living with Fear (1978), 329
Marneros, A., 162
Masdrakis, V., 293–310
Maslach burnout inventory (MBI), 777
Maslow's hierarchy of needs, 431
mass hysteria, 718
Massachusetts General Hospital Handbook of General Hospital Psychiatry, 739
matching: method to overcome confounding, 21–2
maternal deprivation, 540
maternal loss services, 617
maternal mortality, 608
maternal rejection, 447
maternity blues, 615–18
  infanticide, 617–18
  neonaticide, 618
  stillbirth, 616–17
Matsunaga, H., 337
Matte Blanco, I., 422
Matthews, A. M., 329
Mattia, J. L., 451
Matusiewicz, A. K., 436
Maudsley model of anorexia treatment for adults (MANTRA), 570, 582
Maudsley Prescribing Guidelines in Psychiatry (2021), 131, 611
May, S., 390
Mayer-Gross, W., 41, 49
Mayo classification system for TBI severity, 470
Mayo Clinic (Minnesota), 398
MBT, *See* mentalisation-based therapy
MCA, *See* Mental Capacity Act (2005)
McAllister-Williams, H., 162–78
McBride, W. G., 618
McDermott, J. F., 719
McDonald triad for sociopathy, 457
McDougle, C. J., 342
m-chlorophenylpyperazine (mCPP), 342
McKenna, P., 283
MDD, *See* major depressive disorder
MDMA (ecstasy), 116, 123
  key to abbreviation, 509
Meadow, R., 398
Meakin, C. J., 750
meaningful activity, 789, 790
  adult mental health services, 791–3
  definition, 791
  employment support, 791
measles, mumps and rubella (MMR) vaccine, 19
measures of association, 12. *See also* associations (measures of strength)
measures of effect, 12
measures of impact, 13–14
Mechanic, D., 743
mediators, 22, *22*
Medical 203 (US Army, 1945), 47
medical conditions (general): psychosis, 220–1
medical emergencies in eating disorders (MEED), 572, 573, 585
  assessing, 573
  managing, 573
  refeeding, 573
medical history, 51–2
medical outcomes study short form (SF-36), 748
medical treatment: capacity to consent (assessment), 757–8
medically unexplained symptoms (MUS), 391
medically-assisted withdrawal (MAW), 645–7
Medicare and Medicaid (USA), 622
medication, 751
  FND, 381
  monitoring and management, 695–6
  prescription (factors to consider), **720**
  types, 720
Medichec tool (medichec.com), 268
medicine: 'highly pragmatic discipline', 89
Medicines and Healthcare Products Regulatory Agency, 176
medico-legal assessments, 60–1
MEDLINE, 18
Meduna, L., 124
melanchoic depression: clinical presentation (symptom profiles), 76–7
melancholy, 64, 65
  Freud, 65
melatonin, 115, 555, 558
Melbourne, 231
Mellor, C. S., 202, 203
memory
  delusional, 205
  schizophrenia, 210
Mendelian randomisation (MR), 20, 98, 99
  power versus limitations, 92
meningitis, 490, 491
Menninger, K., 656, 673
  on 'rescue fantasies', 674
Menninger, W, 47
menopause, 100, 705
menstrual cycle, 80
mental adjustment to cancer (MAC) scale, 747
Mental Capacity Act (2005), 183, 189, 757, 758, 759, 797
Mental Capacity Act Code of Practice, 759
Mental Deficiency Act (UK, 1913), 40
mental disorders
  definition, 40
  diagnostic systems, 41
  direct side effects of medical treatment, 741
  Kraepelin/Jaspers/NHS, 33
  relation with physical disease, 740–4
  suicide, 662–5
mental health
  converse, 40
  definition (WHO), 39
Mental Health (Patients in Community) Act (1995), 769
Mental Health Act (1959), 768
Mental Health Act (1983), 39, 42, 52, 56, 61, 128, 209, 211, 431, 434, 435, 535, 585, 602, 671, 672, 673, 757–9, 777
  amendments (2007), 781, 797
  detention of patient (application procedure), 759
  in general hospital, 759
  section 117 aftercare, 782
Mental Health Act (2008), 769
Mental Health Act Commission, 672
mental health commissioning, 772–3
mental health intelligence network 'fingertips' tool, 770, 799
Mental Health Investment Standard, 773
mental health measure (Wales), 732
mental health problems
  recognition, diagnosis, classification (primary care), 728
mental health teams: physical health (issues to be addresed), 690
mental health treatment requirement (MHTR), 61
mental ill health: definition, 40
mental illness
  'myth' (antipsychiatry), 38–9
  paradigms (biological versus psychological), 43, 44
mental illness (models), 43–5
  biomedical approach, 44
  case example, 44–5
  interpersonal model, 45
  non-dogmatic holistic approach, 45
  psychodynamic model, 44
  social model, 45
mental illness register, 693
mental programmes (Hofstede), 701
mental state examination, 52–5
  appearance and behaviour, 53
  basic principles, 713–14
  cognitive function, 54
  delusions, 54
  hallucination, 54
  insight, 55
  mood, 53
  passivity phenomena, 54
  speech, 53
  summary, 56
  thoughts, 53

mental state examination (mania and hypomania), 165–6
- appearance, 165
- behaviour, 165
- cognitive abilities, 166
- insight, 166
- mood, 166
- perceptions, 166
- speech, 166
- thinking, 166

Mental Treatment Act (1930), 768
mental wellbeing promotion, 772
mentalisation, 155, 417, 424
mentalisation-based therapy, 426
- personality disorder, 437

Menzies, I. E. P., 418
meprobamate, 39
mercury intoxication, 512
Merskey, H., 401
mesial temporal seizures, 466
meta-analysis: definition, 18
metabolic disorders, 514–16
metabolic syndrome (MS), 235
meta-chlorophenylpiperazine (mCPP), 116
metachromatic leukodystrophy, 515
methadone, 646, 647, 648
- definition, 647

methamphetamine, 34
methanol poisoning, 512
methyl bromide, 513
methylene blue, 34
methylene chloride, 513
methylphenidate, 472, 541
metrazol, 124
Mexico, 636
Meyer, A., 43, 47
- psychobiological approach, 49

MI, *See* myocardial infarction
mianserin, 112, 135
Michelson, D., 741
micro-circuitry: definition, 296
Micronesia, 705
micropsia: definition, 204
microscopy, 35
midazolam, 257
Middle East, 84
Middleton, A., 683
migraine, 193
migrants, 722
- increased risk of psychosis (non-response bias), 23

migration, 228, 233, 721
mild neurocognitive disorder, 501
milk fever, 599, 616
millennium cohort study (MCS), 91
Millon, T., 445
Minamata disease, 512
MIND, 289, 771, 773
mind-body dualism, 718
mindfulness, 192, 288, 381
- ineffectiveness (school settings), 105

mindfulness-based cognitive therapy (MBCT), 153
minerals, 520–2
mini-mental state examination (MMSE), 463, 501, 746
Minnesota Study (1950), 574, 575, 580
minocycline, 123
minor tranquillisers, 39
minority stress theory, 96
mirtazapine, **109**, 112, 130, **132**, 135, 612
- favourable side-effect profile, 113
- pharmacokinetics, 112

missing data, 92
missing heritability, 225
missionary racism, 708
Mistry, H., 714
Misuse of Drugs Act (UK, 1971), 121, 124
mitochondrial disorders, 518–19
mitochondrial encephalomyopathy (MELAS), 518
- full title, 518

mixed depressive and anxiety disorder: clinical presentation (symptom profiles), 76
mixed states: bipolar I disorder, 164–5
Mizrahi, R., 235
moclobemide, **109**, 113, 114, **132**
modafinil, 472, 561
modern electronic patient records, 55
Moffitt, T. E., 446, 447
Moksony, F., 659
Molaison, H., 466
molecular genetics, 198
Moniz, E., 464
monoamine hypothesis, 113
monoamine oxidase (MAO)
- enzyme, 113
- two forms, 113

monoamine oxidase inhibitors, 34, 109, 113–14, 132, 135, 305, 309
- background, 113
- contraindications, 114
- examples, 113
- interactions, 114
- mechanism of action, 113
- pharmacokinetics, 113
- side effects, 113
- toxicity in overdose, 114

monotropism: definition, 529
monozygotic (MZ) twins, 102, 224, 226
Montgomery ruling, 4
Montgomery, S., 348
Montgomery-Asberg depression rating scale (MADRS), 129
month of birth (instrumental variable), 92
Montreal cognitive assessment (MoCA), 463, 501
mood
- bipolar disorder, 166
- mental state examination, 53

mood congruence, 166
mood congruent delusions (types), 69
mood disorders, 199
mood episodes: prophylaxis, 172
Moodkit, 158
mood-monitoring
- bipolar disorder, 190

mood stabilisers, 119–20, 435, **612**
Moore, S., 156
Moorey, S., 147–59
morbid risk, 10, 11
morbidity
- psychosocial stressors, 744
- social factors, 743

Moreira, V., 712
Morel, B., 32, 199
Morgan, C., 228, 230, 233
Morgan, H. G., 6, 664
Morley, S., 394
morphine, 647
Morrison, P., 241–72
Morriss, R., 183–95
Morselli, H., 656, 668
Morton, R.: *Phthisiologia* (1694), 573
Morvan syndrome, 497
Moscow, 35, 784
Mosso, A., *462*
Mota, N. B., 207
mother and baby units (MBUs), 621–3, 624
- assessment and treatment, 623
- diagnoses, 622
- indications for admission, 622
- nurses (functions), 623
- staffing, 622

motivation, 71
motivational interviewing (MI), 648
motor aphasia, 467
motor FND, 370–2
- arm weakness, 371
- dystonia, 371
- facial weakness, 371
- functional Parkinsonism, 371–2
- leg weakness and paralysis, 370–1
- myoclonus, 371
- tics, 371
- tremor, 371

motor side effects (antipsychotics), 263–6
- akathisia, 265
- dystonia, 264–5
- neuroleptic malignant syndrome, 265–6
- Parkinsonism, 264
- tardive dyskinesia, 265

movement disorders, 481–8
- dystonia, 486–7
- Fahr's disease, 488
- Huntington's disease, 485–6
- other, 487–8
- Parkinson's disease, 481–3
- progressive supranuclear palsy, 488
- Sydenham's chorea (St. Vitus's dance), 488
- Tourette syndrome, 483–5
- Wilson's disease, 487–8

Mowrer, O. H., 328
MRI, *See* magnetic resonance imaging
MSE, *See* mental state examination
multi-agency working, 796–7
multi-disciplinary working, 59–60
multifactorial aetiology, 19, 89
multi-infarct dementia, 504
multiple sclerosis, 261, 495–6
multiple sleep latency test (MSLT), 560–1
multivariable modelling techniques, 22
Munafò, M. R., 20
Munchausen by proxy, 398–9
Munchausen syndrome, 397
murder-suicides, 665
Murray, C., 793
Murray, R. M., 224–36
musician's focal dystonia, 487
myocardial infarction, 742, 747, 748, 749
myocarditis, 271
myoclonus dystonia, 487
myoclonus: motor FND, 371
MYRIAD trial, 105

N3 sleep, 555
n-acetyl cysteine, 124
Nagy, E., 156
nalmefene, 455, 649
naloxone, 644, 647
naltrexone, 455, 457, 649
narcissism: characteristics, 445
narcissistic personality disorder, 450
narcolepsy, 560, 561
Narcotics Anonymous, 639, 648
narrative reviews, 18
narrative therapy, 400
narrow-angle glaucoma, 111
nasogastric (NG) feeding, 585
NaSSAs, *See* noradrenergic and specific serotoninergic antidepressants
National Assistance Act (1948), 792
National Association of Parents of Backwards Children (later 'Mencap'), 40
National Association of PICUs, 783
national birth cohort study (1946), 91, 92
national child development study (NCDS), 91
national commissioning for quality and innovation (CQUIN), 770
national comorbidity survey (USA), 327
national comorbidity survey replication (NCS-R, USA), 296
National Confidential Inquiry into Suicide and Homicide (2001, 2014), 657, 661, 664, 669, 729
- inpatient suicide, 672–3

national crime survey (UK): child abuse, 624
national early warning score (NEWS), 258
National Enquiry into Patient Outcome and Death (2017), 740
National Health Service, *See* NHS
National Institute for Health and Care Excellence, *See* NICE
National Institute for Mental Health England: *Personality Disorder* (2003), 414
National Institute of Mental Health (NIMH, USA), 39, 65
national personality disorder programme, 414
national psychiatric morbidity survey (NPMS), 769
National Rifle Association (USA), 680
National Society for Prevention of Cruelty to Children (NSPCC), 626
national strategy for suicide prevention (USA), 682
national survey of health & development (NSHD), 91

national UK research network for behavioural addictions (NUK-BA), 455
national violent death reporting system (USA), 605, 606
nature versus nurture, 224, 329
NAVIGATE programme, 789
necessity doctrine, 758, 759, 782
needle and syringe programmes (NSPs), 644
needle phobia, 755
negative affectivity: definition, 418, 427
negative automatic thoughts, 150
  challenged, 150
  evidence check, 150
negative control outcome, 24
negative therapeutic reaction, 427–8
negative thinking, 150
  advantages and disadvantages, 151
neonatal abstinence syndrome (NAS), 621
neonatal intensive care unit (NICU), 620
neonaticide, 618
  definition, 617
Nepal, 701
Netherlands, 14, 96, 228, 600, 602, 603, 604, 656, 661, 681
neural network theory, 298
neurasthenia, 34
neuroablative treatments for depression, 128
neuroacanthocytosis, 265
neuroanatomical hypothesis, 298
neurobehavioural disorder, 48
neurobiology: PTSD, 316
neuroborreliosis, 493
neurocognitive syndromes, 467–9
  agnosia, 469
  alexia and dyslexia, 468
  aphasia, 467–8
  apraxia, 468–9
  Gerstmann syndrome, 469
  main groups, **467**
neurodegenerative dementias, 501–4
  Alzheimer's disease, 501–3
  dementia with Lewy bodies, 503
neurodiversity, 527, 529
  bipolar disorder, 168
neuroimaging, 16, 461–2
  functional, 379, 461–2
  structural, 379, 461
  techniques (main characteristics), **461**
neuroimaging (OCD), 342–4
  electroencephalography (EEG), 343
  functional imaging, 342–3
  immunological processes, 343–4
  structural imaging, 342
neuroleptic malignant syndrome (NMS), 119
  definition, 265
  motor side effect (antipsychotics), 265–6
neurological diseases
  autoimmune neurological disorders, 495–7
  brain tumours, 475–6
  epilepsy, 476–81
  infectious diseases, 488–95
  movement disorders, 481–7
  movement disorders (other), 487–8
neurological disorders, 469–97
  cerebrovascular disease, 473–5
  traumatic brain injury, 469–73
neurological signs (schizophrenia), 211
  abnormal eye-movements, 211
  abnormal involuntary movements, 211
  cortical signs, 211
neurologists: 'diagnose what they can't treat', 420
neuromodulation: OCD, 349–50
neuromodulatory treatments for depression, 124–7
  deep brain stimulation, 126–7
  electroconvulsive therapy, 124–6
  light therapy, 127
  transcranial magnetic stimulation, 126
  vagal nerve stimulation, 127
neuropharmacology: neuropsychiatric adverse effects, 510–11
neurophysiology, 462
neuropsychiatric disorders, 460–522
  delirium and dementia, 497–505
  neurological disorders, 469–97
  neuropsychiatry (background), 460–9
  toxic, metabolic, endocrine disorders, 505–22
neuropsychiatric inventory (NPI), 464, 501
neuropsychiatry, 2
  definition, 460
neuropsychiatry (background), 460–9
  historical overview, 460–1
  investigations, 461–4
  neurocognitive syndromes, 467–9
  syndromes with regional connections, 464–7
neuropsychiatry (investigations), 463–4
  neuroimaging, 461–2
  neurophysiology, 462
  neuropsychology, 463–4
neuropsychological function: bipolar disorder, 189
neuropsychology, 463–4
neuroscience, 199, 378
neuroscience-based-nomenclature (NbN), 246
neurosis, 34
neurosurgery: OCD, 349–50
neuroticism: definition, 296
neurotransmitters, 327–8, 548
  sleep, 548
  wakefulness, 548
neurotransmitters (OCD), 341–2
  miscellaneous, 342
  pharmacological responses, 342
  platelet studies, 342
  serotonin hypothesis, 341–2
neurovegetative symptoms, 70
neutrophil count, 270
New Haven-Boston Collaborative Depression Project, 153
new knowledge, 46
New South Wales, 749
New Testament: Colossians, 624
New Ways of Working for Psychiatrists (2005), 60, 775, 791
New York, 231, 701, 708
New York: Hillside Hospital, 215
New Zealand, 183, 232, 454, 621, 677
Newton-Howes, G., 407
NHS, 456
  somatisation disorders (annual budget), 376
NHS Benchmarking, 776, 799
NHS Community Mental Health Framework, 415
NHS Digital, 799
NHS England, 59, 415, 535, 623, 696, 740, 760, 770, 773, 774, 786
  five-year forward view (2016), 740, 760
  primary care (policy developments), 735
  standard contract for specialised eating disorder services, 583
NHS Health Check, 693
NHS Improvement, 59, 773
NHS Long Term Plan (2019), 415, 694, 696, 735, 740, 773
NHS Mental Health Dashboard, 773
NHS Plan (2000), 769, 773, 787
NHS Plan [date unspecified], 59
NHS Position Statement on CPA (2021), 770
NHS website, 130
NHSE, *See* NHS England
NICE, 41, 60, 131, 134, 155, 170, 177, 194, 283, 317, 319, 320, 754, 770, 773
  ADHD, 539, 540
  alcohol, 747
  alcohol screening, 644
  anorexia nervosa, 583
  ARFID, 588
  ASPD, 447
  autism, 530
  binge-eating disorder, 592
  bipolar disorder, 183, 434, 435, 436, 664
  bipolar disorder (physical health monitoring recommendations), 195
  bulimia nervosa, 590
  chronic pain, 397
  clozapine (use in pregnancy), 619
  collaborative care approach, 757
  common mental health problems, 728
  complex psychosis, 691, 783, 784
  compulsory treatment, 586
  depression, 73
  depression (mild), 729
  depressive episodes, 128
  eating disorders, 569, 571
  emergency mental health care, 760
  liaison psychology, 760
  MAW treatment (first-line), 646
  obesity, 694
  OCD, 346
  post-natal depression, 611
  pregnancy (eating disorders), 614
  psychiatric disorder in pregnancy, 613
  psychosis (first episode), 789
  psychosis guidelines, 253
  self-harm, 430
  severe mental illness, 730
  stepped models of care, 732
Nicholson, T. R., 366–81
Nicolini, H., 340
nidotherapy, 438
Niemann-Pick disease type C, 515
Nietzsche, F. W., 49
nightmare disorder, 556–7
  assessment, 557
  definition, 556
  psychiatric conditions, 556
  treatment, 557
NIHR Mental Health Policy Research Unit, 420
nimodipine, 123
niqab, 714
Nissl, F., 32
nitrazepam, **646**
nitrous oxide, 513
NMDAR-antibody encephalitis, 497
N-methyl-D-aspartate (NMDA), 111, 308
nociception, 395–6
  definition, 395
nominal aphasia, 468
non-24-hour sleep-wake disorder, 553
non-accidental injury (NAI), 625
non-causal path, *23*, 23, *25*
non-covalent dimer: definition, 176
non-dogmatic holistic approach, 45
non-fluent aphasia, 467
non-medical diagnosis, 60
non-mood congruent hallucinations, 71
non-rapid eye movement sleep, *See* NREM sleep
non-response bias, 15, 23–4
  definition, 23
non-stimulants: ADHD, 541, 542
nonsuicidal self-injury (NSSI), 48, 68, 676, 677
  definition, 68
noradrenergic and specific serotoninergic antidepressants, 112–13
  contraindications, 113
  examples, 112
  mechanism of action, 112
  pharmacokinetics, 112
  side effects, 112
norclozapine, 251
Norström, T., 665
North Africa, 84
Northern Ireland, 757, 773
nortriptyline, 111, 511
Norway, 665
Norwegian twin register, 418
nosology
  benefits, 37
  definition (taxonomy applied to diseases), 37
  dilemma, 31
  psychiatry, 37
not elsewhere defined (NED) conditions, 42
not otherwise specified (NOS) conditions, 42

Nottingham, 230
Novel Psychoactive Treatment: UK Network (NEPTUNE), 261
NREM parasomnias, 555–6
assessment, 556
confusional arousals, 555
psychiatric conditions, 556
sleep terrors, 555
sleep-related eating, 555
sleepwalking, 555
treatment, 556
NREM sleep, 546, 548
NREM1 (N1), 546
NREM2 (N2), 546
NREM3 (N3), 546
nucleus accumbens, 466
Nuevo Metodo di Shockterapie (Cerletti and Bini, 1938), 125
null condition: definition, 26
number needed to treat (NNT), 17, **18**, 104, 644
nurses, 59, 759
nursing care plans, 781
nursing staff, 779, 781
nutrients, 123–4, 519–22
electrolytes and minerals, 520–2
vitamins, 519–20
nutritional iodine deficiency, 521

O'Hara, M. W., 610
obesity, 592
comorbid BED (prevalence, South Australia, 1995-2015), *592*
depression risk factor, 99
holistic approach, *694*
reduction (integrated approach), 694–5
side effect of antipsychotics, 268–9
object relations theory, 154
observational epidemiology, 7
observational studies, 7, 90
causation, 19
cause-and-effect estimates (strengthening), 92–3
threats to validity, 92
observer bias, 24–5, 93
many guises, 24
occasion, 24
way to overcome, 24
obsessions
categories, 345
definition, 334
obsessive-compulsive disorder, 69, 295, 334–59, 394, 547
aetiology, 340–6
age of onset, 340
autism, 533
case examples, 337
course, 340
diagnosis and classification, 334–5
DSM-5 versus ICD-11, **335**
easily mistaken for phobic disorder, 326
epidemiology, 340
female-male ratio, 340
historical perspective, 334
marital status, 340
pharmacotherapy, 348–9
poor insight, 337
post-partum, 614
prevalence, 340
religion, 340
symptoms, 336–7
treatment, 346–50
obsessive-compulsive disorder (aetiology), 340–6
family studies, 341
genetics, 340–1
neuroimaging, 342–4
neurotransmitters, 341–2
psychological theories, 344–6
sociological theories, 346
studying heritability (other methods), 341
twin studies, 341
obsessive-compulsive disorder (differential diagnosis and comorbidity), 337–40
anorexia nervosa and bulimia nervosa, 339
autism, 339
boundary with normality, 337–8
depression, 338
phobic disorders, 338
schizophrenia and other psychoses (with case example), 339
stammering and stuttering, 340
Tourette syndrome, 339
obsessive-compulsive disorder (psychological treatment), 346–50
CBT, 347
CBT (outcome), 347
ERP, 346–7
ERP (outcome), 347
neurosurgery and neuromodulation, 349–50
psychodynamic psychotherapy, 347
obsessive-compulsive personality disorder (OCPD), 339, 451–2
obsessive-compulsive related disorders (OCRDs), 335, 336–50
body dysmorphic disorder, 350–2
DSM-5 versus ICD-11, **335**
hoarding disorder, 352–4
hypochondriasis, 355–9
olfactory reference syndrome, 359
skin-picking disorder, 336–55
trichotillomania, 354–5
types, 335–6
obsessive-compulsive spectrum disorders, 335
obstructive sleep apnoea, 557, 558–9
assessment, 559
psychiatric conditions, 558
treatment, 559
occipital alexia, 468
occipital seizures, 477
occupation
standard mortality ratios for suicide, **667**
suicide risk, 666–7
occupational history, 51
OCD, *See* obsessive-compulsive disorder
OCRDs, *See* obsessive-compulsive related disorders
odds, 10
odds ratios, 13, 102
use in case-control studies, 13
used especially in case-control studies, 12
Odegaard, O., 701
Oedipal complex, 328
oedipism: definition, 678
oestrogen, 608
Office for National Statistics, 606, 657, 667, 769
Office for Science. *See also* Parliamentary Office of Science and Technology
Office for Science: five ways to wellbeing (2008), 772
Öhman, A., 328
O-isopropyl methylphosphonofluoridate (Sarin), 513
olanzapine, 117, 136, 137, 171, 172, 250, 258, 456, 471, 578, 586, 604, 607, **612**, 619, 694, 730, 754
combination with fluoxetine, 117
efficacy, 246, 247
Huntington's disease, 485
long-term prophylaxis, 172
national guidelines, 247
Old Testament, 654
Proverbs, 444
old-age psychiatry, 717
olfactory hallucinations, 54, 204
olfactory reference syndrome, 359
definition, 336
Oliver, J., 627
omega-3 fatty acids, 124
ondansetron, 117, **646**
ONS, *See* Office for National Statistics
open dialogue (OD), 284
OpenGrey, 18
operational criteria, 35
definition, 200
mental disorders, 35
opiates
abrupt discontinuation and symptomatic relief, 646
harm reduction, 644
medically-assisted withdrawal, 646–7
neuropsychiatric manifestations, 510
relapse-prevention medication, 649
stabilisation followed by taper from buprenorphine, 646
withdrawal symptoms (medications), **646**
opioid agonist treatment (OAT), 647–8
opioid substitution treatment (OST), 643, 647
opium, 34
Oppenheim, H., 465, *486*, 486
OPTiMiSE study, 234, 250
OPUS study, 231, 233, 250, 788
oral contraceptives, 177
orbitofrontal syndrome, 465
orexin, 560
organic mental disorder: general hospital setting, 746
organic psychosis (Group I mental disorders), 33
organic psychotic disorders, 260–2
autoimmune encephalitis, 261
CNS infections, 261
drug-induced, 261
epilepsy, 260
general principles, 260
Huntington's disease, 261
inflammatory, 261
stroke, 261
thyroid disorders, 262
traumatic brain injury, 262
organic solvents: toxic effects, 512
organophosphate compounds, 513
orobuccal apraxia, 469
oromandibular dystonia, 486
orthostatic hypotension: definition, 267
Orwell, G., 792
Orygen, 231
OSA, *See* obstructive sleep apnoea
osmotic demyelination syndrome, 522
Othello syndrome, 482
other specific feeding and eating disorders (OSFED), 565, 590
outcome freqency, 19
outcome measurement, 376, 570, 769, 774, 795, 797–8
outcome status: case-control studies, 16
outcomes: 'broad' term, 8
overdose: capacity to consent (to treatment), 758
oxazepam, **612**
oxcarbazepine, 171, 177
Oxford, 400, 584, 677
oximetry, 559
oxycodone, 34
oxytocin, 300
oxytocin receptor gene (OXTR), 376

p factor (transdiagnostic psychopathological factor), 199, 221
P-values, 26
definition, 26
pabrinex, 585
Pacific islands, 378
Padesky, C., 158
paediatric autoimmune neurological syndrome (PANS), 344
paediatric autoimmune neuropsychiatric disorders associated with streptococci (PANDAS), 344
Paffenbarger Jr., R. S, 601
PAFIP-3 trial, 247
pain. *See also* chronic pain
definition, 395
pain disorders
classification, 396–7
management, 397
standard psychiatric approach (assessment items), 397
panel studies, 15
panic, 325, 326, 330
classification of phobic disorders (controversy), 325
panic attack without panic, 373
panic attacks, 474
panic disorder, 614
beta blockers, 307–9
causes, 297–8
diagnosis, 293
epidemiology, 295
triple network model, **298**
panic disorder (beta blockers)
exercise, 308–9
long-term pharmacological treatment, 308
medications after non-response, 308
psychological interventions, 308

short-term pharmacological treatment, 307–8
Papez, J., 465
Papua New Guinea, 494
paracetamol, **646**, 680
paranoid delusions, 58
paranoid personality disorder, 224, 448–9, 630
epidemiolgy and aetiology, 448–9
paraquat, 513, 680
paraquat lung, 513
parasomnias, **555**
definition, 555
NREM parasomnias, 555–6
REM parasomnias, 556–8
parasuicide: WHO definition, 676
parathion, 513
parenting, 420
parenting skills, 623
parietal lesions, 466, 469
parietal lobe, 466–7
parietal seizures, 477
parietal-temporal alexia, 468
Paris, 45, 241, 367
Parker, G., 65, 71
Parkinson plus syndromes, 488
Parkinson, J., 481
Parkinsonism
definition, 264
motor side effect (antipsychotics), 264
Parkinson's dementia, 503, 557
Parkinson's disease, 126, 194, 452, 454, 481–3, 503
CBT, 482
clinical features, 481
definition, 481
dementia, 483
neuropathological hallmark, 481
non-motor symptoms, 482
pharmacotherapy, 482
psychosis (most common form), 482
Parliamentary Office of Science and Technology (POST), 528
paroxetine, 108, 112, 131, 134, 348, 350, 354, **612**
propensity to cause violent episode, 131
side effects, 109
PARRET, 712
Parsons, T., 743
partial agonists, 244
participation mystique, 424
Partners2 study, 734
Partridge, G., 40
passivity phenomenon, 71
paternal age: psychosis risk factor, 227
pathologic laughing and crying scale (PLACS), 464
pathological demand avoidance, 534
pathological intoxication, 509
pathways to psychiatric care model, 726–7
five levels, four filters, *727*
patient attribution (concept), 742
patient health questionnaire (PHQ-9), 129, 464, 746, 750, 795
patient outcomes research team (PORT), 283
patient rated outcome measures (PROMs), 798
patient-level information and costing systems (PLICS), 774
Patterson Inquiry, 58
Paullus, D. L., 445
pauper lunatics, 792
Pavlov, I. P., 44
Pearce, N., 22
peduncular hallucinosis, 475
pellagra, 7, 519
symptoms, 7
United States, 7
Pelto, P. J.: 'tight' versus 'loose' societies, 703
Pemberton, M., 699–722
penicillamine, 487, 519
penicillin, 491
Penttilä, M., 216
people who inject drugs (PWID), 641
Pepper, J., 349
percentage agreement, 8
percentage alcohol by volume (% ABV), 638
percutaneous endoscopic gastrostomy (PEG), 585
Percy Commission (1954-6), 768
Perez, D. L., 379
perfectionism, 345
perinatal mental health services, 604
perinatal nursery nurses, 623
perinatal psychiatry, 2, 598–631, 739
anxiety disorders, 614
child abuse and neglect, 624–31
community perinatal mental health services, 623–4
eating disorders, 614
maternity blues, 615–18
postnatal depression, 606–13
postnatal neonatal adaption syndromes, 615
postpartum OCD, 614
postpartum PTSD, 614–15
psychiatric disorder in pregnancy, 613
psychotropic drugs (teratogenicity), 618–20
puerperal psychoses, 598–606
substance use in pregnancy, 620–3
period prevalence: definition, 10
periodic hypokalaemic paralysis, 521
periodic limb movement disorder, 552–3
assessment, 553
association with mood and anxiety disorders, 552
causes, 552
diagnosis, 552
treatment, 553
peripartum depression, 78
Perry, A., 183
persistent complex bereavement disorder, 48
persistent depressive disorder, 79–80
criteria, 79
four types, 79
onset, 79
persistent postural-perceptual dizziness (PPPD), 374
Bárány Society criteria, **375**
person disorder (shibboleths)
'expresses clinician's dislike of patient', 411
personal history, 50–1
educational history, 51
family history, 51
occupational history, 51
prenatal development and birth, 51
relationship and psychosexual history, 51
summary, 56
personal identity, 373
personalised care, 793–4
black and minority ethnic groups, 793
crisis management, 794
patient choices, 793
peer providers, 793
peer workers (role), 794
physical health care ('key issue'), 794
practical help, 794
social inclusion, 793
statutory teams, 794
treatment, 794
personality deviations (Group III mental disorders), 34
personality difficulty, 409
'subclinical description', 418
subsyndromal form of personality disorder, 404
personality disorder, 2, 51, 128, 404–11, 630
anorexia nervosa patients, 576
assessment by self-rating, 408
borderline as relational psychosis, 417
borderline controversy, 406–7
care and treatment, 417–18
care and treatment (relational practice), 418
cause and onset, 410
classifications (current and immediate past), **408**
clinical approaches, 414–39
common factor theory, 417
comorbidites (prevalence), **420**
core components, 404, 409
course, 410
definition (ICD-11), 404
demographic characteristics, **419**
diagnosis, 404–6
diagnosis (five levels), 404
distress (significant), 406
genetics and environment, 410
ICD-11 classification (reasons), 409
impairment (significant) in functioning, 406
interpersonal dysfunction, 405
lex talionis, 416
maladaptive patterns, 405
mild, moderate, and severe types, 409
odds ratio (aetiological and forensic factors), **419**
persistence, 405–6
prevalence (male-female), **420**
primary care, 729–30
problems in self-function, 405
recognition (importance), 410
relation with trauma, 407–8
severity, **419**
single spectrum of severity, *409*
'stigmatised term', 404
term 'contains profound misunderstanding', 424
term of abuse, 41
therapeutic nihilism, 416–17
treatment (who and what), 416
Type R versus Type S, 406
whole systems approach, 415
personality disorder (aetiology), 421–2
adverse childhood experiences, 421
biological associations, 421
social associations, 421
personality disorder (assessment), 429–31
diagnosis, 429–30
formulation, 430
risk assessment and management, 430–1
personality disorder (care and treatment interventions), 433–9
interventions preferencing exploration, 435–9
interventions preferencing stabilisation, 433–5
organisation of care, 433
personality disorder (care and treatment tasks), 431–3
1. stabilise, 431
2. explore, 432
3. consolidate, 432
personality disorder (containment and boundaries), 426–9
container-contained (Bion), 426–7
drama triangle, 427
grievance (role in avoiding grieving), 427
negative therapeutic reaction, 427–8
rescue phantasy, 427–8
therapeutic relationship, 428–9
personality disorder (developmental psychopathology), 422–5
clinicopathological description, 424–5
core consciousness, psychotic communication, relational psychosis, 423
disruption to expression of personality, 424
explanatory diagram, *424*
gene-environment neurodevelopmental disorder, 422
intrapersonal impact, 423
mammalian systems (social bonding), 423
neglect, self-care systems, negative affective core, 423
primary affects, drives, conscious modification, 423
structural mind, **422**
structured psyche, 422
systems within affective core, 423
personality disorder (formulation), 430
five Ps, 430
power threat meaning framework, 430
personality disorder (interventions preferencing exploration), 435–9
occupational interventions, 435–6
peer support, 436

personality disorder (interventions preferencing exploration) (cont.)
psychological treatments, 436–9
personality disorder (interventions preferencing stabilisation), 433–5
admissions (agreed components), **434**
admissions (to hospital), 434–5
compulson through Mental Health Act, 435
crisis and home treatment teams, 434
crisis planning, 433–4
pharmacological treatments, 435
personality disorder (management and treatment), 425–39
assessment, 429–31
care and treatment tasks, 431–3
initial task, *431*
interventions delivering care and treatment, 433–9
relational approach to personality disorder, 425–9
reworking difficulties, *433*
personality disorder (organisation of care), 433
assessment and allocation, 433
management of planned contacts, 433
management of unplanned contacts, 433
personality disorder (outcomes), 420–1
impact on forensic behaviours, 421
impact on individual's health, 420
impact on parenting, 420
impact on violence, 421
personality disorder (psychological treatments), 436–9
art therapy, 438
CBT, 436
DBT, 436–7
group psychotherapy, 437–8
MBT, 437
nidotherapy, 438
psychodynamic therapy, 437
SFT, 437
short-term interventions, 436
STEPPS, 436
therapeutic community, 438
therapies comparison, 438–9
personality disorder (psychopathological description)
developmental psychopathology, 422–5
personality disorder (management and treatment), 425–39
personality disorder classification, 418–22
personality disorder (recent history), 414–16
Cassel and Henderson Hospitals, 415
personality disorder (relational approach principles), 426–9
containment and boundaries, 426–9
education versus therapy, 429
group versus individual, 429
trauma-informed care, 426
personality disorder (relational approach), 425–9
principles, 426–9
public health model, 426
service structures, 425–6
structured clinical management, 426
personality disorder (shibboleths), 410–11
'grossly over-diagnosed', 411
'redundant diagnosis', 410
'untreatable, so best ignored', 411
personality disorder classification, 418–22
aetiology, 421–2
complex emotional needs, 420
ICD-11, 419–25
outcomes, 420–1
prevalence, 419–20
person-centred care, 4, 37, 48
Person-Centred Care (CR215), 3
personhood, 40, 41
Peru, 636
pervasive refusal syndrome, 375
pesticide compounds, 513
pesticide control: suicide prevention, 680
pesticide poisoning, 657, 680
PET scanning, 422
Peveler, R., 762
phaeochromocytomas, 518
pharmacodynamic interactions, 272
risks, **273**
pharmacodynamics: definition, 271, 720
pharmacogenomics: CYP2D6 enzyme and risperidone, 272
pharmacokinetics: definition, 271, 720
pharmacotherapy (OCD), 348–9
drugs (dosages), 348
drugs (effectiveness), 348
length of treatment, 348
other pharmacological agents, **343**
SRI-refractory patients, 343–8
pharmacotherapy (SRI-refractory OCD patients), 348–9
1. higher dose of SSRI, 349
2. intravenous administration of SRI, 349
3. drug combination, 349
4. novel pharmacological strategies, 349
phenelzine, **109**, 113, 114, **132**
phenothiazine, 241
phenylketonuria, 515
Phillips, D. P., 675
Phinney, J. S., 709, 710
phobias: definition, 324, 474
phobic anxiety disorder: general hospital setting, 746
phobic disorder. *See* specific phobia
phototherapy, 127
physical abuse: child maltreatment, 625–6
physical activity
CMO's guidelines (UK, 2019), *692*
definition, 98
integrated approach, 692
reduces depressive symptomatology, 98–9
physical and psychiatric comorbidity (epidemiology), 744–5
physical and psychiatric comorbidity (impact), 747–50
functional disability and quality of life, 748–9
health care use, 749–50
suicide, 749
survival and disease outcome, 747–8
treatment non-concordance, 749
physical disease
biological factors contributing to psychological change, 740
relation with mental disorder, 740–4
physical disease (psychological response), 741
cognitive approach, 741–2
psychodynamic approach, 742–3
social factors, 743–4
physical disorder
consequence of psychiatric disorder, 741
mistaken for phobic anxiety disorder, 326–7
physical evaluation, 56
physical health care, 688–97
holistic approach to assessment (by psychiatrists), *690*
physical health problems: bidirectional association with depression, 99
physical health: common conditions psychiatrists need to understand, 689–90, 697
physical neglect (indicators), 627
physical treatments for depression (classification), 124–8
neuroablative, 127–8
neuromodulatory, 124–7
physiotherapy: FND, 380
Pick, A., 504
pigs, 492
Pilowsky, L., 243
Pinderhughes, E. B., 708
pindolol, 120–1, 471
contraindications, 121
definition, 306
elimination half-life, 121
mechanism of action, 121
side effects, 121
toxicity in overdose, 121
Pinel, P., 64, 444
Pitt, B., 614
pituitary adenomas, 476
platelet studies: OCD, 342
Plato, 655
pleiotropy, 93
PLMD, *See* periodic limb movement disorder
pneumonia, 269, 271
point prevalence: definition, 10
poisons (environmental), 511–14
Pollard, C., 158
polycystic ovarian syndrome, 176
polydipsia, 522
polygenic risk score for schizophrenia (PRS-Sz), 225, 229
largest study, 229
polygenic risk scores (PRSs), 93, 102, 225
polysomnogram, 546, 549, 551, 553, 557, 558, 559, 560
polyunsaturated fatty acids, 580
polyuria, 522
poor neonatal adaptation (PNA), 613–15
population attributable risk (PAR)
definition, 14
formula, 13
unemployment and suicide, 13–14
population surveys, 65
Porter, R., 768
positive and negative syndrome scale (PANSS), 213, 230, 234
positive memory training approach, 288
positron emission tomography (PET), 243, 247, 297, 343, 344, 462
post-concussion syndrome, 471, 472
posterior cingulate cortex (PCC), 379
post-ictal behavioural symptoms, 478
post-ictal fugues, 478
post-ictal mental state abnormalities, 476
post-ictal psychosis, 478
postnatal depression, 78, 606–13
breast feeding and psychotropic drugs, 611–13
CBT, 608
complex cases, 607–8
consequences, 609
drug therapy, 610–11
effects on infants, 609–10
presentation and symptoms, 606–7
psychotherapy, 610–13
treatment, 610
post-natal neonatal adaption syndromes, 613–15
postpartum depression (PPD), 78
postpartum OCD, 614
postpartum psychosis, 600
postpartum psychotic depression, 599
postpartum psychotic episodes, 78
postpartum PTSD: perinatal psychiatry, 614–15
post-stroke anxiety, 474
post-stroke fatigue: definition, 474
post-traumatic agitation
characteristics, 470
treatment, 471
post-traumatic amnesia, 470
definition, 470
treatment, 471
post-traumatic stress disorder, 295, 314–21, 533
'can mimic' phobic disorder, 326
Covid-19 pandemic, 316
diagnosis and classification, 314–15
DSM-5 criteria, 315
general hospital setting, 747
ICD-11 criteria, 315
neurobiology, 316
outcome, 316
outcome (six-year symptom trajectories), *317*
pharmacological prescribing algorithm, *321*

postpartum, 614–15
prevalence, 315–16
prevention, 317–18
psychological theories, 316–17
symptoms, 314–15
symptoms (main clusters), **314**
traumatic event, 314
treatment, 318–20
treatment (other interventions), 320
treatment (pharmacological), 319–20
post-traumatic stress disorder (psychological treatment), 318–19
CBT without trauma focus, 319
CBT-TF, 318
EMDR, 318–19
RTM, 319
postural orthostatic tachycardia syndrome (POTS), 326, 327
potassium, 521
Potvin, O., 435
Poulter, D., 699–722
poverty, 629
depression factor, 94–5
suicide risk, 666
poverty of thought, 53
Powell, E., 768
power distance, 701, 703
power of attorney, 189
power threat meaning framework (PTMF), 65, 430
PPD. *See* paranoid personality disorder
practical management of personality disorder (model), 425
practice nurses: training about mental health, 735
Prader–Willi syndrome, 355
pragmatic trial designs, 247
prazosin, 557
precision, 27
pre-conception counselling, 604, 611
precuneus, 467
predictive validity, 9
predictive value, 10
formulae, 9
pre-frontal cortex, 464, 465
pregabalin, 304–5
class C controlled substance (2019), 304
pregnancy, 78, 91, 94, 115, 176, 177, 263, 491, 529, 580, 601, 603, 660
alcohol, 620–1
cocaine, 621
environmental risk factors (psychosis), 227
folate deficiency, 519
heroin, 621
iodine deficiency, 521
khat, 621
lithium, 174–5
psychiatric disorder, 613
schizophrenia, 613
smoking, 620
substance use, 620–3
pregnancy prevention programme (PPP), 176
pre-ictal behavioural symptoms, 477
prejudice: definition, 706
premenstrual dysphoric disorder, 48, 80–1
premenstrual syndromes (PMS), 100
premenstrual tension, 607, 611, 616
premorbid personality, 51
present state examination (PSE), 35, 630, 745
prevalence
common error, 11
definition, 10, 91
subtypes, 10
prevalence bias, 16
definition, 24
prevention paradox (Rose, 1981), 104
Prichard, J. C., 444
primary adrenocortical insufficiency, 517
primary care, 59
conclusion, 736
consultation time (limited), 730
definition, 726
education and training, 735–6
epidemiology of mental illness, 726–8
GP education (updating needed), 730
interface with secondary mental health services, 731–5
mental health, 726
mental health problems (recognition, diagnosis, classification), 728
psychiatry, 726–36
psychiatry (scope), 726–8
reactive nature, 730
recognition and management issues, 728–31
schizophrenia, 730
primary care (interface with secondary mental health services), 731–5
collaborative care, 734
co-location, 732
community mental health teams, 731
consultant psychiatrist (typical format of meeting with GP), 733
consultation-liaison model, 733
improving communication, 732
integrated and shared care, 732
link-working, 732
managing demand, 731
NHSE policy developments, 735
restructuring care pathway, 732
traditional ways of working, 731
primary care (recognition and management issues), 728–31
dementia, 731
depression, 728–9
personality disorders, 729–30
severe and enduring mental illness, 730–1
suicide prevention, 729
primary care networks (PCNs), 425, 735
primary care quality framework (2021-2022), 690–1, 695, 696
primary delusion, 54
primary dysthymia, 128
primary dystonia (generalised forms), 487
primary health care teams (PHCT), 733
primary psychotic disorders, 83, 200, 217–21. *See also* schizophrenia
associated with substance use and medical conditions, 220–1
brief psychotic disorder, 217
delusional disorder, 218–19
schizoaffective disorder, 217–18
schizotypal disorder, 220
primary sensory cortex, 466
primary visual cortex, 467
primigravid women, 623
PRIMROSE, 735
prion protein (PrPc), 494
prisons: suicide, 666
problems of daily living, 38, 39
prochlorperazine, **646**
prodrome (term avoided), 188
progesterone, 608, 611
prognostic studies, 15–16
progressive non-fluent aphasia, 504
progressive supranuclear palsy, 488
projective identification, 424
prolactin, 373
promazine, **646**
promethazine, 171, 258, 620, **646**
propensity scoring techniques, 22
propofol, 381
proportion, 10
proportional mortality data (PMR), 667
propranolol, 173, 306, 471
prosopagnosia: definition, 469
Protheroe, C., 603
pseudo-dementia, 500
pseudo-depression, 220
pseudo-hallucinations: definition, 204
pseudo-psychopathy, 220
pseudo-seizures, 481
PSG. *See* polysomnogram
psilocybin, 243, 510
psychedelic-assisted psychotherapy, 124
psychedelics, 124
half-lives, 124
mechanisms of action, 118
side effects, 124
psychiatric assessment
general hospital setting, 750–2
tasks and their order, *58*
psychiatric assessment (communication), 57–61
medico-legal assessments, 60–1
multi-disciplinary working, 59–60
reviewing agreed plan, 58–9
summarising-letter to patients, 58
psychiatric assessment and presenting issues, 50–6
1. history, 50–2
2. mental state examination, 52–5
3. physical assessment and investigations, 55
4. diagnostic formulation and summary, 55
5. risk issues, 55–6
psychiatric assessment and presenting issues (history), 50–2
alcohol and drug history, 52
current social situation, 52
forensic history and history of violence, 52
history of present complaint, 50
medical and psychiatric history, 51–2
personal history, 50–1
pre-morbid personality, 51
psychiatric assessment scheme, 49–61
communicating assessments, 57–61
interviewing style, 57
non-medical diagnosis, 59–60
structure and process, 49
psychiatric assessment scheme: structure and process (summary), 56–7
diagnostic evaluation and formulation, 56
history items, 56
management plan, 56
MSE, 56
physical evaluation, 56
risk assessment, 57
risks (group-based), 57
risks (individual factors), 57
safety assessment, 57
psychiatric disorders
fluctuating course, 16
in pregnancy, 613
Jaspers' classification, *33*
physical disorders as consequence of, 741
psychiatric epidemiology, 16
cohort studies, 15
psychiatric euthanasia, 656
psychiatric formulation, 745
Psychiatric Genomics Consortium (PGC), 225, 588
psychiatric history, 51–2
psychiatric hospital admissions, 14
psychiatric inpatients: suicide, 670–3
psychiatric morbidity surveys, 668, 726
psychiatric nosology, 31, 36
psychiatric nurses: burnout, 777
psychiatric services: benefits (general hospitals), 739
psychiatrists, 397, 400, 411, 439, 796
background, 688
common physical health conditions that need to be understood, 689–90
healing agents on mind of patient, 1
patient suicides, 682
responsibilities (general hospitals), 739
role, 775, 791
training about primary care, 735–6
'treat what they can't diagnose', 420
psychiatrists (holistic assessment)
family history, 689
note-making, 688
social history, 689
systematic enquiry, 689
psychiatry, 35, 406
categorical versus dimensional approaches, 42
comorbidty, 42–3

psychiatry (cont.)
criteria for assessing classification systems (Jablensky and Kendell), 41
formulation and diagnosis, 41–2
general hospital, 2, 739–62
general practice, 2
nature, 2
special responsibility for suicide attempts, 683
taxonomy and nosology, 37
term coined by Reil, 1
psychiatry (primary care), 726–36
scope, 726–8
psychoanalysis, 32, 44, 47
versus 'psychoanalytically-oriented therapies', 154
psychoanalytic theories: OCD, 344
psychodynamic approaches: bipolar disorder treatment, 193
psychodynamic models, 44
psychodynamic therapy, 154–5
FND, 380–1
personality disorder, 437
psychoeducation, 195
apps, 192
bipolar disorder treatment, 191–2
FND, 380
Tourette syndrome, 484
psychogenic nonepileptic attacks, 481
psychogenic: term with 'baggage', 368
psychological debriefing (PD), 317
psychological intervention: influence on outcome, 756–7
psychological skills: required of general clinicians, 755
psychological treatment
assessment, 284
case conceptualisation, 284–5
engagement, 285
FND, 380–1
liaison psychiatry patients, 755–6
negative symptoms, 287
novel CBT interventions, 287–8
psychosis, 283–8
relapse prevention and medication management, 287
work with voices, 285–6
working with delusions, 286–7
psychological wellbeing practitioners (PWP), 734
psychologists: number employed by NHSE, 775
psychology: vulnerability to depression (theories), 101–2
psychomotor excitation: dimension of psychopathology in schizophrenia, 213
psychomotor poverty, 212
dimension of psychopathology in schizophrenia, 213
psycho-oncology, 739
psychopath: medical label (shift to term of abuse), 40
psychopathology, 41
dimensions in schizophrenia, 211–13
non-specific, 213
psychopathy checklist (PCL-22), 445
psychopathy checklist revised (PCL-R-20), 445, **445**, 446
psychopathy: core, 445
psychopharmacology
culture, 720
roots, 241
psychosexual history, 51
psychosis
affective versus non-affective, 198
autism, 533
characteristics, 224
conflation with schizophrenia 'potentially harmful', 221
direct side effect of medical treatment, 741
maintenance treatment and relapse prevention, 248
neurological and medical causes, **260**
rating scales, 285
reverse causation 'longstanding [research] problem', 25
switching medications and optimum dosing, 248
psychosis (acute and first episode treatment), 246–7
expectant management, 246
sedatives, 246
psychosis (causes and outcome), 224–36
environmental risk factors, 227–30
psychosis (course and outcome), 230–6
biological mechanisms, 234–6
low- and middle-income countries, 235–6
onset, 230
outcome, 230–3
risk and mediating factors, 233–4
treatment resistance, 234
psychosis (drug treatment), 241–72
affective comorbidities, 252–4
drug interactions, 271–2
history, 241–2
mechanisms, 242–4
organic psychotic disorders, 260–2
phases, 244–52
schizoaffective disorder, 252–4
side effects, 262–71
specific treatment targets, 254–60
psychosis (outcome), 230–3
antipsychotic medication, 232–3
effects of early intervention, 233
hospitalisation, 232
life expectancy, 231–2
long-term outcome, 230–1
remission and recovery, 230
suicide, 232
systematic review and meta-analysis, 231
psychosis (phases of treatment), 244–52
1. at-risk mental state (ARMS), 244–5
2. first episode and acute psychosis, 246–7
3. maintenance, 247–50
4. treatment-resistant schizophrenia, 250–1
5. ultra-resistant psychosis, 251–2
psychosis (psychosocial management), 282–90
carer support and intervention, 288–9
psychological treatment, 283–8
summary, 289
psychosis (risk and mediating factors), 233–4
childhood adversities, 233
diagnosis, 233
duration of untreated psychosis, 233
migration and social circumstances, 233
recreational drug use, 233–4
psychosis (specific treatment targets), 254–60
catatonia, 259–60
cognition, 255
negative symptoms (pragmatic approach), **255**
rapid tranquilisation, 255–9
psychosis prodrome, 244–5
types, **245**
psychosis risk factors (genetics)
ancestry, 226
classic studies, 224
epigenetics, 226
GWAS, 225
linkage and candidate gene studies, 224
overlap across disorders, 225
polgenic risk scores, 225
rare variants, 225–6
summary, 226–7
Psychosis Work Group (for DSM-5), 200
psychosocial interventions: substance use disorders, 648–9
psychosocial stressors: morbidity, 744
psychotherapy
common clinician errors (suicidal patients), 674–5
culture, 721
definition, 721
focus on ego functioning, 756
goals, 756
suicidal outpatients, 675
suicidal subject, 674
psychotic depression: clinical presentation (symptom profiles), 75–6
psychotic disorders
diagnostic criteria, 200–1
hallmark, 199
spectrum, 198–9
Psychotic Disorders Working Group (for ICD-11), 200, 202, 217
psychotic symptoms (in general population), 229
Psychotropic Drug Directory, 752
psychotropic drugs, 615
database (breast-feeding), **612**
psychotropic drugs (teratogenicity), 618–20
antipsychotics, 618–20
thalidomide scandal, 618
psychotropic medication (liaison psychiatry patients), 752–5
antidepressants, 753–4
antipsychotics, 754–5
anxiolytics, 755
use in medical setting, 753
psychotropic medication (use in medical setting), 753
drug interactions, 753
existing physical disease, 753
prescribing, 753
psylocybin, 124
Public Health England, 39, 454
Public Health Wales, 421
publication bias, 18
assessment using funnel plot, 18
important problem with meta-analysis, 18
puerperal infections, 599
puerperal insanity, 598
puerperal mania, 599
puerperal psychoses, 598–606, 630
aetiology, 601
epidemiology, 601
genetics, 601
link with bipolar disorder, 601
nosology, 600
onset, 598
presentation, 599
prognosis and recurrence, 602–3
prophylaxis, 603
social factors, 602
suicide, 604–6
symptoms, 599
treatment, 602
puerperal psychoses (strategy for relapse prevention), 604
for previous depression, 604
for previous mania, or schizo-mania, 604
puerperal psychotic episodes, 78
puerperal schizophrenia, 599–600
puerperium, 660
Puerto Rico, 677
punding: definition, 482
Purcell, E., 461
purposeful inpatient admission (PIPA), 780
Putnam, J. J., 739
pyrimethamine, 494
pyromania, 457
pyschological theories (OCD), 344–6
behavioural theories (with case examples), 344–5
cognitive theories, 345–6
disgust sensitivity, 345
evolutionary theories, 345
pyschological treatment: evidence, 283–4

QRISK3, 269, 690
QT interval prolongation, 112, 579, 586, 695
cardiac side effect (antipsychotics), 266–7
Quality and Outcomes Framework (2019), 728, 731, 770
Quality Improvement PDSA cycle, *771*
quality of life, 184, 748–9, 756
quatiapine, **612**
querulous litigants, 448
quetiapine, 117, 135, 136, 137, 171, 172, 456, 471, 607
long-term prophylaxis, 172
weight gain, 174
'worst result', 247
quick inventory for depressive symptomatology (QIDS), 464

quick inventory of depression symptomatology clinician rating (QIDS-C), 129
quinine, 491

R.v Pritchard (1836), 61
race, 707, 721, 722
  social construct, 707
race and racism, 706–10
Rachman, S., 345
racial discrimination, 96
racial identity, 707
racism, 96
  WHO definition, 706
radical openness behavioural therapy (RO-BPT), 587
Rado, S. E., 449
RAISE (USA), 284, 789
Ramanuj, P., 739–62
random sampling, 15
randomisation
  method to overcome confounding, 22
  'simple' versus 'balanced' (RCTs), *17*
randomised controlled trials (RCTs), 7, 767
  advantage, 20
  antipsychotics, 247
  balanced randomisation, 17
  'best design for inferring causality', 92
  bipolar disorder, 189
  bipolar disorder, 190
  bipolar disorder (problems), 190
  bipolar disorder (psychoeducation), 191–2
  common complaint, 27
  concealment of allocation, 17
  design, 16–17
  drop-out problem, 17
  inclusion and exclusion criteria, 17
  intention to treat analysis, 17
  key methodological feature, 16
  minimisation, 17
  simple randomisation, 16
  stratified randomisation, 17
rape, 316
Rapee, R. M., 299
rapid assessment interface and discharge (RAID), 740, 760
rapid cycling, 186
  bipolar I disorder, 165
  definition, 165
rapid eye movement sleep. *See* REM sleep
rapid tranquilisation (RT), 255–9
  algorithms, 259
  algorithms (summary), **258**
  antipsychotics, 257–8
  benzodiazepines, 257
  de-escalation, 256
  definition, 256
  general principles, 255–6
  indications, 255
  medication combinations, 258
  medication selection, 256–7
  medications commonly used, **257**
  monitoring, 258–9
  routes of administration, 256
Raspe, R. E., 397
rate differences, 12
  definition and formula, 12
rate ratios, 12, 13
rating scales, 129
rational emotive therapy, 44
Rattansi, A., 708
Ray of Hope, 683
Rayner, R., 328
RBD. *See* REM sleep behaviour disorder
reactions (disorders), 47
reactive states (Group III mental disorders), 34
real world, 43
reality distortion, 221
  dimension of psychopathology in schizophrenia, 213
  schizophrenic symptom, 212
reality testing, 151
reassurance: hypochondriasis, 395
reboxetine, **109**, 115–16, **132**
  contraindications, 116
  interactions, 116
  pharmacokinetics, 115
  side effects, 115
recall bias, 16, 90
  definition, 24
receptive aphasia, 468
reconsolidation of traumatic memories (RTM)
  PTSD, 319
recovering quality of life (ReQoL), 770, 798
recovery
  bipolar disorder, 189
  'broad' versus 'narrow' criteria, 230
  multidimensional concept, 230
recovery rates, **27**
recovery support services (RSS), 650
recovery-orientated integrated systems of care (ROISC), 649–50
  schematic diagram, *651*
recurrent brief depression, 80
  'little impact on clinical practice', 80
recurrent isolated sleep paralysis, 558
  assessment, 558
  psychiatric conditions, 558
  treatment, 558
Redfield, R., 710
reductionism: diagnosis, 37
refeeding syndrome, 521, 582
referral biases, 16
Regier, D. A., 416
regional cerebral blood flow (rCBF), 212
regression (defence mechanism), 743
rehabilitation
  aim, 783
  benefits, 783
  general adult psychiatry services, 783–4
  personal recovery (principal factors), 784
  purpose, 783
  social inclusion, 784
  specialisation, 783
Reid, J. E., 347
Reil, J. C., 1
relapse and remission, 24
relapse signatures, 188
relapse-prevention, 134, 149
  substance use disorders, 649
RELATE, 289
relationship history, 51
relative infant dose (RID), 604, 611, **612**
relative poverty: definition, 94
relentless hope (concept), 416
reliability, 38
  criterion for assessing psychiatric classification systems, 41
  definition, 38
religion, 709
  suicide risk (protective factor), 668
REM parasomnias, 556–8
  nightmare disorder, 556–7
  recurrent isolated sleep paralysis, 558
  REM sleep behaviour disorder, 557–8
REM sleep, 70, 546, 547, 548
REM sleep behaviour disorder, 557–8
  assessment, 557
  cause, 557
  psychiatric conditions, 557
  treatment, 558
Remission in Schizophrenia Working Group (RSWG)
  definition of 'symptomatic remission', 230
renal impairment, 137–8
repetitive transcranial magnetic stimulation (RTMS), 254, 350
Report of Committee of Inquiry into Care of Sharon Campbell (1988), 769
rescue phantasy, 427–8
research diagnostic criteria (RDC), 35, 65
research domain criteria (RDoC), 65
reserpine, 241
residual confounding, 22
resignation syndrome, 375
resilience: 'helpful concept', 189
responsible agency, 438
responsible clinician (RC), 782
restless legs syndrome, 552–3
  assessment, 553
  association with mood and anxiety disorders, 552
  causes, 552
  diagnosis, 552
  relationship with ADHD, 553
  treatment, 553
retardation, 71
RETHINK Mental Illness, 289, 771, 773
retrograde memory, 463
retrospective cohort study, 15
reverse causation, 25
  special form of confounding, 25, *25*
reversible inhibitors of monoamine oxidase A (RIMAs), 307, 309
Rey, H., 428, 433
rhesus monkey, 466
Richards, V., 3–4
risk differences, 12
  definition and formula, 12
risk factor: usage of term, 89
risk issues, 55–6
  dynamic risk, 55
  historical risk, 55
  summary, 57
risk ratios, 13
  definition and formula, 12
risperidone, 117, 171, 172, 243, 450, 471, 586, **612**
  efficacy, 247
  pharmacogenomics, 272
rituals, 344, 345, 346
rivastigmine, 503
RLS. *See* restless legs syndrome
Robbins, J. M., 394
Robins, J., 8, 20, 21, *23*
Robins, L., 447
Robinson, D. G., 215
Rogers, J., 241–72
role disputes, 154
Romanian Orphans, 421
Rorschach test, 207
Rose, G., 104
Rosenweig, S., 417
Ross, E., 683
rostral brainstem, 470
Roth, M., 49, 768
Rothman, K. J., 20
Rowlands, P., 1–4, 30–62, 688–97, 767–99
Roy, A., 678
Roy, C. S., 461
Royal College Centre for Quality Improvement, 797
Royal College of Emergency Medicine, 255, 740
Royal College of General Practitioners (RCGP), 735
Royal College of Physicians, 759, 768
Royal College of Psychiatrists, 2, 58, 130, 349, 414, 415, 420, 425, 426, 572, 622, 623, 754, 759, 768, 775, 783, 799
  ASD diagnostic interview guide, 531
  autism, 534
Royal College of Psychiatrists (curriculum), 3–4
  continued development of training, 4
  generic professional capabilities and specific speciality curricula, 3
  implementation, 3–4
  purpose, 3
  themes, 4
Royal College of Psychiatrists: Perinatal Section (later Faculty), 739
Royal College of Surgeons, 759
Royal Commission on the Care and Control of the Feeble Minded (UK, 1908), 40
Royal Medico-Psychological Association (RMPA), 768
Rüdin, E., 224
rugby league, 682
rumination: definition, 69
Rush, A. J., 147
Russell, L. and M., 414
Russia: vodka sales (1980-2005), 665
Rutz, W., 682
Ryle, J. A., 574

Safeguarding Adults Board, 796, 797
safety and crisis plans, 787
salience network, **298**, 298

Salkovskis, P. M., 395
Sally-Anne test, 528
salt poisoning, 398
Salvation Army, 792
Sam, D. L., 710, 712
Samaritans, 668, 771
Samaritans (organisation), 681
Samoa, 680
sample size, **27**
sampling error, 25
Samson, 654–5
San Francisco: Golden Gate Bridge, 679
SARIs. *See* serotonin antagonists and reuptake inhibitors
Sati Prevention Act (India, 1987), 660
Saul, King, 654, 665
Savage, S. G. H., 601, 602
Scadding, J. G., 36
scale for assessment of negative symptoms (SANS), 230, 234
scale for assessment of positive symptoms (SAPS), 230, 234
Scandinavia, 253, 446, 702, 704, 788
Scharloo, M., 748
schema-focused therapy: personality disorder, 437
schematic memory, 742
schizoaffective disorder, 198, 200, 217–18, 231, 599–600
  antipsychotic drug trials, 253
  diagnosis, 252
  drug treatments, 252–4
  mood stabilisers, 253
  pharmacotherapy principles, **253**
schizoaffective psychosis (Kasanin), 217
schizoid personality disorder, 449
schizophrenia, 1, 11, 15, 24, 25, 622, 694, 701. *See also* primary psychotic disorders
  antidepressants (practical issues), **254**
  case-control studies, 16
  CATIE trial, 247
  clinical features, 198–221
  content of speech (poverty), 206
  course, 198
  definition, 198
  depression 'common', 253
  diagnosis (UK versus USA), 35
  diagnostic criteria, 200–1
  differential diagnosis, 339
  EUFEST trial, 247
  genetic heritability, 102
  hallmark, 199
  ICD-11, 201–2
  inflammatory hypothesis, 741
  link with substance misuse, 43
  low and middle-income countries, 235–6
  origins of concept, 199–200
  pregnancy, 613
  primary care (obstacles), 730
  prognostic factors, 216
  stigmatising label, 41
  suicide, 663
schizophrenia (course and prognosis), 214–17
  1. prodrome and onset, 215
  2. outcome of first episode, 215
  3. medium-term evolution, 215–16
  4. long-term outcome, 216
  5. factors predicting outcome, 216–17
schizophrenia (DSM-5), 201
  course of illness, 201
  dimensional assessments, 201
  duration, 201
  dysfunction (social and occupational), 201
  exclusion of schizoaffective and mood disorder, 201
  exclusion of substance use and general medical conditions, 201
  relationship to pervasive developmental disorder, 201
  subtypes 'not defined', 201
  symptoms (characteristic), 201
schizophrenia (phenomena), 202–11
  catatonia, 208–9
  cognitive impairment, 209–10
  delusions, 204–5
  disorders of affect, 207–8
  disorders of thought, 205–7
  disorders of volition, 208
  hallucinations and illusions, 203–4
  insight (with case example), 211
  neurological signs, 211
  Schneiderian first-rank symptoms, 202–3
  violent behaviour, 209
schizophrenia (psychopathology), 211–13
  characteristic schizophrenic symptoms, 212
  dimensions, 212–13
  three syndromes, 212
  type one versus type two, 212
schizophrenia (subtypes), 213–14
  classical schizophrenia versus integrated psychosis, 214
  deficit versus non-deficit schizophrenia, 213
schizophreniform disorder, 200, 217
schizophrenogenic family, 289
schizotypal disorder, 198, 199, 200, 201, 220, 221
  clinical features, 449–50
Schneider Bakos, D., 437
Schneider, K., 35, 49, 54, 200, 202, 215, 220
Schneiderian first-rank symptoms (schizophrenia), 202–3
  audible thoughts, 202
  delusional perception, 203
  made acts, 203
  made affect, 203
  made will, 203
  somatic passivity, 203
  thought broadcast, 203
  thought insertion, 202
  thought withdrawal, 202
  voices commenting, 202
  voices discussing or arguing, 202
school refusal, 15
Schopenhauer, A., 49
Schou, M., 173
Schwarz, I., 770
scientific term (S), 35
SCOFF questionnaire, 568, 570
Scotland, 61, 530, 583, 617, 638, 732, 757, 773
Scottish Intercollegiate Guidelines Network. *See* SIGN
screening tests (psychiatric), 750–1
screening, brief intervention, and referral to treatment (SBIRT), 755
scurvy, 520
  characteristics, 520
seasonal affective disorder, 78, 127
Seattle, 734
Seattle obstructive lung disease questionnaire (SOLDQ), 748
second opinion appointed doctor (SOAD), 782
secondary analyses, 27
secondary delusions, 53
secondary depression: term 'largely fallen out of use', 84
secondary mental health services: interface with primary care, 731–5
secondary mood syndrome, 84
secondary prevention: definition, 105
secondary psychotic disorders. *See* organic psychotic disorders
second-generation antipsychotics (SGAs), 254, 263, 264, 265, 266, 267, 619
section 136 powers, 60
section 47 enquiry, 625
sedation: antipsychotic side effect, 262–3
sedentary behaviour, 99
Seeman, P., 241
segmental dystonia, 487
selection bias, 16, 23–4, 90
  definition, 23
  non-response bias, 23–4
  prevalence bias, 24
selective mutism, 375
selective serotonin re-uptake inhibitors, 39, 70, 80, 108–10, **109**, **132**, 134, 319, 346, 350, 472, 548, **612**, 619, 630, 754
  background, 108
  BDD, 352
  contraindications, 109
  cytochrome P450 inhibition, **109**
  elimination half-lives, **109**
  examples, 108
  interactions, 109
  mechanism of action, 108
  OCD, 348–9
  pharmacokinetics, 108
  side effects, 108–9
  SSRI activation syndrome, 109–31
  suicidality, 109–30
  terminology, 108
  toxicity in overdose, 110
  violent episodes (out-of-character), 131
selegiline, **109**, 113, **132**, 472, 482
selenium deficiency, 522
self-actualisation, 422, 425
self-awareness, 405
self-care system, 424, 425
self-direction, 405
self-esteem, 187
self-function: problems, 405
self harm, 68, 420, 676–9
  age and gender, 677
  autism, 533
  biological factors, 678
  cases (ratio to completed suicides), 677
  epidemiology, 676–7
  history and definition, 676
  methods, 677
  social factors, 677
self immolation, 678
self injury, 677–8
self mutilation, 677, 678
self poisoning, 657, 677
self-reports: bipolar disorder, 166–7
self-respect, 789
self-worth, 405
Seligman, M. E., 328
Selsick, H., 546–61
Selten, J. P., 228
Seminars in General Adult Psychiatry
  aim, 4
  best way to use book, 2
  second edition (2008), 3
Sen, G., 241
Seneviratne, G., 598–631
sensitivity
  definition, 9
  example with actual numbers, 9–10
  formula, 9
  gold standard, **9**
  sample calculation, **9**
sensorial affects, 423
sensory aphasia, 467
sensory FND, 372
  auditory disorders, 372
  somatosensory dysfunction, 372
  visual dysfunction, 372
separation anxiety disorder
  beta blockers, 309
  causes, 299–300
  epidemiology, 296
SEPEA study, 24
sequenced treatment alternatives to relieve depression (STAR*D), 118, 120, 135
serial 7s test, 463
serious mental illness: general interpretation, 731
serotonin, 678
serotonin and noradrenaline reuptake inhibitors, **109**, 110–11, **132**
  background, 110
  contraindications, 111
  cytochrome P450 inhibition, **110**
  elimination half-lives, **110**
  examples, 110
  interactions, 111
  mechanism of action, 110
  pharmacokinetics, 110
  side effects, 110
  terminological trap, 108
  toxicity in overdose, 111
serotonin antagonists and reuptake inhibitors, 116
serotonin hypothesis: OCD, 341–2
serotonin receptors, 342
serotonin re-uptake inhibitors, 346
  OCD, 347, 348

refractory OCD patients, 348–9
serotonin syndrome, 114
medical emergency, 109
risk, 109, 110
serotonin system, 102
serotonin transporter (SERT), 306
serotonin transporter polymorphism (Caspi), 104
sertraline, 17, 108, 348, 349, 350, 592, 603, 604, **612**, 619, 754
renal impairment cases, 138
risk of abnormalities, 619
titration (gradual), 134
severe mental illness, 43, 94, 689
primary care, 730–1
primary care (template for ten-minute consultation), 730
severe mental illness (integrated approach), 691–6
1. smoking cessation, 691
2. physical activity, 692
3. alcohol use (reduction), 692
4. blood pressure control, 693
5. diabetes (prevention and control), 693
6. blood lipids (control), 693
7. obesity-reduction (diet-improvement), 694
8. atrial fribrillation and cardiac rhythms, 695
9. chronic kidney disease (proper management), 695
10. COPD (proper management), 695
11. medication consequences (monitoring and management), 695
12. cancer-screening (proper access), 696
13. drug misuse, 696
14. vaccination (influenza and Covid-19), 696
sex hormones, 100
sexsomnia, 555
sexual abuse, 624, 629
sexual dysfunction, 263
Sexual Offences Act (UK, 1967), 47
sexual orientation: depression differences, 96
sexual side effects, 109, 114, 116, 117, 118, 130, 134
lithium, 174
sexual trauma, 607
sexual variations, 719
Shaftesbury, Lord, 767, 768
Shakespeare, W.: *Macbeth*, 30
shame, 67–8
suicide, 662
Shape of Training Review, 3
shared care, 732
Sharma, A., 162–78
Shaw, P., 448
Sheffield, 793
shell shock, 367
Shepherd, M., 726
Sherrington, C. S., 462
Shields, J., 224
Shiers, D., 731
shift work disorder, 553
Shneidman, E. S., 674
widening suicidal patient's range of thought, 674
short opiate withdrawal scale (SOWS), 646
short social functioning questionnaire (SSFQ), 411
Shorter, E., 31, 46
SIADH. *See* syndrome of inappropriate antidiuretic hormone
sick role, 40, 743
side effect management: depression treatment, 130–1
side effects, 720
antipsychotic drugs, 262–71
SIGN, 254, 732, 770
eating disorders, 569, 571
significant harm, 629
significant other, 426, 427
Silberman, S.: *Neurotribes* (2015), 528
sildenafil, 130
Simmonds' or Sheehan's disease, 574
simple alcohol withdrawal, 508
simple phobias, 294
Simpson-Angus scale, 264
Singapore, 608, 657, 681
Singer, J., 527, 529
single nucleotide polymorphisms (SNPs), 102, 225
Manhattan plot, *103*
single nucleotide variants (SNVs), 225
single photon emission computed tomography (SPECT), 462
single photon emission tomography (SPET), 243
single point of access, 59
six-month rule, 131
Skapinakis, P., 348
Skellern, E., 415
skin, 269
lithium side effects, 173
Skinner, B. F., 44
skin-picking disorder, 336–55
sleep, 262
factors, 548–9
neurotransmitters, 548
NREM (1), 546
NREM (2), 546
NREM (3), 547
progression across night, 556
psychiatric medications (impact), 548
REM sleep, 547
two-process model, 548–9
sleep architecture, 546
psychiatric conditions, 547–8
psychiatric medications (impact), 548
sleep cycle, 556
hypnogram, *547*
sleep deprivation, 550
sleep diary, 551, 555, 558
sleep disorders, 2, 47, 550–61
central disorders of hypersomnolence, 559–61
circadian rhythm disorders, 553–5
classification, 550
DSWPD, 554–5
insomnia, 550–2
movement disorders, 553
parasomnias, 555–8
sleep-related breathing disorders, 558–9
sleep disturbance: symptom of depressive disorders, 70
sleep history, 551, 555, 558
sleep investigations, 549–50
sleep medicine, 546
sleep problems: association with depression, 99–100
sleep terrors, 555
sleeping pills, 551
sleeping sickness. *See* trypanosomiasis
sleep-related breathing disorders, 558–9
obstructive sleep apnoea, 558–9
sleep-related eating, 555
sleep-related movement disorders, 553
rhythmic movement disorder, 552
RLS and PLMD, 552–3
sleepwalking, 555
Slomian, J., 609
SlowMo app, 283
slowness, 337
slow-wave sleep, 546
small cell carcinoma of lung, 475
Small, D. M., 569
SMART Recovery, 648
SMI. *See* severe mental illness
smiling depression, 71
smoking, 114, 272, 454
integrated approach, 691–2
pregnancy, 620
smoking cessation, *692*
SNOMED coding, 529
SNOMED-CT, 728
snoring, 559
Snow, J., 6
SNRIs. *See* serotonin and noradrenaline re-uptake inhibitors
social adversities: psychosis risk factor, 227–8
social anxiety disorder, **325**, 326
AVPD 'severe variant', 451
causes, 298–9
diagnosis, 294
epidemiology, 295–6
integrated aetiological and maintenance model, *298*
social anxiety disorder (beta blockers), 309
long-term pharmacological treatment, 309
medications after non-response, 309
psychological interventions, 309
short-term pharmacological treatment, 309
social capital, 706
social causation hypothesis, 94
social circumstances: psychosis (risk and mediating factor), 233
social class, 708
psychosis risk factor, 228
social cohesion: definition, 95
social connectedness, 100
social context, 688
social determinants, 721–2
social drift, 25, 94
social functioning questionnaire, 408
social geography: psychosis risk factor, 228
social housing, 793
social interventions, 156
effectiveness (strong evidence), 791
social media, 405, 716, 718
social model, 44, 45
social network, 100
social phobia: identical to social anxiety disorder (*qv*), 294
social relationships: antidote to depression, 100
social support, 100
social workers, 625
social worker's report, 629
societal functions, 40
socioeconomic factors, 608
socioeconomic status (SES), 21, 92, 743, 745
depression differences, 94–5
sociological theories: OCD, 346
sociopath: term proposed by Partridge, 40
Socrates, 655
SOCRATES (pain mnemonic), 751
Socrates, A., 225
sodium channels, 112
sodium valproate, 123
antiepileptic agent (within guidelines), 270
somatic hallucinations, 204
somatisation
definition (Lipowski, 1988), 393
etymology, 393
somatisation disorder, 2, 356, 393. *See also* bodily distress disorder
somatoform disorder, 335
somatoparaphrenia, 475
somatosensory dysfunction, 372
somnolence, 262
South Africa, 228, 236, 601, 620, 660, 706
South America, 494
South Korea, 617, 661, 683
Southampton, 793
South-East Asia, 455, 494, 718
Sowell, T., 707, 721
Spain, 125, 228
Sparta, 618
spasmii, 31
spasmodic torticollis (idiopathic cervical dystonia), 486
specialist supportive clinical management (SSCM), 571, 583
specific outcome (O), 35
specific phobia, 324–31
background, 324
behavioural overview, 328–9
behavioural theories, 328
blood/injection/injury phobia, 328
case example, 324
cognitive theories (with case example), 329
comparison with OCD (with case example), 338
controversy (classification of agoraphobia and panic), 325
definition, 324
diagnosis, 294, 324–5
differential diagnosis and comorbidity, 325–7
epidemiology, 327

specific phobia (cont.)
gender, 327
onset and course, 327
prevalence, 327
psychoanalytic theories, 328
psychological theories, 328
sociological theories, 329
types, **325**
specific phobia (aetiology), 327–8
genetic theories, 327
neurotransmitters, 327–8
specific phobia (treatment), 329–31
behavioural psychotherapy, 329
cognitive therapy, 329–30
combination treatments, 330
pharmacological treatments, 330
specific test (T), 35
specificity
definition, 10
example with actual numbers, 9–10
formula, 9
gold standard, **9**
sample calculation, **9**
speech
bipolar disorder, 166
mental state examination, 53
speech disorders, 374–5
Spickard, P. R., 707
spiders, 324, 329, 338, 345
Spielmeyer, W., 494
spina bifida, 620
Spitzer, R., 35, 47, 48
split-half reliability, 9
Spokes Inquiry, 770
sporadic CJD, 494
Spurzheim, J., 460
squamous cell carcinoma, 475
Sri Lanka, 660, 677, 678, 680, 681
Srinivasan, R., 89–105
SRIs. *See* serotonin re-uptake inhibitors
SSRIs. *See* selective serotonin re-uptake inhibitors
St Louis Criteria, 35
St Vitus's dance, 488
stammering and stuttering, 340
standardised assessment of personality abbreviated scale (SAPAS), 408, 429
standardised mortality ratio (SMR), 666
STAR*D. *See* sequenced treatment alternatives to relieve depression
Stark, M., 427
starvation, 575
state anxiety, 324
State of Mind (charity), 682
statins, 694
statistical abnormality, 36
statistical significance, 26, 27
status epilepticus: definition, 476
Steele-Richardson-Olszewski syndrome, 488
Stein maternity blues scale, 616
Stein, G., 1–2, 30–62, 444–57, 598–631, 654–83
Stein, L. I., 786
Steinhausen, H. C., 591
Stengel, E., 31, 35, 46, 47, 676
Stenger test, 372
Stepniak, B., 229
stereotactic psychosurgery, 127–8
background, 128
examples, 127
mechanism of action, 128
stereotopies: definition, 72
Stern, A., 414, 416, 417, 427
Stevens-Johnson syndrome, 115, 171, 176
Stewart, D., 603
stigma, 8, 37, 38, 96, 185, 192, 193, 199, 236, 340, 405, 409, 410, 429, 489, 568, 682, 683, 717, 719, 785, 793
diagnosis, 40–1
stillbirth, 616–17
counselling, 617
Stillbirth and Neonatal Death Society (SANDS), 617
Stilo, S. A., 224–36
stimulants, 541–2
ADHD, 541, 542
neuropsychiatric manifestations, 509–10
Stone, A. L., 639
Stone, J., 368
Stone, M., 414
Stone, M. H., 664
Stone, T. S., 235
stop overprescribing psychotropic medication (STOMP), 534
Stoudemire, A., 749
STPD. *See* schizotypal personality disorder
Strasbourg, 377
Strategic Clinical Network for Mental Health, South-West, 760
Streltzer, J., 711
stress response, 97–8, 99
stress-diathesis model, 376, 608
stressful life events, 97, 100, 186
stroke
acute management, 474
definition, 473
neuropsychiatric manifestations, **474**
organic psychotic disorders, 261
stroke risk calculator, 695
Stroop task, 210
structural brain disease, 740
structured clinical management (model), 425
structured interview for prodromal syndromes (SIPS), 245
study designs, 14–19
case-control studies, 16
choice, 18–19
cohort studies, 15
cross-sectional studies, 14–15
ecological studies, 14
first question to be asked, 18
prognostic studies, 15–16
publication bias, 18
randomised controlled trials, 16–17
systematic reviews and meta-analysis, 17–18
subacute sclerosing panencephalitis, 492
subgroup analyses, 27
subjective experience of world, 37
subjective personal suffering, 36
subjective wellbeing, 39
submental electromyogram: purpose, 549
sub-Saharan Africa, 488, 490, 491, 616, 705
substance use, 200, 577, 589, 631
comorbidities, 326
pregnancy, 620–3
psychosis, 220–1
psychosis (risk and mediating factor), 233–4
psychosis risk factor, 228–9
substance use (WHO categories)
dependence, 636
harmful, 636
hazardous, 636
substance use disorders, 167, 194, 636–51
assessment, 638–42
definition, 636–8
definitions in practice (example of alcohol), 637–8
five common substances, **640**
node-link map, 649
recovery-orientated integrated systems of care, 649–50
treatment, 642–50
treatment 'black box', 649, *650*
treatment components (integration), 649
treatment stages, 649
substance use disorders (assessment), 638–42
family and personal history, 639–41
forensic history, 641
investigations (key elements), 642
medical history, 641–2
medication, 642
monitoring outcome of treatment, 642
physical examination, 642
presenting problem (history), 639
protective factors, 641
psychiatric history, 639
risk factors, 639
substance use disorders (psychosocial interventions), 648–9
CBT, 648
contingency management, 648
family and social interventions, 648
motivational interviewing (MI), 648
mutual aid, 648
self-help, 648
substance use disorders (treatment), 642–50
brief interventions for alcohol use, 644
FRAMES structure (alcohol), 644
harm reduction, 643–4
medically-assisted withdrawal (MAW), 645–7
opioid agonist treatment (OAT), 647–8
psychosocial interventions, 648–9
relapse-prevention medication, 649
subsyndromal delirium, 498
subsyndromal disorders, 80
Suffolk County Mental Health Project, 231
suicidal behaviour disorder, 48
DSM-5, 676
suicidal ideation, 68
suicidal outpatients: psychotherapy, 675
suicidal patients
common clinician errors, 674–5
psychotherapy, 674
suicidal thoughts, 679
suicidality (assessment), 668–70
difficulties, 669–70
difficulties (description), 669
interviewing, 668–9
potential prompt questions, 669
suicidality: definition, 456
suicide, 2, 7, 67, 85, 193, 420, 431, 439, 454, 513, 591, 654–83
alcohol dependence and harmful drinking, 665
annual worldwide death toll, 654
autism, 533
autistic people, 532
biological factors, 678
carbon monoxide poisoning (UK), 92
central problem in psychiatry, 654
cost-benefit analysis, 157
definitions, 656
Durkheim, 6–7
green spaces (Netherlands), 14
influenced by societal factors, 6
inverse relationship with educational level (Hungary), 659
methods, 656–7
perinatal period, 604–6
perturbation and lethality (Shneidman), 674
physical and psychiatric comorbidity, 749
population attributable risk, 13–14
prisons, 666
psychoanalytic perspectives, 673
psychosis outcome, 232
rate by employment status, **12**
rate of unemployment in case control, **12**
rescue fantasies, 673–4
statistical approach (modern), 656
strong association with violence, 665–6
suggestion and imitation, 675–6
ultimate cause 'psyche-ache' (Shneidman), 674
use of odds ratios in case-control studies, 13
suicide (epidemiology), 659–62
elderly people, 661
marital status, 660
mental illness, 660, 661–2
psychological autopsy studies (diagnostic distribution of suicides), **662**
sex (male predominance), 660
societal factors, 659
young people, 660
suicide (history)
1. biblical times, 654–5

2. ancient Greece, 655
3. early Christians, 655
4. primitive societies, 655–6
5. nineteenth century, 656
suicide (international rates), 657–9
age, 657
Europe versus Middle East, **659**
Germany (Catholic versus Protestant provinces), 659, 668
Hungary, 659
Islam, 659
United Kingdom, 657
WHO data (2019), **658**
suicide (particular mental disorders), 662–5
bipolar disorder, 663
borderline personality disorder, 664–5
comorbidity, 663–4
depression, 662
hopelessness, 662
schizophrenia, 663
shame, 662
suicide (psychiatric inpatients), 670–3
admission procedures, 670
Confidential Enquiry (2001), 671
discharge and leave, 672
hazards in hospital environment, 672
hospital admission, 671
medication, 672
supportive observation, 671
unwilling patient, 672
working with suicidal patient, 671
Suicide Act (1961), 676, 739
suicide bereavement, 683
suicide cards, 679
suicide methods, 671
suicide pacts, 665
suicide risk, 71
economic crises, 667–8
factors, 670
insomnia, 551
occupation, 666–7
overall assessment, 670
poverty, 666
religion and religiosity (protective factor), 668
unemployment, 667–8
suicide survivors, 682–3
suicide verdict, 656, 661
suicide prevention, 672, 679–82, 683
alcohol, 681
charcoal-burning, 681
crisis hotlines, 681–2
educational approaches, 682
jumping from high buildings, 681
means (hindrance to access), 679–80
medication (reduction of availability), 680
pesticide control, 680
primary care, 729
rural China, 680–1
Sukhareva, G., 528
Sullivan, H. S., 451
sulphadiazine, 494
superego, 155
superior mesenteric artery (SMA) syndrome, 580
Supporting People housing, 771
Sure Start, 105
surface dyslexia, 468
Survivors of Bereavement by Suicide (SOBS), 683
Sweden, 6, 191, 232, 378, 539, 601, 602, 605, 608, 616, 663, 665, 680, 681, 682
suicide, 6–7
Switzerland, 45
Sydenham, T., 366, 369
Sydenham's chorea, 488
definition, 343
symptoms checklist 08 (SCL-8), 750
symptoms checklist 20 (SCL-20), 748
syndrome of inappropriate antidiuretic hormone secretion (SIADH), 109, 522
synthetic cannabinoid receptor agonists: UK information, **640**
syphilis, 262, 490–1
cause, 490
congential, 491
dementia, 491
diagnosis, 490
general paresis of insane, 490
stages (four), 490
treatment (historical), 491
treatment (nowadays), 491
Syria, 513, 628
systematic reviews, 18
systemic disturbances, 740
systemic lupus erythematosus, 261, 496–7
systems, 690, 691, 696
systems training for emotional predictability and problem solving (STEPPS), 426, 429, 436
Szasz, T., 38–9, 656

tabes dorsalis, 490
tachycardia, 271
cardiac side effect (antipsychotics), 267
tactile agnosia, 466
tactile hallucinations, 54
taijin kyofusho: definition, 296
Taiwan, 605, 657, 677, 681
talion law, 416, 425
talking treatments, 59, 392, 788, 794–5
tardive dyskinesia
definition, 265
motor side effect (antipsychotics), 265
target population, 15
Task Force for Revision of Personality Disorders (in advance of DSM-5), 408
Tasmania, 680
taxonomy
definition, 37
psychiatry, 37
Tay-Sachs disease, 515–16
TCAs (tricyclic antidepressants). *See* tricyclics
team for assessment of psychiatric services (TAPS), 769
teeth, 174
telemedicine, 732
telephone therapy, 152
TEMPO, 284
temporal lobe, 465–6
temporal lobe epilepsy, 477, 479, 480
temporal lobe epilepsy personality disorder, 479
temporal lobe epilepsy personality syndrome
main features, 480
Tennant, P. W. G., 21
tenofovir, 261
teratogenicity, 175, 618–20
terminal anorexia, 587
test-retest reliability, 8, 38
tetrabenazine, 484
tetrahydrocannabinol (THC), 220, 229, 235, 244
Thai patients, 176
thalidomide scandal, 618
thallium poisoning, 512
thanatos (death instinct), 673
Thatcher, M., 793
therapeutic alliance, 2
therapeutic community, 438
therapeutic concern, 36
therapeutic nihilism, 39
therapeutic relationship, 1, 432, 433, 435, 752, 779
depression cases, 157
therapeutic relationship (boundaries), 428–9
both parties committed, 428
continuity of care, 428
creates opportunity for disclosure, 428
honesty, 428
private but not secret, 428
thiamine, 505, 506, 507, 508, 521. *See also* vitamins
Thiel, A., 339
thinking errors
all-or-nothing, 148
arbitrary inference, 148
labelling, 148
magnification and selective attention, 148
overgeneralisation, 148
thioridazine, 241
thiothixene, 450
thioxanthenes, **612**
third-wave CBT, 153
Thomas, C. S., 708
Thompson, C. E., 707
Thompson, T. L., 749
thought and language disorder (TALD) scale, 207
thought block: definition, 54
thought disorder index (TDI), 207
thought disorders (form of thought), 205–6
categories, symptoms, definitions, **205**
idiosyncracies of thought and language, **205**, 205, 206
idiosyncracies of thought and language (case examples), 206
unstable goals, **205**, 205, 206
unstable goals (case example), 205
weakening of goals, **205**, 206
thought disorders (schizophrenia), 205–7
thought, language and communication (TLC scale), 207
thoughts: mental state examination, 53–4
threats to validity, 20, 28
Thrive service (Kent), 617
Thuwe, I., 601
thyroid disease, 194, 759
thyroid disorders, 262
thyroid function, 119
thyroid hormones, 119–20, 129
mechanism of action, 120
overdoses, 120
side-effect profile, 120
thyroid stimulating hormone (TSH), 172
thyroid: lithium side effects, 173
thyroxine, 120
tics
definition, 483
motor FND, 371
time to change (campaign), 772
tiotropium, 695
tissue damage, 395, 396
TMS. *See* transcranial magnetic stimulation
Todd's paresis, 476
tokophobia: definition, 614
toluene, 513
topiramate, 480, 484, 510, 695
'not always tolerated', 592
Torgersen, S., 452
Tourette syndrome, 349, 483–5
age at onset, 483
comorbidities, 484
course, 483
definition, 483
differential diagnosis, 339
management, 484
pathophysiology, 484
quality of life, 484
tics (types), 483
Tourette, G. G. de la, *483*
Townsend index (1988), 95
toxic, metabolic, endocrine disorders, 505–22
alcohol-related brain damage, 505–9
drug use, 509–10
endocrine disorders, 516–18
environmental poisons and brain intoxicants, 511–14
metabolic disorders, 514–16
mitochondrial disorders, 518–19
neuropsychiatric adverse effects of neuropharmacology, 510–11
nutrients, 519–22
Toxoplasma gondii, 169
toxoplasmosis, 493–4
TRAC mnemonic (trigger, response, alternative coping), 153
traditional causal inference criteria, 19
traditional folk medicines, 718
training, 689
trait anxiety, 324
trait domains: definition, 409
trans people, 96
transcortical aphasia, 32, 468
transcranial alternating current stimulation (TACS), 350
transcranial direct current stimulation (TDCS), 252, 350
transcranial magnetic stimulation, 126, 252, 381
background, 126

transcranial magnetic stimulation (cont.)
bipolar disorder, 177
contraindications, 126
mechanism of action, 126
side effects, 126
transient ischaemic attack: definition, 473
transmissible spongiform encephalopathy. *See* Creutzfeldt-Jakob disease
tranylcypromine, **109**, 113, **132**
TRAP mnemonic (trigger, reaction and avoidance pattern), 153
trauma
psychosis risk factor, 227–8
relation with personality disorder, 407–8
trauma-focused CBT, 284, 400. *See also* CBT with trauma focus
trauma-informed care (TIC), 430
personality disorder, 426
traumatic brain injury, 262, 446, 469–73
acute presentation, 470–1
overview, 469–70
sub-classes, 469
traumatic brain injury (neuropsychiatric aspects), 471–3
mild TBI (post-concussion syndrome), 471
severe TBI (psychiatric sequelae), 471–3
trazodone, **109**, 112, 116, 130, **132**
contraindications, 116
interactions, 116
mechanism of action, 116
pharmacokinetics, 116
side effects, 116
toxicity in overdose, 116
treatment algorithms, 128–38
treatment non-concordance, 749
treatment resistance
definition, 234
psychosis, 234
three crucial elements, 234
unipolar depression (without psychotic symptoms), 135
treatment-resistant schizophrenia (TRS), 250–1
diagnosis, 250
Trélat, U., 444
tremor: motor FND, 371
triangle of care, 288
triangulation, 20
triangulation criteria, 19
trichloroethane, 513
trichloroethylene, 513
trichotillomania, 335, 354–5
definition, 336
epidemiology, 354
management, 355
tricyclicality: definition and terminological problem, 108
tricyclics, **109**, 111–12, 129, **132**, 135, 136, **612**, 619
background, 111
contraindications, 112
cytochrome P450 inhibition, **111**
elimination half-lives, **111**
examples, 111
interactions, 112
mechanism of action, 111
pharmacokinetics, 111
side effects, 111
toxicity in overdose, 112
Trier social stress test, 299
triglycerides, 693
triiodothyronine, 120
TRIUMPH study, 748
Tronick, E., 423
true life, 25
trust, 416
truth, 701, 702
trypanosomiasis, 493
tryptophan, 123, 519
caution, 136
Tseng, W-S., 711, 714, 719
tuberculous meningitis, 491
Tuke, D. H., 30, 32, 34, 43, 48, 64, 689
Tunisia, 241
Turkey, 614
Turna, J., 344
twelve-step fellowships, 639, 648
twilight states (epilepsy), 478
twin studies, 224, 298, 327, 450, 454, 539, 577, 588, 589, 608
gene-environment correlation, 103
genetics of depression, 102
OCD, 341
suicide, 678
Twitter, 676
two-stage screening procedures, 751
Tyagi, H., 349
type 1 disordered eating, 589
type 1 error, 25, **25**, 26, 27, 102
type 2 error, **25**, 26, 27
typhus, 493
Tyrer, P., 404–11

Ucello, P.: St. George and Dragon, 427
ultra-high-risk (UHR) state, 245
uncertainty, 26
unemployment, 13–14, 90, 91, 95
suicide risk, 667–8
UNESCO, 700
unipolar depression, 168, 192, 194
with psychotic symptoms, 136–7
without psychotic symptoms, 134–6
unipolar depression (with psychotic symptoms)
1. first line (rationale), 136
2. second line (rationale), 136–7
3. third line (rationale), 137
4. additional options, 137
unipolar depression (without psychotic symptoms), 134–6
1. first line (rationale), 134
2. second line (rationale), 134–5
3. third line, treatment-resistant (rationale), 135
4. additional options, 135–6
unipolar mania, 165
United Kingdom, 14, 43, 45, 48, 91, 95, 228, 305, 454, 490, 491, 601, 603, 605, 675, 703, 709, 719, 739, 768
ADHD, 539
alcohol consumption, 638
alcohol consumption levels (and associated risks), **637**
austerity programme (2010-2020), 793
autism, 530
block contracts (mental health services), 37
drug consumption, 638
drug misuse (annual cost), 642
fertility rate, 91
infanticide 'rare', 617
mental illnesses (annual cost to economy), 569, 642, 771
prevention gap, 105
primary care, 732
PTSD, 316
schizophrenia diagnosis, 35
United Kingdom BioBank, 592
United Kingdom Clinical Practice Research Datalink, 19
United Kingdom Household Longitudinal Study ('Understanding Society'), 15, 96
United Kingdom National Screening Committee (UK NSC), 493
United Kingdom: Department for Education, 105, 625
United Kingdom: Department of Health, 637, 739
homeless mental illness initiative (early 1990s), 793
United Kingdom: Home Office, 666
United States, 43, 48, 192, 228, 231, 295, 305, 446, 454, 515, 579, 605, 617, 663, 675, 676, 681, 701, 703, 705, 719, 768
depression and ethnicity, 95
eating disorders, 567
FND inpatient health care costs, 376
homelessness, 792
pellagra, 7
schizophrenia diagnosis, 35
suicides (60% by firearms), 657
universal primary prevention, 229
University of Munich, 224
unreliability, 38
urban planning: 'urgent need' for city re-engineering, 229
urbanicity: psychosis risk factor, 228
US Veterans Administration, 748
users: ability to meet needs of (criterion for assessing psychiatric classification system), 41
USSR, 35, 38, 605, 681
utility: criterion for assessing psychiatric classification systems, 41
Utrecht coping list, 748

Vagrancy Act (1824), 792
vagus nerve stimulation (VNS), 127
background, 127
bipolar disorder, 177–8
mechanism of action, 127
side effects, 127
validity, 38
criterion for assessing psychiatric classification systems, 41
versus 'reliability', 37
valproate, 170, 172, 175, 456, 471, **612**, 664
contraindicated in childbearing women, 477, 620
definition, 176
valproate (treatment of bipolar disorder), 176
combinations, 176
dosage, 176
monitoring and testing, 176
pharmacokinetics, 176
selection of patients, 176
side effects, 176
Van Hooff, A. J. L., 665
Varah, C., 681
varenicline: propensity to cause violent episode, 131
Varese, F., 227
variant CJD (vCJD), 494
vascular cognitive impairment, 504
vascular dementia, 504–5
differential diagnosis, 504
vascular depression, 123
VAST-D study, 135
vegan patients, 586
velocardiofacial syndrome (VCFS), 226
Velthorst, E., 231
Venereal Disease Research Laboratory (VDRL), 490
venlafaxine, **109**, 110, 113, 129, 131, **132**, 135, 354, 557, **612**, 754
combination with mirtazapine, 136
diverse effects, 110
side effects, 111
toxicity in overdose, 111
ventral striatum, 466
ventromedial syndrome, 465
verapamil, 123
verbigeration: definition, 72
Vermont, 327
Vermont State Hospital, 216
Verstehen (understanding), 43, 44, 45
vesanii, 31
videotelemetry, 481
Vietnam, 677
Vietnam War, 674
violence, 282, 421, 480
strong association with suicide, 665–6
violent behaviour: schizophrenia, 209
Virchow, R., 35
virtual reality (VR), 283
virtue, 701
visceral affects, 423
visual association cortex, 467
visual dysfunction: sensory FND, 372
visual hallucinations, 54, 71, 204
visual snow syndrome, 372
vitamin deficiencies, 586
vitamins, 519–20
vitamin A (retinol), 520
vitamin B1 (thiamine), 519
vitamin B12 (cobalamin), 520
vitamin B3 (niacin), 519
vitamin B6 (pyridoxine), 519

vitamin B9 (folate), 519
vitamin C (ascorbic acid), 520
vitamin D, 520
VNS. *See* vagus nerve stimulation
voices, 285–6, 289
volition disorders, 208
disjointed volition (with case example), 208
weakened volition, 208
voltage-gated potassium channel (VGKC), 497
vortioxetine, **109**, 116–17, 129, **132**
interactions, 117
mechanism of action, 116
pharmacokinetics, 117
side effects, 117
voxel-based morphometry (VBM), 461
vulnerable adults risk meetings (VARMs), 797
aim, 797
function, 797
local process (example), 797

Wagner, E., 219
wakefulness, 546
neurotransmitters, 548, **548**
Wales, 314, 638, 732, 773
Walker-Smith, D., 768
Wang, J., 745
War Department Technical Bulletin Medical (US Army, 1945), 47
Wardenaar, K. J., 327
Warwick, H. M., 395
Washington DC, 35
Wass. J., 688–97
water intoxication associated with polydipsia and polyuria, 522
Watkins, E. R., 153
Watson, J. B., 44, 328
Watson, S., 162–78
Weber, M., 32, 49
Wechsler adult intelligence scale, 207
weight, 70
weight gain, 271
weighted kappa, 8
Weikard, A., 539
Weiskrantz, L., 467
Weiss, M., 711
Weissman, M., 153, 158
Wells, A., 153, 345
Wernicke encephalopathy, 506, 507, 519
Wernicke, C., 32, *465*, 506
Wernicke's aphasia, 465, 467
Wernicke's area, 468
Wernicke-Korsakoff syndrome, 466, 505, 506, 507, 519
Werther effect (Goethe), 675
Wessely, S., 388
West Midlands, 733
West, M., 416, 423
Western Europe, 84
Westphal variant, 485
Whipple's disease, 492–3
Whipple's triad, 518
white cell counts, 250
Whitehall civil servants, 743
Whiteley index, 394, 395
Whytt, R., 393
Wilcock, J., 731
Wilhelm, S., 351
Williams, A., 616
Williams, K., 64–86
Williams, M., 158
Williams, R., 108–38
Willis, T., 366, 392
Wils, R. S., 233
Wilson, S. K., 487
Wilson's disease, 265
cause, 487
definition, 487
hepatic involvement, 487
pathophysiological process, 487
treatment, 487
Wilson's disease, 487–8
Wing, L., 528
Winnicott, D., 154
Wisconsin, 786, 787
Wisconsin card sorting test, 210
Wisner, K. L., 603
Wittgenstein, L., 41
Witzelsucht, 465
Wolfram disease, 518
women, 84, 91, 170, 194, 306, 307, 339, 352, 355, 366, 376, 445, 450, 451, 456, 457, 565, 663, 739
anonymous birth facility, 618
anxiety disorders, 327
depression (higher prevalence than men), 93
factitious disorders, 398
functional neurological disorder, 369
homelessness, 792
mastectomy, 742
'more likely than men to seek treatment' (most health problems), 93
NMDAR-antibody encephalitis, 497
pesticide-poisoning, 680
RBD, 557
self harm, 676
self-poisoning, 657
sleep problems, 100
somatisation disorder, 390
Wong, Q. J. J., 299
word salad, 53
work and social adjustment scale (WSAS), 795
work place based assessments (WPBAs), 42
workhouses, 792
working memory: definition, 507
World Federation of Societies of Biological Psychiatry (WFSBP), 170, 257, 306
World Health Organization (WHO). *See also* ICD
definition of 'health', 39
World Mental Health Survey, 14, 296, 330
World War I, 367
World War II, 40, 47
worried well, 727
worry, 283
definition, 69
worthlessness, 67–8
writer's cramp, 486
Wunderink, L., 249

Yale-Brown obsessive compulsive scale (Y-BOCS), 346, 347, 348, 349
Yalom, I. D., 155
Yap, P. M., 718
Yarden, P. E., 603
Yates, G., 399
Yemen, 621
yin and yang, 718
York, 768
Young mania rating scale, 168
young people: bipolar disorder, 168
Young, J., 437

Zanarini, M. C., 407
zero suicide (approach), 682
Zimbabwe, 660
Zimmerman, M., 451
zinc deficiency, 522
ziprasidone, 171
absorption with food, 272
zopiclone, **646**
zuclopenthixol, 171, 258